SAUNDERS

COMPREHENSIVE REVIEW FOR

NCLEX-RN

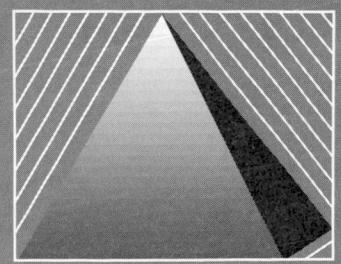

SAUNDERS
COMPREHENSIVE
REVIEW for
NCLEX-RN

LINDA ANNE SILVESTRI, MSN, RN

Assistant Professor of Nursing,
Salve Regina University,
Newport, Rhode Island;
President, Nursing Reviews, Inc., and
Professional Nursing Seminars, Inc.,
Charlestown, Rhode Island

SECOND EDITION

W.B. SAUNDERS COMPANY
An Imprint of Elsevier Science
Philadelphia   London   New York   St. Louis   Sydney   Toronto

SAUNDERS
An Imprint of Elsevier Science

The Curtis Center
Independence Square West
Philadelphia, Pennsylvania 19106

NOTICE:
Pharmacology is an ever-changing field. Standard safety precautions must be followed, but as new research and clinical experience broaden our knowledge, changes in treatment and drug therapy may become necessary or appropriate. Readers are advised to check the most current product information provided by the manufacturer of each drug to be administered to verify the recommended dose, the method and duration of administration, and contraindications. It is the responsibility of the treating appropriately-licensed health care provider, relying on experience and knowledge of the patient, to determine dosages and the best treatment for each individual patient. Neither the Publisher nor the editor assumes any liability for any injury and/or damage to persons or property arising from this publication.

The Publisher

Vice President and Publishing Director, Nursing: Sally Schrefer
Senior Editor: Loren S. Wilson
Senior Developmental Editor: Michele D. Hayden
Project Manager: Patricia Tannian
Production Editor: Steve Hetager
Book Design Manager: Gail Morey Hudson
Cover Designer: Teresa Breckwoldt

Permissions may be sought directly from Elsevier's Health Sciences Rights Department in Philadelphia, USA: phone: (+1)215-238-7869, fax: (+1)215-238-2239, e-mail: healthpermissions@elsevier.com. You may also complete your request on-line via the Elsevier Science homepage (http://www.elsevier.com), by selecting 'Customer Support' and then 'Obtaining Permissions'.

Last digit is the print number: 9   8   7   6   5

To my parents

To my mother

Frances Mary

and in loving memory of my father

Arnold Lawrence

who taught me to always love, care, and be the best that I could be

About the Author

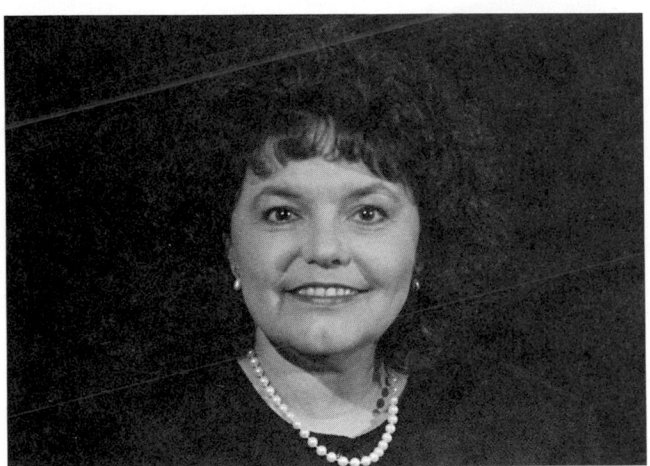

PHOTO BY Laurent W. Valliere.

Linda Anne Silvestri received her diploma in nursing at Cooley Dickinson Hospital School of Nursing in Northampton, Massachusetts. Afterward, she worked at Baystate Medical Center in Springfield, Massachusetts. At Baystate Medical Center, she worked in acute medical-surgical units, the intensive care unit, the emergency department, pediatric units, and other acute care units. She later received an associate degree from Holyoke Community College in Holyoke, Massachusetts, and then received her bachelor of science degree in nursing from American International College in Springfield, Massachusetts.

A native of Springfield, Massachusetts, Linda began her teaching career as an instructor of medical-surgical nursing and leadership-management nursing at Baystate Medical Center School of Nursing in 1981. In 1985, she earned her master of science degree in nursing from Anna Maria College, Paxton, Massachusetts, with a dual major in nursing management and patient education.

Linda relocated to Rhode Island in 1989 and began teaching advanced medical-surgical nursing and psychiatric nursing to RN and LPN students at the Community College of Rhode Island. While she was teaching at the Community College of Rhode Island, a group of students approached Linda, asking her to help them prepare for the NCLEX. On the basis of her experience as a nursing educator and as an NCLEX item writer, she developed a comprehensive review course to prepare nursing graduates for the NCLEX examination. In 1994, Linda began teaching medical-surgical nursing at Salve Regina University in Newport, Rhode Island. She also prepares nursing students at Salve Regina University for the NCLEX-RN examination. Currently, she is matriculated at the University of Rhode Island in the PhD program in nursing. Linda is a member of Sigma Theta Tau.

In 1991, Linda established Professional Nursing Seminars, Inc., and in 2000, she established Nursing Reviews, Inc. Both companies are dedicated to conducting NCLEX-RN and NCLEX-PN review courses and assisting nursing graduates to achieve their goals of becoming registered nurses or licensed practical or vocational nurses.

Today, Linda Silvestri's companies conduct NCLEX review courses throughout New England. She is the successful author of numerous NCLEX-RN and NCLEX-PN review products, including *Saunders Comprehensive Review for NCLEX-RN, Saunders Q & A Review for NCLEX-RN, Saunders Computerized Review for NCLEX-RN, Saunders Instructor's Resource Package for NCLEX-RN, Saunders Comprehensive Review for NCLEX-PN, Saunders Q & A Review for NCLEX-PN,* and *Saunders Instructor's Resource Package for NCLEX-PN.*

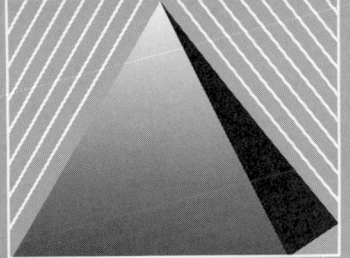

Contributors

Heather Carlson, RN
Graduate, Department of Nursing,
Salve Regina University,
Newport, Rhode Island

Jean DeCoffe, MSN, RN
Assistant Professor of Nursing,
Salve Regina University,
Newport, Rhode Island

Mary Ann Hogan, MSN, RN, CS
Instructor of Nursing,
Holyoke Community College,
Holyoke, Massachusetts

Jo Ann Barnes Mullaney, PhD, RN, CS
Professor of Nursing,
Salve Regina University,
Newport, Rhode Island

Laurent W. Valliere, BS
Vice President,
Professional Nursing Seminars, Inc.,
Charlestown, Rhode Island

The author and publisher would also like to acknowledge the following individuals for contributions to the first edition of this book:

Marion G. Anema, PhD, RN
Dean, Nursing Program,
Professor of Nursing,
Tennessee State University
School of Nursing,
Nashville, Tennessee

Marianne P. Barba, MS, RN, CPC
Care New England,
Coventry, Rhode Island

Carol A. Baxter, EdD, RN
CEO, Baxter Consulting,
Lancaster, Pennsylvania

Eloise M. Brotzman, MSEd, MSN, RNC
Nusing Instructor,
St. Luke's School of Nursing,
Pottsville, Pennsylvania

Reitha Cabaniss, MSN, RN
Nursing Faculty, Health Science Division,
Bevill State Community College,
Jasper, Alabama

Darlene Nebel Cantu, MSN, RNC
Director, School of Professional Nursing,
Baptist Health System;
Adjunct Faculty, San Antonio College,
San Antonio, Texas

Jane Anne Claffy, MSN, RNC
Assistant Professor of Nursing,
Ulster County Community College,
Stone Ridge, New York;
Adjunct Faculty, Avila Institute of Gerontology,
Germantown, New York

Alice D. Coomes, MSN, RN
Assistant Professor of Nursing,
Kentucky Wesleyan College;
Staff Nurse, Owensboro Mercy Health System,
Owensboro, Kentucky

Gloria Coschigano, MSN, RN, CS
Assistant Professor of Nursing,
Westchester Community College,
Valhalla, New York

Jean W. Davis, EdD, RN, CS
Associate Professor of Nursing,
Barry University School of Nursing,
Miami Shores, Florida

Carole A. Devine, MSN, RN
Associate Professor of Nursing,
Community College of Rhode Island
Newport, Rhode Island;
Associate Professor,
University of Rhode Island,
Kingston, Rhode Island

Kerry H. Fater, PhD, RN, CS
Associate Professor of Nursing,
University of Massachusetts—Dartmouth,
North Dartmouth, Massachusetts

Ginette G. Ferszt, PhD, RN, CS
Nursing Faculty, University of Rhode Island,
College of Nursing,
Kingston, Rhode Island

Cathy Fortenbaugh, MSN, RN, AOCN, CNS,C
Oncology Clinical Nurse Specialist,
Pennsylvania Hospital,
Philadelphia, Pennsylvania

Jane H. Freeman, EdD, RN
Professor of Nursing,
Lurleen B. Wallace College of Nursing and Health Sciences,
Jacksonville, Alabama

Rita S. Glazebrook, PhD, RN, CNP
Associate Professor of Nursing,
St. Olaf College;
Director, Minnesota Intercollegiate
Nursing Consortium,
Northfield, Minnesota

Joyce Hammer, MSN, RN
Lecturer of Nursing,
Wayne State University
Detroit, Michigan

Jacqueline L. Harris, MNSc, RN, ONC
Assistant Professor,
Harding University,
Searcy, Arkansas

Mary Kathleen Jackson, BSN, RN, CPN
Instructor of Nursing,
Southeastern Community College,
Whiteville, North Carolina

Gail M. Johnson, EdD, MSN, RN, CNAA, BC
Director, Professional Practice,
Capital Health System,
Trenton, New Jersey

Katherine Lang Jorgensen, MSN, RN, MA
Associate Professor, University of South Dakota,
Department of Nursing,
Vermillion, South Dakota

Elisa Mangosing Lemmon, MSN, RN, C
Program Coordinator,
Riverside School of Professional Nursing,
Riverside Regional Medical Center,
Newport News, Virginia

Teresa Leonard, MSN, RN, CCRN
Assistant Professor of Nursing,
University of North Alabama,
Florence, Alabama

Carol O. Long, PhD, RN
Assistant Professor of Nursing,
Arizona State University,
College of Nursing,
Tempe, Arizona

Marilyn Lusk, MSN, MS, RN
Nursing Faculty,
Mohave Community College,
Kingman, Arizona

Linda Ann Martin, MSN, RN, APN-C
Faculty Coordinator, St. Francis Medical Center,
School of Nursing,
Trenton, New Jersey

Dorothy M. Mathers, MSN, RN
Associate Professor of Nursing,
Pennsylvania College of Technology,
Williamsport, Pennsylvania

Betsy J. Nield, MSN, RNC
Professor of Nursing,
Community College of Rhode Island,
Warwick, Rhode Island

Patricia A. Parsons, MSN, MS, RN
Instructor of Nursing,
Riverland Community College,
Austin, Minnesota

Elizabeth Phillip, MSN, RN
Nursing Faculty,
St. Luke's School of Nursing,
Bethlehem, Pennsylvania

Ethel Pruden, MSN, RN
Assistant Professor,
Armstrong Atlantic State University,
Department of Nursing,
Savannah, Georgia

Marion Sawyier, MSN, RN
Faculty,
Albuquerque Technical-Vocational Institute,
Albuquerque, New Mexico

Nancy Schlapman, PhD, RN
Associate Professor and Coordinator,
Baccalaureate Nursing Program,
Indiana University School of Nursing,
Kokomo, Indiana

Jane Schlickau, MN, RN, ARNP, CTN
Associate Professor of Nursing,
Southwestern College,
Winfield, Kansas

Shellie Simons, MS, RN
Chairperson, Division of Nursing,
Roxbury Community College,
Boston, Massachusetts

Marian I. Stewart, MSN, RN
Associate Professor of Nursing,
Level II Coordinator,
Motlow State Community College,
Lynchburg, Tennessee

Lynn Tesh, MSN, RN
Dean, Curriculum Programs,
Randolph Community College,
Asheboro, North Carolina

Cheryl J. Vitacco-Grab, MSN, RNC
Nursing Instructor,
Lancaster Institute for Health Education,
Lancaster, Pennsylvania

Loretta A. Wack, MSN, PNP, FNP
Associate Professor of Nursing,
Nursing Program Coordinator,
Blue Ridge Community College,
Weyers Cave, Virginia

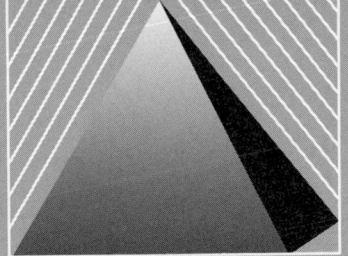

Reviewers

Carolyn Banks, MSN, RN
Nursing Faculty,
Pratt Community College,
Pratt, Kansas

Janice Boundy, PhD, RN
Professor and Coordinator,
Saint Francis College of Nursing,
Peoria, Illinois

Michele Bunning, MSN, RN
Instructor, Good Samaritan Hospital
School of Nursing,
Cincinnati, Ohio

Gina Catena, MS, CNM, NP
Nurse-Midwife,
Bay Care Women's Health Services,
San Rafael, California

Mary Ellen Lashley, PhD, RN, CRNP
Associate Professor, Towson University,
Department of Nursing,
Towson, Maryland

Caron Martin, MSN, RN
Assistant Professor, Northern Kentucky University,
Department of Nursing,
Highland Heights, Kentucky

Debbie Ocedek, MSN, RN
Professor, PN/ADN Program,
Mott Community College,
Flint, Michigan

Sharon Powell-Laney, MSN, RN
Coordinator of Nursing,
Indiana County Technology Center,
Westmoreland County Community College,
Indiana, Pennsylvania

Anita K. Reed, MSN, RN
Instructor of Nursing,
St. Elizabeth School of Nursing,
Lafayette, Indiana

Christine M. Rosner, PhD, RN
Lecturer, Division of Nursing,
Holy Family College,
Philadelphia, Pennsylvania

Linda S. Smith, DSN, RN
Assistant Professor,
Oregon Health Sciences University,
Klamath Falls, Oregon

Ann D. Sumners, PhD, RN
Professor,
North Georgia College and State University,
Department of Nursing,
Dahlonega, Georgia

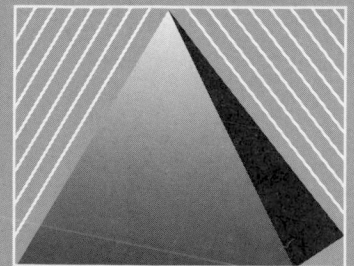

Student Reviewers

Allison Belisle
Salve Regina University,
Newport, Rhode Island

Melissa Caporale
Salve Regina University,
Newport, Rhode Island

Shannon DaCunha
Salve Regina University,
Newport, Rhode Island

Stephanie A. Ferreira
Salve Regina University,
Newport, Rhode Island

Natalie Gendron
Salve Regina University,
Newport, Rhode Island

Jill A. Klein
Villa Julie College,
Stevenson, Maryland

Lauren C. Rodrigues
Salve Regina University,
Newport, Rhode Island

Jinae Selvey
Johns Hopkins University,
School of Nursing,
Baltimore, Maryland

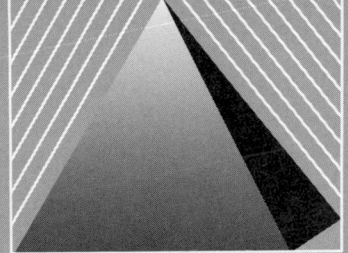

Preface

"To know that even one life has breathed easier because you have lived, this is to have succeeded."
Ralph Waldo Emerson

Welcome to *Saunders Pyramid to Success!*

Saunders Comprehensive Review for NCLEX-RN is one of a series of products designed to assist you in achieving your goal of becoming a registered nurse. *Saunders Comprehensive Review for NCLEX-RN* will provide you with a comprehensive review of all of the nursing content areas specifically related to the new 2001 CAT NCLEX-RN test plan implemented by the National Council of State Boards of Nursing.

ORGANIZATION

Saunders Comprehensive Review for NCLEX-RN contains 21 units and 75 chapters. The chapters are designed to identify specific components of nursing content. Each chapter contains practice questions reflective of the chapter content and of the 2001 CAT NCLEX-RN test plan.

The new test plan identifies a framework based on *Client Needs*. The Client Needs categories include Safe, Effective Care Environment; Health Promotion and Maintenance; Psychosocial Integrity; and Physiological Integrity. *Integrated Concepts and Processes* are also identified as components of the test plan. These include Caring; Communication and Documentation; Cultural Awareness; Nursing Process; Self-Care; and Teaching/ Learning. All of the chapters address the components of the test plan framework.

Unit I: NCLEX-RN Preparation

Chapter 1 addresses all of the information about the 2001 CAT NCLEX-RN test plan and the testing procedures related to the examination. This chapter answers all of those questions that you may have regarding the testing procedures.

Chapter 2 discusses the issue of NCLEX-RN prepara-tion from a nonacademic view and provides a holistic approach to your individual test preparation. This chapter identifies the components of a structured study plan and pattern, anxiety reduction techniques, and personal focus issues.

Nursing students want to hear what other students have to say about their experiences with NCLEX-RN. Students seek a view of what it is really like to take an NCLEX-RN examination. Chapter 3 is written by a nursing student who recently took the NCLEX-RN examination. The chapter addresses the issue of what the examination is all about, and includes the student's "story of success."

Test-taking strategies are an important component of success in taking such an important examination. Chapter 4, "Test-Taking Strategies," includes all of those important strategies that will assist in teaching you how to read a question, how not to read into a question, and how to use the process of elimination and various other methods to select the correct response from the options presented.

Unit II: Issues in Nursing

Unit II addresses relevant nursing issues reflective of the components of the CAT NCLEX-RN test plan. Chapter 5, "Cultural Diversity," discusses cultures and the related factors in nursing care that promote the maintenance of a client's cultural identity. Chapter 6, "Ethical and Legal Issues," provides a review of the ethical and legal considerations important to the practice of nursing and relevant to the components of the test plan. Chapter 7, "Leadership and Management Issues," identifies the leadership and management issues pertinent to the practice of nursing. This chapter includes content related to time management, prioritizing, assignment making, and delegation.

Unit III: Nursing Sciences

The chapters in this unit specifically address areas that students have identified as areas of concern requiring review. Chapter 8, "Fluids and Electrolytes," and Chapter 9, "Acid-Base Balance," highlight the key components of the relevant physiology, and then introduce the necessary nursing assessments and nursing interventions required in caring for a client with an alteration or imbalance. Chapter 10, "Laboratory Values," identifies common laboratory studies, normal values, and significant information related to specific laboratory tests. Chapter 11, "Nutrition," addresses the various food groups and important nutritional components of specific diet therapies. This chapter will assist in your review of the selection of the correct foods or the foods to avoid in certain physiological conditions, because these types of questions are certainly addressed in the CAT NCLEX-RN examination. Chapter 12, "Total Parenteral Nutrition," Chapter 13, "Intravenous Therapy," and Chapter 14, "Administration of Blood Products," stress all of the key components of nursing care in these areas. These chapters focus on the nurse's role in the administration of these therapies and in monitoring for complications.

Unit IV: Fundamental Skills

Chapter 15, "Providing a Safe Environment," addresses nursing care specific to client safety and the measures that promote environmental safety. Chapter 16, "Administering Medication and Intravenous Solutions," includes the important components related to conversion tables and calculation of medication dosages, intravenous (IV) solutions and flow rates, IV medications, and unit doses, such as heparin and insulin. Chapter 17, "Basic Life Support," has been included to assist you in reviewing the steps in cardiopulmonary resuscitation and the Heimlich maneuver and to refresh your memory in regard to the priorities to be addressed in emergency situations. Chapter 18, "Perioperative Nursing Care," addresses the key components of caring for a client requiring surgery. Chapter 19, "Positioning Clients," identifies safe client positions specific to various surgical and diagnostic procedures. Chapter 20, "Care of a Client with a Tube," addresses the various types of tubes, such as chest, gastrointestinal, or renal tubes, which have always been confusing to students, particularly in terms of their purposes and the nursing care involved.

Units V Through VII: Growth and Development and Maternity and Pediatric Nursing

Unit V, "Growth and Development Across the Life Span," addresses the common theories of growth and development used in the profession of nursing. Unit VI, "Maternity Nursing," includes chapters that address maternity issues, the care of the newborn, and maternity and newborn medications. Unit VII, "Pediatric Nursing," focuses on pediatric care and the specifics related to administering medication to a child.

Units VIII Through XVIII: Adult Health

Units VIII through XVIII address the components of adult health. Each of these units discusses a specific body system, including the integumentary, endocrine, gastrointestinal, respiratory, cardiovascular, renal, neurological, musculoskeletal, and immune systems, as well as the eye and the ear and oncology nursing. These chapters incorporate the Integrated Concepts and Processes and all of the Client Needs components of the CAT NCLEX-RN test plan, with a particular emphasis on Physiological Integrity. Each unit includes a pharmacology chapter that provides a comprehensive review of the medications specific to that body system.

Unit XIX: Mental Health Nursing

This unit primarily addresses the Psychosocial Integrity category of the Client Needs component of the test plan. Specific mental health disorders are addressed. This unit includes a chapter that provides a comprehensive review of psychiatric medications.

Unit XX: The Gerontological Client

Unit XX focuses on the variations involved in caring for a gerontological client. This unit reviews the age-related factors and differences that a nurse needs to consider when caring for an elderly client.

Unit XXI: Comprehensive Test

Unit XXI is a comprehensive examination that includes practice questions related to all of the content areas addressed in this book. It consists of 300 questions representative of the percentages identified in the NCLEX-RN test plan.

SPECIAL FEATURES OF THE BOOK
Pyramid Terms

Each content area, either a chapter or a unit, begins with *Pyramid Terms* and their definitions. These important terms are significant to the content of the chapter or unit. In addition, the *Pyramid Terms* appear in bold type throughout the chapter or unit.

Pyramid to Success

The *Pyramid to Success*, a unit or chapter introduction, provides you with an overview of the chapter or unit, guidance and direction regarding the focus of review in the particular content area, and its relative importance to the 2001 CAT NCLEX-RN test plan. Specific nursing content areas, as stipulated in the test plan, are identified. The *Pyramid to Success* reviews the Client Needs and the Integrated Concepts and Processes as they pertain to the content in that unit or chapter. These points are the specific components to keep in mind as you review the unit or chapter.

▲ Pyramid Points

Pyramid Points ▲ are the bullets that are placed next to specific content areas throughout the chapters. The *Pyramid Points* provide you with immediate recognition of content that is important in preparation for CAT NCLEX-RN. These bullets identify areas of content that typically appear on CAT NCLEX-RN.

Practice Questions
Multiple Choice

While they are preparing for the NCLEX-RN, it is crucial for students to answer practice questions. This book contains more than 1800 multiple-choice practice questions in NCLEX format. The accompanying software includes all of the multiple-choice questions from the book, plus an additional 1600 questions, for a total of more than 3400 multiple-choice questions.

Critical Thinking: Free-Text Entry

Each chapter contains one *Critical Thinking: Free-Text Entry* question, for a total of 71. This type of question provides you with practice in prioritizing, decision making, and critical thinking skills.

Images

The accompanying software contains 25 *Image Questions* representative of the 2001 CAT NCLEX-RN test plan. These questions are in NCLEX format, and each question presents an image or picture as a component of the question.

Answer Sections

In each chapter the answer section for the practice questions includes the correct answer, rationale, test-taking strategy, question categories, and one or more references. The structure for the answer section is unique and provides the following information.

The Rationale: The rationale provides you with the significant information regarding both correct and incorrect options.

Test-Taking Strategy: The test-taking strategy provides you with the logical path in selecting the correct option and assists you in selecting an answer to a question on which you must guess. Specific suggestions for review are identified.

Question Categories: Each question is identified on the basis of the categories used by the CAT NCLEX-RN

test plan. Additional content categories are provided with each question to assist you in identifying areas in need of review. The categories identified with each practice question include Level of Cognitive Ability, Client Needs, Integrated Concept/Process, and the specific nursing Content Area. All categories are identified by their full names, so that you do not need to memorize codes or abbreviations.

Reference: A reference, including a page number, is provided so that you can easily find the information that you need to review in your undergraduate nursing textbooks.

PHARMACOLOGY AND MEDICATION CALCULATIONS REVIEW

Students consistently say that pharmacology is an area in which they need assistance. CAT NCLEX-RN 2001 is incorporating pharmacology into the examination to a greater extent than in the past. Therefore, pharmacology chapters have been included for your review and practice. This book includes 13 pharmacology chapters, a medication and intravenous (IV) calculation chapter, and a pediatric medication calculation chapter. Each of these chapters includes practice questions using the same format as described above. This book contains more than 400 pharmacology questions.

NCLEX-RN REVIEW SOFTWARE

Packaged in the back of this book you will find a CD-ROM containing NCLEX-RN review software. This software includes more than 3400 multiple-choice questions. It also includes the image practice questions. This Windows- and Macintosh-compatible program offers three testing modes for review of the multiple-choice questions.

Quiz: Ten randomly chosen questions on a specific selected content area. The answer, rationale, test-taking strategy, question categories, reference, and results appear after you answer all 10 questions.

Study: All questions on a specific selected content area. The answer, rationale, test-taking strategy, question categories, and reference appear after you answer each question.

Examination: One hundred randomly chosen questions from the entire pool of more than 3400 questions. The answer, rationale, test-taking strategy, question categories, reference, and results appear after you answer all 100 questions.

HOW TO USE THIS BOOK

Saunders Comprehensive Review for NCLEX-RN is especially designed to help you with your successful journey to the peak of the *Saunders Pyramid to Success*, becoming a registered nurse. As you begin your journey through this book, you will be introduced to all of the importa points regarding the 2001 CAT NCLEX-RN examination, the process of testing, and the unique and special tips regarding how to prepare yourself for this very important examination.

You should begin your process through the *Saunders Pyramid to Success* by reading all of Unit I in this book and becoming familiar with the important points regarding the CAT NCLEX-RN examination. Read the chapter written by the nursing graduate who recently passed the NCLEX-RN, and note what this graduate has to say about the examination. The test-taking strategy chapter will provide you with important strategies that will guide you in selecting the correct option, or assist you in selecting an answer to a question on which you must guess. Read this chapter, and practice these strategies as you proceed through your journey with this book. Continue your journey by reading each of the chapters in the units that follow. Review the Pyramid Terms and the Pyramid to Success and identify the Client Needs and Integrated Concepts and Processes specific to the test plan in each area. Read each of the chapters, focusing on the Pyramid Points that identify those areas most likely to be tested on CAT NCLEX-RN.

As you read each chapter, identify your strengths and the areas that are in need of further review. Highlight these areas, and test your strengths and abilities by taking all of the practice tests provided at the ends of the chapters. Be sure to read all of the rationales and test-taking strategies. The rationale provides you with the significant information regarding both the correct and incorrect options. The test-taking strategy offers you the logical path to selecting the correct option. The strategy also identifies the content area that you need to review if you had difficulty with the question. Use the reference listed so you can easily find the information that you need to review.

After reviewing all of the chapters in the book, turn to Unit XXI, the Comprehensive Test. Take this examination, and then review each question, answer, and rationale. Identify any areas requiring review; then take the time to review those areas again.

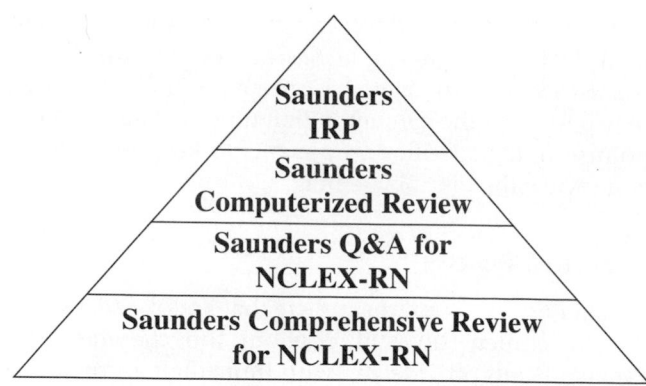

After using this book to review specific content areas, continue on your journey through the *Saunders Pyramid to Success* with the companion book, *Saunders Q & A Review for NCLEX-RN,* for additional practice questions. The companion book and its accompanying software offer you 3500 practice questions in specific areas outlined by the 2001 CAT NCLEX-RN test plan. With practice questions uniquely focused on the Client Needs and the Integrated Concepts and Processes, you can assess your level of competence. To determine your readiness for CAT NCLEX-RN, you will use the next step in the *Saunders Pyramid to Success, Saunders Computerized Review for NCLEX-RN.* This unique software program contains 1500 NCLEX-RN–style questions. The software provides detailed analysis similar to that in standardized nursing examinations. The final component of the *Saunders Pyramid to Success* is *Saunders Instructor's Resource Package for NCLEX-RN.* This manual and CD-ROM accompany the Saunders program of NCLEX-RN review products. Be sure to ask your nursing program director and nursing faculty about this CD-ROM and its use for a review course or for a self-paced review in your school's computer laboratory.

Good luck with your journey through the *Saunders Pyramid to Success.* I wish you continued success throughout your new career as a registered nurse!

Linda Anne Silvestri

To All Future Registered Nurses,

Congratulations to you!

You should be very proud and pleased with yourself on your most recent, well-deserved accomplishment of completing your nursing program to become a registered nurse. I know that you have worked very hard to become successful and that you have proved to yourself that indeed you can achieve your goals.

In my opinion, you are about to enter the most wonderful and rewarding profession that exists. Your willingness, desire, and ability to assist those who need nursing care will bring great satisfaction to your life.

In the profession of nursing, your learning will be a lifelong process. This aspect of the profession makes it stimulating and dynamic. Your learning process will continue to expand and grow as the profession continues to evolve. Your next, very important endeavor will be the learning process involved to achieve success in your examination to become a registered nurse.

I am excited and pleased to be able to provide you with the *Saunders Pyramid to Success* products that will prepare you for your next important professional goal, becoming a registered nurse. I want to thank all of my former nursing students whom I have assisted in preparing for NCLEX-RN for their willingness to offer ideas regarding their needs in preparing for licensure. Student ideas have certainly added a special uniqueness to all of the products available in *Saunders Pyramid to Success*.

Saunders Pyramid to Success products provide you with everything that you need to prepare for the NCLEX-RN. These products include material that is required for NCLEX-RN preparation for all nursing students, regardless of educational background, specific strengths, areas in need of improvement, or clinical experience during the nursing program.

So, let's get started and begin our journey through the *Pyramid to Success*, and welcome to the wonderful profession of nursing!

Sincerely,

Linda Anne Silvestri MSN, RN

Linda Anne Silvestri, MSN, RN

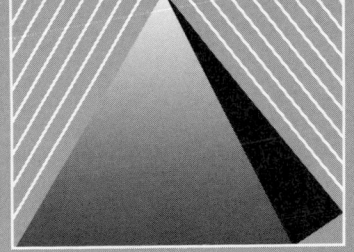

Acknowledgments

Sincere appreciation and warmest thanks are extended to the many individuals who in their own ways have contributed to the publication of this book.

First, I want to thank all of my nursing students at the Community College of Rhode Island in Warwick, who approached me in 1991 and persuaded me to assist them in preparing to take the NCLEX-RN examination. Their enthusiasm and inspiration led to the commencement of my professional endeavors in conducting NCLEX-RN review courses for nursing students. I also thank the numerous nursing students who have attended my review courses for their willingness to share their needs and ideas. Their input has certainly added a uniqueness to this publication.

I wish to acknowledge all of the nursing faculty who taught in my NCLEX-RN review courses. Their commitment, dedication, and expertise have certainly assisted nursing students in achieving success with the NCLEX-RN. In addition, I want to acknowledge Laurent W. Valliere for his contribution to this publication, for teaching in my NCLEX-RN review courses, and for his commitment and dedication in assisting my nursing students to prepare for NCLEX-RN from a nonacademic point of view.

I sincerely acknowledge and thank two very important individuals from Harcourt Health Sciences. I thank Loren Wilson, Senior Editor, for all of her assistance throughout the preparation of this edition and for her continuous enthusiasm, support, and expert professional guidance. And I thank Shelly Hayden, Senior Developmental Editor, for her continuous assistance and for keeping me on track. Her expert organizational skills maintained order in all of the work that I submitted for manuscript production.

A special thank you and acknowledgment go to another important individual, Sarah Miller, my assistant. She provided continuous support and dedication to my work both in the NCLEX review courses and in preparing the second edition of this book.

I want to acknowledge all of the staff at Harcourt Health Sciences for their tremendous assistance throughout the preparation and production of this publication. A special thank you to all of them.

I thank all of the special people in the production department: Steve Hetager, production editor, whose consistent editing assisted in finalizing this publication, Trish Tannian, Project Manager, and Gail Morey Hudson, Book Design Manager.

I sincerely thank Janet Blanner, Marketing Manager, and Linda Morris, Marketing Manager, from the Nursing Marketing Department, whose support, hard work, and special creativity assisted with this publication.

I would also like to acknowledge Patricia Mieg, Educational Sales Representative, who encouraged me to submit my ideas and initial work for the first edition of this book to the W.B. Saunders Company and initiated my meeting with Maura Connor, my former Senior Acquisitions Editor. I want to thank Maura Connor for her professional direction that led me to success as I initially created *Saunders Pyramid to Success* for NCLEX-RN.

I want to acknowledge my parents, who opened my door of opportunity in education. I thank my mother, Frances Mary, for all of her love, support, and assistance as I continuously worked to achieve my professional goals. I thank my father, Arnold Lawrence, who always provided insightful words of encouragement. My memories of his love and support will always remain in my heart.

I also thank my sister, Dianne Elodia, my brother, Lawrence Peter, and my niece, Gina Marie, who were continuously supportive, giving, and helpful during my research and preparation of this publication.

I want to acknowledge all of the contributors, who provided many of the practice questions contained in this publication, and the many faculty and student reviewers for their thoughts and ideas.

I sincerely thank Mary Ann Hogan, MSN, RN, from Holyoke Community College in Holyoke, Massachusetts, who has always encouraged and supported me through my professional endeavors. Her numerous contributions to this publication are a reflection of her dedication to the profession of nursing and to nursing students.

A special thank you to Dr. JoAnn Mullaney from Salve Regina University in Newport, Rhode Island, for her numerous and expert contributions to this publication, and to Heather Carlson, RN, for providing a chapter to this publication regarding her experiences with NCLEX-RN.

I also need to thank Salve Regina University for the opportunity to educate nursing students in the baccalaureate nursing program and for its support during my research and writing of this publication. I would especially like to acknowledge Dr. Louise Murdock and Dr. Ellen McCarty, Co-Chairpersons of the Department of Nursing at Salve Regina University, for their continuous support, academic mentoring, and astute vision regarding the future of the profession of nursing.

I wish to acknowledge the University of Rhode Island, College of Nursing, for providing me with the opportunity for professional growth in my nursing education, particularly Dr. Donna Schwartz-Barcott and Dr. Suzie Kim, my academic advisors in the doctoral program at the university.

I wish to acknowledge the Community College of Rhode Island, which provided me the opportunity to educate nursing students in the Associate Degree of Nursing Program, and a special thank you to Patricia Miller, MSN, RN, and Michelina McClellan, MS, RN, from Baystate Medical Center, School of Nursing, in Springfield, Massachusetts, who were my very first mentors in nursing education.

Last, a very special thank you to all my nursing students, past, present, and future. Your love and dedication to the profession of nursing and your commitment to provide health care will bring never-ending rewards!

Linda Anne Silvestri

Contents

NCLEX Preparation

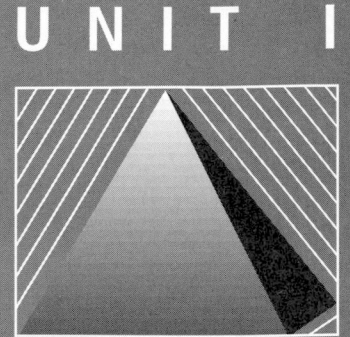

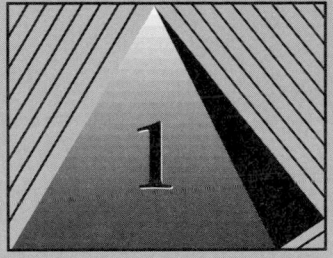

NCLEX-RN

THE PYRAMID TO SUCCESS

Welcome to the Pyramid to Success!

Saunders Comprehensive Review for NCLEX-RN is specially designed to help you begin your successful journey to the peak of the Pyramid, becoming a registered nurse! As you begin your journey, you will be introduced to all of the important points regarding the NCLEX-RN examination and the process of testing and to the unique and special tips regarding how to prepare yourself for this very important examination. You will read what a nursing graduate who recently passed NCLEX-RN has to say about the examination. All those important Test-Taking Strategies are detailed. These details will guide you in selecting the correct option or assist you in selecting an answer to a question you must guess at.

Each of the content areas in this book begins with the Pyramid to Success. The Pyramid to Success addresses specific points related to NCLEX-RN, including the Pyramid Terms and the Client Needs and the Integrated Concepts and Processes as identified in the test plan framework for the examination. Pyramid Terms are key words that are defined and are boldfaced throughout each chapter to direct your attention to those significant NCLEX-RN points. The Client Needs and the Integrated Concepts and Processes specific to the content of the chapter are identified.

Throughout each chapter, you will find Pyramid Point bullets that identify areas most likely to be tested on NCLEX-RN. Read each chapter, and identify your strengths and areas that are in need of further review. Test your strengths and abilities by taking all the practice tests provided in this book. Be sure to read all the rationales and the test-taking strategies. The rationale provides you with significant information regarding both the correct option and incorrect options. The test-taking strategy provides you with the logical path to selecting the correct option. The test-taking strategy also identifies the content area to review, if required. The reference source and page number are provided so that you can easily find the information that you need to review. Each question is coded on the basis of the Level of Cognitive Ability, the Client Needs category, the Integrated Concept and Process, and the nursing content area.

Following the completion of your comprehensive review in this book, continue on your journey though the Pyramid to Success with the companion book, *Saunders Q & A Review for NCLEX-RN*, which provides you with 3500 practice questions based on the NCLEX-RN test plan. Then you are ready for the *Saunders Computerized Review*, a computer disk program that contains 1700 NCLEX-RN–style questions to help you determine your readiness for NCLEX-RN.

Let's begin our journey through the Pyramid to Success!

THE EXAMINATION PROCESS

An important step in the Pyramid to Success is to become as familiar as possible with the examination process. A significant amount of anxiety can occur in candidates facing the challenge of this examination. Knowing what the examination is all about, and knowing what you will encounter during the process of testing, will assist in alleviating fear and anxiety. The information contained in this chapter addresses the procedures related to the development of the NCLEX-RN Test Plan, the components of the Test Plan, and the answers to the questions most commonly asked by nursing students and graduates preparing to take the NCLEX-RN. The information related to the development of the NCLEX-RN Test Plan, the components of the Test Plan, and the testing procedures was adapted from *Test Plan for the National Council Licensure Examination for Registered Nurses*, National Council of State Boards of Nursing, Chicago, 2000, and *The NCLEX Process: Serving as an Anchor for the NCLEX Examination*, National Council of State Boards of Nursing, Chicago, 2000.

DEVELOPMENT OF THE TEST PLAN

As an initial step in the test development process, the National Council of State Boards of Nursing considers the legal scope of nursing practice as governed by state laws and regulations, including the nurse practice act. The National Council uses these laws to define the areas on NCLEX-RN that will assess the competence of candidates for nurse licensure.

The National Council of State Boards of Nursing also conducts a Practice Analysis study to determine the framework for the Test Plan for NCLEX-RN. Since nursing practice continues to change, this study is conducted every 3 years. The results of this study, most recently conducted in 1999, provided the structure for the new test plan implemented in April of 2001.

PRACTICE ANALYSIS STUDY

The participants in this study include newly licensed registered nurses from all types of basic education programs. The participants are provided a list of nursing activities and are asked about the frequency of performing these specific activities, their impact on maintaining client safety, and the setting where the activities were performed. The analysis of the data obtained from this study guides the development of a framework for entry-level nurse performance that incorporates specific client needs and the concepts and processes fundamental to the practice of nursing. The NCLEX-RN Test Plan is derived from this framework.

THE TEST PLAN

The content of NCLEX-RN reflects the activities that a newly licensed entry-level registered nurse must be able to perform in order to provide clients with safe and effective nursing care. The questions are written to address the Levels of Cognitive Ability, Client Needs, and Integrated Concepts and Processes as identified in the Test Plan.

Levels of Cognitive Ability

The NCLEX-RN examination includes questions at the cognitive levels of knowledge, comprehension, application, and analysis. The majority of the questions are written at the application and analysis levels because the practice of nursing requires critical thinking and complex thought processing. This means that the test taker will be required to analyze and/or apply the information provided in the test question (Box 1-1).

Client Needs

In the new Test Plan implemented in April 2001, the National Council of State Boards of Nursing has

---

BOX 1-1

Level of Cognitive Ability

The nurse is caring for a client with a T5 spinal cord injury. The client complains of a severe headache and is feeling anxious. The nurse notes the client is sweating and is bradycardic and hypertensive. Which nursing intervention is most appropriate initially?

1. Check for bladder distention
2. Notify the physician
3. Medicate the client with an analgesic
4. Discuss the client's feelings of anxiety

Answer: 1

This question requires the test taker to analyze the information provided in order to determine the most appropriate initial nursing intervention. The test taker needs to know the signs and symptoms of autonomic dysreflexia and the potential causes, such as a full bladder or bowel.

Level of Cognitive Ability: Analysis

TABLE 1-1

Client Needs and the Percentage of Test Questions

Safe, Effective Care Environment	
Management of Care	7%-13%
Safety and Infection Control	5%-11%
Health Promotion and Maintenance	
Growth and Development Through the Life Span	7%-13%
Prevention and Early Detection of Disease	5%-11%
Psychosocial Integrity	
Coping and Adaptation	5%-11%
Psychosocial Adaptation	5%-11%
Physiological Integrity	
Basic Care and Comfort	7%-13%
Pharmacological and Parenteral Therapies	5%-11%
Reduction of Risk Potential	12%-18%
Physiological Adaptation	12%-18%

---

identified a test plan framework based on *Client Needs*. This framework was selected on the basis of the analysis of the findings in the Practice Analysis study, and because Client Needs provides a structure for defining nursing actions and competencies across all settings for all clients. The National Council of State Boards of Nursing identifies four major categories of Client Needs. These categories are further divided into subcategories, and the percentage of test questions in each subcategory is identified (Table 1-1).

Safe, Effective Care Environment

The Safe, Effective Care Environment category includes two subcategories: Management of Care and Safety and

BOX 1-2

Safe, Effective Care Environment

MANAGEMENT OF CARE

The charge nurse in a medical unit observes that a client is agitated and incoherent. The nurse suspects that the client is experiencing a reaction to medication. In planning a safe environment for this client, the most appropriate intervention is to:

1. Request that the physician order restraints and sedation
2. Ask the family to stay with the client
3. Have a nurse observe the client
4. Use a multidisciplinary approach to plan care

Answer: 4

This question addresses the subcategory, Management of Care, in the Client Needs category, Safe, Effective Care Environment. The nurse has the responsibility to provide safe and effective care. Options 1, 2, and 3 rely on other individuals to care for the client. Option 4 addresses an integrated multidisciplinary health care team approach.

SAFETY AND INFECTION CONTROL

The nurse is caring for a client who is receiving total parenteral nutrition (TPN). Which nursing action will decrease the client's risk of developing an infection from this therapy?

1. Assessing vital signs at 4-hour intervals
2. Instructing the client to perform a Valsalva maneuver during intravenous tubing changes
3. Administering acetaminophen (Tylenol) before changing the central line dressing
4. Using aseptic technique in handling the TPN solution and tubing

Answer: 4

This question addresses the subcategory, Safety and Infection Control, in the Client Needs category, Safe, Effective Care Environment. It addresses content related to asepsis. Option 1 will detect signs of an infection but is not associated with prevention or decreasing the risk of infection. Options 2 and 3 do not relate to infection. Aseptic technique is critical to prevent infection!

BOX 1-3

Health Promotion and Maintenance

GROWTH AND DEVELOPMENT THROUGH THE LIFE SPAN

The nurse is employed in an older adult day care center. Which activity would best promote health and maintenance among these clients?

1. Gardening every day for an hour
2. Cycling three times a week for 20 minutes
3. Sculpting once a week for 40 minutes
4. Walking three to five times a week for 30 minutes

Answer: 4

Rationale: This question addresses the subcategory, Growth and Development Through the Life Span, in the Client Needs category, Health Promotion and Maintenance. One of the best exercises for an older adult is walking, progressing to 30-minute sessions three to five times each week. Swimming and dancing are also beneficial. Exercise and activity are essential for health promotion and maintenance in the older adult and to achieve an optimal level of functioning.

PREVENTION AND EARLY DETECTION OF DISEASE

The nurse has provided instructions to a client regarding measures to prevent the development of thrombophlebitis. Which client statement indicates an understanding of these measures?

1. "I am taking oral contraceptives to avoid pregnancy, which can cause venous stasis."
2. "I avoid sitting or standing in one position for prolonged periods."
3. "I'm glad I don't need to wear those ugly stockings."
4. "I have decreased my fluid consumption to one glass of water a day."

Answer: 2

This question addresses the subcategory, Prevention and Early Detection of Disease, in the Client Needs category, Health Promotion and Maintenance. Avoidance of sitting or standing for a prolonged period of time is one of the measures for the prevention of venous stasis and thrombophlebitis. This option identifies the client's understanding of a health practice that will promote and support wellness.

Infection Control. Management of Care (7% to 13%) addresses content that tests the knowledge, skills, and ability required to provide integrated, cost-effective care to clients by coordinating, supervising, and/or collaborating with members of the multidisciplinary health care team. Safety and Infection Control (5% to 11%) addresses content that tests the knowledge, skills, and ability required to protect clients and health care personnel from environmental hazards (Box 1-2).

Health Promotion and Maintenance

The Health Promotion and Maintenance category includes two subcategories: Growth and Development Through the Life Span and the Prevention and Early Detection of Disease. Growth and Development Through the Life Span (7% to 13%) addresses content that tests the knowledge, skills, and ability required to assist the client and significant others through the normal, expected stages of growth and development from conception through advanced old age. Prevention and Early Detection of Disease (5% to 11%) addresses content that tests the knowledge, skills, and ability required to assist clients to recognize alterations in health and to develop health practices that promote and support wellness (Box 1-3).

Psychosocial Integrity

The Psychosocial Integrity category includes two subcategories: Coping and Adaptation and Psychosocial Adaptation. Coping and Adaptation (5% to 11%) addresses content that tests the knowledge, skills, and ability required to promote the client and/or significant others' ability to cope, adapt, and/or problem solve situations related to illnesses, disabilities, or stressful events. Psychosocial Adaptation (5% to 11%) addresses content that tests the knowledge, skills, and ability required to manage and provide care for clients with maladaptive behaviors or with acute or chronic mental illnesses (Box 1-4).

Physiological Integrity

The Physiological Integrity category includes four subcategories: Basic Care and Comfort, Pharmacological and Parenteral Therapies, Reduction of Risk Potential, and Physiological Adaptation. Basic Care and Comfort (7% to 13%) addresses content that tests the knowledge, skills, and ability required to provide comfort and assistance in the performance of activities of daily living. Pharmacological and Parenteral Therapies (5% to 11%) addresses content that tests the knowledge, skills, and ability required to manage and provide care related to the administration of medications and parenteral therapies. Reduction of Risk Potential (12% to 18%) addresses content that tests the knowledge, skills, and ability required to reduce the likelihood that clients will develop complications or health problems related to existing conditions, treatments, or procedures. Physio-

logical Adaptation (12% to 18%) addresses content that tests the knowledge, skills, and ability required to manage and provide care to clients with acute, chronic, or life-threatening physical health conditions (Box 1-5).

Integrated Concepts and Processes

The National Council of State Boards of Nursing has identified six concepts and processes that are fundamental to the practice of nursing. These concepts and processes are a component of the Test Plan and are incorporated throughout the major categories of Client Needs (Box 1-6).

BOX 1-4

Psychosocial Integrity

COPING AND ADAPTATION

The hospice nurse visits a client dying of ovarian cancer. During the visit, the client says, "If I can just live long enough to attend my daughter's graduation, I'll be ready to die." Which phase of coping is this client experiencing?
1. Isolation
2. Bargaining
3. Depression
4. Acceptance

Answer: 2

This question addresses the subcategory of Coping and Adaptation in the Client Needs category, Psychosocial Integrity. Bargaining is the phase of coping in which the dying person tries to negotiate, as in this case, making deals with God or fate. The content addressed in this question is specific to coping mechanisms.

PSYCHOSOCIAL ADAPTATION

The visiting nurse observes that the elderly male client is confined to his room by his daughter-in-law. When the nurse suggests he walk to the den and join the family, he says, "I'm in everyone's way; my son needs for me to stay here." The most important action for the nurse to take is to:
1. Suggest to the client and daughter-in-law that they consider a nursing home for the client
2. Suggest appropriate resources to the client and daughter-in-law, such as respite care and senior citizens
3. Say nothing as it is best for the nurse to remain neutral and wait to be asked for help
4. Say to the son, "Confining your father to his room is inhuman."

Answer: 2

This question addresses the subcategory, Psychosocial Adaptation in the Client Needs category of Psychosocial Integrity. Caregiver stress and burnout are thought to account for much of the abuse of elderly people. Assisting clients and families to become knowledgeable of available community support systems is a role and responsibility of the nurse. The content addressed in this question is specific to elder abuse/neglect.

BOX 1-5

Physiological Integrity

BASIC CARE AND COMFORT

The client has slight weakness in the right leg. Based on this assessment, the nurse determines that the client would benefit most from the use of a:

1. Walker
2. Wooden crutch
3. Lofstrand crutch
4. Straight leg cane

Answer: 4

This question addresses the subcategory of Basic Care and Comfort in the Client Needs category, Physiological Integrity. A straight leg cane is useful for the client with slight weakness in one leg. In this question, the nurse specifically assists the client in the performance of activities of daily living.

PHARMACOLOGICAL AND PARENTERAL THERAPIES

The nurse is caring for a client with a diagnosis of chronic angina pectoris. The client is receiving sotalol (Betapace), 80 mg PO daily. Which of the following would indicate that the client is experiencing a side effect related to the medication?

1. Difficulty in swallowing
2. Diaphoresis
3. Dry mouth
4. Bradycardia

Answer: 4

This question addresses the subcategory of Pharmacological and Parenteral Therapies in the Client Needs category, Physiological Integrity. Sotalol (Betapace) is a beta-adrenergic blocking agent. Side effects include bradycardia, palpitations, difficulty breathing, irregular heart beat, signs of congestive heart failure, and cold hands and feet. The content addressed in this question is specific to the side effects of a medication.

REDUCTION OF RISK POTENTIAL

The client with acute myocardial infarction receives therapy with alteplase recombinant (tPA). The nurse assesses for complications of this treatment. Which assessment data would the nurse document as indicating a possible complication?

1. Epistaxis
2. Vomiting
3. ST segment elevation on ECG
4. Absent pedal pulses

Answer: 1

This question addresses the subcategory of Reduction of Risk Potential in the Client Needs category, Physiological Integrity. Bleeding is a major side effect of tPA therapy. This question addresses content related to the complication of a treatment.

PHYSIOLOGICAL ADAPTATION

The nurse reviews the blood gas results of a client with Guillain-Barré syndrome. The nurse analyzes the results and determines that the client is experiencing respiratory acidosis. Which of the following validates the nurse's findings?

1. pH 7.45, P_{CO_2} 52 mm Hg
2. pH 7.35, P_{CO_2} 40 mm Hg
3. pH 7.25, P_{CO_2} 50 mm Hg
4. pH 7.50, P_{CO_2} 30 mm Hg

Answer: 3

This question addresses the subcategory of Physiological Adaptation in the Client Needs category, Physiological Integrity. The normal pH is 7.35 to 7.45. The normal P_{CO_2} is 35 to 45 mm Hg. In respiratory acidosis, the pH is down and the P_{CO_2} is up. Options 1 and 4 reflect an elevated pH that indicates an alkalotic condition. Option 2 reflects a normal blood gas result. The content addressed in this question relates to alterations in body systems.

BOX 1-6

Integrated Concepts and Processes

Caring
Communication and Documentation
Cultural Awareness
Nursing Process
Self-Care
Teaching/Learning

ITEM WRITERS

NCLEX-RN item writers are selected by the National Council of State Boards of Nursing after an extensive application process. The item writers are registered nurses who hold a master's degree or a higher degree. Most of the item writers are nursing educators; however, clinical nurse specialists are also selected to participate in this process. These item writers are clinical experts who are currently involved in clinical practice with entry-level registered nurses. Item writers voluntarily submit an application to become an item writer and must meet specific established criteria designated by the National Council in order to be accepted as a participant in the process.

CAT NCLEX-RN

The term NCLEX-RN stands for National Council Licensure Examination for Registered Nurses. CAT NCLEX-RN is a computer-administered examination that the nursing graduate must take and pass in order to practice as a registered nurse. This examination measures the test candidate's knowledge, skills, and abilities required to perform safely and competently as a newly licensed, entry-level registered nurse.

COMPUTERIZED ADAPTIVE TESTING (CAT)

The word CAT stands for Computerized Adaptive Testing. CAT provides a uniqueness to the examination that the candidate will take; the examination adapts to each test taker's skill level. The CAT examination is assembled interactively as the candidate answers the questions. All of the test questions are stored in a large test bank and are categorized on the basis of the test plan structure and the level of difficulty of the question. With the CAT method of testing, an examination is created and tailored to test the candidate's knowledge and abilities while fulfilling Test Plan requirements. The candidate will not waste time answering questions that are far above or below his or her competency level.

When you answer a question on CAT NCLEX-RN, the computer will calculate a competency skill estimate based on the answer that you selected. If you selected a correct answer to a question, the computer scans the test bank and selects a more difficult question. If you selected an incorrect answer, the computer scans the test bank and selects an easier question. This process continues until the test plan requirements are met and a reliable pass or fail decision is made.

THE PROCESS OF REGISTRATION

The initial step in the registration process is that a candidate applies to the state board of nursing in the state in which he or she intends to obtain licensure. (The addresses, telephone numbers, and web sites, if available, of boards of nursing in all states and territories of the United States are provided at the end of this chapter.) You need to obtain information from the board of nursing regarding the specific registration process, as the process may vary from state to state. It is very important that you follow the registration instructions and complete the registration forms precisely and accurately. Registration forms not properly completed, or not accompanied by the proper fees in the required method of payment, will be returned to you and will delay testing. The initial fee for the application process may vary from state to state. Each board of nursing will set its initial license fee according to its own needs. The registration forms will identify the registration and testing service fees. When the board of nursing receives the completed registration form, based on the criteria established by the board, your eligibility is determined, and the board authorizes your admission to the examination.

Once your eligibility to test has been determined by the board of nursing in the jurisdiction in which licensure is requested, the valid NCLEX registration is processed and an Authorization to Test form will be sent to you. You cannot make an appointment until the board of nursing declares eligibility and you receive an Authorization to Test form. The Authorization to Test form will provide a candidate identification number and an authorization number, and these numbers will be needed to make an appointment with the testing center.

SPECIAL TESTING CIRCUMSTANCES

A candidate who is requesting special accommodations should contact the board of nursing prior to submitting a registration form. The board of nursing will provide you with the procedures for the request. The board of nursing must authorize special testing accommodations. Following board of nursing approval, the National Council of State Boards reviews the requested accommodations to ensure that the proposed modification does not affect the psychometric properties of NCLEX or cause a security risk. The National Council of State Boards must also approve the accommodations.

MAKING AN APPOINTMENT TO TEST

The CAT NCLEX-RN examination is administered on a year round basis. You will be provided with a list of testing centers and the telephone numbers. Note the expiration date on the Authorization to Test form. You must schedule and make an appointment before this expiration date. You may take the test at any approved testing center and do not have to test in the same jurisdiction in which you are seeking licensure. An eligible candidate taking NCLEX for the first time will be offered an appointment date within 30 days of the telephone call to the testing center. Repeat candidates will be offered an appointment date within 45 days of the telephone call to the testing center. A confirmation notice will not be sent to you; therefore it is important to note the date and time of the appointment. When you call the test center, it is also important to verify the address and the directions to the testing center.

CANCELING OR RESCHEDULING AN APPOINTMENT

If for any reason you need to cancel or reschedule your appointment to test, the scheduling change must be made before noon, two business days prior to the scheduled appointment. The original appointment must be canceled before a new appointment can be scheduled.

LATE ARRIVALS TO THE TEST CENTER

It is important that you arrive at the testing center 30 minutes before the test is scheduled. Candidates arriving late for the scheduled testing appointment may be required to forfeit the NCLEX appointment. If it is necessary for the appointment to be forfeited, candidates will need to re-register for the examination and pay an additional fee. The board of nursing will be notified that the candidate will not test. A few days before your scheduled date of testing, take the time to drive to the testing center to determine its exact location, the length of time required to arrive to that destination, and any potential obstacles that might delay you, such as road construction, traffic, or parking sites.

THE TESTING CENTER

The test center is designed to ensure complete security of the testing process. Strict candidate identification requirements have been established. To be admitted to the testing center, it is imperative that you bring the Authorization to Test form, along with two forms of identification. You must sign both forms of identification, and one must contain your photograph. The name on the photograph identification must be the same as the name on the Authorization to Test form. Examples of acceptable forms of identification will be included in the information received with the Authorization to Test form. You will be required to sign in and out on the test center log form. Each candidate will be thumbprinted and photographed at the test center, and the photograph will accompany the NCLEX results to confirm the candidate's identity. Personal belongings are not allowed in the testing room. Secure storage will be provided for the candidate; however, storage space is limited, so you must plan accordingly. In addition, the testing center will not assume responsibility for your personal belongings. The testing waiting areas are generally small; therefore friends or family members who accompany you are not permitted to wait in the testing center while you are taking the NCLEX-RN.

Once you have completed the admission process and a brief orientation, the proctor will escort you to the assigned computer. You will be seated at an individual table area with an appropriate work space that includes computer equipment, appropriate lighting, scratch paper, and a pencil. Unauthorized scratch paper may not be brought into or removed from the testing room. Eating, drinking, and smoking are not allowed in the testing room. A video camera is located in the testing room, and full sound and motion videotaping of all test sessions occurs.

Keep your two forms of identification with you at all times. You cannot leave the testing room without the permission of the proctor. If you leave the testing room for any reason, you will be required to show two forms of identification to be readmitted. You must follow the directions given by the test center staff and must remain seated during the test, except when authorized to leave. If you feel that you have a problem with the computer, need more scratch paper, or need the proctor for any reason, you must raise your hand to notify the proctor.

THE COMPUTER

You do not need any computer experience to take the CAT NCLEX-RN examination. A keyboard tutorial is provided and administered to all test takers at the start of the examination. In addition, a proctor is present to assist in explaining the use of the computer to ensure your full understanding of how to proceed.

CAT NCLEX-RN TEST QUESTIONS

The examination is composed of individual (stand alone) test questions. In other words, this examination does not present a case situation followed by several test questions that relate to that case situation. With an individual (stand alone) test question, you can expect that the question will appear on the left-hand side of the screen with the four options on the right-hand side of the screen, or the question will appear across the top of the screen with the four options below (Box 1-7).

Primarily, the test questions will be multiple-choice

BOX 1-7

Appearance of an Individual (Stand Alone) Test Question on the Computer Screen

The most appropriate method for feeding the infant with a cleft lip or palate is:

1. With the head in an upright position
2. With the infant in a lying position
3. With the infant in a side-lying position
4. With the infant prone

The client is admitted with a diagnosis of myasthenia gravis. Pyridostigmine (Mestinon) is prescribed for the client. An adverse effect of this medication is:

1. Muscle cramps
2. Mouth ulcers
3. Depression
4. Unexplained weight gain

(question and four options) questions. You may also be presented with a visual or image type of display and be asked a question about the visual or image. For example, you may be presented with a cardiac rhythm strip and be asked what the nursing action would be if this cardiac rhythm was noted on a client's cardiac monitor. In this example, you would be required to identify the cardiac rhythm and then determine the appropriate nursing action.

Another type of question that you may encounter is the type that will require you to use the mouse component of the computer system. For example, you may be presented with a visual that displays an adult client's thorax. In this visual, you may be asked to "point and click" (using the mouse) on the area where the stethoscope would be placed to take an apical pulse rate.

Finally, you may encounter a question known as a free-text entry. In this type of question, you will be asked to type the answer to the question. For example, you may be provided with intake and output figures for a client receiving a continuous bladder irrigation and then be asked to determine the client's true urine output. Once this is determined, you would need to type your answer in the appropriate area as designated on the computer screen.

When a test question is presented on the computer screen, it must be answered or the test will not move on. This means that you will not be able to skip questions, go back and review questions, or go back and change answers. Students preparing for CAT NCLEX-RN become anxious and frustrated because questions cannot be skipped and returned to at a later time during the examination process. Remember, in a CAT examination, once an answer is recorded, all subsequent questions administered depend, to an extent, on the answer selected for that question. Skipping and returning to earlier questions are not compatible with the logical methodology of a computerized adaptive test. In addition, it is important to recall the number of times you may have changed a correct answer to an incorrect one on a pencil-and-paper nursing examination during your nursing education. The inability to skip questions or go back to change previous answers will not be a disadvantage to you. Actually, you will not fall into that "trap" of changing a correct answer to an incorrect one with CAT. There is no penalty for guessing on CAT NCLEX-RN. Remember, the answer to the question will be right there in front of you. If you need to guess, use your nursing knowledge to its fullest extent, as well as all of the test-taking strategies provided to you in Chapter 4 of this book.

TESTING TIME

The maximum testing time is five hours, and this time period includes the tutorial, sample questions, and all rest breaks. There is no minimum amount of examination time. A mandatory 10-minute break will be taken after 2 testing hours, and an optional 10-minute break can be taken at the end of 3½ hours of testing. The computer screen will notify you of the time for these breaks. You must leave the testing room during breaks. You may leave the room for additional, unscheduled breaks, but no additional testing time will be allowed.

LENGTH OF THE EXAMINATION

The minimum number of questions that you will need to answer in order to meet adequate testing in each area of the test plan is 75. Of these 75 questions, 60 will be real (scored) questions and 15 will be try-out (unscored) questions. The maximum number of questions in the test is 265. Fifteen of the total number of questions that you need to answer will be try-out (unscored) questions.

The try-out questions are questions that may be presented as scored questions on future NCLEX-RN examinations. These try-out questions are not identified as such. In other words, you do not know which questions are the try-out (unscored) questions.

COMPLETING THE EXAM

Once the test is completed, you will complete a brief computer-delivered questionnaire about your testing experience. After this questionnaire is completed, the test proctor will collect all scratch paper, sign you out, and permit you to leave.

PROCESSING RESULTS

Upon completion of the examination, results are transmitted electronically to the data center for scoring. Your results are then transmitted to the board of nursing in the state in which you applied for licensure. The board of nursing will mail the results to the candidate. You should not telephone the testing center, the National Council, or the state board of nursing for results. The results will not be given to candidates over the telephone.

INTERSTATE ENDORSEMENT

Since the CAT NCLEX-RN is a national examination, you can apply to take the examination in any state. Once licensure is received, the registered nurse can apply for Interstate Endorsement. The procedures and requirements for Interstate Endorsement may vary from state to state, and these procedures can be obtained from the state board of nursing in the state in which endorsement is sought.

STATE BOARDS OF NURSING

Alabama Board of Nursing
RSA Plaza, Ste 250
770 Washington Avenue
Montgomery, AL 36130-3900
(334) 242-4060
Web Site: http://www.abn.state.al.us/

Alaska Board of Nursing
Dept. of Comm. and Econ. Development
Div. of Occupational Licensing
3601 C Street, Suite 722
Anchorage, AK 99503
(907) 269-8161
Web Site: http://www.dced.state.ak.us/occ/pnur.htm

American Samoa Health Services
Regulatory Board
LBJ Tropical Medical Center
Pago Pago, AS 96799
(684) 633-1222

Arizona State Board of Nursing
1651 E. Morten Avenue, Suite 150
Phoenix, AZ 85020
(602) 331-8111
Web Site: http://www.azboardofnursing.org/

Arkansas State Board of Nursing
University Tower Building
1123 S. University, Suite 800
Little Rock, AR 72204
(501) 686-2700
Web Site: http://www.state.ar.us/nurse

California Board of Registered Nursing
400 R St., Suite 4030
Sacramento, CA 95814-6239
(916) 322-3350
Web Site: http://www.rn.ca.gov/

Colorado Board of Nursing
1560 Broadway, Suite 880
Denver, CO 80202
(303) 894-2430
Web Site: http://www.dora.state.co.us/nursing/

Connecticut Board of Examiners for Nursing
Division of Health Systems Regulation
410 Capitol Avenue, MS no. 13ADJ
P.O. Box 340308
Hartford, CT 06134-0328
(860) 509-7624
Web Site: http://www.state.ct.us/dph/

Delaware Board of Nursing
861 Silver Lake Blvd
Cannon Building, Suite 203
Dover, DE 19904
(302) 739-4522

District of Columbia Board of Nursing
Department of Health
825 N. Capitol Street, N.E., 2nd Floor
Room 2224
Washington, DC 20002
(202) 442-4778

Florida Board of Nursing
4080 Woodcock Drive, Suite 202
Jacksonville, FL 32207
(904) 858-6940
Web Site: http://www.doh.state.fl.us/mqa/nursing/
    rnhome.htm

Georgia Board of Nursing
237 Coliseum Drive
Macon, GA 31217-3858
(912) 207-1640
Web Site: http://www.sos.state.ga.us/ebd-rn/

Guam Board of Nurse Examiners
P.O. Box 2816
1304 East Sunset Boulevard
Barrgada, GU 96913
(671) 475-0251

Hawaii Board of Nursing
Professional and Vocational Licensing Division
P.O. Box 3469
Honolulu, HI 96801
(808) 586-3000
Web Site: http://www.state.hi.us/dcca/pv/offline/

Idaho Board of Nursing
280 N. 8th Street, Suite 210
P.O. Box 83720
Boise, ID 83720
(208) 334-3110
Web Site: http://www.state.id.us/ibn/ibnhome.htm

Illinois Department of Professional Regulation
James R. Thompson Center
100 West Randolph, Suite 9-300
Chicago, IL 60601
(312) 814-2715
Web Site: http://www.dpr.state.il.us/

Indiana State Board of Nursing
Health Professions Bureau
402 W. Washington Street, Room W041
Indianapolis, IN 46204
(317) 232-2960
Web Site: http://www.state.in.us/hbp/isbn/

Iowa Board of Nursing
RiverPoint Business Park
400 S.W. 8th Street
Suite B
Des Moines, IA 50309-4685
(515) 281-3255
Web Site: http://www.state.ia.us/government/nursing/

Kansas State Board of Nursing
Landon State Office Building
900 S.W. Jackson, Suite 551-S
Topeka, KS 66612
(785) 296-4929
Web Site: http://www.ksbn.org

Kentucky Board of Nursing
312 Whittington Parkway, Suite 300
Louisville, KY 40222
(502) 329-7000
Web Site: http://www.kbn.state.ky.us/

Louisiana State Board of Nursing
3510 N. Causeway Boulevard, Suite 501
Metairie, LA 70003
(504) 838-5332
Web Site: http://www.lsbn.state.la.us/

Maine State Board of Nursing
158 State House Station
Augusta, ME 04333
(207) 287-1133
Web Site: http://www.state.me.us/nursingbd/

Maryland Board of Nursing
4140 Patterson Avenue
Baltimore, MD 21215
(410) 585-1900
Web Site: http://dhmh1d.dhmh.state.md.us/mbn/

Massachusetts Board of Registration in Nursing
Commonwealth of Massachusetts
239 Causeway Street
Boston, MA 02114
(617) 727-9961
Web Site: http://www.state.ma.us/reg/boards/rn/

Michigan CIS/Office of Health Services
Ottawa Towers North
611 W. Ottawa, 4th Floor
Lansing, MI 48933
(517) 373-9102
Web Site: http://www.cis.state.mi.us/bhser/
   genover.htm

Minnesota Board of Nursing
2829 University Avenue SE
Suite 500
Minneapolis, MN 55414
(612) 617-2270
Web Site: http://www.nursingboard.state.mn.us/

Mississippi Board of Nursing
1935 Lakeland Drive, Suite B
Jackson, MS 39216
(601) 987-4188
Web Site: http://www.msbn.state.ms.us/webtest

Missouri State Board of Nursing
3605 Missouri Boulevard
P.O. Box 656
Jefferson City, MO 65102-0656
(573) 751-0681
Web Site: http://www.ecodev.state.mo.us/pr/nursing/

Montana State Board of Nursing
301 South Park
Helena, MT 59620-0513
(406) 444-2071
Web Site: http://www.com.state.mt.us/License/POL/
   index.htm

Nebraska Health and Human Services System
Dept. of Regulation and Licensure, Nursing Section
301 Centennial Mall South, P.O. Box 94986
Lincoln, NE 68509-4986
(402) 471-4376
Web Site: http://www.hhs.state.ne.us/crl/nns.htm

Nevada State Board of Nursing
1755 East Plumb Lane
Suite 260
Reno, NV 89502
(775) 688-2620
Web Site: http://www.nursingboard.state.nv.us

New Hampshire Board of Nursing
78 Regional Drive, Bldg. B
P.O. Box 3898
Concord, NH 03302
(603) 271-2323
Web Site: http://www.state.nh.us/nursing/

New Jersey Board of Nursing
124 Halsey Street, 6th Floor
P.O. Box 45010
Newark, NJ 07101
(973) 504-6586
Web Site: http://www.state.nj.us/lps/ca/medical.htm

New Mexico Board of Nursing
4206 Louisiana Boulevard, NE Suite A
Albuquerque, NM 87109
(505) 841-8340
Web Site: http://www.state.nm.us/clients/nursing

New York State Board of Nursing
89 Washington Avenue
Education Bldg.
2nd Floor, West Wing
Albany, NY 12234
(518) 473-6999
Web Site: http://www.nysed.gov/prof/nurse.htm

North Carolina Board of Nursing
3724 National Drive, Suite 201
Raleigh, NC 27612
(919) 782-3211
Web Site: http://www.ncbon.com/

North Dakota Board of Nursing
919 South 7th Street, Suite 504
Bismarck, ND 58504
(701) 328-9777
Web Site: http://www.ndbon.org/

Ohio Board of Nursing
17 South High Street, Suite 400
Columbus, OH 43215-3413
(614) 466-3947
Web Site: http://www.state.oh.us/nur/

Oklahoma Board of Nursing
2915 N. Classen Boulevard, Suite 524
Oklahoma City, OK 73106
(405) 962-1800

Oregon State Board of Nursing
800 N.E. Oregon Street, Box 25
Suite 465
Portland, OR 97232
(503) 731-4745
Web Site: http://www.osbn.state.or.us/

Pennsylvania State Board of Nursing
124 Pine Street
P.O. Box 2649
Harrisburg, PA 17101
(717) 783-7142
Web Site: http://www.dos.state.pa.us/bpoa/nurbd/
    mainpage.htm

Commonwealth of Puerto Rico
Board of Nurse Examiners
800 Roberto H. Todd Avenue
Room 202, Stop 18
Santurce, PR 00908
(787) 725-8161

Rhode Island Board of Nurse Registration and Nursing
    Education
105 Cannon Building
Three Capitol Hill
Providence, RI 02908
(401) 222-5700
Web Site: http://www.health.state.ri.us

South Carolina State Board of Nursing
110 Centerview Drive
Suite 202
Columbia, SC 29210
(803) 896-4550
Web Site: http://www.llr.state.sc.us/pol/nursing

South Dakota Board of Nursing
4300 South Louise Avenue, Suite C-1
Sioux Falls, SD 57106-3124
(605) 362-2760
Web Site: http://www.state.sd.us/dcr/nursing/

Tennessee State Board of Nursing
426 Fifth Avenue North
1st Floor, Cordell Hull Building
Nashville, TN 37247
(615) 532-5166
Web Site: http://170.142.76.180/bmf-bin/BMFprof
    list.pl

Texas Board of Nurse Examiners
333 Guadalupe, Suite 3-460
Austin, TX 78701
(512) 305-7400
Web Site: http://www.bne.state.tx.us/

Utah State Board of Nursing
Heber M. Wells Bldg., 4th Floor
160 East 300 South
Salt Lake City, UT 84111
(801) 530-6628
Web Site: http://www.commerce.state.ut.us/

Vermont State Board of Nursing
109 State Street
Montpelier, VT 05609-1106
(802) 828-2396
Web Site: http://vtprofessionals.org/nurses/

Virgin Islands Board of Nurse Licensure
Veterans Drive Station
St. Thomas, VI 00803
(340) 776-7397

Virginia State Board of Nursing
6606 W. Broad Street, 4th Fl.
Richmond, VA 23230
(804) 662-9909
Web Site: http://www.dhp.state.va.us/

Washington State Nursing Care Quality Assurance
Commission
Department of Health
1300 Quince Street SE
Olympia, WA 98504-7864
(360) 236-4740
Web Site: http://www.doh.wa.gov/nursing/

West Virginia Board of Examiners for Registered
Professional Nurses
101 Dee Drive
Charleston, WV 25311
(304) 558-3596
Web Site: http://www.state.wv.us/nurses/rn/

Wisconsin Department of Regulation and Licensing
1400 E. Washington Avenue
P.O. Box 8935
Madison, WI 53708
(608) 266-0145
Web Site: http://www.drl.state.wi.us/

Wyoming State Board of Nursing
2020 Carey Avenue, Suite 110
Cheyenne, WY 82002
(307) 777-7601
Web Site: http://nursing.state.wi.us/

Commonwealth Board of Nurse Examiners
Public Health Center
P.O. Box 1458
Saipan, MP 96950
(670) 234-8950

REFERENCES

Hodgson, B. & Kizior, R. (2001). *Saunders nursing drug handbook 2001.* Philadelphia: W.B. Saunders.

National Council of State Boards of Nursing (eds.) (2000). *Test Plan for the National Council Licensure Examination for Registered Nurses.* Chicago: Author.

National Council of State Boards of Nursing (eds.) (2000). *The NCLEX Process: Serving as an Anchor for the NCLEX Examination.* Chicago: Author.

National Council of State Boards of Nursing. Web Site: http://www.ncsbn.org/files/boards/boardscontact.asp

Potter, P., & Perry, A. (2001). *Fundamentals of nursing* (5th ed.). St. Louis: Mosby.

Riley, J. (2000). *Communication in nursing* (4th ed.). St. Louis: Mosby.

Smeltzer, S., & Bare, B. (2000) *Brunner & Suddarth's textbook of medical-surgical nursing* (9th ed.). Philadelphia: Lippincott Williams & Wilkins.

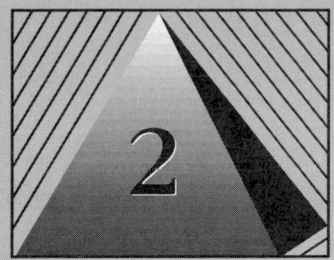

Pathways to Success

LAURENT W. VALLIERE, B.S.

THE PYRAMID TO SUCCESS

Preparing to take the NCLEX-RN examination can produce a great deal of anxiety. You may be thinking that NCLEX-RN is the most important examination that you will ever have to take, and that it reflects the culmination of everything that you have worked so hard for. NCLEX-RN is an important examination because receiving that nursing license means that you can begin your career as a registered nurse. Your success on NCLEX-RN involves expelling all thoughts that allow this examination to appear overwhelming and intimidating. Such thoughts will take complete control over your destiny. A positive attitude, a structured plan for preparation, and maintaining control in your pathway to success will ensure achievement in reaching the peak of the Pyramid to Success (Box 2-1).

BOX 2-1

Pathways to Success

THE FOUNDATION
Maintaining a positive attitude
Thinking about short- and long-term realistic goals
Developing control

THE LIST
Documenting short- and long-term realistic goals
Maintaining control

THE PLAN
Developing a study plan and schedule
Deciding on the place to study
Balancing personal and work obligations with the study schedule
Sharing the study schedule and personal needs with others
Implementing the study plan

POSITIVE PAMPERING
Establishing healthy eating habits
Planning time for exercise and fun activities
Including activities in the schedule that provide positive mental stimulation

FINAL PREPARATION
Reviewing goals
Identifying goals achieved
Remaining focused to complete the plan of study
Writing down the date and time of the examination and posting it next to your name with the letters R.N. following, and the word "YES!"
Planning a test drive to the testing center
Relaxing on the day before the examination

THE DAY OF THE EXAMINATION
Grooming yourself for success
Eating a healthy and nutritious breakfast
Maintaining a confident and positive attitude
Maintaining control
Meeting the challenges of the day
Reaching the peak of the Pyramid to Success

THE FOUNDATION

The foundation of Pathways to Success begins with a positive attitude and developing short- and long-term goals. Both a positive attitude and a list of goals will lead you toward achievement and success. Without these components, the Pathway to Success leads to nowhere and has no end point. You will expend energy and valuable time and will experience exhaustion without any accomplishment. Therefore, it is imperative that you take the time to develop that positive attitude and to establish your short- and long-term goals.

Where do you start? To begin this process, find a location that offers solitude. Sit or lie in a comfortable position, close your eyes, relax, inhale deeply, hold your breath to a count of 4, exhale slowly, and, again, relax. Repeat this breathing exercise several times until you begin to feel relaxed and free from anxiety. Allow your mind to become void of all chatter. Now you are in control and your mind can see for miles. Your highway of life has a multitude of destinations to which you may travel. It is now time for you to plan the order of your journey to the Pyramid to Success.

THE LIST

It is time to create "The List." The List is your set of goals. At this time, you may or may not have a scheduled date for taking the NCLEX-RN examination. Begin by developing the goals you wish to accomplish today, tomorrow, and into the future. Allow yourself the opportunity to list all that is flowing from your uninhibited thought process. Write your goals on a piece of paper. When the List is complete, it is time to bank it away for 2 or 3 days. After 2 or 3 days, retrieve and review the List and begin the process of planning for preparing for the NCLEX-RN examination.

THE PLAN

Now that you have the List in order, look at your goals that relate to studying for the licensing exam. The first task is to decide what study pattern works best for you. Take the time to review what has worked most successfully for you in the past. There are questions that must be addressed in order to develop your plan for study. (Box 2-2)

"The Plan" must include how you will manage your study needs and the demands of your family and friends. Take time to think about how you will balance your everyday commitments with your plan for study. Your family and friends are key players in your life and are going to become a part of your Pyramid to Success. After you have established your study needs, communicate your needs, and the importance of your study plan in achieving your goal of becoming a registered nurse, with your family and friends.

BOX 2-2

Developing a Plan for Study

Do I work better alone or in a group study environment?

If I work best in a group, does the group consist of one, two, or more study partners?

Who are these study partners?

How long should my study sessions last?

Does the time of day that I study make a difference for me?

Do I retain more if I study in the morning?

How does my work schedule affect my study pattern?

How do I balance my family obligations with my need to study?

Do I have a comfortable study area at home or do I need to find an another environment that is conducive to my study needs?

A difficult part of the Plan may be how you will deal with those family and friends who choose not to participate in your Pyramid to Success. What if an individual or individuals choose not to be part of the Pyramid? Then you are faced with a decision. You must weigh all of the factors carefully. You must keep your goals in mind and remember that your need for positive momentum is critical. Your decision may not be an easy one, but must be one that will help you ensure that your goal of becoming a registered nurse is achieved. Remember, a positive momentum and goal achievement need to be shared by all who support you.

The Plan must include a schedule. Establish a realistic schedule that includes your daily, weekly, and future goals, and adhere to it. This consistency will provide advantages to you and to those supporting you. A daily schedule allows you to plan your topic areas for study more carefully. Adherence to the Plan helps you develop a rhythm that can only enhance your retention and positive momentum. Those who are supporting you will share this rhythm and will be able to schedule their activities and life better because you are consistent with your study schedule. You are moving forward, and you are in Control!

POSITIVE PAMPERING

Positive momentum can be maintained only if you are properly balanced. This means that you must continue to care for yourself. Proper exercise, diet, and positive mental stimulation are critical to achieving your goal of becoming a registered nurse. Just as you have developed a schedule for study, you should have a schedule that includes some fun and some form of physical activity. It is your choice—aerobics, running, weight lifting, bowling, or whatever makes you feel good about yourself. Time spent away from the hard study schedule and devoted to some form of fun and physical exercise pays its rewards 100-fold. You will feel alive and more energetic with a schedule that includes these activities.

Establish healthy eating habits. Stay away from fatty foods because they will slow you down. Eat lighter meals and eat more frequently. Include complex carbohydrates in your diet for energy, and be careful not to include too much caffeine in your daily diet. Continue to feel good about yourself, because you are in control. Take the time to pamper yourself with activities that make you feel even better about who you are. Make dinner reservations at your favorite restaurant with someone who is special and is supporting your goal to become a registered nurse. Take walks in a place that has a particular tranquillity that enables you to reflect on the positive momentum that you have achieved and maintained. Whatever it is, wherever it takes you, allow yourself the time to do some Positive Pampering.

FINAL PREPARATION

You have established the foundation of your Pyramid. You have developed your list of goals and your study plan and have maintained your positive momentum. You are moving forward, and you are in control. When you receive your date and time for the NCLEX-RN examination, you may immediately think, "I am not ready!" Stop! Reflect on all that you have achieved. Think about your goal achievement and the organization of the positive life momentum with which you have surrounded yourself. Think about all those individuals who love and support your effort to become a registered nurse. Believe that the challenge that awaits you is one that you have successfully prepared for and will lead you to your goal, becoming a registered nurse!

Take a deep breath, and organize the remaining days so that they support your educational and personal needs. Support your positive momentum with a visual technique. Write your name in large letters, and write the letters R.N. after it. Post one or more of these visual reinforcements in areas that you frequent. This form of motivational technique works for many individuals preparing for this examination.

Through all that you have accomplished to this point, it is imperative that you not fall into the trap of expecting too much of yourself. The idea of perfection must not drive you to a point that causes your positive momentum to hesitate. You must believe in who you are, as you are, and stay focused on your goal. Allow yourself the opportunity to continue to carry out your plan in a manner that is most conducive to who you are, not someone else. The date and time are in hand. Write down the date and time, and underneath write the word "YES." Post this next to your name plus R.N.

You must ensure that you have command over how to get to the testing center. A test run is a must. Time the drive, and allow for road construction or whatever may occur to slow the traffic down. On the test run, when you arrive at the test facility, you may want to walk into it. Walk in and become familiar with the lobby and the surroundings. This may help to alleviate some of the peripheral nervousness associated with entering an unknown building. Remember, you must do whatever it takes to keep yourself in control. If familiarizing yourself with the facility will help you to maintain positive momentum, by all means be sure to do so! Who is in control? You are!

It is time to check your study plan and make the necessary adjustments now that a firm date and time are set. Adjust your review so that it flows to your needs and that your study plan ends 2 days before the examination. Remember that the mind is like a muscle. If it is overworked, it has no strength or stamina. Your strategy is to rest the body and the mind on the day before the examination. Your strategy is to stay in control and allow yourself the opportunity to be absolutely fresh and attentive on the day of the examination. This will help you control the nervousness that is natural, achieve the clear thought processes required, and feel confident that you have done all that is necessary to prepare and conquer this challenge. The day before the examination is to be one of pleasure. Treat yourself to what you enjoy the most.

Relax! You have prepared yourself well for the challenge of tomorrow. Allow yourself a good night's sleep, and wake up on the day of the examination knowing that you are absolutely ready to succeed. Look at your name with R.N. after it and the word "YES!"

THE DAY OF THE EXAMINATION

Wake up believing in yourself and that all you have accomplished is about to propel you to the professional level of registered nurse. Allow yourself plenty of time, eat a nutritious breakfast, and groom yourself for success. You are ready to meet the challenges of the day and overcome any obstacle that may face you. Today will soon be history, and tomorrow will bring you the envelope on which you read your name with the words "Registered Nurse" after it.

Be proud and confident of your achievements. You have worked hard to achieve your goal of becoming a registered nurse. If you believe in yourself and your goals, no one person or obstacle can move you off the pathway that leads to success, to the peak of the Pyramid!

Congratulations and I wish you the very best in your career as a registered nurse!

The NCLEX-RN Examination:
From a Student's Perspective

HEATHER CARLSON, R.N.

First and foremost, I want to congratulate you on your success in completing your nursing program. It is important to remind yourself of this accomplishment as you prepare for the NCLEX-RN examination because your self-confidence and stamina will bring you to the peak of the pyramid to success, becoming a registered nurse!

I was anxious as I sat in front of the computer at the testing center waiting to take the NCLEX-RN examination, an examination that was about to change my life, hopefully for the best. In the testing center, there were approximately ten other individuals typing away at their assigned computers. The room was extremely quiet and still, the kind of stillness that makes one nervous. The computer screen had my photograph on it, and a proctor approached me for the third time to verify that I am who I say I am. The proctor handed me scrap paper and earplugs and wished me "luck" before walking away.

Luck? Is that all I need? A little luck and I become a nurse? It had to be more than that. I have experienced four years of nursing school and hours and hours of learning and studying. I also spent two to three months preparing for the NCLEX-RN examination. Four years of college certainly fills your head with a lot of information. I kept thinking that now all I need to do is to take this examination to prove what I know. I kept saying to myself "Do not stress out," which is certainly always easier said than done. I took a deep breath, wished myself luck (it couldn't hurt), and began to read the first question.

Let me backtrack a little to share with you how I prepared for the most important examination of my life. I began by coming up with a study plan. I knew that my plan had to be a rigid schedule that included when I would wake up, how long I would study, and the other commitments that I needed to meet every day. You may not need to be so rigid, but I am the type of person who needs discipline. I am also a procrastinator and tend to put things on the back burner, so to speak. So the rigid

schedule and the discipline were very important for me. I planned my examination date, and I put my study plan into action.

The nursing school that I attended was very aggressive when it came to preparing for the NCLEX-RN examination. Each week we were required to do practice NCLEX-RN test questions on the computer. I found this method of study very helpful, and this method became the main component of my study plan. I started studying by using the *Saunders Comprehensive Review for NCLEX-RN*. When I completed the book and the practice questions on the CD-ROM that accompanies the book, I began the *Saunders Q & A Review for NCLEX-RN*. Finally, I used the *Saunders Computerized Review for NCLEX-RN*, which really provided me with my "picture of readiness" for the NCLEX-RN examination. I really liked the CD-ROM options and formats for study that accompanied each of these resources. If I had only a limited amount of time on a particular day, I would do ten question quizzes or exams. If I had more time, I would select a 100-question exam. Each day I would answer questions on the computer, keeping notes on information that I hadn't known. After completing the quiz or exam, I would immediately review the areas that I identified as weak ones. I also found the CD-ROMs helpful because each practice question provides a rationale for the correct answer as well as the incorrect answers. The test-taking strategy that is presented with each practice question also provided me with the hints and clues to selecting the correct option. This was particularly helpful if I was unfamiliar with the content being presented or if I had eliminated two of the possible four options and was unsure of the remaining two options.

My study plan also involved having a "study buddy," who was my best friend from nursing school. She was also preparing for the NCLEX-RN examination. We would speak on the telephone every day to ensure that we had achieved our daily goal. We motivated each other and shared the concerns and stressors that accompany preparing for this important examination. This was helpful to me and helped to keep me disciplined.

The night before the NCLEX-RN examination I decided not to study, despite the feelings of panic within me and the feeling that there is still so much to review. Everyone kept telling me how important it was to get a good night's sleep, so that is what I tried to do. I woke up early and prepared myself for success. On the way to the testing center, I tried to ignore the questions flying through my head.

So here I was, sitting in front of the computer, taking the NCLEX-RN examination. The questions were very difficult, but I kept telling myself "That's OK, I want them to be difficult." Some of the answers were basically obvious, while many of the other questions took longer to answer. It is very difficult to stay focused during this examination, but an important thing to remember is that the answer is always right there on the computer screen in front of you. Remember, you can answer this question correctly. My best advice is to read each question carefully, figure out what the question is specifically asking, read every option, and then read the question a second time before making your final selection.

When I found myself on question number seventy-five, I found myself hoping that this would be my last question. Not because it would mean I passed, because we all know that the number of questions asked does not indicate if you've passed or failed. I simply could not be asked another question because it was difficult to stay focused. So, I sat back, took a few deep breaths to move that much-needed oxygen to my brain, selected my answer, and the computer screen went blank. It was over. I immediately wished it would turn back on because I wanted more questions; I wanted to try harder. But it didn't, and I had completed the examination.

As I left the quiet testing room behind, I felt a mix of emotions within me. Did I pass? Did I fail? My mind felt blank and I felt sick. I had absolutely no idea if I had passed or failed. I remembered that in nursing school, after taking an examination, I would have a gut feeling on how I did. Not after this test; I just felt numb. Now I had to wait to find out the results. The wait was very difficult.

Eleven days later while at work, I received a phone call from my brother. He told me that there was an envelope from the board of nursing in the mail and asked if I wanted him to open it? Of course I did, and I waited with a lump in my throat for him to read it. There was a moment of silence; then I heard my parents cheering and he said, "You passed." Wow! I passed. I was now a registered nurse; all my hard work had paid off! I could begin the career that I had worked so hard for!

Looking back on my NCLEX-RN examination experience, I feel that it was not as bad as it had seemed. The mind has a funny way of only remembering the good things. So don't fear the NCLEX-RN examination, because the fear is worse than the reality. My advice is to trust yourself and be confident. Trust in yourself that you are intelligent and well educated. Trust that all of your studying and hard work will pay off. Trust that you will do the best that you can. And, finally, trust that all that is meant to be will somehow fall into place. It did for me, and it will for you. And a little bit of luck never hurt.

Again, congratulations to you and I wish you the best in your career as a registered nurse!

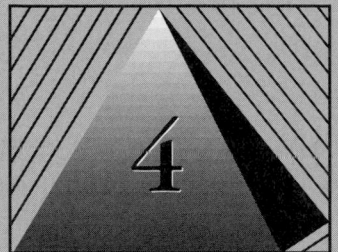

Test-Taking Strategies

I. PYRAMID TO SUCCESS (Box 4-1)

II. HOW TO AVOID READING INTO THE QUESTION

A. Pyramid points
1. Identify the case situation from the stem of the question
2. Identify what the question is asking
3. Look for the key words
4. Read every option
5. Use the process of elimination
6. As you read the question, avoid asking yourself "What if . . . ?"

B. The case situation (Box 4-2)
1. The case situation provides you with the information about a clinical health problem and the information that you need to consider in answering the question
2. Read all of the information and every word in the case situation

C. The stem of the question (Box 4-2)
1. The stem of the question follows the case situation and asks something specific about the case situation
2. Read the stem carefully, and specifically identify exactly what is being asked

D. The options (Box 4-2)
1. The options are all of the answers, and you must select one
2. Read every option carefully and reread the stem of the question to be sure that you understand what is being asked
3. Use the process of elimination
4. Once you have eliminated two incorrect options, reread the stem of the question again to identify specifically what the question is asking, before selecting the correct option

---

BOX 4-1

Pyramid to Success

Read the question and every option thoroughly and carefully!
Ask yourself, "What is the question specifically asking?"
Be alert to key words and true and false response stems!
Eliminate the incorrect options!
Use all of your nursing knowledge, your clinical experiences, and your test-taking skills and strategies to answer the question!

BOX 4-2

Case Situation, Stem, and Options

Case Situation: The nurse is monitoring a child for bleeding following surgery for removal of a brain tumor. The nurse checks the head dressing for the presence of blood and notes a colorless drainage on the back of the dressing.
Stem: Which of the following would be the most appropriate nursing intervention?
Options:
1. Circle the area of drainage and continue to monitor
2. Reinforce the dressing
3. Notify the physician
4. Document the findings and continue to monitor

III. KEY WORDS (Box 4-3)

A. Key words focus your attention on critical ideas in the case situation, the stem, and the options
B. Key words are important to identify because they will assist in eliminating the incorrect options (Box 4-4)
C. Some of the key words may indicate that all of the options are correct, and that it will be necessary to prioritize in order to select the correct option

BOX 4-3

Common Key Words

Early or Late
Best
First
Initial
Immediately
Most Likely or Least Likely
Most Appropriate or Least Appropriate
On the Day of
After Several Days

BOX 4-4

Key Words to Eliminate Incorrect Options

Which of the following is an EARLY sign of shock?
Which of the following is a LATE SIGN of shock?
ON THE DAY OF surgery, following a transurethral resection of the prostate (TURP), the nurse notes that the client's urine is bright red in color. Which of the following nursing actions is MOST APPROPRIATE?
AFTER SEVERAL DAYS, following a transurethral resection of the prostate (TURP), the nurse notes that the client's urine is bright red in color. Which of the following nursing actions is MOST APPROPRIATE?
Noting the key words in each of these situations will assist in directing you to select the correct option.
The EARLY signs of shock are quite different from the LATE signs of shock!
Bright red urine might be expected ON THE DAY OF surgery following a transurethral resection of the prostate (TURP), but would not be expected AFTER SEVERAL DAYS!

BOX 4-5

The Issue of the Question

Fat emulsion is prescribed for the client receiving total parenteral nutrition (TPN). The nurse is preparing to hang the fat emulsion and notes the presence of fat globules in the solution. The most appropriate nursing action is to:
1. Shake the solution to dissolve the globules
2. Call the physician
3. Return the solution to the pharmacy
4. Place the solution in a bath of warm water until the globules dissolve

Answer: 3

Test-Taking Strategy: Focus on the issue, the presence of fat globules in the solution. Thinking about the significance of fat globules in the solution and the potential adverse impact of fat globules entering the client's bloodstream will direct you to the correct option.

IV. THE CLIENT OF THE QUESTION

A. Identify the client of the question
B. The client is the person who is the focus of the question
C. It is important to remember that the client of the question may not necessarily be the person with the health problem; in the test question, the client may be a relative, friend, spouse, significant other, or another member of the health care team
D. After identifying the client of the question, select the option that relates to and most directly addresses that client

V. THE ISSUE OF THE QUESTION (Box 4-5)

A. Identify the issue of the question
B. The issue of the question is the specific subject content that the question is asking about
C. Identifying the issue of the question will assist in eliminating the incorrect options and direct you to selecting the correct option
D. The issue of the question can include
   1. A medication or intravenous (IV) therapy
   2. A side effect of a medication
   3. An adverse or toxic effect of a medication
   4. A treatment or procedure
   5. A complication of a health care problem, treatment, or procedure
   6. A specific nursing action

VI. TRUE OR FALSE RESPONSE STEMS

A. True response stem (Box 4-6)
   1. True response stems use key words that ask you to select an option that is true regarding the case situation in the question
   2. Common key words used in a true response stem
      a. Most or most appropriate
      b. Most likely
      c. Best
      d. Best judgment
      e. Initial
      f. First
      g. Chief
      h. Immediate
B. False response stem (Box 4-7)
   1. False response stems use key words that ask you to select an option that is NOT true regarding the case situation in the question
   2. Common key words used in a false response stem
      a. Except or not
      b. Least likely
      c. Need for further instructions or education
      d. Lowest priority
      e. Incorrect
      f. Unsafe

BOX 4-6

True Response Stem

The nurse is reviewing the laboratory results of a client seen in the health care clinic. The nurse notes that the red blood cell count is decreased. The nurse determines that this finding *most likely* occurs in which of the following conditions?
1. Polycythemia vera
2. Dehydration
3. Severe diarrhea
4. Iron deficiency

Answer: 4

Test-Taking Strategy: Note the key words "most likely." Also, note the relationship between the words "decreased" in the case situation and "deficiency" in the correct option.

BOX 4-7

False Response Stem

The nurse has provided discharge instructions to a client who underwent a right mastectomy with axillary lymph node dissection. Which statement if made by the client indicates a *need for further instruction* regarding home care measures?
1. "I need to be sure to wear thick mitt covers or use thick pot holders when I am cooking."
2. "I should inform all of my other health care providers that I have had this surgical procedure."
3. "It is alright to use a straight razor to shave under my arms."
4. "I need to be sure that I do not have blood pressures or blood drawn from my right arm."

Answer: 3

Test-Taking Strategy: Note the key words "need for further instruction." These key words indicate that you need to select an option that identifies an incorrect client statement. Recalling that edema and infection are the concerns with this client and that the client needs to be instructed in the measures that will avoid trauma to the affected arm will direct you to the correct option.

BOX 4-8

Prioritizing: Maslow's Hierarchy of Needs Theory

The nurse is reviewing the plan of care for a pregnant client with a diagnosis of sickle cell anemia. Which nursing diagnosis, if stated on the plan of care, would the nurse select as receiving the *highest* priority?
1. Anxiety
2. Ineffective individual coping
3. Altered body image
4. Fluid volume deficit

Answer: 4

Test-Taking Strategy: Use Maslow's Hierarchy of Needs theory to prioritize, remembering that physiological needs come first. Using this guideline will direct you to option 4. Fluid volume deficit is a physiological need and is the priority nursing diagnosis.

BOX 4-9

Prioritizing: Use of the ABCs

The client with a diagnosis of cancer is receiving morphine sulfate 10 mg subcutaneously every 3 to 4 hours for pain. When preparing the plan of care for the client, the nurse includes which *priority* action?
1. Monitor the client's temperature
2. Monitor the urine output
3. Encourage the client to cough and deep breath
4. Encourage increased fluids

Answer: 3

Test Taking Strategy: Use the ABCs—airway, breathing, and circulation—as a guide to direct you to the correct option. Recall that morphine sulfate suppresses the cough reflex and the respiratory reflex. The correct option addresses airway.

VII. QUESTIONS THAT REQUIRE PRIORITIZING

A. Identify the key words in the question that indicate the need to prioritize
B. Common key words
   1. Initial
   2. Essential
   3. Vital
   4. Immediate
   5. Highest
   6. Best
   7. Most
   8. Priority
C. Use Maslow's Hierarchy of Needs theory as a guide to prioritize (Box 4-8)
   1. Physiological needs come FIRST; select an option that addresses a physiological need
   2. When a physiological need is not addressed in the question or noted in one of the options, safety needs receive priority; select an option that addresses safety
D. ABCs: airway, breathing, and circulation (Box 4-9)
   1. Use the ABC's when selecting an option
   2. Remember the order of priority: airway, breathing, and circulation
E. Nursing process (Table 4-1)
   1. Guidelines
      a. Use the steps of the nursing process to prioritize
      b. Remember that assessment is the first step in the nursing process
      c. When you are asked to select your first and

TABLE 4-1

Steps of the Nursing Process

Assessment	Use the nursing process to answer questions!
Analysis	Follow the steps of the nursing process to select an option.
Planning	The first step of the nursing process is assessment.
Implementation	When the question asks you what the nurse's initial, first, or most appropriate action is, select the option that relates
Evaluation	to assessment of the client!

BOX 4-11

Assessment: Key Words

Ascertain
Assess
Check
Determine
Find out
Identify
Monitor
Observe
Obtain information

BOX 4-10

Nursing Process: Assessment

The nurse is teaching a client with diabetes mellitus about dietary measures to follow. The client expresses frustration in learning the dietary regimen. The nurse would initially:
1. *Identify* the cause of the frustration
2. Continue with the dietary teaching
3. Notify the physician
4. Tell the client that the diet needs to be followed
Answer: 1
Test-Taking Strategy: Use the steps of the nursing process. Assessment is the first step. Of the four options presented, the only assessment option is option 1. Options 2, 3, and 4 identify the implementation step of the nursing process. The initial action is to identify the cause of the frustration.

BOX 4-12

Nursing Process: Analysis

The nurse is reviewing the laboratory results of a client with a diagnosis of leukemia. The nurse notes that the granulocyte count is decreased. The nurse interprets that the client is at risk for:
1. Infection
2. Bleeding
3. Anemia
4. Dehydration
Answer: 1
Test-Taking Strategy: It is necessary to understand the physiology associated with leukemia and the effects of a decreased granulocyte count to answer this question correctly. Analysis of this information will direct you to the correct option.

initial nursing action, follow the steps of the nursing process to select the correct option
   d. If an option contains the concept of assessment or the collection of client data, select that option
2. Assessment (Box 4-10)
   a. Assessment questions address the process of gathering subjective and objective data relative to the client, confirming that data, and communicating and documenting the data
   b. Remember that assessment is the first step in the nursing process
   c. When you are asked a question regarding your initial or first nursing action, select the option that addresses an assessment action
   d. If an assessment action is not one of the options, follow the steps of the nursing process as your guide to select your initial or first action
   e. When answering questions that focus on assessment, look for key words in the options that reflect assessment (Box 4-11)

3. Analysis (Box 4-12)
   a. Analysis questions are the most difficult questions because they require understanding of the principles of physiological responses and require interpretation of the data on the basis of assessment
   b. Analysis questions require critical thinking and determining the rationale for therapeutic interventions that may be addressed in the case situation
   c. Analysis questions may address the formulation of a nursing diagnosis and the communication and documentation of the results of the process of analysis
4. Planning (Box 4-13)
   a. Planning questions require prioritizing nursing diagnoses, determining goals and outcome criteria for goals of care, developing the plan of care, and communicating and documenting the plan of care
   b. Remember that this is a NURSING examination and the answer to the question most

BOX 4-13

Nursing Process: Planning

The nurse is preparing to care for a client following a gastroscopy procedure. The nurse includes which most appropriate intervention in the nursing care plan?
1. Place the client in a supine position to provide comfort
2. Monitor the client's vital signs every hour for 4 hours
3. Provide saline gargles immediately upon return to the unit to aid in comfort
4. Check the gag reflex by using a tongue depressor to stroke the back of client's throat

Answer: 4

Test-Taking Strategy: Planning questions include developing the plan of care and determining goals and outcome criteria for goals of care. Use of the ABCs—airway, breathing, and circulation—will also assist in answering this question. Option 4 is the only option that addresses airway.

BOX 4-14

Nursing Process: Implementation

The emergency room nurse is caring for a child suspected of epiglottitis. The nurse has ensured that the child has a patent airway. The next priority intervention in the care of this child would be to:
1. Prepare the child for a chest x-ray
2. Assist the physician with intubation
3. Prepare the child for tracheotomy
4. Prepare to administer epinephrine

Answer: 1

Test-Taking Strategy: Implementation questions address the process of organizing and managing care. This question also requires that you prioritize the nursing actions. When epiglottitis is suspected, the priorities are to maintain a patent airway and to obtain a chest x-ray to confirm the diagnosis. If epiglottitis is present, the child is taken promptly to the operating room for tracheal intubation or immediate surgical airway. Epinephrine is not used in the treatment of epiglottitis.

likely involves something that is included in the nursing care plan, rather than the medical plan

5. Implementation (Box 4-14)
   a. This exam is about nursing, so focus on the nursing action rather than on the medical action, unless the question is asking you what prescribed medical action is anticipated
   b. Implementation questions address the process of organizing and managing care, counseling and teaching, providing care to achieve established goals, supervising and coordinating care, and communicating and documenting nursing interventions
   c. On NCLEX-RN, the only client whom you need to be concerned about is the client in the question that you are answering
   d. When you are answering a question, remember that this client is your only assigned client
   e. Answer the question as if the situation were textbook and ideal and the nurse had all the time and resources needed and readily available at the client's bedside
6. Evaluation (Box 4-15)
   a. Evaluation questions focus on comparing the actual outcomes of care with the expected outcomes
   b. Evaluation questions address evaluating the client's ability to implement self-care, health care team members' ability to implement care, and the process of communicating and documenting evaluation findings
   c. Evaluation questions also focus on how the nurse should monitor or make a judgment

BOX 4-15

Nursing Process: Evaluation

The nurse is performing an admission assessment on a child with a seizure disorder. The nurse is interviewing the child's parents to determine their adjustment to caring for their child, who has a chronic illness. Which statement if made by a parent of the child would indicate a need for further teaching?
1. "Our child is involved in a swim program with neighbors and friends."
2. "Our child sleeps in our bedroom at night."
3. "Our baby-sitter just completed cardiopulmonary resuscitation (CPR) training."
4. "We worry about injuries when our child has a seizure."

Answer: 2

Test-Taking Strategy: This is an evaluation question and contains a false response stem as identified by the words "need for further teaching." Option 2 identifies a need to provide the parents with an alternate method to monitor for night seizures. Options 1 and 3 identify parental understanding of the disorder. Option 4 is a common concern.

concerning a client's response to therapy or to a nursing action
   d. In an evaluation question, be alert to false response stems because they are frequently used in evaluation-type questions, and the question may ask for a client statement that indicates either accurate or inaccurate information related to the issue of the question

VIII. CLIENT NEEDS

A. Safe, effective care environment
1. These questions address the provision that the nurse provides and directs care that will ensure an environment that promotes protecting the client, family or significant other(s), and other health care personnel
2. Content addressed in these questions relates to the nursing role of coordinating and integrating cost-effective care, supervising and/or collaborating with members of the multidisciplinary health care team, and environmental safety
3. Be alert to safety needs addressed in a question, and remember the importance of handwashing, call bells, bed positioning, and the appropriate use of side rails

B. Physiological integrity
1. These questions address the provision that the nurse promotes physical health and well-being in the client by providing care and comfort, reducing client risk potential, and managing the client's health alterations
2. Content addressed in these questions relates to basic care and comfort, pharmacological and parenteral therapies, reducing the risk of the development of complications, and managing and providing care to clients with acute, chronic, or life-threatening conditions
3. Remember that physiological needs are a priority and are addressed first
4. Use the ABCs—airway, breathing, and circulation—and the steps of the nursing process when selecting an option addressing physiological integrity

C. Psychosocial integrity
1. These questions address the provision that the nurse provides nursing care that supports and promotes the emotional, mental, and social well-being of the client and significant other(s)
2. Content addressed in these questions relates to promoting the client or significant other's ability to cope, adapt, or problem solve in situations such as illness or stressful events, and providing care to clients with maladaptive behavior or acute or chronic mental illness
3. Communication questions (Table 4-2)
   a. Identify the use of therapeutic communication tools
   b. Use of communication tools indicates a CORRECT option
   c. Use of communication blocks indicates an INCORRECT option
   d. Always focus on the client's feelings first; if an option reflects the client's feelings, select that option as the answer to the question (Box 4-16)

D. Health promotion and maintenance
1. These questions address the provision that the nurse provides and directs care that prevents health problems, provides early detection of health problems, and provides and directs care that incorporates knowledge of expected growth and development principles
2. Content addressed in these questions relates to assisting the client and significant other(s) through the normal stages of growth and development, and assisting the client and significant other(s) to develop health practices that promote wellness and to recognize alterations in health care status

---

TABLE 4-2

Communication Tools and Blocks

Tools	Blocks
Being silent	Giving advice
Offering self for assistance	Showing approval/disapproval
Showing empathy	Using cliches and false reassurance
Focusing	Requesting an explanation "Why?"
Restatement	Devaluing client feelings
Validation/clarification	Being defensive
Giving information	Focusing on inappropriate issues or persons
Dealing with the here and now	Placing the client's issues on "hold"

Always focus on the client's feelings FIRST!
If an answer reflects the client's feelings, select that answer!

BOX 4-16

Focusing on the Client's Feelings

The nurse in the mental health unit is having a conversation with a client diagnosed with post-traumatic stress disorder. The client seems upset and seems to be having difficulty with realistic behavior. The most appropriate nursing response to the client is which of the following?
1. "Don't worry so much."
2. "Everything is going to be all right."
3. "I can see that you are upset about this. Why don't we talk about it?"
4. "Why are you having so much trouble controlling your anxiety?"

Answer: 3

Test-Taking Strategy: Option 3 is the only option that addresses the client's feelings and concerns. Options 1 and 2 provide false reassurance and place the client's feelings on hold. Option 4 is a nontherapeutic communication technique and will increase the client's anxiety.

3. Use the Teaching/Learning Theory if the question addresses client education, remembering that client motivation and client readiness to learn **are** the FIRST priority
4. Be alert to false response stems with questions that address health promotion and maintenance

IX. PYRAMID POINTS (Box 4-17)
A. Unfamiliar content
   1. Answer questions by using your nursing knowledge, clinical experiences, and test-taking skills and strategies
   2. If the content of a question is unfamiliar and you are unable to answer the question by using your nursing knowledge, look for a global option, similar distracters, or similar words, behaviors, thoughts, or feelings in the question and in one of the options
B. Global option (Box 4-18)
   1. When more than one option appears to be correct, look for a global option
   2. A global option is one that is a general statement and may include the ideas of the other options within it
C. Similar distracters
   1. If you don't know the answer, try looking for similar distracters
   2. Remember that there is only ONE correct option
   3. If two options say the same thing or include the same idea, then NEITHER OF THESE OPTIONS can be correct
   4. The answer to the question is the option that is different
D. Similar words, behaviors, thoughts, or feelings
   1. If you do not know the answer, look for a similar word, behavior, thought, or feeling used in the case situation or the stem of the question and in one of the options
   2. If you find a word, behavior, thought, or feeling that is used in the case situation or the stem of the question and is repeated in one of the options, that option MAY be the correct one
E. Pharmacology questions
   1. If you are familiar with the medication, use nursing knowledge to answer the question
   2. Remember that the question will identify both

BOX 4-17

Pyramid Points

If the question asks for an immediate action or response, all options may be correct; therefore, base your selection on priorities

Reword a difficult question, but if you do so, be careful not to change the intent of the question

Relate the situation to something that you are familiar with and try to visualize the client as you go through the case situation and the question

If there are words in the case situation or stem of the question that are unfamiliar, try to figure out the meaning in terms of the context of the sentence or break down the word and use medical terminology skills

If one option includes qualifiers such as GENERALLY, USUALLY, TENDS TO, POSSIBLY, or MAY, and other options do not, select that option

Absolute terminology such as ALWAYS, NEVER, ALL, EVERY, NONE, MUST, and ONLY tend to make an option incorrect

With medication calculations, talk yourself through each step and be sure the answer makes sense; recheck the calculation before selecting an option, particularly if the answer seems like an unusual dosage

Remember, the only client you need to be concerned about is the one in the question you are answering, and answer the question as if the situation were ideal and the nurse had all the time and resources readily available at the client's bedside

Pace yourself, concentrate, and focus on one item at a time; if you find yourself becoming distracted, take a few minutes to breathe deeply and then refocus

SMILE!
BELIEF!
CONFIDENCE!
CONTROL!
SUCCESS!

BOX 4-18

Global Option

The nurse in the emergency room receives a telephone call from emergency medical services and is told that several victims who survived a plane crash will be transported to the hospital. The nurse is told that several victims are suffering from cold exposure because the plane plummeted and submerged into the local river. The initial nursing action of the emergency room nurse is which of the following?

1. Supply the triage rooms with bottles of sterile water and normal saline
2. Call the laundry department and ask the department to send as many warm blankets as possible to the emergency room
3. Call the nursing supervisor to activate the agency disaster plan
4. Call the intensive care unit to request that nurses be sent to the emergency room

Answer: 3

Test-Taking Strategy: Option 3 is the global option. Activating the agency disaster plan will ensure that the interventions in options 1, 2, and 4 will occur.

the generic name and the trade name of the medication

3. If the case situation identifies a diagnosis, then you can make a relationship between the medication and the diagnosis; for example, you can determine that cyclophosphamide (Cytoxan) is an antineoplastic medication if the question refers to a client with breast cancer who is taking this particular medication

4. Try to determine the classification of the medication being addressed to assist in answering the question; identifying the classification will assist in determining a medication action and/or side effects (Cardiazem is a cardiac medication)

5. Use medical terminology, and break the name of the medication into parts; for example, Lopressor can be broken down into Lo and pressor, meaning lowering the blood pressure

6. Look at the prefix and/or suffix of the medication name; "ase" indicates an enzyme, "sone" indicates a steroid; "line" indicates a bronchodilator, and "lol" indicates a beta-blocker

7. General principles to remember
   a. Clients are instructed to avoid alcohol with medications
   b. Capsules and sustained-released medications are not to be crushed
   c. The nurse never adjusts or changes the client's medication dosage and never discontinues a medication
   d. Medications are never administered if the order is difficult to read, is unclear, or identifies a medication dose that is not a normal one

REFERENCES

National Council of State Boards of Nursing (eds.) (2000). *Test Plan for the National Council Licensure Examination for Registered Nurses.* Chicago: Author.

Potter, P., & Perry, A. (2001). *Fundamentals of nursing* (5th ed.). St. Louis: Mosby,

Riley, J. (2000). *Communication in nursing* (4th ed.). St. Louis: Mosby.

Smeltzer, S., & Bare, B. (2000) *Brunner & Suddarth's textbook of medical-surgical nursing* (9th ed.). Philadelphia: Lippincott Williams & Wilkins.

Issues in Nursing

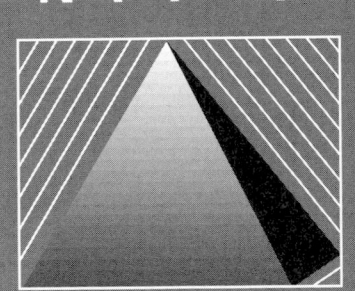

Cultural Diversity

PYRAMID TERMS

acculturation Process of learning norms, beliefs, and behavioral expectations of a group.

belief Something believed as true and accepted by an ethnocultural group.

cultural assimilation Occurs when individuals from a minority group are absorbed by the dominant culture and take on the characteristics of the dominant culture.

cultural competence Having the knowledge, understanding, and skills regarding a diverse culture that allow one to provide acceptable care.

cultural diversity The differences among people that result from ethnic, racial, and cultural variables.

cultural imposition The tendency to impose one's own beliefs, values, and patterns of behavior on individuals from another culture.

culture The structures of knowledge, beliefs, behaviors, ideas, attitudes, values, habits, customs, languages, symbols, rituals, ceremonies, and practices that are unique to a particular group of people.

dominant culture The group whose values prevail within society.

ethnic Relating to a group of people who have had different experiences from those of the dominant culture in terms of status, background, residence, religion, education, or other factors that functionally unify the group.

ethnicity A cultural group's perception of themselves, or the group identity. This self-perception influences how the group members are perceived by others.

ethnocentrism An assumption of cultural superiority and an inability to accept another culture's ways.

minority group An ethnic, racial, or religious group that constitutes less than a numerical majority of the population.

oppression Is based on cultural biases and stems from values, beliefs, traditions, and cultural expectations. Occurs when the rules, modes, and ideals of one group are imposed on another group.

race A grouping of people that is based on biological similarities. Members of a racial group have similar physical characteristics, such as blood group, facial features, and color of skin, hair, and eyes.

racism Discrimination directed toward individuals who are perceived to be inferior because of biological differences. A form of oppression.

stereotyping An expectation that all people within the same racial, ethnic, or cultural group act alike and share the same beliefs and attitudes.

subculture A group of people with characteristic patterns of behavior that distinguish the group from the larger culture or society.

values Principles and standards that have meaning and worth to an individual, family, group, or community.

PYRAMID TO SUCCESS

Often, nurses are caring for clients who come from different ethnic, cultural, or religious backgrounds from their own. Awareness of and sensitivity to the unique health and illness beliefs and practices are essential in the delivery of safe and effective care. Acknowledgment and acceptance of cultural differences with a nonjudgmental attitude are essential in providing culturally sensitive care. The belief underlying the NCLEX-RN Test Plan is that people are unique individuals and define their own systems of daily living, which reflects their values, motives, and lifestyles. The primary Integrated Concepts and Processes addressed in this chapter are Cultural Awareness, Caring, Communication and Documentation.

CLIENT NEEDS
Safe, Effective Care Environment

Acting as a client advocate
Client rights
Confidentiality
Respecting client's control of personal environment and property
Establishing priorities

Ethical practice
Legal responsibilities
Organ donation
Communicating the need for referrals to members of
the health care team

Health Promotion and Maintenance

Disease prevention
Family planning and family systems
Health and wellness
Lifestyle choices

Psychosocial Integrity

Coping mechanisms
Religious and spiritual influences on health
Support systems
End of life
Therapeutic interventions

Physiological Integrity

Basic care and comfort practices
Nutritional preferences (Box 5-1)
Therapeutic procedures
Practices or restrictions related to procedures and
treatments

BOX 5-1

Dietary Preferences

African-Americans
Fried foods
Pork, greens, rice
Some pregnant African-Americans engage in pica
Asian-Americans
Soy sauce
Raw fish
Rice
European (White)–Origin Americans
Carbohydrates (potatoes)
Red meat
Hispanic-Americans
Beans
Fried foods
Spicy foods
Chili
Carbonated beverages
American Indians, Aleuts, Eskimos
Blue cornmeal
Fish
Game
Fruits and berries
Navajos prefer meat and blue cornmeal and tend to
avoid consumption of milk

I. AFRICAN-AMERICANS

A. Communication
  1. Languages include English and Black English
  2. Head nodding does not necessarily mean agreement
  3. Direct eye contact is often viewed as being rude
  4. Nonverbal communication is very important
  5. It is considered to be intrusive to ask personal questions of someone on initial contact or meeting
B. Time orientation and space
  1. Oriented more to the present than the future
  2. Close personal space is important
  3. Touching another's hair is sometimes viewed as offensive
C. Social roles
  1. Large extended-family networks are important
  2. Many single-parent, female-headed households
  3. Religion is usually Protestant (Baptist) (see Box 5-2)
  4. Strong church affiliation with community is important
  5. Social organizations are strong within communities
D. Health and illness
  1. Harmony with nature
  2. No separation of body, mind, and spirit
  3. Illness is a disharmonious state that may be caused by demons or spirits
  4. Illness can be prevented by nutritious meals, rest, and cleanliness
E. Health risks
  1. Sickle cell anemia
  2. Hypertension
  3. Coronary heart disease
  4. Cancer (especially stomach and esophageal)
  5. Lactose intolerance
  6. Coccidioidomycosis
F. Implementation
  1. Avoid **stereotyping**
  2. Do not label Black English as an unacceptable form of language
  3. Clarify meaning of client's verbal and nonverbal behavior
  4. Be flexible and avoid rigidity in scheduling care
  5. Encourage involvement with family
  6. A folk healer or herbalist may be consulted before an individual seeks medical treatment

II. ASIAN-AMERICANS

A. Communication
  1. Languages include Chinese, Japanese, Korean, Vietnamese, English
  2. Silence is valued
  3. Eye contact is considered rude

4. Criticism or disagreement is not expressed verbally
5. Head nodding does not necessarily mean agreement
6. The word "no" is interpreted as disrespect for others

B. Time orientation and space
1. Oriented more to present
2. Social distance is important
3. Usually do not touch others during conversation
4. Touching is unacceptable with members of opposite sex
5. The head is considered to be sacred; therefore touching someone on the head is disrespectful

C. Social roles
1. Devoted to tradition
2. Large extended-family networks
3. Loyalty to immediate and extended family and honor are valued
4. Family unit is very structured and hierarchical
5. Men have the power and authority, and women are expected to be obedient
6. Education is viewed as important

7. Religions include Taoism (Buddhism), Islam, Christianity (see Box 5-2)
8. Social organizations are strong within the community

D. Health and illness
1. Health is a state of physical and spiritual harmony with nature and a balance between positive and negative energy forces (yin and yang)
2. A healthy body is viewed as a gift from ancestors
3. Illness is viewed as an imbalance between yin and yang
4. Yin foods are cold, and yang foods are hot; cold foods are eaten when one has a hot illness, and hot foods are eaten when one has a cold illness
5. Illness is contributed to prolonged sitting or lying, or to overexertion

E. Health risks
1. Hypertension
2. Cancer (stomach and liver)
3. Lactose intolerance
4. Thalassemia
5. Coccidioidomycosis

BOX 5-2

Religions and Dietary Practices

Seventh Day Adventist (Church of God)
Alcohol, coffee, and tea prohibited
Some groups prohibit meat

Baptist
Alcohol prohibited
Discourage consumption of coffee and tea

Buddhism
Alcohol and drug use discouraged
Some sects are vegetarian

Roman Catholicism
Avoid meat on Ash Wednesday and Good Friday
Optional fasting during Lent season
During Lent, discourage meat on Friday
Children and the ill are exempt from fasting

Church of Jesus Christ of Latter-Day Saints (Mormon)
Alcohol, coffee, and tea prohibited
Limited consumption of meat
First Sunday of the month is time for fasting

Hinduism
Beef and veal prohibited
Many individuals are vegetarians
Limited consumption of meat
Fasting occurs on specific days of the week according to which god the person worships
Children are not allowed to participate in fasting
Fasting rituals vary from complete abstinence to consumption of only one meal per day

Islam
Pork prohibited
Any meat product not ritually slaughtered is prohibited

Avoidance of alcohol or drugs
During Ramadan (ninth month of Mohammedan year), fasting occurs during daytime

Jehovah's Witness
Prohibition of any foods to which blood has been added
Can consume animal flesh that has been drained

Judaism
Dietary kosher laws must be adhered to by Orthodox believers
Meats allowed include animals that are vegetable eaters, cloven-hoofed animals, and animals that are ritually slaughtered
Fish that have scales and fins are allowed
Any combination of meat and milk is prohibited
During Yom Kippur, 24-hour fasting
Pregnant women and those who are seriously ill are exempt from fasting
During Passover week, only unleavened bread is eaten

Pentecostal (Assembly of God)
Alcohol is prohibited
Avoid consumption of anything to which blood has been added
Some individuals avoid pork

Russian Orthodox
Abstention from meat and dairy products on Wednesday, Friday, and during Lent
During Lent, all animal products, including dairy products, are forbidden
Fasting during Advent
Exceptions from fasting include illness and pregnancy

F. Implementation
   1. Avoid physical closeness and excessive touching; only touch a client's head when necessary, informing the client before doing so
   2. Limit eye contact
   3. Avoid gesturing with hands
   4. Clarify responses to questions
   5. Be flexible and avoid rigidity in scheduling care
   6. Encourage involvement with family
   7. A healer may be consulted before an individual seeks out traditional treatment

III. EUROPEAN (WHITE)–ORIGIN AMERICANS

A. Communication
   1. Languages include national languages, English
   2. Silence can be used to show respect or disrespect for another, depending on situation
   3. Eye contact is viewed as indicating trustworthiness
B. Time orientation and space
   1. Future oriented
   2. Aloof and tend to avoid close physical contact
   3. Handshakes are used for formal greetings
C. Social roles
   1. The nuclear family is the basic unit; the extended family is also important
   2. The man is the dominant figure
   3. Religion includes Judeo-Christian (see Box 5-2)
   4. Community social organizations are important
D. Health and illness
   1. Health is usually viewed as an absence of disease or illness
   2. Have a tendency to be stoical when expressing physical concerns
   3. Primarily rely on modern Western health care delivery system
E. Health risks
   1. Breast cancer
   2. Heart disease
   3. Diabetes mellitus
   4. Thalassemia
F. Implementation
   1. Monitor and assess client's body language
   2. Respect client's personal space

IV. HISPANIC-AMERICANS

A. Communication
   1. Languages include Spanish and Portuguese, with various dialects
   2. Tend to be verbally expressive, yet confidentiality is important
   3. Eye behavior is significant; for example, the "evil eye" can be given to a child if a person looks at and admires a child without touching the child
   4. Avoiding eye contact indicates respect and attentiveness

5. Direct confrontation is disrespectful, and the expression of negative feelings is impolite
   6. Dramatic body language, such as gestures or facial expressions, is used to express emotion or pain
B. Time orientation and space
   1. Oriented more to present
   2. Comfortable with close proximity to others
   3. Very tactile and use embraces and handshakes
   4. Value the physical presence of others
   5. Politeness and modesty are essential
C. Social roles
   1. The nuclear family is the basic unit; also, there are large extended-family networks
   2. The extended family is highly regarded
   3. Needs of the family take precedence over individual family members' needs
   4. Men are the decision makers and breadwinners, and women are the caretakers and homemakers
   5. Religion includes Catholicism (see Box 5-2)
   6. Strong church affiliation
   7. Social organizations strong within the community
D. Health and illness
   1. Health may be a reward from God or a result of good luck
   2. Health results from a state of balance between "hot and cold" forces and "wet and dry" forces
   3. Illness occurs as a result of God's punishment for sins
   4. Folk medicine traditions
E. Health risks
   1. Lactose intolerance
   2. Diabetes mellitus
   3. Parasites
   4. Coccidioidomycosis
F. Implementation
   1. Communicate with male head of family
   2. Protect privacy
   3. Offer to call priest or other clergy because of the significance of religious practices related to illnesses
   4. Always touch a child when examining him or her
   5. Be flexible and avoid rigidity in scheduling care

V. NATIVE AMERICANS

A. Communication
   1. Languages include English, Navajo, and other tribal languages
   2. Silence indicates respect for the speaker
   3. Speak in a low tone of voice and expect others to be attentive
   4. Eye contact is avoided because it is a sign of disrespect
   5. Body language is important

B. Time orientation and space
1. Oriented more to present
2. Personal space is very important
3. Will lightly touch another person's hand during greetings
▲ 4. Massage is used for the newborn infant to promote bonding between infant and mother
▲ 5. Touching a dead body is prohibited in some tribes
C. Social roles
1. Very family oriented
2. Basic family unit is the extended family, which often includes people from several households
3. In some tribes, grandparents are viewed as family leaders
4. Elders are honored
5. Children are taught to respect traditions
6. The father does all the work outside the home, and the mother assumes responsibility for domestic duties
7. Sacred myths and legends provide spiritual guidance
8. Religion and healing practices are integrated
9. Community social organizations are important
D. Health and illness
1. Health is a state of harmony between the person, the family, and the environment
2. Illness is caused by supernatural forces and disequilibrium between person and environment
3. Traditional health and illness beliefs may continue to be observed; natural and magicoreligious folk medicine tradition
4. Traditional healer: medicine man or woman
▲ E. Health risks
1. Alcohol abuse
2. Accidents
3. Heart disease
4. Diabetes mellitus
5. Tuberculosis
6. Arthritis
7. Lactose intolerance
8. Gallbladder disease
9. American Eskimos are susceptible to glaucoma
▲ F. Implementation
1. Clarify communication
2. Understand that the client may be attentive even when eye contact is absent
3. Be attentive to own use of body language
4. Obtain input from members of extended family
5. Encourage client to personalize space in which health care is delivered; for example, encourage client to bring personal items or objects to the hospital
6. In the home, assess for the availability of running water, and modify infection control and hygiene practices as necessary

VI. PROLONGATION OF LIFE
A. Christian Science religion is unlikely to use medical means to prolong life
B. Jewish faith generally opposes prolonging life after irreversible brain damage

VII. DEATH AND DYING PRACTICES
A. Autopsy may be prohibited, opposed, or discouraged by Eastern Orthodox religions, Muslims, Jehovah's Witnesses, and Orthodox Jews
B. Organ donation is prohibited by Jehovah's Witnesses and Muslims
C. Buddhists in America encourage organ donation and consider it an act of mercy
D. Cremation is discouraged, opposed, or prohibited by the Mormon, Eastern Orthodox, Islamic, and Jewish faiths
E. Hindus prefer cremation and cast the ashes in a holy river

PRACTICE QUESTIONS

1. A nurse in an ambulatory care clinic is performing an admission assessment for an African-American client scheduled for a cataract removal with an intraocular lens implant. Which of the following questions would be inappropriate for the nurse to ask on an initial assessment?
   1. "Do you have any difficulty breathing?"
   2. "Do you have a close family relationship?"
   3. "Do you ever experience chest pain?"
   4. "Do you frequently have episodes of headache?"
2. A nurse is providing discharge instructions to a Chinese client regarding prescribed dietary modifications. During the teaching session, the client continuously turns away from the nurse. Which nursing action is most appropriate?
   1. Continue with the instructions, verifying client understanding
   2. Tell the client about the importance of the instructions for the maintenance of health care
   3. Walk around the client so that the nurse continuously faces the client
   4. Give the client a dietary booklet and return later to continue with the instructions
3. A nurse is preparing a plan of care for a client whose religion is Jehovah's Witness. The client has been told that surgery is necessary. The nurse considers the client's religious preferences in developing the plan of care and documents that:
   1. Surgery is prohibited in this religious group
   2. The administration of blood and blood products is forbidden
   3. Medication administration is not allowed
   4. Faith healing is primarily practiced

4. A nurse is preparing to deliver a food tray to a client whose religion is Jewish. The nurse checks the food on the tray and notes that the client has received a roast beef dinner with whole milk as a beverage. Which action will the nurse take?
   1. Deliver the food tray to the client
   2. Call the dietary department and ask for a new meal tray
   3. Replace the whole milk with fat-free milk
   4. Ask the dietary department to replace the roast beef with pork

5. An ambulatory care nurse is discussing preoperative procedures with a Chinese-American client who is scheduled for surgery the following week. During the discussion, the client continually smiles and nods the head. The nurse interprets this nonverbal behavior as:
   1. The client understands the preoperative procedures
   2. The client is agreeable to the required procedures
   3. Reflecting a cultural value
   4. An acceptance of the treatment

6. A nurse educator is describing the yin and yang theory of the ancient Chinese philosophy of Tao to a group of nursing students. The nurse educator explains that foods are classified as hot and cold in this theory and are transformed into yin and yang energy when metabolized by the body. The nurse educator informs the students that a client who practices this belief:
   1. Consumes cold foods when a "hot" illness is present
   2. Consumes hot foods when a "hot" illness is present
   3. Yin foods are hot
   4. Yang foods are cold

7. A community health nurse has volunteered to assist in providing health care instruction to an American Indian community group. The nurse plans instruction based on the common practices and rituals of this group, knowing that which of the following is not a common characteristic associated with this ethnic group?
   1. Corn is an important component of the diet
   2. Alcohol use is minimal
   3. Fried bread and mutton are prepared in lard
   4. Vitamin D deficiency is a concern

8. A nursing student is discussing cultural diversity issues in a clinical conference. The nursing instructor asks the student to describe ethnocentrism. Which of the following if stated by the student would indicate a lack of understanding of the issue of ethnocentrism?
   1. "It is a tendency to view one's own ways as best."
   2. "It is acting in a manner that is superior to other cultures."
   3. "It is believing that one's own ways are the only acceptable way."
   4. "It is imposing one's beliefs on individuals from another culture."

9. A home health nurse is visiting a client who does not speak English. The nurse attempts to obtain a translator to assist in communication but is unsuccessful in doing so. Which communication technique will not overcome the language barrier during the visit with the client?
   1. Communicating by writing medical terms
   2. Using simple words and avoiding medical terms
   3. Using simple words with simple actions while verbalizing them
   4. Discussing one topic at a time

10. A nurse is preparing to assist a Jewish client with eating lunch. A Kosher meal is delivered to the client. Which nursing action is most appropriate in assisting the client with the meal?
    1. Carefully placing the food from the paper plates to glass plates
    2. Unwrapping the eating utensils for the client
    3. Replacing the plastic utensils with metal eating utensils
    4. Asking the client to unwrap the eating utensils and allowing the client to prepare the meal for eating

11. A nurse is planning the menu for a Chinese client with the hospital dietician. In collaboration with the dietician, the meal plan is designed to include which of the following foods that are generally included in the diet of this cultural group?
    1. Vegetables
    2. Milk
    3. A dessert high in sugar content
    4. Large portions of meat at every meal

12. A nurse is instructing a Native American client of the Navajo culture regarding the procedure for collecting a urine sample. The nurse observes that the client continuously stares at the floor during the instructional session. The nurse interprets this behavior as:
    1. Rude
    2. Lack of interest
    3. Embarrassment
    4. Indicative that the client is paying close attention

13. A clinic nurse is preparing to examine a Hispanic child who was brought to the clinic by the mother. During assessment of the child, the nurse would avoid which of the following?
    1. Asking the mother questions about the child
    2. Admiring the child
    3. Taking the child's temperature
    4. Obtaining an interpreter if necessary

14. A nurse educator is providing inservice education to the nursing staff regarding transcultural

nursing care. A staff member asks the nurse educator to describe the concept of acculturation. The most appropriate response is which of the following?

1. "It is a subjective perspective of the person's heritage and a sense of belonging to a group."
2. "It is a group of individuals in a society that is culturally distinct and has a unique identity."
3. "It is a group that shares some of the characteristics of the larger population group of which it is a part."
4. "It is a process of learning a different culture to adapt to a new or changing environment."

15. A nurse consults with a nutritionist regarding the dietary preferences of a European-American client. Which of the following foods would most likely be requested by the client to be included in the diet?
    1. Red meat
    2. Rice
    3. Fried foods
    4. Raw fish

CRITICAL THINKING: FREE-TEXT ENTRY

A nurse is planning to instruct an African-American client about nutrition to promote health and prevent disease. When developing the plan, the nurse is aware that a common dietary practice of African-Americans is to eat what types of food that places them at risk for disease?

Answer: _____

ANSWERS

1. 2

Rationale: In the African-American culture, it is considered to be intrusive to ask personal questions on the initial contact or meeting. African-Americans are highly verbal and express feelings openly to family or friends, but what transpires within the family is viewed as private. Respiratory, cardiovascular, and neurological assessments include physiological assessments that are the priority assessments.

Test-Taking Strategy: Use Maslow's Hierarchy of Needs theory to answer the question. Note the key words "inappropriate" and "initial." Options 1, 3, and 4 address physiological needs. Option 2 addresses the psychosocial need. Review characteristics of the African-American culture if you had difficulty with this question.

Level of Cognitive Ability: Application
Client Needs: Physiological Integrity
Integrated Concept/Process: Cultural Awareness
Content Area: Fundamental Skills
Reference: Purnell, L., & Paulanka, B. (1998). *Transcultural health care: A culturally competent approach.* Philadelphia: F.A. Davis, p. 55.

2. 1

Rationale: Most Chinese maintain a formal distance with others, which is a form of respect. Many Chinese are uncomfortable with face-to-face communications, especially when there is direct eye contact. If the client turns away from the nurse during a conversation, the most appropriate action is to continue with the conversation. Walking around to the client so that the nurse faces the client is in direct conflict with the cultural practice. Telling the client about the importance of the instructions for the maintenance of health care may be viewed as degrading. The client may view returning later to continue with the explanation as a rude gesture.

Test-Taking Strategy: Use the process of elimination. Eliminate options 2 and 4 first because these actions are nontherapeutic. From the remaining options, option 1 is the most therapeutic. If you had difficulty with this question, review the communication practices of this cultural group.

Level of Cognitive Ability: Application

Client Needs: Psychosocial Integrity
Integrated Concept/Process: Cultural Awareness
Content Area: Fundamental Skills
Reference: Giger, J., & Davidhizar, R. (1999). *Transcultural nursing: Assessment & Intervention* (3rd ed.). St. Louis: Mosby, p. 388.

3. 2

Rationale: Among Jehovah's Witnesses, surgery is not prohibited, but the administration of blood and blood products is forbidden. Administration of medication is an acceptable practice except if the medication is derived from blood products. Faith healing is forbidden in this religious group.

Test-Taking Strategy: Use the process of elimination, recalling that the administration of blood and any associated blood products is forbidden. Review the characteristics of this religious group if you had difficulty with this question.

Level of Cognitive Ability: Application
Client Needs: Psychosocial Integrity
Integrated Concept/Process: Communication and Documentation
Content Area: Fundamental Skills
Reference: Spector, R. (2000). *Cultural diversity in health & illness* (5th ed.). Upper Saddle River, NJ: Prentice Hall, p. 147.

4. 2

Rationale: In the Jewish religion, the dairy-meat combination is not acceptable. Pork and pork products are not allowed in the traditional Jewish religion. The nurse would not deliver the food tray to the client and would ask the dietary department to deliver a new meal tray.

Test-Taking Strategy: Use the process of elimination, recalling that the dairy-meat combination is not acceptable in the Jewish religion. Review the dietary rules of this religious group if you had difficulty with this question.

Level of Cognitive Ability: Application
Client Needs: Physiological Integrity
Integrated Concept/Process: Cultural Awareness
Content Area: Fundamental Skills
Reference: Spector, R. (2000). *Cultural diversity in health & illness* (5th ed.). Upper Saddle River, NJ: Prentice Hall, p. 107.

5. 3

Rationale: Nodding or smiling by a Chinese-American client may only reflect the cultural value of interpersonal harmony. This nonverbal behavior may not be an indication of agreement with the speaker, an acceptance of the treatment, or an understanding of the procedure.

Test-Taking Strategy: Use the process of elimination. Eliminate options 2 and 4 first because they are similar. From the remaining options, select option 3 because it is the most global option. In addition, option 1 is an incorrect interpretation of the client's nonverbal behavior. Review the cultural characteristics of the Chinese-American population if you had difficulty with this question.

Level of Cognitive Ability: Comprehension
Client Needs: Psychosocial Integrity
Integrated Concept/Process: Communication and Documentation
Content Area: Fundamental Skills
Reference: Giger, J., & Davidhizar, R. (1999). *Transcultural nursing: Assessment & Intervention* (3rd ed.). St. Louis: Mosby, p. 15.

6. 1

Rationale: In the yin and yang theory, health is believed to exist when all aspects of the person are in perfect balance. Foods are classified as hot or cold in this theory and are transformed into yin and yang energy when metabolized by the body. Yin foods are cold, and yang foods are hot. Cold foods are eaten when one has a hot illness, and hot foods are eaten when one has a cold illness.

Test-Taking Strategy: Use the process of elimination and knowledge regarding the theory of yin and yang. If you are unfamiliar with this theory, review its elements.

Level of Cognitive Ability: Comprehension
Client Needs: Health Promotion and Maintenance
Integrated Concept/Process: Cultural Awareness
Content Area: Fundamental Skills
Reference: Swanson, J., & Nies, M. (1997). *Community health nursing: Promoting the health of aggregates* (2nd ed.). Philadelphia: W.B. Saunders, pp. 453-454.

7. 2

Rationale: American Indian diets may be deficient in vitamin D because many individuals in this group suffer from lactose intolerance or do not drink milk. Corn is an important staple in the diet of Navajo and other American Indian tribes. Fried bread and mutton are prepared in lard, and these dietary rituals have contributed to the increased risk of gallbladder disease in this population. Alcohol abuse is a concern, and many American Indian tribes exhibit high-risk behaviors related to alcohol abuse.

Test-Taking Strategy: Use the process of elimination. Note the key word "not" in the stem of the question. Knowledge that alcohol abuse is a concern will easily direct you to option 2. Review the common rituals and health care practices in this cultural group if you had difficulty with this question.

Level of Cognitive Ability: Comprehension
Client Needs: Health Promotion and Maintenance
Integrated Concept/Process: Cultural Awareness
Content Area: Fundamental Skills
Reference: Purnell, L., & Paulanka, B. (1998). *Transcultural health care: A culturally competent approach.* Philadelphia: F.A. Davis, pp. 434-436.

8. 4

Rationale: Ethnocentrism is a tendency to view one's own ways of life as the most desirable, acceptable, or best, and to act in a superior manner toward another culture. Cultural imposition is the tendency to impose one's own beliefs, values, and patterns of behavior on individuals from another culture.

Test-Taking Strategy: Use the process of elimination and note the key words "indicate a lack of understanding" in the stem of the question. Also, note the similarity between options 1, 2, and 3. If you had difficulty with this question, review culturally related concepts.

Level of Cognitive Ability: Comprehension
Client Needs: Psychosocial Integrity
Integrated Concept/Process: Cultural Awareness
Content Area: Fundamental Skills
Reference: Harkreader, H. (2000). *Fundamentals of nursing: Caring and clinical judgment.* Philadelphia: W.B. Saunders, p. 60.

9. 1

Rationale: Communicating with the client by writing medical terms does not overcome the language barrier because it is likely that the client will not be able to understand the written language or the medical terms. Options 2, 3, and 4 identify techniques that will assist in overcoming language barriers when an interpreter is not present.

Test-Taking Strategy: Note the key word "not" in the stem of the question. Use the process of elimination and attempt to visualize each of the methods identified in the options to assist in answering the question. Remember that the client may not be able to interpret medical terms or a written language that is different from his own. Review these communication techniques if you had difficulty with this question.

Level of Cognitive Ability: Application
Client Needs: Psychosocial Integrity
Integrated Concept/Process: Communication and Documentation
Content Area: Fundamental Skills
Reference: Riley, J. (2000). *Communication in nursing* (4th ed.). St. Louis: Mosby, p. 65.

10. 4

Rationale: Kosher meals arrive on paper plates and with plastic utensils sealed. Health care providers should not unwrap the utensils or transfer the foodstuffs to another serving dish. Although the nurse may want to be helpful in assisting the client with the meal, the only appropriate option for this client is option 4.

Test-Taking Strategy: Use the process of elimination and knowledge regarding the rituals associated with kosher meals. Options 1 and 3 are similar and can be eliminated first. To choose from the remaining options, it is necessary to be familiar with kosher rituals. If you had difficulty with this question, review the dietary practices of this Jewish client.

Level of Cognitive Ability: Application
Client Needs: Physiological Integrity
Integrated Concept/Process: Cultural Awareness
Content Area: Fundamental Skills
Reference: Purnell, L., & Paulanka, B. (1998). *Transcultural health care: A culturally competent approach.* Philadelphia: F.A. Davis, p. 382.

11. 1

Rationale: The Chinese diet is generally vegetarian, although meat may be served. Native Chinese generally do not drink milk or eat milk products because of a genetic tendency toward lactose intolerance. Most Chinese do not eat desserts high in sugar content, and their desserts are usually fruits.

Test-Taking Strategy: Use the process of elimination and knowledge regarding the food rituals related to the Chinese culture to answer this question. If you had difficulty with this question, review the characteristics of this culture.

Level of Cognitive Ability: Comprehension

Client Needs: Physiological Integrity

Integrated Concept/Process: Cultural Awareness

Content Area: Fundamental Skills

Reference: Purnell, L., & Paulanka, B. (1998). *Transcultural health care: A culturally competent approach.* Philadelphia: F.A. Davis, p. 176.

12. 4

Rationale: Native American clients often stare at the floor when a nurse is talking. This culturally appropriate behavior indicates that the listener is paying close attention to the speaker. In this culture, eye contact is considered a sign of disrespect. Options 1, 2, and 3 are inappropriate interpretations of the client's behavior.

Test-Taking Strategy: Use the process of elimination and knowledge regarding the culturally appropriate behaviors of Navajo clients. If you had difficulty with this question, review the characteristics of this culture.

Level of Cognitive Ability: Comprehension

Client Needs: Psychosocial Integrity

Integrated Concept/Process: Communication and Documentation

Content Area: Fundamental Skills

Reference: Swanson, J., & Nies, M. (1997). *Community health nursing: promoting the health of aggregates* (2nd ed.). Philadelphia: W.B. Saunders, p. 450.

13. 2

Rationale: Hispanic clients may believe in *mal ojo* ("evil eye"). They believe that an individual becomes ill as a result of excessive admiration by another. Options 1 and 3 are appropriate interventions. It is appropriate for the nurse to obtain an interpreter if the child or mother does not speak the same language as the nurse.

Test-Taking Strategy: Use the process of elimination. Note the key word "avoid" in the stem of the question. Options 1 and 4 can be easily eliminated because these are therapeutic and appropriate interventions. There is no reason to avoid taking the child's temperature. If you had difficulty with this question, review the cultural characteristics of the Hispanic population.

Level of Cognitive Ability: Application

Client Needs: Psychosocial Integrity

Integrated Concept/Process: Cultural Awareness

Content Area: Fundamental Skills

Reference: Spector, R. (2000). *Cultural diversity in health & illness* (5th ed.). Upper Saddle River, NJ: Prentice Hall, p. 241.

14. 4

Rationale: Acculturation is a process of learning a different culture to adapt to a new or changing environment. Option 1 describes ethnic identity. Option 2 describes an ethnic group. Option 3 describes a subculture.

Test-Taking Strategy: Knowledge regarding the descriptions and definitions of the foundational concepts related to culture is required to answer this question. Review these concepts if you are unfamiliar with them.

Level of Cognitive Ability: Comprehension

Client Needs: Psychosocial Integrity

Integrated Concept/Process: Cultural Awareness

Content Area: Fundamental Skills

Reference: Kozier, B., Erb, G., Berman, A., & Burke, K. (2000). *Fundamentals of nursing: Concepts, process, and practice* (6th ed.). Upper Saddle River, NJ: Prentice Hall, p. 203.

15. 1

Rationale: European-Americans prefer carbohydrates and red meat. African-American food preferences include pork, greens, rice, and fried foods. Asian-American food preferences include raw fish, rice, and soy sauce.

Test-Taking Strategy: Use the process of elimination and knowledge regarding the food practices and preferences related to the various cultures. Correlate carbohydrates and red meat with European-Americans. This may assist in answering other questions similar to this one. If you had difficulty with this question, review the food preferences associated with the European-American culture.

Level of Cognitive Ability: Comprehension

Client Needs: Physiological Integrity

Integrated Concept/Process: Cultural Awareness

Content Area: Fundamental Skills

Reference: Purnell, L., & Paulanka, B. (1998). *Transcultural health care: A culturally competent approach.* Philadelphia: F.A. Davis, p. 63.

CRITICAL THINKING: FREE-TEXT ENTRY

Answer: Fried foods

Rationale: African-American food preferences include primarily pork, greens, rice, and fried foods. Fried foods are usually prepared in lard. Consumption of foods from the fruit group is minimal. Eating foods that are fried places the African-American client at risk for heart disease.

Test-Taking Strategy: Recalling that African-Americans are at risk for hypertension and coronary artery disease will assist in identifying the types of food that these clients tend to eat. If you had difficulty with this question, review the food preferences associated with the African-American culture.

Level of Cognitive Ability: Comprehension

Client Needs: Physiological Integrity

Integrated Concept/Process: Cultural Awareness

Content Area: Fundamental Skills

Reference: Grodner, M., Anderson, S., & DeYoung, S. (2000). *Foundations and clinical applications of nutrition: A nursing approach.* St. Louis: Mosby, p. 790.

REFERENCES

Clark, M.J. (1999). *Nursing in the community: Dimensions of community health nursing* (3rd ed.). Stamford, Conn: Appleton & Lange.

Giger, J., & Davidhizar, R. (1999). *Transcultural nursing: Assessment & Intervention* (3rd ed.). St. Louis: Mosby.

Grodner, M., Anderson, S., & DeYoung, S. (2000). *Foundations and clinical applications of nutrition: A nursing approach.* St. Louis: Mosby.

Harkreader, H. (2000). *Fundamentals of nursing: Caring and clinical judgment.* Philadelphia: W.B. Saunders.

Kozier, B., Erb, G., Berman, A., & Burke, K. (2000). *Fundamentals of nursing: Concepts, process, and practice* (6th ed.). Upper Saddle River, N.J.: Prentice Hall.

Leahy, J., & Kizilay, P. (1998). *Foundations of nursing practice: A nursing process approach.* Philadelphia: W.B. Saunders.

Luckmann, J. (1997). *Saunders manual of nursing care.* Philadelphia: W.B. Saunders.

Purnell, P., & Paulanka, B. (1998). *Transcultural healthcare: A culturally competent approach.* Philadelphia: F.A. Davis.

Riley, J. (2000). *Communication in nursing* (4th ed.). St. Louis: Mosby.

Spector, R. (2000). *Cultural diversity in health & illness* (5th ed.). Upper Saddle River, N.J.: Prentice Hall.

Swanson, J., & Nies, M. (1997). *Community health nursing: Promoting the health of aggregates* (2nd ed.). Philadelphia: W.B. Saunders.

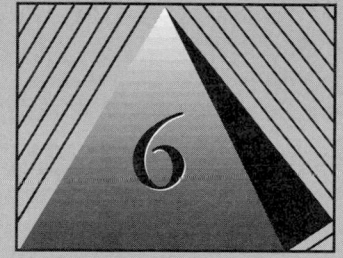

Ethical and Legal Issues

PYRAMID TERMS

advance directive   Written document, recognized by state law, that provides directions concerning the provision of care when a person is unable to make his or her own treatment choices.

advocacy   Acting on the behalf of the client and protecting the client's rights to make his or her own decisions.

consent   Voluntary act by which a person agrees to allow someone else to do something.

ethics   Concerns the distinction between right and wrong on the basis of a body of knowledge, not just on the basis of opinions.

informed consent   The client understands the reason for the proposed intervention, with its benefits and risks, and agrees to the treatment by signing a consent form.

law   A system composed of general rules governing conduct and the procedures for resolving disputes when rules are not followed.

malpractice   Failure to meet the standard of acceptable care, which results in harm to another person.

negligence   Failure to provide care that a reasonable person would ordinarily use in a similar circumstance.

Patient's Bill Of Rights   Includes the rights and responsibilities of clients receiving care.

values   Beliefs and attitudes that may influence behavior and the process of decision making.

▲ PYRAMID TO SUCCESS

Across all settings in the practice of nursing, nurses are frequently confronted with ethical and legal issues related to client care. It is the responsibility of the professional nurse to be aware of the ethical principles, laws, and guidelines related to providing safe and high-quality care to clients. In the Pyramid to Success, focus on ethical practices, the Nurse Practice Act, Client Rights, particularly confidentiality and informed con-

sent, advocacy, documentation, advance directives, death and dying, and organ donation. The primary Integrated Concepts and Processes addressed in this chapter are Nursing Process, Caring, and Communication and Documentation.

CLIENT NEEDS
Safe, Effective Care Environment

Acting as an advocate
Advance directives
Client rights
Confidentiality
Continuous quality improvement
Establishing priorities
Ethical practice
Incident or irregular occurrence reports
Informed consent
Legal responsibilities
Organ donation
Resource management

Health Promotion and Maintenance

Developmental stages and transitions
Family systems
Lifestyle choices

Psychosocial Integrity

Abuse or neglect
Chemical dependency
Coping mechanisms
End of life
Grief and loss
Support systems
Sexual abuse

Physiological Integrity

Alterations in body systems
Palliative or comfort care
Unexpected responses to therapies

I. ETHICS AND VALUES

A. **Ethics:** The branch of philosophy that concerns the distinction between right and wrong on the basis of a body of knowledge, not just on the basis of opinions
B. Morality: Behavior in accordance with customs or tradition, usually reflecting personal or religious beliefs
C. Teleology
   1. Ethical theory states that the value of a situation is determined by its consequences
   2. Principle of Utility states that the act must result in the greatest amount of good for the greatest number of people involved in a situation
D. Deontology: Ethical theory that considers the intrinsic significance of the act itself as the criterion for determination of good
E. Ethical principles: Codes that direct or govern our actions (Box 6-1)
F. **Values:** Beliefs and attitudes that may influence behavior and the process of decision-making
G. **Values** clarification: Process of analyzing one's own **values** to better understand what is truly important
H. Ethical codes
   1. Provide broad principles for determining and evaluating client care
   2. Are not legally binding, but in most states, the Board of Nursing has authority to reprimand nurses for unprofessional conduct that results from violation of the ethical codes
   3. Specific ethical codes
      a. The Code for Nurses developed by the International Council of Nurses
      b. American Nurses Association (ANA) Code of **Ethics**
I. Ethical dilemma
   1. Occurs when there is a conflict between two or more ethical principles
   2. There is no correct decision
   3. The nurse must make a choice between two alternatives that are equally unsatisfactory
   4. Ethical reasoning is the process of thinking through what one ought to do in an orderly and systematic manner to provide justification for actions on the basis of principles
J. **Advocate**
   1. A person who speaks up for or acts on the behalf of the client, protects the client's right to make his or her own decisions, and upholds the principle of fidelity

---

BOX 6-1

Ethical Principles

Autonomy	Respect for an individual's right to self-determination
Nonmaleficence	The obligation to do or cause no harm to another
Beneficence	The duty to do good to others and to maintain a balance between benefits and harms; paternalism is an undesirable outcome of beneficence, in which the health care provider decides what is best for the client and attempts to encourage the client to act against his or her own choices
Justice	The equitable distribution of potential benefits and tasks
Veracity	The obligation to tell the truth
Fidelity	The duty to do what one has promised

---

   2. Represents the client's viewpoint to others
   3. Avoids letting personal **values** influence **advocacy** for the client
   4. Supports the client's decision even when it conflicts with his or her own preferences or choices
K. **Ethics** committees
   1. Multidisciplinary approach to facilitate dialogue regarding ethical dilemmas
   2. Develop and establish policies and procedures for the prevention and resolution of dilemmas

II. REGULATION OF NURSING PRACTICE

A. Nurse practice act
   1. A series of statutes enacted by each state legislature to regulate the practice of nursing in that state
   2. Nurse practice acts set educational requirements for the nurse, distinguish between nursing practice and medical practice, and define the scope of nursing practice
   3. Additional issues covered by nurse practice acts include licensure requirements for protection of the public, grounds for disciplinary action, rights of the nurse licensee if a disciplinary action is taken, and related topics
   4. All nurses are responsible for knowing the provisions of the act for the state or province in which they work
B. Standards of care
   1. Guidelines by which the nurse should practice
   2. Guidelines for determining whether nurses have performed duties in an appropriate manner
   3. If nurses do not perform duties within accepted standards of care, they place themselves in jeopardy of legal action

4. If nurses are named as defendants in a **malprac-tice** lawsuit and it is shown that neither the accepted standards of care outlined by the state or province nursing practice act nor the policies of the employing institution were followed, the nurses' legal liability is clear

C. Employee guidelines
1. Respondent superior: Employer will be held liable for any negligent acts of an employee if the alleged negligent act occurred during the employment relationship and was within the scope of the employee's responsibilities
2. Contracts
   a. Nurses are responsible for carrying out the terms of contractual agreement with the employee agency and the client
   b. The nurse employee relationship is governed by established employee handbooks and client care policies and procedures that create obligations, rights, and duties between those parties
3. Institutional policies
   a. Written policies and procedures of the employing institution that detail how nurses are to perform their duties
   b. Policies and procedures are usually quite specific and are located in manuals in most health care facilities
   c. Although policies are not **laws,** courts generally rule against nurses who violate policies
   d. If the nurse practices nursing in accordance with the client care policies and procedures established by the employer, functions within the job responsibility, and provides care consistently in a nonnegligent manner, the potential for liability is minimized

D. Hospital staffing
1. Nurses should not walk out when staffing is inadequate, because charges of abandonment can be made
2. Nurses in short staffing situations are obligated to make a report to nursing administration

E. Floating
1. An acceptable, legal practice used by hospitals to solve their understaffing problems
2. Legally, a nurse cannot refuse to float unless a union contract guarantees that nurses can work only in a specified area or the nurse can prove lack of knowledge for the performance of assigned tasks
3. Nurses in a floating situation must not assume responsibility beyond their level of experience or qualification
4. Nurses who float should inform the supervisor of any lack of experience in caring for the type of clients on the new nursing unit
5. The nurse should request and be given orientation to the new unit

F. Disciplinary action
1. Boards of nursing may deny, revoke, or suspend any license to practice as a registered nurse, in accordance with their statutory authority
2. Causes for disciplinary action
   a. Unprofessional conduct
   b. Conduct that could adversely affect the health and welfare of the public
   c. Breach of client confidentiality
   d. Failure to use sufficient knowledge, skills, or nursing judgment
   e. Physically or verbally abusing a client
   f. Assuming duties without sufficient preparation
   g. Knowingly delegating to unlicensed personnel nursing care that places the client as risk for injury
   h. Failure to accurately maintain a record for each client
   i. Falsifying a client's record
   j. Leaving a nursing assignment without properly notifying appropriate personnel

III. LEGAL LIABILITY

A. **Laws**
1. Nurses are governed by civil and criminal **law** in roles as providers of services, employees of institutions, and private citizens
2. A nurse has a personal and legal obligation to provide a standard of client care expected of a reasonably competent professional nurse
3. Professional nurses are held responsible (liable) for harm resulting from their negligent acts, or their failure to act

B. Types of **laws** (Box 6-2)

C. **Negligence** and **malpractice**
1. Conduct that falls below the standard of care
2. Can include acts of commission as well as acts of omission
3. If a nurse gives care that does not meet appropriate standards, he or she may be held liable for **negligence**
4. **Malpractice** is **negligence** on the part of a nurse
5. **Malpractice** is determined if the nurse owed a duty to the client and did not carry out the duty, and the client was injured because the nurse failed to perform the duty
6. Proof of liability
   a. Duty: At the time of injury, a duty existed between the plaintiff and the defendant
   b. Breach of duty: The defendant breached duty of care to the plaintiff
   c. Proximate cause: The breach of the duty was the legal cause of injury to the client
   d. Damage or injury: The plaintiff experienced injury or damages or both and can be compensated by **law**

BOX 6-2

Types of Laws

Contract law	Concerned with enforcement of agreements among private individuals
Civil law	Concerned with relationships among people and the protection of a person's rights
	Violation may cause harm to an individual or property, but no grave threat to society exists
Criminal law	Concerned with relationships between individuals and governments and with acts that threaten society and its order; a crime is an offense against society that violates a law and is defined as a misdemeanor (less serious nature) or felony (serious nature)
Tort law	Civil wrong, other than a breach in contract, in which the law allows an injured person to seek damages from a person who caused the injury

D. Professional liability insurance
  1. Nurses need their own liability insurance for protection against **malpractice** lawsuits
  2. Having his or her own insurance provides the nurse protection as an individual and allows the nurse to have an attorney present who has only the nurse's interests in mind
E. Good Samaritan **laws**
  1. Passed by a state legislature
  2. Encourage health care professionals to assist in emergency situations without fear of being sued for the care provided
  3. These **laws** limit liability and offer legal immunity for people helping in an emergency, providing they give reasonable care
  4. Immunity from suit applies only when all conditions of the state **law** are met, such as the health care provider receives no compensation for the care provided and the care given is not intentionally negligent
F. Controlled substances
  1. Adhere to facility policies and procedures concerning administration of controlled substances, which are governed by federal and state **laws**
  2. Controlled substances must be kept securely locked, and only authorized personnel should have access to them

IV. COLLECTIVE BARGAINING
A. Formalized decision-making process between representatives of management and representatives of labor to negotiate wages and conditions of employment
B. When collective bargaining breaks down because an

agreement cannot be reached, the employees usually call a strike
C. Striking presents a moral dilemma to many nurses because nursing practice is a service to people

V. LEGAL RISK AREAS
A. Assault
  1. Occurs when a person puts another person in fear of a harmful or offensive contact
  2. The victim fears and believes that harm will result as a result of the threat
B. Battery: An intentional touching of another's body without the other's **consent**
C. Invasion of privacy: Includes violating confidentiality, intruding on private client or family matters, and sharing client information with unauthorized persons
D. False imprisonment
  1. Occurs when a client is not allowed to leave a health care facility when there is no legal justification to detain the client
  2. Occurs when restraining devices are used without an appropriate clinical need
  3. A client can sign an "Against Medical Advice" form when the client refuses care and is competent to make decisions
  4. Document circumstances in the medical record to avoid allegations by the client that cannot be defended
E. Defamation: Occurs when information is communicated to a third party that causes damage to someone's reputation, either in writing (libel) or verbally (slander)
F. Fraud: Results from a deliberate deception intended to produce unlawful gains

VI. CLIENT RIGHTS
A. Patient's Bill of Rights
  1. Increases health care providers' awareness of the need to treat clients in an ethical and legal manner and encourages protection of rights
  2. Key elements of a client's rights with which nurses should be familiar include **informed consent** and confidentiality
B. Confidentiality
  1. A special relationship exists between two persons, in which information discussed will not be shared with a third party who is not directly involved in the client's care
  2. Nurses are bound to protect client confidentiality by most nurse practice acts, by ethical principles and standards, and by institutional and agency policies and procedures
  3. Treatment records cannot be released to any third party without the client's written **consent** and only after agency policies and procedures have been followed

4. Information release may be mandatory when ordered by a court, or when state statues require reporting of child abuse, communicable diseases, or other associated incidents

C. Privileged communication
1. Information given to a professional person who is forbidden by law from disclosing the information in a court without the consent of the person who provided it
2. The nurse should seek legal counsel in regard to a privileged communication and should become familiar with the rights and privileges of the client and the nurse

▲ D. **Informed consent**
1. **Consent** is the client's approval to have his or her body touched by a specific individual
2. Legally, the client must be mentally competent to give **consent** for procedures
3. Prior to granting a **consent,** the client must be fully informed regarding treatment, tests, surgery, and so on, and must understand both the intended outcome and the potentially harmful results
4. **Consent** must be obtained by the physician, surgeon, or other medical practitioner performing the treatment or procedure
5. In most states, when a nurse is involved in the **informed consent** process, the nurse is only witnessing the signature of the client on the **informed consent** form
6. If a client is determined by a court to be unable to make decisions and is declared incompetent or under a legal disability, a personal guardian is appointed by the court to make decisions
7. An **informed consent** can be waived for urgent medical or surgical intervention as long as institutional policy so indicates
8. Parental or guardian **consent** should be obtained before treatment is initiated for a minor except in an emergency, in situations in which the **consent** of the minor is sufficient, such as treatment of a sexually transmitted disease, or if a court order or other legal authorization has been obtained
9. Minors who are married or emancipated from parents and those seeking treatment for sexually transmitted diseases can sign an informed **consent** form
10. A client has the right to refuse information and waive the **informed consent** and undergo treatment, but this decision must be documented in the medical record

VII. LEGAL SAFEGUARDS
A. Risk management
1. A planned method to identify, analyze, and evaluate risks followed by a plan for reducing the frequency of accidents and injuries

---

BOX 6-3
Telephone Orders

Date and time the entry
Repeat the order to the physician and record the order
Sign the order; begin with t.o. (telephone order), write the physician's name, and then signature the order
If another nurse witnessed the order, that signature follows
The physician needs to countersign the order within a time frame according to agency policy

---

2. Programs are based on a systematic reporting system for incidents or unusual occurrences

B. Incident reports   ▲
1. A tool used as a means of identifying and improving client care
2. Follow specific documentation guidelines
3. Fill out completely, accurately, and factually
4. The report form should not be copied or placed in the client's record
5. No reference should be made to the report form in the client's record
6. Not a substitute for a complete entry in the client's record regarding the incident

C. Physicians' orders   ▲
1. A nurse is obligated to carry out a physician's order except when the nurse believes an order to be inappropriate
2. A nurse carrying out an inaccurate order may be legally responsible for any harm suffered by the client
3. Clarify an unclear or inappropriate order with the physician
4. If no resolution occurs regarding the order in question, contact the nurse manager or supervisor
5. See Box 6-3 concerning telephone orders

D. Documentation   ▲
1. Legally required by accrediting agencies, state licensing **laws,** and state nurse and medical practice acts
2. Follow agency guidelines and procedures (Box 6-4)

E. Client/family teaching
1. Provide complete instructions in a language that client or family can understand
2. Document client and family teaching, what was taught, evaluation of understanding, and who was present during the teaching
3. Inform client of what would happen if information shared during teaching is not followed

BOX 6-4

Documentation Guidelines

NARRATIVE

Use a black pen

Date and time entries

Provide objective, factual, and complete documentation

Document care, medications, treatments, and procedures as soon as possible after completed

Document client responses to interventions

Document consent for or refusal of treatments

Document calls made to other health care providers

Do not document for others or change documentation for other individuals

Sign and title each entry

Use quotes as appropriate for subjective data

Use correct spelling, grammar, and punctuation

Avoid unacceptable abbreviations

Avoid judgmental or evaluative statements, such as "uncooperative client"

Do not leave blank spaces on documentation forms

Follow agency policies when an error is made (draw one line through the error, initial, and date)

Follow agency guidelines regarding late entries

COMPUTERIZED

Use only the user identification (ID) code, name, or password

Never lend access ID to another

Maintain privacy and confidentiality of documented information printed from the computer

VIII. LEGAL DOCUMENTS FOR DECISION MAKING

A. Will
1. Some agencies have specific policies that prohibit a nurse from signing as witness to this legal document for a client
2. If a nurse witnesses a legal document, he or she must document the event and the factual circumstances surrounding the signing in the medical record
3. Documentation should include who was present, any significant comments by the client, and the nurse's observations of the client's conduct during this process

B. **Advance directive**
1. Written document recognized by state **law** that provides directions concerning the provision of care when a person is unable to make his or her own treatment choices
2. Must be made part of the medical record
3. The physician must be notified of its presence so that orders can be written consistent with the client's wishes

C. Living will: Document prepared by a competent adult that provides direction regarding medical care

in the event of the person's incapacitation or otherwise becoming unable to make decisions personally

D. Durable power of attorney
1. Also called health care proxy
2. An authorization that enables any competent individual to name someone to exercise decision-making authority on the individual's behalf under specific circumstances

IX. DEATH AND DYING

A. Right of informed refusal: A competent adult has the right to refuse treatment, even life-sustaining treatment

B. Do not resuscitate (DNR) order
1. A written order must be present and must be reviewed on a regular basis
2. Specific agency guidelines must be followed regarding when and under what circumstances an oral DNR order is acceptable
3. The client or his or her legal representative must provide **informed consent** for the DNR status
4. Both DNR and cardiopulmonary resuscitation (CPR) must be clearly defined so that other treatment, not refused by the client, will be continued

C. Death certificate: The physician is responsible for signing a death certificate

D. Care of the body
1. The nurse is responsible for preparing the body for the morgue or mortuary
2. Follow agency guidelines and the wishes of the family of the deceased
3. Treat the body with dignity

E. Organ transplant: The option to accept an organ transplant can be refused

F. Organ donation
1. Any person 18 years of age or older may become an organ donor by written **consent**
2. Informed choice to donate an organ can take place with the use of a written document signed by the client prior to death, a will, a donor card, or an **advance directive**
3. In the absence of appropriate documentation, a family member or legal guardian may authorize donation of the decedent's organs
4. All 50 states have adopted the Uniform Anatomical Gift Act for cadaveric organ donation

G. Autopsy
1. Medical examination of the body after death for the purpose of determining the cause of death
2. Required by state **law** in certain circumstances, such as a sudden death or a death that occurs under suspicious circumstances
3. If no oral or written instructions were given by the decedent, state **law** determines who has the authority to **consent** to an autopsy requested on a voluntary basis

4. Documentation regarding **consent** must be present before the body can be released for autopsy

H. Assisted suicide

1. Legal support exists for a client to refuse life-sustaining procedures and for health care providers to honor the client's voluntary and informed decision by withdrawing or withholding treatment
2. Taking an active role in assisting a client to die is a criminal offense in most states

X. REPORTING RESPONSIBILITIES

A. Requirements: Nurses are required to report certain communicable diseases or criminal activities such as abuse, gunshot or stab wounds, assaults, homicides, and suicides to the appropriate authorities

B. The impaired nurse

1. If a nurse suspects that a coworker is abusing chemicals, the nurse must report the individual to nursing administration in a confidential manner with the goal of treatment being the priority issue
2. Nursing administration then notifies the board of nursing regarding the nurse's behavior

C. Occupational Safety and Health Act (OSHA)

1. Requires that an employer provide a safe workplace for employees according to regulations
2. Employees can confidentially report working conditions that violate regulations
3. An employee who does not report unsafe working conditions can be retaliated against by the employer

D. Sexual harassment

1. Prohibited by state and federal **laws**
2. Includes unwelcome conduct of a sexual nature
3. Follow agency policies and procedures to handle reporting of a concern or complaint

PRACTICE QUESTIONS

1. A client arrives in the emergency room and is assessed by a nurse. The client is staggering, confused, and verbally abusive. The client complains of a headache from drinking alcohol and is asking for medication. The nurse explains to the client that the physician will need to perform an assessment prior to the administration of medication. When the client becomes verbally abusive, the nurse obtains leather restraints and threatens to place the client in the restraints. With which of the following can the client legally charge the nurse as a result of the nursing action?
   1. Assault
   2. Battery
   3. Negligence
   4. Invasion of privacy

2. A nurse calls a physician in regard to a new medication order because the dosage prescribed is higher than the recommended dosage. The nurse is unable to locate the physician, and the medication is due to be administered. Which of the following actions would the nurse take?
   1. Hold the medication until the physician can be contacted
   2. Administer the dose prescribed
   3. Administer the recommended dose until the physician can be located
   4. Contact the nursing supervisor

3. A nursing graduate is employed as a staff nurse in a local hospital. During orientation the new graduate asks the nurse educator about the need to obtain professional liability insurance. The most appropriate response by the nurse educator is:
   1. "The hospital's liability insurance will cover your actions."
   2. "It is very expensive and not necessary."
   3. "Nurses are encouraged to have their own malpractice insurance."
   4. "The majority of suits are filed against physicians and the hospital."

4. A registered nurse arrives at work and is told to report (float) to the intensive care unit (ICU) for the day because the ICU is understaffed and needs additional nurses to care for the clients. The nurse has never worked in the ICU. Which of the following is the most appropriate nursing action?
   1. Refuse to float to the ICU
   2. Call the hospital lawyer
   3. Call the nursing supervisor
   4. Report to the ICU and identify tasks that can be safely performed

5. A nurse gives an inaccurate dose of a medication to a client. After assessment of the client, the nurse completes an incident report. The nurse notifies the nursing supervisor of the medication error and calls the physician to report the occurrence. The nurse who administered the inaccurate medication dose understands that the:
   1. Error will result in suspension
   2. Incident report is a method of promoting quality care and risk management
   3. Incident will be reported to the board of nursing
   4. Incident will be documented in the personnel file

6. A nurse who works on the night shift enters the medication room and finds a coworker with a tourniquet wrapped around the upper arm. The coworker is about to insert a needle, attached to a syringe containing a clear liquid, into the antecubital area. The most appropriate initial action by the nurse is which of the following?
   1. Call the police

   2. Call security
   3. Lock the coworker in the medication room until help is obtained
   4. Call the nursing supervisor

7. A hospitalized client tells a nurse that a living will is being prepared and that the lawyer will be bringing the will to the hospital today for witness signatures. The client asks the nurse for assistance in obtaining a witness to the will. The most appropriate response to the client is which of the following?
   1. "I will sign as a witness to your signature."
   2. "You will need to find a witness on your own."
   3. "I will call the nursing supervisor to seek assistance regarding your request."
   4. "Whoever is available at the time will sign as a witness for you."

8. A nurse has made an error in documenting an assessment finding on a client and obtains the client's record to correct the error. The nurse corrects the error by:
   1. Trying to erase the error to provide space to write in the correct data
   2. Using whiteout to delete the error and writing in the correct data
   3. Drawing one line through the error, initialing and dating the line, and then documenting the correct information
   4. Documenting a late entry into the client's record

9. A nurse employed in a hospital is waiting to receive a report from the laboratory via the facsimile (Fax) machine. The Fax machine activates, and the nurse expects the report but instead receives a sexually oriented photograph. The most appropriate nursing action is to:
   1. Cut up the photograph and throw it away
   2. Call the laboratory and ask for the name of the individual who sent the photograph
   3. Call the police
   4. Call the nursing supervisor and report the incident

10. A nursing instructor provides a lecture to nursing students regarding the issue of client rights. The instructor asks a nursing student to identify a situation that represents an example of invasion of client privacy. Which of the following if identified by the student indicates an understanding of a violation of this client right?
   1. Performing a procedure without consent
   2. Telling the client that he or she cannot leave the hospital
   3. Threatening to give a client a medication
   4. Observing care provided to the client without the client's permission

11. The nursing staff is sitting in the lounge taking their morning break. A nursing assistant tells the group that she heard that the unit secretary has acquired immunodeficiency syndrome (AIDS). The nursing assistant proceeds to tell the nursing staff that the secretary contracted the disease from her husband, who is supposedly a drug addict. Which legal tort has the nursing assistant violated?
   1. Slander
   2. Libel
   3. Assault
   4. Negligence

12. A nurse hears a client calling out for help. The nurse hurries down the hallway to the client's room and finds a client lying on the floor. The nurse performs a thorough assessment and assists the client back to bed. The nurse notifies the physician of the incident and completes an incident report. Which of the following would the nurse document on the incident report?
   1. The client was found lying on the floor
   2. The client climbed over the side rails
   3. The client fell out of bed
   4. The client became restless and tried to get out of bed

13. A client is brought to the emergency room by the emergency medical services after being hit by a car. The name of the client is not known. The client has sustained a severe head injury and multiple fractures and is unconscious. An emergency craniotomy is required. In regard to informed consent for the surgical procedure, which of the following is the best initial action?
   1. Call the police to identify the client and locate the family
   2. Obtain a court order for the surgical procedure
   3. Ask the emergency medical services team to sign the informed consent
   4. Transport the victim to the operating room for surgery

14. An 87-year-old female is brought to the emergency room for treatment of a fractured arm. On physical assessment, a nurse notes old and new ecchymotic areas on the client's chest and legs. The nurse asks the client how the bruises were sustained. The client, although reluctant, tells the nurse in confidence that her son frequently hits her if supper is not prepared on time when he arrives home from work. Which of the following is the most appropriate nursing response?
   1. "Oh really, I will discuss this situation with your son."
   2. "Do you have any friends who can help you out until you resolve these important issues with your son?"
   3. "Let's talk about the ways you can manage your time to prevent this from happening."
   4. "This is a legal issue, and I need to let you know that I will need to report it."

15. A nurse is working in a long-term care facility and is administering medications to assigned clients. A client refuses to take the prescribed medication, and the nurse threatens the client and tells the client that if the medication is not taken orally, then restraints will be applied and the medication will be given by injection. This statement by the nurse constitutes which legal tort?
    1. Invasion of privacy
    2. Negligence
    3. Assault
    4. Battery

CRITICAL THINKING: FREE-TEXT ENTRY

A nurse is reviewing the physician's orders for a newly admitted client and notes that the physician has prescribed a medication dose that is twice the amount that the client reports is taken prior to admission. The nurse verifies the medication amount taken prior to admission with the client. What is the next most appropriate nursing action?

Answer: _____

ANSWERS

1. **1**
Rationale: An assault occurs when a person puts another person in fear of a harmful or offensive contact. For this intentional tort to be actionable, the victim must be aware of the threat of harmful or offensive contact. Battery is the actual contact with one's body. Negligence involves actions below the standard of care. Invasion of privacy occurs when the individual's private affairs are unreasonably intruded into.
Test-Taking Strategy: Use the process of elimination. Note the key word "threatens" in the question. This key word should easily direct you to option 1. If you had difficulty with this question, review the descriptions associated with the terms in each option.
Level of Cognitive Ability: Comprehension
Client Needs: Safe, Effective Care Environment
Integrated Concept/Process: Communication and Documentation
Content Area: Fundamental Skills
Reference: Harkreader, H. (2000). *Fundamentals of nursing: Caring and clinical judgment.* Philadelphia: W.B. Saunders, p, 24.

2. **4**
Rationale: If the physician writes an order that requires clarification, it is the nurse's responsibility to contact the physician for clarification. If there is no resolution regarding the order because the physician cannot be located, or because the order remains as it was written after the nurse talks with the physician, the nurse should then contact the nurse manager or nursing supervisor for further clarification as to what the next step should be. Under no circumstances should the nurse proceed to carry out the order until clarification is obtained.
Test-Taking Strategy: Use the process of elimination and eliminate options 2 and 3 first because they are similar and unsafe actions. Holding the medication can result in client injury. The nurse needs to take action. Option 4 clearly identifies the required action in this situation. Review nursing responsibilities related to physicians' orders, if you had difficulty with this question.
Level of Cognitive Ability: Application
Client Needs: Safe, Effective Care Environment
Integrated Concept/Process: Nursing Process/Implementation
Content Area: Fundamental Skills
Reference: Kozier, B., Erb, G., Berman, A., & Burke, K. (2000).

Fundamentals of nursing: Concepts, process, and practice (6th ed.). Upper Saddle River, NJ: Prentice Hall, p, 64.

3. **3**
Rationale: Nurses need their own liability insurance for protection against malpractice lawsuits. Nurses erroneously assume that they are protected by an agency's professional liability policies. Usually, when a nurse is sued, the employer is also sued for the nurse's actions or inactions. Even though this is the norm, nurses are encouraged to have their own malpractice insurance.
Test-Taking Strategy: Note that the issue of the question relates to "obtaining professional liability insurance." This issue should easily direct you to option 3. Review liability related to malpractice insurance, if you had difficulty with this question.
Level of Cognitive Ability: Comprehension
Client Needs: Safe, Effective Care Environment
Integrated Concept/Process: Communication and Documentation
Content Area: Fundamental Skills
Reference: Harkreader, H. (2000). *Fundamentals of nursing: Caring and clinical judgment.* Philadelphia: W.B. Saunders, p, 40.

4. **4**
Rationale: Floating is an acceptable, legal practice used by hospitals to solve their understaffing problems. Legally, a nurse cannot refuse to float unless a union contract guarantees that nurses can work only in a specified area or the nurse can prove a lack of knowledge for the performance of assigned tasks. When encountering this situation, nurses should set priorities and identify potential areas of harm to the client.
Test-Taking Strategy: Use the process of elimination, noting the key words "most appropriate." This may indicate that more than one option may be correct. Options 1 and 2 can be eliminated first. From the remaining options, it is premature to call the nursing supervisor. Option 4 is most appropriate. Review nursing responsibilities related to "floating," if you had difficulty with this question.
Level of Cognitive Ability: Application
Client Needs: Safe, Effective Care Environment
Integrated Concept/Process: Nursing Process/Implementation
Content Area: Fundamental Skills
Reference: Leahy, J., & Kizilay, P. (1998). *Foundations of nursing practice: A nursing process approach.* Philadelphia: W.B. Saunders, p. 69.

5. 2

Rationale: Documentation of unusual occurrences, incidents, and accidents, and of the nursing actions taken as a result of an occurrence, is internal to the institution or agency and allows the nurse and administration to review the quality of care and determine any potential risks present. On the basis of the information provided in the question, the nurse's error will not result in suspension, nor will it be documented in the personnel file. The error and the situation presented in the question are not a reason for notifying the board of nursing.

Test-Taking Strategy: Focus on the information provided in the question. Use the process of elimination and knowledge regarding the purpose of incident reports to assist in eliminating options 1, 3, and 4. Note that the correct option is also the global option. If you had difficulty with this question, review the purpose of incident reports.

Level of Cognitive Ability: Comprehension
Client Needs: Safe, Effective Care Environment
Integrated Concept/Process: Communication and Documentation
Content Area: Fundamental Skills
Reference: Kozier, B., Erb, G., Berman, A., & Burke, K. (2000). *Fundamentals of nursing: Concepts, process, and practice* (6th ed.). Upper Saddle River, NJ: Prentice Hall, p. 66.

6. 4

Rationale: Nurse practice acts require reporting impaired nurses. The board of nursing has jurisdiction over the practice of nursing and may develop plans for treatment and supervision of the impaired nurse. This incident needs to be reported to the nursing supervisor, who will then report to the board of nursing and other authorities, such as the police, as required. Option 3 is an inappropriate and unsafe action. Security may be called if a disturbance occurs, but there are no data in the question to support this need, and therefore this is not the initial action.

Test-Taking Strategy: Note the key words "initial action." Eliminate option 3 first because this is an inappropriate and unsafe action. Recall the lines of organization structure to assist in directing you to option 4. If you had difficulty with this question, review the nurse's responsibilities when substance abuse is suspected or occurs in the workplace.

Level of Cognitive Ability: Application
Client Needs: Safe, Effective Care Environment
Integrated Concept/Process: Communication and Documentation
Content Area: Fundamental Skills
Reference: Kozier, B., Erb, G., Berman, A., & Burke, K. (2000). *Fundamentals of nursing: Concepts, process, and practice* (6th ed.). Upper Saddle River, NJ: Prentice Hall, p. 67.

7. 3

Rationale: Living wills are required to be in writing and signed by the client. The client's signature either must be witnessed by specified individuals or must be notarized. Many states prohibit any employee, including a nurse of a facility where the declaring is receiving care, from being a witness. Option 2 is nontherapeutic and not a helpful response. The nurse should seek the assistance of the nursing supervisor.

Test-Taking Strategy: Note the key words "most appropriate." Options 1 and 4 are similar and should be eliminated first. Option 2 is eliminated because it is a nontherapeutic response. Review legal implications associated with wills, if you had difficulty with this question.

Level of Cognitive Ability: Application
Client Needs: Safe, Effective Care Environment
Integrated Concept/Process: Communication and Documentation
Content Area: Fundamental Skills
Reference: Kozier, B., Erb, G., Berman, A., & Burke, K. (2000). *Fundamentals of nursing: Concepts, process, and practice* (6th ed.). Upper Saddle River, NJ: Prentice Hall, p. 58.

8. 3

Rationale: If the nurse makes an error in documenting in the client's record, the nurse should follow agency policies to correct the error. This includes drawing one line through the error, initialing and dating the line, and then documenting the correct information. Erasing data from the client's record and the use of whiteout are prohibited. A late entry is used to document additional information not remembered at the initial time of documentation.

Test-Taking Strategy: Use the process of elimination and principles related to documentation. Recalling that alterations to a client's record are avoided will assist in eliminating options 1 and 2. From the remaining options, focusing on the issue of the question and using knowledge regarding the principles related to documentation will easily direct you to option 3. Review these principles if you had difficulty with this question.

Level of Cognitive Ability: Application
Client Needs: Safe, Effective Care Environment
Integrated Concept/Process: Communication and Documentation
Content Area: Fundamental Skills
Reference: Harkreader, H. (2000). *Fundamentals of nursing: Caring and clinical judgment.* Philadelphia: W.B. Saunders, p. 40.

9. 4

Rationale: Sexual harassment in the workplace is prohibited by state and federal laws. Sexually suggestive jokes, touching, pressuring a coworker for a date, and open displays of sexually oriented photographs or posters are examples of conduct that could be considered sexual harassment by another worker. If the nurse believes that he or she is being subjected to unwelcome sexual conduct, these concerns should be reported to the nursing supervisor immediately. Option 3 is unnecessary at this time. Options 1 and 2 are not the most appropriate actions.

Test -Taking Strategy: Note the key words "most appropriate." This may indicate that one or more than one of the options is partially or totally correct. Use the skills of prioritizing to select the correct option. Remember that it is best to utilize the organizational channels of communication. This will assist in directing you to option 4. Review nursing responsibilities when sexual harassment occurs in the workplace, if you had difficulty with this question.

Level of Cognitive Ability: Application
Client Needs: Safe, Effective Care Environment
Integrated Concept/Process: Communication and Documentation
Content Area: Fundamental Skills

Reference: Leahy, J. & Kizilay, P. (1998). *Foundations of nursing practice: A nursing process approach.* Philadelphia: W.B. Saunders, p, 78.

10. **4**

Rationale: Invasion of privacy takes place when an individual's private affairs are unreasonably intruded into. Telling a client that he or she cannot leave the hospital constitutes false imprisonment. Threatening to give a client a medication constitutes assault. Performing a procedure without consent is an example of battery.

Test-Taking Strategy: The key words in the question are "invasion of client privacy." Focus on these key words to direct you to option 4. If you had difficulty with this question, review those situations that include invasion of privacy.

Level of Cognitive Ability: Comprehension
Client Needs: Safe, Effective Care Environment
Integrated Concept/Process: Caring
Content Area: Fundamental Skills
Reference: Harkreader, H. (2000). *Fundamentals of nursing: Caring and clinical judgment.* Philadelphia: W.B. Saunders, p, 24.

11. **1**

Rationale: Defamation takes place when something untrue is said (slander) or written (libel) about a person, resulting in injury to that person's good name and reputation. An assault occurs when a person puts another person in fear of harmful or offensive contact. Negligence involves the actions of professionals that fall below the standard of care for a specific professional group.

Test-Taking Strategy: Use the process of elimination and eliminate options 3 and 4 first. Recalling that slander constitutes verbal defamation will easily direct you to option 1. If you had difficulty with this question, review the torts identified in each option.

Level of Cognitive Ability: Comprehension
Client Needs: Safe, Effective Care Environment
Integrated Concept/Process: Communication and Documentation
Content Area: Fundamental Skills
Reference: Harkreader, H. (2000). *Fundamentals of nursing: Caring and clinical judgment.* Philadelphia: W.B. Saunders, pp. 23-24.

12. **1**

Rationale: The incident report should contain the client's name, age, and diagnosis. It should contain a factual description of the incident, any injuries experienced by those involved, and the outcome of the situation. Option 1 is the only option that describes the facts as observed by the nurse. Options 2, 3, and 4 are interpretations of the situation and are not factual data as observed by the nurse.

Test-Taking Strategy: Use the process of elimination and read the information contained in the question to select the correct option. Remember to focus on factual information when documenting, and avoid including interpretations. Review documentation principles related to incident reports, if you had difficulty with this question.

Level of Cognitive Ability: Application
Client Needs: Safe, Effective Care Environment
Integrated Concept/Process: Communication and Documentation

Content Area: Fundamental Skills
Reference: Harkreader, H. (2000). *Fundamentals of nursing: Caring and clinical judgment.* Philadelphia: W.B. Saunders, p. 38.

13. **4**

Rationale: Generally, there are only two instances in which the informed consent of an adult client is not needed. One instance is when an emergency is present and delaying treatment for the purpose of obtaining informed consent would result in injury or death to the client. The second instance is when the client waives the right to informed consent. Option 2 will delay emergency treatment, and option 3 is inappropriate. Although option 1 may be pursued, it is not the best initial action.

Test-Taking Strategy: Use the process of elimination. Recalling that an emergency is present, and a delay in treatment for the purpose of obtaining informed consent could result in injury or death, will easily direct you to option 4. Review the issues surrounding informed consent, if you had difficulty with this question.

Level of Cognitive Ability: Application
Client Needs: Safe, Effective Care Environment
Integrated Concept/Process: Communication and Documentation
Content Area: Fundamental Skills
Reference: Craven, R., & Hirnle, C. (2000). *Fundamentals of nursing: Human health and function* (3rd ed.). Philadelphia: Lippincott, p. 99.

14. **4**

Rationale: Confidential issues are not to be discussed with nonmedical personnel or the person's family or friends without the person's permission. Clients should be assured that information is kept confidential, unless it places the nurse under a legal obligation. The nurse must report situations related to child or elderly abuse, gunshot wounds, and certain infectious diseases. Options 1, 2, and 3 do not address the legal implications of the situation and do not ensure a safe environment for the client.

Test-Taking Strategy: Use the process of elimination and knowledge regarding the nursing responsibilities related to reporting obligations. Options 1, 2, and 3 should be eliminated because they are similar in that they do not protect the client from injury. Review the nursing responsibilities related to reporting obligations, if you had difficulty with this question.

Level of Cognitive Ability: Application
Client Needs: Safe, Effective Care Environment
Integrated Concept/Process: Caring
Content Area: Fundamental Skills
Reference: Craven, R., & Hirnle, C. (2000). *Fundamentals of nursing: Human health and function* (3rd ed.). Philadelphia: Lippincott, p. 91.

15. **3**

Rationale: An assault occurs when a person puts another person in fear of harmful or offensive contact. For this intentional tort to be actionable, the victim must be aware of the threat of harmful or offensive contact. Battery is the actual contact with one's body. Negligence involves actions below the standard of care. Invasion of privacy occurs when the individual's private affairs are unreasonably intruded into.

Test-Taking Strategy: Use the process of elimination and knowledge regarding the descriptions of the items in each option. Note the key word "threatens" in the question. This key word should easily direct you to option 3. If you had difficulty with this question, take time to review the descriptions associated with the terms in each option.

Level of Cognitive Ability: Comprehension

Client Needs: Safe, Effective Care Environment

Integrated Concept/Process: Communication and Documentation

Content Area: Fundamental Skills

Reference: Harkreader, H. (2000). *Fundamentals of nursing: Caring and clinical judgment.* Philadelphia: W.B. Saunders, p. 24.

CRITICAL THINKING: FREE-TEXT ENTRY

Answer: Contact the physician

Rationale: If the nurse determines that a physician's order is unclear, or if the nurse has a question about an order, the nurse should contact the physician prior to implementing the order. Under no circumstances should the nurse carry out the order unless the order is clarified by the physician.

Test Taking Strategy: Use prioritizing skills to determine the next most appropriate nursing action. Noting that the nurse verifies the medication amount taken prior to admission with the client will guide you to determine that the physician needs to be contacted. Review guidelines related to physicians' orders if you had difficulty with this question.

Level of Cognitive Ability: Application

Client Needs: Safe, Effective Care Environment

Integrated Concept/Process: Nursing Process/Implementation

Content Area: Fundamental Skills

Reference: Kozier, B., Erb, G., Berman, A., & Burke, K. (2000). *Fundamentals of nursing: Concepts, process, and practice* (6th ed.). Upper Saddle River, NJ: Prentice Hall, p. 64.

REFERENCES

Craven, R., & Hirnle, C. (2000). *Fundamentals of nursing: Human health and function* (3rd ed.). Philadelphia: Lippincott.

Harkreader, H. (2000). *Fundamentals of nursing: Caring and clinical judgment.* Philadelphia: W.B. Saunders.

Kozier, B., Erb, G., Berman, A., & Burke, K. (2000). *Fundamentals of nursing: Concepts, process, and practice* (6th ed.). Upper Saddle River, NJ: Prentice Hall.

Leahy, J., & Kizilay, P. (1998). *Foundations of nursing practice: A nursing process approach.* Philadelphia: W.B. Saunders.

Monahan, F. & Neighbors, M. (1998). *Medical-surgical nursing: Foundations for clinical practice* (2nd ed.). Philadelphia: W.B. Saunders.

Leadership and Management Issues

PYRAMID TERMS

authority   Legitimate power or official right to act.

accountability   A moral concept that involves acceptance by the professional nurse of the consequences of a decision or action.

case management   An interdisciplinary health care delivery system designed to promote appropriate use of hospital personnel and material resources to maximize hospital revenues while providing for optimal outcome of care.

change   A dynamic process that leads to an alteration in behavior.

critical paths   Provide effective clinical management systems for monitoring care and for reducing or controlling the length of hospital stay.

delegation   Process of transferring a selected nursing task in a situation to an individual who is competent to perform that specific task.

empowerment   An interpersonal process of enabling others to do for themselves.

leadership   An interpersonal process that involves motivating and guiding others to achieve goals.

management   The accomplishment of tasks either by oneself or by directing others.

power   Ability to do or act that results in the achievement of desired results.

prioritizing   Deciding which needs or problems require immediate action and which ones could be delayed until a later time because they are not urgent.

responsibility   The duty to act.

variances   Actual deviations or detours from the critical paths.

PYRAMID TO SUCCESS

The professional nurse is both a leader and a manager. As described in the NCLEX-RN Test Plan, the professional nurse needs to provide integrated, cost-effective care to clients by coordinating, supervising, and/or collaborating with members of the multidisciplinary health care team. Pyramid points focus on concepts of leadership and management, case management, resource management, the change process, and the process of delegation. The primary Integrated Concepts and Processes addressed in this chapter include Nursing Process, Communication and Documentation, and Self-Care.

CLIENT NEEDS
Safe, Effective Care Environment

Case management
Concepts of management
Cost-effective measures when providing nursing care
Consultation with members of the health care team
Continuous quality improvement
Delegation of client care
Establishing priorities
Identifying professional practice limitations
Resource management
Supervising the delivery of client care
Variance reports

Health Promotion and Maintenance

Client's ability to perform self-care
Disease prevention
Family systems
Health and wellness
Health screening
Health promotion programs

Psychosocial Integrity

Support systems
Therapeutic interactions

Physiological Integrity

Ensuring that palliative or comfort care is provided to the client

Potential for alterations in body systems

Unexpected responses to therapy and variance reports

I. HEALTH CARE DELIVERY SYSTEMS

A. Managed care
1. Designed to control the cost of health services and promote a continuum of care through the development and use of integrated services
2. Emphasizes the promotion of health, client education and responsible self-care, early identification of disease, and the use of health care resources
3. The practice of prospectively paying predetermined amounts of money to selected providers to maintain the health of a defined population
4. To control health care costs, employers limit employee choices to less costly managed programs or encourage employees to elect managed care options
5. Managed care organizations, through contractual agreements, enter into a variety of relationships with providers to meet the needs of members
6. Less costly to provide this type of care than that associated with acute care and hospitalization
7. Physicians receive a specific monetary amount per member per month to provide care irrespective of services rendered, which provides the incentive to keep the client healthy
8. Requires that physicians authorize specialty care and limit use of hospital-based services to promote efficient, cost-effective care and appropriate use of resources

B. Health maintenance organization (HMO)
1. Offers comprehensive coverage for hospital and physician services in exchange for a fixed, prepaid fee
2. Both an insurance company and a health care delivery system

C. **Case management**
1. Represents an interdisciplinary health care delivery system designed to promote appropriate use of hospital personnel and material resources to maximize hospital revenues while providing the optimal amount of care
2. Provides a care process that assists hospitals and health care providers to standardize the appropriate use of resources
3. Manages client care by managing the client care environment

D. **Critical paths**
1. Developed on the basis of appropriate standards of care
2. Provide effective clinical **management** systems for monitoring care and for reducing or controlling the length of hospital stay
3. Developed through the collaborative efforts of physicians, nurses, pharmacists, and other interdisciplinary caregivers, with the goal of improving the quality and outcomes of care
4. The goal of **critical paths** is to anticipate and recognize negative **variance** early so that appropriate action can be taken and better client outcomes can result
5. **Variances**
   a. Actual deviations or detours from the **critical paths**
   b. Positive **variance** occurs when a client achieves maximum benefit and is discharged earlier than anticipated on his or her **critical path**
   c. Negative **variance** occurs when untoward events prevent a timely discharge, and the length of hospital stay is longer than planned for a client on a specific **critical path**
   d. **Variance** analysis occurs continually as the case manager and other caregivers monitor client outcomes against the **critical path**
   e. Accurate monitoring of **critical paths** with **variance** analysis can estimate the financial impact of client care
   f. If the **variance** is predictable, negotiation with insurers for an additional length of hospital stay can maximize client care revenues

E. Levels of prevention
1. Primary prevention: Relates to heath promotion activities and specific protection against disease or illness
2. Secondary prevention: Focuses on the early diagnosis and prompt treatment of disease
3. Tertiary prevention: Represented by rehabilitative services

F. Health care settings
1. Hospital care
2. Home care
3. Hospice care
4. Long-term care
5. Surgical centers
6. Ambulatory care
7. Public health departments

II. FORMAL ORGANIZATIONS

A. Mission statement: Communicates in broad terms an organization's reason for existence, the geographical area the organization serves, and attitudes and beliefs within which the organization functions
B. Goals and objectives: Measurable activities specific to the development of designated services and programs of an organization
C. Organizational chart: Depicts and communicates

how activities are arranged, how **authority** relationships are defined, and how communication channels are established

D. Procedures and protocols
  1. Guides in defining appropriate courses of action
  2. Procedure defines a task
  3. Protocol signifies the definition of a clinical process

E. Centralization: When decisions are made by a limited number of individuals at the top of the organization, or by managers of a department or unit, and thereafter communicated to the employees

F. Decentralization: **Authority** is distributed throughout the organization to allow for increased **responsibility** and **delegation** in decision making

▲ III. NURSING DELIVERY SYSTEMS
A. Functional nursing
  1. Involves a task approach to client care, with major tasks being delegated by the charge nurse to individual members of the team
  2. Goals are concerned with work productivity at the lowest possible cost
  3. Tasks are generally assigned to the lowest-skilled paid workers who are available to do the work

B. Team nursing
  1. The team is generally led by a registered nurse who is responsible for assessing, developing nursing diagnoses, planning, and evaluating each client's plan of care
  2. Each staff member works fully within the realm of his or her educational and clinical expertise
  3. Each staff member is accountable for client care and outcomes of care delivered in accordance with the licensing and practice scope as determined by hospital policy and state law
  4. Characterized by a high degree of respect for and maturity of team members and a high degree of communication and collaboration between members

C. Primary nursing
  1. Focuses on client outcomes as opposed to nursing tasks
  2. Concerned with keeping the nurse at the bedside, actively involved in client care, while planning goal-directed, individualized care

IV. PROFESSIONAL RESPONSIBILITIES
▲ A. **Accountability**
  1. The process that mandates that individuals are answerable for their actions and have an obligation (or duty) to act
  2. Assuming only the responsibilities that are within one's scope of practice
  3. Not assuming **responsibility** for activities in which competence has not been achieved
  4. Involves admitting mistakes rather than blaming others, and evaluating the outcomes of one's own actions
  5. Includes a **responsibility** to the client to be competent, to render nursing services in accordance with standards of nursing practice, and to adhere to the professional ethic code

B. **Leadership** ▲
  1. The interpersonal process that involves motivating and guiding others to achieve goals
  2. A method of modeling accountable behavior to others

C. **Leadership** styles ▲
  1. Autocratic
    a. Leader focused
    b. Leader maintains strong control, makes the decisions, and solves all problems
    c. Leader dominates the group and commands rather than makes suggestions or seeks input
  2. Democratic
    a. Also called participative **leadership**
    b. Based on the belief that every group member should have input into development of goals and problem solving
    c. Leader acts primarily as a facilitator and a resource person
    d. Leader is concerned for each member of the group
    e. More participative and much less authoritarian than the autocratic **leadership** style
  3. Laissez-faire
    a. Leader assumes a passive, nondirective, and inactive approach
    b. **Leadership** responsibilities are either assumed by the members of the group or completely relinquished
    c. All decision making is left to the group, with the leader giving little if any guidance, support, or feedback
    d. Behavior by the group may be permissible as a result of the leader's lack of limit setting and stated expectations
  4. Situational
    a. Utilizing a combination of styles that is based on current circumstances and events
    b. **Leadership** styles are assumed according to the needs of the group and tasks to be achieved

D. **Leadership** qualities ▲
  1. Communication
    a. Listens actively to others
    b. Communicates in an assertive manner, speaks directly and honestly to others
    c. Differentiates between aggressive, passive, and assertive behavior, to communicate appropriately in a given situation (Box 7-1)
  2. Credibility
    a. Enhances a nurse's **accountability**

BOX 7-1

Types of Behavior

AGGRESSIVE BEHAVIOR
Occurs when an individual meets one's own needs regardless of the impact on others

PASSIVE BEHAVIOR
Giving up one's own rights and not having one's own needs met

ASSERTIVE BEHAVIOR
Occurs when an individual seeks to meet one's own needs while respecting the rights of others

---

BOX 7-2

Managerial Functions

Planning	Determining objectives and identifying methods that lead to achievement of those objectives
Organizing	Using resources (human and material) to achieve predetermined outcomes
Directing	Guiding and motivating others to meet the expected outcomes
Controlling	Using performance standards as criteria for measuring success, and taking corrective action
Decision making	Identifying a problem and deciding which alternative(s) can best achieve the objectives

---

    b. Individuals who perform well are those who can influence others
3. Critical thinking
    a. An individual with an open-minded, questioning attitude
    b. The ineffective leader is one who falls into routine ways of thinking without even being aware of what is happening
4. Initiating action
    a. Initiates measures to solve problems
    b. Puts ideas into action and demonstrates flexibility
    c. If an approach is ineffective, the leader is not hesitant to try another approach
5. Risk taking
    a. Involves taking actions to solve problems
    b. Risk-taking activities are goal directed
6. Persuasiveness and Influence
    a. Motivates and inspires others to achieve goals
    b. Understands how to use **power** effectively and does not dominate, but rather motivates others
    c. Persuasiveness can create enthusiasm, encourage collaboration, and increase cohesiveness among team members
▲ E. **Management:** The accomplishment of tasks either by oneself or by directing others
F. Managerial functions (Box 7-2)
G. Types of managers
    1. Front-line manager
        a. Functions in a role that is closely identified with the actual delivery of client care
        b. Roles include charge nurse, team leader, and client care coordinator
        c. Coordinates the activity of all staff who provide client care, and supervises team members
    2. Middle manager
        a. Roles include unit manager or supervisor

    b. Responsibilities include managing staff, preparing budgets, preparing work schedules, writing and implementing policies that guide client care and unit operations, and maintaining the quality of client services
    3. Nurse executive
        a. Top-level nurse manager; may be the director of nursing services or the vice president for client care services
        b. Supervises multiple departments and works closely with the organization's administrative team
        c. Ensures that all client care provided by nurses is carried out in keeping with the objectives of the health care organization

V. POWER
A. Ability to do or act; results in the achievement of desired results
B. Powerful people are able to modify behavior and influence others to **change,** even when others are resistant to **change**
C. Effective nurse leaders use **power** to improve the ▲ delivery of care and to enhance the profession
D. **Power** that is effective is **power** that is shared
E. Types of **power** (Box 7-3)

VI. EMPOWERMENT
A. An interpersonal process of enabling others to so for themselves
B. Occurs when individuals are better able to influence what happens to them
C. Involves open communication, mutual goal setting, and decision making
D. Nurses can **empower** clients through advocacy

VII. THE CHANGE PROCESS ▲
A. A dynamic process that leads to an alteration in behavior

BOX 7-3

Types of Power

Reward	Ability to provide incentives
Coercive	Ability to punish
Referent	Based on attraction
Expert	Based on having an expert knowledge base and skill level
Legitimate	Based on a position in society
Personal	Derives from a high degree of self-confidence
Informational	Occurs when one person provides explanations why another should behave in a certain way

BOX 7-4

Reasons for Resisting Change

CONFORMITY
Going along with others to avoid conflict

DISSIMILAR BELIEFS AND VALUES
Differences that can impede positive change

HABIT
Routine, set behaviors are often hard to change

SECONDARY GAINS
Benefits or payoff are present and so desirable that there is no incentive to change

THREATS TO SATISFY BASIC NEEDS
Change may be perceived as a threat to self-esteem, security, or survival

FEAR
Fear of failure and fear of the unknown

B. Types of **change**
  1. Planned **change:** A deliberate effort to improve a situation
  2. Unplanned **change**
    a. **Change** that just happens
    b. It is unpredictable and may be imposed by others or by uncontrollable natural events
C. Resistance to **change** (Box 7-4)
  1. Resistance occurs when an individual rejects proposed new ideas without critically thinking about the proposal
  2. **Change** requires energy
  3. There is no guarantee that the **change** activity will lead to positive outcomes
D. Overcoming barriers
  1. Create a flexible and adaptable environment

2. **Change** should be planned and goal directed by people
3. Include all involved in the plan for **change**
4. Focus on the benefits of the **change** in relation to improvement of client care
5. Evaluate the process on an ongoing basis, keeping everyone informed of the progress
6. Provide positive feedback to all involved
7. **Change** takes time; therefore commitment is necessary

VIII. DELEGATION AND ASSIGNMENTS ▲
A. Process of transferring a selected nursing task in a situation to an individual who is competent to perform that specific task
B. Delegation is a tool for nurse leaders that encourages team members to develop skills
C. Professional nurses will be delegating tasks to unlicensed assistive personnel (UAP) and to licensed personnel
D. The nurse practice act defines which aspects of care ▲ can be delegated and which must be performed by the registered nurse
E. Even though a task may be delegated to someone, ▲ the nurse who delegates maintains **accountability** for the overall nursing care of the client
F. Only the task, not the ultimate **accountability**, may ▲ be delegated to another
G. Guidelines for client care assignments ▲
  1. Always ensure client safety
  2. Be aware of individual variations in work abilities
  3. Determine which tasks can be delegated and to whom
  4. Match the task to the delegate on the basis of the Nurse Practice Act and appropriate position descriptions
  5. Provide directions that are clear, concise, accurate, and complete
  6. Validate the person's understanding of the directions
  7. Communicate a feeling of confidence to the delegate, and provide feedback promptly after the task is performed
  8. Maintain continuity of care as much as possible when assigning client care

IX. PRIORITIES OF CARE ▲
A. **Prioritizing:** Deciding which needs or problems require immediate action and which ones could be delayed until a later time because they are not urgent
B. Guidelines for **prioritizing**
  1. The nurse and the client mutually rank the client's needs in order of importance on the basis of the client's' desires, needs, and safety
  2. Priorities are classified as high, intermediate, or low
    a. Client needs that are life threatening or that

could result in harm to the client if they are left untreated are high priorities
   b. Non-emergency and non-life-threatening client needs are intermediate priorities
   c. Client needs that are not directly related to the client's illness or prognosis are low priorities
3. When providing care, the nurse needs to decide which needs or problems require immediate action and which ones could be delayed until a later time because they are not urgent
4. Client problems that involve actual or life-threatening concerns are considered prior to potential health-threatening concerns
5. When **prioritizing** care, the nurse must consider time constraints and available resources
6. Problems identified as important by the client must be given high priority
7. Priority setting may be guided by principles, models, and/or theories, such as Maslow's Hierarchy of Needs
8. Maslow's Hierarchy of Needs identifies the levels of physiological needs, safety, love and belonging, self-esteem, and self-actualization; basic needs are met before moving to other needs in the hierarchy
9. Use the ABCs: airway, breathing, and circulation; client needs related to maintaining a patent airway are always the priority

X. TIME MANAGEMENT
A. Description
   1. A technique designed to assist in completing tasks within a definite time period
   2. Involves efficiency in completing tasks as quickly as possible, and effectiveness in deciding on the most important task to do, and doing it correctly
B. Guidelines
   1. Identify tasks, obligations, and activities, and write them down
   2. Organize the workday; identify which tasks must be completed in specified time frames
   3. Prioritize client needs according to importance
   4. Anticipate the needs of the day, and provide time for unexpected and unplanned tasks that may arise
   5. Focus on beginning the daily tasks working on the most important first, while keeping goals in mind; look at the final goal for the day, which will help to break down tasks into manageable parts
   6. Begin client rounds at the beginning of the shift, collecting data on each assigned client
   7. Delegate tasks when appropriate
   8. Keep a daily hour-by-hour log to assist in providing structure to the tasks that must be accomplished, and cross tasks off the list as they are accomplished

9. Use hospital resources wisely, anticipating resource needs and gathering the necessary supplies before beginning the task
10. Organize paperwork, and continuously document task completion and necessary client data throughout the day
11. At the end of the day, evaluate the effectiveness of time management

PRACTICE QUESTIONS

1. A nurse is reviewing the critical paths of the clients on the nursing unit. In a variance analysis, which of the following would indicate the need for further action and analysis?
   1. A client's family attending a diabetic teaching session
   2. Canceling physical therapy sessions on the weekend
   3. Normal vital signs and absence of wound infection in a postoperative client
   4. A client demonstrating accurate medication administration after teaching

2. A new nursing graduate is attending an agency orientation regarding the nursing model of practice implemented in the facility. The nurse is told that the nursing model is a team nursing approach. The nurse understands that planning of care delivery will be based on which characteristic of this type of nursing model of practice?
   1. A task approach method is used to provide care to clients
   2. A single registered nurse (RN) is responsible for providing nursing care to a group of clients
   3. Managed care concepts and tools are used in providing client care
   4. Nursing personnel are led by an RN leader in providing care to a group of clients

3. A nurse manager has implemented a change in the method of the nursing delivery system from functional to team nursing. A nursing assistant is resistant to the change and is not taking an active part in facilitating the process of change. Which of the following would be the best approach in dealing with the nursing assistant?
   1. Ignore the resistance
   2. Exert coercion with the nursing assistant
   3. Provide a positive reward system for the nursing assistant
   4. Confront the nursing assistant to encourage verbalization of feelings regarding the change

4. A registered nurse (RN) is planning the client assignments for the day. Which of the following is the most appropriate assignment for a nursing assistant?
   1. A client with difficulty swallowing food and fluids

2. A client who requires tap water enemas
3. A client requiring a colostomy irrigation
4. A client receiving continuous tube feedings

5. A registered nurse (RN) employed in a long-term care facility is planning assignments for the clients on a nursing unit. The RN needs to assign four clients and has a licensed practical (vocational) nurse and three nursing assistants on a nursing team. Which of the following clients would the nurse most appropriately assign to the licensed practical (vocational) nurse?
   1. A client who requires a 24-hour urine collection
   2. An elderly client requiring assistance with a bed bath and frequent ambulation
   3. A client who requires a Fleet and an oil retention enema
   4. A client with an abdominal wound that requires irrigations and dressing changes every 3 hours

6. A registered nurse (RN) has received the assignment for the day shift. After making initial rounds and checking all of the assigned clients, which client will the RN plan to care for first?
   1. A client who is ambulatory
   2. A client who has a fever and who is diaphoretic and restless
   3. A client scheduled for physical therapy at 1:00 pm
   4. A postoperative client who has just received pain medication

7. A nurse is assigned to care for four clients. In planning client rounds, which client would the nurse assess first?
   1. A client receiving oxygen via nasal cannula who had difficulty breathing during the previous shift
   2. A postoperative client preparing for discharge
   3. A client scheduled for a chest x-ray
   4. A client requiring daily dressing changes

8. A nurse is giving a bed bath to an assigned client. A nursing assistant enters the client's room and tells the nurse that another assigned client is in pain and needs pain medication. The most appropriate nursing action is which of the following?
   1. Finish the bed bath and then administer the pain medication to the other client
   2. Cover the client, raise the side rails, tell the client that you will return shortly, and administer the pain medication to the other client
   3. Ask the nursing assistant to tell the client in pain that medication will be administered as soon as the bed bath is complete
   4. Ask the nursing assistant to find out when the last pain medication was given to the client

9. A home health care nurse is planning client visits for the day. The nurse is assigned to admit a client who was discharged yesterday from the hospital following a diagnosis of pneumonia. The nurse is also scheduled to visit a client requiring bid ab-dominal dressing changes. The third client to be seen is a client whose spouse is performing daily dressing changes, and the nurse needs to supervise the spouse in performing the dressing change. The fourth client to be seen will be visited by a home health aide (HHA) at 10:00 am, and the nurse needs to orient the aide and provide supervision of client care. The nurse begins the visits at 9:00 am. All clients live within a 5-mile radius. How would the nurse plan the order of the assignments for the day?
   1. The client being visited by the HHA, the client requiring admission, the client regarding supervision of the dressing change, the client requiring bid dressing changes, the client requiring the second bid dressing change
   2. The client requiring admission, the client regarding supervision of the dressing change, the client requiring bid dressing changes, the client being visited by the HHA, the client requiring the second bid dressing change
   3. The client being visited by the HHA, the client requiring bid dressing changes, the client requiring admission, the client regarding supervision of the dressing change, the client requiring the second bid dressing change
   4. The client requiring bid dressing changes, the client being visited by the HHA, the client regarding supervision of the dressing change, the client requiring admission, the client requiring the second bid dressing change

10. A case manager is reviewing the records of the clients in the nursing unit. Which of the following documentations if noted in a client's record would the nurse indicate as a positive variance?
    1. A postoperative client is discharged to home one day earlier than expected
    2. A client is performing colostomy irrigations
    3. A diabetic client is administering insulin injections appropriately
    4. A client with a leg ulcer is demonstrating signs of wound healing

CRITICAL THINKING: FREE-TEXT ENTRY

A nurse on the day shift is assigned to care for three clients. One client has a tracheostomy and is on a mechanical ventilator. Another client is scheduled for a cardiac catheterization at 10:00 AM, and the other client was newly diagnosed with diabetes mellitus and is scheduled for discharge to home. Following report from the night shift, which client will the nurse plan to assess first?

Answer: _____

ANSWERS

1. 2

Rationale: Variances are actual deviations or detours from the critical paths. Variances can be either positive or negative, avoidable or unavoidable, and can be caused by a variety of things. Positive variance occurs when the client achieves maximum benefit and is discharged earlier than anticipated. Negative variance occurs when untoward events prevent a timely discharge. Variance analysis occurs continually in order to anticipate and recognize negative variance early so that appropriate action can be taken.

Test-Taking Strategy: Use the process of elimination, noting the key words "indicate the need for further action and analysis." Options 1, 3, and 4 identify positive outcomes. Option 2 identifies a negative outcome. Review the purpose of variance analysis if you had difficulty with this question.

Level of Cognitive Ability: Analysis
Client Needs: Safe, Effective Care Environment
Integrated Concept/Process: Nursing Process/Evaluation
Content Area: Fundamental Skills
Reference: Rocchiccioli, J., & Tilbury, M. (1998). *Clinical leadership in nursing.* Philadelphia: W.B. Saunders, p. 42.

2. 4

Rationale: In team nursing, nursing personnel are led by an RN leader in providing care to a group of clients. Option 1 identifies functional nursing. Option 2 identifies primary nursing. Option 3 identifies a component of case management.

Test-Taking Strategy: Note that the issue of the question relates to team nursing. Keep this issue in mind, and use the process of elimination. Option 4 is the only option that identifies the concept of a team approach. Review the various types of nursing delivery systems if you had difficulty with this question.

Level of Cognitive Ability: Analysis
Client Needs: Safe, Effective Care Environment
Integrated Concept/Process: Nursing Process/Planning
Content Area: Fundamental Skills
Reference: Kozier, B., Erb, G., Berman, A., & Burke, K. (2000). *Fundamentals of nursing: Concepts, process, and practice* (6th ed.). Upper Saddle River, NJ: Prentice Hall, p. 102.

3. 4

Rationale: Confrontation is an important strategy to meet resistance head-on. Face-to-face meetings to confront the issue at hand will allow verbalization of feelings, identification of problems and issues, and development of strategies to solve the problem. Option 1 will not address the problem. Option 2 may produce additional resistance. Option 3 may provide a temporary solution to the resistance but will not specifically address the concern.

Test-Taking Strategy: Use the process of elimination. Options 1 and 2 can be easily eliminated first. From the remaining options, select option 4 over option 3 because this option specifically addresses the issue and would provide problem-solving measures. If you had difficulty with this question, review the strategies associated with dealing with resistance to change.

Level of Cognitive Ability: Comprehension
Client Needs: Safe, Effective Care Environment
Integrated Concept/Process: Communication and Documentation

Content Area: Fundamental Skills
Reference: Harkreader, H. (2000). *Fundamentals of nursing: Caring and clinical judgment.* Philadelphia: W.B. Saunders, p. 357.

4. 2

Rationale: The nurse must determine the most appropriate assignment on the basis of the skills of the staff member and the needs of the client. In this case, the most appropriate assignment for a nursing assistant would be to care for the client who requires tap water enemas. The nursing assistant is skilled in administering tap water enemas. The client with difficulty swallowing food and fluids is at risk for aspiration. Colostomy irrigations and tube feedings are not performed by unlicensed personnel.

Test-Taking Strategy: Note the key words "most appropriate." Use the process of elimination, recalling the principles of delegation and supervision of the work of others. Remember that work that is delegated to others must be consistent with the individual's level of expertise and licensure or lack of licensure. Review the principles of delegation if you had difficulty with this question.

Level of Cognitive Ability: Application
Client Needs: Safe, Effective Care Environment
Integrated Concept/Process: Nursing Process/Planning
Content Area: Fundamental Skills
Reference: Yoder-Wise, P. (1999). *Leading and managing in nursing* (2nd ed.). St. Louis: Mosby, pp. 310-311.

5. 4

Rationale: When delegating nursing assignments, the nurse needs to consider the skills and educational levels of the nursing staff. Collecting a 24-hour urine, giving a bed bath and assisting with frequent ambulation, and administering enemas can most appropriately be provided by the nursing assistant. The licensed practical nurse (vocational nurse) is skilled in wound irrigations and dressing changes, and this client would most appropriately be assigned to this staff member.

Test-Taking Strategy: Use the process of elimination and knowledge regarding the principles related to delegation and assignment making. Recall that education and job position as described by the nurse practice act and employee guidelines need to be considered in delegating activities and making assignments. Options 1, 2, and 3 can be easily eliminated because a nursing assistant can perform these tasks. If you had difficulty with this question, review the principles related to delegation and assignment making.

Level of Cognitive Ability: Application
Client Needs: Safe, Effective Care Environment
Integrated Concept/Process: Nursing Process/Planning
Content Area: Fundamental Skills
Reference: Rocchiccioli, J., & Tilbury, M. (1998). *Clinical leadership in nursing.* Philadelphia: W.B. Saunders, p. 140.

6. 2

Rationale: The RN would plan to care for the client who has a fever and is diaphoretic and restless first because this client's needs are the priority. It is best to wait for pain medication to take effect before providing care to the postoperative client. The client who is ambulatory and the client scheduled for physical therapy later in the day do not have priority needs related to care.

Test-Taking Strategy: Use the process of elimination and

principles related to prioritizing. Noting the key words "diaphoretic" and "restless" will assist in directing you to this option. Review the principles related to prioritizing if you had difficulty with this question.
Level of Cognitive Ability: Application
Client Needs: Safe, Effective Care Environment
Integrated Concept/Process: Nursing Process/Planning
Content Area: Fundamental Skills
Reference: Harkreader, H. (2000). *Fundamentals of nursing: Caring and clinical judgment.* Philadelphia: W.B. Saunders, p. 242.

7. **1**

Rationale: The airway is always a high priority and the nurse would attend first to the client who has been experiencing an airway problem. The clients described in options 2, 3, and 4 have needs that would be identified as intermediate priorities.
Test-Taking Strategy: Use Maslow's Hierarchy of Needs theory and the ABCs—airway, breathing, and circulation—to answer the question. Remember that airway is always the first priority. Review principles related to prioritizing if you had difficulty with this question.
Level of Cognitive Ability: Application
Client Needs: Safe, Effective Care Environment
Integrated Concept/Process: Nursing Process/Planning
Content Area: Fundamental Skills
Reference: Harkreader, H. (2000). *Fundamentals of nursing: Caring and clinical judgment* Philadelphia: W.B. Saunders, p. 242.

8. **2**

Rationale: The nurse is responsible for the care provided to the assigned clients. The most appropriate action is to provide safety to the client who is receiving the bed bath and prepare to administer the pain medication. Options 1 and 3 delay the administration of medication to the client in pain. Option 4 is not a responsibility of the nursing assistant.
Test-Taking Strategy: Use the process of elimination and principles related to priorities of care. Options 1 and 3 delay the administration of pain medication, and option 4 is not a responsibility of the nursing assistant. The most appropriate action is to plan to administer the medication. Review principles related to priorities of care if you had difficulty with this question.
Level of Cognitive Ability: Application
Client Needs: Safe, Effective Care Environment
Integrated Concept/Process: Nursing Process/Implementation
Content Area: Fundamental Skills
Reference: Leahy, J., & Kizilay, P. (1998). *Foundations of nursing practice: A nursing process approach.* Philadelphia: W.B. Saunders, p. 168.

9. **4**

Rationale: The nurse would plan to see the client requiring bid dressing changes first, since the dressing changes should be spaced as far apart as possible. The nurse would next plan to see the client being visited by the HHA and provide instructions and directions to the HHA regarding care to the client. The nurse would then visit the client regarding supervision of the dressing change, and would perform the admission last since that may take more time than the other

clients. The nurse would then return to the client regarding the second BID dressing.
Test-Taking Strategy: Use the process of elimination, noting the needs of the client and the role of the nurse in caring for each of the clients. Noting that the client requiring bid dressing changes will need to be seen twice will assist in directing you to the correct option. This client should be seen first, since dressing changes should be spaced as far apart as possible. If you had difficulty with this question, review the process of planning care and time management.
Level of Cognitive Ability: Application
Client Needs: Safe, Effective Care Environment
Integrated Concept/Process: Nursing Process/Planning
Content Area: Fundamental Skills
Reference: Rocchiccioli, J., & Tilbury, M. (1998). *Clinical leadership in nursing.* Philadelphia: W.B. Saunders, p. 116.

10. **1**

Rationale: Variances are actual deviations or detours from the critical path. Variances are either positive or negative, avoidable or unavoidable, and may be caused by a variety of things. A positive variance occurs when the client achieved maximum benefits and is discharged earlier than anticipated on his or her critical path. Option 1 is the only option that identifies a positive variance. Options 2, 3, and 4 demonstrate progression on a critical path, but they are not specifically associated with the definition of a positive variance.
Test-Taking Strategy: Use the process of elimination. Note the key word "positive" in the question. This should assist in directing you to selecting the option that identifies the highest level of achievement. If you had difficulty with this question, review variances and critical paths.
Level of Cognitive Ability: Analysis
Client Needs: Safe, Effective Care Environment
Integrated Concept/Process: Communication and Documentation
Content Area: Fundamental Skills
Reference: Rocchiccioli, J., & Tilbury, M. (1998). *Clinical leadership in nursing.* Philadelphia: W.B. Saunders, p. 42.

CRITICAL THINKING: FREE-TEXT ENTRY

Answer: The client that has a tracheostomy and is on a mechanical ventilator
Rationale: Airway is always a high priority and the nurse would assess the client who has a tracheostomy and is on a mechanical ventilator first. The nurse would next assess the client scheduled for the cardiac catheterization followed by the client scheduled for discharge.
Test-Taking Strategy: Use Maslow's Hierarchy of Needs theory and the ABCs—airway, breathing, and circulation. Focus only on the data identified in the question. Remember that airway is always the first priority. Review principles related to prioritizing if you had difficulty with this question.
Level of Cognitive Ability: Application
Client Needs: Safe, Effective Care Environment
Integrated Concept/Process: Nursing Process/Planning
Content Area: Fundamental Skills
Reference: Harkreader, H. (2000). *Fundamentals of nursing: Caring and clinical judgment.* Philadelphia: W.B. Saunders, p. 242.

REFERENCES

Harkreader, H. (2000). *Fundamentals of nursing: Caring and clinical judgment.* Philadelphia: W.B. Saunders.

Kozier, B., Erb, G., Berman, A., & Burke, K. (2000). *Fundamentals of nursing: Concepts, process, and practice* (6th ed.). Upper Saddle River, NJ: Prentice Hall.

Leahy, J. & Kizilay, P. (1998). *Foundations of nursing practice: A nursing process approach.* Philadelphia: W.B. Saunders.

Monahan, F., & Neighbors, M. (1998). *Medical-surgical nursing: Foundations for clinical practice* (2nd ed.). Philadelphia: W.B. Saunders.

Rocchiccioli, J., & Tilbury, M. (1998). *Clinical leadership in nursing.* Philadelphia: W.B. Saunders.

Yoder-Wise, P. (1999). *Leading and managing in nursing* (2nd ed.). St. Louis: Mosby.

UNIT III
Nursing Sciences

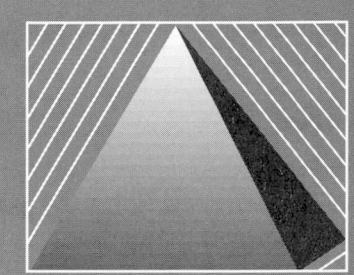

8

Fluids and Electrolytes

PYRAMID TERMS

fluid volume deficit   Dehydration in which the body's fluid intake is not sufficient to meet the body's fluid needs.

fluid volume excess   Fluid intake or fluid retention exceeds the body's fluid needs. Also called overhydration or fluid overload.

homeostasis   The tendency of biological systems to maintain relatively constant conditions in the internal environment while continuously interacting with and adjusting to changes originating within or outside the system.

hypercalcemia   A serum calcium level that exceeds 10 mg/dL

hypocalcemia   A serum calcium level below 8.6 mg/dL

hyperkalemia   A serum potassium level that exceeds 5.1 mEq/L

hypokalemia   A serum potassium level below 3.5 mEq/L

hypermagnesemia   A serum magnesium level that exceeds 2.6 mg/dL.

hypomagnesemia   A serum magnesium level below 1.6 mg/dL.

hypernatremia   A serum sodium level that exceeds 145 mEq/L

hyponatremia   A serum sodium level below 135 mEq/L

hyperphosphatemia   A serum phosphorus level that exceeds 4.5 mg/dL

hypophosphatemia   A serum phosphorus level below 2.7 mg/dL

▲ PYRAMID TO SUCCESS

Pyramid points focus primarily on the assessment of a fluid and electrolyte imbalance, implementation, and evaluating the expected outcomes. Fluids and electrolytes constitute a content area that is sometimes complex and difficult to understand. It is important to understand cell functions and properties and the concepts related to body fluids as outlined in this chapter. Review this content. Pyramid points focus on the common fluid and electrolyte disturbances. As you review this content, focus on the pyramid points related to the causes, assessment findings, and related treatments. In any fluid or electrolyte imbalance, nursing interventions include monitoring the significant laboratory results and monitoring the client's cardiovascular, respiratory, gastrointestinal (GI), neuromuscular, renal, and central nervous system status. The primary Integrated Concepts and Processes addressed in this chapter are Nursing Process, Communication and Documentation, Self-Care, and Teaching/Learning.

CLIENT NEEDS   ▲
Safe, Effective Care Environment

Accident prevention and protection and safety of the client when an imbalance exists, particularly when changes in cardiovascular, respiratory, gastrointestinal (GI), neuromuscular, renal, or central nervous system (CNS) occur, or when the client is at risk for complications such as seizures, respiratory depression, or dysrhythmias

Consultation with members of the health care team

Establishing priorities

Handling hazardous and infectious materials to prevent injury to health care personnel and others

Medical and surgical asepsis and preventing infection in the client when samples for laboratory studies are obtained or when IVs are administered

Standard (universal) precautions to prevent transmission of infection to self and others

Health Promotion and Maintenance

Education related to medication and diet management

Education related to the potential risk for a fluid and electrolyte balance, measures to prevent an imbalance, signs and symptoms of an imbalance, and actions to take if signs and symptoms develop

Health screening and the potential risk for a fluid and electrolyte imbalance

Psychosocial Integrity

Provide support and continuously inform the client of the purposes for prescribed interventions

Reassure the client who is experiencing symptoms related to a fluid and electrolyte imbalance

Physiological Integrity

Assist in managing emergencies

Identify clients who are at risk for a fluid or electrolyte imbalance

Identify the expected and unexpected responses to therapeutic interventions and document accordingly

Monitor for complications related to the imbalance

Monitor laboratory values

▲

I. CONCEPTS OF FLUID AND ELECTROLYTE BALANCE

A. Electrolytes
1. Description: When a substance is dissolved in solution and some of its molecules split or dissociate into electrically charged atoms or ions (Box 8-1)
2. Measurement
   a. To measure volumes of fluids, the metric system is used: liters (L) or milliliters (mL)
   b. The unit of measure that expresses the combining activity of an electrolyte is the milliequivalent (mEq)
   c. One milliequivalent of any cation will always react chemically with one milliequivalent of an anion
   d. Milliequivalents provide information about the number of anions or cations available to combine with other anions or cations
B. Body fluid compartments
1. Description
   a. Fluid in each of the body compartments contains electrolytes
   b. Each compartment has a particular composition of electrolytes, which differs from that of other compartments
   c. To function normally, body cells must have fluids and electrolytes in the right compartments and in the right amounts
   d. Whenever an electrolyte moves out of a cell, another electrolyte moves in to take its place
   e. The numbers of cations and anions must be the same for **homeostasis** to exist
   f. Compartments are separated by semipermeable membranes
2. Intracellular compartment
   a. Refers to all fluid inside the cells
   b. Most of the body fluids are inside the cells
3. Extracellular compartment: Fluid outside the cells

BOX 8-1

Cell Properties

ATOM

The smallest part of an element that still has the properties of the element.

Composed of particles known as the proton (positive charge), neutron (neutral), and electron (negative charge).

Protons and neutrons are in the nucleus of the atom; therefore, the nucleus is positively charged.

Electrons carry a negative charge and revolve around the nucleus.

As long as the number of electrons is the same as the number of protons, there is no net charge on the atom; that is, it is neither positive or negative.

Atoms may gain, lose, or share electrons and then no longer are neutral.

MOLECULE

Two or more atoms that combine to form a substance.

ION

An atom that carries an electrical charge because it has either gained or lost electrons.

Some ions carry a negative electrical charge, and some carry a positive charge.

CATION

An ion that carries a positive charge and has given away or lost electrons.

The result is fewer electrons than protons, and the result is a positive charge.

ANION

An ion that has gained electrons and therefore carries a negative charge.

When an ion has gained or taken on electrons, it assumes a negative charge and the result is a negatively charged ion.

---

4. Intravascular compartment: Fluid that is within blood vessels
5. Interstitial fluids: Fluid between the cells and blood vessels
C. Third-spacing
1. The accumulation and sequestration of trapped extracellular fluid in an actual or potential body space as a result of disease or injury
2. The trapped fluid represents a volume loss and is unavailable for normal physiological processes
3. Fluid may be trapped in body spaces such as the pericardial, pleural, peritoneal, or joint cavities; the bowel; or the abdomen; or within soft tissues after trauma or burns
4. Assessing the intravascular fluid loss is difficult; it may not be reflected in weight changes or intake

and output (I&O) records, and may not become apparent until after organ malfunction occurs

D. Edema
  1. An excess accumulation of fluid in the interstitial spaces
  2. Localized edema occurs as a result of traumatic injury from accidents or surgery, local inflammatory processes, or burns
  3. Generalized edema, also called anasarca, is an excessive accumulation of fluid in the interstitial space throughout the body as a result of a condition such as cardiac, renal, or liver failure

E. Body fluid
  1. Description
    a. Provides transportation of nutrients to the cells and carries waste products from the cells
    b. Total body fluid amounts to about 60% of body weight
    c. A loss of 10% of body fluid in the adult is serious
    d. A loss of 20% of the body fluid in the adult is fatal
  2. Constituents of body fluids
    a. Body fluids consist of water and dissolved substances
    b. The largest single fluid constituent of the body is water
    c. Some substances, such as glucose, urea, and creatinine, do not dissociate in solution; that is, they do not separate from their complex forms into simpler substances when they are in solutions
    d. Other substances do dissociate; for example, when sodium chloride (NaCl) is in a solution, it dissociates or separates into two parts or elements

F. Body fluid transport
  1. Diffusion
    a. The movement of particles in all directions through a solution
    b. The process by which a solute (substance that is dissolved) may spread through a solution or solvent (solution in which the solute is dissolved)
    c. Diffusion of a solute will spread the molecules from an area of high concentration to an area of lower concentration
    d. A permeable membrane will allow substances to pass through it without restriction
    e. A selectively permeable membrane will allow some solutes to pass through without restriction but will prevent other solutes from passing freely
    f. Diffusion occurs within fluid compartments and from one compartment to another, if the barrier between the compartments is permeable to the diffusing substances

  2. Osmosis
    a. Osmotic pressure is the force that draws the water from a less concentrated solution through a selectively permeable membrane into a more concentrated solution
    b. If a membrane is permeable to water but not to all the solutes present, it is a selective or semipermeable membrane
    c. When the solvent or water moves across the membrane, the process is called osmosis
    d. Osmosis is the diffusion of solvent molecules across a membrane in response to a concentration gradient, usually from a solution of lesser to one of greater solute concentration
    e. When there is a more concentrated solution on one side of a selectively permeable membrane and a less concentrated solution on the other side, a pull called osmotic pressure draws the water through the membrane to the more concentrated side or the side with more solute
  3. Filtration
    a. Filtration is the movement of solutes and solvents by hydrostatic pressure
    b. The movement is from an area of greater pressure to an area of lesser pressure
  4. Hydrostatic pressure
    a. The force exerted by the weight of a solution
    b. When there is a difference in the hydrostatic pressure on two sides of a membrane, water and diffusible solutes move out of the solution that has the higher hydrostatic pressure by the process of filtration
    c. At the arterial end of the capillary, the hydrostatic pressure is greater than the osmotic pressure; therefore, fluids and diffusible solutes move out of the capillary
    d. At the venous end, the osmotic pressure or pull is greater than the hydrostatic pressure, and fluids and some solutes move into the capillary
    e. The excess fluid and solutes remaining in the interstitial spaces are returned to the intravascular compartment by the lymph channels
  5. Osmolality
    a. Refers to the number of osmotically active particles per kilogram of water
    b. In the body, osmotic pressure is measured in milliosmols
    c. The normal osmolality of plasma is 280 to 294 mOsm/kg

G. Movement of body fluid
  1. Description
    a. Cell membranes separate the interstitial fluid from the intravascular fluid
    b. Cell membranes are selectively permeable; that is, the cell membrane and the capillary

wall will allow water and some solutes free passage through them

c. Several forces affect the movement of water and solutes through the walls of cells and capillaries

d. The greater the number of particles in the concentrated solution, the more pull there will be to move the water through the membrane

e. If the body loses more electrolytes than fluids, as can happen in diarrhea, then the extracellular fluid will contain fewer electrolytes or less solute than the intracellular fluid (ICF)

f. Fluids and electrolytes must be kept in balance for health; when they remain out of balance, death can occur

2. Isotonic solutions (Table 8-1)

a. When the solutions on both sides of a selectively permeable membrane have established equilibrium or are equal in concentration, they are then isotonic

b. An example of an isotonic solution is 0.9% sodium chloride, which is referred to as isotonic saline solution or normal saline solution

c. Isotonic solutions are isotonic to human cells, and thus there will be very little osmosis

d. Other solutions that are isotonic are 5% dextrose in water, 5% dextrose in 0.225% saline, and lactated Ringer's solution

3. Hypotonic solutions (Table 8-1)

a. When a solution contains a lower concentration of salt or solute than other solutions, it is hypotonic

b. A hypotonic solution has less salt or more water than an isotonic solution

c. 0.45% normal saline and distilled water are examples of hypotonic solutions

d. Hypotonic solutions are hypotonic to the cells; therefore, osmosis would continue in an attempt to bring about balance or equality

4. Hypertonic solutions (Table 8-1)

a. A solution that has a higher concentration of solutes than another solution is a hypertonic solution

b. Hypertonic solutions include 10% dextrose in water, 5% dextrose in 0.9% saline, 5% dextrose in 0.45% saline, and 5% dextrose in lactated Ringer's solution

5. Osmotic pressure

a. The force that draws the solvent from a solution with more solvent activity through a selectively permeable membrane to a solution with less solvent activity

b. The amount of osmotic pressure is determined by the relative number of particles of solute on the side of greater concentration

TABLE 8-1

Tonicity of Intravenous Fluids

Solution	Tonicity
0.45% saline (½ NS)	Hypotonic
0.9% saline (NS)	Isotonic
5% dextrose in water (5% D/W)	Isotonic
5% dextrose in 0.225% saline (5% D/¼ NS)	Isotonic
Lactated Ringer's solution	Isotonic
5% dextrose in lactated Ringer's solution	Hypertonic
5% dextrose in 0.45% saline (5% D/½ NS)	Hypertonic
5% dextrose in 0.9% saline (5% D/NS)	Hypertonic
10% dextrose in water (10% D/W)	Hypertonic

c. When the solutions on each side of a selectively permeable membrane are equal in concentration, they are isotonic

d. A hypotonic solution has less solute than an isotonic solution, whereas a hypertonic solution contains more solute

e. If the selectively permeable membrane will allow the solvent to pass through but will not allow the solute through freely, the solvent will move to the side of greater solute concentration

6. Active transport

a. If an ion is to move through a membrane from an area of low concentration to an area of high concentration, an active transport system is necessary

b. An active transport system moves molecules or ions uphill against concentration and osmotic pressure

c. Metabolic processes in the cell supply the energy for active transport

d. Substances that are actively transported through the cell membrane include ions of sodium, potassium, calcium, iron, and hydrogen, some of the sugars, and the amino acids

H. Body fluid excretion (Box 8-2)

1. Description

a. Fluids leave the body by several routes, including the skin, lungs, GI tract, and kidneys

b. The kidneys excrete the largest quantity of fluid

c. As long as all organs are functioning normally, the body is able to maintain balance in its fluid content

2. Skin

a. Water is lost through the skin by diffusion in the amount of 300 to 400 mL per day and by perspiration

---

BOX 8-2

Daily Body Fluid Excretion

Skin by diffusion = 350 mL
Skin by perspiration = 100 mL
Lungs = 350 mL
Feces = 200 mL
Kidneys = 1400 mL

---

b. The amount of water lost by perspiration will vary according to the temperature of the environment and of the body, but the average amount of loss is 100 mL per day

c. Water lost through the skin by diffusion is called insensible loss (individual is unaware of losing that water)

3. Lungs

a. Water is lost from the lungs through expired air that is saturated with water vapor

b. The amount of water lost from the lungs will vary with the rate and the depth of respiration

c. The average amount of water lost from the lungs is 300 to 400 mL per day

d. Water lost from the lungs is called insensible loss

4. GI tract

a. Large quantities of water are secreted into the GI tract, but almost all of this fluid is reabsorbed

b. A very large volume of electrolyte-containing liquids moves into the GI tract and then returns again into the extracellular fluid (ECF)

c. The average amount of water lost in the feces is 200 mL per day, equal to the amount of water gained through the oxidation of foods

d. Severe diarrhea will result in the loss of large quantities of fluids and electrolytes

5. Kidneys

a. Play a major role in regulating fluid and electrolyte balance

b. Normal kidneys can adjust the amount of water and electrolytes leaving the body

c. The quantity of fluid excreted by the kidneys is determined by the amount of water ingested and the amount of waste and solutes excreted

d. The usual urine output is approximately 1400 mL per day; however, this will vary greatly depending on fluid intake, amount of perspiration, and other factors

I. Body fluid replacement

1. Description: Water enters the body through three sources: oral liquids, water in foods, and water formed by oxidation of foods

2. Amounts

a. The average total amount of water taken into the body by all three sources is 2400 mL per day

b. About 10 mL of water is released by the metabolism of each 100 calories of fat, carbohydrates, or proteins

3. Electrolytes

a. Electrolytes are present in both foods and liquids

b. With a normal diet, an excess of essential electrolytes is taken in and the unused electrolytes are excreted

J. Maintaining fluid and electrolyte balance

1. Description

a. **Homeostasis** is a term that indicates the relative stability of the internal environment

b. Concentration and composition of body fluids must be nearly constant

c. In the client, when one of the substances, either fluids or electrolytes, is deficient, it must be replaced either normally by the intake of food and water or by therapy such as IVs and/or medications

d. When the client has an excess of fluid or electrolytes, therapy is directed toward assisting the body to eliminate the excess

2. Kidneys: Play a major role in controlling all types of balance in fluid and electrolytes

3. Adrenal glands: Through the secretion of aldosterone, the adrenal glands also aid in controlling extracellular fluid volume by regulating the amount of sodium reabsorbed by the kidneys

4. Antidiuretic hormone (ADH): ADH from the pituitary gland regulates the osmotic pressure of extracellular fluid by regulating the amount of water reabsorbed by the kidney

II. FLUID VOLUME DEFICIT

A. Description

1. Dehydration in which the body's fluid intake is not sufficient to meet the body's fluid needs

2. The goal of treatment is to restore fluid volume, replace electrolytes as needed, and eliminate the cause of the **fluid volume deficit**

B. Types

1. Isotonic dehydration

a. Water and dissolved electrolytes are lost in equal proportions

b. Known as hypovolemia and is the most common type of dehydration

c. Results in decreased circulating blood volume and inadequate tissue perfusion

2. Hypertonic dehydration

a. Water loss exceeds electrolyte loss

b. The clinical problems that occur result from alterations in the concentrations of specific plasma electrolytes

c. Fluid moves from the intracellular compartment into the plasma and interstitial fluid spaces, causing cellular dehydration and shrinkage

3. Hypotonic dehydration
   a. Electrolyte loss exceeds water loss
   b. The clinical problems that occur result from fluid shifts between compartments, causing a decrease in plasma volume
   c. Fluid moves from the plasma and interstitial fluid spaces into the cells, causing a plasma volume deficit and causing the cells to swell

▲ C. Causes
   1. Isotonic dehydration
      a. Inadequate intake of fluids and solutes
      b. Fluid shifts between compartments
      c. Excessive losses of isotonic body fluids
   2. Hypertonic dehydration: Conditions that increase fluid loss, such as excessive perspiration, hyperventilation, ketoacidosis, prolonged fevers, diarrhea, early-stage renal failure, and diabetes insipidus
   3. Hypotonic dehydration
      a. Chronic illness
      b. Excessive fluid replacement (hypotonic)
      c. Renal failure
      d. Chronic malnutrition

▲ D. Assessment
   1. Cardiovascular
      a. Thready, increased pulse rate
      b. Decreased blood pressure and postural hypotension
      c. Flat neck and hand veins in dependent positions
      d. Diminished peripheral pulses
   2. Respiratory: Increased rate and depth of respirations
   3. Neuromuscular
      a. Decreased central nervous system activity, from lethargy to coma
      b. Fever
   4. Renal
      a. Decreased urinary output
      b. Increased specific gravity
   5. Integumentary
      a. Dry and scaly skin
      b. Poor turgor, tenting present
      c. Dry and fissured mouth, paste-like coating present
   6. GI
      a. Decreased motility and diminished bowel sounds
      b. Constipation
      c. Thirst
   7. Hypotonic dehydration: Skeletal muscle weakness
   8. Hypertonic dehydration
      a. Hyperactive deep tendon reflexes

   b. Increased sensation of thirst
   c. Pitting edema

E. Implementation
   1. Monitor cardiovascular, respiratory, neuromuscular, renal, integumentary, and GI status
   2. Prevent further fluid losses and increase fluid compartment volumes to normal ranges
   3. Provide oral rehydration therapy if possible; IV fluid replacement if the dehydration is severe
   4. Generally, isotonic dehydration is treated with isotonic fluid solutions; hypertonic dehydration with hypotonic fluid solutions; and hypotonic dehydration with hypertonic fluid solutions
   5. Administer medications as prescribed to correct the cause, such as antidiarrheal, antimicrobial, antiemetic, or antipyretic
   6. Administer oxygen as prescribed
   7. Monitor electrolyte values, and prepare to administer medication to treat an imbalance if present

III. FLUID VOLUME EXCESS

A. Description
   1. Fluid intake or fluid retention exceeds the body's fluid needs
   2. Also called overhydration or fluid overload
   3. The goal of treatment is to restore fluid balance, correct electrolyte imbalances if present, and eliminate or control the underlying cause of the overload

B. Types
   1. Isotonic overhydration
      a. Known as hypervolemia and results from excessive fluid in the extracellular fluid compartment
      b. Only the extracellular fluid compartment is expanded, and fluid does not shift between the extracellular and intracellular compartments
      c. Causes circulatory overload and interstitial edema; when severe or when it occurs in a client with poor cardiac function, congestive heart failure and pulmonary edema can result
   2. Hypertonic overhydration
      a. Occurrence is rare and is caused by an excessive sodium intake
      b. Fluid is drawn from the intracellular fluid compartment; the extracellular fluid volume expands, and the intracellular fluid volume contracts
   3. Hypotonic overhydration
      a. Known as water intoxication
      b. The excessive fluid moves into the intracellular space, and all body fluid compartments expand
      c. Electrolyte imbalances occur as a result of dilution

C. Causes
  1. Isotonic overhydration
     a. Poorly controlled IV therapy
     b. Renal failure
     c. Long-term corticosteroid therapy
  2. Hypertonic overhydration
     a. Excessive sodium ingestion
     b. Rapid infusion of hypertonic saline
     c. Excessive sodium bicarbonate therapy
  3. Hypotonic overhydration
     a. Early renal failure
     b. Congestive heart failure
     c. Syndrome of inappropriate antidiuretic hormone
     d. Poorly controlled IV therapy
     e. Replacement of isotonic fluid loss with hypotonic fluids
     f. Irrigation of wounds and body cavities with hypotonic fluids
▲ D. Assessment
  1. Cardiovascular
     a. Bounding, increased pulse rate
     b. Peripheral pulses full
     c. Elevated blood pressure; decreased pulse pressure
     d. Elevated central venous pressure
     e. Distended neck and hand veins
     f. Engorged venous varicosities
  2. Respiratory
     a. Increased respiratory rate
     b. Shallow respirations
     c. Dyspnea
     d. Moist crackles on auscultation
  3. Neuromuscular
     a. Altered level of consciousness
     b. Headache
     c. Visual disturbances
     d. Skeletal muscle weakness
     e. Paresthesias
  4. Integumentary
     a. Pitting edema in dependent areas
     b. Skin pale and cool to touch
  5. GI: Increased motility
  6. Isotonic overhydration
     a. Liver enlargement
     b. Ascites
  7. Hypotonic overhydration
     a. Polyuria
     b. Diarrhea
     c. Nonpitting edema
     d. Dysrhythmias
     e. Projectile vomiting
E. Implementation
  1. Monitor cardiovascular, respiratory, neuromuscular, integumentary, and GI status
  2. Prevent further fluid overload, and restore normal fluid balance

  3. Administer diuretics; osmotic diuretics are typically prescribed first to prevent severe electrolyte imbalances
  4. Restrict fluid and sodium intake
  5. Monitor I&O and weight
  6. Monitor electrolyte values, and prepare to administer medication to treat an imbalance if present

IV. HYPOKALEMIA ▲
A. Description
  1. A serum potassium level below 3.5 mEq/L (Box 8-3)
  2. Potassium deficit is potentially life threatening because every body system is affected
B. Causes ▲
  1. Actual total body potassium loss
     a. Inappropriate or excessive use of medications such as diuretics, digitalis, or corticosteroids
     b. Increased secretion of aldosterone, such as in Cushing's syndrome
     c. Vomiting; diarrhea
     d. Wound drainage, particularly GI
     e. Prolonged nasogastric suction
     f. Heat-induced excessive diaphoresis
     g. Renal disease impairing reabsorption of potassium
  2. Inadequate potassium intake: NPO
  3. Movement of potassium from ECF to ICF
     a. Alkalosis
     b. Hyperinsulinism
     c. Hyperalimentation or total parenteral nutrition
  4. Dilution of serum potassium
     a. Water intoxication
     b. IV therapy with potassium-poor solutions

BOX 8-3

Potassium

NORMAL VALUE
3.5 mEq/L to 5.1 mEq/L

COMMON FOOD SOURCES
Avocado
Raisins
Pork, beef, veal
Cantaloupe
Spinach
Bananas
Fish
Oranges
Strawberries
Mushrooms
Carrots
Potatoes
Tomatoes

▲ C. Assessment
1. Cardiovascular
    a. Thready, weak pulse; variable pulse rate
    b. Peripheral pulses difficult to palpate
    c. Orthostatic hypotension
    d. ECG changes: ST depression; flat or inverted T wave; prominent U wave; heart block (Table 8-2)
2. Respiratory
    a. Shallow, ineffective respirations that result from profound weakness of the skeletal muscles of respiration
    b. Diminished breath sounds
3. Neuromuscular
    a. Anxiety, lethargy, confusion, coma
    b. Skeletal muscle weakness; eventual flaccid paralysis
    c. Loss of tactile discrimination
    d. Deep tendon hyporeflexia
4. GI
    a. Decreased motility, hypoactive to absent bowel sounds
    b. Nausea, vomiting, constipation, abdominal distension
    c. Paralytic ileus
5. Renal
    a. Decreased specific gravity
    b. Increased urinary output

▲ D. Implementation
1. Monitor cardiovascular, respiratory, neuromuscular, GI, and renal status
2. Monitor electrolyte values
3. Administer potassium supplements orally or IV as prescribed
4. Oral potassium supplements
    a. May cause nausea and vomiting; they should not be taken on an empty stomach; if the client complains of abdominal pain, distention, nausea, vomiting, diarrhea, or GI bleeding, the oral potassium may need to be discontinued
    b. Liquid potassium chloride has an unpleasant taste and should be taken with juice or another liquid
5. IV potassium
    a. Potassium is never given by IV push or by the intramuscular or subcutaneous route
    b. A dilution of no more than 1 mEq/10 mL of solution is recommended
    c. When potassium is added to an IV solution, shake the bag and invert it to ensure that the potassium is evenly distributed throughout the IV solution
    d. The maximum recommended infusion rate is 5 to 10 mEq/hr, never to exceed 20 mEq/hour under any circumstances
    e. A client receiving more than 10 mEq/hr should be placed on a cardiac monitor, and the infusion should be controlled by an infusion device
    f. Monitor for cardiac changes during the administration of potassium; place the client on a cardiac monitor
    g. Can cause phlebitis; therefore, the nurse assesses the IV site every 2 hours for signs of infiltration; if infiltration occurs, the IV is stopped immediately
    h. Assess renal function before administering potassium; monitor I & O during administration
6. Institute safety measures for the client experiencing muscle weakness
7. If the client is taking a potassium-losing diuretic, it may be discontinued; a potassium-sparing diuretic may be prescribed
8. Instruct client about foods that are high in potassium content (Box 8-3)
9. Instruct client about foods that are high in fiber to prevent constipation

V. HYPERKALEMIA ▲
A. Description: A serum potassium level that exceeds 5.1 mEq/L (Box 8-3)
B. Causes ▲
1. Excessive potassium intake
    a. Overingestion of potassium-containing foods or medications such as potassium chloride or salt substitutes
    b. Rapid infusion of potassium-containing IV solutions
2. Decreased potassium excretion
    a. Potassium-sparing diuretics
    b. Renal failure
    c. Adrenal insufficiency, such as in Addison's disease

TABLE 8-2

Electrocardiographic Changes in Electrolyte Imbalances

HYPOKALEMIA	HYPERKALEMIA
ST depression	Tall T waves
Flat or inverted T wave	Widened QRS complex
Prominent U wave	Prolonged PR interval
Heart block	Flattened or absent P waves
	Heart block
HYPOCALCEMIA	**HYPERCALCEMIA**
Prolonged ST interval	Shortened ST segment
Prolonged QT interval	Widened T wave
HYPOMAGNESEMIA	**HYPERMAGNESEMIA**
Tall T waves	Prolonged PR interval
Depressed ST segment	Widened QRS complexes

3. Movement of potassium from ICF to ECF
   a. Tissue damage
   b. Acidosis
   c. Hyperuricemia
   d. Hypercatabolism

C. Assessment
1. Cardiovascular
   a. Irregular heart rate; slow, weak pulse rate
   b. Decreased blood pressure
   c. ECG changes: Tall T waves; widened QRS complexes; prolonged PR intervals; flattened or absent P waves; heart block (Table 8-2)
   d. Dysrhythmias
2. Respiratory: Profound weakness of the skeletal muscles causes respiratory failure
3. Neuromuscular
   a. Early: Muscle twitches, cramps, paresthesias (tingling and burning followed by numbness in the hands and feet and around the mouth)
   b. Late: Profound weakness, ascending flaccid paralysis in the arms and legs (trunk, head, and respiratory muscles become affected when the serum potassium level reaches a lethal level)
4. GI
   a. Increased motility, hyperactive bowel sounds
   b. Diarrhea

D. Implementation
1. Monitor cardiovascular, respiratory, neuromuscular, renal, and GI status; place client on a cardiac monitor
2. Discontinue IV potassium (keep IV catheter patent), and hold oral potassium supplements
3. Initiate a potassium-restricted diet
4. Prepare to administer potassium-excreting diuretics if renal function is not impaired
5. If renal function is impaired, prepare to administer sodium polystyrene sulfonate (Kayexalate), a cation exchange resin that promotes GI sodium absorption and potassium excretion
6. Prepare the client for dialysis and blood ultrafiltration if potassium levels are dangerously high
7. Prepare for the IV administration of 100 mL of 10% to 20% glucose with 10 to 20 units of regular insulin to move excess potassium into the cells
8. Monitor renal function
9. When blood transfusions are prescribed for a client with a potassium imbalance, the client should receive fresh blood if possible; transfusions of stored blood may elevate the potassium level because the breakdown of older blood cells releases potassium
10. Teach the client to avoid foods high in potassium (Box 8-3)
11. Instruct the client to avoid the use of salt substitutes or other potassium-containing substances

VI. HYPONATREMIA

A. Description
1. A serum sodium level below 135 mEq/L (Box 8-4)
2. Sodium imbalances are usually associated with fluid volume imbalances

B. Causes
1. Increased sodium excretion
   a. Excessive diaphoresis
   b. High-ceiling diuretics
   c. Wound drainage, especially GI
   d. Decreased secretion of aldosterone
   e. Hyperlipidemia
   f. Renal disease
2. Inadequate sodium intake
   a. Nothing by mouth
   b. Low-salt diet
3. Dilution of serum sodium
   a. Excessive ingestion of hypotonic fluids or irrigation with hypotonic fluids
   b. Renal failure
   c. Freshwater drowning
   d. Syndrome of inappropriate antidiuretic hormone secretion
   e. Hyperglycemia
   f. Congestive heart failure

C. Assessment
1. Cardiovascular
   a. Symptoms vary with changes in vascular volume
   b. Normovolemic: Rapid pulse rate; normal blood pressure
   c. Hypovolemic: Thready, weak, rapid pulse rate;

BOX 8-4

Sodium

NORMAL VALUE
135 to 145 mEq/L

COMMON FOOD SOURCES
Table salt
Soy sauce
Cured pork
Cottage cheese
American cheese
Milk
Butter
White and whole-wheat bread
Ketchup
Mustard
Bacon
Frankfurters
Lunch meat
Canned food
Processed food
Snack food

hypotension; flat neck veins; central venous pressure is normal or low

d. Hypervolemic: Rapid, bounding pulse; blood pressure normal or elevated; central venous pressure is normal or elevated

2. Respiratory
   a. Shallow, ineffective respiratory movements as a late manifestation related to skeletal muscle weakness
   b. Signs of pulmonary edema, such as rapid, shallow respirations, and moist rales
3. Neuromuscular
   a. Generalized skeletal muscle weakness that is worse in the extremities
   b. Diminished deep tendon reflexes
4. Cerebral function
   a. Headache
   b. Personality changes
5. GI
   a. Increased motility and hyperactive bowel sounds
   b. Nausea
   c. Abdominal cramping and diarrhea
6. Renal
   a. Decreased specific gravity
   b. Increased urinary output

D. Implementation
   1. Monitor cardiovascular, respiratory, neuromuscular, cerebral, renal, and GI status
   2. If hyponatremia is accompanied by a fluid deficit (hypovolemia), IV saline infusions are administered to restore both sodium content and fluid volume
   3. If hyponatremia is accompanied by fluid excess (hypervolemia), osmotic diuretics are administered to promote the excretion of water rather than sodium
   4. If the cause is inappropriate or excessive secretion of antidiuretic hormone (ADH), medications that antagonize ADH, such as lithium and demeclocycline (Declomycin), are administered
   5. Instruct client to increase oral sodium intake, and inform the client about the foods to include in the diet (Box 8-4)
   6. If the client is taking lithium, monitor lithium level because **hyponatremia** can cause diminished lithium excretion and result in toxicity

VII. HYPERNATREMIA

A. Description: A serum sodium level that exceeds 145 mEq/L (Box 8-4)

B. Causes
   1. Decreased sodium excretion
      a. Corticosteroids
      b. Cushing's syndrome
      c. Renal failure
      d. Hyperaldosteronism

2. Increased sodium intake: Excessive oral sodium ingestion or excessive administration of sodium-containing IV fluids
3. Decreased water intake: NPO
4. Increased water loss: Increased rate of metabolism; fever; hyperventilation; infection; excessive diaphoresis; watery diarrhea; dehydration

C. Assessment
   1. Cardiovascular
      a. Decreased myocardial contractility and diminished cardiac output
      b. Heart rate and blood pressure respond to vascular volume
   2. Respiratory: Pulmonary edema if hypervolemia is present
   3. Neuromuscular
      a. Early: Spontaneous muscle twitches; irregular muscle contractions
      b. Late: Skeletal muscle weakness; deep tendon reflexes diminished or absent
   4. Central nervous
      a. Altered cerebral function is the most common manifestation of **hypernatremia**
      b. Normovolemia or hypovolemia: Agitation, confusion, seizures
      c. Hypervolemia: Lethargy, stupor, coma
   5. Renal
      a. Increased specific gravity
      b. Decreased urinary output
   6. Integumentary
      a. Dry, flaky skin
      b. Presence or absence of edema, depending on fluid volume changes

D. Implementation
   1. Monitor cardiovascular, respiratory, neuromuscular, cerebral, renal, and integumentary status
   2. If the cause is fluid loss, prepare to administer IV infusions of glucose and water, such as 5% dextrose in water
   3. If the cause is inadequate renal excretion of sodium, prepare to administer diuretics that promote sodium loss
   4. Prepare the client for dialysis and ultrafiltration if sodium levels are dangerously high
   5. Restrict sodium and fluid intake as prescribed (Box 8-4)

VIII. HYPOCALCEMIA

A. Description: A serum calcium level below 8.6 mg/dL (Box 8-5)

B. Causes
   1. Inhibition of calcium absorption from the GI tract
      a. Inadequate oral intake of calcium
      b. Lactose intolerance
      c. Malabsorption syndromes such as celiac sprue or Crohn's disease

BOX 8-5
Calcium

NORMAL VALUE
8.6 to 10.0 mg/dL

COMMON FOOD SOURCES
Yogurt, low-fat
Milk
Rhubarb
Collard greens
Cheese
Tofu
Spinach
Broccoli
Green beans
Carrots

d. Inadequate intake of vitamin D
e. End-stage renal disease
2. Increased calcium excretion
   a. Renal failure, polyuric phase
   b. Diarrhea
   c. Steatorrhea
   d. Wound drainage, especially GI
3. Conditions that decrease the ionized fraction of calcium
   a. Hyperproteinemia
   b. Alkalosis
   c. Medications such as calcium chelators or binders
   d. Acute pancreatitis
   e. **Hyperphosphatemia**
   f. Immobility
   g. Removal or destruction of the parathyroid glands
C. Assessment
   1. Cardiovascular
      a. Decreased myocardial contractility and heart rate
      b. Hypotension
      c. Diminished peripheral pulses
      d. ECG changes: Prolonged ST interval; prolonged QT interval (Table 8-2)
   2. Respiratory: Not directly affected; however, respiratory failure or arrest can result from decreased respiratory movement because of muscle tetany or seizures
   3. Neuromuscular
      a. Irritable skeletal muscles: twitches, cramps, tetany, seizures
      b. Painful muscle spasms in the calf or foot during periods of inactivity
      c. Paresthesias followed by numbness that may affect the lips, nose, and ears in addition to the limbs
      d. Positive Trousseau's and Chvostek's signs

e. Hyperactive deep tendon reflexes
f. Anxiety, irritability, psychosis
4. GI
   a. Increased gastric motility; hyperactive bowel sounds
   b. Abdominal cramping, diarrhea
D. Implementation
   1. Monitor cardiovascular, respiratory, neuromuscular, and GI status; place client on a cardiac monitor
   2. Administer oral calcium supplements or intravenous (IV) calcium
   3. When administering IV calcium, warm injection to body temperature before administration; administer slowly; monitor for ECG changes; observe for infiltration; and monitor for **hypercalcemia** and **hypomagnesemia**
   4. Administer medications that increase calcium absorption
      a. Aluminum hydroxide reduces serum phosphorus levels, causing the countereffect of increasing calcium levels
      b. Vitamin D aids in the absorption of calcium from the intestinal tract
   5. Administer medications that reduce nerve and skeletal muscle excitability
   6. Provide a quiet environment to reduce environmental stimuli
   7. Initiate seizure precautions
   8. Keep 10% calcium gluconate available for treatment of acute calcium deficit
   9. Move client carefully, and monitor for signs of a fracture
   10. Instruct client to take oral calcium supplements 1 to 2 hours after meals or at bedtime to maximize intestinal absorption
   11. Instruct client to consume foods high in calcium (Box 8-5)

IX. HYPERCALCEMIA
A. Description: A serum calcium level that exceeds 10 mg/dL (Box 8-5)
B. Causes
   1. Increased calcium absorption
      a. Excessive oral intake of calcium
      b. Excessive oral intake of vitamin D
   2. Decreased calcium excretion
      a. Renal failure
      b. Use of thiazide diuretics
   3. Increased bone resorption of calcium
      a. Hyperparathyroidism
      b. Hyperthyroidism
      c. Malignancy
      d. Immobility
      e. Use of glucocorticoids
   4. Hemoconcentration
      a. Dehydration

b. Use of lithium
c. Adrenal insufficiency
C. Assessment
1. Cardiovascular
a. Increased heart rate in early phase; bradycardia and cardiac arrest in late phases
b. Increased blood pressure
c. Bounding, full peripheral pulses
d. ECG changes: Shortened ST segment; widened T wave (Table 8-2)
e. Clot formation in vessels or organs in which blood flow is slow or blocked
2. Respiratory: Ineffective respiratory movement as a result of profound skeletal muscle weakness
3. Neuromuscular
a. Profound muscle weakness
b. Diminished or absent deep tendon reflexes
c. Disorientation, lethargy, coma
4. Renal
a. Increased urinary output leading to dehydration
b. Formation of renal calculi
5. GI
a. Decreased motility and hypoactive bowel sounds
b. Anorexia, nausea, abdominal distention, constipation
D. Implementation
1. Monitor cardiovascular, respiratory, neuromuscular, renal, and GI status; place client on a cardiac monitor
2. IV infusions of solutions containing calcium are discontinued, as well as oral medications containing calcium or vitamin D
3. Thiazide diuretics are discontinued and are replaced with diuretics that enhance the excretion of calcium
4. Administer an IV infusion of normal saline as prescribed to help restore serum calcium levels
5. Administer medications as prescribed that inhibit calcium resorption from the bone, such as phosphorus, calcitonin (Calcimar), biphosphonates (etidronate), and prostaglandin synthesis inhibitors (aspirin, nonsteroidal anti-inflammatory drugs)
6. Prepare the client with severe **hypercalcemia** for dialysis or blood ultrafiltration, if medications fail to reduce the serum calcium level
7. Move client carefully and monitor for signs of a fracture
8. Monitor for flank or abdominal pain, and strain urine to check for the presence of urinary stones
9. Instruct client who is at risk for **hypercalcemia** regarding the sources of calcium (Box 8-5)

X. HYPOMAGNESEMIA
A. Description: A serum magnesium level below 1.6 mg/dL (Box 8-6)

B. Causes
1. Insufficient magnesium intake
a. Malnutrition and starvation
b. Diarrhea
c. Steatorrhea
d. Celiac disease
e. Crohn's disease
2. Increased magnesium secretion
a. Medications such as diuretics, aminoglycoside antibiotics, cisplatin, amphotericin B, cyclosporine
b. Citrate (blood products)
c. Ethanol ingestion
3. Intracellular movement of magnesium
a. Hyperglycemia
b. Insulin administration
c. Sepsis
d. Alkalosis
C. Assessment
1. Cardiovascular
a. ECG changes: Tall T waves; depressed ST segments (Table 8-2)
b. Dysrhythmias
c. Hypertension
2. GI
a. Decreased motility
b. Decreased bowel sounds
c. Anorexia, nausea, abdominal distention
3. Respiratory: Shallow respirations
4. Neuromuscular
a. Fasciculations; twitches; paresthesias
b. Positive Trousseau's and Chvostek's signs
c. Hyperreflexia
d. Tetany; seizures
5. Central Nervous
a. Irritability
b. Confusion; psychosis

BOX 8-6
Magnesium
NORMAL VALUE
1.6 to 2.6 mg/dL

COMMON FOOD SOURCES
Green leafy vegetables such as spinach and broccoli
Avocado
Canned white tuna fish
Low fat yogurt
Cooked rolled oats
Milk
Peas
Potatoes
Pork, beef, chicken
Raisins
Peanut butter
Cauliflower

D. Implementation
1. Monitor cardiovascular, GI, respiratory, neuromuscular, and central nervous system status; place client on a cardiac monitor
2. Because **hypocalcemia** frequently accompanies **hypomagnesemia,** interventions also aim to restore normal serum calcium levels
3. Medications that contribute to **hypomagnesemia** are discontinued
4. Magnesium sulfate (MgSO$_4$) by the IV route is administered in severe cases (intramuscular injections cause pain and tissue damage)
5. Initiate seizure precautions
6. Monitor serum magnesium levels every 12 to 24 hours when client is receiving magnesium by IV
7. Monitor for reduced deep tendon reflexes, suggesting **hypermagnesemia,** during administration of magnesium
8. Oral preparations of magnesium may cause diarrhea and increase magnesium loss
9. Instruct client in regard to increasing the intake of foods that contain magnesium (Box 8-6)

XI. HYPERMAGNESEMIA
A. Description: A serum magnesium level that exceeds 2.6 mg/dL (Box 8-6)
B. Causes
1. Increased magnesium intake
   a. Magnesium-containing antacids and laxatives
   b. IV magnesium replacement
2. Decreased renal excretion of magnesium as a result of renal insufficiency
C. Assessment
1. Cardiovascular
   a. Bradycardia
   b. Peripheral vasodilation
   c. Hypotension
   d. Dysrhythmias
   e. ECG changes: Prolonged PR interval; widened QRS complexes (Table 8-2)
2. Respiratory: respiratory insufficiency when the skeletal muscles of respiration are involved
3. Neuromuscular
   a. Diminished or absent deep tendon reflexes
   b. Skeletal muscle weakness
4. Central nervous: Drowsiness and lethargy that progresses to coma
D. Implementation
1. Monitor cardiovascular, respiratory, neuromuscular, and central nervous system status; place client on cardiac monitor
2. Oral and parenteral magnesium-containing medications are discontinued
3. Administer magnesium-free IV fluids as prescribed to reduce serum magnesium levels
4. Administer high-ceiling (loop) diuretics as prescribed to increase renal excretion
5. Administer calcium when cardiac manifestations

are severe, to reverse the cardiac effects of hypermagnesemia
6. Instruct client in regard to restricting dietary intake of magnesium-containing foods (Box 8-6)
7. Instruct client in regard to avoiding the use of laxatives and antacids containing magnesium

XII. HYPOPHOSPHATEMIA
A. Description
1. A serum phosphorus level below 2.7 mg/dL (Box 8-7)
2. A decrease in the serum phosphorus level is accompanied by an increase in the serum calcium level
B. Causes
1. Insufficient phosphorus intake: Malnutrition and starvation
2. Increased phosphorus excretion
   a. Hyperparathyroidism
   b. Renal failure
   c. Malignancy
   d. Use of aluminum hydroxide–based or magnesium-based antacids
3. Intracellular shift
   a. Hyperglycemia
   b. Hyperalimentation
   c. Respiratory alkalosis
C. Assessment
1. Cardiovascular
   a. Decreased contractility and cardiac output
   b. Slowed peripheral pulses
   c. Reversible cardiomyopathy
2. Respiratory: Shallow respirations
3. Neuromuscular
   a. Weakness
   b. Rhabdomyolysis
   c. Decreased deep tendon reflexes
   d. Decreased bone density that can cause fractures and alterations in bone shape
4. Central nervous
   a. Irritability
   b. Confusion
   c. Seizures

BOX 8-7

Phosphorus

NORMAL VALUE
2.7 to 4.5 mg/dL

COMMON FOOD SOURCES
Fish
Pork, beef, chicken
Organ meats
Nuts
Whole-grain breads and cereals

5. Hematological
   a. Decreased platelet aggregation and increased bleeding
   b. Immunosuppression
D. Implementation
   1. Monitor cardiovascular, respiratory, neuromuscular, central nervous system, and hematologic status
   2. Medications that contribute to **hypophosphatemia** are discontinued
   3. Administer oral phosphorus along with a vitamin D supplement
   4. IV phosphorus is administered only when serum phosphorus levels fall below 1 mg/dL and when the client has serious clinical manifestations
   5. IV phosphorus is administered slowly because of the risks associated with **hyperphosphatemia**
   6. Assess renal system before administering phosphorus
   7. Move client carefully, and monitor for signs of a fracture
   8. Instruct client regarding the use of antacids
   9. Instruct client to increase intake of phosphorus-containing foods while decreasing the intake of calcium-containing foods (Boxes 8-5 and 8-7)

XIII. HYPERPHOSPHATEMIA
A. Description
   1. A serum phosphorus level that exceeds 4.5 mg/dL (Box 8-7)
   2. Elevated serum phosphorus levels are tolerated well by most body systems
   3. An increase in the serum phosphorus level is accompanied by a decrease in the serum calcium level
   4. The problems that occur in **hyperphosphatemia** center on the **hypocalcemia** that results when serum phosphorus levels increase
B. Causes
   1. Decreased renal excretion resulting from renal insufficiency
   2. Tumor lysis syndrome
   3. Increased intake of phosphorus, including dietary intake or overuse of phosphate-containing laxatives or enemas
   4. Hypoparathyroidism
C. Assessment: Refer to assessment of **hypocalcemia**
D. Implementation
   1. Interventions entail the management of **hypocalcemia**
   2. Administer phosphate-binding medications that increase fecal excretion of phosphorus by binding phosphorus from food in the GI tract
   3. Instruct client to avoid phosphate-containing medications, including laxatives and enemas
   4. Instruct client to decrease the intake of food that is high is phosphorus (Box 8-7)
   5. Instruct client in how to take phosphate-binding

medications, emphasizing that they should be taken with meals or immediately after meals

PRACTICE QUESTIONS

1. A nurse is reading a physician's progress notes in the client's record and reads that the physician has documented "insensible fluid loss of approximately 800 mL daily." The nurse understands that this type of fluid loss can occur through:
   1. The gastrointestinal (GI) tract
   2. Urinary output
   3. Wound drainage
   4. The skin
2. A nurse is assigned to care for a group of clients. On review of the clients' medical records, the nurse determines that which client is at risk for fluid volume deficit?
   1. A client with a colostomy
   2. A client receiving frequent wound irrigations
   3. A client with congestive heart failure (CHF)
   4. A client with decreased kidney function
3. A nurse is caring for a client who has been taking diuretics on a long-term basis. A fluid volume deficit is suspected. Which assessment finding would be noted in a client with this condition?
   1. Rales
   2. Increased blood pressure
   3. Decreased hematocrit
   4. Decreased central venous pressure (CVP)
4. A nurse is assigned to care for a group of clients. On review of the clients' medical records, the nurse determines that which client is at risk for a fluid volume excess?
   1. The client with renal failure
   2. The client with an ileostomy
   3. The client on diuretics
   4. The client on gastrointestinal (GI) suctioning
5. The nurse is caring for a client with congestive heart failure (CHF). On assessment, the nurse notes that the client is dyspneic and that rales are heard on auscultation. The nurse suspects fluid volume excess. What additional signs would the nurse expect to note in this client if fluid volume excess is present?
   1. A decreased central venous pressure
   2. Flat neck and hand veins
   3. An increase in blood pressure
   4. Weight loss
6. A nurse is preparing to care for a client with a potassium deficit. The nurse reviews the client's record and determines that the client is at risk for developing the potassium deficit because the client:
   1. Is on nasogastric (NG) suction
   2. Has a history of renal disease
   3. Has a history of Addison's disease
   4. Is taking a potassium-sparing diuretic

7. A nurse reviews a client's electrolyte laboratory report and notes that the potassium level is 3.2 mEq/L. Which of the following would the nurse note on the ECG as a result of the laboratory value?
   1. Elevated T waves
   2. Absent P waves
   3. Elevated ST segment
   4. U waves

8. A nurse prepares to administer IV potassium chloride as prescribed to a client with hypokalemia. Which of the following would not be a part of the nurse's plan in regard to the preparation and administration of the potassium?
   1. Prepare the medication for bolus administration
   2. Obtain a controlled IV infusion pump
   3. Dilute in appropriate amount of normal saline
   4. Monitor urine output during administration

9. A nurse instructs a client at risk for hypokalemia about the foods high in potassium that should be included in the daily diet. The nurse determines that the client understands the food sources of potassium if the client states that the food item lowest in potassium is:
   1. Spinach
   2. Carrots
   3. Avocado
   4. Apples

10. A nurse caring for a group of clients reviews the electrolyte laboratory results and notes a potassium level of 5.5 mEq/L on one client's laboratory reports. The nurse understands that which client is at most risk for the development of a potassium value at this level?
    1. The client who has sustained a traumatic burn
    2. The client with Cushing's syndrome
    3. The client with colitis
    4. The client who has been overusing laxatives

11. A nurse reviews the electrolyte results of an assigned client and notes that the potassium level is 5.4 mEq/L. Which of the following would the nurse expect to note on the ECG as a result of the laboratory value?
    1. Tall T waves
    2. Prominent U wave
    3. ST depression
    4. Inverted T wave

12. A nurse caring for a group of clients reviews the electrolyte laboratory results and notes a sodium level of 130 mEq/L on one client's laboratory reports. The nurse understands that which client is at most risk for the development of a sodium value at this level?
    1. The client who is taking diuretics
    2. The client who is taking corticosteroids
    3. The client with renal failure
    4. The client with hyperaldosteronism

13. A nurse is caring for a client with acute congestive heart failure who is receiving high doses of a high-ceiling diuretic. On assessment, the nurse notes that the client has flat neck veins, generalized muscle weakness, and diminished deep tendon reflexes. The nurse suspects hyponatremia. What additional signs would the nurse expect to note in this client if hyponatremia is present?
    1. Dry, flaky skin
    2. Decreased urinary output
    3. Increased specific gravity of the urine
    4. Hyperactive bowel sounds

14. A nurse is caring for a client with a nasogastric (NG) tube. NG tube irrigations are prescribed to be performed once every shift. The client's serum electrolyte results indicate a potassium level of 4.5 mEq/L and a sodium level of 132 mEq/L. On the basis of these laboratory findings, the nurse selects which solution to use for the NG tube irrigation?
    1. Tap water
    2. Distilled water
    3. Sterile water
    4. Normal saline

15. A nurse is reviewing laboratory results and notes that a client's serum sodium level is 150 mEq/L. The nurse reports the serum sodium level to the physician, and the physician prescribes dietary instructions based on the sodium level. Which food item does the nurse instruct the client to avoid?
    1. Low-fat yogurt
    2. Cauliflower
    3. Processed oat cereals
    4. Peas

16. A nurse is reviewing a client's laboratory reports and notes that the serum calcium level is 4.0 mg/dL. The nurse understands that which condition most likely caused this serum calcium level?
    1. Prolonged bed rest
    2. Excessive administration of vitamin D
    3. Renal insufficiency
    4. Hyperparathyroidism

17. A nurse is assessing a client with a suspected diagnosis of hypocalcemia. Which of the following assessment signs/symptoms would not be an indication of this diagnosis?
    1. Hypoactive bowel sounds
    2. Paresthesias
    3. Hyperactive deep tendon reflexes
    4. Positive Trousseau's sign

18. A nurse caring for a client with hypocalcemia would expect to note which of the following changes on the electrocardiogram (ECG)?
    1. Prominent U wave
    2. Widened T wave
    3. Shortened ST segment
    4. Prolonged QT interval

19. A nurse caring for a client with severe malnutrition reviews the laboratory results and notes a

magnesium level of 1.0 mg/dL. Which ECG change would the nurse expect to note based on the magnesium level?

1. Prominent U waves
2. Depressed ST segment
3. Widened QRS complexes
4. Prolonged PR interval

20. A nurse reviews the serum phosphorus level and notes that the client's level is 2.0 mg/dL. Which condition most likely caused this serum phosphorus level?

1. Alcoholism

2. Hypoparathyroidism
3. Tumor lysis syndrome
4. Renal insufficiency

CRITICAL THINKING: FREE-TEXT ENTRY

A nurse is caring for a client with a diagnosis of hyperthyroidism. Laboratory studies are performed and the serum calcium level is 12.0 mg/dL. Is this calcium level high or low, and what is the normal serum calcium level?

Answer: _____

ANSWERS

1. 4
Rationale: Sensible losses are those of which the person is aware, such as through wound drainage, GI tract losses, and urination. Insensible losses may occur without the person's awareness. Insensible losses occur daily through the skin and the lungs.
Test-Taking Strategy: Use the process of elimination, noting the similarity between options 1, 2, and 3. Note that the issue of the question is fluid loss. In options 1, 2 and 3, these types of losses can be measured for accurate output. Fluid loss through the skin cannot be accurately measured, only approximated. If you had difficulty with this question, review the difference between sensible and insensible fluid loss.
Level of Cognitive Ability: Comprehension
Client Needs: Physiological Integrity
Integrated Concept/Process: Communication and Documentation
Content Area: Fundamental Skills
Reference: Ignatavicius, D., Workman, M., & Mishler, M. (1999). *Medical-surgical nursing across the health care continuum* (3rd ed.). Philadelphia: W.B. Saunders, p. 220.

2. 1
Rationale: Causes of a fluid volume deficit include vomiting, diarrhea, conditions that cause increased respirations or increased urinary output, insufficient IV fluid replacement, draining fistulas, and the presence of an ileostomy or colostomy. A client with CHF or decreased kidney function or a client receiving frequent wound irrigations is at risk for fluid volume excess.
Test-Taking Strategy: Read the question carefully, noting that it asks for the client at risk for a deficit. Read each option and think about the fluid imbalance that can occur in each. Use the process of elimination. The clients presented in options 2, 3, and 4 retain fluid. The only condition that can cause a deficit is the condition noted in option 1. If you had difficulty with this question, review the causes of fluid volume deficit.
Level of Cognitive Ability: Analysis
Client Needs: Physiological Integrity
Integrated Concept/Process: Nursing Process/Assessment
Content Area: Fundamental Skills
Reference: LeMone, P., & Burke, K. (2000). *Medical-surgical nursing: Critical thinking in client care* (2nd ed.). Upper Saddle River, NJ: Prentice-Hall, p. 106.

3. 4
Rationale: Assessment findings in a client with a fluid volume deficit include increased respirations and heart rate, decreased CVP, weight loss, poor skin turgor, dry mucous membranes, decreased urine volume, increased specific gravity of the urine, increased hematocrit, and altered level of consciousness. The normal CVP is between 4 and 11 mm H_2O. A client with dehydration has a low CVP. The assessment findings in options 1, 2, and 3 are seen in a client with fluid volume excess.
Test-Taking Strategy: Use the process of elimination and focus on the issue, fluid volume deficit. Eliminate options 1 and 2 first. Rales are noted in fluid volume excess, as is increased blood pressure. From the remaining options, recall that central venous pressure reflects the pressure under which blood is returned to the superior vena cava and right atrium. Therefore, pressure (volume) would be decreased in a fluid volume deficit. If you had difficulty with this question, review the assessment findings noted in fluid volume deficit.
Level of Cognitive Ability: Analysis
Client Needs: Physiological Integrity
Integrated Concept/Process: Nursing Process/Assessment
Content Area: Fundamental Skills
Reference: Smeltzer, S., & Bare, B. (2000). *Textbook of medical-surgical nursing* (9th ed). Philadelphia: Lippincott Williams & Wilkins, p. 209.

4. 1
Rationale: The causes of fluid volume excess include decreased kidney function, congestive heart failure (CHF), the use of hypotonic fluids to replace isotonic fluid losses, excessive irrigation of wounds and body cavities, and excessive ingestion of sodium. The client with an ileostomy, the client on diuretics, and the client on GI suctioning are at risk for fluid volume deficit.
Test-Taking Strategy: Use the process of elimination and focus on the issue, fluid volume excess. Read each option and think about the fluid imbalance that can occur in each. The clients presented in options 2, 3, and 4 lose fluid. The only condition that can cause an excess is the condition noted in option 1. If you had difficulty with this question, review the causes of fluid volume excess.
Level of Cognitive Ability: Analysis
Client Needs: Physiological Integrity
Integrated Concept/Process: Nursing Process/Assessment

Content Area: Fundamental Skills
Reference: Phipps, W., Sands, J., & Marek, J. (1999). *Medical-surgical nursing: Concepts & clinical practice* (6th ed.). St. Louis: Mosby, p. 406.

5. **3**

Rationale: Assessment findings associated with fluid volume excess include cough, dyspnea, rales, tachypnea, tachycardia, an elevated BP and a bounding pulse, an elevated central venous pressure (CVP), weight gain, edema, neck and hand vein distention, altered level of consciousness, and a decreased hematocrit. Options 1, 2, and 4 identify signs noted in fluid volume deficit.

Test-Taking Strategy: Use the process of elimination and knowledge regarding the assessment findings in fluid volume excess. Note the similarities in options 1, 2, and 4. Each of these signs reflects a decrease. Option 3 reflects an increase. Remember that CVP reflects the pressure under which blood is returned to the superior vena cava and right atrium. Pressure (volume) would be elevated in fluid volume excess. If you had difficulty with this question, review the assessment findings noted in fluid volume excess.

Level of Cognitive Ability: Analysis
Client Needs: Physiological Integrity
Integrated Concept/Process: Nursing Process/Assessment
Content Area: Fundamental Skills
Reference: Phipps, W., Sands, J., & Marek, J. (1999). *Medical-surgical nursing: Concepts & clinical practice* (6th ed.). St. Louis: Mosby, p. 406.

6. **1**

Rationale: Potassium-rich GI fluids are lost through GI suction, placing the client at risk for hypokalemia. The client with renal disease or Addison's disease and the client taking a potassium-sparing diuretic are at risk for hyperkalemia.

Test-Taking Strategy: Use the process of elimination. Note that the issue is a potassium deficit. Option 1 is the only option that identifies a loss of body fluid. If you had difficulty with this question, review the causes of hypokalemia.

Level of Cognitive Ability: Analysis
Client Needs: Physiological Integrity
Integrated Concept/Process: Communication and Documentation
Content Area: Fundamental Skills
Reference: Lewis, S., Heitkemper, M., & Dirksen, S. (2000). *Medical-surgical nursing: Assessment and management of clinical problems* (5th ed.). St. Louis: Mosby, p. 336.

7. **4**

Rationale: A serum potassium level below 3.5 mEq/L is indicative of hypokalemia. Potassium deficit is a relatively common electrolyte imbalance and is potentially life threatening. ECG changes include inverted T waves, ST segment depression, heart block, and prominent U waves.

Test-Taking Strategy: Use the process of elimination. From the information in the question, you need to determine that the client is experiencing hypokalemia. From this point, it is necessary to know the ECG changes that are expected when hypokalemia exists. If you had difficulty with this question, review the ECG changes that occur in hypokalemia.

Level of Cognitive Ability: Analysis
Client Needs: Physiological Integrity
Integrated Concept/Process: Nursing Process/Analysis

Content Area: Fundamental Skills
Reference: Lewis, S., Heitkemper, M., & Dirksen, S. (2000). *Medical-surgical nursing: Assessment and management of clinical problems* (5th ed.). St. Louis: Mosby, p. 336.

8. **1**

Rationale: Potassium chloride administered by IV must always be diluted in IV fluid and infused via a pump or controller. The usual concentration of IV potassium chloride is 20 to 40 mEq/L. Potassium chloride is never given by bolus (IV push). Giving potassium chloride by IV push can result in cardiac arrest. Dilution in normal saline is recommended, and dextrose solution is avoided because this type of solution increases intracellular potassium shifting. The IV bag containing the potassium chloride is always agitated before hanging. The IV site is monitored closely because potassium chloride is very irritating to the veins and the risk of phlebitis exists. Urinary output is monitored during administration, and the physician is contacted if the urinary output is less than 30 mL/hr.

Test-Taking Strategy: Use the process of elimination and knowledge regarding the administration of IV potassium chloride. Noting the key word "not" in the stem of the question will easily direct you to option 1. Review the administration of potassium chloride if you had difficulty with this question.

Level of Cognitive Ability: Application
Client Needs: Physiological Integrity
Integrated Concept/Process: Nursing Process/Planning
Content Area: Pharmacology
Reference: Ignatavicius, D., Workman, M., & Mishler, M. (1999). *Medical-surgical nursing across the health care continuum* (3rd ed.). Philadelphia: W.B. Saunders, p. 246.

9. **4**

Rationale: A medium apple provides approximately 159 mg of potassium. Spinach (3½ oz) provides 470 mg. A large carrot provides 341 mg and a medium avocado provides 1097 mg of potassium.

Test-Taking Strategy: Use the process of elimination and knowledge regarding the potassium content of foods to answer this question. Take the time to learn the foods that are high and low in potassium content if you had difficulty with this question.

Level of Cognitive Ability: Analysis
Client Needs: Health Promotion and Maintenance
Integrated Concept/Process: Teaching/Learning
Content Area: Fundamental Skills
Reference: Ignatavicius, D., Workman, M., & Mishler, M. (1999). *Medical-surgical nursing across the health care continuum* (3rd ed.). Philadelphia: W.B. Saunders, p. 222.

10. **1**

Rationale: A serum potassium level greater than 5.1 mEq/L is indicative of hyperkalemia. Clients who experience cellular shifting of potassium in the early stages of massive cell destruction, such as in trauma, burns, or sepsis or with metabolic or respiratory acidosis, are at risk for hyperkalemia. The client with Cushing's syndrome or colitis and the client who has been overusing laxatives are at risk for hypokalemia.

Test-Taking Strategy: Use the process of elimination. Eliminate option 3 and 4 first because they are similar, both being reflective of a GI loss. Remembering that cell destruction causes potassium shifts may assist in directing you to the

correct option. Remember that Cushing's syndrome presents a risk for hypokalemia and that Addison's disease presents a risk for hyperkalemia. If you had difficulty with this question, review the risk factors associated with hyperkalemia.
Level of Cognitive Ability: Analysis
Client Needs: Physiological Integrity
Integrated Concept/Process: Nursing Process/Assessment
Content Area: Fundamental Skills
Reference: Lewis, S., Heitkemper, M., & Dirksen, S. (2000). *Medical-surgical nursing: Assessment and management of clinical problems* (5th ed.). St. Louis: Mosby, p. 336.

11. **1**
Rationale: A serum potassium level above 5.4 mEq/L is indicative of hyperkalemia. ECG changes include flat P waves, prolonged PR intervals, widened QRS complexes, and tall T waves.
Test-Taking Strategy: Use the process of elimination. From the information in the question, you need to determine that this condition is a hyperkalemic one. From this point, it is necessary to know the ECG changes that are expected when hyperkalemia exists. If you had difficulty with this question, review the normal serum potassium level and the ECG changes that occur in hyperkalemia.
Level of Cognitive Ability: Analysis
Client Needs: Physiological Integrity
Integrated Concept/Process: Nursing Process/Analysis
Content Area: Fundamental Skills
Reference: Lewis, S., Heitkemper, M., & Dirksen, S. (2000). *Medical-surgical nursing: Assessment and management of clinical problems* (5th ed.). St. Louis: Mosby, p. 336.

12. **1**
Rationale: Hyponatremia is evidenced by a serum sodium level of less than 135 mEq/L. Hyponatremia can occur in the client taking high-ceiling diuretics. The client taking corticosteroids and the client with renal failure or hyperaldosteronism are at risk for hypernatremia.
Test-Taking Strategy: Use the process of elimination. First determine that the client is experiencing hyponatremia. Next, it is necessary to know the causes of hyponatremia to direct you to option 1. Review the normal serum sodium level and the causes of hyponatremia if you had difficulty with this question.
Level of Cognitive Ability: Analysis
Client Needs: Physiological Integrity
Integrated Concept/Process: Nursing Process/Assessment
Content Area: Fundamental Skills
Reference: Ignatavicius, D., Workman, M., & Mishler, M. (1999). *Medical-surgical nursing across the health care continuum* (3rd ed.). Philadelphia: W.B. Saunders, p. 253.

13. **4**
Rationale: Hyperactive bowel sounds are indicative of hyponatremia. Options 1, 2, and 3 are signs of hypernatremia. In hyponatremia, increased urinary output and decreased specific gravity of the urine would be noted. Dry, flaky skin occurs in fluid volume deficit.
Test-Taking Strategy: Use the process of elimination. Knowledge regarding the signs of hyponatremia is needed to answer the question. If you had difficulty with this, review the assessment signs associated with both hyponatremia and hypernatremia.

Level of Cognitive Ability: Analysis
Client Needs: Physiological Integrity
Integrated Concept/Process: Nursing Process/Assessment
Content Area: Fundamental Skills
Reference: Ignatavicius, D., Workman, M., & Mishler, M. (1999). *Medical-surgical nursing across the health care continuum* (3rd ed.). Philadelphia: W.B. Saunders, p. 250.

14. **4**
Rationale: A potassium level of 4.5 mEq/L is within normal range. A sodium level of 132 mEq/L is low, indicating hyponatremia. In clients with hyponatremia, normal (isotonic) saline should be used rather than water for GI or urinary tract irrigations.
Test-Taking Strategy: Use the process of elimination. Eliminate options 1, 2, and 3 because they are similar (sterile water, distilled water, and tap water). Also, recalling that the serum sodium level indicates hyponatremia will direct you to option 4. If you had difficulty with this question, review the care of the client experiencing hyponatremia.
Level of Cognitive Ability: Analysis
Client Needs: Physiological Integrity
Integrated Concept/Process: Nursing Process/Implementation
Content Area: Fundamental Skills
Reference: Lewis, S., Heitkemper, M., & Dirksen, S. (2000). *Medical-surgical nursing: Assessment and management of clinical problems* (5th ed.). St. Louis: Mosby, p. 335.

15. **3**
Rationale: The normal serum sodium level is 135 to 145 mEq/L. A serum sodium level of 150 mEq/L is indicative of hypernatremia. On the basis of this finding, the nurse would instruct the client to avoid foods high in sodium. Low-fat yogurt, cauliflower, and peas are good food sources of phosphorus. Processed foods are high in sodium content.
Test-Taking Strategy: First it is necessary to determine that the client has hypernatremia. Next, note the key word "avoid" in the stem of the question. Eliminate options 2 and 4 first because these are vegetables. From the remaining two options, note the word "processed" in option 3. Processed foods tend to be higher in sodium content. Review foods high in sodium content if you had difficulty with this question.
Level of Cognitive Ability: Application
Client Needs: Health Promotion and Maintenance
Integrated Concept/Process: Teaching/Learning
Content Area: Fundamental Skills
Reference: Ignatavicius, D., Workman, M., & Mishler, M. (1999). *Medical-surgical nursing across the health care continuum* (3rd ed.). Philadelphia: W.B. Saunders, pp. 221, 224.

16. **1**
Rationale: The normal serum calcium level is 8.6 to 10.0 mg/dL. A client with a serum calcium level of 4.0 mg/dL is experiencing hypocalcemia. The excessive administration of vitamin D and hyperparathyroidism are causative factors associated with hypercalcemia. End-stage renal disease rather than renal insufficiency is a cause of hypocalcemia. Prolonged bed rest is a cause of hypocalcemia. Although immobilization can initially cause hypercalcemia, the long-term effect of prolonged bed rest is hypocalcemia.
Test-Taking Strategy: Note the key words "most likely." First, it is necessary to determine that the client is experiencing hypocalcemia. This should assist in eliminating option 2.

Next, recall the causative factors associated with hypocalcemia to direct you to option 1. If you had difficulty with question, review the causative factors associated with hypocalcemia.
Level of Cognitive Ability: Analysis
Client Needs: Physiological Integrity
Integrated Concept/Process: Nursing Process/Analysis
Content Area: Fundamental Skills
Reference: Ignatavicius, D., Workman, M., & Mishler, M. (1999). *Medical-surgical nursing across the health care continuum* (3rd ed.). Philadelphia: W.B. Saunders, pp. 255, 258.

17. **1**
Rationale: Hypoactive bowel sounds are noted in hypercalcemia. Signs of hypocalcemia include paresthesias followed by numbness, hyperactive deep tendon reflexes, and a positive Trousseau's or Chvostek's sign. Additional signs of hypocalcemia include increased neuromuscular excitability, muscle cramps, twitching, tetany, seizures, irritability, and anxiety. GI symptoms include increased gastric motility, hyperactive bowel sounds, abdominal cramping, and diarrhea.
Test-Taking Strategy: Note the key word "not" in the stem of the question. Use the process of elimination, noting that options 2, 3, and 4 are similar in that they all reflect a hyperactivity of the neuromuscular system. The option that is different is option 1. Review the assessment signs and symptoms noted in hypocalcemia if you had difficulty with this question.
Level of Cognitive Ability: Analysis
Client Needs: Physiological Integrity
Integrated Concept/Process: Nursing Process/Assessment
Content Area: Fundamental Skills
Reference: Ignatavicius, D., Workman, M., & Mishler, M. (1999). *Medical-surgical nursing across the health care continuum* (3rd ed.). Philadelphia: W.B. Saunders, pp. 256, 259.

18. **4**
Rationale: ECG changes that occur in a client with hypocalcemia include a prolonged ST or QT interval. A shortened ST segment and a widened T wave are seen in hypercalcemia. Prominent U waves are seen in hypokalemia.
Test-Taking Strategy: Use the process of elimination and knowledge regarding the ECG changes that occur in calcium imbalances. Remember that hypocalcemia causes a prolonged ST or QT interval. If you had difficulty with this question, review the ECG changes that occur in these conditions.
Level of Cognitive Ability: Analysis
Client Needs: Physiological Integrity
Integrated Concept/Process: Nursing Process/Analysis
Content Area: Fundamental Skills
Reference: Ignatavicius, D., Workman, M., & Mishler, M. (1999). *Medical-surgical nursing across the health care continuum* (3rd ed.). Philadelphia: W.B. Saunders, pp. 244, 256, 259.

19. **2**
Rationale: The normal magnesium level is 1.6 to 2.6 mg/dL. A magnesium level of 1.0 mg/dL indicates hypomagnesemia. In hypomagnesemia, the nurse would note tall T waves and a depressed ST segment. Options 3 and 4 would be noted in a client experiencing hypermagnesemia. Prominent U waves are seen in hypokalemia.
Test-Taking Strategy: First it is necessary to determine that the client is experiencing hypomagnesemia. Next, identify the ECG changes that occur in this condition. If you had difficulty with this question, review the normal magnesium level and the ECG changes that occur in both hypomagnesemia and hypermagnesemia.
Level of Cognitive Ability: Analysis
Client Needs: Physiological Integrity
Integrated Concept/Process: Nursing Process/Analysis
Content Area: Fundamental Skills
Reference: Ignatavicius, D., Workman, M., & Mishler, M. (1999). *Medical-surgical nursing across the health care continuum* (3rd ed.). Philadelphia: W.B. Saunders, pp. 262-263.

20. **1**
Rationale: The normal serum phosphorus level is 2.7 to 4.5 mg/dL. The client is experiencing hypophosphatemia. Causative factors relate to malnutrition or starvation, and the use of aluminum hydroxide–based or magnesium-based antacids. Malnutrition is associated with alcoholism. Hypoparathyroidism, renal insufficiency, and tumor lysis syndrome are causative factors of hyperphosphatemia.
Test-Taking Strategy: First it is necessary to determine that the client is experiencing hypophosphatemia. From this point, it is necessary to know the causes of hypophosphatemia. If you had difficulty with this question, review the causative factors associated with hypophosphatemia.
Level of Cognitive Ability: Analysis
Client Needs: Physiological Integrity
Integrated Concept/Process: Nursing Process/Analysis
Content Area: Fundamental Skills
Reference: Ignatavicius, D., Workman, M., & Mishler, M. (1999). *Medical-surgical nursing across the health care continuum* (3rd ed.). Philadelphia: W.B. Saunders, p. 260.

CRITICAL THINKING: FREE-TEXT ENTRY

Answer: The normal serum calcium level is 8.6 to 10.0 mg/dL; therefore a level of 12.0 mg/dL is high.
Rationale: The normal serum calcium level is 8.6 to 10.0 mg/dL. This client is experiencing hypercalcemia.
Test-Taking Strategy: It is necessary to know the normal serum calcium level to answer this question. If you are unfamiliar with this level, review and learn it.
Level of Cognitive Ability: Comprehension
Client Needs: Physiological Integrity
Integrated Concept/Process: Nursing Process/Assessment
Content Area: Fundamental Skills
Reference: Ignatavicius, D., Workman, M., & Mishler, M. (1999). *Medical-surgical nursing across the health care continuum* (3rd ed.). Philadelphia: W.B. Saunders, p. 258.

REFERENCES

Ignatavicius, D., Workman, M., & Mishler, M. (1999). *Medical-surgical nursing across the health care continuum* (3rd ed.). Philadelphia: W.B. Saunders.

LeMone, P., & Burke, K. (2000). *Medical-surgical nursing: Critical thinking in client care* (2nd ed.). Upper Saddle River, NJ: Prentice-Hall.

Lewis, S., Heitkemper, M., & Dirksen, S. (2000). *Medical-surgical nursing: Assessment and management of clinical problems* (5th ed.). St. Louis: Mosby.

Phipps, W., Sands, J., & Marek, J. (1999). *Medical-surgical nursing: Concepts & clinical practice* (6th ed.). St. Louis: Mosby.

Smeltzer, S., & Bare, B. (2000) *Textbook of medical-surgical nursing* (9th ed). Philadelphia: Lippincott Williams & Wilkins.

Acid-Base Balance

PYRAMID TERMS

Allen test   Testing for collateral circulation to the hand by evaluating the patency of the radial and ulnar arteries.

respiratory acidosis   The total concentration of buffer base is lower than normal, with a relative increasing hydrogen ion (H^+) concentration; thus a greater number of H^+ ions are circulating in the blood than can be absorbed by the buffer system. Caused by primary defects in the function of the lungs or by changes in normal respiratory patterns as a result of secondary problems. Any condition that causes an obstruction of the airway or depresses respiratory status can cause respiratory acidosis.

respiratory alkalosis   A deficit of carbonic acid (H_2CO_3) or a decease in H^+ concentration. Results from the accumulation of base or from a loss of acid without a comparable loss of base in the body fluids. Due to conditions that cause overstimulation of the respiratory status.

metabolic acidosis   The total concentration of buffer base is lower than normal, with a relative increase in the H^+ concentration. It occurs as a result of losing buffer bases or retaining too many acids without sufficient bases. It occurs in conditions such as renal failure and diabetic ketoacidosis, from the production of lactic acid, and from the ingestion of toxins, such as aspirin.

metabolic alkalosis   A deficit or loss of H^+ or acids or an excess of base (bicarbonate). Results from the accumulation of base or from a loss of acid without a comparable loss of base in the body fluids. Caused by conditions resulting in hypovolemia, the loss of gastric fluid, excessive bicarbonate intake, the massive transfusion of whole blood, and hyperaldosteronism.

PYRAMID TO SUCCESS

Acid-base imbalance is a content area that is sometimes viewed as complex and difficult to understand. It is important to understand the description of each imbalance and then review the causes of each disorder, correlating the pathophysiology with each cause. From this point, note the assessment signs related to each disorder and the treatment associated with the clinical manifestations. Maintenance of a patent airway is a priority. The nurse also needs to monitor vital signs, neurological status, intake and output, laboratory values, and arterial blood gas values. Safety and seizure precautions need to be initiated. The primary Integrated Concepts and Processes addressed in this chapter are Nursing Process, Communication and Documentation, Self-Care, and Teaching/Learning.

CLIENT NEEDS
Safe, Effective Care Environment

Accident prevention
Establishing priorities
Informed consent for invasive procedures
Medical and surgical asepsis
Providing safety to the client during implementation of various treatments for the acid-base imbalance
Standard (universal) precautions

Health Promotion and Maintenance

Client and family education about prevention, early detection, and treatment measures for health disorders
Disease prevention
Health and wellness
Identifying clients at risk for an acid-base imbalance
Techniques of physical assessment

Psychosocial Integrity

Emotional support of the client and family
Sensory/perceptual alterations
Support systems
Therapeutic interactions

Physiological Integrity

Administering and monitoring medications, IV fluids, and other therapeutic interventions

Alterations in body systems

Basic care and comfort

Diagnostic tests

Expected effects of pharmacological and parenteral therapies

Laboratory values

Medical emergencies

Monitoring for changes in status and for complications

Obtaining arterial blood gas (ABG) values

Providing wound care when blood is obtained for an ABG study

Reducing the likelihood that an acid-base imbalance will occur

---

I. HYDROGEN IONS, ACIDS, AND BASES

A. Hydrogen ions (H^+)
  1. Vital to life
  2. Expressed as pH
  3. Circulate in the body in two forms:
     a. Volatile hydrogen of carbonic acid
     b. Nonvolatile form of hydrogen and organic acids
B. Acids
  1. Produced as end products of metabolism
  2. Contain hydrogen ions
  3. Hydrogen ion donors, which means that acids give up H^+ to neutralize or decrease the strength of an acid or to form a weaker base
  4. The strength of an acid is determined by the number of hydrogen ions it contains
  5. The number of hydrogen ions in body fluid determines its acidity, alkalinity, or neutrality
  6. The lungs excrete 13,000 to 30,000 mEq of volatile hydrogen per day in the form of carbonic acid (H_2CO_3) as carbon dioxide (CO_2)
  7. The kidneys excrete 50 mEq of nonvolatile acids per day
C. Bases
  1. Contain no H^+; hydrogen ion acceptors
  2. Accept H^+ from acids to neutralize or decrease the strength of a base or to form a weaker acid

II. REGULATORY SYSTEMS FOR HYDROGEN ION CONCENTRATION IN THE BLOOD

A. Buffers
  1. The fastest-acting regulatory system
  2. Provide immediate protection against changes in H^+ concentration in the extracellular fluid
  3. Reactors that function only to keep the pH within the narrow limits of stability when too much acid or base is released into the system
  4. Absorb or release H^+ as needed

  5. Serve as a transport mechanism that carries excess H^+ to the lungs
  6. Once the primary buffer systems react, they are consumed, and this leaves the body less able to withstand further stress until they are replaced
B. Primary buffer systems in extracellular fluid
  1. Hemoglobin (Hgb) system
     a. In the red blood cells (RBCs)
     b. Maintains acid-base balance by a process called chloride shift
     c. Chloride shifts in and out of the cells in response to the level of oxygen (O_2) in the blood
     d. For each chloride ion that leaves an RBC, a bicarbonate ion enters
     e. For each chloride ion that enters an RBC, a bicarbonate ion leaves
  2. Plasma proteins system
     a. Functions in conjunction with the liver to vary the amount of H^+ in the chemical structure of protein
     b. Plasma proteins have the ability to attract or release H^+
  3. Carbonic acid/bicarbonate system
     a. Maintains a pH of 7.4 with a ratio of 20 parts bicarbonate to 1 part carbonic acid (20:1)
     b. This ratio (20:1) determines H^+ concentration of body fluid
     c. Carbonic acid concentration is controlled by the excretion of CO_2 by the lungs; the rate and depth of respiration change in response to changes in CO_2
     d. Bicarbonate concentration is controlled by the kidneys, which selectively retain or secrete bicarbonates in response to the body needs
  4. Phosphate Buffer System
     a. Present in the cells and body fluids
     b. Especially active in the kidneys
     c. Acts like bicarbonate and clears spare H^+
C. Lungs
  1. Body's second defense that interacts with the buffer system to maintain acid-base balance
  2. In acidosis, the pH goes down and the respiratory rate and depth go up in an attempt to blow off acids; the carbonic acid created by the neutralizing action of bicarbonate can be carried to the lungs, where it is reduced to CO_2 and water and exhaled; thus H^+ are inactivated and excreted
  3. In alkalosis, the pH goes up and the respiratory rate and depth go down; the CO_2 is retained, and the carbonic acid builds to neutralize and decrease the strength of excess bicarbonate
  4. The action of the lungs is reversible in controlling an excess or deficit
  5. The lungs can hold H^+ until the deficit is corrected or can inactivate H^+, changing them to water molecules to be exhaled as CO_2, thus correcting the excess

6. The process of correcting a deficit or excess takes 10 to 30 seconds to complete
7. The lungs are capable of inactivating only H⁺ carried by H_2CO_3; excess H⁺ created by other problems must be excreted by the kidneys

D. Kidneys
1. The ultimate correction of acid-base disturbances is dependent on the kidneys, even though the renal excretion of acids and alkali occurs more slowly
2. Compensation requires a few hours to several days; however, it is more thorough and selective than that of other regulators
3. In acidosis, the pH goes down, and excess H⁺ are secreted into the tubules and combine with buffers for excretion in the urine
4. In alkalosis, the pH goes up, and bicarbonate ions move into the tubules, combine with sodium, and are excreted in the urine
5. Selective regulation of bicarbonate in the kidneys
   a. The kidneys restore bicarbonate by the release of H⁺ and by holding bicarbonate ions
   b. Extra H+ are excreted in the urine in the form of phosphoric acid
   c. The alteration of certain amino acids in the renal tubules results in a diffusion of ammonia into the kidneys, and the ammonia combines with extra H⁺ and is excreted in the urine

▲ E. Potassium
1. Plays an exchange role in maintaining acid-base balance
2. The body changes the potassium (K) level by drawing H⁺ into the cell or by pushing them out of the cell
▲ 3. The K level changes to compensate for H⁺ level changes
   a. In acidosis, the body protects itself from the acid state by moving H⁺ into the cell; therefore, K moves out to make room for H⁺; the serum K level goes up
   b. In alkalosis, the cells release H⁺ into the blood in an attempt to increase the acidity of the blood and combat alkalinity; the K moves into the cells, and the serum K level goes down

▲ **III. RESPIRATORY ACIDOSIS**
A. Description: The total concentration of buffer base is lower than normal, with a relative increasing H⁺ concentration; thus, a greater number of H⁺ are circulating in the blood than can be absorbed by the buffer system
B. Causes
1. Due to primary defects in the function of the lungs or changes in normal respiratory patterns
2. Any condition that causes an obstruction of the airway or depresses respiratory status can cause **respiratory acidosis**

3. Hypoventilation: Carbon dioxide (CO_2) is retained and the H⁺ increase, leading to the acid state; carbonic acid is retained and the pH goes down
4. Medications: Sedatives, narcotics, and anesthetics depress the respiratory center, leading to hypoventilation; carbon dioxide is retained and the H⁺ increases
5. Bronchitis: Inflammation causes airway obstruction, resulting in inadequate oxygenation
6. Atelectasis: Excessive mucus collection, with the collapse of alveolar sacs caused by mucus plugs, infectious drainage, or anesthetic medications, results in decreased respirations
7. Brain trauma: Excessive pressure on the respiratory center or medulla oblongata depresses respirations
8. Emphysema: Loss of elasticity of alveolar sacs restricts air flow in and out, primarily out, leading to an increased CO_2 level
9. Asthma: Spasms resulting from allergens, irritants, or emotions cause the smooth muscles of the bronchioles to constrict
10. Pulmonary edema: Extracellular accumulation of fluid in acute congestive heart failure (CHF) causes disturbances in alveolar diffusion and perfusion
11. Bronchiectasis: Bronchi become dilated as a result of inflammation, and destructive changes and weakness in the walls of the bronchi occur

C. Assessment
1. In an attempt to compensate, the respiratory ▲ rate and depth increase
2. Headache
3. Restlessness
4. Mental status changes, such as drowsiness and confusion
5. Visual disturbances
6. Diaphoresis
7. Cyanosis as the hypoxia becomes more acute
8. Hyperkalemia ▲
9. Rapid, irregular pulse
10. Dysrhythmias leading to ventricular fibrillation

D. Implementation
1. Monitor for signs of respiratory distress
2. Administer oxygen as prescribed
3. Place client in semi-Fowler's position unless contraindicated
4. Encourage and assist the client to turn, cough, and deep breathe
5. Prepare to administer respiratory treatments as prescribed
6. Encourage hydration to thin secretions unless excess fluid intake is contraindicated
7. Suction client if necessary
8. Reduce restlessness by improving ventilation rather than by the administration of tranquiliz-

ers, sedatives, or narcotics, because they further depress respirations

9. Monitor electrolyte values, particularly the K level
10. Administer antibiotics for infection or other medications as prescribed

IV. RESPIRATORY ALKALOSIS

A. Description: A deficit of H_2CO_3 and a decrease in H^+ concentration; results from the accumulation of base or from a loss of acid without a comparable loss of base in the body fluids
B. Causes
   1. Due to conditions that cause overstimulation of the respiratory status
   2. Hyperventilation: Rapid respirations cause the blowing off of CO_2, leading to a decrease in H_2CO_3
   3. Hysteria: Often neurogenic in nature and related to a psychoneurosis; however, this condition leads to vigorous breathing and excessive exhaling of CO_2
   4. Overventilation by mechanical ventilators: The administration of O_2 and the depletion of CO_2 can occur from mechanical ventilation; the client may be hyperventilated
   5. Conditions that increase metabolism, such as fever
   6. Pain or brain trauma: Causes overstimulation of the respiratory center in the brainstem, with resultant carbonic acid deficit
   7. Salicylates: Stimulate the respiratory center, causing hyperventilation
   8. Hypoxia: Causes respiratory stimulation with resultant carbonic acid deficit
C. Assessment
   1. Initially the hyperventilation and respiratory stimulation will cause abnormal rapid respirations (tachypnea); in an attempt to compensate, respiratory rate and depth then go down
   2. Headache
   3. Lightheadedness, vertigo
   4. Mental status changes
   5. Paresthesias, such as tingling of the fingers and toes
   6. Hypokalemia, hypocalcemia
   7. Tetany, convulsions
D. Implementation
   1. Provide emotional support and reassurance to the client
   2. Encourage appropriate breathing patterns
   3. Assist with breathing techniques and breathing aids as prescribed
      a. Voluntary holding of breath
      b. Rebreathe exhaled CO_2
      c. Rebreathing mask as prescribed
      d. Carbon dioxide breaths as prescribed

4. Provide cautious care with ventilator clients so that they are not forced to take breaths too deeply or rapidly
5. Monitor electrolyte values, particularly K and calcium levels
6. Administer medications as prescribed
7. Prepare to administer calcium gluconate for tetany as prescribed

V. METABOLIC ACIDOSIS

A. Description: The total concentration of buffer base is lower than normal, with a relative increase in the H^+ concentration; occurs as a result of losing too many bases and holding too many acids without sufficient bases
B. Causes
   1. Diabetes mellitus/diabetic ketoacidosis: An insufficient supply of insulin causes increased fat metabolism, leading to an excess accumulation of ketones or other acids; the bicarbonate then ends up being exhausted
   2. Renal insufficiency/failure
      a. Increased waste products of protein metabolism are retained
      b. Excessive acids build up, and bicarbonate is unable to maintain acid-base balance
   3. Insufficient metabolism of carbohydrates: When an insufficient supply of O_2 is available for the proper burning of carbohydrates, glucose, and water, lactic acid increases and lactic acidosis results
   4. Excessive ingestion of acetylsalicylic acid (aspirin): Causes an increase in the H^+ concentration
   5. Severe diarrhea: Intestinal and pancreatic secretions are normally alkaline; therefore, excessive loss of base leads to acidosis
   6. Malnutrition: Improper metabolism of nutrients causes fat catabolism, leading to an excess build-up of ketones and acids
   7. High-fat diet: A high intake of fat causes a much too rapid accumulation of the waste products of fat metabolism, leading to a build-up of ketones and acids
C. Assessment
   1. In an attempt to blow off the extra CO_2 and compensate for the acidosis, hyperpnea with Kussmaul's respirations occurs
   2. Headache
   3. Nausea, vomiting, diarrhea
   4. Fruity-smelling breath as a result of improper fat metabolism
   5. Central nervous system depression: mental dullness, drowsiness, stupor, coma
   6. Twitching, convulsions
   7. Hyperkalemia
D. Implementation
   1. Assess level of consciousness (LOC) for central nervous system (CNS) depression

2. Monitor I & O and assist with fluid and electrolyte replacement as prescribed
3. Prepare to administer IV solutions such as normal saline, 5% dextrose and ½ normal saline, sodium lactate, or bicarbonate to increase the buffer base
4. Initiate safety and seizure precautions
5. Monitor the serum K level closely; when acidosis is being treated, K will move back into the cell and the serum K level will drop

E. Implementation in diabetes mellitus/diabetic keto-acidosis
1. Insulin is given to hasten the movement of serum glucose into the cell, thereby decreasing the concurrent ketosis
2. When glucose is being properly metabolized, the body will stop converting fats to glucose
3. Monitor for circulatory collapse caused by polyuria, which may result from the hyperglycemic state, because polyuria or diuresis may lead to extracellular volume deficit

F. Implementation in renal failure
1. In renal failure, dialysis may be used to remove protein and waste products, thereby lessening the acidosis state
2. A diet low in protein and high in calories will decrease the amount of protein waste products resulting from protein catabolism; this in turn will lessen the acidosis

▲ VI. METABOLIC ALKALOSIS

A. Description: A deficit of H_2CO_3 and a decease in hydrogen ion concentration; results from the accumulation of base or from a loss of acid without a comparable loss of base in the body fluids

B. Causes
1. Results from a malfunction of metabolism leading to an increased amount of available basic solution in the blood and a decrease in available acids in the blood
2. Ingestion of excess sodium bicarbonate: Causes an increase in the amount of base in the blood
▲ 3. Excessive vomiting or gastrointestinal suctioning: Leads to an excessive loss of acids
▲ 4. Diuretics: The loss of H^+ and chloride causes a compensatory increase in the bicarbonate in the blood
5. Hyperaldosteronism: Increased renal tubular reabsorption of sodium occurs, with the resultant loss of hydrogen ions
6. Massive transfusion of whole blood: The citrate anticoagulant used for the storage of blood is metabolized to bicarbonate

C. Assessment
▲ 1. In an attempt to compensate, respiratory rate and depth go down to conserve CO_2
2. Nausea, vomiting, diarrhea

3. Restlessness
4. Numbness and tingling in the extremities
5. Twitching in the extremities
6. Hypokalemia
7. Hypocalcemia
8. Dysrhythmias: tachycardia

D. Implementation
1. Monitor potassium and calcium serum blood levels
2. Institute safety precautions
3. Prepare to administer medications as prescribed to promote the kidney excretion of bicarbonate
4. Prepare to replace potassium chloride as prescribed

VII. ARTERIAL BLOOD GASES (Box 9-1) ▲

A. Obtaining an arterial blood gas specimen
1. Obtain vital signs
2. Determine whether the client has an arterial line in place
3. Perform the **Allen test** to determine the presence of collateral circulation (Box 9-2)
4. Assess factors that may affect the accuracy of the results, such as changes in the O_2 settings, suctioning within the last 20 minutes, and client activities
5. Provide emotional support to the client
6. Assist with the specimen draw by preparing a heparinized syringe
7. Apply pressure immediately to the puncture site ▲ following the blood draw; maintain pressure for 5 minutes, or for 10 minutes if the client is taking anticoagulants

---

BOX 9-1

Normal Blood Gas Values

pH 7.35-7.45
Pco_2 35-45 mm Hg
HCO_3 22-27 mEq/L
Po_2 80-100 mm Hg

BOX 9-2

Performing the Allen Test

Apply direct pressure over the client's ulnar and radial arteries simultaneously

While pressure is applied, ask the client to open and close the hand repeatedly; the hand should blanch

Release pressure from the ulnar artery while compressing the radial artery and assess the color of the extremity distal to the pressure point

If pinkness fails to return within 6 seconds, the ulnar artery is insufficient, indicating that the radial artery should not be used for obtaining a blood specimen

BOX 9-3

Analyzing Arterial Blood Gas Results

If you can remember the following pyramid points and steps, you will be able to analyze any blood gas report!

PYRAMID POINTS
In acidosis, the pH is down.
In alkalosis, the pH is up.
The respiratory function indicator is the Pco_2.
The metabolic function indicator is the HCO_3.

PYRAMID STEPS
Pyramid Step 1
Look at the blood gas report. Look at the pH. Is it up or down? If it is up, it reflects alkalosis. If it is down, it reflects acidosis.
Pyramid Step 2
Look at the Pco_2. Is it up or down? If it reflects an opposite response to the pH, then you know that the condition is a respiratory imbalance. If it does not reflect an opposite response to the pH, then move on to Pyramid Step 3.
Pyramid Step 3
Look at the HCO_3. Does the HCO_3 reflect a corresponding response with the pH? If it does, then the condition is a metabolic imbalance.
Pyramid Step 4
Remember, compensation has occurred if the pH is in a normal range of 7.35-7.45. If the pH is not within normal range, look at the respiratory or metabolic function indicators.
Respiratory Imbalances:
If the condition is a respiratory imbalance, look at the HCO_3 to determine the state of compensation.
If the HCO_3 is normal, then the condition is uncompensated. If the HCO_3 is abnormal, then the condition is partial compensation.
Metabolic Imbalances:
If the condition is a metabolic imbalance, look at the Pco_2 to determine the state of compensation.
If the Pco_2 is normal, then the condition is uncompensated. If the Pco_2 is abnormal, then the condition is partial compensation.

8. Appropriately label the specimen, and transport it on ice to the laboratory
9. On the laboratory form, record the client's temperature and the type of supplemental oxygen that the client is receiving
B. Respiratory imbalances
   1. Remember, the respiratory function indicator is the Pco_2
   2. In a respiratory imbalance, you will find an opposite response between the pH and the Pco_2; in other words, the pH will be up with a Pco_2 down (alkalosis), or the pH will be down with an elevated Pco_2 (acidosis)
   3. Look at the pH and the Pco_2 to determine if the condition is a respiratory problem

4. **Respiratory acidosis:** The pH is down; the Pco_2 is up
5. **Respiratory alkalosis:** The pH is up; the Pco_2 is down
C. Metabolic imbalances
   1. Remember, the metabolic function indicator is the bicarbonate (HCO_3)
   2. In a metabolic imbalance, you will find a corresponding response between the pH and the HCO_3; in other words, the pH will be up and the HCO_3 will be up (alkalosis), or the pH will be down and the HCO_3 will be down (acidosis)
   3. Look at the pH and the HCO_3 to determine if the condition is a metabolic problem
   4. **Metabolic acidosis:** The pH is down; the HCO_3 is down
   5. **Metabolic alkalosis:** The pH is up; the HCO_3 is up
D. Compensation
   1. **Respiratory acidosis** and **respiratory alkalosis**
      a. When compensation has occurred, the pH will be within normal limits
      b. The blood gas result reflects partial compensation if the HCO_3 is abnormal
      c. The blood gas result reflects an uncompensated condition if the HCO_3 is normal
   2. **Metabolic acidosis** and **metabolic alkalosis**
      a. When compensation has occurred, the pH will be within normal limits
      b. The blood gas result reflects partial compensation if the Pco_2 is abnormal
      c. The blood gas result reflects an uncompensated condition if the Pco_2 is normal
E. Analyzing arterial blood gas results (Box 9-3)

PRACTICE QUESTIONS

1. A nurse plans care for a client with chronic obstructive pulmonary disease (COPD) knowing that the client is most likely to experience what type of acid-base imbalance?
   1. Respiratory acidosis
   2. Respiratory alkalosis
   3. Metabolic acidosis
   4. Metabolic alkalosis
2. A nurse reviews the blood gas results of a client with Guillain-Barré syndrome. The nurse analyzes the results and determines that the client is experiencing respiratory acidosis. Which of the following validates the nurse's findings?
   1. pH 7.50, Pco_2 52 mm Hg
   2. pH 7.35, Pco_2 40 mm Hg
   3. pH 7.25, Pco_2 50 mm Hg
   4. pH 7.50, Pco_2 30 mm Hg
3. A nurse is caring for a client who is on a mechanical ventilator. Blood gas results indicate a pH of 7.50 and a Pco_2 of 30 mm Hg. The nurse has

determined that the client is experiencing respiratory alkalosis. Which laboratory value would most likely be noted in this condition?
1. Sodium level of 145 mEq/L
2. Potassium level of 3.0 mEq/L
3. Magnesium level of 2.0 mg/dL
4. Phosphorus level of 4.0 mg/dL

4. A nurse reviews the arterial blood gas results of a client and notes the following: pH of 7.45, P_{CO_2} of 30 mm Hg, and HCO_3 of 22 mEq/L. The nurse analyzes these results as indicating:
1. Metabolic acidosis, compensated
2. Metabolic alkalosis, uncompensated
3. Respiratory alkalosis, compensated
4. Respiratory acidosis, uncompensated

5. A client is scheduled for blood to be drawn from the radial artery for an arterial blood gas (ABG) determination. Before the blood is drawn, an Allen test is performed to determine the adequacy of the:
1. Popliteal circulation
2. Ulnar circulation
3. Femoral circulation
4. Carotid circulation

6. A nurse is caring for a client with a nasogastric tube that is attached to low suction. The nurse monitors the client, knowing that the client is at risk for which acid-base disorder?
1. Respiratory acidosis
2. Respiratory alkalosis
3. Metabolic acidosis
4. Metabolic alkalosis

7. A nurse caring for a client with an ileostomy understands that the client is at most risk for developing which acid-base disorder?
1. Respiratory acidosis
2. Respiratory alkalosis
3. Metabolic acidosis
4. Metabolic alkalosis

8. A nurse is caring for a client with diabetic ketoacidosis and documents that the client is experiencing Kussmaul's respirations. Based on this documentation, which of the following did the nurse observe?
1. Respirations that are abnormally deep, regular, and increased in rate
2. Respirations that are regular but abnormally slow
3. Respirations that are labored and increased in depth and rate
4. Respirations that cease for several seconds

9. A nurse understands that the excessive use of oral antacids containing bicarbonate can result in which acid-base disturbance?
1. Respiratory alkalosis
2. Respiratory acidosis
3. Metabolic acidosis
4. Metabolic alkalosis

10. A nurse is caring for a client with renal failure. Blood gas results indicate a pH of 7.30, a P_{CO_2} of 32 mm Hg, and an HCO_3 of 20 mEq/L. The nurse has determined that the client is experiencing metabolic acidosis. Which of the following laboratory values would the nurse expect to note?
1. Sodium level of 145 mEq/L
2. Magnesium level of 2.0 mg/dL
3. Potassium level of 5.2 mEq/L
4. Phosphorus level of 4.0 mg/dL

CRITICAL THINKING: FREE-TEXT ENTRY

A nurse reviews the arterial blood gas (ABG) results of an assigned client and notes that the laboratory report indicates a pH of 7.30, P_{CO_2} of 58 mm Hg, P_{O_2} of 80 mm Hg, and HCO_3 of 27 mEq/L. The nurse interprets that the client has which acid-base disturbance?

Answer: _____

ANSWERS

1. **1**

Rationale: Respiratory acidosis is most often due to hypoventilation. Chronic respiratory acidosis is most commonly caused by COPD. In end-stage disease, pathological changes lead to airway collapse, air trapping, and disturbance of ventilation-perfusion (V/Q) relationships. Options 2, 3, and 4 are incorrect options.

Test-Taking Strategy: Use the process of elimination. Note the key words "most likely." Remembering that hypoventilation results in respiratory acidosis will direct you to option 1. Review the causes of respiratory acidosis if you had difficulty with this question.

Level of Cognitive Ability: Analysis

Client Needs: Physiological Integrity

Integrated Concept/Process: Nursing Process/Analysis

Content Area: Fundamental Skills

Reference: Lewis, S., Heitkemper, M., & Dirksen, S. (2000). *Medical-surgical nursing: Assessment and management of clinical problems* (5th ed.). St. Louis: Mosby, p. 344.

2. **3**

Rationale: The normal pH is 7.35 to 7.45. The normal P_{CO_2} is 35 to 45 mm Hg. In respiratory acidosis, the pH is down and the P_{CO_2} is up. Option 1 identifies an alkalotic condition. Option 2 identifies normal values. Option 4 identifies respiratory alkalosis.

Test-Taking Strategy: Use the process of elimination. Remember that in a respiratory imbalance you will find an opposite

response between the pH and the PCO$_2$. Also remember that the pH is down in an acidotic condition. Options 1 and 4 reflect an elevated pH, which indicates an alkalotic condition. Option 2 reflects a normal blood gas result. Option 3 is the only option that reflects an acidotic condition. Review blood gas analysis if you had difficulty with this question.
Level of Cognitive Ability: Analysis
Client Needs: Physiological Integrity
Integrated Concept/Process: Nursing Process/Assessment
Content Area: Fundamental Skills
Reference: Smeltzer, S., & Bare, B. (2000). *Textbook of medical-surgical nursing* (9th ed.). Philadelphia: Lippincott Williams & Wilkins, pp. 232-234.

3. 2
Rationale: Clinical manifestations of respiratory alkalosis include headache, tachypnea, paresthesias, tetany, vertigo, convulsions, hypokalemia, and hypocalcemia. Options 1, 3, and 4 identify normal laboratory values. Option 2 identifies the presence of hypokalemia.
Test-Taking Strategy: Use the process of elimination and knowledge regarding the clinical manifestations of respiratory alkalosis and normal laboratory values to answer the question. The only abnormal laboratory value is the potassium level, option 2. Review the clinical manifestations of respiratory alkalosis and normal laboratory values if you had difficulty with this question.
Level of Cognitive Ability: Analysis
Client Needs: Physiological Integrity
Integrated Concept/Process: Nursing Process/Assessment
Content Area: Fundamental Skills
Reference: Phipps, W., Sands, J., & Marek, J. (1999). *Medical-surgical nursing: Concepts & clinical practice* (6th ed.). St. Louis: Mosby, p. 437.

4. 3
Rationale: The normal pH is 7.35 to 7.45. In respiratory condition, an opposite effect will be seen between the pH and the PCO$_2$. In this situation, the pH is at the high end of the normal value and the PCO$_2$ is low. In an alkalotic condition, the pH is up. Therefore, the values identified in the question indicate a respiratory alkalosis. Compensation occurs when the pH returns to a normal value. Since the pH is in the normal range at the high end, compensation has occurred.
Test-Taking Strategy: Remember that in a respiratory imbalance you will find an opposite response between the pH and the PCO$_2$ as indicated in the question. Therefore, options 1 and 2 can be eliminated. Also remember that the pH is up in an alkalotic condition and compensation occurs as evidenced by a normal pH. Option 3 reflects a respiratory alkalotic condition and compensation, and describes the blood gas values as indicated in the question. Review the steps related to reading blood gas values if you had difficulty with this question.
Level of Cognitive Ability: Analysis
Client Needs: Physiological Integrity
Integrated Concept/Process: Nursing Process/Analysis
Content Area: Fundamental Skills
Reference: LeMone, P., & Burke, K. (2000). *Medical-surgical nursing: Critical thinking in client care* (2nd ed.). Upper Saddle River, NJ: Prentice-Hall, p. 153.

5. 2
Rationale: Before radial puncture for obtaining an arterial specimen for ABGs, an Allen test should be performed to determine adequate ulnar circulation. Failure to determine the presence of adequate collateral circulation could result is severe ischemic injury to the hand, if damage to the radial artery occurs with arterial puncture. Options 1, 3, and 4 are incorrect options.
Test-Taking Strategy: Use the process of elimination and knowledge regarding the purpose and procedure for the Allen test. Remember that the purpose of this test is to assess the adequacy of the ulnar circulation. Review the purpose and procedure of the Allen test if you had difficulty with this question.
Level of Cognitive Ability: Comprehension
Client Needs: Physiological Integrity
Integrated Concept/Process: Nursing Process/Assessment
Content Area: Fundamental Skills
Reference: Lewis, S., Heitkemper, M., & Dirksen, S. (2000). *Medical-surgical nursing: Assessment and management of clinical problems* (5th ed.). St. Louis: Mosby, p. 1920.

6. 4
Rationale: Loss of gastric fluid via nasogastric suction or vomiting causes metabolic alkalosis as a result of the loss of hydrochloric acid. Options 1, 2, and 3 are incorrect.
Test-Taking Strategy: Remembering that hydrochloric acid is lost when the client is on nasogastric suction will direct you to the option identifying an alkalotic condition. Since the question addresses a situation other than a respiratory one, the acid-base disorder would be a metabolic condition. If you had difficulty with this question, review the causes of metabolic alkalosis.
Level of Cognitive Ability: Analysis
Client Needs: Physiological Integrity
Integrated Concept/Process: Nursing Process/Analysis
Content Area: Fundamental Skills
Reference: Ignatavicius, D., Workman, M., & Mishler, M. (1999). *Medical-surgical nursing across the health care continuum* (3rd ed.). Philadelphia: W.B. Saunders, p. 301.

7. 3
Rationale: Intestinal secretions high in bicarbonate may be lost through enteric drainage tubes or an ileostomy or with diarrhea. These conditions result in metabolic acidosis. Options 1, 2, and 4 are incorrect because they do not occur in the client with an ileostomy.
Test-Taking Strategy: Use the process of elimination. Note that the client's condition described in the question is a gastrointestinal disorder. This will direct you toward a metabolic disorder. Remembering that intestinal fluids are primarily alkaline will assist you in selecting the correct option. When excess bicarbonate is lost, acidosis will result. If you had difficulty with this question, review the causes of metabolic acidosis.
Level of Cognitive Ability: Analysis
Client Needs: Physiological Integrity
Integrated Concept/Process: Nursing Process/Analysis
Content Area: Fundamental Skills
Reference: LeMone, P., & Burke, K. (2000). *Medical-surgical nursing: Critical thinking in client care* (2nd ed.). Upper Saddle Rver, NJ: Prentice-Hall, p. 133.

8. 1

Rationale: Kussmaul's respirations are abnormally deep, regular, and increased in rate. In bradypnea, respirations are regular but abnormally slow. In hyperpnea, respirations are labored and increased in depth and rate. Apnea is described as respirations that cease for several seconds.

Test-Taking Strategy: Use the process of elimination and knowledge of the description of Kussmaul's respirations. Recalling that this type of respiration occurs in diabetic ketoacidosis will easily direct you to option 1. Review the characteristics of this type of respiration if you had difficulty with this question.

Level of Cognitive Ability: Comprehension

Client Needs: Physiological Integrity

Integrated Concept/Process: Communication and Documentation

Content Area: Fundamental Skills

Reference: Lewis, S., Heitkemper, M., & Dirksen, S. (2000). *Medical-surgical nursing: Assessment and management of clinical problems* (5th ed.). St. Louis: Mosby, p. 569.

9. 4

Rationale: Increases in base components occur as a result of oral or parenteral intake of bicarbonates, carbonates, acetates, citrates, or lactates. Excessive use of oral antacids containing bicarbonate can cause a metabolic alkalosis. Options 1, 2, and 3 are incorrect.

Test-Taking Strategy: Use the process of elimination. Eliminate options 1 and 2 first because a respiratory condition is not addressed in the question. From the remaining options, remembering that antacids contain bicarbonate and that an excess oral intake will increase bicarbonate will assist in directing you to option 4. Review the causes of metabolic alkalosis if you had difficulty with the question.

Level of Cognitive Ability: Comprehension

Client Needs: Physiological Integrity

Integrated Concept/Process: Nursing Process/Assessment

Content Area: Fundamental Skills

Reference: Ignatavicius, D., Workman, M., & Mishler, M. (1999). *Medical-surgical nursing across the health care continuum* (3rd ed.). Philadelphia: W.B. Saunders, p. 301.

10. 3

Rationale: Clinical manifestations of metabolic acidosis include hyperpnea with Kussmaul's respirations; headache; nausea, vomiting, diarrhea; fruity-smelling breath resulting from improper fat metabolism; central nervous system depression, including mental dullness, drowsiness, stupor, and coma; twitching; and convulsions. Hyperkalemia will occur.

Test-Taking Strategy: Use the process of elimination and knowledge regarding the clinical manifestations of metabolic acidosis and normal laboratory values to answer the question. The only abnormal laboratory value is the potassium level, option 3. Review the clinical manifestations of metabolic acidosis and normal laboratory values if you had difficulty with this question.

Level of Cognitive Ability: Analysis

Client Needs: Physiological Integrity

Integrated Concept/Process: Nursing Process/Assessment

Content Area: Fundamental Skills

Reference: Ignatavicius, D., Workman, M., & Mishler, M. (1999). *Medical-surgical nursing across the health care continuum* (3rd ed.). Philadelphia: W.B. Saunders, p. 299.

CRITICAL THINKING: FREE-TEXT ENTRY

Answer: Respiratory acidosis

Rationale: The normal pH is 7.35 to 7.45. The normal P_{CO_2} is 35 to 45 mm Hg. In respiratory acidosis the pH is low and the P_{CO_2} is elevated.

Test-Taking Strategy: Remember that in a respiratory imbalance you will find an opposite response between the pH and the P_{CO_2}. Also remember that the pH is down in an acidotic condition. Review interpretation of blood gas results if you had difficulty with this question.

Level of Cognitive Ability: Analysis

Client Needs: Physiological Integrity

Integrated Concept/Process: Nursing Process/Analysis

Content Area: Fundamental Skills

Reference: LeMone, P., & Burke, K. (2000). *Medical-surgical nursing: Critical thinking in client care* (2nd ed.). Upper Saddle River, NJ: Prentice-Hall, p. 153.

REFERENCES

Ignatavicius, D., Workman, M., & Mishler, M. (1999). *Medical-surgical nursing across the health care continuum* (3rd ed.). Philadelphia: W.B. Saunders.

LeMone, P., & Burke, K. (2000). *Medical-surgical nursing: Critical thinking in client care* (2nd ed.). Upper Saddle River, NJ: Prentice-Hall.

Lewis, S., Heitkemper, M., & Dirksen, S. (2000). *Medical-surgical nursing: Assessment and management of clinical problems* (5th ed.). St. Louis: Mosby.

Phipps, W., Sands, J., & Marek, J. (1999). *Medical-surgical nursing: Concepts & clinical practice* (6th ed.). St. Louis: Mosby.

Smeltzer, S., & Bare, B. (2000) *Textbook of medical-surgical nursing* (9th ed). Philadelphia: Lippincott Williams & Wilkins.

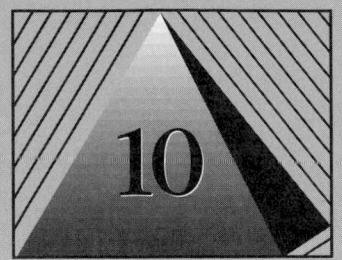

Laboratory Values

10

PYRAMID TERMS

capillary puncture Preferred for a peripheral blood smear

plasma The fluid ground substance; what remains after the cells have been removed from a sample of whole blood

serum Blood plasma from which clotting agents have been removed

venipuncture Puncture into a vein to obtain a blood specimen for testing; the antecubital veins are the veins of choice because of ease of access

▲ PYRAMID TO SUCCESS

This chapter identifies the normal adult values for the most common laboratory tests. If you are familiar with the normal values, you will be able to determine if an abnormality exists when a laboratory value is presented in a question. It is unlikely that a question on NCLEX-RN will simply ask you what a normal value may be. The questions on NCLEX-RN related to laboratory values will require you to identify whether the laboratory value is normal or abnormal, and then you will be required to think critically about the effects of the laboratory value in terms of the client. Pyramid points focus on knowledge of the normal values for the most common laboratory tests, therapeutic serum medication levels of commonly prescribed medications, and determination of the need to implement specific actions based on the findings. Remember that most blood samples should not be drawn during hemodialysis. When a question is presented on NCLEX-RN regarding a specific laboratory value, note the disorder presented in the question and the associated body organ that is affected as a result of the disorder. This process will assist you in determining the correct answer. For example, if the question is asking you about the immune status of a client receiving chemotherapy, assessment of laboratory values will focus on the white

blood cell count and the neutrophils. You are required to analyze these results as possibly being low, and determine the specific client need, which in this case would be the risk for infection. In the client receiving chemotherapy who has a low white blood cell count, your plan centers on the immune system and protecting that client from infection. Implementation focuses on preventive interventions related to infection, perhaps protective isolation measures. Evaluation may focus on maintenance of a normal temperature in the client. The primary Integrated Concepts and Processes addressed in this chapter are Nursing Process, Communication and Documentation, Self-Care, and Teaching/Learning. Box 10-1 lists the abbreviations found in laboratory values.

CLIENT NEEDS
Safe, Effective Care Environment

Informed consent for specific procedures
Verifying the identity of the client
Medical and surgical asepsis
Principles of infection control
Standard (universal) and other precautions

BOX 10-1	
Pyramid Abbreviations	
g/dL	grams per deciliter
μg/dL	micrograms per deciliter
mg/dL	milligrams per deciliter
mEq/L	milliequivalents per liter
U/L	units per liter
mm/hr	millimeters per hour
IU/L	International Units per liter
μg/mL	micrograms per milliliter
ng/mL	nanograms per milliliter
μU/mL	microunits per milliliter
mL/kg	milliliters per kilogram

Procedures for handling hazardous and infectious materials

Health Promotion and Maintenance

Client preparation for laboratory test
Post-test procedures
Signs and symptoms that indicate the need to notify the health care provider
Importance of follow-up laboratory studies
Community resources available for the follow-up

Psychosocial Integrity

Communicate purpose of test to client
Provide emotional support during testing
Identify support systems
Communication with the client regarding laboratory results
Describe specific interventions or home care measures required on the basis of the results

Physiological Integrity

Comfort interventions
Normal values for the most common laboratory tests
Therapeutic serum medication levels of commonly prescribed medications
Reporting significant laboratory values
Determining the need to implement specific actions based on the laboratory results
Monitoring for clinical manifestations associated with an abnormal laboratory value
Monitoring for potential complications related to a test

TABLE 10-1

Normal Adult Electrolyte Values

Sodium	135-145 mEq/L
Potassium	3.5-5.1 mEq/L
Chloride	98-107 mEq/L
Bicarbonate (venous)	22-29 mEq/L

I. **ELECTROLYTES** (Table 10-1)
   A. **Serum** sodium (Na)
      1. Description
         a. A major cation of extracellular fluid
         b. Maintains osmotic pressures and acid-base balance and assists in transmission of nerve impulses
         c. Absorbed from the small intestine and excreted in the urine in amounts dependent on dietary intake
         d. Minimum daily requirement of Na is 15 mEq
      2. Nursing consideration: Drawing blood samples proximal to IV infusion of sodium chloride will falsely elevate results
   B. **Serum** potassium (K)
      1. Description
         a. A major intracellular cation; regulates cellular water balance, electrical conduction in muscle cells, and acid-base balance
         b. The body obtains K through dietary ingestion,
and the kidneys either preserve or excrete K, depending upon cellular need
         c. K levels are used to evaluate cardiac function, renal function, gastrointestinal (GI) function, and the need for IV replacement therapy
      2. Nursing considerations
         a. Use of a tourniquet and pumping the hand prior to venous sampling can increase the value
         b. Do not draw blood from a site where an IV infusion exists
         c. If the client is receiving K, note on the laboratory form
         d. Clients with elevated WBC counts and platelet counts may have falsely elevated K levels
   C. **Serum** chloride
      1. Description
         a. A hydrochloric acid salt that is the most abundant body anion in the extracellular fluid
         b. Functions in counterbalancing cations, such as sodium, and acts as a buffer during oxygen and carbon dioxide exchange in red blood cells
         c. Aids in digestion and maintaining osmotic pressure and water balance
      2. Nursing considerations
         a. Draw blood from an extremity that does not have saline infusing into it
         b. Do not allow the client to clench/unclench the hand prior to blood draw
         c. Any condition accompanied by prolonged vomiting, diarrhea, or both will alter levels

II. **COAGULATION STUDIES**
   A. Activated partial thromboplastin time (aPTT)
      1. Description
         a. Evaluates how well the coagulation sequence is functioning by measuring the amount of time it takes for recalcified, citrated **plasma** to clot after partial thromboplastin is added to it
         b. Screens for deficiencies and inhibitors of all factors except VII and XIII
         c. Most commonly used to monitor heparin therapy and screen for coagulation disorders
      2. Value: 20 to 36 seconds, depending on the type of activator used

3. Nursing considerations
   a. If the client is receiving intermittent heparin therapy, draw sample 1 hour prior to next scheduled dose
   b. Do not draw samples from an arm into which heparin is infusing
   c. Transport specimen to laboratory immediately
   d. The aPTT should be between 1.5 and 2.5 times normal when the client is receiving heparin therapy; if the value is prolonged, initiate bleeding precautions

B. Prothrombin time (PT) and international normalized ratio (INR)
   1. Description
      a. Prothrombin is a vitamin K–dependent glycoprotein, produced by the liver, that is necessary for firm fibrin clot formation
      b. Each laboratory establishes a normal value or control based on the method used to perform the test (PT)
      c. The PT measures the amount of time it takes for clot formation and is used to monitor response to warfarin sodium (Coumadin) therapy or to screen for dysfunction of the extrinsic system resulting from liver disease, vitamin K deficiency, or disseminated intravascular coagulation (DIC)
      d. A PT value within 2 seconds (plus or minus) of the control is considered normal
      e. The INR standardized the PT ratio and is calculated in the laboratory setting by raising the observed PT ratio to the power of the International Sensitivity Index specific to the thromboplastin reagent used
   2. Values
      a. PT: 9.6 to 11.8 seconds (adult male) and 9.5 to 11.3 seconds (adult female)
      b. INR: 2.0 to 3.0 for standard warfarin sodium (Coumadin) therapy
      c. INR: 3.0 to 4.5 for high-dose warfarin sodium (Coumadin) therapy
   3. Nursing considerations
      a. Baseline PT should be drawn before anticoagulation therapy is started
      b. Note time of collection on laboratory form
      c. Provide direct pressure to the site for 3 to 5 minutes if a coagulation defect is present
      d. Concurrent warfarin sodium (Coumadin) therapy with heparin therapy can lengthen PT for up to 5 hours after dosing
      e. Diets high in green leafy vegetables can increase the absorption of vitamin K, which shortens the PT
      f. A PT greater than 30 seconds places the client at risk for hemorrhage

g. Oral anticoagulation therapy usually maintains the PT at 1.5 to 2 times the laboratory control value

C. Clotting time
   1. Description: Measures the time required for the interaction of all factors involved in the clotting process
   2. Value: 8 to 15 minutes
   3. Nursing considerations
      a. The client should not receive heparin therapy for 3 hours prior to specimen collection
      b. The test result is prolonged by any anticoagulant therapy, test tube agitation, or high temperature changes that may affect the specimen

D. Platelet count
   1. Description
      a. Platelets function in hemostatic plug formation, clot retraction, and coagulation factor activation
      b. Platelets are produced by the bone marrow to function in hemostasis
   2. Value: 150,000 to 400,000 cells/μL
   3. Nursing considerations
      a. Monitor the site for bleeding in clients with known thrombocytopenia
      b. High altitudes, chronic cold weather, and exercise increase platelet counts
      c. Bleeding precautions should be instituted in clients with a low platelet count

III. SERUM GASTROINTESTINAL STUDIES

A. Albumin
   1. Description
      a. A main **plasma** protein of blood
      b. Maintains oncotic pressure and transports bilirubin, fatty acids, medications, hormones, and other substances that are insoluble in water
   2. Value: 3.4 to 5 g/dL
   3. Nursing considerations
      a. Draw from an extremity the does not have an IV infusing into it
      b. Instruct the client to consume a low-fat diet on the day of the test

B. Alkaline phosphatase
   1. Description
      a. An enzyme normally found in bone, liver, intestine, and placenta
      b. The level rises during periods of bone growth, liver disease, and bile duct obstruction
   2. Value: 4.5 to 13 King-Armstrong units/dL
   3. Nursing considerations
      a. The client may be requested to fast 10 to 12 hours prior to test
      b. Hepatotoxic medications administered within

12 hours prior to specimen collection invalidate the test

c. Transport specimen to laboratory immediately

C. Ammonia
1. Description
   a. A waste product from nitrogen breakdown during protein metabolism
   b. Metabolized by the liver and excreted by the kidneys as urea
   c. Elevated levels resulting from hepatic dysfunction may lead to encephalopathy
   d. Not a reliable indicator of hepatic coma
2. Value: 35 to 65 μg/dL
3. Nursing considerations
   a. Instruct client to fast, except for water, and to refrain from smoking for 8 to10 hours prior to the test
   b. Place the specimen in an ice water bath
   c. Transport to the laboratory immediately

D. Amylase
1. Description
   a. An enzyme, produced by the pancreas and salivary glands, that aids in the digestion of complex carbohydrates and is excreted by the kidneys
   b. In acute pancreatitis, the amylase level is greatly increased; the level starts rising in 3 to 6 hours after the onset of pain, peaks at about 24 hours, and returns to normal in 2 to 3 days after the onset of pain
2. Value: 25 to 151 IV/L
3. Nursing considerations
   a. On the laboratory form, list medications that the client has taken 24 hours prior to the test.
   b. Note that many medications may cause false-positive or false-negative results
   c. Results are invalidated if the specimen was obtained less than 72 hours after cholecystography with radiopaque dyes

E. Bilirubin
1. Description
   a. Produced by the liver, spleen, and bone marrow and is also a by-product of hemoglobin breakdown
   b. Total bilirubin levels can be broken down into direct bilirubin, which is primarily excreted via the intestinal tract, and indirect bilirubin, which circulates primarily in the bloodstream
   c. Total bilirubin levels rise with any type of jaundice, whereas direct and indirect levels rise depending on the etiology of the jaundice
2. Values
   a. Bilirubin, direct: 0 to 0.3 mg/dL
   b. Bilirubin, indirect: 0.1 to 1.0 mg/dL
   c. Bilirubin, total: less than 1.5 mg/dL

3. Nursing considerations
   a. Instruct the client to eat a diet low in yellow foods, such as carrots, yams, yellow beans, and pumpkins, for 3 to 4 days before sampling
   b. Instruct the client to fast for 4 hours before sampling
   c. Note that results will be elevated with the use of alcohol, morphine, theophylline, ascorbic acid, or aspirin
   d. Note that results are invalidated if the client has received a radioactive scan within 24 hours prior to the test

F. Lipase
1. Description
   a. A pancreatic enzyme that changes fats and triglycerides into fatty acids and glycerol
   b. Elevated lipase levels occur in pancreatic disorders; elevations may not occur until 24 to 36 hours after the onset of illness and may remain for up to 14 days
2. Value: 10 to 140 U/L
3. Nursing considerations
   a. Endoscopic retrograde cholangiopancreatography (ERCP) may increase lipase activity
   b. Traumatic **venipuncture** can inhibit lipase activity

G. Lipids
1. Description
   a. Blood lipids consist primarily of cholesterol, triglycerides, and phospholipids
   b. Lipid assessment includes total cholesterol, high-density lipoprotein (HDL), low-density lipoprotein (LDL), and triglycerides
   c. Cholesterol is present in all body tissues and is a major component of low-density lipoproteins (LDL), brain and nerve cells, cell membranes, and some gallstones
   d. Triglycerides constitute a major part of very low-density lipoproteins (VLDL) and a small part of low-density lipoproteins (LDL)
   e. Triglycerides are synthesized in the liver from fatty acids, protein, and glucose, and are obtained from the diet
2. Values:
   a. Cholesterol: 140 to 199 mg/dL
   b. LDL: less than 130 mg/dL
   c. HDL: 30 to 70 mg/dL
   d. Triglycerides: less than 200 mg/dL
3. Nursing considerations
   a. Oral contraceptives may increase the levels of lipids in the **serum**
   b. Instruct the client to abstain from foods and fluid, except for water, for 12 to 14 hours and from alcohol for 24 hours prior to the test
   c. Instruct the client that the evening meal prior

to the test should be free of high-cholesterol foods

    d. Cholesterol levels tend to decrease temporarily with major illness or surgery

H. Protein

  1. Description

    a. Reflects the total amount of albumin and globulins in the **serum**

    b. Regulates osmotic pressure and comprises coagulation factors for hemostasis, enzymes, hormones, tissue growth and repair, and pH buffers

  2. Value: 6.0 to 8.0 g/dL

  3. Nursing considerations

    a. Do not draw in an extremity with an IV infusion

    b. Instruct the client to avoid a high-fat diet for 8 hours prior to the test

I. Uric acid

  1. Description

    a. Formed as the purines, adenine and guanine, and is continuously metabolized during the formation and degradation of DNA and RNA, and from the metabolism of dietary purines

    b. Elevated amounts deposit in joints and soft tissue and cause gout

    c. Conditions of fast cell turnover, as well as slowed renal excretion of uric acid, may cause uricemia

    d. Elevated amounts of urinary uric acid precipitate into urate stones in the kidneys

  2. Values

    a. Male: 4.5 to 8 mg/dL

    b. Female: 2.5 to 6.2 mg/dL

  3. Nursing considerations

    a. Instruct the client to fast for 8 hours prior to test

    b. Aminophylline, caffeine, and vitamin C may cause falsely elevated results

IV. GLUCOSE STUDIES

A. Fasting blood glucose (FBS)

  1. Description

    a. Glucose is a monosaccharide found in fruits and is formed from the digestion of carbohydrates and the conversion of glycogen by the liver

    b. Glucose is the body's main source of cellular energy and is essential for brain and erythrocyte function

    c. FBS levels are used to help diagnose diabetes mellitus and hypoglycemia (Table 10-2)

  2. Nursing considerations

    a. Instruct the client to fast for 8 to 12 hours prior to test

    b. Instruct a client with diabetes mellitus to withhold morning insulin or oral hypo-

TABLE 10-2	
Normal Adult Glucose Values	
Glucose, fasting	70-110 mg/dL
Glucose monitoring (capillary blood)	60-110 mg/dL
Glucose tolerance test, oral	
Baseline fasting	70-110 mg/dL
30 minute fasting	110-170 mg/dL
60 minute fasting	120-170 mg/dL
90 minute fasting	100-140 mg/dL
120 minute fasting	70-120 mg/dL
Glucose, 2-hour postprandial	<140 mg/dL

glycemic medication until after the blood is drawn

B. Glucose tolerance test (GTT) (Table 10-2)

  1. Description

    a. Aids in the diagnosis of diabetes mellitus

    b. If the glucose levels peak at higher than normal at 1 and 2 hours after injection or ingestion of glucose and are slower than normal to return to fasting levels, then diabetes mellitus is confirmed

  2. Nursing considerations

    a. Instruct the client to eat a high-carbohydrate (200 to 300 g) diet for 3 days before the test

    b. Instruct the client to avoid alcohol, coffee, and smoking for 36 hours before testing

    c. Instruct the client to fast for 10 to 16 hours prior to the test

    d. Instruct the client to avoid strenuous exercise for 8 hours before and after the test

    e. Instruct the client with diabetes mellitus to withhold morning insulin or oral hypoglycemic medication

    f. Instruct the client that the test will take 3 to 5 hours, requires intravenous or oral administration of glucose, and multiple blood samples

C. Glycosylated hemoglobin

  1. Description

    a. Glycosylated hemoglobin is blood glucose bound to hemoglobin

    b. HbA1c (glycosylated hemoglobin A) is a reflection of how well blood glucose levels have been controlled for up to the prior 4 months

    c. Hyperglycemia in diabetics is usually a cause of an increase in HbA1c

  2. Values

    a. Values are expressed as a percentage of total hemoglobin

    b. Diabetic with good control: 7.5% or less

    c. Diabetic with fair control: 7.6% to 8.9%

    d. Diabetic with poor control: 9% or greater

3. Nursing consideration: Fasting is not required prior to the test

V. RENAL FUNCTION STUDIES

A. **Serum** creatinine
   1. Description
      a. A very specific indicator of renal function, revealing the balance between creatinine formation and excretion
      b. Increased levels indicate a slowing of the glomerular filtration rate
   2. Value: 0.6-1.3 mg/dL
   3. Nursing considerations: Instruct the client to avoid excessive exercise for 8 hours and excessive red meat intake for 24 hours before the test

▲ B. Blood urea nitrogen (BUN)
   1. Description
      a. Urea nitrogen is the nitrogen portion of urea, a substance formed in the liver through an enzymatic protein breakdown process
      b. Urea is normally freely filtered through the renal glomeruli, with a small amount reabsorbed in the tubules and the remainder excreted in the urine
      c. Elevated values may be a result of prerenal, renal, or postrenal causes
   2. Value: 8 to 25 mg/dL
   3. Nursing considerations: Both creatinine levels and urea nitrogen levels should be analyzed when renal function is evaluated

VI. SERUM ENZYMES/CARDIAC MARKERS

▲ A. Creatine kinase (CK)
   1. Description
      a. An enzyme found in muscle and brain tissue; reflects tissue catabolism resulting from cell trauma
      b. The test is performed to detect myocardial or skeletal muscle damage or central nervous system damage; normal CK is 26-174 U/L
      c. Isoenzymes include CK-MB (cardiac), CK-BB (brain), and CK-MM (muscles)
      d. CK-MB is found mainly in cardiac muscle, CK-BB is found mainly in brain tissue, and CK-MM is found mainly is skeletal muscle
   2. Values
      a. CK-MB: 0% to 5% of total
      b. CK-MM: 95% to 100% of total
      c. CK-BB: 0%
   3. Nursing considerations
      a. If the test is to evaluate skeletal muscle, instruct the client to avoid strenuous physical activity for 24 hours prior to the test
      b. Instruct the client to avoid ingestion of alcohol for 24 hours prior to the test
      c. Invasive procedures and IM injections may falsely elevate CK levels

TABLE 10-3

Normal Adult Lactate Dehydrogenase

Lactate dehydrogenase	140-280 U/L
Lactate dehydrogenase isoenzymes	
LDH_1	14%-26%
LDH_2	29%-39%
LDH_3	20%-26%
LDH_4	8%-16%
LDH_5	6%-16%

B. Lactate dehydrogenase (LD or LDH)
   1. Description
      a. The isoenzymes that are particularly affected with acute myocardial infarction are LDH_1 and LDH_2
      b. This enzyme begins to elevate approximately 24 hours after myocardial infarction and peaks in 48 to 72 hours; thereafter it returns to normal, usually within 7 to 14 days (Table 10-3)
      c. The presence of an LD flip (when LD_1 is higher than LD_2) is helpful in diagnosing a myocardial infarction
   2. Nursing considerations
      a. LDH isoenzymes should be interpreted in view of the clinical findings
      b. Testing should be repeated on 3 consecutive days

C. Troponins
   1. Description
      a. Troponin is a regulatory protein found in striated muscle
      b. The troponins function together in the contractile apparatus for striated muscle in skeletal muscle and in the myocardium
      c. Increased amounts of troponins are released into the bloodstream when an infarction causes damage to the myocardium
      d. Serial measurements are important to compare with a baseline test
   2. Values:
      a. Troponin I: less than 0.6 ng/mL; greater than 1.5 ng/mL is consistent with a myocardial infarction
      b. Troponin T: greater than 0.1 to 0.2 ng/mL is consistent with a myocardial infarction
   3. Nursing consideration: Client does not need to be fasting

VII. ERYTHROCYTE STUDIES

A. Erythrocyte sedimentation rate
   1. Description
      a. The rate at which erythrocytes settle out of anticoagulated blood in 1 hour

b. Not diagnostic of any particular disease but indicates that a disease process is ongoing

2. Value: 0 to 30 mm/hour, depending on age of client

3. Nursing consideration: Fasting is not necessary, but a fatty meal may cause **plasma** alterations

B. Hemoglobin and hematocrit
   1. Description
      a. Hemoglobin is the main component of erythrocytes and serves as the vehicle for the transportation of oxygen and carbon dioxide
      b. Hemoglobin determinations are important in identifying anemia
      c. Hematocrit represents red blood cell mass and is an important measurement in the identification of anemia or polycythemia (Table 10-4)
   2. Nursing consideration: Fasting is not required

C. **Serum** iron
   1. Description
      a. Iron is mostly found in hemoglobin
      b. Iron acts as a carrier of oxygen from the lungs to the tissues and indirectly aids in return of carbon dioxide to the lungs
      c. Aids in diagnosing anemias and hemolytic disorders
   2. Values
      a. Male: 65-175 µg/dL
      b. Female: 50-170 µg/dL
   3. Nursing consideration: Level will be increased if the client has ingested iron prior to test

D. Red blood cell (RBC) count
   1. Description
      a. RBCs function in hemoglobin transport, which results in delivery of oxygen to the body tissues
      b. RBCs are formed by red bone marrow, have a life span of 120 days, and are removed from the blood by the liver, spleen, and bone marrow
      c. Aids in diagnosing anemias and blood dyscrasias
      d. Evaluates the body's ability to produce red blood cells in sufficient numbers

TABLE 10-4

Normal Adult Hemoglobin and Hematocrit Levels

Hemoglobin	
Male	14-16.5 g/dL
Female	12-15 g/dL
Hematocrit	
Male	42%-52%
Female	35%-47%

2. Values
   a. Female: 4 to 5.5 million/µL
   b. Male: 4.5 to 6.2 million/µL
3. Nursing consideration: Fasting is not required

VIII. ELEMENTS

A. Calcium
   1. Description
      a. A cation that is absorbed into the bloodstream from dietary sources and functions in bone formation, nerve impulse transmission, and contraction of myocardial and skeletal muscles
      b. Aids in blood clotting by converting prothrombin to thrombin
   2. Value: 8.6 to 10.0 mg/dL
   3. Nursing considerations
      a. Instruct the client to eat a diet with normal calcium levels (800 mg/day) for 3 days before test
      b. Instruct the client that fasting may be required for 8 hours prior to the test

B. Magnesium
   1. Description
      a. Used as an index to determine metabolic activity and renal function
      b. Magnesium is needed in the blood-clotting mechanism, regulates neuromuscular activity, acts as a cofactor that modifies the activity of many enzymes, and has an effect on the metabolism of calcium
   2. Value: 1.6 to 2.6 mg/dL
   3. Nursing considerations
      a. Prolonged use of magnesium products will cause increased levels
      b. Long-term total parenteral nutrition therapy or excessive loss of body fluids may cause decreased levels

C. Phosphorus
   1. Description
      a. Important in bone formation, energy storage and release, urinary acid-base buffering, and carbohydrate metabolism
      b. Absorbed from food and excreted by the kidneys
      c. High concentrations of phosphorus are stored in bone and skeletal muscle
   2. Value: 2.7 to 4.5 mg/dL
   3. Nursing considerations: Instruct the client to fast prior to the test

IX. THYROID STUDIES
   1. Description
      a. Performed if a thyroid disorder is suspected
      b. Helpful to differentiate primary thyroid disease from secondary causes and from abnormalities in thyroxine-binding globulin levels

2. Values
   a. Thyroid-stimulating hormone (thyrotropin; TSH): 0.2 to 5.4 uU/mL
   b. Thyroxine (T_4): 5.0 to 12.0 µg/dL
   c. Thyroxine, free (FT_4): 0.8 to 2.4 ng/dL
   d. Triiodothyronine (T_3): 80 to 230 ng/dL
3. Nursing consideration: Test results are invalid if client has undergone a radionuclide scan within 7 days prior to the test

X. WHITE BLOOD CELL (WBC) COUNT

1. Description
   a. White blood cells function in the body's immune defense system
   b. The WBC count assesses each leukocyte distribution
2. Value: 4500 to 11,000/µL (Table 10-5)
3. Nursing considerations
   a. A "shift to the left" means that there is an increased number of immature neutrophils in the peripheral blood
   b. A low total WBC count with a left shift indicates a recovery from bone marrow depression or an infection of such intensity that the demand for neutrophils in the tissue is greater than the capacity of the bone marrow to release them into the circulation
   c. A high total WBC count with a left shift indicates an increased release of neutrophils by the bone marrow in response to an overwhelming infection or inflammation
   d. A "shift to the right" means that cells have more than the usual number of nuclear segments; found in liver disease, Down's syndrome, or megaloblastic and pernicious anemia

XI. HEPATITIS TESTS

A. Description
   1. Tests include radioimmune assay (RIA), enzyme-linked immunosorbent assay (ELISA), and microparticle enzyme immunoassay (MEIA)
   2. Serologic tests for specific hepatitis virus markers assist in defining the specific type of hepatitis

TABLE 10-5

Normal Adult White Blood Cell Differential

Neutrophils	56% or 1800-7800/µL
Bands	3% or 0-700/µL
Eosinophils	2.7% or 0-450/µL
Basophils	0.3% or 0-200/µL
Lymphocytes	34% or 1000-4800/µL
Monocytes	4% or 0-800/µL

B. Values
   1. The presence of IgM antibody to hepatitis A virus (IgM anti-HAV) and the total antibody to hepatitis A virus (total anti-HAV) identify the disease
   2. Detection of core antigen (HBcAg), envelope antigen (HBeAg), and surface antigen (HBsAg), or their corresponding antibodies, constitutes hepatitis B assessment
   3. Hepatitis C is confirmed by the presence of antibodies to hepatitis C (anti-HCV)
   4. Serologic hepatitis delta virus (HDV) determination is made by detection of the hepatitis D antigen (HDAg) early in the course of the infection and by detection of anti-HDV antibody in the later disease stages
   5. Specific serologic tests for hepatitis E virus (HEV) include detection of IgM and IgG antibodies to hepatitis E (anti-HEV)
   6. Hepatitis G (HGV) has been found in some blood donors, IV drug users, hemodialysis clients, and clients with hemophilia; however, HGV does not appear to cause significant liver disease
C. Nursing consideration: If the RIA technique is being used, the injection of radionuclides within 1 week prior to the test may falsely elevate results

XII. HUMAN IMMUNODEFICIENCY VIRUS (HIV) AND ACQUIRED IMMUNODEFICIENCY SYNDROME (AIDS) TESTING

A. Description
   1. Detects HIV types 1 and 2 (HIV-1/2), which cause AIDS
   2. Tests used to determine the presence of antibodies to HIV-1 include ELISA, Western blot (WB), and indirect fluorescent antibody (IFA)
   3. A single reactive ELISA test by itself cannot be used to diagnose AIDS and should be repeated in duplicate with the same blood sample; if the result is repeatedly reactive, follow-up tests using WB or IFA should be done
   4. A positive WB or IFA is considered confirmatory for HIV
   5. A positive ELISA that fails to be confirmed by WB or IFA should not be considered negative, and repeat testing should take place in 3 to 6 months
B. Nursing considerations
   1. Maintain issues of confidentiality surrounding HIV and AIDS testing
   2. Follow prescribed state regulations and protocols related to reporting positive test results

XIII. URINE TESTS (Table 10-6)

XIV. THERAPEUTIC SERUM MEDICATION LEVELS
(Table 10-7)

TABLE 10-6

Normal Adult Values: Urine Tests

Name of Test	Value
Chloride	110-250 mEq/24 hr
Magnesium	7.3-12.2 mg/dL/day
Potassium	25-125 mEq/24 hr
Protein	40-150 mg/24 hr
Sodium	40-220 mEq/24 hr
Uric acid	250-750 mg/24 hr
pH	4.5-7.8
Specific gravity	1.016 to 1.022

TABLE 10-7

Therapeutic Serum Medication Levels

Medication	Therapeutic Range
Acetaminophen (Tylenol)	10-20 µg/mL
Amikacin (Amikin)	25-30 µg/mL
Amitriptyline (Elavil)	120-150 ng/mL
Carbamazepine (Tegretol)	5-12 µg/mL
Chloramphenicol (Chloromycetin)	10-20 µg/mL
Desipramine (Norpramin)	150-300 ng/mL
Digitoxin (Crystodigin)	15-25 ng/mL
Digoxin (Lanoxin)	0.5-2.0 ng/mL
Disopyramide (Norpace)	2-5 µg/mL
Ethosuximide (Zarontin)	40-100 µg/mL
Gentamicin (Garamycin)	5-10 µg/mL
Imipramine (Tofranil)	150-300 ng/mL
Lidocaine (Xylocaine)	1.5-5.0 µg/mL
Lithium (Lithobid)	0.5-1.3 mEq/L
Magnesium sulfate	4-7 mg/dL
Nortriptyline (Aventyl)	50-150 ng/mL
Phenobarbital (Luminal)	10-30 µg/mL
Phenytoin (Dilantin)	10-20 µg/mL
Primidone (Mysoline)	5-20 µg/mL
Procainamide (Pronestyl)	4-10 µg/mL
Propranolol (Inderal)	50-100 ng/mL
Quinidine (Quinaglute, Cardioquin)	2-5 µg/mL
Salicylate	100-250 µg/mL
Theophylline (Aminophylline, Theo-Dur)	10-20 µg/mL
Tobramycin (Nebcin)	5-10 µg/mL
Valproic acid (Depakene)	50-100 µg/mL

PRACTICE QUESTIONS

1. A nurse is assigned to a 40 year-old client who has a diagnosis of chronic pancreatitis. The nurse reviews the laboratory result, anticipating a laboratory report that indicates a serum amylase level of:
   1. 45 U/L
   2. 100 U/L
   3. 300 U/L
   4. 500 U/L

2. A client is suspected of having a myocardial infarction. A nurse assesses for elevations in which of the following isoenzyme values reported with the creatinine phosphokinase (CPK) level?
   1. MM
   2. MB
   3. BB
   4. MK

3. An adult client has had laboratory work done as part of a routine physical examination. A nurse interprets that the client may have a mild degree of renal insufficiency if which of the following serum creatinine levels is found?
   1. 0.2 mg/dL
   2. 0.5 mg/dL
   3. 1.9 mg/dL
   4. 3.5 mg/dL

4. A client with a history of a seizure disorder who has been compliant with medication therapy is admitted to the hospital with seizure activity. Phenytoin (Dilantin) is administered to the client by the IV push route, and subsequently a serum phenytoin level is drawn. A nurse evaluates that the medication therapy has been most effective if the laboratory result is:
   1. 3 µg/mL
   2. 8 µg/mL
   3. 16 µg/mL
   4. 24 µg/mL

5. A client who takes theophylline (Theo-Dur) for chronic obstructive pulmonary disease (COPD) is seen in the urgent care center for respiratory distress. Just before therapy is initiated, a baseline theophylline level is drawn. Once the client is stabilized, a nurse begins discharge teaching. The nurse would be especially vigilant to include information about complying with medication therapy if the client's baseline result was:
   1. 10 µg/mL
   2. 12 µg/mL
   3. 15 µg/mL
   4. 18 µg/mL

6. A nurse checks the laboratory result for a serum digoxin level that was drawn for a client earlier in the day and notes that the result is 2.4 ng/mL. Which of the following is the most important action on the part of the nurse?
   1. Record the normal value on the client's flowsheet
   2. Administer the next dose of the medication as scheduled
   3. Check the client's last pulse rate
   4. Notify the physician

7. A client is receiving a continuous IV infusion of heparin in the treatment of deep vein thrombosis. The client's activated partial thromboplastin time (aPTT) level is 65 seconds. The client's baseline

before the initiation of therapy was 30 seconds. A nurse anticipates that which action is needed?

1. Shutting off the heparin infusion
2. Decreasing the rate of the heparin infusion
3. Leaving the rate of the heparin infusion as is
4. Increasing the rate of the heparin infusion

8. A client with atrial fibrillation who is receiving maintenance therapy of warfarin sodium (Coumadin) has a prothrombin time (PT) of 30 seconds. On the basis of the PT level, a nurse anticipates which of the following orders?

1. Holding the next dose of warfarin sodium
2. Administering the next dose of warfarin sodium
3. Increasing the next dose of warfarin sodium
4. Adding a dose of heparin

9. An adult client who has had pre-admission testing before surgery has had serum electrolytes drawn. A nurse would report which of the following abnormal values to the surgeon's office preoperatively?

1. Sodium, 148 mEq/L
2. Potassium, 3.8 mEq/L
3. Chloride, 101 mEq/L
4. Bicarbonate, 26 mEq/L

10. A client with a history of cardiac disease is due for a morning dose of furosemide (Lasix). A nurse plans to report which serum potassium level before administering the dose of furosemide?

1. 3.8 mEq/L
2. 3.2 mEq/L
3. 4.8 mEq/L
4. 4.2 mEq/L

11. An adult client with a history of gastrointestinal (GI) bleeding has a platelet count of 300,000 cells/uL. Which action by a nurse is most appropriate upon reading this report?

1. Report the abnormally low count
2. Report the abnormally high count
3. Place the client on bleeding precautions
4. Place the normal report in the client's medical record

12. An adult client with hepatic cirrhosis has been following a diet with optimal amounts of protein, since neither an excess nor a deficiency of protein has been helpful. The nurse evaluates the client's status as being most satisfactory if the total protein level is which of the following values, in the normal range?

1. 0.4 g/dL
2. 3.7 g/dL
3. 6.4 g/dL
4. 9.8 g/dL

13. A client is seen in the urgent care center for complaints of chest pain that began three days ago. Since that time, the client has not been feeling well and fatigues easily. A nurse would suspect myocardial infarction at the time of chest pain if which of

the following isoenzymes for lactic dehydrogenase (LDH) came back positive?

1. LDH_1
2. LDH_3
3. LDH_4
4. LDH_5

14. An adult client was diagnosed with acute pancreatitis nine days ago. A nurse interprets that the client is recovering from this episode if the serum lipase level drops to which of the following values, which is just underneath the upper limit of normal?

1. 20 U/L
2. 80 U/L
3. 135 U/L
4. 350 U/L

15. An adult female client has a hemoglobin level of 10.8 g/dL. A nurse interprets that this result is most likely due to which of the following conditions noted in the client's history?

1. Chronic obstructive pulmonary disease (COPD)
2. Heart failure
3. Dehydration
4. Iron deficiency anemia

16. A client with diabetes mellitus has a glycosylated hemoglobin A1C level of 9%. On the basis of this test result, a nurse plans to teach the client about the need to:

1. Avoid infection
2. Take in adequate fluids
3. Prevent hyperglycemia
4. Prevent hypoglycemia

17. A nurse is caring for a client with a diagnosis of cancer who is immunosuppressed. A nurse would consider implementing neutropenic precautions if the client's white blood cell (WBC) count was:

1. 2,000/μL
2. 5,800/μL
3. 8,400/μL
4. 11,500/μL

18. A 22-year-old young adult has a cholesterol blood test done at a screening clinic sponsored by a local health club. A nurse volunteering at the screening teaches the client that diet and exercise should be used as health measures to keep the total cholesterol level below:

1. 140 mg/dL
2. 200 mg/dL
3. 250 mg/dL
4. 300 mg/dL

19. A 78-year-old client has been admitted for urinary tract infection and dehydration. A nurse evaluates that the client has received adequate volume replacement if the blood urea nitrogen (BUN) level drops to:

1. 35 mg/dL
2. 29 mg/dL

3. 15 mg/dL
4. 3 mg/dL

20. A client arrives in the emergency room complaining of chest pain that began 4 hours ago. A troponin T blood specimen is obtained, and the results indicate a level of 0.6 ng/mL. The nurse interprets that this result indicates:

1. A normal level
2. A level that indicates the presence of possible angina
3. A low value indicating possible gastritis
4. A level that indicates a myocardial infarction

CRITICAL THINKING: FREE-TEXT ENTRY

A nurse reviews the fasting blood glucose level of a client with diabetes mellitus who is scheduled for surgery. The nurse plans to report an abnormal level to the physician.

What is the normal range for the blood glucose level?

Answer: _____

ANSWERS

1. 3
Rationale: The normal serum amylase level is 25 to 151 IU/L. With chronic cases of pancreatitis, the rise in serum amylase levels usually does not exceed three times the normal value. In acute pancreatitis, the value may exceed five times the normal value. Option 1 indicates a low value. Option 2 is within normal limits. Option 4 is an extremely elevated level seen in acute pancreatitis.
Test-Taking Strategy: Use the process of elimination. Note the key word "chronic" in the question. It is necessary to understand the effects of chronic pancreatitis on the amylase level. Review these effects if you had difficulty with this question.
Level of Cognitive Ability: Analysis
Client Needs: Physiological Integrity
Integrated Concept/Process: Nursing Process/Analysis
Content Area: Adult Health/Gastrointestinal
Reference: Corbett, J. (2000). *Laboratory tests and diagnostic procedures* (5th ed.). Upper Saddle River, NJ: Prentice-Hall, p. 297.

2. 2
Rationale: CPK is a cellular enzyme that can be fractionated into three isoenzymes. The MB band reflects CPK from cardiac muscle. This is the level that elevates with myocardial infarction. The MM band reflects CPK from skeletal muscle. The BB band reflects CPK from the brain. There is no MK band.
Test-Taking Strategy: To answer this question correctly, it is necessary to have specific knowledge of the isoenzymes that are produced with elevations in this enzyme (CPK). If necessary, review this important laboratory value for detecting myocardial infarction.
Level of Cognitive Ability: Comprehension
Client Needs: Physiological Integrity
Integrated Concept/Process: Nursing Process/Assessment
Content Area: Adult Health/Cardiovascular
Reference: Phipps, W., Sands, J., & Marek, J. (1999). *Medical-surgical nursing: Concepts & clinical practice* (6th ed.). St. Louis: Mosby, p. 643.

3. 3
Rationale: The normal serum creatinine level for adults is 0.6 to 1.3 mg/dL. The client with a mild degree of renal insufficiency would have a slightly elevated level. A creatinine

level of 0.2 mg/dL is low, and a level of 0.5 mg/dL is just below normal. A creatinine level of 3.5 mg/dL may be associated with acute or chronic renal failure.
Test-Taking Strategy: Note the key word "mild." This tells you that the correct option will be an abnormal value, but perhaps not the most abnormal of all the options. Recall the normal value for this common laboratory test to direct you to option 3. Review the normal value for this laboratory test if you had difficulty with this question.
Level of Cognitive Ability: Analysis
Client Needs: Physiological Integrity
Integrated Concept/Process: Nursing Process/Analysis
Content Area: Adult Health/Renal
Reference: LeMone, P., & Burke, K. (2000). *Medical-surgical nursing: Critical thinking in client care* (2nd ed.). Upper Saddle River, NJ: Prentice-Hall, p. 958.

4. 3
Rationale: The therapeutic range for serum phenytoin (Dilantin) level is 10 to 20 µg/mL. If the level is below the therapeutic range, the client may continue to experience seizure activity. If the level is too high, the client could experience phenytoin toxicity.
Test-Taking Strategy: Use the process of elimination. Recalling that the therapeutic range is 10 to 20 µg/mL will direct you to option 3. Learn this therapeutic range if you had difficulty with this question.
Level of Cognitive Ability: Analysis
Client Needs: Physiological Integrity
Integrated Concept/Process: Nursing Process/Evaluation
Content Area: Adult Health/Neurological
Reference: Hodgson, B., & Kizior, R. (2001). *Saunders nursing drug handbook 2001.* Philadelphia: W.B. Saunders, p. 825.

5. 1
Rationale: The therapeutic range for the serum theophylline (or aminophylline) level is 10 to 20 µg/mL. If the level is below the therapeutic range, the client may experience frequent exacerbations of the disorder. Although all of the options identify values within the therapeutic range, option 1 is the option that reflects a need for compliance with medication.
Test-Taking Strategy: Use the process of elimination. Note the key words "especially vigilant." Recalling the therapeutic level of theophylline will direct you to option 1. Review this therapeutic range if you had difficulty with this question.

Level of Cognitive Ability: Analysis
Client Needs: Physiological Integrity
Integrated Concept/Process: Teaching/Learning
Content Area: Adult Health/Respiratory
Reference: Hodgson, B. & Kizior, R. (2001). *Saunders nursing drug handbook 2001.* Philadelphia: W.B. Saunders, pp. 44-47.

6. **4**
Rationale: The normal therapeutic range for digoxin is 0.5 to 2.0 ng/mL. A value of 2.4 exceeds the therapeutic range and could be toxic to the client. The most important action is to notify the physician, who may give further orders about holding further doses of digoxin. Option 1 is incorrect because the value is not normal. The next dose should not be administered automatically. Checking the client's last pulse rate is not incorrect, but may have limited value in this situation. Depending on the time that has elapsed since the last assessment, it may be more useful to do a current assessment of the client's status.
Test-Taking Strategy: Use the process of elimination and note the key words "most important action." To choose correctly, it is necessary to be familiar with the therapeutic range for this medication and to note that the value of 2.4 ng/mL is a toxic one. If this question was difficult, review the information on this commonly used medication and measurement of its therapeutic serum level.
Level of Cognitive Ability: Analysis
Client Needs: Safe, Effective Care Environment
Integrated Concept/Process: Nursing Process/Implementation
Content Area: Adult Health/Cardiovascular
Reference: Hodgson, B,. & Kizior, R. (2001). *Saunders nursing drug handbook 2001.* Philadelphia: W.B. Saunders, pp. 324-326.

7. **3**
Rationale: The normal aPTT varies between 20 and 36 seconds, depending on the type of activator used in testing. The therapeutic dose of heparin for treatment of deep vein thrombosis is to keep the aPTT between 1.5 and 2.5 times normal. Thus, the client's aPTT is within the therapeutic range, and the dose should remain unchanged.
Test-Taking Strategy: To answer this question accurately, it is necessary to be familiar with both the normal aPTT level and the therapeutic level needed following institution of heparin therapy. Remember that the normal range is 20 to 36 seconds and that the aPTT should be between 1.5 and 2.5 times normal when the client is on heparin therapy. If this question was difficult, review this important content area.
Level of Cognitive Ability: Analysis
Client Needs: Physiological Integrity
Integrated Concept/Process: Nursing Process/Analysis
Content Area: Adult Health/Cardiovascular
Reference: Ignatavicius, D., Workman, M., & Mishler, M. (1999). *Medical-surgical nursing across the health care continuum* (3rd ed.). Philadelphia: W.B. Saunders, p. 874.

8. **1**
Rationale: The normal PT is 9.6 to 11.8 seconds (adult male) or 9.5 to 11.3 seconds (adult female). A therapeutic PT level is 1.5 to 2.0 times greater than the client's control level. Since the value stated is high (and perhaps near the critical range), the nurse should anticipate that the client would not receive further doses at this time.

Test-Taking Strategy: Use the process of elimination, recalling that the normal PT is 9.6 to 11.8 seconds (adult male) or 9.5 to 11.3 seconds (adult female) and that a therapeutic PT level is 1.5 to 2.0 times greater than the client's control level. If this question was difficult, review this important content area.
Level of Cognitive Ability: Analysis
Client Needs: Physiological Integrity
Integrated Concept/Process: Nursing Process/Analysis
Content Area: Adult Health/Cardiovascular
Reference: Corbett, J. (2000). *Laboratory tests and diagnostic procedures* (5th ed.). Upper Saddle River, NJ: Prentice-Hall, p. 307.

9. **1**
Rationale: The normal serum electrolyte ranges for adults are as follows: sodium, 135 to 145 mEq/L; potassium, 3.5 to 5.1 mEq/L; chloride, 98 to 107 mEq/L; bicarbonate (venous), 22-29 mEq/L. The only abnormal value identified above is the serum sodium. The nurse reports any abnormal preoperative laboratory value to the surgeon's office.
Test-Taking Strategy: Use the process of elimination and knowledge of the normal serum electrolyte values to direct you to option 1. If this question was difficult, memorize these common laboratory values.
Level of Cognitive Ability: Comprehension
Client Needs: Physiological Integrity
Integrated Concept/Process: Communication and Documentation
Content Area: Fundamental Skills
Reference: Ignatavicius, D., Workman, M., & Mishler, M. (1999). *Medical-surgical nursing across the health care continuum* (3rd ed.). Philadelphia: W.B. Saunders, p. 221.

10. **2**
Rationale: The normal serum potassium level in the adult is 3.5 to 5.1 mEq/L. Option 2 is the only value that falls below the therapeutic range. Administering furosemide to a client with a low potassium level and a cardiac history could precipitate ventricular dysrhythmias. Options 1, 3, and 4 are within the normal range.
Test-Taking Strategy: Use the process of elimination and knowledge of the normal serum potassium level to answer this question. This will assist you in identifying the value that is not within normal range. If this question was difficult memorize this common laboratory value.
Level of Cognitive Ability: Analysis
Client Needs: Physiological Integrity
Integrated Concept/Process: Communication and Documentation
Content Area: Adult Health/Cardiovascular
Reference: Ignatavicius, D., Workman, M., & Mishler, M. (1999). *Medical-surgical nursing across the health care continuum* (3rd ed.). Philadelphia: W.B. Saunders, p. 221.

11. **4**
Rationale: A normal platelet count ranges from 150,000 to 400,000cells/µL. The nurse should place the report containing the normal laboratory value in the client's medical record. A platelet count of 300,000 cells/µL is not an elevated count. It is also not a low count; therefore, it is not necessary to place the client on bleeding precautions.
Test-Taking Strategy: Use the process of elimination. Remember that options that are similar are not likely to be correct.

With this in mind, eliminate options 1 and 3 first. To discriminate between the final two options, it is necessary to be familiar with the normal range for this laboratory test. Since this is a common hematological study, the normal range is worth memorizing.

Level of Cognitive Ability: Application
Client Needs: Physiological Integrity
Integrated Concept/Process: Nursing Process/Implementation
Content Area: Adult Health/Gastrointestinal
Reference: Lewis, S., Heitkemper, M., & Dirksen, S. (2000). *Medical-surgical nursing: Assessment and management of clinical problems* (5th ed.). St. Louis: Mosby, p. 730.

12. 3

Rationale: The normal range for total serum protein level in the adult client is 6.0 to 8.0 g/dL. The client with cirrhosis often has low total protein levels as a result of inadequate nutrition. Excess protein is not helpful, though, since a function of the liver is to metabolize protein. Protein metabolism may not be done well by a diseased liver. Options 1 and 2 identify low values, and option 4 identifies a high protein value.

Test-Taking Strategy: Use the process of elimination. Note the key words "normal range." Familiarity with the normal total protein level will direct you to option 3. If necessary, review this important laboratory range.

Level of Cognitive Ability: Analysis
Client Needs: Physiological Integrity
Integrated Concept/Process: Nursing Process/Evaluation
Content Area: Adult Health/Gastrointestinal
Reference: Corbett, J. (2000). *Laboratory tests and diagnostic procedures* (5th ed.). Upper Saddle River, NJ: Prentice-Hall, p. 737.

13. 1

Rationale: The isoenzymes that are particularly affected with acute myocardial infarction are LDH_1 and LDH_2. The LDH begins to elevate approximately 24 hours after myocardial infarction and peaks in 48 to 72 hours. Thereafter, it returns to normal, usually within 7 to 14 days.

Test-Taking Strategy: Use the process of elimination. It is necessary to be familiar with the cardiac isoenzymes for LDH. Review this important laboratory data if you had difficulty with this question.

Level of Cognitive Ability: Analysis
Client Needs: Physiological Integrity
Integrated Concept/Process: Nursing Process/Analysis
Content Area: Adult Health/Cardiovascular
Reference: Phipps, W., Sands, J., & Marek, J. (1999). *Medical-surgical nursing: Concepts & clinical practice* (6th ed.). St. Louis: Mosby, p. 643.

14. 3

Rationale: The normal serum lipase level is 10 to 140 U/L. The client who is recovering from acute pancreatitis usually has elevated lipase levels for approximately 10 days after the onset of symptoms. This makes lipase a valuable test in monitoring the client's pancreatic function, since serum amylase levels usually return to normal 3 days after the onset of symptoms. Option 3 is the only option that contains a value just underneath the upper limit of normal.

Test-Taking Strategy: Use the process of elimination and knowledge of the serum lipase level to answer this question.

Note the key words "just underneath the upper limit of normal." Review the range for this laboratory study if you had difficulty with this question.

Level of Cognitive Ability: Analysis
Client Needs: Physiological Integrity
Integrated Concept/Process: Nursing Process/Evaluation
Content Area: Adult Health/Gastrointestinal
Reference: Fischbach, F. (2000). *A manual of laboratory & diagnostic tests* (6th ed.). Philadelphia: Lippincott Williams & Wilkins, p. 436.

15. 4

Rationale: The normal hemoglobin level for an adult female client is 12 to 15 g/dL. Iron deficiency anemia can result in lower hemoglobin levels. Heart failure and COPD may increase the hemoglobin level as a result of the need of the body for more oxygen-carrying capacity. Dehydration may increase the hemoglobin level by hemoconcentration.

Test-Taking Strategy: Use the process of elimination. Evaluate each of the options in terms of whether each is likely to raise or lower the hemoglobin level. Review the normal hemoglobin level if you had difficulty with this question.

Level of Cognitive Ability: Analysis
Client Needs: Physiological Integrity
Integrated Concept/Process: Nursing Process/Analysis
Content Area: Fundamental Skills
Reference: Lewis, S., Heitkemper, M., & Dirksen, S. (2000). *Medical-surgical nursing: Assessment and management of clinical problems* (5th ed.). St. Louis: Mosby, p. 739.

16. 3

Rationale: In the glycosylated hemoglobin A1C, 7.5% indicates good control, 7.6% to 8.9% indicates fair control, and 9% or higher indicates poor control. This test measures the amount of glucose that has become permanently bound to the red blood cells from circulating glucose. Elevations in blood glucose will cause elevations in the amount of glycosylation. Thus, the test is useful in identifying clients who have periods of hyperglycemia that are undetected in other ways. Elevations indicate continued need for teaching related to prevention of hyperglycemic episodes.

Test-Taking Strategy: Use the process of elimination and knowledge regarding the values for this test and their significance to answer the question. If you had difficulty with this question or are unfamiliar with this important test, be sure to review.

Level of Cognitive Ability: Analysis
Client Needs: Health Promotion and Maintenance
Integrated Concept/Process: Teaching/Learning
Content Area: Adult Health/Endocrine
Reference: Corbett, J. (2000). *Laboratory tests and diagnostic procedures* (5th ed.). Upper Saddle River, NJ: Prentice-Hall, p. 196.

17. 1

Rationale: The normal WBC count ranges from 4500 to 11,000/µL. The client who is immunosuppressed has a decrease in the number of circulating WBCs. The nurse implements neutropenic precautions when the client's values fall sufficiently below the low normal level. The specific value for implementing neutropenic precautions is usually determined by agency policy. Options 2, 3, and 4 are normal values.

Test-Taking Strategy: Use the process of elimination. Recalling that the normal WBC count is 4500 to 11,000/μL will easily direct you to option 1. Review this common hematological test if you had difficulty with this question.
Level of Cognitive Ability: Analysis
Client Needs: Safe, Effective Care Environment
Integrated Concept/Process: Nursing Process/Analysis
Content Area: Adult Health/Oncology
Reference: Corbett, J. (2000). *Laboratory tests and diagnostic procedures* (5th ed.). Upper Saddle River, NJ: Prentice-Hall, p. 49.

18. **2**
Rationale: The client should be counseled to keep the total cholesterol level under 200 mg/dL. This will aid in prevention of atherosclerosis, which can lead to a number of cardiovascular disorders later in life. Options 3 and 4 are elevated values and place the client at risk for cardiovascular disease. Although option 1 is a low cholesterol level, the realistic value to assist in preventing cardiovascular disease is identified in option 2.
Test-Taking Strategy: Recalling that the cholesterol level ranges from 140 to 199 mg/dL and noting the issue of the question will direct you to option 2. Because of the importance of the health problems resulting from atherosclerosis and cardiovascular disease, it would be a helpful value to have memorized.
Level of Cognitive Ability: Application
Client Needs: Health Promotion and Maintenance
Integrated Concept/Process: Self-Care
Content Area: Adult Health/Cardiovascular
Reference: Fischbach, F. (2000). *A manual of laboratory & diagnostic tests* (6th ed.). Philadelphia: Lippincott Williams & Wilkins, p. 467.

19. **3**
Rationale: The normal BUN is 8 to 25 mg/dL. Values such as those in options 1 and 2 reflect continued dehydration. Option 4 reflects a lower than normal value, which may occur with fluid volume overload, among other conditions.
Test-Taking Strategy: Use the process of elimination and knowledge of the normal BUN level to answer the question. Option 3 is the only option that identifies a normal value. Learn this normal value if you had difficulty with this question.
Level of Cognitive Ability: Analysis
Client Needs: Physiological Integrity
Integrated Concept/Process: Nursing Process/Evaluation

Content Area: Adult Health/Renal
Reference: Corbett, J. (2000). *Laboratory tests and diagnostic procedures* (5th ed.). Upper Saddle River, NJ: Prentice-Hall, p. 91.

20. **4**
Rationale: Troponin is a regulatory protein found in striated muscle. The troponins function together in the contractile apparatus for striated muscle in skeletal muscle and in the myocardium. Increased amounts of troponins are released into the bloodstream when an infarction causes damage to the myocardium. A troponin T that is greater than 0.1 to 0.2 ng/mL is consistent with a myocardial infarction. A normal troponin I level is less than 0.6 ng/mL, while a level greater than 1.5 ng/mL is consistent with a myocardial infarction.
Test-Taking Strategy: Note that the issue of the question relates to the troponin T. Knowledge that a level that is greater than 0.1 to 0.2 ng/mL is consistent with a myocardial infarction will easily direct you to option 4. Review this important diagnostic test if you are unfamiliar with it.
Level of Cognitive Ability: Analysis
Client Needs: Physiological Integrity
Integrated Concept/Process: Nursing Process/Analysis
Content Area: Adult Health/Cardiovascular
Reference: Corbett, J. (2000). *Laboratory tests and diagnostic procedures* (5th ed.). Upper Saddle River, NJ: Prentice-Hall, p. 297.

CRITICAL THINKING: FREE-TEXT ENTRY

Answer: 70 to 110 mg/dL
Rationale: The normal range for the fasting blood glucose level is 70 to 110 mg/dL. Levels outside of this range need to be reported to the physician, particularly in a client scheduled for surgery.
Test-Taking Strategy: It is necessary to know the normal range for the fasting blood glucose level. Learn this normal range if you were unable to answer this question.
Level of Cognitive Ability: Comprehension
Client Needs: Physiological Integrity
Integrated Concept/Process: Nursing Process/Planning
Content Area: Adult Health/Endocrine
Reference: Fischbach, F. (2000). *A manual of laboratory & diagnostic tests* (6th ed.). Philadelphia: Lippincott Williams & Wilkins, p. 367.

REFERENCES

Corbett, J. (2000). *Laboratory tests and diagnostic procedures* (5th ed.). Upper Saddle River: NJ: Prentice-Hall.

Fischbach, F. (2000). *A manual of laboratory & diagnostic tests* (6th ed.). Philadelphia: Lippincott Williams & Wilkins.

Hodgson, B. & Kizior, R. (2001). *Saunders nursing drug handbook 2001* Philadelphia: W.B. Saunders.

Ignatavicius, D., Workman, M., & Mishler, M. (1999). *Medical-surgical nursing across the health care continuum* (3rd ed.). Philadelphia: W.B. Saunders.

LeMone, P., & Burke, K. (2000). *Medical-surgical nursing: Critical thinking in client care* (2nd ed.). Upper Saddle River, NJ: Prentice-Hall.

Lewis, S., Heitkemper, M., & Dirksen, S. (2000). *Medical-surgical nursing: Assessment and management of clinical problems* (5th ed.). St. Louis: Mosby.

Phipps, W., Sands, J., & Marek, J. (1999). *Medical-surgical nursing: Concepts & clinical practice* (6th ed.). St. Louis: Mosby.

11

Nutrition

PYRAMID TERMS

absorption   Passage of digested nutrients through the wall of the stomach or small intestine into the blood or lymph system.

anorexia   A lack of appetite with no desire to eat.

digestion   The breakdown of carbohydrates, fats, and proteins into monosaccharides, fatty acids, and amino acids.

enteral nutrition   Administering nutrition with liquefied foods into the gastrointestinal (GI) tract via a tube.

malnutrition   Deficiency of the nutrients required for development and maintenance of the human body.

metabolism   Ongoing chemical process within the body that converts digested nutrients into energy for the functioning of body cells.

nutrients   Include carbohydrates, fats/lipids, proteins, vitamins, minerals, and water. Must be supplied in adequate amounts to provide energy, growth, development, and maintenance of the human body.

▲ PYRAMID TO SUCCESS

Nutrition is a basic need that must be met for all clients. Nurses must have the knowledge required to educate and care for healthy clients, as well as clients with nutritional needs or disorders requiring alterations in dietary measures. NCLEX-RN will address the dietary measures required for basic needs and for particular body system alterations. When presented with a question related to nutrition, consider the client's diagnosis and the particular requirement or restriction necessary for treatment of the disorder. Pyramid points focus on the common types of therapeutic diets, nutrients contained in food items, and enteral feedings. The Integrated Concepts and Processes addressed in this chapter include Nursing Process, Caring, Communication and Documentation, Cultural Awareness, Self-Care, and Teaching/Learning.

CLIENT NEEDS   ▲
Safe, Effective Care Environment

Consultation with members of the health care team
Dietary consultation and referral
Informed consent for invasive procedures
Medical and surgical asepsis
Standard (universal) and other precautions

Health Promotion and Maintenance

Dietary teaching
Disease prevention
Health and wellness
Health promotion programs
Cultural preferences related to lifestyle choices
Techniques of physical assessment

Psychosocial Integrity

Coping mechanisms
Religious and spiritual influences on health

Physiological Integrity

Alteration in body systems
Elimination patterns
Monitoring enteral feedings and the client's ability to tolerate feedings
Monitoring laboratory values
Monitoring fluid and electrolyte balance
Nutrition and oral hydration

I. NUTRIENTS

A. Carbohydrates (Table 11-1)
   1. The preferred source of energy
   2. Include sugars, starches, and cellulose, and provide 4 cal/g
   3. Promote normal fat **metabolism,** spare protein, and enhance lower GI function
   4. Major food sources include milk, grains, fruits, and vegetables
   5. Inadequate carbohydrate intake affects **metabolism**

B. Fats (Table 11-2)
   1. Provide a concentrated source and a stored form of energy
   2. Protect internal organs and maintain body temperature
   3. Enhance **absorption** of the fat-soluble vitamins
   4. Provide 9 cal/g
   5. Inadequate fat intake leads to clinical manifestations of sensitivity to cold, skin lesions, increased risk of infection, and amenorrhea in women
   6. Diets high in fat can lead to obesity and increase the risk of cardiac disease and some cancers

C. Proteins (Box 11-1)
   1. Made from amino acids, critical to all aspects of growth and development of body tissues, and provide 4 cal/g
   2. Build and repair body tissues, regulate fluid balance, maintain acid-base balance, produce antibodies, provide energy, and produce enzymes and hormones
   3. Essential amino acids (EAAs) are required in the diet because the body cannot manufacture them
   4. High-quality proteins or complete proteins such as eggs, dairy products, meat, fish, and poultry contain adequate amounts of EAAs
   5. Foods that do not contain the EAAs in sufficient amounts are lower-quality or incomplete proteins
   6. Inadequate protein can cause protein energy **malnutrition,** and severe wasting of fat and muscle tissue

D. Vitamins (Box 11-2)
   1. Facilitate **metabolism** of proteins, fats, and

TABLE 11-1

Carbohydrate Food Sources

GLUCOSE	FRUCTOSE	CELLULOSE	LACTOSE
Grapes	Honey	Bran	Milk
Oranges	Fruits	Apples	
Dates		Beans	
Corn		Cabbage	
Carrots			

SUCROSE	STARCH
Granulated table sugar	Wheat
Molasses	Corn
Apricots	Oats
Peaches	Rye
Plums	Barley
Honeydew and cantaloupe	Potatoes and pasta
Peas and corn	Beets, carrots, and peas

TABLE 11-2

Fat Food Sources

SATURATED FATS	MONOUNSATURATED FATS
Beef	Duck and goose
Luncheon Meats	Eggs
Hard yellow cheeses	Olive and peanut oils
Butter	

POLYUNSATURATED FATS	CHOLESTEROL
Safflower oil	Animal products
Corn oil	Egg yolks
Sunflower oil	Liver and organ meats

BOX 11-1

Protein Food Sources

Meats
Dairy products
Cereal products
Dried beans

BOX 11-2

Food Sources of Vitamins

WATER SOLUBLE
Vitamin C (ascorbic acid): Citrus fruits, tomatoes, broccoli, cabbage
Vitamin B_1 (thiamine): Pork and nuts, whole grain cereals, and legumes
Vitamin B_2 (riboflavin): Milk, lean meats, fish, grains
Niacin: Meats, poultry, fish, beans, peanuts, grains
Vitamin B_6 (pryidoxine): Yeast, corn, meat, poultry, fish
Vitamin B_{12} (cobalamin): Meat, liver
Folic acid: Green, leafy vegetables; liver, beef and fish; legumes; grapefruit and oranges

FAT SOLUBLE
Vitamin A: Liver, egg yolk, whole milk, green or orange vegetables, fruits
Vitamin D: Fortified milk, fish oils, cereals
Vitamin E: Vegetable oils; green, leafy vegetables; cereals; apricots, apples, and peaches
Vitamin K: Green, leafy vegetables; cauliflower and cabbage

BOX 11-3
Food Sources of Minerals

CALCIUM
Yogurt, low-fat
Milk
Rhubarb
Collard greens
Cheese
Tofu
Spinach
Broccoli
Green beans
Carrots

CHLORIDE
Salt

MAGNESIUM
Green leafy vegetables
Avocado
Canned white tuna fish
Low fat yogurt
Cooked rolled oats
Milk
Peas
Potatoes
Pork, beef, chicken
Raisins
Peanut butter
Cauliflower

PHOSPHORUS
Fish
Pork, beef, chicken
Organ meats
Nuts
Whole-grain breads and cereals

POTASSIUM
Avocado
Raisins
Pork, beef, veal
Cantaloupe
Spinach
Bananas
Fish
Oranges
Strawberries
Mushrooms
Carrots
Potatoes
Tomatoes

SODIUM
Table salt
Soy sauce
Cured pork
Cottage cheese
American cheese
Milk
Butter
White and whole-wheat bread
Ketchup
Mustard
Bacon
Frankfurters
Lunch meat
Canned food
Processed food
Snack food

IRON
Liver, meats, egg yolk, dark-green vegetables, breads and cereals

ZINC
Meats, eggs, leafy vegetables, protein-rich foods

carbohydrates; act as catalysts for metabolic functions; promote life and growth processes; and maintain and regulate body functions

2. Fat-soluble vitamins A, D, E, and K can be stored in the body, so an excess can cause toxicity
3. The B vitamins and vitamin C are water soluble, are not stored in the body, and can be excreted in the urine
4. Vitamin K acts as a catalyst for facilitating blood-clotting factors, especially prothrombin
5. Vitamin C produces collagen, a vital component in wound healing
6. Vitamin A maintains eyesight and epithelial linings

E. Minerals (Box 11-3)

1. Components of hormones, cells, tissues, and bones
2. Act as catalysts for chemical reactions and enhancers of cell function
3. Almost all foods contain some form of minerals
4. A deficiency of minerals can occur in chronically ill or hospitalized clients

II. **FOOD GUIDE PYRAMID** (Fig. 11-1)
A. Groups six broad families of foods with similar kinds of **nutrients** together
B. Levels of the pyramid
   1. Level one (base of the pyramid)
      a. Bread, cereal, rice, and pasta group
      b. Daily recommendation is 6 to 11 servings

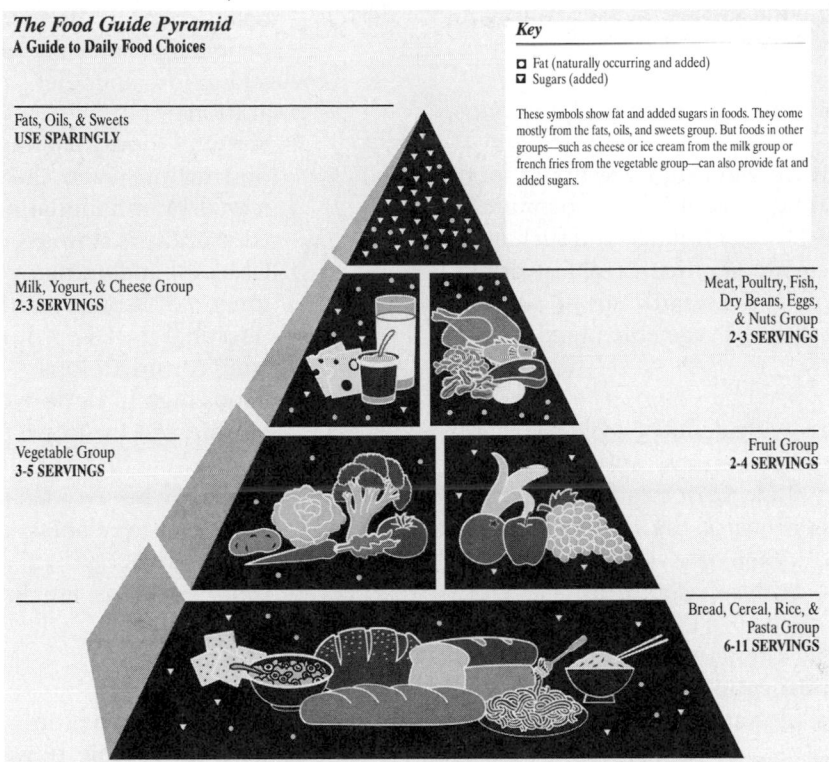

FIG. 11-1   Food guide pyramid: a guide to daily food choices and number of servings. (From Phipps W, Sands J, Marek J: *Medical-surgical nursing: concepts and clinical practice,* ed 6, St Louis, 1999, Mosby.)

2. Level two
   a. Vegetables and fruit group
   b. Daily recommendation is 3 to 5 servings of vegetables and 2 to 4 servings of fruit
3. Level three
   a. Includes the milk, yogurt, and cheese group and the meats, poultry, fish, dry beans and peas, eggs, and nuts group
   b. Daily recommendation is 2 to 3 servings for each group
   c. The recommendation for the milk group depends on the various life stage of the individual
4. Peak of the pyramid
   a. Includes fats, oils, and sweets group
   b. Foods are high in fats, sugar, or alcohol and are to be eaten sparingly because they are kilocalorie-dense, nutrient-sparse foods

III. THERAPEUTIC DIETS
A. Clear liquid diet
   1. Indications
      a. Serves a primary function of providing fluids and electrolytes to prevent dehydration
      b. Initial feeding after complete bowel rest
      c. Used initially to feed a malnourished person or a person who has not had any oral intake for some time
      d. Bowel preparation for surgery or tests
      e. Postsurgical diet
      f. Diarrhea
   2. Nursing considerations
      a. Clear liquid is deficient in energy and most **nutrients**
      b. The body digests and absorbs clear liquids easily
      c. Contributes to little or no residue in the GI tract
      d. Can be unappetizing and boring
      e. Client should not stay on a clear liquid diet for more than a day or two
      f. Consists of foods that are relatively transparent to light, and are clear and liquid at room and body temperature
      g. Foods include such items as water, bouillon, clear broth, carbonated beverages, gelatin, hard candy, lemonade, popcicles, and either regular or decaffeinated coffee or tea
      h. The nurse should limit the amount of caffeine consumed by the client because caffeine can cause an upset stomach and sleeplessness
      i. Client may have salt or sugar
      j. Dairy products are not allowed
B. Full liquid diet
   1. Indication: May be used as a second diet after

clear liquids following surgery, or for a client who is unable to chew or swallow

2. Nursing considerations
   a. Nutritionally deficient in energy and most **nutrients**
   b. Includes both clear and opaque liquid foods and those that liquefy at body temperature
   c. Foods include all clear liquids, and such items as plain ice cream, sherbet, breakfast drinks, milk, pudding and custard, soups that are strained, and strained vegetable juices

C. Soft diet
1. Indications
   a. Used in clients with dental problems, clients with poor-fitting dentures, and clients who have difficulty chewing or swallowing
   b. Used for ulcerations of the mouth or gums, oral surgery, broken jaw, plastic surgery of head or neck, or dysphasia, or for the stroke client
   c. Therapeutic for clients with impaired **digestion** and/or **absorption** as a result of conditions such as ulcerative colitis and Crohn's disease
2. Nursing considerations
   a. Clients with mouth sores should be served foods at cooler temperatures
   b. Clients who have difficulty chewing and swallowing because of a reduced flow of saliva can increase salivary flow by sucking on sour candy
   c. Encourage the client to eat a variety of foods
   d. Provide plenty of fluids with meals to ease chewing and swallowing of foods
   e. Sucking fluids through a straw may be easier than drinking them from a cup or glass
   f. All foods and seasonings are permitted; however, liquid, chopped, or puréed foods or regular foods with a soft consistency are best tolerated
   g. Avoid foods than contain nuts or seeds, which can easily become trapped in the mouth and cause discomfort
   h. Raw fruits and vegetables, fried foods, and whole grains are avoided

D. Bland diet
1. Indication: May be used for the client with gastritis, ulcers, reflux esophagitis, congestive heart failure (CHF), or myocardial infarction (MI)
2. Nursing considerations
   a. Bland foods are less likely to form gas than regular diets
   b. Eliminate foods that stimulate gastric acid secretions
   c. Eliminate foods that are irritating to the gastric mucosa
   d. Foods to be avoided include alcohol; caffeine and caffeine-containing beverages such as cola, cocoa, coffee, and tea; fried foods; pepper and spicy foods

E. Low-residue/low-fiber diet
1. Indications
   a. Supplies foods that are least likely to form an obstruction when the intestinal tract is narrowed by inflammation or scarring or when GI motility is slowed
   b. Used for inflammatory bowel disease, ileostomy, colostomy, partial obstructions of the intestinal tract, enteritis, or diarrhea
2. Nursing considerations
   a. Foods high in carbohydrate are usually low in residue and include white bread, cereals, and pasta
   b. Foods to be avoided are raw fruits (except bananas), vegetables, seeds, plant fiber, and whole grains
   c. Dairy products are limited to two servings a day

F. High-fiber diet
1. Indications
   a. Used in constipation
   b. Used in irritable bowel syndrome when the primary symptom is alternating constipation and diarrhea
   c. Helps regulate blood glucose in clients with diabetes mellitus
   d. Helps control blood cholesterol in clients with heart disease
2. Nursing considerations
   a. Provides 20 to 25 grams of dietary fiber daily
   b. Adds volume and weight to the stool and speeds the movement of undigested materials through the intestine
   c. Consists of fruits and vegetables

G. Fat-controlled diet (Table 11-2)
1. Indications
   a. Indicated for atherosclerosis, diabetes, hyperlipidemia, hypertension, MI, nephrotic syndrome, and renal failure
   b. Reduces the risk of heart disease
2. Nursing consideration: Limit both the total amount of fats and amounts of polyunsaturated, monounsaturated, and saturated fats and cholesterol

H. High-calorie diet
1. Indications: Severe stress, burns, cancer, human immunodeficiency virus (HIV) infections, acquired immunodeficiency syndrome (AIDS), chronic obstructive pulmonary disease (COPD), respiratory failure, or any other type of debilitating disease
2. Nursing considerations
   a. The high-calorie diet should also be high in protein because the purpose of the diet is to build or maintain lean body mass
   b. Add fats to foods whenever possible

c. Add nuts and dried fruits such as raisins to desserts or cereals if the client can tolerate and eat these foods

d. Add sugar to food, and provide high-calorie desserts

e. Encourage snacks between meals, such as milkshakes and instant breakfasts

I. Sodium-restriction diet

▲ 1. Indications: Hypertension, CHF, kidney diseases, cardiac diseases, and cirrhosis of the liver

2. Nursing considerations (Box 11-4)

a. The amount of sodium allowed varies from 250 mg to about 4 g of sodium daily

b. A no-added-salt diet includes no salt at the table and lightly salting foods during cooking

c. Cereals allowed on a sodium-restricted diet include dried or instant cereals, puffed wheat, puffed rice, and shredded wheat

J. Protein-restriction diet

▲ 1. Indications: Acute renal failure, chronic renal disease, cirrhosis of the liver, and hepatic coma

2. Nursing considerations

a. Provide enough protein to maintain nutritional status but not an amount that will allow the build-up of waste products from protein **metabolism** (40 to 60 g of protein daily)

b. The smaller the amount of protein allowed, the more important it becomes that all protein included in the diet be of high quality

c. An adequate total energy intake from foods is critical for clients on protein-restricted diets (protein will be used for energy, rather than for protein synthesis)

d. Special low-protein products, such as pastas, bread, cookies, wafers, and gelatin made with wheat starch, can improve energy intake and add variety to the diet

e. Carbohydrates in powdered or liquid forms can also provide additional energy

f. Vegetables and fruits contain some protein, and for very low-protein diets, these foods must be calculated into the diet

▲ g. Foods are limited from the milk, meat, bread, and starch exchange

K. High-protein diet

▲ 1. Indications: Tissue building, burns, liver disease, and maternity clients

2. Nursing considerations

a. High-protein diets correct protein loss or assist with tissue repair by increasing the intake of protein food sources

b. Increase foods such as meat, fish, fowl, and ▲ dairy products

c. The client may need protein supplements

L. Low-calcium diet

1. Indication: To prevent renal calculi (Table 11-3)

2. Nursing Considerations: Decrease the total intake ▲ of calcium to prevent further stone formation; avoid whole grains, milk and dairy products, and green, leafy vegetables

M. High-calcium diet

1. Indications: Calcium is needed during bone growth and in adulthood to prevent osteoporosis

2. Nursing considerations

a. Primary dietary sources of calcium are dairy products (refer to Chapter 8, Box 8-5, for food items high in calcium)

b. Clients experiencing lactose intolerance need to regularly incorporate sources of calcium other than dairy products into their dietary patterns

N. Low-purine diet

1. Indication: Used to treat gout

2. Nursing Considerations

a. Purine is a precursor for uric acid that forms stones and crystals

b. The client needs to avoid consuming fish such ▲ as anchovies, herring, mackerel, sardines, and scallops

c. The client needs to avoid consuming glandu- ▲ lar meats, gravies, meat extracts, wild game, goose, and sweetbreads

---

TABLE 11-3

Diets For Renal Calculi

ALKALINE ASH DIET

Purpose: To increase pH

Foods:

Milk

Fruits except cranberries, blueberries, plums, and prunes

Rhubarb

Vegetables

Small amounts of beef, halibut, veal, trout, and salami allowed

ACID ASH DIET

Purpose: To decrease pH

Foods:

Eggs

Meat

Cranberries, blueberries, plums, prunes

Fish

Poultry

Oysters

BOX 11-4

Sodium-Free Spices and Flavorings

Allspice, almond extract, bay leaves, caraway seeds, cinnamon, curry powder, garlic powder or garlic, ginger, lemon extract, maple extract, marjoram, mustard powder, and nutmeg

O. High-iron diet
1. Indication: Used in anemia
2. Nursing Considerations
   a. Replaces iron deficit from inadequate intake or loss
   b. Includes organ meats, meat, egg yolks, whole wheat products, leafy vegetables, dried fruit, legumes
P. Diet for diverticular disease
1. Symptomatic diverticulitis: fiber is avoided because a high-fiber diet is irritating to the bowel
2. Asymptomatic diverticular disease: a high-fiber diet is consumed to prevent constipation
3. The client should maintain a liberal fluid intake of 2500 to 3000 mL/day, unless contraindicated
4. Seeds and nuts should be avoided because they become trapped in the diverticula and cause irritation
5. Gas-forming foods should be avoided (Box 11-5)
Q. Fluid restriction (Box 11-6)
1. Indications: Acute renal failure-oliguric phase, chronic renal disease, cirrhosis of the liver, CHF, hepatic coma, and MI
2. Nursing considerations: Usually this diet restricts those foods that are composed largely of water, such as carbonated beverages, coffee, juices, milk, tea, water, frozen yogurt, gelatin, ice cream, ice milk, Popsicles, sherbet, soup, cream, and liquid medications
R. Carbohydrate-controlled diet
1. Indications
   a. Helps maintain normal glucose levels in clients with disorders that cause blood glucose levels to rise or fall abnormally
   b. Used for diabetes mellitus, hypoglycemia, lactose intolerance, galactosemia, dumping syndrome, and obesity
2. Nursing considerations
   a. Adjust energy intake from foods so as to provide specific amounts and types of carbohydrates
   b. The exchange list system is used most frequently to plan carbohydrate-controlled diets
S. Miscellaneous diets: Refer to Chapter 8, Boxes 8-3, 8-4, 8-6, and 8-7, for foods high in potassium, sodium, magnesium, and phosphorus

IV. THE EXCHANGE SYSTEM
A. Starches and breads
1. One bread is equal to 15 g of carbohydrate, 3 g of protein, trace of fat, and 80 calories
2. Equal to $3/4$ cup ready-to-eat cereal, $1/3$ cup cooked beans, $1/2$ cup corn
B. Meats
1. One lean meat is equal to 7 g of protein, 3 g of fat, and 55 calories
2. One meat exchange is equal to 1 ounce
3. One ounce of lean meat is equal to 1 ounce of chicken meat without skin, 1 ounce of any fish, $1/4$ cup canned tuna, 1 ounce low-fat cheese
4. Medium-fat meats
   a. One medium-fat meat is equal to 7 g of protein, 5 g of fat, and about 75 calories
   b. One ounce medium-fat meat is equal to 1 ounce lean meat in protein content but has 5 g of fat
   c. Equal to 1 ounce pork loin, 1 egg, $1/4$ cup creamed cottage cheese
5. High-fat meats
   a. One high-fat meat is equal to 7 g of protein, 8 g of fat, and 100 calories
   b. A hotdog counts as 1 high-fat meat exchange plus 1 fat exchange
   c. One ounce high-fat meat is equal to 1 ounce lean meat in protein content but includes an extra 1 fat
   d. Equal to 1 ounce ham, 1 ounce cheddar cheese, 1 small hotdog
   e. Peanut butter is like a meat in terms of its protein content
   f. One tablespoon peanut butter is equal to 1 high-fat meat
   g. One tablespoon peanut butter is equal to 7 g of protein, 8 g of fat, and 100 calories
C. Vegetables
1. One vegetable is equal to 5 g of carbohydrate, 2 g of protein, and 25 calories
2. One-half cup of carrots is equal to $1/2$ cup of greens, $1/2$ cup of Brussels sprouts, $1/2$ cup of beets
D. Fruits
1. One fruit is equal to 15 g of carbohydrate and 60 calories
2. One-half banana is equal to one small apple, $1/2$ grapefruit, $1/2$ cup orange juice

---

BOX 11-5

Gas-Forming Foods

Apples, artichokes, barley, beans, bran, broccoli, Brussels sprouts, cabbage, celery, cherries, coconuts, eggplant, figs, honey, melons, milk, molasses, nuts, onions, radishes, soybeans, wheat and yeast

---

BOX 11-6

Measures to Relieve Thirst

Chew gum or suck hard candy
Freeze fluids so they take longer to consume
Add lemon juice to water to make it more refreshing
Gargle with refrigerated mouthwash

E. Milks
   1. One milk is equal to 12 g of carbohydrate, 8 g of protein, trace of fat, and 90 calories
   2. One cup nonfat milk is equal to 1 cup of nonfat plain yogurt, 1 cup of nonfat buttermilk, ½ cup evaporated nonfat milk
F. Fats
   1. One fat is equal to 5 g of fat and 45 calories
   2. One teaspoon (tsp) of butter is equal to 1 tsp margarine, 1 tsp any oil, 1 tablespoon salad dressing, 1 strip of bacon, 5 large olives, 10 whole peanuts
G. Legumes
   1. Similar to meats, are rich in protein and iron, and are lower in fat than meat
   2. Contain starch
   3. One cup of legumes is equal to 1 lean meat plus 2 starches
   4. One cup of legumes is equal to 30 g of carbohydrates, 13 g of protein, 3 g of fat, and 215 calories

V. ENTERAL NUTRITION

A. Description: Provides liquefied foods into the GI tract via a tube
B. Indications
   1. When the GI tract is functional but oral intake is not feasible
   2. Used for clients with swallowing problems, burns, major trauma, liver failure, or severe **malnutrition**
C. Nursing considerations
   1. Clients with lactose intolerance need to be placed on lactose-free formulas
   2. Refer to Chapter 20 for information regarding the administration of GI tube feedings

PRACTICE QUESTIONS

1. A nurse has provided dietary instructions to a client with renal calculi who must learn to eat an alkaline ash diet. The nurse determines that the client has properly understood the information presented if the client chooses which of the following selections from a diet menu?
   1. Chicken, potatoes, and cranberries
   2. Peanut butter sandwich, milk, and prunes
   3. Spinach salad, milk, and a banana
   4. Linguini with shrimp, tossed salad, and a plum
2. A client with hypertension has been told that it is necessary to maintain a diet low in sodium. A nurse who is teaching this client about foods that are allowed would plan to include which food item in a list provided to the client?
   1. Tomato soup
   2. Summer squash
   3. Instant oatmeal
   4. Boiled shrimp

3. A client has been diagnosed with gout. In developing a dietary plan for the client, a nurse plans to include which item on a list of foods to be avoided?
   1. Liver
   2. Chocolate
   3. Carrots
   4. Tapioca
4. A clear liquid diet has been prescribed for a client who is recovering from gastric surgery. A nurse would check with the dietary department to ensure that the nursing unit kitchen is stocked with which food item that is allowed in this diet?
   1. Chicken broth
   2. Sherbet
   3. Orange juice
   4. Ice cream
5. A female adult client with diabetes mellitus has been instructed in the dietary exchange system. The client tells a nurse that she would like to eat 8 ounces of nonfat yogurt with breakfast. The nurse determines that the client understands the principles of the exchange system if the client states that she will:
   1. Not eat ice cream for one week
   2. Omit 8 oz. of skim milk at that meal
   3. Omit salad dressing and butter for the day
   4. Eat only half of a meat exchange at supper
6. A nurse is planning to teach a client with heart disease about the necessity of following a low-fat diet. The nurse develops a list of high-fat foods to avoid. Which food item would the nurse plan to include in this list?
   1. Broccoli
   2. Oranges
   3. Cream cheese
   4. Broiled haddock
7. A client is recovering from abdominal surgery and has a large abdominal wound. A nurse encourages the client to eat which food item that is naturally high in vitamin C to promote wound healing?
   1. Chicken
   2. Bananas
   3. Oranges
   4. Milk
8. A nurse is caring for a client with cirrhosis of the liver. To minimize the effects of the disorder, the nurse teaches the client about foods that are high in thiamine. The nurse determines that the client has the best understanding of the dietary measures to follow if the client states an intention to increase the intake of:
   1. Pork
   2. Milk
   3. Chicken
   4. Broccoli

9. A client who has developed atrial fibrillation that is not responding to medication therapy has been placed on warfarin sodium (Coumadin). A nurse is doing discharge dietary teaching with the client. The nurse would plan to teach the client to avoid which of the following foods while taking this medication?
   1. Cherries
   2. Potatoes
   3. Spaghetti
   4. Broccoli

10. A client who has recently been started on enteral feedings begins to complain of abdominal cramping, followed by passage of two liquid stools. A nurse notes that the client has abdominal distention as well. The nurse reviews the nutritional content on the label of the can of feeding to see if it has which of the following ingredients?
   1. Maltose
   2. Lactose
   3. Sucrose
   4. Fructose

CRITICAL THINKING: FREE-TEXT ENTRY

Spironolactone (Aldactone), a diuretic, is prescribed for a client with congestive heart failure. A nurse provides dietary instructions to the client and instructs the client to avoid foods that are high in which electrolyte?

Answer: _____

ANSWERS

1. **3**
Rationale: In an alkaline ash diet, all fruits are allowed except cranberries, blueberries, prunes, and plums. Options 1, 2, and 4 represent an acid ash diet.
Test-Taking Strategy: Use the process of elimination. Remembering that cranberries, blueberries, prunes, and plums are not allowed in an alkaline ash diet will easily direct you to option 3. Review the foods allowed in this diet if you had difficulty with this question.
Level of Cognitive Ability: Analysis
Client Needs: Health Promotion and Maintenance
Integrated Concept/Process: Teaching/Learning
Content Area: Adult Health/Renal
Reference: Phipps, W., Sands, J., & Marek, J. (1999). *Medical-surgical nursing: Concepts & clinical practice* (6th ed.). St. Louis: Mosby, p. 1431.

2. **2**
Rationale: Foods that are lower in sodium include fruits and vegetables (option 2), because they do not contain physiologic saline. Highly processed or refined foods (options 1 and 3) are higher in sodium unless their food labels specifically state "low sodium." Salt-water fish and shellfish are high in sodium.
Test-Taking Strategy: Use the process of elimination. Begin to answer this question by eliminating option 4, knowing that salt-water fish and shellfish are high in sodium. Next, elimination options 1 and 3 because they are processed foods. Review the foods that are high in sodium if you had difficulty with this question.
Level of Cognitive Ability: Application
Client Needs: Health Promotion and Maintenance
Integrated Concept/Process: Teaching/Learning
Content Area: Adult Health/Cardiovascular
Reference: Grodner, M., Anderson, S., & DeYoung, S. (2000). *Foundations and clinical applications of nutrition: A nursing approach.* St. Louis: Mosby, p. 226.

3. **1**
Rationale: Liver should be omitted from the diet of a client who has gout because of its high purine content. The food items identified in the other options contain negligible amounts of purines and may be consumed freely by the client with gout.
Test-Taking Strategy: Use the process of elimination. Recalling that high-purine foods need to be avoided will direct you to option 1. Review foods high in purine if you had difficulty with this question.
Level of Cognitive Ability: Application
Client Needs: Health Promotion and Maintenance
Integrated Concept/Process: Teaching/Learning
Content Area: Adult Health/Musculoskeletal
Reference: Grodner, M., Anderson, S., & DeYoung, S. (2000). *Foundations and clinical applications of nutrition: A nursing approach.* St. Louis: Mosby, p. 786.

4. **1**
Rationale: A clear liquid diet consists of foods that are relatively transparent. The food items in options 2, 3, and 4 would be included in a full liquid diet.
Test-Taking Strategy: Remember that a clear liquid diet consists of foods that are relatively transparent. By the process of elimination you should easily select option 1 because it is the only food item that is transparent. Review food items allowed on a clear liquid diet and a full liquid diet if you had difficulty with this question.
Level of Cognitive Ability: Application
Client Needs: Physiological Integrity
Integrated Concept/Process: Nursing Process/Planning
Content Area: Adult Health/Gastrointestinal
Reference: Grodner, M., Anderson, S., & DeYoung, S. (2000). *Foundations and clinical applications of nutrition: A nursing approach.* St. Louis: Mosby, p. 461.

5. **2**
Rationale: Yogurt belongs to the milk exchange. On the exchange system, foods are exchanged within that food group only. Salad dressing and butter belong to the fat exchange. Meats are a separate exchange. Ice cream is not recommended for use in the diabetic diet because it is high in fat and sugar. The exchange system is used within a meal, not between meals (options 3 and 4) or spread out over extended periods of time (option 1).
Test-Taking Strategy: Familiarity with the various foods in the

diabetic diet and the exchange system is needed to answer this question. However, note the relationship between the words "with breakfast" in the question and "at that meal" in the correct option. Review foods and categories in the exchange system if you had difficulty with this question.
Level of Cognitive Ability: Analysis
Client Needs: Health Promotion and Maintenance
Integrated Concept/Process: Teaching/Learning
Content Area: Adult Health/Endocrine
Reference: LeMone, P., & Burke, K. (2000). *Medical-surgical nursing: Critical thinking in client care* (2nd ed.). Upper Saddle River, NJ: Prentice-Hall, p. 746.

6. **3**
Rationale: Fruits and vegetables tend to be lower in fat because they do not come from animal sources. Fish is also naturally lower in fat. Cream cheese is a high-fat food.
Test-Taking Strategy: Use the process of elimination and focus on the issue of the question, the high-fat food. Options 1 and 2 can be easily eliminated. From the remaining two options, remember that cheese is high in fat content. Review foods that are high in fat content if you had difficulty with this question.
Level of Cognitive Ability: Application
Client Needs: Health Promotion and Maintenance
Integrated Concept/Process: Teaching/Learning
Content Area: Adult Health/Cardiovascular
Reference: Lewis, S., Heitkemper, M., & Dirksen, S. (2000). *Medical-surgical nursing: Assessment and management of clinical problems* (5th ed.). St. Louis: Mosby, p. 850.

7. **3**
Rationale: Citrus fruits and juices are especially high in Vitamin C. Bananas are high in potassium. Meats and dairy products are two food groups that are high in the B vitamins.
Test-Taking Strategy: Note the key words "naturally high" in the stem of the question. Use the process of elimination, recalling that citrus fruits and juices are high in vitamin C. Review the foods high in vitamin C if you are unfamiliar with them.
Level of Cognitive Ability: Application
Client Needs: Health Promotion and Maintenance
Integrated Concept/Process: Teaching/Learning
Content Area: Fundamental Skills
Reference: Harkreader. H. (2000). *Fundamentals of nursing: Caring and clinical judgment.* Philadelphia: W.B. Saunders. p. 684.

8. **1**
Rationale: The client with cirrhosis needs to consume foods high in thiamine. Thiamine is present in a variety of foods of plant and animal origin. Pork products are especially rich in this vitamin. Other good food sources include nuts, whole grain cereals, and legumes. Milk contains vitamins A, D, and B_2. Poultry contains niacin. Broccoli contains vitamins C, E, K, and folic acid.
Test-Taking Strategy: Note the key words "best understanding" in the stem of the question. This may indicate that more than one option may be a food that contains thiamine. Remembering that pork products are especially rich in thiamine will easily direct you to option 1. Review food items high in thiamine if you had difficulty with this question.
Level of Cognitive Ability: Analysis
Client Needs: Health Promotion and Maintenance

Integrated Concept/Process: Teaching/Learning
Content Area: Adult Health/Gastrointestinal
Reference: Harkreader. H. (2000). *Fundamentals of nursing: Caring and clinical judgment.* Philadelphia: W.B. Saunders, p. 683.

9. **4**
Rationale: Anticoagulant medications work by antagonizing the action of vitamin K, which is needed for clotting. When a client is taking an anticoagulant, foods high in vitamin K are often omitted from the diet. Vitamin K is found in green, leafy vegetables such as broccoli. The other options listed are foods that are lower in vitamin K.
Test-Taking Strategy: Knowledge about the relationship between warfarin sodium and vitamin K is needed to answer this question. Note the key word "avoid" in the stem of the question. This tells you that the correct option is a food that is high in vitamin K. Remember that green, leafy vegetables are high in vitamin K. If you had difficulty with this question, review the foods high in vitamin K.
Level of Cognitive Ability: Analysis
Client Needs: Physiological Integrity
Integrated Concept/Process: Teaching/Learning
Content Area: Pharmacology
Reference: Grodner, M., Anderson, S., & DeYoung, S. (2000). *Foundations and clinical applications of nutrition: A nursing approach.* St. Louis: Mosby, p. 199.

10. **2**
Rationale: Several tube feeding formulas contain lactose. A client with an unreported history of lactose intolerance would develop symptoms such as these in response to nutritional therapy with these formulas. If the client is diagnosed as lactose intolerant, a lactose-free formula should be prescribed by the physician. This will resolve the client's symptoms and promote adequate nutrition for the client.
Test-Taking Strategy: The issue of the question is the ability to associate the symptoms experienced by the client with the symptoms of lactose intolerance. If you had difficulty with this question, review the symptoms of lactose intolerance and the nursing considerations related to enteral feedings.
Level of Cognitive Ability: Analysis
Client Needs: Physiological Integrity
Integrated Concept/Process: Nursing Process/Assessment
Content Area: Fundamental Skills
Reference: Lewis, S., Heitkemper, M., & Dirksen, S. (2000). *Medical-surgical nursing: Assessment and management of clinical problems* (5th ed.). St. Louis: Mosby, p. 1058.

CRITICAL THINKING: FREE-TEXT ENTRY

Answer: The client should avoid foods high in potassium.
Rationale: Spironolactone is a potassium-sparing diuretic and the client should avoid foods high in potassium. If foods high in potassium are not avoided, the client could develop hyperkalemia.
Test-Taking Strategy: Knowledge that spironolactone is a potassium-sparing diuretic will direct your thinking to the need for the client to avoid consuming foods high in potassium. If you had difficulty answering this question, review this medication and the client teaching points related to its administration.
Level of Cognitive Ability: Application

Client Needs: Physiological Integrity
Integrated Concept/Process: Teaching/Learning
Content Area: Adult Health/Cardiovascular
References: Grodner, M., Anderson, S., & DeYoung, S. (2000). *Foundations and clinical applications of nutrition: A nursing approach.* St. Louis: Mosby, p. 461.
Hodgson, B., & Kizior, R. (2001). *Saunders nursing drug handbook 2001.* Philadelphia: W.B. Saunders, pp. 942-944.

REFERENCES

Grodner, M., Anderson, S., & DeYoung, S. (2000). *Foundations and clinical applications of nutrition: A nursing approach.* St. Louis: Mosby.

Harkreader. H. (2000). *Fundamentals of nursing: Caring and clinical judgment.* Philadelphia: W.B. Saunders.

Hodgson, B., & Kizior, R. (2001). *Saunders nursing drug handbook 2001.* Philadelphia: W.B. Saunders.

Ignatavicius, D., Workman, M., & Mishler, M. (1999). *Medical-surgical nursing across the health care continuum* (3rd ed.). Philadelphia: W.B. Saunders.

Lewis, S., Heitkemper, M., & Dirksen, S. (2000). *Medical-surgical nursing: Assessment and management of clinical problems* (5th ed.). St. Louis: Mosby.

LeMone, P., & Burke, K. (2000). *Medical-surgical nursing: Critical thinking in client care* (2nd ed.). Upper Saddle River, NJ: Prentice-Hall.

Phipps, W., Sands, J., & Marek, J. (1999). *Medical-surgical nursing: Concepts & clinical practice* (6th ed.). St. Louis: Mosby.

Smeltzer, S., & Bare, B. (2000) *Brunner & Suddarth's textbook of medical-surgical nursing* (9th ed.). Philadelphia: Lippincott Williams & Wilkins.

Total Parenteral Nutrition (TPN)

PYRAMID TERMS

fat emulsion (lipids) Administered during parenteral nutrition therapy to prevent fatty acid deficiency.

malnutrition Poor nourishment resulting from an improper diet or from some defect in metabolism that prevents the body from using its food properly.

parenteral nutrition The administration of nutrition through a central or peripheral intravenous catheter.

peripheral parenteral nutrition (PPN) Parenteral nutrition administered through a peripheral vein in an extremity.

total parenteral nutrition (TPN) Parenteral nutrition administered through a central vein, such as the subclavian vein; also called hyperalimentation or central venous or central parenteral nutrition.

▲ PYRAMID TO SUCCESS

The NCLEX-RN test plan addresses TPN as related content in the Client Needs area of Physiological Integrity, Pharmacological and Parenteral Therapies. Pyramid points focus on the administration of TPN and fat emulsions, nursing interventions, and the interventions required in monitoring for complications. Pyramid points also focus on home care instructions for the client receiving TPN at home. The primary Integrated Concepts and Processes addressed in this chapter are Nursing Process, Communication and Documentation, Self-Care, and Teaching/Learning.

▲ CLIENT NEEDS
Safe, Effective Care Environment

Consultation with members of the health care team
Dietary consultation
Handling hazardous and infectious materials
Home health care referral
Informed consent for venous access and placement of the catheter

Medical and surgical asepsis to prevent infection
Standard (universal) and other precautions

Health Promotion and Maintenance

Health and wellness related to nutrition
Client and family education regarding the administration of TPN at home
Client and family education regarding monitoring for complications

Psychosocial Integrity

Role changes related to the need to receive TPN
Support systems in the home to assist with the administration of TPN

Physiological Integrity

Nutritional needs
Providing comfort and assistance in the performance of activities of daily living
Rest and sleep
Central venous access device
TPN
Laboratory values
Monitoring for potential complications
Monitoring for expected effects
Documentation

I. TOTAL PARENTERAL NUTRITION (TPN)
A. Description
1. Supplies necessary nutrients via veins
2. Supplies carbohydrates in the form of dextrose, fats in special emulsified form, proteins in the form of amino acids, vitamins, minerals, and water

3. Prevents subcutaneous fat and muscle protein from being catabolized by the body for energy

B. Indications
   1. Clients whose gastrointestinal (GI) tracts are severely dysfunctional or nonfunctional and are unable to process nutrients normally
   2. Clients who can take some oral nutrition, but not enough to meet the body's needs
   3. Clients with multiple GI surgeries, GI trauma, severe intolerance to enteral feedings, or intestinal obstructions, or when the bowel needs to rest for healing
   4. Clients with acquired immunodeficiency syndrome (AIDS), cancer, or **malnutrition,** or clients receiving chemotherapy

C. Components
   1. Carbohydrates
      a. Mainly in the form of glucose; ranges from a 5% glucose solution for **peripheral parenteral nutrition** to a 50% to 70% glucose (hypertonic) solution for **central parenteral nutrition**
      b. The strength of the glucose solution prescribed depends on the client's nutritional needs and on agency protocols
      c. Provides 60% to 70% of caloric (energy) needs
   2. Amino acids: Provide 3% to 15% of the total calories
   3. **Lipid (fat emulsion)**
      a. Provides up to 30% of caloric (energy) needs
      b. Provides nonprotein calories and prevents or corrects fatty acid deficiency
   4. Vitamins
   5. Minerals and trace elements
   6. Water
   7. Electrolytes
   8. Insulin may be added to control the blood glucose level because of the high concentration of glucose solution in the TPN
   9. Heparin may be added to reduce the build-up of a fibrinous clot at the catheter tip

II. INTRAVENOUS SITES
A. **Central parenteral nutrition (CPN)**
   1. **TPN** is administered through a central venous access when the client requires a larger concentration of carbohydrates (greater than 10% glucose)
   2. The subclavian or internal jugular veins are used when **TPN** is a short-term intervention (less than 4 weeks)
   3. When **TPN** is anticipated for an extended period (greater than 4 weeks), a more permanent catheter, such as a peripherally inserted central catheter (PICC) line, a tunneled catheter, or an implanted vascular access device, is used

B. **Peripheral parenteral nutrition (PPN)**
   1. Administered through a peripheral vein
   2. Used for short periods (5 to 7 days) and when the client needs only small concentrations of carbohydrates, fats, and proteins
   3. Used to deliver isotonic or mildly hypertonic solutions; the delivery of highly hypertonic solutions into peripheral veins can cause sclerosis, phlebitis, or swelling

III. LIPIDS (FAT EMULSION)
A. An isotonic solution that can be administered through a peripheral vein
B. Administered to prevent or correct fatty acid deficiency
C. Commercial lipid emulsions are formulations of safflower oil, soybean oil, or a combination of these two, with glycerol added for tonicity and egg phospholipid added as an emulsifying agent
D. Assess client for an allergy to eggs or any of the components of the lipid emulsion solution
E. Examine bottle for separation of emulsion into layers or fat globules or for the accumulation of froth; if observed, do not use and return the solution to the pharmacy
F. Do not put additives into the **fat emulsion** solution
G. Do not use an IV filter because particles in the **fat emulsion** are too large to pass through filters
H. If the **fat emulsion** has been added to the **parenteral nutrition** solution, a 1.2-micron (μ) filter or a larger filter should be used to allow the **fat emulsion** to pass through
I. Use vented IV tubing because the solution is supplied in a glass container for administration
J. Infuse solution initially at 1.0 mL/min, monitor vital signs every 10 minutes, and observe for adverse reactions for the first 30 minutes of the infusion; if signs of an adverse reaction occur, stop the infusion and notify the physician (Box 12-1)
K. If no adverse reaction occurs, adjust flow to prescribed rate

---

BOX 12-1

Signs of an Adverse Reaction to Lipids

Chills
Fever
Flushing
Diaphoresis
Dyspnea
Cyanosis
Chest and back pain
Nausea and vomiting
Headache
Pressure over the eyes
Vertigo
Sleepiness
Thrombophlebitis

L. Monitor serum **lipids** 4 hours after discontinuing infusion
M. Monitor liver function tests for evidence of impaired liver function indicating the liver's inability to metabolize the **lipids**

IV. FILTERS
A. **TPN** and **PPN** must be administered through tubing with an in-line filter to remove crystals from the solution
B. A 0.22-micron (μ) filter is sufficient for administering solutions without lipid additives
C. **Lipids** are administered through separate tubing attached below the filter of the main IV administration because particles in the **fat emulsion** are too large to pass through filters
D. If the **parenteral nutrition** solution has **lipids** added to it, a 1.2-micron (μ) filter or a larger filter should be used

V. COMPLICATIONS (Box 12-2)
A. Description
1. Pneumothorax and air embolism are associated with central line placement; air embolism is also associated with tubing changes
2. Other complications include infection (catheter related), fluid overload, and metabolic alterations such as hyperglycemia and hypoglycemia; these complications are usually due to the **parenteral nutrition** solution itself
B. Pneumothorax (Box 12-3)
1. Monitor for signs of pneumothorax
2. After insertion of the catheter, obtain a portable chest x-ray to confirm correct catheter placement and to detect the presence of a pneumothorax; **parenteral nutrition** is not initiated until correct catheter placement is verified and the absence of pneumothorax is verified
3. After confirmation of catheter placement and the absence of pneumothorax, **parenteral nutrition** is initiated
C. Air embolism (Box 12-4)
1. Instruct the client in the Valsalva maneuver for tubing/cap changes
2. For tubing/cap changes, place client in a head down position with the head turned in the opposite direction of insertion site (increases intrathoracic venous pressure)
3. Check all catheter connections and tape tubing connections
4. If an air embolism is suspected:
   a. Place the client in a left side-lying position with the head lower than the feet (to trap air in right side of the heart)
   b. Notify physician
   c. Administer oxygen as prescribed
D. Infection (Box 12-5)
1. Use strict aseptic technique; because the **TPN** solution is a high-concentrate glucose, it is a medium for bacterial growth
2. Monitor temperature; in the event of fever, sepsis should be suspected
3. Assess IV site for redness, swelling, tenderness, or drainage
4. Change **TPN** solution every 12 to 24 hours or according to agency protocol
5. Change IV tubing every 24 hours or according to agency protocol
6. Change dressing at the IV site every 48 hours or according to agency protocol

BOX 12-2
Complications of Total Parenteral Nutrition

Pneumothorax
Air embolism
Infection
Fluid overload
Hyperglycemia
Hypoglycemia

BOX 12-3
Signs of a Pneumothorax

Chest or shoulder pain
Sudden shortness of breath
Tachycardia
Absence of breath sounds on affected side

BOX 12-4
Signs of an Air Embolism

Respiratory distress
Apprehension
Chest pain
Dyspnea
Hypotension
Rapid and weak pulse
Churning heart murmur

BOX 12-5
Signs of an Infection

Fever
Chills
Erythema or drainage at the insertion site
Elevated white blood cell count
Septic shock

BOX 12-6

Signs of Fluid Overload

Bounding pulse
Jugular vein distension
Headache
Increased blood pressure
Crackles on lung auscultation
Weight gain greater than desired

BOX 12-7

Signs of Hyperglycemia

Elevated blood glucose level
Excessive thirst
Diuresis
Fatigue
Restlessness
Confusion
Weakness
Kussmaul's respirations
Coma, when severe

BOX 12-8

Signs of Hypoglycemia

Blood glucose level less than 70 mg/dL
Shakiness
Weakness
Anxious
Diaphoresis
Hunger

---

7. If signs of infection occur at the site:
   a. The IV line must be removed and restarted at a different site
   b. Remove the tip of the IV catheter and send to the laboratory for culture
   c. Prepare the client for blood cultures
E. Fluid overload (Box 12-6)
   1. Occurs if the client receives the IV solution too rapidly
   2. **TPN** is always delivered via an electronic infusion device
   3. Never increase the infusion rate to "catch up" if the IV infusion gets behind
   4. Monitor intake and output
   5. Weigh daily (ideal weight gain is 1 to 3 pounds per week)
F. Hyperglycemia (Box 12-7)
   1. Assess the client for a history of glucose intolerance
   2. Assess the client's medication history (corticosteroids may increase the blood glucose level)
   3. Begin infusion at a slow rate, usually 40 mL/hour, as prescribed
   4. Never increase the infusion rate to "catch up" if the IV infusion gets behind
   5. Monitor blood glucose levels every 4 to 6 hours or according to agency protocol
   6. Start sliding scale insulin therapy as prescribed

G. Hypoglycemia (Box 12-8)
   1. Continue blood glucose monitoring
   2. Gradually decrease infusion when discontinuing **TPN**
   3. When an infusion of hypertonic glucose is stopped, an infusion of 10% dextrose should be instituted and maintained for 1 to 2 hours to prevent hypoglycemia
   4. Assess blood glucose level 1 hour after discontinuing **TPN**
   5. Prepare for the administration of glucose if hypoglycemia occurs

VI. ADDITIONAL NURSING CONSIDERATIONS ▲
A. Always check the **TPN** solution with the physician's order to ensure that the prescribed components are contained in the solution
B. To prevent infection and solution incompatibility, IV medications and blood are not given through the **TPN** line
C. Monitor partial thromboplastin time (PTT) and prothrombin time (PT) for clients receiving anticoagulants
D. Monitor electrolytes, albumin, and liver and renal function tests
E. In severely dehydrated clients, the albumin level may drop initially as the treatment restores hydration
F. With severely malnourished clients, monitor for "refeeding syndrome" (a rapid drop in potassium, magnesium, and phosphate serum levels)
G. Abnormal liver function values may indicate intolerance to or an excess of **fat emulsions,** or problems with metabolism with glucose and protein
H. Abnormal renal function tests indicate an excess of amino acids
I. **TPN** solutions should be stored under refrigeration and administered within 24 hours from the time that they were prepared (remove from refrigerator 0.5 to 1 hour before use)
J. **TPN** solutions that are cloudy or darkened should not be used and should be returned to the pharmacy

VII. HOME CARE INSTRUCTIONS (Box 12-9) ▲

BOX 12-9

Home Care Instructions

How to administer and maintain TPN fluids

How to change a sterile dressing

Instruct to obtain weight daily at the same time in the same clothes

Stress that a weight gain of more than 3 pounds per week may indicate excessive fluid intake and should be reported

Check urine for sugar and acetone or check capillary blood glucose level and report abnormalities immediately

Check for signs and symptoms of infection, thrombosis, air embolism, and catheter displacement

Instruct in the importance of reporting signs and symptoms of complications

Symptoms of an air embolus should be taught to another person in the client's home

For symptoms of thrombosis, the client should report edema of the arm or catheter insertion site, neck pain, and jugular vein distention

Leaking of fluid from the insertion site or pain or discomfort as the fluids are infused may indicate displacement of the catheter; this must be reported immediately

PRACTICE QUESTIONS

1. A client has been discharged to home on total parenteral nutrition (TPN). With each visit, a home care nurse assesses which of the following parameters most closely in monitoring this therapy?
   1. Temperature and weight
   2. Temperature and blood pressure
   3. Pulse and weight
   4. Pulse and blood pressure

2. A nurse is caring for a group of adult clients on an acute care medical-surgical nursing unit. The nurse understands that which of the following clients would be the least likely candidate for total parenteral nutrition (TPN)?
   1. A 66-year-old client with extensive burns
   2. A 42-year-old client who had an open cholecystectomy
   3. A 35-year-client with persistent nausea and vomiting from chemotherapy
   4. A 27-year-old client with severe exacerbation of regional enteritis (Crohn's disease)

3. A nurse is planning to hang the first bag of total parenteral nutrition (TPN) solution via the central line of an assigned client. The nurse plans to obtain which of the following most essential pieces of equipment before hanging the solution?
   1. Electronic infusion pump
   2. Blood glucose meter
   3. Urine test strips
   4. Noninvasive blood pressure monitor

4. A home care nurse is monitoring a client's response to total parenteral nutrition (TPN). The client's weight 1 week ago was 114 pounds. The nurse determines that the client is not gaining weight too rapidly if this morning's weight was:
   1. 116 pounds
   2. 119 pounds
   3. 120 pounds
   4. 122 pounds

5. A nurse is assigned to a client receiving TPN who had a blood glucose measurement done at 06:00. The nurse documents on the client's clinical worksheet for the day that the blood glucose level should be checked at which of the following times?
   1. 08:00
   2. 12:00
   3. 16:00
   4. 18:00

6. A client is receiving nutrition by means of total parenteral nutrition (TPN). A nurse monitors the client for complications of the therapy and assesses the client for which of the following signs of hyperglycemia?
   1. Nausea, vomiting, and oliguria
   2. Sweating, chills, and abdominal pain
   3. Fever, weak pulse, and thirst
   4. Weakness, thirst, and increased urine output

7. At 8:00 A.M. a nurse checks the amount of solution left in a total parenteral nutrition (TPN) infusion bag for an assigned client. It is a 3000 mL bag with 1000 mL remaining. The solution is running at a rate of 100 mL/hr. The bag was hung the previous day at 12:00 noon. The nurse plans to change the infusion bag and tubing today at:
   1. 12:00 noon
   2. 2:00 P.M.
   3. 4:00 P.M.
   4. 8:00 P.M.

8. A nurse is changing the central line dressing of a client receiving total parenteral nutrition (TPN). The nurse notes that the catheter insertion site appears reddened. The nurse next assesses which of the following items?
   1. Tightness of tubing connections
   2. Client's temperature
   3. Expiration date on the bag
   4. Time of last dressing change

9. A nurse is preparing to hang a fat emulsion. The nurse notes that fat globules are visible at the top of the solution. The nurse takes which of the following actions?
   1. Runs the bottle of solution under warm water
   2. Rolls the bottle of solution gently

3. Shakes the bottle of solution vigorously
4. Obtains a different bottle of solution

10. A client is being weaned from total parenteral nutrition (TPN) and is expected to begin taking solid food today. The ongoing solution rate has been 100 mL/hr. A nurse anticipates that which of the following orders regarding the TPN solution will accompany the diet order?
    1. Discontinue the TPN
    2. Continue current infusion rate orders for TPN
    3. Decrease TPN rate to 50 mL/hr
    4. Hang 1000 mL 0.9% normal saline

11. A nurse is preparing to change the total parenteral nutrition (TPN) solution bag and tubing. The client's central venous line is located in the right subclavian vein. The nurse asks the client to do which of the following most essential items during the tubing change?
    1. Take a deep breath, hold it, and bear down
    2. Exhale slowly and evenly
    3. Turn the head to the right
    4. Breathe normally

12. A client with total parenteral nutrition (TPN) infusing has disconnected the tubing from the central line catheter. A nurse assesses the client and suspects an air embolism. The nurse should immediately place the client in which of the following positions?
    1. On the left side with the head higher than the feet
    2. On the left side with the head lower than the feet
    3. On the right side with the head higher than the feet
    4. On the right side with the head lower than the feet

13. A client receiving total parenteral nutrition (TPN) complains of a headache. A nurse notes that the client has an increased blood pressure, bounding pulse, jugular vein distention, and crackles bilaterally. The nurse interprets that the client is experiencing which complication of TPN therapy?
    1. Hyperglycemia
    2. Air embolism
    3. Sepsis
    4. Fluid overload

14. A client receiving TPN suddenly spikes a fever. A nurse notifies the physician and the physician initially orders that the solution and tubing be changed. The nurse should do which of the following with the discontinued materials?
    1. Return them to the hospital pharmacy
    2. Send them to the laboratory for culture
    3. Save them for return to the manufacturer
    4. Discard them in the unit trash

15. A nurse enters the room of a client receiving total parenteral nutrition (TPN) and discovers that the electronic infusion pump has been shut off. After checking the line for patency and restarting the infusion, the nurse assesses the client for which of the following signs and symptoms?
    1. Weakness, thirst, and excessive urination
    2. Fever and chills
    3. Weakness, shakiness, diaphoresis, and complaints of hunger
    4. Dyspnea and hypotension

16. A nurse is making initial rounds at the beginning of the shift. The total parenteral nutrition (TPN) bag of an assigned client is empty. Which of the following solutions readily available on the nursing unit should the nurse hang until another TPN solution is mixed and delivered to the nursing unit?
    1. 5% dextrose in water
    2. 5% dextrose in 0.9% sodium chloride
    3. 5% dextrose in Ringer's lactate
    4. 10% dextrose in water

17. At the beginning of a shift, a nurse assesses a client receiving TPN with fat emulsion piggybacked to the line. The nurse notes that the fat emulsion tubing has an in-line 0.22-micron (μ) filter. Which of the following actions by the nurse is most appropriate?
    1. Inspect the filter for clogging
    2. Remove the filter
    3. Leave the system alone
    4. Check the line for patency

18. A nurse is monitoring the status of a client's fat emulsion infusion. The nurse notes that the infusion is 1 hour behind. Which of the following actions by the nurse is most appropriate?
    1. Adjust the infusion rate to run wide open until the solution is back on time
    2. Leave the fat emulsion infusion rate as it is
    3. Adjust the infusion rate to catch up over the next 2 hours
    4. Adjust the infusion rate to catch up over the next hour

19. A client receiving total parenteral nutrition (TPN) in the home setting has a weight gain of 5 pounds in 1 week. The nurse next assesses the client to detect the presence of which of the following?
    1. Crackles on auscultation of the lungs
    2. Thirst
    3. Decreased blood pressure
    4. Polyuria

20. A nurse is caring for a restless client who is beginning nutritional therapy with total parenteral nutrition (TPN). The nurse should plan to ensure that which of the following is done to prevent the client from injury?
    1. Monitor blood glucose levels every 12 hours
    2. Tape all connections in the TPN system
    3. Monitor the temperature once daily
    4. Calculate daily intake and output (I&O)

CRITICAL THINKING: FREE-TEXT ENTRY

A nurse is preparing to administer lipid emulsion to a client who has just been started on total parenteral nutrition (TPN). Prior to administering the lipid emulsion, the nurse asks the client about allergies. The nurse would withhold the lipid emulsion and contact the physician if the client identified an allergy to what particular food item?

Answer: _____

ANSWERS

1. 1
Rationale: The client receiving TPN at home should have the temperature monitored as a means of detecting infection, which is a potential complication of this therapy. An infection could also result in sepsis, since the catheter is in a blood vessel. The client's weight is monitored as a measure of the effectiveness of this nutritional therapy and to detect fluid overload. The pulse and blood pressure are important parameters to assess, but they do not relate specifically to the effects of TPN.
Test-Taking Strategy: Note the key words "TPN" and "most closely," which tell you that more than one or all of the options may be partially or totally correct. Remember also that when there are multiple parts to an option, all of the parts must be correct in order for that option to be correct. Recalling that infection and fluid overload are complications of TPN and that weight is monitored as a measure of the effectiveness of this nutritional therapy will direct you to option 1. Review these important assessments if you had difficulty with this question.
Level of Cognitive Ability: Application
Client Needs: Health Promotion and Maintenance
Integrated Concept/Process: Nursing Process/Assessment
Content Area: Fundamental Skills
Reference: Craven, R. & Hirnle, C. (2000). *Fundamentals of nursing: Human health and function* (3rd ed.). Philadelphia: Lippincott Williams & Wilkins, p. 580.

2. 2
Rationale: TPN is indicated in clients whose gastrointestinal (GI) tracts are not functional, or who cannot take in a diet enterally for extended periods of time. Examples of these conditions include those of the clients identified in options 1, 3, and 4. Other clients would be those who have had extensive surgery, have multiple fractures, are septic, or have advanced cancer or acquired immunodeficiency syndrome (AIDS). The client with the open cholecystectomy is not a candidate because this client would resume a diet within a few days following surgery.
Test-Taking Strategy: Note the key words "TPN" and "least likely," which tell you that the correct option is the client who does not require this type of nutritional support. Use nursing knowledge of these various conditions and baseline knowledge of the purposes of TPN to make your selection. Review the indications for TPN if you had difficulty with this question.
Level of Cognitive Ability: Comprehension
Client Needs: Physiological Integrity
Integrated Concept/Process: Nursing Process/Assessment
Content Area: Fundamental Skills
Reference: Phipps, W., Sands, J., & Marek, J. (1999). *Medical-surgical nursing: Concepts & clinical practice* (6th ed.). St. Louis: Mosby, p. 1364.

3. 1
Rationale: The nurse obtains an electronic infusion pump before hanging a TPN solution. Because of the high glucose content, it is necessary to use an infusion pump to ensure that the solution does not infuse too rapidly or fall too far behind. Because the client's blood glucose is monitored every 4 to 6 hours during administration of TPN, a blood glucose meter will also be needed, but this is not the most essential item needed prior to hanging of the solution. Urine test strips (to measure glucose) are rarely used since the advent of blood glucose monitoring. A noninvasive blood pressure monitor is unnecessary for this procedure.
Test-Taking Strategy: Note the key words "most essential." They tell you that the correct option identifies the item that is needed to start the infusion. Use the process of elimination and knowledge of the procedure for initiating TPN to answer the question. Review these procedures if you had difficulty with this question.
Level of Cognitive Ability: Application
Client Needs: Safe, Effective Care Environment
Integrated Concept/Process: Nursing Process/Planning
Content Area: Fundamental Skills
Reference: Phipps, W., Sands, J., & Marek, J. (1999). *Medical-surgical nursing: Concepts & clinical practice* (6th ed.). St. Louis: Mosby, p. 1364.

4. 1
Rationale: The client receiving TPN should not gain more than 3 pounds per week, with optimal weight gain being 1 to 3 pounds per week. The weight goal for the client on TPN is individual and depends on the client's metabolic needs and baseline weight (whether underweight, overweight, or at optimal weight). The correct option identifies a reasonable weight gain of 2 pounds per week. Options 2, 3, and 4 indicate a weekly weight gain that is greater than expected.
Test-Taking Strategy: Use the process of elimination and recall that the optimal weekly weight gain for the client on TPN is 1 to 3 pounds weekly. Review the expected outcomes of TPN if you had difficulty with this question.
Level of Cognitive Ability: Analysis
Client Needs: Health Promotion and Maintenance
Integrated Concept/Process: Nursing Process/Evaluation
Content Area: Fundamental Skills
Reference: Smith, S., Duell, D., & Martin, B. (2000). *Clinical nursing skills: Basic to advanced skills* (5th ed.). Upper Saddle River, NJ: Prentice-Hall Health, p. 900.

5. 2
Rationale: The client's blood glucose level should be monitored every 4 to 6 hours during TPN. Depending on agency policy, this may be done every 8 hours instead. It is unnecessary to monitor the blood glucose level every 2 hours (option 1). Monitoring every 10 or 12 hours (options 3 and 4) is insufficient.

Test-Taking Strategy: Use the process of elimination. Recalling that the client on TPN should have the blood glucose level monitored every 4 to 6 hours and knowledge of military time will direct you to the correct option. If you had difficulty with this question, review the nursing interventions related to the administration of TPN.
Level of Cognitive Ability: Application
Client Needs: Physiological Integrity
Integrated Concept/Process: Communication and Documentation
Content Area: Fundamental Skills
Reference: Smith, S., Duell, D., & Martin, B. (2000). *Clinical nursing skills: Basic to advanced skills* (5th ed.). Upper Saddle River, NJ: Prentice-Hall Health, p. 900.

6. **4**
Rationale: The high glucose concentration in TPN places the client at risk for hyperglycemia. Signs of hyperglycemia include excessive thirst, fatigue, restlessness, confusion, weakness, Kussmaul's respirations, diuresis, and coma, when hyperglycemia is severe. If the client presents with these symptoms, the blood glucose level should be checked immediately. Options 1, 2, and 3 do not identify signs specific to hyperglycemia.
Test-Taking Strategy: Use the process of elimination. Remember that in order for an option to be correct, all of the parts of that option must be correct. Begin to answer this question by eliminating options 2 and 3 because chills and fever are indicative of infection. Choose option 4 over option 1 because the client with hyperglycemia has increased urine output rather than decreased urine output. Review the signs of hyperglycemia if you had difficulty with this question.
Level of Cognitive Ability: Comprehension
Client Needs: Physiological Integrity
Integrated Concept/Process: Nursing Process/Assessment
Content Area: Fundamental Skills
Reference: Smith, S., Duell, D., & Martin, B. (2000). *Clinical nursing skills: Basic to advanced skills* (5th ed.). Upper Saddle River, NJ: Prentice-Hall Health, p. 900.

7. **1**
Rationale: TPN solution should be changed every 24 hours because the TPN solution is a high-concentrate glucose, and is a medium for bacterial growth. Infection control is also aided by use of aseptic technique with bag and tubing changes. Most agencies recommend that tubing be changed every 24 hours along with the bag, although some agencies recommend changing tubing every 48 to 72 hours. Specific agency policies should always be adhered to. Options 2, 3, and 4 identify insufficient time frames and present the risk for infection.
Test-Taking Strategy: Use the process of elimination. Recalling that the infusion bag should be changed every 24 hours will easily direct you to the correct option. Review the principles related to the prevention of infection in the client receiving TPN if you had difficulty with this question.
Level of Cognitive Ability: Application
Client Needs: Safe, Effective Care Environment
Integrated Concept/Process: Nursing Process/Planning
Content Area: Fundamental Skills
Reference: Smith, S., Duell, D., & Martin, B. (2000). *Clinical nursing skills: Basic to advanced skills* (5th ed.). Upper Saddle River, NJ: Prentice-Hall Health, p. 900.

8. **2**
Rationale: Redness at the catheter insertion site is a possible indication of infection. The nurse would next assess for other signs of infection. Of the options given, the temperature is the next item to assess. The tightness of tubing connections should be assessed each time the TPN is checked; loose connections would result in leakage, not skin redness. The expiration date on the bag is a viable alternative, but that also should be checked at the time the solution is hung, and with each shift change. The time of the last dressing change should be checked with each shift change.
Test-Taking Strategy: Note the key word "next." This question requires that you prioritize on the basis of the information provided in the question. Also note the relationship between "site appears reddened" in the question and the word "temperature" in the correct option. Focusing on the issue of infection will easily direct you to option 2. Review the signs of infection in the client receiving TPN if you had difficulty with this question.
Level of Cognitive Ability: Application
Client Needs: Physiological Integrity
Integrated Concept/Process: Nursing Process/Assessment
Content Area: Fundamental Skills
Reference: Lewis, S., Heitkemper, M., & Dirksen, S. (2000). *Medical-surgical nursing: Assessment and management of clinical problems* (5th ed.). St. Louis: Mosby, p. 1062.

9. **4**
Rationale: The nurse should examine the bottle of fat emulsion for separation of emulsion into layers or fat globules, or for the accumulation of froth. The nurse should not hang a fat emulsion if any of these observations are made and should return the solution to the pharmacy. Options 1, 2, and 3 are inappropriate actions.
Test-Taking Strategy: Use the process of elimination. Remember that options that are similar are not likely to be correct. With this in mind, eliminate options 2 and 3 first. Discriminate between the final two options by recalling the significance of fat globules in the solution. Also, think about the potential adverse impact of fat globules entering the client's bloodstream. Review the procedure for administering fat emulsion if you had difficulty with this question.
Level of Cognitive Ability: Application
Client Needs: Safe, Effective Care Environment
Integrated Concept/Process: Nursing Process/Implementation
Content Area: Fundamental Skills
Reference: Smith, S., Duell, D., & Martin, B. (2000). *Clinical nursing skills: Basic to advanced skills* (5th ed.). Upper Saddle River, NJ: Prentice-Hall Health, p. 899.

10. **3**
Rationale: When a client begins taking a diet after a period of receiving parenteral nutrition, the TPN is gradually decreased. TPN that is discontinued abruptly can cause hypoglycemia. Clients often have anorexia after being without food for some time, and the digestive tract is also not used to producing the digestive enzymes that will be needed. Gradually decreasing the infusion rate allows the client to remain adequately nourished during the transition to a normal diet and prevents the occurrence of hypoglycemia. Even before clients are started on a solid diet, they are given clear liquids followed by full liquids to further ease the transition. A solution of normal

saline will not provide the glucose needed during the transition of discontinuing the TPN and could also cause the client to experience hypoglycemia.

Test-Taking Strategy: Use the process of elimination and note the key word "weaned" in the question. Recalling the effects of TPN and the complications that occur will easily direct you to option 3. If you had difficulty with this question, review the concepts related to discontinuing TPN solution.

Level of Cognitive Ability: Analysis
Client Needs: Physiological Integrity
Integrated Concept/Process: Nursing Process/Analysis
Content Area: Fundamental Skills
Reference: Smith, S., Duell, D., & Martin, B. (2000). *Clinical nursing skills: Basic to advanced skills* (5th ed.). Upper Saddle River, NJ: Prentice-Hall Health, p. 900.

11. 1
Rationale: The client should be asked to perform the Valsalva maneuver during tubing changes. This helps to avoid air embolism during tubing changes. This is commonly achieved by asking the client to take a deep breath, hold it, and bear down. If the IV line is on the right, the client turns the head to the left. This position will increase intrathoracic pressure. Options 2 and 4 are inappropriate and could cause the potential for an air embolism during the tubing change.

Test-Taking Strategy: Note the key words "most essential." Use the process of elimination, recalling that air embolism is a complication that can occur during tubing changes. Review the procedure for TPN bag and tubing change if you had difficulty with this question.

Level of Cognitive Ability: Application
Client Needs: Physiological Integrity
Integrated Concept/Process: Nursing Process/Implementation
Content Area: Fundamental Skills
Reference: Craven, R. & Hirnle, C. (2000). *Fundamentals of nursing: Human health and function* (3rd ed.). Philadelphia: Lippincott Williams & Wilkins, p. 581.

12. 2
Rationale: When air embolism is suspected, the client should be placed in a left side-lying position. The head should be lower than the feet. This position is used to try to minimize the effect of the air traveling as a bolus to the lungs by trapping it in the right side of the heart. Options 1, 3, and 4 are incorrect positions if an air embolism is suspected.

Test-Taking Strategy: Use the process of elimination and recall the concept that the goal is to trap air in the right side of the heart. If you had difficulty with this question, review the immediate interventions when air embolism is suspected.

Level of Cognitive Ability: Application
Client Needs: Physiological Integrity
Integrated Concept/Process: Nursing Process/Implementation
Content Area: Fundamental Skills
Reference: Smeltzer, S., & Bare, B. (2000) *Brunner & Suddarth's textbook of medical-surgical nursing* (9th ed.). Philadelphia: Lippincott Williams & Wilkins, p. 853.

13. 4
Rationale: The client's signs and symptoms are consistent with fluid overload. The increased intravascular volume increases the blood pressure, while the pulse rate increases as the heart tries to pump the extra fluid volume. The volume also causes neck vein distention, and shifting of fluid into the alveoli,

resulting in lung crackles. The signs and symptoms presented in the question are not indicative of hyperglycemia, air embolism, or sepsis.

Test-Taking Strategy: Use the process of elimination, focusing on the signs and symptoms presented in the question. Recalling the signs of fluid overload will easily direct you to option 4. If you had difficulty with this question, review the signs of fluid overload.

Level of Cognitive Ability: Analysis
Client Needs: Physiological Integrity
Integrated Concept/Process: Nursing Process/Analysis
Content Area: Fundamental Skills
Reference: Craven, R. & Hirnle, C. (2000). *Fundamentals of nursing: Human health and function* (3rd ed.). Philadelphia: Lippincott Williams & Wilkins, p. 502.

14. 2
Rationale: When the client who is receiving TPN spikes a temperature, a catheter-related infection should be suspected. The solution and tubing should be changed, and the discontinued materials should be cultured for infectious organisms. The other options are incorrect.

Test-Taking Strategy: Use the process of elimination. Identifying the issue of the question, infection, and correlating the elevated temperature with infection of the IV line should direct you to option 2. Review the procedure when infection is suspected in the client receiving TPN if you had difficulty with this question.

Level of Cognitive Ability: Application
Client Needs: Safe, Effective Care Environment
Integrated Concept/Process: Nursing Process/Implementation
Content Area: Fundamental Skills
Reference: Phipps, W., Sands, J., & Marek, J. (1999). *Medical-surgical nursing: Concepts & clinical practice* (6th ed.). St. Louis: Mosby, p. 1365.

15. 3
Rationale: If the pump that is infusing TPN becomes shut off for a period of time, the nurse assesses the client for signs and symptoms of hypoglycemia. These include weakness, shakiness, headache, anxiety, diaphoresis, and complaints of hunger. The blood glucose level will be less than 70 mg/dL. The other signs and symptoms described are those of hyperglycemia (option 1), infection (option 2), and air embolism (option 4).

Test-Taking Strategy: Use the process of elimination and focus on the issue of the question that the infusion pump has been shut off. Recall that the client is at risk for hypoglycemia when the TPN is stopped or discontinued. Next, recalling the signs of hypoglycemia will direct you to option 3. Review the complications associated with TPN and the signs of the complications, if you had difficulty with this question.

Level of Cognitive Ability: Analysis
Client Needs: Physiological Integrity
Integrated Concept/Process: Nursing Process/Assessment
Content Area: Fundamental Skills
Reference: Phipps, W., Sands, J., & Marek, J. (1999). *Medical-surgical nursing: Concepts & clinical practice* (6th ed.). St. Louis: Mosby, p. 1365.

16. 4
Rationale: The solution containing the highest amount of glucose should be hung until the new TPN becomes available.

Since TPN solutions contain high glucose concentrations, the 10% dextrose in water solution is the best of the choices presented. The solution selected should be one that minimizes the risk of hypoglycemia. Options 1, 2, and 3 will not be as effective in minimizing the risk of hypoglycemia.

Test-Taking Strategy: Use the process of elimination, recalling that this particular client is at risk for hypoglycemia. With this in mind, you would then select the solution that minimizes this risk to the client. Also, remember that options that are similar are not likely to be correct. Each of the incorrect options represents a solution commonly stocked on the nursing unit and contains 5% dextrose. Review the nursing actions to prevent hypoglycemia in the client receiving TPN if you had difficulty with this question.

Level of Cognitive Ability: Application
Client Needs: Physiological Integrity
Integrated Concept/Process: Nursing Process/Implementation
Content Area: Fundamental Skills
Reference: Phipps, W., Sands, J., & Marek, J. (1999). *Medical-surgical nursing: Concepts & clinical practice* (6th ed.). St. Louis: Mosby, p. 1365.

17. **2**

Rationale: The most appropriate action by the nurse is to remove the filter. A 0.22-micron (μ) filter is appropriate for the administration of TPN, and fat emulsion should be administered without a filter. If fat emulsion is mixed into the TPN solution, then a 1.2-micron (μ) filter or a larger filter should be used to allow the fat emulsion to pass through.

Test-Taking Strategy: Use the process of elimination recalling that fat emulsion should be administered without a filter. If you had difficulty with this question, review the procedure for the administration of fat emulsion.

Level of Cognitive Ability: Application
Client Needs: Safe, Effective Care Environment
Integrated Concept/Process: Nursing Process/Implementation
Content Area: Fundamental Skills
Reference: Lewis, S., Heitkemper, M., & Dirksen, S. (2000). *Medical-surgical nursing: Assessment and management of clinical problems* (5th ed.). St. Louis: Mosby, pp. 1061, 1065.

18. **2**

Rationale: The nurse should not increase the rate of a fat emulsion to make up the difference if the infusion falls behind. Doing so could place the client at risk for fat overload. The same principle applies to total parenteral nutrition (TPN); increasing the rate suddenly in this case could cause hyperglycemia and fluid overload.

Test-Taking Strategy: Note the key words "most appropriate." Remember also that options that are similar are not likely to be correct. This guides you to eliminate options 3 and 4 first. Choose option 2 over option 1, recalling that the nurse never increases the infusion rate or adjusts an infusion rate to run wide open if an infusion is behind. Review these safety principles if you had difficulty with this question.

Level of Cognitive Ability: Application
Client Needs: Safe, Effective Care Environment
Integrated Concept/Process: Nursing Process/Implementation
Content Area: Fundamental Skills
Reference: Smith, S., Duell, D., & Martin, B. (2000). *Clinical nursing skills: Basic to advanced skills* (5th ed.). Upper Saddle River, NJ: Prentice-Hall Health, p. 901.

19. **1**

Rationale: Optimal weight gain on TPN is 1 to 3 pounds per week. The client who has a weight gain of 5 pounds per week while receiving TPN is likely to have fluid retention that can result in fluid overload. Signs of fluid overload include a bounding pulse, jugular vein distention, headache, increased blood pressure, crackles on lung auscultation, and weight gain greater than desired. Options 2 and 4 are associated with hyperglycemia. Option 3 is likely to be noted in a fluid volume deficit.

Test-Taking Strategy: Focus on the issue of the question, a weight gain of 5 pounds in 1 week. This should direct your thinking to the potential for fluid overload. With this in mind, use the process of elimination, selecting the option that identifies the signs of fluid overload. If you had difficulty with this question, review the signs and symptoms of the complications associated with the administration of TPN.

Level of Cognitive Ability: Analysis
Client Needs: Physiological Integrity
Integrated Concept/Process: Nursing Process/Assessment
Content Area: Fundamental Skills
Reference: Smith, S., Duell, D., & Martin, B. (2000). *Clinical nursing skills: Basic to advanced skills* (5th ed.). Upper Saddle River, NJ: Prentice-Hall Health, p. 900.

20. **2**

Rationale: The nurse should plan to tape all connections in the tubing. This will help prevent the restless client from pulling the connections apart accidentally. The nurse should also monitor I & O, but this does not specifically relate to a risk for injury as presented in the question. Also, options 1 and 3 do not relate to a risk for injury as presented in the question. In addition, the client's temperature and blood glucose levels are monitored more frequently than the time frames identified in the options, to detect signs of infection and hyperglycemia respectively.

Test-Taking Strategy: Note the key words "restless," "ensure," "prevent," and "injury." Focus on the issue of the question, and use the process of elimination to direct you to option 2. Review the precautions related to TPN if you had difficulty with this question.

Level of Cognitive Ability: Application
Client Needs: Safe, Effective Care Environment
Integrated Concept/Process: Nursing Process/Planning
Content Area: Fundamental Skills
Reference: Craven, R., & Hirnle, C. (2000). *Fundamentals of nursing: Human health and function* (3rd ed.). Philadelphia: Lippincott Williams & Wilkins, p. 580.

CRITICAL THINKING: FREE-TEXT ENTRY

Answer: Egg protein
Rationale: Lipid emulsions are a 10% or 20% combination of triglycerides, egg phospholipids, glycerol, and water. Clients who are allergic to egg protein may have an acute or allergic reaction to lipid emulsion.

Test-Taking Strategy: Recalling that egg phospholipids are a component of lipid emulsions will assist in answering this question. Review the nursing responsibilities related to the administration of lipid emulsions if you had difficulty with this question.

Level of Cognitive Ability: Application

Client Needs: Safe, Effective Care Environment
Integrated Concept/Process: Nursing Process/Implementation
Content Area: Fundamental Skills

Reference: Altman, G., Buchsel, P., & Coxon, V. (2000). *Delmar's fundamental & advanced nursing skills.* Albany, N.Y.: Delmar, p. 1026; 1050.

REFERENCES

Altman, G., Buchsel, P., & Coxen, V. (2000). *Delmar's fundamental & advanced nursing skills.* Albany, N.Y.: Delmar, pp. 1026, 1050.

Craven, R. & Hirnle, C. (2000). *Fundamentals of nursing: Human health and function* (3rd ed.). Philadelphia: Lippincott Williams & Wilkins.

Lewis, S., Heitkemper, M., & Dirksen, S. (2000). *Medical-surgical nursing: Assessment and management of clinical problems* (5th ed.). St. Louis: Mosby.

Phipps, W., Sands, J., & Marek, J. (1999). *Medical-surgical nursing: Concepts & clinical practice* (6th ed.). St. Louis: Mosby.

Smeltzer, S., & Bare, B. (2000) *Brunner & Suddarth's textbook of medical-surgical nursing* (9th ed). Philadelphia: Lippincott Williams & Wilkins.

Smith, S., Duell, D., & Martin, B. (2000). *Clinical nursing skills: Basic to advanced skills* (5th ed.). Upper Saddle River, NJ: Prentice-Hall Health.

Intravenous Therapy

PYRAMID TERMS

air embolism Caused by a bolus of air that enters the vein through an inadequately primed intravenous (IV) line, from a loose connection, or during tubing change or removal of the IV.

catheter embolism Occurs as the result of breakage of the tip of the catheter during IV insertion or removal.

hypertonic Refers to solutions that are more concentrated or have a higher osmolality than body fluids.

hypotonic Refers to solutions that are more dilute or have a lower osmolality than body fluids.

infiltration Seepage of IV fluid out of the vein and into the surrounding interstitial spaces.

isotonic Refers to solutions that have the same osmolality as body fluids.

phlebitis An inflammation of the vein that can occur as a result of either mechanical or chemical (medication) trauma or a local infection.

▲ PYRAMID TO SUCCESS

Professional nurses are responsible for managing and providing care to clients receiving IV therapy. Pyramid points focus on the safety measures required to initiate and maintain an IV. It is critical for the nurse to assess the client for allergies, including latex sensitivity, prior to initiating an IV. Additional nursing responsibilities include monitoring for complications related to the IV, and the initiation of measures required when an IV complication occurs. Pyramid points focus on the signs and symptoms of infection, infiltration, phlebitis, circulatory overload, and air embolism, and the treatment measures associated with each. The primary Integrated Concepts and Processes addressed in this chapter include Nursing Process, Communication and Documentation, Teaching/Learning, and Self-Care.

CLIENT NEEDS ▲
Safe, Effective Care Environment

Informed consent for invasive procedures
Establishing priorities
Consultation with members of the health care team
Medical and surgical asepsis during handling of equipment and supplies
Standard (universal) precautions
Applying principles of infection control
Error prevention in administering IV's
Handling hazardous or infectious materials

Health Promotion and Maintenance

Health and wellness
Lifestyle choices related to home care of IV
Teaching client and family regarding care of IV
Evaluation of client's home environment for self-care modifications
Client's ability to perform self-care

Psychosocial Integrity

Assessment of coping mechanisms
Support systems in the home for caring for IV
Client's emotional response to treatment

Physiological Integrity

Intravenous therapy
Parenteral therapies
Central venous access devices
Expected effects of IV therapy
Monitoring laboratory values for fluid and electrolyte imbalances
Monitoring for complications of IV therapy
Immediate interventions if a complication occurs

I. INTRAVENOUS THERAPY

A. Purpose and uses
1. Used to sustain clients who are unable to take substances orally
2. Replaces water, electrolytes, and nutrients more rapidly than oral administration
3. Provides immediate access to the vascular system for the rapid delivery of specific solutions without the time required for gastrointestinal (GI) tract absorption
4. Provides a vascular route for the administration of medication or blood components

B. Types of solutions (Table 13-1)
1. **Isotonic**
   a. Solutions with the same osmolality as body fluids
   b. Increase extracellular fluid (ECF) volume
   c. These solutions do not enter the cells because there is no osmotic force to shift the fluids
2. **Hypotonic**
   a. Solutions that are more dilute or have a lower osmolality than body fluids
   b. Cause movement of water into cells by osmosis
   c. These solutions should be administered slowly to prevent cellular edema
3. **Hypertonic**
   a. Solutions that are more concentrated or have a higher osmolality than body fluids
   b. Concentrate ECF and cause movement of water from cells into the ECF by osmosis
4. Crystalloids
   a. Solutions that contain electrolytes
   b. May be used for fluid volume replacement
5. Colloids
   a. Also called plasma expanders
   b. Pull fluid from the interstitial compartment into the vascular compartment
   c. Used to increase the vascular volume rapidly, such as in hemorrhage or severe hypovolemia

II. INTRAVENOUS DEVICES

A. IV cannulas
1. Steel needles or butterfly sets
   a. A wing-tip needle with a metal cannula, plastic or rubber wings, and a plastic catheter or hub
   b. The needle is 0.5 to 1.5 in length, with needle gauge sizes from 16 to 26
   c. Used when the infusion time will be short
   d. **Infiltration** is more common with these devices
   e. The butterfly infusion set is commonly used in children and elderly people, whose veins are likely to be small or fragile
2. Plastic cannulas
   a. May be either an over-the-needle device or an in-needle catheter; primarily used for short-term therapy
   b. Over-the-needle device consists of a plastic catheter mounted over a needle; after venipuncture, the catheter is guided off the needle and into the vein
   c. Over-the-needle device is preferred for rapid infusion and is more comfortable for the client
   d. In-needle catheter: after venipuncture, it is guided through the needle into the vein, and the needle is removed from the catheter
   e. The in-needle catheter can cause **catheter embolism** if the tip of the cannula breaks

B. IV gauges
1. The smaller the gauge number, the larger the outside diameter of the cannula
2. The size used depends on the solution to be administered and the diameter of the available vein
3. Larger gauges allow a higher fluid rate than smaller ones and allow the administration of higher concentrations of solutions
4. For rapid emergency fluid administration, blood products, or anesthetics, a large gauge is used, such as a 14-, 16-, 18-, or 19-gauge needle
5. For peripheral fat infusions (lipids), a 20- or 21-gauge is used
6. For standard IV fluid and clear liquid IV medications, a 22- or 24-gauge is used
7. If the client has very small veins, a 24- to 25-gauge is used

C. IV containers (Fig. 13-1)
1. Container may be glass or plastic

TABLE 13-1

Types of Intravenous Solutions

Solution	Tonicity
0.45% saline (½ NS)	Hypotonic
0.9% saline (NS)	Isotonic
0.225% saline (¼ NS)	Hypotonic
0.33% saline (⅓ NS)	Hypotonic
3% saline (3% NS)	Hypertonic
5% saline (5% NS)	Hypertonic
5% dextrose in water (D_5W)	Isotonic
10% dextrose in water ($D_{10}W$)	Hypertonic
5% dextrose in 0.9% saline (5% D/NS)	Hypertonic
5% dextrose in 0.45% saline (5% D/½ NS)	Hypertonic
5% dextrose in 0.225% saline (5% D/¼ NS)	Isotonic
Lactated Ringer's (RL) solution	Isotonic
5% dextrose in lactated Ringer's solution	Hypertonic
Dextran	Colloid
Albumin	Colloid

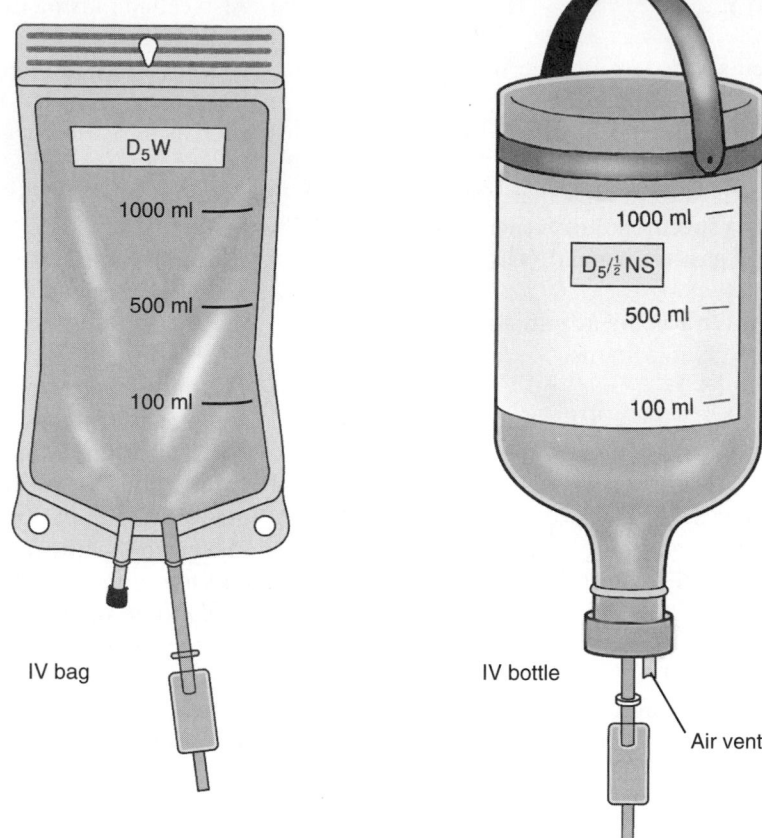

FIG. 13-1   Intravenous containers. (From Kee JL, Marshall SM: *Clinical calculations: with applications to general and specialty areas,* ed 4, Philadelphia, WB Saunders.)

2. Squeeze the plastic bag to ensure intactness and assess glass bottle for any cracks before hanging
3. Do not write on the plastic IV bag with a marking pen because it may be absorbed into the solution
4. Use a label and a ballpoint pen for marking the bag, placing the label onto the bag

D. Intravenous tubing (Fig. 13-2)
   1. Contains a spike end for the bag or bottle, a drop chamber, a roller clamp, a Y-site, and an adapter end for attachment to the needle
   2. Add extension tubing for children, clients who are restless, or clients who have special mobility needs
   3. Use shorter secondary tubing for piggyback solutions, connecting them to the injection sites nearest to the drip chamber
   4. Use special tubing for medication that absorbs into plastic
   5. Vented and nonvented tubing
      a. A vent allows air to enter the IV container as the fluid leaves
      b. A vented adapter can be used to add a vent to a nonvented IV tubing system
      c. Use nonvented tubing for flexible containers
      d. Use vented tubing for glass or rigid plastic containers to allow air to enter and displace the fluid as it leaves; fluid will not flow from a rigid IV container unless it is vented

E. Drip chambers (Fig. 13-3)
   1. Microdrip chamber
      a. Normally this has a short vertical metal piece where the drop forms
      b. Delivers between 50 and 60 drops per milliliter (mL)
      c. Read the tubing package to determine how many drops per mL are delivered (drop factor)
      d. Used if fluid will be infused at a slow rate (less than 50 mL per hour)
      e. Used if the solution contains potent medication that needs to be titrated, such as in a critical care setting or in pediatrics
   2. Macrodrip chamber
      a. Used if the solution is thick or is to infuse rapidly
      b. Drop factor varies from 10 to 20 drops per milliliter
      c. Read the tubing package to determine how many drops per mL are delivered (drop factor)

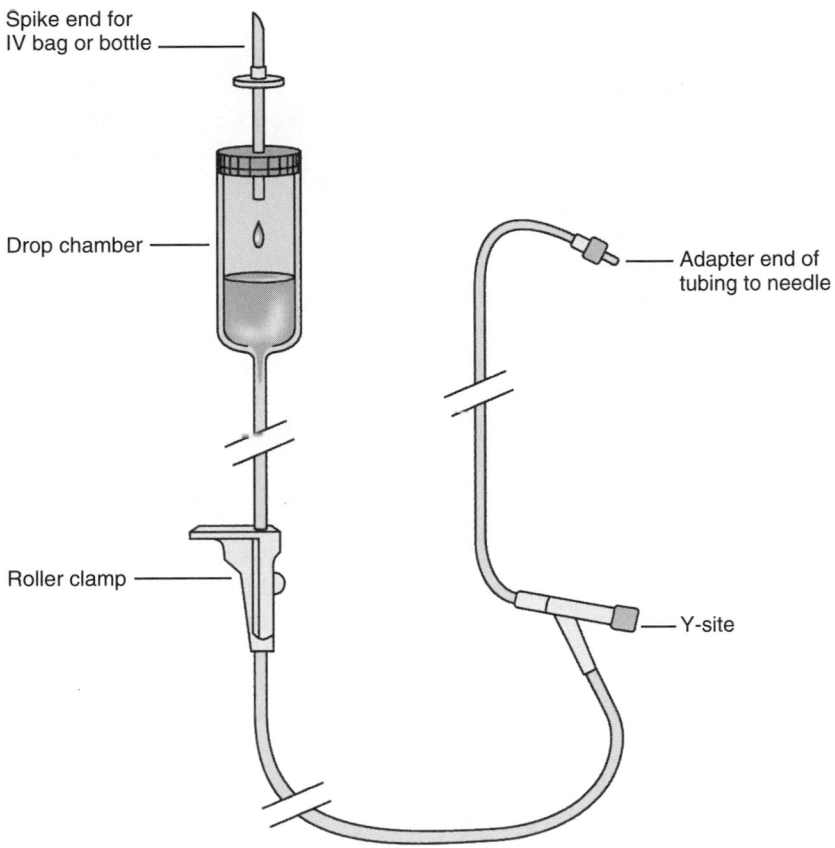

FIG. 13-2   Intravenous tubing. (From Kee JL, Marshall SM: *Clinical calculations: with applications to general and specialty areas,* ed 4, Philadelphia, WB Saunders.)

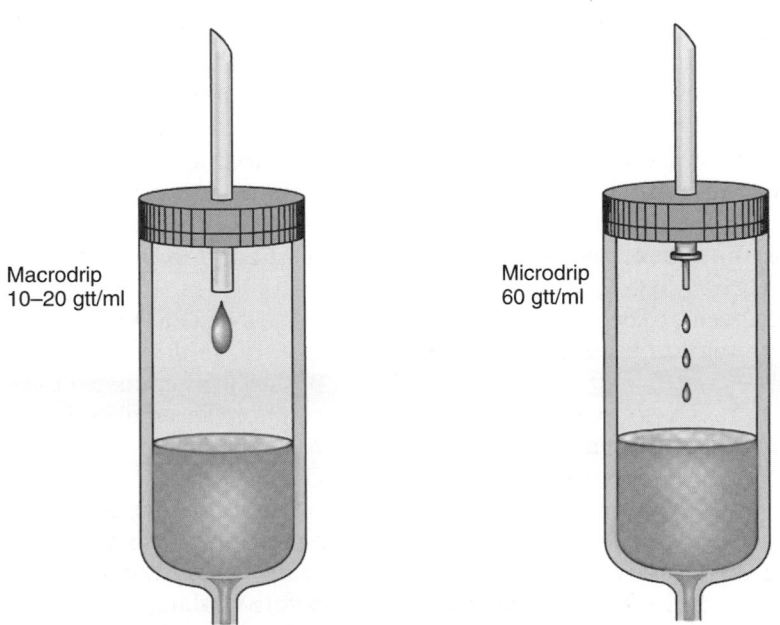

FIG. 13-3   Macrodrip and microdrip sizes. (From Kee JL, Marshall SM: *Clinical calculations: with applications to general and specialty areas,* ed 4, Philadelphia, 2000, WB Saunders.)

F. Filters
  1. Provide protection by preventing particles from entering the client's veins
  2. Used in IV lines to trap small particles such as undissolved antibiotics or salt, or medications that have precipitated in solution
  3. Assess the agency policy regarding the use of filters
  4. A 0.22-micron filter is used for most solutions, a 1.2-micron for solutions containing lipids or albumin, and a special filter for blood components
  5. Change filters every 24 to 72 hours (depending on agency policy) to prevent bacterial growth
G. Needleless systems
  1. Include recessed needles, plastic cannulas, and one-way valves; decrease the exposure to contaminated needles
  2. Do not administer total parenteral nutrition (TPN) or blood products through a one-way valve
H. Intermittent infusion sets
  1. Used when intravascular accessibility is desired for intermittent administration of medications by either IV push or IV piggyback
  2. An IV lock is attached for intermittent infusion devices
  3. Patency is maintained by periodic flushing with normal saline (NS) solution (sodium chloride and normal saline are interchangeable names)
  4. When administering medication, flush with 1 to 2 mL (depending on agency policy) of NS to confirm placement of the IV cannula; administer the prescribed medication, and then flush the cannula again with 1 to 2 mL (depending on agency policy) of NS to maintain patency

III. LATEX ALLERGY
A. Assess the client for an allergy to latex
B. IV supplies that contain latex include IV catheters, IV tubing, IV ports (particularly IV rubber injection ports), rubber stoppers on multidose vials, and adhesive tape
C. Latex-safe IV supplies need to be used, such as polyvinyl chloride IV tubing and Jelko or Deseret IV catheters
D. A three-way stopcock, rather than a rubber injection port, needs to be used on plastic tubing
E. Refer to Chapter 67 for additional information regarding latex allergy

IV. SELECTION OF A PERIPHERAL IV SITE
A. Veins in the hand, forearm, and antecubital fossa are suitable sites
B. Veins in the lower extremities are not suitable because of the risk of thrombus formation and possible pooling of medication in areas of decreased venous return (Box 13-1)

BOX 13-1

Peripheral Intravenous Sites to Avoid

Edematous extremity
An arm that is weak, traumatized, or paralyzed
The arm on the same side as a mastectomy
An arm that has an arteriovenous fistula or shunt for dialysis

---

C. Veins in the scalp and feet may be suitable sites for infants
D. The most frequently used sites are the veins of the forearm, because the bones of the forearm act as a natural support and splint
E. Assess the veins of both arms very closely before selecting a site
F. Start the IV infusion distally to provide the option of proceeding up the extremity if the vein is ruptured or **infiltration** occurs; if **infiltration** occurs from the antecubital vein, the lower veins usually cannot be used for further puncture sites
G. Determine the client's dominant side, and select the opposite side for a venipuncture site
H. Bending the elbow on the arm with an IV may easily obstruct the flow of solution, causing **infiltration** that could lead to thrombophlebitis
I. Avoid checking the blood pressure on the arm receiving the IV infusion
J. Do not place restraints over the venipuncture site
K. Use an armboard when the venipuncture site is located in an area of flexion

V. ADDING MEDICATION TO AN IV
A. Assess for compatibility of medication and solution
B. When adding medication to the bag, mix the bag end-to-end several times before hanging it, to disperse the medication
C. Ensure that medication can be mixed in soft plastic, because some medications absorb into the soft plastic and should be mixed only in glass

VI. ADMINISTERING IV SOLUTIONS
A. The IV solution should be checked against the physician's orders for the type, amount, percent of solution, and rate of flow
B. Assess the health status and medical disorders of the client
C. Identify client conditions that contraindicate use of a particular IV solution
D. Wash hands thoroughly before inserting an IV and before working with an IV
E. Use sterile technique when inserting an IV and when changing the dressing over the IV site
F. When inserting an IV, clean the skin with an antimicrobial solution, using an inner to outer circular motion

G. Prime the tubing to remove air from system

H. Change the venipuncture site every 48 to 72 hours, depending on agency policy

I. Change the IV dressing every 72 hours, when the dressing is wet or contaminated, or as specified by the agency policy

J. Change the IV tubing every 24 to 72 hours, depending on agency policy

K. Label the tubing, dressing, and solution bags clearly, indicating the date and time when changed

L. Do not let an IV bag or bottle hang for more than 24 hours because of the potential for sepsis

M. Do not allow the IV tubing to touch the floor because of the potential for bacterial contamination

N. Before adding medications or solutions, swab access ports with 70% alcohol, another equally effective solution, or as specified by the agency policy

VII. IV PRECAUTIONS

A. On insertion, an IV can cause initial pain and discomfort for the client

B. An IV provides a route of entry for microorganisms into the body

C. Medications enter the blood immediately, and any adverse reactions or allergic responses can occur immediately

D. Fluid (circulatory) overload or electrolyte imbalances can occur from an excessive or too rapid infusion of IV fluids

E. Incompatibilities between certain solutions and medications can occur

▲ F. Clients with respiratory, cardiac, renal, or liver diseases, elderly clients, and very young persons cannot tolerate an excessive fluid volume, and the risk of fluid overload exists with these clients

▲ G. A client with congestive heart failure is usually not given a solution containing saline because this type of fluid encourages the retention of water and would therefore exacerbate heart failure by increasing the fluid overload

▲ H. A client with diabetes mellitus does not typically receive dextrose (glucose) solutions

I. Lactated Ringer's solution contains potassium and should not be administered to clients with renal failure

VIII. COMPLICATIONS (Table 13-2)

A. Infection
   1. Description
      a. The entry of microorganisms into the body through the venipuncture site
      b. Venipuncture interrupts the integrity of the skin, the first line of defense against infection
      c. The longer the therapy continues, the greater the risk of infection
      d. Infection can occur locally at the IV insertion site or systemically from the entry of microorganisms into the body

TABLE 13-2

Signs of Complications of Intravenous Therapy

Complication	Signs
Infection	Local: redness, swelling, and drainage at site
	Systemic: chills, fever, malaise, headache, nausea, vomiting, backache, tachycardia
Tissue damage	Skin color changes, sloughing of the skin, discomfort at site
Phlebitis	Heat, redness, tenderness at site
	Not swollen or hard
	IV infusion sluggish
Thrombophlebitis	Hard and cordlike vein
	Heat, redness, tenderness at site
	IV infusion sluggish
Infiltration	Edema, pain, and coolness at site
	May or may not have a blood return
Catheter embolism	Decrease in BP
	Pain along vein
	Weak, rapid pulse
	Cyanosis of nail beds
	Loss of consciousness
Circulatory overload	Increased BP
	Distended jugular veins
	Rapid breathing
	Dyspnea
	Moist cough and crackles
Electrolyte overload	Signs depend on the specific electrolyte imbalance
Hematoma	Ecchymosis, immediate swelling and leakage of blood at the site, and hard and painful lumps at the site
Air embolism	Tachycardia
	Dyspnea
	Hypotension
	Cyanosis
	Decreased level of consciousness

   2. At-risk clients
      a. Immunocompromised clients with diseases such as cancer or acquired immunodeficiency syndrome (AIDS)
      b. Clients receiving treatments, such as chemotherapy, that have altered or lowered the white blood cell (WBC) count
      c. Elderly clients, because aging alters the effectiveness of the immune system
   3. Prevention and implementation
      a. Assess client for predisposition to or risk for infection
      b. Maintain strict asepsis when caring for the IV site
      c. Monitor for signs of local infection, such as redness, swelling, and drainage at the IV site
      d. Monitor for signs of systemic infection, such as chills, fever, malaise, headache, nausea, vomiting, backache, and tachycardia

e. Monitor white blood cell counts

f. Check fluid containers for cracks, leaks, cloudiness, or other evidence of contamination

g. Change tubing and site dressing every 24 to 72 hours according to agency policy

h. Use antimicrobial ointment at the IV site

i. Label the IV site, bag or bottle, and tubing with the date and time to ensure that it is changed on time according to agency policy

j. Ensure that the IV solution is not hanging for more than 24 hours

k. If infection occurs, discontinue the IV, place a sterile cover on the venipuncture device for possible culture, and notify the physician

l. Prepare to obtain blood cultures as prescribed if infection occurs

m. Restart an IV in the opposite arm to differentiate sepsis (systemic infection) from local infection at the IV site

n. Document the assessment of the finding related to infection

B. Tissue damage

1. Description

a. Tissues most commonly damaged include the skin, veins, and the subcutaneous tissue

b. Tissue damage can be uncomfortable and can cause permanent negative effects

2. Prevention and implementation

a. Use a careful and gentle approach when applying a tourniquet

b. Avoid tapping the skin over the vein when starting an IV

c. Monitor for ecchymosis when penetrating the skin with the cannula

d. Assess for any allergies to tape or dressing adhesives

e. Monitor for skin color changes, sloughing of the skin, or discomfort at the IV site

f. Notify the physician if tissue damage is suspected

g. Document the assessment of the tissue damage and its effects

C. **Phlebitis** and thrombophlebitis

1. Description

a. An inflammation of the vein that can occur from either mechanical or chemical (medication) trauma or as a result of a local infection

b. **Phlebitis** can cause the development of a clot (thrombophlebitis)

2. Prevention and implementation

a. Use an IV cannula smaller than the vein, and avoid very small veins when administering irritating solutions

b. Avoid using the lower extremities as an access area for the IV

c. Avoid venipuncture over an area of flexion

d. Anchor the cannula and a loop of tubing securely with tape

e. Use an armboard or a splint if the client is restless or active

f. Change the venipuncture site every 48 to 72 hours, depending on agency policy

g. If **phlebitis** occurs, remove the IV device immediately and restart it in the opposite extremity

h. Notify the physician if **phlebitis** is suspected, and apply warm, moist compresses as prescribed

i. If thrombophlebitis occurs, never irrigate the IV catheter; remove the IV, notify the physician, and restart the IV in the opposite extremity

j. Document the assessment of the **phlebitis** or thrombophlebitis and its effects

D. **Infiltration**

1. Description

a. A form of tissue damage; also called extravasation

b. Seepage of the intravenous fluid out of the vein and into the surrounding interstitial spaces

c. Occurs when an access device has become dislodged or perforates the wall of the vein, or when vein back pressure occurs as a result of a clot or venospasm

2. Prevention and implementation

a. Avoid venipuncture over an area of flexion

b. Anchor the cannula and a loop of tubing securely with tape

c. Use an armboard or a splint if the client is restless or active

d. Assess the IV site for pain, edema, or coolness, comparing it with the opposite extremity

e. Monitor the IV rate for a decrease or a stop in flow

f. Evaluate the IV site for **infiltration** by occluding the vein proximal to the IV site; if the IV fluid continues to flow, the cannula is probably outside the vein (infiltrated); if the IV flow stops after occlusion of the vein, the IV device is still in the vein

g. Lower the IV fluid container below the IV site, and monitor for the appearance of blood in the IV tubing; if blood appears, the IV device is in the vein

h. If **infiltration** has occurred, the IV device is removed immediately

i. Do not rub an infiltrated area, which can cause the development of a hematoma

j. If **infiltration** has occurred, elevate the extremity and apply compresses (warm or cool, depending on the IV solution that was infusing and the physician's order) over the affected area

k. Document the assessment of the **infiltration,** its effects, and the action taken

E. **Catheter embolism**
   1. Description: The tip of the catheter breaks off during IV insertion or removal, resulting in the possibility of an embolus
   2. Prevention and implementation
      a. Monitor for signs of **catheter embolism,** including a decrease in blood pressure (BP), pain along the vein, weak and rapid pulse, cyanosis of nail beds, and loss of consciousness
      b. Remove the catheter carefully
      c. Inspect the catheter when removed
      d. If the catheter tip has broken off, place a tourniquet high on the limb of the IV site, notify the physician immediately, prepare to obtain an x-ray, and prepare the client for surgery to remove the catheter pieces if prescribed

F. Circulatory overload
   1. Description
      a. Also known as fluid overload
      b. Results from the administration of fluids too rapidly or in a client at risk for fluid overload
   2. Prevention and implementation
      a. Identify clients at risk for circulatory overload
      b. Calculate and monitor the drip (flow) rate frequently
      c. Use an infusion controller device, and frequently check the drip rate or pump setting, particularly in clients at risk for overload
      d. Add a time strip to the IV bag or bottle
      e. Monitor for signs of circulatory overload, including increased BP, distended jugular veins, rapid breathing, dyspnea, moist cough, and crackles
      f. If circulatory overload occurs, decrease the flow rate to a minimum at a keep vein open (KVO) rate, elevate the head of the bed, keep the client warm, assess for edema, and notify the physician
      g. Document the assessment and actions taken

G. Electrolyte overload
   1. Description: An electrolyte imbalance caused by too rapid or excessive infusion or by use of an inappropriate intravenous solution
   2. Prevention and implementation
      a. Assess laboratory value reports
      b. Verify the correct solution
      c. Calculate and monitor the flow rate
      d. Use an infusion controller device, and frequently check the flow rate or pump setting
      e. Add a time strip to the IV bag or bottle
      f. Place a colored sticker on the bag or bottle if a medication, such as potassium chloride, has been added to the IV solution
      g. Monitor for signs of electrolyte imbalance, and notify the physician if they occur

H. Hematoma
   1. Description: The collection of blood in the tissues after an unsuccessful venipuncture or after the venipuncture site is discontinued
   2. Prevention and implementation
      a. When starting an IV, avoid piercing the posterior wall of the vein
      b. Do not apply a tourniquet to the extremity immediately after an unsuccessful venipuncture
      c. When discontinuing an IV, apply pressure to the site for at least 1 minute and elevate the extremity; apply pressure longer for clients with a bleeding disorder or on anticoagulants
      d. Monitor for ecchymosis, immediate swelling and leakage of blood at the site, and hard and painful lumps at the site
      e. If a hematoma develops, elevate the extremity and apply pressure and ice as prescribed

I. **Air embolism**
   1. Description: A bolus of air enters the vein through an inadequately primed IV line, from a loose connection, during tubing change, or during removal of the IV
   2. Prevention and implementation
      a. Prime tubing with fluid before use, and monitor for any air bubbles in the tubing
      b. Secure all connections
      c. Replace the IV fluid before the bag or bottle is dry
      d. Monitor for signs of **air embolism,** including tachycardia, dyspnea, hypotension, cyanosis, and decreased level of consciousness; a possible "mill wheel murmur," a continuous loud, turning sound over the precordium that results from air in the right ventricle, may be heard
      e. If air embolus is suspected, clamp the tubing, turn the client on the left side with the head of the bed lowered (Trendelenburg's position) to trap the air in the right atrium, and notify the physician

IX. CENTRAL VENOUS CATHETERS (Fig. 13-4)

A. Description
   1. Used to deliver hyperosmolar solutions, to measure central venous pressure, or to infuse total parenteral nutrition (TPN) or multiple IV infusions or medications
   2. Catheter position is determined by x-ray after insertion
   3. May have a single, double, or triple lumen
   4. May be inserted peripherally and threaded through the basilic or cephalic vein into the superior vena cava, inserted centrally through the internal jugular or subclavian veins, or surgically tunneled through subcutaneous tissue into the cephalic vein

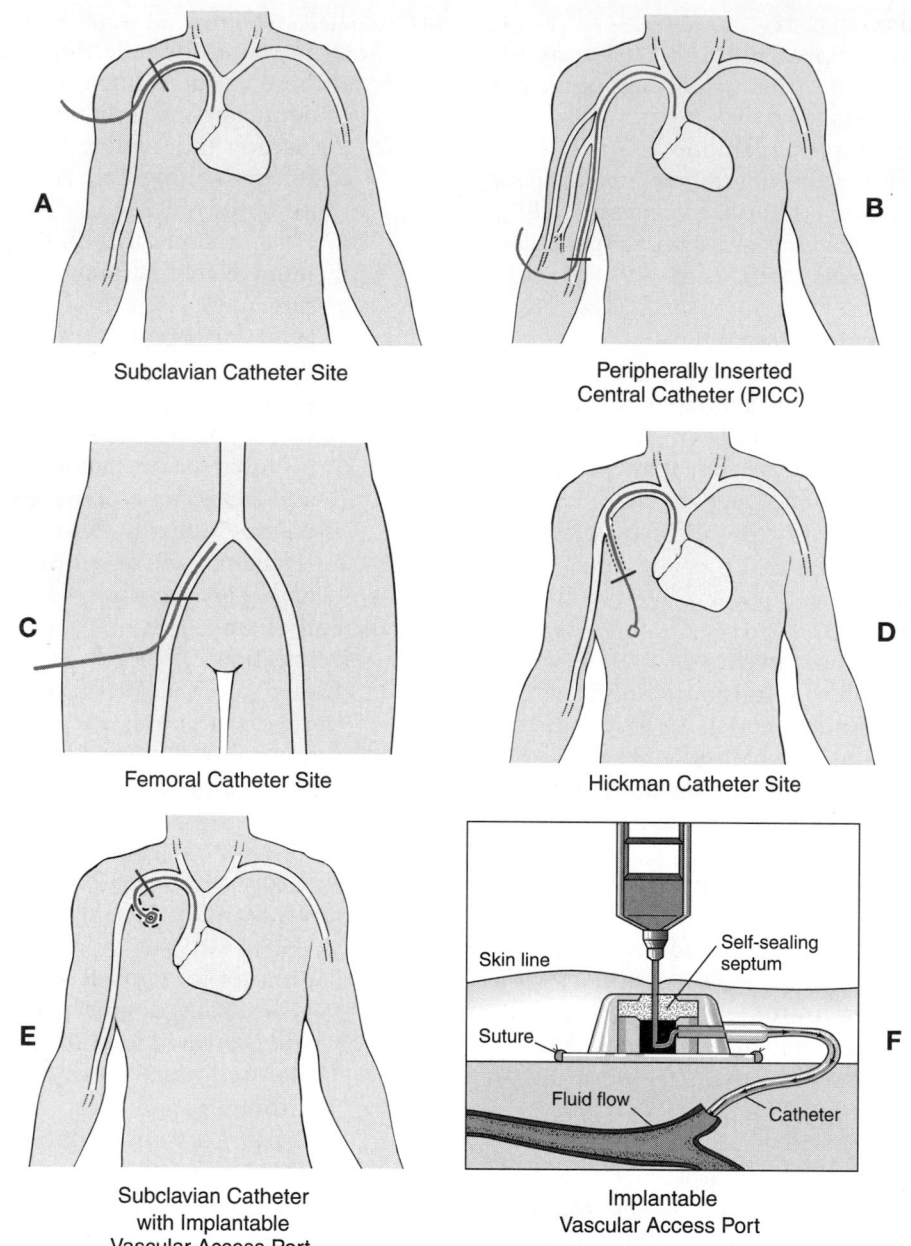

FIG. 13-4 Central venous access site(s). **A,** Subclavian catheter. **B,** Peripherally inserted central catheter (PICC). **C,** Femoral catheter. **D,** Hickman catheter. **E,** Subclavian catheter with implantable vascular access port. **F,** Implantable vascular access port. (From Kee JL, Marshall SM: *Clinical calculations: with applications to general and specialty areas,* ed 4, Philadelphia, 2000, WB Saunders. **F** redrawn from Winters B: Implantable vascular access devices, *Oncology Nursing Forum* 11(6):25-30, 1984.)

5. With multilumen catheters, more than one medication can be administered at the same time without incompatibility problems, and there is only one insertion site for care

6. For central line insertion, tubing change, and line removal, place the client in Trendelenburg position if not contraindicated, or supine position, and instruct the client to perform Valsalva maneuver to increase pressure in the central veins when the IV system is open

B. Tunneled central venous catheters
   1. A more permanent type of catheter, such as the Hickman, Broviac, or Groshong catheter, that is used for long-term IV therapy
   2. May be single lumen or multilumen
   3. Inserted in the operating room, and the catheter

is threaded into the lower part of the vena cava at the entrance of the right atrium

4. The catheter will be fitted with an intermittent infusion device to allow access as needed and to keep the system closed and intact

▲ 5. Patency is maintained by flushing with a diluted heparin solution as per agency policy

6. Groshong catheters require only normal saline flush to maintain patency

C. Vascular access ports (implantable port)

1. Surgically implanted under the skin, such as a Port-a-Cath, Mediport, or Infusaport; used for long-term administration of repeated IV therapy

▲ 2. For access, requires palpation and injection through the skin into the self-sealing port with a noncoring needle such as a Huber-point needle

▲ 3. Patency is maintained by periodic flushing with a diluted heparin solution per agency policy

D. Peripherally inserted central catheter (PICC) line

1. Used for long-term IV therapy, frequently in the home

2. The basilic vein is usually used, but the median cubital and cephalic veins in the antecubital area can also be used

3. Threaded so that the catheter tip may terminate in either the axillary or the subclavian vein or the superior vena cava

4. A small amount of bleeding may occur at the time of insertion and continue for 24 hours, but bleeding thereafter is not expected

5. **Phlebitis** is a common complication

6. Insertion is below the heart level; therefore, **air embolism** is not common

PRACTICE QUESTIONS

1. A nurse has an order to hang an IV bag of 1000 mL 5% dextrose in water with 20 mEq potassium chloride (KCl). The nurse should plan to do which of the following immediately after injecting the KCl into the port of the IV bag?
   1. Attach the tubing to the client
   2. Check the solution for yellowish discoloration
   3. Rotate the bag gently
   4. Place the time tape on the IV

2. A nurse is inserting an intravenous line into a client's vein. After the initial stick, the nurse continues to advance the catheter if the nurse notes that:
   1. The catheter advances easily
   2. There is blood return in the backflash chamber of the catheter
   3. The vein is distended under the needle
   4. The client does not complain of discomfort

3. A client is scheduled for insertion of a peripherally inserted central catheter (PICC). The nurse has explained the advantages of this catheter to the client. Which statement if made by the client indicates a need for further explanation?
   1. "There is less pain and discomfort."
   2. "This type of catheter is very reliable."
   3. "It is reasonable in cost."
   4. "It is specifically designed for short-term use."

4. A nurse is planning to provide a list of instructions to a client being discharged to home with a peripherally inserted central catheter (PICC). The nurse would avoid writing which of the following incorrect items on the instruction sheet?
   1. Keep activity level to a minimum while this catheter is in place
   2. Keep the insertion site protected when in the shower or bath
   3. Have a repair kit available in the home for use if needed
   4. Wear a Medic-Alert tag or bracelet

5. A nurse is assessing the IV dressing of a client with a peripheral intravenous infusion running. The date on the dressing is 7/25 (July 25). The nurse documents on the client's record that the dressing should be changed on which of the following dates?
   1. 7/26
   2. 7/28
   3. 7/30
   4. 8/1

6. A nurse is making initial rounds on the nursing unit to assess the condition of assigned clients. The nurse notes that a client's IV site is cool, pale, and swollen, and the solution is not infusing. The nurse concludes that which of the following complications has been experienced by the client?
   1. Thrombosis
   2. Infection
   3. Infiltration
   4. Phlebitis

7. A client rings the call bell and complains of pain at the site of an IV infusion. A nurse assesses the site and determines that the client has developed phlebitis. The nurse would plan to avoid which of the following actions in the care of this client?
   1. Apply warm moist packs to the site
   2. Start a new IV line in a proximal portion of the same vein
   3. Discontinue the IV catheter at that site
   4. Notify the physician

8. A client had a 1000-mL bag of 5% dextrose in 0.9% sodium chloride hung at 15:00. A nurse making rounds at 15:45 finds the client to be complaining of a pounding headache and to be dyspneic, experiencing chills, apprehensive, and the pulse rate is increased. The IV bag has 400 mL remaining. The nurse should take which of the following actions first?
   1. Sit the client up in bed
   2. Call the physician

3. Slow the IV infusion
4. Remove the IV catheter

9. A nurse notes that the site of a client's peripheral IV catheter is reddened, warm, painful, and slightly edematous proximal to the insertion point of the IV catheter. After taking appropriate steps to care for the client, the nurse documents in the medical record that the client experienced:
    1. Hypersensitivity to the IV solution
    2. Allergic reaction to the IV catheter material
    3. Infiltration of the IV line
    4. Phlebitis of the vein

10. A physician has written an order to discontinue an intravenous line. A nurse obtains which of the following supplies from the unit supply area for use in applying pressure to the site after removing the IV catheter?
    1. Band-Aid
    2. Sterile 2 × 2 gauze
    3. Alcohol swab
    4. Betadine swab

11. A client has just undergone insertion of a central venous catheter at the bedside. A nurse would be sure to check the results of which of the following before increasing the flow rate of the IV solution attached to the line from KVO (keep vein open) to 100 mL/hour?
    1. Serum electrolytes
    2. Serum osmolality
    3. Portable chest x-ray
    4. Intake and output record

12. A nurse is preparing a continuous intravenous (IV) infusion at the medication cart. As the nurse goes to attach the distal end of the IV tubing to a needleless device, the tubing drops and hits the top of the medication cart. Which of the following is the appropriate action by the nurse?
    1. Wipe the distal end of the tubing with Betadine

2. Scrub the needleless device with an alcohol swab
3. Attach a new needleless device
4. Obtain new IV tubing

13. A nurse is preparing to insert an IV angiocatheter into a client's inner forearm. Before cannulating the vein, the nurse cleanses the entry site by using which of the following motions?
    1. Scrubbing from the wrist toward the elbow
    2. Scrubbing from the elbow toward the wrist
    3. Using a circular motion from the center outward
    4. Using a circular motion inward toward the center

14. A client is hypovolemic and plasma expanders are not available. A nurse anticipates that which of the following solutions available on the nursing unit will be prescribed by the physician?
    1. 5% dextrose in 0.45% sodium chloride
    2. 5% dextrose in water
    3. 0.9% sodium chloride
    4. 0.45% sodium chloride

15. A nurse hears an attending physician asking an intern to prescribe a hypotonic IV solution for a client. Which of the following IV solutions would the nurse expect the intern to prescribe?
    1. 0.45% saline (½NS)
    2. 5% dextrose in water (5% D/W)
    3. 10% dextrose in water (10% D/W)
    4. 5% dextrose in 0.9% saline (5% D/NS)

CRITICAL THINKING: FREE-TEXT ENTRY

A nurse is completing a time tape for a 1000-mL IV bag that is scheduled to infuse over 8 hours. The nurse has just placed the 11:00 A.M. marking at the 500-mL level. The nurse would place the mark for 12:00 noon at which numerical level (mL) on the time tape?

Answer: _____

ANSWERS

1. **3**
Rationale: After adding a medication to a bag of IV solution, the nurse should agitate or rotate the bag gently to mix the medication evenly in the solution. The nurse should then attach a completed medication label. The nurse can then place a time tape on the bag if this has not been done. The IV solution should have been checked for discoloration before the medication was added to the solution. The tubing is attached to the client last.
Test-Taking Strategy: Use the process of elimination. Note the key words "immediately after injecting." They imply a correct time sequence, and you need to prioritize. Visualize and think through the steps of adding medication to an IV bag, and make your choice accordingly. Review the procedure for adding KCl to an IV bag if you had difficulty with this question.

Level of Cognitive Ability: Application
Client Needs: Physiological Integrity
Integrated Concept/Process: Nursing Process/Implementation
Content Area: Fundamental Skills
Reference: Altman, G., Buchsel, P., & Coxon, V. (2000). *Delmar's fundamental & advanced nursing skills.* Albany, N.Y.: Delmar, p. 597.

2. **2**
Rationale: The IV catheter has successfully entered the lumen of the vein when there is blood backflash in the IV catheter. The vein should have been distended by the tourniquet before the vein was cannulated. Client discomfort varies with the client, the site, and the nurse's insertion technique, and is not a reliable measure of catheter placement. The nurse should not advance the catheter until placement in the vein is verified by blood return.

Test-Taking Strategy: Use the process of elimination, focusing on the issue of the question, correct placement of an IV catheter. Noting the key words "blood return" in option 2 will direct you to this option. Review the steps for inserting an IV catheter if you had difficulty with this question.
Level of Cognitive Ability: Application
Client Needs: Physiological Integrity
Integrated Concept/Process: Nursing Process/Implementation
Content Area: Fundamental Skills
Reference: Craven, R., & Hirnle, C. (2000). *Fundamentals of nursing: Human health and function* (3rd ed.). Philadelphia: Lippincott, p. 566.

3. **4**
Rationale: PICC catheters are intended to be used for clients needing long-term catheter placement. They are reasonable in cost because they do not need routine replacement, as do traditional peripheral IV catheters. The catheter is more comfortable for the client because there is no repeated venipuncture with catheter change. The catheter is also very reliable. It is less likely to infiltrate and can be used for administration of a number of different types of medications.
Test-Taking Strategy: Use the process of elimination, noting the key words "need for further explanation." Noting the key words "short-term" in option 4 will assist in directing you to this option. Review the characteristics of a PICC catheter if you had difficulty with this question.
Level of Cognitive Ability: Analysis
Client Needs: Physiological Integrity
Integrated Concept/Process: Teaching/Learning
Content Area: Fundamental Skills
Reference: Phipps, W., Sands, J., & Marek, J. (1999). *Medical-surgical nursing: Concepts & clinical practice* (6th ed.). St. Louis: Mosby, pp. 575–576.

4. **1**
Rationale: The client should be taught that there are only minor activity restrictions with this type of catheter. The client should protect the site during bathing, and should carry or wear a Medic-Alert identification. The client should have a repair kit in the home for PRN use, since it is a long-term catheter.
Test-Taking Strategy: Use the process of elimination. Note the key word "avoid." Recalling that the PICC line is used for long-term use will assist in directing you to option 1. It is unreasonable that activity needs to be kept to a minimum with such a catheter. Review home care instructions for a client with a PICC line if you had difficulty with this question.
Level of Cognitive Ability: Application
Client Needs: Health Promotion and Maintenance
Integrated Concept/Process: Self-Care
Content Area: Fundamental Skills
Reference: Leahy, J., & Kizilay, P. (1998). *Foundations of nursing practice: A nursing process approach.* Philadelphia: W.B. Saunders, p. 814.

5. **2**
Rationale: The IV site dressing should be changed every 48 to 72 hours, which is every 2 to 3 days. With an insertion date of 7/25, the due date for change, depending on agency policy, would be either 7/27 or 7/28. It would be unnecessary, uncomfortable, and not cost effective to change the site dressing on a daily basis (option 1). Changing the site dressing every 5 or 7 days (options 3 and 4) would place the client at higher risk for infection or other catheter complications.

Test-Taking Strategy: Use the process of elimination. Recalling that the IV site dressing should be changed every 48 to 72 hours will easily direct you to option 2. Review the standard accepted guidelines for intravenous site maintenance if you had difficulty with this question.
Level of Cognitive Ability: Comprehension
Client Needs: Safe, Effective Care Environment
Integrated Concept/Process: Communication and Documentation
Content Area: Fundamental Skills
Reference: Harkreader, H. (2000). *Fundamentals of nursing: Caring and clinical judgment.* Philadelphia: W.B. Saunders, p. 770.

6. **3**
Rationale: An infiltrated IV is one that has dislodged from the vein and is lying in subcutaneous tissue. Pallor, coolness, and swelling are the result of IV fluid being deposited in the subcutaneous tissue. When the pressure in the tissues exceeds the pressure in the tubing, the flow of the IV solution will stop. The corrective action is to remove the catheter and start a new IV line at another site. The other three options are likely to be accompanied by warmth at the site, not coolness.
Test-Taking Strategy: Use the process of elimination, focusing on the clinical manifestations identified in the question. Noting the key word "cool" in the question will direct you to option 3. Review the signs of infiltration if you had difficulty with this question.
Level of Cognitive Ability: Analysis
Client Needs: Physiological Integrity
Integrated Concept/Process: Nursing Process/Assessment
Content Area: Fundamental Skills
Reference: Harkreader, H. (2000). *Fundamentals of nursing: Caring and clinical judgment.* Philadelphia: W.B. Saunders, p. 774.

7. **2**
Rationale: The nurse should discontinue the IV at the phlebitic site, and apply warm moist compresses to the area to speed resolution of the inflammation. Since phlebitis has occurred, the nurse also notifies the physician about the IV complication. The nurse should restart the IV in a vein other than the one that has developed phlebitis.
Test-Taking Strategy: Use the process of elimination. Note the key word "avoid." This tells you that the correct option is an incorrect nursing action. Recalling that the nurse should restart the IV in a vein other than the one that has developed phlebitis will easily direct you to option 2. Review nursing interventions related to phlebitis if you had difficulty with this question.
Level of Cognitive Ability: Application
Client Needs: Physiological Integrity
Integrated Concept/Process: Nursing Process/Planning
Content Area: Fundamental Skills
Reference: Craven, R., & Hirnle, C. (2000). *Fundamentals of nursing: Human health and function* (3rd ed.). Philadelphia: Lippincott, p. 573.

8. **3**
Rationale: The client's symptoms are compatible with circulatory overload. This may be verified by noting that 600 mL has infused in the course of 45 minutes. The first action of the nurse is to slow the infusion. Other actions may follow in rapid sequence. The nurse may elevate the head of the bed to aid the client's breathing, if necessary. The physician is also

notified immediately. The IV catheter does not need to be removed; it may continue to be needed once the complication has been managed.

Test-Taking Strategy: Use the process of elimination. Note the key word "first." This tells you that more than one or all of the options are likely to be correct actions, and the nurse needs to prioritize them according to a time sequence. You must be able to recognize the signs of circulatory overload. From this point, select the option that provides the intervention specific to circulatory overload. Review nursing actions related to this complication if you had difficulty with this question.

Level of Cognitive Ability: Analysis
Client Needs: Physiological Integrity
Integrated Concept/Process: Nursing Process/Implementation
Content Area: Fundamental Skills
Reference: Harkreader, H. (2000). *Fundamentals of nursing: Caring and clinical judgment.* Philadelphia: W.B. Saunders, p. 774.

9. 4
Rationale: Phlebitis at an IV site can be distinguished by client discomfort at the site, as well as by redness, warmth, and swelling proximal to the catheter. If phlebitis occurs, the IV line should be discontinued, and a new IV line should be inserted at a different site. Coolness at the site would be noted if the IV was infiltrated. An allergic reaction produces a rash, redness, and itching. A major reaction, such as hypersensitivity, can cause coughing, dyspnea, a swollen tongue, and cyanosis.

Test-Taking Strategy: Use the process of elimination. Remember that options that are similar are not likely to be correct. In this situation, options 1 and 2 are similar and are therefore eliminated. Choose option 4 over option 3 after recalling the signs of common IV complications. Review the signs and symptoms of phlebitis if you had difficulty with this question.

Level of Cognitive Ability: Analysis
Client Needs: Physiological Integrity
Integrated Concept/Process: Communication and Documentation
Content Area: Fundamental Skills
Reference: Craven, R., & Hirnle, C. (2000). *Fundamentals of nursing: Human health and function* (3rd ed.). Philadelphia: Lippincott, p. 573.

10. 2
Rationale: A dry sterile dressing such as a sterile 2 × 2 is used to apply pressure to the discontinued IV site. This material is absorbent, sterile, and nonirritating. A Betadine swab or an alcohol swab would irritate the opened puncture site and would not stop the blood flow. A Band-Aid may be used to cover the site once hemostasis has occurred.

Test-Taking Strategy: Use the process of elimination. Note the key words "applying pressure." Visualize this procedure, thinking about each of the items identified in the options to direct you to option 2. Review this basic procedure if you had difficulty with this question.

Level of Cognitive Ability: Application
Client Needs: Safe, Effective Care Environment
Integrated Concept/Process: Nursing Process/Planning
Content Area: Fundamental Skills
Reference: Craven, R., & Hirnle, C. (2000). *Fundamentals of*

nursing: Human health and function (3rd ed.). Philadelphia: Lippincott, p. 577.

11. 3
Rationale: Before beginning administration of large volumes of IV solution, the nurse should assess whether the results of chest x-ray reveal that the central catheter is in the proper place. This is necessary to prevent infusion of IV fluid into pulmonary or subcutaneous tissues. The other options represent items that are useful for the nurse to be aware of in the general care of this client, but they do not relate to this procedure.

Test-Taking Strategy: Use the process of elimination. Note the key words "central venous catheter at the bedside." Recalling the potential complications associated with insertion of central venous lines will easily direct you to option 3. Review the principles of care for a central venous catheter after insertion if you had difficulty with this question.

Level of Cognitive Ability: Application
Client Needs: Safe, Effective Care Environment
Integrated Concept/Process: Nursing Process/Assessment
Content Area: Fundamental Skills
Reference: Potter, P., & Perry, A. (2001). *Fundamentals of nursing* (5th ed.). St. Louis: Mosby, p. 1372.

12. 4
Rationale: The nurse should obtain a new IV tubing because contamination has occurred and could cause systemic infection to the client. Wiping the port with Betadine is insufficient and would be contraindicated anyway, since the catheter will be attached directly to an angiocatheter in the client's vein. The needleless device has not been contaminated and does not need replacement or cleansing.

Test-Taking Strategy: Use the process of elimination and knowledge of basic infection control measures and intravenous therapy concepts to answer this question. There is clearly only one correct option. Review aseptic technique if you had difficulty with this question.

Level of Cognitive Ability: Application
Client Needs: Safe, Effective Care Environment
Integrated Concept/Process: Nursing Process/Implementation
Content Area: Fundamental Skills
Reference: Leahy, J., & Kizilay, P. (1998). *Foundations of nursing practice: A nursing process approach.* Philadelphia: W.B. Saunders, p. 813.

13. 3
Rationale: The nurse cleans the skin by using a circular motion from inward to outward. This is the standard accepted aseptic technique to carry microorganisms away from the insertion site. It is the same technique used in cleansing any area requiring surgical asepsis. Options 1, 2, and 4 are incorrect procedures.

Test-Taking Strategy: Use the process of elimination and basic principles of asepsis to answer the question. Knowledge of these principles allows you to choose correctly even without specific knowledge of IV insertion techniques. Review the basic principles of asepsis if you had difficulty with this question.

Level of Cognitive Ability: Application
Client Needs: Safe, Effective Care Environment
Integrated Concept/Process: Nursing Process/Implementation
Content Area: Fundamental Skills

Reference: Craven, R., & Hirnle, C. (2000). *Fundamentals of nursing: Human health and function* (3rd ed.). Philadelphia: Lippincott, p. 566.

14. **1**

Rationale: 5% dextrose in 0.45% sodium chloride is a hypertonic solution. An advantage of hypertonic solutions is that they may be used to treat hypovolemia when plasma expanders are not readily available. Options 2 and 3 are isotonic solutions. Option 4 is a hypotonic solution.

Test-Taking Strategy: Use the process of elimination. Noting the key word "hypovolemic" will assist in directing you to option 1 if you are familiar with the IV solutions that are hypertonic. If this question was difficult, review the nature and purposes of hypertonic, isotonic, and hypotonic IV solutions.

Level of Cognitive Ability: Analysis
Client Needs: Physiological Integrity
Integrated Concept/Process: Nursing Process/Analysis
Content Area: Fundamental Skills
Reference: Leahy, J., & Kizilay, P. (1998). *Foundations of nursing practice: A nursing process approach.* Philadelphia: W.B. Saunders, p. 811.

15. **1**

Rationale: Hypotonic solutions contain a lower concentration of salt or more water than an isotonic solution. 0.45% saline (½NS) is hypotonic and is probably the only hypotonic solution used in clinical situations. 5% dextrose in water (5% D/W) is an isotonic solution. 10% dextrose in water (10% D/W) and 5% dextrose in 0.9% saline (5% D/NS) are hypertonic solutions. Distilled water is another example of a hypotonic solution.

Test-Taking Strategy: Use the process of elimination. Note the similarities in options 2, 3, and 4. All of these solutions contain dextrose. Option 1 is different from the other options. Select the option that is different. If you had difficulty with this question, review the tonicity of the various IV solutions.

Level of Cognitive Ability: Comprehension
Client Needs: Physiological Integrity
Integrated Concept/Process: Nursing Process/Planning
Content Area: Fundamental Skills
Reference: LeMone, P., & Burke, K. (2000). *Medical-surgical nursing: Critical thinking in client care* (2nd ed.). Upper Saddle River, NJ: Prentice-Hall, p. 110.

CRITICAL THINKING: FREE-TEXT ENTRY

Answer: 375 mL

Rationale: If the IV is scheduled to run over 8 hours, then the hourly rate is 125 mL per hour. Using 500 mL as the reference point, the next hourly marking would be at 375 mL, which is 125 mL less than 500.

Test-Taking Strategy: Use basic principles related to pharmacology math and IV administration to answer this question. If this question was difficult, review the concepts related to marking an IV solution by using a time tape.

Level of Cognitive Ability: Application
Client Needs: Safe, Effective Care Environment
Integrated Concept/Process: Nursing Process/Implementation
Content Area: Fundamental Skills
Reference: Leahy, J., & Kizilay, P. (1998). *Foundations of nursing practice: A nursing process approach.* Philadelphia: W.B. Saunders, p. 818.

REFERENCES

Altman, G., Buchsel, P., & Coxon, V. (2000). *Delmar's fundamental & advanced nursing skills.* Albany, N.Y.: Delmar.

Craven, R., & Hirnle, C. (2000). *Fundamentals of nursing: Human health and function* (3rd ed.). Philadelphia: Lippincott.

Harkreader, H. (2000). *Fundamentals of nursing: Caring and clinical judgment.* Philadelphia: W.B. Saunders.

Leahy, J., & Kizilay, P. (1998). *Foundations of nursing practice: A nursing process approach.* Philadelphia: W.B. Saunders.

Phipps, W., Sands, J., & Marek, J. (1999). *Medical-surgical nursing: Concepts & clinical practice* (6th ed.). St. Louis: Mosby.

Potter, P. & Perry, A. (2001). *Fundamentals of nursing* (5th ed.). St. Louis: Mosby.

Administration of Blood Products

PYRAMID TERMS

ABO A type of antigen system. The ABO type of the donor should be compatible with the recipient's. Type A can match with types A or O; type B can match with types B or O; type O can match only with type O; type AB can match with A, B, or O.

autologous donation A donation of the client's own blood before a scheduled procedure.

blood salvage An autologous donation that involves suctioning blood from body cavities, joint spaces, or other closed body sites during a procedure.

crossmatching The testing of the donor's blood and the recipient's blood for compatibility.

compatibility Determined by two different types of antigen systems, ABO and Rh, present on the membrane surface of the red blood cells (RBCs).

circulatory overload A complication resulting from the infusion of blood at a rate too rapid for the size, cardiac status, or clinical condition of the recipient.

designated donor A compatible donor who has been selected by the recipient.

disease transmission Diseases can be transmitted through blood transfusions, with the most common disease transmitted being hepatitis C. The incidence of transmission of human immunodeficiency virus (HIV) has been rare since routine donor testing was implemented in 1985.

fresh-frozen plasma Administered to increase the level of clotting factors in clients with such a deficiency.

iron overload A delayed transfusion complication; it can occur in clients receiving more than 100 units of blood over a period of time.

platelets Administered to clients with low platelet counts and to thrombocytopenic clients who are actively bleeding or scheduled for an invasive procedure.

red blood cells (RBCs) Used to replace erythrocytes lost as a result of trauma or surgical interventions, or in clients with bone marrow suppression.

Rh Represents a type of antigen system. Rh-negative blood can be given to an Rh-negative or an Rh-positive recipient.

septicemia The presence of infective agents or their toxins in the bloodstream. Septicemia is a serious disease and must be treated promptly; otherwise the infection leads to circulatory collapse, profound shock, and death.

transfusion reaction A hemolytic transfusion reaction is caused by blood type or Rh incompatibility. An allergic transfusion reaction is most often seen in clients with a history of allergy. A febrile transfusion reaction most commonly occurs in clients with antibodies directed against the transfused white blood cells (WBCs). A bacterial transfusion reaction is seen after transfusion of contaminated blood products.

whole blood Whole blood is composed of RBCs, plasma, and plasma proteins; it is administered primarily to treat hypovolemic shock resulting from hemorrhage.

PYRAMID TO SUCCESS

Pyramid points focus on the safe administration of blood components, managing and providing care related to the procedure for administering blood components, and monitoring for complications. Focus is on the safe procedure for administering blood and on the signs and symptoms of transfusion reaction. Pyramid points also focus on the immediate interventions if a transfusion reaction occurs, and evaluation and documentation of expected and unexpected effects of the therapy. The primary Integrated Concepts and Processes addressed in this chapter are Nursing Process, Caring, Communication and Documentation, Cultural Awareness, and Teaching/Learning.

CLIENT NEEDS
Safe, Effective Care Environment

Client rights
Continuity of care and close supervision during transfusion
Establishing priorities

Ethical practice and legal responsibilities

Handling hazardous and infectious materials

Informed consent for the administration of blood products

Medical and surgical asepsis

Standard (universal) and other precautions

Health Promotion and Maintenance

Client education about the signs of a transfusion reaction

Lifestyle choices related to receiving a blood transfusion

Psychosocial Integrity

Religious, spiritual, and cultural considerations related to blood administration

Therapeutic interactions with the client regarding the procedure for blood administration

Physiological Integrity

Documenting the client's response to receiving the blood product

Managing medical emergencies if a transfusion reaction or other complication occurs

Monitoring for complications related to blood administration

Monitoring laboratory values

Monitoring for expected effects

Safe administration of blood and blood products

Venous access devices for blood administration

I. TYPES OF BLOOD COMPONENTS

A. **RBCs**
1. Used to replace erythrocytes
2. Packed **RBCs** are usually supplied in 250-mL unit bags; however, they can be supplied in 250- to 350- or 350- to 400-mL bags; always check the unit for the volume of the blood component
3. Each unit increases the hemoglobin by 1 g/dL and hematocrit by 2% to 3%; the change in laboratory values takes 4 to 6 hours to appear
4. Evaluation of an effective response is based on the resolution of the symptoms of anemia and an increase in the erythrocyte count

B. **Whole blood**
1. Rarely used; treatment with a specific blood component is usually prescribed
2. Used to resolve hypovolemic shock resulting from hemorrhage
3. Contains **RBCs,** plasma, and plasma proteins, and each unit normally contains 500 mL; always check the bag for the volume of the blood component

4. Evaluation of an effective response is based on the resolution of the symptoms of hypovolemia

C. **Platelets**
1. **Platelets** are used to treat thrombocytopenia and **platelet** dysfunctions
2. **Crossmatching** is not required but is usually done (**platelet** concentrates contain few **RBCs)**
3. The volume in a unit of **platelets** may vary from 50 to 70 mL per unit to 200 to 400 mL per unit; always check the bag for the volume of the blood component
4. **Platelets** are administered immediately upon receipt from the blood bank and are given rapidly, usually over 15 to 30 minutes
5. Evaluation of an effective response is based on improvement in the **platelet** count, and **platelet** counts are normally evaluated 1 hour and 18 to 24 hours after the transfusion

D. **Fresh-frozen plasma**
1. **Fresh-frozen plasma** may be used to provide clotting factors or volume expansion; it contains no platelets
2. It is infused within 6 hours of thawing, while clotting factors are still viable, and is infused as rapidly as possible
3. **Rh** compatibility and **ABO** compatibility are required for the transfusion of plasma products
4. A unit normally contains 200 to 250 mL; always check the bag for the volume of the blood component
5. Evaluation of an effective response is assessed by monitoring coagulation studies, particularly the prothrombin time (PT) and the partial thromboplastin time (PTT), and resolution of hypovolemia

II. TYPES OF BLOOD DONATIONS

A. **Autologous**
1. A donation of the client's own blood before a scheduled procedure; it reduces the risk of disease transmission and potential transfusion complications
2. Not an option for a client with leukemia or bacteremia
3. A donation can be made every 3 days if the hemoglobin remains at or above 11g/dL
4. Donations should begin within 5 weeks of the transfusion date and end at least 3 days before the date of transfusion

B. **Blood salvage**
1. An **autologous donation** that involves suctioning blood from body cavities, joint spaces, or other closed body sites
2. Blood may need to be "washed," a special process that removes tissue debris before reinfusion

C. **Designated donation**
1. Occurs when recipients select their own compatible donors

2. It does not reduce the risk of contracting infections transmitted by the blood; however, recipients feel more comfortable identifying their donors

III. COMPATIBILITY

▲ A. Client blood samples are drawn and labeled at the bedside when drawn; the client is asked to state his or her name, which is compared with the name on the identification bracelet
B. The recipient's **ABO** type and **Rh** type are identified
C. An antibody screen is done to determine the presence of antibodies other than anti-A and anti-B
D. **Crossmatch testing** is done, in which donor **RBCs** are combined with recipient's serum and Coombs' serum; **crossmatch** is compatible if no **RBC** agglutination has occurred
▲ E. In an emergency, O-negative **RBCs** and AB plasma can be safely administered to most clients without serologic testing

IV. INFUSION CONTROLLERS AND PUMPS

A. Infusion controllers and pumps may be used to administer blood products if they are designed to function with opaque solutions; however, the negative pressure exerted by the cassette of the machine can cause **RBC** hemolysis
B. Always consult manufacturer guidelines for the controller or pump
C. Special manual pressure cuffs may be used to increase the flow rate but should not exceed 300 mm Hg
D. Standard sphygmomanometer cuffs are not to be used to increase flow rate because they do not exert uniform pressure against all parts of the bag

V. BLOOD WARMERS

A. Blood warmers may be used to prevent hypothermia and adverse reactions when several units of blood are being administered
B. Special warmers have been designed for this purpose, and only devices specifically tested and approved for this use can be used
▲ C. Do not warm blood products in a microwave or in hot water

VI. PRECAUTIONS AND NURSING RESPONSIBILITIES (Box 14-1)

VII. COMPLICATIONS

▲ A. **Transfusion reactions**
1. Signs of an immediate **transfusion reaction**
   a. Chills and diaphoresis
   b. Muscle aches, back pain, or chest pain
   c. Rashes, hives, itching, and swelling
   d. Rapid, thready pulse
   e. Dyspnea, cough, wheezing, or rales
   f. Pallor and cyanosis
   g. Apprehension
   h. Tingling and numbness
   i. Headache
   j. Nausea, vomiting, abdominal cramping, and diarrhea
2. Signs of **transfusion reaction** in an unconscious client:
   a. Weak pulse
   b. Fever
   c. Tachycardia or bradycardia
   d. Hypotension
   e. Visible hemoglobinuria
   f. Oliguria or anuria
3. Delayed **transfusion reactions**
   a. Reactions can occur days to years after a transfusion
   b. Signs include fever, mild jaundice, and decreased hematocrit
4. Implementation
   a. Stop the transfusion immediately
   b. Keep the IV line open with 0.9% NS
   c. Notify the physician immediately
   d. Remain with the client, observing signs and symptoms and monitoring VS as often as every 5 minutes
   e. Prepare to administer emergency medications such as antihistamines, vasopressors, fluids, and steroids as prescribed
   f. Obtain a urine specimen for laboratory studies
   g. Return blood bag, tubing, attached labels, and transfusion record to the blood bank

B. **Circulatory overload**
1. Description: Caused by infusion of blood at a rate too rapid for the client to tolerate
2. Assessment
   a. Cough, dyspnea, chest pain, rales, and pulmonary edema
   b. Headache
   c. Hypertension
   d. Tachycardia and a rapid, bounding pulse
   e. Distended neck veins
3. Implementation
   a. Slow the rate of infusion
   b. Place the client in upright position, with the feet in a dependent position
   c. Notify the physician
   d. Administer oxygen, diuretics, and morphine sulfate as prescribed
   e. Monitor for dysrhythmias
   f. Phlebotomy may also be a method of prescribed treatment

C. **Septicemia**
1. Description: Occurs with the transfusion of blood contaminated with microorganisms
2. Assessment
   a. Rapid onset of chills and a high fever
   b. Vomiting

BOX 14-1

Precautions and Nursing Responsibilities

GENERAL PRECAUTIONS

A large volume of refrigerated blood infused rapidly through a central catheter into the ventricle of the heart can cause cardiac dysrhythmias.

No solution other than NS should be added to blood components.

Medications are never added to blood transfusions.

To avoid the risk of septicemia, infusions (1 unit) should not exceed 4 hours.

The blood administration set should be changed every 4 to 6 hours or according to institution policy to reduce the risk of septicemia.

Always check the blood bag for the date of expiration; components expire at midnight on the day marked on the bag unless otherwise specified.

Inspect the blood bag for leaks, abnormal color, clots, excessive air, and bubbles.

Blood must be administered within 30 minutes from its being received at the blood bank, as this is the maximal allowable time out of monitored storage.

NEVER refrigerate blood in refrigerators other than those used in blood banks; if the blood is not administered within 30 minutes, return it to blood bank.

The recommended rate of infusion varies with the blood component being transfused and depends on client's condition; generally, blood is infused as quickly as the client's condition allows.

Components containing few RBCs and platelets may be infused rapidly, but caution should be taken to avoid circulatory overload.

Vital signs (VS) and lung sounds should be taken before the transfusion and again after the first 15 minutes and every hour until 1 hour after the transfusion has been discontinued.

BLOOD BANK PRECAUTIONS

Blood will be released from the blood bank only to personnel as specified by agency policy.

The name and identification (ID) number of the intended recipient must be provided to the blood bank, and a documented permanent record of this information is maintained.

Blood should be transported from the blood bank to only one client at a time to prevent blood delivery to the wrong client.

CLIENT IDENTITY AND COMPATIBILITY

The most critical phase of the transfusion is confirming product compatibility and verifying client identity.

Two RNs need to check the physician's order, the client's identity, and the ID band and number, verifying that the name and number are identical to those on the blood component tag.

At the bedside, the client is asked to state his or her name, and the nurse compares it with the name on the ID bracelet.

The blood bag tag, label, and requisition form are assessed to ensure that ABO and Rh types are compatible.

The blood bag label is checked to ensure that the correct components have been issued; if there are any inconsistencies or questions, notify the blood bank immediately.

CLIENT ASSESSMENT

Determine whether the client has ever experienced any previous reactions to blood transfusions.

Ensure that an informed consent has been obtained.

Check the client's vital signs; assess renal, circulatory, and respiratory status and ability to tolerate IV fluids.

If the temperature is elevated, notify the physician before beginning the transfusion; a fever may be a cause for delaying the transfusion in addition to masking a possible symptom of an acute transfusion reaction.

ADMINISTERING THE TRANSFUSION

Maintain standard (universal) precautions.

Insert an IV and infuse normal saline (NS); maintain at a keep vein open (KVO) rate; a central catheter is an acceptable venous access option for blood transfusions.

An 18- or 19-gauge IV needle will be needed to achieve a maximum flow rate of blood products and prevent damage to RBCs; if a smaller-gauge needle must be used, RBCs may be diluted with NS.

Blood products should be infused through administration sets designed specifically for blood; use a Y tubing or straight tubing blood administration set that contains a filter designed to trap fibrin clots and other debris that accumulate during blood storage.

Premedicate the client with acetaminophen (Tylenol) or diphenhydramine hydrochloride (Benadryl) as prescribed if the client has a history of adverse reactions; if prescribed, oral medications should be administered 30 minutes before the transfusion is started, and IV medications may be given immediately before the transfusion is started.

Instruct the client to report anything unusual immediately.

Determine rate of infusion by physician order or, if not specified, by institution policy.

Begin the transfusion slowly under close supervision; if no reaction is noted within the first 15 minutes, the flow can be increased to the prescribed rate.

During the transfusion, monitor the client for signs and symptoms of transfusion reaction; the first 15 minutes of the transfusion are the most critical, and the nurse must stay with client.

If a major ABO incompatibility exists or a severe allergic reaction occurs, it is usually evident within the first 50 mL of the transfusion.

Document the client's tolerance to the administration of the blood product.

Monitor appropriate laboratory values and document effectiveness of treatment related to the specific type of blood product.

REACTIONS TO THE TRANSFUSION

Stop the transfusion, change the IV tubing down to the IV site, keep the IV line open with NS, notify the physician and blood bank, and return the blood bag and tubing to the blood bank.

Do not leave the client alone, and monitor for any life-threatening symptoms.

Obtain appropriate laboratory samples according to agency policies, such as blood and urine samples (free hemoglobin indicates that RBCs were hemolyzed).

    c. Diarrhea

    d. Hypotension

    e. Shock

  3. Implementation

    a. Notify the physician

    b. Obtain blood cultures and cultures of the blood bag

    c. Administer oxygen, IV fluids, antibiotics, vasopressors, and steroids as ordered

D. **Iron overload**

  1. Description: Can occur in clients receiving more than 100 units of blood over a period of time

  2. Assessment

    a. Vomiting

    b. Diarrhea

    c. Hypotension

    d. Altered hematological values

  3. Implementation

    a. Deferoxamine (Desferal), administered by IV or subcutaneously, removes accumulated iron via the kidneys

    b. Urine turns red as iron is excreted after administration of Desferal; treatment is discontinued when serum iron levels return to normal

E. **Disease transmission**

  1. The most common disease transmitted is hepatitis C, manifested by anorexia, nausea, vomiting, dark urine, and jaundice; it usually occurs within 4 to 6 weeks after the transfusion

  2. The transmission of HIV has become rare since routine donor testing was implemented in 1985

F. Hypocalcemia and citrate intoxication

  1. Citrate in transfused blood binds with calcium and is excreted

  2. Assess serum calcium before and after transfusion

  3. Monitor for signs of hypocalcemia

  4. Slow the transfusion and notify the physician if signs of hypocalcemia occur

G. Hyperkalemia

  1. Stored blood liberates potassium through hemolysis

  2. The older the blood, the greater the risk of hyperkalemia; therefore, clients at risk for hyperkalemia, such as renal insufficiency or renal failure clients, should receive fresh blood

  3. Assess the date on the blood as well as the serum potassium before and after transfusion

  4. Monitor the potassium level and for signs of hyperkalemia

  5. Slow the transfusion and notify the physician if signs of hyperkalemia occur

PRACTICE QUESTIONS

1. A nurse has just obtained a unit of blood from the blood bank to transfuse to a client as ordered. Before preparing the blood for transfusion, the nurse next plans to look for which of the following members of the health care team to assist in checking the unit of blood?

  1. Blood bank technician

  2. Registered nurse (RN)

  3. Medical student

  4. Phlebotomist

2. A nurse has obtained a unit of blood from the blood bank and has properly checked the blood bag with another nurse. Just before beginning the transfusion, the nurse assesses which of the following items?

  1. Vital signs

  2. Latest hematocrit level

  3. Skin color

  4. Urine output

3. A nurse has just received an order to transfuse a unit of packed red blood cells for an assigned client. In planning coverage for the client assignment, the nurse asks if another nurse will be available to check on the other assigned clients for how long when the unit of blood is hung?

  1. 5 minutes

  2. 15 minutes

  3. 30 minutes

  4. 45 minutes

4. A client has an order to receive a unit of packed red blood cells. A nurse would obtain which of the following IV solutions from the IV storage area to hang with the blood product at the client's bedside?

  1. 0.9% sodium chloride

  2. Lactated Ringer's

  3. 5% dextrose in 0.9% sodium chloride

  4. 5% dextrose in 0.45% sodium chloride

5. A nurse is assigned to care for a client who was just admitted to the hospital for the treatment of iron overload. The nurse reviews the physician's admission orders and anticipates that the physician will prescribe which medication to treat the iron overload?

  1. Granisetron (Kytril)

  2. Deferoxamine (Desferal)

  3. Ketoconazole (Nizoral)

  4. Terbinafine hydrochloride (Lamisil)

6. A client with severe blood loss resulting from multiple trauma requires rapid transfusion of several units of blood. A nurse asks another health team member to obtain which of the following devices for use during the transfusion procedure to help reduce the risk of cardiac dysrhythmias?

  1. Cardiac monitor

  2. Pulse oximetry

  3. Blood warming device

  4. Infusion controller

7. A nurse enters a client's room to assess the client, who began receiving a blood transfusion 45 min-

utes earlier. The client is flushed and dyspneic. On assessment, the nurse auscultates the presence of crackles in the lung bases. The client states that he was just going to ring the call bell for the nurse. The nurse determines that this client is most likely experiencing which of the following complications of blood transfusion therapy?
1. Hypovolemia
2. Transfusion reaction
3. Fluid overload
4. Bacteremia

8. A nurse determines that a client is having a transfusion reaction. As the nurse is stopping the unit of packed red blood cells (RBCs) that is currently infusing, the nurse plans to take which of the following actions next?
1. Run normal saline at a KVO (keep vein open) rate
2. Change the solution to 5% dextrose in water
3. Remove the IV line
4. Obtain a culture of the tip of the catheter device removed from the client

9. A nurse has discontinued a unit of blood that was infusing into a client, because the client has experienced a transfusion reaction. After documenting the incident appropriately, the nurse sends the blood bag to which of the following areas according to agency protocol?
1. Infection Control Department
2. Blood Bank
3. Risk Management
4. Environmental Services

10. A nurse has just received a unit of packed red blood cells (PRBCs) from the blood bank for transfusion to an assigned client. The nurse is careful to select tubing especially made for blood products, knowing that this tubing is manufactured with:
1. A microdrip chamber
2. Tinted tubing to protect the blood from light
3. An air vent
4. An in-line filter

11. Packed red blood cells have been prescribed for a client with low hemoglobin and hematocrit. A nurse measuring a client's temperature prior to hanging a blood transfusion finds it to be 100.6° F orally. The nurse does which of the following as the most appropriate nursing action?
1. Administer an antihistamine and begin the transfusion
2. Administer two tablets of acetaminophen (Tylenol) and begin the transfusion
3. Begin the transfusion as prescribed
4. Delay hanging the blood and notify the physician

12. A nurse has received an order to transfuse a client with a unit of packed red blood cells. Before explaining the procedure to the client, the nurse asks which of the following initial questions?
1. "Why do you think that you need the transfusion?"
2. "Do you know the complications and risks of a transfusion?"
3. "Have you ever had a transfusion before?"
4. "Have you ever gone into shock for any reason in the past?"

13. A nurse is signing for a unit of packed blood cells at the hospital blood bank. After putting the pen down, the nurse glances at the clock, which reads 1:00. The nurse calculates that the transfusion must be started by:
1. 1:30
2. 1:45
3. 2:00
4. 2:15

14. A client has received a transfusion of platelets. The nurse evaluates that the client is benefiting most from this therapy if the client exhibits which of the following?
1. Decline of temperature to normal
2. Decreased oozing of blood from puncture sites and gums
3. Increased hemoglobin level
4. Increased hematocrit level

15. A nurse listening to morning report learns that an assigned client received a unit of granulocytes the previous evening. The nurse makes a note to assess the results of which of the following daily serum laboratory studies to assess the effectiveness of the transfusion?
1. White blood cell (WBC) count
2. Erythrocyte count
3. Hemoglobin level
4. Hematocrit level

16. A client ordered to receive a transfusion has experienced a rash with pruritus during previous transfusions. The client asks the nurse if it is safe to receive the transfusion. In formulating a response, the nurse incorporates the understanding that which of the following medications will most likely be ordered before the transfusion is begun?
1. Diphenhydramine (Benadryl)
2. Acetylsalicylic acid (ASA, aspirin)
3. Acetaminophen (Tylenol)
4. Ibuprofen (Motrin)

17. A nurse who is about to begin a blood transfusion knows that blood cells start to deteriorate after a certain period of time. The nurse checks which of the following items carefully before beginning the transfusion to ensure that this has not happened?
1. Blood identification number
2. Expiration date
3. Blood group and type
4. Presence of clots

18. A nurse overhears a physician stating that a client who is in hypovolemic shock requires plasma expansion. The nurse anticipates receiving an order to transfuse which of the following blood products to this client?
    1. Cryoprecipitate
    2. Packed red blood cells
    3. Albumin
    4. Platelets
19. A client is told by a physician that a blood transfusion is needed, and that a blood sample must be drawn first for blood typing and cross-match. After the physician leaves, the client asks the nurse, "What exactly is a blood type, anyway?" The nurse incorporates which of the following statements into a response?
    1. "The blood type represents an antibody that normally circulates in the blood plasma."
    2. "The blood type represents an antigen that normally circulates in the blood plasma."
    3. "The blood type represents an antigen found on the surface of the red blood cells."
    4. "The blood type represents an antibody found on the surface of the red blood cells."

20. A client requiring upcoming surgery is extremely anxious about the possible need for blood transfusion during or after surgery. The nurse advises the client to do which of the following as the most effective way to eliminate the risk of cross-infection?
    1. Take iron supplements before surgery to boost hemoglobin levels
    2. Request that any donated blood be screened twice by the blood bank
    3. Ask a friend or family member to donate blood ahead of time
    4. Donate autologous blood prior to the surgery

CRITICAL THINKING: FREE-TEXT ENTRY

A nurse has an order to transfuse a unit of packed red blood cells to a client who does not currently have an IV line inserted. When obtaining supplies from the IV supply area to start the IV, the nurse selects an angiocatheter that is at least which gauge size?

Answer: _____

ANSWERS

1. 2
Rationale: Two RN's or one RN and a licensed practical nurse (depending on agency policy) must together check the label on the blood product against the client's identification number, blood group, and complete name. This minimizes the risk of error in checking information on the blood bag, and thereby minimizes the risk of harm or injury to the client. A blood bank technician will verify data with the nurse when the blood is obtained from the blood bank but will not verify information on the nursing unit or at the client's bedside. The other options are also incorrect.
Test-Taking Strategy: Use the process of elimination and specific knowledge of blood administration methods and techniques. Remember that two RN's or one RN and a licensed practical nurse (depending on agency policy) must together check the blood product. Review the procedures related to checking blood prior to administration if you had difficulty with this question.
Level of Cognitive Ability: Application
Client Needs: Safe, Effective Care Environment
Integrated Concept/Process: Nursing Process/Planning
Content Area: Fundamental Skills
Reference: Potter, P. & Perry, A. (2001). *Fundamentals of nursing* (5th ed.). St. Louis: Mosby, p. 1243.
2. 1
Rationale: A change in vital signs during the transfusion may indicate that a transfusion reaction is occurring. This is why the nurse assesses vital signs prior to the procedure, every 15 minutes for the first half-hour, and every half-hour thereafter. The other options do not identify assessments that are required just prior to beginning a transfusion.

Test-Taking Strategy: Use the process of elimination. Note the key words "just before beginning the transfusion." This tells you that more than one of the options may be partially or totally correct and that the correct option needs to be assessed for possible comparison during the transfusion. Use the ABCs—airway, breathing, and circulation—to direct you to option 1. Review the nursing interventions for preparing to administer a blood transfusion if you had difficulty with this question.
Level of Cognitive Ability: Application
Client Needs: Physiological Integrity
Integrated Concept/Process: Nursing Process/Assessment
Content Area: Fundamental Skills
Reference: Potter, P., & Perry, A. (2001). *Fundamentals of nursing* (5th ed.). St. Louis: Mosby, p. 1242.
3. 2
Rationale: The nurse must remain with the client for the first 15 minutes of a transfusion, which is the most frequent period during which a transfusion reaction may occur. This enables the nurse to quickly detect a reaction and intervene quickly. The nurse engages in safe nursing practice by obtaining coverage for the other clients during this time. Options 1, 3, and 4 are incorrect.
Test-Taking Strategy: Use the process of elimination and knowledge regarding blood transfusion procedures to answer this question. Remember, the client must be directly monitored for the first 15 minutes of the transfusion. Review the nursing responsibilities involved in beginning a blood transfusion if you had difficulty with this question.
Level of Cognitive Ability: Application
Client Needs: Physiological Integrity
Integrated Concept/Process: Nursing Process/Planning

Content Area: Fundamental Skills
Reference: Potter, P., & Perry, A. (2001). *Fundamentals of nursing* (5th ed.). St. Louis: Mosby, p.1243.

4. **1**

Rationale: Sodium chloride 0.9% (normal saline, NS) is an isotonic solution that is standardly used both to precede and to follow infusion of blood products. Dextrose is not used because it could result in clumping and subsequent hemolysis of red blood cells. Lactated Ringer's is not the solution of choice with this procedure.

Test-Taking Strategy: Use the process of elimination and eliminate options 3 and 4 first because they are similar in that both solutions contain dextrose. From the remaining options, remember that NS is the solution that is compatible with red blood cells. If this question was difficult, review the procedures related to the administration of blood.
Level of Cognitive Ability: Application
Client Needs: Physiological Integrity
Integrated Concept/Process: Nursing Process/Implementation
Content Area: Fundamental Skills
Reference: Altman, G., Buchsel, P., & Coxon, V. (2000). *Delmar's fundamental & advanced nursing skills.* Albany, N.Y.: Delmar, p. 981.

5. **2**

Rationale: Deferoxamine (Desferal) is an antidote used to treat iron toxicity. Granisetron (Kytril) is an antimetic. Ketoconazole (Nizoral) and terbinafine hydrochloride (Lamisil) are antifungal medications.

Test-Taking Strategy: Use the process of elimination and knowledge of the classifications of the medications identified in the options. Eliminate options 3 and 4 first because they are both antifungal medications. From the remaining options it is necessary to know that granisetron is an antiemetic and that deferoxamine is the medication used to treat iron toxicity. Review the medications identified in the options if you had difficulty with this question.
Level of Cognitive Ability: Analysis
Client Needs: Physiological Integrity
Integrated Concept/Process: Nursing Process/Analysis
Content Area: Fundamental Skills
Reference: Hodgson, B., & Kizior, R. (2001). *Saunders nursing drug handbook 2001.* Philadelphia: W.B. Saunders, pp. 289, 479, 565, 967.

6. **3**

Rationale: If several units of blood are to be administered, a blood warmer should be used. Rapid transfusion of cool blood places the client at risk for cardiac dysrhythmias. To prevent this occurrence, the nurse warms the blood as needed, using a blood warming device. Electronic infusion devices are not helpful in this case, since the infusion must be rapid, and infusion devices are generally used to control the flow rate. In addition, not all infusion devices are made to handle blood or blood products. Pulse oximetry and cardiac monitoring equipment are useful for the early assessment of complications, but do not reduce the occurrence of cardiac dysrhythmias.

Test-Taking Strategy: Use the process of elimination. Note that the key words "rapid" and "reduce the risk." They tell you that the infusions will infuse quickly and that the correct option is the one that will minimize the risk of cardiac dysrhythmias

occurring. Eliminate option 1 and 2 first because these items are used to assess for rather than reduce the risk of complications. From the remaining options, use knowledge related to the complications of transfusion therapy and note the relationship between the words "several units of blood" in the question and "blood warming device" in the correct option. Review the concepts related to the use of a blood warmer if you had difficulty with this question.
Level of Cognitive Ability: Application
Client Needs: Physiological Integrity
Integrated Concept/Process: Nursing Process/Planning
Content Area: Fundamental Skills
Reference: Altman, G., Buchsel, P., & Coxon, V. (2000). *Delmar's fundamental & advanced nursing skills.* Albany, N.Y.: Delmar, p. 984.

7. **3**

Rationale: With fluid overload, the client has the presence of crackles in addition to dyspnea. An allergic reaction, which is one type of blood transfusion reaction, would produce symptoms such as flushing, dyspnea, itching, and a generalized rash. With bacteremia, the client should have a fever, which is not part of the clinical picture presented. Hypovolemia is not a complication of a blood transfusion.

Test-Taking Strategy: Use the process of elimination, noting the key words "most likely." Read the question carefully, and focus on the symptoms identified in the question. Eliminate option 1 first because it is not a complication of a blood transfusion. Next eliminate option 4 because there are no data in the question that indicate that the client has an elevated temperature. From the remaining options, focusing on the key words "crackles in the lung bases" will direct you to option 3. Review the complications of blood transfusion therapy if you had difficulty with this question.
Level of Cognitive Ability: Analysis
Client Needs: Physiological Integrity
Integrated Concept/Process: Nursing Process/Analysis
Content Area: Fundamental Skills
Reference: Craven, R., & Hirnle, C. (2000). *Fundamentals of nursing: Human health and function* (3rd ed.). Philadelphia: Lippincott, p. 584.

8. **1**

Rationale: If the nurse suspects a transfusion reaction, the transfusion is stopped and normal saline is infused at a KVO rate pending further physician orders. This maintains a patent IV access line and aids in maintaining the client's intravascular volume. The nurse would not discontinue the IV line, because then there would be no IV access route. Obtaining a culture of the tip of the catheter device removed from the client is incorrect. First, the catheter should not be removed. Second, cultures are performed when infection, not transfusion reaction, is suspected. Normal saline is the solution of choice over solutions containing dextrose because saline does not cause RBCs to clump.

Test-Taking Strategy: Use the process of elimination, noting the key word "next." Knowing that the IV should not be removed or discontinued assists in eliminating options 3 and 4. Recalling that normal saline, not dextrose, is used when administering a unit of blood will direct you to option 1. Review care to the client when a transfusion reaction occurs if you had difficulty with this question.

Level of Cognitive Ability: Application
Client Needs: Physiological Integrity
Integrated Concept/Process: Nursing Process/Planning
Content Area: Fundamental Skills
Reference: Potter, P., & Perry, A. (2001). *Fundamentals of nursing* (5th ed.). St. Louis: Mosby, p. 1243.

9. **2**

Rationale: The nurse returns the blood transfusion bag containing any remaining blood to the blood bank. This allows the blood bank to complete any follow-up testing procedures needed once a transfusion reaction has been documented. The other options are incorrect.

Test-Taking Strategy: Use the process of elimination and specific knowledge related to routine transfusion-related procedures to answer the question. Recalling that blood is issued from the blood bank may help you to eliminate each of the incorrect options. Review nursing responsibilities if a transfusion reaction occurs if you had difficulty with this question.

Level of Cognitive Ability: Application
Client Needs: Safe, Effective Care Environment
Integrated Concept/Process: Nursing Process/Implementation
Content Area: Fundamental Skills
Reference: Potter, P., & Perry, A. (2001). *Fundamentals of nursing* (5th ed.). St. Louis: Mosby, p. 1243.

10. **4**

Rationale: The tubing used for blood administration has an in-line filter. This helps ensure that any particles larger than the size of the filter are caught in the filter and are not infused into the client. The tubing should be macrodrip, not microdrip, to allow blood to flow freely through the drip chamber. An air vent is unnecessary, since the blood bag is not made of glass. Option 2 is incorrect, and, in addition, blood does not need to be protected from light.

Test-Taking Strategy: Use the process of elimination. Read each option carefully, and visualize the process of blood administration. Remember that tubing used for blood administration has an in-line filter. Review concepts related to tubing used for blood administration if you had difficulty with this question.

Level of Cognitive Ability: Application
Client Needs: Safe, Effective Care Environment
Integrated Concept/Process: Nursing Process/Implementation
Content Area: Fundamental Skills
Reference: Harkreader, H. (2000). *Fundamentals of nursing: Caring and clinical judgment.* Philadelphia: W.B. Saunders, p. 1131.

11. **4**

Rationale: If the client has a temperature greater than 100° F, the unit of blood should not be hung until the physician is notified and has the opportunity to give further orders. It is likely that the physician will prescribe that the blood be administered regardless of the temperature, but it is not within the realm of the nurse's scope of practice to make that determination. The other options are incorrect.

Test-Taking Strategy: Use the process of elimination. Eliminate options 1, 2, and 3 because they all indicate beginning the transfusion. Review the nursing responsibilities prior to administering a blood transfusion if you had difficulty with this question.

Level of Cognitive Ability: Application
Client Needs: Physiological Integrity
Integrated Concept/Process: Nursing Process/Implementation
Content Area: Fundamental Skills
Reference: Smith, S., Duell, D., & Martin, B. (2000). *Clinical nursing skills: Basic to advanced skills* (5th ed.). Upper Saddle River, NJ: Prentice-Hall Health, p. 876.

12. **3**

Rationale: Asking the client about personal experience with transfusion therapy provides a good starting point for client teaching about this procedure. Options 2 and 4 are not helpful because they may elicit a fearful response from the client. Although it is important to determine whether the client knows the reason for the transfusion, option 1 is not an appropriate statement in terms of eliciting information from the client regarding an understanding of the need for the transfusion.

Test-Taking Strategy: Use the process of elimination. Note that the key words in the question are "initial question." This tells you that the correct option is the best starting point for discussion about the transfusion therapy. Options 2 and 4 have emotionally laden trigger words, including "risks" and "gone into shock," respectively, which make them incorrect. From the remaining options, focus on the key words and use therapeutic communication techniques to direct you to option 3. Review pretransfusion assessment procedures if you had difficulty with this question.

Level of Cognitive Ability: Comprehension
Client Needs: Physiological Integrity
Integrated Concept/Process: Nursing Process/Assessment
Content Area: Fundamental Skills
Reference: Potter, P., & Perry, A. (2001). *Fundamentals of nursing* (5th ed.). St. Louis: Mosby, p. 1242.

13. **1**

Rationale: Blood must be hung within 30 minutes after obtaining it from the blood bank. After that time, the blood temperature will be in excess of 50° F and could be unsafe for use. For this reason options 2, 3, and 4 are incorrect.

Test-Taking Strategy: Use the process of elimination. It is necessary to know that blood must be hung within 30 minutes after obtaining it from the blood bank to answer this question correctly. Review the standard procedures related to safe blood administration if you had difficulty with this question.

Level of Cognitive Ability: Application
Client Needs: Physiological Integrity
Integrated Concept/Process: Nursing Process/Planning
Content Area: Fundamental Skills
Reference: Smeltzer, S., & Bare, B. (2000). *Brunner & Suddarth's textbook of medical-surgical nursing* (9th ed). Philadelphia: Lippincott Williams & Wilkins, p. 782.

14. **2**

Rationale: Platelets are necessary for proper blood clotting. The client with insufficient platelets may exhibit frank bleeding, or oozing of blood from puncture sites, wounds, and mucous membranes. A temperature would decline to normal after infusion of granulocytes if those cells were then instrumental in fighting infection in the body. Increased hemoglobin and hematocrit would be seen when the client has received a transfusion of red blood cells.

Test-Taking Strategy: Use the process of elimination and

knowledge regarding the potential uses and benefits of the various types of blood product transfusions. Eliminate options 3 and 4 first because they are similar. From the remaining options, recalling that platelets are necessary for proper blood clotting will easily direct you to option 2. If this question was difficult, review the key types of blood products available for transfusion.

Level of Cognitive Ability: Analysis
Client Needs: Physiological Integrity
Integrated Concept/Process: Nursing Process/Evaluation
Content Area: Fundamental Skills
Reference: Ignatavicius, D., Workman, M., & Mishler, M. (1999). *Medical-surgical nursing across the health care continuum* (3rd ed.). Philadelphia: W.B. Saunders, p. 985.

15. **1**
Rationale: The client who has neutropenia may receive a transfusion of granulocytes, or WBCs. These are often clients with severe infections who are unresponsive to antibiotic therapy. The nurse notes the results of follow-up WBC counts to evaluate the effectiveness of therapy. The nurse also continues to monitor the client for signs and symptoms of infection. Erythrocyte count and hemoglobin and hematocrit levels are measured after transfusion of whole blood or packed red blood cells.
Test-Taking Strategy: Use the process of elimination. Recalling that granulocytes are a component of white blood cells will assist in directing you to option 1. In addition, note that options 2, 3, and 4 are similar in that these options all refer to erythrocytes. Review the key points related to types of blood products if you had difficulty with this question.
Level of Cognitive Ability: Analysis
Client Needs: Physiological Integrity
Integrated Concept/Process: Nursing Process/Evaluation
Content Area: Fundamental Skills
Reference: Ignatavicius, D., Workman, M., & Mishler, M. (1999). *Medical-surgical nursing across the health care continuum* (3rd ed.). Philadelphia: W.B. Saunders, p. 985.

16. **1**
Rationale: A urticaria reaction is characterized by a rash accompanied by pruritus. This type of transfusion reaction is prevented by pretreating the client with an antihistamine, such as diphenhydramine. Acetaminophen and acetylsalicylic acid are analgesics, while ibuprofen is a nonsteroidal antiinflammatory drug.
Test-Taking Strategy: Use the process of elimination, recalling the classifications of the medications noted in each option. Recalling that diphenhydramine is an antihistamine will easily direct you to option 1. Review the measures implemented to prevent a transfusion reaction if you had difficulty with this question.
Level of Cognitive Ability: Analysis
Client Needs: Physiological Integrity
Integrated Concept/Process: Nursing Process/Analysis
Content Area: Pharmacology
Reference: Smeltzer, S., & Bare, B. (2000) *Brunner & Suddarth's textbook of medical-surgical nursing* (9th ed). Philadelphia: Lippincott Williams & Wilkins, p. 784.

17. **2**
Rationale: The nurse notes the expiration date on the unit of blood to ensure that the blood is fresh. Blood cells begin to degenerate over time, so safe storage is limited to 35 days. Careful notation of the expiration date by the nurse is an essential part of the verification process that is done before hanging a unit of blood. Also noted are the blood identification (unit) number, blood group and type, and client's name. The nurse also inspects the unit of blood for clots, and returns the unit to the blood bank if found.
Test-Taking Strategy: Use the process of elimination and note that the key word in this question is "deteriorates." To answer this question correctly, you must know which part of the pretransfusion verification procedure relates to the "freshness" of the unit of blood. Keeping this issue in mind should allow you to eliminate each of the incorrect options systematically. Review the procedure for checking blood if you had difficulty with this question.
Level of Cognitive Ability: Application
Client Needs: Physiological Integrity
Integrated Concept/Process: Nursing Process/Implementation
Content Area: Fundamental Skills
Reference: Harkreader, H. (2000). *Fundamentals of nursing: Caring and clinical judgment.* Philadelphia: W.B. Saunders, p. 1130.

18. **3**
Rationale: Albumin may be used as a plasma expander. Cryoprecipitate is useful in treating bleeding from hemophilia or disseminated intravascular coagulopathy because it is rich in clotting factors. Packed red blood cells replace erythrocytes and are not a plasma expander. Platelets are used when the client's platelet count is low.
Test-Taking Strategy: Use the process of elimination, noting the key words "requires plasma expansion." Recalling the composition of each of the blood components identified in the options will direct you to option 3. If you had difficulty with this question, review the various blood component therapies.
Level of Cognitive Ability: Analysis
Client Needs: Physiological Integrity
Integrated Concept/Process: Nursing Process/Analysis
Content Area: Fundamental Skills
Reference: Smeltzer, S., & Bare, B. (2000). *Brunner & Suddarth's textbook of medical-surgical nursing* (9th ed). Philadelphia: Lippincott Williams & Wilkins, p. 779.

19. **3**
Rationale: The major blood types are A, B, AB, and O. The blood type indicates an antigen that is found on the surface of the red blood cells (RBCs). Each blood type also has the ability to form antibodies to agglutinate the antigens that are lacking. These antibodies are actually formed only when that specific antigen has gained entry into the body. For example, a person with type B blood has B antigen on the RBCs, and has agglutinins to cause clumping of A antigens.
Test-Taking Strategy: Use the process of elimination and specific knowledge related to the meaning of blood groups. If you had difficulty with this question, review these basic concepts.
Level of Cognitive Ability: Analysis
Client Needs: Physiological Integrity
Integrated Concept/Process: Nursing Process/Analysis
Content Area: Fundamental Skills

Reference: Phipps, W., Sands, J., & Marek, J. (1999). *Medical-surgical nursing: Concepts & clinical practice* (6th ed.). St. Louis: Mosby, pp. 2175-2177.

20. **4**

Rationale: Donating autologous blood to be reinfused as needed during or after surgery eliminates the risk of cross-infection from contaminated blood. The next most effective way is to ask a family member to donate blood prior to surgery. Blood banks do not provide extra screening on request. Preoperative iron supplements are helpful for iron deficiency anemia but are not most helpful in replacing blood lost during the surgery.

Test-Taking Strategy: Use the process of elimination. Note that the question contains the key words "most effective." This tells you that more than one or all of the options may be partially or totally correct. Recalling that an autologous transfusion is the collection of the client's own blood will easily direct you to option 4. Review the concepts related to disease transmission and blood donation procedures if you had difficulty with this question.

Level of Cognitive Ability: Application
Client Needs: Physiological Integrity
Integrated Concept/Process: Nursing Process/Implementation

Content Area: Fundamental Skills
Reference: Potter, P., & Perry, A. (2001). *Fundamentals of nursing* (5th ed.). St. Louis: Mosby, p. 1242.

CRITICAL THINKING: FREE-TEXT ENTRY

Answer: 18- or 19-gauge catheter

Rationale: The IV catheter used for a blood transfusion should be at least an 18 or 19 gauge. Blood has a thicker and stickier consistency than IV solutions, and using an 18- or 19-gauge catheter ensures that the bore of the catheter is large enough to prevent damage to the blood cells.

Test-Taking Strategy: Think about the consistency of blood. Focus on the need to insert an IV catheter that has a bore large enough to allow the passage of the blood as it infuses. If this question was difficult, review the concepts related to the administration of blood.

Level of Cognitive Ability: Application
Client Needs: Physiological Integrity
Integrated Concept/Process: Nursing Process/Implementation
Content Area: Fundamental Skills
Reference: Harkreader, H. (2000). *Fundamentals of nursing: Caring and clinical judgment.* Philadelphia: W.B. Saunders, p. 1130.

REFERENCES

Altman, G., Buchsel, P., & Coxon, V. (2000). *Delmar's fundamental & advanced nursing skills.* Albany, N.Y.: Delmar.

Craven, R., & Hirnle, C. (2000). *Fundamentals of nursing: Human health and function* (3rd ed.). Philadelphia: Lippincott.

Harkreader, H. (2000). *Fundamentals of nursing: Caring and clinical judgment.* Philadelphia: W.B. Saunders.

Hodgson, B., & Kizior, R. (2001). *Saunders nursing drug handbook 2001.* Philadelphia: W.B. Saunders.

Ignatavicius, D., Workman, M., & Mishler, M. (1999). *Medical-surgical nursing across the health care continuum* (3rd ed.). Philadelphia: W.B. Saunders.

Phipps, W., Sands, J., & Marek, J. (1999). *Medical-surgical nursing: Concepts & clinical practice* (6th ed.). St. Louis: Mosby.

Potter, P., & Perry, A. (2001). *Fundamentals of nursing* (5th ed.). St. Louis: Mosby.

Smeltzer, S., & Bare, B. (2000) *Brunner & Suddarth's textbook of medical-surgical nursing* (9th ed.). Philadelphia: Lippincott Williams & Wilkins.

Smith, S., Duell, D., & Martin, B. (2000). *Clinical nursing skills: Basic to advanced skills* (5th ed.). Upper Saddle River, NJ: Prentice-Hall Health.

Fundamental Skills

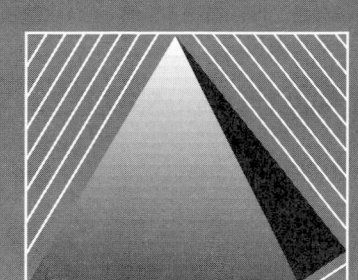

Providing a Safe Environment

PYRAMID TERMS

chemical restraints Medications given to inhibit a specific behavior or movement.

nosocomial infections Infections acquired in the hospital or other health care facility that were not present or incubating at the time of the client's admission; also referred to as hospital-acquired infections.

physical restraints Devices that are applied to restrict a client's movement.

poison Any substance that impairs health or destroys life when ingested, inhaled, or otherwise absorbed by the body.

standard (universal) precautions Guidelines used by all health care providers with all clients to reduce the risk of infection for clients and caregivers.

transmission-based precautions Guidelines that are used in addition to standard precautions; used for specific syndromes that are highly suggestive of infections until a diagnosis is confirmed.

▲ PYRAMID TO SUCCESS

Safety and Infection Control is a subcategory of the Client Needs component "Safe, Effective Care Environment" of the test plan for NCLEX-RN. Pyramid points focus on maintaining environmental safety, preventing accidents, the use of restraints, and priority nursing actions in the event of an emergency or a disaster. Pyramid points also focus on standard (universal) and transmission-based precautions and the measures required to handle hazardous or infectious materials. The primary Integrated Concepts and Processes addressed in this chapter include Nursing Process, Communication and Documentation, and Teaching/Learning.

CLIENT NEEDS
Safe, Effective Care Environment

Establishing priorities
Client rights and informed consent
Maintaining precautions to prevent accidents
Standard (universal) and transmission-based precautions
Handling hazardous and infectious materials
Guidelines regarding the use of restraints
Disaster planning

Health Promotion and Maintenance

Home safety assessment
Assisting clients and families to identify environmental hazards in the home
Client and family education regarding accident prevention
Client and family education to prevent the spread of infection
Client and family education regarding measures to be implemented in an emergency

Psychosocial Integrity

Cultural and religious lifestyles
Sensory/perceptual alterations
Support systems

Physiological Integrity

Providing comfort and assistance to the client
Assisting the client with activities of daily living (ADLs)
Use of assistive devices to prevent injury

Managing and providing care to clients with infectious diseases

Priority nursing actions in an emergency

I. ENVIRONMENTAL SAFETY

A. Fire safety (Box 15-1)
1. Keep open spaces free of clutter
2. Clearly mark fire exits
3. Know the locations of all fire alarms, exits, and extinguishers (Table 15-1; Box 15-2)
4. Know the telephone number for reporting fires
5. Know the agency's fire drill and evacuation plan
6. Never use the elevator in the event of a fire
▲ 7. Turn off oxygen and appliances in the vicinity of the fire
8. In the event of a fire, if a client is on life support, maintain the client's respiratory status manually with an Ambu-bag until the client is moved away from the threat of the fire
9. In the event of a fire, ambulatory clients can be directed to walk by themselves to a safe area, and in some cases may be able to assist in moving clients in wheelchairs
10. Bedridden clients are generally moved from the scene of a fire by stretcher, their beds, or wheelchair
11. If a client must be carried from the area of a fire, appropriate transfer techniques need to be used
12. If fire department personnel are at the scene of the fire, they can help evacuate clients
B. Electrical safety
1. Electrical equipment must be maintained in good working order and should be grounded
▲ 2. Use a three-pronged electrical cord
3. In a three-pronged electrical cord, the third, longer prong of the cord is the ground; the other two prongs carry the power to the piece of electrical equipment
▲ 4. Any electrical equipment that the client brings into the health care facility must be inspected for safety prior to use
▲ 5. Check electrical cords and outlets for exposed, frayed, or damaged wires
6. Avoid overloading any circuit
7. Read warning labels on all equipment; never operate unfamiliar equipment
8. Use safety extension cords only when absolutely necessary, and tape them to the floor with electrical tape
9. Never run electrical wiring under carpets
10. Never pull a plug by using the cord; always grasp the plug itself
11. Never use electrical appliances near sinks, bathtubs, or other water sources
12. Always disconnect a plug from the outlet before cleaning equipment or appliances

---

BOX 15-1

Priority Actions in the Event of a Fire

Remember the mnemonic RACE to set priorities in the event of a fire:
R: Rescue: Remove all clients from the vicinity of a fire.
A: Alarm: Activate the fire alarm; report a fire before attempting to extinguish it.
C: Confine: Close doors and windows when a fire is detected.
E: Extinguish: Extinguish the fire, using the appropriate fire extinguisher.

TABLE 15-1

Fire Extinguishers

Type	Class of Fires
Type A: Water	Wood, draperies, upholstery, paper, and rubbish
Type B or C: Carbon Dioxide or dry chemical	Flammable liquids or gases, grease, and electrical
Type A, B, or C: Multipurpose or dry chemical	Any fire

BOX 15-2

Using a Fire Extinguisher

Remember the mnemonic PASS to use a fire extinguisher:
P: Pull the pin.
A: Aim at the base of the fire.
S: Squeeze the handles.
S: Sweep the fire from side to side.

---

13. If a client receives an electrical shock, turn off ▲ the electricity before touching the client
C. Radiation safety
1. Know the health care agency's protocols and guidelines
2. Label potentially radioactive material
3. To reduce exposure to radiation:
a. The time spent near the source should be limited
b. The distance from the source should be as great as possible
c. A shielding device such as a lead apron should be used
4. Monitor radiation exposure with a film badge
5. Place the client who has a radiation implant in a private room
6. Never touch dislodged implants ▲
7. Wear gloves when handling body discharges
D. Disposal of infectious wastes
1. Handle all infectious materials as a hazard

2. Dispose of waste in designated areas only, using proper containers for disposal
3. Ensure that infectious material is properly labeled
▲ 4. Needles should not be recapped, bent, or broken
5. Dispose of all sharps immediately after use in closed, puncture-resistant disposal containers that are leak proof and labeled or color coded

E. Falls (see Box 15-3 for measures to prevent falls)

▲ F. Restraints
1. Protective devices used to limit the physical activity of a client or to immobilize a client or an extremity
2. **Physical restraints:** Restrict client movement through the application of a device
3. **Chemical restraints:** Medications given to inhibit a specific behavior or movement
▲ 4. Implementation
   a. When **restraints** are necessary, the physician's orders should state the type of restraint, identify specific client behaviors for which restraints are to be used, and identify a limited time frame for use
   b. Physicians' orders for **restraints** should be renewed within a specific time frame according to the agency's policy
   c. **Restraints** are not to be ordered PRN
   d. The reason for the **restraints** should be given to the client and the family, and their permission should be sought
   e. **Restraints** should not interfere with any treatments or affect the client's health problem
   f. Use a clove hitch knot so that the restraint can be changed and released easily
   g. Ensure that there is enough slack on the straps to allow some movement of the body part
   h. Secure restraint to the bed frame, not to the side rails
   i. Assess skin integrity and neurovascular and circulatory status every 30 minutes, and release the **restraint** to permit muscle exercise and promote circulation
   j. Continually assess the need for **restraints** (Box 15-4)
▲ 5. Alternatives to **restraints**
   a. Orient client and family to surroundings
   b. Explain all procedures and treatments to client and family
   c. Encourage family and friends to stay with the client, and utilize sitters for clients who need supervision
   d. Assign confused and disoriented clients to rooms near the nurses' station
   e. Provide appropriate visual and auditory stimuli to the client, such as clocks, calendars, television, and a radio
   f. Place familiar items, such as family pictures, near the client's bedside.
   g. Maintain toileting routines

BOX 15-3

Measures to Prevent Falls

Assess the client's risk for falling.
Assign the client at risk for falling to a room near the nurses' station.
Alert all personnel to the client's risk for falling.
Orient the client to physical surroundings.
Instruct the client to seek assistance when getting up.
Explain use of the call bell system.
Keep the bed in the low position with side rails up if required.
Lock all beds, wheelchairs, and stretchers.
Keep personal items within reach.
Eliminate clutter and obstacles in the client's room.
Provide adequate lighting.
Reduce bathroom hazards.
Maintain the client's toileting schedule throughout the day.

BOX 15-4

Documentation Points with the Use of a Restraint

Reason for restraint
Method of restraint
Date and time of application of restraint
Duration of use of restraint and client's response
Release from restraint with periodic exercise and circulatory, neurovascular, and skin assessment
Assessment of continued need for restraint
Evaluation of client's response

---

   h. Eliminate bothersome treatments, such as tube feedings, as soon as possible
   i. Evaluate all medications that the client is receiving
   j. Use relaxation techniques with the client
   k. Institute exercise and ambulation schedules as the client's condition allows

G. **Poisons**
1. Any substance that impairs health or destroys life when ingested, inhaled, or otherwise absorbed by the body
2. Specific antidotes or treatments are available for only some types of **poisons**
3. The capacity of body tissue to recover from a **poison** determines the reversibility of the effect
4. **Poison** can impair the respiratory, circulatory, central nervous, hepatic, gastrointestinal (GI), and renal systems of the body
5. The toddler, the preschooler, and the young school-aged child must be protected from accidental poisoning
6. In older adults, diminished eyesight and impaired memory may result in accidental ingestion of poisonous substances or an overdose of prescribed medications

7. A **Poison** Control Center phone number should be visible on the telephone itself in homes with small children; in all cases of expected poisoning, the number should be called immediately

8. Implementation
   a. Remove any obvious materials from the mouth, eyes, or body area immediately
   b. Identify the type and amount of substance ingested
   c. Call the **Poison** Control Center before attempting an intervention
   d. If the victim vomits or vomiting is induced, save the vomitus if requested to do so, and deliver it to the **Poison** Control Center
   e. If instructed by the **Poison** Control Center to take the person to the emergency department, call an ambulance
   f. Vomiting is never induced following ingestion of lye, household cleaners, grease, or petroleum products
   g. Vomiting is never induced in an unconscious victim

II. DISASTERS
A. Know the agency's disaster plan
B. Internal disasters are those in which the agency is in danger
C. External disasters occur in the community, and victims will be brought to the health care facility for care
D. When the health care agency is notified of a disaster, plans specified in agency policy must be carried out

III. NOSOCOMIAL INFECTIONS
A. Also referred to as hospital-acquired infections
B. Infections acquired in a hospital or other health care facility that were not present or incubating at the time of a client's admission
C. Illness impairs the body's normal defense mechanisms
D. The hospital environment provides exposure to a variety of virulent organisms that the client has not been exposed to in the past; therefore, the client has not developed resistance to these organisms
E. Infections can be transmitted by health care personnel who fail to practice proper handwashing procedures or fail to change gloves between client contacts

IV. STANDARD (UNIVERSAL) PRECAUTIONS
A. Description
   1. Must be practiced with all clients in any setting, regardless of the diagnosis or presumed infectiousness
   2. Promotes handwashing and the use of gloves, masks, eye protection, and gowns, when appropriate, for client contact
   3. These precautions apply to blood; all body fluids,

secretions, and excretions except sweat, regardless of whether they contain blood; nonintact skin; and mucous membranes

B. Implementation
   1. Handle all blood and body fluids from all clients as if they were contaminated
   2. Hands are washed between client contacts; after contact with blood, body fluids, secretions, or excretions, and after contact with equipment or articles contaminated by them; and immediately after gloves are removed
   3. Gloves are worn when blood, body fluids, secretions, excretions, nonintact skin, mucous membranes, or contaminated items are touched; gloves should be removed and hands washed between client care contacts
   4. Masks, eye protection, or face shields are worn if client care activities may generate splashes or sprays of blood or body fluid
   5. Gowns are worn if soiling of clothing is likely from blood or body fluid; wash hands after removing a gown
   6. Client care equipment is properly cleaned and reprocessed, and single-use items are discarded
   7. Contaminated linen is placed in leakproof bags and handled to prevent skin and mucous membrane exposure
   8. All sharp instruments and needles are discarded in a puncture-resistant container; needles are disposed of uncapped, or a mechanical device for recapping is used if necessary
   9. Spills of blood or body fluids are cleaned with a solution of bleach and water (diluted 1:10) or agency-approved disinfectant
   10. A private room is unnecessary unless the client's hygiene is unacceptable; the nurse should consult with the infection-control professional

V. TRANSMISSION-BASED PRECAUTIONS
A. Airborne precautions
   1. Diseases
      a. Measles
      b. Chickenpox (varicella)
      c. Disseminated varicella zoster
      d. Pulmonary or laryngeal tuberculosis (TB)
   2. Barrier protection for airborne precautions
      a. Single room maintained under negative pressure; door kept closed except when someone is entering or exiting the room
      b. Negative air-flow pressure in the room, with a minimum of 6 to 12 air exchanges per hour depending on the health care agency
      c. Mask or respiratory protection device
   3. Barrier protection for TB
      a. Includes airborne precautions and the additional following precautions
      b. Use of ultraviolet germicide irradiation or

BOX 15-5

Common Drug-Resistant Nosocomial Infections

Vancomycin resistant enterococci (VRE)
Methicillin-resistant *Staphylococcus aureus* (MRSA)
Multidrug-resistant (MDR) tuberculosis

HEPA filter, which may reduce the number of droplet nuclei
  c. Use of personal respiratory protective devices (masks), capable of filtration of 95% efficiency, when personnel enter the isolation room; ability to fit-test masks to obtain a face-seal leakage of less than or equal to 10%
  d. Place a mask on the client when the client is out of the room; the client leaves the room only if necessary
B. Droplet precautions
  1. Diseases
    a. Diphtheria (pharyngeal)
    b. Rubella
    c. Streptococcal pharyngitis
    d. Mycoplasma pneumonia or menigococcal pneumonia or sepsis
    e. Scarlet fever in infants and younger children
    f. Pertussis
    g. Mumps
    h. Pneumonic plague
  2. Barrier protection
    a. Private room or cohort client
    b. Use of a mask
    c. Place a mask on the client when the client is out of the room; the client leaves the room only if necessary
C. Contact precautions
  1. Diseases
    a. Respiratory syncytial virus (RSV)
    b. *Shigella* and other enteric pathogens
    c. Major wound infections
    d. Herpes simplex
    e. Scabies
    f. Varicella zoster (disseminated)
    g. Colonization or infection with multidrug-resistant organism (Box 15-5)
  2. Barrier protection
    a. Private room or cohort client
    b. Use of gloves and a gown by health care personnel when in contact with the client

PRACTICE QUESTIONS

1. A nurse enters a client's room and finds that the wastebasket is on fire. The nurse immediately assists the client out of the room. The next nursing action would be to:
   1. Confine the fire by closing the room door
   2. Activate the fire alarm
   3. Call for help
   4. Extinguish the fire

2. A nurse enters the nursing lounge and discovers that a chair is on fire. She activates the alarm, closes the lounge door, and obtains the fire extinguisher to extinguish the fire. The nurse pulls the pin on the fire extinguisher. The next appropriate action in the use of the fire extinguisher is to:
   1. Squeeze the handle on the extinguisher
   2. Aim at the base of the fire
   3. Sweep the fire from side to side with the extinguisher
   4. Sweep the fire from top to bottom with the extinguisher

3. A home care nurse performs a home safety assessment and discovers that a client is using a space heater to heat her apartment. Which of the following instructions would the nurse provide to the client regarding the use of the space heater?
   1. A space heater should not be used in an apartment
   2. The space heater needs to be placed at least 3 feet from anything that can burn
   3. The space heater should be placed in the hallway at night
   4. The space heater should be kept at a low setting at all times

4. A nurse is preparing to initiate an IV containing a high dose of potassium chloride and plans to use an IV infusion pump. The nurse brings the pump to the bedside, prepares to plug the pump cord into the wall, and notes that there is no available receptacle in the wall socket. Which of the following is the most appropriate nursing action?
   1. Use an extension cord from the nurses' lounge for the pump plug
   2. Initiate the IV without the use of a pump
   3. Plug in the pump cord in the available plug above the room sink
   4. Contact the electrical maintenance department for assistance

5. A nurse obtains an order from a physician to restrain a client by using a jacket restraint. The nurse instructs a nursing assistant to apply the restraint to the client. Which of the following observations, if made by the nurse, would indicate inappropriate application of the restraint by the nursing assistant?
   1. A clove hitch knot in the restraint straps
   2. Restraint straps are safely secured to the side rails
   3. The jacket restraint is secure, and two fingers can easily slide between the restraint and the client's skin
   4. The jacket restraint straps do not tighten when force is applied against it

6. A nurse is giving report to a nursing assistant who will be caring for a client who has hand restraints.

The nurse instructs the nursing assistant to assess the skin integrity of the restrained hands:
1. Every 30 minutes
2. Every 2 hours
3. Every 3 hours
4. Every 4 hours

7. A nurse is planning care for a client with an internal radiation implant. Which of the following is not an appropriate component for the nurse to include in the plan of care?
   1. Placing the client in a semiprivate room at the end of the hallway
   2. Wearing gloves when emptying the client's bedpan
   3. Keeping all linens in the room until the implant is removed
   4. Wearing a lead apron when providing direct care to the client

8. A mother calls the home care nurse and tells the nurse that her 3-year-old child has just ingested liquid furniture polish. The home care nurse would direct the mother to immediately:
   1. Administer Ipecac to induce vomiting
   2. Bring the child to the emergency room
   3. Call an ambulance
   4. Call the Poison Control Center

9. An emergency room nurse receives a telephone call and is informed that a tornado has hit a local residential area and that numerous casualties have occurred. The victims will be brought to the emergency room. The initial nursing action is which of the following?
   1. Prepare the triage rooms
   2. Obtain additional supplies from the central supply department
   3. Activate the agency disaster plan
   4. Obtain additional nursing staff to assist in treating the casualties

10. A nurse is caring for a client with a nosocomial infection caused by methicillin-resistant *Staphylococcus aureus* (MRSA). Contact precautions are initiated. The nurse prepares to provide colostomy care to the client. The nurse obtains which of the following protective items required to perform this procedure?
    1. Gloves, gown, and goggles
    2. Gloves and goggles
    3. Gloves, gown, and shoe protectors
    4. Gloves and a gown

CRITICAL THINKING: FREE-TEXT ENTRY

A nurse employed on a medical unit in a hospital receives a telephone call from the admission office and is told that a client with a diagnosis of mycoplasmal pneumonia will be admitted to the nursing unit. The nurse prepares for the admission and obtains the necessary supplies to place the client on which type of transmission-based precautions?

Answer: _____

ANSWERS

1. 2

Rationale: The order of priority in the event of a fire is to rescue the clients who are in immediate danger. The next step is to activate the fire alarm. The fire is then confined by closing all doors, and, last, the fire is extinguished.

Test-Taking Strategy: Remember the mnemonic RACE to prioritize in the event of a fire. R = Rescue clients in immediate danger; A = Alarm, sound the alarm; C = Confine the fire by closing all doors; E = Extinguish or evacuate. If you had difficulty with this question, review the principles related to fire safety.

Level of Cognitive Ability: Application
Client Needs: Safe, Effective Care Environment
Integrated Concept/Process: Nursing Process/Implementation
Content Area: Fundamental Skills
Reference: Potter, P., & Perry, A. (2001). *Fundamentals of nursing* (5th ed.). St. Louis: Mosby, p. 1044.

2. 2

Rationale: A fire can be extinguished by smothering it with a blanket or by the use of a fire extinguisher. To use the extinguisher, the pin is pulled first. The extinguisher should then be aimed at the base of the fire. The handle of the extinguisher is then squeezed, and the fire is extinguished by sweeping from side to side to coat the area evenly.

Test-Taking Strategy: Remember the mnemonic PASS to prioritize in the use of a fire extinguisher. P = Pull the pin; A = Aim at the base of the fire; S = Squeeze the handle; S = Sweep from side to side to coat the area evenly. If you had difficulty with this question, review the steps in the appropriate use of a fire extinguisher.

Level of Cognitive Ability: Application
Client Needs: Safe, Effective Care Environment
Integrated Concept/Process: Nursing Process/Implementation
Content Area: Fundamental Skills
Reference: Potter, P., & Perry, A. (2001). *Fundamentals of nursing* (5th ed.). St. Louis: Mosby, p. 1045.

3. 2

Rationale: Space heaters need to be used appropriately because they present a great risk of fire. A space heater needs to be placed at least 3 feet from anything that can burn. Placing a heater in a hallway does not guarantee that it will be 3 feet from anything that can burn. A low setting does not reduce the risk of fire. A space heater can be used in an apartment if there is ample space and safety precautions are followed.

Test-Taking Strategy: Use the process of elimination, keeping

in mind the issue related to fire safety. Note that option 2 is the only option that specifically defines a safety measure related to the use of a space heater. Review fire safety prevention measures in the home if you had difficulty with this question.
Level of Cognitive Ability: Application
Client Needs: Safe, Effective Care Environment
Integrated Concept/Process: Teaching/Learning
Content Area: Fundamental Skills
Reference: Leahy, J., & Kizilay, P. (1998). *Foundations of nursing practice: A nursing process approach.* Philadelphia: W.B. Saunders, p. 392.

4. 4
Rationale: The nurse needs to utilize hospital resources for assistance. A regular extension cord should not be used because it poses the risk of fire. The use of electrical appliances near a sink also presents a hazard. An IV that contains a high dose of potassium chloride should be administered by the use of a pump.
Test-Taking Strategy: Use the process of elimination. Noting the key words "high dose" in the question will assist in eliminating option 2. Recalling safety issues related to electrical hazards will assist in eliminating options 1 and 3. If you had difficulty with this question, review the interventions related to electrical safety.
Level of Cognitive Ability: Application
Client Needs: Safe, Effective Care Environment
Integrated Concept/Process: Nursing Process/Implementation
Content Area: Fundamental Skills
Reference: Leahy, J., & Kizilay, P. (1998). *Foundations of nursing practice: A nursing process approach.* Philadelphia: W.B. Saunders, p. 389.

5. 2
Rationale: A clove hitch knot should be used for applying a restraint because it does not tighten when force is applied against it and allows quick and easy removal of the restraint in the case of an emergency. The restraint straps are secured to the bed frame and never to the side rail, to avoid accidental injury in the event that the side rail is released. The jacket restraint should be secure, and one to two fingers should easily slide between the restraint and the client's skin.
Test-Taking Strategy: Use the process of elimination. Note the key words "indicate inappropriate application." This indicates that you are looking for an option that identifies an inaccurate measure related to the application of restraints. Read each option carefully. The words "secured to the side rails" in option 2 should direct your attention as an inappropriate action. Review guidelines related to the application of restraints if you had difficulty with this question.
Level of Cognitive Ability: Analysis
Client Needs: Safe, Effective Care Environment
Integrated Concept/Process: Nursing Process/Evaluation
Content Area: Fundamental Skills
Reference: Harkreader, H. (2000). *Fundamentals of nursing: Caring and clinical judgment.* Philadelphia: W.B. Saunders, p. 671.

6. 1
Rationale: The nurse should instruct the nursing assistant to assess restraints and skin integrity every 30 minutes. Agency guidelines regarding the use of restraints should always be followed.

Test-Taking Strategy: Use the process of elimination. In this situation, it is best to select the option that identifies the most frequent time frame. Review the guidelines related to the use of restraints if you had difficulty with this question.
Level of Cognitive Ability: Application
Client Needs: Safe, Effective Care Environment
Integrated Concept/Process: Teaching/Learning
Content Area: Fundamental Skills
Reference: Harkreader, H. (2000). *Fundamentals of nursing: Caring and clinical judgment.* Philadelphia: W.B. Saunders, p. 671.

7. 1
Rationale: A private room with a private bath is essential if a client has an internal radiation implant. This is necessary to prevent accidental exposure of other clients to radiation. Options 2, 3, and 4 are accurate interventions for a client with a radiation implant.
Test-Taking Strategy: Use the process of elimination. Note the key words "not an appropriate." Option 2 can be eliminated first because this is a component of standard precautions for all clients. Options 3 and 4 can be eliminated next because they directly relate to radiation safety. Review radiation safety principles if you had difficulty with this question.
Level of Cognitive Ability: Application
Client Needs: Safe, Effective Care Environment
Integrated Concept/Process: Nursing Process/Planning
Content Area: Fundamental Skills
Reference: Craven, R., & Hirnle, C. (2000). *Fundamentals of nursing: Human health and function* (3rd ed.). Philadelphia: Lippincott, p. 651.

8. 4
Rationale: If a poisoning occurs, the Poison Control Center should be contacted immediately. Vomiting should not be induced if the victim is unconscious or if the substance ingested is a strong corrosive or petroleum product. Bringing the child to the emergency room or calling an ambulance would not be the initial action because this would delay treatment. The Poison Control Center may advise the mother to bring the child to the emergency room, and if this is the case, the mother should call an ambulance.
Test-Taking Strategy: Use the process of elimination. Note the key word "immediately" in the stem of the question. Eliminate options 2 and 3 because these options will delay treatment. Recalling that vomiting should not be induced if a corrosive substance was ingested will assist in eliminating option 1. Review poison control measures if you had difficulty with this question.
Level of Cognitive Ability: Application
Client Needs: Safe, Effective Care Environment
Integrated Concept/Process: Nursing Process/Implementation
Content Area: Fundamental Skills
Reference: Potter, P., & Perry, A. (2001). *Fundamentals of nursing* (5th ed.). St. Louis: Mosby, p. 1047.

9. 3
Rationale: In an external disaster, many victims may be brought to the emergency room for treatment. Although options 1, 2, and 4 may be components of preparing for the casualties, the initial nursing action must be to activate the disaster plan.
Test-Taking Strategy: Use the process of elimination in

determining the priority action. Note the key word "initial" in the stem of the question. Note that option 3 is the global option. Review procedures related to management of a disaster if you had difficulty with this question.

Level of Cognitive Ability: Application
Client Needs: Safe, Effective Care Environment
Integrated Concept/Process: Nursing Process/Implementation
Content Area: Fundamental Skills
Reference: Craven, R., & Hirnle, C. (2000). *Fundamentals of nursing: Human health and function* (3rd ed.). Philadelphia: Lippincott, p. 653.

10. 1
Rationale: Goggles are worn to protect the mucous membranes of the eyes during interventions that may produce splashes of blood, body fluids, secretions, or excretions. In addition, contact precautions require the use of gloves, and a gown should be worn if direct client contact is anticipated. Shoe protectors are not necessary.

Test-Taking Strategy: Note the key words "contact precautions" and "colostomy." Use the process of elimination in determining the necessary items required in caring for this client. If you had difficulty with this question, review transmission-based precautions.

Level of Cognitive Ability: Application

Client Needs: Safe, Effective Care Environment
Integrated Concept/Process: Nursing Process/Planning
Content Area: Fundamental Skills
Reference: Potter, P., & Perry, A. (2001). *Fundamentals of nursing* (5th ed.). St. Louis: Mosby, pp. 858-859.

CRITICAL THINKING: FREE-TEXT ENTRY

Answer: Droplet precautions
Rationale: Droplet precautions are required for a client with mycoplasmal pneumonia because this type of pneumonia is transmitted by droplet nuclei larger than 5 μm. Barrier protection includes placing the client in a private room or with a cohort client. A mask is worn by the nurse when in the client's room.

Test-Taking Strategy: Focus on the diagnosis of the client, and recall that pneumonia is transmitted by droplets larger than 5 μm. If you are unfamiliar with transmission-based precautions, review these isolation procedures.

Level of Cognitive Ability: Application
Client Needs: Safe, Effective Care Environment
Integrated Concept/Process: Nursing Process/Planning
Content Area: Fundamental Skills
Reference: Potter, P., & Perry, A. (2001). *Fundamentals of nursing* (5th ed.). St. Louis: Mosby, pp. 858-859.

REFERENCES

Craven, R., & Hirnle, C. (2000). *Fundamentals of nursing: Human health and function* (3rd ed.). Philadelphia: Lippincott.

Harkreader, H. (2000). *Fundamentals of nursing: Caring and clinical judgment.* Philadelphia: W.B. Saunders.

Leahy, J., & Kizilay, P. (1998). *Foundations of nursing practice: A nursing process approach.* Philadelphia: W.B. Saunders.

Potter, P., & Perry, A. (2001). *Fundamentals of nursing* (5th ed.). St. Louis: Mosby.

Administering Medication and Intravenous Solutions

PYRAMID TERMS

conversion Conversion is the first step in the calculation of a medication problem.

generic name The common or chemical name of a medication; printed on the label in smaller letters, usually under the trade name.

milliequivalent Milliequivalent, abbreviated mEq, is an expression of the number of grams of a medication contained in 1 mL of a normal solution.

parenteral Parenteral always means injection route. Injections are administered by intravenous (IV), intramuscular (IM), and subcutaneous (SQ, SC) routes.

percentage solutions Percentage solutions express the number of grams of a medication per 100 mL of solution.

reconstitution Powders must be dissolved with a sterile diluent before use, and usually sterile water or normal saline is used. The dissolving procedure is called reconstitution.

ratio solutions Ratio solutions express the number of grams of a medication per total milliliters of solution.

trade name Also called the brand name; printed on the label in large bold letters.

unit Unit, abbreviated as U or u, is measurement of a medication in terms of its action, not its physical weight.

▲ PYRAMID TO SUCCESS

When a medication or intravenous calculation question is presented, a nurse should always use the appropriate formula to solve the problem. Shortcuts should not be used in making these calculations. The problem and the answer should be expressed in the correct units of measure. Be careful with decimal points. It is important to place the decimal points in the correct places, or the answer will be incorrect. When solving a medication calculation problem, the nurse determines whether the answer is within reason and makes sense. In the clinical setting, the nurse should always seek assistance if he or she is unsure of the accuracy of a calculation.

On CAT NCLEX-RN, you may be provided with an optional drop-down calculator for calculating dosages. Even if you use the calculator to calculate dosages, it is important to check the calculation before selecting the answer to the question. REMEMBER, on CAT NCLEX-RN, the correct answer will be on the screen. Following the formula, placing the decimal points in the correct places, and checking the accuracy of the calculation will ensure selection of the correct answer. Remember, practice makes perfect!

The Integrated Concepts and Processes addressed in this chapter are Nursing Process, Caring, Communication and Documentation, Cultural Awareness, Self-Care, and Teaching/Learning.

CLIENT NEEDS
Safe, Effective Care Environment

Client rights
Error prevention
Handling hazardous or infectious materials
Intravenous fluid and medication calculations
Medical and surgical asepsis
Medication calculations
Referrals for home care
Standard (universal) and other precautions

Health Promotion and Maintenance

Client teaching regarding prescribed medication(s) or
  IV therapy
Disease prevention
Lifestyle choices
Physical assessment of client

BOX 16-1

Medication Administration

Assess medication order

Ask client about a history of allergies

Assess client's current condition and the purpose for the medication or intravenous solution

Determine client's understanding regarding the purpose of the prescribed medication or need for IV solution

Teach client about the medication and about self-administration at home

Identify and address concerns (social, cultural, religious) that the client may have about taking the medication

Assess the need for conversion when preparing a dose of medication for administration to the client

Assess the five rights: right medication, right dose, right client, right route, and right time

Assess vital signs prior to administering medication

Document the administration of the prescribed therapy and client's response to the therapy

Psychosocial Integrity

Religious and spiritual influences on health

Support systems

Therapeutic interactions

Use of coping mechanisms

Physiological Integrity

Actions of medications and IV therapy

Administration of medications and IV therapy

Adverse effects of and contraindications to medication or IV therapy

Alterations in body systems

Expected effects of pharmacological therapy

Laboratory values

Unexpected responses to therapy

TABLE 16-1

Metric System

Abbreviations	Equivalents
meter: m	1 mg = 1000 mcg or 0.001 g
liter: L	1 g = 1000 mg
gram: g, gm, Gm	1 mL = 0.001 L or 1 cc
milligram: mg, mgm	1 kg = 1000 g
microgram: μg, mcg	1 mcg = 0.000001 g
kilogram: kg, Kg	1 cc = 1 mL or 0.001 L
milliliter: mL	1 kg = 2.2 lb
cubic centimeter: cc	1 L = 1000 mL

TABLE 16-2

Apothecary and Household Systems

Abbreviations	Equivalents
grain: gr	gr 1 = 60 mg
dram: dr	gr 5 = 300 mg
ounce: oz	gr 15 = 1000 mg or 1 g
minim: min, M, or m	gr 1/150 = 0.4 mg
quart: qt	1 oz = 30 mL
pint: pt	1 dr = 4 mL
drops: gtt	1 T = 15 mL or 3 tsp
tablespoon: T or tbs	1 t or tsp = 5 mL
teaspoon: t or tsp	1 min = 1 gtt
pound: lb	15 min = 1 mL
	60 min = 1 dr
	8 dr = 1 oz
	1 qt = 1000 mL or 1 L
	1 qt = 2 pt or 32 oz
	1 pt = 16 oz
	16 oz = 1 lb
	2.2 lbs = 1 kg

I. MEDICATION ADMINISTRATION (Box 16-1)

II. DRUG MEASUREMENT SYSTEMS (Table 16-1)

A. Metric system
   1. The basic units of metric measures are meter, liter, and gram
      a. Meter measures length
      b. Liter measures volume
      c. Gram measures weight
B. Apothecary and household systems (Table 16-2)
   1. The apothecary and household systems are the oldest of the medication measurement systems
   2. The four apothecary measures sometimes used are grain, minim, dram, and ounce
      a. Grain measures weight
      b. Minim, dram, and ounce measure volume
   3. The three household measures commonly used are tablespoon, teaspoon, and drop
C. Additional common drug measures
   1. **Milliequivalent**
      a. Abbreviated mEq
      b. Is an expression of the number of grams of a medication contained in 1 mL of a normal solution
      c. Example: Potassium
   2. **Unit**
      a. Abbreviated as U or u; measures a medication in terms of its action, not its physical weight
      b. Examples: Penicillin, heparin sodium, insulin

III. CONVERSIONS

A. Conversion between metric units (Box 16-2)
   1. The metric system is a decimal system; therefore, conversions between the units in this system can be done by either dividing or multiplying by 1000 or by moving the decimal point three places to the right or three places to the left

BOX 16-2

Conversion Between Metric Units

1. PROBLEM:
Convert 2 grams to milligrams.
Solution:
Change a larger unit to a smaller unit.
2.000 grams = 2000 mg (moving decimal 3 places to right)

2. PROBLEM:
Convert 250 mL to liters.
Solution:
Change a smaller unit to a larger unit.
250 mL = 0.250 L or 0.25 L (moving decimal 3 places to left)

BOX 16-3

Calculating Equivalents Between Two Systems

Calculating equivalents between two systems may be done by using the method of ratio and proportion!

PROBLEM:
The physician orders nitroglycerin, gr 1/150. The medication label reads 0.4 mg per tablet. The nurse prepares to administer how many tablets to the client?
gr 1 : 60 mg = gr 1/150 : x mg
$60 \times 1/150 = x$
x = 0.4 mg (1 tablet)

TABLE 16-3

Celsius and Fahrenheit Temperature

Fahrenheit to Celsius
To convert Fahrenheit to Celsius, subtract 32 and divide result by 1.8
Formula: $C = (F - 32) \div 1.8$
Celsius to Fahrenheit
To convert Celsius to Fahrenheit, multiply by 1.8 and add 32
Formula: $F = 1.8 \, C + 32$

IV. **CELSIUS AND FAHRENHEIT TEMPERATURE** (Table 16-3)
  A. To convert Fahrenheit to Celsius, subtract 32 and divide result by 8
  B. To convert Celsius to Fahrenheit, multiply by 1.8 and add 32

V. **MEDICATION LABELS**
  A. A medication label will contain both the **generic name** and the **trade name** of the medication
  B. The **generic name** is the common or chemical name of a medication; the **generic name** is not capitalized
  C. The **trade name,** also called brand name, is printed on the medication label in large bold letters
  D. Each medication has only one official name but may have several trade names, each for the exclusive use of the company that manufactures the medication
  E. Always check expiration dates on medication labels ▲

VI. **MEDICATION ORDERS** (Box 16-4)
  A. In a medication order, the name of the medication is written first, followed by the dosage, route, and frequency
  B. If there are any questions about or inconsistencies in the written order, the person who wrote the order must be contacted immediately, and the order must be verified

VII. **ORAL MEDICATIONS**
  A. Scored tablets contain an indented mark to be used for possible breakage into partial dosages; when necessary, scored tablets (those marked for division) can be divided into halves or quarters
  B. Enteric-coated tablets and sustained-released capsules delay absorption until the medication reaches the small intestine; these medications should not be crushed
  C. Capsules contain a powered or oily medication in a gelatin cover
  D. Oral liquids are supplied in solution form and contain a specific amount of medication in a given amount of solution, as stated on the label
  E. The medicine cup
    1. Has a capacity of 30 mL or 1 ounce

▲
  2. In the metric system, to convert larger to smaller, multiply by 1000 or move the decimal point three places to the right
  3. In the metric system, to convert smaller to larger, divide by 1000 or move the decimal point three places to the left
  B. Conversion between apothecary, household, and metric systems
    1. Conversions between the metric and apothecary and household measures are equivalent not equal measures
    2. Conversion to equivalent measures between systems is necessary when a medication order is written in one system but the medication label is stated in another
    3. Medications are not always ordered and prepared in the same system of measurement; it is therefore necessary to convert units from one system to another
    4. Conversion is the first step in the calculation of dosages
    5. Calculating equivalents between two systems may be done by using the method of ratio and proportion (Box 16-3)

THREE MILLILITER SYRINGE

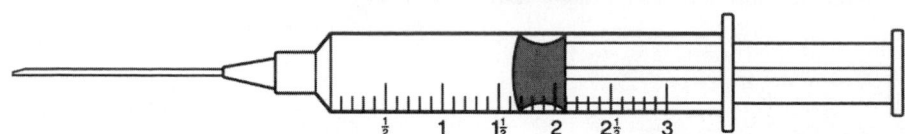

FIG. 16-1 Three-milliliter syringe with 0.1-mL markings. (From Kee JF, Marshall SM: *Clinical calculations: with applications to general and specialty areas,* ed. 4, Philadelphia, 2000, WB Saunders.)

BOX 16-4

Medication Orders

Name of client
Date and time when order is written
Name of medication to be given
Dosage of medication
Medication route
Time and frequency of administration
Signature of person writing the order

---

2. Is used for oral liquids
3. Is calibrated to measure teaspoons, tablespoons, and drams
4. To pour accurately, hold the medication cup at eye level, and then line up the measure that is needed and pour

F. Volumes of less than 5 mL are measured by using a syringe with the needle removed
G. A calibrated dropper is used for giving medicine to children or for adding small amounts of liquid to water or juice; calibrations are in milliliters, cubic centimeters, drops, or minims

VIII. PARENTERAL MEDICATIONS

A. **Parenteral** always means injection route, and **parenteral** medications are administered by intravenous (IV), intramuscular (IM), or subcutaneous (SC) injection
B. **Parenteral** medications are packaged in single-use ampules, in single- and multiple-use rubber-stoppered vials, and in premeasured syringes and cartridges
C. The nurse should not administer more than 3 mL per IM or SC injection site, as volumes larger than 3 mL are difficult for a single injection site to absorb
D. Always question excessively large or small volumes of medication
E. The standard 3-mL (cc) syringe is used to measure most injectable medications; it is calibrated in tenths (0.1) of a milliliter (Fig. 16-1)
F. The calibrations on a syringe are read from the top black ring on the syringe, not the raised middle section and not the bottom ring

G. Prefilled medication cartridge and cartridge holder/syringe (Fig. 16-2)
1. Tubex and Carpuject are trade names of two widely used, reusable, metal or plastic cartridge holders
2. The medication cartridge slips into the cartridge holder, which provides a plunger for injection of the medication
3. The medication cartridge is prefilled with sterile medication and is labeled with the medication name and dosage
4. The medication cartridge is routinely overfilled with 0.1 to 0.2 mL of medication to allow for manipulation of the holder to expel air from the needle prior to injection
5. The medication cartridge is designed to provide sufficient capacity to allow for the addition of a second medication when combined dosages are prescribed
6. The prefilled medication cartridge is to be used once and discarded; if a nurse is to give less than a full single dose provided, the nurse needs to discard the extra amount before giving the client the injection, following agency policies and procedures

H. Standard medication doses for adults are to be rounded to the nearest tenth (0.1) of an mL or cc and measured on the mL scale; for example, 1.25 mL is rounded to 1.3 mL
I. When volumes larger than 3 mL are required, a 5-, 6-, 10-, or 12-mL syringe may be used; these syringes are calibrated in fifths (Fig. 16-3)
J. Syringes larger than 12 mL are calibrated in full mL measures
K. Tuberculin syringe (Fig. 16-4)
1. Holds a total capacity of 1 mL or cc and is used to measure small or critical amounts of medication, such as allergen extract, vaccine, or a child's medication
2. It is calibrated in hundredths (0.01) of an mL, with each one tenth (0.1) marked on the metric scale
L. Insulin syringe (Fig. 16-5)
1. The standard U-100 insulin syringe is used to measure U-100 insulin only; it is calibrated for a total of 100 units, or 1 mL (cc)

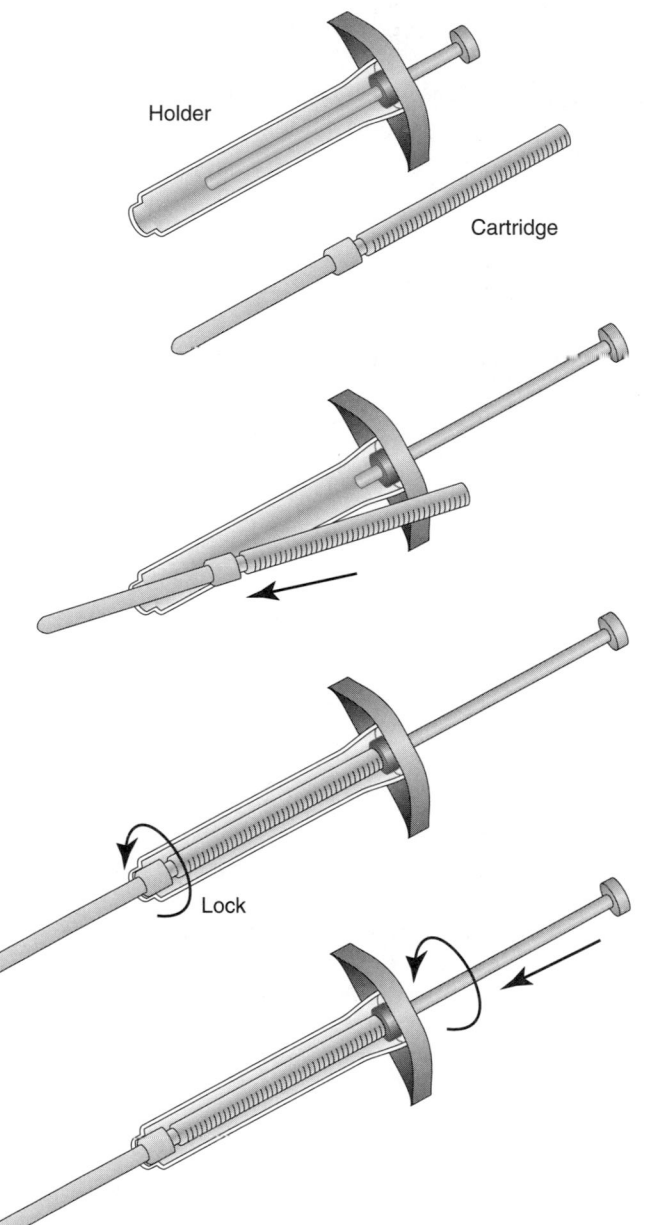

FIG. 16-2   Cartridge-type syringe. (From Leahy JM, Kizilay PE, eds: *Foundations of nursing practice: a nursing process approach,* Philadelphia, 1998, WB Saunders.)

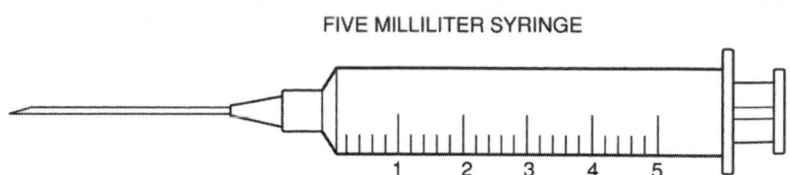

FIG. 16-3   Five-milliliter syringe with 0.2-mL markings. (From Kee J, Hayes E: *Pharmacology: a nursing process approach,* ed. 3, Philadelphia, 2000, WB Saunders.)

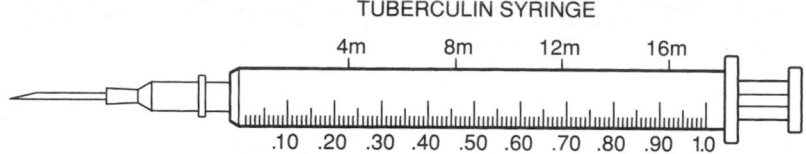

FIG. 16-4 Tuberculin syringe. (From Kee J, Hayes E: *Pharmacology: a nursing process approach,* ed. 3, Philadelphia, 2000, WB Saunders.)

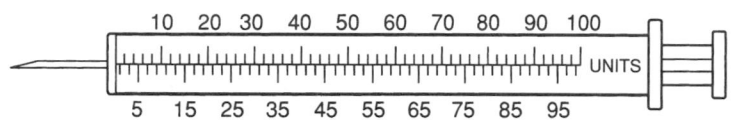

FIG. 16-5 Insulin syringe. (From Kee J, Hayes E: *Pharmacology: a nursing process approach,* ed. 3, Philadelphia, 2000, WB Saunders.)

2. Insulin should not be measured in any other type of syringe
3. When the insulin order states to combine Regular and NPH insulin, remember "R.N.": draw "R"egular insulin first, and then draw the "N"PH insulin

IX. INJECTABLE MEDICATIONS IN POWDER FORM

A. Some medications become unstable when stored in solution form and are therefore packaged in powder form
B. Powders must be dissolved with a sterile diluent before use; usually sterile water or normal saline is used. The dissolving procedure is called **reconstitution** (Box 16-5)

X. CALCULATING THE CORRECT DOSAGE
(Table 16-4)

A. When calculating dosages of oral medications, check the calculation and question an order if the calculation calls for more than three tablets
B. When calculating dosages of **parenteral** medications, check the calculation and question an order if the amount to be given is too large a dose
C. Regardless of the source of an error, if a nurse gives an incorrect dose, he or she is legally responsible for the action
D. Be sure that all measures are in the same system, and that all units are in the same size, converting when necessary; carefully consider what is the reasonable amount of the medication that should be administered
E. Round standard injection doses to tenths and measure in a 3-mL syringe
F. Round small, critical, or children's doses to hundredths and measure in the 1-mL tuberculin syringe

---

BOX 16-5

Reconstitution

In reconstituting the medication, locate the instructions on the label or in the vial package insert, and read and follow the directions carefully.
Instructions will state the volume of diluent to be used and the resulting volume of the reconstituted medication.
Often the powdered medication adds volume to the solution in addition to the amount of diluent added.
When reconstituting a multiple-dose vial, label the medication vial with the date and time of preparation, your initials, and the date of expiration.
It is also important to label the strength per volume.
The total volume of the prepared solution will always exceed the volume of the diluent added.

TABLE 16-4

Formula for Calculating a Medication Dosage

$$\frac{D \text{ (Desired)}}{A \text{ (Available)}} \times Q \text{ (Quantity)} = x$$

D (Desired) = The dosage that the physician ordered
A (Available) = The dosage strength as stated on the medication label
Q (Quantity) = The volume that the dosage strength is available in, such as tablets, capsules, or mL

XI. CALCULATING DOSAGES EXPRESSED AS RATIO OR PERCENT

A. **Percentage solutions**
1. Express the number of grams of the medication per 100 mL of solution

TABLE 16-5

Formulas for Intravenous Calculations

Flow Rates

$$\frac{\text{Total volume} \times \text{gtt factor}}{\text{Time in minutes}} = \text{gtt per min}$$

Infusion Time

$$\frac{\text{Total volume to infuse}}{\text{mL per hour being infused}} = \text{Infusion time}$$

2. Example: Calcium gluconate 10% = 10 g of pure medication per 100 mL of solution
B. **Ratio solutions**
   1. Express the number of grams of the medication per total milliliters of solution
   2. Example: Epinephrine 1:1000 = 1 g of pure medication per 1000 mL solution

XII. INTRAVENOUS FLOW RATES

A. Monitor IVs every 30 minutes for adults and every 15 minutes for children
B. If an IV is running behind schedule, collaborate with the physician to determine the client's ability to tolerate an increased flow rate, particularly clients with cardiac, pulmonary, renal, or neurological conditions
C. The nurse should never arbitrarily speed up an IV to catch up if the IV is running behind schedule
D. Whenever an IV rate is increased, the nurse should assess the client for increased heart rate, increased respirations, or increased lung congestion, which could indicate fluid overload
E. IV fluids are most frequently ordered on the basis of milliliters (mL) per hour to be administered
F. The volume per hour ordered is administered by adjusting the rate at which the IV infuses, which is counted in drops (gtt) per minute
G. Most flow rate calculations involve changing milliliters per hour into drops per minute
H. IV tubing
   1. Calibrated in gtt per milliliter, and this calibration is needed for calculating flow rates
   2. A standard or macrodrip set is used for routine adult IV administrations; depending on the manufacturer and type of tubing, it will require 10, 15, or 20 gtt to equal 1 mL
   3. A minidrip or microdrip set is used when more exact measurements are needed, such as in intensive care units and pediatric units
   4. In a minidrip or microdrip set, 60 gtt is equal to 1 mL
   5. The calibration, in gtt per mL, is written on the IV tubing package

XIII. INTRAVENOUS CALCULATIONS (Table 16-5)

BOX 16-6

Infusions Ordered by Unit Dosage per Hour

Calculation of these problems requires a two-step process:
1. Determine the amount of medication per 1 mL
2. Determine the infusion rate or mL per hour

PROBLEM:
Order: Continuous heparin sodium by IV drip, 1000 units per hour
Available: IV bag of 500 mL D$_5$W with 25,000 units of heparin sodium
How many milliliters per hour are required to administer the correct dose?
Solution:
STEP 1: Calculate the units per mL

$$\frac{\text{Known amount of medication in solution}}{\text{Total volume of diluent}} =$$
$$\text{Amount of medication per mL}$$

$$\frac{25,000 \text{ units}}{500 \text{ mL}} = 50 \text{ units per 1 mL}$$

STEP 2: Calculate mL per hour

$$\frac{\text{Dose per hour desired}}{\text{Concentration per mL}} = \text{Infusion rate or mL per hour}$$

$$\frac{1000 \text{ units}}{50 \text{ units}} = 20 \text{ mL per hour}$$

PROBLEM:
Order: Continuous Regular Insulin by IV at 10 units per hour
Available: IV bag of 100 mL NS with 50 units Regular Insulin
How many mL per hour are required to administer the correct dose?
Solution:
STEP 1:

$$\frac{\text{Known amount of medication in solution}}{\text{Total volume of diluent}} =$$
$$\text{Amount of medication per mL}$$

$$\frac{50 \text{ units}}{100 \text{ mL}} = 0.5 \text{ units per 1 mL}$$
1 mL = 0.5 units

STEP 2:

$$\frac{\text{Dose per hour desired}}{\text{Concentration per mL}} = \text{Infusion rate or mL per hour}$$

$$\frac{10 \text{ units}}{0.5 \text{ units per mL}} = 20 \text{ mL per hour}$$

XIV. ELECTRONIC IV FLOW RATE REGULATORS

A. Controller
   1. Works on the same principle of gravity as a regular IV drip, with the rate of flow being maintained by rapid compression and decompression of the IV tubing by the machine

2. The desired flow rate is set on the controller in milliliters per hour
3. Because controllers work by gravity, the height of the solution bag is critical; it must be maintained at a minimum of 36 inches above the controller
4. The nurse should continue to assess the amount of IV solution in the IV container and monitor the controller to ensure proper functioning of the machine

B. Pump
1. A pump is different from a controller in that it physically pumps fluids against resistance
2. Gravity is not a factor in the use of a pump, and the height of the IV solution container is not a critical factor
3. The flow rate on a pump is set in milliliters per hour
4. The nurse should continue to assess the amount of IV solution in the IV container and monitor the pump to ensure proper functioning of the machine

XV. CALCULATING INFUSIONS ORDERED BY UNIT DOSAGE PER HOUR (Box 16-6)
A. The most common medications that will be ordered by **unit** dosage per hour and to run by continuous infusion are heparin sodium and Regular insulin
B. Calculation of these infusions requires a two-step process
1. Determine the amount of medication per 1 mL
2. Determine the infusion rate or milliliters per hour

PRACTICE QUESTIONS

1. A physician orders 1000 mL of NS to infuse over 12 hours. The drop factor is 15 drops per 1 mL. A nurse prepares to set the flow rate at how many drops per minute?
   1. 15 drops per minute
   2. 17 drops per minute
   3. 21 drops per minute
   4. 23 drops per minute

2. A physician orders an intravenous (IV) dose of 400,000 units of penicillin G benzathine (Bicillin). The label on the 10-mL ampule sent from the pharmacy reads penicillin G benzathine (Bicillin), 300,000 units per mL. A nurse prepares how much medication to administer the correct dose?
   1. 1.3 mL
   2. 1.5 mL
   3. 10 mL
   4. 13 mL

3. A physician's order reads potassium chloride (KCl) 30 mEq, to be added to 1000 mL NS and to be administered over a 10-hour period. The label on the medication bottle reads 40 mEq (KCl) per

20 mL. A nurse prepares how many mL of potassium chloride (KCl) to administer the correct dose of medication?
   1. 10 mL
   2. 15 mL
   3. 20 mL
   4. 50 mL

4. A physician orders 3000 mL of D₅W to infuse over a 24-hour period. The drop factor is 10 drops per 1 mL. A nurse sets the flow rate at how many drops per minute?
   1. 15 drops per minute
   2. 17 drops per minute
   3. 21 drops per minute
   4. 24 drops per minute

5. A physician's order reads clindamycin phosphate (Cleocin Phosphate) 0.3 g in 50 mL NS to be administered IV over 30 minutes. The medication label reads clindamycin phosphate (Cleocin Phosphate) 900 mg in 6 mL. A nurse prepares how many milliliters of the medication to administer the correct dose?
   1. 1 mL
   2. 2 mL
   3. 3 mL
   4. 5 mL

6. A physician's order reads phenytoin (Dilantin) 0.2 g PO bid. The medication label states 100-mg capsules. A nurse prepares how many capsule(s) to administer one dose?
   1. 1 capsule
   2. 2 capsules
   3. 3 capsules
   4. 4 capsules

7. A physician orders 1000 mL of ½ NS to infuse over 8 hours. The drop factor is 15 drops per 1 mL. The nurse sets the flow rate at how many drops per minute?
   1. 20 drops per minute
   2. 22 drops per minute
   3. 28 drops per minute
   4. 31 drops per minute

8. A physician orders 2000 mL of 5% dextrose and ½ NS to infuse over 24 hours. The drop factor is 15 drops per 1 mL. A nurse sets the flow rate at how many drops per minute?
   1. 15 drops per minute
   2. 17 drops per minute
   3. 21 drops per minute
   4. 28 drops per minute

9. A physician orders heparin sodium (Liquaemin), 1300 units per hour by continuous IV infusion. The pharmacy prepares the medication and delivers an IV bag labeled heparin sodium (Liquaemin) 20,000 units per 250 mL D₅W. An infusion pump must be used to administer the medication. The nurse sets

the infusion pump at how many milliliters per hour to deliver 1300 units per hour?
1. 12 mL
2. 16 mL
3. 20 mL
4. 22 mL

10. A physician's order reads cyanocobalamin (vitamin B_{12}) 1000 µg IM. The medication label reads cyanocobalamin (vitamin B_{12}) 0.5 mg per mL. A nurse prepares the medication and administers how many mL to the client?
1. 0.5 mL
2. 1 mL
3. 2 mL
4. 3 mL

11. A physician orders 3000 mL of D_5W to be administered over a 24-hour period. A nurse determines that how many milliliters per hour will be administered to the client?
1. 50 mL per hour
2. 75 mL per hour
3. 100 mL per hour
4. 125 mL per hour

12. Gentamicin sulfate (Garamycin), 80 mg in 100 mL NS, is to be administered over 30 minutes. The drop factor is 10 drops per mL. A nurse sets the flow rate at how many drops per minute?
1. 18 drops
2. 23 drops
3. 33 drops
4. 43 drops

13. A physician's order reads levothyroxine (Synthroid), 150 mcg PO daily. The medication label reads Synthroid, 0.1 mg per tablet. A nurse administers how many tablet(s) to the client?
1. 1 tablet
2. 1.5 tablets
3. 2 tablets
4. 2.5 tablets

14. Cefuroxime axetil (Ceftin), 1 g in 50 mL NS, is to be administered over 30 minutes. The drop factor is 15 drops per mL. A nurse sets the flow rate at how many drops per minute?
1. 15 drops
2. 25 drops
3. 20 drops
4. 22 drops

15. A physician orders 1000 mL D_5W to infuse at a rate of 125 mL per hour. A nurse determines that it will take many hours for 1 liter to infuse?
1. 8 hours
2. 10 hours
3. 12 hours
4. 15 hours

16. A physician orders 500 mL of NS to infuse over 5 hours. The drop factor is 10 drops per 1 mL. A nurse sets the flow rate at how many drops per minute?
1. 15 drops
2. 17 drops
3. 20 drops
4. 22 drops

17. A physician orders 1 unit of packed red blood cells to infuse over 4 hours. The unit of blood contains 250 mL. The drop factor is 10 drops per 1 mL. A nurse prepares to set the flow rate at how many drops per minute?
1. 10 drops
2. 15 drops
3. 17 drops
4. 20 drops

18. A physician orders 3000 mL of NS to infuse over 24 hours. The drop factor is 15 drops per 1 mL. The nurse prepares to set the flow rate at how many drops per minute?
1. 17 drops per minute
2. 20 drops per minute
3. 24 drops per minute
4. 31 drops per minute

19. A physician's order reads morphine sulfate, gr 1/8 IM stat. The medication ampule reads morphine sulfate, 10 mg per mL. A nurse prepares how many milliliters to administer the correct dose?
1. 0.5 mL
2. 0.75 mL
3. 0.85 mL
4. 1.5 mL

20. A physician orders Regular insulin, 8 units per hour by continuous IV infusion. The pharmacy prepares the medication and the delivers an IV bag labeled 100 units of Regular insulin in 100 mL NS. An infusion pump must be used to administer the medication. The nurse sets the infusion pump at how many milliliters per hour to deliver 8 units per hour?
1. 1 mL
2. 4 mL
3. 8 mL
4. 10 mL

CRITICAL THINKING: FREE-TEXT ENTRY

The physician orders meperidine (Demerol) 60 mg and atropine sulfate gr 1/150 IM for a preoperative client. The medications are compatible and will be mixed into one syringe. The label on the meperidine (Demerol) bottle states 100 mg per mL. The label on the atropine sulfate bottle states 0.4 mg per mL. How many mL of meperidine (Demerol) and how many mL of atropine sulfate will be prepared for administration?

Answer: _____

ANSWERS

1. 3

Rationale: Use the IV flow rate formula.

Formula:

$$\frac{\text{Total volume in mL} \times \text{drop factor}}{\text{Time in minutes}} =$$

Flow rate in drops per minute

$$\frac{1000 \text{ mL} \times 15 \text{ drops}}{720 \text{ minutes}} = \frac{15,000}{720} = 20.8, \text{ or } 21 \text{ drops per minute}$$

Test-Taking Strategy: Use the formula for calculating IV flow rates when answering the question. Be careful with the multiplication and division. Using the formula carefully will direct you to the correct option. Review IV infusion rates if you had difficulty with this question.

Level of Cognitive Ability: Application

Client Needs: Physiological Integrity

Integrated Concept/Process: Nursing Process/Planning

Content Area: Fundamental Skills

Reference: Potter, P., & Perry, A. (2001). *Fundamentals of nursing* (5th ed.). St. Louis: Mosby, p.1229.

2. 1

Rationale: Use the medication formula.

Formula:

$$\frac{\text{Desired}}{\text{Available}} \times \text{mL} = \text{mL per dose}$$

$$\frac{400,000 \text{ units}}{300,000 \text{ units}} \times 1 \text{ mL} = \text{mL per dose}$$

$$\frac{400,000}{300,000} = 1.3 \text{ mL}$$

Test-Taking Strategy: Follow the formula for the calculation of the correct dose. It is not necessary to perform a conversion with this problem. Label each figure, including the answer. Recheck your work, and make sure that the answer makes sense. If you had difficulty with this question, review medication calculation problems.

Level of Cognitive Ability: Application

Client Needs: Physiological Integrity

Integrated Concept/Process: Nursing Process/Planning

Content Area: Fundamental Skills

Reference: Harkreader, H. (2000). *Fundamentals of nursing: Caring and clinical judgment.* Philadelphia: W.B. Saunders, p. 548.

3. 2

Rationale: Use the medication calculation formula.

Formula:

$$\frac{\text{Desired}}{\text{Available}} \times \text{mL} = \text{mL per dose}$$

$$\frac{30 \text{ mEq}}{40 \text{ mEq}} \times 20 \text{ mL} = 15 \text{ mL}$$

Test-Taking Strategy: Follow the formula for the calculation of the correct dose. It is not necessary to perform a conversion with this problem. Label each figure, including the answer. Recheck your work, and make sure that the answer makes sense. If you had difficulty with this question, review medication calculation problems.

Level of Cognitive Ability: Application

Client Needs: Physiological Integrity

Integrated Concept/Process: Nursing Process/Planning

Content Area: Fundamental Skills

Reference: Harkreader, H. (2000). *Fundamentals of nursing: Caring and clinical judgment.* Philadelphia: W.B. Saunders, p. 548.

4. 3

Rationale: Use the IV flow rate formula.

Formula:

$$\frac{\text{Total volume in mL} \times \text{drop factor}}{\text{Time in minutes}} =$$

Flow rate in drops per minute

$$\frac{3000 \text{ mL} \times 10 \text{ drops}}{1440 \text{ minutes}} = \frac{30,000}{1440} = 20.8, \text{ or } 21 \text{ drops per minute}$$

Test-Taking Strategy: Use the formula for calculating IV flow rates when answering the question. Be careful with multiplication and division. Using the formula carefully will direct you to the correct option. Review IV infusion rates if you had difficulty with this question.

Level of Cognitive Ability: Application

Client Needs: Physiological Integrity

Integrated Concept/Process: Nursing Process/Implementation

Content Area: Fundamental Skills

Reference: Potter, P., & Perry, A. (2001). *Fundamentals of nursing* (5th ed.). St. Louis: Mosby, p. 1229.

5. 2

Rationale: It is necessary to convert 0.3 g to mg. In the metric system, to convert larger to smaller multiply by 1000, or move the decimal 3 places to the right. Therefore, 0.3 g = 300 mg. Following conversion from g to mg, use the formula to calculate the correct dose.

Formula:

$$\frac{\text{Desired}}{\text{Available}} \times \text{mL} = \text{mL per dose}$$

$$\frac{300 \text{ mg}}{900 \text{ mg}} \times 6 \text{ mL} = \frac{1800}{900} = 2 \text{ mL}$$

Test-Taking Strategy: In this medication calculation problem, it is necessary to first convert grams to milligrams. Next, follow the formula for the calculation of the correct dose. Recheck your work, and make sure that the answer makes sense. If you had difficulty with this question, review medication calculation problems.

Level of Cognitive Ability: Application

Client Needs: Physiological Integrity

Integrated Concept/Process: Nursing Process/Planning

Content Area: Fundamental Skills

Reference: Harkreader, H. (2000). *Fundamentals of nursing: Caring and clinical judgment.* Philadelphia: W.B. Saunders, pp. 547-548.

6. 2

Rationale: It is necessary to convert 0.2 g to mg. In the metric system, to convert larger to smaller multiply by 1000 or move the decimal 3 places to the right. Therefore, 0.2 g = 200 mg. After conversion from g to mg, use the formula to calculate the correct dose.

Formula:

$$\frac{Desired}{Available} \times Capsules = Capsules\ per\ dose$$

$$\frac{200\ mg}{100\ mg} \times 1\ capsule = 2\ capsules$$

Test-Taking Strategy: In this medication calculation problem, it is necessary to first convert grams to milligrams. Once you have done the conversion and reread the medication calculation problem, you will know that two capsules is the correct answer. Follow the formula for the calculation of the correct dose. Recheck your work, and make sure that the answer makes sense. If you had difficulty with this question, review medication calculation problems.
Level of Cognitive Ability: Application
Client Needs: Physiological Integrity
Integrated Concept/Process: Nursing Process/Planning
Content Area: Fundamental Skills
Reference: Harkreader, H. (2000). *Fundamentals of nursing: Caring and clinical judgment.* Philadelphia: W.B. Saunders, pp. 547-548.

7. **4**
Rationale: Use the IV flow rate formula.
Formula:

$$\frac{Total\ volume\ in\ mL \times drop\ factor}{Time\ in\ minutes} =$$

$$Flow\ rate\ in\ drops\ per\ minute$$

$$\frac{1000\ mL \times 15\ drops}{480\ minutes} = \frac{15,000}{480} = 31.2,\ or\ 31\ drops\ per\ minute$$

Test-Taking Strategy: Use the formula for calculating IV flow rates when answering the question. Be careful with the multiplication and division. Using the formula carefully will direct you to the correct option. Review IV infusion rates if you had difficulty with this question.
Level of Cognitive Ability: Application
Client Needs: Physiological Integrity
Integrated Concept/Process: Nursing Process/Implementation
Content Area: Fundamental Skills
Reference: Potter, P., & Perry, A. (2001). *Fundamentals of nursing* (5th ed.). St. Louis: Mosby, p. 1229.

8. **3**
Rationale: Use the IV flow rate formula.
Formula:

$$\frac{Total\ volume\ in\ mL \times drop\ factor}{Time\ in\ minutes} =$$

$$Flow\ rate\ in\ drops\ per\ minute$$

$$\frac{2000\ mL \times 15\ drops}{1440\ minutes} = \frac{30,000}{1440} = 20.8,\ or\ 21\ drops\ per\ minute$$

Test-Taking Strategy: Use the formula for calculating IV flow rates when answering the question. Be careful with the multiplication and division. Using the formula carefully will direct you to the correct option. Review IV infusion rates if you had difficulty with this question.
Level of Cognitive Ability: Application
Client Needs: Physiological Integrity
Integrated Concept/Process: Nursing Process/Implementation

Content Area: Fundamental Skills
Reference: Potter, P., & Perry, A. (2001). *Fundamentals of nursing* (5th ed.). St. Louis: Mosby, p. 1229.

9. **2**
Rationale: Calculation of this problem requires a two step process. First you need to determine the amount of heparin sodium in 1 mL. The next step is to determine the infusion rate, or milliliters per hour.
Formula:
Step 1:

$$\frac{Known\ amount\ of\ medication}{Total\ volume\ of\ diluent} =$$

$$Amount\ of\ medication\ per\ mL$$

$$\frac{20,000\ units}{250\ mL} = 80\ units\ per\ mL$$
$$1\ mL = 80\ units$$

Step 2:
Formula:

$$\frac{Dose\ per\ hour\ desired}{Concentration\ per\ mL} = Infusion\ rate\ or\ mL\ per\ hour$$

$$\frac{1300\ units}{80\ units\ per\ mL} = 16.25,\ or\ 16\ mL\ per\ hour$$

Test-Taking Strategy: Read the question carefully, noting that two steps are required to solve this medication problem. If you had difficulty with this question, learn these steps now. These steps can be used for similar medication problems related to the administration of heparin sodium or Regular insulin by IV infusion.
Level of Cognitive Ability: Application
Client Needs: Physiological Integrity
Integrated Concept/Process: Nursing Process/Implementation
Content Area: Fundamental Skills
Reference: Kee, J., & Marshall, S. (2000). *Clinical calculations: With applications to general and specialty areas* (4th ed.). Philadelphia: W.B. Saunders, pp. 240-241.

10. **3**
Rationale: It is necessary to convert 1000 μg to mg. In the metric system, to convert smaller to larger divide by 1000 or move the decimal 3 places to the left. Therefore, 1000 μg = 1.0 mg. Next, use the formula to calculate the correct dose.
Formula:

$$\frac{Desired}{Available} \times mL = mL\ per\ dose$$

$$\frac{1.0\ mg}{0.5\ mg} \times 1\ mL = \frac{1.0}{0.5} = 2\ mL$$

Test-Taking Strategy: In this medication calculation problem, it is necessary to first convert micrograms to milligrams. Next, follow the formula for the calculation of the correct dose. Label each figure, including the answer. Recheck your work, and make sure that the answer makes sense. If you had difficulty with this question, review medication calculation problems.
Level of Cognitive Ability: Application
Client Needs: Physiological Integrity

Integrated Concept/Process: Nursing Process/Implementation
Content Area: Fundamental Skills
Reference: Harkreader, H. (2000). *Fundamentals of nursing: Caring and clinical judgment.* Philadelphia: W.B. Saunders, pp. 547-548.

11. 4

Rationale: Use the IV formula to determine milliliters per hour.

Formula:

$$\frac{\text{Total volume in mL}}{\text{Number of hours}} = \text{Number of mL per hour}$$

$$\frac{3000 \text{ mL}}{24 \text{ hours}} = 125 \text{ mL per hour}$$

Test-Taking Strategy: Read the question carefully, noting that the question is asking about milliliters per hour to be administered to the client. Use the formula for calculating milliliters per hour to direct you to the correct option. Review the IV formula for calculating milliliters per hour if you had difficulty with this question.
Level of Cognitive Ability: Analysis
Client Needs: Physiological Integrity
Integrated Concept/Process: Nursing Process/Analysis
Content Area: Fundamental Skills
Reference: Potter, P., & Perry, A. (2001). *Fundamentals of nursing* (5th ed.). St. Louis: Mosby, p. 1229.

12. 3

Rationale: Use the IV flow rate formula.

Formula:

$$\frac{\text{Total volume in mL} \times \text{Drop factor}}{\text{Time in minutes}} =$$

Flow rate in drops per minute

$$\frac{100 \text{ mL} \times 10 \text{ drops}}{30 \text{ minutes}} = \frac{1000}{30} = 33.3, \text{ or } 33 \text{ drops per minute}$$

Test-Taking Strategy: Use the formula for calculating IV flow rates when answering the question. Be careful with the multiplication and division. Using the formula carefully will direct you to the correct option. Review IV infusion rates if you had difficulty with this question.
Level of Cognitive Ability: Application
Client Needs: Physiological Integrity
Integrated Concept/Process: Nursing Process/Implementation
Content Area: Fundamental Skills
Reference: Potter, P., & Perry, A. (2001). *Fundamentals of nursing* (5th ed.). St. Louis: Mosby, p. 1229.

13. 2

Rationale: It is necessary to convert 150 mcg to mg. In the metric system, to convert smaller to larger divide by 1000 or move the decimal 3 places to the left. Therefore, 150 mcg = 0.15 mg. Next, use the formula to calculate the correct dose.

Formula:

$$\frac{\text{Desired}}{\text{Available}} \times \text{Tablet} = \text{Tablets per dose}$$

$$\frac{0.15 \text{ mg}}{0.1 \text{ mg}} \times 1 \text{ tablet} = 1.5 \text{ tablets}$$

Test-Taking Strategy: In this medication calculation problem, it is necessary to first convert micrograms to milligrams. Next,

follow the formula for the calculation of the correct dose. Label each figure, including the answer. Recheck your work, and make sure that the answer makes sense. If you had difficulty with this question, review medication calculation problems.
Level of Cognitive Ability: Application
Client Needs: Physiological Integrity
Integrated Concept/Process: Nursing Process/Implementation
Content Area: Fundamental Skills
Reference: Harkreader, H. (2000). *Fundamentals of nursing: Caring and clinical judgment.* Philadelphia: W.B. Saunders, pp. 547-548.

14. 2

Rationale: Use the IV flow rate formula.

Formula:

$$\frac{\text{Total volume in mL} \times \text{Drop factor}}{\text{Time in minutes}} =$$

Flow rate in drops per minute

$$\frac{50 \text{ mL} \times 15 \text{ drops}}{30 \text{ minutes}} = \frac{750}{30} = 25 \text{ drops per minute}$$

Test-Taking Strategy: Use the formula for calculating IV flow rates when answering the question. Be careful with the multiplication and division. Using the formula carefully will direct you to the correct option. Review IV infusion rates if you had difficulty with this question.
Level of Cognitive Ability: Application
Client Needs: Physiological Integrity
Integrated Concept/Process: Nursing Process/Implementation
Content Area: Fundamental Skills
Reference: Potter, P., & Perry, A. (2001). *Fundamentals of nursing* (5th ed.). St. Louis: Mosby, p. 1229.

15. 1

Rationale: It is necessary to determine that 1 liter = 1000 mL. Next, use the formula for determining infusion time in hours.

Formula:

$$\frac{\text{Total volume in mL}}{\text{mL per hour}} = \text{Infusion time in hours}$$

$$\frac{1000 \text{ mL}}{125 \text{ mL}} = 8 \text{ hours}$$

Test-Taking Strategy: Read the question carefully, noting that the question is asking about infusion time in hours. First, convert 1 liter to milliliters. Next, use the formula for determining infusion time in hours. Review the IV formula for calculating infusion time if you had difficulty with this question.
Level of Cognitive Ability: Analysis
Client Needs: Physiological Integrity
Integrated Concept/Process: Nursing Process/Analysis
Content Area: Fundamental Skills
Reference: Potter, P., & Perry, A. (2001). *Fundamentals of nursing* (5th ed.). St. Louis: Mosby, p. 1229.

16. 2

Rationale: Use the IV flow rate formula.

Formula:

$$\frac{\text{Total volume in mL} \times \text{Drop factor}}{\text{Time in minutes}} =$$

Flow rate in drops per minute

$$\frac{500 \text{ mL} \times 10 \text{ drops}}{300 \text{ minutes}} = \frac{5000}{300} = 16.6, \text{ or } 17 \text{ drops per minute}$$

Test-Taking Strategy: Use the formula for calculating IV flow rates when answering the question. Be careful with the multiplication and division. Using the formula carefully will direct you to the correct option. Review IV infusion rates if you had difficulty with this question.
Level of Cognitive Ability: Application
Client Needs: Physiological Integrity
Integrated Concept/Process: Nursing Process/Implementation
Content Area: Fundamental Skills
Reference: Potter, P., & Perry, A. (2001). *Fundamentals of nursing* (5th ed.). St. Louis: Mosby, p. 1229.
17. **1**
Rationale: Use the IV flow rate formula.
Formula:

$$\frac{\text{Total volume in mL} \times \text{Drop factor}}{\text{Time in minutes}} =$$

Flow rate in drops per minute

$$\frac{250 \text{ mL} \times 10 \text{ drops}}{240 \text{ minutes}} = \frac{25,000}{240} = 10.4, \text{ or } 10 \text{ drops per minute}$$

Test-Taking Strategy: Use the formula for calculating IV flow rates when answering the question. Be careful with the multiplication and division. Using the formula carefully will direct you to the correct option. Review IV infusion rates if you had difficulty with this question.
Level of Cognitive Ability: Application
Client Needs: Physiological Integrity
Integrated Concept/Process: Nursing Process/Planning
Content Area: Fundamental Skills
Reference: Potter, P., & Perry, A. (2001). *Fundamentals of nursing* (5th ed.). St. Louis: Mosby, p. 1229.
18. **4**
Rationale: Use the IV flow rate formula.
Formula:

$$\frac{\text{Total volume in mL} \times \text{Drop factor}}{\text{Time in minutes}} =$$

Flow rate in drops per minute

$$\frac{3000 \text{ mL} \times 15 \text{ drops}}{1440 \text{ minutes}} = \frac{45,000}{1440} = 31.2, \text{ or } 31 \text{ drops per minute}$$

Test-Taking Strategy: Use the formula for calculating IV flow rates when answering the question. Be careful with the multiplication and division. Using the formula carefully will direct you to the correct option. Review IV infusion rates if you had difficulty with this question.
Level of Cognitive Ability: Application
Client Needs: Physiological Integrity
Integrated Concept/Process: Nursing Process/Planning
Content Area: Fundamental Skills
Reference: Potter, P., & Perry, A. (2001). *Fundamentals of nursing* (5th ed.). St. Louis: Mosby, p. 1229.
19. **2**
Rationale: It is necessary to convert gr 1/8 to mg. After converting gr to mg, use the formula to calculate the correct dose.

Conversion:
60 mg: gr 1 :: x mg : gr 1/8
1x = 1/8 × 60/1
x = 60/ 8 = 7.5 mg
Formula:

$$\frac{\text{Desired}}{\text{Available}} \times \text{Tablet} = \text{Tablets per dose}$$

$$\frac{7.5 \text{ mg}}{10 \text{ mg}} \times 1 \text{ mL} = \frac{7.5}{10} = 0.75 \text{ mL}$$

Test-Taking Strategy: In this medication calculation problem, it is necessary to first convert grains to milligrams. Next, follow the formula for the calculation of the correct dose. Label each figure, including the answer. Recheck your work, and make sure that the answer makes sense. If you had difficulty with this question, review medication calculation problems.
Level of Cognitive Ability: Application
Client Needs: Physiological Integrity
Integrated Concept/Process: Nursing Process/Planning
Content Area: Fundamental Skills
Reference: Harkreader, H. (2000). *Fundamentals of nursing: Caring and clinical judgment.* Philadelphia: W.B. Saunders, pp. 547-548.
20. **3**
Rationale: Calculation of this problem requires a two-step process. First you need to determine the amount of Regular insulin in 1 mL. The next step is to determine the infusion rate, or milliliters per hour.
Formula:
Step 1:

$$\frac{\text{Known amount of medication}}{\text{Total volume of diluent}} =$$

Amount of medication per mL

$$\frac{100 \text{ units}}{100 \text{ mL}} = 1 \text{ unit per mL}$$

1 mL = 1 unit

Step 2:
Formula:

$$\frac{\text{Dose per hour desired}}{\text{Concentration per mL}} = \text{Infusion rate or mL per hour}$$

$$\frac{8 \text{ units}}{1 \text{ unit per mL}} = 8 \text{ mL per hour}$$

Test-Taking Strategy: Read the question carefully, noting that two steps are required to solve this medication problem. If you had difficulty with this question, learn these steps now. These steps can be used for similar medication problems related to the administration of heparin sodium or Regular insulin by IV infusion.
Level of Cognitive Ability: Application
Client Needs: Physiological Integrity
Integrated Concept/Process: Nursing Process/Implementation
Content Area: Fundamental Skills
Reference: Kee, J., & Marshall, S. (2000). *Clinical calculations: With applications to general and specialty areas* (4th ed.). Philadelphia: W.B. Saunders, pp. 240-241.

CRITICAL THINKING: FREE-TEXT ENTRY

Answer: Meperidine (Demerol) = 0.6 mL; atropine sulfate = 1 mL

Rationale: Use the formula for calculating the mL of meperidine to be administered. Next, convert atropine sulfate gr 1/150 to mg. After converting gr to mg, use the formula to calculate the correct dose.

Meperidine (Demerol):
Formula:

$$\frac{\text{Desired}}{\text{Available}} \times \text{mL} = \text{mL per dose}$$

$$\frac{60 \text{ mg}}{100 \text{ mg}} \times 1 \text{ mL} = 0.6 \text{ mL}$$

Atropine Sulfate:
Conversion:

60 mg : gr 1 :: x mg : gr 1/150
1x = 1/150 × 60/1
x = 60/150 = 0.4 mg

Formula:

$$\frac{\text{Desired}}{\text{Available}} \times \text{mL} = \text{mL per dose}$$

$$\frac{0.4 \text{ mg}}{0.4 \text{ mg}} \times 1 \text{ mL} = 1 \text{ mL}$$

Test-Taking Strategy: This medication calculation requires determining the mL to be administered for two medications, meperidine (Demerol) and atropine sulfate. First, calculate the mL for the meperidine. To calculate the mL of atropine sulfate to be administered, it is necessary to first convert grains to milligrams. Next, follow the formula for the calculation of the correct dose. Label each figure, including the answer. Recheck your work, and make sure that the answer makes sense. If you had difficulty with this question, review medication calculation problems.

Level of Cognitive Ability: Application
Client Needs: Physiological Integrity
Integrated Concept/Process: Nursing Process/Implementation
Content Area: Fundamental Skills
Reference: Kee, J., & Marshall, S. (2000). *Clinical calculations: With applications to general and specialty areas* (4th ed.). Philadelphia: W.B. Saunders, p. 158.

REFERENCES

Harkreader, H. (2000). *Fundamentals of nursing: Caring and clinical judgment.* Philadelphia: W.B. Saunders.

Kee, J., & Marshall, S. (2000). *Clinical calculations: With applications to general and specialty areas* (4th ed.). Philadelphia: W.B. Saunders.

Potter, P., & Perry, A. (2001). *Fundamentals of nursing* (5th ed.). St. Louis: Mosby.

Basic Life Support

PYRAMID TERMS

automated external defibrillator (AED) Converts ventricular fibrillation into a perfusing rhythm and allows for early defibrillation by first responders.

basic life support (BLS) Providing oxygen to the brain, heart and other vital organs until help arrives.

cardiopulmonary resuscitation (CPR) An interchangeable term for basic life support.

head tilt–chin lift Preferred method to open a victim's airway.

Heimlich maneuver Method of rescue to remove foreign objects from a choking victim.

jaw thrust maneuver Method used to open a victim's airway if a neck injury is suspected.

▲ PYRAMID TO SUCCESS

The Pyramid to Success focuses on the emergency measures related to performing basic life support. Focus on the points related to the breaths and compression ratio with one-man and two-man adult CPR and CPR in the infant and the child. Pyramid points focus on airway management in CPR and on performing the Heimlich maneuver. Focus on the correct hand placements for cardiac compressions and on the differences between the adult, the child, and the infant. Remember, prior to initiating CPR, determining unresponsiveness is the initial action. Remember the ABCs—airway, breathing, and circulation—when performing CPR. The primary Integrated Concepts and Processes addressed in this chapter include Nursing Process, Caring, Communication and Documentation, Cultural Awareness, and Teaching/Learning.

▲ CLIENT NEEDS
Safe, Effective Care Environment

Advanced directives regarding the client's documented requests

Advocacy regarding the client's wishes

Client rights
Establishing priorities
Ethical and legal responsibilities
Standard (universal) and other precautions

Health Promotion and Maintenance

Health promotion programs
Teaching significant other to perform BLS
Techniques of physical assessment

Psychosocial Integrity

Potential end-of-life issues
Emotional support to significant other
Religious and spirtual influences
Therapeutic interactions

Physiological Integrity

Alterations in cardiopulmonary system
Handling medical emergencies
Use of special equipment
Administration of emergency medications and IVs
Documentation of response to BLS

▲

I. **BASIC LIFE SUPPORT (BLS)** (Box 17-1)
A. Providing oxygen to the brain, heart, and other vital organs until help arrives
B. Also known as **cardiopulmonary resuscitation (CPR)**

II. **ADULT BLS**
A. Description: An adult can be defined as a person ▲ who is 8 years of age or older
B. Airway
    1. Remember that assessment is the first step of the ▲

BOX 17-1

The ABCs of Basic Life Support (BLS)

A: Airway
B: Breathing
C: Circulation
Each step of the ABCs of BLS begins with assessment!

---

nursing process; assessing a victim of sudden illness or accident for unconsciousness is the initial action; assess for 5 to10 seconds

2. Gently shake the victim's shoulders and ask "Are you OK?"; be alert to the potential for a head or neck injury
3. Activate emergency medical system (EMS): "phone first," children ≥8 years of age and adults; "phone last," children <8 years
4. Place the victim in a supine position on a firm, flat surface (logroll the victim, using spine precautions)
   a. One-person rescue: The rescuer is positioned on his or her knees, parallel to victim's sternum and facing the victim
   b. Two-person rescue: One rescuer faces the victim, kneeling parallel to victim's head; the second rescuer moves to opposite side and faces the victim, kneeling parallel to the victim's sternum
   c. The rescuers apply gloves and face shield, if available
5. Open the airway
6. The **head tilt–chin lift** is the preferred method for opening the airway; if there is a neck injury, the **jaw thrust maneuver** is used to open the airway
7. Look for any foreign material, liquids, or solids in the victim's mouth; wipe out any foreign material with a hooked index or middle finger

C. Breathing
1. Assess breathing, maintaining an open airway
2. The rescuer places his or her ear over the victim's nose and mouth and looks for the chest to rise and fall, listens for air moving in and out of the lungs, and feels for the flow of air
3. Breathing victim
   a. Place the victim on his or her side if no cervical trauma is suspected; logroll the victim onto his or her side as a unit (without twisting) to help maintain an open airway
   b. If trauma or injury is suspected, the victim should not be moved
4. Nonbreathing victim
   a. Maintain the **head tilt–chin lift**; pinch the nostrils closed, and give two, slow full ventilations (breaths) of 2 seconds per breath

(use resuscitation bag or face shield if available, ensuring an adequate air seal); allow victim to exhale between breaths
   b. Give 10 to 12 ventilations per minute
   c. If unsuccessful at giving the breath or ventilation, reposition the victim's head and try again (improper chin and head position is the most common cause of difficulty in ventilating the victim)
   d. If still unsuccessful, check the victim's mouth for a foreign body or for loose dentures (remove dentures only if they interfere with the mouth seal), clear the airway, and try to ventilate again
   e. Be alert to gastric distention when giving ventilations
5. Mouth to nose: Recommended when it is impossible to ventilate through the victim's mouth, the mouth cannot be opened, the mouth is seriously injured, or a tight mouth-to-mouth seal is difficult to achieve
6. Mouth to Stoma: Used for the victim who has had a laryngectomy or has a temporary tracheostomy; to be effective, an adequate seal over the victim's mouth and nose is necessary

D. Circulation
1. Assess circulation; always check for the absence of a pulse before beginning chest compressions on the victim
2. Maintain an open airway and palpate for a carotid pulse for 5 to 10 seconds
3. If there is a pulse, continue to give 10 to 12 ventilations per minute
4. Recheck the pulse after 1 minute; if there is no pulse, start chest compressions

E. Chest compressions
1. Hand placement
   a. Correct hand placement for chest compressions is crucial
   b. Hand placement is on the lower half of the sternum
   c. With the hand closest to the victim's feet, locate the lower margin of the rib cage
   d. Move the fingertips along the margin to the notch where the ribs meet the sternum
   e. Place the middle finger on the notch and the index finger next to middle finger
   f. Place the heel of the opposite hand next to the index finger, and place the other hand on top
2. Complications of chest compressions
   a. Laceration of internal organs
   b. Punctured lungs
   c. Fractured ribs or sternum

III. ADULT ONE-MAN BLS

A. The ratio is 15:2; that is, 15 chest compressions to 2 ventilations

B. The rate of compressions is 100 a minute at a depth of 1.5 to 2 inches
C. Perform four complete cycles; then reassess the victim
D. Check the carotid pulse after the first four cycles of **CPR** and every few minutes thereafter; if no pulse is felt, continue **CPR**

IV. ADULT TWO-MAN BLS
A. One person is at the victim's side performing chest compressions; one person is at the victim's head, maintaining an open airway, monitoring the carotid pulse, and doing the rescue breathing
B. The adult ratio for two-man **BLS** is 15 to 2; that is, 15 compressions at a rate of 100 per minute, and 2 ventilations at 2 seconds per breath
C. When the second rescuer arrives at the scene, he or she must identify himself or herself and tell the first rescuer that he or she knows two-man **CPR**
D. The second rescuer then activates EMS, if this has not been done, and then returns to the scene to help
E. The second rescuer can perform one-man **CPR** if the first rescuer is fatigued; or, the first rescuer finishes 15 compressions, gives 2 ventilations, moves to the head, opens the airway, and checks the carotid pulse
F. If there is no pulse, the first rescuer announces "No pulse, continue **CPR**"
G. The second rescuer locates the landmark for chest compressions
H. The two rescuers begin **CPR** at a ratio of 15 compressions to 2 ventilations
I. At the end of 1 minute, the ventilator checks for a pulse and checks for breathing; if there is none, the ventilator says "No pulse, continue **CPR**"
J. When the compressor becomes tired, the compressor should change positions with minimal interruption of chest compressions
K. The rescuer ventilating the victim assumes responsibility for monitoring for signs of circulation and breathing

V. PEDIATRIC DIFFERENCES
A. Description
  1. A child can be defined as a person between 1 and 8 years of age
  2. An infant can be defined as a person under 1 year of age
B. Airway: Assess unresponsiveness
C. Breathing
  1. Breathing victim: Keep the airway open
  2. Nonbreathing victim
    a. Give two ventilations at 1 to 1.5 seconds per breath
    b. With the infant, provide ventilations by mouth to mouth and nose

c. With the larger child, provide ventilations by mouth to mouth
d. With the infant or the child, give 20 ventilations per minute
e. Activate EMS as soon as possible
D. Circulation
  1. Assess circulation
  2. If the victim is older than 1 year, assess circulation via the carotid pulse
  3. If the victim is younger than 1 year, assess circulation via the brachial pulse
  4. The ratio is 5 compressions to 1 ventilation
  5. Reassess every few minutes
  6. Infant chest compressions
    a. The imaginary line between the nipples is located over the breastbone (sternum)
    b. The index finger of the hand farthest from the infant's head is placed just under the intermammary line where it intersects the sternum
    c. The area of compression is one fingerwidth below this intersection, at the location of the middle and ring fingers
    d. With the use of 2 or 3 fingers, the breast bone is compressed 0.5 to 1 inch at 100 times per minute
    e. Two-thumb encircling hands technique is the preferred two-rescuer technique
  7. Chest compressions for a child
    a. The location for hand placement is the same as for an adult
    b. Depress the chest 1 to 1.5 inches at 100 times per minute with the heel of one hand

VI. THE CHOKING VICTIM AND HEIMLICH MANEUVER
A. Conscious adult
  1. Ask the victim, "Are you choking?" (the victim will not be able to speak or cough if he or she is choking)
  2. If the victim's airway is partially obstructed, a crowing sound is heard; encourage the victim to cough
  3. Relieve the obstruction by the **Heimlich maneuver** (Box 17-2)
  4. Perform the **Heimlich maneuver** until the object is dislodged or the victim becomes unconscious
B. Unconscious adult
  1. Assess unconsciousness
  2. Call for help; activate EMS as soon as possible
  3. Perform tongue-jaw lift technique; fingersweep to remove object
  4. Open the airway
  5. Attempt ventilation
  6. Reposition the head if unsuccessful; reattempt ventilation

---

BOX 17-2

Heimlich Maneuver

Stand behind the victim

Place arms around the victim's waist

Make a fist

Place the thumb side of the fist just above the umbilicus (belly button) and well below the xiphoid process

Perform five quick in and up thrusts (between the umbilicus and the xiphoid process)

Use chest thrusts for the markedly obese or for the advanced pregnancy victim

---

7. Relieve the obstruction by the **Heimlich maneuver** with five thrusts; then fingersweep the mouth
8. To perform the **Heimlich maneuver,** straddle the victim's thighs, place the heel of one hand on top of the other between umbilicus and xiphoid process, and give five thrusts in and up with the heel of the bottom hand
9. Reattempt ventilation
10. Repeat the sequence of tongue-jaw lift, fingersweep, breaths, and **Heimlich maneuver** until successful
11. Be sure to assess the victim's pulse and respirations
12. Perform **CPR** if required

C. Choking child or infant
1. Choking is suspected in infants and children experiencing acute respiratory distress associated with coughing, gagging, or stridor (high-pitched noisy breathing)
2. Allow the victim to continue to cough if the cough is forceful
3. If the cough is ineffective or the victim develops increased respiratory difficulty accompanied by a high-pitched noise while inhaling, help is needed
4. Conscious child
   a. Assess for obstruction by asking the child, "Are you choking?"
   b. Relieve the obstruction by the **Heimlich maneuver** until the obstruction is dislodged or the child becomes unconscious
5. Unconscious child
   a. Assess unconsciousness
   b. Open the airway by the tongue-jaw lift
   c. Check for breathing and look for a foreign object
   d. Attempt ventilation
   e. If unsuccessful, reposition the head; reattempt ventilation
   f. Relieve the obstruction by using the **Heimlich maneuver,** giving five abdominal thrusts, and

fingersweep the mouth only if the object is seen
   g. Assess airway for foreign object and reattempt ventilation
   h. Repeat the sequence
   i. Assess pulse and respirations and perform **CPR** if required
6. Conscious infant
   a. Assess for obstruction and note breathing problems
   b. Relieve the obstruction by five back blows and five chest thrusts
   c. Straddle the infant over the arm, place the infant's head lower than the trunk, and support the head firmly, holding the jaw
   d. Give five back blows with the heel of the hand between the shoulder blades
   e. Turn the infant; place the head lower than the trunk
   f. Give five chest thrusts at the same location as for chest compressions
   g. Check for the object and remove if seen
   h. Blind fingersweeps are avoided in infants and small children, since the object may be pushed back farther into the airway, causing further obstruction
   i. Continue until the object is removed or the infant becomes unconscious
7. Unconscious infant
   a. Assess unconsciousness by gentle taps
   b. Open the airway by the tongue-jaw lift
   c. Check for breathing and look for a foreign object
   d. Attempt ventilation
   e. Reposition the head if unsuccessful; reattempt ventilation
   f. Relieve the obstruction by five back blows and five chest thrusts
   g. Fingersweep the mouth only if the object is seen
   h. Reattempt ventilation and repeat the sequence
   i. Activate EMS after 1 minute of unresponsiveness
   j. Perform **CPR** if required

VII. PREGNANT OR OBESE VICTIM
A. **Heimlich maneuver**
1. Place arms under the woman's axilla and across the chest
2. Place the thumb side of a clenched fist against the middle of the sternum, and place the other hand over the fist
3. Perform backward chest thrusts until the foreign body is expelled or until the woman becomes unconscious
4. If she becomes unconscious, place her on her back; a wedge, such as a pillow or rolled blanket,

should be placed under the right abdominal flank and hip to displace the uterus to the left side of the abdomen

5. If unable to ventilate, position the hands as for chest compressions and deliver chest thrusts firmly to remove the obstruction

B. Defibrillation in the pregnant client: If defibrillation is needed, place the paddles one rib interspace higher than usual because the heart is displaced slightly by the enlarged uterus

VIII. AUTOMATED EXTERNAL DEFIBRILLATOR (AED)

A. Description
   1. Used to convert ventricular fibrillation into a perfusing rhythm
   2. Differentiates nonventricular fibrillation rhythms and allows for early defibrillation by first responders

B. Implementation
   1. Attach **AED** leads to the victim
   2. Turn on the **AED** and push the button to activate the analyzer
   3. Follow instructions given for the **AED**, usually to "assess," "stand back," "shock," and "reassess"
   4. Evaluate for return of the pulse, and if the victim is pulseless, repeat defibrillation as directed up to three times; if defibrillation is still ineffective, perform **CPR** for 1 minute, and then deliver another series of three shocks (Box 17-3)

PRACTICE QUESTIONS

1. A nurse on the day shift walks into a client's room and finds the client unresponsive. The client is not breathing and does not have a pulse. The nurse immediately calls out for help. The next nursing action is which of the following?
   1. Ventilate with a mouth-to-mask device
   2. Start chest compressions
   3. Give the client oxygen
   4. Open the airway

2. A nurse is performing cardiopulmonary resuscitation (CPR) on an adult client. When performing chest compressions, the nurse understands that correct hand placement is located over the:
   1. Lower third of the sternum
   2. Upper half of the sternum
   3. Upper third of the sternum
   4. Lower half of the sternum

3. A nurse witnesses a neighbor's husband sustain a fall from the roof of his house. The nurse rushes to the victim and determines the need to open the airway. The nurse opens the airway in this victim by using which most appropriate method?
   1. Head tilt–chin lift
   2. Flexed position
   3. Modified head tilt–chin lift
   4. Jaw thrust maneuver

4. A nurse is preparing to do the Heimlich maneuver on a 3-year-old conscious child. The nurse performs this maneuver by placing the hands between the:
   1. Umbilicus and the groin
   2. Groin and the abdomen
   3. Umbilicus and the xiphoid process
   4. Lower abdomen and the chest

5. A nurse is performing basic life support (BLS) on a 7-year-old child. The nurse delivers how many breaths per minute to the child?
   1. 12
   2. 16
   3. 18
   4. 20

6. A nurse is performing cardiopulmonary resuscitation (CPR) on an infant. When performing chest compressions, the nurse understands that the compression rate is at least:
   1. 60 times per minute
   2. 80 times per minute
   3. 100 times per minute
   4. 160 times per minute

7. A nursing instructor teaches a group of students about basic life support (BLS). The instructor asks a student to identify the most appropriate location to assess the pulse of an infant under 1 year of age. Which of the following, if stated by the student, would indicate that the student understands the appropriate assessment procedure?
   1. Brachial
   2. Carotid
   3. Popliteal
   4. Radial

8. A nurse is teaching cardiopulmonary resuscitation (CPR) to a group of community members. The nurse asks a member of the group to describe the reason why blind fingersweeps are avoided in infants. The nurse determines that the person understands this reason if the person makes which statement?
   1. "The object may be forced back farther into the throat."

2. "The mouth is too small to see the object."

3. "The object may have been swallowed."

4. "The infant may bite down on the finger"

9. A nurse is performing cardiopulmonary resuscitation (CPR) on an adult client. The nurse understands that when chest compressions are performed, the sternum should be depressed:
   1. $\frac{1}{2}$ to $\frac{3}{4}$ inch
   2. $\frac{3}{4}$ to 1 inch
   3. $1\frac{1}{2}$ to 2 inches
   4. $2\frac{1}{2}$ to 3 inches

10. A nursing instructor asks a nursing student to describe the procedure for performing the Heimlich maneuver on an unconscious pregnant woman at 8 months' gestation. The student describes the procedure correctly if the student states to:
   1. Perform abdominal thrusts until the object is dislodged

2. Place the hands in the pelvis to perform the thrusts

3. Place a rolled blanket under the right abdominal flank and hip area

4. Perform left lateral abdominal thrusts until the object is dislodged

CRITICAL THINKING: FREE-TEXT ENTRY

A nurse is using an automated external defibrillator (AED) on a victim who collapsed while shopping at a local mall. The nurse follows the instructions on the AED and repeats the defibrillation three times as directed. The defibrillation attempts are unsuccessful. What is the nurse's next action while waiting for emergency medical services to arrive?

Answer: _____

ANSWERS

1. **4**

Rationale: The next nursing action would be to open the airway. Ventilation cannot be initiated unless the airway is opened. Chest compressions are started after the airway is opened and ventilation is initiated. Oxygen may be helpful at some point, but the airway is opened first.

Test-Taking Strategy: Use the process of elimination. Visualize the steps of basic life support to answer the question. Recalling the ABCs—airway, breathing, and circulation—will assist in directing you to option 4. Review the steps of BLS if you had difficulty with this question.

Level of Cognitive Ability: Application

Client Needs: Physiological Integrity

Integrated Concept/Process: Nursing Process/Implementation

Content Area: Adult Health/Cardiovascular

Reference: Potter, P., & Perry, A. (2001). *Fundamentals of nursing* (5th ed.). St. Louis: Mosby, p. 1184.

2. **4**

Rationale: If a pulse is not present, chest compressions will need to be initiated. Proper hand placement for chest compressions is determined by locating the notch where the rib margin meets the sternum, and placing the middle finger on this notch and the index finger next to it. Then, the heel of the opposite hand is placed on the lower half of the sternum close to the index finger. The first hand is removed and placed on top of the hand on the sternum, and chest compressions are begun. This location is the lower half of the sternum.

Test-Taking Strategy: Use the process of elimination. Eliminate options 2 and 3 first because these locations would be ineffective. Visualize the procedure and consider the anatomical location of the heart to answer this question. If you had difficulty with this question, review the landmarks for chest compressions.

Level of Cognitive Ability: Application

Client Needs: Physiological Integrity

Integrated Concept/Process: Nursing Process/Implementation

Content Area: Adult Health/Cardiovascular

Reference: American Heart Association (1997-1999). Special resuscitation situations. *Basic life support for health care providers.* Dallas: Author, pp. 5-14.

3. **4**

Rationale: If a neck injury is suspected, the jaw thrust maneuver is used to open the airway. The head tilt–chin lift produces hyperextension of the neck and could cause complications if a neck injury is present. A flexed position is an inappropriate position for opening the airway.

Test-Taking Strategy: Use the process of elimination. Eliminate options 1 and 3 first because they are similarly stated. Next, eliminate option 2, since this position would not open the airway. If you had difficulty with this question, review the appropriate methods to open an airway.

Level of Cognitive Ability: Application

Client Needs: Safe, Effective Care Environment

Integrated Concept/Process: Nursing Process/Implementation

Content Area: Adult Health/Neurological

Reference: American Heart Association (1997-1999). Special resuscitation situations. *Basic life support for health care providers.* Dallas: Author, pp. 5-9.

4. **3**

Rationale: To perform the Heimlich maneuver on a child, the rescuer stands behind the victim and places the arms directly under the victim's axillae and around the victim. The thumb side of one fist is placed against the victim's abdomen in the midline slightly above the umbilicus and well below the tip of the xiphoid process. The fist is grasped with the other hand, and up to five thrusts are delivered. Care must be taken not to touch the xiphoid process or the lower margins of the rib cage because force applied to these structures may damage internal organs.

Test-Taking Strategy: Use the process of elimination, noting the age of the child. Eliminate options 1 and 2 first because they are similar. From the remaining options, consider the anatomical location and the effect of the maneuver in dislodging an obstruction. If you had difficulty with this question, review the correct hand placement for the Heimlich maneuver.

Level of Cognitive Ability: Application
Client Needs: Safe, Effective Care Environment
Integrated Concept/Process: Nursing Process/Implementation
Content Area: Child Health
Reference: Wong, D. (1999). *Whaley & Wong's nursing care of infants and children* (6th ed.). St. Louis: Mosby, p. 1453.

5. **4**

Rationale: In a child between the ages of 1 and 8 years, 20 breaths per minute are delivered. Initially, the nurse would give the child two breaths at 1 to 1.5 seconds per breath. Options 1, 2, and 3 are incorrect.

Test-Taking Strategy: Use the process of elimination and note the age of the child. Knowledge regarding the normal respiratory rate in a child at this age will assist in directing you to option 4. If you had difficulty with this question, review BLS for a child.

Level of Cognitive Ability: Application
Client Needs: Physiological Integrity
Integrated Concept/Process: Nursing Process/Implementation
Content Area: Child Health
Reference: Wong, D. (1999). *Whaley & Wong's nursing care of infants and children* (6th ed.). St. Louis: Mosby, p. 1447.

6. **3**

Rationale: In an infant, the rate of chest compressions is at least 100 times per minute. Options 1 and 2 identify rates that are too low, and option 4 identifies a rate that is too high.

Test-Taking Strategy: Use the process of elimination, considering the normal heart rate of an infant. Eliminate options 1 and 2 because of the low rates identified in the options. Eliminate option 4 because this rate would be much too rapid for an infant. If you had difficulty with this question, review CPR for an infant.

Level of Cognitive Ability: Application
Client Needs: Physiological Integrity
Integrated Concept/Process: Nursing Process/Implementation
Content Area: Child Health
Reference: Wong, D. (1999). *Whaley & Wong's nursing care of infants and children* (6th ed.). St. Louis: Mosby, p. 1447.

7. **1**

Rationale: To assess a pulse in an infant (under 1 year of age), the pulse should be checked at the brachial artery. The infant's relatively short, fat neck makes palpation of the carotid artery difficult. The popliteal and radial pulses are also difficult to palpate in an infant.

Test-Taking Strategy: Use the process of elimination and knowledge regarding circulatory assessment in an infant. Options 3 and 4 can be easily eliminated. Consider the body structure of an infant to assist in directing you to option 1. Review cardiac assessment and BLS for an infant if you had difficulty with this question.

Level of Cognitive Ability: Analysis
Client Needs: Physiological Integrity
Integrated Concept/Process: Teaching/Learning
Content Area: Child Health
Reference: Wong, D. (1999). *Whaley & Wong's nursing care of infants and children* (6th ed.). St. Louis: Mosby, p. 1447.

8. **1**

Rationale: Blind fingersweeps are not recommended for infants and children because of the risk of forcing the object farther down into the airway. Options 2, 3, and 4 are not directly related to the issue of the question.

Test-Taking Strategy: Use the ABCs—airway, breathing, and circulation—to answer this question. Option 1 addresses the concern of airway patency. If you had difficulty with this question, review obstructed airway management for an infant or a child.

Level of Cognitive Ability: Analysis
Client Needs: Health Promotion and Maintenance
Integrated Concept/Process: Teaching/Learning
Content Area: Child Health
Reference: American Heart Association (1997-1999). Pediatric basic life support. *Basic life support for health care providers.* Dallas: Author, pp. 6-11.

9. **3**

Rationale: When performing CPR on an adult client, the sternum should be depressed 1.5 to 2 inches. Options 1 and 2 identify compression depths that would be ineffective in an adult. Option 4 identifies a depth that could cause injury to the client.

Test-Taking Strategy: Use the process of elimination. Note the key word "adult" in the question. Consider the normal body structure of an adult to assist in answering the question. If you had difficulty with this question, review adult BLS.

Level of Cognitive Ability: Application
Client Needs: Physiological Integrity
Integrated Concept/Process: Nursing Process/Implementation
Content Area: Adult Health/Cardiovascular
Reference: Potter, P., & Perry, A. (2001). *Fundamentals of nursing* (5th ed.). St. Louis: Mosby, p. 1187.

10. **3**

Rationale: To perform the Heimlich maneuver on a woman in an advanced stage of pregnancy, the woman is placed on her back. A wedge, such as a pillow or rolled blanket, should be placed under the right abdominal flank and hip to displace the uterus to the left side of the abdomen. Options 1, 2, and 4 are incorrect and can cause harm to the woman and the fetus.

Test-Taking Strategy: Use the process of elimination and note that the client is an unconscious pregnant woman at 8 months' gestation. Recall the concepts associated with hypotension and vena cava syndrome to assist in directing you to option 3. Review the principles associated with performing the Heimlich maneuver on a pregnant woman if you had difficulty with this question.

Level of Cognitive Ability: Analysis
Client Needs: Safe, Effective Care Environment
Integrated Concept/Process: Nursing Process/Evaluation
Content Area: Maternity
Reference: Lowdermilk, D., Perry, S., & Bobak, I. (2000). *Maternity & women's health care* (7th ed.). St. Louis: Mosby, p. 895.

CRITICAL THINKING: FREE-TEXT ENTRY

Answer: Perform cardiopulmonary resuscitation (CPR)
Rationale: If the attempt at defibrillation is ineffective, the

nurse performs CPR for 1 minute and then another series of three shocks is delivered.

Test-Taking Strategy: Focus on the key words "next action" and the issue, that defibrillation attempts have been unsuccessful. Also note that the nurse is waiting for emergency medical services to arrive. Use the ABCs—airway, breathing, and circulation—to direct your thinking to the need to perform CPR.

Level of Cognitive Ability: Application
Client Needs: Physiological Integrity
Integrated Concept/Process: Nursing Process/Implementation
Content Area: Adult Health/Cardiovascular
Reference: Ignatavicius, D., Workman, M., & Mishler, M. (1999). *Medical-surgical nursing across the health care continuum* (3rd ed.). Philadelphia: W.B. Saunders, p. 798.

REFERENCES

American Heart Association (1997-1999). Pediatric basic life support. *Basic life support for health care providers.* Dallas: Author.

American Heart Association and International Liaison Committee on Resuscitation (2000). *Guidelines 2000 for Cardiopulmonary Resuscitation and Emergency Cardiovascular Care.* Dallas: Author.

Ignatavicius, D., Workman, M., & Mishler, M. (1999). *Medical-surgical nursing across the health care continuum* (3rd ed.). Philadelphia: W.B. Saunders.

Lowdermilk, D., Perry, S., & Bobak, I. (2000). *Maternity & women's health care* (7th ed.). St. Louis: Mosby.

Potter, P., & Perry, A. (2001). *Fundamentals of nursing* (5th ed.). St. Louis: Mosby.

Wong, D. (1999). *Whaley & Wong's nursing care of infants and children* (6th ed.). St. Louis: Mosby.

Perioperative Nursing Care

PYRAMID TERMS

atelectasis   A collapsed or airless state of the lung that may be the result of airway obstruction caused by accumulated secretions or failure of the client to deep breathe. It is the most common postoperative complication and usually occurs 1 to 2 days after surgery.

extended postoperative stage   The period of at least 1 to 4 days after surgery.

immediate postoperative stage   The period of 1 to 4 hours after surgery.

intermediate postoperative stage   The period of 4 to 24 hours after surgery.

wound dehiscence   Opening of the wound edges.

wound evisceration   Protrusion of internal organs and tissues through an opening in the wound edges.

▲ PYRAMID TO SUCCESS

Pyramid points focus on teaching the client and family or significant other in the preoperative stage, preparing the client for the operative procedure, ensuring that prescribed preoperative tests and procedures such as x-rays or laboratory studies have been performed, and ensuring that the results of the tests and procedures are within expected ranges and are documented. In the postoperative stage, pyramid points focus on monitoring for surgical complications and on the implementation of initial nursing measures if a complication arises. Pyramid points also focus on preparing the client for discharge, teaching related to the prescribed treatments, and the mobilization of home care support services as needed. The Integrated Concepts and Processes addressed in this chapter include Nursing Process, Caring, Communication and Documentation, Cultural Awareness, Self-Care, and Teaching/Learning.

CLIENT NEEDS
Safe, Effective Care Environment

Advance directives
Client rights
Establishing priorities
Informed consent for the surgical procedure
Informing the client of the surgical process
Preventing a surgical infection
Providing safety to the medicated client
Referral to home care and other support services
Surgical asepsis
Standard (universal) precautions

Health Promotion and Maintenance

Client and family teaching related to the prescribed discharge plan
Expected body image changes
Health and wellness teaching to prevent complications
Promoting lifestyle choices
Techniques of physical assessment

Psychosocial Integrity

Assessment of psychosocial concerns
Assisting the client to develop coping methods
Promoting an environment that will allow the client to express concerns
Support systems
Therapeutic interactions
Unexpected body image changes

Physiological Integrity

Safe administration of preoperative and postoperative medications

Safe administration of IV fluids and blood products as prescribed

Providing respiratory therapy

Providing basic care and comfort

Monitoring for surgical complications

Monitoring for wound infection

Monitoring for unexpected responses to treatments and procedures

Initiating nursing interventions when surgical complications arise

I. PREOPERATIVE CARE

A. Obtaining informed consent
  1. The surgeon is responsible for obtaining the consent for surgery
  2. No sedation should be administered to the client before he or she signs the consent
  3. Minors may need a parent or legal guardian to sign the consent form
  4. Older clients may need a legal guardian to sign the consent form
  5. The nurse may witness the client's signing of the consent form, but the nurse must be sure that the client has understood the surgeon's explanation of the surgery
  6. The nurse needs to document the witnessing of the signing of the consent form, after the client acknowledges understanding the procedure

B. Nutrition
  1. Assess the physician's orders regarding the NPO status prior to surgery
  2. Solid foods and liquids are withheld for 6 to 8 hours before general anesthesia and for 3 hours before surgery with local anesthesia, to avoid aspiration
  3. Prepare to initiate an IV and administer IV fluids as prescribed
  4. Prepare to administer total parenteral nutrition (TPN) to clients who are malnourished, have protein or metabolic deficiencies, or cannot ingest foods

C. Elimination
  1. If the client is to have intestinal or abdominal surgery, an enema or laxative or both may be prescribed the night before surgery
  2. The client should void immediately before surgery
  3. Prepare to insert a Foley catheter if prescribed
  4. If there is a Foley catheter in place, it should be emptied immediately before surgery and the amount and quality of urine output documented

D. Surgical site
  1. Prepare to clean the surgical site with a mild antiseptic soap the night before surgery, as prescribed
  2. Prepare to shave the operative site as prescribed
  3. Hair should be shaved only if it will interfere with the surgical procedure and only if prescribed
  4. Shaving of hair, if prescribed, should be done in the direction of hair growth and with a sharp razor, and caution should be used to prevent cuts or epidermal damage

E. Preoperative client teaching
  1. Inform the client about what to expect postoperatively
  2. Inform the client to notify the nurse if any pain is experienced postoperatively and that pain medication will be prescribed to be given as the client requests
  3. Inform the client that requesting a narcotic after surgery will not make the client a drug addict
  4. Demonstrate the use of a client-controlled analgesia pump if its use is prescribed
  5. Instruct the client to use the noninvasive pain relief techniques, such as relaxation, distraction techniques, and guided imagery, before the pain occurs and as soon as the pain is noticed
  6. The client should be instructed not to smoke for at least 24 hours before surgery
  7. Instruct the client in deep breathing and coughing techniques, the use of incentive spirometry, and the importance of performing the techniques postoperatively to prevent the development of pneumonia and **atelectasis** (Box 18-1 and Fig. 18-1)
  8. Instruct the client in leg and foot exercises to prevent venous stasis of blood and facilitate venous blood return (Box 18-1 and Fig. 18-2)
  9. Instruct the client in how to splint an incision and to turn and reposition (Box 18-1 and Fig. 18-3)
  10. Inform the client of any invasive devices that may be needed after surgery, such as nasogastric tube, drain, Foley catheter, epidural catheter, intravenous or subclavian lines
  11. Instruct the client not to pull on any of the invasive devices, as they will be removed as soon as possible

F. Psychosocial preparation
  1. Be alert to the client's anxiety level
  2. Answer any questions or concerns the client may have regarding surgery
  3. Allow time for privacy for the client to prepare for surgery psychologically
  4. Provide support and assistance as needed

G. Preoperative checklist
  1. Ensure that the client is wearing an identification bracelet
  2. Assess for allergies (refer to Chapter 67 for information on latex allergy)
  3. Review the preoperative checklist to be sure that each item is addressed before the client is transported to surgery

BOX 18-1

Client Teaching

DEEP BREATHING AND COUGHING EXERCISES

Instruct the client that a sitting position gives the best lung expansion for coughing and deep breathing exercises.

Instruct the client to breathe deeply three times, inhaling through the nostrils and exhaling slowly through pursed lips.

Instruct the client that the third breath should be held for three seconds; then the client should cough deeply three times.

The client should perform this exercise every 2 hours.

INCENTIVE SPIROMETRY

Instruct the client to assume a sitting position.

Instruct the client to place the mouth tightly around the mouthpiece.

Instruct the client to inhale slowly to raise and maintain the flow rate indicator between the 600 and 900 marks.

Instruct the client to hold the breath for 5 seconds, and then to exhale through pursed lips.

Instruct the client to repeat this process ten times every hour.

LEG AND FOOT EXERCISES

Gastrocnemius (calf) pumping: Instruct the client to move both ankles by pointing the toes up and then down.

Quadriceps (thigh) setting: Instruct the client to press the back of the knees against the bed, and then to relax the knees; this contracts and relaxes the thigh and calf muscles to prevent thrombus formation.

Foot circles: Instruct the client to rotate each foot in a circle.

Hip and knee movements: Instruct the client to flex the knee and thigh and to straighten the leg and hold the position for 5 seconds before lowering (not performed if the client is having abdominal surgery or if the client has a back problem).

SPLINTING THE INCISION

If the surgical incision is abdominal or thoracic, instruct the client to place a pillow, or one hand with the other hand on top, over the incisional area.

During deep breathing and coughing, the client presses gently against the incisional area to splint or support it.

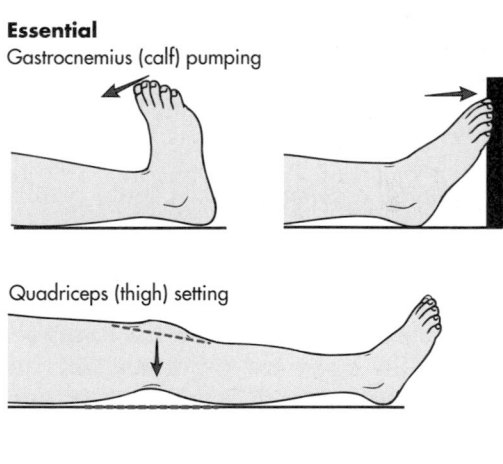

Essential
Gastrocnemius (calf) pumping

Quadriceps (thigh) setting

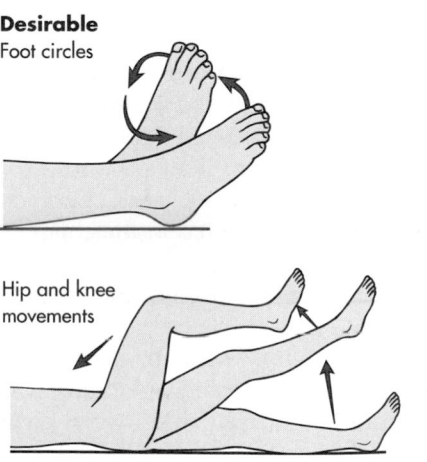

Desirable
Foot circles

Hip and knee movements

FIG. 18-1 Incentive spirometer. (From Phipps WJ, Sands JK, Marek JF: *Medical-surgical nursing: concepts and clinical practice,* ed 6, St Louis, 1999, Mosby.)

FIG. 18-2 Postoperative leg exercises. (From Lewis SL, Collier IC, Heitkemper MM, Dirksen SR: *Medical-surgical nursing: assessment and management of clinical problems,* ed 5, St Louis, 2000, Mosby.)

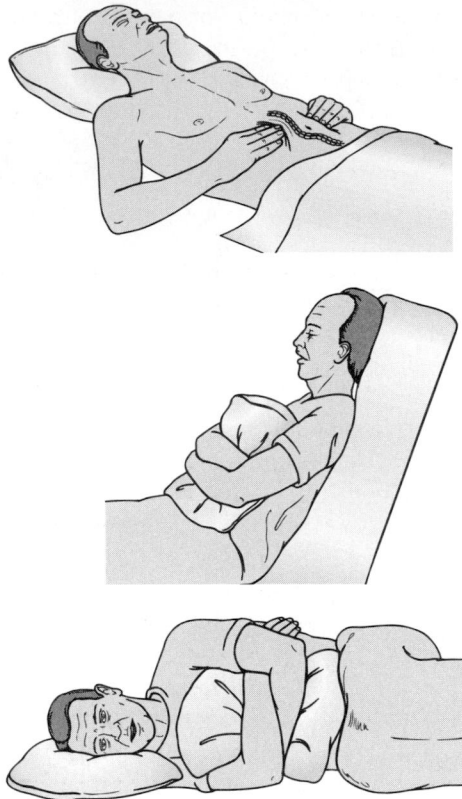

FIG. 18-3 Techniques for splinting wound when coughing. (From Lewis SL, Collier IC, Heitkemper MM, Dirksen SR: *Medical-surgical nursing: assessment and management of clinical problems,* ed 5, St Louis, 2000, Mosby.)

4. Ensure that informed consent forms were signed for the operative procedure, for any blood transfusions, for disposal of a limb, or for surgical sterilization procedures
5. Ensure that a history and physical exam were completed and documented in the client's record
6. Ensure that consultations prescribed were completed and documented in the client's record
7. Ensure that prescribed laboratory results are documented in the client's record
8. Ensure that the ECG and chest radiograph reports are documented in the client's record
9. Ensure that a blood type and screen or type and cross-match is performed and documented in the client's record
10. Remove jewelry, makeup, dentures, hairpins, nail polish, glasses, and prostheses
11. Document that valuables were given to the client's family members or locked in the hospital safe
12. Document the last time the client ate or drank
13. Document that the client has voided prior to surgery

14. Document that the prescribed preoperative medication was given (Box 18-2)
15. Monitor and document the client's vital signs
H. Preoperative medications
   1. Prepare to administer preoperative medications

BOX 18-2

Medications That Can Affect the Surgical Client

ANTIBIOTICS
Potentiate the action of anesthetic agents.
If taken for 2 weeks before surgery, aminoglycosides such as gentamycin (Garamycin), tobramycin (Nebcin), and neomycin (Mycifradin) may cause mild respiratory depression as a result of depressed neuromuscular transmission.

ANTIDYSRHYTHMICS
Reduce cardiac contractility and impair cardiac conduction during anesthesia.

ANTICOAGULANTS
Alter normal clotting factors and increase the risk of hemorrhaging.
Aspirin (acetylsalicylic acid, ASA) and ibuprofen (Motrin, Advil) are commonly used medications that can alter clotting mechanisms.
These medications should be discontinued at least 48 hours before surgery.

ANTICONVULSANTS
Long-term use of certain anticonvulsants can alter the metabolism of anesthetic agents.

ANTIHYPERTENSIVES
Can interact with anesthetic agents and cause bradycardia, hypotension, and impaired circulation.

CORTICOSTEROIDS
Cause adrenal atrophy and reduce the body's ability to withstand stress.
Before and during surgery, dosages may be temporarily increased.

INSULIN
The need for insulin after surgery in a diabetic either may be reduced because the client's nutritional intake is decreased or may be increased because of the stress response and IV administration of glucose solutions.

DIURETICS
Potentiate electrolyte imbalances after surgery.

ANTIDEPRESSANTS
May lower the blood pressure during anesthesia.

ANTICHOLINERGICS
Medications with anticholinergic effects increase the potential for confusion.

as prescribed, or on call to the operating room immediately before surgery

2. Instruct the client that he or she will feel drowsy shortly after the medications are administered
3. After administering the preoperative medications, keep the client in bed with the side rails up
4. Place the call bell next to the client; instruct the client not to get out of bed and to call for assistance if needed

I. Arrival in the operating room
1. When the client arrives in the operating room, the operating room nurse will verify the identification bracelet with the client's verbal response and will review the client's chart
2. The operating room nurse will confirm the operative procedure and the site to be operated on
3. The client's chart will be checked for completeness and reviewed for informed consent forms, a history and physical examination, and allergic reaction information
4. Physicians' orders will be reviewed, and that they were carried out will be verified
5. The IV line may be initiated at this time if prescribed
6. The anesthesia team will administer the prescribed anesthesia

II. POSTOPERATIVE CARE
A. Immediate stage
1. Description: The period of 1 to 4 hours after surgery
2. Respiratory system
   a. Monitor vital signs
   b. Monitor airway patency and adequate ventilation, since prolonged mechanical ventilation during anesthesia may affect postoperative lung function
   c. Remember that extubated clients who are lethargic may not be able to maintain an airway
   d. Monitor for secretions, and remove them by suctioning if the client is unable to clear the airway by coughing
   e. Observe chest movement for symmetry and the use of accessory muscles
   f. Monitor oxygen administration if prescribed
   g. Monitor pulse oximetry
   h. Encourage deep breathing and coughing exercises as soon as possible
   i. Note the rate, depth, and quality of respirations; the respiratory rate should be greater than 10 and less than 30 breaths per minute
   j. Assess breath sounds
   k. Stridor, wheezing, or crowing can indicate partial obstruction, bronchospasm, or laryngospasm; crackles or rhonchi may indicate pulmonary edema
   l. Monitor the client for signs of **atelectasis,** pneumonia, or pulmonary embolism
3. Cardiovascular system
   a. Assess the client's color and check capillary refill
   b. Assess peripheral pulses and for peripheral edema
   c. Monitor for bleeding
   d. Assess pulse for rate and rhythm; a bounding pulse may indicate hypertension, fluid overload, or excitement
   e. Monitor for signs of hypertension and hypotension
   f. Monitor for cardiac dysrhythmias
   g. Assess for Homans' sign, particularly in clients positioned in lithotomy position during surgery, as these clients may be predisposed to developing deep vein thrombosis
4. Musculoskeletal system
   a. Assess the client for moving extremities
   b. Assess physician's orders regarding client positioning or restrictions
   c. Unless contraindicated, place client in a low-Fowler's position after surgery to increase the size of the thorax for lung expansion
   d. Avoid positioning the client in a supine position until pharyngeal reflexes have returned
   e. If the client is comatose or semicomatose, position on the side and keep an oral airway in place
5. Neurological system
   a. Assess level of consciousness
   b. Frequent periodic attempts to awaken the client should continue until the client awakens
   c. Orient the client to environment
   d. Speak in a soft tone, and filter out extraneous noises in the environment
   e. Maintain body temperature and prevent heat loss by providing the client with warm blankets and raising the room temperature as necessary
6. Temperature control
   a. Monitor temperature
   b. Monitor for signs of hypothermia that may result from anesthesia, a cool operating room, and exposure of the skin and internal organs during surgery
   c. Apply warm blankets and continue oxygen as prescribed if the client is shivering
7. Integumentary system
   a. Assess surgical site, drains, and wound dressings
   b. Monitor for and document any drainage or bleeding from the surgical site
   c. Assess skin for redness, abrasions, or break-

down that may have resulted from surgical positioning

8. Fluid and electrolyte balance
   a. Monitor IV administration as prescribed
   b. Record I & O
   c. Monitor for signs of hypocalcemia, hyperglycemia, and metabolic and respiratory acidosis or alkalosis
9. Gastrointestinal system
   a. Monitor for nausea and vomiting
   b. Maintain patency of nasogastric tube if present
   c. Monitor for abdominal distension
   d. Monitor for return of bowel sounds
10. Renal system
    a. Assess bladder for distention
    b. Monitor color, quantity, and quality of urine output if a Foley catheter is present
    c. Expect the client to void 6 to 8 hours after the surgical procedure, depending on the type of anesthesia administered
11. Pain management
    a. Assess for pain
    b. Assess the type of anesthetic used and preoperative medication that the client received, and note whether the client received any pain medications in the postanesthesia period
    c. Inquire about the type and location of pain
    d. Ask the client to rate the degree of pain on a scale of 1 to 10, with 10 being the most severe
    e. Monitor for objective data related to pain, such as facial expressions, body gestures, increased pulse rate, increased blood pressure, and increased respirations
    f. Inquire about the effectiveness of the last pain medication
    g. Administer pain medication as prescribed
    h. If a narcotic has been prescribed, during the initial administration, assess the client every 30 minutes for respiratory rate and pain relief
    i. Use noninvasive measures to relieve postoperative pain, including distraction, comfort measures, positioning, backrubs, and providing a quiet and restful environment
    j. Document effectiveness of pain medication

B. Intermediate stage
   1. Description: The period of 4 to 24 hours after surgery
   2. Respiratory system
      a. Monitor vital signs
      b. Continue assessments as during the immediate stage
      c. Monitor patency of airway, verifying that the lungs are clear on auscultation
      d. Encourage deep breathing and coughing

3. Cardiovascular system
   a. Monitor circulatory status, such as peripheral pulses, capillary refill, and the absence of edema, numbness, and tingling
   b. Encourage the use of antiembolism stockings, if prescribed, to promote venous return, strengthen muscle tone, and prevent pooling of secretions in the lungs
4. Musculoskeletal system
   a. Assess for movement in all extremities and encourage ambulation
   b. Before ambulation, instruct the client to sit at the edge of the bed with the feet supported
   c. If the client is unable to get out of bed, turn client every 1 to 2 hours
5. Neurological system
   a. Assess level of consciousness
   b. Maintain orientation to the environment
6. Integumentary system
   a. Assess surgical site and drains
   b. Monitor temperature and wound for signs of infection
   c. Maintain a dry and intact dressing
   d. Reinforce wound with a sterile dressing if necessary, and notify the physician if bleeding occurs from the site
   e. Change dressings as prescribed, noting the amount of bleeding or drainage, odor, and intactness of sutures or staples
   f. Use an abdominal binder for obese and debilitated individuals to prevent rupture of the incision (Fig. 18-4)
   g. Drains should be patent, and there should be minimal bleeding or drainage
   h. Prepare to assist with the removal of drains as prescribed by the physician when the drainage amount becomes insignificant
7. Gastrointestinal system
   a. Monitor I & O
   b. Monitor for nausea and vomiting
   c. Turn the client to a side-lying position if vomiting occurs, and have suctioning equipment available and ready to use
   d. Administer frequent mouth care
   e. Maintain the NPO status until the gag reflex returns and peristalsis returns
   f. Continue IV fluids as prescribed until the client can tolerate fluids
   g. When oral fluids are permitted, start with ice chips and water
   h. Ensure that the client advances to clear liquids and then to a regular diet as prescribed
   i. Assess for bowel sounds in all four quadrants
   j. Monitor the client for gas pains and encourage ambulation
8. Renal system
   a. Monitor urinary output (should be greater than 30 mL per hour)

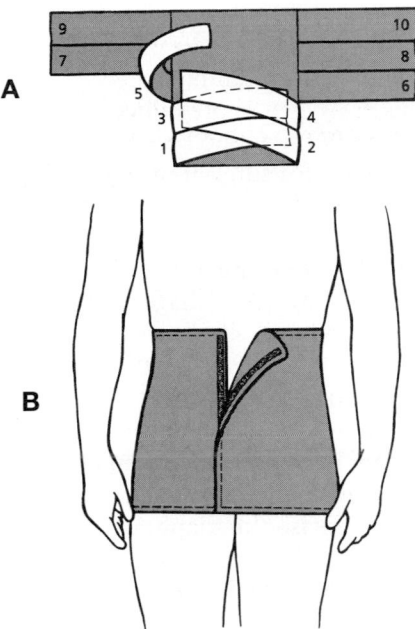
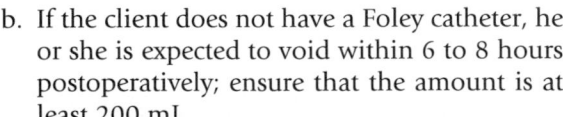

FIG. 18-4   Abdominal binders. **A,** Scultetus. **B,** Straight. (From Elkin ME, Perry AG, Potter PA: *Nursing interventions and clinical skills,* ed 2, St Louis, 2000, Mosby.)

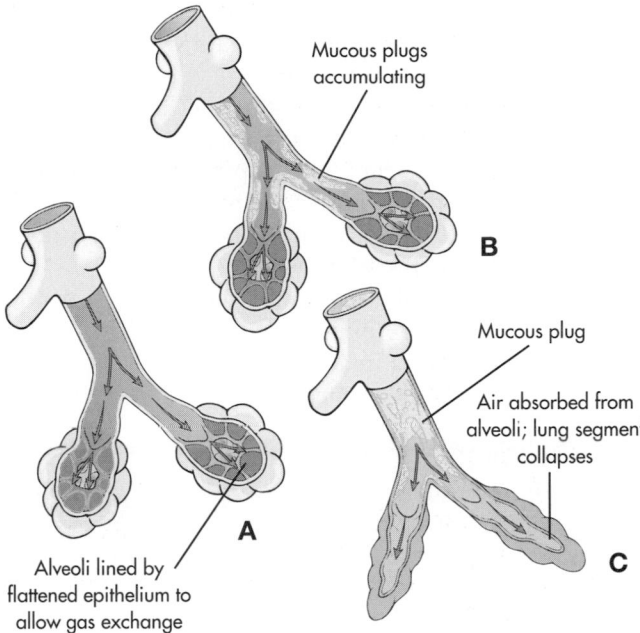

FIG. 18-5   Postoperative atelectasis. **A,** Normal bronchiole and alveoli. **B,** Mucus plug in bronchiole. **C,** Collapse of alveoli as a result of atelectasis following absorption of air. (From Lewis SL, Collier IC, Heitkemper MM, Dirksen SR: *Medical-surgical nursing: assessment and management of clinical problems,* ed 5, St Louis, 2000, Mosby.)

b. If the client does not have a Foley catheter, he or she is expected to void within 6 to 8 hours postoperatively; ensure that the amount is at least 200 mL

9. Pain management: Continue with assessments and interventions as during the immediate stage

C. Extended stage

1. Description: The period of at least 1 to 4 days postoperatively

2. Implementation

a. Continue to assess and observe the client's body systems during this stage

b. Monitor for signs of infection, such as redness, swelling, and tenderness at the surgical site, fever, and leukocytosis

c. Encourage active range of motion exercises every 2 hours

d. Continue to encourage ambulation, which will promote peristalsis and the passage of flatus

e. Increase ambulation every day to increase muscle strength

f. Encourage the client to perform as many of activities of daily living as possible

g. Instruct the client to eat foods that are high in protein and vitamin C content to promote wound healing

III. PNEUMONIA AND ATELECTASIS (Box 18-3 and Fig. 18-5)

A. Description

1. Pneumonia: An inflammation of the alveoli

BOX 18-3

Postoperative Complications

Pneumonia and atelectasis
Hypoxia
Pulmonary embolism
Hemorrhage
Shock
Thrombophlebitis
Urinary retention
Constipation
Paralytic ileus
Wound infection
Wound dehiscence
Wound evisceration

---

caused by an infectious process; may develop 3 to 5 days postoperatively as a result of infection, aspiration, or immobility

2. **Atelectasis:** A collapse of the alveoli with retained mucous secretions; the most common postoperative complication; usually occurs 1 to 2 days postoperatively

B. Assessment

1. Assess for factors that may increase the risk of pneumonia and **atelectasis**

2. Dyspnea and increased respiratory rate

3. Crackles over involved lung area

4. Elevated temperature
5. Productive cough and chest pain

C. Implementation
1. Assess lung and breath sounds
2. Reposition the client every 1 to 2 hours
3. Encourage the client to deep breathe and cough and to use the incentive spirometer
4. Provide chest physiotherapy (CPT) postural drainage as prescribed
5. Suction to clear secretions if the client is unable to cough
6. Encourage fluid intake
7. Encourage early ambulation

▲ **IV. HYPOXIA** (Box 18-3)
A. Description: An inadequate concentration of oxygen in arterial blood
B. Assessment
1. Restlessness
2. Dyspnea
3. Hypertension
4. Tachycardia
5. Diaphoresis
6. Cyanosis
C. Implementation
1. Monitor for signs of hypoxia
2. Eliminate the cause of hypoxia
3. Monitor lung sounds and pulse oximetry
4. Administer oxygen as prescribed
5. Encourage deep breathing and coughing and use of the incentive spirometer
6. Turn and reposition the client

V. PULMONARY EMBOLISM (Box 18-3)
A. Description: An embolus blocking the pulmonary artery and disrupting blood flow to one or more lobes of the lung
B. Assessment
1. Dyspnea
2. Sudden sharp chest or upper abdominal pain
3. Cyanosis
4. Tachycardia
5. A drop in blood pressure
C. Implementation
1. Notify the physician immediately
2. Monitor vital signs
3. Administer oxygen and medications as prescribed

VI. HEMORRHAGE (Box 18-3)
A. Description: The loss of a large amount of blood externally or internally in a short period of time
B. Assessment
1. Restlessness
2. Weak and rapid pulse
3. Hypotension
4. Tachypnea
5. Cool, clammy skin
6. Reduced urine output

C. Implementation
1. Provide pressure to the site of bleeding
2. Notify the physician immediately
3. Administer oxygen as prescribed
4. Administer IV fluids and blood as prescribed
5. Prepare client for surgical procedure if necessary

VII. SHOCK (Box 18-3) ▲
A. Description: Loss of circulatory fluid volume, which is usually caused by hemorrhage
B. Assessment: Similar to assessment findings in hemorrhage
C. Implementation
1. If shock develops, elevate the legs
2. If the client had spinal anesthesia, do not elevate the legs any higher than placing them on the pillow; otherwise the diaphragm muscles could be impaired
3. Determine and treat the cause of shock
4. Administer oxygen as prescribed
5. Monitor level of consciousness
6. Monitor vital signs for increased pulse or decreased blood pressure
7. Monitor I & O
8. Assess color, temperature, turgor, and moisture of skin and mucous membranes
9. Administer IV fluids, blood, and colloid solutions as prescribed

VIII. THROMBOPHLEBITIS (Box 18-3)
A. Description
1. Inflammation of a vein, often accompanied by clot formation
2. Veins in the legs are most commonly affected
B. Assessment
1. Vein inflammation
2. Aching or cramping pain
3. Vein feels hard and cordlike and is tender to touch
4. Elevated temperature
5. Positive Homans' sign
C. Implementation
1. Monitor legs for swelling, inflammation, pain, tenderness, venous distention, and cyanosis
2. Elevate the extremity 30 degrees without allowing any pressure on the popliteal area
3. Encourage the use of antiembolism stockings as prescribed; remove stockings twice a day to wash and inspect the legs
4. Use intermittent pulsatile compression device as prescribed (Fig. 18-6)
5. Perform passive range of motion every 2 hours if the client is on bed rest
6. Encourage early ambulation as prescribed
7. Do not allow the client to dangle the legs
8. Instruct the client not to sit in one position for an extended period of time
9. Administer heparin sodium or warfarin (Coumadin) as prescribed

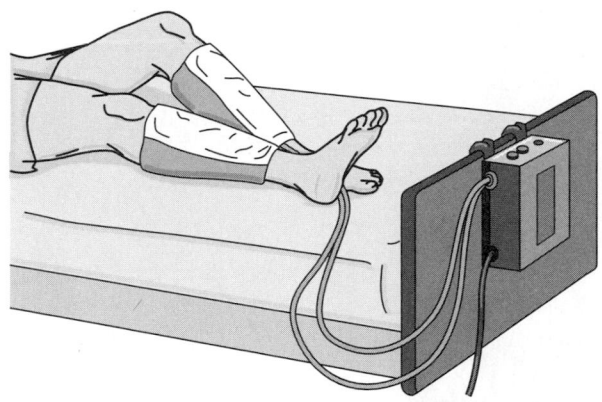

FIG. 18-6 Intermittent pulsatile compression device (IPC). (From Phipps WJ, Sands JK, Marek JF: *Medical-surgical nursing: concepts and clinical practice*, ed 6, St Louis, 1999, Mosby.)

IX. URINARY RETENTION (Box 18-3)
A. Description
   1. Involuntary accumulation of urine in the bladder as a result of loss of muscle tone
   2. Due to the effects of anesthetics and narcotic analgesics
   3. Appears 6 to 8 hours after surgery
B. Assessment
   1. Inability to void
   2. Restlessness and diaphoresis
   3. Lower abdominal pain and a distended bladder
   4. Hypertension
   5. On percussion, the bladder sounds like a drum
C. Implementation
   1. Monitor for voiding
   2. Assess for distended bladder
   3. Encourage ambulation when prescribed
   4. Encourage fluid intake unless contraindicated
   5. Assist the client to void by helping to stand
   6. Provide privacy
   7. Pour warm water over the perineum or allow the client to hear running water to promote voiding
   8. Catheterize the client as prescribed after all noninvasive techniques have been attempted

X. CONSTIPATION (Box 18-3)
A. Description
   1. Infrequent passage of stool
   2. When the client resumes a solid diet postoperatively, failure to pass stool within 48 hours is a cause for concern
B. Assessment
   1. Abdominal distention
   2. Absence of bowel movements
   3. Anorexia, headache, and nausea
C. Implementation
   1. Assess bowel sounds

   2. Encourage fluid intake up to 3000 mL per day unless contraindicated
   3. Encourage early ambulation
   4. Encourage consumption of fiber foods unless contraindicated
   5. Administer stool softeners and laxatives as prescribed
   6. Provide privacy and adequate time for bowel elimination

XI. PARALYTIC ILEUS (Box 18-3)
A. Description
   1. Failure of appropriate forward movement of bowel contents
   2. May occur as a result of anesthetic medications or manipulation of the bowel during the surgical procedure
B. Assessment
   1. Nausea and vomiting immediately postoperatively
   2. Abdominal distention
   3. Absence of bowel sounds, bowel movement, or flatus
C. Implementation
   1. Monitor I & O
   2. Maintain NPO status until bowel sounds return
   3. Maintain patency of NG tube if in place
   4. Encourage ambulation
   5. Administer IV fluids or TPN as prescribed
   6. Administer medications as prescribed to increase GI motility and secretions
   7. If ileus occurs, it is first treated nonsurgically by bowel decompression by insertion of an NG tube attached to intermittent to constant suction

XII. WOUND INFECTION (Box 18-3)
A. Description
   1. Caused by poor aseptic technique or a contaminated wound before surgical exploration
   2. Usually occurs 3 to 6 days after surgery
   3. Purulent material may exit from the drains or separated wound edges
B. Assessment
   1. Fever and chills
   2. Warm, tender, painful, and inflamed incision site
   3. Edematous skin at incision and tight skin sutures
   4. Elevated white blood cell count
C. Implementation
   1. Monitor temperature
   2. Monitor incision site for approximation of suture line, edema, or bleeding, and signs of infection
   3. Maintain patency of drains, and assess drainage amount, color, and consistency
   4. Keep drain and tubes away from incision line, and maintain asepsis
   5. Change dressing as prescribed
   6. Administer antibiotics as prescribed

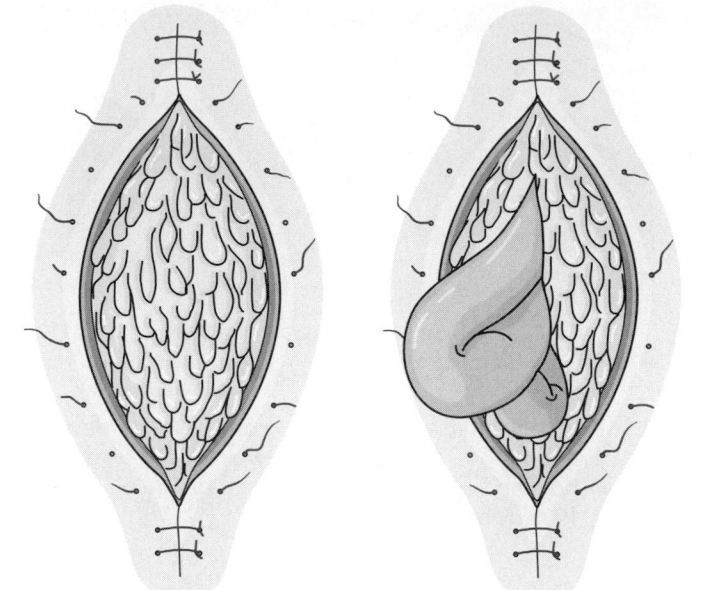

FIG. 18-7 **A,** Wound dehiscence. **B,** Wound evisceration. (From Phipps WJ, Sands JK, Marek JF: *Medical-surgical nursing: concepts and clinical practice,* ed 6, St Louis, 1999, Mosby.)

XIII. WOUND DEHISCENCE (Box 18-3 and Fig. 18-7)

A. Description
   1. Separation of the wound edges at the suture line
   2. Usually occurs 6 to 8 days after surgery
B. Assessment
   1. Increased drainage
   2. Opened wound edges
   3. Appearance of underlying tissues through the wound
C. Implementation
   1. Notify the physician immediately
   2. Cover the wound with a sterile normal saline dressing
   3. Place the client in low-Fowler's position with knees bent to prevent abdominal tension on an abdominal suture line
   4. Prevent wound infection
   5. Administer antiemetics as prescribed to prevent vomiting and further strain on the abdominal incision
   6. Instruct the client to splint the abdominal incision when coughing

XIV. WOUND EVISCERATION (Box 18-3 and Fig. 18-7)

A. Description
   1. Protrusion of the internal organs and tissues through an opening in the wound edges
   2. Most common among obese clients, clients who have had abdominal surgery, or those who have poor wound-healing ability
   3. Usually occurs 6 to 8 days after surgery
   4. Wound evisceration is an emergency
B. Assessment

   1. Discharge of serosanguinous fluid from a previously dry wound
   2. The appearance of loops of bowel or other abdominal contents through the wound
   3. The client may report feeling a popping sensation after coughing or turning
C. Implementation
   1. Notify the physician immediately
   2. Cover the wound with a sterile normal saline dressing
   3. Place the client in low-Fowler's position with knees bent to prevent abdominal tension
   4. Prevent wound infection
   5. Administer antiemetics as prescribed to prevent vomiting and further strain on the incision
   6. Instruct the client to splint the incision when coughing

XV. AMBULATORY SURGERY

A. Criteria for client discharge
   1. Is alert and oriented
   2. Has voided
   3. Has no respiratory distress
   4. Is able to ambulate, swallow, and cough
   5. Has minimal pain
   6. Is not vomiting
   7. Has minimal, if any, bleeding from incision site
   8. A responsible adult is available to drive the client home
   9. The surgeon has signed a release form
B. Discharge teaching (Box 18-4)
   1. Should be performed prior to the date of the scheduled procedure

BOX 18-4

Postoperative Discharge Teaching

Assess the client's readiness to learn, educational level, and desire to change or modify lifestyle.

Assess the need for resources needed for home care.

Demonstrate care to the incision and how to change the dressing.

Instruct the client to cover the incision with plastic if showering is allowed.

Be sure the client is provided with a 48-hour supply of dressings for home use.

Instruct the client on the importance of returning to the physician's office for follow-up.

Instruct the client that sutures are usually removed in the physician's office 7 to 10 days after surgery.

Inform the client that staples are removed 7 to 14 days after surgery and that the skin may become slightly reddened when they are ready to be removed.

Steri-Strips may be applied to provide extra support after the sutures are removed.

Instruct the client on the use of medications, their purpose, doses, administration, and side effects.

Instruct the client on diet and to drink 6 to 8 glasses of liquid a day.

Instruct the client on activity levels and to resume normal activities gradually.

Instruct the client to avoid lifting for 6 weeks if a major surgical procedure was performed.

Instruct the client with an abdominal incision not to lift anything weighing 10 pounds or more and not to engage in any activities that involve pushing or pulling.

Clients usually can return to work in 6 to 8 weeks as prescribed by the physician.

Instruct the client on the signs and symptoms of complications and when to call a physician.

2. Provide written instructions to the client and family regarding the specifics of care
3. Instruct the client and family about postoperative complications that can occur
4. Provide appropriate resources for home care support
5. Instruct the client not to drive for 24 hours if he or she has had general anesthesia
6. Instruct the client to call the surgeon, ambulatory center, or emergency department if postoperative problems occur
7. Instruct the client to keep follow-up appointments with the surgeon

PRACTICE QUESTIONS

1. A client with a perforated gastric ulcer is scheduled for emergency surgery. The client cannot sign the operative consent form because of sedation from narcotic analgesics that have been administered. The nurse should take which of the following most appropriate actions in the care of this client?
   1. Obtain a telephone consent from a family member and have the consent witnessed by two persons
   2. Obtain a court order for the surgery
   3. Send the client to surgery without the consent form being signed
   4. Have the hospital chaplain sign the informed consent immediately
2. A preoperative client expresses anxiety to a nurse about upcoming surgery. Which response by the nurse is most likely to stimulate further discussion between the client and the nurse?
   1. "I will be happy to explain the entire surgical procedure to you."
   2. "Let me tell you about the care you'll receive after surgery and the amount of pain you can anticipate."
   3. "If it's any help, everyone is nervous before surgery."
   4. "Can you share with me what you've been told about your surgery?"
3. A nurse is conducting preoperative teaching with a client about the use of an incentive spirometer in the postoperative period. The nurse would include which piece of information in discussions with the client?
   1. Keep a loose seal between the lips and the mouthpiece
   2. Inhale as rapidly as possible
   3. After maximum inspiration, hold the breath for 10 seconds and exhale
   4. The best results are achieved when sitting at least half-way or fully upright
4. A nurse has conducted preoperative teaching for a client scheduled for surgery in 1 week's time. The client has a history of arthritis and has been taking acetylsalicylic acid (aspirin, ASA). The nurse determines that the client needs additional teaching if the client states:
   1. "I need to continue to take the aspirin as prescribed until the day of surgery."
   2. "Aspirin can cause bleeding after surgery."
   3. "Aspirin can cause my ability to clot blood to be abnormal."
   4. "I need to discontinue the aspirin 48 hours before the scheduled surgery."
5. A nurse is preparing a preoperative client for transfer to the operating room (OR). The nurse should take which of the following actions in the care of this client at this time?
   1. Administer all the daily medications
   2. Ensure that the client has voided
   3. Verify that the client has not eaten for the last 24 hours
   4. Practice postoperative breathing exercises

6. A nurse in a surgical unit receives a postoperative client from the post-anesthesia care unit (PACU). After the initial assessment of the client, the nurse plans to continue with postoperative assessment activities:
   1. Every 5 minutes for the first half-hour, every 15 minutes for 2 hours, every 30 minutes for 4 hours, and then every hour as needed
   2. Every 15 minutes for the first hour, every 30 minutes for 2 hours, every hour for 4 hours, and then every 4 hours as needed
   3. Every 30 minutes for the first hour, every hour for 2 hours, and then every 4 hours as needed
   4. Every hour for 2 hours, and then every 4 hours as needed

7. A nurse receives a telephone call from the postanesthesia care unit (PACU) stating that a client is being transferred to the surgical unit. The nurse plans do which of the following first upon arrival of the client?
   1. Assess the patency of the airway
   2. Assess the vital signs (VS) to compare with preoperative measurements
   3. Check the dressing to assess for bleeding
   4. Check tubes or drains for patency

8. A nurse has just reassessed the condition of a postoperative client who was admitted 1 hour ago to the surgical unit. The nurse plans to most carefully monitor which of the following parameters during the next hour?
   1. Serous drainage on the surgical dressing
   2. Blood pressure of 100/70 mm Hg
   3. Urinary output of 20 mL/hour
   4. Temperature of 37.6° C. (99.6° F.)

9. A postoperative client asks a nurse why it is so important to deep breathe and cough after surgery. In formulating a response, the nurse incorporates the understanding that retained pulmonary secretions in a postoperative client can lead to:
   1. Fluid imbalance
   2. Carbon dioxide retention
   3. Pulmonary edema
   4. Pneumonia

10. A client is admitted to a surgical unit postoperatively with a wound drain in place. Which action would the nurse avoid in the care of the drain?
    1. Check the drain for patency
    2. Curl the drain tightly and tape firmly to body
    3. Maintain aseptic technique when emptying the drain
    4. Observe for bright red bloody drainage

11. A nurse assesses a client's surgical incision for signs of infection. Which finding by the nurse would be interpreted as a normal finding at the surgical site?
    1. Red, hard skin
    2. Purulent drainage
    3. Serous drainage
    4. Warm, tender skin

12. When performing a surgical dressing change of a client's abdominal dressing, a nurse notes an increase in the amount of drainage and separation of the incision line. The underlying tissue is visible to the nurse. The nurse should plan to do which of the following in the initial care of this wound?
    1. Leave the incision open to the air to dry the area
    2. Apply a Betadine-soaked sterile dressing
    3. Irrigate the wound and apply a sterile dry dressing
    4. Apply a sterile dressing soaked with normal saline

13. A nurse is monitoring the status of a postoperative client. The nurse would become most concerned with which of the following signs, which could indicate an evolving complication?
    1. Blood pressure of 110/70 mm Hg and a pulse of 86 beats per minute
    2. Increasing restlessness
    3. Hypoactive bowel sounds in all four quadrants
    4. A negative Homans' sign

14. A nurse is reviewing a physician's order sheet for a preoperative client that states that the client must be NPO after midnight. The nurse would telephone the physician to clarify whether which of the following medications should be given to the client and not withheld?
    1. Conjugated estrogen (Premarin)
    2. Prednisone (Deltasone)
    3. Cyclobenzaprine (Flexeril)
    4. Ferrous sulfate

15. A client who underwent preadmission testing had serum laboratory studies drawn, including a complete blood count, electrolytes, coagulation studies, and a creatinine level. Which of the following laboratory results would be reported to the surgeon's office by the nurse, knowing that it could cause surgery to be postponed?
    1. Platelets, 210,000/mm^3
    2. Serum creatinine, 0.8 mg/100 mL
    3. Sodium (Na$^+$), 141 mEq/L
    4. Hemoglobin (Hgb), 8.9 g/dL

16. A nurse is developing a plan of care for a preoperative client who has a latex allergy. Which of the following interventions would be included in the plan?
    1. Apply a cloth barrier to the client's arm under a blood pressure (BP) cuff when taking the BP
    2. Use medications that are from ampules with rubber stoppers
    3. Avoid using medications from glass ampules
    4. Avoid using IV tubing that is made of polyvinyl chloride

17. A nurse is developing a plan of care for a client scheduled for surgery. The nurse would include

which of the following activities in the nursing care plan for the client on the day of surgery?
1. Remove nail polish from fingernails and toenails
2. Report immediately any slight increase in blood pressure or pulse
3. Verify that the client has not eaten for the last 24 hours
4. Avoid oral hygiene and rinsing with mouthwash

18. A nurse is developing a list of home care instructions for a client being discharged after a laparoscopic cholecystectomy. Which of the following instructions would be least appropriate to include in the postoperative discharge plan of care?
1. Wound care
2. Activity restrictions
3. Follow-up care
4. Deep breathing exercises

19. A nurse is monitoring a postoperative client after abdominal surgery for signs of complications. The nurse assesses the client for the presence of Homans' sign and determines that this sign is positive if which of the following is noted?
1. Pain with dorsiflexion of the foot
2. Incisional pain

3. Absent bowel sounds
4. Crackles on auscultation of the lungs

20. An operating room nurse is positioning a client on the operating room table so as to prevent the client's extremities from dangling over the sides of the table. A nursing student who is observing for the day asks the nurse why this is so important. The nurse responds that this is done primarily to avoid:
1. A drop in blood pressure
2. Muscle fatigue in the extremities
3. An increase in pulse rate
4. Nerve and muscle damage

CRITICAL THINKING: FREE-TEXT ENTRY

A nurse is caring for a client scheduled for abdominal surgery and administers the preoperative medications as prescribed. The nurse then raises the side rails on the stretcher, places the safety strap across the client, places the call bell near the client, and instructs the client to call for assistance. Shortly thereafter, the client calls the nurse and reports the need to urinate. What action would the nurse take to meet this client's need?

Answer: _____

ANSWERS

1. **1**

Rationale: Every effort must be made to obtain permission from a responsible family member to perform surgery if the client is unable to sign the consent form. A telephone consent must be witnessed by 2 persons who hear the family member's oral consent. The two witnesses then sign the consent with the name of the family member, noting that an oral consent was obtained. Consent is not informed if it is obtained from a client who is confused, unconscious, mentally incompetent, or under the influence of sedatives. In emergencies, a client may be unable to sign and family members may not be available. In this type of a situation, a physician is legally permitted to perform surgery without consent. Options 2 and 4 are not appropriate. In addition, actions that delay treatment in an emergency are not appropriate.

Test-Taking Strategy: Use the process of elimination. Note the key words "most appropriate" in the question. Eliminate options 2 and 4 first. Option 2 will delay necessary surgery and option 4 is inappropriate. Select option 1 over option 3 because it is the most appropriate of the options presented and it is legally acceptable to obtain a telephone permission from a family member if it is witnessed by two persons. Review the implications surrounding informed consent, if you had difficulty with this question.

Level of Cognitive Ability: Application
Client Needs: Safe, Effective Care Environment
Integrated Concept/Process: Nursing Process/Implementation
Content Area: Fundamental Skills
Reference: Potter, P., & Perry, A. (2001). *Fundamentals of nursing* (5th ed.). St. Louis: Mosby, p. 1677.

2. **4**

Rationale: Explanations should begin with the information that the client knows. By providing the client with individualized explanations of care and procedures, the nurse can assist the client in handling anxiety and fear for a smooth preoperative experience. Clients who are calm and emotionally prepared for surgery withstand anesthesia better and experience fewer postoperative complications. Options 1, 2, and 3 will produce anxiety in the client.

Test-Taking Strategy: Use the process of elimination. Note that the stem of the question contains the key words "most likely" and "stimulate further discussion." Use the steps of the nursing process and therapeutic communication techniques. Option 4 addresses assessment and is the only therapeutic response. If this question was difficult, review the fundamental principles of communication.

Level of Cognitive Ability: Application
Client Needs: Psychosocial Integrity
Integrated Concept/Process: Communication and Documentation
Content Area: Fundamental Skills
Reference: Harkreader, H. (2000). *Fundamentals of nursing: Caring and clinical judgment.* Philadelphia: W.B. Saunders, pp. 320-321.

3. **4**

Rationale: For optimal lung expansion with the incentive spirometer, the client should assume the semi-Fowler's or high-Fowler's position. The mouthpiece should be covered completely and tightly while the client inhales slowly with a constant flow through the unit. The breath should be held for 5 seconds before exhaling slowly.

Test-Taking Strategy: Use the process of elimination and knowledge of the procedure for using the incentive spirometer. Options 1, 2, and 3 are incorrect steps with regard to incentive spirometer use. If you had difficulty with this question, review the correct procedure related to the use of an incentive spirometer.
Level of Cognitive Ability: Application
Client Needs: Health Promotion and Maintenance
Integrated Concept/Process: Teaching/Learning
Content Area: Fundamental Skills
Reference: Smith, S., Duell, D., & Martin, B. (2000). *Clinical nursing skills: Basic to advanced skills* (5th ed.). Upper Saddle River, NJ: Prentice-Hall Health, pp. 739-740.

4. 1
Rationale: Anticoagulants alter normal clotting factors and increase the risk of bleeding after surgery. Aspirin has properties that can alter the clotting mechanism and should be discontinued at least 48 hours before surgery.
Test-Taking Strategy: Use the process of elimination. Note the key words "the client needs additional teaching." Options 2 and 3 are eliminated first because they are similar. From the remaining options, recalling that aspirin has properties that can alter the clotting mechanism will direct you to option 1. If you had difficulty with this question, review medications that affect the client preparing for surgery.
Level of Cognitive Ability: Analysis
Client Needs: Physiological Integrity
Integrated Concept/Process: Teaching/Learning
Content Area: Pharmacology
Reference: Potter, P., & Perry, A. (2001). *Fundamentals of nursing* (5th ed.). St. Louis: Mosby, p. 1668.

5. 2
Rationale: The nurse should ensure that the client has voided, if a Foley catheter is not in place. The nurse does not administer all daily medications just prior to sending a client to the OR. Rather, the physician writes a specific order outlining which medications may be given with a sip of water. The client has nothing by mouth for 8 hours prior to surgery, not 24 hours. The time of transfer to the OR is not the time to practice breathing exercises. This should have been accomplished earlier.
Test-Taking Strategy: Use the process of elimination. Note that the question contains the key words "at this time." This tells you that you must prioritize your answer according to a time line. With this in mind, eliminate options 1 and 3 first because they are incorrect. Choose correctly between the remaining two options either by knowing that the client must empty the bladder or by knowing that the client is likely to be anxious at this time, making it inappropriate to practice breathing exercises. Review preoperative nursing interventions if you had difficulty with this question.
Level of Cognitive Ability: Application
Client Needs: Physiological Integrity
Integrated Concept/Process: Nursing Process/Implementation
Content Area: Fundamental Skills
Reference: Potter, P., & Perry, A. (2001). *Fundamentals of nursing* (5th ed.). St. Louis: Mosby, p. 1689.

6. 2
Rationale: When the postoperative client arrives from the PACU, an initial assessment is performed. Common time frames for continuing postoperative assessment activities are every 15 minutes the first hour, every 30 minutes for 2 hours, every hour for 4 hours, and then every 4 hours as needed. Options 3 and 4 identify time frames that are too infrequent and will not provide adequate assessment of the postoperative client. Option 1 identifies close time frames that are unnecessary.
Test-Taking Strategy: Use the process of elimination. Eliminate option 1 first because the time frames are so close. By the time that the nurse completed the assessment, the 5 minutes would have lapsed and the nurse would have to immediately perform the assessment again. This is unnecessary and unreasonable. Eliminate options 3 and 4 because they identify time frames that are too infrequent and will not provide adequate assessment of the postoperative client. Review postoperative assessment procedures if you had difficulty with this question.
Level of Cognitive Ability: Application
Client Needs: Physiological Integrity
Integrated Concept/Process: Nursing Process/Planning
Content Area: Fundamental Skills
Reference: Harkreader, H. (2000). *Fundamentals of nursing: Caring and clinical judgment.* Philadelphia: W.B. Saunders, p. 1538.

7. 1
Rationale: The first action of the nurse is to assess the patency of the airway and respiratory function. The nurse then takes VS followed by checking the dressing and the tubes or drains. If the airway is not patent, immediate measures must be taken for the survival of the client.
Test-Taking Strategy: Use the principles of prioritization when answering this question. Remember the ABCs—airway, breathing, and circulation. Ensuring airway patency is the first action to be taken; therefore option 1 is correct. Options 2, 3, and 4 are all nursing actions that should be performed after a patent airway has been established.
Level of Cognitive Ability: Application
Client Needs: Physiological Integrity
Integrated Concept/Process: Nursing Process/Planning
Content Area: Fundamental Skills
Reference: Harkreader, H. (2000). *Fundamentals of nursing: Caring and clinical judgment.* Philadelphia: W.B. Saunders, p. 1538.

8. 3
Rationale: Urine output should be maintained at a minimum of 30 mL/hour for an adult. An output of less than 30 mL for each of two consecutive hours should be reported to the physician. A temperature above 37.7° C (100° F) or below 36.1° C (97° F) and a falling systolic blood pressure under 90 mm Hg are usually considered reportable at once. The client's preoperative or baseline blood pressure is used to make informed postoperative comparisons. Moderate or light serous drainage from the surgical site is considered normal.
Test-Taking Strategy: To answer this question correctly, you must know the normal ranges for temperature, blood pressure, urinary output, and wound drainage. Through the process of elimination, you can then determine that the urinary output is the only observation that is not within the normal range. Review these basic postoperative assessment findings, if you had difficulty with this question.
Level of Cognitive Ability: Analysis

Client Needs: Physiological Integrity
Integrated Concept/Process: Nursing Process/Planning
Content Area: Fundamental Skills
Reference: Craven, R., & Hirnle, C. (2000). *Fundamentals of nursing: Human health and function* (3rd ed.). Philadelphia: Lippincott, p. 620.

9. 4
Rationale: The most common postoperative respiratory problems are atelectasis, pneumonia, and pulmonary emboli. Pneumonia is inflammation of lung tissue that causes productive cough, dyspnea, and crackles. Pulmonary edema usually results from left-sided heart failure and can be caused by medications or fluid overload. Carbon dioxide retention results from inability to exhale carbon dioxide in conditions such as chronic obstructive pulmonary disease. Fluid imbalance can be a deficit or excess related to fluid loss or overload.
Test-Taking Strategy: Use the process of elimination. Focus on the relationship between the words "deep breathe and cough" in the question and "pneumonia" in the correct option. Review the common postoperative complications, if you had difficulty with this question.
Level of Cognitive Ability: Application
Client Needs: Physiological Integrity
Integrated Concept/Process: Teaching/Learning
Content Area: Fundamental Skills
Reference: Potter, P., & Perry, A. (2001). *Fundamentals of nursing* (5th ed.). St. Louis: Mosby, p. 1709.

10. 2
Rationale: A postoperative drain should not be curled tightly or obstructed in any way. This could prevent the drain from functioning properly. The tube/drain should be checked for patency to provide an exit for the fluid/blood to promote healing. Aseptic technique must be used for emptying the drainage container or changing the dressing, to avoid contamination of the wound. Usually the drainage from the wound is pale, red, and watery. Active bleeding will be bright red.
Test-Taking Strategy: Use the process of elimination, noting the key word "avoid." Remember that surgical drains need to remain patent so that accumulated secretions can escape from the wound bed. If you had difficulty with this question, review nursing care for the client with a surgical drain.
Level of Cognitive Ability: Application
Client Needs: Physiological Integrity
Integrated Concept/Process: Nursing Process/Implementation
Content Area: Fundamental Skills
Reference: Potter, P., & Perry, A. (2001). *Fundamentals of nursing* (5th ed.). St. Louis: Mosby, p. 1712.

11. 3
Rationale: Serous drainage is an expected finding at a surgical site. The other options indicate signs of wound infection. Signs and symptoms of infection include warm, red, and tender skin around the incision. Purulent material may exit from drains or from separated wound edges. It may be caused by poor aseptic technique and a contaminated wound before surgical exploration. Wound infection usually appears 3 to 6 days after surgery. The client may also have a fever and chills.
Test-Taking Strategy: Use the process of elimination, noting the key words "normal finding." Recalling the signs of a wound infection and noting these key words will easily direct

you to option 3. Review the signs of a wound infection if you had difficulty with this question.
Level of Cognitive Ability: Analysis
Client Needs: Physiological Integrity
Integrated Concept/Process: Nursing Process/Assessment
Content Area: Fundamental skills
Reference: Potter, P., & Perry, A. (2001). *Fundamentals of nursing* (5th ed.). St. Louis: Mosby, p. 1710.

12. 4
Rationale: Wound dehiscence is the separation of wound edges at the suture line. Signs and symptoms include increased drainage and the appearance of underlying tissues. It usually occurs 6 to 8 days after surgery. The client should be instructed to remain quiet and to avoid coughing or straining. The client should be positioned to prevent further stress on the wound. Sterile dressings soaked with sterile normal saline should be used to cover the wound. The physician must be notified after this initial dressing is applied to the wound.
Test-Taking Strategy: Use the process of elimination. Eliminate option 1 first because this action would dry the wound and also present a risk of infection to the underlying tissues. Eliminate options 2 and 3 next because a dry dressing and a dressing soaked with Betadine will irritate the exposed body tissues. Review initial nursing care when dehiscence or evisceration occurs, if you had difficulty with this question.
Level of Cognitive Ability: Application
Client Needs: Physiological Integrity
Integrated Concept/Process: Nursing Process/Planning
Content Area: Fundamental Skills
Reference: Phipps, W., Sands, J., & Marek, J. (1999). *Medical-surgical nursing: Concepts & clinical practice* (6th ed.). St. Louis: Mosby, p. 547.

13. 2
Rationale: Increasing restlessness is a sign that requires continuous and close monitoring, because it could indicate a potential complication, such as hemorrhage and shock. Hypoactive bowel sounds heard in all four quadrants are a normal occurrence, as is a negative Homans' sign. (A positive Homans' sign may be indicative of thrombophlebitis). A blood pressure of 110/70 mm Hg with a pulse of 86 beats per minute is within normal limits.
Test-Taking Strategy: Use the process of elimination, noting the key words "indicate an evolving complication." Eliminate each of the incorrect options because they are normal expected findings. If you had difficulty with this question, review the normal expected postoperative findings and the signs and symptoms of postoperative complications.
Level of Cognitive Ability: Analysis
Client Needs: Physiological Integrity
Integrated Concept/Process: Nursing Process/Analysis
Content Area: Fundamental Skills
Reference: Potter, P., & Perry, A. (2001). *Fundamentals of nursing* (5th ed.). St. Louis: Mosby, pp. 1704-1705.

14. 2
Rationale: Prednisone is a corticosteroid. With prolonged use, corticosteroids cause adrenal atrophy, which reduces the body's ability to withstand stress. When stress is severe, corticosteroids are essential to life. Before and during surgery, dosages may be temporarily increased. Cyclobenzaprine (Flexeril) is a skeletal muscle relaxant. Ferrous sulfate is an oral

iron preparation used to treat iron deficiency anemia. Conjugated estrogen (Premarin) is an estrogen used for hormonal replacement therapy in postmenopausal women. The other three medications may be withheld before surgery without undue effects on the client.

Test-Taking Strategy: Use the process of elimination and knowledge about medications that may have special implications for the surgical client. Remember that when stress is severe, corticosteroids are essential to life. Review the effects of corticosteroids if you had difficulty with this question.

Level of Cognitive Ability: Analysis
Client Needs: Safe, Effective Care Environment
Integrated Concept/Process: Nursing Process/Implementation
Content Area: Pharmacology
Reference: Potter, P., & Perry, A. (2001). *Fundamentals of nursing* (5th ed.). St. Louis: Mosby, p. 1168.

15. **4**

Rationale: Routine screening tests include a complete blood count, serum electrolyte analysis, coagulation studies, and serum creatinine tests. The complete blood count includes the hemoglobin analysis. All of these values are within normal range except the hemoglobin. If a client has a low hemoglobin level, the surgery could likely be postponed by the surgeon.

Test-Taking Strategy: Use the process of elimination and knowledge of the normal laboratory values. The only option that identifies an abnormal laboratory value is option 4. Review these laboratory values, if you had difficulty answering this question.

Level of Cognitive Ability: Analysis
Client Needs: Physiological Integrity
Integrated Concept/Process: Nursing Process/Analysis
Content Area: Fundamental Skills
Reference: Potter, P., & Perry, A. (2001). *Fundamentals of nursing* (5th ed.). St. Louis: Mosby, p. 1673.

16. **1**

Rationale: If a client has a latex allergy, a cloth barrier should be applied to the client's arm under a BP cuff to prevent skin contact with the cuff. It is safe to use medications from glass ampules and unsafe to use medications from ampules with rubber stoppers. Latex-safe IV tubing made of polyvinyl chloride should be used for the client with a latex allergy.

Test-Taking Strategy: Use the process of elimination, focusing on the issue of the question, latex allergy. Recalling the causes of a latex allergy will easily direct you to option 1. Review nursing interventions for the client with a latex allergy if you had difficulty with this question.

Level of Cognitive Ability: Application
Client Needs: Safe, Effective Care Environment
Integrated Concept/Process: Nursing Process/Planning
Content Area: Fundamental Skills
Reference: Harkreader, H. (2000). *Fundamentals of nursing: Caring and clinical judgment.* Philadelphia: W.B. Saunders, p. 1521.

17. **1**

Rationale: Nail polish needs to be removed from the client's fingernails and toenails so that capillary refill of the nailbeds and circulation can be adequately assessed. A slight increase in blood pressure and pulse is common during the preoperative period and is usually the result of anxiety. The client usually has a restriction of food and fluids for 8 hours prior to surgery instead of 24 hours. Oral hygiene is allowed, but the client should not swallow any water.

Test-Taking Strategy: Use the process of elimination and read each option carefully. Eliminate option 2 because of the words "immediately" and "slight." Eliminate option 3, knowing that the client should be NPO for 8 hours prior to surgery. From the remaining options, use the ABCs—airway, breathing, and circulation. Option 1 is necessary so that circulation can be adequately assessed. Review general preoperative care if you had difficulty with this question.

Level of Cognitive Ability: Application
Client Needs: Physiological Integrity
Integrated Concept/Process: Nursing Process/Planning
Content Area: Fundamental Skills
Reference: Potter, P., & Perry, A. (2001). *Fundamentals of nursing* (5th ed.). St. Louis: Mosby, pp. 1685, 1689.

18. **4**

Rationale: The type of planning and instruction required varies with each individual and the type of surgery. Specific instructions that the client needs to receive prior to discharge should include wound care, activity restrictions, dietary instructions, postoperative medication instructions, personal hygiene, and follow-up appointments. Deep breathing exercises are taught in the preoperative period.

Test-Taking Strategy: Use the process of elimination, noting the key words "least appropriate." Options 1, 2, and 3 are similar and refer to information that needs to be taught postoperatively. Option 4 refers to information that should be taught preoperatively. Review the client education points related to discharge teaching both preoperatively and postoperatively, if you had difficulty with this question.

Level of Cognitive Ability: Application
Client Needs: Health Promotion and Maintenance
Integrated Concept/Process: Self Care
Content Area: Fundamental Skills
Reference: Potter, P., & Perry, A. (2001). *Fundamentals of nursing* (5th ed.). St. Louis: Mosby, p. 1679.

19. **1**

Rationale: To elicit Homans' sign, the nurse would dorsiflex the client's foot and assess the client for pain in the calf area. If pain is present, a positive Homans' sign is present, which is an indication of thrombophlebitis. Incisional pain is an expected occurrence after abdominal surgery. Absent bowel sounds may occur in the immediate postoperative period. Crackles on auscultation of the lungs may be an indication of a respiratory complication.

Test-Taking Strategy: Use the process of elimination and knowledge of the significance of a positive Homans' sign. Knowing that a positive Homans' sign is indicative of thrombophlebitis will easily direct you to option 1. Review this assessment technique if you had difficulty with this question.

Level of Cognitive Ability: Analysis
Client Needs: Health Promotion and Maintenance
Integrated Concept/Process: Nursing Process/Assessment
Content Area: Fundamental Skills
Reference: Harkreader, H. (2000). *Fundamentals of nursing: Caring and clinical judgment.* Philadelphia: W.B. Saunders, p. 1544.

20. **4**

Rationale: The client's extremities should not be allowed to dangle over the sides of the table because this may impair circulation to the local area or cause nerve and muscle damage. It is part of the operating room nurse's role to ensure that the safety needs of the client are met, which includes proper positioning.

Test-Taking Strategy: Use the process of elimination and knowledge regarding the basic principles related to positioning. Recalling that the client is anesthetized will easily direct you to option 4. Review the nurse's role during surgery if you had difficulty with this question.

Level of Cognitive Ability: Application
Client Needs: Safe, Effective Care Environment
Integrated Concept/Process: Nursing Process/Implementation
Content Area: Fundamental Skills
Reference: Potter, P., & Perry, A. (2001). *Fundamentals of nursing* (5th ed.). St. Louis: Mosby, p. 1699.

CRITICAL THINKING: FREE-TEXT ENTRY

Answer: Assist the client onto a bedpan

Rationale: Because preoperative medications cause sedation, the client should not be allowed to leave the bed or stretcher after the medications are administered. To ensure safety, the nurse would assist the client to use a bedpan.

Test-Taking Strategy: Focus on the issue, that the client has received preoperative medications. Recall that the client should not be allowed to leave the bed or stretcher after preoperative medications are administered. With this in mind, think about the action that would meet this client's need. Review the principles related to administering preoperative medications if you had difficulty with this question.

Level of Cognitive Ability: Application
Client Needs: Safe, Effective Care Environment
Integrated Concept/Process: Nursing Process/Implementation
Content Area: Fundamental Skills
Reference: Potter, P., & Perry, A. (2001). *Fundamentals of nursing* (5th ed.). St. Louis: Mosby, p. 1692.

REFERENCES

Craven, R., & Hirnle, C. (2000). *Fundamentals of nursing: Human health and function* (3rd ed.). Philadelphia: Lippincott.

Harkreader, H. (2000). *Fundamentals of nursing: Caring and clinical judgment.* Philadelphia: W.B. Saunders.

Reference: Phipps, W., Sands, J., & Marek, J. (1999). *Medical-surgical nursing: Concepts & clinical practice* (6th ed.). St. Louis: Mosby.

Potter, P., & Perry, A. (2001). *Fundamentals of nursing* (5th ed.). St. Louis: Mosby.

Smith, S., Duell, D., & Martin, B. (2000). *Clinical nursing skills: Basic to advanced skills* (5th ed.). Upper Saddle River, NJ: Prentice-Hall Health.

19

Positioning Clients

PYRAMID TERMS

Fowler's position   The client is supine and the head of the bed is elevated to 45 degrees.

low Fowler's position (semi-Fowler's)   The client is supine and the head of the bed is elevated to 30 degrees.

high Fowler's position   The client is supine and the head of bed is elevated to 90 degrees.

lateral (side-lying) position   The client is lying on the side, and the head and shoulders are aligned with the hips and the spine and are parallel to the edge of the mattress. The head, neck, and upper arm are supported by a pillow. The lower shoulder is pulled forward slightly and, along with the elbow, flexed at 90 degrees. The legs are flexed or extended. A pillow is placed to support the back.

lithotomy position   The client is lying on the back with the hips and knees flexed at right angles and the feet in stirrups.

prone position   The client is lying on the abdomen with head turned to the side. The shoulders are abducted and rotated 90 degrees, with arms flexed at the elbows and palms facing downward along the side of the head. The legs are extended and slightly separated. The feet should extend over the bottom of the mattress, with the ankles at a 90-degree angle or supported at a 90-degree angle with sandbags.

supine (dorsal recumbent) position   The client is lying on the back. The head and shoulders are usually slightly elevated with a small pillow. The arms and legs are extended, and the legs are slightly abducted.

Sims' position (semi-prone)   The client is lying on the side with the body turned prone at 45 degrees. The spine is parallel to the mattress, and shoulders and hips are aligned. The face is supported by a small pillow. The lower arm is behind the body, with the shoulder retracted and hyperextended, and the elbow is slightly flexed. The lower leg is extended, with the upper leg flexed at the hip and knee to a 45- to 90-degree angle. The ankles are supported at 90 degrees.

PYRAMID TO SUCCESS

Nursing responsibility includes positioning clients in a safe and appropriate manner to provide safety and comfort. Knowledge regarding the client position required for a certain procedure or condition is expected (Fig. 19-1). It is the nurse's responsibility to reduce the likelihood and prevent the development of complications related to an existing condition, prescribed treatment, or medical or surgical procedure. It is imperative that the nurse review the physician's orders after treatments or procedures and take note of instructions regarding positioning and mobility. The primary Integrated Concepts and Processes addressed in this chapter include Nursing Process, Caring, Communication and Documentation, and Teaching/Learning.

CLIENT NEEDS
Safe, Effective Care Environment

Accident prevention
Appropriate positioning
Establishing priorities
Environmental and personal safety
Informed consent
Medical and surgical asepsis
Protective measures
Use of restraints

Health Promotion and Maintenance

Instructions regarding the need for prescribed therapies
Techniques of physical assessment

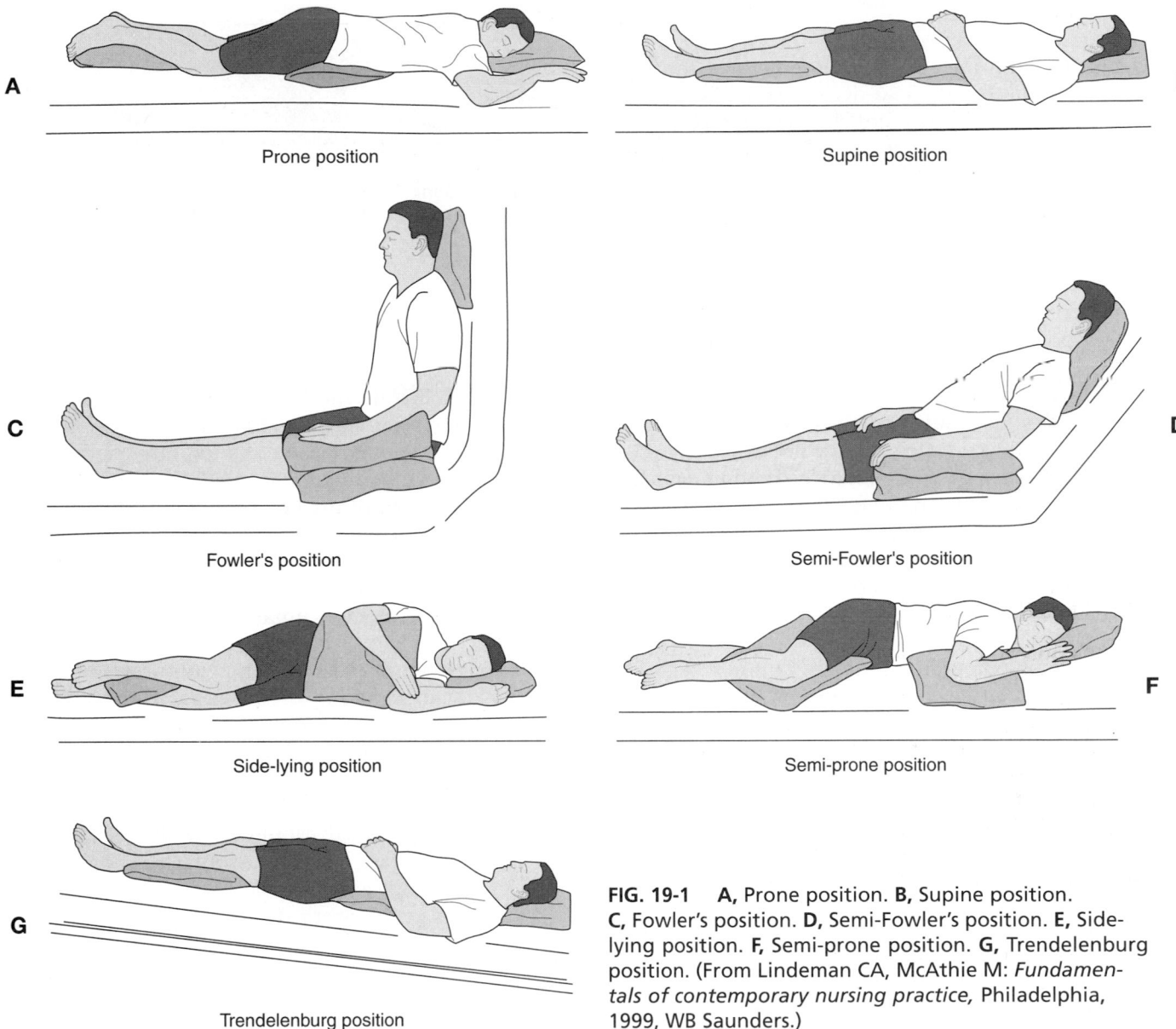

FIG. 19-1 **A,** Prone position. **B,** Supine position. **C,** Fowler's position. **D,** Semi-Fowler's position. **E,** Side-lying position. **F,** Semi-prone position. **G,** Trendelenburg position. (From Lindeman CA, McAthie M: *Fundamentals of contemporary nursing practice,* Philadelphia, 1999, WB Saunders.)

Psychosocial Integrity

Assisting the client to use coping mechanisms
Keeping the family informed of client progress
Providing support to the client
Therapeutic interactions

Physiological Integrity

Comfort measures for rest and sleep
Immobility
Preventing complications
Providing nutrition and oral intake
Providing personal hygiene as needed
Use of assistive devices

I. PROVIDING SAFETY AND COMFORT

A. Integumentary system
  1. Autograft: After surgery, the site is immobilized for 3 to 7 days to provide the time needed for the graft to adhere and attach to the wound bed
  2. Burns of the face and head: Elevate the head of the bed to prevent or reduce facial, head, and tracheal edema
  3. Circumferential burns of the extremities: Elevate the extremities above the level of the heart to prevent or reduce dependent edema
  4. Skin graft: Elevate and immobilize the graft site to prevent movement and shearing of the graft and disruption of tissue; avoid weight bearing

B. Reproductive system
   1. Mastectomy
      a. Position the client with the head of the bed elevated at least 30 degrees (**semi-Fowler's**), with the affected arm elevated on a pillow to promote lymphatic fluid return after the removal of axillary lymph nodes
      b. Turn the client only to the back and unaffected side
   2. Perineal and vaginal procedures: place the client in lithotomy position
C. Endocrine system
   1. Hypophysectomy: Elevate the head of the bed to prevent increased intracranial pressure
   2. Thyroidectomy
      a. Place in **semi-Fowler's position** to reduce swelling and edema in the neck area
      b. Sandbags or pillows may be used to support the client's head or neck
D. Gastrointestinal system
   1. Hemorrhoidectomy: Assist the client to a **lateral (side-lying) position** to prevent pain and bleeding
   2. Liver biopsy
      a. During procedure
         (1) Position client **supine,** with the right side of the upper abdomen exposed
         (2) The client's right arm is raised and extended over the left shoulder behind the head
         (3) The liver is located on the right side, and this position provides for maximal exposure of the right intercostal space
      b. After procedure
         (1) Assist the client into a right **lateral (side-lying) position**
         (2) Place a small pillow or folded towel under the puncture site for at least 3 hours to provide pressure to the site and prevent bleeding
   3. Intestinal tubes (Miller-Abbott, Cantor, and Harris tubes)
      a. After insertion, to facilitate movement of the tube, the client's position is rotated as prescribed; position 2 hours on the right side, 2 hours on the back with the head elevated, and 2 hours on the left side
      b. If prescribed by the physician and according to agency policies and procedures, advance the tube 2 to 4 inches at a time to facilitate movement of the tube
   4. Nasogastric tube
      a. Insertion
         (1) Position the client in **high-Fowler's** with the head tilted forward
         (2) This position will close the trachea and open the esophagus

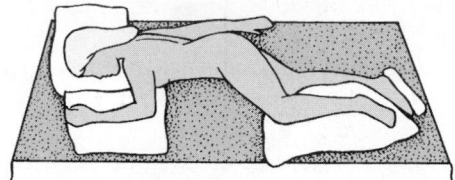

FIG. 19-2   Sims' (semiprone) position. (From Potter PA, Perry AG: *Fundamentals of nursing,* ed 5, St Louis, 2001, Mosby.)

      b. Irrigations and tube feedings
         (1) Elevate the head of the bed 30 degrees (**semi-Fowler's**) to prevent aspiration
         (2) Maintain head elevation for 1 hour after an intermittent feeding
         (3) Head of the bed should remain elevated for continuous feedings
   5. Rectal enemas/irrigations: Place client in left **Sims' position** to allow the solution to flow by gravity in the natural direction of the colon (Fig. 19-2)
   6. Sengstaken-Blakemore and Minnesota tubes: Maintain elevation of the head of the bed to enhance lung expansion and reduce portal blood flow, permitting effective compression of the varices
E. Respiratory system
   1. Chronic obstructive pulmonary disease: In advanced disease, place in a sitting position, leaning forward, with the client's arms over several pillows or an overbed table; this position will assist the client to breathe easier
   2. Laryngectomy (radical neck dissection): Place the client in **semi-Fowler's** or **Fowler's position** to maintain a patent airway and minimize edema
   3. Bronchoscopy postprocedure: Place the client in a **semi-Fowler's** position to prevent choking or aspiration resulting from an impaired ability to swallow
   4. Postural drainage: the lung segment to be drained should be in the uppermost position
   5. Thoracentesis
      a. During procedure: To facilitate removal of fluid from the chest wall, position the client sitting on the edge of the bed and leaning over the bedside table, with the feet supported on a stool, or lying in bed on the unaffected side with the head of the bed elevated 45 degrees (**Fowler's**)
      b. After procedure: Assist the client to a position of comfort
   6. Thoracotomy: Check physician's orders regarding positioning

F. Cardiovascular system
 1. Abdominal aneurysm resection
   a. After surgery, limit elevation of the head of the bed to 45 degrees (**Fowler's**) to avoid flexion of the graft
   b. Turn the client from side to side regularly
 2. Amputation of the lower extremity
   a. During the first 24 hours after amputation, elevate the foot of the bed (but not the stump itself) to reduce edema; then keep the bed flat to prevent hip flexion contractures
   b. Consult with the physician, and then position the client **prone** every 3 to 4 hours for a 20- to 30-minute period to stretch muscles and prevent flexion contractures of the hip
   c. When the client is in the **prone position,** keep the client's legs close together to prevent abduction
   d. Teach the client to contract the gluteal muscles of the buttocks
 3. Arterial vascular grafting of an extremity
   a. To promote graft patency after the procedure, bed rest is maintained for at least 24 hours, and the affected extremity is kept straight
   b. Limit movement and avoid flexion of the hip and knee
 4. Cardiac catheterization
   a. After cardiac catheterization, the extremity in which the catheter was inserted is kept straight for 4 to 6 hours
   b. If the femoral artery was used, strict bed rest is enforced for 6 to 12 hours; the client may turn from side to side
   c. The affected leg is kept straight and the head elevated no greater than 30 degrees until hemostasis is adequately achieved
 5. Congestive heart failure and pulmonary edema: Position the client upright, preferably with the legs dangling over the side of the bed, to decrease venous return and lung congestion
 6. Peripheral arterial disease
   a. Obtain the physician's order for positioning
   b. Because swelling can prevent arterial blood flow, clients may be advised to elevate their feet at rest, but they should not raise their legs above the level of the heart because extreme elevation slows arterial blood flow
 7. Thrombophlebitis
   a. Place the client on bed rest, with an elevation of the affected extremity
   b. No knee gatch or pillow is placed under the knees
 8. Vein ligation and stripping
   a. Elevate the feet above the level of the heart
   b. Instruct the client to avoid leg dangling and chair sitting

G. Sensory system
 1. Cataract Surgery
   a. Postoperatively, elevate the head of the bed 30 to 45 degrees (**semi-Fowler's** to **Fowler's**)
   b. Turn the client to the back or the nonoperative side to prevent the development of edema at the operative site
 2. Retinal reattachment
   a. Obtain physician's order regarding positioning
   b. If gas as a gas tamponade is used to flatten the retina, the client may have to be specially positioned to make the gas bubble float into the best position
   c. Some clients must lie face down or on the side for days at a time

H. Neurological system
 1. Autonomic dysreflexia: Elevate the head of the bed to a **high-Fowler's position** to assist with adequate ventilation and assist in the prevention of hypertensive stroke
 2. Cerebral aneurysm: Complete bed rest with the head of the bed elevated 30 to 45 degrees (**semi-Fowler's** to **Fowler's**) to prevent pressure on the aneurysm site
 3. Cerebral angiography
   a. Maintain bed rest for 6 to 24 hours as prescribed
   b. The extremity into which the contrast medium was injected is kept straight and immobilized for approximately the length of the bed rest
 4. Cerebrovascular accident (CVA)
   a. In clients with hemorrhagic strokes, the head of the bed is elevated to 30 degrees to reduce intracranial pressure and to facilitate venous drainage
   b. For clients with ischemic strokes, the head of the bed is kept flat
   c. Maintain the head in a midline, neutral position to facilitate venous drainage from the head
   d. Avoid extreme hip and neck flexion; extreme hip flexion may increase intrathoracic pressure, whereas extreme neck flexion prohibits venous drainage from the brain
 5. Craniotomy
   a. The client should NOT be positioned on the site that was operated on, especially if the bone flap has been removed, because the brain has no bony covering on the affected site
   b. Elevate the head of the bed 30 to 45 degrees (**semi-Fowler's** to **Fowler's**) and maintain the head in a midline, neutral position to facilitate venous drainage from the head
   c. Avoid extreme hip and neck flexion; extreme

hip flexion may increase intrathoracic pressure, whereas extreme neck flexion prohibits venous drainage from the brain

6. Laminectomy
   a. Logroll the client, by turning the client all at once, to keep the back as straight as possible
   b. When the client is out of bed, the client's back is kept straight and the client is placed in a straight-backed chair, with the feet resting comfortably on the floor

7. Increased intracranial pressure
   a. Elevate the head of the bed 30 to 45 degrees (**semi-Fowler's** to **Fowler's**) and maintain the head in a midline, neutral position to facilitate venous drainage from the head
   b. Avoid extreme hip and neck flexion; extreme hip flexion may increase intrathoracic pressure, whereas extreme neck flexion prohibits venous drainage from the brain

8. Lumbar puncture
   a. During procedure: Assist the client to the **lateral (side-lying) position,** with the back bowed at the edge of the examining table, the knees flexed up to the abdomen, and the head bent so that the chin is resting on the chest
   b. After procedure: Place the client in the **supine (dorsal recumbent) position** for 4 to 12 hours

9. Myelogram postprocedure
   a. If water-soluble dye is used, the head of the bed should be elevated for at least 8 hours to keep the dye from irritating the cerebral meninges
   b. If an oil-based dye is used, position the client flat in bed 6 to 8 hours after the dye is removed, to prevent leakage of cerebrospinal fluid

10. Spinal cord injury
    a. Immobilize the client on a spinal backboard, with the head in a neutral position, to prevent incomplete injury from becoming complete
    b. Prevent head flexion, rotation, or extension; the head is immobilized with a firm, padded cervical collar
    c. Maintain traction and alignment of the head by placing the hand on either side of the head by the client's ears
    d. Logroll the client; no part of the body should be twisted or turned, nor should the client be allowed to assume a sitting position

I. Musculoskeletal system
   1. Hip surgery
      a. Avoid extreme positions and acute flexion of the operative hip, and keep the affected leg abducted

      b. Place a pillow between the client's legs to maintain abduction; instruct the client not to cross the legs
      c. Prevent external rotation of the operative leg by placing a trochanter roll beside the external aspect of the thigh, and elevate the heels
      d. Check the physician's orders regarding elevation of the head of the bed
      e. Turn the client only after checking the physician's orders, as many clients are permitted to turn to the nonoperative side and to the back only

PRACTICE QUESTIONS

1. A client has just returned to a nursing unit after an above-the-knee amputation of the right leg. A nurse places the client in which of the following most appropriate positions?
   1. Supine with the stump flat on the bed
   2. Supine with the stump elevated
   3. Reverse Trendelenburg
   4. Prone

2. A nurse is caring for a client with a severe burn. The client is scheduled for an autograft to be placed on the lower extremity. The nurse develops a postoperative plan of care for the client and includes which of the following in the plan?
   1. Maintain surgical extremity in a flat position
   2. Keep surgical extremity covered with a blanket
   3. Maintain the client in a prone position
   4. Elevate and immobilize the grafted extremity

3. A nurse is preparing to care for a client who has returned to the nursing unit following cardiac catheterization performed through the femoral artery. The nurse plans to ensure which most appropriate client position/activity following the procedure?
   1. Bed rest with head elevation at 60 degrees
   2. Bed rest with head elevation no greater than 30 degrees
   3. Bed rest with bathroom privileges only
   4. Bed rest in high-Fowlers position

4. A nurse is providing instructions to a client and the family regarding home care after right eye cataract removal. Which statement, if made by the client, would indicate effective teaching?
   1. "I will not sleep on my right side."
   2. "I will not sleep on my left side."
   3. "I will not sleep with my head elevated."
   4. "I will not wear my glasses until my physician says it is OK."

5. A nurse assists a physician in performing a liver biopsy. After the biopsy, the nurse plans to place the client in which of the following positions?
   1. Supine
   2. Prone

3. A left side-lying position with a small pillow or folded towel under the puncture site
4. A right side-lying position with a small pillow or folded towel under the puncture site

6. A nurse is administering a cleansing enema to a client with a fecal impaction. Before administering the enema, the nurse places the client in which of the following positions?
   1. On the left side of the body, with the head of the bed elevated 45 degrees
   2. On the right side of the body, with the head of the bed elevated 45 degrees
   3. Left Sims' position
   4. Right Sims' position

7. A client is being prepared for a thoracentesis. A nurse assists the client to which of the following positions for the procedure?
   1. Lying in bed on the affected side, with the head of the bed elevated 45 degrees
   2. Lying in bed on the unaffected side, with the head of the bed elevated 45 degrees
   3. Prone with the head turned to the side and supported by a pillow
   4. Sims' position with the head of the bed flat

8. A nurse assists a physician with the insertion of a Harris tube in a client with a bowel obstruction. Following insertion of the tube, the nurse assists the client to which of the following positions initially?
   1. Prone

2. Supine with the head flat
3. Right side
4. Sims'

9. A client is diagnosed with deep vein thrombophlebitis. A nurse develops a plan of care for the client and includes which client position/activity in the plan?
   1. Bed rest with the affected extremity in a dependent position
   2. Out-of-bed activities as desired
   3. Bed rest with the affected extremity kept flat
   4. Bed rest with elevation of the affected extremity

10. A nurse is preparing to care for a client who has had a supratentorial craniotomy. The nurse plans to place the client in which position?
    1. Prone
    2. Supine
    3. Semi-Fowler's
    4. Dorsal recumbent

CRITICAL THINKING: FREE-TEXT ENTRY

A nurse is caring for a client with congestive heart failure. The client suddenly becomes anxious and restless, has a sudden onset of breathlessness, and becomes cyanotic. The nurse suspects pulmonary edema and immediately places the client in what position?

Answer: _____

ANSWERS

1. **2**
Rationale: The stump is elevated for the first 24 hours following surgery to promote venous return and decrease edema, which will increase mobility. After the first 24 hours, the stump is placed flat on the bed to reduce hip contracture. Edema is also controlled by stump-wrapping techniques. Options 1, 3, and 4 are inappropriate positions for the client immediately after surgery.
Test-Taking Strategy: Use the process of elimination. A key issue in this question is that the client has just returned from surgery. Using basic principles related to immediate postoperative care will assist in directing you to option 2. If you had difficulty with this question, review postoperative positioning following amputation.
Level of Cognitive Ability: Application
Client Needs: Physiological Integrity
Integrated Concept/Process: Nursing Process/Implementation
Content Area: Fundamental Skills
Reference: LeMone, P., & Burke, K. (2000). *Medical-surgical nursing: Critical thinking in client care* (2nd ed.). Upper Saddle River, NJ: Prentice-Hall, p. 1608.

2. **4**
Rationale: Autografts placed over joints or on lower extremities are elevated and immobilized following surgery for 3 to 7 days, depending on the surgeon's preference. This period of immobilization allows the autograft time to adhere and attach to the wound bed, and the elevation minimizes edema. Keeping the client in a prone position and covering the extremity with a blanket can disrupt the graft site.
Test-Taking Strategy: Use the process of elimination. Options 2 and 3 can be eliminated first because both a blanket and a prone position can easily disrupt a graft. From the remaining options, recall the principles related to gravity and edema to assist in directing you to option 4. Review care to the client following an autograft if you had difficulty with this question.
Level of Cognitive Ability: Application
Client Needs: Physiological Integrity
Integrated Concept/Process: Nursing Process/Planning
Content Area: Fundamental Skills
Reference: Smeltzer, S., & Bare, B. (2000) *Brunner & Suddarth's textbook of medical-surgical nursing* (9th ed). Philadelphia: Lippincott Williams & Wilkins, p. 1519.

3. **2**
Rationale: After cardiac catheterization, the extremity in which the catheter was inserted is kept straight for 4 to 6 hours. If the femoral artery was used, strict bed rest is enforced for 6 to 12 hours. The client may turn from side to side. The affected leg is kept straight and the head is elevated no greater than 30 degrees until hemostasis is adequately achieved.
Test-Taking Strategy: Use the process of elimination. Knowing that the head of the bed should not be elevated more than 30

degrees will assist in eliminating options 1 and 4. Remembering that bathroom privileges are not allowed in the immediate post-catheterization period will assist in eliminating option 3. If you had difficulty with this question, review care after cardiac catheterization.

Level of Cognitive Ability: Application
Client Needs: Safe, Effective Care Environment
Integrated Concept/Process: Nursing Process/Planning
Content Area: Fundamental Skills
Reference: Smeltzer, S., & Bare, B. (2000) *Brunner & Suddarth's textbook of medical-surgical nursing* (9th ed). Philadelphia: Lippincott Williams & Wilkins, p. 558.

4. 1
Rationale: After cataract surgery, the client should not sleep on the side of the body that was operated on. The client should also be placed in a semi-Fowler's position to assist in minimizing edema and an increase in intraocular pressure. During the day, the client may wear glasses or a protective shield; at night, the protective shield alone is sufficient.

Test-Taking Strategy: Use the process of elimination. Remember to instruct the client to remain off the operative side. This will assist you with answering questions related to cataract surgery. Review postoperative instructions for the client following cataract surgery if you had difficulty with this question.

Level of Cognitive Ability: Analysis
Client Needs: Health Promotion and Maintenance
Integrated Concept/Process: Teaching/Learning
Content Area: Fundamental Skills
Reference: Ignatavicius, D., Workman, M., & Mishler, M. (1999). *Medical-surgical nursing across the health care continuum* (3rd ed.). Philadelphia: W.B. Saunders, p. 1178.

5. 4
Rationale: After a liver biopsy, the client is assisted to assume a right side-lying position with a small pillow or folded towel under the puncture site for 2 hours. This position compresses the liver against the chest wall at the biopsy site.

Test-Taking Strategy: Use the process of elimination and knowledge regarding the anatomy of the body to answer this question. Remember that the liver is on the right side of the body, and that the application of pressure on the right side will minimize the escape of blood or bile through the puncture site. Review care to the client following a liver biopsy if you had difficulty with this question.

Level of Cognitive Ability: Application
Client Needs: Physiological Integrity
Integrated Concept/Process: Nursing Process/Planning
Content Area: Fundamental Skills
Reference: Altman, G., Buchsel, P., & Coxon, V. (2000). *Delmar's fundamental & advanced nursing skills.* Albany, N.Y.: Delmar, p. 1320.

6. 3
Rationale: For administering an enema, the client is placed in a left Sims' position so that the enema solution can flow by gravity in the natural direction of the colon. The head of the bed is not elevated in the Sims' position.

Test-Taking Strategy: Use the process of elimination and knowledge regarding the anatomy of the bowel to answer the question. This will assist in eliminating options 2 and 4. Attempt to visualize the procedure for administering an enema

and eliminate option 1 because the head of the bed should be flat during enema administration. Review the procedure for administering an enema if you had difficulty with this question.

Level of Cognitive Ability: Application
Client Needs: Physiological Integrity
Integrated Concept/Process: Nursing Process/Implementation
Content Area: Fundamental Skills
Reference: Potter, P., & Perry, A. (2001). *Fundamentals of nursing* (5th ed.). St. Louis: Mosby, p. 1463.

7. 2
Rationale: To facilitate removal of fluid from the chest wall, the client is positioned sitting at the edge of the bed leaning over the bedside table with the feet supported on a stool, or lying in bed on the unaffected side with the head of the bed elevated 30 to 45 degrees. The prone and Sims' positions are inappropriate positions for this procedure.

Test-Taking Strategy: Use the process of elimination. Eliminate option 1 first because if the client was lying on the affected side, it would be very difficult to perform the procedure. Option 4 can be eliminated next because the Sims' position is primarily used for rectal enemas or irrigations. Next, visualize the prone position. In the prone position, the client is lying on the abdomen, which is not an appropriate position for this procedure. Review the procedure for a thoracentesis if you had difficulty with this question.

Level of Cognitive Ability: Application
Client Needs: Physiological Integrity
Integrated Concept/Process: Nursing Process/Implementation
Content Area: Fundamental Skills
Reference: Smeltzer, S., & Bare, B. (2000) *Brunner & Suddarth's textbook of medical-surgical nursing* (9th ed.). Philadelphia: Lippincott Williams & Wilkins, p. 398.

8. 3
Rationale: The Harris tube is a single-lumen, mercury-weighted tube. The weight of the mercury tube carries the tube by gravity. After insertion, to facilitate movement of the tube, the client is positioned 2 hours on the right side, 2 hours on the back with the head elevated, and 2 hours on the left.

Test-Taking Strategy: Use the process of elimination. Knowledge of the anatomy of the gastrointestinal tract and the Harris tube will easily direct you to option 3. If you had difficulty with this question, review nursing care related to the client with a Harris tube.

Level of Cognitive Ability: Application
Client Needs: Physiological Integrity
Integrated Concept/Process: Nursing Process/Implementation
Content Area: Fundamental Skills
Reference: Phipps, W., Sands, J., & Marek, J. (1999). *Medical-surgical nursing: Concepts & clinical practice* (6th ed.). St. Louis: Mosby, p. 1346.

9. 4
Rationale: Elevation of the affected leg facilitates blood flow by the force of gravity and also decreases venous pressure, which in turn relieves edema and pain. Bed rest is indicated to prevent emboli and to prevent pressure fluctuations in the venous system that occur with walking.

Test-Taking Strategy: Use the process of elimination. Focus on the client's diagnosis and think about the principles related to gravity flow and edema to answer the question. If you had

difficulty with this question, review nursing care for clients with a venous disorder.
Level of Cognitive Ability: Application
Client Needs: Physiological Integrity
Integrated Concept/Process: Nursing Process/Planning
Content Area: Fundamental Skills
Reference: Ignatavicius, D., Workman, M., & Mishler, M. (1999). *Medical-surgical nursing across the health care continuum* (3rd ed.). Philadelphia: W.B. Saunders, p. 873.

10. **3**
Rationale: After supratentorial surgery (surgery above the brain's tentorium), the client's head is usually elevated 30 degrees to promote venous outflow through the jugular veins. Options 1, 2, and 4 are incorrect positions after this surgery.
Test-Taking Strategy: Use the process of elimination and knowledge regarding supratentorial surgery and craniotomy to answer this question. A helpful strategy is to remember: supra, above the brain's tentorium, head up. If you had difficulty with this question, review positioning after craniotomy surgery.
Level of Cognitive Ability: Application
Client Needs: Physiological Integrity

Integrated Concept/Process: Nursing Process/Planning
Content Area: Fundamental Skills
Reference: Ignatavicius, D., Workman, M., & Mishler, M. (1999). *Medical-surgical nursing across the health care continuum* (3rd ed.). Philadelphia: W.B. Saunders, p. 1142.

CRITICAL THINKING: FREE-TEXT ENTRY

Answer: Upright with the legs dangling over the side of the bed
Rationale: Positioning the client upright with the legs dangling over the side of the bed has an immediate effect of decreasing venous return and decreasing lung congestion.
Test-Taking Strategy: Think about the physiological occurrence in pulmonary edema. Recalling that the lung congestion that occurs results in severe hypoxemia will assist in determining the optimal position for the client.
Level of Cognitive Ability: Application
Client Needs: Physiological Integrity
Integrated Concept/Process: Nursing Process/Implementation
Content Area: Fundamental Skills
Reference: Smeltzer, S., & Bare, B. (2000). *Brunner & Suddarth's textbook of medical-surgical nursing* (9th ed.). Philadelphia: Lippincott Williams & Wilkins, p. 662.

REFERENCES

Altman, G., Buchsel, P., & Coxon, V. (2000). *Delmar's fundamental & advanced nursing skills.* Albany, NY: Delmar.

Ignatavicius, D., Workman, M., & Mishler, M. (1999). *Medical-surgical nursing across the health care continuum* (3rd ed.). Philadelphia: W.B. Saunders.

LeMone, P., & Burke, K. (2000). *Medical-surgical nursing: Critical thinking in client care* (2nd ed.). Upper Saddle River, NJ: Prentice-Hall.

Phipps, W., Sands, J., & Marek, J. (1999). *Medical-surgical nursing: Concepts & clinical practice* (6th ed.). St. Louis: Mosby.

Potter, P., & Perry, A. (2001). *Fundamentals of nursing* (5th ed.). St. Louis: Mosby.

Smeltzer, S., & Bare, B. (2000) *Brunner & Suddarth's textbook of medical-surgical nursing* (9th ed.). Philadelphia: Lippincott Williams & Wilkins.

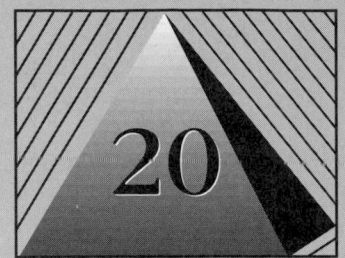

Care of a Client with a Tube

20

PYRAMID TERMS

chest tube Returns negative pressure to the intrapleural space; used to remove abnormal accumulations of air and fluid from the pleural space.

endotracheal tube Used to maintain a patent airway; indicated when a client needs mechanical ventilation.

gastrointestinal (GI) intubation Refers to the insertion of a tube into the stomach or intestine.

intestinal tube Passed nasally and designed so that it enters the small intestine through the pyloric sphincter because of the weight of a small bag of mercury at the end of the tube; used to decompress the bowel or to remove intestinal contents.

Sengstaken-Blakemore tube Triple-lumen gastric tube with an inflatable esophageal balloon, an inflatable gastric balloon, and a gastric aspiration lumen; used as a treatment modality for a client with esophageal varices.

tracheostomy Artificial opening created into the trachea to establish an airway.

PYRAMID TO SUCCESS

The Pyramid to Success focuses on the common types of tubes used in the clinical setting. NCLEX-RN is likely to address content areas related to the appropriate care of certain tubes and the immediate interventions required if a complication arises. Focus on the specific assessment points related to the specific type of tube. Review procedures for insertion of a particular tube, verifying correct placement, and administering medications or feedings, if appropriate. Pyramid points also focus on interventions associated with complications or emergencies that may occur. The primary Integrated Concepts and Processes addressed in this chapter include Nursing Process, Caring, Communication and Documentation, and Teaching/Learning.

CLIENT NEEDS
Safe, Effective Care Environment

Advance directives
Advocacy related to client's concerns
Client rights
Consultations with members of the health care team
Establishing priorities
Handling infectious materials
Informed consent for invasive procedure
Medical and surgical asepsis
Standard (universal) precautions

Health Promotion and Maintenance

Client and family education regarding care at home
Disease prevention
Lifestyle changes
Techniques of physical assessment

Psychosocial Integrity

Home care services
Sensory/perceptual alterations
Situational role changes
Support systems
Therapeutic interactions
Unexpected body image changes

Physiological Integrity

Diagnostic tests to confirm accurate placement of tube
Emergency interventions for complications
Laboratory values
Measures to ensure basic care and comfort
Medication administration

Nutrition and oral hydration
Potential complications associated with the tube
Respiratory care

I. NASOGASTRIC (NG) TUBES (Fig. 20-1)

A. Description
   1. Short tubes used to intubate the stomach
   2. Inserted from nose to stomach
B. Types of tubes
   1. Levine
      a. Single-lumen nasogastric tube
      b. Used to remove gastric contents via intermittent suction, or to provide tube feedings
   2. Salem sump
      a. Double-lumen nasogastric tube with an air vent
      b. Used for decompression with continuous suction
      c. Air vent is not to be clamped and is to be kept above the level of the stomach
      d. If leakage occurs through the air vent, instill 30 mL of air into the air vent and irrigate the main lumen with normal saline (NS)
C. Intubation procedures
   1. Place the client in high-Fowler's position
   2. Measure from tip of nose to earlobe to xiphoid process to determine the length of insertion, and mark with tape
   3. Lubricate tube about 3 inches with a water-soluble jelly only (oil-soluble is not used), to prevent the development of pneumonia if the tube accidentally slips into the bronchus
   4. Instruct the client to bend the head forward, which closes the epiglottis and opens the esophagus
   5. Insert into nostril; advance backward and through the nasopharynx
   6. Have the client take a sip of water, and advance the tube as the client swallows
   7. Do not force the tube
   8. If the client experiences any respiratory distress (coughing or choking) during insertion, pull back on the tube and wait until the distress subsides
   9. Advance until the taped mark is reached; tape in place when correct placement is confirmed
   10. If feedings are prescribed, x-ray confirmation should be done before feedings are initiated.
   11. When **GI** tubes are attached to suction, suction may be continuous or intermittent, with a pressure not exceeding 25 mm Hg as prescribed by the physician
D. Assessing placement
   1. Note that the most reliable method to determine placement is by x-ray, which should be performed after initial placement
   2. Assess tube placement every 4 hours and before administering feedings or medications
   3. Assess tube placement by aspirating gastric contents and measuring the pH, which should be 4 or less (pH values greater than 6 indicate intestinal placement)
   4. Inserting 5 to10 mL of air into the NG tube and listening for the rush of air over the stomach with a stethoscope is an alternative method for assessing placement, but is not as reliable as an x-ray or checking gastric pH
E. Assessing residual
   1. Check residual volumes every 4 hours, before each feeding, and before giving medications
   2. Aspirate all stomach contents (residual) and measure amount
   3. Reinstill residual feeding to prevent excessive fluid and electrolyte losses, unless the residual volume appears abnormal
F. Irrigating
   1. Performed every 4 hours to check the patency of the tube
   2. Assess placement before irrigating
   3. Gently instill 30 to 50 mL of water or normal saline (NS) (depending on agency policy) with an irrigation syringe
   4. Pull back on the syringe plunger to withdraw the fluid to check patency; repeat if tube remains sluggish
G. Removal of an NG tube: Ask the client to take a deep breath and hold; remove the tube slowly and evenly over the course of 3 to 6 seconds (coil the tube around the hand as it is being removed)

II. GI TUBE FEEDINGS

A. Tubes
   1. Nasogastric: Nose to stomach
   2. Nasoduodenal/nasojejunal: Nose to duodenum or jejunum
   3. Gastrostomy: Stomach
   4. Jejunostomy: Jejunum
B. Types of administration
   1. Bolus
      a. Resembles normal meal feeding patterns
      b. Approximately 300 to 400 mL of formula is administered over a 30- to 60-minute period every 3 to 6 hours
   2. Continuous
      a. Administered continually for 24 hours
      b. An infusion pump regulates the flow
   3. Cyclical
      a. Administered in either the daytime or the nighttime for 8 to 16 hours
      b. An infusion pump regulates the flow
      c. Feedings at night allow for more freedom during the day

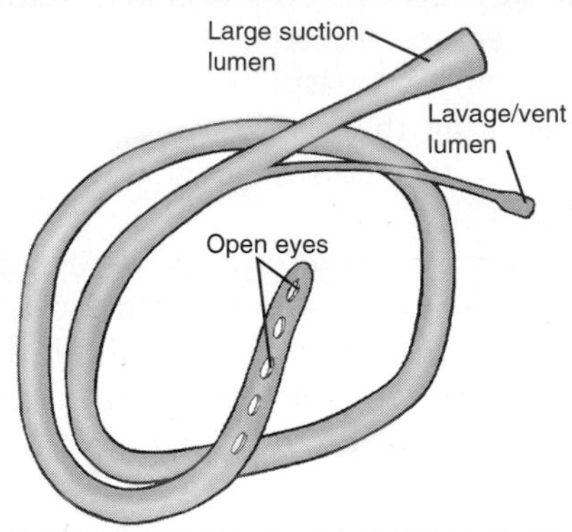

Lavacuator tube

An orogastric tube with a large suction lumen and a smaller lavage/vent lumen that provides continuous suction because irrigating solution enters the lavage lumen while stomach contents are removed through the suction lumen. Used to remove toxic substances from the stomach.

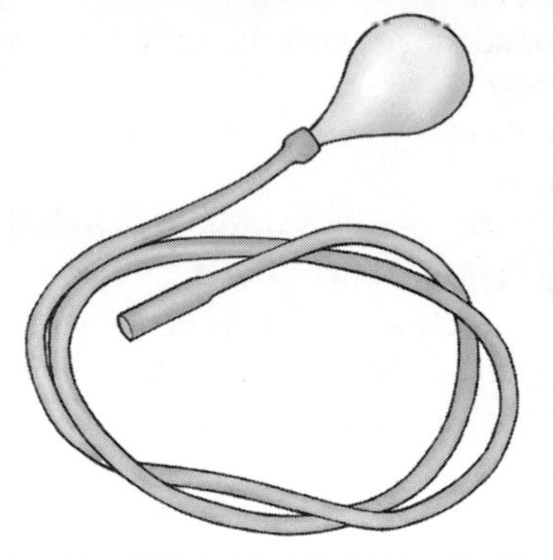

Large suction lumen

Lavage/vent lumen

Open eyes

Cantor tube

A single-lumen long tube with a small inflatable bag at the distal end. Five to ten mL of mercury are injected with a needle (gauge 21 or smaller or balloon may leak) and syringe into the bag prior to insertion of the tube.

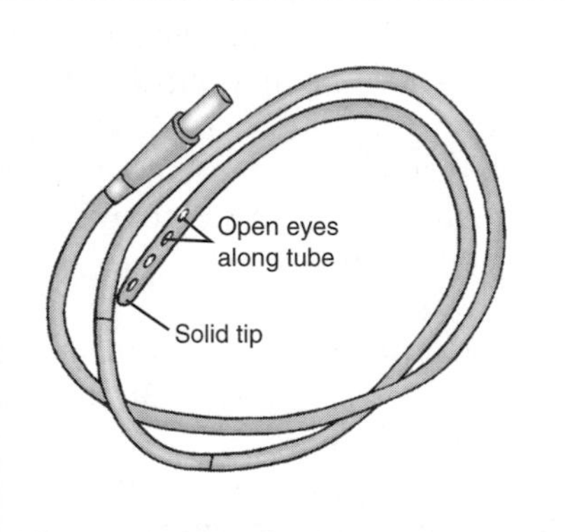

Levin tube

A plastic or rubber single-lumen tube with a solid tip that may be inserted into the stomach via the nose or mouth. Used to drain fluid and gas from the stomach. Single lumen must be used for irrigation and drainage, so continuous irrigation is not possible.

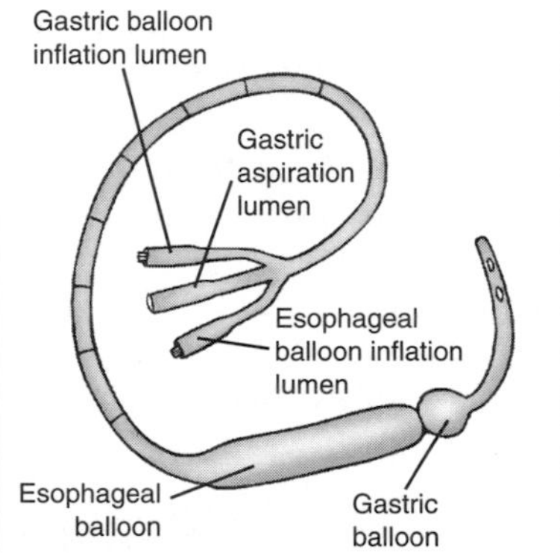

Open eyes along tube

Solid tip

Sengstaken-Blakemore tube

A three-lumen tube. Two ports inflate an esophageal and a gastric balloon for tamponade, and the third is used for nasogastric suction. This tube does not provide esophageal suction, but a nasogastric tube may be inserted in the opposite naris or the mouth and allowed to rest on top of the esophageal balloon. Esophageal suction is then possible, reducing the risk of aspiration.

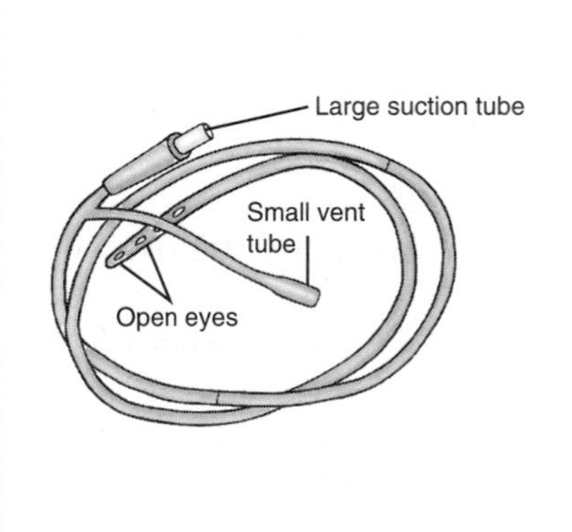

Gastric balloon inflation lumen

Gastric aspiration lumen

Esophageal balloon inflation lumen

Esophageal balloon

Gastric balloon

Salem sump tube

A short double-lumen tube. The small vent tube within the large suction tube prevents mucosal suction damage by maintaining the pressure in open eyes at the distal end of the tube at less than 25 mm Hg.

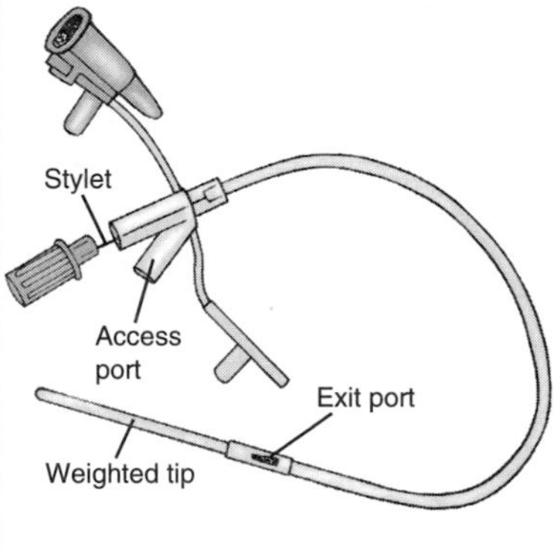

Large suction tube

Small vent tube

Open eyes

Weighted flexible feeding tube with stylet

Access port with irrigation adaptor allows maintenance of the tube without disconnecting the feeding set.

Stylet

Access port

Exit port

Weighted tip

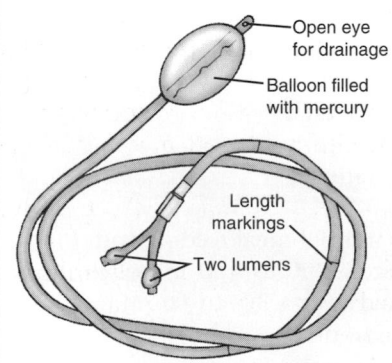

Open eye for drainage

Balloon filled with mercury

Length markings

Two lumens

Miller-Abbott tube

A long double-lumen tube used to drain and decompress the small intestine. One lumen leads to a balloon that is filled with mercury once it is in the stomach; the second is for irrigation and drainage.

FIG. 20-1 Comparison of design and function of selected gastrointestinal tubes. (From Monahan FD, Neighbors M: *Medical-surgical nursing: foundations for clinical practice,* Philadelphia, 1998, WB Saunders.)

▲ C. Administering feedings
1. Position the client in high-Fowler's and on the right side if comatose
2. Warm feeding to room temperature to prevent diarrhea and cramps
3. Aspirate all stomach contents (residual), measure the amount, and return the contents to the stomach to prevent electrolyte imbalances
4. Check physician's order and agency policy regarding residual amounts; usually if the residual is less than 100 to 150 mL, feeding is administered; if the residual is greater than 150 mL, hold the feeding
5. Assess tube placement by aspirating gastric contents and measuring the pH (should be 4 or less)
6. Assess bowel sounds; hold feeding and notify the physician if bowel sounds are absent
7. Use a feeding pump for continuous or cyclic feedings
8. For bolus feeding, leave the client in a high-Fowler's position for 30 minutes after feeding
9. For a continuous feeding, keep the client in a semi-Fowler's position at all times
D. Precautions
1. Change the feeding container and tubing every 24 hours
2. Do not hang more solution than will be required for a 4-hour period, to prevent bacterial growth
3. Check the expiration date on the formula before administering
4. Shake the formula well prior to inserting into container
5. Always assess placement of the tube prior to feeding
6. Always assess bowel sounds; do not administer any feedings if bowel sounds are absent
7. If an obstruction occurs, try flushing with water, saline, cranberry juice, ginger ale, or cola, if not contraindicated, after checking placement
8. Add a drop of methyline blue to the feeding, particularly with clients who have **endotracheal** or tracheal tubes; suspect tracheoesophageal fistula when blue gastric contents appear in tracheal excretion, and if this is noted, notify the physician immediately
9. Administer feeding at prescribed rate, or via gravity flow (intermittent, bolus feedings) with a 60-mL syringe with the plunger removed
10. Gently flush with 30 to 50 mL of water or normal saline (depending on agency policy) with the irrigation syringe after the feeding
▲ E. Prevention of complications
1. Diarrhea
a. Use fiber-containing feedings

b. Administer feeding slowly and at room temperature
2. Aspiration
a. Verify tube placement
b. Do not administer feeding if residual is greater than 150 mL
c. Keep the head of the bed elevated
d. If aspiration occurs, suction as needed, assess respiratory rate, auscultate lung sounds, monitor temperature for aspiration pneumonia, and prepare to obtain chest radiograph
3. Clogged tube
a. Use liquid forms of medication, if possible
b. Flush the tube with 30 to 50 mL of water or NS (depending on agency policy) before and after medication administration and before and after bolus feeding
c. Flush with water every 4 hours for continuous feeding
4. Vomiting
a. Administer feedings slowly, and for bolus feedings, make the feeding last for 30 minutes
b. Measure abdominal girth
c. Do not allow feeding to run dry
d. Do not allow air to enter the tubing
e. Administer feeding at room temperature
f. Elevate the head of the bed
g. Administer antiemetics as prescribed
h. If client vomits, place in side-lying position

III. MEDICATIONS VIA NG OR GASTROSTOMY TUBE ▲
A. Crush medications or use elixir forms of medications
B. Ensure that the medication ordered can be crushed or that the capsule can be opened
C. Dissolve crushed medication or capsule contents in 5 to 10 mL of water
D. Check placement and residual prior to instilling medications
E. Draw up the medication into a catheter tip syringe, clear excess air, and insert medication into the tube
F. Flush with 30 to 50 mL of water or NS (depending on agency policy)
G. Clamp the tube for 30 to 60 minutes (depending on medication and agency policy)

IV. INTESTINAL TUBES (Fig. 20-1)
A. Description
1. Passed nasally into the small intestine
2. Used to decompress the bowel or to remove intestinal contents
3. Enters the small intestine through the pyloric sphincter because of the weight of a small bag of mercury at the end

B. Types of tubes
1. Cantor and Harris tubes
    a. Single-lumen tube with a reservoir for 5 to 10 mL of mercury located at its tip, below the level of the drainage holes
    b. Mercury is inserted before the tube is passed through the nose, making the procedure uncomfortable
    c. The Harris tube is also used for lavage and suction
2. Miller-Abbott tube
    a. Double-lumen tube
    b. One lumen is for the instillation of mercury once the tube is in the stomach, and the other is for irrigation or drainage

C. Implementation
1. Assess physician's orders and agency policy for advancement and removal of tube
2. Position client on the right side to facilitate passage of the mercury weights within the tube through the pylorus of the stomach and into the small intestine
3. Do not secure the tube to the face with tape until it has reached final placement (may take several hours) in the intestines
4. X-ray is performed to verify desired placement
5. Monitor drainage from the tube
6. If the tube becomes blocked, notify the physician; a small amount of air injected into the lumen may be prescribed to clear the tube
7. Assess the abdomen and measure abdominal girth
8. To remove the tube, the mercury and air are removed from the balloon portion of the tube with a 5-mL syringe; the tube is gradually removed (6 inches every hour) as prescribed by the physician
9. Dispose of the mercury in the appropriate manner as per agency policy

V. ESOPHAGEAL AND GASTRIC TUBES (Fig. 20-1)
A. Description
1. Used to apply pressure against esophageal veins to control bleeding
2. Not used if the client has ulceration or necrosis of the esophagus or has had previous esophageal surgery
B. **Sengstaken-Blakemore tube**
1. Triple-lumen gastric tube with an inflatable esophageal balloon, an inflatable gastric balloon, and a gastric aspiration lumen
2. The gastric balloon applies pressure at the cardioesophageal junction to directly compress gastric varices and to decrease blood flow to esophageal varices; traction is applied to maintain the gastric balloon in place

3. The esophageal balloon directly compresses esophageal varices
4. If bleeding is not stopped with inflation of the gastric balloon, the esophageal balloon is inflated to 25 to 45 mm Hg
5. An x-ray of upper abdomen and chest confirms placement
6. Gastric contents are aspirated by gastric lavage or intermittent suction via the gastric aspiration port
7. With the **Sengstaken-Blakemore tube,** a nasogastric tube is also inserted in the opposite naris to collect secretions that accumulate above the esophageal balloon
C. Minnesota tube
1. Four-lumen gastric tube
2. A modified **Sengstaken-Blakemore** tube with an additional lumen for aspirating esophagopharyngeal secretions
D. Implementation
1. Check patency and integrity of all balloons prior to insertion
2. Label each lumen
3. Place the client in the upright or Fowler's position for insertion
4. Immediately after insertion, prepare for x-ray to verify placement
5. Maintain head elevation once the tube is in place
6. Double-clamp the balloon ports to prevent air leaks
7. Keep scissors at the bedside at all times; monitor for respiratory distress, and if it occurs, cut tubes to deflate balloons
8. To prevent ulceration or necrosis of the esophagus, release esophageal pressure as prescribed and per agency policy
9. Monitor for increased bloody drainage, which may indicate persistent bleeding
10. Monitor for signs of esophageal rupture, which includes a drop in blood pressure, increased heart rate, back and upper abdominal pain; esophageal rupture is an emergency and must be reported to the physician immediately

VI. LAVAGE TUBES
A. Description: Used to remove toxic substances from the stomach
B. Types of tubes
1. Lavacuator
    a. An orogastric tube with a large suction lumen and a smaller lavage/vent lumen that provides continuous suction
    b. Irrigation solution enters the lavage lumen while stomach contents are removed through the suction lumen
2. Ewald's: Reusable single-lumen large tube used for rapid one-time irrigation and evacuation

VII. URINARY AND RENAL TUBES
A. Routine urinary catheter care
  1. Use gloves and wash perineal area with warm soapy water
  2. With nondominant hand, pull back the labia or foreskin to expose the meatus (in the adult male, return foreskin to its normal position)
  3. Cleanse along the catheter with soap and water
  4. Anchor catheter to the thigh
  5. Maintain catheter bag below the level of the bladder
B. Ureteral and nephrostomy tubes
  1. Never clamp
  2. Maintain patency
  3. Monitor output closely
  4. Urine output of less than 30 mL per hour or lack of output for more than 15 minutes should be reported to the physician immediately
  5. Irrigate only if prescribed by a physician, using strict aseptic technique
  6. To irrigate, a maximum of 5 mL of sterile normal saline is instilled slowly and gently
  7. If patency cannot be established with prescribed irrigation, notify the physician immediately

VIII. RESPIRATORY SYSTEM TUBES
A. **Endotracheal (ET) tubes** (Fig. 20-2)
  1. Description
    a. Used to maintain a patent airway

b. Indicated when the client needs mechanical ventilation
c. If the client requires an artificial airway for longer than 10 to 14 days, a **tracheostomy** may be created to avoid mucosal and vocal cord damage that can be caused by the **endotracheal tube**
d. The cuff (located at the distal end of the tube), when inflated, produces a seal between the trachea and the cuff to prevent aspiration and ensure delivery of a set tidal volume when mechanical ventilation is used; an inflated cuff also prevents air from passing to the vocal cords, nose, or mouth
e. The pilot balloon permits air to be inserted into the cuff, prevents air from escaping, and is used as a guideline for determining the presence or absence of air in the cuff
f. The universal adapter enables attachment of the tube to mechanical ventilation tubing or other types of oxygen delivery systems
  2. Orotracheal
    a. Allows use of a larger-diameter tube and reduces the work of breathing
    b. Indicated when the client has a nasal obstruction or a predisposition to epistaxis
    c. Uncomfortable and can be manipulated by the tongue, causing airway obstruction; an

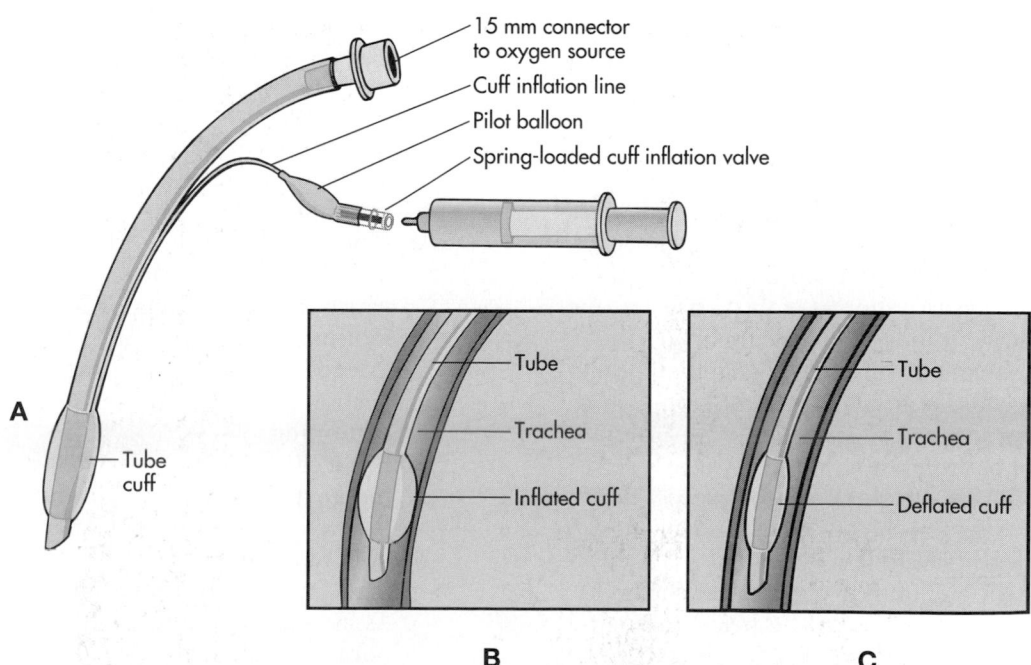

FIG. 20-2   A, Parts of a cuffed endotracheal tube. **B,** Tube in place with the cuff inflated. **C,** Tube in place with the cuff deflated. (From Beare PG, Myers JL: *Adult health nursing,* ed 3, St Louis, 1998, Mosby.)

oral airway may be needed to keep the client from biting on the tube

3. Nasotracheal
   a. Smaller-sized tube; increases resistance and increases client's work of breathing
   b. Discouraged in clients with bleeding disorders
   c. More comfortable for the client, and the client is unable to manipulate with the tongue

4. Implementation
   a. Placement is confirmed by chest x-ray (correct placement is 1 to 2 cm above the carina)
   b. Placement is assessed by auscultating both sides of chest while manually ventilating with a resuscitation (Ambu) bag (if breath sounds and chest wall movement are absent of the left side, the tube may be in the right main stem bronchus)
   c. Auscultation over the stomach is performed to rule out esophageal intubation
   d. If the tube is in the stomach, louder breath sounds will be heard over the stomach than over the chest, and abdominal distention will be present
   e. Secure the tube with adhesive tape immediately after intubation
   f. Monitor the position of the tube at the lip or nose
   g. Monitor skin and mucous membranes
   h. Suction only when needed
   i. The oral tube needs to be moved to the opposite side of the mouth daily to prevent pressure and necrosis of the lip and mouth area, prevent nerve damage, and facilitate inspection and cleaning of the mouth; moving the tube to the opposite side of the mouth should be done by two health care providers
   j. To prevent dislodgment, prevent pulling or tugging on the tube; suction, coughing, and speaking attempts by the client place extra stress on the tube and can cause dislodgment
   k. Keep a resuscitation (Ambu) bag at the bedside at all times
   l. Assess the pilot balloon to ensure that the cuff is inflated; maintain cuff inflation, which creates a seal and allows complete mechanical control of respiration
   m. Monitor cuff pressures at least every 8 hours; they should not exceed at 20 mm Hg

5. Minimal leak technique
   a. Inflate the cuff until a seal is established
   b. No harsh sound should be heard through a stethoscope placed over the trachea when the client breathes in, but a slight air leak on peak inspiration is present and heard
   c. The client cannot make verbal sounds, and no air is felt coming out of the client's mouth

6. Minimal occluding volume
   a. Provides an adequate seal in the trachea at the lowest possible cuff pressure
   b. Same procedure as minimal leak technique, without an air leak

7. Extubation
   a. Hyperoxygenate the client, and suction the **ET tube** and the oral cavity
   b. Place the client in semi-Fowler's position
   c. The cuff is deflated; have the client inhale, and at peak inspiration, remove the tube, suctioning the airway through the tube as it is pulled out
   d. After removal, instruct the client to cough and deep breathe to assist in removing accumulated secretions in the throat
   e. Apply oxygen therapy as prescribed
   f. Monitor for respiratory difficulty; contact the physician if respiratory difficulty occurs
   g. Inform the client that hoarseness or a sore throat is normal and that he or she should limit talking if it occurs

B. **Tracheostomy** (Fig. 20-3)
   1. Description
      a. A tracheotomy is a surgical incision into the trachea for the purpose of establishing an airway
      b. A **tracheostomy** is the stoma or opening that results from the tracheotomy (Table 20-1)
      c. The **tracheostomy** can be temporary or permanent
   2. Implementation
      a. Assess respirations and for bilateral breath sounds
      b. Monitor arterial blood gases (ABGs) and pulse oximetry
      c. Encourage coughing and deep breathing
      d. Maintain a semi-Fowler's to high-Fowler's position
      e. Monitor for bleeding, difficulty with breathing, absence of breath sounds, and crepitus, which are indications of hemorrhage, pneumothorax, and subcutaneous emphysema
      f. Provide respiratory treatments as prescribed
      g. Suction PRN; hyperoxygenate the client before suctioning
      h. If the client is allowed to eat, sit client up for meals, and ensure that the cuff is inflated (if the tube is not capped) for meals and for 1 hour after meals
      i. Monitor cuff pressures as prescribed
      j. Assess the stoma and secretions for blood or purulent drainage
      k. Follow the physician's orders and agency policy for cleaning the **tracheostomy** site and inner cannula; usually one-half strength hydrogen peroxide is used

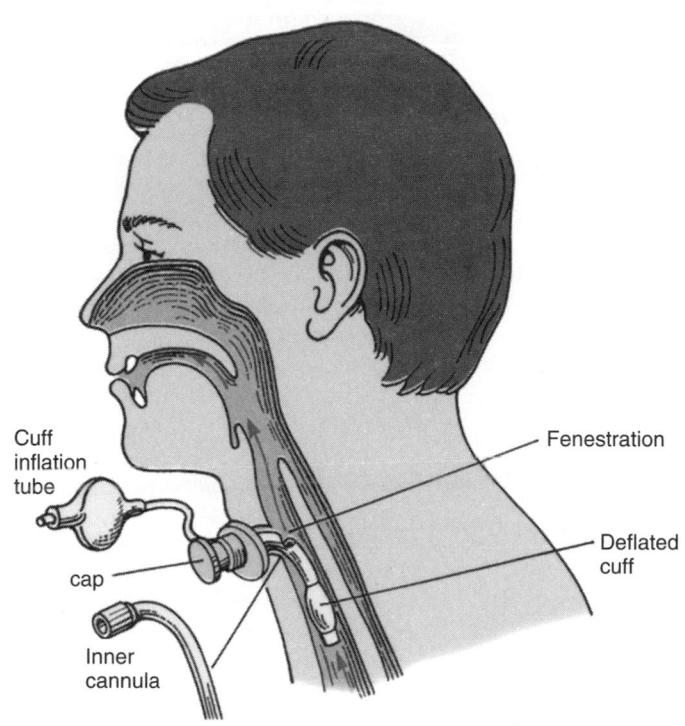

Cuff
inflation
tube

cap

Inner
cannula

Fenestration

Deflated
cuff

FIG. 20-3 Trach tube (fenestrated) with inner cannula removed and cap in place to allow speech. Tubes without opening interfere with speech. (From Elkin M, Perry AG, Potter PA: *Nursing interventions and clinical skills,* St Louis, 2000, Mosby.)

TABLE 20-1

Types of Tracheostomy Tubes

Type	Description	Type	Description
Double-lumen tube	• The double-lumen tube has three major parts: • Outer cannula—fits into the stoma and keeps the airway open. The face plate indicates the size and type of tube and has small holes on both sides for securing the tube with tracheostomy ties. • Inner cannula—fits snugly into the outer cannula and locks into place. Provides the universal adaptor for use with the ventilator and other respiratory therapy equipment. Some may be removed, cleaned, and reused; others are disposable. • Obturator—is a stylet with a blunt end used to facilitate direction of the tube when inserting or changing a tracheostomy tube. It is removed immediately after tube placement and is always kept with the client and at the bedside in case of accidental decannulation.	Fenestrated tube Cuffed fenestrated tube	• The fenestrated tube has a precut opening (fenestration) in the upper posterior wall of the outer cannula. It is used to wean the client from a tracheostomy by ensuring that the client can tolerate breathing through his or her natural airway before the entire tube is removed. This tube allows the client to speak. • The cuffed fenestrated tube facilitates mechanical ventilation and speech. It is often used for clients with spinal cord paralysis or neuromuscular disease who do not require ventilation all the time. When not on the ventilator, the client can have the cuff deflated and the tube capped for speech. A cuffed fenestrated tube is never used in weaning from a tracheostomy because the cuff, even fully deflated, may partially obstruct the airway.

From Ignatavicius D, Workman M, Mishler M: *Medical-surgical nursing across the health care continuum,* ed 3, Philadelphia, 1999, WB Saunders.

Continued

TABLE 20-1

Types of Tracheostomy Tubes—cont'd

Type	Description	Type	Description
Single-lumen tube	• The single-lumen tube is a long tube used for clients with long or extra thick necks. Often called a "bull neck trach" because of the long distance from the skin to the trachea or the longer length of the trachea in large people. More intensive nursing care is required with this tube because there is no inner cannula to ensure a patent lumen.	Metal tracheostomy tube	• The metal tracheostomy tube is used for permanent tracheostomy. It is a cuffless double-lumen tube and can be cleaned and reused indefinitely. A special adaptor attaches a manual resuscitation bag. Popular types are the Jackson and Holinger tubes.
Cuffed tube	• A cuff, when inflated, seals the airway. Used with mechanical ventilation, in preventing aspiration of oral or gastric secretions, or for tube feeding. A pilot balloon attached to the outside of the tube indicates the presence or absence of air in the cuff.	Talking tracheostomy tube	• The talking tracheostomy tube provides a means of communication for the client who is using a ventilator on a long-term basis. An extra air channel allows air to flow up through the vocal cords so that the client can speak with the cuff inflated. The air can cause drying of the vocal cords from constant dry airflow. Examples are the Pitt Trach Speaking Tube (National Catheter Corporation) and Communitrach (Implant Technologies, Inc.).
Cuffless tube	• The cuffless tube is a plastic, silicone-like (Silastic), or metal tube, usually double lumen. Used for long-term airway management in those clients who require a tracheostomy, who can protect themselves from aspiration, and who do not require mechanical ventilation. Many people can speak with this tube in place.		

From Ignatavicius D, Workman M, Mishler M: *Medical-surgical nursing across the health care continuum,* ed 3, Philadelphia, 1999, WB Saunders.

BOX 20-1

Complications of a Tracheostomy

TUBE OBSTRUCTION
Assessment
Difficulty in breathing
Noisy respirations
Difficulty in inserting the suction catheter
Thick, dry secretions
Unexplained peak pressures if client is on a mechanical ventilator
Implementation
Assist the client to cough and deep breath
Provide humidification and suctioning
Clean the inner cannula regularly
Instill normal saline into the tracheostomy tube as prescribed to loosen secretions (check agency policy regarding the instillation of normal saline)

TUBE DISLODGMENT
Prevention
Securing the tube in place
Minimizing manipulation and traction on the tube
Ensuring that the client does not pull on the tube
Implementation
Ensure that a tracheostomy tube of the same type and size is at the client's bedside

Be familiar with institutional policy regarding replacement of a tracheostomy tube as a nursing procedure

During the first 72 hours following surgical placement of the tracheostomy:
The nurse manually ventilates the client by using a manual resuscitation (Ambu) bag while another nurse calls the resuscitation team for help

After 72 hours following surgical placement of the tracheostomy:
Extend the client's neck and open the tissues of the stoma to secure the airway
Grasp the retention sutures (if they are present) to spread the opening
Use a tracheal dilator (curved clamp) to hold the stoma open
Prepare to insert tracheostomy tube; place obturator into tracheostomy tube, replace the tube, and remove the obturator
Maintain ventilation by resuscitation (Ambu) bag
Assess airflow and bilateral breath sounds
If unable to secure an airway, call the resuscitation team and the anesthesiologist

TABLE 20-2

Complications of Tracheostomy

Complications and Description	Signs and Symptoms	Management	Prevention
Tracheomalacia: constant pressure exerted by the cuff causes tracheal dilation and erosion of cartilage.	• An increased amount of air is required in the cuff to maintain the seal. • A larger tracheostomy tube is required to prevent an air leak at the stoma. • Food particles are seen in tracheal secretions. • The client does not receive tidal volume on the ventilator.	• No special management is needed unless bleeding occurs.	• Use an uncuffed tube as soon as possible. • Monitor cuff pressure and air volumes closely and detect changes.
Tracheal stenosis: narrowed tracheal lumen is due to scar formation from irritation of tracheal mucosa by the cuff.	• Stenosis usually seen after the cuff is deflated or the tracheostomy tube is removed. • The client has increased coughing; inability to expectorate secretions; or difficulty in breathing or talking.	• Tracheal dilation or surgical intervention is used.	• Prevent pulling of and traction on the tracheostomy tube. • Properly secure the tube in the midline position. • Maintain proper cuff pressure. • Minimize oronasal intubation time.

Tracheoesophageal fistula (TEF): excessive cuff pressure causes erosion of the posterior wall of the trachea. A hole is created between the trachea and the anterior esophagus. The client at highest risk also has a nasogastric tube present.	• Similar to tracheomalacia:
	  • Food particles are seen in tracheal secretions.
	  • Increased air in cuff is needed to achieve a seal.
	• The client has increased coughing and choking while eating.
	• The client does not receive the set tidal volume on the ventilator.
		• Manually administer oxygen by mask to prevent hypoxemia.
		• A small soft feeding tube is used instead of a nasogastric tube for tube feedings. A gastrostomy or jejunostomy may be performed.
		• Monitor the client with a nasogastric tube closely; assess for TEF and aspiration.
			• Maintain cuff pressure.
			• Monitor the amount of air needed for inflation and detect changes.
			• Progress to deflated cuff or cuffless tube as soon as possible.

Trachea–innominate artery fistula: a malpositioned tube causes its distal tip to push against the lateral wall of the tracheostomy. Continued pressure causes necrosis and erosion of the innominate artery. **This is a medical emergency.**	• The tracheostomy tube pulsates in synchrony with the heart beat. • There is exsanguination from the stoma. • This is a life-threatening complication.	• Remove the tracheostomy tube immediately. • Apply direct pressure to the innominate artery at the stoma site. • Prepare the client for immediate repair surgery.	• Correct the tube size, length, and midline position. • Prevent pulling or tugging on the tracheostomy tube. • Immediately notify the physician of pulsating tube.

From Ignatavicius D, Workman M, Mishler M: *Medical-surgical nursing across the health care continuum,* ed 3, Philadelphia, 1999, WB Saunders.

l. Administer humidified oxygen as prescribed, as the normal humidification process is bypassed in a client with a **tracheostomy**

m. Obtain assistance in changing **tracheostomy** ties; after placing the new ties, cut and remove the old ties holding the **tracheostomy** in place

n. Never insert a decannulation plug into a **tracheostomy** tube until the cuff is deflated and the inner cannula is removed; prior insertion prevents airflow to the client

o. Keep a resuscitation (Ambu) bag, obturator, clamps, and a tracheotomy set at the bedside

3. Complications of a **tracheostomy** (Box 20-1 and Table 20-2)

IX. CHEST TUBE DRAINAGE SYSTEM (Fig. 20-4)

A. Description

1. Returns negative pressure to the intrapleural space

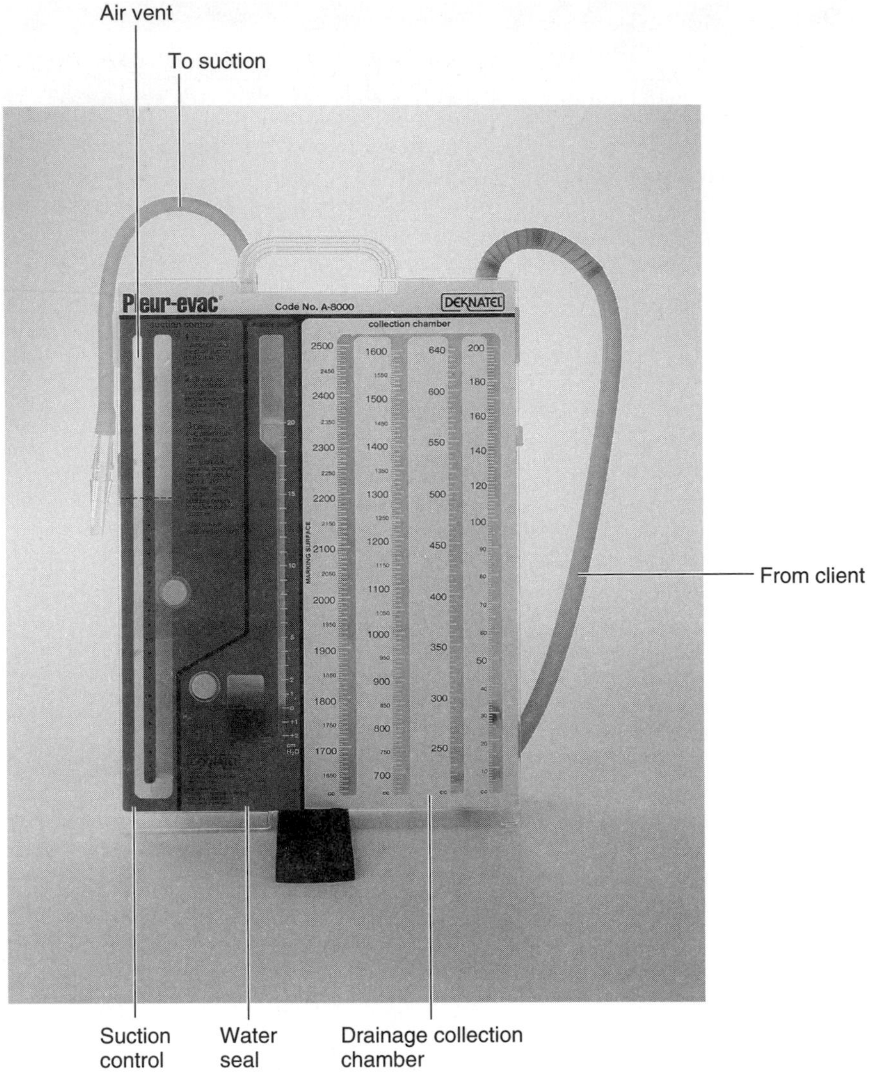

FIG. 20-4 The Pleur-Evac drainage system, a commercial three-bottle chest drainage device. (From Ignatavicius D, Workman M, Mishler M: *Medical-surgical nursing across the health care continuum,* ed 3, Philadelphia, 1999, WB Saunders.)

Labels on figure: Air vent; To suction; From client; Suction control; Water seal; Drainage collection chamber; Pleur-evac; Code No. A-8000; DEKNATEL; collection chamber

2. Used to remove abnormal accumulations of air and fluids from the pleural space
B. Collection chamber
   1. Where the **chest tube** from the client connects to the system
   2. Drainage from the tube drains into and collects in a series of calibrated columns in this chamber
C. Water seal chamber
   1. The tip of the tube is underwater, allowing fluid and air to drain from the pleural space and preventing air from entering the pleural space
   2. Water oscillates (moves up as the client inhales and moves down as the client exhales)
   3. Bubbling indicates an air leak in the **chest tube** system
D. Suction control chamber
   1. Provides the suction, which can be controlled to provide negative pressure to the chest
   2. This chamber is filled with various levels of water

to achieve the desired level of suction; without this control, lung tissue could be sucked into the **chest tube**
   3. Gentle bubbling in this chamber indicates that there is suction, and it does not indicate that air is escaping from the pleural space
E. Dry suction system (Fig. 20-5)
   1. Because this is a dry suction system, absence of bubbling is noted in the suction control chamber
   2. A knob on the collection device is used to set the prescribed amount of suction; then the wall suction source dial is turned until a small orange floater valve appears in the window on the device (when the orange floater valve is in the window, the correct amount of suction is applied)
F. Implementation
   1. Collection chamber
      a. Monitor drainage; notify the physician if drainage is greater than 100 mL per hour or if

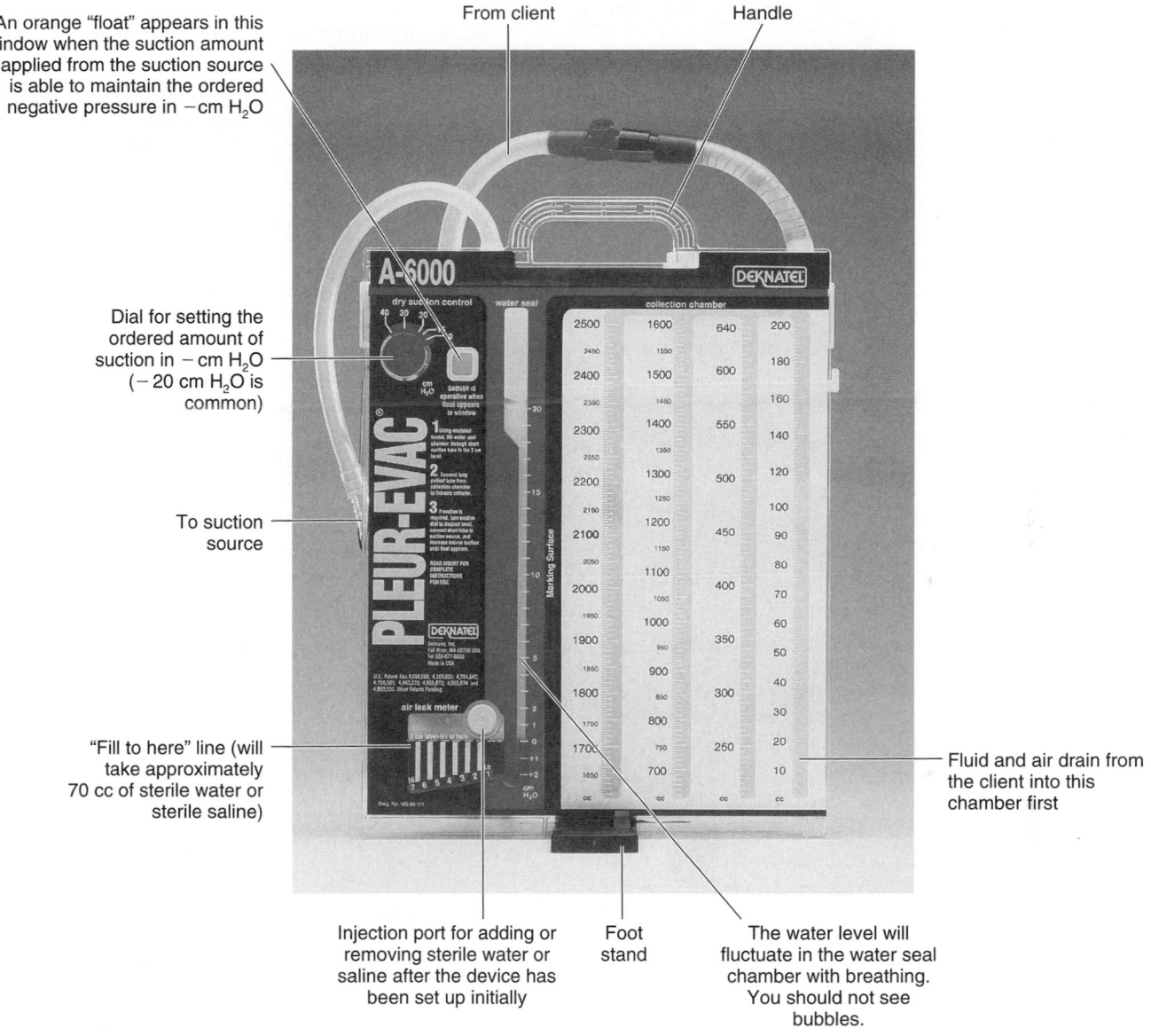

An orange "float" appears in this window when the suction amount applied from the suction source is able to maintain the ordered negative pressure in −cm H₂O

From client

Handle

Dial for setting the ordered amount of suction in − cm H₂O (− 20 cm H₂O is common)

To suction source

"Fill to here" line (will take approximately 70 cc of sterile water or sterile saline)

Fluid and air drain from the client into this chamber first

Injection port for adding or removing sterile water or saline after the device has been set up initially

Foot stand

The water level will fluctuate in the water seal chamber with breathing. You should not see bubbles.

FIG. 20-5   The A-6000 dry suction control Pleur-Evac chest drainage system. (Courtesy Deknatel, Inc, Fall River, Mass.) (From Ignatavicius D, Workman M, Mishler M: *Medical-surgical nursing across the health care continuum,* ed 3, Philadelphia, 1999, WB Saunders.)

drainage becomes bright red or increases suddenly
   b. Mark the **chest tube** drainage in the collection chamber at 1- to 4-hour intervals, using a piece of tape
2. Water seal chamber
   a. Monitor for fluctuation of the fluid level in the water seal chamber
   b. Fluctuation in the water seal chamber stops if the tube is obstructed, if a dependent loop exists, if the suction is not working properly, or if the lung has re-expanded
   c. If the client has a known pneumothorax, intermittent bubbling in the water seal

chamber is expected as air is drained from the chest, but continuous bubbling indicates of an air leak in the system
   d. Notify the physician if there is continuous bubbling in the water seal chamber
3. Suction control chamber: Gentle bubbling should be noted in the suction control chamber (vigorous bubbling indicates an air leak, and the physician should be notified)
4. An occlusive sterile dressing is maintained at the insertion site
5. A chest radiograph assesses the position of the tube and determines whether the lung has re-expanded

6. Assess respiratory status and auscultate lung sounds
7. Monitor for signs of extended pneumothroax or hemothorax
8. Keep the drainage system below the level of the chest and the tubes free of kinks, dependent loops, or other obstructions
9. Ensure that all connections are secure
10. Encourage coughing and deep breathing
11. Change the client's position frequently to promote drainage and ventilation
12. Do not strip or milk a **chest tube** unless specifically directed to do so by a physician and if the agency policy allows
13. Keep a clamp and a sterile occlusive dressing at the bedside at all times
14. Never clamp a **chest tube** without a written order from the physician; also, determine agency policy for clamping **chest tubes**
15. If the drainage system cracks or breaks, insert the tube into a bottle of sterile water, remove the cracked or broken system, and replace it with a new system
16. If the **chest tube** is accidentally pulled out of the chest, pinch the skin opening together, apply an occlusive sterile dressing, cover the dressing with overlapping pieces of 2-inch tape, and call the physician immediately
17. When the **chest tube** is removed, the client is asked to take a deep breath and hold it, and the tube is removed; a dry sterile dressing, petroleum gauze dressing, or Telfa dressing (depending on the physician's preference) is taped in place after removal of the **chest tube**
18. Depending on the physician's preference, when the **chest tube** is removed, the client may be asked to take a deep breath, exhale, and bear down (Valsalva's maneuver)

PRACTICE QUESTIONS

1. A nurse orientee is preparing to insert a nasogastric (NG) tube, and a nurse educator is observing the procedure. Which of the following supplies if obtained by the nurse orientee would indicate a need for further education regarding this procedure?
   1. Half-inch or one-inch tape
   2. Oil-soluble lubricant
   3. A glass of tap water with a straw
   4. A 50-mL catheter tip syringe
2. A registered nurse is observing a new orientee who is inserting a nasogastric (NG) tube in an adult client. The new orientee is determining the length of tube insertion. Which of the following observations indicates accurate measurement of the length of the tube to be inserted?
   1. The new orientee places the tube at the tip of the

nose and measures by extending the tube to the earlobe and then down to the xiphoid process
   2. The new orientee places the tube at the tip of the nose and measures by extending the tube to the earlobe and then down to the top of the sternum
   3. The new orientee marks the tube at 10 inches
   4. The new orientee marks the tube at 32 inches
3. A nurse is inserting a nasogastric (NG) tube in an adult client. During the procedure the client begins to cough and has difficulty breathing. Which of the following is the most appropriate nursing action?
   1. Remove the tube and reinsert when the respiratory distress subsides
   2. Pull back on the tube and wait until the respiratory distress subsides
   3. Quickly insert the tube
   4. Notify the physician immediately
4. A nurse is assessing for correct placement of a nasogastric (NG) tube. The nurse aspirates the stomach contents and checks the contents for pH. The nurse verifies correct tube placement if which pH value is noted?
   1. 7.5
   2. 7.35
   3. 7.0
   4. 4.0
5. A nurse is preparing to remove a nasogastric (NG) tube from a client. The nurse would instruct the client to do which of the following just before the nurse removes the tube?
   1. To perform a Valsalva maneuver
   2. To take and hold a deep breath
   3. To exhale
   4. To inhale and exhale quickly
6. A nurse is preparing to administer medication through a nasogastric tube (NG) that is connected to suction. To administer the medication accurately, the nurse would:
   1. Aspirate the NG tube after medication administration to maintain patency
   2. Position the client supine to assist in medication absorption
   3. Clamp the NG tube for 30 minutes following administration of the medication
   4. Change the suction setting to low intermittent suction for 30 minutes after medication administration
7. A nurse assists a physician with the insertion of a Miller-Abbott tube. After insertion of the tube, the nurse would assist the client to which of the following positions?
   1. On the right side
   2. On the left side
   3. Prone
   4. Left lateral Sims'
8. A nurse is preparing to care for a client with esophageal varices who has just had a Sengstaken-Blakemore tube inserted. The nurse gathers sup-

plies, knowing that which of the following items must be kept at the bedside at all times?
1. An irrigation set
2. A pair of scissors
3. A Kelly clamp
4. An obturator

9. A nurse is inserting an indwelling urinary catheter into the urethra of a male client. As the nurse inflates the balloon, the client complains of discomfort. The most appropriate nursing action is to:
   1. Remove the syringe from the balloon; discomfort is normal and temporary
   2. Aspirate the fluid, advance the catheter farther, and reinflate the balloon
   3. Aspirate the fluid, withdraw the catheter slightly, and reinflate the balloon
   4. Aspirate the fluid, remove the catheter and insert a new catheter

10. A nurse is inserting an indwelling urinary catheter into a male client. As the catheter is inserted into the urethra, urine begins to flow into the tubing. At this point, the nurse:
    1. Immediately inflates the balloon
    2. Withdraws the catheter approximately 1 inch and inflates the balloon
    3. Inserts the catheter until resistance is met and inflates the balloon
    4. Inserts the catheter 2.5 to 5 cm and inflates the balloon

11. A nurse is assisting a physician with the insertion of a chest tube. The nurse monitors the client and notes fluctuation of the fluid level in the water seal chamber after the tube is inserted. On the basis of this assessment, which of the following actions would be most appropriate?
    1. Inform the physician
    2. Encourage the client to deep breathe
    3. Continue to monitor, as this is an expected finding
    4. Reinforce the occlusive dressing

12. A nurse is caring for a client with a chest tube. The nurse turns the client to the side, and the chest tube accidentally disconnects. The initial nursing action is to:
    1. Call the physician
    2. Place the tube in a bottle of sterile water
    3. Immediately replace the chest tube system
    4. Place a sterile dressing over the disconnection site

13. A nurse is assisting a physician with the removal of a chest tube. The nurse most appropriately instructs the client to:
    1. Stay very still
    2. Inhale and exhale quickly
    3. Exhale as the tube is pulled out
    4. Perform the Valsalva maneuver

14. A nurse is changing the tapes on a tracheostomy tube. The client coughs and the tube is dislodged. The initial nursing action is to:
    1. Cover the tracheostomy site with a sterile dressing to prevent infection
    2. Call the physician to reinsert the tube
    3. Grasp the retention sutures to spread the opening
    4. Call the respiratory therapy department to reinsert the tracheotomy

15. A nurse is caring for a client immediately after removal of the endotracheal tube following radical neck dissection. The nurse plans to report which of the following signs immediately if experienced by the client?
    1. Stridor
    2. Occasional pink-tinged sputum
    3. Respiratory rate of 24 breaths per minute
    4. A few basilar crackles on the right

CRITICAL THINKING: FREE-TEXT ENTRY

A nurse is caring for a client who is receiving feedings via a nasogastric tube. The client suddenly begins to vomit, and the nurse quickly places the client in a high-Fowler's position. The client is coughing and having difficulty breathing, and the nurse suspects that the client has aspirated the feeding. What is the nurse's next action?

Answer: _____

ANSWERS

1. **2**

Rationale: Water-soluble lubricant is used to lubricate 3 to 4 inches of the tube at the insertion end. An oil lubricant is not used because if the tube accidentally goes into the bronchus, pneumonia can develop. Half-inch tape is used to secure the tube after correct placement is verified. A 50-mL catheter tip syringe is used to aspirate gastric contents to confirm placement. The client will be asked to take a sip of water through a straw to help with the passage of the tube.

Test-Taking Strategy: Use the process of elimination. Note the key words "indicate a need for further education." Attempt to visualize the procedure as you answer the question. Remember that water-soluble lubricant must be used to lubricate the tube. If you had difficulty with this question, review the procedure for inserting an NG tube.
Level of Cognitive Ability: Analysis
Client Needs: Physiological Integrity
Integrated Concept/Process: Nursing Process/Evaluation
Content Area: Adult Health/Gastrointestinal

Reference: Potter, P., & Perry, A. (2001). *Fundamentals of nursing* (5th ed.). St. Louis: Mosby, p. 1474.

2. 1

Rationale: Measuring the length of tube needed is done by placing the tube at the tip of the client's nose and extending the tube to the earlobe and then down to the xiphoid process. The average length for an adult is about 22 to 26 inches.

Test-Taking Strategy: Use the process of elimination. Attempt to visualize this procedure. Eliminate options 3 and 4 first because 10 inches is short and 32 inches is rather lengthy. Remember the abbreviation NEX, which stands for nose, earlobe, xiphoid process, to assist in answering questions similar to this one. Review the procedure for measuring the length of an NG tube for insertion if you had difficulty with this question.

Level of Cognitive Ability: Analysis
Client Needs: Safe, Effective Care Environment
Integrated Concept/Process: Nursing Process/Evaluation
Content Area: Adult Health/Gastrointestinal
Reference: Potter, P., & Perry, A. (2001). *Fundamentals of nursing* (5th ed.). St. Louis: Mosby, p. 1474.

3. 2

Rationale: During the insertion of an NG tube, if the client experiences difficulty breathing or any respiratory distress, withdraw the tube slightly, stop the tube advancement, and wait until the distress subsides. Options 1 and 4 are unnecessary. Quickly inserting the tube is not an appropriate action because, in this situation, it may be likely that the tube has entered the bronchus.

Test-Taking Strategy: Use the process of elimination. Options 3 and 4 can be eliminated first. Visualizing the procedure and anticipating potential complications will assist in eliminating option 1 as an unnecessary action. Review the cautions related to inserting an NG tube if you had difficulty with this question.

Level of Cognitive Ability: Application
Client Needs: Physiological Integrity
Integrated Concept/Process: Nursing Process/Implementation
Content Area: Adult Health/Gastrointestinal
Reference: Potter, P., & Perry, A. (2001). *Fundamentals of nursing* (5th ed.). St. Louis: Mosby, p. 1476.

4. 4

Rationale: If the NG tube is in the stomach, the pH of the contents will be acidic. Gastric aspirates have acidic pH values and should be 4 or less. Option 1 indicates an alkaline pH. Option 2 indicates a neutral pH. Option 3 indicates a slightly acidic pH.

Test-Taking Strategy: Use the process of elimination and note the key word "verifies." Recalling that gastric contents are acidic will easily direct you to option 4. If you had difficulty with this question, review the procedure for assessing NG tube placement.

Level of Cognitive Ability: Analysis
Client Needs: Physiological Integrity
Integrated Concept/Process: Nursing Process/Analysis
Content Area: Adult Health/Gastrointestinal
Reference: Potter, P., & Perry, A. (2001). *Fundamentals of nursing* (5th ed.). St. Louis: Mosby, p. 1476.

5. 2

Rationale: When the nurse removes an NG tube, the client is instructed to take and hold a deep breath. This will close the epiglottis, and the airway will be temporarily obstructed during the tube removal. This allows for easy withdrawal through the esophagus into the nose. The nurse removes the tube with one very smooth continuous pull.

Test-Taking Strategy: Use the process of elimination and focus on the issue, removing an NG tube. Visualize the procedure as a guide, considering what each action identified in the options would produce. Review the procedure for removing an NG tube, if you had difficulty with this question.

Level of Cognitive Ability: Application
Client Needs: Physiological Integrity
Integrated Concept/Process: Nursing Process/Implementation
Content Area: Adult Health/Gastrointestinal
Reference: Potter, P., & Perry, A. (2001). *Fundamentals of nursing* (5th ed.). St. Louis: Mosby, p. 1479.

6. 3

Rationale: If a client has an NG tube connected to suction, the nurse should wait up to 30 minutes before reconnecting the tube to the suction apparatus to allow adequate time for medication absorption. Aspirating the NG tube will remove the medication just administered. Low intermittent suction will also remove the medication just administered. The client should not be placed in the supine position because of the risk for aspiration.

Test-Taking Strategy: Use the process of elimination. Eliminate options 1 and 4 first because these actions are similar and will produce the same effect. Recalling that the client should not be placed in a supine position will assist in eliminating option 2. If you had difficulty with this question, review the procedure for administering medications through an NG tube.

Level of Cognitive Ability: Application
Client Needs: Physiological Integrity
Integrated Concept/Process: Nursing Process/Implementation
Content Area: Adult Health/Gastrointestinal
Reference: Leahy, J., & Kizilay, P. (1998). *Foundations of nursing practice: A nursing process approach.* Philadelphia: W.B. Saunders, p. 464.

7. 1

Rationale: A Miller-Abbott tube is an intestinal tube that has a double lumen, one for a mercury balloon and the other for suction or drainage. After insertion, the tube is allowed to advance over several hours. The client is positioned on the right side to facilitate passage through the pylorus of the stomach and into the small intestine.

Test-Taking Strategy: Use the process of elimination. Eliminate options 2 and 4 because they are similar. From the remaining options, recalling the purpose of this tube and the anatomy of the body will assist in directing you to option 1. If you had difficulty with this question, review care to the client with a Miller-Abbott tube.

Level of Cognitive Ability: Application
Client Needs: Physiological Integrity
Integrated Concept/Process: Nursing Process/Implementation
Content Area: Adult Health/Gastrointestinal
Reference: Smith, S., Duell, D., & Martin, B. (2000). *Clinical nursing skills: Basic to advanced skills* (5th ed.). Upper Saddle River, NJ: Prentice-Hall Health, p. 654.

8. 2

Rationale: When the client has a Sengstaken-Blakemore tube, a pair of scissors must be kept at the client's bedside at all times. The client needs to be observed for sudden respiratory distress, which occurs if the gastric balloon ruptures and the entire tube moves upward. If this occurs, the nurse immediately cuts all balloon lumens and removes the tube. An obturator and a Kelly clamp are kept at the bedside of a client with a tracheostomy. An irrigation set may be kept at the bedside, but it is not the priority item.

Test-Taking Strategy: Use the process of elimination and knowledge regarding the structure, function, and placement of a Sengstaken-Blakemore tube to answer this question. Note the key word "must" in the stem of the question. This should assist in eliminating options 1, 3, and 4. If you had difficulty with this question, review nursing care for a client with a Sengstaken-Blakemore tube.

Level of Cognitive Ability: Application
Client Needs: Safe, Effective Care Environment
Integrated Concept/Process: Nursing Process/Planning
Content Area: Adult Health/Gastrointestinal
Reference: Ignatavicius, D., Workman, M., & Mishler, M. (1999). *Medical-surgical nursing across the health care continuum* (3rd ed.). Philadelphia: W.B. Saunders, p. 1473.

9. **2**

Rationale: If the balloon is malpositioned in the urethra, inflating the balloon could produce trauma, and pain will occur. If pain occurs, the fluid should be aspirated and the catheter inserted a little farther in order to provide sufficient space to inflate the balloon. The catheter's balloon is behind the opening at the insertion tip. Inserting the catheter the extra distance will ensure that the balloon is inflated inside the bladder and not in the urethra. There is no need to remove the catheter and insert a new one. Pain when the balloon is inflated is not normal.

Test Taking Strategy: Use the process of elimination, noting the issue of the question, the client's complain of discomfort. Attempt to visualize this procedure and the anatomy of the urinary system to answer this question. If you had difficulty with this question, review the procedure for inserting a urinary catheter.

Level of Cognitive Ability: Application
Client Needs: Physiological Integrity
Integrated Concept/Process: Nursing Process/Implementation
Content Area: Adult Health/Renal
Reference: Altman, G., Buchsel, P., & Coxon, V. (2000). *Delmar's fundamental & advanced nursing skills.* Albany, N.Y.: Delmar, p. 697.

10. **4**

Rationale: The catheter's balloon is behind the opening at the insertion tip. The catheter is inserted 2.5 to 5 cm after urine begins to flow in order to provide sufficient space to inflate the balloon. Inserting the catheter the extra distance will ensure that the balloon is inflated inside the bladder and not in the urethra. Inflating the balloon in the urethra could produce trauma.

Test-Taking Strategy: Knowledge of the proper procedure for inserting an indwelling urinary catheter will assist you in answering this question. Note the key words "urine begins to flow." Options 2 and 3 can easily be eliminated. Eliminate option 1 next because of the word "immediately." If you had difficulty with this question, review the procedure for bladder catheterization.

Level of Cognitive Ability: Application
Client Needs: Safe, Effective Care Environment

Integrated Concept/Process: Nursing Process/Implementation
Content Area: Adult Health/Renal
Reference: Potter, P., & Perry, A. (2001). *Fundamentals of nursing* (5th ed.). St. Louis: Mosby, p. 1419.

11. **3**

Rationale: The presence of fluctuation of the fluid level in the water seal chamber indicates a patent drainage system. With normal breathing, the water level rises with inspiration and falls with expiration. Fluctuation stops if the tube is obstructed, if a dependent loop exists, if the suction is not working properly, or if the lung has re-expanded. Options 1, 2, and 4 are incorrect.

Test-Taking Strategy: Use the process of elimination, focusing on the issue, fluctuation of the fluid level in the water seal chamber. Recalling that this is an expected finding will direct you to the correct option. Review the expected and unexpected assessment findings in the care of a client with a chest tube if you had difficulty with this question.

Level of Cognitive Ability: Analysis
Client Needs: Physiological Integrity
Integrated Concept/Process: Nursing Process/Implementation
Content Area: Adult Health/Respiratory
Reference: Smeltzer, S., & Bare, B. (2000). *Brunner & Suddarth's textbook of medical-surgical nursing* (9th ed.). Philadelphia: Lippincott Williams & Wilkins, p. 518.

12. **2**

Rationale: If the chest drainage system is disconnected, the end of the tube is placed in a bottle of sterile water held below the level of the chest. After this initial action, the nurse then replaces the system. Placing a sterile dressing over the disconnection site will not prevent complications resulting from the disconnection. The physician may need to be notified, but this is not the initial action.

Test-Taking Strategy: Use the process of elimination. Note the key word "initial" in the stem of the question. This indicates that a nursing action is required that will prevent a serious complication as a result of the disconnection. Eliminate options 1 and 3, as these actions delay required and immediate intervention. Knowledge of the complications that can occur from a disconnection will easily direct you to option 2. Review interventions related to the complications of a chest tube if you had difficulty with this question.

Level of Cognitive Ability: Application
Client Needs: Physiological Integrity
Integrated Concept/Process: Nursing Process/Implementation
Content Area: Adult Health/Respiratory
Reference: Lewis, S., Heitkemper, M., & Dirksen, S. (2000). *Medical-surgical nursing: Assessment and management of clinical problems* (5th ed.). St. Louis: Mosby, p. 648.

13. **4**

Rationale: When the chest tube is removed, the client is asked to perform the Valsalva maneuver (take a deep breath, exhale, and bear down), the tube is quickly withdrawn, and an airtight dressing is taped in place. An alternative instruction is to ask the client to take a deep breath and hold the breath while the tube is removed. Options 1, 2, and 3 are incorrect client instructions.

Test-Taking Strategy: Use the process of elimination. Visualize the procedure and the client instructions as you select an option. If you had difficulty with this question, review the procedure for removal of a chest tube.

Level of Cognitive Ability: Application
Client Needs: Physiological Integrity
Integrated Concept/Process: Nursing Process/Implementation
Content Area: Adult Health/Respiratory
Reference: Smeltzer, S., & Bare, B. (2000). *Brunner & Suddarth's textbook of medical-surgical nursing* (9th ed.). Philadelphia: Lippincott Williams & Wilkins, p. 518.

14. 3
Rationale: If the tube is accidentally dislodged, the initial nursing action is to grasp the retention sutures and spread the opening. If agency policy permits, the nurse then attempts to immediately replace the tube. Covering the tracheostomy site will block the airway. Options 2 and 4 will delay treatment in this emergency situation.
Test-Taking Strategy: Use the process of elimination. Eliminate options 2 and 4 first because they are similar and will delay the immediate intervention needed. Eliminate option 1 because this action will block the airway. If you had difficulty with this question, review the intervention required if a tracheostomy tube dislodges.
Level of Cognitive Ability: Application
Client Needs: Physiological Integrity
Integrated Concept/Process: Nursing Process/Implementation
Content Area: Adult Health/Respiratory
Reference: Lewis, S., Heitkemper, M., & Dirksen, S. (2000). *Medical-surgical nursing: Assessment and management of clinical problems* (5th ed.). St. Louis: Mosby, p. 595.

15. 1
Rationale: The nurse reports stridor to the physician immediately. This is a high-pitched, coarse sound that is heard with the stethoscope over the trachea. It indicates airway edema, and places the client at risk for airway obstruction. Options 2, 3, and 4 are not signs that require immediate notification of the physician.

Test Taking Strategy: Use the process of elimination. Recall that the prime danger after removal of an artificial airway is the client's ability to maintain a patent airway and breathe independently. In comparing each of the options with this risk in mind, eliminate options 2, 3, and 4. Since stridor indicates laryngeal edema and possible airway obstruction, it is the symptom that must be reported immediately. Review care to the client following removal of an endotracheal tube if you had difficulty with this question.
Level of Cognitive Ability: Analysis
Client Needs: Physiological Integrity
Integrated Concept/Process: Nursing Process/Planning
Content Area: Adult Health/Respiratory
Reference: Lewis, S., Heitkemper, M., & Dirksen, S. (2000). *Medical-surgical nursing: Assessment and management of clinical problems* (5th ed.). St. Louis: Mosby, p. 1937.

CRITICAL THINKING: FREE-TEXT ENTRY

Answer: Suction the client
Rationale: If the client aspirates the feeding, the nurse would suction the client. The client's respiratory status would be monitored closely until a normal respiratory pattern resumed.
Test-Taking Strategy: Focus on the information provided in the question. Use the ABCs—airway, breathing, and circulation. If a client aspirates a feeding, suctioning is necessary to provide a patent airway. Review care to the client receiving tube feedings if you had difficulty with this question.
Level of Cognitive Ability: Application
Client Needs: Physiological Integrity
Integrated Concept/Process: Nursing Process/Implementation
Content Area: Adult Health/Respiratory
Reference: Smith, S., Duell, D., & Martin, B. (2000). *Clinical nursing skills: Basic to advanced skills* (5th ed.). Upper Saddle River, NJ: Prentice-Hall Health, p. 477.

REFERENCES

Altman, G., Buchsel, P., & Coxon, V. (2000). *Delmar's fundamental & advanced nursing skills.* Albany, N.Y.: Delmar.

Elkin, M., Perry, A., & Potter, P. (2000). *Nursing interventions and clinical skills* (2nd ed.). St. Louis: Mosby.

Ignatavicius, D., Workman, M., & Mishler, M. (1999). *Medical-surgical nursing across the health care continuum* (3rd ed.). Philadelphia: W.B. Saunders.

Leahy, J., & Kizilay, P. (1998). *Foundations of nursing practice: A nursing process approach.* Philadelphia: W.B. Saunders.

Lewis, S., Heitkemper, M., & Dirksen, S. (2000). *Medical-surgical nursing: Assessment and management of clinical problems* (5th ed.). St. Louis: Mosby.

Monahan, F., & Neighbors, M. (1998). *Medical-surgical nursing: Foundations for clinical practice* (2nd ed.). Philadelphia: W.B. Saunders.

Potter, P., & Perry, A. (2001). *Fundamentals of nursing* (5th ed.). St. Louis: Mosby.

Smeltzer, S., & Bare, B. (2000). *Brunner & Suddarth's textbook of medical-surgical nursing* (9th ed.). Philadelphia: Lippincott Williams & Wilkins.

Smith, S., Duell, D., & Martin, B. (2000). *Clinical nursing skills: Basic to advanced skills* (5th ed.). Upper Saddle River, NJ: Prentice-Hall Health.

UNIT V

Growth and Development Across the Life Span

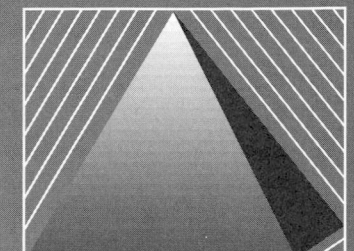

PYRAMID TERMS

accommodation The ability to change a schema in order to introduce new ideas, objects, or experiences.

assimilation The ability to incorporate new ideas, objects, and experiences into the framework of one's thoughts.

conscious Includes all experiences that are within an individual's awareness and that the individual is able to control.

ego One's "sense of self"; provides such functions as problem solving, mobilization of defense mechanisms, reality testing, and the capability of functioning independently. The mediator between the id and the superego.

id Source of all primitive drives and instincts; is thought of as the reservoir of all psychic energy.

schema Refers to an individual's cognitive structure or framework of thought.

schemata Categories that an individual forms in his or her mind to organize and understand the world.

subconscious Often called the preconscious; includes experiences, thoughts, feelings, or desires that might not be in immediate awareness but can be recalled to consciousness; helps repress unpleasant thoughts or feelings.

superego Internal representative of the values, ideals, and moral standards of society.

unconscious Includes memories, feelings, thoughts, or wishes that are repressed and that are not available to the conscious mind.

▶ PYRAMID TO SUCCESS

Normal growth and development proceed in an orderly, systematic, and predictable pattern, which provides a basis for identifying and assessing an individual's abilities. Understanding the path of growth and development across the life span assists the nurse in identifying appropriate and expected human behavior. The Pyramid to Success focuses on Sigmund Freud's Theory of Psychosexual Development, Jean Piaget's Theory of Cognitive Development, Erik Erikson's Psychosocial Theory, and Lawrence Kohlberg's Theory of Moral Development. The Integrated Concepts and Processes addressed in this unit include Nursing Process, Caring, Communication and Documentation, Cultural Awareness, Self-Care, and Teaching/Learning.

CLIENT NEEDS
Safe, Effective Care Environment

Advocacy
Client rights
Confidentiality
Consultation with members of the health care team
Establishing priorities
Ethical practice
Legal responsibilities
Referrals
Respect for client and family needs on the basis of their preferences

Health Promotion and Maintenance

Aging process
Developmental stages and transition
Family planning and family systems
Health and wellness
Health care beliefs and preferences
Lifestyle choices

Psychosocial Integrity

Coping mechanisms
End of life
Mental health concepts
Religious and spiritual influences on health
Support systems

Physiological Integrity

Basic care and comfort

Health care preferences

Incorporating interventions compatible with client's cultural, religious, and health care beliefs, education level, and language

Practices or restrictions related to procedures and treatments

Providing care using a nonjudgmental approach

REFERENCES

Craven, R., & Hirnle, C. (2000). *Fundamentals of nursing: Human health and function* (3rd ed.). Philadelphia: Lippincott Williams & Wilkins.

Lewis, S., Heitkemper, M., & Dirksen, S. (2000). *Medical-surgical nursing: Assessment and management of clinical problems* (5th ed.). St. Louis: Mosby.

Lowdermilk, D., Perry, S., & Bobak, I. (2000). *Maternity & women's health care* (7th ed.). St. Louis: Mosby.

National Council of State Boards of Nursing (eds.) (2000). *Test Plan for the National Council Licensure Examination for Registered Nurses.* Chicago: Author.

Phipps, W., Sands, J., & Marek, J. (1999). *Medical-surgical nursing: Concepts & clinical practice* (6th ed.). St. Louis: Mosby.

Olds, S., London. M., & Ladewig, P. (2000). *Maternal-newborn nursing: A family and community-based approach* (6th ed.). Upper Saddle River, N.J.: Prentice-Hall Health.

Varcarolis, E. (1998). *Foundations of psychiatric mental health nursing* (3rd ed.). Philadelphia: W.B. Saunders.

Wong, D. (1999). *Whaley & Wong's nursing care of infants and children* (6th ed.). St. Louis: Mosby.

21

Theories of Growth and Development

I. PSYCHOSOCIAL DEVELOPMENT AND ERIK ERIKSON

A. The theory
1. Describes the human life cycle as a series of eight **ego** developmental stages from birth to death
2. Each stage presents a psychosocial crisis, the goal of which is to integrate physical, maturation, and societal demands
3. Focuses on psychosocial tasks that are accomplished throughout the life cycle
4. The **ego** is separate and liberated from the **id,** developing across the course of the complete life cycle
5. **Ego** development is influenced by family, social, and developmental factors

B. Psychosocial development
1. A lifelong series of conflicts affected by social and cultural factors
2. Each conflict must be resolved for the child or adult to progress emotionally
3. Unsuccessful resolution leaves the individual emotionally handicapped

C. Stages of psychosocial development (Table 21-1)

II. COGNITIVE DEVELOPMENT AND JEAN PIAGET

A. The theory
1. Defines cognitive acts as ways in which the mind organizes and adapts to its environment
2. **Schema:** Refers to an individual's cognitive structure or framework of thought
3. **Schemata**
   a. Categories that an individual forms in his or her mind to organize and understand the world

   b. A young child has only a few **schemata** with which to understand the world, and gradually these are increased
   c. Adults use a wide variety of **schemata** to understand the world
4. **Assimilation**
   a. The ability to incorporate new ideas, objects, and experiences into the framework of one's thoughts
   b. The growing child will perceive and give meaning to new information according to what is already known and understood
5. **Accommodation**
   a. The ability to change a **schema** in order to introduce new ideas, objects, or experiences
   b. Changes the mental structure so that new experiences can be added

B. Stages of cognitive development
1. Sensorimotor stage
   a. 0 to 2 years
   b. Development proceeds from reflex activity to imagining and solving problems through the senses and movement
2. Preoperational stage
   a. 2 to 7 years
   b. Learning to think in terms of past, present, and future
   c. The child moves from knowing the world through sensation and movement to prelogical thinking and finding solutions to problems
3. Concrete operational
   a. 7 to 11 years
   b. Able to classify, order, and sort facts
   c. The child moves from prelogical thought to solving concrete problems through logic

TABLE 21-1

Erik Erikson's Stages of Psychosocial Development

Age	Psychosocial Crisis	Task
Infancy (0-18 months)	Trust vs. Mistrust	Attachment to the mother

Resolution of Crisis
Trust in people; faith and hope about the environment and the future
Unsuccessful Resolution of Crisis
General difficulties relating to people effectively; suspicion; trust-fear conflict, fear of the future

Age	Psychosocial Crisis	Task
Early childhood (18 months to 3 years)	Autonomy vs. Shame and Doubt	Gaining some basic control over self and environment

Resolution of Crisis
Sense of self-control and adequacy; will power
Unsuccessful Resolution of Crisis
Independence-fear conflict; severe feelings of self-doubt

Age	Psychosocial Crisis	Task
Late childhood (3-6 years)	Initiative vs. Guilt	Becoming purposeful and directive

Resolution of Crisis
Ability to initiate one's own activities; sense of purpose
Unsuccessful Resolution of Crisis
Aggression-fear conflict; sense of inadequacy or guilt

Age	Psychosocial Crisis	Task
School age (6-12 years)	Industry vs. Inferiority	Developing social, physical, and school skills

Resolution of Crisis
Competence; ability to learn and work
Unsuccessful Resolution of Crisis
Sense of inferiority; difficulty learning and working

Age	Psychosocial Crisis	Task
Adolescence (12-20 years)	Identity vs. Role Confusion	Developing sense of identity

Resolution of Crisis
Sense of personal identity
Unsuccessful Resolution of Crisis
Confusion about who one is; identity submerged in relationships or group memberships

Age	Psychosocial Crisis	Task
Early adulthood (20-35 years)	Intimacy vs. Isolation	Establishing intimate bonds of love and friendship

Resolution of Crisis
Ability to love deeply and commit oneself
Unsuccessful Resolution of Crisis
Emotional isolation, egocentricity

Age	Psychosocial Crisis	Task
Middle adulthood (35-65 years)	Generativity vs. Stagnation	Fulfilling life goals that involve family, career, and society

Resolution of Crisis
Ability to give and care for others
Unsuccessful Resolution of Crisis
Self-absorption; inability to grow as a person

Age	Psychosocial Crisis	Task
Later (65 years to death)	Integrity vs. Despair	Looking back over one's life and accepting its meaning

Resolution of Crisis
Sense of integrity and fulfillment
Unsuccessful Resolution of Crisis
Dissatisfaction with life

BOX 21-1

Moral Development and Lawrence Kohlberg

LEVEL ONE: PRECONVENTIONAL

Stage 0 (0-2 years)

The infant has no awareness of right or wrong.

Stage 1 (2-3 years)

At this stage children cannot reason as mature members of society.

Children view the world in a selfish way, with no real understanding of right or wrong.

The child obeys rules and demonstrates acceptable behavior to avoid punishment, to avoid displeasing those who are in power, and because he or she fears punishment from a superior force as a parent.

A toddler typically is at the first substage of the preconventional stage, involving punishment and obedience orientation, in which the toddler makes judgments on the basis of avoiding punishment, or obtaining a reward.

Physical punishment and withholding privileges tend to give the toddler a negative view of morals.

Withdrawing love and affection as punishment leads to feelings of guilt in the toddler.

Appropriate discipline includes providing simple explanations why certain behaviors are unacceptable, praising appropriate behavior, and using distractions when the toddler is headed for danger.

Stage 2 (4-7 years)

The child conforms to rules to obtain rewards or have favors returned.

The child's moral standards are those of others, and the child's observes them to either avoid punishment or obtain rewards.

A preschooler is in the preconventional stage of moral development.

In this stage, conscience emerges and the emphasis is on external control.

LEVEL TWO: CONVENTIONAL

The child conforms to rules to please others.

The child has increased awareness of others' feelings.

A concern for social order begins to emerge.

A child views good behavior as that which those in authority will approve.

If the behavior is not acceptable, the child feels guilty.

Stage 3 (7-10 years)

Conformity occurs to avoid disapproval or dislike by others.

This stage involves living up to what is expected by individuals close to you or what individuals generally expect of others in their roles as son, brother, friend, and so on.

Being good is important and is interpreted as having good motives and showing concern about others.

It also means maintaining mutual relationships, such as trust, loyalty, respect, and gratitude.

Stage 4 (10-12 years)

The child has more concern with society as a whole.

Emphasis is on obeying laws to maintain social order.

Moral reasoning develops as the child shifts the focus of living to society.

The school-aged child is at the conventional level of the role conformity stage and has an increased desire to please others.

The child observes and to some extent internalizes the standards of others.

The child wants to be considered "good" by those individuals whose opinions matter to the child.

LEVEL THREE: POSTCONVENTIONAL

The individual focuses on individual rights and principles of conscience.

The focus is a concern regarding what is best for all.

Stage 5

Being aware that people hold a variety of values and opinions and that most values and rules are relative to the group.

The adolescent in this stage gives as well as takes, and does not expect to get something without paying for it.

Stage 6

Conformity is based on universal principles of justice and occurs to avoid self-condemnation.

This stage involves following self-chosen ethical principles.

The development of the postconventional level of morality occurs in the adolescent at about age 13 years, marked by the development of an individual conscience and a defined set of moral values.

The adolescent can now acknowledge a conflict between two socially accepted standards and try to decide between them.

Control of conduct is now internal, both in standards observed and in reasoning about right and wrong.

---

4. Formal operations
   a. 11 years to adulthood
   b. Able to think abstractly and logically
   c. Logical thinking is expanded to include solving abstract and concrete problems

III. MORAL DEVELOPMENT AND LAWRENCE KOHLBERG

A. Moral development

 1. A complicated process involving the acceptance of the values and rules of society in a way that shapes behavior

2. Classified in a series of levels and behaviors

B. Levels of moral development (Box 21-1)

IV. PSYCHOSEXUAL DEVELOPMENT AND SIGMUND FREUD

A. Components of the theory
   1. Levels of awareness
   2. Agencies of the mind (**id, ego, superego**)

3. Concept of anxiety and defense mechanisms
4. Psychosexual stages of development

B. Levels of awareness
   1. Conscious level of awareness
      a. The **conscious** mind is logical and is regulated by the Reality Principle
      b. Includes all experiences that are within an individual's awareness and that the individual is able to control
      c. Includes all information that is easily remembered and immediately available to an individual
   2. Preconscious level of awareness
      a. Called the **subconscious**
      b. Includes experiences, thoughts, feelings, or desires that might not be in immediate awareness but can be recalled to consciousness
      c. The **subconscious** can help repress unpleasant thoughts or feelings and can examine and censor certain wishes and thinking
   3. Unconscious level of awareness
      a. The **unconscious** is not logical and is governed by the Pleasure Principle, which refers to seeking immediate tension reduction
      b. Memories, feelings, thoughts, or wishes are repressed and are not available to the **conscious** mind
      c. These repressed memories, thoughts, or feelings, if made prematurely **conscious**, can cause anxiety

C. Agencies of the mind
   1. **Id, ego,** and **superego**
      a. The three systems of personality
      b. The psychological processes that follow different operating principles
      c. In a mature and well-adjusted personality, they work together as a team under the leadership of the **ego**
   2. The **id**
      a. Source of all drives
      b. Is present at birth
      c. Includes genetic inheritance, reflexes, capacities to respond, instincts, basic drives, needs, and wishes that motivate an individual
      d. It operates according to the Pleasure Principle
      e. The **id** does not tolerate uncomfortable states and seeks to discharge the tension and return to a more comfortable, constant level of energy
      f. The **id** acts immediately in an impulsive, irrational way and pays no attention to the consequences of its actions, and therefore often behaves in ways harmful to self and others
      g. The "primary" process is a psychological activity in which the **id** attempts to reduce tension

      h. The "primary" process can include hallucinating or forming an image of the object that will satisfy its needs and remove the tension
      i. The "primary" process by itself is not capable of reducing tension; therefore, a "secondary" psychological process must develop if the individual is to survive; when this occurs, the structure of the second system of the personality, the **ego,** begins to take form
   3. The **ego**
      a. The functions of the **ego** include reality testing and problem solving
      b. Begins its development during the fourth or fifth month of life
      c. The **ego** emerges out of the **id** and acts as an intermediary between the **id** and the external world
      d. Emerges because the needs, wishes, and demands of the **id** require appropriate exchanges with the outside world of reality
      e. Distinguishes between things in the mind and things in the external world
      f. Reality testing is a function of the **ego,** and the **ego** uses realistic thinking
      g. The **ego** follows the Reality Principle and operates by means of the "secondary" process—that is, realistic thinking
      h. The aim of the Reality Principle is to satisfy the **id's** impulses in the external world with an object that is suitable; the Reality Principle determines whether an experience is true or false and whether it has external existence or not
      i. The **ego** devises a plan and tests the plan by some kind of action to see if it will work
   4. The **superego**
      a. A necessary part of socialization that develops during the phallic stage of 3 to 6 years of age
      b. It develops from the interactions with one's parents during the extended period of childhood dependency
      c. It includes the internalization of the values, ideals, and moral standards of society
      d. The child internalizes the moral standards of parents and society
      e. The **superego** consists of the conscience and the **ego** ideal
      f. The conscience refers to the capacity for self-evaluation and criticism
      g. When moral codes are violated, the conscience punishes the individual by instilling guilt
      h. What parents approve of, and what they reward the child for doing, become incorporated as the **ego** ideal by the mechanism of introjection
      i. The **superego** strives for perfection rather than

BOX 21-2

Freud's Psychosexual Stages of Development

ORAL STAGE (0-1 YEARS)

During this stage, the infant is concerned with his or her own gratification.

The infant is all id, operating on the Pleasure Principle and striving for immediate gratification of needs.

When the infant experiences gratification of basic needs, a sense of trust and security begins.

The ego begins to emerge as the infant begins to see self as separate from the mother; this marks the beginning of the development of a sense of self.

ANAL STAGE (1-3 YEARS)

Toilet training occurs during this period, and the child gains pleasure both from the elimination of the feces and from their retention.

The conflict of this stage is between those demands from society and the parents and the sensations of pleasure associated with the anus.

The child begins to gain a sense of control over instinctive drives and learns to delay immediate gratification to gain a future goal.

PHALLIC STAGE (3-6 YEARS)

The child experiences both pleasurable and conflicting feelings associated with the genital organs.

The pleasures of masturbation and the fantasy life of children set the stage for the Oedipus complex.

The child's unconscious sexual attraction to and wish to possess the parent of the opposite sex, the hostility and desire to remove the parent of the same sex, and the subsequent guilt for these wishes is the conflict the child faces.

The conflict is resolved when the child identifies with the parent of the same sex.

The emergence of the superego is both the solution to and the result of these intense impulses.

LATENCY STAGE (6-12 YEARS)

A tapering off of conscious biological and sexual urges.

The sexual impulses are channeled and elevated into a more culturally accepted level of activity.

Growth of ego functions and the ability to care about and relate to others outside the home is the task of this stage of development.

GENITAL STAGE (12 YEARS AND BEYOND)

Emerges at adolescence with the onset of puberty when the genital organs mature.

The individual gains gratification from his or her own body.

During this stage, the individual develops satisfying sexual and emotional relationships with members of the opposite sex.

The individual plans life goals and gains a strong sense of personal identity.

---

pleasure and represents the ideal rather than the real

  j. Living up to one's **ego** ideal results in the individual feeling proud and increases self-esteem

D. Anxiety and defense mechanisms

  1. The **ego** develops defenses or defense mechanisms to fight off anxiety

  2. Defense mechanisms operate on an **unconscious** level, except for suppression, so the individual is not aware of their operation

  3. Defense mechanisms deny, falsify, or distort reality to make it less threatening

  4. An individual cannot survive without defense mechanisms; however, if they become too extreme in distorting reality, then interference in healthy adjustment and personal growth may occur

E. Psychosexual stages of development (Box 21-2)

  1. Human development proceeds through a series of stages from infancy to adulthood

  2. Each stage is characterized by the inborn tendency of all individuals to reduce tension and seek pleasure

  3. Each stage is associated with a particular conflict that must be resolved before the child can move successfully to the next stage

  4. Experiences during the early stages determine an individual's adjustment patterns and the personality traits that the individual has as an adult

PRACTICE QUESTIONS

1. A maternity nurse is providing instructions to a new mother regarding the psychosocial development of the newborn infant. Using Erikson's psychosocial development theory, the nurse would instruct the mother to:

   1. Allow the newborn infant to signal a need

   2. Anticipate all of the needs of the newborn infant

   3. Avoid the newborn infant during the first 10 minutes of crying

   4. Attend to the newborn infant immediately when crying

2. A mother of a 3-year-old tells a clinic nurse that the child is constantly rebelling and having temper tantrums. The nurse most appropriately tells the mother to:

   1. Punish the child every time the child says "no," to change the behavior

2. Allow the behavior because this is normal at this age period
3. Set limits on the child's behavior
4. Ignore the child when this behavior occurs

3. A home health nurse visits a 70-year-old woman on a weekly basis. At each visit the client reminisces about past life experiences in a positive way. The home health nurse interprets this behavior as:
   1. A normal psychosocial response
   2. Requiring a psychiatric consultation
   3. A mental status alteration
   4. A sensory deficit requiring social activities

4. The mother of an 8-year-old child tells the clinic nurse that she is concerned about the child because the child seems to be more attentive to friends than anything else. The most appropriate nursing response would be which of the following?
   1. "You need to be concerned."
   2. "You need to monitor the child's behavior closely."
   3. "At this age, the child is developing his own personality."
   4. "You need to provide more praise to the child to stop this behavior."

5. The mother of a 4-year-old child calls the clinic nurse and expresses concern because the child has been masturbating. The most appropriate response by the nurse is which of the following?
   1. "The child is very young to begin this behavior and should be brought to the clinic."
   2. "This is not normal behavior, and the child should be seen by the physician."
   3. "This is a normal behavior at this age."
   4. "Children usually begin this behavior at age 8 years."

6. A nursing instructor asks a nursing student to present a clinical conference to peers regarding Freud's psychosexual stages of development, specifically the anal stage. The student plans the conference, knowing that which of the following most appropriately relates to this stage of development?
   1. This stage is associated with toilet training
   2. This stage is associated with pleasurable and conflicting feelings about the genital organs
   3. This stage is characterized by a tapering off of conscious biological and sexual urges
   4. This stage is characterized by the gratification of self

7. A mother of a 5-year-old child tells the nurse that the child scolds the floor or a table if the child hurts herself on the object. According to Piaget's theory

of cognitive development, this behavior is identified as:
   1. Object permanence
   2. Egocentric speech
   3. Animism
   4. Global organization

8. A nursing instructor asks a nursing student to describe the formal operations stage of Piaget's cognitive developmental theory. The most appropriate response by the nursing student is:
   1. "The child has the ability to think abstractly."
   2. "The child develops logical thought patterns."
   3. "The child has difficulty separating fantasy from reality."
   4. "The child begins to understand the environment."

9. A clinic nurse is preparing to discuss the concepts of moral development with a mother. The nurse understands that according to Kohlberg's theory of moral development, in the preconventional level, moral development is thought to be motivated by which of the following?
   1. The parents' behavior
   2. Peer pressure
   3. Social pressures
   4. Punishment and reward

10. A nurse educator is preparing to conduct a session to the nursing staff regarding the theories of growth and development. The nurse educator plans to discuss Kohlberg's theory of moral development and understands that which of the following is not a component of the theory?
   1. Moral development progresses in relationship to cognitive development
   2. Individuals move through all six stages in a sequential fashion
   3. It provides a framework for understanding how individuals determine a moral code to guide their behavior
   4. A person's ability to make moral judgments develops over a period of time

CRITICAL THINKING: FREE-TEXT ENTRY

The nurse is developing a plan of care for an adolescent who is hospitalized and is placed in skeletal traction. The nurse incorporates interventions in the plan of care that address the psychosocial development of the adolescent. What is the chief developmental task of the adolescent according to Erik Erikson?

Answer: _____

ANSWERS

1. 1

Rationale: According to Erikson, the caregiver should not try to anticipate the newborn infant's needs at all times, but must allow the newborn infant to signal needs. If a newborn infant is not allowed to signal a need, he or she will not learn how to control the environment. Erikson believed that a delayed or prolonged response to a newborn infant's signal would inhibit the development of trust and lead to mistrust of others.

Test-Taking Strategy: Use the process of elimination. Eliminate options 2, 3, and 4 because of the absolute terms "all," "avoid," and "immediately" in these options. Review Erikson's stages of psychosocial development if you had difficulty with this question

Level of Cognitive Ability: Application
Client Needs: Psychosocial Integrity
Integrated Concept/Process: Teaching/Learning
Content Area: Child Health
Reference: Leahy, J., & Kizilay, P. (1998). *Foundations of nursing practice: A nursing process approach.* Philadelphia: W.B. Saunders, p. 264.

2. 3

Rationale: According to Erikson, the child focuses on independence between ages 1 and 3 years. Gaining independence often means that the child has to rebel against the parents' wishes. Saying things like "no" or "mine" and having temper tantrums are common during this period of development. Being consistent and setting limits on the child's behavior are necessary elements.

Test-Taking Strategy: Use the process of elimination. Options 2 and 4 can be eliminated first because they are similar. Next, eliminate option 1 because this action is likely to produce a negative response during this normal developmental pattern. Review psychosocial development of the toddler according the Erikson, if you had difficulty with this question.

Level of Cognitive Ability: Application
Client Needs: Psychosocial Integrity
Integrated Concept/Process: Teaching/Learning
Content Area: Child Health
Reference: Ball, J. & Bindler, R. (1999). *Pediatric nursing: Caring for children* (2nd ed.). Stamford, Conn: Appleton & Lange, p. 36.

3. 1

Rationale: According the Erikson, late adulthood is the period of old age. The adult reminisces about past life experiences, viewing them in a positive way. The adult needs to feel good about accomplishments, see successes in life, and feel that he or she has made a contribution to society.

Test-Taking Strategy: Use the process of elimination. Note the similarity in options 2, 3, and 4 in that all of these options indicate an abnormal response. Review Erikson's theory of psychosocial development of late adulthood if you had difficulty with this question.

Level of Cognitive Ability: Analysis
Client Needs: Psychosocial Integrity
Integrated Concept/Process: Caring
Content Area: Fundamental Skills
Reference: Craven, R., & Hirnle, C. (2000). *Fundamentals of nursing: Human health and function* (3rd ed.). Philadelphia: Lippincott, p. 266.

4. 3

Rationale: According to Erikson, during school age years (ages 6 to 12 years), the child begins to move toward peers and friends and away from the parents for support. The child also begins to develop special interests that reflect his or her own developing personality instead of the parents.

Test-Taking Strategy: Use the process of elimination and knowledge of Erikson's psychosocial development theory related to middle childhood. Options 1 and 2 can be easily eliminated first. Eliminate option 4 next because although praising the child for accomplishments is important at this age, the behavior that the child is exhibiting is normal. Review psychosocial development related to this age group according to Erikson if you had difficulty with this question.

Level of Cognitive Ability: Application
Client Needs: Psychosocial Integrity
Integrated Concept/Process: Caring
Content Area: Child Health
Reference: Varcarolis, E. (1998). *Foundations of psychiatric mental health nursing* (3rd ed.). Philadelphia: W.B. Saunders, p. 44.

5. 3

Rationale: According to Freud's psychosexual stages of development, between the ages of 3 and 6, the child is in the phallic stage. At this time, the child devotes much energy to examining his or her genitalia, masturbating, and expressing interest in sexual concerns.

Test-Taking Strategy: Use the process of elimination. Eliminate options 1 and 2 first because they are similar. Focus on the issue of the question and note the words "age 8 years" in option 4 to assist in eliminating this option. If you had difficulty with this question, review Freud's psychosocial stages of development.

Level of Cognitive Ability: Application
Client Needs: Psychosocial Integrity
Integrated Concept/Process: Caring
Content Area: Child Health
Reference: Varcarolis, E. (1998). *Foundations of psychiatric mental health nursing* (3rd ed.). Philadelphia: W.B. Saunders, p. 40.

6. 1

Rationale: Generally, toilet training occurs during this period. According to Freud, the child gains pleasure both from the elimination of feces and from their retention. Option 2 relates to the phallic stage. Option 3 relates to the latency period. Option 4 relates to the oral stage.

Test-Taking Strategy: Use the process of elimination. Note the relationship between the words "anal" in the question and "toilet training" in the correct option. If you had difficulty with this question, review Freud's psychosocial stages of development.

Level of Cognitive Ability: Comprehension
Client Needs: Psychosocial Integrity
Integrated Concept/Process: Nursing Process/Planning
Content Area: Child Health
Reference: Wong, D. (1999). *Whaley & Wong's nursing care of infants and children* (6th ed.). St. Louis: Mosby, p. 132.

7. 3

Rationale: Animism means that all inanimate objects are given living meaning. Object permanence, the realization that something out of sight still exists, occurs in the later stages of the sensorimotor stage of development. Egocentric speech occurs when the child talks just for fun and cannot see another's point of view. Global organization means that if any part of an object or situation changes, the whole thing has changed. Options 2 and 4 occur during the preoperational stage.

Test-Taking Strategy: Use the process of elimination. Attempt to make a relationship between the behavior identified in the question and the correct option. This will assist in directing you to option 3. If you had difficulty with this question, review the concepts of Piaget's theory of cognitive development.

Level of Cognitive Ability: Comprehension
Client Needs: Psychosocial Integrity
Integrated Concept/Process: Nursing Process/Assessment
Content Area: Child Health
Reference: Potter, P., & Perry, A. (2001). *Fundamentals of nursing* (5th ed.). St. Louis: Mosby, pp. 199.

8. **1**
Rationale: In the formal operations stage, the child has the ability the think abstractly and logically. Option 2 identifies the concrete operations stage. Option 3 identifies the preoperational stage. Option 4 identifies the sensorimotor stage.

Test-Taking Strategy: Use the process of elimination and knowledge regarding the characteristics of Piaget's cognitive developmental theory to answer this question. If you had difficulty with this question, review these concepts.

Level of Cognitive Ability: Comprehension
Client Needs: Psychosocial Integrity
Integrated Concept/Process: Communication and Documentation
Content Area: Child Health
Reference: Bowden, V., Dickey, S, & Greenberg, C. (1998). *Children and their families: The continuum of care.* Philadelphia: W.B. Saunders, p. 210.

9. **4**
Rationale: In the preconventional stage, morals are thought to be motivated by punishment and reward. If the child is obedient and is not punished, then he or she is being moral. The child sees actions as either good or bad. If the child's actions are good, the child is praised. If the child's actions are bad, the child is punished.

Test-Taking Strategy: Use the process of elimination. Eliminate options 2 and 3 because they are similar. Knowledge that the preconventional stage occurs between the ages of 2 and 7 years

will assist in directing you to option 4. If you had difficulty with this question, review Kohlberg's theory of moral development.
Level of Cognitive Ability: Comprehension
Client Needs: Psychosocial Integrity
Integrated Concept/Process: Nursing Process/Planning
Content Area: Child Health
Reference: Potter, P., & Perry, A. (2001). *Fundamentals of nursing* (5th ed.). St. Louis: Mosby, pp. 158, 167.

10. **2**
Rationale: Kohlberg's theory states that individuals move through the six stages of development in a sequential fashion but that not everyone reaches stages 5 and 6 in his or her development of personal morality. Options 1, 3, and 4 are correct statements regarding Kohlberg's theory.

Test-Taking Strategy: Use the process of elimination. Note the key word "not" in the stem of the question. Also, note the absolute term "all" in option 2. If you had difficulty with this question, review Kohlberg's theory.
Level of Cognitive Ability: Comprehension
Client Needs: Psychosocial Integrity
Integrated Concept/Process: Nursing Process/Planning
Content Area: Fundamental Skills
Reference: Potter, P., & Perry, A. (2001). *Fundamentals of nursing* (5th ed.). St. Louis: Mosby, pp. 167-179.

CRITICAL THINKING: FREE-TEXT ENTRY

Answer: Identity vs. Role Confusion
Rationale: Adolescence is a period of major physical changes. The adolescent is aware of these changes and is very concerned with the way he or she appears to others. Adolescents are trying to learn who they are. Role confusion occurs when the adolescent is unable to see himself or herself as separate or unique from others and does not establish a direction or career goal in life.

Test-Taking Strategy: It is necessary to know the psychosocial stages of development according to Erik Erikson in order to answer this question. Review this theory if you are unfamiliar with it.
Level of Cognitive Ability: Comprehension
Client Needs: Psychosocial Integrity
Integrated Concept/Process: Nursing Process/Planning
Content Area: Fundamental Skills
Reference: Leahy, J., & Kizilay, P. (1998). *Foundations of nursing practice: A nursing process approach.* Philadelphia: W.B. Saunders, p. 266.

REFERENCES

Ball, J., & Bindler, R. (1999). *Pediatric nursing: Caring for children* (2nd ed.). Stamford, Conn: Appleton & Lange.

Bowden, V., Dickey, S, & Greenberg, C. (1998). *Children and their families: The continuum of care.* Philadelphia: W.B. Saunders.

Craven, R., & Hirnle, C. (2000). *Fundamentals of nursing: Human health and function* (3rd ed.). Philadelphia: Lippincott.

Leahy, J., & Kizilay, P. (1998). *Foundations of nursing practice: A nursing process approach.* Philadelphia: W.B. Saunders.

Potter, P., & Perry, A. (2001). *Fundamentals of nursing* (5th ed.). St. Louis: Mosby.

Varcarolis, E. (1998). *Foundations of psychiatric mental health nursing* (3rd ed.). Philadelphia: W.B. Saunders.

Wong, D. (1999). *Whaley & Wong's nursing care of infants and children* (6th ed.). St. Louis: Mosby.

Maternity Nursing

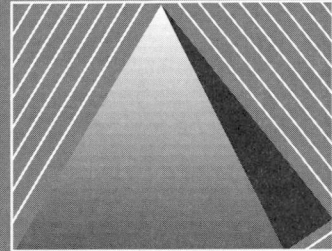

PYRAMID TERMS

amniotic fluid Fluid that surrounds and protects the fetus; consists of 500 to 1000 mL by the end of pregnancy. The fetus floats in the amniotic fluid, which serves as a cushion against injury from sudden blows or movements and helps maintain a constant body temperature for the fetus. The fetus voids into the amniotic fluid and also drinks and breathes the fluid.

ballottement Rebounding of the fetus against the examiner's finger on palpation. When the cervix is tapped, the fetus floats upward in the amniotic fluid. A rebound is felt by the examiner when the fetus falls back.

Chadwick's sign Bluish coloration of the mucous membranes of cervix, vagina, and vulva; occurs at approximately 6 weeks of pregnancy and is a probable sign of pregnancy.

delivery Actual event of birth; the expulsion or extraction of the neonate

fertilization Takes place when sperm and ovum unite; occurs within 12 hours of ovulation and within 2 to 3 days of insemination, the average duration of viability for the ovum and sperm.

Goodell's sign Softening of the cervix; occurs at the beginning of the second month of gestation and is a probable sign of pregnancy.

gravida A pregnant woman; called gravida I (primagravida) during the first pregnancy, gravida II (secundigravida) during the second, and so on.

Hegar's sign Compressibility and softening of the lower uterine segment; occurs at about week 6 of gestation; a probable sign of pregnancy.

implantation Zygote propels toward the uterus and implants in the uterine wall 6 to 8 days after ovulation.

Infant A baby born alive; also from 28 days of age until the first birthday.

labor Coordinated sequence of involuntary uterine contractions resulting in effacement and dilation of cervix, followed by expulsion of the products of conception.

lochia Discharge from the uterus that consists of blood from the vessels of the placental site and debris from the decidua; lasts for approximately 2 to 3 weeks after delivery.

Nagele's rule Determines the estimated date of confinement (EDC). Add 7 days to the first day of the last menstrual period (LMP). Subtract 3 months and add 1 year.

neonate A human offspring from the time of birth to the 28th day of life; also called newborn.

newborn A human offspring from the time of birth to the 28th day of life; also called neonate.

parity The number of pregnancies that have been carried to viability.

placenta Provides for the exchange of nutrients and waste products between the fetus and the mother; produces hormones to maintain pregnancy; develops by the third month of gestation; also called afterbirth.

quickening First perception of fetal movement, appearing usually in the 16th to 18th week of pregnancy.

PYRAMID TO SUCCESS

The Pyramid to Success focuses on the physiological and psychosocial aspects related to the experience of pregnancy. Pyramid points begin with instructing the pregnant client in measures that will promote a healthy environment for both the mother and the fetus. Focus on the importance of antepartum follow-up, nutrition, and the interventions for common discomforts that occur during pregnancy. Review the purpose of the commonly prescribed diagnostic tests and procedures in the antepartum period. Focus on disorders that can occur during pregnancy, particularly pregnancy-induced hypertension (PIH) and diabetes. Review the labor and delivery process and the immediate interventions for conditions in which the mother or fetal status is compromised, such as prolapsed cord or altered fetal heart rate. Review fetal effects from the mother with human immunodeficiency virus (HIV) or acquired immunodeficiency syndrome (AIDS) or the substance abuse mother. Focus on the normal expectations of the postpartum period and the complications that can occur. Pyramid points also focus on the normal physical assessment findings in the neonate and the early identification of disorders in the neonate. The Integrated Concepts and Processes addressed in this unit include Nursing Process, Caring, Communication and Documentation, Cultural Awareness, Self-Care, and Teaching/Learning.

▲ CLIENT NEEDS

Safe, Effective Care Environment

Confidentiality
Consultations with members of the health care team
Continuity of care
Establishing priorities
Handling infectious materials
Informed consent for procedures
Medical and surgical asepsis
Parent rights
Referrals
Standard (universal) precautions during delivery of care

Health Promotion and Maintenance

Birthing and parenting issues
Concepts of wellness
Expected body image changes
Family planning and family systems
Growth and development and health care screening
Lifestyle choices
Reproduction and human sexuality
Teaching regarding antepartum, intrapartum, and post-
  partum care
Techniques of physical assessment

Psychosocial Integrity

Cultural, religious, and spiritual influences regarding
  birth and motherhood
Coping mechanisms
Situational role changes

Support systems
Therapeutic interactions

Physiological Integrity

Alterations in body systems
Commonly prescribed diagnostic tests and procedures
Interventions for unexpected events during pregnancy
Labor and delivery process
Normal expectations during pregnancy
Nutrition
Physiological changes that occur during pregnancy
Risk identification during pregnancy

REFERENCES

Herlihy, B., & Maebius, N. (2000). *The human body in health and illness.* Philadelphia: W.B. Saunders.

Ladewig, P., London. M., & Olds, S. (1998). *Maternal-newborn nursing care: The nurse, the family, and the community* (4th ed.). Menlo Park, Calif.: Addison-Wesley Longman.

Lowdermilk, D., Perry, S., & Bobak, I. (2000). *Maternity & women's health care* (7th ed.). St. Louis: Mosby.

National Council of State Boards of Nursing (eds.) (2000). *Test Plan for the National Council Licensure Examination for Registered Nurses.* Chicago: Author.

Olds, S., London. M., & Ladewig, P. (2000). *Maternal-newborn nursing: A family and community-based approach* (6th ed.). Upper Saddle River, N.J.: Prentice-Hall Health.

Sherwen, L., Scoloveno, M.A., & Weingarten, C. (1999). *Maternity nursing: Care of the childbearing family* (3rd ed.). Stamford, Conn: Appleton & Lange.

Wong, D. (1999). *Whaley & Wong's nursing care of infants and children* (6th ed.). St. Louis: Mosby.

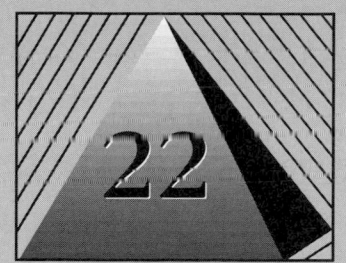

Female Reproductive System

I. REPRODUCTIVE STRUCTURES
A. Ovaries
1. Formation and expulsion of ova
2. Secrete estrogen and progesterone
B. Fallopian tubes
1. Muscular tubes (oviducts) approximate to the ovaries and connect to the uterus
2. Propel the ova from the ovaries to the uterus
C. Uterus
1. A muscular pear-shaped cavity in which the fetus develops
2. The cavity from which menstruation occurs
D. Cervix
1. Internal os opens into the body of the uterine cavity
2. Cervical canal is located between the internal os and the external os
3. External os opens into the vagina
E. Vagina
1. Mucous membrane–lined channel through the muscles of the pelvic floor
2. Known as the birth canal
3. Provides a passage between the cervical os and the external environment
   a. Passageway for menstrual blood flow
   b. Passageway for fetus

II. MENSTRUAL CYCLE (Table 22-1)
A. Ovarian hormones
1. Include the follicle-stimulating hormone (FSH) and luteinizing hormone (LH)
2. Released by the anterior pituitary gland
3. Produce changes in the ovaries
4. Secretion of ovarian hormones leads to changes in the endometrium
5. The menstrual cycle, the regularly recurring physiological changes in the endometrium that culminate in its shedding, may vary in length, with the average length being approximately 28 days
B. Ovarian changes
1. Preovulatory phase
2. Luteal phase
C. Uterine changes
1. Menstrual phase
2. Proliferative phase
3. Secretory phase

III. FEMALE PELVIS AND MEASUREMENTS
A. True pelvis
1. Lies below the pelvic brim
2. Consists of the pelvic inlet, midpelvis, and pelvic outlet
B. False pelvis
1. Shallow portion above the pelvic brim
2. Supports the abdominal viscera
C. Types of pelvis
1. Gynecoid
   a. Normal female pelvis
   b. Transversely rounded or blunt
   c. Most favorable for successful **labor** and birth
2. Android
   a. Wedge-shaped or angulated
   b. Seen in males
   c. Not favorable for **labor**
   d. Narrow pelvic planes can cause slow descent and midpelvis arrest
3. Anthropoid
   a. Oval shaped
   b. The outlet is adequate, with a normal or moderately narrow pubic arch
4. Platypelloid
   a. Flat in shape with an oval inlet

TABLE 22-1

Menstrual Cycle

OVARIAN CHANGES

Preovulatory Phase

The hypothalamus releases gonadotropin-releasing hormone (GnRH) through the portal system to the anterior pituitary system.

Secretion of FSH by the anterior lobe of the pituitary gland stimulates growth of follicles.

Most follicles die, leaving one to mature into a large graafian follicle.

Estrogen produced by the follicle stimulates increased secretions of LH by the anterior lobe of the pituitary gland.

The follicle ruptures and releases an ovum into the peritoneal cavity.

Luteal Phase

Begins with ovulation.

Body temperature drops and then rises by 0.5° to 1° F around the time of ovulation.

Corpus luteum is formed from follicle cells that remain in the ovary following ovulation.

Corpus luteum secretes estrogen and progesterone during the remaining 14 days of the cycle.

Corpus luteum degenerates if the ovum is not fertilized, and secretion of estrogen and progesterone declines.

The decline of estrogen and progesterone stimulates the anterior pituitary to secrete more FSH and LH, initiating a new reproductive cycle.

UTERINE CHANGES

Menstrual Phase

Consists of 4 to 6 days of bleeding as endometrium breaks down owing to decreased amount of estrogen and progesterone.

FSH rises, enabling the beginning of a new cycle.

Proliferative Phase

Estrogen stimulates proliferation and growth of endometrium.

This phase lasts about 9 days.

As estrogen increases, it suppresses secretion of FSH and increases secretion of LH.

LH stimulates ovulation and the development of the corpus luteum.

Ovulation occurs between day 12 and day 16.

Estrogen is high and progesterone is low.

Secretory Phase

This phase lasts about 12 days.

Follows ovulation.

Initiated in response to the increase in LH.

Graafian follicle replaced by corpus luteum.

Corpus luteum secretes progesterone and estrogen.

Progesterone prepares the endometrium for pregnancy should a fertilized ovum be implanted.

---

b. Transverse diameter is wide but anteroposterior diameter is short, making the outlet inadequate

D. Pelvic inlet diameters
  1. Anteroposterior diameters
    a. Diagonal conjugate: distance from the lower margin of the symphysis pubis to the sacral promontory; is at least 12.5 cm
    b. True conjugate or conjugate vera: distance from the upper margin of the symphysis pubis to the sacral promontory; is at least 11.5 cm
    c. Obstetric conjugate: the smallest front-to-back distance through which the fetal head must pass in moving through the pelvic inlet; is about 11 cm
  2. Transverse diameter: The largest of the pelvic inlet diameters; is located at right angles to the true conjugate and is about 13.5 cm
  3. Oblique (diagonal) diameter: Cannot be measured clinically; is about 12.5 cm
  4. Posterior sagittal diameter: Extends from the point where the anteroposterior and transverse diameters cross each other to the middle of the sacral promontory; is about 4.5 cm

E. Pelvic cavity (midplane/midpelvis) diameters
  1. Plane of greatest dimensions
    a. Anteroposterior diameter: 12.75 cm
    b. Transverse diameter: 12.5 cm
  2. Plane of least dimensions
    a. Anteroposterior diameter: 12.0 cm
    b. Transverse diameter: 10.5 cm
    c. Posterior sagittal diameter: 4.5 to 5.0 cm
F. Pelvic outlet diameters
    a. Bi-ischial or intertuberous diameter: 10 cm
    b. Obstetric anteroposterior diameter: 11.5 cm
    c. Transverse diameter: 11 cm
    d. Posterior sagittal diameter: 9.0 cm
    e. Anterior sagittal diameter: 6.0 cm

IV. FERTILIZATION AND IMPLANTATION

A. **Fertilization**
  1. Occurs in the upper region of the fallopian tubes
  2. Occurs within 12 hours of ovulation and within 2 to 3 days of insemination, the average durations of viability for the ovum and sperm
  3. Takes place when sperm and ovum unite
  4. Once **fertilized,** the membrane of the ovum undergoes changes that prevent the entry of other sperm

TABLE 22-2

Fetal Development

Embryonic Stage	Fetal Period
Week 1	*Week 16*
Free-floating blastocyst	Active movements are present
Weeks 2 to 3	Fetal skin is transparent
2 mm in length	Lanugo hair begins to develop
Groove formed along middle of back	Skeletal ossification occurs
Beginning of blood circulation	Sex of fetus can be determined at this time
Heart tubular in shape	*Week 20*
Week 5	19 cm in length
4 to 6 mm in length	465 g in weight
0.4 g in weight	Lanugo covers the entire body
Double heart chambers visible	Fetus has nails
Heart beginning to beat	Muscles developed
Limb buds	Enamel and dentin are depositing
Week 8	Heart beat detected by fetoscope
3 cm in length	*Week 24*
2 g in weight	28 cm in length
Eyelids begin to fuse	780 g in weight
Circulatory system through umbilical cord well established	Hair on head well formed
Every organ system present	Skin reddish and wrinkled
Week 12	Reflex hand grasp
8 cm in length	Vernix caseosa covers entire body
45 g in weight	Has ability to hear
Face well formed	*Week 28*
Limbs long and slender	38 cm in length
Kidneys begin to form urine	1200 g in weight
Spontaneous movements occur	Limbs are well flexed
Heart tones detected by electronic devices between 8 and 12 weeks	Brain develops rapidly
Sex visually recognizable	Eyelids open and close
	Lungs sufficiently developed to provide gas exchange (lecithin forming)
	If born, neonate can breathe at this time
	Week 32
	30 cm in length
	2000 g in weight
	Bones are fully developed
	Subcutaneous fat collected
	L/S (lecithin/sphingomyelin) ratio switching to 1.2:1
	Week 36
	42 to 48 cm length
	2500 g in weight
	Skin pink, body rounded
	Less wrinkled
	Lanugo disappearing
	L/S ratio $\geq$ 2:1
	Week 40
	48 to 52 cm in length
	3000 to 3600 g in weight
	Skin pinkish and smooth
	Lanugo present on upper arms and shoulders
	Vernix caseosa decreases
	Fingernails extend beyond fingertips
	Sole (plantar) creases down to heel
	Testes in scrotum
	Labia majoria well developed

5. Each reproductive cell carries 23 chromosomes
6. Sperm carry an X and a Y chromosome; XY: male, XX: female

▲ B. **Implantation**
1. Zygote propels toward the uterus
2. Implants 6 to 8 days after ovulation
3. Blastocyst secretes chorionic gonadotropin to ensure that the corpus luteum remains viable and secretes estrogen and progesterone for the first 2 to 3 months of gestation

V. FETAL DEVELOPMENT (Table 22-2)
A. Embryonic stage: From conception to 12 weeks
B. Fetal period: From third month to gestation

VI. FETAL ENVIRONMENT
A. Amnion
1. Encloses the amniotic cavity
2. Inner membrane that forms about the second week of embryonic development
3. Forms a fluid-filled sac that surrounds the embryo and later the fetus
B. Chorion
1. Outer membrane
2. Becomes vascularized and forms the fetal part of the **placenta**

▲ C. **Amniotic fluid**
1. Consists of 500 to 1000 mL by the end of pregnancy
2. Surrounds, cushions, and protects the fetus and allows for fetal movement
3. Maintains the body temperature of the fetus
4. Consists largely of fetal urine, and is therefore a measure of fetal kidney function
5. The fetus drinks, swallows, and urinates the **amniotic fluid** and breathes the **amniotic fluid** into its lungs

▲ D. **Placenta**
1. Provides for exchange of nutrients and waste products between fetus and mother
2. Develops by the third month
3. Dependent upon maternal circulation
4. Produces hormones to maintain pregnancy and assumes full responsibility for the production of these hormones by the 12th week of gestation
5. Large particles such as bacteria cannot pass through the **placenta**
6. In addition to nutrients, drugs, antibodies, and viruses can pass through the **placenta**
7. In the third trimester, transfer of maternal immunoglobulin provides fetus passive immunity to certain diseases for the first few months after birth
8. By week 8, genetic testing can be done

VII. FETAL CIRCULATION
A. Umbilical cord
1. Contains two arteries and one vein

2. Arteries carry deoxygenated blood and waste products from the fetus
3. The vein carries oxygenated blood and provides oxygen and nutrients to the fetus
B. Fetal heart rate
1. 120 to 160 beats per minute
2. Approximately twice the maternal heart rate
C. Fetal circulation bypass
1. Present because of nonfunctioning lungs
2. Bypasses must close following birth to allow blood to flow through the lungs and the liver
3. Ductus arteriosus connects the pulmonary artery to the aorta, bypassing lungs
4. Ductus venosus connects the umbilical vein and the inferior vena cava, bypassing liver
5. Foramen ovale is the opening between right and left atria of heart, bypassing lungs

PRACTICE QUESTIONS

1. A nurse is conducting a prenatal teaching class and is reviewing the functions of the female reproductive system. A client in the class asks the nurse about the function of the fallopian tubes. The nurse tells the client that:
   1. Estrogen and progesterone are secreted from the fallopian tubes
   2. The fallopian tubes are the passageway for the fetus
   3. The fetus develops in the fallopian tubes
   4. Fertilization occurs in the fallopian tubes

2. A nursing instructor is discussing the menstrual cycle with a group of nursing students. The instructor asks a nursing student to describe the follicle-stimulating hormone (FSH) and the luteinizing hormone (LH). The nursing student accurately responds by stating that:
   1. FSH and LH are released from the anterior pituitary gland
   2. FSH and LH are secreted by the corpus luteum of the ovary
   3. FSH and LH are secreted by the adrenal glands
   4. FSH and LH stimulate the formation of milk during pregnancy

3. A nurse employed in a prenatal clinic reviews a client's chart and notes that the physician documents that the client has a gynecoid pelvis. The nurse plans care for this client, knowing that this type of pelvis:
   1. Is not favorable for labor
   2. Has a narrow pubic arch
   3. Is a wide pelvis with a short diameter
   4. Is the most favorable for labor and birth

4. A client asks a nurse about the purpose of the placenta. The nurse responds most appropriately by telling the client that the placenta:
   1. Prevents antibodies and viruses from passing to the fetus

2. Cushions and protects the fetus
3. Provides an exchange of nutrients and waste products between the mother and the fetus
4. Maintains the body temperature of the fetus

5. A nurse is describing the process of fetal circulation to a client during a prenatal visit. The nurse accurately tells the client that fetal circulation consists of:
   1. Two umbilical veins and one umbilical artery
   2. Two umbilical arteries and one umbilical vein
   3. Arteries carrying oxygenated blood to the fetus
   4. Veins carrying deoxygenated blood to the fetus

6. A nursing student is assigned to a client in labor. A nursing instructor asks the student to describe fetal circulation, specifically the ductus venosus. The nursing instructor determines that the student understands fetal circulation if the student states that the ductus venosus:
   1. Connects the pulmonary artery to the aorta
   2. Is an opening between the right and left atria
   3. Connects the umbilical artery to the inferior vena cava
   4. Connects the umbilical vein to the inferior vena cava

7. A nurse is caring for a client during the prenatal period. The client tells that nurse that she wants to know the sex of the fetus as soon as it can be determined. The nurse responds to the client, knowing that the sex of the fetus can be visually recognizable as early as week:
   1. 4
   2. 6
   3. 8
   4. 12

8. A nurse prepares to assess a fetal heart beat. The nurse uses a fetoscope, knowing that the fetal heart beat can first be heard with a fetoscope at gestational week:
   1. 5
   2. 10
   3. 16
   4. 20

9. During a prenatal visit, a nurse assesses the fetal heart rate. The nurse determines that the fetal heart rate is normal if which of the following is noted?
   1. 80 beats per minute
   2. 100 beats per minute
   3. 150 beats per minute
   4. 180 beats per minute

10. A high school nurse is conducting a session with female adolescents regarding the menstrual cycle. The nurse tells the adolescents that the normal duration of the menstrual cycle is about:
    1. 14 days
    2. 28 days
    3. 30 days
    4. 45 days

CRITICAL THINKING: FREE-TEXT ENTRY

A client who has just been told that she is pregnant asks a clinic nurse when the fetus's heart will be developed and beating. The nurse tells the client that the fetal heart is beating at what gestational week?

Answer: _____

ANSWERS

1. **4**
Rationale: Each fallopian tube is a hollow, muscular tube that transports a mature oocyte for final maturation and fertilization. Fertilization typically occurs near the boundary between the ampulla and isthmus of the tube. Estrogen is a hormone produced by the ovarian follicles, corpus luteum, adrenal cortex, and placenta during pregnancy. Progesterone is a hormone secreted by the corpus luteum of the ovary, adrenal glands, and placenta during pregnancy. The vagina is the passageway for the fetus, and the fetus develops in the uterus.
Test-Taking Strategy: Use the process of elimination and knowledge of the anatomy and physiology of the female reproductive system. Remember that fertilization occurs in the fallopian tubes. If you had difficulty with this question, review anatomy and physiology of the reproductive system.
Level of Cognitive Ability: Comprehension
Client Needs: Physiological Integrity
Integrated Concept and Process: Teaching/Learning
Content Area: Maternity

Reference: Olds, S., London. M., & Ladewig, P. (2000). Maternal-newborn nursing: A family and community-based approach (6th ed.). Upper Saddle River, N.J.: Prentice-Hall Health, pp. 130-132.

2. **1**
Rationale: FSH and LH, when stimulated by GnRH from the hypothalamus, are released from the anterior pituitary gland to stimulate follicular growth and development, growth of the graafian follicle, and the production of progesterone. Options 2, 3, and 4 are incorrect.
Test-Taking Strategy: Use the process of elimination. Remember that FSH and LH are released from the anterior pituitary gland. If you had difficulty with this question, review the menstrual cycle.
Level of Cognitive Ability: Analysis
Client Needs: Physiological Integrity
Integrated Concept/Process: Nursing Process/Evaluation
Content Area: Maternity
Reference: Herlihy, B., & Maebius, N. (2000). The human body in health and illness. Philadelphia: W.B. Saunders, p. 464.

3. 4
Rationale: A gynecoid pelvis is a normal female pelvis and is the most favorable for successful labor and birth. An android pelvis would not be favorable for labor because of the narrow pelvic planes. An anthropoid pelvis has an outlet that is adequate, with a normal or moderately narrow pubic arch. The platypelloid pelvis has a wide transverse diameter, but the anteroposterior diameter is short, making the outlet inadequate.
Test-Taking Strategy: Use the process of elimination and knowledge regarding pelvic types to answer this question. Remember that the gynecoid pelvis is the normal female pelvis. Review pelvic types if you had difficulty with this question.
Level of Cognitive Ability: Comprehension
Client Needs: Physiological Integrity
Integrated Concept/Process: Nursing Process/Planning
Content Area: Maternity
Reference: Olds, S., London. M., & Ladewig, P. (2000). *Maternal-newborn nursing: A family and community-based approach* (6th ed.). Upper Saddle River, N.J.: Prentice-Hall Health, pp. 136-137, 473.

4. 3
Rationale: The placenta provides an exchange of nutrients and waste products between the mother and the fetus. The amniotic fluid surrounds, cushions, and protects the fetus and maintains the body temperature of the fetus. Nutrients, drugs, antibodies, and viruses can pass through the placenta.
Test-Taking Strategy: Use the process of elimination and knowledge regarding the purpose of the placenta and amniotic fluid. Remember that the placenta provides nutrients. If you had difficulty with this question, review the structure and function of the placenta and amniotic fluid.
Level of Cognitive Ability: Comprehension
Client Needs: Physiological Integrity
Integrated Concept/Process: Teaching/Learning
Content Area: Maternity
Reference: Sherwen, L., Scoloveno, M.A., & Weingarten, C. (1999). *Maternity nursing: Care of the childbearing family* (3rd ed.). Stamford, Conn.: Appleton & Lange, p. 356.

5. 2
Rationale: Blood pumped by the embryo's heart leaves the embryo through two umbilical arteries. Once oxygenated, the blood is then returned by one umbilical vein. Arteries carry deoxygenated blood and waste products from the fetus, and veins carry oxygenated blood and provide oxygen and nutrients to the fetus.
Test-Taking Strategy: Use the process of elimination and knowledge regarding fetal circulation to answer this question. Remember that there are three umbilical vessels within an umbilical cord (two arteries and one vein). If you had difficulty with this question, review fetal circulation.
Level of Cognitive Ability: Comprehension
Client Needs: Physiological Integrity
Integrated Concept/Process: Teaching/Learning
Content Area: Maternity
Reference: Herlihy, B., & Maebius, N. (2000). *The human body in health and illness.* Philadelphia: W.B. Saunders, pp. 314-316.

6. 4
Rationale: The ductus venosus connects the umbilical vein to the inferior vena cava. Options 1, 2, and 3 are incorrect. The foramen ovale is a temporary opening between the right and left atria. The ductus arteriosus joins the aorta and the pulmonary artery.
Test-Taking Strategy: Use the process of elimination and knowledge regarding fetal circulation to answer this question. Remember that the ductus venosus connects the umbilical vein to the inferior vena cava. Review fetal circulation if you had difficulty with this question.
Level of Cognitive Ability: Analysis
Client Needs: Physiological Integrity
Integrated Concept/Process: Nursing Process/Evaluation
Content Area: Maternity
Reference: Herlihy, B., & Maebius, N. (2000). *The human body in health and illness.* Philadelphia: W.B. Saunders, pp. 314-316.

7. 4
Rationale: By the end of the 12th week, the external genitalia of the fetus have developed to such a degree that the sex of the fetus can be visually determined. Options 1, 2, and 3 are incorrect.
Test-Taking Strategy: Use the process of elimination and knowledge regarding fetal development to answer this question. It is important to remember that the sex of the fetus can be visually recognizable by gestational week 12. If you had difficulty with this question, review fetal development.
Level of Cognitive Ability: Comprehension
Client Needs: Physiological Integrity
Integrated Concept/Process: Teaching/Learning
Content Area: Maternity
Reference: Sherwen, L., Scoloveno, M.A., & Weingarten, C. (1999). *Maternity nursing: Care of the childbearing family* (3rd ed.). Stamford, Conn.: Appleton & Lange, p. 357.

8. 4
Rationale: The fetal heart beat can first be heard with a fetoscope at 18 to 20 weeks of gestation. If a Doppler ultrasound device is used, the fetal heart rate can be detected as early as 8 to 12 weeks of gestation. Options 1, 2, and 3 are incorrect.
Test-Taking Strategy: Use the process of elimination and knowledge regarding assessment of fetal heart sounds to answer this question. Note the key word "fetoscope" in the question. If you had difficulty with this question, review fetal heart assessment.
Level of Cognitive Ability: Comprehension
Client Needs: Physiological Integrity
Integrated Concept/Process: Nursing Process/Implementation
Content Area: Maternity
Reference: Lowdermilk, D., Perry, S., & Bobak, I. (2000). *Maternity & women's health care* (7th ed.). St. Louis: Mosby, p. 402.

9. 3
Rationale: The normal fetal heart rate is 120 to 160 beats per minute. If the fetal heart rate is less than 120 or more than 160 beats per minute with the uterus at rest, the fetus may be in distress. Options 1 and 2 indicate bradycardia. Option 4 indicates tachycardia.
Test-Taking Strategy: Use the process of elimination and knowledge regarding the normal fetal heart to answer this question. Remember that the normal fetal heart rate is 120 to 160 beats per minute. Review fetal heart rate if you had difficulty with this question.
Level of Cognitive Ability: Comprehension

Client Needs: Physiological Integrity
Integrated Concept/Process: Nursing Process/Assessment
Content Area: Maternity
Reference: Sherwen, L., Scoloveno, M.A., & Weingarten, C. (1999). *Maternity nursing: Care of the childbearing family* (3rd ed.). Stamford, Conn.: Appleton & Lange, p. 781.

10. **2**

Rationale: The normal duration of the menstrual cycle is about 28 days, although it may range from 20 to 45 days. Significant deviations from the 28-day cycle are associated with reduced fertility. The first day of the menstrual period is counted as day 1 of the woman's cycle.

Test-Taking Strategy: Use the process of elimination and knowledge regarding the duration of the menstrual cycle to answer this question. Note the key words "normal duration" in the question. This will assist in eliminating options 1, 3, and 4. If you had difficulty with this question, review the menstrual cycle.

Level of Cognitive Ability: Application
Client Needs: Physiological Integrity
Integrated Concept/Process: Teaching/Learning

Content Area: Maternity
Reference: Gorrie, T., McKinney, E., & Murray, S. (1998). *Foundations of maternal-newborn nursing* (2nd ed.). Philadelphia: W.B. Saunders, p. 67.

CRITICAL THINKING: FREE-TEXT ENTRY

Answer: Week 5

Rationale: The fetal heart is beating and developing four chambers by gestational week 5.

Test-Taking Strategy: Knowledge regarding the weekly development of the fetus is required to answer this question. Review fetal development in relation to the fetal heart beat if you had difficulty with this question.

Level of Cognitive Ability: Application
Client Needs: Physiological Integrity
Integrated Concept/Process: Teaching/Learning
Content Area: Maternity
Reference: Gorrie, T., McKinney, E., & Murray, S. (1998). *Foundations of maternal-newborn nursing* (2nd ed.). Philadelphia: W.B. Saunders, p. 105.

REFERENCES

Gorrie, T., McKinney, E., & Murray, S. (1998). *Foundations of maternal-newborn nursing* (2nd ed.). Philadelphia: W.B. Saunders.

Herlihy, B., & Maebius, N. (2000). *The human body in health and illness.* Philadelphia: W.B. Saunders.

Lowdermilk, D., Perry, S., & Bobak, I. (2000). *Maternity & women's health care* (7th ed.). St. Louis: Mosby.

Olds, S., London. M., & Ladewig, P. (2000). *Maternal-newborn nursing: A family and community-based approach* (6th ed.). Upper Saddle River, N.J.: Prentice-Hall Health.

Sherwen, L., Scoloveno, M.A., & Weingarten, C. (1999). *Maternity nursing: Care of the childbearing family* (3rd ed.). Stamford, Conn.: Appleton & Lange.

Obstetrical Assessment

I. GESTATION
A. Estimated date of confinement (EDC)
B. Lasts approximately 280 days
C. **Nagele's rule** for estimating EDC (Box 23-1)
   1. For **Nagele's rule** to be accurate requires that the woman have a regular 28-day menstrual cycle
   2. Add 7 days to the first day of the last menstrual period (LMP), subtract 3 months, and then add 1 year to that date

II. GRAVIDITY AND PARITY
A. **Gravidity**
   1. **Gravida** refers to a pregnant woman
   2. **Gravidity** refers to the number of pregnancies
   3. **Nulligravida** is a woman who has never been pregnant
   4. **Primigravida** is a woman who is pregnant for the first time
   5. **Multigravida** is a woman in at least her second pregnancy
B. **Parity**
   1. **Parity** is the number of births (not the number of fetuses; e.g., twins) past 20 weeks' gestation, whether the fetus was born alive or not
   2. **Nullipara** is a woman who has not had a birth at more than 20 weeks of gestation

---

BOX 23-1

Nagele's Rule for Estimating EDC

First day of LMP: September 11, 2002
Add 7 days: September 18, 2002
Subtract 3 months: June 18, 2002
Add 1 year: June 18, 2003
EDC: June 18, 2003

---

3. **Primipara** is a woman who has had one birth that occurs after the 20th week of gestation
4. **Multipara** is a woman who has had two or more pregnancies resulting in viable offspring

III. PREGNANCY SIGNS
A. Presumptive signs
   1. Amenorrhea
   2. Nausea and vomiting
   3. Increased size and increased feeling of fullness in breasts
   4. Pronounced nipples
   5. Urinary frequency
   6. **Quickening:** First perception of fetal movement; may occur as early as the 14th to 16th week of gestation
   7. Fatigue
   8. Discoloration and thickening of the vaginal mucosa
B. Probable signs
   1. Uterine enlargement
   2. **Hegar's sign:** Softening and thinning of the lower uterine segment that occurs about week 6
   3. **Goodell's sign:** Softening of the cervix that occurs at the beginning of the second month
   4. **Chadwick's sign:** Bluish coloration of the mucous membranes of cervix, vagina, and vulva that occurs about week 6
   5. **Ballottement:** Rebounding of the fetus against the examiner's fingers on palpation
   6. Braxton Hicks contractions
   7. Positive pregnancy test measuring for human chorionic gonadotropin (hCG)
C. Positive signs
   1. Fetal heart rate by Doppler at 8 to 12 weeks and by fetoscope at 20 weeks of gestation
   2. Active fetal movements palpable by examiner
   3. Outline of fetus via radiography or ultrasound

IV. FUNDAL HEIGHT (Box 23-2)
A. Performed to evaluate fetus's gestational age
B. During the second and third trimesters (weeks 18 to 30), fundal height in centimeters approximately equals the fetus's age in weeks ± 2 cm
C. At 16 weeks, the fundus can be found halfway between the symphysis pubis and the umbilicus
D. At 20 to 22 weeks, the fundus is at the umbilicus
E. At 36 weeks, the fundus is at the xiphoid process

▲ V. MATERNAL RISK FACTORS
A. German measles (rubella)
  1. The risk of maternal and fetal or congenital infection is related to the trimester of placental infection
  2. Maternal infection during the first 8 weeks of gestation carries the highest rate of maternal and fetal infection
B. Sexually transmitted diseases
  1. Syphilis
    a. May cross the **placenta**
    b. Usually leads to spontaneous abortions
    c. Increases the incidence of mental subnormality and physical deformities
  2. Genital herpes
    a. May cross the **placenta**
    b. Fetus is contaminated after membranes rupture or with vaginal **delivery**
  3. Gonorrhea
    a. Fetus is contaminated at the time of **delivery**
    b. May result in postpartum infection
    c. Risks to the **neonate** include ophthalmia neonatorum, pneumonia, and sepsis
▲ C. Human immunodeficiency virus (HIV)
  1. The virus is transmitted through blood, blood products, and other bodily fluids such as urine, semen, and vaginal fluid
  2. Repeated exposure to HIV during pregnancy through unsafe sex practices or intravenous drug use can increase the risk of transmission to the fetus
▲ D. Substance abuse
  1. Many substances cross the **placenta;** therefore no drugs, including over-the-counter medications, should be taken unless prescribed by physician
  2. Substances commonly abused include alcohol, cocaine, crack, marijuana, amphetamines, barbiturates, and heroin

  3. Substance abuse threatens normal fetal growth and successful term completion of the pregnancy
  4. Substance abuse places the pregnancy at risk for fetal growth retardation, abruptio placentae, and fetal bradycardia
  5. Physical signs of drug abuse may include dilated or contracted pupils, fatigue, track marks, skin abscesses, inflamed nasal mucosa, and inappropriate behavior by the mother
  6. Alcohol during pregnancy may lead to fetal alcohol syndrome and can cause jitteriness, physical abnormalities, congenital anomalies, and growth deficits
  7. Smoking leads to low birth weights, a higher incidence of birth defects, and stillbirths
E. Adolescent pregnancy
  1. Factors that result in adolescent pregnancy include the early onset of menarche, changing sexual behaviors in this age group, faulty family development, poverty, and the lack of knowledge of reproduction and birth control
  2. The major concerns related to adolescent pregnancy include poor nutritional status, emotional and behavioral difficulties, lack of support systems, increased risk of stillbirth, low-birth-weight **newborn infants,** fetal mortality, cephalopelvic disproportion, and the increased risk of maternal complications such as hypertension, anemia, prolonged **labor,** and infections

PRACTICE QUESTIONS

1. A client arrives at a prenatal clinic for the first prenatal assessment. The client tells a nurse that the first day of her last menstrual period was September 19, 2002. Using Nagele's rule, the nurse determines the estimated date of confinement (EDC) as:
    1. July 26, 2003
    2. June 12, 2002
    3. June 26, 2003
    4. July 12, 2002
2. A nurse is collecting data during an admission assessment of a client who is pregnant with twins. The client has a healthy 5-year-old child and tells the nurse that she does not have a history of any type of abortion or fetal demise. The nurse would document which gravida and para status for this client?
    1. Gravida III, Para II
    2. Gravida II, Para II
    3. Gravida I, Para I
    4. Gravida II, Para I
3. A nurse is performing an assessment of a primipara who is being evaluated in a clinic during her second trimester of pregnancy. Which of the following indicates an abnormal physical finding necessitating further testing?
    1. Consistent increase in fundal height

BOX 23-2

Measuring Fundal Height

1. Place client in supine position
2. Place end of tape measure at level of symphysis pubis
3. Stretch tape to top of uterine fundus
4. Note and record measurement

2. Fetal heart rate of 180 beats per minute
3. Braxton Hicks contractions
4. Quickening

4. A nurse is providing instructions to a pregnant client with genital herpes about the measures that need to be implemented to protect the fetus. The nurse tells the client that:
   1. Daily administration of acyclovir (Zovirax) is necessary during the entire pregnancy
   2. Total abstinence from sexual intercourse is necessary during the entire pregnancy
   3. Sitz baths need to be taken every 4 hours while awake if vaginal lesions are present
   4. A cesarean section will be necessary if vaginal lesions are present at the time of labor

5. A nurse is performing an assessment of a pregnant client who is at 28 weeks of gestation. The nurse measures the fundal height in centimeters and expects the findings to be which of the following?
   1. 22 cm
   2. 28 cm
   3. 36 cm
   4. 40 cm

6. A pregnant client is seen in a health care clinic for a regular prenatal visit. The client tells the nurse that she is experiencing irregular contractions. The nurse determines that the client is experiencing Braxton Hicks contractions. On the basis of this finding, which nursing action is most appropriate?
   1. Instruct the client to maintain bed rest for the remainder of the pregnancy
   2. Instruct the client that these are common and may occur throughout the pregnancy
   3. Contact the physician
   4. Call the maternity unit and inform them that the client will be admitted in a prelabor condition

7. A nurse is reviewing the record of a client who has just been told that a pregnancy test is positive. The physician has documented the presence of Goodell's sign. The nurse determines that this sign is indicative of:
   1. A softening of the cervix
   2. A soft blowing sound that corresponds to the maternal pulse during auscultation of the uterus

3. The presence of human chorionic gonadotropin (hCG) in the urine
4. The presence of fetal movement

8. A nursing instructor asks a nursing student to describe the process of quickening. Which of the following statements if made by the student indicates an understanding of this term?
   1. "It is the irregular, painless contractions that occur throughout pregnancy."
   2. "It is the soft blowing sound that can be heard when the uterus is auscultated."
   3. "It is the fetal movement that is felt by the mother."
   4. "It is the thinning of the lower uterine segment."

9. A nurse midwife is performing an assessment of a pregnant client and is assessing the client for the presence of ballottement. Which of the following would the nurse implement to test for the presence of ballottement?
   1. Auscultating for fetal heart sounds
   2. Palpating the abdomen for fetal movement
   3. Assessing the cervix for thinning
   4. Initiating a gentle upward tap on the cervix

10. A pregnant client asks the nurse in the clinic when she will be able to start feeling the fetus move. The nurse responds by telling the mother that fetal movements will be noted between:
    1. 6 and 8 weeks of gestation
    2. 8 and 10 weeks of gestation
    3. 10 and 12 weeks of gestation
    4. 14 and 16 weeks of gestation

CRITICAL THINKING: FREE-TEXT ENTRY

A nurse is assisting a health care provider in performing a physical assessment of a client who is six weeks pregnant. The health care provider tells the nurse that Hegar's sign is present. After the examination, the client asks the nurse to describe Hegar's sign. What does the nurse tell the client?

Answer: _____

ANSWERS

1. **3**

Rationale: Accurate use of Nagele's rule requires that the woman have a regular 28-day menstrual cycle. Add 7 days to the first day of the last menstrual period (LMP), subtract 3 months, and then add 1 year to that date. First day of the LMP: September 19, 2002; add 7 days: September 26, 2002; subtract 3 months: June 26, 2002; add 1 year: June 26, 2003.

Test-Taking Strategy: Use the process of elimination and knowledge regarding the use of Nagele's rule to answer this question. Use caution when following steps to determine the EDC. Avoid taking shortcuts, particularly when math is involved. Read all of the options carefully, noting the dates and years in the options, before selecting an option. Review Nagele's rule if you had difficulty with this question.
Level of Cognitive Ability: Analysis

Client Needs: Health Promotion and Maintenance
Integrated Concept/Process: Nursing Process/Assessment
Content Area: Maternity
Reference: Lowdermilk, D., Perry, S., & Bobak, I. (2000). *Maternity & women's health care* (7th ed.). St. Louis: Mosby, pp. 381-382.

2. **4**
Rationale: Gravida is a term that refers to a woman who is or has been pregnant, regardless of the duration of the pregnancy. Para (parity) is a term that means the number of births (not the number of fetuses) past 20 weeks' gestation, whether the fetus was born alive or not. Therefore, option 4 is the only correct option for a woman who is currently pregnant with twins and has had one other pregnancy past 20 weeks of gestation. Options 1, 2, & 3 are incorrect on the basis of the above definitions.
Test-Taking Strategy: Use the process of elimination. Knowledge and understanding of the terms gravida and para will easily direct you to option 4. If you had difficulty answering this question, review these definitions.
Level of Cognitive Ability: Application
Client Needs: Health Promotion and Maintenance
Integrated Concept/Process: Nursing Process/Assessment
Content Area: Maternity
Reference: Sherwen, L., Scoloveno, M.A., & Weingarten, C. (1999). *Maternity nursing: Care of the childbearing family* (3rd ed.). Stamford, Conn.: Appleton & Lange, pp. 428-429.

3. **2**
Rationale: The normal fetal heart rate is 120 to 160 beats per minute. Options 1, 3, and 4 are normal expected findings.
Test-Taking Strategy: Use the process of elimination. Note the key words "indicates an abnormal physical finding." Recalling that the normal fetal heart rate is 120 to 160 beats per minute will easily direct you to option 2. Review normal assessment findings in pregnancy if you had difficulty with this question.
Level of Cognitive Ability: Analysis
Client Needs: Physiological Integrity
Integrated Concept/Process: Nursing Process/Assessment
Content Area: Maternity
Reference: Sherwen, L., Scoloveno, M.A., & Weingarten, C. (1999). *Maternity nursing: Care of the childbearing family* (3rd ed.). Stamford, Conn.: Appleton & Lange, p. 781.

4. **4**
Rationale: For women with active lesions, either recurrent or primary at the time of labor, delivery should be by cesarean section to prevent the fetus from being in contact with the genital herpes. The safety of acyclovir has not been established during pregnancy, and it should be used only when a life-threatening infection is present. Clients should be advised to abstain from sexual contact while the lesions are present. If it is an initial infection, they should continue to abstain until they become culture negative, because prolonged viral shedding may occur in such cases. Keeping the genital area clean and dry will promote healing.
Test-Taking Strategy: Use the process of elimination. Eliminate options 1 and 2 first because of the absolute word "entire" in these options. From the remaining options, recalling that the lesions should be kept clean and dry to promote healing will assist in eliminating option 3. If you had difficulty with this

question, review the content related to genital herpes as a maternal risk factor.
Level of Cognitive Ability: Application
Client Needs: Safe, Effective Care Environment
Integrated Concept/Process: Teaching/Learning
Content Area: Maternity
Reference: Ladewig, P., London. M., & Olds, S. (1998). *Maternal-newborn nursing care: The nurse, the family, and the community* (4th ed.). Menlo Park, Calif.: Addison Wesley Longman, p. 315.

5. **2**
Rationale: During the second and third trimesters (weeks 18 to 30), fundal height in centimeters approximately equals the fetus's age in weeks ± 2 cm. At 16 weeks, the fundus can be located halfway between the symphysis pubis and the umbilicus. At 20 to 22 weeks, the fundus is at the umbilicus, and at 36 weeks, the fundus is at the xiphoid process.
Test-Taking Strategy: Use the process of elimination. Remember that during the second and third trimesters (weeks 18 to 30), fundal height in centimeters approximately equals the fetus's age in weeks ± 2 cm. If you are unfamiliar with this assessment technique, review this content area.
Level of Cognitive Ability: Analysis
Client Needs: Health Promotion and Maintenance
Integrated Concept/Process: Nursing Process/Assessment
Content Area: Maternity
Reference: Lowdermilk, D., Perry, S., & Bobak, I. (2000). *Maternity & women's health care* (7th ed.). St. Louis: Mosby, p. 401.

6. **2**
Rationale: Braxton Hicks contractions are irregular, painless contractions that may occur intermittently throughout pregnancy. Since Braxton Hicks contractions may occur and are normal in some pregnant women during pregnancy, options 1, 3, and 4 are unnecessary and inappropriate actions.
Test-Taking Strategy: Use the process of elimination. Options 3 and 4 are similar and can be eliminated first. From the remaining options, knowing that Braxton Hicks contractions are common and can occur throughout pregnancy will assist in directing you to option 2. If you had difficulty with this question, review the physiology associated with Braxton Hicks contractions.
Level of Cognitive Ability: Application
Client Needs: Health Promotion and Maintenance
Integrated Concept/Process: Teaching/Learning
Content Area: Maternity
Reference: Lowdermilk, D., Perry, S., & Bobak, I. (2000). *Maternity & women's health care* (7th ed.). St. Louis: Mosby, p. 399.

7. **1**
Rationale: In the early weeks of pregnancy, the cervix becomes softer as a result of pelvic vasoconstriction, which causes Goodell's sign. Cervical softening is noted by the examiner during pelvic examination. A soft blowing sound that corresponds to the maternal pulse may be auscultated over the uterus and is due to blood circulation through the placenta. hCG is noted in maternal urine in a positive urine pregnancy test. Goodell's sign does not indicate the presence of fetal movement.

Test-Taking Strategy: Use the process of elimination and knowledge regarding the physiological findings in Goodell's sign to answer this question. Remember that Goodell's sign refers to a softening of the cervix. If you had difficulty with this question, review the changes in the cervix that occur during pregnancy.
Level of Cognitive Ability: Analysis
Client Needs: Health Promotion and Maintenance
Integrated Concept/Process: Nursing Process/Analysis
Content Area: Maternity
Reference: Lowdermilk, D., Perry, S., & Bobak, I. (2000). *Maternity & women's health care* (7th ed.). St. Louis: Mosby, p. 339.

8. **3**
Rationale: Quickening is fetal movement and may occur as early as the 14th to 16th week of gestation, and the expectant mother first notices subtle fetal movements that gradually increase in intensity. A soft blowing sound that corresponds to the maternal pulse may be auscultated over the uterus, and this in known as uterine souffle. This sound is due to the blood circulation to the placenta and corresponds to the maternal pulse. Braxton Hicks contractions are irregular, painless contractions that may occur throughout pregnancy. A thinning of the lower uterine segment occurs about the sixth week of pregnancy and is called Hegar's sign.
Test-Taking Strategy: Use the process of elimination and knowledge regarding the term "quickening" to answer this question. Remember that quickening is fetal movement. If you are unfamiliar with this sign associated with pregnancy, review this content area.
Level of Cognitive Ability: Analysis
Client Needs: Health Promotion and Maintenance
Integrated Concept/Process: Teaching/Learning
Content Area: Maternity
Reference: Lowdermilk, D., Perry, S., & Bobak, I. (2000). *Maternity & women's health care* (7th ed.). St. Louis: Mosby, p. 340.

9. **4**
Rationale: Ballottement is a technique of palpating a floating structure by bouncing it gently and feeling it rebound. In the technique used to palpate the fetus, the examiner places a finger in the vagina and taps gently upward, causing the fetus to rise. The fetus tthen sinks, and a gentle tap is felt on the finger. Options 1, 2, and 3 are incorrect.
Test-Taking Strategy: Use the process of elimination. Recalling that ballottement is a technique of palpating a floating

structure by bouncing it gently and feeling it rebound will easily direct you to option 4. Review this assessment technique if you had difficulty with this question.
Level of Cognitive Ability: Application
Client Needs: Health Promotion and Maintenance
Integrated Concept/Process: Nursing Process/Implementation
Content Area: Maternity
Reference: Lowdermilk, D., Perry, S., & Bobak, I. (2000). *Maternity & women's health care* (7th ed.). St. Louis: Mosby, p. 340.

10. **4**
Rationale: Quickening is fetal movement and may occur as early as the 14th to 16th week of gestation. The expectant mother first notices subtle fetal movements during this time, which gradually increase in intensity. Options 1, 2, and 3 are incorrect.
Test-Taking Strategy: Use the process of elimination and knowledge regarding the occurrence of quickening. In this situation, it is best to select the option that indicates the greatest length of gestational time. Review the process of quickening if you had difficulty with this question.
Level of Cognitive Ability: Application
Client Needs: Health Promotion and Maintenance
Integrated Concept/Process: Teaching/Learning
Content Area: Maternity
Reference: Lowdermilk, D., Perry, S., & Bobak, I. (2000). *Maternity & women's health care* (7th ed.). St. Louis: Mosby, p. 340.

CRITICAL THINKING: FREE-TEXT ENTRY

Answer: Softening and thinning of the lower uterine segment that occur about week 6
Rationale: At about the sixth week of pregnancy, the lower uterine segment becomes soft and thin. This is known as Hegar's sign.
Test-Taking Strategy: It is necessary to know the description of the changes that occur in the cervix and lower uterine segment to answer this question. Review the signs of pregnancy if you are unfamiliar with them.
Level of Cognitive Ability: Application
Client Needs: Health Promotion and Maintenance
Integrated Concept/Process: Teaching/Learning
Content Area: Maternity
Reference: Gorrie, T., McKinney, E., & Murray, S. (1998). *Foundations of maternal-newborn nursing* (2nd ed.). Philadelphia: W.B. Saunders, p. 138.

REFERENCES

Gorrie, T., McKinney, E. & Murray, S. (1998). *Foundations of maternal-newborn nursing* (2nd ed.). Philadelphia: W.B. Saunders.

Ladewig, P., London. M., & Olds, S. (1998). *Maternal-newborn nursing care: The nurse, the family, and the community* (4th ed.). Menlo Park, Calif.: Addison Wesley Longman.

Lowdermilk, D., Perry, S., & Bobak, I. (2000). *Maternity & women's health care* (7th ed.). St. Louis: Mosby.

Olds, S., London. M., & Ladewig, P. (2000). *Maternal-newborn nursing: A family and community-based approach* (6th ed.). Upper Saddle River, N.J.: Prenticee-Hall Health.

Sherwen, L., Scoloveno, M.A., & Weingarten, C. (1999). *Materntiy nursing: Care of the childbearing family* (3rd ed.). Stamford, Conn.: Appleton & Lange.

Prenatal Period

I. PHYSIOLOGICAL MATERNAL CHANGES

A. Cardiovascular system
1. Circulating blood volume increases, plasma increases, total volume increases by 40% to 50%
2. Total red cell volume increases
3. Physiological anemia occurs as the plasma increase exceeds the increase in red blood cell (RBC) production
4. Heart size increases with left ventricle hypertrophy
5. Heart is elevated upward and to the left because of displacement of the diaphragm as the uterus enlarges
6. Pulse may increase about 10 beats per minute
7. Blood pressure may decline in the second trimester
8. Iron requirements are increased
9. Retention of sodium and water may occur

B. Respiratory
1. Oxygen consumption increases by 15% to 20%
2. Diaphragm is elevated because of the enlarged uterus
3. Respiratory rate remains unchanged
4. Shortness of breath may be experienced

C. Gastrointestinal system
1. Nausea and vomiting may occur as a result of the secretion of human chorionic gonadotropin (hCG), and subsides by the third month
2. Poor appetite may occur because of the decreased gastric motility
3. Alterations in taste and smell
4. Constipation as a result of decreased gastrointestinal (GI) motility or pressure of the uterus
5. Flatulence and heartburn because of decreased GI motility and slow emptying of the stomach
6. Hemorrhoids as a result of increased venous pressure

7. Gum tissue may become swollen and easily bleed
8. Ptyalism (excessive secretion of saliva)

D. Renal system
1. Frequency of urination occurs in the first and third trimesters as a result of pressure of the enlarging uterus on the bladder
2. Decreased bladder tone is caused by hormonal changes
3. Decreased bladder capacity
4. Renal function increases
5. Renal threshold for glucose may be reduced

E. Endocrine system
1. Basal metabolic rate rises
2. Anterior lobe of the pituitary gland enlarges
3. Thyroid enlarges slightly, and thyroid activity increases
4. Aldosterone levels gradually increase
5. Parathyroid increases in size

F. Reproductive system
1. Uterus
   a. Uterus enlarges from a weight of 60 g to a weight of 1000 g
   b. Size and number of blood vessels and lymphatics increase
   c. Irregular contractions occur
2. Cervix
   a. Becomes shorter, more elastic, and larger in diameter
   b. Endocervical glands secrete a thick mucus plug, which is expelled from the canal when dilation begins
   c. Increased vascularization causes a softening and blue-purple discoloration known as **Chadwick's sign,** which occurs at approximately 6 weeks of gestational age
3. Ovaries
   a. The maturation of new follicles is blocked
   b. The ovaries cease ovum production

4. Vagina
   a. Hypertrophy and thickening of the muscle
   b. Increase in vaginal secretions, and secretions are usually thick, white, and acidic
5. Breasts
   a. Breast size increases
   b. Nipples become more pronounced
   c. Areola becomes darker in color
   d. Superficial veins become prominent
   e. Hypertrophy of the Montgomery follicles occurs
   f. Colostrum may appear from the breast

G. Skin
   1. Pigmentation increases
   2. A dark streak down the midline of the abdomen may appear (linea nigra)
   3. Chloasma, or mask of pregnancy, may occur over the forehead, cheeks, and nose
   4. Reddish-purple stretch marks (striae) may occur on the abdomen, breasts, thighs, and upper arms
   5. Vascular spider nevi may occur on the neck, chest, face, arms, and legs
   6. Rate of hair growth may decrease

H. Skeletal system
   1. Center of gravity changes
   2. Postural changes occur as the increased weight of the uterus causes a forward pull of the bony pelvis

I. Metabolism
   1. Metabolic function increases
   2. Body weight increases
   3. The average expected weight gain during pregnancy is 2 to 4 pounds in the first trimester and approximately 1 pound per week in the second and third trimesters
   4. Water retention is increased, which can contribute to weight gain

II. PSYCHOLOGICAL MATERNAL CHANGES

A. Ambivalence
   1. Occurs early in pregnancy, even when the pregnancy is planned
   2. Mother may experience dependence-independence conflict and ambivalence related to role changes
   3. Father may experience ambivalence related to the new role he is assuming, the increased financial responsibilities, and sharing the wife's attention with the child

B. Acceptance: Factors that may be related to acceptance of the pregnancy are the woman's readiness for the experience and her identification with the motherhood role

C. Emotional lability
   1. May be manifested by frequency in the change of emotional states or extremes in emotional states
   2. These emotional changes are common, and the mother may feel that these changes are abnormal

D. Body image changes
   1. The changes in a woman's perception of her image during pregnancy occurs gradually and may be either positive or negative
   2. The physical changes and symptoms that the woman experiences during pregnancy contribute to her body image

III. DISCOMFORTS OF PREGNANCY

A. Nausea and vomiting
   1. Occur in the first trimester
   2. Due to elevated hCG levels and changes in carbohydrate metabolism
   3. Implementation
      a. Eating dry crackers before arising
      b. Eating small, frequent, low-fat meals during the day
      c. Drinking liquids between meals
      d. Avoiding fried foods
      e. Avoiding all antiemetics throughout pregnancy

B. Syncope
   1. Usually occurs in the first trimester
   2. May be hormonally triggered or caused by the increased blood volume, anemia, fatigue, or sudden position changes
   3. Implementation
      a. Sitting with the feet elevated
      b. Changing positions slowly
      c. Changing the position to the left side to relieve the pressure of the uterus on the inferior vena cava

C. Urinary urgency and frequency
   1. Usually occur in the first and third trimesters
   2. Due to pressure of the uterus on the bladder
   3. Implementation
      a. Drinking 2 quarts of fluid per day
      b. Limiting fluid intake in the evening
      c. Voiding at regular intervals
      d. Sleeping on the side at night
      e. Wearing perineal pads if necessary

D. Breast tenderness
   1. Can occur from the first through the third trimesters
   2. Due to increased levels of estrogen and progesterone
   3. Implementation
      a. Encouraging the use of a supportive bra with nonelastic straps
      b. Avoiding the use of soap on the nipples and areola area to prevent drying

E. Increased vaginal discharge
   1. Can occur from the first through the third trimesters
   2. Due to hyperplasia of vaginal mucosa and increased mucus production
   3. Implementation
      a. Proper cleansing and hygiene

b. Wearing cotton underwear

c. Avoiding douching

d. Advising the client to consult the physician or health care provider if infection is suspected

F. Nasal stuffiness

1. Occurs during the first through the third trimesters

2. Occurs as a result of increased estrogen, which causes swelling of the nasal tissues and dryness

3. Implementation

a. Encouraging the use of a humidifier

b. Avoiding the use of nasal sprays or antihistamines

G. Fatigue

1. Occurs usually in the first and third trimesters

2. Usually a result of hormonal changes

3. Implementation

a. Arranging frequent rest periods throughout the day

b. Obtaining regular exercise

c. Avoiding eating and drinking foods containing stimulants throughout pregnancy

H. Heartburn

1. Occurs in the second and the third trimesters

2. Results from increased progesterone levels, decreased GI motility and esophageal reflux, and displacement of the stomach by the enlarging uterus

3. Implementation

a. Eating small, frequent meals

b. Sitting upright for 30 minutes following a meal

c. Drinking milk between meals

d. Avoiding fatty and spicy food

e. Avoiding antacids and histamine receptor antagonists throughout pregnancy

f. Administering antacids (Maalox or Mylanta) only when recommended by the physician or health care provider

I. Ankle edema

1. Usually occurs in the second and the third trimesters

2. Occurs as a result of vasodilation, venous stasis, and increased venous pressure below the uterus

3. Implementation

a. Elevating the legs at least twice a day

b. Sleeping on the left side

c. Wearing supportive stockings

d. Avoiding sitting or standing in one position for long periods of time

e. Avoiding the use of diuretics during pregnancy

J. Varicose veins

1. Usually occur in the second and the third trimesters

2. Occur as a result of weakening walls of the veins or valves and venous congestion

3. Implementation

a. Wearing support hose

b. Elevating the feet when sitting

c. Lying with the feet and hips elevated

d. Moving about while standing to improve circulation

e. Avoiding pressure on the lower thighs

f. Avoiding leg crossing

g. Avoiding long periods of standing or sitting

h. Avoiding constricting articles of clothing

K. Headaches

1. Usually occur in the second and third trimesters

2. Occur as a result of changes in blood volume and vascular tone

3. Implementation

a. Changing position slowly

b. Applying a cool cloth to the forehead

c. Eating a small snack

d. Using acetaminophen (Tylenol) sparingly and only if prescribed by the physician or health care provider

L. Hemorrhoids

1. Usually occur in the second and third trimesters

2. Occur as a result of increased venous pressure and/or constipation

3. Implementation

a. Soaking in a warm sitz bath

b. Sitting on a soft pillow

c. Eating high-fiber foods and avoiding constipation

d. Drinking sufficient fluids

e. Increasing exercise, such as walking

f. Applying ointments, suppositories, or compresses as prescribed

M. Constipation

1. Usually occurs in the second and third trimesters

2. Occurs as a result of decreased intestinal motility, the displacement of the intestines, and taking iron supplements

3. Implementation

a. Eating high-fiber foods

b. Drinking plenty of fluids

c. Exercising regularly

d. Avoiding mineral oil or castor oil laxatives and using psyllium (Metamucil), senna (Senokot), or Milk of Magnesia at bedtime sparingly, only as prescribed by the physician or health care provider

N. Backache

1. Usually occurs in the second and third trimesters

2. Occurs from an exaggerated lumbosacral curve resulting from the enlarged uterus

3. Implementation

a. Encouraging rest

b. Using good body mechanics and improving posture

c. Wearing low-heeled shoes

d. Performing pelvic lift exercises and exercises such as squatting, sitting, and pelvic rocking

e. Sleeping on a firm mattress

O. Leg cramps
1. Usually occur in the second and third trimesters
2. Occur as a result of an altered calcium-phosphorus balance and pressure of the uterus on nerves, or from fatigue
3. Implementation
   a. Getting regular exercise, especially walking
   b. Elevating the feet and dorsiflexing the feet when resting
   c. Increasing calcium intake
P. Shortness of breath
1. Can occur in the second and third trimesters
2. Occurs as a result of pressure on the diaphragm
3. Implementation
   a. Allowing frequent rest periods
   b. Sleeping with the head elevated or on the side
   c. Avoiding overexertion

IV. LABORATORY TESTS (Box 24-1)
▲ A. Blood type and Rh factor
1. ABO typing is performed to determine the woman's blood type
2. Rh typing is done to determine the presence or absence of Rh antigen (Rh positive or Rh negative)
3. If the client is Rh negative and has a negative antibody screen, the client will need repeat antibody screens and should receive Rh immune globulin at 28 weeks' gestation
▲ B. Rubella titer
1. If the client has a negative titer, indicating susceptibility to the rubella virus, the client should receive the appropriate immunization postpartum
2. The client must be using effective birth control at the time of the immunization and must be counseled not to become pregnant for 3 months following immunization
C. Hemoglobin and hematocrit levels
1. Hemoglobin and hematocrit levels will drop during gestation as a result of increased plasma volume
2. An increase in the hematocrit level may indicate the development of pregnancy-induced hypertension (PIH)
3. A decrease in the hemoglobin level below 10 g/dL or in the hematocrit level below 30 g/dL indicates anemia
D. Papanicolaou smear: Done during the initial prenatal examination to screen for cervical neoplasia

E. Gonorrhea culture: Done during the initial prenatal examination to screen for gonorrhea; may be repeated during the third trimester in high-risk clients
F. Syphilis screening: Done during the initial prenatal examination to screen for syphilis; may be repeated during the third trimester in high-risk clients
G. Herpes cultures
1. Indicated for clients with a positive history or those with active lesions
2. Performed to determine the route of **delivery**
3. Weekly cultures may be done at the 35th or 36th week of pregnancy until **delivery**
H. Chlamydia culture
1. Indicated if the client is in a high-risk group
2. Indicated if **infants** from previous pregnancies have developed neonatal conjunctivitis or pneumonia
I. Sickle cell screening
1. Indicated for clients at risk for sickle cell disease
2. A positive test may indicate a need for further screening
J. Tuberculin skin test ▲
1. The health care provider may prefer to perform this skin test after **delivery**
2. A positive skin test indicates the need for a chest radiograph (using an abdominal lead shield) to rule out active disease; in a pregnant client, a chest radiograph will not be performed until after 20 weeks of gestation (after fetal organs are formed)
3. Converters to positive may be referred for treatment with medication following **delivery**
K. Hepatitis B surface antigens ▲
1. Recommended for all women because of the prevalence of the disease in the general population
2. Vaccination for hepatitis B antigen may be specifically indicated for:
   a. Health care workers
   b. Clients born in Asia, Africa, Haiti, or the Pacific islands
   c. Clients with previously undiagnosed jaundice or chronic liver disease
   d. IV drug abusers
   e. Clients with tattoos
   f. Clients with histories of blood transfusions
   g. Clients with histories of multiple episodes of sexually transmitted diseases
   h. Clients who have been previously rejected as blood donors
   i. Clients with histories of dialysis or renal transplantation
   j. Clients from households having hepatitis B–infected members or hemodialysis clients
L. Urinalysis and urine culture
1. A urine specimen for glucose and protein determinations should be obtained at every prenatal visit

---

BOX 24-1

Prenatal Visits

Every 4 weeks for first 28 to 32 weeks
Every 2 weeks from 32 to 36 weeks
Every week from 36 to 40 weeks

2. Glycosuria is a common result of decreased renal threshold that occurs during pregnancy
3. If glycosuria persists, this may indicate diabetes
4. White blood cells in the urine may indicate infection
5. Ketonuria may result from insufficient food intake or vomiting
6. Levels of 2+ to 4+ protein in the urine may indicate infection or pregnancy-induced hypertension (PIH)

V. DIAGNOSTIC TESTS

A. Ultrasound
  1. Outlines and identifies fetal and maternal structures
  2. Assists to confirm gestational age and estimated date of **delivery**
  3. May be done abdominally or transvaginally during pregnancy
  4. Implementation
    a. If the abdominal ultrasound is being performed, the woman usually needs to have a full bladder to obtain a better image of the fetus
    b. Inform the client that the test presents no known risks to the client or the fetus
B. Alpha-fetoprotein screening (AFP)
  1. Assesses the quantity of fetal serum proteins; if elevated, is associated with open neural tube and abdominal wall defects
  2. Can detect spina bifida and Down's syndrome
  3. Implementation
    a. Explain that the level is determined by a single maternal blood sample drawn at 15 to 18 weeks' gestation
    b. If the level is elevated and the gestation is less than 18 weeks, a second sample is drawn
    c. An ultrasound is performed for elevated levels to rule out fetal abnormalities or multiple gestation
C. Chorionic villus sampling (CVS)
  1. Aspiration of a small sample of chorionic villus tissue at 8 to 12 weeks' gestation
  2. Test is performed for the purpose of detecting genetic abnormalities; obtain consent
  3. Implementation
    a. Instruct the client to drink water to fill the bladder before the procedure, to aid in positioning the uterus for catheter insertion
    b. Instruct the client to report bleeding, infection, or leakage of fluid at insertion site after the procedure
    c. Rh-negative women may be given RhoGAM for risks related to the procedure
D. Kick counts (fetal movement counting)
  1. Mother sits quietly or lies down on the left side for 1 hour after meals and counts fetal kicks for 30 minutes

2. Instruct the client to notify the physician or health care provider if there are fewer than 3 kicks in 1 hour
E. Amniocentesis
  1. Aspiration of **amniotic fluid** done from 14 weeks of pregnancy and on
  2. Performed to determine genetic disorders, the sex of the fetus, and fetal lung maturity
  3. Risks
    a. Maternal hemorrhage
    b. Infection
    c. Rh isoimmunization
    d. Abruptio placentae
    e. **Amniotic fluid** emboli
  4. Implementation
    a. Obtain informed consent
    b. Instruct the client to empty the bladder before the procedure
    c. Prepare the client for ultrasound, which is performed to locate the **placenta**
    d. Obtain baseline vital signs and fetal heart rate (FHR), and monitor every 15 minutes
    e. Position the client supine
    f. Instruct the client that if chills, fever, leakage of fluid at the needle insertion site, decreased fetal movement, or uterine contractions occur, she is to notify the physician or health care provider
F. Fern test
  1. A microscopic slide test to determine the presence of **amniotic fluid** leakage
  2. By use of sterile technique, a specimen is obtained from the external os of the cervix and vaginal pool
  3. Fluid is examined on a slide under a microscope
  4. A fernlike pattern occurring from the salts of **amniotic fluid** indicates the presence of **amniotic fluid**
  5. Implementation
    a. Position the client in the dorsal lithotomy position
    b. Instruct the client to cough to cause the fluid to leak from the uterus if the membranes are ruptured
G. Nitrazine test
  1. Use of a Nitrazine test strip to detect the presence of **amniotic fluid** in vaginal secretions
  2. Vaginal secretions have a pH of 4.5 to 5.5 and do not affect the yellow Nitrazine strip or swab
  3. **Amniotic fluid** has a pH of 7.0 to 7.5 and turns the yellow Nitrazine blue
  4. Implementation
    a. Position the client in dorsal lithotomy position
    b. Touch the test tape to the fluid
    c. Assess the test tape for a blue-green, blue-gray, or deep blue color, which indicates that the membranes are probably ruptured

---

BOX 24-2

Nonstress Test (NST)

DESCRIPTION

Performed to assess placental function and oxygenation

Determines fetal well-being

Evaluates fetal heart rate (FHR) in response to fetal movement

IMPLEMENTATION

External ultrasound transducer and the tocodynamometer (toco) are applied to the mother, and a tracing of at least 20 minutes' duration is obtained so that the FHR and the uterine activity can be observed

Obtain baseline blood pressure (BP) and monitor BP frequently

Position mother in the left lateral position to avoid vena cava compression

The mother may be asked to press a button every time she feels fetal movement; the monitor records a mark at each point of fetal movement, which is used as a reference point to assess FHR response

RESULTS

Reactive Nonstress Test (Normal/Negative)

Indicates a healthy fetus

Two or more FHR accelerations of at least 15 beats per minute, lasting at least 15 seconds from the beginning of the acceleration to the end, in association with fetal movement, during a 20-minute period

Nonreactive Nonstress Test (Abnormal)

No accelerations or accelerations of less than 15 beats per minute or lasting less than 15 seconds in duration for a 40-minute observation

Unsatisfactory

Cannot be interpreted because of the poor quality of the FHR tracing

---

BOX 24-3

Contraction Stress Test

DESCRIPTION

Assesses placental oxygenation and function

Determines fetal ability to tolerate labor and determines fetal well-being

Fetus is exposed to the stressor of contractions to assess the adequacy of placental perfusion under simulated labor conditions

Performed if the nonstress test is abnormal

IMPLEMENTATION

The external fetal monitor is applied to the mother, and a 20- to 30-minute baseline strip is recorded

The uterus is stimulated to contract either by the administration of a dilute dose of oxytocin (Pitocin) or by having the mother use nipple stimulation until three palpable contractions with a duration of 40 seconds or more in a 10-minute period have been achieved

Frequent maternal BP readings are done, and the mother is monitored closely while increasing doses of oxytocin are given

RESULTS

Negative Contraction Stress Test

Represented by no late or variable decelerations of the FHR

Positive Contraction Stress Test (Abnormal)

Represented by late or variable decelerations of the FHR with 50% or more of the contractions in the absence of hyperstimulation of the uterus

Equivocal

Contains decelerations but with less than 50% of the contractions, or the uterine activity shows a hyperstimulated uterus

Unsatisfactory

Adequate uterine contractions cannot be achieved, or the FHR tracing is not of sufficient quality for adequate interpretation

---

H. Nonstress test (Box 24-2)

I. Contraction stress test (Box 24-3)

◤ **VI. NUTRITION** (Box 24-4)

◤ A. General guidelines

  1. The average expected weight gain during pregnancy is 2 to 4 pounds in the first trimester, and approximately 1 pound per week in the second and third trimesters

  2. Instruct the client to choose foods from the Food Guide Pyramid

  3. An increase of about 300 calories per day is needed during pregnancy

  4. A diet consisting of 2500 calories per day, depending on age, should meet the nutritional demands of pregnancy

  5. Calorie needs are greater in the last two trimesters than in the first

  6. An increase of about 500 calories per day is needed during lactation

  7. Encourage a diet high in folic acid with folic acid supplements

  8. A diet rich in folic acid is necessary for all women of childbearing age to prevent neural tube defect in the fetus during the first trimester of pregnancy

  9. Increase calories, proteins, vitamins, calcium, and other minerals as required

BOX 24-4

Cultural Considerations in Nutrition

Asian, Chinese, and Japanese
Important foods in diet include seafood, rice, vegetables, and fresh fruits
Milk and cheese are used infrequently
Orthodox Jewish
Poultry and some meat of cattle, sheep, goats, and deer are permissible; pork and pork products are not permissible
Milk and cheese may not be eaten with or within 6 hours of a meat meal
Mexican
Food products include corn, chili peppers, and beans
Milk is used infrequently

10. Drink at least 8 to 10 (8-oz) glasses of fluid each day, of which 4 to 6 glasses are water
11. Sodium is not restricted unless specifically prescribed by the physician or health care provider

B. Vegetarianism
   1. During pregnancy, it is necessary to obtain ample and complete proteins from dairy products and eggs
   2. An adequate pure vegetarian diet contains protein from unrefined grains such as brown rice and whole wheat; legumes such as beans, split peas, and lentils; nuts in large quantities; and a variety of cooked and fresh vegetables and fruits
   3. Seeds may provide protein if the quantity consumed is large enough
   4. Vegetarians do not eat any animal products; therefore a daily supplement of 4 μg of vitamin B$_{12}$ is necessary
   5. Complete protein may be obtained by eating any of the following food combinations at the same time:
      a. Legumes and whole grain cereals
      b. Nuts and whole grain cereals
      c. Nuts and legumes

C. Lactose intolerance
   1. Lactose consumed by an individual with an intolerance can cause abdominal distention, discomfort, nausea, vomiting, cramps, and loose stools
   2. Milk may be tolerated in cooked form, such as in custards or fermented dairy products
   3. Cheese and yogurt are sometimes tolerated
   4. Lactase, an enzyme, may be prescribed and is available as a tablet to be chewed before ingesting milk or milk products or as a liquid to add to milk
   5. Lactase-treated milk or lactose-free products are also available commercially

D. Pica
   1. Defined as eating substances that are not ordinarily considered edible or to have nutritive value
   2. Practiced in poverty-stricken areas where diets tend to be inadequate, but pica may also be found at other socioeconomic levels
   3. Substances most commonly ingested are dirt, clay, starch, and freezer frost
   4. Iron deficiency anemia occurs as a result of pica

PRACTICE QUESTIONS

1. A physician has prescribed transvaginal ultrasonography for a woman in the first trimester of pregnancy. The woman asks the nurse about the procedure. The nurse accurately provides which of the following information to the client?
   1. The procedure takes about 2 hours
   2. Transmission gel is spread over the abdomen, and a transducer will be moved over the abdomen to obtain the picture
   3. It will be necessary to drink 1 to 2 quarts of water prior to the examination
   4. The transvaginal probe encased in a disposable cover and coated with a gel is inserted into the vagina

2. A clinic nurse has instructed a pregnant client in measures to prevent varicose veins during pregnancy. Which statement if made by the client indicates a need for further education?
   1. "I should wear support hose."
   2. "I should be wearing flat nonslip shoes that have an arch support."
   3. "I should wear pantyhose."
   4. "I can wear knee-high hose as long as I don't leave them on longer than 8 hours."

3. A maternity client calls a clinic and tells a nurse that she is experiencing leg cramps and is awakened by the cramps at night. To provide relief from the leg cramps, the nurse tells the client to:
   1. Dorsiflex the foot while extending the knee when the cramps occur
   2. Dorsiflex the foot while flexing the knee when the cramps occur
   3. Plantar flex the foot while flexing the knee when the cramps occur
   4. Plantar flex the foot while extending the knee when the cramps occur

4. A clinic nurse is providing instructions to the pregnant client regarding measures that will assist in alleviating heartburn. Which statement if made by the client indicates an understanding of the measures to alleviate heartburn?
   1. "I should lie down for an hour after eating."
   2. "I should avoid between-meal snacks."
   3. "I should substitute spices for cooking rather than using salt."

4. "I should avoid eating gas-producing foods and fatty foods."

5. A nurse in a health care clinic is instructing a pregnant woman in how to perform "kick counts." Which statement if made by the pregnant woman indicates a need for further education?
   1. "I should place my hands on the largest part of my abdomen and concentrate on the fetal movements to count the kicks."
   2. "I will record the number of movements or kicks."
   3. "I need to lie flat on my back to perform the procedure."
   4. "A count of fewer than three fetal movements in 1 hour indicates the need to contact the physician."

6. A clinic nurse is instructing a pregnant client regarding dietary measures to promote a healthy pregnancy. The nurse instructs the client to have an adequate intake of fluid on a daily basis. Which statement if made by the mother indicates an understanding of the daily fluid requirement?
   1. "I should drink at least 8 to 10 glasses of fluid each day, of which 4 to 6 glasses are water."
   2. "I should drink 12 glasses of fruit juices or milk every day."
   3. "I should drink 8 to 10 glasses of liquid a day, and I can count all of the diet soft drinks that I consume."
   4. "I should drink 12 glasses of liquid a day, and I can include the coffee or tea that I drink in the count."

7. A nurse is instructing a pregnant client regarding measures to increase sources of iron in the diet. The nurse instructs the client to consume which of the following foods, which contains the highest source of dietary iron?
   1. Milk
   2. Dark, green leafy vegetables
   3. Potatoes
   4. Cantaloupe

8. A nurse is providing instructions regarding treatment for hemorrhoids to a client who is in the second trimester of pregnancy. Which statement if made by the mother indicates a need for further instruction?
   1. "I can apply ice packs to the hemorrhoids to reduce the swelling."
   2. " I should apply heat packs to the hemorrhoids to help the hemorrhoids shrink."
   3. "I should avoid straining during bowel movements."
   4. "I can gently replace the hemorrhoids into the rectum."

9. A nurse is providing instructions to a client in the first trimester of pregnancy regarding measures to

assist in reducing breast tenderness. Which instruction would the nurse provide to the client?
   1. To avoid wearing a bra
   2. To wash the nipples and areola area daily with soap, and massage the breasts with lotion
   3. To wear tight-fitting blouses or dresses to provide support
   4. To wash the breasts with warm water and keep them dry

10. A nonstress test is prescribed for a pregnant client, and the client asks the nurse about the procedure. The nurse tells the client that:
    1. The test is an invasive procedure and requires that an informed consent be signed
    2. The test will take about 2 hours and will require close monitoring for 2 hours after the procedure is completed
    3. An ultrasound transducer that records fetal heart activity is secured over the abdomen where the fetal heart is heard most clearly
    4. The fetus is challenged or stressed by uterine contractions to obtain the necessary information

11. A nurse has assisted in performing a nonstress test on a pregnant client and is reviewing the documentation related to the results of the test. The nurse notes that the physician has documented the test results as reactive. The nurse interprets that this result indicates:
    1. Normal findings
    2. Abnormal findings
    3. The need for further evaluation
    4. That the findings on the monitor were difficult to interpret

12. A nonstress test is performed on a client who is pregnant, and the results of the test indicate nonreactive findings. The physician prescribed a contraction stress test. The test is performed, and the nurse notes that the physician has documented the results as negative. The nurse interprets this finding as indicating:
    1. A high risk for fetal demise
    2. A normal test result
    3. The need for a cesarean delivery
    4. An abnormal test result

13. A nurse is reviewing a nutritional plan of care with a pregnant client and is identifying the food items that are highest in folic acid. The nurse determines that the client understands which foods supply the highest amounts of folic acid if the client states that she will include which of the following in the daily diet?
    1. A banana
    2. Leafy, green vegetable
    3. Milk
    4. Yogurt

14. A pregnant client tells a nurse that she has been

craving "unusual foods." The nurse gathers additional assessment data from the client and discovers that the client has been ingesting daily amounts of white clay dirt from her backyard. Laboratory studies are performed on the client. The nurse reviews the laboratory results and determines that which of the following indicates a physiological consequence of this client's practice?

1. Hematocrit, 38%
2. Hemoglobin, 9.1 g/dL
3. Glucose, 86 mg/dL
4. White blood cell count, 12,400/mm^3

15. A pregnant client who is at 30 weeks' gestation comes to a clinic for a routine visit. A nurse performs an assessment on the client. Which observation made by the nurse during the assessment indicates a need for teaching?
    1. The client is wearing panty hose
    2. The client is wearing flat shoes
    3. The client is wearing nonslip shoes
    4. The client is wearing knee-high hose

16. A nurse is developing a plan of care for a pregnant client who is complaining of intermittent episodes of constipation. The nurse includes in the plan of care measures to prevent the episodes of constipation and plans to tell the client to:
    1. Take a mild stool softener daily in the evening
    2. Drink 6 glasses of water per day
    3. Consume a low-roughage diet
    4. Use a Fleet enema when the episodes occur

17. A pregnant client visits a clinic for a scheduled prenatal appointment. On assessment, the client tells the nurse that she frequently has a backache. The nurse provides instructions to the client regarding measures that will assist in relieving the backache. Which statement made by the client indicates a need for further education regarding the measures to relieve the backache?
    1. "I need to try to maintain good posture."
    2. "I should do more exercises to strengthen my back muscles."
    3. "I should sleep on a firm mattress."
    4. "I should wear low-heeled shoes."

18. A nurse is providing instructions to a pregnant client who is scheduled for an amniocentesis. The nurse tells the client that:
    1. A fever is expected following the procedure because of the trauma to the abdomen
    2. Strict bed rest is required following the procedure
    3. An informed consent will need to be signed prior to the procedure
    4. Hospitalization is necessary for 24 hours following the procedure

19. A pregnant client in the first trimester calls a nurse at a health care clinic and reports that she has noticed a thin, colorless, vaginal drainage. The nurse most appropriately tells the mother:
    1. To come to the clinic immediately
    2. To report to the emergency room at the maternity center immediately
    3. That the vaginal discharge may be bothersome but is a normal occurrence
    4. To use tampons if the discharge is bothersome, but to be sure to change the tampons every 2 hours

20. A pregnant client asks a nurse about the types of exercises that are allowable during the pregnancy. The nurse would instruct the client that the safest exercise to engage in is which of the following?
    1. Bicycling with the legs in the air
    2. Swimming
    3. Scuba diving
    4. Low-weight gymnastics

CRITICAL THINKING: FREE-TEXT ENTRY

A pregnant client has a rubella titer drawn and the results show a negative titer, indicating susceptibility to the rubella virus. The client is told that she will receive a rubella virus vaccine in the postpartum period following delivery. The nurse provides the client with what specific information about becoming pregnant after receiving the vaccine?

Answer: _____

ANSWERS

1. **4**

Rationale: Transvaginal ultrasonography allows clear visibility of the uterus, gestational sac, embryo, and deep pelvic structures, such as the ovaries and fallopian tubes. The woman is placed in a lithotomy position and a transvaginal probe, encased in a disposable cover and coated with a gel that provides for lubrication and promotes conductivity, is inserted into the vagina. The woman may feel more comfortable if she is allowed to insert the probe. The procedure takes about 10 to 15 minutes. Options 2 and 3 identify components of the abdominal ultrasound.

Test-Taking Strategy: Use the process of elimination. Note the key words "transvaginal ultrasonography." Also, note the relationship of the name of the test as stated in the question and the description in the correct option. If you had difficulty with this question, review the procedure for transvaginal ultrasonography.

Level of Cognitive Ability: Application
Client Needs: Physiological Integrity
Integrated Concept/Process: Communication and Documentation
Content Area: Maternity
Reference: Lowdermilk, D., Perry, S., & Bobak, I. (2000). *Maternity & women's health care* (7th ed.). St. Louis: Mosby, p. 798.

2. **4**
Rationale: Varicose veins often develop in the lower extremities during pregnancy. Any constrictive clothing, such as knee-high hose, impedes venous return from the lower legs and places the client at risk for developing varicosities. The client should be encouraged to wear support hose or pantyhose. Flat nonslip shoes with proper support are important to assist the pregnant women to maintain proper posture and balance and minimize falls.
Test-Taking Strategy: Use the process of elimination. Note the key words "a need for further education." Focus on the issue of the question as it relates to preventing varicose veins. Recall that anything that constricts the lower vessels and impedes venous return from the lower legs will place the client at risk for varicosities. If you had difficulty with this question, review measures to prevent varicose veins.
Level of Cognitive Ability: Analysis
Client Needs: Health Promotion and Maintenance
Integrated Concept/Process: Teaching/Learning
Content Area: Maternity
Reference: Lowdermilk, D., Perry, S., & Bobak, I. (2000). *Maternity & women's health care* (7th ed.). St. Louis: Mosby, p. 416.

3. **1**
Rationale: Leg cramps occur when the pregnant woman stretches the leg and plantar flexes the foot. Dorsiflexion of the foot while extending the knee stretches the affected muscle, prevents the muscle from contracting, and stops the cramping. Options 2, 3, and 4 are not measures that will provide relief from the leg cramps.
Test-Taking Strategy: Use the process of elimination. Focus on the issue of the question, to provide relief from the leg cramps. Attempt to visualize each of the descriptions in the options to assist in directing you to option 1. If you had difficulty with this question, review measures that assist in alleviating muscle cramps.
Level of Cognitive Ability: Application
Client Needs: Health Promotion and Maintenance
Integrated Concept/Process: Teaching/Learning
Content Area: Maternity
Reference: Sherwen, L., Scoloveno, M.A., & Weingarten, C. (1999). *Maternity nursing: Care of the childbearing family* (3rd ed.). Stamford, Conn.: Appleton & Lange, p. 575.

4. **4**
Rationale: Lying down is likely to lead to reflux of stomach contents, especially immediately following a meal. The client should be instructed to avoid spices along with salt because spices will trigger heartburn. Salt will produce edema. The client should be encouraged to eat between-meal snacks and instructed that eating smaller, more frequent portions is preferred over eating three large meals, to control heartburn. The client should also limit or avoid gas-producing and fatty foods.

Test-Taking Strategy: Use the process of elimination and note the key words "indicates an understanding." Knowledge that the client needs to limit or avoid gas-producing and fatty foods will assist in directing you to option 4. Review the measures that will alleviate heartburn in the pregnant client if you had difficulty with this question.
Level of Cognitive Ability: Analysis
Client Needs: Health Promotion and Maintenance
Integrated Concept/Process: Teaching/Learning
Content Area: Maternity
Reference: Lowdermilk, D., Perry, S., & Bobak, I. (2000). *Maternity & women's health care* (7th ed.). St. Louis: Mosby, p. 415.

5. **3**
Rationale: The woman should lie on her side to perform kick counts. Lying flat on the back is not necessary to perform this procedure, can cause discomfort, and presents a risk of vena caval syndrome. The woman is instructed to place her hands on the largest part of the abdomen and concentrates on the fetal movements. The woman records the number of movements felt during a specified time period. A count of fewer than three fetal movements in 1 hour indicates the need to contact the physician.
Test-Taking Strategy: Use the process of elimination, noting the key words "a need for further education." If you are unfamiliar with this procedure, recalling that the risk of vena caval syndrome exists when the client lies on her back will direct you to option 3. Review the procedure for kick counts if you had difficulty with this question.
Level of Cognitive Ability: Analysis
Client Needs: Health Promotion and Maintenance
Integrated Concept/Process: Teaching/Learning
Content Area: Maternity
Reference: Lowdermilk, D., Perry, S., & Bobak, I. (2000). *Maternity & women's health care* (7th ed.). St. Louis: Mosby, pp. 796, 977.

6. **1**
Rationale: The nurse should instruct the client to have an adequate fluid intake on a daily basis to assist in digestion and in the management of constipation. The pregnant woman should consume at least 8 to 10 (8-oz) glasses of fluid each day, of which 4 to 6 glasses are water. Because of their sodium content, diet soft drinks should be consumed in moderation. Caffeinated beverages have a diuretic effect, which may be counterproductive to increasing fluid intake.
Test-Taking Strategy: Use the process of elimination. Knowledge that diet soft drinks and caffeine-containing products should be avoided will assist in eliminating options 3 and 4. Recalling that water needs to be included in the daily fluid intake will assist in directing you to option 1. If you had difficulty with this question, review client instructions regarding water and fluid intake during pregnancy.
Level of Cognitive Ability: Analysis
Client Needs: Health Promotion and Maintenance
Integrated Concept/Process: Teaching/Learning
Content Area: Maternity
Reference: Ladewig, P., London. M., & Olds, S. (1998). *Maternal-newborn nursing care: The nurse, the family, and the community* (4th ed.). Menlo Park, Calif.: Addison Wesley Longman, p. 245.

7. 2

Rationale: Dietary sources of iron include lean meats, liver, shellfish, dark green leafy vegetables, legumes, whole grains and enriched grains, cereals, and molasses. Milk is high in calcium and also contains phosphorus. Cantaloupe and potatoes are high in vitamin C.

Test-Taking Strategy: Use the process of elimination and knowledge of the dietary sources of iron to assist in answering the question. Remember that dark, green leafy vegetables are high in iron. If you had difficulty with this question, review food items high in iron.

Level of Cognitive Ability: Application

Client Needs: Health Promotion and Maintenance

Integrated Concept/Process: Teaching/Learning

Content Area: Maternity

Reference: Ladewig, P., London. M., & Olds, S. (1998). *Maternal-newborn nursing care: The nurse, the family, and the community* (4th ed.). Menlo Park, Calif.: Addison Wesley Longman, p. 243.

8. 2

Rationale: Measures that provide relief from hemorrhoids include avoiding constipation and straining during bowel movements, applying ice packs to reduce the hemorrhoidal swelling, gently replacing the hemorrhoids into the rectum, using stool softeners, ointments, or sprays as prescribed, and assuming certain positions to relieve pressure on the hemorrhoids. Heat packs will increase the blood flow to the area and worsen the discomfort from hemorrhoids.

Test-Taking Strategy: Use the process of elimination, noting the key words "need for further instruction." Use knowledge of the principles regarding heat and cold to assist in directing you to option 2. If you had difficulty with this question, review the measures for the treatment of hemorrhoids.

Level of Cognitive Ability: Analysis

Client Needs: Health Promotion and Maintenance

Integrated Concept/Process: Teaching/Learning

Content Area: Maternity

Reference: Sherwen, L., Scoloveno, M.A., & Weingarten, C. (1999). *Maternity nursing: Care of the childbearing family* (3rd ed.). Stamford, Conn.: Appleton & Lange, p. 523.

9. 4

Rationale: The pregnant woman should be instructed to wash the breasts with warm water and keep them dry. The woman should be instructed to avoid using soap on the nipples and areola area to prevent the drying of tissues. Wearing a supportive bra with wide adjustable straps can decrease breast tenderness. Tight-fitting blouses or dresses will cause discomfort. The woman is instructed to wear soft-textured clothing to decrease nipple tenderness and to use breast pads inside the bra to prevent leakage if colostrum is a problem.

Test-Taking Strategy: Use the process of elimination. Focus on the issue of the question, reducing breast tenderness, and visualize each of the measures identified in the options. If you had difficulty with this question, review treatment measures for the client with breast tenderness.

Level of Cognitive Ability: Application

Client Needs: Health Promotion and Maintenance

Integrated Concept/Process: Teaching/Learning

Content Area: Maternity

Reference: Lowdermilk, D., Perry, S., & Bobak, I. (2000). *Maternity & women's health care* (7th ed.). St. Louis: Mosby, p. 414.

10. 3

Rationale: The nonstress test takes about 20 to 30 minutes. The test is termed "nonstress" because it consists of monitoring only; the fetus is not challenged or stressed by uterine contractions to obtain the necessary data. It is a noninvasive test, and an ultrasound transducer that records fetal heart activity is secured over the maternal abdomen where the fetal heart is heard most clearly. A tocotransducer that detects uterine activity and fetal movement is also secured to the maternal abdomen. Fetal heart activity and movements are recorded.

Test-Taking Strategy: Use the process of elimination. Focus on the name of the test and the procedure for this test to eliminate options 1, 2, and 4. If you are unfamiliar with this test or had difficulty answering this question, review this procedure.

Level of Cognitive Ability: Application

Client Needs: Physiological Integrity

Integrated Concept/Process: Teaching/Learning

Content Area: Maternity

Reference: Gorrie, T., McKinney, E., & Murray, S. (1998). *Foundations of maternal-newborn nursing* (2nd ed.). Philadelphia: W.B. Saunders, p. 235.

11. 1

Rationale: A reactive nonstress test is a normal result. To be considered reactive, the baseline fetal heart rate (FHR) must be within normal range (110 to 160 beats per minute) with good long-term variability. In addition, there must be two or more FHR accelerations of at least 15 beats per minute, each with a duration of at least 15 seconds, in a 20-minute interval.

Test-Taking Strategy: Use the process of elimination and knowledge regarding the interpretation of the results of the nonstress test. Note that options 2, 3, and 4 are similar. If you had difficulty with this question and are unfamiliar with the interpretation of the results of a nonstress test, review this content.

Level of Cognitive Ability: Analysis

Client Needs: Physiological Integrity

Integrated Concept/Process: Communication and Documentation

Content Area: Maternity

Reference: Sherwen, L., Scoloveno, M.A., & Weingarten, C. (1999). *Maternity nursing: Care of the childbearing family* (3rd ed.). Stamford, Conn.: Appleton & Lange, p. 555.

12. 2

Rationale: Contraction stress test results may be interpreted as negative (normal), positive (abnormal), or equivocal. A negative test result indicates that no late decelerations occurred in the fetal heart rate, although the fetus was stressed by three contractions of at least 40 seconds' duration in a 10-minute period.

Test-Taking Strategy: Use the process of elimination, noting that options 1, 3, and 4 are similar in that they indicate an abnormal test result finding. If you had difficulty with this question and are unfamiliar with the interpretation of the results of a contraction stress test, review this content.

Level of Cognitive Ability: Analysis

Client Needs: Physiological Integrity

Integrated Concept/Process: Documentation and Communication

Content Area: Maternity

Reference: Gorrie, T., McKinney, E., & Murray, S. (1998). *Foundations of maternal-newborn nursing* (2nd ed.). Philadelphia: W.B. Saunders, p. 237.

13. **2**

Rationale: Leafy, green vegetables are rich in folate (folic acid). Bananas provide potassium; milk and yogurt supply calcium.

Test-Taking Strategy: Use the process of elimination and knowledge regarding the food sources that are high in folic acid. Eliminate options 3 and 4 first because they are similar. Remember that leafy, green vegetables are high in folic acid. Review these foods if you had difficulty with this question.

Level of Cognitive Ability: Comprehension

Client Needs: Physiological Integrity

Integrated Concept/Process: Teaching/Learning

Content Area: Maternity

Reference: Grodner, M., Anderson, S., & DeYoung, S. (2000). *Foundations and clinical applications of nutrition: A nursing approach.* St. Louis: Mosby, p. 181.

14. **2**

Rationale: Pica cravings often lead to iron deficiency anemia, resulting in a lowered hemoglobin. The laboratory values in options 1, 3, and 4 are within normal limits for the pregnant woman.

Test-Taking Strategy: Use the process of elimination, recalling that pica results in anemia. This will assist in eliminating options 3 and 4. From the remaining options, recall the normal laboratory values in a pregnant client to assist in directing you to option 2. Review the physiological effects of pica and the normal laboratory values in a pregnant client, if you had difficulty with this question.

Level of Cognitive Ability: Analysis

Client Needs: Physiological Integrity

Integrated Concept/Process: Nursing Process/Analysis

Content Area: Maternity

Reference: Lowdermilk, D., Perry, S., & Bobak, I. (2000). *Maternity & women's health care* (7th ed.). St. Louis: Mosby, p. 365.

15. **4**

Rationale: Varicose veins often develop in the lower extremities during pregnancy. Any constricting clothing such as knee-high hose impede venous return from the lower legs and thus place the client at higher risk for developing varicosities. Clients should be encouraged to wear panty hose or support hose. Flat, nonslip shoes with proper support are important to assist the pregnant woman to maintain proper posture and balance and minimize the risk for falls.

Test-Taking Strategy: Use the process of elimination, noting the key words "indicates a need for teaching." Remembering that the pregnant client is at risk for developing varicosities and recalling the measures to prevent their occurrence will direct you to option 4. Review the measures that will assist in preventing varicosities, if you had difficulty with this question.

Level of Cognitive Ability: Comprehension

Client Needs: Physiological Integrity

Integrated Concept/Process: Nursing Process/Assessment

Content Area: Maternity

Reference: Lowdermilk, D., Perry, S., & Bobak, I. (2000).

Maternity & women's health care (7th ed.). St. Louis: Mosby, p. 416.

16. **2**

Rationale: The nurse should instruct the client to drink 6 glasses of water per day and to consume a diet that includes roughage to prevent the constipation. The client should not take stool softeners, laxatives, mineral oil, other medications, or enemas without first consulting with the physician or other health care provider.

Test-Taking Strategy: Use the process of elimination and recall the basic principles related to the prevention of constipation. Also remember that the client is a pregnant client. Review measures to prevent constipation in the pregnant client if you had difficulty with this question.

Level of Cognitive Ability: Application

Client Needs: Health Promotion and Maintenance

Integrated Concept/Process: Teaching/Learning

Content Area: Maternity

Reference: Lowdermilk, D., Perry, S., & Bobak, I. (2000). *Maternity & women's health care* (7th ed.). St. Louis: Mosby, p. 415.

17. **2**

Rationale: Some of the measures that will assist in relieving a backache include maintaining good posture and body mechanics; resting and avoiding fatigue; wearing low-heeled shoes; and sleeping on a firm mattress. The back discomfort that occurs in a pregnant client is often due to the exaggerated lumbar and cervicothoracic curves caused by a change in the center of gravity resulting from the enlarged uterus. Performing more exercises to strengthen the back muscles could be harmful to a pregnant client.

Test-Taking Strategy: Use the process of elimination, focusing on the key words "need for further education." Use knowledge regarding the principles related to relieving a backache to assist in directing you to the correct option. Review these measures if you had difficulty with this question.

Level of Cognitive Ability: Analysis

Client Needs: Health Promotion and Maintenance

Integrated Concept/Process: Teaching/Learning

Content Area: Maternity

Reference: Lowdermilk, D., Perry, S., & Bobak, I. (2000). *Maternity & women's health care* (7th ed.). St. Louis: Mosby, p. 415.

18. **3**

Rationale: Since amniocentesis is an invasive procedure, informed consent will need to be obtained prior to the procedure. After the procedure, the client is instructed to rest, but may resume light activity after the cramping subsides. The client is instructed to keep the puncture site clean and to report any complications such as vaginal discharge, severe, persistent cramping, and the onset of fever. Amniocentesis is an outpatient procedure and may be done in a physician's private office or in a special prenatal testing unit. Hospitalization is not necessary following the procedure.

Test-Taking Strategy: Use the process of elimination. Simply recalling that this procedure is an invasive one will direct you to option 3. If you had difficulty with this question, review the procedure related to amniocentesis.

Level of Cognitive Ability: Application

Client Needs: Physiological Integrity

Integrated Concept/Process: Teaching/Learning
Content Area: Maternity
Reference: Sherwen, L., Scoloveno, M.A., & Weingarten, C. (1999). *Maternity nursing: Care of the childbearing family* (3rd ed.). Stamford, Conn.: Appleton & Lange, p. 514.

19. **3**
Rationale: Leukorrhea begins during the first trimester. Many women notice a thin, colorless, or yellow vaginal discharge throughout pregnancy. Some clients become distressed about this condition. This occurrence does not require that the client report to the health care clinic or the emergency room immediately. If vaginal discharge is profuse, panty liners may be used, but the woman should not wear tampons because of the risk of infection. If panty liners are used, they should be changed frequently.
Test-Taking Strategy: Use the process of elimination. Eliminate options 1 and 2 first because they are similar. From the remaining options, recalling that either this manifestation is a normal physiological occurrence or that tampons should be avoided will assist in directing you to the correct option. Review the normal occurrences related to vaginal discharge in a pregnant woman, if you had difficulty with this question.
Level of Cognitive Ability: Application
Client Needs: Health Promotion and Maintenance
Integrated Concept/Process: Nursing Process/Implementation
Content Area: Maternity
Reference: Sherwen, L., Scoloveno, M.A., & Weingarten, C. (1999). *Maternity nursing: Care of the childbearing family* (3rd ed.). Stamford, Conn.: Appleton & Lange, p. 453.

20. **2**
Rationale: Nonweight bearing exercises are preferable to weight bearing exercises during pregnancy. Exercises to avoid are shoulder standing and bicycling with the legs in the air because the knee-chest position should be avoided. Competitive or high-risk sports such as scuba diving, water skiing, downhill skiing, horseback riding, basketball, volleyball, and gymnastics should be avoided. Nonweight bearing exercises such as swimming are allowable.
Test-Taking Strategy: Use the process of elimination. Identify those activities or exercises that could cause or produce an injury to the fetus. This should easily direct you to option 2. If you had difficulty with this question, review the teaching points related to exercising for a client who is pregnant.
Level of Cognitive Ability: Application
Client Needs: Health Promotion and Maintenance
Integrated Concept/Process: Teaching/Learning
Content Area: Maternity
Reference: Lowdermilk, D., Perry, S., & Bobak, I. (2000). *Maternity & women's health care* (7th ed.). St. Louis: Mosby, p. 408.

CRITICAL THINKING: FREE-TEXT ENTRY

Answer: The client is counseled not to become pregnant for 3 months following immunization.
Rationale: The client must be using effective birth control at the time of the immunization. The client is counseled not to become pregnant for 3 months following immunization because there is a possible risk to the fetus from the live virus vaccine.
Test-Taking Strategy: Focus on the issue, specific information about becoming pregnant. Recalling that the rubella vaccine is a live virus vaccine will assist in answering this question. Review client instructions following this immunization if you had difficulty with this question.
Level of Cognitive Ability: Application
Client Needs: Health Promotion and Maintenance
Integrated Concept/Process: Teaching/Learning
Content Area: Maternity
Reference: Gorrie, T., McKinney, E., & Murray, S. (1998). *Foundations of maternal-newborn nursing* (2nd ed.). Philadelphia: W.B. Saunders, pp. 442, 735.

REFERENCES

Gorrie, T., McKinney, E., & Murray, S. (1998). *Foundations of maternal-newborn nursing* (2nd ed.). Philadelphia: W.B. Saunders.

Grodner, M., Anderson, S., & DeYoung, S. (2000). *Foundations and clinical applications of nutrition: A nursing approach.* St. Louis: Mosby.

Ladewig, P., London. M., & Olds, S. (1998). *Maternal-newborn nursing care: The nurse, the family, and the community* (4th ed.). Menlo Park, Calif.: Addison Wesley Longman.

Lowdermilk, D., Perry, S., & Bobak, I. (2000). *Maternity & women's health care* (7th ed.). St. Louis: Mosby.

Olds, S., London. M., & Ladewig, P. (2000). *Maternal-newborn nursing: A family and community-based approach* (6th ed.). Upper Saddle River, N.J.: Prenticee-Hall Health.

Sherwen, L., Scoloveno, M.A., & Weingarten, C. (1999). *Maternity nursing: Care of the childbearing family* (3rd ed.). Stamford, Conn.: Appleton & Lange.

Risk Conditions Related to Pregnancy

I. ABORTION

A. Description: Termination of pregnancy before the fetus is viable (20 weeks or a weight of 500 g)

B. Types
1. Spontaneous: Pregnancy ends because of natural causes
2. Induced: Therapeutic or elective reasons for terminating the pregnancy
3. Threatened: Developing spontaneous abortion
4. Inevitable: Threatened loss that cannot be prevented
5. Incomplete: Loss of some products of conception and retention of others
6. Complete: Loss of all products of conception
7. Missed: Retention of products of conception in utero after fetal death
8. Habitual: Spontaneous abortions in three or more successive pregnancies

C. Assessment
1. Spontaneous vaginal bleeding
2. Passage of clots or tissue through the vagina
3. Low uterine cramping or contractions
4. Hemorrhage and shock

D. Implementation
1. Maintain bed rest
2. Monitor vital signs
3. Monitor cramping and bleeding
4. Count perineal pads to evaluate blood loss
5. Save expelled tissues and clots
6. Provide IV fluids as prescribed to prevent shock
7. Prepare client for dilatation and curretage as prescribed for incomplete abortion

II. ACQUIRED IMMUNODEFICIENCY SYNDROME (AIDS)

A. Description
1. The human immunodeficiency virus (HIV) is a causative factor in the development of AIDS
2. HIV infection is a progressive, severe weakening of the immune system that makes an individual highly susceptible to other infections and certain types of cancer
3. The virus attacks the lymphocytes and produces immune deficiency by destroying the T-helper lymphocytes; this interferes with cell-mediated immunity
4. Develops slowly over years
5. Women infected with HIV virus may first demonstrate symptoms at the time of pregnancy or possibly develop life-threatening infections because normal pregnancy involves some suppression of the maternal immune system
6. Zidovudine (AZT) is recommended for the prevention of maternal-fetal HIV transmission and reduces the transmission risk if given late in pregnancy, during **labor,** and to the **newborn infant** for the first 6 weeks of life; zidovudine is administered orally at 14 to 34 weeks' gestation, intravenously during **labor,** and in the form of syrup to the **neonate** after birth

B. Transmission
1. All body fluids from an infected host, except perspiration, have been shown to contain the virus
2. Blood, semen, and breast milk have higher concentrations of the virus than urine, saliva, vomitus, and stool
3. HIV can cross some membranes such as the **placental** barrier, the blood-brain barrier, vaginal mucosa, and (in the **neonate**) the walls of the gastrointestinal tract
4. Sexual contact
5. Transfusion with blood or blood products
6. Occupational exposure, such as in health care workers
7. Shared needles during drug use and use of dirty needles

8. Perinatal transmission from infected mother to fetus or **newborn** via transplacental transmission, via contamination with maternal blood during birth, or through breast milk
C. Risks to the mother
   1. The mother with HIV is managed as high risk
   2. Frequent complaints of fatigue, shortness of breath, nausea, back pain, urinary frequency, and headaches
   3. More vulnerable to postpartum infections
   4. May need longer courses of antibiotics for infection
D. Diagnosis
   1. Client may be infected with the virus but has not yet produced antibodies, thereby testing negative but being capable of infecting others
   2. Clients who by history may be at risk for possible HIV but test negative for the HIV antibody should be retested; it usually takes 6 to 12 weeks for a host to manufacture detectable HIV antibodies
   3. Enzyme-linked immunosorbent assay (ELISA) screening test for AIDS antibody is a very sensitive test but not highly specific; a positive ELISA test indicates the need for further testing using the Western blot
E. Assessment (Table 25-1)
F. Implementation
   1. Prenatal period
      a. Prevention of opportunistic infections
      b. Instruct the client on good handwashing procedure
      c. Avoid persons who are ill
      d. Avoid exposure to cat feces, cat or dog litter, or fish tanks
      e. Avoid undercooked meats, raw eggs, and unpasteurized milk
      f. Prevent further exposure to HIV through sexual contact or the use of needles
      g. Initiate recovery from substance abuse
      h. Avoid procedures that increase the risk of perinatal transmission, such as amniocentesis and fetal scalp sampling
   2. Intrapartal period
      a. Note that if the fetus has not been exposed to HIV in utero, the highest risk exists during **delivery** through the birth canal
      b. Never use scalp electrodes
      c. Avoid episiotomy to decrease the amount of maternal blood in and around the birth canal
      d. Avoid the administration of oxytocin (Pitocin), since oxytocin contractions can be strong, inducing vaginal tears or necessitating the need for episiotomy
      e. Minimize the **neonate's** exposure to maternal blood and body fluids
      f. Place heavy absorbent pads under the mother's hips to absorb **amniotic fluid** and maternal blood
      g. Promptly remove the **neonate** from the mother's blood following **delivery**
      h. Suction the **infant** promptly
      i. Prepare to administer zidovudine (AZT) intravenously as prescribed during **labor** and **delivery**
   3. Postpartum period
      a. Monitor for signs of infection, such as an increased temperature and white blood cell (WBC) count
      b. Place the mother in protective isolation to prevent infection if the mother is experiencing a suppressed immune response
      c. Restrict breastfeeding
      d. Instruct the mother in how to take the temperature and to identify symptoms necessitating immediate follow-up
      e. Urge the mother to refrain from donating blood or body organs
      f. Advise the mother to avoid sharing toothbrushes, razors, or other materials potentially contaminated with blood
G. The **neonate** and HIV
   1. Description
      a. The fetus of an HIV antibody–positive woman should be monitored closely throughout the pregnancy
      b. Serial ultrasound screenings should be done to identify intrauterine growth restriction
      c. Weekly nonstress testing after 32 weeks of

TABLE 25-1

Assessment of the Stages of AIDS

Stage 1	Stage 2	Stage 3	Stage 4
Fever	Active but asymptomatic and	Symptomatic	Advanced HIV infection
Myalgia	may remain so for years	Evidence of immune dysfunction	Vulnerable to common bacterial
Lymphadenopathy	May experience an outbreak of	All body systems can present with	infections
Headache	herpes zoster (shingles)	signs of immune dysfunction	Development of opportunistic
	May experience a transient	Integumentary and gynecological	infections
	thrombocytopenia	problems are common	Serious immune compromise

gestation and biophysical profiles may be necessary

d. **Neonates** born to HIV-positive clients may test positive because the mother's positive antibodies may persist for as long as 18 months after birth

e. The use of antiviral medication, reduction of **neonate** exposure to maternal blood and body fluids, and early identification of HIV in pregnancy reduce the risk of transmission to the **neonate**

f. All **neonates** acquire maternal antibody to HIV infection, but not all acquire infection

2. Transmission
   a. Across the **placental** barrier
   b. During the process of **labor** and **delivery**
   c. Via breast milk

3. Implementation
   a. Bathe **neonate** carefully before any invasive procedure, such as the administration of vitamin K, heel sticks, or venipunctures
   b. **Neonate** can room with mother
   c. Prepare to administer zidovudine (AZT) to the **newborn infant** as prescribed for the first 6 weeks of life
   d. All HIV-exposed **newborn infants** should be treated with medication to prevent infection by *Pneumocystis carinii*
   e. Note that an HIV culture is recommended at age 1 month and after 4 months of age; **infants** at risk for HIV infection should be seen by the physician at birth, 1 week, 2 weeks, 1 month, 2 months, and 4 months of life
   f. **Infants** at risk for HIV infection need to receive all recommended immunizations at the regular schedule; no live immunizations should be administered
   g. Note that the **neonate** may be asymptomatic for the first several years of life; monitor for early signs of immune deficiency, such as an enlarged spleen or liver, lymphadenopathy, and impairment in growth and development

III. ANEMIA

A. Description
   1. A condition that can develop as a result of iron deficiency, with a hemoglobin below 10 g/dL or a hematocrit below 30 g/dL
   2. Anemia predisposes the client to postpartum infection and hemorrhage

B. Assessment
   1. Fatigue
   2. Headache
   3. Pallor
   4. Tachycardia
   5. Hemoglobin below 10 g/dL and hematocrit below 30 g/dL

C. Implementation
   1. Monitor hemoglobin and hematocrit levels every 2 weeks
   2. Administer and instruct the client about iron and folic acid supplements
   3. Instruct the client to take iron with a source of vitamin C and to avoid taking iron with tea
   4. Instruct the client to eat foods high in iron, folic acid, and protein
   5. Teach the client to monitor for signs and symptoms of infection
   6. Prepare to administer injectable iron as prescribed in severe cases
   7. Prepare to administer transfusions if prescribed, although they are rarely necessary
   8. Prepare for the administration of oxytoxic medications as prescribed postpartum to prevent hemorrhage

IV. CARDIAC DISEASE

A. Description
   1. The inability to cope with the added plasma volume and the increased cardiac output
   2. Blood volume is at a maximum during the last weeks of the second trimester

B. Assessment
   1. Signs and symptoms of cardiac decompensation, particularly during the second trimester
   2. Cough
   3. Peripheral edema
   4. Signs of pulmonary edema
   5. Anginal-type pain
   6. Dyspnea and fatigue
   7. Palpitations and tachycardia
   8. Signs of respiratory infection

C. Implementation
   1. Monitor vital signs, fetal heart rate (FHR), and condition of fetus
   2. Monitor for signs of respiratory infection
   3. Avoid exposure to infection
   4. Plan activity level and stress the need for sufficient rest
   5. Encourage adequate nutrition to prevent anemia
   6. Administer antibiotics as prescribed
   7. Administer cardiac medications as prescribed
   8. Maintain bed rest for the client as prescribed during the last weeks of pregnancy
   9. During **labor**
      a. Monitor vital signs frequently
      b. Place the client on a cardiac monitor and on an external fetal monitor
      c. Maintain bed rest, with mother lying on side or in semirecumbent position
      d. Administer oxygen as prescribed
      e. Monitor for signs of pulmonary edema and heart failure
      f. Provide emotional support

V. CHORIOAMNIONITIS

A. Description
1. A bacterial infection of the amniotic cavity, which can occur as a result of premature rupture of the membrane, vaginitis, amniocentesis, or intrauterine procedures
2. Chorioamnionitis causes the development of postpartum endometritis and causes perinatal mortality and maternal morbidity
B. Assessment
1. Uterine tenderness and contractions
2. Elevated temperature
3. Maternal or fetal tachycardia
4. Foul odor to **amniotic fluid**
5. Leukocytosis
C. Implementation
1. Monitor maternal vital signs and FHR
2. Monitor for uterine tenderness, contractions, and fetal activity
3. Monitor results of blood culture
4. Prepare for amniocentesis to obtain amniotic fluid for Gram stain and leukocyte count
5. Administer antibiotics as prescribed after cultures are obtained
6. Administer oxytoxic medications as prescribed to increase uterine tone
7. Prepare for the **delivery** of the fetus
8. Prepare for neonatal cultures after **delivery**

VI. CHRONIC HYPERTENSION

A. Description
1. Hypertension that occurs before pregnancy, is diagnosed before the 20th week of gestation, or is diagnosed for the first time during pregnancy and persists beyond the 42nd day postpartum
2. The condition predisposes the client to pregnancy-induced hypertension (PIH)
3. Can cause abruptio placentae and intrauterine growth retardation
B. Assessment
1. Headaches
2. Visual changes
3. Blood pressure (BP) of 140/90 mm Hg or greater
4. Delayed fetal growth
5. Oligohydramnios
C. Implementation
1. Monitor blood pressure
2. Monitor fetal activity and fetal growth
3. Encourage frequent rest periods, instructing the client to lie in the left lateral position
4. Administer antihypertensive medications as prescribed for diastolic pressures greater than 100 mm Hg
5. Monitor intake and output (I & O)
6. Evaluate renal function through prescribed studies such as blood urea nitrogen (BUN), serum creatinine, and 24-hour urine levels for creatinine clearance and protein

VII. DIABETES MELLITUS

A. Description
1. A chronic metabolic disease caused by a disturbance in normal production of insulin
2. Pregnancy places demands on carbohydrate metabolism and causes insulin requirements to increase
B. Insulin-dependent diabetes mellitus
1. Maternal glucose crosses the **placenta** but insulin does not
2. During the first trimester, maternal insulin needs decrease
3. The fetus produces its own insulin and pulls glucose from the mother, which predisposes the mother to hypoglycemic reactions
4. During the second and third trimesters, increases in **placental** hormones cause an insulin-resistant state, requiring an increase in the client's insulin dose
5. After **placental delivery, placental** hormone levels drop abruptly and insulin requirements decrease
C. Diabetes mellitus in pregnancy
1. Diabetes mellitus is more difficult to control during pregnancy
2. Premature **delivery** is more frequent
3. The **newborn infant** of a diabetic mother may be large in size but will have functions related to gestational age rather than size
4. The **newborn infant** of a diabetic mother is subject to hypoglycemia, hyperbilirubinemia, respiratory distress syndrome, and congenital anomalies
5. Stillborn and neonatal mortality rates are higher in pregnancies of a diabetic woman
6. Conditions that can occur as a result of diabetes mellitus include:
   a. Acidosis
   b. Infection
   c. Pregnancy-induced hypertension
   d. Hemorrhage
   e. Polyhydramnios
   f. Fetal death
D. Gestational diabetes mellitus
1. Occurs during the second or third trimester
2. Occurs in pregnancy in clients not previously diagnosed as diabetic and occurs when the pancreas cannot respond to the demand for more insulin
3. Pregnant women should be screened for glucose levels at the 26th week of gestation
4. A 3-hour glucose tolerance test will be performed to confirm diabetes mellitus
5. Oral hypoglycemic agents are never used during pregnancy

6. Frequently can be treated by diet alone; however, insulin may be needed for some clients
7. Most gestational diabetics convert to normal after **delivery**; however, these individuals have an increased risk of developing diabetes mellitus in their lifetimes

E. Predisposing conditions to gestational diabetes
   1. Over age 35
   2. Obesity
   3. Multiple gestation
   4. Family history of diabetes mellitus

F. Assessment
   1. Excessive thirst
   2. Hunger
   3. Weight loss
   4. Blurred vision
   5. Frequent urination
   6. Recurrent urinary tract infections and vaginal yeast infections
   7. Glycosuria and ketonuria
   8. Signs of pregnancy-induced hypertension
   9. Polyhydramnios
   10. Fetus large for gestational age

G. Implementation
   1. Screen clients between the 24th and 28th weeks of pregnancy
   2. Prenatal visits bimonthly for 6 months and weekly thereafter
   3. The goal of therapy is to maintain the blood glucose in a narrow, low range of 65 to 130 mg/dL
   4. Monitor for signs of hypoglycemia; episodes of mild or moderate hypoglycemia can be treated with oral intake of 10 to 15 g of simple carbohydrate
   5. Observe for signs of hyperglycemia
   6. Assess insulin needs
   7. Monitor and maintain blood glucose levels according to gestational week
   8. Monitor for glycosuria and ketonuria
   9. Monitor weight
   10. Insulin administration if diet cannot control blood glucose levels
   11. Assess for signs of preeclampsia, which include hypertension, proteinuria, and edema
   12. Check for increased temperature and signs of infection
   13. Instruct the client to report burning and pain on urination or vaginal discharge or itching
   14. Assess fetal status and monitor for signs of premature **labor**
   15. Assess for signs of polyhydramnios
   16. Increase calorie intake to 2200 to 2500 daily as prescribed, with adequate insulin therapy so that glucose will move into the cells
   17. Calories in diet should consist of 50% to 60% carbohydrates, 12% to 20% protein, and 20% to 30% fat

H. Implementation during **labor**
   1. Monitor fetal status continuously for signs of distress and, if noted, prepare the client for immediate cesarean section
   2. Carefully regulate insulin and provide IV glucose as prescribed, since **labor** depletes glycogen

I. Implementation during the postpartum period
   1. Observe client closely for an insulin reaction, since a precipitous drop in insulin requirements is usual
   2. The client may not require insulin for the first 24 hours
   3. Reregulate insulin needs as prescribed after the first day, according to blood glucose testing
   4. Assess dietary needs on the basis of blood glucose and insulin requirements
   5. Monitor for signs of infection or postpartum hemorrhage

VIII. DISSEMINATED INTRAVASCULAR COAGULATION (DIC)

A. Description
   1. A condition in the mother's body that results in an exaggerated clotting process that increases the formation of clots in microcirculation
   2. Thromboplastin from **placental** tissue and clots enter the bloodstream through open vessels at the **placenta**l site and initiate an exaggeration of the normal clotting process
   3. The rapid and extensive formation of clots causes the platelets and clotting factors to be depleted; this results in bleeding and the potential vascular occlusion of organs from thromboembolus formation

B. Predisposing conditions
   1. Abruptio placentae
   2. Intrauterine fetal death
   3. **Amniotic fluid** embolism
   4. PIH
   5. Liver disease
   6. Sepsis

C. Assessment
   1. Uncontrolled bleeding
   2. Bruising, purpura, petechiae, and ecchymosis
   3. Presence of occult blood
   4. Hematuria, hematemesis, or vaginal bleeding
   5. Signs of shock
   6. Decreased fibrinogen level, platelet count, and hematocrit level
   7. Increased prothrombin time (PT) and partial thromboplastin time (PTT), clotting time, and fibrin degradation products

D. Implementation
   1. Monitor vital signs
   2. Administer oxygen
   3. Assess for bleeding and signs of shock
   4. Administer heparin as prescribed to prevent clot

formation and increase available fibrinogen, coagulation factors, and platelets

    5. Administer blood or blood products as prescribed, such as fresh-frozen plasma and/or platelets

IX. ECTOPIC PREGNANCY

A. Description: A pregnancy that occurs in an other than uterine site, with **implantation** usually occurring in fallopian tubes

B. Assessment
  1. Pain unilaterally, with cramping and tenderness
  2. Mass in the adnexa or cul-de-sac
  3. Nausea and vomiting
  4. Slight, dark vaginal bleeding
  5. Fever
  6. Tachycardia
  7. Leukocytosis
  8. Low hemoglobin and hematocrit levels, elevated erythrocyte sedimentation rate
  9. Profound shock if rupture occurs

C. Implementation
  1. Obtain assessment data rapidly
  2. Obtain vital signs
  3. Initiate measures to prevent rupture and shock
  4. Monitor bleeding
  5. Obtain blood specimen for type and cross-match
  6. Prepare for methotrexate therapy if prescribed, for unruptured masses smaller than 4 cm, to induce abortion and preserve the fallopian tube
  7. Prepare the client for laparotomy and removal of the pregnancy and tube, if necessary, or repair of tube
  8. Administer antibiotics and RhoGAM as prescribed
  9. Encourage follow-up care
  10. Encourage counseling for future pregnancies

X. ENDOMETRITIS

A. Description
  1. An infection of the lining of the uterus following **delivery;** caused by bacteria that invade the uterus at the **placental** site
  2. The infection may spread and involve the entire endometrium and cause peritonitis, pelvic thrombophlebitis, or cellulitis

B. Assessment
  1. Chills and fever
  2. Increased pulse
  3. Decreased appetite
  4. Headache
  5. Backache
  6. Prolonged, severe afterpains
  7. Tender, large uterus
  8. Foul odor to **lochia** or reddish-brown **lochia**
  9. Ileus
  10. Elevated WBC count with a left shift and immature formed cells

C. Implementation
  1. Monitor vital signs
  2. Position client in Fowler's position to facilitate drainage of **lochia**
  3. Provide a private room for client
  4. Inform the mother that it is not necessary to isolate the **newborn infant** from the mother
  5. Instruct the client in proper handwashing techniques
  6. Initiate wound and skin precautions as necessary
  7. Monitor I & O and encourage fluids
  8. Administer IV antibiotics as prescribed
  9. Administer comfort measures such as back rubs and positioning changes, and pain medications as prescribed
  10. Administer oxytoxic medications as prescribed to improve uterine tone

XI. FETAL DEATH IN UTERO (FDIU)

A. Description
  1. The death of a fetus after the 20th week of gestation and before birth
  2. DIC can develop if the dead fetus is retained in the uterus for 3 to 4 weeks or more

B. Assessment
  1. Absence of fetal movement
  2. Absence of fetal heart tones
  3. Maternal weight loss
  4. Lack of fetal growth or decrease in fundal height
  5. Lack of cardiac activity and other characteristics suggestive of fetal death noted on the ultrasound

C. Implementation
  1. Prepare for the **delivery** of the fetus
  2. Support the client's decision about **labor,** birth, and the postpartum period
  3. Facilitate the grieving process
  4. Allow the parents to hold the **infant** after birth
  5. Allow the parents to name the **infant**
  6. Accept such behaviors as anger and hostility from parents
  7. Refer parents to an appropriate support group

XII. HEPATITIS B

A. Description
  1. An inflammation of the liver caused by the hepatitis B virus
  2. Maternal fetal risk in uncomplicated hepatitis B is not generally increased unless infection occurs in the third trimester or in the immediate postpartum period
  3. Intrapartum risks include increased risk for prematurity, premature **delivery,** and vertical fetal transmission

B. Transmission to fetus and **neonate**
  1. Transplacental
  2. Intrapartum exposure to infected blood, **amniotic fluid,** or vaginal secretions

3. Through postpartum exposure
4. Through breastfeeding

C. Risk to fetus and **neonate**
   1. Infections in early life are usually asymptomatic
   2. The **neonate** is identified as an HBsAg carrier
   3. Chronic hepatitis
   4. Associated with glomerulonephritis and nephritis

D. Implementation
   1. Minimize the number of vaginal examinations
   2. Minimize the risk for intrapartum ascending infections
   3. Double-glove for extended periods of blood contact
   4. Administer antibiotics as prescribed during **labor** to decrease the risk of transmission to the **neonate,** especially if the membranes are ruptured
   5. Remove maternal blood from the **neonate** immediately after birth
   6. Protect the **neonate's** scalp integrity
   7. Suction the **neonate** immediately after birth
   8. Bathe the **neonate** prior to invasive procedures
   9. Clean and dry the face and eyes before instilling eye prophylaxis
   10. Discourage kissing until the mother and the **neonate** have been treated
   11. Support breastfeeding after maternal and neonatal treatment; breastfeeding is not contraindicated if an infected mother and **newborn infant** are treated
   12. Immune globulin and vaccine are given to all HbsAg-positive neonates within 2 to 12 hours of **delivery,** at least before 24 hours, and not more than 7 days after birth
   13. Inform the mother that HBV vaccine will be administered to the **neonate,** with the first dose given before the **newborn infant** leaves the hospital; the second dose at 1 month; and the third dose at 6 months
   14. If the mother is identified positive more than 1 month after **delivery,** her HbsAg-negative **infant** should be treated

XIII. HEMATOMA

A. Description
   1. The formation of a hematoma following the escape of blood into the tissues of the reproductive sac after the **delivery**
   2. Predisposing conditions include operative **delivery** with forceps or injury to a blood vessel
   3. A life-threatening condition

B. Assessment
   1. Abnormal, severe pain
   2. Pressure in perineal area
   3. Palpable, sensitive tumor in perineal area, with discolored skin

4. Inability to void
5. Decreased hemoglobin and hematocrit levels
6. Signs of shock, such as pallor, tachycardia, and hypotension, if significant blood loss has occurred

C. Implementation
   1. Monitor vital signs
   2. Monitor client for abnormal pain, especially when forceps **delivery** has occurred
   3. Apply ice to the hematoma site
   4. Administer analgesics as prescribed
   5. Monitor I & O
   6. Encourage fluids and voiding; prepare for urinary catheterization if client is unable to void
   7. Administer blood replacements as prescribed
   8. Monitor for signs of infection, such as increased temperature, pulse rate, and WBC count
   9. Administer antibiotics as prescribed, since infection is common following hematoma formation
   10. Prepare for incision and evacuation of hematoma if necessary

XIV. HYDATIDIFORM MOLE

A. Description
   1. A developmental anomaly of the **placenta** that changes chorionic villi into a mass of clear vesicles
   2. Presents as an edematous grapelike cluster that may be nonmalignant or may develop into choriocarcinoma

B. Assessment
   1. Fetal heart rate not detectable
   2. Vaginal bleeding, which usually occurs by week 12, of a bright red or dark brown color; may be slight, profuse, or intermittent
   3. Symptoms of PIH, such as an elevated blood pressure, edema, and proteinuria, which may be present before week 20
   4. Fundal height is greater than expected for date
   5. Elevated human chorionic gonadotropin (hCG) levels
   6. Ultrasound shows a characteristic snowstorm pattern

C. Implementation
   1. Monitor vital signs
   2. Prepare mother for uterine evacuation
   3. Monitor for postprocedure hemorrhage and infection
   4. Prepare for hysterectomy if necessary
   5. Monitor hCG levels for 1 year
   6. Administer chemotherapeutic agents if necessary and as prescribed
   7. Instruct parents regarding birth control measures so that pregnancy can be prevented during the 1-year follow-up

XV. HYPEREMESIS GRAVIDARUM

A. Description: Intractable nausea and vomiting that persist beyond the first trimester and cause disturbances in nutrition, electrolytes, and fluid balance

B. Assessment
1. Nausea most pronounced on arising; however, it can occur at other times during the day
2. Persistent vomiting
3. Weight loss
4. Signs of dehydration
5. Electrolyte imbalances
6. Ketonuria
7. Increased hematocrit levels

C. Implementation
1. Monitor vital signs
2. Monitor fetal heart rate, fetal activity, and fetal growth
3. Monitor for signs of dehydration and electrolyte imbalances
4. Monitor daily weight
5. Monitor I & O and calorie count
6. Restrict PO intake until vomiting subsides; begin on a dry diet, alternating liquids and solids in small quantities, and advance diet slowly
7. Monitor urine for ketones
8. Monitor electrolytes, hemoglobin, and hematocrit levels
9. Administer IV fluids and electrolytes as prescribed
10. Administer antiemetics as prescribed

XVI. INCOMPETENT CERVIX

A. Description
1. Premature dilatation of the cervix, which occurs most often in the 4th or 5th month of pregnancy
2. Is associated with cervical trauma as a result of previous surgery or birth
3. Treatment is surgical

B. Assessment
1. Vaginal bleeding at 18 to 28 weeks of gestation
2. Fetal membranes visible through the cervix

C. Implementation
1. Monitor vital signs
2. Monitor fetal heart rate
3. Provide bed rest
4. Prepare for surgical procedure
   a. Pursestring around cervix is called McDonald's procedure
   b. Stitch through cervix is called Shirodkar's procedure
5. Monitor for postprocedure complications such as rupture of the membranes or contractions of the uterus
6. Maintain bed rest for 24 hours postprocedure
7. Report any postprocedure vaginal bleeding or increased uterine contractions immediately to physician or health care provider

XVII. INFECTIONS

A. Toxoplasmosis (protozoa)
1. Produces symptoms of acute, flu-like infection in mother
2. Transmitted through raw meat or handling cat litter of infected cats
3. Organism is transmitted across the **placenta**
4. Spontaneous abortion likely to occur early in pregnancy

B. Rubella
1. Organism is transmitted across the **placenta**
2. Extremely teratogenic in first trimester
3. Causes congenital defects of eyes, heart, ears, and brain
4. Women with low rubella titers should be vaccinated at least 3 months before becoming pregnant or following a **delivery**

C. Cytomegalovirus (CMV)
1. Produces flu-like or mononucleosis-like symptoms in the mother
2. Transmitted through the respiratory or sexual route
3. Organism is transmitted across the **placenta,** or the fetus may be infected through the birth canal
4. May cause fetal death, retardation, heart defects, deafness
5. No effective treatment available

D. Genital herpes
1. Affects the external genitalia, vagina, and cervix
2. Causes draining, painful vesicles
3. Virus is lethal to fetus if it is inoculated during vaginal **delivery**
4. **Delivery** of the fetus is usually by cesarean section if active lesions are present in the vagina; **delivery** may be performed vaginally if the lesions are in the anal, perineal, or inner thigh area (strict precautions are necessary to protect the fetus during **delivery**)
5. No vaginal examinations are done in the presence of active vaginal herpetic lesions
6. Maintain isolation procedures during hospitalization if the disease is active
7. **Neonate** and mother may be separated during the active period, or other special precautionary measures may be used to avoid transmission to **neonate**

XVIII. MULTIPLE GESTATION

A. Description
1. Results from double ovulation (fraternal or dizygotic) or a splitting of the fertilized egg (identical or monozygotic)
2. Complications include spontaneous abortion, anemia, congenital anomalies, hyperemesis gravidarum, intrauterine growth retardation, PIH, polyhydramnios, postpartum hemorrhage, pre-

mature rupture of membranes, and preterm **labor** and **delivery**

B. Assessment
1. Excessive fetal activity
2. Uterus large for gestational age
3. Palpation of three or four large parts in the uterus
4. Auscultation of more than one fetal heart rate
5. Excessive weight gain

C. Implementation
1. Monitor vital signs
2. Monitor fetal heart rates, fetal activity, and fetal growth
3. Monitor for cervical changes
4. Prepare client for ultrasound as prescribed
5. Monitor for anemia; administer supplemental iron and vitamins as prescribed
6. Monitor for preterm **labor** and treat preterm **labor** promptly
7. Prepare for cesarean section for abnormal presentations
8. Prepare to administer oxytoxic medications after **delivery** to prevent postpartum hemorrhage from uterine overdistension

XIX. PREGNANCY-INDUCED HYPERTENSION (PIH)

A. Description
1. An acute hypertensive state that develops after the 20th week of gestation
2. The condition can be mild or severe and can progress to seizures (eclampsia) (Box 25-1)
3. The classic signs of preeclampsia are hypertension, generalized edema, and proteinuria

B. Predisposing conditions
1. Primigravida
2. Teenagers and women over 35 years of age
3. Poor nutrition
4. Low socioeconomic status
5. Chronic hypertension
6. Diabetes mellitus
7. Chronic renal disease
8. History of PIH

C. Complications of PIH
1. Abruptio placentae
2. DIC

3. Thrombocytopenia
4. **Placental** insufficiency
5. Intrauterine fetal death

D. Mild preeclampsia
1. Assessment
   a. Hypertension of 15 to 30 mm Hg above baseline
   b. Weight gain of 1 lb or more per week in last trimester
   c. Mild, generalized edema
   d. Proteinuria of 1+
2. Implementation
   a. Provide bed rest and position client in left lateral position
   b. Monitor blood pressure and weight
   c. Monitor neurological status, since changes can indicate cerebral hypoxia or impending seizure
   d. Monitor deep tendon reflexes and for the presence of clonus, as hyperreflexia indicates increased central nervous system irritability (Box 25-2)
   e. Provide adequate fluids

BOX 25-2

Assessment of Reflexes

Patellar
Position the client with legs dangling over the edge of the examining table or lying on back with legs slightly flexed.
Strike the patellar tendon just below the kneecap with the percussion hammer.
Normal Response: Extension or kicking out of leg.

Biceps
Position your thumb over the client's biceps tendon, supporting the client's elbow with the palm of the hand.
Strike a downward blow over the client's thumb with the percussion hammer.
Normal Response: Flexion of the arm at the elbow.

Clonus
Position the client with legs dangling over the edge of the examining table.
Support the leg with one hand and sharply dorsiflex the client's foot with the other hand.
Maintain the dorsiflexed position for a few seconds; then release the foot.
Normal Response (Negative Clonus Response)
Foot will remain steady in the dorsiflexed position.
No rhythmic oscillations or jerking of the foot will be felt.
When released, the foot will drop to a plantar flexed position with no oscillations.
Abnormal Response (Positive Clonus Response)
Rhythmic oscillations when the foot is dorsiflexed.
Similar oscillations will be noted when the foot drops to the plantar flexed position.

BOX 25-1

Signs of Worsening PIH or Impending Seizures

BP 160/110 mm Hg or above
Epigastric pain
Decreased urinary output
Visual changes
Headache
Excessive proteinuria

f. Monitor I & O; a urinary output of 30 mL per hour indicates adequate renal perfusion

g. Increase dietary protein and carbohydrates with no added salt

h. Administer medications as prescribed to lower blood pressure to prevent a cerebrovascular accident; however, blood pressure should not be lowered drastically because **placental** perfusion can be compromised

E. Severe preeclampsia

1. Assessment

a. Severe hypertension, 30 to 40 mm Hg above baseline while on bed rest

b. Massive, generalized edema and weight gain

c. Proteinuria 4+

d. Less than 400 mL urine output in 24 hours

e. Severe headache

f. Dizziness

g. Blurred vision and spots before eyes

h. Nausea and vomiting

i. Epigastric pain

j. Central nervous system irritability

2. Implementation

a. Administer magnesium sulfate as prescribed; plan for the administration of magnesium sulfate for 24 to 48 hours postpartum as prescribed

b. Administer antihypertensives such as hydralazine (Apresoline) as prescribed, to prevent a cerebrovascular accident

c. Prepare for the induction of **labor**

F. Eclampsia

1. Assessment

a. Severe edema

b. Proteinuria 4+

c. Sudden large increase in weight

d. BP greater than 160/110 mm Hg

e. Cyanosis

f. Fetal distress

g. Seizures

h. Coma

2. Implementation

a. Protect the client from injury

b. Administer oxygen

c. Monitor fetal heart rate and contractions

d. Initiate seizure precautions

e. Administer seizure medications as prescribed

f. Prepare for **delivery** after stabilization of the client

XX. PYELONEPHRITIS

A. Description

1. Results from bacterial infections that extend upward from the bladder through the blood vessels and lymphatics

2. Frequently follows untreated urinary tract infections and is associated with increased incidence

of anemia, low birth weight, PIH, premature **labor** and **delivery,** and premature rupture of the membranes

B. Assessment

1. Flank pain

2. Burning or painful urination

3. Increased frequency of urination

4. Chills, malaise, nausea

5. Increased temperature, pulse rate, and fetal heart rate

6. Vomiting

7. Uterine contractions

8. Elevated WBC count

C. Implementation

1. Monitor vital signs

2. Monitor fetal heart rate and for contractions

3. Encourage fluids; monitor I & O

4. Monitor renal function

5. Administer antibiotics as prescribed

6. Administer antipyretics such as acetaminophen (Tylenol) as prescribed

7. Obtain urine cultures every 2 to 4 weeks after resolution of infection

XXI. SEXUALLY TRANSMITTED DISEASES (STD)

A. Chlamydia

1. Description

a. Common, sexually transmitted pathogen associated with an increased risk for premature births, stillbirths, neonatal conjunctivitis, and **newborn** chlamydial pneumonia

b. In the nonpregnant state, can cause salpingitis, pelvic abscesses, chronic pelvic pain, and infertility

c. Incubation period is 5 to 10 days or longer, up to 28 days

d. Diagnostic test is culture for *Chlamydia trachomatis*

2. Assessment

a. Increased vaginal discharge and itching

b. Low-grade temperature

c. Right upper quadrant abdominal pain

d. Bleeding between periods

e. Pain with coitus

f. Dysuria

g. Rectal pain or discharge

h. Mucopurulent cervicitis

i. Cervix that bleeds easy

j. In the **newborn,** conjunctivitis and pneumonia

3. Implementation

a. Screen the client to determine whether high risk; instruct the client in the importance of rescreening, because reinfection can occur as the client nears term

b. Instruct the client about the prescribed medication for treatment of the STD

TABLE 25-2

Assessment of the Stages of Syphilis

Primary Stage	Secondary Stage	Tertiary Stage
Most infectious stage Appearance of ulcerative, painless lesions produced by spirochetes at the point of entry into the body	Highly infectious stage Lesions appear about 3 weeks after the primary stage and may occur anywhere on the skin and mucous membranes Generalized lymphadenopathy occurs	Spirochetes enter the internal organs and cause permanent damage; symptoms may occur 10 to 30 years following the occurrence of an untreated primary lesion Invades the CNS, causing meningitis, ataxia, general paresis, and progressive mental deterioration Affects the aortic valve and aorta

    c. Instruct the mother about medication for the **neonate** if prescribed

    d. Administer appropriate eye prophylaxis to the **neonate** as prescribed

    e. Monitor neonate for signs and symptoms of pneumonia if at risk

    f. Ensure that the sexual partner is treated

B. Syphilis

  1. Description

    a. A chronic infectious disease caused by the organism *Treponema pallidum*

    b. Transmission is by intimate physical contact with syphilitic lesions, which are usually found on the skin or the mucous membranes of the mouth and genitals

    c. The incubation period is 2 to 6 weeks following exposure

    d. The infection may cause abortion or premature **labor** and is passed to the fetus after the 4th month of pregnancy as congenital syphilis

  2. Assessment (Table 25-2)

  3. Implementation

    a. Obtain serum test for syphilis on first prenatal visit; prepare to repeat the test just before the fourth month, as the disease may be acquired after the initial visit

    b. Instruct the client that treatment of her partner is necessary if infection occurs

    c. Prepare to administer procaine penicillin G to mother as prescribed

C. Gonorrhea

  1. Description

    a. Infection, caused by *Neisseria gonorrhoeae*, that causes inflammation of the mucous membranes of the genital and urinary tracts

    b. Transmission of organism is by sexual intercourse

    c. Infection may be transmitted to the baby's eyes during **delivery**, causing blindness (ophthalmia neonatorum)

  2. Assessment

    a. Female: Usually asymptomatic; vaginal discharge, urinary frequency, and pain possible

    b. Male: Fever, painful urination, pelvic pain, epididymitis with pain, tenderness, and swelling

  3. Implementation

    a. Obtain culture for gonorrhea on the first prenatal visit; prepare to repeat culture, as infection may occur during pregnancy

    b. Administer prophylactic antibiotics: erythromycin or 1% silver nitrate to the **newborn infant**

    c. Instruct the client that treatment of her partner is necessary if infection occurs

D. Genital warts

  1. Description

    a. Caused by human papillomavirus (HPV); affects the cervix, urethra, anus, penis, and scrotum

    b. Appears 1 to 2 months after exposure

    c. Transmitted through sexual contact

    d. There is no cure for HPV

  2. Assessment

    a. Small to large wartlike growths on genitals

    b. Cervical cell changes noted because HPV is associated with cervical malignancies

  3. Implementation

    a. Encourage yearly Papanicolaou smear

    b. Limit sexual contacts and use condoms

    c. Instruct the client regarding potential treatment, including cytotoxic agents, cryotherapy, electrocautery, and surgical excision to remove the lesions

XXII. TUBERCULOSIS

A. Description

  1. A highly communicable disease caused by *Mycobacterium tuberculosis*

  2. It is transmitted by the airborne route

3. Tuberculosis has an insidious onset, and many clients are not aware of symptoms until the disease is well advanced

▲ 4. A multidrug-resistant strain (MDR-TB) of TB can exist as a result of improper compliance or noncompliance with treatment programs and the development of mutations in the tubercle bacilli

B. Transmission
   1. Transplacental transmission is rare
   2. Can occur during birth through aspiration of infected **amniotic fluid**
   3. **Neonate** can become infected from contact with infected individuals

C. Risk to mother: Active disease during pregnancy has been associated with an increase in hypertensive disorders of pregnancy

D. Diagnosis
   1. If a chest radiograph is required for the mother, it is done only after 20 weeks gestation, and a lead shield for the abdomen is required
   2. TB skin testing is safe during pregnancy
   3. Many immigrants have false positive PPDs as a result of the immunizations received in their home countries; therefore, immigrants are more likely to require a chest radiograph after 20 weeks' gestation to assist in confirming the diagnosis

E. Assessment
   1. Maternal
      a. May be asymptomatic
      b. Fever and chills
      c. Night sweats
      d. Weight loss
      e. Fatigue
      f. Cough, hemoptysis, or green or yellow sputum
      g. Dyspnea
      h. Pleural pain
   2. **Neonate**
      a. Fever
      b. Lethargy
      c. Poor feeding
      d. Failure to thrive
      e. Respiratory distress
      f. Hepatosplenomegaly
      g. Meningitis
      h. Disease may spread to all major organs

F. Implementation
   1. Mother
      a. Administration of isoniazid (INH), ethambutol (Myambutol), and rifampin (Rifadin) for 6 to 12 months during and after pregnancy
      b. Pyridoxine should be administered with INH to pregnant women to prevent the development of peripheral neuropathy caused by the INH
      c. Note that teratogenicity is unknown with rifampin
      d. Promote breastfeeding only if the mother is noninfectious
      e. Breastfeeding is not contraindicated with isoniazid (INH), ethambutol, or rifampin
      f. Note that pregnancy and immunosuppression are contraindications to bacille Calmette-Guérin (BCG) administration
   2. **Neonate**
      a. If born to a mother with active TB, should be treated with INH for 3 months
      b. **Neonates** born to infected mothers with active disease can be vaccinated with BCG; note that a Mantoux test turns positive after BCG is given
      c. Isolate and separate the **neonate** from the mother during active disease until the mother is known to be noninfectious, after a minimum of 3 weeks of medication therapy

XXIII. URINARY TRACT INFECTION (UTI)

A. Description: The most common medical complication of pregnancy, but, if untreated, the client can develop pyelonephritis

B. Predisposing conditions
   1. History of UTI
   2. Sickle cell trait
   3. Poor hygiene
   4. Anemia
   5. Diabetes mellitus
   6. Pregnancy

C. Assessment
   1. May be asymptomatic during pregnancy
   2. Burning and pain on urination
   3. Increased frequency of urination
   4. Lower abdominal pain and costovertebral angle tenderness
   5. Fever
   6. Proteinuria, hematuria, bacteruria, WBCs in urine

D. Implementation
   1. Monitor vital signs
   2. Monitor fetal heart rate
   3. Increase fluid intake
   4. Monitor I & O
   5. Monitor urine for consistency and odor
   6. Monitor for signs and symptoms of pyelonephritis (dip test urine with each prenatal visit)
   7. Obtain urine for culture and sensitivity
   8. Provide heat to lower abdomen or back
   9. Administer antibiotics as prescribed
   10. Instruct the client to complete the course of antibiotics if prescribed
   11. Instruct the client regarding the need to repeat the culture after treatment is completed

PRACTICE QUESTIONS

1. A pregnant client in the last trimester has been admitted to the hospital with a diagnosis of severe preeclampsia. A nurse monitors for complications associated with the diagnosis and assesses the client for:
   1. Any bleeding, such as in the gums, petechiae, and purpura
   2. Enlargement of the breasts
   3. Periods of fetal movement followed by quiet periods
   4. Complaints of feeling hot when the room is cool

2. A nurse in a maternity unit is reviewing the records of the clients on the unit. Which of the clients would the nurse identify as being at most risk for developing disseminated intravascular coagulation (DIC)?
   1. A gravida IV who delivered 8 hours ago and has lost 500 mL of blood
   2. A gravida II who has just been diagnosed with dead fetus syndrome
   3. A primigravida with mild preeclampsia
   4. A primigravida who delivered a 10-pound baby 3 hours ago

3. A client in the first trimester of pregnancy arrives at a health care clinic and reports that she has been experiencing vaginal bleeding. A threatened abortion is suspected, and a nurse instructs the client regarding management of care. Which statement if made by the client indicates a need for further education?
   1. "I will maintain strict bed rest throughout the remainder of the pregnancy."
   2. "I will avoid sexual intercourse until the bleeding has stopped, and for 2 weeks following the last evidence of bleeding."
   3. "I will count the number of perineal pads used on a daily basis and note the amount and color of blood on the pad."
   4. "I will watch for the evidence of the passage of tissue."

4. A prenatal nurse is providing instructions to a group of pregnant clients regarding measures to prevent toxoplasmosis. Which statement if made by one of the clients indicates a need for further instructions?
   1. "I need to cook meat thoroughly."
   2. "I need to avoid touching mucous membranes of the mouth or eyes while handling raw meat."
   3. "I need to drink unpasteurized milk only."
   4. "I need to avoid contact with materials that are possibly contaminated with cat feces."

5. A pregnant woman reports to a health care clinic, complaining of loss of appetite, weight loss, and fatigue. Following assessment of the woman, tuberculosis is suspected. A sputum culture is obtained and identifies *Mycobacterium tuberculosis*. The nurse provides instructions to the mother regarding therapeutic management of the tuberculosis. The nurse tells the client that:
   1. Medication will not be started until after delivery of the fetus
   2. Isoniazid (INH) plus rifampin (Rifadin) will be required for a total of 9 months
   3. The newborn infant will need to receive medication therapy immediately following birth
   4. Therapeutic abortion is required

6. A clinic nurse has provided home care instructions to a client with a history of cardiac disease who has just been told that she is pregnant. Which of the following statements if made by the client indicates a need for further education?
   1. "During the pregnancy, I need to avoid contact with other individuals as much as possible to prevent infection."
   2. "I need to avoid excessive weight gain to prevent increased demands on my heart."
   3. "It is best that I rest on my left side to promote blood return to the heart."
   4. "I need to try to avoid stressful situations because stress increases the workload on the heart."

7. A nurse is providing instructions to a maternity client with a history of cardiac disease regarding appropriate dietary measures. Which of the following statements if made by the client indicates an understanding of the measures to take?
   1. "I need to increase my fluid intake and intake of high-fiber foods."
   2. "I need to maintain a low-calorie diet to prevent any weight gain."
   3. "I need to lower my blood volume by limiting my fluids."
   4. "I do not need to be concerned about sodium intake during pregnancy."

8. A clinic nurse is performing a psychosocial assessment of a client who has been told that she is pregnant. Which of the following assessment findings would indicate to the nurse that the client is at high risk for contracting human immunodeficiency virus (HIV)?
   1. A past history of IV drug use
   2. A history of one sexual partner for the past 10 years
   3. No history of any sexually transmitted diseases
   4. A significant other who is heterosexual

9. A nurse in a maternity unit is providing emotional support to a client and her husband who are preparing to be discharged from the hospital after giving birth to a dead fetus. Which statement if made by the client indicates a component of the normal grieving process?
   1. "We would really like to attend a support group."
   2. "We're OK and we are going to try to have another baby immediately."
   3. "We never want to have a baby again."

   4. "We are going to try to adopt a child immediately."

10. A nurse assists a pregnant client with cardiac disease to identify resources to help her care for her 18-month-old child during the last trimester of pregnancy. The nurse encourages the pregnant client to use these resources primarily to:
    1. Help the mother prepare for labor and delivery
    2. Reduce excessive maternal stress and fatigue
    3. Prepare the 18-month-old child for maternal separation during hospitalization
    4. Avoid exposure to potential pathogens and resulting infections

11. A nurse evaluates a hepatitis B–positive client's ability to safely bottle feed her infant during postpartum hospitalization. Which maternal action best exemplifies the client's knowledge of potential disease transmission to the infant?
    1. The client tests the temperature of the formula prior to initiating feeding
    2. The client holds the infant properly during feeding and burping
    3. The client washes and dries her hands prior to and following self-pericare and asks for a pair of gloves prior to feeding
    4. The client requests that the window be closed prior to feeding

12. A nurse is providing instructions to a human immunodeficiency virus (HIV)–positive pregnant client regarding care to the newborn infant following delivery. The client asks the nurse about the feeding options that are available. Which statement will the nurse provide to the client regarding feeding the newborn infant?
    1. "You will be able to breast feed for 6 months; then will need to switch to bottle feeding."
    2. "You will be able to breast feed for 9 months; then will need to switch to bottle feeding."
    3. "You will need to feed the newborn infant by nasogastric tube feeding."
    4. "You will need to bottle feed the newborn infant."

13. During the intrapartum period, a nurse is caring for a laboring client with sickle cell disease. The nurse ensures that the client receives appropriate IV fluid intake and oxygen consumption primarily to:
    1. Stimulate the labor process
    2. Avoid the necessity of a cesarean delivery
    3. Prevent dehydration and hypoxemia
    4. Eliminate the need for analgesic administration

14. A home care nurse visits a pregnant client with a diagnosis of mild preeclampsia who is being monitored for pregnancy-induced hypertension (PIH). Which assessment finding indicates a worsening of the preeclampsia and the need to notify the physician?
    1. Blood pressure reading is at the prenatal baseline

   2. Urinary output has increased
   3. The client complains of a headache and blurred vision
   4. Dependent edema has resolved

15. A client with a 38-week twin gestation is admitted to a birthing center in early labor. One of the fetuses is a breech presentation. Of the following interventions, which will the nurse list as the lowest priority in planning the nursing care of this client?
    1. Attach electronic fetal monitoring
    2. Prepare the client for a possible cesarean section
    3. Measure fundal height
    4. Visually examine the perineum and vaginal opening

16. A stillborn was delivered in the birthing suite a few hours ago. After the birth, the family has remained together, holding and touching the baby. Which statement by the nurse would further assist the family in their initial period of grief?
    1. "Don't worry, there is nothing you could do to prevent this from happening."
    2. "We need to take the baby from you now so that you can get some sleep."
    3. "What have you named your lovely baby?"
    4. "We will see to it that you have an early discharge so that you don't have to be reminded of this experience."

17. A nurse implements a teaching plan for a pregnant client who is newly diagnosed with gestational diabetes mellitus. Which statement if made by the client indicates a need for further education?
    1. "I need to stay on the diabetic diet."
    2. "I will perform glucose monitoring at home."
    3. "I need to avoid exercise because of the negative effects on insulin production."
    4. "I need to be aware of any infections and report signs of infection immediately to my health care provider."

18. A primigravada is receiving magnesium sulfate for the treatment of pregnancy-induced hypertension. The nurse who is caring for the client is performing assessments every 30 minutes. Which assessment finding would be of most concern to the nurse?
    1. Urinary output of 20 mL since the previous assessment
    2. Deep tendon reflexes of 2+
    3. Respiratory rate of 10 breaths per minute
    4. Fetal heart rate of 120 beats per minute

19. A nurse is caring for a pregnant client with preeclampsia. The nurse prepares a plan of care for the client and documents in the plan that if the client progresses from preeclampsia to eclampsia, the nurse's first action is to:
    1. Administer IV magnesium sulfate
    2. Assess the blood pressure and fetal heart rate
    3. Clear and maintain an open airway
    4. Administer oxygen by facemask

20. A client has just had surgery to deliver a nonviable fetus resulting from abruptio placenta. As a result of the abruptio placenta, the client develops disseminated intravascular coagulopathy (DIC) and is told about the complication. The client begins to cry and screams "God, just let me die now!" Which nursing diagnosis should direct care for this client?
    1. Hopelessness related to loss of baby and personal health
    2. Knowledge deficit related to disease process
    3. Self-esteem disturbance related to being ill
    4. Grief related to loss of the baby

CRITICAL THINKING: FREE-TEXT ENTRY

A home care nurse is monitoring a pregnant client with pregnancy-induced hypertension who is at risk for preeclampsia. At each home care visit, the nurse assesses the client for which three classic signs of preeclampsia?

Answer: _____

ANSWERS

1. **1**
Rationale: Severe preeclampsia can trigger disseminated intravascular coagulation (DIC) because of the widespread damage to vascular integrity. Bleeding is an early sign of DIC and should be reported to the health care provider if noted on assessment. Options 2, 3, and 4 are all normal occurrences in the last trimester of pregnancy.
Test-Taking Strategy: Use the process of elimination and knowledge regarding the normal physiological occurrences in pregnancy to answer the question. Eliminate options 2, 3, and 4 because they are all normal occurrences in the last trimester of pregnancy. Review the assessment findings in DIC if you had difficulty with this question.
Level of Cognitive Ability: Analysis
Client Needs: Physiological Integrity
Integrated Concept/Process: Nursing Process/Assessment
Content Area: Maternity
Reference: Lowdermilk, D., Perry, S., & Bobak, I. (2000). *Maternity & women's health care* (7th ed.). St. Louis: Mosby, p. 858.

2. **2**
Rationale: Dead fetus syndrome is considered a risk factor for DIC. Hemorrhage is a risk factor with DIC; however, a loss of 500 mL is not considered hemorrhage. Severe preeclampsia is considered a risk factor for DIC; a mild case is not. Delivering a large baby is not considered a risk factor for DIC.
Test-Taking Strategy: Use the process of elimination and knowledge regarding the risk factors associated with DIC to answer this question. Recalling that dead fetus syndrome is a risk factor for DIC will assist in directing you to option 2. If you had difficulty answering this question, review these risk factors.
Level of Cognitive Ability: Analysis
Client Needs: Physiological Integrity
Integrated Concept/Process: Nursing Process/Analysis
Content Area: Maternity
Reference: Lowdermilk, D., Perry, S., & Bobak, I. (2000). *Maternity & women's health care* (7th ed.). St. Louis: Mosby, p. 858.

3. **1**
Rationale: Strict bed rest throughout the remainder of the pregnancy is not required. The woman is advised to curtail sexual activities until bleeding has ceased, and for 2 weeks following the last evidence of bleeding or as recommended by the physician or other health care provider. The woman is instructed to count the number of perineal pads used on a daily basis and to note the quantity and color of blood on the pad. The woman should also watch for the evidence of the passage of tissue.
Test-Taking Strategy: Use the process of elimination to assist in answering the question. Note the key words "need for further education" in the stem of the question. Noting the word "strict" in option 1 will assist in directing you to this option. Review therapeutic management for a threatened abortion, if you had difficulty with this question.
Level of Cognitive Ability: Analysis
Client Needs: Health Promotion and Maintenance
Integrated Concept/Process: Teaching/Learning
Content Area: Maternity
Reference: Gorrie, T., McKinney, E., & Murray, S. (1998). *Foundations of maternal newborn nursing* (2nd ed.). Philadelphia: W.B. Saunders, p. 674.

4. **3**
Rationale: All pregnant woman should be advised to do the following to prevent the development of toxoplasmosis. Women should be instructed to cook meats thoroughly, particularly pork, beef, and lamb; avoid touching mucous membranes of the mouth or eyes while handling raw meat; thoroughly wash all kitchen surfaces that come in contact with uncooked meat; wash the hands thoroughly after handling raw meat; avoid uncooked eggs and unpasteurized milk; wash fruits and vegetables before consumption; and avoid contact with materials that are possibly contaminated with cat feces, such as cat litter boxes, sand boxes, or garden soil.
Test-Taking Strategy: Note the key words "need for further instructions." Also, note the absolute term "only" in option 3. If you are unfamiliar with the measures to prevent toxoplasmosis, review this content.
Level of Cognitive Ability: Analysis
Client Needs: Health Promotion and Maintenance
Integrated Concept/Process: Teaching/Learning
Content Area: Maternity
Reference: Gorrie, T., McKinney, E., & Murray, S. (1998). *Foundations of maternal newborn nursing* (2nd ed.). Philadelphia: W.B. Saunders, p. 739.

5. **2**
Rationale: More than one medication may be used to prevent growth of resistant organisms in the pregnant woman with tuberculosis. Treatment must continue for a prolonged period of time. The preferred treatment for the pregnant woman is INH plus rifampin daily for a total of 9 months. Ethambutol is

added initially if medication resistance is suspected. Pyridoxine (vitamin B_6) is often administered with isoniazid to prevent fetal neurotoxicity. The infant will be tested at birth and may be started on preventive isoniazid therapy. Skin testing should be repeated at 3 months on the infant, and isoniazid may be stopped if the skin test result remains negative. If the skin test result converts to positive, a full course of isoniazid would be given.

Test-Taking Strategy: Knowledge regarding the therapeutic management for the mother with tuberculosis and for the newborn infant is required to answer this question. If you had difficulty with this question, review treatment measures for the mother with tuberculosis.

Level of Cognitive Ability: Application
Client Needs: Physiological Integrity
Integrated Concept/Process: Teaching/Learning
Content Area: Maternity
Reference: Gorrie, T., McKinney, E., & Murray, S. (1998). *Foundations of maternal newborn nursing* (2nd ed.). Philadelphia: W.B. Saunders, p. 738.

6. **1**
Rationale: To avoid infections, visitors with active infections should not be allowed to visit the client. Otherwise restrictions are not required. Stress causes increased heart workload, and the client should be instructed to avoid stress. Too much weight gain can place further demands on the heart. Resting should be on the left side to promote blood return.

Test-Taking Strategy: Use the process of elimination. Note the key words "cardiac disease" and "need for further education" in the question. Using principles related to the therapeutic management of cardiac disease in general will assist in directing you to option 1. If you had difficulty with this question, review the measures for the pregnant client with cardiac disease.

Level of Cognitive Ability: Analysis
Client Needs: Health Promotion and Maintenance
Integrated Concept/Process: Teaching/Learning
Content Area: Maternity
Reference: Gorrie, T., McKinney, E., & Murray, S. (1998). *Foundations of maternal newborn nursing* (2nd ed.). Philadelphia: W. B. Saunders, p. 724.

7. **1**
Rationale: Constipation can cause the client to use the Valsalva maneuver. This maneuver can cause blood to rush to the heart and overload the cardiac system. Therefore, high-fiber foods are important. A low-calorie diet is not recommended during pregnancy. Diets low in fluid can cause a decrease in blood volume that can deprive the fetus of nutrients. Therefore, adequate fluid intake and high-fiber foods are important. Sodium should be restricted by some degree as prescribed by the physician because this will cause an overload to the circulating blood volume and contribute to cardiac complications.

Test-Taking Strategy: Use the process of elimination. Think about the physiology of the cardiac system, the maternal and fetus needs, and the factors that increase the workload on the heart to answer the question. If you had difficulty with this question, review nursing measures for the pregnant client with cardiac disease.

Level of Cognitive Ability: Analysis

Client Needs: Health Promotion and Maintenance
Integrated Concept/Process: Teaching/Learning
Content Area: Maternity
Reference: Gorrie, T., McKinney, E., & Murray, S. (1998). *Foundations of maternal newborn nursing* (2nd ed.). Philadelphia: W. B. Saunders, p. 724.

8. **1**
Rationale: HIV is transmitted by intimate sexual contact and the exchange of body fluids, exposure to infected blood, and transmission from an infected woman to her fetus. Women who fall into the high-risk category for HIV infection include those with persistent and recurrent sexually transmitted diseases, those with a history of multiple sexual partners, and those who have used IV drugs. A heterosexual partner, particularly a partner who has had only one sexual partner in 10 years, is not a high risk factor for the development of HIV.

Test-Taking Strategy: Use the process of elimination, recalling that that exchange of blood and body fluids places the client at high risk for HIV infection. This will assist in directing you to the correct option. If you had difficulty with this question, review the risk factors for HIV.

Level of Cognitive Ability: Analysis
Client Needs: Health Promotion and Maintenance
Integrated Concept/Process: Nursing Process/Assessment
Content Area: Maternity
Reference: Gorrie, T., McKinney, E., & Murray, S. (1998). *Foundations of maternal newborn nursing* (2nd ed). Philadelphia: W. B. Saunders, p. 738.

9. **1**
Rationale: A support group can help the parents work through their pain by nonjudgmental sharing of feelings. Option 1 identifies a statement that would indicate positive normal grieving. Although the other options may indicate reactions of the client and significant other, they are not specifically a part of the normal grieving process.

Test-Taking Strategy: Use the process of elimination. Read all of the options carefully before selecting an answer and focus on the issue of the question, the normal grieving process. Note the similarity between options 2, 3, and 4 in that they all relate to childbearing. If you had difficulty with this question, review the components of the normal grieving process.

Level of Cognitive Ability: Analysis
Client Needs: Psychosocial Integrity
Integrated Concept/Process: Caring
Content Area: Maternity
Reference: Gorrie, T., McKinney, E., & Murray, S. (1998). *Foundations of maternal newborn nursing* (2nd ed.). Philadelphia: W.B. Saunders, p. 663.

10. **2**
Rationale: A variety of factors can cause increased emotional stress during pregnancy, resulting in further cardiac complications. The client with known cardiac disease is at greater risk for such complications. The use of resources will assist the client to avoid emotional stress, thus reducing additional cardiac compromise during the last trimester. These resources are not intended to minimize potential risk of maternal infection or prepare the client and/or family for the subsequent labor, delivery, and hospitalization.

Test-Taking Strategy: Focus on the issue of the question, noting the client's diagnosis. Also note the key word "primarily" in the stem of the question. Use Maslow's Hierarchy of Needs theory and focus on the client's condition to assist in directing you to option 2. Review considerations in caring for the pregnant client with cardiac disease if you had difficulty with this question.

Level of Cognitive Ability: Analysis
Client Needs: Health Promotion and Maintenance
Integrated Concept/Process: Self-Care
Content Area: Maternity
Reference: Gorrie, T., McKinney, E., & Murray, S. (1998). *Foundations of maternal newborn nursing* (2nd ed.). Philadelphia: W B. Saunders, pp. 722-727.

11. 3
Rationale: Hepatitis B virus (HBV) is highly contagious when transmitted by direct contact with blood and body fluids of infected persons. The rationale for identifying childbearing women with this disease is to provide adequate protection of the fetus and the newborn infant, to minimize transmission to other humans, and to reduce further maternal morbidity for the mother. Option 3 provides the best evaluation of maternal understanding of disease transmission. Options 1 and 2 are appropriate feeding techniques for bottle feeding, but do not minimize disease transmission for hepatitis B. Option 4 will not affect disease transmission.

Test-Taking Strategy: Focus on the issue of the question, "disease transmission to the infant." This focus and the process of elimination will easily direct you to option 3. Review measures to prevent transmission of hepatitis if you had difficulty with this question.

Level of Cognitive Ability: Analysis
Client Needs: Safe, Effective Care Environment
Integrated Concept/Process: Self-Care
Content Area: Maternity
Reference: Dickason, E., Silverman, B., & Kaplan, J. (1998). *Maternal-infant nursing care* (3rd ed.). St. Louis: Mosby, pp. 697-699.

12. 4
Rationale: Perinatal transmission of HIV can occur during the antepartal period, during labor and birth, or in the postpartum period if the mother is breastfeeding. Women who carry HIV are advised not to breastfeed. There is no physiological reason why the newborn infant needs to be fed by nasogastric tube.

Test-Taking Strategy: Use the process of elimination and knowledge regarding the transmission of HIV to assist in answering the question. Eliminate options 1 and 2 first because these options are similar in that they both address breastfeeding. From the remaining options, select option 4, knowing that it is not necessary to feed the infant by nasogastric tube. Review feeding options for the newborn infant of an HIV client, if you had difficulty with this question.

Level of Cognitive Ability: Application
Client Needs: Safe, Effective Care Environment
Integrated Concept/Process: Teaching/Learning
Content Area: Maternity
Reference: Sherwen, L., Scoloveno, M.A., & Weingarten, C. (1999). *Maternity nursing: Care of the childbearing family* (3rd ed.). Stamford, Conn.: Appleton & Lange, p. 998.

13. 3
Rationale: A variety of conditions, including dehydration, hypoxemia, infection, and exertion, can stimulate the sickling

process during the intrapartum period. Maintaining adequate IV fluid intake and the administration of oxygen via facemask will help to ensure a safe environment for maternal and fetal health during labor. These measures will not stimulate the labor process, avoid the need for a cesarean delivery, or eliminate the need for analgesic administration.

Test-Taking Strategy: Note the relationship between "appropriate IV fluid intake and oxygen consumption" in the question and "prevent dehydration and hypoxemia" in the correct option. This relationship and knowledge regarding the care measures for sickle cell anemia will easily direct you to option 3. Review these care measures if you had difficulty with this question.

Level of Cognitive Ability: Application
Client Needs: Physiological Integrity
Integrated Concept/Process: Nursing Process/Implementation
Content Area: Maternity
Reference: Gorrie, T., McKinney, E., & Murray, S. (1998). *Foundations of maternal newborn nursing* (2nd ed.). Philadelphia: W.B. Saunders, pp. 727-729.

14. 3
Rationale: If the client complains of a headache and blurred vision, the physician should be notified because these are signs of worsening preeclampsia. Options 1, 2, and 4 are all normal signs.

Test-Taking Strategy: Use the process of elimination, noting the key word "worsening" in the stem of the question. Eliminate options 1, 2, and 4 because these options indicate normal findings. Review the signs that indicate a worsening of preeclampsia, if you had difficulty with this question.

Level of Cognitive Ability: Analysis
Client Needs: Physiological Integrity
Integrated Concept/Process: Nursing Process/Assessment
Content Area: Maternity
Reference: Lowdermilk, D., Perry, S., & Bobak, I. (2000). *Maternity & women's health care* (7th ed.). St. Louis: Mosby, p. 817.

15. 3
Rationale: Option 3 is a low priority because fundal height should be measured at each antepartal clinic visit, not in the intrapartum period. Options 1, 2, and 4 are all high priorities. Intrapartal management and assessment require careful attention to maternal and fetal status. The fetuses should be monitored by dual electronic fetal monitoring, and any signs of distress need to be reported to the physician or health care provider. A cesarean section may be necessary if a fetus is breech. The nurse should visually examine the perineum and vaginal opening for signs of the cord, which sometimes will prolapse through the cervix.

Test-Taking Strategy: Use the process of elimination and note the key words "lowest priority." Also note that the client is in early labor. With this in mind, think about the nursing interventions associated with early labor. Review care to the pregnant client with a twin pregnancy and a breech presentation if you had difficulty with this question.

Level of Cognitive Ability: Application
Client Needs: Physiological Integrity
Integrated Concept/Process: Nursing Process/Planning
Content Area: Maternity

Reference: Sherwen, L., Scoloveno, M.A., & Weingarten, C. (1999). *Maternity nursing: Care of the childbearing family* (3rd ed.). Stamford, Conn.: Appleton & Lange, p. 770.

16. 3

Rationale: Nurses should be able to explore measures that assist the family to create memories of the newborn infant so that the existence of the child is confirmed and the parents can complete the grieving process. Option 3 provides this support and demonstrates a caring and empathetic response. Options 1, 2, & 4 are blocks to communication and devalue the parents' feelings.

Test-Taking Strategy: Use the process of elimination and therapeutic communication techniques to answer the question. Option 3 is the only option that reflects use of therapeutic communication techniques. Review these techniques and the nursing strategies in caring for parents who experience perinatal death if you had difficulty with this question.

Level of Cognitive Ability: Application
Client Needs: Psychosocial Integrity
Integrated Concept/Process: Caring
Content Area: Maternity
Reference: Sherwen, L., Scoloveno, M.A., & Weingarten, C. (1999). *Maternity nursing: Care of the childbearing family* (3rd ed.). Stamford, Conn.: Appleton & Lange, pp. 330-331.

17. 3

Rationale: Exercise is safe for the client with gestational diabetes mellitus and is helpful in lowering the blood glucose level. Dietary modifications are the mainstay of treatment, and the client is placed on a standard diabetic diet. Many women are taught to perform blood glucose monitoring. If the woman is not performing the blood glucose monitoring at home, then it will be performed at the clinic or health care provider's office. Signs of infection need to be reported to the health care provider.

Test-Taking Strategy: Use the process of elimination, noting the key words "need for further education." Noting these key words and the absolute term "avoid" in option 3 will assist in answering the question. If you had difficulty with this question, review the teaching points for a client with gestational diabetes mellitus.

Level of Cognitive Ability: Application
Client Needs: Health Promotion and Maintenance
Integrated Concept/Process: Teaching/Learning
Content Area: Maternity
Reference: Lowdermilk, D., Perry, S., & Bobak, I. (2000). *Maternity & women's health care* (7th ed.). St. Louis: Mosby, p. 879.

18. 3

Rationale: Magnesium sulfate depresses the respiratory rate. If the respiratory rate is less than 12 breaths per minute, the physician or other health care provider needs to be notified and continuation of the medication needs to be reassessed. A urinary output of 20 mL in a 30-minute period is adequate; less that 30 mL in 1 hour needs to be reported. Deep tendon reflexes of 2+ are normal. The fetal heart tone is within normal limits for a resting fetus.

Test-Taking Strategy: Use the process of elimination. Note the key words "most concern" in the stem of the question. Knowledge of the normal and abnormal assessment findings will easily direct you to option 3. Review care to the client

receiving magnesium sulfate if you had difficulty with this question.

Level of Cognitive Ability: Analysis
Client Needs: Physiological Integrity
Integrated Concept/Process: Nursing Process/Assessment
Content Area: Maternity
Reference: Lowdermilk, D., Perry, S., & Bobak, I. (2000). *Maternity & women's health care* (7th ed.). St. Louis: Mosby, p. 831.

19. 3

Rationale: The immediate care during a seizure (eclampsia) is to ensure a patent airway. Options 1, 2, and 4 are all actions that follow or will be implemented after the seizure has ceased.

Test-Taking Strategy: Note the key words "first action" in the stem of the question. Use the ABCs—airway, breathing, and circulation—to answer the question. Remember that the airway is always the first priority. Review care to the client with eclampsia if you had difficulty with this question.

Level of Cognitive Ability: Application
Client Needs: Physiological Integrity
Integrated Concept/Process: Nursing Process/Implementation
Content Area: Maternity
Reference: Lowdermilk, D., Perry, S., & Bobak, I. (2000). *Maternity & women's health care* (7th ed.). St. Louis: Mosby, p. 834.

20. 1

Rationale: By seeing no way out of the situation except for death, the client meets the criteria for hopelessness. A person who lacks hope feels that life is too much to handle. Option 2 is a possible nursing diagnosis later, but there are not enough data to support it at this point. The data given do not support the nursing diagnosis of self-esteem disturbance. Option 4 is a possible nursing diagnosis at a later time; however, at this time the diagnosis of hopelessness should take precedence.

Test-Taking Strategy: Use the process of elimination. When answering a question regarding a nursing diagnosis, focus on the issue of the question and only on the data in the question. There are no data to support options 2, 3, or 4.

Level of Cognitive Ability: Analysis
Client Needs: Psychosocial Integrity
Integrated Concept/Process: Nursing Process/Analysis
Content Area: Maternity
Reference: Sherwen, L., Scoloveno, M.A., & Weingarten, C. (1999). *Maternity nursing: Care of the childbearing family* (3rd ed.). Stamford, Conn.: Appleton & Lange, p. 613.

CRITICAL THINKING: FREE-TEXT ENTRY

Answer: Hypertension, generalized edema, and proteinuria
Rationale: The three classic signs of preeclampsia are hypertension, generalized edema, and proteinuria.
Test-Taking Strategy: It is necessary to know the classic signs of preeclampsia to answer this question. If you had difficulty with this question, review preeclampsia and learn these signs.
Level of Cognitive Ability: Application
Client Needs: Health Promotion and Maintenance
Integrated Concept/Process: Nursing Process/Assessment
Content Area: Maternity
Reference: Gorrie, T., McKinney, E., & Murray, S. (1998). *Foundations of maternal newborn nursing* (2nd ed.). Philadelphia: W.B. Saunders, p. 693.

REFERENCES

Dickason, E., Silverman, B., & Kaplan, J. (1998). *Maternal-infant nursing care* (3rd ed.). St. Louis: Mosby.

Gorrie, T., McKinney, E., & Murray, S. (1998). *Foundations of maternal newborn nursing* (2nd ed.). Philadelphia: W.B. Saunders.

Lowdermilk, D., Perry, S., & Bobak, I. (2000). *Maternity & women's health care* (7th ed.). St. Louis: Mosby.

Sherwen, L., Scoloveno, M.A., & Weingarten, C. (1999). *Maternity nursing: Care of the childbearing family* (3rd ed.). Stamford, Conn.: Appleton & Lange.

26

Labor and Delivery

I. THE PROCESS OF LABOR

A. **Labor**
   1. Coordinated sequence of involuntary uterine contractions
   2. Results in effacement and dilation of the cervix, followed by expulsion of the products of conception
B. **Delivery:** Actual event of birth
C. Passenger: The fetus
D. Attitude
   1. The relationship of the fetal body parts to one another
   2. Normal intrauterine attitude is flexion, in which the fetal back is rounded, the head is forward on the chest, and the arms and legs are folded in against the body
E. Lie
   1. Relationship of the spine of the fetus to the spine of the mother
   2. Longitudinal or vertical
      a. Fetal spine is parallel to the mother's spine
      b. Fetus is either cephalic or breech presentation
   3. Transverse or horizontal
      a. Fetal spine is at a right angle, or perpendicular, to the mother's spine
      b. Presenting part is the shoulder
      c. **Delivery** by cesarean section
   4. Oblique
      a. Fetal spine is at a slight angle from a true horizontal lie
      b. **Delivery** is by cesarean section if uncorrectable
F. Presentation
   1. Presenting part: Portion of the fetus that enters the pelvis first
   2. Cephalic
      a. The most common presentation
      b. Fetal head presents first

   3. Breech
      a. Buttocks present first
      b. **Delivery** by cesarean section may be required, although it is often possible to deliver vaginally
   4. Shoulder
      a. Fetus is in a transverse lie, or the arm, back, abdomen, or side could present
      b. If the fetus does not spontaneously rotate or if it is not possible to turn the fetus manually, a cesarean section may be performed
G. Position: Relationship of assigned area of the presenting part or landmark to the maternal pelvis (Box 26-1)
H. Station
   1. The measurement of the progress of descent in centimeters above or below the midplane from the presenting part to the ischial spine
   2. Station 0: at ischial spine
   3. Minus station: above ischial spine
   4. Plus station: below ischial spine
I. Powers
   1. The forces acting to expel the fetus

BOX 26-1

Fetal Positions

ROA : Right occiput anterior
LOA: Left occiput anterior
ROP: Right occiput posterior
LOP: Left occiput posterior
ROT: Right occiput transverse
LOT: Left occiput transverse
RMA: Right mentum anterior
LMA: Left mentum anterior
RMP:Right mentum posterior
LSA: Left sacrum anterior
LSP: Left sacrum posterior

2. Effacement: Shortening and thinning of the cervix during the first stage of **labor**
3. Dilation: Enlargement of cervical os and cervical canal during first stage

II. MECHANISMS OF LABOR (Box 26-2)
A. Assessment
1. Lightening or dropping: Fetus descends into the pelvis about 2 weeks prior to **delivery** for a primipara; the fetus may engage into the pelvis after **labor** commences for a multipara
2. Braxton Hicks contractions increase
3. Show
4. Vaginal mucosa congested and vaginal mucus increases
5. Brownish or blood-tinged cervical mucus passed
6. Cervix ripens, becomes soft, partly effaced, and may begin to dilate
7. Sudden burst of energy

BOX 26-2

Mechanisms of Labor

Engagement
Mechanism by which the fetus nestles into the pelvis
Also termed lightening or dropping

Descent
The process that the fetal head undergoes as it begins its journey through the pelvis
A continuous process from the time of engagement until birth, and is assessed by the measurement called station

Flexion
Process of the fetal head's nodding forward toward the fetal chest

Internal Rotation
Internal rotation of the fetus; most commonly from the occiput transverse position, assumed at engagement into the pelvis, to the occiput anterior position while continuously descending

Extension
Enables the head to emerge when the fetus is in a cephalic position
Begins after the head crowns
Is complete when the head passes under the symphysis pubis and occiput, and the anterior fontanel, brow, face, and chin pass over the sacrum and coccyx and are over the perineum

Restitution
Realignment of the fetal head with the body after the head emerges

External Rotation
The shoulders externally rotate after the head emerges and restitution occurs, so that the shoulders are in the anteroposterior diameter of the pelvis

Expulsion
The birth of the entire body

---

8. Loss of 1 to 3 pounds from water loss resulting from fluid shifts produced by the changes in progesterone and estrogen levels
9. Spontaneous rupture of membranes
B. True **labor**
1. Contractions increase in duration and intensity
2. Cervical dilation and effacement are progressive
C. False **labor**
1. Exaggeration of normal contractions
2. Does not produce dilation, effacement, or descent
3. Contractions are irregular without progression
4. Walking has no effect on contractions and often relieves false **labor**

III. LEOPOLD'S MANEUVERS
A. Description: To determine position, presentation, and engagement
B. Preparation
1. Ask the mother to empty the bladder
2. Warm hands and apply them to the mother's abdomen with firm and gentle pressure
C. First maneuver
1. Determines which part of the fetus is in the fundus
2. Place palms on each side of the upper abdomen and palpate around the fundus
3. If the head is in the fundus, one would feel a hard, round, movable object
4. The buttocks will feel soft and have an irregular shape and are more difficult to move
D. Second maneuver
1. Move hands downward over each side of the abdomen, applying firm, even pressure
2. The fetus's back, which is a smooth, hard surface, should be felt on one side of the abdomen
3. Irregular knobs and lumps, which may be the hands, feet, elbows, and knees, will be felt on the opposite side of the abdomen
E. Third maneuver
1. Confirms fetal position
2. Place hand above the symphysis pubis
3. Bring thumb and fingers together and grasp the part of fetus between them (may be either the head or the buttocks)
F. Fourth maneuver
1. Used in the late stage of pregnancy to determine how far the fetus has descended into the pelvic inlet
2. Place hands on the sides of the lower abdomen, close to the midline
3. Slide hands downward and press inward
4. If it has been determined that the buttocks are in the fundus, then feel for the head
5. If the head cannot be felt, it has probably descended

▲ **IV. BREATHING TECHNIQUES**

A. Abdominal breathing
1. Used until **labor** is more advanced
2. The abdomen moves outward during inhalation and downward during exhalation
3. The rate remains slow, with approximately six to nine breaths per minute

B. Pant-pant-blow
1. Used in advanced **labor**
2. A more rapid pattern, consisting of two short blows from the mouth followed by a longer blow
3. All exhalations are a blowing motion

▲ **V. FETAL MONITORING**

A. Description
1. Displays fetal heart rate (FHR)
2. Monitors uterine activity
3. Assesses frequency, duration, and intensity of contractions
4. Assesses FHR in relation to maternal contractions
5. Baseline FHR is measured between contractions; the normal FHR is 120 to 160 beats per minute

B. External fetal monitoring
1. Noninvasive and performed by the use of a tocotransducer or Doppler ultrasonic transducer
2. Perform Leopold's maneuvers to determine on which side the fetal back is located, and place the ultrasound transducer over this area (fasten with a belt)
3. Place the tocotransducer over the fundus of the uterus where contractions feel the strongest (fasten with a belt)
4. Allow the client to assume a comfortable position, avoiding vena cava compression

C. Internal fetal monitoring
1. Invasive and requires rupturing of the membranes and attaching an electrode to the presenting part of the fetus
2. Mother must be dilated 2 to 3 cm to perform internal monitoring

D. Periodic patterns in the FHR
1. Fetal bradycardia and tachycardia
    a. Bradycardia: FHR is less than 120 beats per minute
    b. Tachycardia: FHR is greater than 160 beats per minute
    c. Change position of the mother and administer oxygen
    d. Notify the physician
2. Variability (Box 26-3)
    a. The fluctuations in the baseline FHR
    b. Short-term variability: changes in the FHR from one beat to the next (beat to beat); may be decreased by medications, fetal sleep, tachycardia, prematurity, hypoxia of the cen-

tral nervous system (CNS), or abnormalities of the CNS, heart, or both
    c. Long-term variability: broader fluctuations that are apparent over 1-minute intervals; vary with fetal sleep (diminish during sleep and increase when the fetus awakens)
    d. An FHR that fluctuates 6 to 25 beats per minute is considered reassuring
    e. Reassuring short-term variability: the beat-to-beat rate changes that occur over 1 minute of baseline FHR are at least 6 beats per minute (BPM) but lower than 25 BPM
    f. Reassuring long-term variability: there are three to six broad cycles of rate changes within the 6- to 25-BPM range
3. Accelerations
    a. Brief, temporary increases in the FHR of at least 15 beats above the baseline, lasting at least 15 seconds
    b. Usually a reassuring sign, reflecting a responsive, nonacidotic fetus
    c. Usually occur with fetal movement
    d. May be nonperiodic (having no relation to contractions) as well as periodic
    e. May occur with uterine contractions, vaginal examinations, or mild cord compression or when the fetus is in a breech presentation
4. Early decelerations
    a. Decrease in FHR below baseline; the rate at the lowest point of the deceleration usually remains above 100 BPM
    b. Occur during contractions as the fetal head is pressed against the woman's pelvis or soft tissues, such as the cervix, and return to the baseline FHR by the end of the contraction
    c. Tracing shows a uniform shape and mirror image of uterine contractions
    d. Not associated with fetal compromise and require no intervention
5. Late decelerations
    a. A nonreassuring pattern that reflects impaired **placental** exchange or uteroplacental insufficiency

---

BOX 26-3

Variability

Minimal Variability
Fetal heart rate fluctuates 3 to 5 beats per minute
Absent Variability
Fetal heart rate fluctuates 0 to 2 beats per minute
Sinusoidal Pattern
Presence of a uniform, long-term variability with no short-term variability in fetal heart rate

b. Look similar to early decelerations but begin well after the contraction begins, and return to baseline after the contraction ends

c. The degree of fall in the rate from baseline is not related to the amount of uteroplacental insufficiency

d. Interventions include improving **placental** blood flow and fetal oxygenation

6. Variable decelerations

a. Caused by conditions that restrict flow through the umbilical cord

b. Do not have the uniform appearance of early and late decelerations

c. Their shape, duration, and degree of fall below baseline rate are variable; they fall and rise abruptly with the onset and relief of cord compression

d. May also be nonperiodic, occurring at times unrelated to contractions

e. Baseline rate and variability are considered when variable decelerations are evaluated

f. Significant when the FHR repeatedly decreases to less than 70 BPM and persists at that level for at least 60 seconds before returning to the baseline

7. Hypertonic uterine activity

a. Assessment of uterine activity includes frequency, duration, intensity of the contractions, and uterine resting tone

b. The uterus should relax between contractions for 60 seconds or longer

c. Uterine contraction intensity is about 50 to 75 mm Hg (with the intrauterine uterine catheter) during **labor,** and may reach 110 mm Hg with pushing during the second stage

d. The average resting tone is 5 to 15 mm Hg

e. In hypertonic uterine activity, the uterine resting tone between contractions is high, reducing uterine blood flow and decreasing fetal oxygen supply

8. Interventions for nonreassuring patterns (Box 26-4)

a. Identify the cause (assess for cord prolapse)

b. Discontinue oxytocin (Pitocin) if infusing as prescribed

c. Change the mother's position (avoid the supine position for patterns associated with cord compression)

d. Administer oxygen by face mask at 8 to 10 L per minute

e. Increase IV fluids as prescribed

f. Notify the physician or nurse midwife as soon as possible

g. Prepare to initiate continuous electronic fetal monitoring with internal devices if not contraindicated

---

BOX 26-4

Nonreassuring Patterns

Tachycardia
Bradycardia
Decreased or absent variability
Late decelerations
Variable decelerations falling to less than 70 BPM for longer than 60 seconds
Prolonged decelerations
Hypertonic uterine activity

---

h. Prepare to obtain a fetal scalp pH monitor to determine a blood pH value

i. Prepare for cesarean **delivery** if necessary

VI. STAGES OF LABOR

A. Stage I latent phase

1. Assessment

a. Cervical dilation of 1 to 4 cm

b. Uterine contractions every 15 to 30 minutes, 15 to 30 seconds in duration and of mild intensity

c. Mother talkative and eager to be in **labor**

2. Implementation

a. Encourage mother and partner to participate in care

b. Assist with comfort measures, changes of position, and ambulation

c. Keep mother and partner informed of progress

d. Offer fluids and ice chips

e. Encourage voiding every 1 to 2 hours

B. Stage I active phase

1. Assessment

a. Cervical dilation of 4 to 7 cm

b. Uterine contractions every 3 to 5 minutes, 30 to 60 seconds in duration and of moderate intensity

c. Mother may experience feelings of helplessness

d. Mother becomes restless and anxious as contractions become stronger

2. Implementation

a. Encourage maintenance of effective breathing patterns

b. Provide a quiet environment

c. Keep mother and partner informed of progress

d. Promote comfort with backrubs, sacral pressure, pillow support, and position changes

e. Instruct partner in effleurage

f. Offer fluids and ice chips and ointment for dry lips

g. Encourage voiding every 1 to 2 hours

C. Stage I transition phase
 1. Assessment
    a. Cervical dilation of 8 to 10 cm
    b. Uterine contractions every 2 to 3 minutes, 45 to 90 seconds in duration and of strong intensity
    c. Mother becomes tired, is restless and irritable, and feels out of control
 2. Implementation
    a. Encourage rest between contractions
    b. Wake mother at beginning of contraction so she can begin breathing pattern
    c. Keep mother and partner informed of progress
    d. Provide privacy
    e. Offer fluids and ice chips and ointment for dry lips
    f. Encourage voiding every 1 to 2 hours
D. Implementation throughout stage I
    a. Monitor maternal vital signs
    b. Monitor FHR via ultrasound Doppler, fetoscope, or electronic fetal monitor
    c. Assess FHR before, during, and after a contraction, noting that the normal FHR is 120 to 160 beats per minute
    d. Monitor uterine contractions by palpation or monitor, determining frequency, duration, and intensity
    e. Assess status of cervical dilation and effacement
    f. Assess fetal station presentation and position by Leopold's maneuvers
    g. Assist with pelvic examination and prepare for a Nitrazine test and a fern test
    h. Assess the color of the **amniotic fluid** if the membranes have ruptured, because meconium-stained fluid can indicate fetal distress
E. Stage 2
 1. Assessment
    a. Cervical dilation is complete
    b. Progress of **labor** is measured by descent of fetal head through the birth canal (change in fetal station)
    c. Uterine contractions occur every 2 to 3 minutes, lasting 60 to 75 seconds, and the intensity is strong
    d. Increase in bloody show occurs
    e. Mother feels urge to bear down; assist mother in pushing efforts
 2. Implementation
    a. Perform assessments every 5 minutes
    b. Monitor maternal vital signs
    c. Monitor FHR via ultrasound Doppler, fetoscope, or electronic fetal monitor
    d. Assess FHR before, during, and after a contraction, noting that normal fetal heart rate is 120 to 160 beats per minute

    e. Monitor uterine contractions by palpation or monitor, determining frequency, duration, and intensity
    f. Provide mother with encouragement and praise and provide for rest between contractions
    g. Keep mother and partner informed of progress
    h. Maintain privacy
    i. Provide ice chips and ointment for dry lips
    j. Assist mother into a position that promotes comfort and assists pushing efforts, such as lithotomy, semisitting, kneeling, side-lying, or squatting
    k. Monitor for signs of approaching birth, such as perineal bulging or visualization of the fetal head
    l. Prepare for birth
F. Stage 3
 1. Assessment
    a. Contractions occur until **placenta** is born
    b. **Placental** separation and expulsion occur
    c. Birth of **placenta** occurs 5 to 30 minutes after birth of the baby
    d. Schultze's mechanism: Center portion of **placenta** separates first, and its shiny fetal surface emerges from the vagina
    e. Duncan's mechanism: Margin of **placenta** separates, and the dull, red, rough maternal surface emerges from the vagina first
 2. Implementation
    a. Assess maternal vital signs
    b. Assess uterine status
    c. Provide parents with an explanation regarding birth of the **placenta**
    d. Following birth of **placenta**, uterine fundus remains firm and is located 2 fingerbreadths below the umbilicus
    e. Examine **placenta** for cotyledons and membranes to verify that it is intact
    f. Assess mother for shivering and provide warmth
    g. Promote parental-neonatal attachment
G. Stage 4
 1. Description: the period of time from 1 to 4 hours after **delivery**
 2. Assessment
    a. Blood pressure returns to prelabor level
    b. Pulse is slightly lower than during **labor**
    c. Fundus remains contracted, in the midline, 1 to 2 fingerbreadths below the umbilicus
    d. **Lochia** is moderate or scant and is red
 3. Implementation
    a. Maternal assessments every 15 minutes for 1 hour, every 30 minutes for 1 hour, and hourly for 2 hours

b. Provide warm blankets

c. Apply icepacks to the perineum

d. Massage the uterus if needed and teach the mother to massage the uterus

e. Provide breastfeeding support as needed

f. Refer to Chapter 30 for information on caring for the **newborn**

VII. ANESTHESIA

A. Local anesthesia

1. Used for blocking pain during episiotomy

2. Administered just before the birth of baby

3. No effect on the fetus

B. Paracervical block

1. Used in the first stage of **labor**

2. Provides a rapid block of uterine pain

3. No effect on the perineal area

4. No effect on the ability to bear down

5. May cause fetal bradycardia

C. Pudendal block

1. Administered just before the birth of the baby

2. Injection site at pudendal nerve through a transvaginal route

3. Blocks perineal area for episiotomy

4. Effect lasts about 30 minutes

5. No effect on contractions or fetus

D. Epidural block

1. Injection site in epidural space at L3-L4

2. Administered after **labor** is established or just before a scheduled cesarean birth

3. Relieves pain from contractions and numbs vagina and perineum

4. May cause hypotension

5. Does not cause headache because the dura mater is not penetrated

6. Assess maternal blood pressure

7. Maintain the mother in side-lying position or place a rolled blanket beneath the right hip to displace the uterus from the vena cava

8. Administer IV fluids as prescribed

9. Increase fluids as prescribed if hypotension occurs

E. Spinal block

1. Injection site in spinal subarachnoid space at L3-L5

2. Administered just before birth

3. Relieves uterine and perineal pain and numbs vagina, perineum, and lower extremities

4. May cause maternal hypotension

5. May cause postpartum headache

6. The mother must lie flat 8 to 12 hours following spinal injection

7. Place a rolled blanket under the right hip to displace the uterus from the vena cava

8. Administer IV fluids as prescribed

F. General anesthesia

1. May be used for some surgical interventions

2. The mother is not awake

3. Presents a danger of respiratory depression and vomiting

VIII. OBSTETRICAL PROCEDURES

A. Bishop score (Box 26-5)

1. Used to determine maternal readiness for **labor**

2. Evaluates cervical status and fetal position

3. Indicated before the induction of **labor**

4. The five factors are assigned a score of 0 to 3, and the total score is calculated

5. A score of 6 or more indicates a readiness for **labor** induction

B. Induction

1. A deliberate initiation of uterine contractions that stimulates **labor**

2. Elective induction may be accomplished by oxytocin (Pitocin) infusion

3. Obtain baseline tracing of uterine contractions and FHR

4. Increase IV dosage of oxytocin as prescribed only after assessing contractions, FHR, and maternal blood pressure and pulse

5. Do not increase rate of oxytocin once the desired contraction pattern is obtained (contraction frequency of 2 to 3 minutes and lasting 60 seconds)

6. Discontinue oxytocin as prescribed if contraction frequency is less than 2 minutes or duration is more than 90 seconds, or if fetal distress is noted

C. Amniotomy

1. Artificial rupture of membranes (AROM); performed by the physician to stimulate **labor**

2. Performed if the fetus is at "0" or "+" station

3. Increases risk of prolapsed cord and infection

4. Monitor FHR before and after AROM

5. Record time of AROM, FHR, and characteristics of fluid

6. Meconium-stained **amniotic fluid** may be associated with fetal distress

7. Bloody **amniotic fluid** may indicate abruptio placentae or fetal trauma

8. An unpleasant odor to **amniotic fluid** is associated with infection

9. Polyhydramnios is associated with maternal diabetes and certain congenital disorders

10. Oligohydramnios is associated with intrauter-

BOX 26-5

Factors of the Bishop Score

Dilation of cervix
Effacement of cervix
Consistency of cervix
Position of cervix
Station of presenting part

ine growth retardation (IUGR) and congenital disorders

11. Expect more variable decelerations after rupture of the membranes, as a result of cord compression during contractions

12. Limit client activity if prescribed

D. External version
1. External manipulation of the fetus from an abnormal position into a normal presentation
2. Indicated for an abnormal presentation that exists after the 34th week
3. Monitor vital signs
4. If the mother is Rh-negative, ensure that RH immune globulin was given at 28 weeks' gestation
5. Prepare for nonstress test to evaluate fetal well-being
6. IV fluids and tocolytic therapy may be administered to relax the uterus and permit easier manipulation of fetus
7. Ultrasound is used during the procedure to evaluate fetal position and **placental** placement and guide direction to the fetus
8. Abdominal wall is manipulated to direct fetus into a cephalic presentation if possible
9. Monitor blood pressure to identify vena cava compression
10. Monitor for unusual pain
11. Following the procedure
   a. Perform nonstress test to evaluate fetal well-being
   b. Monitor for uterine activity, bleeding, ruptured membranes, and decreased fetal activity
   c. With Rh-negative clients, perform Kleihauer-Betke test as prescribed to detect the presence and amount of fetal blood in the maternal circulation and to identify clients who need additional Rh immune globulin

E. Episiotomy
1. Incision made into perineum to enlarge vaginal outlet and facilitate **delivery**
2. Check episiotomy site
3. Institute measures to relieve pain
4. Provide ice pack during the first 24 hours
5. Instruct the client in the use of sitz baths
6. Apply analgesic spray or ointment as prescribed
7. Provide perineal care, using clean technique
8. Instruct the client in the proper care of the incision
9. Instruct the client to dry the perineal area from front to back and to blot the area rather than wipe it
10. Instruct the client to shower rather than bathe in a tub
11. Apply a peripad without touching the inside surface of the pad

12. Report any bleeding or discharge to the physician

F. Forceps **delivery**
1. Two double-crossed, spoonlike articulated blades that are used to assist in the **delivery** of the fetal head
2. Reassure the mother and explain the need for forceps
3. Monitor mother and fetus during **delivery**
4. Check **neonate** and mother after **delivery** for any possible injury
5. Assist with repair of any lacerations

G. Vacuum extraction
1. A caplike suction device is applied to the fetal head to facilitate extraction
2. Suction is used to assist in **delivery** of the fetal head
3. Traction is applied during uterine contractions until descent of the fetal head is achieved
4. The suction device should not be kept in place any longer than 25 minutes
5. Monitor FHR every 5 minutes if external fetal monitoring is not used
6. Assess **newborn infant** at birth and throughout postpartum period for signs of cerebral trauma
7. Monitor for developing cephalohematoma
8. Caput succedaneum is normal and will resolve in 24 hours

H. Cesarean **delivery**
1. **Delivery** of the fetus usually through a transabdominal, low-segment incision of the uterus
2. Preoperative
   a. If planned, prepare the mother and partner
   b. If an emergency, quickly explain the need and procedure to the mother and partner
   c. Obtain informed consent
   d. Make sure that the preoperative diagnostic tests are done, including the Rh factor
   e. Prepare to insert an IV line and a Foley catheter
   f. Prepare the abdomen as prescribed
   g. Monitor the mother and fetus continuously for signs of **labor**
   h. Provide emotional support
   i. Administer preoperative medications as prescribed
3. Postoperative
   a. Monitor vital signs
   b. Provide pain relief
   c. Encourage turning, coughing, and deep breathing
   d. Encourage ambulation
   e. Monitor for signs of infection and bleeding
   f. Burning and pain on urination may indicate a bladder infection
   g. A tender uterus and foul-smelling **lochia** may indicate endometritis

h. A productive cough or chills may indicate pneumonia

i. A positive Homans' sign, pain, or edema of extremity may indicate thrombophlebitis

PRACTICE QUESTIONS

1. A nurse is caring for a client in labor. The nurse documents that the client is beginning the second stage of labor when which of the following assessments is noted?
   1. The client begins to expel clear vaginal fluid
   2. The contractions are regular
   3. The membranes have ruptured
   4. The cervix is completely dilated

2. A nurse in the labor room is caring for a client in the active stage of labor. The nurse is assessing the fetal patterns and notes a late deceleration on the monitor strip. The most appropriate nursing action is to:
   1. Place the mother in a supine position
   2. Document the findings and continue to monitor the fetal patterns
   3. Administer oxygen via face mask
   4. Increase the rate of the intravenous (IV) oxytocin (Pitocin) infusion

3. A nurse is performing an assessment of a client who is scheduled for a cesarean delivery. Which assessment finding would indicate a need to contact the physician?
   1. Fetal heart rate of 180 beats per minute
   2. White blood cell (WBC) count of 12,000/mm^3
   3. Maternal pulse rate of 85 beats per minute
   4. Hemoglobin of 11.0 g/dL

4. A client in labor is transported to the delivery room and is prepared for a cesarean delivery. The client is transferred to the delivery room table, and the nurse places the client in the:
   1. Trendelenburg position with the legs in stirrups
   2. Semi-Fowler's position with a pillow under the knees
   3. Prone position with the legs separated and elevated
   4. Supine position with a wedge under the right hip

5. A nurse has provided discharge instructions to a client who delivered a healthy newborn infant by cesarean delivery. Which statement if made by the client indicates a need for further education?
   1. "I will notify the physician if I develop a fever."
   2. "I will lift nothing heavier than the newborn infant for at least 2 weeks."
   3. "I will begin abdominal exercises immediately."
   4. "I will turn on my side and push up with my arms to get out of bed."

6. A nurse is caring for a client in labor and prepares to auscultate the fetal heart rate (FHR) by using a Doppler ultrasound device. The nurse most accurately determines that the fetal heart sounds are heard by:
   1. Noting if the heart rate is above 140 beats per minute
   2. Placing the diaphragm of the Doppler on the mother's abdomen
   3. Performing Leopold maneuvers first to determine the location of the fetal heart
   4. Palpating the maternal radial pulse while listening to the fetal heart rate

7. A nurse is caring for a client in labor who is receiving oxytocin (Pitocin) by intravenous infusion to stimulate uterine contractions. Which assessment finding would indicate to the nurse that the infusion needs to be discontinued?
   1. Three contractions occurring within a 10-minute period
   2. A fetal heart rate of 90 beats per minute
   3. Adequate resting tone of the uterus palpated between contractions
   4. Increased urinary output

8. A nurse is preparing to care for a client in labor. The physician has prescribed an intravenous infusion of oxytocin (Pitocin). The nurse ensures that which of the following is implemented prior to initiating the infusion?
   1. Placing the client on complete bed rest
   2. Continuous electronic fetal monitoring
   3. An intravenous infusion of antibiotics
   4. Placing a code cart at the client's bedside

9. A nurse is monitoring a client in active labor and notes that the client is having contractions every 3 minutes that last 45 seconds. The nurse notes that the fetal heart rate between contractions is 100 beats per minute. Which of the following nursing actions is most appropriate?
   1. Encourage the client's coach to continue to encourage breathing techniques
   2. Encourage the client to continue pushing with each contraction
   3. Continue monitoring the fetal heart rate
   4. Notify the physician or nurse-midwife

10. A nurse is caring for a client in labor and is monitoring the fetal heart rate patterns. The nurse notes the presence of episodic accelerations on the electronic fetal monitor tracing. Which of the following actions is most appropriate?
    1. Document the findings and tell the mother that the monitor indicates fetal well-being
    2. Take the mother's vital signs and tell the mother that bed rest is now required to conserve oxygen
    3. Notify the physician or nurse-midwife of the findings
    4. Reposition the mother and check the monitor for changes in the fetal tracing

11. A nurse is admitting a pregnant client to the labor room and attaches an external electronic fetal monitor to the client's abdomen. After attachment of the electronic fetal monitor, the initial nursing assessment is which of the following?
    1. Identifying the types of accelerations
    2. Assessing the baseline fetal heart rate
    3. Determining the frequency of the contractions
    4. Determining the intensity of the contractions

12. A nurse is reviewing the record of a client in the labor room and notes that the nurse midwife has documented that the fetus is at minus one station. The nurse determines that the fetal presenting part is:
    1. 1 cm above the ischial spine
    2. 1 fingerbreadth below the symphysis pubis
    3. 1 inch below the coccyx
    4. 1 inch below the iliac crest

13. A pregnant client is admitted to the labor room. An assessment is performed, and the nurse notes that the client's hemoglobin and hematocrit levels are low, indicating anemia. Which nursing diagnosis does the nurse include in the plan of care?
    1. Anxiety
    2. Low self-esteem
    3. Risk for cerebrovascular accident (CVA)
    4. Potential for postpartum infection

14. A nurse assists in the vaginal delivery of a newborn infant. After the delivery, the nurse observes the umbilical cord lengthen and a spurt of blood from the vagina. The nurse documents these observations as signs of:
    1. Hematoma
    2. Placenta previa
    3. Uterine atony
    4. Placental separation

15. A client arrives at a birthing center in active labor. Her membranes are still intact. A nurse-midwife prepares to perform an amniotomy. A nurse who is assisting the nurse-midwife explains to the client that after this procedure, she will most likely have:
    1. Less pressure on her cervix
    2. Increased efficiency of contractions
    3. Decreased number of contractions
    4. The need for increased maternal blood pressure (BP) monitoring

16. A nurse is monitoring a client in labor. The nurse suspects umbilical cord compression if which of the following is noted on the external monitor tracing during a contraction?
    1. Early decelerations
    2. Variable decelerations
    3. Late decelerations
    4. Short-term variability

17. A nurse explains the purpose of effleurage to a client in early labor. The nurse tells the client that effleurage is:
    1. A form of biofeedback to enhance bearing down efforts during delivery
    2. Light stroking of the abdomen to facilitate relaxation during labor and provide tactile stimulation to the fetus
    3. The application of pressure to the sacrum to relieve a backache
    4. Performed to stimulate uterine activity by contracting a specific muscle group while other parts of the body rest

18. A client in labor has been pushing effectively for 1 hour and is 8 cm dilated. A nurse determines that the client's primary physiological need at this time is to:
    1. Change positions frequently
    2. Ambulate
    3. Consume oral food and fluids
    4. Rest between contractions

19. A low-risk client is dilated 10 cm and feeling the urge to push with contractions. At this time during labor, the nurse should plan to assess and document the fetal heart rate at least:
    1. Before each contraction
    2. Every 15 minutes
    3. Every 30 minutes
    4. Hourly

20. A nurse is caring for a client in the second stage of labor. The client is experiencing uterine contractions every 2 minutes. The client cries out in pain with the pushing efforts. The nurse recognizes this behavior as:
    1. Exhaustion
    2. Fear of losing control
    3. Involuntary grunting
    4. Valsalva's maneuver

CRITICAL THINKING: FREE-TEXT ENTRY

A nurse is monitoring a client in labor, and the client's membranes rupture spontaneously. What is the initial nursing action?

Answer: _____

ANSWERS

1. 4

Rationale: The second stage of labor begins when the cervix is completely dilated and ends with birth of the neonate. Options 1, 2, and 3 are not specific assessment findings of the second stage of labor.

Test-Taking Strategy: Use the process of elimination. Eliminate options 1 and 3 first because they are similar. From the remaining options, recalling that regular contractions occur prior to the second stage of labor will easily direct you to option 4. Review the stages of labor if you had difficulty with this question.

Level of Cognitive Ability: Analysis
Client Needs: Physiological Integrity
Integrated Concept/Process: Communication and Documentation
Content Area: Maternity
Reference: Lowdermilk, D., Perry, S., & Bobak, I. (2000). *Maternity & women's health care* (7th ed.). St. Louis: Mosby, p. 457.

2. 3

Rationale: Late decelerations are due to uteroplacental insufficiency as the result of decreased blood flow and oxygen to the fetus during the uterine contractions. This causes hypoxemia; therefore, oxygen is necessary. The supine position is avoided because it decreases uterine blood flow to the fetus. The client should be turned onto her side to displace pressure of the gravid uterus on the inferior vena cava. An IV oxytocin infusion is discontinued when a late deceleration is noted. The oxytoxin would cause further hypoxemia because of increased uteroplacental insufficiency resulting from stimulation of contractions by this medication. Option 2 would delay necessary treatment.

Test-Taking Strategy: Use the ABCs—airway, breathing, and circulation—and knowledge related to the significance of a late deceleration to answer this question. Review content related to late deceleration if you had difficulty with this question.

Level of Cognitive Ability: Application
Client Needs: Physiological Integrity
Integrated Concept/Process: Nursing Process/Implementation
Content Area: Maternity
Reference: Lowdermilk, D., Perry, S., & Bobak, I. (2000). *Maternity & women's health care* (7th ed.). St. Louis: Mosby, p. 500.

3. 1

Rationale: A normal fetal heart rate is 120 to 160 beats per minute. A count of 180 beats per minute could indicate fetal distress and would warrant physician notification. WBC counts in a normal pregnancy begin to rise in the second trimester and peak in the third trimester, with a normal range of 11,000 to 15,000/mm^3, up to 18,000/mm^3. During the immediate postpartum period the count may be as high as 25,000 to 30,000/mm^3 as a result of increased leukocytosis during delivery. By full term, a normal maternal hemoglobin range is 11 to 13 g/dL as a result of the hemodilution caused by an increase in plasma volume during pregnancy. The maternal pulse rate during pregnancy increases 10 to 15 beats per minute over pre-pregnancy readings to facilitate increased cardiac output, oxygen transport, and kidney filtration.

Test-Taking Strategy: Use the process of elimination, noting the key words "indicate a need to contact the physician." Knowledge regarding the normal and abnormal findings in the pregnant client and the fetus will direct you to option 1. If you are unfamiliar with these normal and abnormal findings, review this content.

Level of Cognitive Ability: Analysis
Client Needs: Safe, Effective Care Environment
Integrated Concept/Process: Communication and Documentation
Content Area: Maternity
Reference: Lowdermilk, D., Perry, S., & Bobak, I. (2000). *Maternity & women's health care* (7th ed.). St. Louis: Mosby, pp. 493, 1155.

4. 4

Rationale: Vena cava and descending aorta compression by the pregnant uterus impedes blood return from the lower trunk and extremities. This leads to decreasing cardiac return, cardiac output, and blood flow to the uterus and subsequently the fetus. The best position to prevent this would be side-lying with the uterus displaced off the abdominal vessels. Positioning for abdominal surgery necessitates a supine position; however, a wedge placed under the right hip provides displacement of the uterus. Trendelenburg positioning places pressure from the pregnant uterus on the diaphragm and lungs, decreasing respiratory capacity and oxygenation. A semi-Fowler's or prone position is not practical for this type of abdominal surgery.

Test-Taking Strategy: Knowledge regarding vena cava syndrome and the appropriate position to prevent this syndrome is required to answer this question. Use the process of elimination, visualizing each of the positions identified in the options and considering the effect that the position may have on the mother and the fetus. If you had difficulty with this question, review care of the mother requiring cesarean delivery.

Level of Cognitive Ability: Application
Client Needs: Physiological Integrity
Integrated Concept/Process: Nursing Process/Implementation
Content Area: Maternity
Reference: Lowdermilk, D., Perry, S., & Bobak, I. (2000). *Maternity & women's health care* (7th ed.). St. Louis: Mosby, p. 1006.

5. 3

Rationale: Abdominal exercises should not start immediately following abdominal surgery and the client should wait at least 3 to 4 weeks postoperatively to allow for healing of the incision. Options 1, 2, and 4 are appropriate instructions for the client following a cesarean delivery.

Test-Taking Strategy: Use the process of elimination. Note the key words "indicates a need for further education." Keep in mind that the client had a cesarean delivery and noting the absolute term "immediately" in option 3 will assist in directing you to this option. Review home care instructions for the client following cesarean delivery if you had difficulty with this question.

Level of Cognitive Ability: Analysis
Client Needs: Health Promotion and Maintenance
Integrated Concept/Process: Teaching/Learning
Content Area: Maternity

Reference: Sherwen, L., Scoloveno, M.A., & Weingarten, C. (1999). *Maternity nursing: Care of the childbearing family* (3rd ed.). Stamford, Conn.: Appleton & Lange, p. 807.

6. **4**

Rationale: The nurse should simultaneously palpate the maternal radial or carotid pulse and auscultate the FHR to differentiate the two. If the fetal and maternal heart rates are similar, the nurse may mistake the maternal heart rate for the FHR. Noting if the heart rate is above 140 beats per minute or placing the diaphragm of the Doppler on the mother's abdomen will not ensure accuracy in obtaining the FHR. Leopold maneuvers may help the examiner locate the position of the fetus but will not ensure a distinction between the two rates.

Test-Taking Strategy: Use the process of elimination and focus on the key words "most accurately determines." Option 4 is the only option that identifies an action that will directly distinguish the maternal heart rate from the FHR. Review FHR monitoring if you had difficulty with this question.

Level of Cognitive Ability: Analysis
Client Needs: Physiological Integrity
Integrated Concept/Process: Nursing Process/Implementation
Content Area: Maternity
Reference: Olds, S., London. M., & Ladewig, P. (2000). *Maternal-newborn nursing: A family and community-based approach* (6th ed.). Upper Saddle River, N.J.: Prentice-Hall Health, p. 518.

7. **2**

Rationale: A normal fetal heart rate is 120 to 160 beats per minute. Bradycardia or late or variable decelerations indicate fetal distress and the need to discontinue the oxytocin. The goal of labor augmentation is to achieve three good-quality contractions (appropriate intensity and duration) in a 10-minute period. The uterus should return to resting tone between contractions, and there should be no evidence of fetal distress. Increased urinary output is unrelated to the use of oxytocin.

Test-Taking Strategy: Use the process of elimination and note the key words "infusion needs to be discontinued." Eliminate option 4 first because it is unrelated to the use of oxytocin. Next eliminate option 3 because of the key words "adequate resting tone." From the remaining options, knowing that the normal fetal heart rate is 120 to 160 beats per minute will easily direct you to option 2. Review monitoring the client receiving an oxytocin infusion if you had difficulty with this question.

Level of Cognitive Ability: Analysis
Client Needs: Physiological Integrity
Integrated Concept/Process: Nursing Process/Analysis
Content Area: Maternity
Reference: Olds, S., London. M., & Ladewig, P. (2000). *Maternal-newborn nursing: A family and community-based approach* (6th ed.). Upper Saddle River, N.J.: Prentice-Hall Health, p. 661.

8. **2**

Rationale: Continuous electronic fetal monitoring should be implemented during an intravenous infusion of oxytocin. There are no data in the question that indicate the need for complete bed rest or the need for antibiotics. It is not necessary to place a code cart at the bedside of a client receiving an oxytocin infusion.

Test-Taking Strategy: Use the process of elimination and the ABCs—airway, breathing, and circulation—to assist in answering the question. Option 2 is the only option that addresses oxygenation and circulation. If you had difficulty with this question, review the nursing considerations related to the administration of oxytocin.

Level of Cognitive Ability: Application
Client Needs: Physiological Integrity
Integrated Concept/Process: Nursing Process/Planning
Content Area: Maternity
Reference: Olds, S., London. M., & Ladewig, P. (2000). *Maternal-newborn nursing: A family and community-based approach* (6th ed.). Upper Saddle River, N.J.: Prentice-Hall Health, p. 660.

9. **4**

Rationale: A normal fetal heart rate is 120 to 160 beats per minute. Fetal bardycardia between contractions may indicate the need for immediate medical management and the physician or nurse mid-wife needs to be notified. Options 1, 2, and 3 are not appropriate nursing actions in this situation.

Test-Taking Strategy: Use the process of elimination. Knowledge that the normal fetal heart rate is 120 to 160 beats per minute will easily assist you in recognizing that fetal bradycardia is present. If you had difficulty with this question, review the expected and unexpected findings during the labor process.

Level of Cognitive Ability: Application
Client Needs: Physiological Integrity
Integrated Concept/Process: Nursing Process/Implementation
Content Area: Maternity
Reference: Lowdermilk, D., Perry, S., & Bobak, I. (2000). *Maternity & women's health care* (7th ed.). St. Louis: Mosby, p. 493.

10. **1**

Rationale: Accelerations are transient increases in the fetal heart rate that often accompany contractions or are caused by fetal movement. Episodic accelerations are thought to be a sign of fetal well-being and adequate oxygen reserve. Options 2, 3, and 4 are inaccurate nursing actions and are unnecessary.

Test-Taking Strategy: Use the process of elimination. Note that options 2, 3, and 4 are similar in that they indicate the need for further intervention. Knowing that accelerations indicate fetal well-being will easily direct you to option 1. Review the significance of episodic accelerations if you had difficulty with this question.

Level of Cognitive Ability: Application
Client Needs: Physiological Integrity
Integrated Concept/Process: Nursing Process/Implementation
Content Area: Maternity
Reference: Lowdermilk, D., Perry, S., & Bobak, I. (2000). *Maternity & women's health care* (7th ed.). St. Louis: Mosby, p. 496.

11. **2**

Rationale: Assessing the baseline fetal heart rate is important so that abnormal variations of the baseline rate will be identified if they occur. The intensity of contractions is assessed by an internal fetal monitor, not an external fetal monitor. Options 1 and 3 are important to assess but not as the first priority. Fetal heart rate is evaluated by assessing both baseline and periodic changes. Periodic changes occur in response to intermittent stress of uterine contractions and the baseline beat-to-beat variability of the fetal heart rate.

Test-Taking Strategy: Use the process of elimination. Note the key word "initial" in the stem of the question. Use the ABCs—airway, breathing, and circulation. Fetal heart rate reflects the ABCs. Review the concepts related to external fetal monitoring if you had difficulty with this question.

Level of Cognitive Ability: Application
Client Needs: Physiological Integrity
Integrated Concept/Process: Nursing Process/Assessment
Content Area: Maternity
Reference: Olds, S., London. M., & Ladewig, P. (2000). *Maternal-newborn nursing: A family and community-based approach* (6th ed.). Upper Saddle River, N.J.: Prentice-Hall Health, p. 523.

12. 1
Rationale: Station is the relationship of the presenting part to an imaginary line drawn between the ischial spines, is measured in centimeters, and is noted as a negative number above the line and a positive number below the line. At minus one station, the fetal presenting part is 1 cm above the ischial spines.

Test-Taking Strategy: Use the process of elimination. Knowledge that station is measured in centimeters and utilizes the ischial spines as a reference point will assist in answering this question. Note that options 2, 3, and 4 are similar in the use of "below," which would be represented by a positive measurement in determining station. Review stations of the presenting part if you had difficulty with this question.

Level of Cognitive Ability: Analysis
Client Needs: Physiological Integrity
Integrated Concept/Process: Nursing Process/Analysis
Content Area: Maternity
Reference: Lowdermilk, D., Perry, S., & Bobak, I. (2000). *Maternity & women's health care* (7th ed.). St. Louis: Mosby, p. 448.

13. 4
Rationale: Anemic women have a greater likelihood of cardiac failure during labor, postpartum infection, and/or poor wound healing. Anemia does not specifically present a risk for CVA. Both anxiety and low self-esteem are unrelated to physiological integrity.

Test-Taking Strategy: Use the process of elimination and Maslow's Hierarchy of Needs theory. Eliminate options 1 and 2 first because they are not physiological needs. From the remaining options, eliminate option 3 because it is a medical diagnosis. Review the risks associated with anemia in pregnancy if you had difficulty with this question.

Level of Cognitive Ability: Analysis
Client Needs: Physiological Integrity
Integrated Concept/Process: Nursing Process/Analysis
Content Area: Maternity
Reference: Lowdermilk, D., Perry, S., & Bobak, I. (2000). *Maternity & women's health care* (7th ed.). St. Louis: Mosby, p. 363.

14. 4
Rationale: As the placenta separates, it settles downward into the lower uterine segment. The umbilical cord lengthens, and a sudden trickle or spurt of blood appears. Options 1, 2, and 3 are incorrect interpretations.

Test-Taking Strategy: Use the process of elimination. Options 1, 2, and 3 are similar in that they identify complications of pregnancy. Option 4 indicates a normal finding following delivery of the newborn infant vaginally. Review this stage of labor if you had difficulty with this question.

Level of Cognitive Ability: Comprehension
Client Needs: Physiological Integrity
Integrated Concept/Process: Communication and Documentation
Content Area: Maternity
Reference: Gorrie, T., McKinney, E., & Murray, S. (1998). *Foundations of maternal-newborn nursing* (2nd ed.). Philadelphia: W.B. Saunders, p. 289.

15. 2
Rationale: Amniotomy (artificial rupture of the membranes [AROM]) can be used to induce labor when the condition of the cervix is favorable (ripe) or to augment labor if the progress begins to slow. Rupturing of membranes allows the fetal head to contact the cervix more directly and may increase the efficiency of contractions. It is not necessary to perform increased maternal BP monitoring following this procedure. The fetal heart rate, however, needs to be monitored frequently.

Test-Taking Strategy: Use the process of elimination. Recalling that AROM is performed to augment labor if the progress begins to slow will easily direct you to option 2. Review the purpose of AROM if you had difficulty with this question.

Level of Cognitive Ability: Application
Client Needs: Physiological Integrity
Integrated Concept/Process: Communication and Documentation
Content Area: Maternity
Reference: Lowdermilk, D., Perry, S., & Bobak, I. (2000). *Maternity & women's health care* (7th ed.). St. Louis: Mosby, p. 993.

16. 2
Rationale: Variable decelerations occur if the umbilical cord becomes compressed, thus reducing blood flow between the placenta and the fetus. Early decelerations result from pressure on the fetal head during a contraction. Late decelerations are an ominous pattern in labor because it suggests uteroplacental insufficiency during a contraction. Short-term variability refers to the beat-to beat range in the fetal heart rate.

Test-Taking Strategy: Use the process of elimination, focusing on the key issue, umbilical cord compression. Recalling that variable decelerations occur if the umbilical cord becomes compressed will easily direct you to option 2. Review the findings in umbilical cord compression if you had difficulty with this question.

Level of Cognitive Ability: Analysis
Client Needs: Physiological Integrity
Integrated Concept/Process: Nursing Process/Assessment
Content Area: Maternity
Reference: Ladewig, P., London. M., & Olds, S. (1998). *Maternal-newborn nursing care: The nurse, the family, and the community* (4th ed.). Menlo Park, Calif.: Addison-Wesley Longman, p. 384.

17. 2
Rationale: Effleurage is a specific type of cutaneous stimulation involving light stroking of the abdomen and is used prior to

transition to promote relaxation and relieve mild to moderate pain. It provides tactile stimulation to the fetus. Options 1, 3, and 4 are inaccurate descriptions of effleurage.
Test-Taking Strategy: Use the process of elimination. Focus on the key words "in early labor" to eliminate option 1. Eliminate option 3 because not all clients in labor experience backache. Eliminate option 4 because it focuses on stimulation of uterine activity rather than relaxation. Review the components of effleurage if you had difficulty with this question.
Level of Cognitive Ability: Comprehension
Client Needs: Psychosocial Integrity
Integrated Concept/Process: Teaching/Learning
Content Area: Maternity
Reference: Olds, S., London. M., & Ladewig, P. (2000). *Maternal-newborn nursing: A family and community-based approach* (6th ed.). Upper Saddle River, N.J.: Prentice-Hall Health, p. 219.

18. **4**
Rationale: The birth process expends a great deal on energy. Encouraging rest between contractions conserves maternal energy, facilitating voluntary pushing efforts with contractions. Uteroplacental perfusion is also enhanced, which promotes fetal tolerance of the stress of labor. Changing positions frequently is not the primary physiological need. Ambulation is encouraged during early labor. Ice chips should be provided. Food and fluids are likely to be withheld at this time.
Test-Taking Strategy: Use the process of elimination. Focusing on the key words "pushing effectively" will assist in directing you to option 4. Review care to the client in the transition stage of labor if you had difficulty with this question.
Level of Cognitive Ability: Analysis
Client Needs: Physiological Integrity
Integrated Concept/Process: Nursing Process/Analysis
Content Area: Maternity
Reference: Olds, S., London. M., & Ladewig, P. (2000). *Maternal-newborn nursing: A family and community-based approach* (6th ed.). Upper Saddle River, N.J.: Prentice-Hall Health, p. 560.

19. **2**
Rationale: The second stage of labor begins when the cervix is completely dilated (10 cm). Maternal pulse, blood pressure, and fetal heart rate are assessed every 5 to 15 minutes; some agency protocols recommend assessment after each contraction. Options 3 and 4 represent lengthy time intervals for assessment in this stage of labor.
Test-Taking Strategy: Use the process of elimination and focus on the data in the question, dilated 10 cm. Noting the key words "at least" will assist in directing you to the option that identifies the most frequent time frame. Review care of the client in the second stage of labor if you had difficulty with this question.
Level of Cognitive Ability: Application
Client Needs: Physiological Integrity
Integrated Concept/Process: Nursing Process/Planning
Content Area: Maternity
Reference: Olds, S., London. M., & Ladewig, P. (2000). *Maternal-newborn nursing: A family and community-based approach* (6th ed.). Upper Saddle River, N.J.: Prentice-Hall Health, p. 563.

20. **2**
Rationale: Pains, helplessness, panicking, and fear of losing control are possible behaviors in the second stage of labor. Options 1, 3, and 4 are not indicative of the description provided in the question.
Test-Taking Strategy: Use the process of elimination, focusing on the information provided in the question. Recalling that during the second stage of labor the woman may feel out of control will direct you to option 2. Review maternal behavioral responses during the second stage of labor if you had difficulty with this question.
Level of Cognitive Ability: Analysis
Client Needs: Psychosocial Integrity
Integrated Concept/Process: Nursing Process/Assessment
Content Area: Maternity
Reference: Olds, S., London. M., & Ladewig, P. (2000). *Maternal-newborn nursing: A family and community-based approach* (6th ed.). Upper Saddle River, N.J.: Prentice-Hall Health, p. 560.

CRITICAL THINKING: FREE-TEXT ENTRY

Answer: Assess the fetal heart rate
Rationale: When the membranes rupture in the birth setting, the nurse immediately assesses the fetal heart rate to detect changes associated with prolapse or compression of the umbilical cord.
Test-Taking Strategy: Use the principles of prioritizing to answer this question. Remember the ABCs—airway, breathing, and circulation. Fetal heart rate is associated with fetal breathing and circulation. If you had difficulty with this question, review initial nursing actions when ruptured membranes occur.
Level of Cognitive Ability: Application
Client Needs: Physiological Integrity
Integrated Concept/Process: Nursing Process/Implementation
Content Area: Maternity
Reference: Lowdermilk, D., Perry, S., & Bobak, I. (2000). *Maternity & women's health care* (7th ed.). St. Louis: Mosby, p. 536.

REFERENCES

Gorrie, T., McKinney, E., & Murray, S. (1998). *Foundations of maternal-newborn nursing* (2nd ed.). Philadelphia: W.B. Saunders.

Ladewig, P., London. M., & Olds, S. (1998). *Maternal-newborn nursing care: The nurse, the family, and the community* (4th ed.). Menlo Park, Calif.: Addison-Wesley Longman.

Lowdermilk, D., Perry, S., & Bobak, I. (2000). *Maternity & women's health care* (7th ed.). St. Louis: Mosby.

Olds, S., London. M., & Ladewig, P. (2000). *Maternal-newborn nursing: A family and community-based approach* (6th ed.). Upper Saddle River, N.J.: Prentice-Hall Health.

Sherwen, L., Scoloveno, M.A., & Weingarten, C. (1999). *Maternity nursing: Care of the childbearing family* (3rd ed.). Stamford, Conn.: Appleton & Lange.

Problems with Labor and Delivery

I. DYSTOCIA

A. Description
   1. Difficult **labor** that is prolonged or more painful
   2. Occurs because of problems caused by uterine contractions, the fetus, or the bones and tissues of the maternal pelvis
   3. Contractions may be hypotonic or hypertonic
   4. Fetus may be excessively large, malpositioned, or in an abnormal presentation
   5. Can result in maternal dehydration, infection, fetal injury or death

B. Assessment
   1. Excessive abdominal pain
   2. Abnormal contraction pattern
   3. Fetal distress
   4. Maternal or fetal tachycardia
   5. Lack of progress in **labor**

C. Implementation
   1. Assess fetal heart rate (FHR); monitor for fetal distress
   2. Monitor uterine contractions
   3. Monitor maternal temperature and heart rate
   4. Assist with pelvic examination, measurements, ultrasounds, and other procedures
   5. Administer prophylactic antibiotics as prescribed to prevent infection
   6. Administer IV fluids as prescribed
   7. Monitor intake & output (I & O)
   8. Assess for dehydration
   9. Instruct the mother in breathing techniques and relaxation exercises
   10. Fetal monitoring if oxytocin (Pitocin) is prescribed
   11. Monitor color of **amniotic fluid**
   12. Provide rest and comfort as with a normal **delivery**, such as backrubs and position changes
   13. Assess mother's fatigue and pain and administer sedatives and pain medications as prescribed
   14. Assess for prolapse of the cord after rupture of the membranes
   15. If prolapse occurs
       a. Place mother in Trendelenburg's or knee-chest position to minimize pressure on the cord
       b. Administer oxygen
       c. Notify the physician
       d. Prepare for emergency cesarean section

II. PRECIPITOUS LABOR AND DELIVERY

A. Description: **Labor** lasts less than 3 hours
B. Implementation
   1. Stay with the mother at all times
   2. Provide emotional support and keep the mother calm
   3. Encourage the mother to pant between contractions
   4. Prepare for rupturing membranes when head crowns if they are not already ruptured
   5. Do not try to keep fetus from being delivered
   6. If **delivery** is necessary:
      a. Apply gentle pressure to fetal head upward toward the vagina to prevent damage to the fetal head and vaginal lacerations
      b. Deliver fetus between contractions, checking for the cord around the neck
      c. Use restitution to deliver the posterior shoulder
      d. Use gentle downward pressure to move the anterior shoulder under the pubic symphysis

e. Clear the **neonate's** mouth

f. Dry and cover the **neonate** to keep the body warm

g. Allow **placenta** to separate naturally

h. Place **newborn infant** on mother's abdomen or breast to induce uterine contractions

III. PRETERM LABOR

A. Description

1. **Labor** occurring after the 20th week but before the 37th week

2. Contractions occurring at least once every 10 minutes and lasting 30 seconds or longer

3. Documented cervical change or cervical effacement of 80% or dilatation of 2 cm

B. Assessment

1. Increased or bloody discharge

2. Backache

3. Pressure and cramping

4. Palpable uterine contractions

5. Diarrhea

C. Implementation

1. Maintain bed rest, a quiet environment, and a lateral recumbent position

2. Administer tocolytic agents as prescribed to suppress **labor**

3. Prepare for the administration of betamethasone to stimulate fetal lung maturity when preterm **delivery** appears inevitable

4. If magnesium sulfate is prescribed:

a. Assess effects of medication on **labor** and fetus

b. Monitor FHR

c. Monitor maternal reflexes

d. Have antidote (calcium gluconate) available at bedside

e. Monitor vital signs

f. Monitor for hypotension

g. Auscultate lungs and monitor for an increased respiratory rate and fluid overload, which may indicate pulmonary edema

IV. RUPTURE OF UTERUS

A. Description: Complete or incomplete separation of the uterine tissue as a result of rupture of the uterus from the stress of **labor**

B. Complete rupture of the uterus

1. Pain, which is shearing, excruciating, diffuse or localized

2. Contractions may stop or fail to progress

3. Relaxation between contractions is incomplete

4. Rigid abdomen

5. Signs of maternal shock

6. Absent FHR

7. Fetus palpated outside the uterus

C. Incomplete rupture of the uterus

1. Abdominal pain that occurs during contractions

2. Cervix fails to dilate

3. Slight vaginal bleeding

4. Absent FHR

D. Implementation

1. Monitor maternal vital signs and FHR

2. Prepare client for cesarean section or hysterotomy with hysterectomy

3. Provide emotional support for client and partner

4. Monitor for and treat signs of shock

V. PLACENTA PREVIA

A. Description

1. Improperly implanted **placenta** in the lower uterine segment near or over the internal cervical os

2. Total: The internal os is entirely covered by the **placenta** when the cervix is fully dilated

3. Partial: Incomplete coverage of the internal os

4. Marginal: Only an edge of the **placenta** extends to the internal os but may extend onto the os during dilation of the cervix during **labor**

5. Low-lying **placenta**: The **placenta** is implanted in the lower uterine segment but does not reach the os

B. Assessment

1. Painless bleeding as early as 7 months; bleeding may be mild to hemorrhage

2. Soft uterus

3. Abnormal fetal position of breech or transverse lie

4. High presenting part

5. Uterine contractions

6. Anemia

C. Implementation

1. Monitor maternal vital signs, FHR, and fetal activity

2. Assess bleeding, including amount and quality

3. Maintain bed rest

4. Place client in left lateral position

5. Administer IV fluids as prescribed

6. Monitor and treat signs of shock

7. Avoid vaginal examination if bleeding is occurring

8. Prepare for ultrasound for **placental** localization

9. Administer iron supplements or blood transfusions as prescribed to maintain a hematocrit level above 30%

10. Prepare to administer Rh immune globulin if the mother is Rh negative and has not been given the injection at 28 weeks' gestation

11. Prepare for premature birth or cesarean section

VI. ABRUPTIO PLACENTAE

A. Description: Premature separation of the **placenta** from the uterine wall after the 20th week of gestation and before the fetus is delivered

B. Assessment
1. Painful vaginal bleeding
2. Hypertonic to tetanic, enlarged uterus
3. Boardlike rigidity of abdomen
4. Abnormal or absent fetal heart tones
5. Hypotension
6. Tachycardia
7. Pallor
8. Cool, moist skin
9. Bloody **amniotic fluid**
10. Rising fundal height from blood trapped behind the **placenta**
11. Signs of shock
12. Manifestations of coagulopathy
C. Implementation
1. Monitor maternal vital signs and FHR
2. Assess for vaginal bleeding, abdominal pain, and increase in fundal height
3. Maintain bed rest
4. Administer oxygen as prescribed
5. Monitor and report any uterine activity
6. Administer IV fluids as prescribed
7. Monitor I & O, because a urine output of less than 30 mL/hour indicates decreased renal perfusion
8. Administer blood products as prescribed
9. Monitor blood studies for impending signs of disseminated intravascular coagulation (DIC), which include decreased fibrinogen, hematocrit level, and platelet count and increased prothrombin time (PT), partial thromboplastin time (PTT), clotting time, and fibrin degradation products
10. Prepare for the **delivery** of the fetus as quickly as possible, with vaginal **delivery** preferable if the fetus is healthy and stable and the presenting part is in the pelvis; emergency cesarean section is performed if the fetus is alive but shows signs of distress
11. Perform Kleihauer-Betke test after **delivery** for Rh-negative clients because fetal maternal hemorrhage is common
12. Monitor for signs of DIC in the postpartum period

▲ **VII. PROLAPSED CORD**
A. Description: The umbilical cord is displaced, either between the presenting part and the amnion or protruding through the cervix, causing compression of the cord and compromising fetal circulation
B. Assessment
1. A feeling that something is coming through the vagina
2. Umbilical cord is seen or palpated
3. FHR is irregular and slow

4. Fetal heart monitor will show variable deceleration or bradycardia after rupture of the membranes
5. If fetal hypoxia is severe, violent fetal activity may occur and then cease
C. Implementation
1. Relieve cord pressure immediately
2. Reposition mother; turn side to side or her hips may be elevated to shift the fetal presenting part toward her diaphragm
3. Elevate fetal presenting part that is lying on the cord by applying finger pressure with a sterile gloved hand
4. Do not attempt to push the cord into the uterus
5. Monitor FHR
6. Assess fetus for hypoxia
7. Administer oxygen by face mask to the mother as prescribed
8. Prepare for emergency cesarean birth

VIII. INVERTED UTERUS
A. Description: Uterus turns inside out, usually during **delivery** or after **delivery** of the **placenta**
B. Assessment
1. Hemorrhage
2. Severe pain
3. Signs of shock
C. Implementation
1. Monitor vital signs
2. Monitor for signs of shock
3. Prepare the client for a return of the uterus to the correct position via the vagina

IX. AMNIOTIC FLUID EMBOLISM
A. Description
1. The escape of **amniotic fluid** into the maternal circulation
2. The debris containing **amniotic fluid** deposits in the pulmonary arterioles and is usually fatal to the mother
B. Assessment
1. Sudden chest pain
2. Dyspnea
3. Cyanosis
4. Pulmonary edema
C. Implementation
1. Institute emergency measures to maintain life
2. Administer oxygen as prescribed
3. Monitor vital signs
4. Monitor for hemorrhage
5. Prepare to administer digoxin (Lanoxin) as prescribed for failing cardiac function
6. Prepare to administer fibrinogen as prescribed to replace depleted reserves
7. Prepare to administer heparin sodium as prescribed

8. Prepare to administer blood transfusions as prescribed
9. Prepare for forceps **delivery** if the cervix is dilated

X. VENA CAVA SYNDROME (SUPINE HYPOTENSIVE SYNDROME)
A. Description
1. Occurs when the venous return to the heart is impaired by the weight of the uterus
2. Results in partial occlusion of the vena cava
B. Assessment
1. Signs of shock, such as tachycardia and hypotension
2. Sweating
3. Nausea and vomiting
4. Respiratory distress
5. Fetal distress
C. Implementation
1. Position client by turning to the left side to shift weight of the fetus off the inferior vena cava
2. Administer oxygen as prescribed
3. Monitor vital signs and FHR
4. Assess for shock caused by reduced cardiac output

XI. FETAL DISTRESS
A. Assessment
1. Fetal heart rate above 160 or below 120 beats per minute
2. Meconium-stained **amniotic fluid**
3. Fetal hyperactivity
4. Variable deceleration pattern
5. Late deceleration
6. Fetal pH below 7.2
B. Implementation
1. Position mother by turning to the left side; elevate legs
2. Administer oxygen via face mask as prescribed
3. Discontinue oxytocin (Pitocin) as prescribed
4. Increase IV fluids as prescribed to correct hypotension
5. Monitor vital signs
6. Prepare for emergency cesarean section

PRACTICE QUESTIONS

1. A nurse in a labor room is monitoring a client with dysfunctional labor for signs of fetal or maternal compromise. Which of the following assessment findings would alert the nurse to a compromise?
   1. Persistent nonreassuring fetal heart rate
   2. Maternal fatigue
   3. Progressive changes in the cervix
   4. Coordinated uterine contractions
2. A nurse is assigned to care for a client with hypotonic uterine dysfunction and signs of a slowing labor. The nurse is reviewing the physician's orders and would expect to note which of the following prescribed treatments for this condition?
   1. Medication that will provide sedation
   2. Increased hydration
   3. Oxytocin (Pitocin) infusion
   4. Administration of a tocolytic medication
3. A nurse in a labor room is preparing to care for a client with hypertonic uterine dysfunction. The nurse is told that the client is experiencing uncoordinated contractions that are erratic in their frequency, duration, and intensity. The priority nursing intervention in caring for the client is to:
   1. Monitor the oxytocin (Pitocin) infusion closely
   2. Provide pain relief measures
   3. Prepare the client for an amniotomy
   4. Promote ambulation every 30 minutes
4. A nurse is providing emergency measures to a client in labor who has been diagnosed with a prolapsed cord. The mother becomes anxious and frightened and says to the nurse, "Why are all of these people in here? Is my baby going to be alright?" Which of the following nursing diagnoses would be most appropriate for this client at this time?
   1. Fear
   2. Powerlessness
   3. Ineffective individual coping
   4. Sensory overload
5. A nurse has developed a plan of care for a client experiencing dystocia and includes several nursing interventions in the plan of care. The nurse prioritizes the plan of care and selects which of the following nursing interventions as the highest priority?
   1. Keeping the significant other informed of the progress of the labor
   2. Providing comfort measures
   3. Monitoring the fetal heart rate
   4. Changing the client's position frequently
6. A maternity nurse is preparing to care for a pregnant client in labor who will be delivering twins. The nurse prepares to monitor the fetal heart rates by placing the external fetal monitor:
   1. Over the fetus that is most anterior to the mother's abdomen
   2. Over the fetus that is most posterior to the mother's abdomen
   3. So that each fetal heart rate is monitored separately
   4. So that one fetus is monitored for a 15-minute period followed by a 15-minute fetal monitoring period for the second fetus
7. A nurse is preparing a plan of care for a client who just delivered a dead fetus. The most appropriate initial intervention in planning to meet the emo-

tional needs of the client and her spouse is which of the following?
1. Encourage the client to talk about the dead fetus
2. Allow the client and the spouse to hold the baby
3. Allow family members to name the baby
4. Assess the client and the spouse's perception of the event

8. A nurse in the postpartum unit is caring for a client who has just delivered a newborn infant following a pregnancy with a placenta previa. The nurse reviews the plan of care and prepares to monitor the client for which of the following risks associated with placenta previa?
1. Disseminated intravascular coagulation
2. Chronic hypertension
3. Infection
4. Hemorrhage

9. A nurse in a delivery room is assisting with the delivery of a newborn infant. After the delivery of the newborn, the nurse assists in delivering the placenta. Which observation would indicate that the placenta has separated from the uterine wall and is ready for delivery?
1. The umbilical cord shortens in length and changes in color
2. A soft and boggy uterus
3. Maternal complaints of severe uterine cramping
4. Changes in the shape of the uterus

10. A nurse in a labor room is performing a vaginal assessment on a pregnant client in labor. The nurse notes the presence of the umbilical cord protruding from the vagina. Which of the following would be the initial nursing action?
1. Place the client in the Trendelenburg position
2. Call the delivery room to notify the staff that the client will be transported immediately
3. Gently push the cord into the vagina
4. Find the closest telephone and stat page the physician

11. A maternity nurse is caring for a client with abruptio placenta and is monitoring the client for disseminated intravascular coagulopathy (DIC). Which assessment finding is least likely to be associated with DIC?
1. Swelling of the calf of one leg
2. Prolonged clotting times
3. Decreased platelet count
4. Petechiae, oozing from injection sites, and hematuria

12. A nurse is assessing a pregnant client in the second trimester of pregnancy who was admitted to the maternity unit with a suspected diagnosis of abruptio placentae. Which of the following assessment findings would the nurse not expect to note if this condition is present?
1. Acute abdominal pain

2. A hard boardlike abdomen
3. Uterine tenderness
4. Painless bright red vaginal bleeding

13. A maternity nurse is preparing for the admission of a client in the third trimester of pregnancy who is experiencing vaginal bleeding and has a suspected diagnosis of placenta previa. The nurse anticipates the client's needs and prepares a plan of care. Which of the following would not be a component of the plan for this client?
1. Prepare the client for an ultrasound
2. Obtain equipment for external electronic fetal heart rate monitoring
3. Obtain equipment for a manual pelvic exam
4. Prepare to draw a hemoglobin and hematocrit blood sample

14. An ultrasound is performed on a client at term gestation who is experiencing moderate vaginal bleeding. The results of the ultrasound indicate that abruptio placentae is present. On the basis of these findings, the nurse would prepare the client for:
1. Complete bed rest for the remainder of the pregnancy
2. Delivery of the fetus
3. Strict monitoring of intake and output
4. The need for weekly monitoring of coagulation studies until the time of delivery

15. A nurse in a labor room is assisting with the vaginal delivery of a newborn infant. The nurse would monitor the client closely for the risk of uterine rupture if which of the following occurred?
1. Hypotonic contractions
2. Forceps delivery
3. Schultz presentation
4. Weak bearing down efforts

16. A clinic nurse is performing a prenatal assessment on a pregnant client. The nurse would implement teaching related to the risk of abruptio placentae if which of the following information was obtained on assessment?
1. The client has a history of hypertension
2. The client performs moderate exercise on a regular daily schedule
3. The client is 28 years of age
4. This is the second pregnancy

17. A nurse is performing an initial assessment on a client who has just been told that a pregnancy test is positive. Which assessment finding would indicate that the client is at risk for preterm labor?
1. The client is a 35-year-old primigravida
2. The client is a 20-year-old primigravida of average weight and height
3. The client's hemoglobin level is 13.5 g/dL
4. The client has a history of cardiac disease

18. A nurse is monitoring a client who is in the active stage of labor. The client has been experiencing contractions that are short, irregular, and weak. The nurse documents that the client is experiencing which type of labor dystocia?
    1. Hypotonic
    2. Precipitous
    3. Hypertonic
    4. Preterm labor

19. A nurse is caring for a client who is experiencing a precipitous birth. The nurse is waiting for the physician to arrive. When the infant's head crowns, the nurse would instruct the client to:
    1. Bear down
    2. Push with each contraction
    3. Breathe rapidly
    4. Hold her breath

20. After a precipitous delivery, a nurse notes that the new mother is passive and only touches her newborn infant briefly with her fingertips. The nurse would do which of the following to help the woman process what has happened?
    1. Encourage the mother to breastfeed soon after birth
    2. Tell the mother that it is important to hold the newborn infant
    3. Document a complete account of the mother's reaction on the birth record
    4. Support the mother in her reaction to the newborn infant

CRITICAL THINKING: FREE-TEXT ENTRY

A nurse is caring for a client in labor. The client tells the nurse that she feels like something is coming through the vagina. The nurse performs an assessment and notes the presence of the umbilical cord protruding from the vagina. The nurse immediately places the client in what position?

Answer: _____

ANSWERS

1. **1**

Rationale: Signs of a fetal or maternal compromise include a persistent nonreassuring fetal heart rate, fetal acidosis, and the passage of meconium. Maternal exhaustion and infection can occur if the labor is prolonged but do not indicate fetal or maternal compromise. Progressive changes in the cervix and coordinated uterine contractions are a reassuring pattern in labor.

Test-Taking Strategy: Focus on the issue of the question, signs of fetal or maternal compromise. Use the process of elimination, noting that options 2, 3, and 4 are normal expectations during labor. Review the assessment findings that indicate fetal or maternal compromise if you had difficulty with this question.

Level of Cognitive Ability: Analysis
Client Needs: Physiological Integrity
Integrated Concept/Process: Nursing Process/Assessment
Content Area: Maternity
Reference: Gorrie, T., McKinney, E., & Murray, S. (1998). *Foundations of maternal newborn nursing* (2nd ed.). Philadelphia: W.B. Saunders, p. 746.

2. **3**

Rationale: Therapeutic management for hypotonic uterine dysfunction includes oxytocin augmentation and amniotomy to stimulate a labor that slows. A cesarean birth will be performed if no progress in labor occurs. Options 1, 2, and 4 identify therapeutic measures for a client with hypertonic dysfunction.

Test-Taking Strategy: Focus on the key word "hypotonic" to assist in answering the question. Use the process of elimination and identify the option that will assist to stimulate labor. This should easily direct you to option 3. If you had difficulty with this question, review the therapeutic management for hypotonic uterine dysfunction.

Level of Cognitive Ability: Analysis
Client Needs: Physiological Integrity
Integrated Concept/Process: Communication and Documentation
Content Area: Maternity
Reference: Gorrie, T., McKinney, E., & Murray, S. (1998). *Foundations of maternal newborn nursing* (2nd ed.). Philadelphia: W.B. Saunders. p. 747.

3. **2**

Rationale: Management of hypertonic labor depends on the cause. Relief of pain is the primary intervention to promote a normal labor pattern. An amniotomy and an oxytocin infusion are not treatment measures for hypertonic dysfunction; however, these treatments may be used in clients with hypotonic dysfunction. The client with hypertonic uterine dysfunction would not be encouraged to ambulate every 30 minutes, but would be encouraged to rest.

Test-Taking Strategy: Use the process of elimination, focusing on the key word "hypertonic." This key word and knowledge of the therapeutic management for this condition will easily assist in directing you to option 2. Options 1, 3, and 4 are therapeutic measures for hypotonic dysfunction. If you had difficulty with this question, review the therapeutic management for hypertonic uterine dysfunction.

Level of Cognitive Ability: Application
Client Needs: Physiological Integrity
Integrated Concept/Process: Nursing Process/Implementation
Content Area: Maternity
Reference: Lowdermilk, D., Perry, S., & Bobak, I. (2000). *Maternity & women's health care* (7th ed.). St. Louis: Mosby, p. 982.

4. 1

Rationale: The mother is anxious and frightened, and the most appropriate nursing diagnosis for the client at this time is Fear. There are no data in the question to support a nursing diagnosis of Powerlessness, Ineffective Individual Coping, or Sensory Overload, although these nursing diagnoses may be considered for this client at some point during the hospitalization experience.

Test-Taking Strategy: When answering questions related to nursing diagnosis, focus specifically on the data provided in the question. Note the relationship between the words "frightened" in the question and "Fear" in the correct option. Review maternal psychosocial responses when a prolapsed cord occurs if you had difficulty with this question.

Level of Cognitive Ability: Analysis
Client Needs: Psychosocial Integrity
Integrated Concept/Process: Nursing Process/Analysis
Content Area: Maternity
Reference: Olds, S., London. M., & Ladewig, P. (2000). *Maternal-newborn nursing: A family and community-based approach* (6th ed.). Upper Saddle River, N.J.: Prentice-Hall Health, p. 644.

5. 3

Rationale: The priority is to monitor the FHR. Although providing comfort measures, changing the client's position frequently, and keeping the significant other informed of the progress of the labor are components of the plan of care, the fetal status would be the priority.

Test-Taking Strategy: Note the key words "highest priority." Use Maslow's Hierarchy of Needs theory and the ABCs—airway, breathing, and circulation—to assist in answering the question. Review priority nursing interventions for the client with dystocia if you had difficulty with this question.

Level of Cognitive Ability: Application
Client Needs: Physiological Integrity
Integrated Concept/Process: Nursing Process/Planning
Content Area: Maternity
Reference: Olds, S., London. M., & Ladewig, P. (2000). *Maternal-newborn nursing: A family and community-based approach* (6th ed.). Upper Saddle River, N.J.: Prentice-Hall Health, p. 611.

6. 3

Rationale: In a client with a multifetal pregnancy, each fetal heart rate is monitored separately. Options 1, 2, and 4 are incorrect because these actions would provide information regarding the status of only one fetus at one time.

Test-Taking Strategy: Use the process of elimination. Note that options 1, 2, and 4 are similar in that they all relate to monitoring only one fetus at one time. Review care of the client with a multifetal pregnancy if you had difficulty with this question.

Level of Cognitive Ability: Application
Client Needs: Physiological Integrity
Integrated Concept/Process: Nursing Process/Planning
Content Area: Maternity
Reference: Gorrie, T., McKinney, E., & Murray, S. (1998). *Foundations of maternal newborn nursing* (2nd ed.). Philadelphia: W.B. Saunders, p. 752.

7. 4

Rationale: The most appropriate initial intervention in planning to meet the emotional needs of the client and her spouse is to assess their perception of the event. Although options 1, 2, and 3 are likely to be components of the plan of care, the initial intervention in planning is to assess the perception of the event.

Test-Taking Strategy: Note the key word "initial" in the stem of the question. Use the process of elimination and the steps of the nursing process to assist in answering the question. Remember that assessment is the first step in the nursing process. Review nursing interventions when fetal demise occurs if you had difficulty with this question.

Level of Cognitive Ability: Application
Client Needs: Psychosocial Integrity
Integrated Concept/Process: Nursing Process/Planning
Content Area: Maternity
Reference: Lowdermilk, D., Perry, S., & Bobak, I. (2000). *Maternity & women's health care* (7th ed.). St. Louis: Mosby, p. 1148.

8. 4

Rationale: Because the placenta is implanted in the lower uterine segment, which does not contain the same intertwining musculature as the fundus of the uterus, this site is more prone to bleeding. Options 1, 2, and 3 are not risks that are specifically related to placenta previa.

Test-Taking Strategy: Use the process of elimination, focusing on the issue of the question, placenta previa. Recalling that bleeding is a primary concern in this client will easily direct you to option 4. Review the complications associated with placenta previa if you had difficulty with this question.

Level of Cognitive Ability: Application
Client Needs: Physiological Integrity
Integrated Concept/Process: Nursing Process/Planning
Content Area: Maternity Reference: Lowdermilk, D., Perry, S., & Bobak, I. (2000). *Maternity & women's health care* (7th ed.). St. Louis: Mosby, p. 852.

9. 4

Rationale: Signs of placental separation include lengthening of the umbilical cord, a sudden gush of dark blood from the introitus, a firmly contracted uterus, and the uterus changing from a discoid to a globular shape. The client may experience vaginal fullness, but not severe uterine cramping.

Test-Taking Strategy: Use the process of elimination, reading each option carefully. Recalling that the placenta is attached to the uterine wall will assist in directing you to option 4. Review the findings associated with placental separation if you had difficulty with this question.

Level of Cognitive Ability: Analysis
Client Needs: Physiological Integrity
Integrated Concept/Process: Nursing Process/Assessment
Content Area: Maternity
Reference: Lowdermilk, D., Perry, S., & Bobak, I. (2000). *Maternity & women's health care* (7th ed.). St. Louis: Mosby, p. 570.

10. 1

Rationale: When cord prolapse occurs, prompt actions are taken to relieve cord compression and increase fetal oxygenation. The mother should be positioned with the hips higher than the head to shift the fetal presenting part toward the diaphragm. The nurse should push the call light to summon help, and other staff members should call the physician and notify the delivery room. If the cord is protruding from the vagina, no attempt should be made to replace it because to do so could traumatize it and further reduce blood flow. The examiner may, however, place a gloved hand into the vagina and hold the presenting part off of the umbilical cord. Oxygen at 8 to 10 liters per minute by face mask is administered to the mother to increase fetal oxygenation.

Test-Taking Strategy: Use the process of elimination, noting the key words "umbilical cord protruding from the vagina." Options 2 and 4 can be eliminated first because these actions delay necessary and immediate treatment. Knowledge that the cord should not be pushed back into the vagina will easily direct you to option 1. Review priority nursing measures for prolapsed cord if you had difficulty with this question.

Level of Cognitive Ability: Application
Client Needs: Physiological Integrity
Integrated Concept/Process: Nursing Process/Implementation
Content Area: Maternity
Reference: Lowdermilk, D., Perry, S., & Bobak, I. (2000). *Maternity & women's health care* (7th ed.). St. Louis: Mosby, p. 1015.

11. 1
Rationale: DIC is a state of diffuse clotting in which clotting factors are consumed. This leads to widespread bleeding. Platelets are decreased because they are consumed by the process; coagulation studies show no clot formation (and are thus normal to prolonged); and fibrin plugs may clog the microvasculature diffusely, rather than in an isolated area. The presence of petechiae, oozing from injection sites, and hematuria are signs associated with the presence of DIC. Swelling and pain in the calf of one leg are more likely to be associated with thrombophlebitis.

Test-Taking Strategy: Use the process of elimination. Note the key words "least likely" in the stem of the question. Knowledge that DIC is a widespread problem rather than a localized one will easily direct you to option 1. Review the signs related to DIC if you had difficulty with this question.

Level of Cognitive Ability: Analysis
Client Needs: Physiological Integrity
Integrated Concept/Process: Nursing Process/Assessment
Content Area: Maternity
Reference: Olds, S., London. M., & Ladewig, P. (2000). *Maternal-newborn nursing: A family and community-based approach* (6th ed.). Upper Saddle River, N.J.: Prentice-Hall Health, p. 636.

12. 4
Rationale: Painless bright red vaginal bleeding in the second or third trimester of pregnancy is a sign of placenta previa. In abruptio placentae, acute abdominal pain is present. Uterine tenderness accompanies placental abruption, especially with a central abruption and trapped blood behind the placenta. The abdomen will feel hard and boardlike upon palpation as the blood penetrates the myometrium and causes uterine irritability. Observation of the fetal monitoring often reveals increased uterine resting tone, caused by failure of the uterus to relax in an attempt to constrict blood vessels and control bleeding.

Test-Taking Strategy: Note the key word "not" in the stem of the question. Remember that the difference between placenta previa and abruptio placentae involves the presence of uterine pain and tenderness with an abruption, as opposed to painless bleeding with a previa. Options 1, 2, and 3 describe the

presence of abruptio placenta, while option 4 is the only one that describes placenta previa. Review the signs of abruptio placentae if you had difficulty with this question.

Level of Cognitive Ability: Analysis
Client Needs: Physiological Integrity
Integrated Concept/Process: Nursing Process/Assessment
Content Area: Maternity
Reference: Lowdermilk, D., Perry, S., & Bobak, I. (2000). *Maternity & women's health care* (7th ed.). St. Louis: Mosby, p. 856.

13. 3
Rationale: Manual pelvic examinations are contraindicated when vaginal bleeding is apparent in the third trimester until a diagnosis is made and placental previa is ruled out. Digital examination of the cervix can lead to maternal and fetal hemorrhage. A diagnosis of placental previa is made by ultrasound. The hemoglobin and hematocrit levels are monitored, and external electronic fetal heart rate monitoring is initiated. Electronic fetal monitoring (external) is crucial in evaluating the status of the fetus who is at risk for severe hypoxia.

Test-Taking Strategy: Use the process of elimination and knowledge of the pathophysiology associated with placenta previa. Note the key word "not" in the stem of the question. Also, note that option 3 is the only procedure that is invasive to the pregnancy and endangers the physiological safety of the client and the fetus. Review care of the client with placenta previa if you had difficulty with this question.

Level of Cognitive Ability: Application
Client Needs: Physiological Integrity
Integrated Concept/Process: Nursing Process/Planning
Content Area: Maternity
Reference: Lowdermilk, D., Perry, S., & Bobak, I. (2000). *Maternity & women's health care* (7th ed.). St. Louis: Mosby, p. 852.

14. 2
Rationale: The goal of management in abruptio placentae is to control the hemorrhage and deliver the fetus as soon as possible. Delivery is the treatment of choice if the fetus is at term gestation or if the bleeding is moderate to severe and mother or fetus is in jeopardy. Since delivery of the fetus is necessary, options 1, 3, and 4 are incorrect regarding management of the client with abruptio placentae.

Test-Taking Strategy: Use the process of elimination and knowledge regarding the management of abruptio placentae to answer the question. Note the key words "term gestation" and "moderate vaginal bleeding." Knowing that the goal is to deliver the fetus will easily direct you to option 2. If you had difficulty with this question or are unfamiliar with the management of abruptio placentae, review this content.

Level of Cognitive Ability: Application
Client Needs: Physiological Integrity
Integrated Concept/Process: Nursing Process/Planning
Content Area: Maternity
Reference: Lowdermilk, D., Perry, S., & Bobak, I. (2000). *Maternity & women's health care* (7th ed.). St. Louis: Mosby, p. 856.

15. 2
Rationale: Excessive fundal pressure, forceps delivery, violent bearing down efforts, tumultuous labor, and shoulder dystocia can place a woman at risk for traumatic uterine rupture.

Hypotonic contractions and weak bearing down efforts do not alone add to the risk of rupture because they do not add to the stress on the uterine wall. Schultz presentation is the expulsion of the placenta with the fetal side presenting first and is not associated with uterine rupture.

Test-Taking Strategy: Use the process of elimination. Read each option carefully, and select the option that provides an additional source of pressure to the uterus and would be most likely to add to the risk of rupturing or "tearing" the uterus. Option 2 is the only option that would provide an additional source of pressure to the uterus. Review the risks associated with uterine rupture if you had difficulty with this question.

Level of Cognitive Ability: Analysis
Client Needs: Physiological Integrity
Integrated Concept/Process: Nursing Process/Assessment
Content Area: Maternity
Reference: Lowdermilk, D., Perry, S., & Bobak, I. (2000). *Maternity & women's health care* (7th ed.). St. Louis: Mosby, p. 1015.

16. 1
Rationale: Abruptio placentae is associated with conditions characterized by poor uteroplacental circulation, such as hypertension, smoking, and alcohol or cocaine abuse. It is also associated with physical and mechanical factors such as overdistension of the uterus that occurs with multiple gestation or polyhydramnios. In addition, a short umbilical cord, physical trauma, and increased maternal age and parity are risk factors.

Test-Taking Strategy: Use the process of elimination, focusing on the risk factors associated with abruptio placentae. Eliminate options 2, 3, and 4 because they are not situations that would present a risk for this condition. Review the risk factors associated with abruptio placentae if you had difficulty with this question.

Level of Cognitive Ability: Analysis
Client Needs: Health Promotion and Maintenance
Integrated Concept/Process: Nursing Process/Assessment
Content Area: Maternity
Reference: Lowdermilk, D., Perry, S., & Bobak, I. (2000). *Maternity & women's health care* (7th ed.). St. Louis: Mosby, p. 855.

17. 4
Rationale: Several factors are associated with preterm labor. These include a history of past medical conditions, present and past obstetric problems, social and environmental factors, and demographic factors such as race and age. Other risk factors include a multifetal pregnancy, which contributes to overdistention of the uterus; anemia, which decreases oxygen supply to the uterus; and age less than 18 years or first pregnancy over the age of 40.

Test-Taking Strategy: Use the process of elimination and note that option 4 is the only option that identifies an abnormal condition. Options 1, 2, and 3 are all average and normal findings. Review the risk factors for preterm labor if you had difficulty with this question.

Level of Cognitive Ability: Analysis
Client Needs: Physiological Integrity
Integrated Concept/Process: Nursing Process/Assessment
Content Area: Maternity
Reference: Olds, S., London. M., & Ladewig, P. (2000).

Maternal-newborn nursing: A family and community-based approach (6th ed.). Upper Saddle River, N.J.: Prentice-Hall Health, p. 399.

18. 1
Rationale: Hypotonic labor contractions are short, irregular, and weak and usually occur during the active phase of labor. Hypertonic dysfunction usually occurs during the latent phase of labor. Precipitous labor is that which lasts in its entirety for 3 hours or less. Preterm labor is the onset of labor after 20 weeks gestation and before the beginning of the 37th week of gestation.

Test-Taking Strategy: Use the process of elimination. Note the relationship between the words "short, irregular, and weak" in the question and "hypotonic" in the correct option. If you are unfamiliar with dysfunctional labor (dystocia), review this content.

Level of Cognitive Ability: Application
Client Needs: Physiological Integrity
Integrated Concept/Process: Communication and Documentation
Content Area: Maternity
Reference: Gorrie, T., McKinney, E., & Murray, S. (1998). *Foundations of maternal newborn nursing* (2nd ed.). Philadelphia: W.B. Saunders, p. 746.

19. 3
Rationale: During a precipitous birth, when the infant's head crowns, the nurse instructs the client to breathe rapidly to decrease the urge to push. The client is not instructed to push or bear down. Holding the breath decreases the amount of oxygen both to the mother and to the fetus.

Test-Taking Strategy: Use the process of elimination, focusing on the key words "precipitous birth." Option 4 can be eliminated first because this action decreases the amount of oxygen both to the mother and to the fetus. Next, eliminate options 1 and 2 because they are similar. Review the nursing interventions in the care of a client experiencing a precipitous birth if you had difficulty with this question.

Level of Cognitive Ability: Application
Client Needs: Physiological Integrity
Integrated Concept/Process: Nursing Process/Implementation
Content Area: Maternity
Reference: Olds, S., London. M., & Ladewig, P. (2000). *Maternal-newborn nursing: A family and community-based approach* (6th ed.). Upper Saddle River, N.J.: Prentice-Hall Health, p. 577.

20. 4
Rationale: Women who have experienced precipitous labor often describe feelings of disbelief that their labor progressed so rapidly. To assist the woman to process what has happened, it is best to support the mother in her reaction to the newborn infant. Options 1, 2, and 3 do not acknowledge the mother's feelings.

Test-Taking Strategy: Use therapeutic communication techniques. Option 4 is the only option that acknowledges the mother's feelings. If you had difficulty with this question, review these techniques and care to the mother following a precipitous birth.

Level of Cognitive Ability: Application
Client Needs: Psychosocial Integrity
Integrated Concept/Process: Nursing Process/Implementation

Content Area: Maternity
Reference: Lowdermilk, D., Perry, S., & Bobak, I. (2000). *Maternity & women's health care* (7th ed.). St. Louis: Mosby, p. 989.

CRITICAL THINKING: FREE-TEXT ENTRY

Answer: The client may be turned side to side or the hips are elevated to shift the fetal presenting part toward her diaphragm, thus relieving cord compression
Rationale: If cord prolapse or compression is suspected, the client is immediately repositioned. Cord compression needs to be relieved so that adequate fetal oxygenation occurs. The client may be turned side to side or the hips are elevated to shift the fetal presenting part toward her diaphragm, thus relieving cord compression.

Test-Taking Strategy: Focus on the issue, the presence of the umbilical cord protruding from the vagina. Recalling that cord compression needs to be relieved immediately will assist in identifying the position in which the mother should be placed. Review immediate nursing interventions if prolapsed cord is suspected, if you had difficulty with this question.
Level of Cognitive Ability: Application
Client Needs: Physiological Integrity
Integrated Concept/Process: Nursing Process/Implementation
Content Area: Maternity
Reference: Gorrie, T., McKinney, E., & Murray, S. (1998). *Foundations of maternal-newborn nursing* (2nd ed.). Philadelphia: W.B. Saunders, p. 356.

REFERENCES

Gorrie, T., McKinney, E., & Murray, S. (1998). *Foundations of maternal-newborn nursing* (2nd ed.). Philadelphia: W.B. Saunders.

Ladewig, P., London. M., & Olds, S. (1998). *Maternal-newborn nursing care: The nurse, the family, and the community* (4th ed.). Menlo Park, Calif.: Addison-Wesley Longman.

Lowdermilk, D., Perry, S., & Bobak, I. (2000). *Maternity & women's health care* (7th ed.). St. Louis: Mosby.

Olds, S., London. M., & Ladewig, P. (2000). *Maternal-newborn nursing: A family and community-based approach* (6th ed.). Upper Saddle River, N.J.: Prentice-Hall Health.

Sherwen, L., Scoloveno, M.A., & Weingarten, C. (1999). *Maternity nursing: Care of the childbearing family* (3rd ed.). Stamford, Conn.: Appleton & Lange.

28

The Postpartum Period

I. POSTPARTUM

A. Description: Period when the reproductive tract returns to the normal, nonpregnant state

B. Postpartum period: Starts immediately after **delivery** and is completed usually by week 6 following **delivery**

II. PHYSIOLOGICAL MATERNAL CHANGES

A. Involution
1. Description
   a. The rapid decrease in the size of the uterus as it returns to the nonpregnant state
   b. Clients who breastfeed may experience a more rapid involution
2. Assessment
   a. Weight of the uterus decreases from 2 pounds to 2 ounces in 6 weeks
   b. Endometrium regenerates
   c. Fundus steadily descends into the pelvis
   d. Fundal height decreases about 1 fingerbreadth (1 cm) per day
   e. By 10 days postpartum, uterus cannot be palpated abdominally
   f. Note that a flaccid fundus indicates uterine atony and should be massaged until firm; a tender fundus indicates an infection

B. **Lochia**
1. Description: Discharge from the uterus that consists of blood from the vessels of the **placental** site and debris from the decidua
2. Assessment
   a. Rubra: Bright red discharge that occurs from **delivery** day to day 3
   b. Serosa: Brownish pink discharge that occurs from days 4 to 10
   c. Alba: White discharge that occurs from days 10 to 14
   d. Normally, the discharge has a fleshy odor
   e. Discharge decreases daily in amount
   f. Discharge may increase with ambulation
   g. Weigh the perineal pad before and after use and identify the amount of time between pad changes to most accurately determine the amount of **lochial** flow

C. Cervix: Cervical involution, and after 1 week the muscle begins to regenerate

D. Vagina: Vaginal distention decreases, although muscle tone is never restored completely to the pregravid state

E. Ovarian function and menstruation
1. Ovarian function depends on the rapidity with which the pituitary function is restored
2. Menstrual flow resumes within 8 weeks in nonbreastfeeding mothers
3. Menstrual flow usually resumes within 3 to 4 months in breastfeeding mothers
4. Breastfeeding mothers may experience amenorrhea during the entire period of lactation
5. Women may ovulate without menstruating, so breastfeeding should not be considered a form of birth control

F. Breasts
1. Breasts continue to secrete colostrum
2. A decrease in estrogen and progesterone levels after **delivery** stimulates increased prolactin levels, which promote breast milk production
3. Breasts become distended with milk on the third day
4. Engorgement occurs in 48 to 72 hours in nonbreastfeeding mothers
5. Breastfeeding will relieve engorgement

G. Urinary tract
  1. May have urinary retention as a result of loss of elasticity and tone, loss of sensation in the bladder from trauma, medications, anesthesia, and lack of privacy
  2. Diuresis usually begins within the first 12 hours after **delivery**
H. Gastrointestinal tract
  1. Women are usually very hungry after **delivery**
  2. Constipation can occur
  3. Hemorrhoids are common
I. Vital signs
  1. Temperature may be elevated during the first 24 hours because of dehydration
  2. Bradycardia is common during the first week, with a range of 50 to 70 beats per minute
  3. Blood pressure remains unchanged

III. POSTPARTUM IMPLEMENTATION

A. Assessment
  1. Monitor vital signs
  2. Assess height, consistency, and location of the fundus
  3. Monitor color, amount, and odor of **lochia**
  4. Assess breasts for engorgement
  5. Monitor perineum for swelling or discoloration
  6. Monitor episiotomy for healing
  7. Assess incisions or dressings of cesarean birth client
  8. Monitor bowel status
  9. Monitor I & O
  10. Encourage frequent voiding
  11. Encourage ambulation
  12. Administer RhoGam as prescribed within 72 hours postpartum to the Rh-negative client who has given birth to an Rh-positive **neonate**
  13. Assess bonding with the **newborn infant**
  14. Assess emotional status
B. Client teaching
  1. Initiate counseling of the client in discharge instructions
  2. Demonstrate **newborn** care skills as necessary
  3. Provide the opportunity for the mother to bathe the **newborn infant**
  4. Instruct in feeding technique
  5. Instruct the mother to avoid heavy lifting for at least 3 weeks
  6. Instruct the mother to plan at least one rest period per day
  7. Instruct the mother that contraception should begin after **delivery** or with the initiation of coitus (coitus should be postponed at least until the **lochia** ceases)
  8. Instruct the mother in the importance of follow-up, which should be scheduled at 4 to 6 weeks
  9. Instruct the mother to report any signs of chills, fever, increased **lochia,** or depressed feelings to the physician immediately

IV. POSTPARTUM DISCOMFORTS

A. Afterbirth pains
  1. Occur as a result of contractions of the uterus
  2. Are more common in multiparas, breastfeeding mothers, clients treated with oxytocin (Pitocin), and clients who had an overdistended uterus during **pregnancy,** such as with carrying twins
B. Perineal discomfort
  1. Apply ice packs to the perineum during the first 24 hours to reduce swelling
  2. After the first 24 hours, apply warmth by sitz baths
C. Episiotomy
  1. Instruct the client to administer perineal care after each voiding
  2. Encourage the use of an analgesic spray as prescribed
  3. Administer analgesics as prescribed if comfort measures are unsuccessful
D. Breast discomfort from engorgement
  1. Encourage wearing of a support bra at all times, even while the client is sleeping
  2. Encourage the use of ice packs if the client is not breastfeeding
  3. Encourage the use of warm soaks before feeding for the breastfeeding mother
  4. Administer analgesics as prescribed if comfort measures are unsuccessful
E. Postpartum blues (Box 28-1)
  1. Condition is caused by physiological and emotional stress
  2. The mother may feel upset and depressed at times
  3. Verbalization should be encouraged
  4. Postpartum blues may progress to postpartum depression if unresolved

V. NUTRITIONAL COUNSELING

A. Discuss caloric intake for breastfeeding and non-breastfeeding mothers
B. Nutritional needs depend on prepregnancy weight, ideal weight for height, and whether the mother is breastfeeding
C. If the mother is breastfeeding, calorie needs increase by approximately 500 calories per day, and the mother may require increased fluids and the continuance of prenatal vitamins and minerals

VI. BREASTFEEDING

A. General principles/considerations
  1. Put the baby to breast as soon as the mother and baby's conditions are stable (on **delivery** table if possible)
  2. Stay with the mother each time she nurses until she feels secure or confident with the baby and her feelings

BOX 28-1

Rubin's Postpartum Phases of Regeneration

Taking-In Phase: First 3 Days

Mother focuses on her own primary needs, such as sleep and food

Important for the nurse to listen and to help the mother interpret the events of delivery to make them more meaningful

Not an optimum time to teach the mother about baby care

Taking Hold Phase: Days 3 to 10

More in control of independence

Begins to assume the tasks of mothering

An optimum time to teach the mother about baby care

Letting Go Phase

Mother may feel deep loss over separation of the baby from part of the body and may grieve over the loss

Mother may be caught in a dependent/independent role, wanting to feel safe and secure yet wanting to make decisions

Teenage mothers need special consideration because of the conflict taking place within them as part of adolescence

---

3. Uterine cramping may occur the first day after **delivery** while the mother is nursing, when oxytocin simulation causes the uterus to contract
4. Use general hygiene and wash the breasts once daily
5. Do not use soap on the breasts, as it tends to remove natural oils, which increases the chance of cracked nipples
6. Bra should be well fitted and supporting
7. Breasts may leak between feedings or during coitus; place breast pad in bra
8. Calories should be increased by 500 per day, and the diet should include additional fluids; prenatal vitamins should be taken as prescribed
9. Baby's stools will be light yellow, watery, and frequent
10. Medications should be avoided unless prescribed
11. Gas-producing foods and caffeine should be avoided
12. Hormonal contraceptives may cause a decrease in the milk supply and are best avoided during the first 6 weeks after birth
13. Oral contraceptives containing estrogen are not recommended for breastfeeding mothers; progestin-only birth control pills are less likely to interfere with the milk supply
14. Baby will develop his or her own feeding schedule

B. Breastfeeding procedure for mother
1. Wash hands and assume a comfortable position
2. Start with the breast that the last feeding ended with

3. Brush the **newborn infant's** lower lip with nipple
4. Tickle the lips to have the baby open the mouth wide
5. Guide the nipple and surrounding areola into the baby's mouth
6. After the baby has nursed, release suction by depressing the **newborn infant's** chin or inserting a clean finger into the baby's mouth
7. Burp the baby after the first breast
8. Repeat the procedure on the second breast until the baby stops nursing
9. Burp the baby again
10. Instruct the mother to listen for audible sucking and swallowing

C. Engorgement
1. Breastfeed frequently
2. Apply warm packs before feeding
3. Apply ice packs between feedings

D. Cracked nipples
1. Expose nipples to air for 10 to 20 minutes after feeding
2. Rotate the position of the baby for each feeding
3. Be sure that the baby is latched on to the areola, not just the nipple

PRACTICE QUESTIONS

1. A postpartum nurse is preparing to care for a woman who has just delivered a healthy newborn infant. In the immediate postpartum period the nurse plans to take the woman's vital signs:
   1. Every 30 minutes during the first hour and then every hour for the next 2 hours
   2. Every 15 minutes during the first hour and then every 30 minutes for the next 2 hours
   3. Every hour for the first 2 hours and then every 4 hours
   4. Every 5 minutes for the first 30 minutes and then every hour for the next 4 hours

2. A postpartum nurse is taking the vital signs of a woman who delivered a healthy newborn infant 4 hours ago. The nurse notes that the mother's temperature is 100.2° F. Which of the following actions would be most appropriate?
   1. Retake the temperature in 15 minutes
   2. Notify the physician
   3. Document the findings
   4. Increase hydration by encouraging oral fluids

3. A nurse is assessing a client who is 6 hours postpartum after delivering a full-term healthy newborn infant. The client complains to the nurse of feelings of faintness and dizziness. Which of the following nursing actions would be most appropriate?
   1. Obtain hemoglobin and hematocrit levels
   2. Instruct the mother to request help when getting out of bed
   3. Elevate the mother's legs

   4. Inform the nursery room nurse to avoid bringing the newborn infant to the mother until the feelings of lightheadedness and dizziness have subsided

4. A nurse is preparing to perform a fundal assessment on a postpartum client. The initial nursing action in performing this assessment is which of the following?
   1. Ask the client to turn on her side
   2. Ask the client to lie flat on her back with the knees and legs flat and straight
   3. Ask the mother to urinate and empty her bladder
   4. Massage the fundus gently prior to determining the level of the fundus

5. A nurse is assessing the lochia discharge on a 1 day postpartum woman. The nurse notes that the lochia is red and has a foul-smelling odor. The nurse determines that this assessment finding is:
   1. Normal
   2. Indicates the presence of infection
   3. Indicates the need for increasing oral fluids
   4. Indicates the need for increasing ambulation

6. When performing a postpartum assessment on a client, a nurse notes the presence of clots in the lochia. The nurse examines the clots and notes that they are larger than 1 cm. Which of the following nursing actions is most appropriate?
   1. Document the findings
   2. Notify the physician
   3. Reassess the client in 2 hours
   4. Encourage increased oral intake of fluids

7. A nurse in a postpartum unit is instructing a mother regarding lochia and the amount of expected lochia drainage. The nurse instructs the mother that the normal amount of lochia may vary but should never exceed the need for:
   1. 1 peripad a day
   2. 2 peripads a day
   3. 3 peripads a day
   4. 8 peripads a day

8. A nurse is performing a postpartum assessment on a client who is preparing to breastfeed. Which of the following breast assessment findings would the nurse determine to be the most effective for breastfeeding?
   1. Flat nipples
   2. Inverted nipples
   3. Erectile nipples
   4. Nipples that are level with the skin surface

9. A postpartum nurse is providing instructions to a woman after delivery of a healthy newborn infant. The nurse instructs the mother that she should expect normal bowel elimination to return:
   1. On the day of delivery
   2. Three days postpartum
   3. Seven days postpartum
   4. Within 2 weeks postpartum

10. A nursing student is preparing to perform a cardiovascular assessment on a postpartum woman. A nursing instructor asks the student about the procedure to elicit Homans' sign. Which response by the nursing student would indicate an understanding of this assessment technique?
   1. "I will ask the woman to raise the legs up to the waist and then to slowly lower the legs."
   2. "I will ask the woman to extend her legs flat on the bed, and I will grasp the foot and gently dorsiflex it forward."
   3. "I will ask the woman to extend the legs flat on the bed, and I will grasp the foot and sharply extend it backward."
   4. "I will ask the woman to raise the legs and to try to lower them against pressure from my hand."

CRITICAL THINKING: FREE-TEXT ENTRY

A postpartum nurse is monitoring the amount of lochial flow in a client following delivery. The nurse implements which procedure to most accurately determine the amount of lochial flow?

Answer: _____

ANSWERS

1. **2**
Rationale: During the immediate postpartum period, vital signs are taken every 15 minutes in the first hour after birth, every 30 minutes for the next 2 hours, and every hour for the next 2 to 6 hours. Vital signs are monitored thereafter every 4 hours for 24 hours and every 8 to 12 hours for the remainder of the hospital stay.
Test-Taking Strategy: Use the process of elimination, noting that the nurse is caring for the client in the immediate postpartum period. Read each option carefully. It is not necessary to take vital signs every 5 minutes unless an alteration in physiological integrity has occurred during the labor period. Options 1 and 3 can be eliminated next because the time frames are not frequent enough to monitor the immediate postpartum status. If you had difficulty with this question, review postpartum assessment procedures.
Level of Cognitive Ability: Application
Client Needs: Physiological Integrity
Integrated Concept/Process: Nursing Process/Planning
Content Area: Maternity
Reference: Lowdermilk, D., Perry, S., & Bobak, I. (2000). *Maternity & women's health care* (7th ed.). St. Louis: Mosby, p. 591.

2. **4**

Rationale: The mother's temperature may be taken every 4 hour hours while she is awake. Temperatures up to 100.4° F (38° C) in the first 24 hours after birth are often related to the dehydrating effects of labor. The most appropriate action is to increase hydration by encouraging oral fluids, which should bring the temperature to a normal reading. Although the nurse would also document the findings, the most appropriate action would be to increase the hydration. It is not necessary to contact the physician. Taking the temperature in another 15 minutes is not the most appropriate action.

Test-Taking Strategy: Use the process of elimination and knowledge regarding the physiological findings in the immediate postpartum period to assist in answering this question. Note the key words "most appropriate" in the stem of the question. Recalling that a temperature elevation is often related to the dehydrating effects of labor will direct you to the correct option. Review normal postpartum assessment findings if you had difficulty with this question.

Level of Cognitive Ability: Application
Client Needs: Physiological Integrity
Integrated Concept/Process: Nursing Process/Implementation
Content Area: Maternity
Reference: Lowdermilk, D., Perry, S., & Bobak, I. (2000). *Maternity & women's health care* (7th ed.). St. Louis: Mosby, p. 587.

3. **2**

Rationale: Orthostatic hypotension may be evident during the first 8 hours after birth. Feelings of faintness or dizziness are signs that caution the nurse to beware for the client's safety. The nurse should advise the mother to get help the first few times the mother gets out of bed. Option 1 requires a physician's order. Option 3 is not the most appropriate or helpful action. Option 4 is unnecessary.

Test-Taking Strategy: Use the process of elimination and focus on the issue of the question, client safety. Option 4 is inappropriate and should be eliminated first. Elevating the client's legs is not an appropriate nursing intervention. From the remaining options recall that safety is a primary issue. This should assist in directing you to the correct option. If you had difficulty with this question, review postpartum nursing interventions.

Level of Cognitive Ability: Application
Client Needs: Safe, Effective Care Environment
Integrated Concept/Process: Nursing Process/Implementation
Content Area: Maternity
Reference: Sherwen, L., Scoloveno, M.A., & Weingarten, C. (1999). *Maternity nursing: Care of the childbearing family* (3rd ed.). Stamford, Conn.: Appleton & Lange, p. 863.

4. **3**

Rationale: Before fundal assessment is started, the nurse should ask the mother to empty her bladder so that an accurate assessment can be done. When the nurse is performing fundal assessment, the woman is asked to lie flat on her back with the knees flexed. Massaging the fundus is not appropriate unless the fundus is boggy or soft, and then it should be massaged gently until firm.

Test-Taking Strategy: Use the process of elimination. Note the key words "initial nursing action" in the stem of the question. Attempt to visualize the procedure when answering the

question. This should easily direct you to option 3. If you had difficulty with this question, review fundal assessment in the postpartum period.

Level of Cognitive Ability: Application
Client Needs: Physiological Integrity
Integrated Concept/Process: Nursing Process/Implementation
Content Area: Maternity
Reference: Sherwen, L., Scoloveno, M.A., & Weingarten, C. (1999). *Maternity nursing: Care of the childbearing family* (3rd ed.). Stamford, Conn.: Appleton & Lange, p. 858.

5. **2**

Rationale: Lochia, the discharge present after birth, is red for the first 1 to 3 days and gradually decreases in amount. Normal lochia has a fleshy odor. Foul-smelling or purulent lochia usually indicates infection, and these findings are not normal. Encouraging the woman to drink fluids or increase ambulation is not an accurate nursing intervention.

Test-Taking Strategy: Use the process of elimination, noting the key words "foul-smelling." This should easily direct you to option 2. If you had difficulty with this question, review normal assessment findings of lochia in the postpartum woman.

Level of Cognitive Ability: Analysis
Client Needs: Physiological Integrity
Integrated Concept/Process: Nursing Process/Analysis
Content Area: Maternity
Reference: Sherwen, L., Scoloveno, M.A., & Weingarten, C. (1999). *Maternity nursing: Care of the childbearing family* (3rd ed.). Stamford, Conn.: Appleton & Lange, p. 858.

6. **2**

Rationale: Normally there may be a few small clots in the first 1 to 2 days after birth, from pooling of the blood in the vagina. Clots larger than 1 cm are considered abnormal. The cause of these clots, such as uterine atony or retained placental fragments, needs to be determined and treated to prevent further blood loss. Although the findings would be documented, the most appropriate action is to notify the physician. Reassessing the client in 2 hours would delay necessary treatment. Increasing oral intake of fluids would not be an appropriate action in this situation.

Test-Taking Strategy: Use the process of elimination, focusing on the key words "larger than 1 cm." Knowledge regarding the presence of clots in the postpartum period and their significance will direct you to option 2. If you had difficulty with this question, review normal postpartum findings in the woman.

Level of Cognitive Ability: Application
Client Needs: Physiological Integrity
Integrated Concept/Process: Nursing Process/Implementation
Content Area: Maternity
Reference: Lowdermilk, D., Perry, S., & Bobak, I. (2000). *Maternity & women's health care* (7th ed.). St. Louis: Mosby, p. 935.

7. **4**

Rationale: The normal amount of lochia may vary with the individual but should never exceed 4 to 8 peripads a day. The average number of peripads used is 6 per day.

Test-Taking Strategy: Use the process of elimination and knowledge regarding the normal amount of lochia drainage in the postpartum period to answer the question. Noting the key words "should never exceed" will assist in directing you to option 4. If you had difficulty with this question, review postpartum assessment.

Level of Cognitive Ability: Application
Client Needs: Health Promotion and Maintenance
Integrated Concept/Process: Teaching/Learning
Content Area: Maternity
Reference: Sherwen, L., Scoloveno, M.A., & Weingarten, C. (1999). *Maternity nursing: Care of the childbearing family* (3rd ed.). Stamford, Conn.: Appleton & Lange, p. 859.

8. **3**
Rationale: For the breastfeeding woman, the nurse should note the presence of an erectile nipple that the infant can easily latch on to. The nurse should also observe and palpate for nipple soreness, breast tenderness, engorgement, mastitis, the presence of colostrum, and the presence of leaking milk. A flat or inverted nipple is more difficult for the infant to grasp and may require interventions for breastfeeding to be successful. Nipples that are level with the skin surface are the same as flat nipples.
Test-Taking Strategy: Use the process of elimination, noting the issue of the question, breastfeeding and assessment of the breasts. Eliminate options 1 and 4 first because they are similar. From the remaining options, thinking about the process of breastfeeding will easily direct you to option 3. If you had difficulty with this question, review preparing the postpartum client for breastfeeding.
Level of Cognitive Ability: Analysis
Client Needs: Physiological Integrity
Integrated Concept/Process: Nursing Process/Evaluation
Content Area: Maternity
Reference: Gorrie, T., McKinney, E., & Murray, S. (1998). *Foundations of maternal-newborn nursing* (2nd ed.). Philadelphia: W.B. Saunders. p. 996.

9. **2**
Rationale: After birth, the woman's abdomen should be auscultated in all four quadrants to determine the return of bowel sounds. Normal bowel elimination usually returns 2 to 3 days postpartum. Surgery, anesthesia, and the use of narcotics and pain control agents also contribute to the longer period of altered bowel functions. Options 1, 3, and 4 are incorrect.
Test-Taking Strategy: Use the process of elimination and general principles related to postpartum care to assist in answering this question. Eliminate options 3 and 4 first because of the length of time stated in these options. From the remaining options, eliminate option 1 because it would seem unreasonable that bowel function would return that quickly in the postpartum woman. Review normal gastrointestinal functions in the postpartum client if you had difficulty with this question.
Level of Cognitive Ability: Application

Client Needs: Physiological Integrity
Integrated Concept/Process: Teaching/Learning
Content Area: Maternity
Reference: Lowdermilk, D., Perry, S., & Bobak, I. (2000). *Maternity & women's health care* (7th ed.). St. Louis: Mosby, p. 586.

10. **2**
Rationale: To elicit Homans' sign, the nurse asks the woman to extend her legs flat on the bed. The nurse grasps the foot and dorsiflexes it forward. If this causes any discomfort or resistance, the nurse should notify the physician or midwife that Homans' sign is present. Options 1, 3, and 4 are incorrect descriptions of this assessment technique.
Test-Taking Strategy: Knowledge regarding the assessment technique to elicit Homans' sign is required to answer this question. Use the process of elimination and visualize this technique to assist in directing you to option 2. If you had difficulty with this question, review the technique to elicit Homans' sign.
Level of Cognitive Ability: Analysis
Client Needs: Health Promotion and Maintenance
Integrated Concept/Process: Nursing Process/Evaluation
Content Area: Maternity
Reference: Olds, S., London. M., & Ladewig, P. (2000). *Maternal-newborn nursing: A family and community-based approach* (6th ed.). Upper Saddle River, N.J.: Prentice-Hall Health, p. 925.

CRITICAL THINKING: FREE-TEXT ENTRY

Answer: Weighing the perineal pad before and after use and identifying the amount of time between pad changes
Rationale: The most accurate method for determining the amount of lochial flow is to weigh the perineal pads before and after use. Once these two weights are noted, the amount of lochial flow can be accurately determined. Each gram increase in the weight is roughly equivalent to 1 milliliter of blood loss. To obtain an accurate estimate of lochial flow, the time factor must be incorporated into the analysis.
Test Taking Strategy: Note the key words "to most accurately determine the amount." Recalling the need to weigh the perineal pads and to identify the time factor between pad changes will assist in answering the question. Review postpartum assessment measures if you had difficulty with this question.
Level of Cognitive Ability: Application
Client Needs: Physiological Integrity
Integrated Concept/Process: Nursing Process/Assessment
Content Area: Maternity
Reference: Lowdermilk, D., Perry, S., & Bobak, I. (2000). *Maternity & women's health care* (7th ed.). St. Louis: Mosby, p. 582.

REFERENCES

Gorrie, T., McKinney, E., & Murray, S. (1998). *Foundations of maternal-newborn nursing* (2nd ed.). Philadelphia: W.B. Saunders.

Ladewig, P., London. M., & Olds, S. (1998). *Maternal-newborn nursing care: The nurse, the family, and the community* (4th ed.). Menlo Park, Calif.: Addison-Wesley Longman.

Lowdermilk, D., Perry, S., & Bobak, I. (2000). *Maternity & women's health care* (7th ed.). St. Louis: Mosby.

Olds, S., London. M., & Ladewig, P. (2000). *Maternal-newborn nursing: A family and community-based approach* (6th ed.). Upper Saddle River, N.J.: Prentice-Hall Health.

Sherwen, L., Scoloveno, M.A., & Weingarten, C. (1999). *Maternity nursing: Care of the childbearing family* (3rd ed.). Stamford, Conn.: Appleton & Lange.

Postpartum Complications

I. CYSTITIS
A. Description: An infection of the bladder
B. Assessment
   1. Burning and pain on urination
   2. Lower abdominal pain
   3. Increased frequency of urination
   4. Costovertebral angle tenderness
   5. Fever
   6. Proteinuria, hematuria, bacteriuria, white blood cells in the urine
C. Implementation
   1. Palpate bladder for distention
   2. Palpate fundus
   3. Obtain urine specimen for culture and sensitivity if prescribed
   4. Institute measures to assist the client to void
   5. Encourage frequent and complete emptying of the bladder
   6. Force fluids to 3000 mL per day
   7. Administer antibiotics as prescribed after the urine culture is obtained
   8. Instruct the client in the methods of prevention and treatment of cystitis

II. HEMATOMA
A. Description
   1. Localized collection of blood into the tissues of the reproductive sac after the **delivery**
   2. Predisposing conditions include operative **delivery** with forceps and injury to a blood vessel
   3. Can be a life-threatening condition
B. Assessment
   1. Abnormal severe pain
   2. Pressure in the perineal area
   3. Sensitive, bulging mass in the perineal area with discolored skin
   4. Inability to void
   5. Decreased hemoglobin and hematocrit (H & H) levels
   6. Signs of shock, such as pallor, tachycardia, and hypotension, if significant blood loss has occurred
C. Implementation
   1. Monitor vital signs
   2. Monitor client for abnormal pain, especially when forceps **delivery** has occurred
   3. Place ice at the hematoma site
   4. Administer analgesics as prescribed
   5. Monitor intake and output (I & O)
   6. Encourage fluids and voiding
   7. Prepare for urinary catheterization if the client is unable to void
   8. Administer blood products as prescribed
   9. Monitor for signs of infection, such as increased temperature, pulse rate, and WBC count
   10. Administer antibiotics as prescribed, as infection is common following hematoma formation
   11. Prepare for incision and evacuation of hematoma if necessary

III. HEMORRHAGE
A. Description: Bleeding of 500 mL or more following **delivery**
B. Assessment
   1. Early
      a. Hemorrhage occurs during the first 24 hours after **delivery**
      b. Caused by uterine atony, lacerations, or inversion of the uterus
   2. Late
      a. Hemorrhage occurs after the first 24 hours following **delivery**
      b. Caused by retained **placental** fragments
C. Implementation
   1. Massage fundus, with care not to overmassage

2. Notify physician or health care provider if hemorrhage occurs
3. Monitor vital signs and fundus every 5 to 15 minutes
4. Remain with the client
5. Assess and estimate blood loss by pad count
6. Assess level of consciousness
7. Administer fluids and monitor I & O
8. Monitor H & H levels
9. Maintain asepsis, since hemorrhage predisposes to infection
10. Prepare for the administration of oxytocin (Pitocin) if prescribed
11. Prepare for the administration of blood transfusions if prescribed

IV. INFECTION
A. Description: Any infection of the reproductive organs that occurs within 28 days of **delivery** or abortion
B. Assessment
  1. Fever
  2. Chills
  3. Anorexia
  4. Pelvic discomfort or pain
  5. Vaginal discharge
  6. Elevated WBC count
C. Implementation
  1. Monitor vital signs and temperature every 2 to 4 hours
  2. Make the mother as comfortable as possible; position for comfort and to promote drainage
  3. Keep the mother warmed if chilled
  4. Isolate the baby from the mother only if the mother can infect the baby
  5. Provide nutritious, high-calorie, protein diet
  6. Force fluids to 3000 to 4000 mL per day, if not contraindicated
  7. Encourage frequent voiding and monitor I & O
  8. Monitor culture results if cultures were prescribed
  9. Administer antibiotics according to organism, as prescribed

▲ V. MASTITIS
A. Description
  1. Inflammation of the breast as a result of infection
  2. Primarily seen in breastfeeding mothers 2 to 3 weeks after **delivery** but may occur at any time during lactation
B. Assessment
  1. Localized heat and swelling
  2. Pain
  3. Elevated temperature
  4. Complaints of flu-like symptoms
C. Implementation
  1. Instruct the mother in good handwashing and breast hygiene techniques

2. Promote comfort
3. Apply heat or cold to site as prescribed
4. Maintain lactation in breastfeeding mothers
5. Encourage manual expression of breast milk or use of breast pump every 4 hours
6. Encourage mother to support breasts by wearing a supportive bra
7. Administer analgesics as prescribed
8. Administer antibiotics as prescribed

VI. PULMONARY EMBOLISM
A. Description: The passage of thrombus, often originating in one of the uterine or other pelvic veins, into the lungs, where it disrupts the circulation of the blood
B. Assessment
  1. Dyspnea, tachypnea, and tachycardia
  2. Cough and rales
  3. Hemoptysis
  4. Pleuritic chest pain
  5. Feeling of impending doom
C. Implementation
  1. Administer oxygen as prescribed
  2. Position client with the head of the bed elevated to promote comfort
  3. Monitor vital signs frequently
  4. Frequently assess respiratory rate and breath sounds
  5. Monitor for signs of respiratory distress and for signs of increasing hypoxemia
  6. Administer IV fluids as prescribed
  7. Administer anticoagulants as prescribed
  8. Prepare to assist physician to administer streptokinase to dissolve the clot if prescribed

VII. SUBINVOLUTION
A. Description: Incomplete involution or failure of the uterus to return to its normal size and condition
B. Assessment
  1. Uterine pain on palpation
  2. Uterus is larger than expected
  3. Greater than normal vaginal bleeding
C. Implementation
  1. Assess vital signs
  2. Assess uterus and fundus
  3. Monitor for vaginal bleeding
  4. Elevate the legs to promote venous return
  5. Encourage frequent voiding
  6. Monitor H & H
  7. Prepare to administer methylergonovine maleate (Methergine) as prescribed

VIII. THROMBOPHLEBITIS
A. Description
  1. A condition in which a clot forms in a vessel wall as a result of the inflammation of the vessel wall
  2. A partial obstruction of the vessel can occur

TABLE 29-1

Assessment of the Types of Thrombophlebitis

Superficial	Femoral	Pelvic
Tenderness and pain in the affected lower extremity	Chills and fever	Severe chills
	Malaise	Dramatic body temperature changes
Warm and pinkish red color over thrombus area	Pain, stiffness, and swelling of the affected leg	Occurrence of pulmonary embolism may be the first sign
Palpable thrombus that feels bumpy and hard	Shiny, white skin over the affected area	
	Positive Homans' sign	
	Diminished peripheral pulses	

  3. Increased blood-clotting factors in the postpartum period place the client at risk
B. Types
  1. Superficial thrombophlebitis
  2. Femoral thrombophlebitis
  3. Pelvic thrombophlebitis
C. Assessment (Table 29-1)
D. Implementation
  1. Assess the lower extremities for edema, tenderness, varices, and increased skin temperature
  2. Evaluate the legs for Homans' sign by extending the legs with the knees slightly flexed and dorsiflexing the foot
  3. Maintain bed rest
  4. Elevate the affected leg
  5. Apply a bed cradle and keep bedclothes off affected leg
  6. Never massage the leg
  7. Monitor for manifestations of pulmonary embolism
  8. Superficial thrombophlebitis
    a. Provide bed rest
    b. Apply hot packs to the affected site as prescribed
    c. Apply elastic stockings
    d. Administer analgesics as prescribed
  9. Femoral thrombophlebitis
    a. Provide bed rest
    b. Elevate affected leg
    c. Apply moist heat continuously to affected area if prescribed to alleviate discomfort
    d. Administer analgesics as prescribed
    e. Administer antibiotics if prescribed
    f. Prepare to administer intravenous heparin sodium to prevent further thrombus formation if prescribed
  10. Pelvic thrombophlebitis
    a. Provide bed rest
    b. Administer analgesics as prescribed
    c. Administer antibiotics if prescribed
    d. Prepare to administer intravenous heparin sodium
E. Client education (Box 29-1)

BOX 29-1

Client Education for Thrombophlebitis

Avoid pressure behind the knees
Avoid prolonged sitting
Avoid constrictive clothing
Avoid crossing the legs
Never massage the leg
Know how to apply support hose if prescribed
Understand the importance of anticoagulant therapy as prescribed
Understand the importance of follow-up with the health care provider

PRACTICE QUESTIONS

1. A nurse is caring for a postpartum woman who has received epidural anesthesia and is monitoring the woman for the presence of a vulvar hematoma. Which of the following assessment findings would best indicate the presence of a hematoma?
   1. Complaints of a tearing sensation
   2. Complaints of intense pain
   3. Changes in vital signs
   4. Signs of heavy bruising
2. A nurse is developing a plan of care for a postpartum woman with a small vulvar hematoma. The nurse includes which specific intervention in the plan for this client?
   1. Assess vital signs every 4 hours
   2. Inform health care provider of assessment findings
   3. Measure fundal height every 4 hours
   4. Prepare an ice pack for application to the area
3. A new mother received an epidural during labor and had a forceps delivery after pushing for 2 hours. At 6 hours postpartum, her systolic blood pressure has dropped 20 points, her diastolic blood pressure has dropped 10 points, and her pulse is 120 beats per minute. The client is very anxious and restless. Upon further assessment, a vulvar hematoma is

verified. After notifying the health care provider, the nurse immediately plans to:

1. Monitor fundal height
2. Apply perineal pressure
3. Prepare the client for surgery
4. Reassure the client

4. After surgical evacuation and repair of a paravaginal hematoma, the 3 days postpartum mother is discharged. A nurse knows that the new mother needs further discharge instructions when the new mother states:

1. "Because I am so sore, I will nurse the baby while lying on my side."
2. "I will probably need my mother to help me with housekeeping."
3. "My husband and I will not have intercourse until the stitches are healed."
4. "The only medications I will take are prenatal vitamins and stool softeners."

5. A nurse is monitoring a new mother in the postpartum period for signs of hemorrhage. Which of the following signs if noted in the mother would be an early sign of excessive blood loss?

1. A temperature of 100.4° F
2. An increase in the pulse rate from 88 to 102 beats per minute
3. An increase in the respiratory rate from 18 to 22 breaths per minute
4. A blood pressure change from 130/88 to 124/80 mm Hg

6. A nurse is preparing to assess the uterine fundus of a client in the immediate postpartum period. When the nurse locates the fundus, she notes that the uterus feels soft and boggy. Which of the following nursing interventions would be most appropriate initially?

1. Massage the fundus until it is firm
2. Elevate the mother's legs
3. Push on the uterus to assist in expressing clots
4. Encourage the mother to void

7. A postpartum nurse is assessing a mother who delivered a healthy newborn infant by cesarean section. The nurse is assessing for signs and symptoms of superficial venous thrombosis. Which of the following signs or symptoms would the nurse note if superficial venous thrombosis were present?

1. Paleness of the calf area
2. Enlarged, hardened veins
3. Coolness of the calf area
4. Palpable dorsalis pedis pulses

8. A nurse is developing a plan of care for a postpartum client who was diagnosed with superficial venous thrombosis. Which of the following interventions would not be a component of the plan of care?

1. Elevation of the affected extremity
2. Maintaining bed rest

3. Applying warm pads to the affected area
4. Administering the prescribed anticoagulants

9. A client in a postpartum unit complains of sudden sharp chest pain. The nurse notes that the client is tachycardic and the respiratory rate is elevated. The nurse suspects a pulmonary embolism. The initial nursing action would be which of the following?

1. Assess the client's blood pressure
2. Initiate an IV line
3. Administer oxygen at 8 to 10 liters per minute by face mask
4. Prepare to administer morphine sulfate

10. A nurse is providing instructions to a mother who has been diagnosed with mastitis. Which of the following statements if made by the mother indicates a need for further education?

1. "I need to take antibiotics, and I should begin to feel better in 24 to 48 hours."
2. "I can use analgesics to assist in alleviating some of the discomfort."
3. "I need to wear a supportive bra to relieve the discomfort."
4. "I need to stop breastfeeding until this condition resolves."

11. A nurse is monitoring a postpartum client in the fourth stage of labor. Which of the following findings if noted by the nurse would indicate a complication related to a laceration of the birth canal?

1. The presence of dark red lochia
2. The saturation of more than one peripad per hour
3. Palpation of the uterus as a firm contracted ball
4. Palpation of the fundus at the level of the umbilicus

12. A nurse is developing a plan of care for a new mother recovering from a cesarean delivery. To prevent thrombophlebitis, the nurse plans to encourage the woman to:

1. Ambulate frequently
2. Apply warm moist packs to the legs
3. Remain on bed rest
4. Elevate the legs

13. A postpartum client is being treated for deep venous thrombophlebitis. A nurse understands that the client's response to treatment will be evaluated by regularly assessing the client for:

1. Dysuria, ecchymosis, and vertigo
2. Epistaxis, hematuria, and dysuria
3. Hematuria, ecchymosis, and epistaxis
4. Hematuria, ecchymosis, and vertigo

14. A nurse suspects that a postpartum client with femoral thrombophlebitis has developed a pulmonary embolism. The immediate nursing action would be to:

1. Administer oxygen by face mask as prescribed at 8 to 10 liters per minute
2. Elevate the head of the bed to 30 to 45 degrees

3. Initiate an IV line if one is not already in place
4. Monitor vital signs

15. A nurse performs an assessment on a client who is 4 hours postpartum. The nurse notes that the client has cool, clammy skin and is restless and excessively thirsty. The nurse prepares to immediately:
    1. Assess for hypovolemia and notify the health care provider
    2. Begin hourly pad counts and reassure the client
    3. Begin fundal massage and start oxygen by mask
    4. Elevate the head of the bed and assess vital signs

16. A nurse is assessing a client in the fourth stage of labor and notes that the fundus is firm but that bleeding is excessive. The initial nursing action would be which of the following?
    1. Massage the fundus
    2. Place the mother in the Trendelenburg position
    3. Notify the physician
    4. Record the findings

17. A new mother is seen in a health care clinic 2 weeks after giving birth to a healthy newborn infant. The mother is complaining that she feels as though she has the flu and complains of fatigue and aching muscles. On further assessment, the nurse notes a localized area of redness on the left breast, and the mother is diagnosed with mastitis. The mother asks the nurse about the condition. The most appropriate nursing response is which of the following?
    1. "The infection can occur at any time during breastfeeding."
    2. "The infection is most common for women who have breastfed in the past."
    3. "The infection usually involves both breasts."
    4. "The infection usually is caused by wearing a supportive bra."

18. A nurse is providing instructions to a mother who is breastfeeding her newborn infant regarding measures to prevent postpartum mastitis. Which of the following if stated by the mother would indicate a need for further instructions?
    1. "I should change the breast pads frequently."

2. "I should wash the nipples daily with soap and water."
3. "I should wash my hands well before breastfeeding."
4. "I should breastfeed every 2 to 3 hours."

19. A home care nurse visits a client who delivered a healthy newborn infant via vaginal delivery. An episiotomy was performed, and the woman has developed a wound infection at the episiotomy site. The nurse provides instructions to the mother regarding care related to the infection. Which of the following statements if made by the mother would indicate a need for further instructions?
    1. "I need to take the antibiotics as prescribed."
    2. "I need to apply warm compresses to provide comfort."
    3. "I need to take warm sitz baths to promote healing."
    4. "I need to isolate the infant for 48 hours after the initiation of the antibiotics."

20. A nurse is caring for a postpartum client with a diagnosis of deep vein thrombosis who is receiving a continuous intravenous infusion of heparin sodium. Which of the following laboratory results will the nurse specifically review to determine if an effective and appropriate dose of the heparin is being delivered?
    1. Prothrombin time
    2. International Normalized Ratio
    3. Activated partial thromboplastin time
    4. Platelet count

CRITICAL THINKING: FREE-TEXT ENTRY

A nurse is assessing the fundus in a postpartum woman. The nurse notes that the uterus is soft and spongy. What is the most appropriate initial nursing action?

Answer: _____

ANSWERS

1. **3**

Rationale: Because the woman has had epidural anesthesia and is anesthetized, she cannot feel pain, pressure, or a tearing sensation. Changes in vital signs indicate hypovolemia in the anesthetized postpartum woman with vulvar hematoma. Option 4 (heavy bruising) may be visualized, but vital sign changes indicate hematoma caused by blood collection in the perineal tissues.

Test-Taking Strategy: Use the process of elimination, noting the key words "epidural anesthesia." With this in mind,

eliminate options 1 and 2. From the remaining options, use the ABCs—airway, breathing, and circulation—to direct you to option 3. Review the signs of a vulvar hematoma in a woman who had epidural anesthesia if you had difficulty with this question.

Level of Cognitive Ability: Analysis
Client Needs: Physiological Integrity
Integrated Concept/Process: Nursing Process/Assessment
Content Area: Maternity
Reference: Lowdermilk, D., Perry, S., & Bobak, I. (2000). *Maternity & women's health care* (7th ed.). St. Louis: Mosby, p. 1023.

2. **4**

Rationale: Application of ice will reduce swelling caused by hematoma formation in the vulvar area. Options 1, 2, and 3 are not interventions that are specific to the plan of care for a client with a small vulvar hematoma.

Test-Taking Strategy: Use the process of elimination, noting the key words "small" and "specific intervention" in the question. This focus will assist in directing you to option 4. Review nursing care of the client with a hematoma if you had difficulty with this question.

Level of Cognitive Ability: Application

Client Needs: Physiological Integrity

Integrated Concept/Process: Nursing Process/Planning

Content Area: Maternity

Reference: Olds, S., London. M., & Ladewig, P. (2000). *Maternal-newborn nursing: A family and community-based approach* (6th ed.). Upper Saddle River, N.J.: Prentice-Hall Health, p. 984.

3. **3**

Rationale: The use of an epidural, prolonged second-stage labor, and forceps delivery are predisposing factors for hematoma formation, and a collection of up to 500 mL of blood can occur in the vaginal area. Although the other options may be implemented, the immediate action would be to prepare the client for surgery to stop the bleeding.

Test-Taking Strategy: Use the process of elimination and note the key word "immediately." Focus on the clinical manifestations identified in the question to direct you to option 3. Review nursing content related to vulvar hematomas if you had difficulty with this question.

Level of Cognitive Ability: Application

Client Needs: Physiological Integrity

Integrated Concept/Process: Nursing Process/Planning

Content Area: Maternity

Reference: Olds, S., London. M., & Ladewig, P. (2000). *Maternal-newborn nursing: A family and community-based approach* (6th ed.). Upper Saddle River, N.J.: Prentice-Hall Health, p. 984.

4. **4**

Rationale: The postoperative client will need an antibiotic because she is at increased risk for infection as a result of the break in skin integrity and collection of blood at the hematoma site. Options 1, 2, and 3 indicate that the mother understands the home care measures following surgical evacuation and repair of a paravaginal hematoma.

Test-Taking Strategy: Use the process of elimination, noting the key words "needs further discharge instructions." Recalling that the client is at increased risk for infection because of the break in skin integrity and collection of blood at the hematoma site will easily direct you to option 4. Review treatment plans associated with hematoma if you had difficulty with this question.

Level of Cognitive Ability: Analysis

Client Needs: Health Promotion and Maintenance

Integrated Concept/Process: Teaching/Learning

Content Area: Maternity

Reference: Olds, S., London. M., & Ladewig, P. (2000). *Maternal-newborn nursing: A family and community-based approach* (6th ed.). Upper Saddle River, N.J.: Prentice-Hall Health, p. 984.

5. **2**

Rationale: During the fourth stage of labor, the maternal blood pressure, pulse, and respiration should be checked every 15 minutes during the first hour. A rising pulse is an early sign of excessive blood loss because the heart pumps faster to compensate for reduced blood volume. The blood pressure will fall as the blood volume diminishes, but a decreased blood pressure would not be the earliest sign of hemorrhage. A slight rise in temperature is normal in the postpartum period.

Test-Taking Strategy: Use the process of elimination, noting the key word "early" in the stem of the question. Think about the physiological occurrences of shock and the expected findings in the postpartum period. This should assist in directing you to option 2. Review signs of early hemorrhage if you had difficulty with this question.

Level of Cognitive Ability: Analysis

Client Needs: Physiological Integrity

Integrated Concept/Process: Nursing Process/Analysis

Content Area: Maternity

Reference: Gorrie, T., McKinney, E., & Murray, S. (1998). *Foundations of maternal-newborn nursing* (2nd ed.). Philadelphia: W.B. Saunders, p. 330.

6. **1**

Rationale: If the uterus is not firmly contracted, the first intervention is to massage the fundus until it is firm and to express clots that may have accumulated in the uterus. Pushing on an uncontracted uterus can invert the uterus and cause massive hemorrhage. Elevating the client's legs and encouraging the client to void will not assist in managing uterine atony. If the uterus does not remain contracted as a result of the uterine massage, the problem may be a distended bladder and the nurse should assist the mother to urinate, but this would not be the initial action.

Test-Taking Strategy: Use the process of elimination. Note the key word "initially" in the stem of the question. Focus on the issue of the question and knowledge regarding the therapeutic management for uterine atony to assist in directing you to the correct option. If you had difficulty with this question, review therapeutic management for the client with uterine atony.

Level of Cognitive Ability: Application

Client Needs: Physiological Integrity

Integrated Concept/Process: Nursing Process/Implementation

Content Area: Maternity

Reference: Gorrie, T., McKinney, E., & Murray, S. (1998). *Foundations of maternal-newborn nursing* (2nd ed.). Philadelphia: W.B. Saunders, p. 785.

7. **2**

Rationale: Thrombosis of superficial veins is usually accompanied by signs and symptoms of inflammation. These include swelling of the involved extremity as well as redness, tenderness, and warmth. It also may be possible to palpate the enlarged, hard vein. Clients sometimes experience pain when they walk.

Test-Taking Strategy: Use the process of elimination, eliminating option 4 first because this is a normal and expected finding. Next eliminate options 1 and 3 because they are similar. If you had difficulty with this question, review the clinical manifestations associated with venous thrombosis.

Level of Cognitive Ability: Analysis

Client Needs: Physiological Integrity
Integrated Concept/Process: Nursing Process/Assessment
Content Area: Maternity
Reference: Gorrie, T., McKinney, E., & Murray, S. (1998). *Foundations of maternal-newborn nursing* (2nd ed.). Philadelphia: W.B. Saunders, p. 793.

8. 4
Rationale: Thrombosis that is limited to the superficial veins of the saphenous system is treated with analgesics, rest, and elastic support stockings. Elevation of the lower extremity to improve venous return may also be recommended. Warm packs may be applied to the affected area to promote healing. There is no need for anticoagulants or antiinflammatory agents unless the condition persists. After 5 to 7 days of bed rest, and when symptoms disappear, the woman may ambulate gradually.
Test-Taking Strategy: Use the process of elimination, focusing on the diagnosis of superficial venous thrombosis. Note the key word "superficial" in the stem of the question. Knowledge that anticoagulants are not used in this disorder will assist in directing you to option 4. Review therapeutic management of superficial venous thrombosis if you had difficulty with this question.
Level of Cognitive Ability: Application
Client Needs: Physiological Integrity
Integrated Concept/Process: Nursing Process/Planning
Content Area: Maternity
Reference: Gorrie, T., McKinney, E., & Murray, S. (1998). *Foundations of maternal-newborn nursing* (2nd ed.). Philadelphia: W.B. Saunders, p. 793.

9. 3
Rationale: If pulmonary embolism is suspected, oxygen should be administered at 8 to 10 liters per minute by face mask. Oxygen is used to decrease hypoxia. The woman is also kept on bed rest with the head of the bed slightly elevated to reduce dyspnea. Morphine may be prescribed for the client, but this action would not be the initial nursing action. An IV line will also be required, and vital signs need to be monitored, but these actions would follow the administration of the oxygen.
Test-Taking Strategy: Use the process of elimination, noting the key words "initial" in the stem of the question. Use the ABCs—airway, breathing, and circulation—to assist in directing you to option 3. If you had difficulty with this question, review therapeutic management of the client with pulmonary embolism.
Level of Cognitive Ability: Application
Client Needs: Physiological Integrity
Integrated Concept/Process: Nursing Process/Implementation
Content Area: Maternity
Reference: Gorrie, T., McKinney, E., & Murray, S. (1998). *Foundations of maternal-newborn nursing* (2nd ed.). Philadelphia: W.B. Saunders, p. 796.

10. 4
Rationale: In most cases, the mother can continue to breastfeed with both breasts. If the affected breast is too sore, the mother can pump the breast gently. Regular emptying of the breast is important to prevent abscess formation. Antibiotic therapy assists in resolving the mastitis within 24 to 48 hours. Additional supportive measures include ice packs, breast supports, and analgesics.

Test-Taking Strategy: Use the process of elimination, noting the key words "need for further education." Knowledge regarding the therapeutic management associated with mastitis will assist in eliminating options 1, 2, and 3. Review measures for the client with mastitis if you had difficulty with this question.
Level of Cognitive Ability: Analysis
Client Needs: Physiological Integrity
Integrated Concept/Process: Teaching/Learning
Content Area: Maternity
Reference: Gorrie, T., McKinney, E., & Murray, S. (1998). *Foundations of maternal-newborn nursing* (2nd ed.). Philadelphia: W.B. Saunders, p. 801.

11. 2
Rationale: In the first 24 hours after birth, the uterus will feel like a firmly contracted ball roughly the size of a large grapefruit. It should be easily located at the level of the umbilicus. Lochia should be dark red and moderate in amount. Saturation of more than one peripad per hour is considered excessive even in the early postpartum period.
Test-Taking Strategy: Use the process of elimination, focusing on the issue of the question. Eliminate those options that indicate normal physiological findings in the fourth stage of labor. Noting the key word "saturation" in option 2 will assist in directing you to this option. Review the normal findings in the fourth stage of labor if you had difficulty with this question.
Level of Cognitive Ability: Analysis
Client Needs: Physiological Integrity
Integrated Concept/Process: Nursing Process/Assessment
Content Area: Maternity
Reference: Gorrie, T., McKinney, E., & Murray, S. (1998). *Foundations of maternal-newborn nursing* (2nd ed.). Philadelphia: W.B. Saunders, p. 784.

12. 1
Rationale: Stasis is believed to be a predisposing factor in the development of thrombophlebitis. Because cesarean delivery is also a risk factor for thrombophlebitis, new mothers should ambulate early and frequently to promote circulation and prevent stasis. Options 2, 3, and 4 are interventions for the client diagnosed with thrombophlebitis.
Test-Taking Strategy: Use the process of elimination, noting the key words "prevent thrombophlebitis." Eliminate options 2, 3, and 4 because they are similar and are interventions for the client who has been diagnosed with thrombophlebitis. Review content related to the prevention of thrombophlebitis in the postoperative period if you had difficulty with this question.
Level of Cognitive Ability: Application
Client Needs: Health Promotion and Maintenance
Integrated Concept/Process: Teaching/Learning
Content Area: Maternity
Reference: Olds, S., London. M., & Ladewig, P. (2000). *Maternal-newborn nursing: A family and community-based approach* (6th ed.). Upper Saddle River, N.J.: Prentice-Hall Health, p. 938.

13. 3
Rationale: The treatment for deep venous thrombophlebitis is anticoagulant therapy. The nurse assesses for bleeding, which is an adverse effect of anticoagulants. This includes hematuria,

ecchymosis, and epistaxis. Dysuria and vertigo (options 1, 2, and 4) are not specifically associated with bleeding.

Test-Taking Strategy: Use the process of elimination. Recall that deep venous thrombophlebitis is treated with anticoagulant therapy and that bleeding is an adverse effect. Eliminate options 1, 2, and 4 because dysuria and vertigo are not specifically associated with bleeding. Review the treatment for deep venous thrombophlebitis and the adverse effects of treatment if you had difficulty with this question.

Level of Cognitive Ability: Analysis
Client Needs: Physiological Integrity
Integrated Concept/Process: Nursing Process/Evaluation
Content Area: Maternity
Reference: Sherwen, L., Scoloveno, M.A., & Weingarten, C. (1999). *Maternity nursing: Care of the childbearing family* (3rd ed.). Stamford, Conn.: Appleton & Lange, p. 906.

14. **1**

Rationale: Because pulmonary circulation is compromised in the presence of an embolus, cardiorespiratory support is initiated by oxygen administration. Although options 2, 3, and 4 may be implemented, they are not the immediate nursing action.

Test-Taking Strategy: Use the process of elimination, noting the key words "immediate nursing action." This question requires that you prioritize your actions. Use the ABCs—airway, breathing, and circulation—to direct you to option 1. Review immediate interventions for the client who has developed a pulmonary embolism if you had difficulty with this question.

Level of Cognitive Ability: Application
Client Needs: Physiological Integrity
Integrated Concept/Process: Nursing Process/Implementation
Content Area: Maternity
Reference: Gorrie, T., McKinney, E., & Murray, S. (1998). *Foundations of maternal-newborn nursing* (2nd ed.). Philadelphia: W.B. Saunders, p. 796.

15. **1**

Rationale: Symptoms of hypovolemia include cool, clammy, pale skin, sensations of anxiety or impending doom, restlessness, and thirst. When these symptoms are present, the nurse should further assess for hypovolemia and notify the health care provider. Option 2 will delay necessary treatment. There is no indication in the question of the cause of the hypovolemia or that the client is hemorrhaging and that fundal massage is needed. The head of the bed is not elevated in a hypovolemic condition.

Test-Taking Strategy: Use the process of elimination and focus on the data provided in the question. Note the key word "immediately." Use the steps of the nursing process to select the correct option. Option 1 is the only option that addresses assessment. Review the interventions for the client experiencing hypovolemia if you had difficulty with this question.

Level of Cognitive Ability: Analysis
Client Needs: Physiological Integrity
Integrated Concept/Process: Nursing Process/Planning
Content Area: Maternity
Reference: Gorrie, T., McKinney, E., & Murray, S. (1998). *Foundations of maternal-newborn nursing* (2nd ed.). Philadelphia: W.B. Saunders, p. 790.

16. **3**

Rationale: If bleeding is excessive, the cause may be laceration of the cervix or birth canal. Massaging the fundus if it is firm will not assist in controlling the bleeding. The Trendelenburg position is to be avoided because it may interfere with cardiac function. Although the nurse would record the findings, the initial nursing action would be to contact the physician.

Test-Taking Strategy: Read the question carefully, noting the issue of the question and the clinical manifestations identified in the question. Use the process of elimination and eliminate option 1 first, because if the uterus is firm, it would not be necessary to perform fundal massage. Knowing that the Trendelenburg position is not advised will assist in eliminating this option. From the remaining options, noting the key words "bleeding is excessive" will assist in directing you to option 3. Review the interventions related to a client who is hemorrhaging if you had difficulty with this question.

Level of Cognitive Ability: Application
Client Needs: Safe, Effective Care Environment
Integrated Concept/Process: Nursing Process/Implementation
Content Area: Maternity
Reference: Gorrie, T., McKinney, E., & Murray, S. (1998). *Foundations of maternal-newborn nursing* (2nd ed.). Philadelphia: W.B. Saunders, pp. 787, 789.

17. **1**

Rationale: Mastitis is an infection of the lactating breasts and occurs most often during the second and third weeks after birth, although it may develop at any time during breastfeeding. It is more common in mothers nursing for the first time, and usually affects one breast. A supportive bra will not cause mastitis; however, constriction of the breasts from a bra that is too tight may interfere with emptying of all the ducts and may also lead to infection.

Test-Taking Strategy: Use the process of elimination. Focus on the diagnosis presented in the question to assist in directing you to the correct option. If you are unfamiliar with the etiology and characteristics associated with mastitis, review this content.

Level of Cognitive Ability: Application
Client Needs: Health Promotion and Maintenance
Integrated Concept/Process: Teaching/Learning
Content Area: Maternity
Reference: Gorrie, T., McKinney, E., & Murray, S. (1998). *Foundations of maternal-newborn nursing* (2nd ed.). Philadelphia: W.B. Saunders, p. 800.

18. **2**

Rationale: Mastitis is generally caused by an organism that enters through an injured area of the nipples such as a crack or blister. Measures to prevent the development of mastitis include changing nursing pads when they are wet and avoiding continuous pressure on the breasts. Soap is drying and could lead to cracking of the nipples, and the mother should be instructed to avoid the use of soap on the nipples during breastfeeding. The mother is taught about the importance of handwashing and that she should breastfeed every 2 to 3 hours.

Test-Taking Strategy: Use the process of elimination. Note the key words "a need for further instructions" in the stem of the question. Recalling that the use of soap is drying to the skin, could cause cracking, and thus provide an entry point for

organisms will easily direct you to option 2. Review these measures if you had difficulty with this question.
Level of Cognitive Ability: Analysis
Client Needs: Health Promotion and Maintenance
Integrated Concept/Process: Teaching/Learning
Content Area: Maternity
Reference: Gorrie, T., McKinney, E., & Murray, S. (1998). *Foundations of maternal-newborn nursing* (2nd ed.). Philadelphia: W.B. Saunders, pp. 800-801.

19. **4**
Rationale: Broad-spectrum antibiotics will be prescribed for the mother, and the mother should be instructed to take the antibiotics as prescribed. Analgesics are often necessary, and warm compresses or sitz baths may be used to provide comfort in the area. The infant is not routinely isolated from the mother with a wound infection, but the mother must be taught how to protect the infant from contact with contaminated articles.
Test-Taking Strategy: Use the process of elimination, noting the key words "need for further instructions." Eliminate options 2 and 3 first because they are similar. Knowing that the infant does not need to be isolated from the mother will assist in directing you to the correct option. Review care to the client with a wound infection from an episiotomy sire if you had difficulty with this question.
Level of Cognitive Ability: Analysis
Client Needs: Health Promotion and Maintenance
Integrated Concept/Process: Teaching/Learning
Content Area: Maternity
Reference: Gorrie, T., McKinney, E., & Murray, S. (1998). *Foundations of maternal-newborn nursing* (2nd ed.). Philadelphia: W.B. Saunders, p. 800.

20. **3**
Rationale: Anticoagulation therapy may be used to prevent the extension of thrombus by delaying the clotting time of the blood. Activated partial thromboplastin time should be monitored, and a heparin dose should be adjusted to maintain a therapeutic level of 1.5 to 2.5 times the control. The prothrombin time and the International Normalized Ratio are used to monitor coagulation time when warfarin (Coumadin) is used. The platelet count cannot be used to determine an adequate dosage for the heparin infusion.
Test-Taking Strategy: Knowledge regarding the administration of heparin and the laboratory tests specific to monitoring for an appropriate and effective dose is required to answer this question. Remember that the activated partial thromboplastin time is used to monitor the effectiveness of a heparin infusion. If you are unfamiliar with the administration of heparin and the specific laboratory tests that are monitored, review this content.
Level of Cognitive Ability: Analysis
Client Needs: Physiological Integrity
Integrated Concept/Process: Nursing Process/Analysis
Content Area: Maternity
Reference: Gorrie, T., McKinney, E., & Murray, S. (1998). *Foundations of maternal-newborn nursing* (2nd ed.). Philadelphia: W.B. Saunders, p. 794.

CRITICAL THINKING: FREE-TEXT ENTRY

Answer: Massage the fundus gently until firm
Rationale: If the fundus is boggy (soft), the initial nursing action is to massage the fundus gently until firm. The physician will need to be notified if uterine massage is not helpful.
Test-Taking Strategy: Note the key words "most appropriate initial nursing action." Noting that the fundus is soft and spongy will assist in identifying the initial nursing action. Review nursing interventions related to this occurrence if you had difficulty with this question.
Level of Cognitive Ability: Application
Client Needs: Physiological Integrity
Integrated Concept/Process: Nursing Process/Implementation
Content Area: Maternity
Reference: Olds, S., London. M., & Ladewig, P. (2000). *Maternal-newborn nursing: A family and community-based approach* (6th ed.). Upper Saddle River, N.J.: Prentice-Hall Health, p. 921.

REFERENCES

Gorrie, T., McKinney, E., & Murray, S. (1998). *Foundations of maternal-newborn nursing* (2nd ed.). Philadelphia: W.B. Saunders.

Ladewig, P., London. M., & Olds, S. (1998). *Maternal-newborn nursing care: The nurse, the family, and the community* (4th ed.). Menlo Park, Calif.: Addison-Wesley Longman.

Lowdermilk, D., Perry, S., & Bobak, I. (2000). *Maternity & women's health care* (7th ed.). St. Louis: Mosby.

Olds, S., London. M., & Ladewig, P. (2000). *Maternal-newborn nursing: A family and community-based approach* (6th ed.). Upper Saddle River, N.J.: Prentice-Hall Health.

Sherwen, L., Scoloveno, M.A., & Weingarten, C. (1999). *Maternity nursing: Care of the childbearing family* (3rd ed.). Stamford, Conn.: Appleton & Lange.

30

Care of the Newborn

▲ **I. INITIAL CARE OF THE NEWBORN**

A. Assessment
1. Observe or assist with initiation of respirations
2. Assess Apgar score
3. Note characteristics of cry
4. Monitor for nasal flaring, grunting, retractions, abnormal respirations
5. Obtain vital signs
6. Observe **newborn** for signs of hypothermia or hyperthermia
7. Assess for gross anomalies

B. Implementation
1. Suction mouth, then nares, with bulb syringe
2. Dry **newborn** and stimulate crying by rubbing
3. Maintain temperature stability; wrap **newborn** in warm blankets and place a stockinette cap on **newborn's** head
4. Keep **newborn** with mother to facilitate bonding
5. Place **newborn** at mother's breast if breastfeeding is planned, or place on mother's abdomen
6. Place **newborn** in warmer
7. Position **newborn** on side or abdomen or in modified Trendelenburg position to facilitate drainage of mucus
8. Ensure **newborn's** proper identification
9. Footprint **newborn** and fingerprint mother on identification sheet, per agency policies and procedures
10. Place matching identification bracelets on mother and **newborn**

▲ C. Apgar scoring system
1. Perform and record the Apgar score at 1 minute and at 5 minutes
2. If the score is less than 7 at 5 minutes, the Apgar score should be performed at 10 minutes

3. Assess each of five items to be scored, and assign value of 0 (very poor) to 2 (excellent) for each item
4. Add the points to determine the **newborn's** total score
   a. A score of 7 to 10 indicates a healthy **newborn**
   b. A score of 3 to 6 is considered moderately depressed
   c. A score of 0 to 2 is severely depressed
5. Five vital indicators (Table 30-1)
6. Implementation (Table 30-2)

II. INITIAL PHYSICAL EXAMINATION ▲

A. General guidelines
1. Keep **newborn** warm during the examination
2. Begin with general observations; then perform assessments that are least disturbing to the **newborn** first
3. Initiate nursing interventions for abnormal findings
4. Document all abnormal findings

B. Vital signs ▲
1. Heart rate: 100 to 170 beats per minute (apical); assess for a full minute because of irregularities after birth
2. Respirations: 30 to 80 breaths per minute; assess for a full minute
3. Axillary temperature: 96.8 to 99° F
4. Blood pressure: 73/55 mm Hg

C. Body measurements
1. Length: 45 to 55 cm (18 to 22 inches)
2. Weight: 2500 to 4300 g (5.5 to 9.5 pounds)
3. Head circumference: 33 to 35.5 cm (13 to 14 inches)
4. Chest circumference: 30 to 33 cm (12 to 13 inches) and should be equal to or 2 to 3 cm less than the head circumference

TABLE 30-1

Apgar Scoring

Indicator	0 Points	1 Point	2 Points
Heart rate	Absent	Less than 100	More than 100
Respiratory rate	Absent	Slow, irregular weak cry	Good vigorous cry
Muscle tone	Flaccid, limp	Some flexion of extremities	Good flexion, active motion
Reflex irritability	No response	Weak cry and grimace	Vigorous cry, cough, sneeze
Skin color	Blue	Body skin normal, extremities blue	Body and extremity skin color normal

TABLE 30-2

Apgar Score Implementation

Score	Implementation
7 to 10	Rarely needs resuscitation
3 to 6	Requires resuscitation
	Suction
	Dry quickly
	Maintain warmth
	Ventilate 30 to 50 times a minute until heart rate is above 100, color is pink, and spontaneous respirations begin
	Provide oxygen
	Careful observation needed during the first few days of life
0 to 2	Requires intensive resuscitation
	Clear airway
	Insert endotracheal tube
	Use Ambu bag if necessary
	Ventilate with 100% oxygen at 40 to 60 breaths per minute
	Initiate full CPR as needed
	Maintain body temperature
	Support parents

▲ D. Head
  1. 25% of the body length (cephalocaudal development)
  2. Bones of the skull are not fused
  3. Palpable sutures (connective tissue between the skull bones)
  4. Fontanels: Unossified membranous tissue at the junction of the sutures (Table 30-3)
  5. Molding: Asymmetry of the head as a result of pressure in the birth canal; disappears in about 72 hours
  6. Masses from birth trauma
    a. Caput succedaneum: Edema of the soft tissue over bone (crosses over suture line); subsides within a few days
    b. Cephalhematoma: Swelling caused by bleeding into an area between the bone and its periosteum (does not cross over suture line); usually absorbed within 6 weeks with no treatment

  7. Head lag
    a. Common when pulling **newborn** to a sitting position
    b. When prone, **newborn** should be able to lift the head slightly and turn the head from side to side
E. Eyes
  1. Slate gray (light skin) or brown-gray (dark skin)
  2. Symmetrical and clear
  3. Pupils equal, round, react to light by accommodation
  4. Blink reflex present
  5. Eyes cross because of weak extraocular muscles
  6. Able to track and fixate momentarily
  7. Red reflex present
  8. Eyelids often edematous as a result of pressure during the birth process and the effects of eye medication
F. Ears
  1. Symmetrical
  2. Firm cartilage with recoil
  3. Pinna should be on or above line drawn from canthus of eye
  4. Low-set ears associated with Down's syndrome
G. Nose
  1. Flat, broad, in center of face
  2. Obligatory nose breathing
  3. Occasional sneezing to remove obstructions
H. Mouth
  1. Pink, moist gums
  2. Soft and hard palates intact
  3. Epstein's pearls (small, white cysts) may be present on hard palate
  4. Uvula in midline
  5. Tongue moves freely, is symmetrical, has short frenulum
  6. Sucking and crying movements symmetrical
  7. Able to swallow
  8. Gag reflex present
I. Neck
  1. Short and thick
  2. Head held in midline
  3. Trachea on midline
  4. Good range of motion (ROM) and is able to flex and extend

TABLE 30-3

Fontanels

Fontanel	Characteristics	Closure
Anterior	Soft, flat, diamond shaped 3 to 4 cm wide by 2 to 3 cm long	Closes between 12 and 18 months of age
Posterior	Triangular 0.5 to 1 cm wide Located between occipital and parietal bones	Closes between birth and 2 to 3 months of age

J. Chest
1. Appears circular since anteroposterior and lateral diameters are about equal
2. Respirations appear diaphragmatic
3. Bronchial sounds heard on auscultation
4. Nipples prominent and often edematous
5. Milky secretion (witch's milk) common
6. Breast tissue present
7. Clavicles need to be palpated to assess for fractures

▲ K. Skin
1. Pinkish red (light-skinned **newborn**) to pinkish brown or pinkish yellow (dark-skinned **newborn**)
2. Vernix caseosa
3. Lanugo
4. Milia
5. Dry, peeling skin
6. Dark red color common in premature **newborns**
7. Cyanosis common with hypothermia, infection, and hypoglycemia, and with cardiac, respiratory, or neurological abnormalities
8. Acrocyanosis is a normal phenomenon and may be due to compromised peripheral circulation
9. Assess for ecchymosis and petechiae resulting from the trauma of birth
10. Assess skin turgor over the abdomen to determine hydration status
11. Observe for forceps marks
12. Harlequin sign
   a. Deep red color develops over one side of the **newborn's** body while the other side remains pale; is due to vasomotor disturbance
   b. Skin resembles a clown's suit
13. Birthmarks (Table 30-4)

▲ L. Abdomen
▲ 1. Umbilical cord
   a. Three vessels, two arteries and one vein, in cord; if fewer than three vessels are noted, notify the physician
   b. Small, thin cord may be associated with poor fetal growth
   c. Assess for intact cord, and ensure that clamp is secured
   d. Cord should be clamped for at least the first 24 hours after birth; clamp can be removed when the cord is dried and occluded

TABLE 30-4

Birthmarks

Birthmark	Characteristics
Telangiectatic nevi (stork bites)	Pale pink or red, flat, dilated capillaries On eyelids, nose, lower occipital bone, and nape of neck Blanch easily More noticeable during crying periods Disappear by age 2 years
Nevus flammeus (port-wine stain)	Capillary angioma directly below epidermis Nonelevated, sharply demarcated, red to purple, dense areas of capillaries Commonly appears on face Does not fade with time May require surgery in the future
Nevus vasculosus (strawberry mark)	Capillary hemangioma Raised, clearly delineated, dark red, with a rough surface Common in head region Disappears by age 7 to 9 years
Mongolian spots	Bluish black pigmentation On lumbar dorsal area and buttocks Gradually fade during first and second years of life Common in Asian and dark-skinned races

   e. Note any bleeding or drainage from the cord
   f. Triple dye may be applied for initial cord care because it minimizes microorganisms and promotes drying; use a cotton-tipped applicator to paint the dye, one time, on the cord and on 1 inch of surrounding skin
   g. Application of 70% isopropyl alcohol to the cord with each diaper change and at least two or three times a day to minimize microorganisms and promote drying
   h. If symptoms of infection such as moistness, oozing, discharge, and a reddened base occur, antibiotic treatment is prescribed

2. Gastrointestinal
   a. Monitor cord for meconium staining
   b. Assess for umbilical hernia
   c. Note abdominal depression associated with diaphragmatic hernia
   d. Assess for abdominal distension associated with obstruction, mass, or sepsis
   e. Monitor bowel sounds, which should occur within 1 to 2 hours after birth
3. Anus
   a. Anal opening patent
   b. First-stool meconium should pass within first 24 hours

M. Genitals
   1. Female
      a. Labia edematous, clitoris enlarged
      b. Smegma present (thick, white mucus discharge)
      c. Pseudomenstruation possible (blood-tinged mucus)
      d. Hymen tag may be visible
      e. First voiding should occur within 24 hours
   2. Male
      a. Prepuce (foreskin) covers glans penis
      b. Scrotum edematous
      c. Meatus at tip of penis
      d. Testes descended but may retract with cold
      e. Assess for hernia or hydrocele
      f. First voiding should occur within 24 hours

N. Spine
   1. Straight
   2. Posture flexed
   3. Supports head momentarily when prone
   4. Arms and legs flexed
   5. Chin flexed on upper chest
   6. Sporadic movements that are well coordinated
   7. A degree of hypotonicity or hypertonicity is indicative of central nervous system (CNS) damage

O. Extremities
   1. Flexed
   2. Full ROM; movements symmetrical
   3. Fists clenched
   4. Fingers and toes should be 10 each in number and separate
   5. Legs bowed
   6. Major gluteal folds even
   7. Creases on soles of feet
   8. Assess for fractures (especially clavicle) or dislocations (hip)
   9. Assess for hip dysplasia; when thighs are rotated outward, no clicks should be heard
   10. Pulses palpable (radial, brachial, femoral)
   11. Slight tremors are common but could be a sign of hypoglycemia or drug withdrawal

III. BODY SYSTEMS ASSESSMENT

A. Cardiovascular system
   1. Keep **newborn** warm
   2. Take apical heart rate for 1 full minute
   3. Listen for murmurs
   4. Palpate pulses
   5. Assess for cyanosis; blanch skin on trunk and extremities to assess circulation
   6. Observe for cardiac distress when **newborn** is feeding

B. Respiratory system
   1. Position **newborn** on side
   2. Suction as necessary: use a bulb syringe for upper airway suctioning (compress bulb before insertion) and a French catheter for deeper suctioning
   3. Observe for respiratory distress and hypoxemia
      a. Nasal flaring
      b. Increasingly severe retractions
      c. Grunting
      d. Cyanosis
      e. Bradycardia and periods of apnea lasting longer than 15 seconds
   4. Administer oxygen via hood if necessary and as prescribed

C. Hepatic system
   1. Normal or physiological jaundice appears after the first 24 hours in full-term **neonates** and after the first 48 hours in premature **neonates;** jaundice occurring prior to this time (pathological jaundice) may indicate early hemolysis of red blood cells (RBCs) and must be reported to the physician
   2. Physiological jaundice peaks about the fifth day of life (indirect bilirubin levels: 6 to 7 mg/dL)
   3. Monitor serum bilirubin levels
   4. Feed early to stimulate intestinal activity and to keep the bilirubin level low
   5. If **neonate** is being breastfed, temporarily discontinue breastfeeding for 48 hours if bilirubin levels exceed 15 to 20 mg/dL and if prescribed by the physician
   6. Prevent chilling, as hypothermia can cause acidosis that interferes with bilirubin conjugation and excretion
   7. Liver stores iron passed from the mother for 5 to 6 months
   8. Glycogen storage occurs in the liver
   9. **Neonate** is at risk for hemorrhagic disorders; coagulation factors synthesized in the liver are dependent on vitamin K, which is not synthesized until intestinal bacteria are present
   10. Handle **neonate** carefully and monitor for any bruising or bleeding episodes
   11. Watch for meconium stool and subsequent stools
   12. Administer one dose of vitamin K (Aqua-MEPHYTON), 0.5 to 1.0 mg IM, to the **neonate** in the lateral aspect of the middle third of the vastus lateralis muscle as prescribed, to prevent hemorrhagic disorders
   13. Assess **newborn's** hemoglobin and blood glucose levels

D. Renal system
1. The immature kidneys are unable to concentrate urine
2. A weight loss of 5% to 15% during the first week of life occurs as a result of voiding and limited intake
3. Weigh **newborn** daily
4. Monitor intake and output (I & O); weigh diapers if necessary
5. Measure specific gravity of urine if necessary
6. Assess for signs of dehydration (dry mucous membranes, sunken eyeballs, poor skin turgor, sunken fontanels)

E. Immune system
1. Passive immunity via the **placenta** (IgG)
2. Passive immunity from colostrum (IgA)
3. Elevations in IgM indicate infection in utero
4. Use aseptic technique when caring for the **newborn**
5. Observe universal (standard) precautions when handling the **newborn**
6. Ensure meticulous handwashing
7. Wear gowns when caring for the **newborn**
8. Ensure that an infection-free staff cares for the **newborn**
9. Monitor **newborn's** temperature
10. Observe for any cracks or openings in the skin
11. Administer eye medication within 1 hour after birth to prevent ophthalmia neonatorum
   a. Eye prophylaxis may be delayed until an hour or so after birth so that eye contact and parent-**infant** attachment and bonding are facilitated
   b. Erythromycin (0.5%) and tetracycline (1%) ophthalmic ointment or drops are both bacteriostatic and bactericidal and provide prophylaxis against *Neisseria gonorrhoeae* and *Chlamydia trachomatis*
   c. Silver nitrate (1%) solution may be prescribed, but its use is minimal because it does not protect against chlamydial infection and can cause chemical conjunctivitis
12. Provide cord care
   a. Umbilical clamp can be removed after 24 hours
   b. Teach mother how to perform cord care
   c. Keep the cord clean and dry by wiping with alcohol after each diaper change and at least two or three times a day
   d. Keep diaper from covering cord; fold diaper below cord
   e. Assess cord for odor, swelling, or discharge
   f. Sponge bathe the **newborn** until the cord falls off (within 2 weeks)
13. Provide circumcision care
   a. Apply petroleum jelly gauze to the penis except when a Plastibell is used
   b. Remove petroleum jelly gauze, if applied, after first voiding following circumcision
   c. Observe for swelling, infection, or bleeding from the circumcision site
   d. Teach mother care of circumcision site
   e. Cleanse the penis after each voiding by squeezing warm water over the penis
   f. A milky covering over the glans penis is normal and should not be disrupted
   g. Monitor for urinary retention

F. Metabolic system and gastrointestinal system
1. **Newborns** are able to digest simple carbohydrates but are unable to digest fats because of the lack of lipase
2. Proteins may be only partially broken down, so they may serve as antigens and provoke an allergic reaction
3. The **newborn** has a small stomach capacity (about 90 mL) with rapid intestinal peristalsis (bowel emptying time is 2.5 to 3 hours)
4. Breastfeeding can usually begin immediately after birth; bottle-fed **newborns** may be offered a few milliliters of sterile water or 5% dextrose 1 to 4 hours after birth prior to a feeding with formula
5. Observe feeding reflexes, such as rooting, sucking, and swallowing
6. Assist mother with breastfeeding or formula feeding
7. Burp **newborn** during and after feeding
8. Assess for regurigation or vomiting
9. Position **newborn** on right side after feeding
10. Observe for normal stool and the passage of meconium
   a. Meconium stool, which is greenish black with a thick, sticky, tar-like consistency, is usually passed within the first 24 hours of life
   b. Transitional stool, the second type of stool excreted by the **newborn,** is greenish brown and of looser consistency than meconium
   c. Soft, yellow stools are noted in breastfed **newborns;** seedy, yellow stools in formula-fed **newborns**
11. Perform **newborn** phenylketonuria (PKU) screening test before discharge and as an outpatient after sufficient protein intake occurs; the **newborn** should be on formula or breast milk for 24 hours before screening, and screening must be repeated in 7 to 14 days

G. Neurological system
1. **Newborn** head size is proportionally larger than that of adults because of cephalocaudal development
2. Myelinization of nerve fibers is incomplete, so primitive reflexes are present
3. Fontanels are open to allow for brain growth
4. Assess for an abnormal head size and a bulging or depressed anterior fontanel
5. Measure and graph head circumference in relation to chest circumference and length

6. Assess **newborn's** movements, noting symmetry, posture, and abnormal movements
7. Observe for jitteriness, marked tremors, and seizures
8. Test **newborn's** reflexes
9. Assess for lethargy
10. Assess pitch of cry

▲ H. Thermal regulatory system
1. **Newborns** do not shiver to produce heat
2. **Newborns** have brown fat deposits, which produce heat
3. Heat is dissipated through vasodilation
4. Prevent heat loss resulting from evaporation by keeping **newborn** dry and well-wrapped with a blanket
5. Prevent heat loss resulting from radiation by keeping **newborn** away from cold objects and outside walls
6. Prevent heat loss resulting from convection by shielding the **newborn** from drafts
7. Prevent heat loss resulting from conduction by performing all treatments on a warm, padded surface
8. Keep temperature in room warm
9. Take **newborn's** axillary temperature every hour for the first 4 hours of life, every 4 hours for the remainder of the first 24 hours, and then every shift

▲ I. Reflexes
1. Sucking and rooting
   a. Touch the **newborn's** lip, cheek, or corner of the mouth with a nipple
   b. **Newborn** turns head toward the nipple, opens the mouth, takes hold of the nipple, and sucks
   c. Usually disappears after 3 to 4 months but may persist for up to 1 year
2. Swallowing reflex
   a. Occurs spontaneously after sucking and obtaining fluids
   b. **Newborn** swallows in coordination with sucking without gagging, coughing, or vomiting
3. Tonic neck or fencing
   a. While the **newborn** is falling asleep or sleeping, gently and quickly turn the head to one side
   b. As the **newborn** faces the left side, the left arm and leg extend outward while the right arm and leg flex
   c. When the head is turned to the right side, the right arm and leg extend outward while the left arm and leg flex
   d. Usually disappears within 3 to 4 months
4. Palmar-plantar grasp
   a. Place a finger in the palm of the **newborn's** hand; then place a finger at the base of the toes

b. The **newborn's** fingers curl around the examiner's fingers, and the **newborn's** toes curl downward
   c. Palmar response lessens within 3 to 4 months
   d. Plantar response lessens within 8 months
5. Moro reflex
   a. Hold the **newborn** in a semisitting position; then allow the head and trunk to fall backward to at least a 30-degree angle
   b. The **newborn** symmetrically abducts and extends the arms
   c. The **newborn** fans the fingers out and forms a C with the thumb and the forefinger
   d. The **newborn** adducts the arms to an embracing position and returns to a relaxed flexion state
   e. Present at birth; a complete response may occur up to 8 weeks
   f. A body jerk motion occurs from 8 to 18 weeks
   g. No response may be noted by 6 months as long as neurological maturation has not been delayed
   h. A persistent response lasting more than 6 months may indicate the occurrence of brain damage during pregnancy
6. Startle reflex
   a. The response is best elicited if the **newborn** is a least 24 hours old
   b. The examiner makes a loud noise or claps hands to elicit the response
   c. The **newborn's** arms adduct while the elbows flex
   d. The hands stay clenched
   e. The reflex should disappear within 4 months
7. Pull-to-sit
   a. Pull the **newborn** up from the wrist while the **newborn** is in the prone position
   b. The head will lag until the **newborn** is in an upright position; then the head will be level with the chest and shoulders momentarily before falling forward
   c. The head will then lift for a few minutes
   d. The response depends on the **newborn's** general muscle tone and condition as well as maturity levels
8. Babinski sign—plantar
   a. Beginning at the heel of the foot, gently stroke upward along the lateral aspect of the sole; then the examiner moves the finger along the ball of the foot
   b. The **newborn's** toes hyperextend while the big toe dorsiflexes
   c. Reflex disappears after the **newborn** is 1 year old
   d. Absence of this reflex indicates the need for a neurological examination

9. Stepping or walking
   a. Hold the **newborn** in a vertical position, allowing one foot to touch a table surface
   b. The **newborn** simulates walking, alternately flexing and extending the feet
   c. The reflex is usually present for 3 to 4 months
10. Crawling
    a. Place the **newborn** on the abdomen
    b. The **newborn** begins making crawling movements with the arms and legs
    c. The reflex usually disappears after about 6 weeks

▲ **IV. PARENT TEACHING**
A. Formula feeding
   1. Teach sterilization techniques if the water supply is located in areas where the purification process of the water is questionable
   2. Remind the mother not to heat the bottle of formula in a microwave oven
   3. Inform the mother that formula is a sufficient diet for the first 4 to 6 months
   4. Assess the mother's ability to burp the **newborn**
B. Breastfeeding
   1. Assess the **newborn's** ability to attach to the mother's breast and suck
   2. Teach the mother about engorgement
   3. Teach the mother how to pump her breasts and how to store breast milk properly
   4. Inform the mother that breast milk is a sufficient and superior diet for the first 4 to 6 months
   5. Give the mother the phone numbers of the local organizations that offer support to breastfeeding mothers
C. Bathing
   1. Bathe the **newborn** in a warm room before feeding
   2. Have all equipment for bathing available
   3. Use a mild soap (not on the face)
   4. Proceed from the cleanest area to the dirtiest
   5. Clean eyes from the inner canthus outward
   6. Special care should be taken to clean under the folds of the neck, underarms, groin, and genitals
   7. Make bath time enjoyable for both the **newborn** and the mother
D. Clothing
   1. Assess diaper and clothing needs for the **newborn** with the mother
   2. Instruct the mother that the **newborn's** head should be covered in cold weather to prevent heat loss
   3. Instruct the mother to layer the **newborn's** clothing in cooler weather
E. Cord care: Refer to cord care under Body Systems Assessment
F. Circumcision: Refer to circumcision care under Body Systems Assessment

G. Uncircumcised **newborn**
   1. Inform the mother that the foreskin and glans are two similar layers of cells that separate from each other and that the separation process is normally complete between 3 and 5 years of age
   2. Instruct the mother not to pull back the foreskin but to allow for the natural separation to occur
   3. Inform the mother that as the process of separation occurs, sterile sloughed cells build up between the layers of the foreskin and the glans, and that when retraction occurs, daily gentle washing of the glans with soap and water is sufficient to maintain adequate cleanliness

V. PRETERM NEWBORN
A. Description
   1. A **neonate** born before 37 weeks of gestation
   2. The primary concern relates to immaturity of all body systems
B. Assessment
   1. Respirations irregular with periods of apnea
   2. Body temperature is below normal
   3. **Newborn** has poor suck and swallow reflexes
   4. Bowel sounds are diminished
   5. Increased or decreased urinary output
   6. Extremities are thin, with minimal creasing on soles and palms
   7. **Newborn** extends extremities and does not maintain flexion
   8. Lanugo, on skin and in the hair on the **newborn's** head, is present in woolly patches
   9. Skin is thin, with visible blood vessels and minimal subcutaneous fat pads
   10. Skin may appear jaundiced
   11. Testes are undescended in boys
   12. Labia are narrow in girls
C. Implementation
   1. Monitor vital signs every 2 to 4 hours
   2. Maintain cardiopulmonary functions
   3. Administer oxygen and humidification as prescribed
   4. Monitor I & O and electrolyte balance
   5. Monitor daily weight
   6. Maintain **newborn** in a warming device
   7. Position every 1 to 2 hours, and handle **newborn** carefully
   8. Avoid exposure to infections
   9. Provide **newborn** with appropriate stimulation, such as touch

VI. POST-TERM NEWBORN
A. Description: A **neonate** born after 42 weeks of gestation
B. Assessment
   1. Hypoglycemia
   2. Parchment-like skin (dry and cracked) without lanugo

3. Fingernails long and extended over ends of fingers
4. Profuse scalp hair
5. Body is long and thin
6. Extremities show wasting of fat and muscle
7. Meconium staining may be present on nails and umbilical cord

C. Implementation
1. Provide normal **newborn** care
2. Monitor for hypoglycemia
3. Maintain **newborn's** temperature
4. Monitor for meconium aspiration

VII. SMALL FOR GESTATIONAL AGE

A. Description: A **neonate** who is plotted at or below the 10th percentile on the intrauterine growth curve
B. Assessment
1. Fetal distress
2. Gestational age and physical maturity
3. Lowered or elevated body temperature
4. Physical abnormalities
5. Hypoglycemia
6. Signs of polycythemia
   a. Ruddy appearance
   b. Cyanosis
   c. Jaundice
7. Signs of infection
8. Signs of aspiration of meconium

C. Implementation
1. Maintain airway
2. Maintain body temperature
3. Observe for signs of respiratory distress
4. Monitor for infection and initiate measures to prevent sepsis
5. Monitor blood glucose levels and for signs of hypoglycemia
6. Initiate early feedings and monitor for signs of aspiration
7. Provide stimulation, such as touch and cuddling

VIII. LARGE FOR GESTATIONAL AGE

A. Description: A **neonate** who is plotted at or above the 90th percentile on the intrauterine growth curve
B. Assessment
1. Gestational age
2. Birth trauma or injury
3. Respiratory distress
4. Hypoglycemia

C. Implementation
1. Monitor vital signs
2. Monitor blood glucose levels and for signs of hypoglycemia
3. Initiate early feedings
4. Monitor for infection and initiate measures to prevent sepsis
5. Provide stimulation, such as touch and cuddling

IX. RESPIRATORY DISTRESS SYNDROME (RDS)

A. Description: A serious lung disorder caused by immaturity and inability to produce surfactant, resulting in hypoxia and acidosis
B. Assessment
1. Tachypnea
2. Flaring nares
3. Expiratory grunting
4. Retractions
5. Decreased breath sounds
6. Apnea
7. Pallor and cyanosis
8. Hypothermia
9. Poor muscle tone

C. Implementation
1. Monitor color, respiratory rate, and degree of effort in breathing
2. Support respirations as prescribed
3. Monitor arterial blood gases (ABGs) and oxygen saturation levels (ABGs from umbilical artery)
4. Monitor ABGs so that oxygen administered to the **newborn** is at the lowest possible concentration necessary to maintain adequate arterial oxygenation
5. Schedule any premature **newborn** who required oxygen support for an eye examination before discharge to assess for retinal damage
6. Suction every 2 hours or more often as necessary
7. Position **newborn** on side or back, with neck slightly extended
8. Prepare to administer surfactant replacement therapy (instilled into the endotracheal tube)
9. Administer respiratory therapy (percussion and vibration) as prescribed; use padded small plastic cup or small oxygen mask for percussion; use padded electric toothbrush for vibration
10. Provide nutrition
11. Support bonding
12. Prepare parents for short- to long-term period of oxygen dependency if necessary
13. Encourage mother to pump breasts for future breastfeeding if she so desires
14. Encourage as much parental participation in **newborn's** care as condition allows

X. HYPERBILIRUBINEMIA

A. Description
1. At any serum bilirubin level, the appearance of jaundice during the first day of life indicates a pathological process
2. Evaluation is indicated when serum levels are over 12 mg/dL in the term **newborn**
3. Therapy is aimed at preventing kernicterus, which results in permanent neurological damage resulting from the deposition of bilirubin in the brain cells

B. Assessment
 1. Jaundice
 2. Elevated serum bilirubin levels
 3. Enlarged liver
 4. Poor muscle tone
 5. Lethargy
 6. Poor sucking reflex
C. Implementation
 1. Monitor for the presence of jaundice
   a. Examine the **newborn's** skin color in natural light
   b. Press finger over a bony prominence or tip of the **newborn's** nose to press out capillary blood from the tissues
   c. Note that jaundice starts at the head first, spreads to the chest, then the abdomen, then the arms and legs, followed by the hands and feet, which are the last to be jaundiced
 2. Keep **newborn** well hydrated to maintain blood volume
 3. Facilitate early, frequent feeding to hasten passage of meconium and encourage excretion of bilirubin
 4. Report to the physician any signs of jaundice in the first 24 hours and any abnormal signs and symptoms
 5. Prepare for phototherapy, and monitor the **newborn** closely during the treatment
D. Phototherapy
 1. Description
   a. Use of intense florescent lights to reduce serum bilirubin levels in the **newborn**
   b. Injury from treatment, such as eye damage, dehydration, or sensory deprivation, can occur
 2. Implementation
   a. Expose as much of the **newborn's** skin as possible
   b. Cover the genital area, and monitor genital area for skin irritation or breakdown
   c. Cover the **newborn's** eyes with eye shields or patches; make sure eyelids are closed when shields or patches are applied
   d. Remove the shields or patches at least once per shift to inspect the eyes for infection or irritation and to allow eye contact
   e. Measure the quantity of light every 8 hours
   f. Monitor skin temperature closely
   g. Increase fluids to compensate for water loss
   h. Expect loose green stools and green urine
   i. Monitor the **newborn's** skin color with the florescent light turned off, every 4 to 8 hours
   j. Monitor the skin for bronze baby syndrome, a grayish brown discoloration of the skin
   k. Reposition **newborn** every 2 hours
   l. Provide stimulation
   m. After treatment, continue monitoring for signs

of hyperbilirubinemia, as rebound elevations are normal after therapy is discontinued

XI. ERYTHROBLASTOSIS FETALIS

A. Description
 1. Destruction of RBCs that results from an antigen-antibody reaction
 2. Characterized by hemolytic anemia or hyperbilirubinemia
 3. Exchange of fetal and maternal blood takes place primarily when the **placenta** separates at birth
 4. Rh antigens from the baby's blood enter the maternal bloodstream
 5. The mother produces anti-Rh antibodies against the fetal blood cells
 6. Antibodies are harmless to the mother but attach to the erythrocytes in the fetus and cause hemolysis
 7. Sensitization is rare with the first pregnancy
 8. ABO incompatibility is usually less severe
B. Assessment
 1. Anemia
 2. Jaundice that develops rapidly after birth and before 24 hours
 3. Edema
C. Implementation
 1. Administer $Rh_o(D)$ immune globulin to the mother during the first 72 hours after **delivery** if the Rh-negative mother delivers an Rh-positive fetus but remains unsensitized
 2. Assist with exchange transfusion after birth or intrauterine transfusion as prescribed
 3. The baby's blood is replaced with Rh-negative blood to stop the destruction of the baby's red blood cells; the Rh-negative blood is replaced with the baby's own blood gradually
 4. Reassure the mother that the **newborn** will suffer no untoward effects from the condition

XII. SEPSIS

A. Description: Generalized infection resulting from the presence of bacteria in the blood
B. Assessment
 1. Pallor
 2. Tachypnea, tachycardia
 3. Poor feeding
 4. Abdominal distention
 5. Temperature instability
C. Implementation
 1. Assess for periods of apnea or irregular respirations
 2. If apnea is present, stimulate by gently rubbing chest or foot
 3. Administer oxygen as prescribed
 4. Monitor vital signs
 5. Maintain warmth in an Isolette
 6. Provide isolation as necessary

7. Assess for a fever
8. Monitor I & O and obtain daily weight
9. Monitor for diarrhea
10. Assess feeding and sucking reflex, which may be poor
11. Assess for jaundice
12. Assess for irritability and lethargy
13. Administer antibiotics as prescribed and observe carefully for toxicity, because a **newborn's** liver and kidneys are immature

XIII. TORCH SYNDROME

A. Description
   1. Refers to infections of the fetus or **newborn**
   2. Caused by one of the following
      a. Toxoplasmosis
      b. **Other** viruses
      c. Rubella
      d. Cytomegalovirus
      e. Herpes
B. Infections (Table 30-5)

XIV. SYPHILIS

A. Description
   1. Sexually transmitted disease
   2. Congenital syphilis can result in premature **delivery**, skin lesions, abnormal skeletal development
   3. The organism *Treponema pallidum*, a spirochete, is able to cross the **placenta** throughout pregnancy and infect the fetus, usually after 18 weeks' gestation
   4. Risks include preterm birth, stillbirth, and low birth weight
   5. Congenital effects are irreversible and may include CNS damage and hearing loss
B. Assessment
   1. Hepatosplenomegaly
   2. Joint swelling
   3. Palmar rash
   4. Anemia
   5. Jaundice
   6. Snuffles
   7. Ascites
   8. Pneumonitis
   9. Cerebrospinal fluid changes
C. Implementation
   1. Monitor **newborn** for signs of syphilis
   2. Monitor for palmar rash and snuffles
   3. Prepare **newborn** for serological testing if prescribed
   4. Administer antibiotic therapy as prescribed
   5. Use universal (standard) precautions and drainage/secretion precautions with suspected congenital syphilis
   6. Wear gloves when handling **neonate** until 24 hours of antibiotic therapy has been administered

TABLE 30-5

Infections Included in TORCH Syndrome

Infection	Characteristics
Toxoplasmosis	Protozoan infection
	Produces no serious effects in the mother
	Can be transmitted to the fetus
	Can result in severe physical and developmental abnormalities
	Common carriers include cat feces and raw beef
Other infections	Such as syphilis
Rubella	Systemic viral infection
	Causes congenital rubella syndrome, which includes congenital heart disease, cataracts, growth retardation, and pneumonia if the mother becomes infected within the first trimester
	Deafness and some learning disabilities can occur if the mother becomes infected during the first trimester
Cytomegalovirus	A viral infection that persists in the body indefinitely, with periods of reactivation without symptoms
	Can infect the fetus or infant during delivery or after birth through breast milk, blood transfusions, or contact with infected secretions
	May cause microcephaly, blindness, deafness, and mental and motor retardation
Herpes simplex	Sexually transmitted disease caused by a virus
	Periods of reactivation
	Neonate is commonly infected during delivery by direct contact with lesions in the genital tract
	Can cause neurological impairment or death

7. Provide psychological support to the mother, and provide instructions regarding follow-up care to the **newborn**

XV. THE ADDICTED NEWBORN

A. Description: **Newborn** who has become passively addicted to drugs that have passed through the **placenta**
B. Addicting drugs
   1. Heroin
      a. **Newborn** may appear normal at birth with a low birth weight
      b. Withdrawal occurs within 12 to 24 hours and may last 5 to 7 days
   2. Methadone
      a. Withdrawal occurs within 1 to 2 days to 1

week or more, is most evident at 48 to 72 hours, and may last 6 days to 8 weeks
  b. **Newborn** appears very ill
  c. May develop jaundice as a result of prematurity
3. Cocaine
  a. Causes decreased interactive behavior
  b. Feeding problems are present
  c. Irregular sleep patterns and diarrhea occur

C. Assessment
  1. Irritability
  2. Tremors
  3. Hyperactivity and hypertonicity
  4. Respiratory distress
  5. Vomiting
  6. High-pitched cry
  7. Sneezing
  8. Fever
  9. Diarrhea
  10. Excessive sweating
  11. Poor feeding
  12. Extreme sucking of fists
  13. Convulsions

D. Implementation
  1. Monitor respiratory and cardiac status frequently
  2. Monitor temperature and vital signs
  3. Hold **newborn** firm and close to the body during feeding and when giving care
  4. Initiate seizure precautions (pad sides of crib)
  5. Provide small frequent feedings and allow a longer period for feeding
  6. Monitor I & O
  7. Administer IV hydration if prescribed
  8. Protect **neonate's** skin from injury that can be caused by the constant rubbing from hyperactive jitters
  9. Swaddle **newborn**
  10. Place **newborn** in a quiet room and reduce stimulation
  11. Allow mother to ventilate feelings of anxiety and guilt
  12. Refer mother for treatment of substance abuse problem

XVI. FETAL ALCOHOL SYNDROME
A. Description
  1. Caused by maternal alcohol use during pregnancy
  2. Most serious cause of teratogenesis
  3. Causes mental and physical retardation
B. Assessment
  1. Facial changes
    a. Short palpebral fissures
    b. Hypoplastic philtrum
    c. Short, upturned nose
    d. Flat midface

  e. Thin upper lip
  f. Low nasal bridge
  2. Abnormal palmar creases
  3. Respiratory distress (apnea, cyanosis)
  4. Congenital heart disorders
  5. Irritability, hypersensitivity to stimuli
  6. Tremors
  7. Poor feeding
  8. Seizures

C. Implementation
  1. Monitor for respiratory distress
  2. Position **newborn** on side to facilitate drainage of secretions
  3. Keep resuscitation equipment at the bedside
  4. Monitor for hypoglycemia
  5. Assess suck and swallow reflex
  6. Administer small feedings and burp well
  7. Suction as necessary
  8. Monitor I & O
  9. Monitor weight and head circumference
  10. Decrease environmental stimuli

XVII. NEWBORN WITH ACQUIRED IMMUNODEFICIENCY SYNDROME (AIDS)
A. Description
  1. The fetus of a human immunodeficiency virus (HIV) antibody–positive woman should be monitored closely throughout the pregnancy
  2. Serial ultrasound screenings should be done during pregnancy to identify intrauterine growth restriction
  3. Weekly nonstress testing after 32 weeks of gestation and biophysical profiles may be necessary during pregnancy
  4. **Neonates** born to HIV-positive clients may test positive because the mother's positive antibodies may persist for as long as 18 months after birth
  5. The use of antiviral medication, the reduction of **neonate** exposure to maternal blood and body fluids, and the early identification of HIV in pregnancy reduce the risk of transmission to the **newborn**
  6. All **neonates** born to HIV-positive mothers acquire maternal antibody to HIV infection, but not all acquire the infection
  7. The **neonate** may be asymptomatic for the first several years of life
B. Transmission
  1. Across **placental** barrier
  2. During **labor** and **delivery**
  3. Breast milk
C. Assessment
  1. May have no outward signs for the first several months of life
  2. Signs of immune deficiency
  3. Hepatomegaly
  4. Splenomegaly

5. Lymphadenopathy
6. Impairment in growth and development
D. Implementation
   1. Cleanse **newborn's** skin carefully before any invasive procedure, such as the administration of vitamin K, heel sticks, or venipunctures
   2. Circumcisions are not done on **newborns** with HIV-positive mothers until the **newborn's** status is determined
   3. **Newborn** can room with mother
   4. All HIV-exposed **newborns** should be treated with medication to prevent infection by *Pneumocystis carinii*
   5. Zidovudine (AZT) may be administered as prescribed for the first 6 weeks of life
   6. Monitor for early signs of immune deficiency, such as enlarged spleen or liver, lymphadenopathy, and impairment in growth and development
   7. **Newborns** at risk for HIV infection should be seen by the physician at birth and at 1 week, 2 weeks, 1 month, and 2 months of life
   8. Inform the mother that an HIV culture is recommended at age 1 month and after 4 months of age
E. Immunizations
   1. **Newborns** at risk for HIV infection need to receive all recommended immunizations at the regular schedule
   2. Immunizations with live vaccines, such as oral polio and measles-mumps-rubella (MMR), should not be done until the **newborn's, infant's,** or child's status is confirmed
   3. If a child is infected, live vaccine will not be given

▲ **XVIII. NEWBORN OF DIABETIC MOTHER**
A. Description
   1. **Neonate** born to an insulin-dependent mother or gestational diabetic mother
   2. High incidence of congenital anomalies
   3. High incidences of hypoglycemia, respiratory distress, hypocalcemia, and hyperbilirubinemia
B. Assessment
   1. Excessive size and weight as a result of excess fat and glycogen in tissues
   2. Edema or puffiness in the face and cheeks
   3. Signs of hypoglycemia, such as twitching, difficulty in feeding, lethargy, apnea, seizures, and cyanosis
   4. Hyperbilirubinemia
   5. Signs of respiratory distress, such as tachypnea, cyanosis, retractions, grunting, and nasal flaring
C. Implementation
   1. Monitor for signs of respiratory distress
   2. Monitor bilirubin and blood glucose levels
   3. Monitor weight
   4. Feed early, with 10% glucose in water, breast milk, or formula as prescribed

5. Administer IV glucose to treat hypoglycemia if necessary and as prescribed
6. Monitor for edema
7. Monitor for tremors, seizures, apnea, and acidosis

XIX. HYPOGLYCEMIA   ▲
A. Description
   1. Abnormally low level of glucose in the blood (less than 30 mg/dL in the first 72 hours or below 45 mg/dL after the first 3 days of life)
   2. Normal blood glucose level is 40 to 60 mg/dL in a 1-day-old **neonate** and 50 to 90 mg/dL in a **neonate** older than 1 day
B. Assessment
   1. Increased respiratory rate
   2. Twitching, nervousness, or tremors
   3. Unstable temperature
   4. Cyanosis
C. Implementation
   1. Prevent low blood glucose through early feedings
   2. Administer glucose orally or by IV as prescribed
   3. Monitor blood glucose levels as prescribed
   4. Monitor for feeding problems
   5. Monitor for apneic periods
   6. Assess for shrill or intermittent cries
   7. Evaluate lethargy and poor muscle tone

PRACTICE QUESTIONS

1. A nurse instructs a mother in how to bathe a newborn infant. The nurse tells the mother to:
   1. Start with the dirtiest area first
   2. Begin with the eyes and face
   3. Begin with the feet and work upward
   4. Only wash the diaper area, since this is the only part of the infant that gets soiled
2. A nurse in a delivery room is assisting with the delivery of a newborn infant. After the delivery, the nurse prepares to prevent heat loss in the newborn infant resulting from evaporation by:
   1. Warming the crib pad
   2. Turning on the overhead radiant warmer
   3. Closing the doors to the room
   4. Drying the infant with a warm blanket
3. A nurse is providing instructions to a new mother regarding cord care for a newborn infant. Which statement if made by the mother indicates a need for further education?
   1. "I should cleanse the cord two or three times a day."
   2. "The cord will fall off in 1 to 2 weeks."
   3. "Alcohol may be used to clean the cord."
   4. "I need to fold the diaper above the cord to prevent infection."
4. The mother of a newborn infant calls a clinic and reports to a nurse that when cleansing the umbilical

cord, the mother noticed that the cord was moist and that discharge was present. The most appropriate nursing instruction to the mother is which of the following?

1. To increase the number of times that the cord is cleansed per day
2. To monitor the cord for another 24 to 48 hours and to call the clinic if the discharge continues
3. To bring the infant to the clinic
4. That this is a normal occurrence

5. A nurse is assessing a newborn infant following circumcision and notes that the circumcised area is red with a small amount of bloody drainage. Which of the following nursing actions would be most appropriate?

1. Document the findings
2. Contact the physician
3. Circle the amount of bloody drainage on the dressing and reassess in 30 minutes
4. Reinforce the dressing

6. A nurse has provided instructions to a mother of a male newborn infant who is not circumcised about measures to clean the penis. Which statement if made by the mother indicates an understanding of how to clean the newborn infant's penis?

1. "I need to retract the foreskin and clean the penis every time I give my infant a bath."
2. "I should gently retract the foreskin as far as it will go on the penis and then pull the skin back over the penis after cleaning."
3. "I should retract the foreskin and clean the penis every time I change the diaper."
4. "I need to avoid pulling back the foreskin to clean the penis because this may cause adhesions."

7. A nurse in a newborn nursery is monitoring a preterm newborn infant for respiratory distress syndrome (RDS). Which assessment signs if noted in the newborn infant would alert the nurse to the possibility of this syndrome?

1. Hypotension and bradycardia
2. Tachypnea and retractions
3. Acrocyanosis and grunting
4. The presence of a barrel chest with acrocyanosis

8. A nurse is assessing the reflexes of a newborn infant. In eliciting the Moro reflex, the nurse would perform which of the following?

1. Stimulate the perioral cavity of the newborn infant with a finger
2. Clap the hand or slap on the newborn infant's mattress
3. Stimulate the pads of the newborn infant's hands by firm pressure
4. Stimulate the newborn infant's ball of the foot by firm pressure

9. A nurse in a newborn nursery is performing an assessment of a newborn infant. The nurse is preparing to measure the head circumference of the infant. The nurse would most appropriately:

1. Wrap the tape measure around the infant's head and measure just above the eyebrows
2. Place the tape measure under the infant's head at the base of the skull and wrap around to the front just above the eyes
3. Place the tape measure under the infant's head, wrap around the occiput, and measure just above the eyes
4. Place the tape measure at the back of the infant's head, wrap around across the ears, and measure across the infant's mouth

10. A postpartum nurse is providing instructions to the mother of a newborn infant with hyperbilirubinemia who is being breastfed. Which of the following instructions would the nurse provide to the mother?

1. Switch to bottle feeding the baby during the period of high bilirubin levels and to feed less frequently
2. Stop the breast feedings and switch to bottle feeding permanently
3. Provide bottled water feedings between the breastfeeding sessions
4. Continue to breastfeed every 2 to 4 hours

11. A nurse in the newborn nursery is caring for a neonate. On assessment, the infant is exhibiting signs of cyanosis, tachypnea, nasal flaring, and grunting. Respiratory distress syndrome (RDS) is diagnosed, and the physician prescribes surfactant replacement therapy. The nurse would prepare to administer this therapy by:

1. Subcutaneous injection
2. Intravenous injection
3. Instillation of the preparation into the lungs through an endotracheal tube
4. Intramuscular injection

12. A nurse is assessing a newborn infant who was born to a mother who is addicted to drugs. Which of the following assessment findings would the nurse not expect to note during the assessment of this newborn?

1. Irritability
2. Difficulty in consoling the newborn
3. Lethargy
4. Incessant crying

13. A nurse is preparing to administer an injection of vitamin K to a newborn. In preparing to administer the injection, the nurse would select which of the following injection sites?

1. The lateral aspect of the middle third of the vastus lateralis muscle
2. The medial aspect of the upper third of the vastus lateralis muscle
3. The lower aspect of the rectus femoris muscle
4. The gluteal muscle

14. A 4-day-old newborn infant is receiving photo-therapy at home for a bilirubin level of 14 mg/dL. The nurse should plan to include which of the following in the plan of care during the home visit to the mother of the newborn infant?
   1. Having minimal contact with the newborn infant to prevent stimulation
   2. Advising the mother to limit newborn infant oral intake during phototherapy
   3. Applying lotions to exposed newborn infant's skin
   4. Assessing skin integrity and fluid and electrolyte status of the newborn infant

15. A nurse notes hypotonia, irritability, and a poor sucking reflex in a full-term newborn infant upon admission to the nursery. The nurse suspects fetal alcohol syndrome (FAS) and is aware that which of the following additional sign(s) would be consistent with FAS?
   1. Head circumference appropriate for gestational age
   2. Birth weight of 6 pounds 14 ounces
   3. Length of 19 inches
   4. Abnormal palmar creases

16. A nurse is preparing a plan of care for a newborn infant with fetal alcohol syndrome (FAS). The nurse would include which of the following priority interventions in the plan of care?
   1. Monitor the newborn infant's response to feedings and weight gain pattern
   2. Encourage frequent handling of the newborn infant by staff and parents
   3. Maintain the newborn infant in a brightly lighted area of the nursery
   4. Allow the newborn infant to establish own sleep/rest pattern

17. A nurse administers erythromycin ointment (0.5%) to the eyes of a newborn infant. The mother asks the nurse why this is performed. The nurse explains to the mother that this is routinely done to:
   1. Minimize the spread of microorganisms to the newborn infant from invasive procedures during labor
   2. Protect the newborn infant's eyes from possible infections acquired while hospitalized
   3. Prevent ophthalmia neonatorum from occurring after delivery in a newborn infant born to a woman with an untreated gonococcal infection
   4. Prevent cataracts in the newborn infant born to a woman who is rubella susceptible

18. A nurse prepares to administer a vitamin K injection to a newborn infant. The mother asks the nurse why her newborn infant needs the injection. The best response by the nurse would be:
   1. "Your infant needs vitamin K to develop immunity."
   2. "The vitamin K will protect your infant from being jaundiced."
   3. "Newborn infants are deficient in vitamin K, and this injection prevents your infant from abnormal bleeding."
   4. "Newborn infants have sterile bowels, and vitamin K promotes the growth of bacteria in the bowel."

19. A nurse develops a plan of care for a human immunodeficiency virus (HIV)–infected mother and her newborn infant. The nurse includes which intervention in the plan of care?
   1. Instruct the breastfeeding mother regarding the treatment of the nipples with nystatin ointment
   2. Monitor the newborn infant's vital signs routinely
   3. Maintain standard (universal) precautions at all times while caring for the newborn
   4. Initiate referral to evaluate for blindness, deafness, learning, or behavioral problems

20. A nurse in a newborn nursery receives a telephone call to prepare for the admission of a 43-week-gestation newborn infant with Apgar scores of 1 and 4. In planning for admission of this infant, the nurse's highest priority should be to:
   1. Connect the resuscitation bag to the oxygen outlet
   2. Turn on the apnea and cardiorespiratory monitors
   3. Set up the intravenous line with 5% dextrose in water
   4. Set the radiant warmer control temperature at 36.5° C (97.6° F)

CRITICAL THINKING: FREE-TEXT ENTRY

A nurse is caring for a post-term, small-for-gestational age (SGA) newborn infant immediately after admission to the nursery. The priority nursing action would be to monitor the results of what serum laboratory study?

Answer: _____

ANSWERS

1. 2

Rationale: Bathing should start at the eyes and face, usually the cleanest area. Next, the external ear and the areas behind the ears are cleansed. The infant's neck should be washed because formula, lint, or breast milk will often accumulate in the folds of the neck. Hands and arms are then washed. The infants legs are washed, and the diaper area is washed last.

Test-Taking Strategy: Use the process of elimination. Remember the basic techniques of bathing a client to assist in answering this question. Always start with the cleanest area of the body first and proceed to the dirtiest area. Use techniques related to washing an adult to assist in answering this question. If you had difficulty with this question, review home care measures related to the care of the newborn infant.

Level of Cognitive Ability: Application
Client Needs: Health Promotion and Maintenance
Integrated Concept/Process: Teaching/Learning
Content Area: Maternity
Reference: Olds, S., London. M., & Ladewig, P. (2000). *Maternal-newborn nursing: A family and community-based approach* (6th ed.). Upper Saddle River, N.J.: Prentice-Hall Health, pp. 996-997.

2. 4

Rationale: Evaporation of moisture from a wet body dissipates heat along with the moisture. Keeping the newborn infant dry by drying the wet newborn infant at birth will prevent hypothermia via evaporation. Hypothermia caused by conduction occurs when the newborn infant is on a cold surface, such as a cold pad or mattress, and heat from the newborn infant's body is transferred to the colder object. Warming the crib pad will assist in preventing hypothermia by conduction. Convection occurs as air moves across the newborn infant's skin from an open door and heat is transferred to the air. Radiation occurs when heat from the newborn infant radiates to a colder surface.

Test-Taking Strategy: Use the process of elimination. Note the key word "evaporation" in the question to assist in selecting the correct option. Knowledge that evaporation of moisture from a wet body dissipates heat along with the moisture will assist in directing you to option 4. Review these heat loss concepts if you had difficulty with this question.

Level of Cognitive Ability: Application
Client Needs: Physiological Integrity
Integrated Concept/Process: Nursing Process/Planning
Content Area: Maternity
Reference: Sherwen, L., Scoloveno, M.A., & Weingarten, C. (1999). *Maternity nursing: Care of the childbearing family* (3rd ed.). Stamford, Conn.: Appleton & Lange, p. 922.

3. 4

Rationale: The cord should be kept clean and dry to decrease bacterial growth. The diaper should be folded below the cord to keep urine away from the cord. The cord should be cleansed two or three times a day with alcohol or other prescribed agents. Cord care is required until the cord dries up and falls off between 7 and 14 days.

Test-Taking Strategy: Use the process of elimination. Read each option carefully, and attempt to visualize the descriptions in each of the options. Also note the key words "need for further education" in the stem of the question. Knowing that option 4 suggests folding the diaper above the cord should assist in directing you to this option because the cord can become saturated and contaminated with urine with this method of diapering. Review concepts related to cord care if you had difficulty with this question.

Level of Cognitive Ability: Analysis
Client Needs: Health Promotion and Maintenance
Integrated Concept/Process: Teaching/Learning
Content Area: Maternity
Reference: Gorrie, T., McKinney, E., & Murray, S. (1998). *Foundations of maternal-newborn nursing* (2nd ed.). Philadelphia: W.B. Saunders, p. 574.

4. 3

Rationale: Symptoms of infection are moistness, oozing, discharge, and a reddened base around the cord. If symptoms of infection occur, the mother should be instructed to notify a health care provider. If these symptoms occur, antibiotics are necessary. Options 1, 2, and 4 are inappropriate nursing interventions for the description given in the question.

Test-Taking Strategy: Use the process of elimination. Focus on the clinical manifestations provided in the question to assist in directing you to the correct option. Noting the key word "discharge" in the question will assist in directing you to the option that indicates that the newborn needs to be seen by the health care provider. Review interventions related to cord care, if you had difficulty with this question.

Level of Cognitive Ability: Application
Client Needs: Physiological Integrity
Integrated Concept/Process: Nursing Process/Implementation
Content Area: Maternity
Reference: Olds, S., London. M., & Ladewig, P. (2000). *Maternal-newborn nursing: A family and community-based approach* (6th ed.). Upper Saddle River, N.J.: Prentice-Hall Health, p. 967.

5. 1

Rationale: The penis is normally red during the healing process. A yellow exudate may be noted in 24 hours, and this is part of normal healing. The nurse would expect that the area would be red with a small amount of bloody drainage. If the bleeding is excessive, the nurse would apply gentle pressure with a sterile gauze. If bleeding is not controlled, then the blood vessel may need to be ligated and the nurse would notify the physician. Since the findings identified in the question are normal, the nurse would document the assessment.

Test-Taking Strategy: Use the process of elimination. Note the key words "small amount of bloody drainage." This should assist in directing you to the option that this is a normal occurrence following circumcision. If you had difficulty with this question, review the expected findings following this procedure.

Level of Cognitive Ability: Application
Client Needs: Physiological Integrity
Integrated Concept/Process: Communication and Documentation
Content Area: Maternity
Reference: Lowdermilk, D., Perry, S., & Bobak, I. (2000). *Maternity & women's health care* (7th ed.). St. Louis: Mosby, p. 748.

6. **4**

Rationale: In male newborn infants, prepuce is continuous with the epidermis of the glans and is not retractable. If retraction is forced, this may cause adhesions to develop. The mother should be told to allow separation to occur naturally, which usually occurs between 3 years and puberty. Most foreskins are retractable by 3 years of age and should be pushed back gently at this time for cleaning once a week. Options 1, 2, and 3 identify an action that addresses retraction of the foreskin.

Test-Taking Strategy: Use the process of elimination. Note that options 1, 2, and 3 are similar in that they all identify retracting the foreskin. Option 4 is the option that is different. If you had difficulty with this question, review teaching points related to cleaning the penis of a newborn male infant who is uncircumcised.

Level of Cognitive Ability: Analysis
Client Needs: Health Promotion and Maintenance
Integrated Concept/Process: Teaching/Learning
Content Area: Maternity
Reference: Olds, S., London. M., & Ladewig, P. (2000). *Maternal-newborn nursing: A family and community-based approach* (6th ed.). Upper Saddle River, N.J.: Prentice-Hall Health, p. 967.

7. **2**

Rationale: The newborn infant with respiratory distress syndrome may present with clinical signs of cyanosis, tachypnea or apnea, nasal flaring, chest wall retractions, or audible grunts. Acrocyanosis is the bluish discoloration of the hands and feet, is associated with immature peripheral circulation, and is not uncommon in the first few hours of life. Options 1, 3, and 4 do not indicate clinical signs of RDS.

Test-Taking Strategy: Use the process of elimination. Recalling that acrocyanosis may be a normal sign in a newborn infant will assist in eliminating options 3 and 4. From the remaining options, it is necessary to be familiar with the signs of respiratory distress syndrome. Also, note the relationship between the diagnosis and the signs noted in option 2. If you had difficulty with this question, review the signs of RDS.

Level of Cognitive Ability: Analysis
Client Needs: Physiological Integrity
Integrated Concept/Process: Nursing Process/Assessment
Content Area: Maternity
Reference: Ladewig, P., London. M., & Olds, S. (1998). *Maternal-newborn nursing care: The nurse, the family, and the community* (4th ed.). Menlo Park, Calif.: Addison-Wesley Longman, p. 679.

8. **2**

Rationale: The Moro reflex is elicited by a loud noise such as a hand clap or a slap on the mattress to startle the newborn infant. Symmetric extension and abduction of the arms are seen; fingers fan out and form a C with the thumb and forefinger; slight tremor may be noted; the arms are adducted in an embracing motion and then return to a relaxed flexion and movement. Legs may follow a similar pattern of response. This reflex disappears at 6 months of age. The rooting reflex is elicited by stimulating the perioral area with the finger. The palmar grasp reflex is elicited by stimulating the palm of the hand by firm pressure, and the plantar grasp reflex is elicited by stimulating the ball of the foot by firm pressure.

Test-Taking Strategy: Use the process of elimination. Options 3 and 4 are similar and should be eliminated first. Focusing on the issue of the question, the Moro reflex, will assist in directing you to option 2. Review assessment of neonatal reflexes if you had difficulty with this question.

Level of Cognitive Ability: Application
Client Needs: Health Promotion and Maintenance
Integrated Concept/Process: Nursing Process/Assessment
Content Area: Maternity
Reference: Lowdermilk, D., Perry, S., & Bobak, I. (2000). *Maternity & women's health care* (7th ed.). St. Louis: Mosby, p. 690.

9. **3**

Rationale: To measure head circumference, the nurse should place the tape measure under the infant's head, wrap the tape around the occiput, and measure just above the eyebrows so that the largest area of the occiput is included. Options 1, 2, and 4 are incorrect methods to measure the head circumference.

Test-Taking Strategy: Use the process of elimination. Attempt to visualize each of the descriptions in the options. Remembering that the largest area of the occiput is included in the measurement will assist in directing you to option 3. If you had difficulty with this question, review measuring head circumference in a newborn infant.

Level of Cognitive Ability: Application
Client Needs: Health Promotion and Maintenance
Integrated Concept/Process: Nursing Process/Implementation
Content Area: Maternity
Reference: Ball, J., & Bindler, R. (1999). *Quick reference to pediatric clinical skills.* Stamford, Conn.: Appleton & Lange, p. 19.

10. **4**

Rationale: Breastfeeding should be initiated within 2 hours after birth and every 2 to 4 hours thereafter. The infant should not be fed less frequently. It is not necessary to stop breastfeeding permanently. Supplementation with water does not reduce hyperbilirubinemia and should be discouraged because supplemental feedings with water do not promote stool excretion.

Test-Taking Strategy: Use the process of elimination. Note the similarities between options 1, 2, and 3. These options discourage the continuation of breastfeeding and are therefore similar. Review client instructions related to hyperbilirubinemia in the newborn infant if you had difficulty with this question.

Level of Cognitive Ability: Application
Client Needs: Health Promotion and Maintenance
Integrated Concept/Process: Teaching/Learning
Content Area: Maternity
Reference: Olds, S., London. M., & Ladewig, P. (2000). *Maternal-newborn nursing: A family and community-based approach* (6th ed.). Upper Saddle River, N.J.: Prentice-Hall Health, p. 893.

11. **3**

Rationale: The aim of therapy in respiratory distress syndrome is to support the disease until the disease runs its course with the subsequent development of surfactant. The infant may benefit from surfactant replacement therapy. In surfactant replacement, an exogenous surfactant preparation is instilled into the lungs through an endotracheal tube. Options 1, 2, and 4 identify incorrect methods of administering surfactant.

Test Taking Strategy: Knowledge regarding surfactant replacement therapy is required to answer this question. If you are unfamiliar with the administration of this therapy, review this procedure.
Level of Cognitive Ability: Application
Client Needs: Physiological Integrity
Integrated Concept/Process: Nursing Process/Planning
Content Area: Maternity
Reference: Lowdermilk, D., Perry, S., & Bobak, I. (2000). *Maternity & women's health care* (7th ed.). St. Louis: Mosby. p. 315.
12. **3**
Rationale: A newborn infant born to a woman using drugs is irritable. The infant is easily overloaded by sensory stimulation. The infant may cry incessantly and be difficult to console. The infant would hyperextend and posture rather than cuddle when being held.
Test-Taking Strategy: Use the process of elimination. Note the key word "not" in the stem of the question. Note that options 1, 2, and 4 are similar in that they indicate hyperactivity of the newborn. Review assessment findings in the newborn infant born to a drug-addicted mother if you had difficulty with this question.
Level of Cognitive Ability: Analysis
Client Needs: Physiological Integrity
Integrated Concept/Process: Nursing Process/Assessment
Content Area: Maternity
Reference: Lowdermilk, D., Perry, S., & Bobak, I. (2000). *Maternity & women's health care* (7th ed.). St. Louis: Mosby, p. 1063.
13. **1**
Rationale: The preferred injection site for vitamin K in the newborn infant is the lateral aspect of the middle third of the vastus lateralis muscle in the infant's thigh. This muscle is the preferred injection site because it is free of major blood vessels and nerves and is large enough to absorb the medication.
Test-Taking Strategy: Use the process of elimination and knowledge regarding the preferred injection site for a newborn infant. If you had difficulty with this question, review the procedure for administering vitamin K to the newborn infant.
Level of Cognitive Ability: Application
Client Needs: Physiological Integrity
Integrated Concept/Process: Nursing Process/Planning
Content Area: Maternity
Reference: Ball, J., & Bindler, R. (1999). *Quick reference to pediatric clinical skills.* Stamford, Conn.: Appleton & Lange, p. 51.
14. **4**
Rationale: Assessing skin integrity and fluid and electrolyte status of the newborn infant is an essential component of phototherapy. Contact with the newborn infant is important. Lotions are not used to minimize skin breakdown and to enhance the therapeutic effect of light in subcutaneous tissue. Adequate oral fluids are essential to prevent dehydration, since diarrhea is a common side effect of therapy. In addition, safe care for the newborn infant during phototherapy requires shielding the eyes with a soft eye shield to prevent retinal damage, keeping the newborn's skin exposed except for a diaper, and changing position frequently.

Test-Taking Strategy: Use the process of elimination and knowledge regarding phototherapy. Note that option 4 addresses the first step of the nursing process, assessment. If you had difficulty with this question, review care to the newborn infant receiving phototherapy.
Level of Cognitive Ability: Application
Clients Needs: Physiological Integrity
Integrated Concept/Process: Teaching/Learning
Content Area: Maternity
Reference: Lowdermilk, D., Perry, S., & Bobak, I. (2000). *Maternity & women's health care* (7th ed.). St. Louis: Mosby, pp. 744-745.
15. **4**
Rationale: Features of newborn infants diagnosed with FAS include craniofacial abnormalities, intrauterine growth retardation (IUGR), cardiac abnormalities, abnormal palmar creases, and respiratory distress. Options 1, 2, and 3 are normal assessment findings in the full-term newborn infant.
Test-Taking Strategy: Use the process of elimination and knowledge regarding normal assessment findings in the full-term newborn infant to answer this question. Note that options 1, 2, and 3 are similar and represent normal assessment findings in the full-term newborn infant. If you had difficulty with this question, review the content related to normal newborn infant assessment findings and FAS.
Level of Cognitive Ability: Analysis
Client Needs: Physiological Integrity
Integrated Concept/Process: Nursing Process/Assessment
Content Area: Maternity
Reference: Lowdermilk, D., Perry, S., & Bobak, I. (2000). *Maternity & women's health care* (7th ed.). St. Louis: Mosby, p. 1060.
16. **1**
Rationale: A primary nursing goal for the newborn infant diagnosed with FAS is to establish nutritional balance following delivery. These newborn infants may exhibit hyperirritability, vomiting, diarrhea, or an uncoordinated sucking and swallowing ability. A quiet environment with minimal stimuli and handling will help establish appropriate sleep/rest cycles in the newborn infant as well. Options 2, 3, and 4 are inappropriate interventions.
Test-Taking Strategy: Use the process of elimination. Recalling that these newborn infants may exhibit hyperirritability, vomiting, diarrhea, or an uncoordinated sucking and swallowing ability will easily direct you to option 1. Review care to the newborn infant with FAS if you had difficulty with this question.
Level of Cognitive Ability: Application
Client Needs: Physiological Integrity
Integrated Concept/Process: Nursing Process/Planning
Content Area: Maternity
Reference: Sherwen, L., Scoloveno, M.A., & Weingarten, C. (1999). *Maternity nursing: Care of the childbearing family* (3rd ed.). Stamford, Conn.: Appleton & Lange, p. 1025.
17. **3**
Rationale: Erythromycin ophthalmic ointment (Ilotycin ophthalmic) 0.5% is used as a prophylactic treatment for ophthalmia neonatorum, which is caused by the bacterium *Neisseria gonorrhoeae.* Preventive treatment of gonorrhea is

required by law. Options 1, 2, and 4 are not the purposes for administering this medication to the newborn infant.

Test-Taking Strategy: Use the process of elimination and knowledge of the purpose of administering erythromycin ophthalmic ointment to the newborn infant. If you had difficulty with this question, review initial care to the newborn infant.

Level of Cognitive Ability: Application
Client Needs: Health Promotion and Maintenance
Integrated Concept/Process: Teaching/Learning
Content Area: Maternity
Reference: Olds, S., London. M., & Ladewig, P. (2000). *Maternal-newborn nursing: A family and community-based approach* (6th ed.). Upper Saddle River, N.J.: Prentice-Hall Health, p. 762.

18. **3**
Rationale: Vitamin K is necessary for the body to synthesize coagulation factors. Vitamin K is administered to the newborn infant to prevent abnormal bleeding. It promotes liver formation of the clotting factors II, VII, IX, and X. Newborn infants are vitamin K deficient because the bowel does not have the bacteria necessary for synthesizing fat-soluble vitamin K. The normal flora in the intestinal tract produces vitamin K. The newborn infant's bowel does not support the normal production of vitamin K until bacteria adequately colonize it. The bowel becomes colonized by bacteria as food is ingested. Vitamin K does not promote the development of immunity or prevent the infant from becoming jaundiced.

Test-Taking Strategy: Use the process of elimination. Note the key word "best." Because jaundice and immunity are not related to the action of vitamin K, eliminate options 1 and 2. From the remaining options, recall the action of vitamin K to direct you to option 3. If you had difficulty with this question, review the purpose of vitamin K injection.

Level of Cognitive Ability: Application
Client Needs: Physiological Integrity
Integrated Concept/Process: Teaching/Learning
Content Area: Maternity
Reference: Olds, S., London. M., & Ladewig, P. (2000). *Maternal-newborn nursing: A family and community-based approach* (6th ed.). Upper Saddle River, N.J.: Prentice-Hall Health, p. 761.

19. **3**
Rationale: The newborn infant born of an HIV-infected mother must be cared for with strict attention to standard (universal) precautions. This prevents the transmission of HIV from the newborn infant, if infected, to others, and prevents transmission of other infectious agents to the possibly immunocompromised newborn infant. HIV-infected mothers should not breastfeed. Options 2 and 4 are not specifically associated with the care of a potentially HIV-infected newborn infant.

Test-Taking Strategy: Use the process of elimination and knowledge regarding care of a newborn infant born to an HIV-infected woman. Eliminate options 2 and 4 first because

they are not specifically associated with the care of a potentially HIV-infected newborn infant. Recalling that HIV-infected mothers should not breastfeed will easily direct you to option 3. Review care of an infant born to an HIV-infected woman if you had difficulty with this question.

Level of Cognitive Ability: Application
Client Needs: Safe, Effective Care Environment
Integrated Concept/Process: Nursing Process/Planning
Content Area: Maternity
Reference: Olds, S., London. M., & Ladewig, P. (2000). *Maternal-newborn nursing: A family and community-based approach* (6th ed.). Upper Saddle River, N.J.: Prentice-Hall Health, p. 840.

20. **1**
Rationale: The highest priority on admission to the nursery for a newborn with low Apgar scores is airway, which would involve preparing respiratory resuscitation equipment. The remaining options are also important, although they are of somewhat lower priority. The newborn infant will be placed on a cardiorespiratory monitor. Setting up an IV with 5% dextrose in water would provide circulatory support. The radiant warmer will provide an external heat source, which is necessary to prevent further respiratory distress.

Test-Taking Strategy: Use the process of elimination and note the key words "highest priority." This question asks you to prioritize care on the basis of information about a newborn infant's condition. Use the ABCs—airway, breathing, and circulation. A method of planning for airway support is to have the resuscitation bag connected to an oxygen source. Review care to the newborn infant with low Apgar scores if you had difficulty with this question.

Level of Cognitive Ability: Application
Client Needs: Safe, Effective Care Environment
Integrated Concept/Process: Nursing Process/Planning
Content Area: Maternity
Reference: Sherwen, L., Scoloveno, M.A., & Weingarten, C. (1999). *Maternity nursing: Care of the childbearing family* (3rd ed.). Stamford, Conn.: Appleton & Lange, pp. 931-932, 1087.

CRITICAL THINKING: FREE-TEXT ENTRY

Answer: Blood glucose levels
Rationale: The most common metabolic complication in the SGA newborn infant is hypoglycemia, which can produce central nervous system abnormalities and mental retardation if not corrected immediately.

Test-Taking Strategy: Recalling that the most common metabolic complication in the SGA newborn infant is hypoglycemia will assist in answering the question. Review the SGA newborn content if you had difficulty with this question.

Level of Cognitive Ability: Analysis
Client Needs: Physiological Integrity
Integrated Concept/Process: Nursing Process/Assessment
Content Area: Maternity
Reference: Lowdermilk, D., Perry, S., & Bobak, I. (2000). *Maternity & women's health care* (7th ed.). St. Louis: Mosby, p. 1127.

REFERENCES

Ball, J., & Bindler, R. (1999). *Quick reference to pediatric clinical skills.* Stamford, Conn.: Appleton & Lange.

Gorrie, T., McKinney, E., & Murray, S. (1998). *Foundations of maternal-newborn nursing* (2nd ed.). Philadelphia: W.B. Saunders.

Ladewig, P., London. M., & Olds, S. (1998). *Maternal-newborn nursing care: The nurse, the family, and the community* (4th ed.). Menlo Park, Calif.: Addison-Wesley Longman.

Lowdermilk, D., Perry, S., & Bobak, I. (2000). *Maternity & women's health care* (7th ed.). St. Louis: Mosby.

Olds, S., London. M., & Ladewig, P. (2000). *Maternal-newborn nursing: A family and community-based approach* (6th ed.). Upper Saddle River, N.J.: Prentice-Hall Health.

Sherwen, L., Scoloveno, M.A., & Weingarten, C. (1999). *Maternity nursing: Care of the childbearing family* (3rd ed.). Stamford, Conn.: Appleton & Lange.

Maternity and Newborn Medications

I. OXYTOCIC MEDICATION: OXYTOCIN (PITOCIN)

A. Description
1. Stimulates the smooth muscle of the uterus and induces contraction of the myocardium
2. Promotes milk letdown
3. Routes of administration include intranasal, intramuscular (IM), and intravenous (IV)
4. Minimal cervical change is usually noted until the active phase of **labor** is achieved

B. Uses
1. Induce or augment **labor**
2. Control postpartum bleeding
3. Promote milk letdown and facilitate breastfeeding (intranasal route)
4. Induce or complete an abortion

C. Adverse reactions and contraindications
1. Rare, but may include allergies, dysrhythmias, changes in blood pressure (BP), uterine rupture, and water intoxication; intranasal administration may cause nasal vasoconstriction
2. May produce uterine hypertonicity resulting in fetal or maternal injury
3. High doses may cause hypotension, with rebound hypertension
4. Postpartum hemorrhage can occur because the uterus may become atonic when the medication wears off
5. Should not be used in a client who cannot deliver vaginally or in a client with hypertonic uterine contractions

D. Implementation
1. Monitor maternal vital signs (every 15 minutes), especially the blood pressure (BP) and heart rate, weight, intake and output (I & O), level of consciousness (LOC), and lung sounds
2. Monitor frequency, duration, force of contractions, and resting uterine tone every 15 minutes

3. Monitor fetal heart rate (FHR) every 15 minutes and notify the health care provider if significant changes occur; an internal fetal scalp electrode should be used
4. Administered by IV infusion via an infusion monitoring device; carefully monitor dose being administered
5. Administered via a Y-setup or via stopcock, with normal saline in the primary line
6. Do not leave the client unattended while the oxytocin is infusing
7. Administer oxygen if prescribed
8. Monitor for hypertonic contractions
9. Stop the medication if uterine hyperstimulation or a nonreassuring FHR occurs; turn the client on her side, increase the IV rate (normal saline), and administer oxygen via facemask
10. Notify the health care provider if uterine hyperstimulation or nonreassuring FHR occurs
11. Monitor for signs of water intoxication
12. Have emergency equipment available
13. Document the dose of the medication and the time the medication was started, increased, maintained, and discontinued
14. Keep the family informed of the client's progress

II. ERGOT ALKALOIDS (Box 31-1)

A. Description
1. Directly stimulate uterine muscle and increase the force and frequency of contractions
2. Produce a firm tetanic contraction of the uterus
3. Produce arterial vasoconstriction and can cause vasospasm of the coronary arteries
4. Not administered before the **delivery** of the **placenta**
5. May be administered by the oral or IM route; for IV use in an emergency, either medication may be administered undiluted

Ergot Alkaloids

Ergonovine (Ergotrate)
Methylergonovine (Methergine)

Uterine Relaxants

Ritodrine (Yutopar)
Terbutaline (Bricanyl)

B. Uses
   1. Postpartum hemorrhage
   2. Postabortal hemorrhage resulting from atony or involution
C. Adverse reactions and contraindications
   1. Nausea
   2. Uterine cramping
   3. Can cause bradycardia, dysrhythmias, myocardial infarction, and severe hypertension
   4. High doses are associated with peripheral vasospasm or vasoconstriction, angina, miosis, confusion, respiratory depression, seizures, or unconsciousness; uterine tetany can occur
   ▲ 5. Contraindicated during pregnancy
   6. Contraindicated in clients with significant cardiovascular disease, peripheral vascular disease, hypertension, eclampsia, or preeclampsia
D. Implementation
   1. Monitor maternal vital signs, weight, I & O, LOC, and lung sounds
   2. Monitor the BP closely; the medication produces vasoconstriction, and if a rise in BP is noted, withhold the medication and notify the health care provider
   3. Monitor uterine contractions (frequency, strength, and duration)
   4. Assess for chest pain, headache, shortness of breath, itching, pale or cold hands or feet, nausea, diarrhea, or dizziness
   5. Notify the health care provider if chest pain occurs
   6. Assess the extremities for color, warmth, movement, and pain
   7. Assess vaginal bleeding
   8. Administer analgesics as prescribed; may be required because the medication produces painful uterine contractions

III.   UTERINE RELAXANTS (Box 31-2)
A. Description
   1. Produce uterine relaxation
   2. Ritodrine is the preferred medication of choice to control premature **labor**
   3. Ritodrine may be used orally or IV
   4. Ritodrine is usually administered IV when premature **labor** begins; when contractions have been controlled for 12 to 24 hours, the client may be started on oral ritodrine and the IV infusion may be discontinued

   5. Contractions may resume when the client is on oral therapy
B. Uses
   1. Ritodrine is used to halt spontaneous **labor** when it appears after the 20th week of pregnancy and before the 36th week
   2. Terbutaline, primarily used to control bronchospasm, is an alternative medication for the control of premature **labor**
C. Adverse reactions and contraindications
   1. Ritodrine
      a. Heart palpitations, tachycardia, nausea and vomiting, trembling, flushing, and headache
      b. Fetal tachycardia
      c. High doses can cause cardiovascular symptoms and pulmonary edema
      d. Contraindicated in clients with preexisting cardiac disease
   2. Terbutaline
      a. Hypokalemia, pulmonary edema, and hypoglycemia may occur if given during **labor**
      b. Hypoglycemia may be found in **neonate**
D. Implementation
   1. Monitor vital signs, uterine contractions, and FHR every 5 minutes when initiating therapy, every 15 to 30 minutes when the client is stable, and every 4 hours when the client is taking oral maintenance doses
   2. An infusion monitoring device is used when administered by IV
   3. Monitor for pulmonary edema; assess lung sounds for rales
   4. Monitor potassium and glucose levels
   5. Instruct the client to contact the health care provider if 4 to 6 contractions per hour occur

IV.   PROSTAGLANDINS (BOX 31-3)
A. Description
   1. Potent stimulators of the myometrium
   2. Dinoprostone is administered as a gel or suppository directly into the vagina
   3. Carboprost can be administered by deep IM injection
B. Uses
   1. Abortifacient
   2. Induce abortion during the second trimester, when the uterus is resistant to oxytocin
   3. Dinoprostone is also used to soften and promote dilation of the cervix to facilitate vaginal **delivery**

BOX 31-3

Prostaglandins

Carboprost (Hemabate)
Dinoprostone (Cervidil)

C. Adverse reactions and contraindications
   1. Significant gastrointestinal side effects, including diarrhea, nausea, vomiting, and stomach cramps
   2. Fever, chills, and flushing
   3. Anaphylaxis, dysrhythmias, bronchoconstriction, chest pain, hypertension, and peripheral vasoconstriction
   4. Contraindicated in clients with significant cardiovascular disease or those with a history of asthma or pulmonary disease
   5. High doses can cause uterine cramping and tetany
D. Implementation
   1. Monitor maternal vital signs, especially the BP and heart rate, weight, I & O, LOC, and lung sounds
   2. Monitor frequency, duration, force of uterine contractions, and resting uterine tone frequently; palpate the fundus
   3. Monitor vaginal bleeding
   4. Remain with the client for 30 minutes after administration to monitor for anaphylaxis; signs include shortness of breath or difficulty breathing, tachycardia, hives, tightness in the chest, or swelling of the face
   5. Maintain client in a supine position for 30 minutes following administration of the medication
   6. Keep side rails up; have a suction machine at the bedside
   7. Administer antidiarrheal and antiemetic medications as prescribed

V. MAGNESIUM SULFATE
A. Description
   1. A central nervous system (CNS) depressant and anticonvulsant
   2. Causes smooth muscle relaxation
   3. Antidote: calcium gluconate
B. Uses
   1. Prevent and control seizures in preeclamptic and eclamptic clients
   2. Treat preterm **labor**
C. Adverse reactions and contraindications
   1. Can cause reduced respiratory rate, decreased reflexes, flushing, hypotension, and decreased heart rate
   2. Continuous IV infusion increases the risk of magnesium toxicity in the **neonate**

3. IV administration should not be used for 2 hours preceding **delivery**
   4. Magnesium sulfate is continued for the first 12 to 24 hours postpartum if it is used for preeclampsia
   5. High doses can cause loss of deep tendon reflexes, heart block, respiratory paralysis, and cardiac arrest
   6. Contraindicated in the client with heart block, myocardial damage, or renal failure
   7. Used with caution in the client with severe renal impairment
D. Implementation
   1. Monitor maternal vital signs, especially respirations, every 30 to 60 minutes
   2. Call the health care provider if respirations are less than 12, indicating respiratory depression
   3. Assess renal function and ECG for cardiac function
   4. Monitor magnesium levels, as the target range is 4 to 7 mEq/L; if a rise in the magnesium level occurs, notify the health care provider
   5. Administered by IV infusion via an infusion monitoring device; carefully monitor dose being administered
   6. Keep calcium gluconate on hand in case of a magnesium sulfate overdose, because calcium gluconate antagonizes the effect of magnesium sulfate
   7. Monitor deep tendon reflexes hourly for signs of developing toxicity
   8. Test patellar reflex or knee jerk reflex before administering repeat parenteral doses (used as an indicator of CNS depression; suppressed reflex may be a sign of impending respiratory arrest)
   9. Patellar reflex must be present and respiratory rate must be greater than 16 breaths per minute before each parenteral dose
   10. Monitor I & 0 hourly; output should be maintained at 30 mL per hour because the medication is eliminated through the kidneys

VI. MEPERIDINE HYDROCHLORIDE (DEMEROL)
A. Description
   1. Narcotic analgesic
   2. Administered by IM or IV route
   3. Antidote: naloxone (Narcan)
B. Use: Relieve moderate to severe pain associated with **labor**
C. Adverse reactions and contraindications
   1. Dizziness, nausea, vomiting, sedation, decreased BP, decreased respirations, diaphoresis, flushed face, decreased urination
   2. May be administered with promethazine (Phenergan) to prevent nausea
   3. High dosages may result in respiratory depression, skeletal muscle flaccidity, cold, clammy

skin, cyanosis, extreme somnolence progressing to convulsions, stupor, and coma

4. Used cautiously in clients delivering preterm **infants**
5. Not administered in early **labor** because it may slow the **labor** process
6. Not administered in advanced **labor** (within 1 hour of **delivery**) if the **neonate** is to be delivered before the medication is adequately removed from the fetal circulation (may cause respiratory depression)
7. Regular use of opiates during pregnancy may produce withdrawal symptoms in the **neonate** (irritability, excessive crying, tremors, hyperactive reflexes, fever, vomiting, diarrhea, yawning, sneezing, and seizures)

D. Implementation
1. Monitor vital signs, particularly respiratory status; if respirations are 12 per minute or lower, withhold medication and contact the health care provider
2. Monitor for BP changes (hypotension); maintain in a recumbent position
3. Have antidote available

▲ **VII. Rh$_o$(D) IMMUNE GLOBULIN (RDIG)**

A. Description
1. Prevention of anti-Rh (D) antibody formation is most successful if the medication is administered twice: at 28 weeks of gestation and again within 72 hours after **delivery**
2. Should be administered within 72 hours after potential or actual exposure to Rh-positive blood; must be given with each subsequent exposure or potential exposure to Rh-positive blood
3. Of no benefit once the client has developed a positive antibody titer to the Rh antigen

B. Use: Prevent isoimmunization in Rh-negative clients who are exposed or potentially exposed to Rh-positive red blood cells by transfusion, termination of pregnancy, amniocentesis, chorionic villus sampling (CVS), abdominal trauma, or bleeding during pregnancy or the birth process

▲ C. Adverse reactions and contraindications
1. Slight rise in temperature
2. Tenderness at the injection site
3. Contraindicated for Rh-positive women
4. Contraindicated in clients with a history of systemic allergic reactions to preparations containing human immunoglobulins
5. Not administered to a **newborn infant**

D. Implementation
1. Administer to mother by IM injection at 28 weeks' gestation and within 72 hours after **delivery**
2. Never administer by the IV route
3. Monitor for temperature elevation
4. Monitor injection site for tenderness

VIII. BETAMETHASONE (CELESTONE)

A. Description
1. Corticosteroid
2. Increases production of surfactant

B. Use: For client in preterm **labor** between 28 and 32 weeks whose **labor** can be inhibited for 48 hours without jeopardizing mother or fetus

C. Adverse reactions and contraindications
1. Decreases mother's resistance to infection
2. Breastfeeding is contraindicated during medication administration

D. Implementation
1. Monitor maternal vital signs
2. Monitor mother for signs of infection
3. Monitor white blood cell count

IX. LUNG SURFACTANTS (Box 31-4)   ▲

A. Description
1. Replenish surfactant and restore surface activity to the lungs
2. Administered by the intratracheal route

B. Use: Prevent or treat respiratory distress syndrome (hyaline membrane disease) in premature **infants**

C. Adverse reactions and contraindications
1. Side effects include transient bradycardia and oxygen desaturation
2. Administered with caution in those at risk for circulatory overload

D. Nursing implementation   ▲
1. Instill through catheter inserted into **infant's** endotracheal tube; avoid suctioning for at least 2 hours after administration
2. Monitor for bradycardia and decreased oxygen saturation during administration
3. Assess lung sounds for rales and moist breath sounds

X. EYE PROPHYLAXIS FOR THE NEONATE   ▲

A. Description
1. Erythromycin (0.5% Ilotycin) and tetracycline (1%) ophthalmic ointment or drops are both bacteriostatic and bactericidal and provide prophylaxis against *Neisseria gonorrhoeae* and *Chlamydia trachomatis*
2. Silver nitrate (1%) solution may be prescribed, but its use is minimal because it does not protect against chlamydial infection and can cause chemical conjunctivitis
3. Preventive treatment of gonorrhea is required by law

B. Use: as a prophylactic measure to protect against *Neisseria gonorrhoeae* and *Chlamydia trachomatis*
C. Adverse reaction: Silver nitrate (1%) solution can cause chemical conjunctivitis
D. Implementation
1. Cleanse the **neonate's** eyes before instilling drops or ointment
2. Instill into each of the **neonate's** conjunctival sacs within 1 hour after **delivery**; eye prophylaxis may be delayed until an hour or so after birth so that eye contact and parent-**infant** attachment and bonding are facilitated
3. Do not flush the eyes after instillation

XI. VITAMIN K (AquaMEPHYTON)
A. Description
1. Necessary for aiding in the production of active prothrombin
2. **Newborns** are deficient in vitamin K for the first 5 to 8 days of life because of the lack of intestinal flora that is necessary to absorb vitamin K
B. Use: For prophylaxis and to treat hemorrhagic disease of the **newborn**
C. Adverse reaction: Can cause hyperbilirubinemia in the **newborn**
D. Implementation
1. Protect the medication from light
2. Administer during the early neonatal period
3. Administer in the vastus lateralis muscle of the thigh
4. Monitor for bruising at the injection site and for bleeding from the cord
5. Monitor for jaundice and monitor bilirubin level because the medication can cause hyperbilirubinemia in the **newborn**

PRACTICE QUESTIONS

1. Epidural analgesia is administered to a woman for pain relief following a cesarean birth. The nurse assigned to care for the woman ensures that which medication is readily available if respiratory depression occurs?
   1. Betamethasone (Celestone)
   2. Morphine sulfate
   3. Merperidine hydrochloride (Demerol)
   4. Naloxone (Narcan)
2. Rh$_o$(D) immune globulin (RDIG) (anti-Rh$_o$(D) gamma globulin) is prescribed for a woman following delivery of a newborn infant. The nurse provides information to the woman about the purpose of the medication. The nurse determines that the woman understands the purpose of the medication if the woman states that RDIG will protect her next baby from which of the following?
   1. Being affected by Rh incompatibility

2. Having Rh positive blood
3. Developing a rubella infection
4. Developing physiological jaundice

3. Methylergonovine (Methergine) is prescribed for a postpartum woman to treat postpartum hemorrhage. Before administration of methylergonovine, the priority nursing assessment is to check the:
   1. Amount of lochia
   2. Blood pressure
   3. Deep tendon reflexes
   4. Uterine tone
4. A nurse is preparing to administer beractant (Survanta) to a premature infant who has respiratory distress syndrome (hyaline membrane disease). The nurse plans to administer the medication by which of the following routes?
   1. Subcutaneous
   2. Intratracheal
   3. Intramuscular
   4. Intradermal
5. A nurse is caring for a client who is receiving pitocin (Oxytocin) for the induction of labor. The nurse discontinues the pitocin infusion if which one of the following is noted on assessment of the client?
   1. Drowsiness
   2. Fatigue
   3. Early decelerations of the fetal heart rate
   4. Uterine hyperstimulation
6. A pregnant client is receiving magnesium sulfate for the management of preeclampsia. A nurse determines that the client is experiencing toxicity from the medication if which of the following is noted on assessment?
   1. Presence of deep tendon reflexes
   2. Serum magnesium level of 6 mEq/L
   3. Proteinuria of +3
   4. Respirations of 10 per minute
7. A woman with preeclampsia is receiving magnesium sulfate. The nurse assigned to care for the client determines that the magnesium sulfate therapy is effective if:
   1. Ankle clonus is noted
   2. The blood pressure decreases
   3. Seizures do not occur
   4. Scotomas are present
8. Methylergonovine (Methergine) is prescribed for a client with postpartum hemorrhage. Prior to administering the medication, a nurse contacts the health care provider who prescribed the medication if which of the following conditions is documented in the client's medical history?
   1. Peripheral vascular disease
   2. Hypothyroidism
   3. Hypotension
   4. Diabetes mellitus
9. Vitamin K (AquaMEPHYTON) is prescribed for a

neonate. A nurse prepares the medication and selects which muscle site to administer the medication?

1. Deltoid
2. Triceps
3. Vastus lateralis
4. Biceps

10. A nursing instructor asks a nursing student to describe the procedure for administering erythromycin (0.5% Ilotycin) ointment to the eyes of a neonate. The instructor determines that the student needs to further research this procedure if the student states:

1. "I will cleanse the neonate's eyes before instilling ointment."
2. "I will flush the eyes after instilling the ointment."
3. "I will instill the eye ointment into each of the neonate's conjunctival sacs within 1 hour after birth."
4. "Administration of the eye ointment may be delayed until an hour or so after birth so that eye contact and parent-infant attachment and bonding can occur."

CRITICAL THINKING: FREE-TEXT ENTRY

A nurse is caring for a pregnant client with severe preeclampsia who is receiving IV magnesium sulfate. The nurse ensures that what medication, the antidote to magnesium sulfate, is in the client's room?

Answer: _____

ANSWERS

1. 4

Rationale: Narcotics are used for epidural analgesia. An adverse reaction of epidural analgesia is a delayed respiratory depression. Naloxone (Narcan) is a narcotic antagonist, which reverses the effects of narcotics and is given for respiratory depression. Morphine sulfate and meperidine hydrochloride are narcotics. Celestone is a corticosteroid administered to enhance fetal lung maturity.

Test-Taking Strategy: Use the process of elimination, focusing on the issue of the question, the antidote for respiratory depression. Eliminate options 2 and 3 first, knowing that these medications are narcotics. Next eliminate option 1, knowing that this medication is a corticosteroid. Review the purpose and actions of these medications if you had difficulty with this question.

Level of Cognitive Ability: Application
Client Needs: Safe, Effective Care Environment
Integrated Concept/Process: Nursing Process/Planning
Content Area: Maternity
Reference: Hodgson, B., & Kizior, R. (2001). *Saunders nursing drug handbook 2001.* Philadelphia: W.B. Saunders, pp. 719-721.

2. 1

Rationale: Rh incompatibility can occur when an Rh-negative mother becomes sensitized to the Rh antigen. Sensitization may develop when an Rh-negative woman becomes pregnant with a fetus who is Rh positive. During pregnancy and at delivery, some of the baby's Rh-positive blood can enter the maternal circulation, causing the woman's immune system to form antibodies against Rh-positive blood. Administration of RDIG prevents the woman from developing antibodies against Rh-positive blood by providing passive antibody protection against the Rh antigen.

Test-Taking Strategy: Use the process of elimination. Options 3 and 4 can be easily eliminated first. From the remaining options, note the relationship between the name of the medication, Rh₀(D) immune globulin, and the word "incompability" in the correct option. Review the purpose of this medication if you had difficulty with this question.

Level of Cognitive Ability: Analysis
Client Needs: Health Promotion and Maintenance
Integrated Concept/Process: Teaching/Learning
Content Area: Maternity
Reference: Hodgson, B., & Kizior, R. (2001). *Saunders nursing drug handbook 2001.* Philadelphia: W.B. Saunders, p. 1328.

3. 2

Rationale: Methylergonovine, an ergot alkaloid, is an agent that is used to prevent or control postpartum hemorrhage by contracting the uterus. It causes continuous uterine contractions and may elevate blood pressure. A priority assessment before the administration of the medication is to check the blood pressure. The physician should be notified if hypertension is present. Although options 1, 3, and 4 may be components of the postpartum assessment, option 2, blood pressure, is specifically related to the administration of this medication.

Test-Taking Strategy: Use the process of elimination. Eliminate options 1 and 4 first because they are similar and related to one another. From the remaining options, use the ABCs—airway, breathing, and circulation. Blood pressure is a method of assessing circulation. Review the adverse effects of this medication if you had difficulty with this question.

Level of Cognitive Ability: Analysis
Client Needs: Safe, Effective Care Environment
Integrated Concept/Process: Nursing Process/Assessment
Content Area: Maternity
Reference: Clark, J., Queener, S., & Karb, V. (2000). *Pharmacologic basis of nursing practice* (6th ed.). St. Louis: Mosby, pp. 834, 838.

4. 2

Rationale: Respiratory distress is common in premature neonates and may be due to lung immaturity as a result of surfactant deficiency. The mainstay of treatment is the administration of exogenous surfactant. It is administered by the intratracheal route. Options 1, 3, and 4 are not routes of administration for this medication.

Test-Taking Strategy: Use the process of elimination. Note the relationship between the diagnosis "respiratory distress syndrome" and the correct option, "intratracheal." Review this medication if you had difficulty with this question.

Level of Cognitive Ability: Application
Client Needs: Physiological Integrity
Integrated Concept/Process: Nursing Process/Planning
Content Area: Maternity
Reference: Bowden, V., Dickey, S, & Greenberg, C. (1998). *Children and their families: The continuum of care.* Philadelphia: W.B. Saunders, p. 743.

5. **4**
Rationale: Pitocin stimulates uterine contractions and is one of the common pharmacological methods to induce labor. An adverse reaction associated with administration of the medication is hyperstimulation of uterine contractions. Therefore, pitocin infusion must be stopped when there are any signs of uterine hyperstimulation. Drowsiness and fatigue may be due to the labor experience. Early decelerations of the fetal heart rate are a reassuring sign and do not indicate fetal distress.

Test-Taking Strategy: Use the process of elimination, focusing on the issue, an adverse reaction to pitocin. Options 1 and 2 can be easily eliminated first. From the remaining options, recalling that early decelerations of the fetal heart rate are a reassuring sign will easily direct you to option 4. Review the nursing responsibilities associated with this medication if you had difficulty with this question.

Level of Cognitive Ability: Application
Client Needs: Physiological Integrity
Integrated Concept/Process: Nursing Process/Implementation
Content Area: Maternity
Reference: Clark, J., Queener, S., & Karb, V. (2000). *Pharmacologic basis of nursing practice* (6th ed.). St. Louis: Mosby, p. 834.

6. **4**
Rationale: Magnesium toxicity can occur from magnesium sulfate therapy. Signs of magnesium sulfate toxicity relate to central nervous system (CNS) depressant effects of the medication and include respiratory depression, loss of deep tendon reflexes, and sudden drop in fetal heart rate and/or maternal heart rate and blood pressure. Therapeutic serum levels of magnesium are 4 to 7 mEq/L. Proteinuria of 3+ is likely to be noted in a client with preeclampsia.

Test-Taking Strategy: Use the process of elimination and eliminate option 1 first because it is a normal finding. Next eliminate option 2, knowing that the therapeutic serum level of magnesium is between 4 and 7 mEq/L. From the remaining options, recalling that proteinuria of +3 would be noted in a client with preeclampsia will direct you to the correct option. Review the adverse effects of magnesium sulfate if you had difficulty with this question.

Level of Cognitive Ability: Analysis
Client Needs: Physiological Integrity
Integrated Concept/Process: Nursing Process/Assessment
Content Area: Maternity
Reference: Hodgson, B., & Kizior, R. (2001). *Saunders nursing drug handbook 2001.* Philadelphia: W.B. Saunders, p. 619.

7. **3**
Rationale: For a client with preeclampsia, the goal of care is directed at preventing eclampsia (seizures). Magnesium sulfate is an anticonvulsant; it is not an antihypertensive agent. Although a decrease in blood pressure may be noted initially, this effect is usually transient. Ankle clonus indicates hyperreflexia and may precede the onset of eclampsia. Scotomas are areas of complete or partial blindness. Visual disturbances, such as scotomas, often precede an eclamptic seizure.

Test-Taking Strategy: Use the process of elimination. Knowing that magnesium sulfate is an anticonvulsant will easily direct you to option 3. Review this medication if you had difficulty with this question.

Level of Cognitive Ability: Analysis
Client Needs: Physiological Integrity
Integrated Concept/Process: Nursing Process/Evaluation
Content Area: Maternity
Reference: Hodgson, B., & Kizior, R. (2001). *Saunders nursing drug handbook 2001.* Philadelphia: W.B. Saunders, p. 617.

8. **1**
Rationale: Methylergonovine is an ergot alkaloid used for postpartum hemorrhage. Ergot alkaloids are avoided in clients with significant cardiovascular disease, peripheral disease, hypertension, eclampsia, or preeclampsia. These conditions are worsened by the vasoconstrictive effects of the ergot alkaloids. Options 2, 3, and 4 are not contraindications related to the use of ergot alkaloids.

Test-Taking Strategy: Use the process of elimination. Recalling that ergot alkaloids produce vasoconstriction will easily direct you to option 1. Review the effects of this medication and the associated contraindications if you had difficulty with this question.

Level of Cognitive Ability: Analysis
Client Needs: Safe, Effective Care Environment
Integrated Concept/Process: Communication and Documentation
Content Area: Maternity
Reference: Clark, J., Queener, S., & Karb, V. (2000). *Pharmacologic basis of nursing practice* (6th ed.). St. Louis: Mosby, p. 835.

9. **3**
Rationale: Newborns are deficient in vitamin K for the first 5 to 8 days of life because of the lack of intestinal flora that is necessary to absorb vitamin K. Vitamin K is administered to the neonate to aid in the production of active prothrombin and to prevent hemorrhagic disease. It is administered in the vastus lateralis muscle. Options 1, 2, and 4 are incorrect administration sites.

Test-Taking Strategy: Use the process of elimination. Visualize the procedure for administering an injection to a neonate to assist in directing you to option 3. Review this procedure if you had difficulty with this question.

Level of Cognitive Ability: Application
Client Needs: Physiological Integrity
Integrated Concept/Process: Nursing Process/Implementation
Content Area: Maternity
Reference: Wong, D. (1999). *Whaley & Wong's nursing care of infants and children* (6th ed.). St. Louis: Mosby, p. 330.

10. **2**
Rationale: Eye prophylaxis protects the neonate against *Neisseria gonorrhoeae* and *Chlamydia trachomatis.* The eyes are

not flushed after instillation of the medication because the flush will wash away the administered medication. Options 1, 3, and 4 are correct statements regarding the procedure for administering eye medication to the neonate.

Test-Taking Strategy: Use the process of elimination, noting the key words "needs to further research." Eliminate options 3 and 4 first because they are similar. From the remaining options, visualize the effect of each. This will direct you to option 2. Review the procedure for administering eye medication to the neonate if you had difficulty with this question.

Level of Cognitive Ability: Analysis
Client Needs: Safe, Effective Care Environment
Integrated Concept/Process: Teaching/Learning
Content Area: Maternity
Reference: Wong, D. (1999). *Whaley & Wong's nursing care of infants and children* (6th ed.). St. Louis: Mosby, p. 329.

CRITICAL THINKING: FREE-TEXT ENTRY

Answer: Calcium gluconate
Rationale: Calcium gluconate is the medication that acts as an antidote to magnesium sulfate. It should be placed in the room of the client receiving IV magnesium sulfate.
Test-Taking Strategy: It is necessary to know the antidote for magnesium sulfate to answer this question. If you are unfamiliar with the guidelines for the administration of this medication, review this content.
Level of Cognitive Ability: Application
Client Needs: Physiological Integrity
Integrated Concept/Process: Nursing Process/Implementation
Content Area: Maternity
Reference: Gorrie, T., McKinney, E., & Murray, S. (1998). *Foundations of maternal-newborn nursing* (2nd ed.). Philadelphia: W.B. Saunders, p. 696.

REFERENCES

Bowden, V., Dickey, S, & Greenberg, C. (1998). *Children and their families: The continuum of care.* Philadelphia: W.B. Saunders.

Clark, J., Queener, S., & Karb, V. (2000). *Pharmacologic basis of nursing practice* (6th ed.). St. Louis: Mosby.

Gorrie, T., McKinney, E., & Murray, S. (1998). *Foundations of maternal-newborn nursing* (2nd ed.). Philadelphia: W.B. Saunders.

Hodgson, B., & Kizior, R. (2001). *Saunders nursing drug handbook 2001.* Philadelphia: W.B. Saunders.

Lowdermilk, D., Perry, S., & Bobak, I. (2000). *Maternity & women's health care* (7th ed.). St. Louis: Mosby.

Olds, S., London. M., & Ladewig, P. (2000). *Maternal-newborn nursing: A family and community-based approach* (6th ed.). Upper Saddle River, N.J.: Prentice-Hall Health.

Wong, D. (1999). *Whaley & Wong's nursing care of infants and children* (6th ed.). St. Louis: Mosby.

Pediatric Nursing

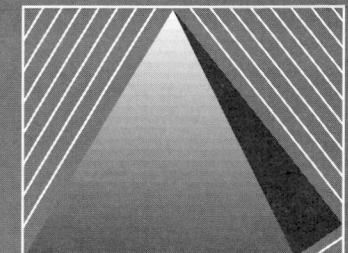

PYRAMID TERMS

abuse   Nonaccidental physical injury or the nonaccidental act of omission by a parent or person responsible for the care of a child.

active immunity   The protection, which can last months, years, or even a lifetime, that forms in response to exposure to antigens in nature or vaccines.

atresia   Congenital absence or closure of a body orifice.

attenuated vaccines   Vaccines derived from microorganisms or viruses whose virulence has been weakened as a result of passage through another host.

cephalocaudal   Characterized by growth and development that proceeds from head to toe.

chronological age   Age in years.

developmental age   Age based on functional behavior and ability to adapt to the environment. It does not necessarily correspond to chronological age.

encopresis   Fecal incontinence after age 4.

functional age   The age equivalent at which a child is actually able to perform specific self-care or related tasks.

growth   Measurable physical and physiological changes that occur over time.

growth spurts   Brief periods of rapid increase in growth rate.

hereditary   Involving the transmission of genetic characteristics from parent to offspring.

inactivated vaccines   Vaccines that contain killed microorganisms.

intelligence   What an individual can do relative to learning, thinking, and problem solving.

learning   Behavior changes that occur as a result of both maturation and experience with the environment.

nasal flaring   A serious sign of air hunger; a widening of the nares to enable an infant or child to take in more oxygen.

passive immunity   Antibody transfer from a person with active immunity to a person who does not have that antibody.

puberty   The period of time during which the adolescent experiences a growth spurt, develops secondary sex characteristics, and achieves reproductive maturity.

regression   Behavior that is more appropriate to an earlier stage of development and is often used to cope with stress or anxiety.

regurgitation   An abnormal backward flow of body fluid.

retractions   An abnormal movement of the chest walls during inspiration.

separation anxiety   Distress and apprehension caused by being removed from parents, home, or familiar surroundings.

shunt   Movement of blood or body fluid through an abnormal anatomic or surgically created opening.

stenosis   The narrowing or constriction of an opening.

stridor   A shrill harsh sound heard during inspiration or expiration, or both, that is produced by the flow of air through a narrowed segment of the respiratory tract.

wheezing   High-pitched musical whistles heard with or without a stethoscope.

PYRAMID TO SUCCESS

Pyramid points focus on psychosocial, cognitive, psychosexual, and moral stages of growth and development. Growth and development include physical characteristics, nutritional behaviors, skills, play, and specific safety measures relevant to a particular age group. Pyramid points focus on safety and the age-appropriate measures to ensure a safe and hazard-free environment for the child. Additional pyramid points focus on acute disorders that can occur in children. Focus on specific feeding techniques, positioning techniques, and interventions that will provide and maintain adequate airway, breathing, and circulation patterns in the child. On the NCLEX RN, be alert to the age of the child, if the age is presented in a question. The Integrated Concepts and Processes addressed in this unit include Nursing Process, Caring, Communication and Documentation, Cultural Awareness, Self-Care, and Teaching/Learning.

CLIENT NEEDS
Safe, Effective Care Environment

Accident prevention
Confidentiality
Continuity of care

Environmental and personal safety related to the developmental age of the child
Establishing priorities
Informed consent in regard to minors
Parent and child rights
Protection of the child and other contacts to prevent illness
Protective measures
Spread and control of infectious agents, particularly with regard to communicable diseases

Health Promotion and Maintenance

Developmental stages
Disease prevention
Family systems
Health promotion programs
Immunizations and communicable diseases
Instructions to the child and parents regarding care at home

Psychosocial Integrity

Child abuse and neglect
Communication
Cultural, religious, and spiritual differences
End of life issues
Family and support systems
Grief and loss
Play

Physiological Integrity

Age-appropriate normal body structure and function
Comfort measures
Elimination
Intrusive procedures
Medication administration
Nutrition
Responses to therapies
Rest and sleep

REFERENCES

Ball, J., & Bindler (1999). *Pediatric nursing: Caring for children* (2nd ed.). Stamford, Conn.: Appleton & Lange.

Bowden V., Dickey, S., & Greenberg, C. (1998). *Children and their families: The continuum of care.* Philadelphia: W.B. Saunders.

National Council of State Boards of Nursing (eds.) (2000). *Test plan for the National Council Licensure Examination for Registered Nurses.* Chicago: Author.

Wong, D. (1999). *Whaley & Wong's nursing care of infants and children* (6th ed.). St. Louis: Mosby.

Growth and Development

I. THE HOSPITALIZED INFANT AND TODDLER

A. **Separation anxiety**
1. Protest
   a. Cries, screams, searches for a parent; avoids and rejects contact with strangers
   b. Verbal attack on others
   c. Physical fighting; kicks, fights, hits, pinches
2. Despair
   a. Withdrawn, depressed, uninterested in the environment
   b. Loss of newly learned skills
3. Detachment
   a. Is uncommon and is sometimes called denial
   b. Superficially, the toddler appears to have adjusted to the loss
   c. During this phase, the toddler again becomes more interested in the environment, plays with others, and seems to form new relationships; this behavior is a form of resignation and is not a sign of contentment
   d. The toddler detaches from the parents in an effort to escape the emotional pain of desiring the parent's presence
   e. The toddler copes by forming shallow relationships with others, becoming increasingly self-centered, and attaching primary importance to material objects
   f. This is the most serious phase because reversal of the potential adverse effects is less likely to occur once detachment is established; in most situations, the temporary separation imposed by hospitalization does not cause such prolonged parental absence that the toddler enters into detachment

B. Fear of injury and pain: Affected by previous experiences, separation from parents, and preparation for the experience

C. Loss of control
1. Hospitalization with its own set of rituals and routines can severely disrupt the life of a toddler
2. The lack of control is often exhibited in behaviors related to feeding, toileting, playing, and bedtime
3. The toddler may demonstrate **regression**

D. Implementation
1. Provide swaddling and soft talking to the infant
2. Provide opportunities for sucking and oral stimulation for the infant using a pacifier if the infant is NPO
3. Provide stimulation if appropriate for the infant, using objects of contrasting colors and textures
4. Provide routines and rituals as close as possible to what the toddler is used to at home
5. Provide choices as much as possible to the toddler, to provide some control
6. Approach the toddler with a positive attitude
7. Allow the toddler to express feelings of protest
8. Encourage the toddler to talk about parents or others in their lives
9. Accept regressive behavior without ridiculing the toddler
10. Provide the toddler with favorite and comforting objects
11. Allow the toddler as much mobility as possible
12. Anticipate temper tantrums from the toddler, and maintain a safe environment for physical acting out
13. Employ pain-reduction techniques as appropriate

II. THE HOSPITALIZED PRESCHOOLER

A. **Separation anxiety**
1. Generally less obvious and less serious than in the toddler
2. As stress increases, the preschooler's ability to separate from the parents decreases

3. Protest
   a. Less direct and aggressive than the toddler
   b. May displace feelings onto others
4. Despair
   a. Similar to the toddler
   b. Quietly withdrawn, depressed, uninterested in the environment
   c. Loss of newly learned skills
   d. The preschooler becomes generally uncooperative, refusing to eat or take medication
   e. The preschooler repeatedly asks when the parents will be visiting
5. Detachment: Similar to the toddler
B. Fear of injury and pain
   1. The preschooler has a general lack of understanding of body integrity
   2. Fears invasive procedures and mutilation
   3. Imagines things to be much worse than they are
   4. Preschoolers believe that they are ill because of something they did or thought
C. Loss of control
   1. Likes familiar routines and rituals and may show **regression** if not allowed to maintain some control
   2. Has attained a good deal of independence and self-care at home and may expect that to continue in the hospital
D. Implementation
   1. Provide a safe and secure environment
   2. Take time for communication
   3. Allow the preschooler to express anger
   4. Acknowledge fears and anxieties
   5. Accept regressive behavior; assist the preschooler in moving from regressive to appropriate behaviors according to age
   6. Encourage rooming-in or leave favorite toy
   7. Allow mobility and provide play and diversional activities
   8. Place the preschooler with other children of the same age if possible
   9. Encourage the preschooler to be independent
   10. Explain procedures simply, on the preschooler's level
   11. Avoid intrusive procedures when possible
   12. Allow wearing underpants

III. THE HOSPITALIZED SCHOOL-AGED CHILD
A. **Separation anxiety**
   1. Accustomed to periods of separation from the parents, but as stressors are added the separation becomes more difficult
   2. More concerned with missing school and the fear that their friends will forget them
   3. Usually do not see the stage of behavior of protest, despair, and detachment with school-aged children

B. Fear of injury and pain
   1. Fear bodily injury and pain
   2. Fear of illness itself, disability, death, and intrusive procedures in genital areas
   3. Uncomfortable with any type of sexual examination
   4. Groans or whines, holds rigidly still, communicates about pain
C. Loss of control
   1. Is usually highly social, independent, and involved with activities
   2. Seeks information and asks relevant questions about tests and procedures and the illness
   3. Associates his or her actions with the cause of the illness
   4. May feel helpless and dependent if physical limitations occur
D. Implementation
   1. Encourage rooming-in
   2. Focus on the school-aged child's abilities and needs
   3. Encourage the school-aged child to become involved with his or her own care
   4. Accept **regression** but encourage independence
   5. Provide choices to the school-aged child
   6. Allow expression of feelings both verbally and nonverbally
   7. Acknowledge fears and concerns and allow for discussion
   8. Explain all procedures, using body diagrams or outlines
   9. Provide privacy
   10. Avoid intrusive procedures if possible
   11. Allow the school-aged child to wear underpants
   12. Involve the school-aged child in activities appropriate to developmental level and conditions
   13. Provide individualized recreation
   14. Encourage the school-aged child to contact friends
   15. Provide for educational needs
   16. Employ appropriate interventions to relieve pain

IV. THE HOSPITALIZED ADOLESCENT
A. **Separation anxiety**
   1. Not sure whether they want their parents with them when they are hospitalized
   2. Separation from friends is a source of anxiety
   3. Become upset if friends go on with their lives, excluding them
B. Fear of injury and pain
   1. Fear of being different from others and their peers
   2. May give the impression that they are not afraid even though they are terrified
   3. Become guarded when any areas related to sexual development are examined

C. Loss of control
  1. Behaviors exhibited include anger, withdrawal, and uncooperativeness
  2. Seek help and then reject it
D. Implementation
  1. Encourage questions about appearance and effects of the illness on the future
  2. Explore feelings about the hospital and the significance the illness might have for relationships
  3. Encourage to wear own clothes and perform normal grooming
  4. Allow favorite foods to be brought in to the hospital if possible
  5. Provide privacy
  6. Use medical terminology and body diagrams to prepare for procedures
  7. Introduce to other adolescents in the nursing unit
  8. Encourage maintaining contact with peer groups
  9. Provide for educational needs
  10. Identify formation of future plans
  11. Help develop positive coping mechanisms

V. COMMUNICATION APPROACHES

 A. General guidelines
  1. Allow the child to feel comfortable with the nurse
  2. Communicate through the use of objects
  3. Allow the child to express fears and concerns
  4. Speak clearly and in a quiet, unhurried voice
  5. Offer choices when possible
  6. Be honest with the child
  7. Set limits with the child as appropriate
B. Infant
  1. Infants respond to nonverbal communication behaviors of adults, such as holding, rocking, patting, and touching
  2. Use a slow approach and allow the infant to get to know the nurse
  3. Use a calm, soft, soothing voice
  4. Be responsive to cries
  5. Talk and read to infants
  6. Allow security objects such as blankets and pacifiers if the infant has them
C. Toddler
  1. Approach toddler cautiously
  2. Remember that toddlers accept verbal communications of others literally
  3. Learn the toddler's words for common items and use them in conversations
  4. Use short, concrete terms
  5. Prepare the toddler for procedures immediately before the event
  6. Repeat explanations and descriptions
  7. Use play for demonstrations

  8. Use visual aids such as picture books, puppets, and dolls
  9. Allow the toddler to handle the equipment or instruments; explain what the equipment or instrument does and how it feels
  10. Encourage the use of comfort objects
D. Preschooler
  1. Seek opportunities to offer choices
  2. Speak in simple sentences
  3. Be concise and limit the length of explanations
  4. Allow asking questions
  5. Describe procedures as they are about to be performed
  6. Use play to explain procedures and activities
  7. Allow handling the equipment or instruments, which will ease fear and help to answer questions
E. School-aged child
  1. Establish limits
  2. Provide reassurance to help in alleviating fears and anxieties
  3. Engage in conversations that encourage thinking
  4. Use medical play techniques
  5. Use photographs, books, dolls, and videos to explain procedures
  6. Explain in clear terms
  7. Allow time for composure and privacy
F. Adolescent
  1. Remember that the adolescent may be preoccupied with body image
  2. Encourage and support independence
  3. Provide privacy
  4. Use photographs, books, and videos to explain procedures
  5. Engage in conversations about adolescents' interests
  6. Avoid becoming too abstract, too detailed, and too technical
  7. Avoid responding to less than desirable social behaviors by prying, confrontation, or judgmental attitudes

VI. DEVELOPMENTAL CHARACTERISTICS

A. Infant
  1. Physical
     a. Height increases by ¾ inch per month
     b. Weight is doubled at 5 to 6 months and tripled at 12 months
     c. At birth, head circumference is 2 cm greater than chest circumference
     d. By 1 to 2 years of age, head circumference and chest circumference are equal
     e. Anterior fontanel (soft and flat in a normal infant) closes at 12 to 18 months
     f. Posterior fontanel (soft and flat in a normal infant) closes by 2 to 3 months

g. Ten upper and 10 lower deciduous teeth by 1 to 2 years of age

h. Lower central incisors present by 6 to 8 months

i. Reflexes such as rooting, tonic neck, palmar grasp, Moro, and stepping disappear by 4 months of age, with sucking lasting through infancy

j. Sleeps most of the time

2. Vital signs (Table 32-1)

3. Nutrition

a. The infant may breastfeed or bottle feed, depending on the mother's choice

b. Calorie requirements are 110 to 120 kcal/kg/day

c. Give no more than 30 ounces of formula per day

d. Iron stores from birth are depleted by 4 months

e. Do not give skim milk, because fatty acids are required

f. Introduce solid foods at 4 to 6 months

g. Introduce solid foods one at a time, with sequence as follows: rice cereal; fruits and vegetables, starting with yellow and then green; meats; and then egg yolks, avoiding egg whites

h. Avoid nuts, foods with seeds, raisins, and popcorn

i. Never mix food and/or medications with formula

j. Avoid adding honey to milk or water to prevent botulism

k. By 12 to 14 months the child should drink from a cup

4. Skills (Table 32-2)

5. Play
a. Solitary
b. Birth to 3 months: verbal, visual, and tactile stimuli
c. 4 to 6 months: initiates actions and recognizes new experiences
d. 6 to 12 months: aware of self, imitates, repeats pleasurable actions
e. Enjoys soft stuffed animals, crib mobiles with contrasting colors, squeeze toys, rattles, musical toys, water toys during the bath, large picture books, and push toys after he or she begins to walk

6. Safety
a. Baby-proof home
b. Infants who weigh up to 20 pounds should be restrained in a car seat in a semireclined, rear-facing position
c. Use safety straps for infant seats
d. Guard infant when on bed or changing table

TABLE 32-1

Vital Signs

Newborn Infant	1-Year-Old
Temperature: axillary, 96.8° to 99° F	Temperature: axillary, 96.8° to 99° F
Apical rate: 100-170 beats per minute	Apical rate: 90-130 beats per minute
Respirations: 30-80 breaths per minute	Respirations: 20-40 breaths per minute
BP: 73/55 mm Hg	BP: 90/56 mm Hg

TABLE 32-2

Infant Skills

2-3 Months	4-5 Months	6-7 Months
Smiles	Grasps objects	Creeps
Turns head side to side	Switches objects from hands	Sits with support
Cries	Rolls over for the first time	Imitates
Follows objects	Enjoys social interaction	Exhibits fear of strangers
Holds head in midline	Begins to show memory	Holds arms out
	Aware of unfamiliar surroundings	Frequent mood swings
		Waves bye-bye

8-9 Months	10-11 Months
Sits steadily unsupported	Can change from prone to sitting position
Crawls	Walks while holding onto furniture
May stand while holding on	Stands securely
Begin to stand without help	Entertains self for periods of time
12 -13 Months	**14-15 Months**
Walks with one hand held	Walks alone
Can take a few steps without falling	Can crawl upstairs
	Shows emotions such as anger and affection
	Will explore away from mother in familiar surroundings

e. Use gates to protect infant from stairs

f. Never shake or vigorously jiggle a baby's head

g. Be sure that bath water is not hot; do not leave unattended in bath

h. Do not hold infant while drinking or working near hot liquids

i. Cool vaporizers should be used instead of steam, to prevent burn injuries

j. Avoid food that is round and similar to the size of the airway, to prevent choking

k. Be sure toys have no small pieces

l. Hanging toys or mobiles over the crib should be well out of reach, to prevent strangulation

m. Avoid placing large toys in the crib because an older infant may use them as steps to climb

n. Cribs should be positioned away from curtains and blind cords

o. Cover electrical outlets

p. Remove hazardous objects from low, reachable places

q. Remove chemicals, poisons, and plants from infant's reach

r. Keep syrup of ipecac and the poison control number available

B. Toddler

1. Physical

a. Height and weight increase in a steplike fashion, reflecting **growth spurts** and lags

b. Head circumference increases about 1 inch between ages 1 and 2; thereafter, head circumference increases about $\frac{1}{2}$ inch per year until age 5

c. Anterior fontanel closes between ages 12 to 18 months

d. Weight gain is slower than in infancy; by age 2, the average weight is 27 pounds

e. Normal height changes include a **growth** of about 3 inches per year; the average height of the toddler is 34 inches at age 2 years

f. Lordosis is evident, with a "pot belly"

g. The toddler should see a dentist soon after the first teeth erupt, usually around 1 year of age; flouride supplements may be necessary if the water is not fluoridated

h. A toddler should never be allowed to fall asleep with a bottle containing milk, juice, soda pop, or sweetened water because of the risk of bottle-mouth caries; if a bottle is allowed at nap time or bedtime, it should contain only water

i. Typically sleeps through the night and has one daytime nap and discontinues the daytime nap at about age 3

j. A consistent bedtime ritual helps prepare the toddler for sleep

k. Security objects at bedtime may assist in sleep

2. Vital signs (Box 32-1)

3. Nutrition

a. Calorie requirements are 100 kcal/kg/day

b. Most toddlers prefer to feed themselves

c. The toddler generally does best by eating several small nutritious meals each day rather than three large meals

d. Offer a limited number of foods at any one time

e. Limit concentrated sweets and empty calories

f. At risk for aspiration of small foods that are not easily chewed, such as peanuts and popcorn

g. Physiological anorexia is normal, owing to the alternating periods of fast and slow **growth**

h. Sit the toddler in a high chair at the family table

i. Allow sufficient time to eat, but remove food when toddler begins playing with it

j. The toddler drinks well from a cup held with both hands

k. The toddler is skillful at handling finger foods

l. Avoid using food as a reward or punishment

4. Skills

a. The toddler begins to walks with one hand held by age 12 to 13 months

b. Runs by age 2 years and walks backward and hops on one foot by age 3 years

c. The toddler usually cannot alternate feet when climbing stairs

d. The toddler begins to master fine-motor skills for building, undressing, and drawing lines

e. Often uses "no" even when the toddler means "yes," to assert independence

f. Begins to use short sentences and has a vocabulary of about 300 words by age 2

g. Tends to ask many "why" questions

5. Bowel and bladder control

a. Signs that a toddler is ready for toilet training include muscle coordination with walking, communicating with parents, awareness of a wet or soiled diaper, holding urine for 2 hours, and interest in pleasing parents

b. Bowel control develops before bladder control

c. By age 3, the toddler achieves fairly good bowel and bladder control

d. The toddler may stay dry during the day but may need a diaper at night until about age 4

BOX 32-1

The Toddler's Vital Signs

Temperature: axillary, 97.5° to 98.6° F
Apical rate: 80-120 beats per minute
Respirations: 20-30 breaths per minute
Blood pressure: average, 92/55 mm Hg

6. Play
   a. The major socializing mechanism is parallel play, and therapeutic play can begin at this age
   b. Has a short attention span, causing the toddler to change toys often
   c. Explores body parts of self and others
   d. Typical toys include push/pull toys, blocks, sand, finger paints and bubbles, large balls, crayons, trucks and dolls, containers, Play-Doh, toy telephones, cloth books, wooden puzzles

▲ 7. Safety
   a. Toddlers are eager to explore the world around them
   b. The toddler should be supervised at play
   c. Once toddlers are able to sit up alone; they should be restrained in an upright, forward-facing position in a car seat when they reach a body weight of 9 kg (20 pounds), and a car seat should be used until they weigh at least 40 pounds, regardless of age.
   d. Lock car doors
   e. Use back burners on the stove to prepare a meal, and turn pot handles inward and toward the middle of the stove
   f. Keep dangling cords from small appliances away from toddlers
   g. Place inaccessible locks on windows and doors, and keep furniture away from windows
   h. Secure screens on all windows
   i. Place gates at stairways
   j. Do not permit to sleep or play in an upper bunk bed
   k. Never leave the toddler alone near a bathtub, pail of water, swimming pool, or any other body of water
   l. Keep toilet lids closed
   m. Keep all medicines, poisons, household plants, and toxic products high and locked out of reach
   n. Keep syrup of ipecac and the poison control number available

C. Preschooler
   1. Physical
      a. Grows 2½ to 3 inches per year
      b. Average height is 37 inches at age 3; 40½ inches at age 4; and 43 inches at age 5
      c. Gains 5 pounds per year; average weight of 32 pounds at age 5
      d. Requires about 12 hours of sleep each day
      e. A security object and a night-light assist with sleeping
      f. At the beginning of the preschool period, the eruption of the deciduous (primary) teeth is complete
      g. Dental care is essential, and the preschooler requires assistance with brushing and flossing

---

BOX 32-2

The Preschooler's Vital Signs

Temperature: axillary, 97.5° to 98.6° F
Apical rate: 70-110 beats per minute
Respirations: 16-22 breaths per minute
Blood pressure: average, 95/57 mm Hg

---

of teeth; fluoride supplements may be necessary if the water is not fluoridated
   2. Vital signs (Box 32-2)
   3. Nutrition
      a. Daily calorie requirement is about 1700 kcal/per day
      b. Exhibits food fads and strong taste preferences
      c. By 5 years old, tends to focus on social aspects of eating, table conversations, manners, and willingness to try new foods
   4. Skills
      a. Has good posture
      b. Develops fine-motor coordination
      c. Can hop, skip, and run more smoothly
      d. Athletic abilities begin to develop
      e. Demonstrates increased skills in balancing
      f. Alternates feet when climbing stairs
      g. Can tie shoelaces
      h. May talk continuously and ask many "why" questions
      i. Vocabulary increases to about 900 words by age 3 and 2100 words by age 5
      j. By age 3 usually talks in three- or four-word sentences and speaks in short phrases
      k. By age 4 speaks five- or six-word sentences and by age 5 speaks in longer sentences that contain all parts of speech
      l. Can be readily understood by others and can clearly understand what others are saying
   5. Bowel and bladder control   ▲
      a. By age 4, the preschooler has daytime control of bowel and bladder but may experience bed-wetting accidents at night
      b. By age 5, the preschooler achieves both bowel and bladder control, although accidents may occur in stressful situations
   6. Play
      a. Cooperative
      b. Imaginary playmates
      c. Likes to build and create things, and play is simple and imaginative
      d. Understands sharing and is able to interact with peers
      e. Requires regular socialization with age mates
      f. Play activities include a large space for running and jumping
      g. Likes dress-up clothes, paints, paper, and crayons for creative expressions

h. Swimming and sports aid with **growth** development

i. Puzzles and toys aid with fine-motor development

7. Safety

a. Preschoolers are active and inquisitive

b. Because of their magical thinking, they may believe that daring feats seen in cartoons are possible and they may attempt them

c. Can learn simple safety practices because they can follow simple and verbal directions and their attention span is lengthened

d. Once the child has outgrown the car safety seat (weight more than 40 pounds), the preschooler should be placed and restrained in a booster seat (until the preschooler weighs 60 pounds or his or her head is higher than the vehicle back seat), which raises the child high enough to allow the car seat belt to be correctly positioned over the child's chest and pelvis

e. Teach the preschooler basic safety rules to ensure safety when playing in a playground near swings and ladders

f. Never allow the preschooler to play with matches or lighters

g. The preschooler should be taught what to do in the event of a fire or if clothes catch fire; fire drills should be practiced with preschooler

h. Guns should be stored unloaded and secured under lock and key; the preschooler should be taught to leave an area immediately if a gun is seen, and to tell an adult

i. The preschooler should be taught never to point a toy gun at another person

j. Teach the preschooler that if another person touches his or her body in an inappropriate way to tell an adult

k. Teach the preschooler to avoid speaking to strangers and never to accept a ride, toys, or gifts from a stranger

l. Teach the preschooler his or her full name, address, parents' names, and telephone number

m. Keep syrup of ipecac and the poison control number available

n. Teach the preschooler how to dial 911 in an emergency situation

D. School-aged child

1. Physical

a. Girls usually grow faster than boys

b. **Growth** of about 2 inches per year between ages 6 and 12

c. Height ranges from 45 inches at age 6 to 59 inches at age 12

d. Weight gain of 4½ to 6½ pounds per year

e. Average weight of 46 pounds at age 6 and 88 pounds at age 12

BOX 32-3

The School-Aged Child's Vital Signs

Temperature: oral, 97.5° to 98.6° F
Apical rate: 60-100 beats per minute
Respirations: 16-20 breaths per minute
Blood pressure: average, 107/64 mm Hg

---

f. The first permanent (secondary) teeth erupt around age 6, and deciduous teeth are gradually lost

g. Regular dentist visits are necessary, and the school-aged child needs to be supervised with brushing and flossing teeth; fluoride supplements may be necessary if the water is not fluoridated

h. For school-aged children with mixed and permanent dentition, the best toothbrush is one with soft nylon bristles and an overall length of about 6 inches

i. Sleep requirements range from 10 to 12 hours a night

2. Vital signs (Box 32-3)

3. Nutrition

a. Increased **growth** needs

b. Balanced diet from foods in the Food Group Pyramid

c. May still be a picky eater but willing to try new foods

4. Skills

a. Refinement of fine-motor skills

b. Continued development of gross-motor skills

c. Increase in strength and endurance

5. Play

a. Play is more competitive

b. Rules and rituals are important aspects of play and games

c. Enjoys drawing, collecting items, dolls, pets, guessing games, board games, listening to the radio, TV, reading, and videos and computer games

d. Participation in team sports

e. Participates in secret clubs, gang activities, scout organizations

6. Safety

a. Experiences less fear in play activities and frequently imitates real life by using tools and household items

b. Adjust car seat belts so that the lap belt fits snugly over the bony pelvis and the shoulder harness is positioned across the chest

c. Place the shoulder harness of the seat belt behind the shoulder if it crosses the face or soft tissue of the neck

d. Major causes of injuries include bicycles,

skateboards, and team sports as the child is increasing motor abilities and independence

  e. Children should always wear a helmet when riding a bike or using inline skates or skateboards
  f. Teach the school-aged child water safety rules
  g. Instruct the school-aged child to avoid teasing or playing roughly with animals
  h. Never allow the school-aged child to play with matches or lighters
  i. The school-aged child should be taught what to do in the event of a fire or if clothes catch fire; fire drills should be practiced with the school-aged child
  j. Guns should be stored unloaded and secured under lock and key; the school-aged child should be taught to leave an area immediately if a gun is seen, and to tell an adult
  k. Teach the school-aged child that if another person touches his or her body in an inappropriate way to tell an adult
  l. Teach the school-aged child to avoid speaking to strangers and never to accept a ride, toys, or gifts from a stranger
  m. Teach the school-aged child traffic safety rules
  n. Teach the school-aged child how to dial 911 in an emergency situation
  o. Keep syrup of ipecac and the poison control number available

E. Adolescent
  1. Physical
  a. In girls, **puberty** begins between ages 8 and 14
  b. In boys, **puberty** begins between the ages of 9 and 16
  c. Body mass increases to adult size
  d. Sebaceous and sweat glands become active and fully functional
  e. Body hair distribution occurs
  f. Increase in height, weight, breast development, and pelvic girth in girls
  g. Menstrual periods occur about 2½ years after the onset of **puberty**
  h. In boys, increase in height, weight, muscle mass, and penis and testicle size
  i. Voice deepens in boys
  j. Normal weight gain during **puberty**
    (1.) Girls gain 15 to 55 pounds
    (2.) Boys gain 15 to 65 pounds
  k. Careful brushing and care of the teeth are important, and many adolescents must wear braces
  l. Sleep patterns include a tendency to stay up late; therefore, in an attempt to catch up on missed sleep, adolescents sleep late at every opportunity
  2. Vital signs (Box 32-4)

BOX 32-4

The Adolescent's Vital Signs

Temperature: oral, 97.5° to 98.6° F
Apical rate: 55-90 beats per minute
Respirations: 12-20 breaths per minute
Blood pressure: average, 121/70 mm Hg

---

  3. Nutrition
  a. Average daily requirements in girls: 38 to 48 kcal/kg/day
  b. Average daily requirements in boys: 42 to 60 kcal/kg/day
  c. Teaching about the Food Guide Pyramid is important
  d. Typically eat whenever they have a break in activities
  e. Calcium and protein needed to aid in bone and muscle **growth**
  4. Skills
  a. Gross- and fine-motor skills are well developed
  b. Strength and endurance increase
  5. Play
  a. Games and athletics are the most common forms of play
  b. Competition and strict rules are important
  c. Enjoy activities such as sports, videos, movies, reading, parties, hobbies, computer games, music, and experimenting as with makeup and hairstyles
  6. Safety
  a. Risk takers
  b. Have a natural urge to experiment and be independent
  c. Instruct in the dangers related to drugs and alcohol
  d. Help to recognize that there are choices when difficult or potentially dangerous situations arise
  e. Advocate the use of seat belts
  f. Instruct in the consequences of injuries that motor vehicle accidents can cause
  g. Instruct in water safety and emphasize that they should enter the water feet first as opposed to diving, especially when the depth of the water is unknown
  h. Instruct about the dangers associated with guns, violence, and gangs

PRACTICE QUESTIONS

1. The parents of a 2-year-old arrive at a hospital to visit their child. The child is in the playroom

when the parents arrive. When the parents enter the playroom, the child does not readily approach the parents. The nurse interprets this behavior as indicating that:
1. The child is withdrawn
2. The child is self-centered
3. The child has adjusted to the hospitalized setting
4. This is a normal pattern

2. A mother arrives at a clinic with her toddler and tells a nurse that she has a difficult time getting the child to go to bed at night. Which of the following is most appropriate for the nurse to suggest to the mother?
1. Inform the child of bedtime a few minutes before it is time for bed
2. Allow the child to have temper tantrums
3. Allow the child to set bedtime limits
4. Avoid a nap during the day

3. A mother of a 3-year-old asks a clinic nurse about appropriate and safe toys for the child. The nurse tells the mother that the most appropriate toy for a 3-year-old is which of the following?
1. A farm set
2. A golf set
3. A jack set with marbles
4. A wagon

4. A clinic nurse provides information to the mother of a toddler regarding toilet training. Which statement if made by the mother indicates a need for further information regarding the toilet training?
1. "The child will not be ready to toilet train until the age of about 18 to 24 months."
2. "Bladder control is usually achieved before bowel control."
3. "The child shouldn't be forced to sit on the potty for long periods."
4. "The ability of the child to remove clothing is a sign of physical readiness."

5. The mother of a 3-year-old is concerned because the child is still insisting on a bottle at nap time and at bedtime. Which of the following is the most appropriate suggestion to the mother?
1. Do not allow the child to have the bottle
2. Allow the bottle during naps but not at bedtime
3. Allow the bottle if it contains juice
4. Allow the bottle if it contains water

6. A nurse assesses the vital signs of a 12-month-old infant with a respiratory infection. The respiratory rate is 35 breaths per minute. On the basis of this finding, which action is most appropriate?
1. Notify the physician
2. Administer oxygen
3. Reassess the respiratory rate in 15 minutes
4. Document the findings

7. A nurse prepares to take the blood pressure (BP) of a school-aged child. To obtain an accurate measurement, the nurse ensures that the BP cuff covers:
1. One half of the distance between the antecubital fossa and the shoulder
2. One third of the distance between the antecubital fossa and the shoulder
3. Two thirds of the distance between the antecubital fossa and the shoulder
4. One quarter of the distance between the antecubital fossa and the shoulder

8. A nurse provides instructions to the parents of a newborn infant regarding car travel and safety seats. Which of the following is the most appropriate information related to the safety of the infant?
1. Restrain in a car seat in the front seat in a semireclined, rear-facing position
2. Restrain in a car seat in the front seat in a semireclined, forward-facing position
3. Restrain in a car seat in the back seat in a semireclined, rear-facing position
4. Restrain in a car seat in the back seat in a semireclined, forward-facing position

9. A nurse is monitoring a 3-month-old infant for signs of increased intracranial pressure (ICP). On palpation of the fontanels, the nurse notes that the anterior fontanel is soft and flat. On the basis of this finding, which action should the nurse take next?
1. Elevate the head of the bed to 90 degrees
2. Notify the physician
3. Increase oral fluids
4. Document the finding

10. A nurse is evaluating the developmental level of a 2-year-old. Which of the following does the nurse expect to observe in this child?
1. Uses a fork to eat
2. Uses a straw and a cup
3. Uses a knife for cutting food
4. Pours own milk into a cup

11. A nurse is preparing to care for a 5-year-old who has been placed in traction following a fracture of the femur. The nurse plans care, knowing that which of the following is the most appropriate activity for this child?
1. Large picture books
2. A radio
3. Crayons and a coloring book
4. A sports video

12. The mother of a 16-year-old tells a nurse that she is concerned because the child sleeps about 8 hours every night and until noontime every weekend. The most appropriate nursing response is which of the following?
1. "The child probably is anemic and should eat more foods containing iron."
2. "Adolescents need that amount of sleep every night."

3. "The child shouldn't be staying up so late at night."
4. "If the child eats properly, that shouldn't be happening."

13. A 4-year old child diagnosed with leukemia is hospitalized for chemotherapy. The child is fearful of the hospitalization. Which nursing intervention would be most appropriate to alleviate the child's fears?
    1. Advise the family to visit only during the scheduled visiting hours
    2. Encourage play with other children of the same age
    3. Provide a private room, allowing the child to bring the favorite toys from home
    4. Encouraging the child's parents to stay with the child

14. A 16-year-old is admitted to the hospital for acute appendicitis, and an appendectomy is performed. Which of the following nursing interventions is most appropriate to facilitate normal growth and development?
    1. Allow the family to bring in the child's favorite computer games
    2. Encourage the parents to room-in with the child
    3. Encourage the child to rest and read
    4. Allow the child to participate in activities with other individuals in the same age group when the condition permits

15. A nurse prepares to administer digoxin (Lanoxin) to a 3-year-old child with a diagnosis of congestive heart failure. The nurse notes that the apical rate is 110 beats per minute. On the basis of this finding, which nursing action is most appropriate?
    1. Administer the digoxin
    2. Recheck the apical rate in 15 minutes
    3. Notify the physician
    4. Hold the medication

16. A 2-year-old child is treated in the emergency room for a burn to the chest and abdomen. The child sustained the burn by grabbing a cup of hot coffee that was left on the kitchen counter. The nurse reviews safety principles with the parents prior to discharge. Which statement, if made by the parents, indicates an understanding of the measures to provide safety in the home?
    1. "I guess my children need to understand what the word 'hot' means."
    2. "We will install a safety gate as soon as we get home so the children can't get into the kitchen."
    3. "We will be sure that the children stay in their rooms when we work in the kitchen."

4. "We will be sure not to leave hot liquids unattended."

17. A clinic nurse provides instructions to a parent of a toddler experiencing physiologic anorexia. Which statement if made by the parent indicates a need for further education?
    1. "I will not force-feed my child."
    2. "I will limit the juice intake to less than 12 ounces per day."
    3. "I will feed my child if she will not eat."
    4. "At mealtime, I will offer less than my child may eat and let my child ask for more."

18. A mother of a 4-year-old expresses concern because her hospitalized child has begun thumb sucking. The mother states that this behavior began 2 days after hospital admission. The most appropriate nursing response is which of the following?
    1. "A 4-year-old is too old for this type of behavior."
    2. "Your child is acting like a baby."
    3. "The doctor will need to notified."
    4. "It is best to ignore the behavior."

19. A clinic nurse assesses the communication patterns of a 4-month-old infant. The nurse determines that the infant is demonstrating the highest level of developmental achievement expected if the infant:
    1. Uses simple words such as "mama"
    2. Uses monosyllabic babbling
    3. Links syllables together
    4. Coos when comforted

20. The mother of a toddler asks a nurse when it is safe to place the car safety seat in a face-forward position. The best nursing response is which of the following?
    1. When the toddler weighs 20 pounds
    2. The seat should not be placed in a face-forward position unless there are safety locks in the car
    3. The seat should never be placed in a face-forward position because of the risk of the child unbuckling the harness
    4. When the weight of the toddler is greater than 40 pounds

CRITICAL THINKING: FREE-TEXT ENTRY

The mother of a preschooler asks a clinic nurse when it will be safe to allow the child to use the car seat belts, rather than the booster seat, for traveling in the car. The nurse provides the mother with what information?

Answer: _____

ANSWERS

1. 4

Rationale: The phases through which young children progress when separated from their parents include protest, despair, and denial or detachment. In the stage of protest, when the parents return, the child readily goes to them. In the stage of despair, the child may not readily approach them, or may cling to a parent. In denial or detachment, when the parents return, the child becomes cheerful, interested in the environment and new persons (seemingly unaware of the lost parents), friendly with the staff, and interested in developing superficial relationships. Options 1, 2, and 3 are incorrect interpretations of the child's behavior.

Test-Taking Strategy: Use the process of elimination and knowledge regarding the phases of separation anxiety to answer the question. In addition, focusing on the data in the question will assist in eliminating options 1, 2, and 3. Review the concepts related to the hospitalized toddler and separation anxiety if you had difficulty with this question.

Level of Cognitive Ability: Analysis
Client Needs: Psychosocial Integrity
Integrated Concept/Process: Nursing Process/Analysis
Content Area: Child Health
Reference: Bowden V., Dickey, S., & Greenberg, C. (1998). *Children and their families: The continuum of care.* Philadelphia: W.B. Saunders, pp. 465-466.

2. 1

Rationale: Toddlers often resist going to bed. Bedtime protests may be reduced by establishing a consistent before-bedtime routine and enforcing consistent limits regarding the child's bedtime behavior. Informing the child of bedtime a few minutes before it is time for bed is the most appropriate option. Firm consistent limits are needed for temper tantrums or when toddlers try stalling tactics. Most toddlers take an afternoon nap and until their second birthday may also require a morning nap.

Test-Taking Strategy: Use the process of elimination. Note the key words "most appropriate." Eliminate options 2, 3, and 4 by using concepts related to growth and development. Remember that preparing the toddler for an event will minimize resistive behavior. Review concepts related to sleep patterns and the toddler if you had difficulty with this question.

Level of Cognitive Ability: Application
Client Needs: Health Promotion and Maintenance
Integrated Concept/Process: Teaching/Learning
Content Area: Child Health
Reference: Wong, D. (1999). *Whaley & Wong's nursing care of infants and children* (6th ed.). St. Louis: Mosby, p. 593.

3. 4

Rationale: Toys for the toddler must be strong, safe, and too large to swallow or place in the ear or nose. Toddlers need supervision at all times. Push/pull toys, large balls, large crayons, trucks, and dolls are some of the appropriate toys. A farm set, a golf set, and jacks with marbles may contain items that the child could swallow.

Test-Taking Strategy: Use the process of elimination and focus on the issue, the appropriate toy for a 3-year-old. Options 1, 2, and 3 can be easily eliminated because they contain items that could be swallowed by the child. Remember that large and strong toys are safest for the toddler. Review the principles related to play activities and the toddler if you had difficulty with this question.

Level of Cognitive Ability: Application
Client Needs: Safe, Effective Care Environment
Integrated Concept/Process: Teaching/Learning
Content Area: Child Health
Reference: Ball, J., & Bindler, R. (1999). *Pediatric nursing: Caring for children* (2nd ed.). Stamford, Conn.: Appleton & Lange, p. 67.

4. 2

Rationale: Bowel control is usually achieved before bladder control. The physical ability to control the anal and urethral sphincters is achieved sometime after the child is walking, probably between the ages of 18 and 24 months. The child should not be forced to sit for long periods. The ability to remove clothing is one of the physical signs of readiness.

Test-Taking Strategy: Use the process of elimination and knowledge of the concepts related to readiness for toilet training. Note the key words "indicates a need for further information." Look for the option that indicates that the nurse needs to provide additional information to the mother regarding the toilet training. Review the concepts related to readiness for toilet training if you had difficulty with this question.

Level of Cognitive Ability: Analysis
Client Needs: Physiological Integrity
Integrated Concept/Process: Teaching/Learning
Content Area: Child Health
Reference: Wong, D. (1999). *Whaley & Wong's nursing care of infants and children* (6th ed.). St. Louis: Mosby, p. 673.

5. 4

Rationale: A toddler should never be allowed to fall asleep with a bottle containing milk, juice, soda pop, or sweetened water because of the risk of bottle-mouth caries. If a bottle is allowed at nap time or bedtime, it should contain only water.

Test-Taking Strategy: Use the process of elimination. Eliminate options 1 and 2 first because they are similar. From the remaining options, recalling that bottle-mouth caries is a concern in a child will assist in directing you to option 4. Review dental health principles related to children if you had difficulty with this question.

Level of Cognitive Ability: Application
Client Needs: Health Promotion and Maintenance
Integrated Concept/Process: Teaching/Learning
Content Area: Child Health
Reference: Wong, D. (1999). *Whaley & Wong's nursing care of infants and children* (6th ed.). St. Louis: Mosby, p. 686.

6. 4

Rationale: The normal respiratory rate in a 12-month-old infant is 20 to 40 breaths per minute. The normal apical rate is 80 to 130 beats per minute, and the average blood pressure is 90/53 mm Hg. The nurse would document the findings.

Test-Taking Strategy: Knowledge regarding the normal vital signs of an infant is required to answer this question. If you had difficulty with this question, review these normal parameters.

Level of Cognitive Ability: Application
Client Needs: Physiological Integrity
Integrated Concept/Process: Communication and Documentation

Content Area: Child Health
Reference: Ball, J., & Bindler, R. (1999). *Quick reference to pediatric clinical skills.* Stamford, Conn.: Appleton & Lange, pp. 20-22.

7. 3
Rationale: The size of the BP cuff is important. Cuffs that are too small will cause falsely elevated values, and those that are too large will cause inaccurate low values. The cuff should cover two thirds of the distance between the antecubital fossa and the shoulder.
Test-Taking Strategy: Use the process of elimination. Attempt to visualize the placement measurements described in each of the options. This will assist in directing you to option 3. If you had difficulty with this question, review the procedure for taking BP in a child.
Level of Cognitive Ability: Comprehension
Client Needs: Health Promotion and Maintenance
Integrated Concept/Process: Nursing Process/Implementation
Content Area: Child Health
Reference: Ball, J., & Bindler, R. (1999). *Quick reference to pediatric clinical skills.* Stamford, Conn.: Appleton & Lange, p. 21.

8. 3
Rationale: The infant should be placed in a car safety seat restraint in the back seat of the car, in a rear-facing position, until the infant weighs 20 pounds. The infant should never be placed in a forward-facing position or in the front seat.
Test-Taking Strategy: Visualize each of the descriptions in the options, with a focus of safety in mind. Use the process of elimination. Eliminate options 1 and 2 because of the words "front seat." Next, eliminate option 4 because of the words "forward-facing." If you had difficulty with this question, review the car safety measures for the infant.
Level of Cognitive Ability: Application
Client Needs: Safe, Effective Care Environment
Integrated Concept/Process: Teaching/Learning
Content Area: Child Health
Reference: Wong, D. (1999). *Whaley & Wong's nursing care of infants and children* (6th ed.). St. Louis: Mosby, pp. 352, 610.

9. 4
Rationale: The anterior fontanel is diamond shaped and located on the top of the head. It should be soft and flat in a normal infant, and it normally closes by 12 to 18 months of age. The nurse would document the finding, since it is normal.
Test-Taking Strategy: Use the process of elimination. Note the key words "soft and flat." This should provide you with the clue that this is a normal finding. A bulging or tense fontanel may result from crying or increased ICP. If you had difficulty with this question, review normal assessment findings in an infant.
Level of Cognitive Ability: Application
Client Needs: Physiological Integrity
Integrated Concept/Process: Communication and Documentation
Content Area: Child Health
Reference: Wong, D. (1999). *Whaley & Wong's nursing care of infants and children* (6th ed.). St. Louis: Mosby, p. 321.

10. 2
Rationale: By age 2 years, the child can use a straw and a cup and can use a spoon correctly but with some spilling. By ages 3

to 4, the child begins to use a fork. By the end of the preschool period, the child should be able to pour milk into a cup and begin to use a knife for cutting.
Test-Taking Strategy: Note the age of the child and use the process of elimination. Option 3 can be easily eliminated. Next, think about the fine-motor skills that need to be developed in selecting the correct option. With this in mind, eliminate options 1 and 4. If you had difficulty with this question, review the developmental skills of a 2-year-old.
Level of Cognitive Ability: Analysis
Client Needs: Health Promotion and Maintenance
Integrated Concept/Process: Nursing Process/Assessment
Content Area: Child Health
Reference: Wong, D. (1999). *Whaley & Wong's nursing care of infants and children* (6th ed.). St. Louis: Mosby, p. 681.

11. 3
Rationale: In the preschooler, play is simple and imaginative, and includes activities such as crayons and coloring books, puppets, felt and magnetic boards, and Play-Doh. Large picture books are most appropriate for the infant. A radio and a sports video are most appropriate for the adolescent.
Test-Taking Strategy: Use the process of elimination. Note the age of the child, and think about the age-related activity that would be most appropriate. Eliminate options 3 and 4, knowing that they are most appropriate for the adolescent. From the remaining options, the word "large" in option 1 should provide you with the clue that this activity would be more appropriate for a child younger than age 5. If you had difficulty with this question, review the appropriate activities for a preschooler.
Level of Cognitive Ability: Analysis
Client Needs: Psychosocial Integrity
Integrated Concept/Process: Nursing Process/Planning
Content Area: Child Health
Reference: Ball, J., & Bindler, R. (1999). *Pediatric nursing: Caring for children* (2nd ed.). Stamford, Conn.: Appleton & Lange, p. 192.

12. 2
Rationale: The adolescent needs 8 to 8½ hours of sleep per night. During this age, with an increase in social activities, school commitments, and possibly work activities, it is important that the adolescent receive enough sleep at night. Options 1, 3, and 4 are inaccurate and inappropriate nursing responses.
Test-Taking Strategy: Use the process of elimination and focus on the issue of the question. Note the key words "most appropriate." There is no indication in the question that a physiological alteration is present; therefore eliminate option 1. Use therapeutic communication techniques to direct you to option 2. Review adolescent sleep patterns if you had difficulty with this question.
Level of Cognitive Ability: Application
Client Needs: Health Promotion and Maintenance
Integrated Concept/Process: Communication and Documentation
Content Area: Child Health
Reference: Bowden V., Dickey, S., & Greenberg, C. (1998). *Children and their families: The continuum of care.* Philadelphia: W.B. Saunders, p. 320.

13. 4

Rationale: Although the preschooler may already be spending some time away from parents at a day care center or preschool, illness adds a stressor that makes separation more difficult. The child may repeatedly ask when parents will be coming for a visit or may be constantly wanting to call the parents. Options 1 and 3 will increase stress related to separation anxiety. Option 2 is unrelated to the issue of the question and, in addition, may not be appropriate for a child at risk for immunocompromise.

Test-Taking Strategy: Note that the issue relates to the child's fear. Use the process of elimination. Options 1 and 3 will further increase anxiety and fear, and should be eliminated. Bearing the issue of the question in mind and considering the child's diagnosis will assist in eliminating option 2. Review interventions to prevent or minimize separation anxiety if you had difficulty with this question.

Level of Cognitive Ability: Application
Client Needs: Psychosocial Integrity
Integrated Concept/Process: Caring
Content Area: Child Health
Reference: Wong, D. (1999). *Whaley & Wong's nursing care of infants and children* (6th ed.). St. Louis: Mosby, p. 1142.

14. 4

Rationale: Adolescents often are not sure whether they want their parents with them when they are hospitalized. Because of the importance of the peer group, separation from friends is a source of anxiety. Ideally, the members of the peer group will support their ill friend. Options 1, 2, and 3 isolate the child from the peer group.

Test-Taking Strategy: Consider the psychosocial needs of the adolescent when answering the question. Options 1, 2, and 3 are similar in that they isolate the child from his or her own peer group. If you had difficulty with this question, review the psychosocial needs of the adolescent.

Level of Cognitive Ability: Application
Client Needs: Psychosocial Integrity
Integrated Concept/Process: Caring
Content Area: Child Health
Reference: Wong, D. (1999). *Whaley & Wong's nursing care of infants and children* (6th ed.). St. Louis: Mosby, pp. 1193-1194.

15. 1

Rationale: The normal apical heart rate for a 3-year-old is 80 to 120 beats per minute. Since the apical rate is within the normal range, options 2, 3, and 4 are inappropriate.

Test-Taking Strategy: Use the process of elimination and knowledge of the normal apical rate for a 3-year-old to answer the question. Recalling that a heart rate of 100 beats per minute is within the normal range will direct you to option 1. Review the normal vital signs for a 3-year-old if you had difficulty with this question.

Level of Cognitive Ability: Application
Client Needs: Physiological Integrity
Integrated Concept/Process: Nursing Process/Implementation
Content Area: Child Health
Reference: Ball, J., & Bindler, R. (1999). *Quick reference to pediatric clinical skills.* Stamford, Conn.: Appleton & Lange, p. 20.

16. 4

Rationale: Toddlers, with their increased mobility and development of motor skills, can reach hot water or hot objects placed on counters and stoves, and open fires or stove burners above their eye level. Parents should be encouraged to remain in the kitchen when preparing a meal, to use the back burners on the stove, and to turn pot handles inward and toward the middle of the stove. Hot liquids should never be left unattended, and the toddler should always be supervised. The statements in options 1, 2, and 3 do not indicate an understanding of the principles of safety.

Test-Taking Strategy: Use the process of elimination, noting the key words "indicates an understanding." Option 1 can be easily eliminated. Options 2 and 3 are similar in that they isolate the child from the environment. Option 4 is the only option that reflects an understanding of safety principles by the parents. Review these safety principles if you had difficulty with this question.

Level of Cognitive Ability: Analysis
Client Needs: Safe, Effective Care Environment
Integrated Concept/Process: Teaching/Learning
Content Area: Child Health
Reference: Wong, D. (1999). *Whaley & Wong's nursing care of infants and children* (6th ed.). St. Louis: Mosby, p. 691.

17. 3

Rationale: A toddler has the skills required to feed himself or herself. The parent needs to be instructed not to feed children who can feed themselves, or to force-feed a child. To increase nutritious intake at mealtime, juice intake needs to be limited to less than 12 ounces per day. At mealtime, it is best to offer less than the toddler may eat and let the child ask for more food.

Test-Taking Strategy: Note the key words "a need for further education." Bearing in mind that the goal is to provide a nutritious intake should assist in directing you to option 3. In addition, feeding a child if he or she will not eat will impair independence. Review interventions that will promote nutrition in the toddler if you had difficulty with this question.

Level of Cognitive Ability: Analysis
Client Needs: Physiological Integrity
Integrated Concept/Process: Teaching/Learning
Content Area: Child Health
Reference: Wong, D. (1999). *Whaley & Wong's nursing care of infants and children* (6th ed.). St. Louis: Mosby, p. 680.

18. 4

Rationale: In the hospitalized preschooler, it is best to accept regression if it occurs. Regression is most often due to the stress of the hospitalization. Parents may be overly concerned about regression and should be told that their child may continue the behavior at home. When regression does occur, the best approach is to ignore it while praising existing patterns of appropriate behavior. There is no need to call the physician. Options 1 and 2 are inappropriate.

Test-Taking Strategy: Use the process of elimination. Note the key words "most appropriate." Options 1 and 2 are clearly inappropriate and are eliminated first. Option 3 may cause increased concern in the mother. If you had difficulty with this question, review the psychosocial issues related to the hospitalized preschool child.

Level of Cognitive Ability: Application
Client Needs: Psychosocial Integrity
Integrated Concept/Process: Communication and Documentation

Content Area: Child Health
Reference: Wong, D. (1999). *Whaley & Wong's nursing care of infants and children* (6th ed.). St. Louis: Mosby, p. 680.

19. 2

Rationale: Using monosyllabic babbling occurs between 3 and 6 months of age. Using simple words such as "mama" occurs between 9 and 12 months of age. Linking syllables together when communicating occurs between 6 and 9 months of age. Cooing begins at birth and continues until 2 months of age.
Test-Taking Strategy: Use the process of elimination and knowledge of language and communication developmental milestones to answer the question. Focus on the age of the infant to assist in directing you to the correct option. Review the patterns of infant communication if you had difficulty with this question.
Level of Cognitive Ability: Analysis
Client Needs: Health Promotion and Maintenance
Integrated Concept/Process: Nursing Process/Assessment
Content Area: Child Health
Reference: Wong, D. (1999). *Whaley & Wong's nursing care of infants and children* (6th ed.). St. Louis: Mosby, p. 680.

20. 1

Rationale: The transition point for switching to the forward-facing position is defined by the manufacturer of the safety seat but is generally at a body weight of 9 kg (20 pounds). The car safety seat should be used until the child weighs at least 40 pounds, regardless of age. Options 2, 3, and 4 are incorrect.
Test-Taking Strategy: Use the process of elimination and focus on the issue of the question. Eliminate options 2 and 3 first because of the absolute words "not" and "never." From the remaining options, use knowledge regarding car safety and the toddler to answer the question. Review these safety principles if you had difficulty with this question.
Level of Cognitive Ability: Application
Client Needs: Safe, Effective Care Environment
Integrated Concept/Process: Teaching/Learning
Content Area: Child Health
Reference: Wong, D. (1999). *Whaley & Wong's nursing care of infants and children* (6th ed.). St. Louis: Mosby, p. 687.

CRITICAL THINKING: FREE-TEXT ENTRY

Answer: The preschooler is restrained in a booster seat until the preschooler weighs 60 pounds or his or her head is higher than the vehicle back seat.
Rationale: At this developmental level, the child's head is high enough to allow a car seat belt to be correctly positioned over the child's chest and pelvis.
Test-Taking Strategy: Focus on the issue of the question and the developmental level of the child, the preschooler, to answer the question. Review the principles and guidelines related to car safety if you had difficulty with this question.
Level of Cognitive Ability: Application
Client Needs: Safe, Effective Care Environment
Integrated Concept/Process: Teaching/Learning
Content Area: Child Health
Reference: Wong, D. (1999). *Whaley & Wong's nursing care of infants and children* (6th ed.). St. Louis: Mosby, pp. 687-690.

REFERENCES

Ball, J., & Bindler, R. (1999). *Pediatric nursing: Caring for children* (2nd ed.). Stamford, Conn.: Appleton & Lange.

Ball, J., & Bindler, R. (1999). *Quick reference to pediatric clinical skills.* Stamford, Conn.: Appleton & Lange.

Bowden V., Dickey, S., & Greenberg, C. (1998). *Children and their families: The continuum of care.* Philadelphia: W.B. Saunders.

Ladewig, P., London, M., & Olds, S. (1998). *Maternal-newborn care: The nurse, the family, and the community* (4th ed.). Menlo Park, Calif.: Addison-Wesley.

Wong, D. (1999). *Whaley & Wong's nursing care of infants and children* (6th ed.). St. Louis: Mosby.

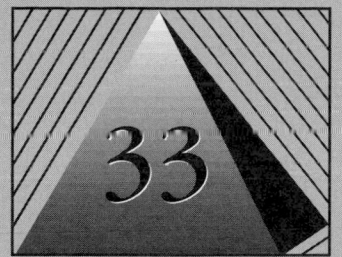

Neurological, Cognitive, and Psychosocial Disorders

I. HEAD INJURY

A. Description
1. The pathological result of any mechanical force to the skull, scalp, meninges, or brain
2. Manifestations depend on the type of injury and the subsequent amount of increased intracranial pressure (ICP)

B. Assessment (ICP)
1. Early Signs
   a. Headache
   b. Visual disturbances, diplopia
   c. Nausea and vomiting
   d. Dizziness or vertigo
   e. Slight change in vital signs
   f. Change in pupillary response and equality
   g. Sunsetting eyes
   h. Slight change in level of consciousness (LOC)
   i. Infant: bulging fontanel; wide sutures, increased head circumference; dilated scalp veins; high-pitched cry
2. Late signs
   a. Significant decrease in LOC
   b. Cushing's triad: increased systolic blood pressure and widened pulse pressure; bradycardia; and irregular respirations
   c. Decorticate posturing: Adduction of the arms at the shoulders, the arms being flexed on the chest with the wrists flexed and the hands fisted, and the lower extremities being extended and adducted; seen with severe dysfunction of the cerebral cortex (Fig. 33-1)
   d. Decerebrate posturing: Rigid extension and pronation of the arms and the legs; a sign of dysfunction at the level of the midbrain (Fig. 33-1)
   e. Fixed and dilated pupils

C. Implementation
1. Monitor the airway
2. Assess injuries; immobilize the neck if a cervical injury is suspected
3. Monitor vital signs and neurological function
4. Monitor for decreased responsiveness to pain (a significant sign of altered LOC)
5. Initiate seizure precautions
6. Maintain an NPO status or provide clear liquids if prescribed, until it is determined that vomiting will not occur
7. Administer oxygen and IV fluids as prescribed
8. Monitor IV fluids carefully to avoid aggravating any cerebral edema and to minimize the possibility of overhydration
9. Elevate the head of the bed 15 to 30 degrees if not contraindicated
10. Position so that the head is maintained midline to facilitate venous drainage and avoid jugular vein compression; turning side to side is contraindicated because of the risk of jugular vein compression
11. Assess wound dressings for the presence of drainage and monitor for nose or ear drainage, which could indicate leakage of cerebrospinal fluid (CSF); drainage that is positive indicates leakage of CSF from a skull fracture
12. Administer tepid sponge baths or place on a hypothermia blanket if hyperthermia occurs
13. Suctioning through the nares is contraindicated because of the high risk of a secondary infection and the probability of the catheter entering the brain through a fracture
14. Administer acetaminophen (Tylenol) for headache; anticonvulsants for seizures; antibiotics if a laceration is present; and tetanus toxoid as appropriate

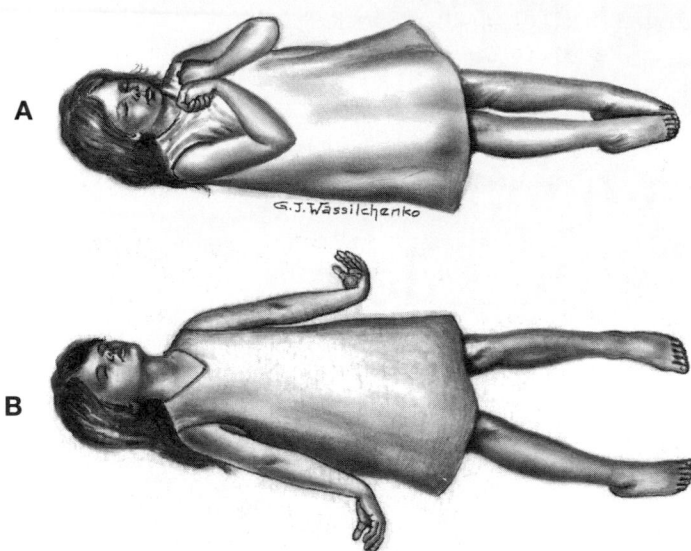

FIG. 33-1 **A,** Decorticate posturing. **B,** Decerebrate posturing. (From Wong DL et al: *Whaley & Wong's nursing care of infants and children,* ed 6, St Louis, 1999, Mosby.)

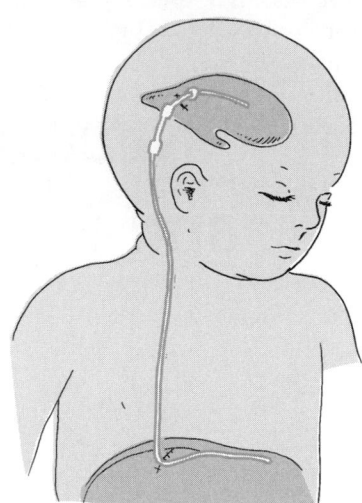

FIG. 33-2 Ventriculoperitoneal shunt. Catheter is threaded beneath the skin. (From Wong DL et al: *Whaley & Wong's nursing care of infants and children,* ed 6, St Louis, 1999, Mosby.)

BOX 33-1

Signs of Brainstem Involvement

Deep, rapid, or intermittent and gasping respirations
Wide fluctuations or noticeable slowing of the pulse
Widening pulse pressure or extreme fluctuations in
blood pressure

---

15. Sedating medications are withheld during the acute phase of the injury
16. Monitor for signs of brainstem involvement (Box 33-1)
17. Epidural hematoma: monitor for asymmetric pupils (one dilated, unreactive pupil in a comatose child is a neurosurgical emergency that may require evacuation of the hematoma)

II. HYDROCEPHALUS
A. Description
   1. An imbalance of CSF absorption or production, caused by malformations, tumors, hemorrhage, infections, or trauma
   2. Results in head enlargement and increased ICP
B. Types
   1. Communicating
      a. Occurs as a result of impaired absorption within the subarachnoid space
      b. Interference of CSF within the ventricular system does not occur
   2. Noncommunicating: obstruction of CSF flow within the ventricular system occurs

C. Assessment
   1. Infant
      a. Increased head circumference
      b. Bones of the head are thin and widely separated and produce a cracked-pot sound (Macewen sign) on percussion
      c. Anterior fontanel tense, bulging, and non-pulsating
      d. Scalp veins dilated
      e. Frontal bossing
      f. Sunsetting eyes
   2. Child
      a. Behavior changes such as irritability and lethargy
      b. Headache upon awakening
      c. Nausea and vomiting
      d. Ataxia
      e. Nystagmus
   3. Late signs: A high, shrill cry and seizure activities
D. Surgical implementation
   1. The goal of surgical treatment is to prevent further CSF accumulation by bypassing the blockage and draining the fluid from the ventricles to a location where it may be reabsorbed
   2. Ventriculoperitoneal **shunt** (VP **shunt**): CSF drains into the peritoneal cavity from the lateral ventricle (Fig. 33-2)
   3. Atrioventricular **shunt** (AV **shunt**): CSF drains into the right atrium of the heart from the lateral ventricle, bypassing the obstruction (used in older children and in children with abdominal pathology)

E. Implementation postoperatively
1. Monitor vital signs and neurological signs
2. Position on the unoperated side to prevent pressure on the shunt valve
3. The child is kept flat as prescribed to avoid rapid reduction of intracranial fluid
4. Observe for increased ICP; if increased ICP occurs, elevate the head of the bed to 15 to 30 degrees to enhance gravity flow through the **shunt**
5. Monitor for signs of infection and assess dressings for drainage
6. Measure head circumference
7. Monitor I & O
8. Provide comfort measures; administer medications as prescribed, which may include diuretics, antibiotics, or anticonvulsants
9. Instruct parents in how to recognize **shunt** infection or malfunction
10. In a toddler, headache and a lack of appetite are the earliest common signs of **shunt** malfunction

III. SPINA BIFIDA
A. Description
1. Central nervous system (CNS) defect that occurs as a result of neural tube failure to close during embryonic development
2. Associated deficits include sensory motor disturbance, dislocated hips, clubfoot, and hydrocephalus
3. Defect closure is usually done during infancy
B. Types
1. Spina bifida occulta
   a. Posterior vertebral arches fail to close in the lumbosacral area
   b. Spinal cord remains intact and usually is not visible
   c. Meninges are not exposed on the skin surface
   d. Neurological deficits are not usually present
2. Spina bifida cystica
   a. Protrusion of the spinal cord and/or its meninges
   b. Results in incomplete closure of the vertebral and neural tubes, resulting in a sac-like protrusion in the lumbar or sacral area, with varying degrees of nervous tissue involvement
   c. Can include meningocele, myelomeningocele, lipomeningocele, and lipomeningomyelocele
3. Meningocele
   a. Protrusion involves meninges and a sac-like cyst that contains CSF in the midline of the back, usually in the lumbosacral area
   b. No involvement of the spinal cord
   c. Neurological deficits are usually not present

4. Myelomeningocele
   a. Protrusion of meninges, CSF, nerve roots, and a portion of the spinal cord
   b. The sac (defect) is covered by a thin membrane that is prone to leakage or rupture
   c. Neurological deficits are evident
C. Assessment
1. Depends on the spinal cord involvement
2. Visible spinal defect
3. Flaccid paralysis of the legs
4. Altered bladder and bowel function
5. Hip and joint deformities
D. Implementation
1. Evaluate the sac and measure the lesion
2. Perform neurological assessment
3. Monitor for increased ICP, which might indicate developing hydrocephalus
4. Measure head circumference; assess the anterior fontanel for fullness
5. Protect the sac; cover with a sterile, moist (normal saline), nonadherent dressing to maintain the moisture of the sac and contents, and change the dressing every 2 to 4 hours as prescribed
6. Place in a prone position to minimize tension on the sac and the risk of trauma; the head is turned to one side for feeding
7. Change the dressing covering the sac whenever soiled, because of the risk of infection; diapering may be contraindicated until the defect has been repaired
8. Use aseptic technique to prevent infection
9. Assess the sac for redness, clear or purulent drainage, abrasions, irritation, and signs of infection
10. Early signs of infection include elevated temperature (axillary), irritability, lethargy, and nuchal rigidity
11. Assess for physical impairments such as hip and joint deformities
12. Prepare the child and family for surgery
13. Administer antibiotics as prescribed to prevent infection
14. Administer anticholinergics to improve urinary continence and laxatives to achieve bowel continence in the child, and antispasmodics to control bladder spasms

IV. REYE'S SYNDROME
A. Description
1. Acute encephalopathy that follows a viral illness and is characterized pathologically by cerebral edema and fatty changes in the liver
2. The exact cause is not clear
3. It is recommended that aspirin not be administered to children with varicella or influenza because of its association with Reye's syndrome

4. Acetaminophen (Tylenol) is considered the medication of choice for pediatric clients
5. The goal of treatment is to maintain effective cerebral perfusion and control increasing ICP

B. Assessment
1. History of systemic viral illness 4 to 7 days before the onset of symptoms
2. Malaise
3. Nausea and vomiting
4. Progressive neurological deterioration

C. Implementation
1. Assess neurological status
2. Monitor for altered level of consciousness and signs of increased ICP
3. Monitor I & O
4. Provide rest and decrease stimulation in the environment
5. Monitor for signs of bleeding and signs of impaired coagulation, such as a prolonged bleeding time

V. MENINGITIS

A. Description
1. An infectious process of the CNS caused by bacteria and viruses that may be acquired as a primary disease or as a result of complications of neurosurgery, trauma, infection of the sinus or ears, or systemic infections
2. Diagnosis is made by testing CSF obtained by lumbar puncture, which shows increased pressure, cloudy CSF, high protein, and low glucose
3. Meningococcal meningitis occurs in epidemic form and is the only type readily transmitted by droplet infection from nasopharyngeal secretions
4. Viral meningitis is associated with viruses such as mumps, paramyxovirus, herpes virus, and enterovirus

B. Assessment
1. Signs and symptoms vary, depending on the type, the age of the child, and the duration of the preceding illness; there is no one classic sign or symptom
2. Fever, chills
3. Vomiting, diarrhea
4. Poor feeding or anorexia
5. Nuchal rigidity
6. Poor or high-pitched cry
7. Altered level of consciousness, such as lethargy or irritability
8. Bulging anterior fontanel in the infant
9. Kernig's sign and Brudzinski's sign in children and adolescents
10. Muscle or joint pain
11. Petechial or purpuric rashes (meningococcal infection)

C. Implementation
1. Provide isolation and maintain for at least 24 hours after antibiotics are initiated
2. Administer antibiotics as prescribed
3. Perform neurological assessment
4. Assess for personality changes and irritability
5. Monitor I & O
6. Assess nutritional status
7. Determine close contacts of the child with meningitis, because the contacts will need prophylactic treatment

VI. SEIZURE DISORDERS

A. Description
1. Sudden, transient alterations in brain function resulting from excessive levels of electrical activity in the brain
2. Classified as either partial or generalized, or unclassified, depending on the area of the brain involved

B. Assessment
1. Obtain information from the parents about the time of onset, precipitating events, and behavior before and after the seizure
2. Determine the child's history related to seizures

C. Seizure precautions (Box 33-2)

D. Implementation (Box 33-3)

VII. CEREBRAL PALSY (CP)

A. Description
1. Disorder characterized by impaired movement and posture resulting from an abnormality in the extrapyramidal or pyramidal motor system
2. The most common clinical type is spastic CP, which represents an upper motor neuron type of muscle weakness

B. Assessment
1. Extreme irritability and crying
2. Feeding difficulties
3. Stiff and rigid arms or legs
4. Delayed gross development

BOX 33-2

Seizure Precautions

Raise the side rails when the child is sleeping or resting
Pad the side rails and other hard objects
Place a waterproof mattress or pad on the bed or crib
Instruct the child to wear or carry medical identification
Instruct the child in precautions to take during potentially hazardous activities
Instruct the child to swim with a companion
Instruct the child to use a protective helmet and padding during bicycle riding, skateboarding, inline skating
Alert caregivers to the need for any special precautions

5. Abnormal motor performance
6. Alterations of muscle tone
7. Abnormal posturing, such as opisthotonic (exaggerated arching of the back)
8. Persistence of primitive infantile reflexes

C. Implementation
1. The goal of management is early recognition and intervention to maximize the child's abilities
2. A multidisciplinary team approach is implemented to meet the many needs of the child
3. Therapeutic management includes physical therapy, occupational therapy, speech therapy, education, and recreation
4. Assess the child's developmental level and **intelligence**
5. Encourage early intervention and participation in school programs
6. Prepare for using mobilizing devices to help prevent or reduce deformities
7. Encourage communication and interaction with the child on a functional level, not **chronological age** level
8. Provide a safe environment such as by removing sharp objects, using a protective helmet if the child falls frequently, and implementing seizure precautions if necessary
9. Provide safe, appropriate toys for age and developmental level
10. Position upright after meals
11. Administer medications as prescribed to decrease spasticity

---

BOX 33-3

Emergency Treatment for Seizures

Ensure airway patency
Time the seizure episode
If the child is standing or sitting, ease the child down to the floor
Place a pillow or folded blanket under the child's head; if no bedding is available, place own hands under the child's head or place the child's head in own lap
Loosen restrictive clothing
Remove eyeglasses from the child if present
Clear area of any hazards or hard objects
Allow seizure to proceed and end without interference
If vomiting occurs, turn child to one side as a unit
Do not restrain the child, place anything in the child's mouth, or give any food or liquids to the child
Prepare to administer medications as prescribed
Remain with the child until the child fully recovers
Observe for incontinence, which may have occurred during the seizure
Document the occurrence

---

12. Surgical interventions are reserved for the child who does not respond to more conservative measures or for the child whose spasticity causes progressive deformity

VIII. MENTAL RETARDATION

A. Description
1. Subaverage general intellectual functioning along with a deficit in adaptation in behavior
2. Down syndrome is a congenital condition that results in moderate to severe retardation and has been linked to an extra group G chromosome, chromosome 21 (trisomy 21)

B. Assessment
1. Deficits in cognitive skills and level of adaptive functioning
2. Delays in fine- and gross-motor skills
3. Speech delays
4. Decreased spontaneous activity
5. Nonresponsiveness
6. Irritability
7. Poor eye contact during feeding

C. Implementation
1. Medical strategies are focused at correcting structural deformities and treating associated behaviors
2. Implement community and educational services, using a multidisciplinary approach
3. Promote care skills as much as possible
4. Assist with communication and socialization skills
5. Facilitate appropriate playtime
6. Initiate safety precautions as necessary
7. Assist the family with decisions regarding care
8. Provide information regarding support services and community agencies

IX. AUTISM

A. Description
1. A severe mental disorder beginning in infancy or toddlerhood
2. Apparent to the parents before the age of 3
3. Characterized by impairment in reciprocal social interaction and in verbal and nonverbal communication
4. The cause is unknown and the prognosis may be poor
5. Diagnosis is established on the basis of symptoms and through the use of specialized autism assessment tools
6. Also called infantile autism

B. Assessment
1. Disturbance in the rate and appearance of physical, social, and language skills
2. Abnormal responses of body sensations
3. Abnormal ways of relating to people, objects, and

events; the child is self-absorbed and unable to relate to others

4. There are no delusions, hallucinations, or incoherence, and the facies is intelligent and responsive

5. The child may play happily alone for hours, but have temper tantrums if interrupted

6. Language disturbance often includes repetition of previously heard speech and reversal of the pronouns "I" and "you"

7. If the child can talk, he or she uses speech not for communication but to repeat words or phrases meaninglessly

8. The child may develop an unusual attachment to a significant object and display frequent rocking, spinning, twirling, or other bizarre behaviors

C. Implementation

1. Determine the child's routines, habits, and preferences, and maintain consistency as much as possible

2. Determine the specific ways in which the child communicates

3. Facilitate communication through the use of picture boards

4. Evaluate the child for safety

5. Implement safety precautions as necessary for self-injurious behaviors such as head banging

6. Monitor for stress and anxiety

7. Avoid placing demands on the child

8. Initiate referrals to special programs as required

9. Provide support to parents

X. ATTENTION-DEFICIT HYPERACTIVITY DISORDER (ADHD)

A. Description

1. A developmental disorder characterized by developmentally inappropriate degrees of inattention, overactivity, and impulsivity

2. One of the most common reasons for referral of children to mental health services

3. Childhood problems include lowered intellectual development, some minor physical abnormalities, sleeping disturbances, behavioral or emotional disorders, and difficulty in social relationships

4. Diagnosis is established on the basis of self-reports, parent and teacher reports, and psychological assessments

B. Assessment

1. Fidgets with hands or feet or squirms in the seat

2. Easily distracted with external or internal stimuli

3. Difficulty with following through on instructions

4. Poor attention span

5. Shifts from one uncompleted activity to another

6. Talks excessively

7. Interrupts or intrudes on others

8. Engages in physically dangerous activities without considering the possible consequences

C. Implementation

1. Provide environmental and physical safety measures

2. Enhance capabilities and self-esteem

3. Encourage support groups for parents

4. Administer prescribed medication; the most commonly prescribed medications include methylphenidate hydrochloride (Ritalin), pemoline (Cylert), and dextroamphetamine sulfate (Dexadrine)

5. Instruct the child and parents regarding medication administration

6. Inform the child and parents that positive effects of the medication may be seen within 1 to 2 weeks if taken as prescribed

XI. TOURETTE'S DISORDER

A. Description: Appears between ages 2 and 15 and is characterized by recurrent involuntary and rapid movements affecting various parts of the body, accompanied by vocal noises such as barks, grunts, or profanities

B. Implementation

1. Establish a trusting one-to-one relationship

2. Protect the child from harm by providing a helmet or protective padding

3. Allow the child to have a favorite toy or other object

4. Provide positive reinforcement for appropriate behaviors

5. Maintain eye contact

6. Assess suicide potential

7. Remove dangerous objects from the environment

8. Set limits on socially inappropriate or manipulative behaviors

9. Encourage the child to confront tension and frustration before they emerge as inappropriate behaviors

10. Provide noncompetitive group situations

XII. CHILD ABUSE

A. Description: Involves emotional or physical **abuse** or neglect, as well as sexual exploitation or molestation by caretakers or other individuals

B. Assessment

1. Physical **abuse**
   a. Unexplained bruises, burns, or fractures
   b. Bald spots on the scalp
   c. Apprehensive child
   d. Extreme aggressiveness or withdrawal
   e. Fear of parents
   f. Lack of crying when approached by a stranger

2. Physical neglect
   a. Inadequate weight gain
   b. Poor hygiene
   c. Consistent hunger

d. Inconsistent school attendance
e. Constant fatigue
f. Reports of lack of child supervision
g. Delinquency
3. Emotional **abuse**
a. Speech disorders
b. Habit disorders such as sucking, biting, and rocking
c. Psychoneurotic reactions
d. **Learning** disorders
e. Suicide attempts
4. Sexual **abuse**
a. Difficulty walking or sitting
b. Torn, stained, or bloody underclothing
c. Pain, swelling, or itching of the genitals
d. Bruises, bleeding, or lacerations in the genital or anal area
e. Unwillingness to change clothes or unwillingness to participate in gym activities
f. Poor peer relations
g. Delinquency
h. Changes in sleep performance
i. Self-disruptive behavior
C. Implementation
1. Support the child during a thorough physical assessment
2. Assess injuries
3. Report case of suspected **abuse**
4. Place the child in an environment that is safe, thereby preventing further injury
5. Document in an objective manner information related to the suspected **abuse**
6. Assess parents' strengths and weaknesses, normal coping mechanisms, and presence or absence of support systems
7. Assist the family in identifying stressors, support systems, and resources
8. Refer the family to appropriate support groups

PRACTICE QUESTIONS

1. A nurse is performing an admission assessment on a 6-month-old infant with a diagnosis of hydrocephalus. The nurse assesses for the major sign associated with hydrocephalus when the nurse:
   1. Tests the urine for protein
   2. Takes the apical pulse
   3. Palpates the anterior fontanel
   4. Takes the blood pressure
2. A nurse has provided discharge instructions to the parents of an infant who had a ventriculoperitoneal (VP) shunt procedure performed for the treatment of hydrocephalus. Which statement if made by the parents indicates an accurate understanding of the presence of a shunt complication?
   1. "If the infant has a high-pitched cry, I should call the doctor."
   2. "I should position my infant on the side with the shunt when sleeping."
   3. "My infant will pass urine more often now that the shunt is in place."
   4. "I should call my doctor if my infant refuses baby food."
3. A nurse is performing an admission assessment on a newborn infant with a diagnosis of spina bifida (meningomyelocele). The nurse assesses for a major symptom associated with this type of spina bifida when the nurse:
   1. Checks the capillary refill of the nailbeds of the upper extremities
   2. Tests the urine for blood
   3. Palpates the abdomen for masses
   4. Checks for responses to painful stimuli from the torso downward
4. A mother arrives at an emergency room with her 5-year-old child. The mother states that the child fell off a bunk bed. A head injury is suspected, and a nurse is continuously assessing the child for signs of increased intracranial pressure (ICP). Which of the following would indicate a late sign of increased ICP in this child?
   1. Bulging fontanel
   2. Dilated scalp veins
   3. Nausea
   4. Widened pulse pressure
5. A nurse is caring for a newborn infant with spina bifida (meningomyelocele type) who is scheduled for surgical closure of the sac. In the preoperative period, the priority nursing action would be to monitor the:
   1. Blood pressure
   2. Moisture of the normal saline dressing covering the sac
   3. Specific gravity of the urine
   4. Anterior fontanel for depression
6. A child is diagnosed with Reye's syndrome. A nurse develops a nursing care plan for the child and includes which intervention in the plan?
   1. Providing a quiet atmosphere with dimmed lighting
   2. Assessing hearing loss
   3. Monitoring urine output
   4. Changing body position every 2 hours
7. A physician prescribes home health nurse visits for a child discharged home with Reye's syndrome. During a home visit, a nurse instructs the parents about the residual effects of Reye's syndrome. Which statement if made by the parents would indicate a need for further instruction?
   1. "We need to decrease the stimuli at home to prevent intracranial pressure."
   2. "We need to give frequent, small, nutritious meals to decrease the amount of vomiting."

3. "We need to have the child nap during the day to provide rest."

4. "We need to check for jaundiced skin and eyes every day."

8. A nurse develops a plan of care for a child at risk for generalized tonic-clonic seizures. In the plan of care, the nurse initiates seizure precautions and documents that which items need to be placed at the child's bedside?
   1. Suctioning equipment and an airway
   2. Oxygen with a tracheotomy set
   3. Emergency cart
   4. Airway and a tracheotomy set

9. A nurse is caring for a child recently diagnosed with cerebral palsy. The parents of the child ask the nurse about the disorder. The nurse bases her response on the understanding that cerebral palsy is:
   1. A chronic disability characterized by impaired muscle movement and posture
   2. An infectious disease of the central nervous system
   3. An inflammation of the brain as a result of a viral illness
   4. A congenital condition that results in moderate to severe retardation

10. A nurse is developing a plan of care for a child with cerebral palsy. The nurse includes interventions in the plan of care, understanding that a primary goal is to:
    1. Eliminate the cause of the disorder
    2. Prevent the occurrence of emotional disturbances
    3. Maximize the child's assets and minimize the limitations caused by the disorder
    4. Cure the disorder

11. A nurse is caring for a child diagnosed with Down syndrome. In describing the disorder to the parents, the nurse bases the explanation on the fact that Down syndrome is a condition characterized by:
    1. Above average intellectual functioning with deficits in adaptive behavior
    2. Average intellectual functioning and the absence of deficits in adaptive behavior
    3. Moderate to severe retardation, congenital nature, and linkage to an extra chromosome 21, group G
    4. Subaverage intellectual functioning with the absence of deficits in adaptive behavior

12. A nurse is assigned to care for an 8-year-old child with a diagnosis of a basilar skull fracture. The nurse reviews the physician's orders and contacts the physician to question which order?
    1. Clear liquid intake only
    2. Maintain a patent IV line
    3. Daily weight
    4. Suction PRN

13. A lumbar puncture is performed on a child suspected of having bacterial meningitis. Cerebrospinal fluid (CSF) is obtained for analysis. A nurse reviews the results of the CSF analysis and determines that which of the following results would verify the diagnosis?
    1. Cloudy CSF, decreased protein, and decreased glucose
    2. Cloudy CSF, elevated protein, and decreased glucose
    3. Clear CSF, elevated protein, and decreased glucose
    4. Clear CSF, decreased pressure, and elevated protein

14. A nurse is planning care for a child with acute bacterial meningitis. On the basis of the mode of transmission of this infection, which of the following would be included in the plan of care?
    1. No precautions are required as long as antibiotics have been started
    2. Maintain enteric precautions
    3. Maintain respiratory isolation precautions for at least 24 hours after the initiation of antibiotics
    4. Maintain neutropenic precautions

15. A clinic nurse is observing a child diagnosed with autistic disorder. The nurse would expect to observe which characteristic of this disorder?
    1. Normal responses to sensory stimuli
    2. Normal social play
    3. Lack of social interaction
    4. Normal verbal but abnormal nonverbal communication

16. An emergency room nurse is performing an assessment on a child suspected of being sexually abused. Which assessment data obtained by the nurse would most likely support this suspicion?
    1. Poor hygiene
    2. Bald spots on the scalp
    3. Fear of the parents
    4. Difficulty walking

17. A nurse performs an admission assessment on a child and suspects physical abuse. On the basis of this suspicion, the primary legal nursing responsibility is which of the following?
    1. Document the child's physical assessment findings accurately and thoroughly
    2. Report the case in which the abuse is suspected to the local authorities
    3. Refer the family to the appropriate support groups
    4. Assist the family in identifying resources and support systems

18. A maternity nurse employed in a newborn nursery receives a telephone call from the delivery room and is told that a newborn with spina bifida (meningomyelocele type) will be transported to the

nursery. The maternity nurse prepares for the arrival of the newborn and places which of the following priority items at the newborn's bedside?
1. A blood pressure cuff
2. A rectal thermometer
3. A specific gravity urinometer
4. A bottle of sterile normal saline

19. A nurse is performing an assessment of a 7-year-old child who is suspected of having episodes of absence seizures. Which of the following assessment questions to the mother will assist in providing information that will identify the symptoms associated with this type of seizure?
1. "Does the child have a blank expression during these episodes?"
2. "Does the muscle twitching occur on one side of the body?"
3. "Does twitching occur in the face and neck?"
4. "Does the muscle twitching occur on both sides of the body?"

20. A nurse is reviewing the record of a child with increased intracranial pressure and notes that the child has exhibited signs of decerebrate posturing. On assessment of the child, the nurse would expect to note which of the following if this type of posturing was present?
1. Abnormal flexion of the upper extremities and extension of the lower extremities
2. Rigid extension and pronation of the arms and legs
3. Rigid pronation of all extremities
4. Flaccid paralysis of all extremities

CRITICAL THINKING: FREE-TEXT ENTRY

A nurse is caring for a child who sustained a head injury after falling from a tree. On assessment of the child, the nurse notes the presence of a watery discharge from the child's nose. What is the nurse's initial action?

Answer: _____

ANSWERS

1. **3**
Rationale: In infants with hydrocephalus, the head grows at an abnormal rate, and the first sign of the disorder may be bulging fontanels without head enlargement. A bulging, tense, and nonpulsatile anterior fontanel indicates an increase in cerebrospinal fluid collection in the cerebral ventricle. A method of assessing fluid collection in the cranial cavity is to palpate the anterior fontanel. Proteinuria, apical pulse, and blood pressure changes are not specific to hydrocephalus.
Test-Taking Strategy: Use the process of elimination and the principles associated with excessive fluid buildup in the cranial cavity when answering the question. In addition, correlate "hydrocephalus" in the question with "anterior fontanel" in option 3. If you had difficulty with this question, review the signs associated with hydrocephalus.
Level of Cognitive Ability: Analysis
Client Needs: Physiological Integrity
Integrated Concept/Process: Nursing Process/Assessment
Content Area: Child Health
Reference: Wong, D. (1999). *Whaley & Wong's nursing care of infants and children* (6th ed.). St. Louis: Mosby, p. 497.

2. **1**
Rationale: If the shunt is broken or malfunctioning, the fluid from the ventricle part of the brain will not be diverted to the peritoneal cavity. The cerebrospinal fluid will build up in the cranial area. The result is intracranial pressure, which then causes a high-pitched cry in the infant. The infant should not have pressure placed on the shunt side. Skin breakdown and possible compressions to the apparatus could result. This type of shunt affects the gastrointestinal system, not the genitourinary system. Option 4 is only a concern if the infant becomes malnourished or dehydrated, which could then raise the body temperature. Otherwise, refusing baby food has no direct relationship to the shunt functioning.
Test-Taking Strategy: Use the process of elimination, noting the key words "presence of a shunt complication." Recalling that shunt malfunction is a complication, and that if it occurs, the infant will exhibit signs of increased intracranial pressure, will direct you to the correct option. Remember that a high-pitched cry in an infant indicates a concern or problem. If you had difficulty with this question, review the assessment findings that indicate a complication with a shunt.
Level of Cognitive Ability: Analysis
Client Needs: Health Promotion and Maintenance
Integrated Concept/Process: Teaching/Learning
Content Area: Child Health
Reference: Ball, J., & Bindler, R. (1999). *Pediatric nursing: Caring for children* (2nd ed.). Stamford, Conn.: Appleton & Lange, pp. 758; 783.

3. **4**
Rationale: Newborn infants with spina bifida (meningomyelocele type) demonstrate lack of innervation from below the site of the sac that contains the meninges and spinal cord and excess cerebrospinal fluid. They therefore show diminished or no responses to painful stimuli in these areas below the sac. Options 1, 2, and 3 are incorrect because the area above the sac is not affected. The capillary refill is normal. The urine will not have blood present. If the kidneys are affected, proteinuria could be present but is not generally noted in the newborn period. No abdominal masses are present besides the sac on the back area, externally protruding from the vertebral deformity.

Test-Taking Strategy: Use the process of elimination, recalling that diminished or absent innervation occurs in the area below the sac. If you had difficulty with this question, review the symptoms associated with meningomyelocele.
Level of Cognitive Ability: Analysis
Client Needs: Physiological Integrity
Integrated Concept/Process: Nursing Process/Assessment
Content Area: Child Health
Reference: Wong, D. (1999). *Whaley & Wong's nursing care of infants and children* (6th ed.). St. Louis: Mosby, p. 486.
4. **4**
Rationale: Late signs of increased ICP include a significant decrease in level of consciousness, Cushing's triad (increased systolic blood pressure and widened pulse pressure, bradycardia, and irregular respirations), and fixed and dilated pupils. A bulging fontanel and dilated scalp veins are early signs of increased ICP and would be noted in an infant, not a 5-year-old child. Nausea is an early sign of increased ICP.
Test-Taking Strategy: Use the process of elimination. Note the age of the child and the key word "late." Options 1 and 2 can be eliminated first because these signs would be noted in an infant, not a 5-year-old child. Focusing on the key word "late" will direct you to option 4. If you had difficulty with this question, review the early and late signs of increased ICP in an infant and in a child.
Level of Cognitive Ability: Analysis
Client Needs: Physiological Integrity
Integrated Concept/Process: Nursing Process/Assessment
Content Area: Child Health
Reference: Ball, J., & Bindler, R. (1999). *Pediatric nursing: Caring for children* (2nd ed.). Stamford, Conn.: Appleton & Lange, p. 758.
5. **2**
Rationale: The infant is usually placed in an incubator or a radiant warmer so that temperature can be maintained without clothing or covers that might irritate the delicate lesion. A sterile normal saline dressing is placed over the sac to maintain moisture of the sac and its contents and to prevent tearing or breakdown of the skin integrity at the site. Any opening in the sac greatly increases the risk of infection of the central nervous system. When an overhead warmer is used, the dressings over the defect require more frequent moistening because of the drying effect of the radiant heat. Blood pressure is difficult to assess during the newborn period and is not the best indicator of infection. Urine concentration is not well developed in the newborn stage of development. Depression of the anterior fontanel is a sign of dehydration. In spina bifida, monitoring for an increase in intracranial pressure is the priority, and it would be identified by the presence of a bulging anterior fontanel, among other signs.
Test-Taking Strategy: Note the key words "preoperative period" and "priority nursing action." Use the process of elimination, recalling the importance of the care of the sac in the preoperative period. Eliminate options 1 and 3 first. Although blood pressure and specific gravity are common preoperative assessments, they are not reliable indicators of the status of a newborn. Knowledge that an increase in intracranial pressure is a concern will assist in eliminating option 4. Review preoperative care for the infant with a meningomyelocele if you had difficulty with this question.

Level of Cognitive Ability: Application
Client Needs: Physiological Integrity
Integrated Concept/Process: Nursing Process/Implementation
Content Area: Child Health
Reference: Wong, D. (1999). *Whaley & Wong's nursing care of infants and children* (6th ed.). St. Louis: Mosby, p. 490.
6. **1**
Rationale: In Reye's syndrome, supportive care is directed toward monitoring and managing cerebral edema. Decreasing stimuli in the environment by providing a quiet environment with dimmed lighting would decrease the stress on the cerebral tissue and neuron responses. Hearing loss and urine output are not affected. Changing the body position every 2 hours would not affect the cerebral edema directly. The child should be in a head-elevated position to decrease the progression of the cerebral edema and promote drainage of cerebrospinal fluid.
Test-Taking Strategy: Use the process of elimination. Knowledge that cerebral edema is a concern for the child with Reye's syndrome will easily direct you to option 1. If you had difficulty with this question, review the appropriate plan of nursing care for the child with Reye's syndrome.
Level of Cognitive Ability: Application
Client Needs: Physiological Integrity
Integrated Concept/Process: Nursing Process/Planning
Content Area: Child Health
Reference: Bowden, V., Dickey, S, & Greenberg, C. (1998). *Children and their families: The continuum of care.* Philadelphia: W.B. Saunders, p. 1403.
7. **2**
Rationale: The vomiting that occurs in Reye's syndrome is caused by cerebral edema and is a symptom of increased intracranial pressure. Small frequent meals will not affect the amount of vomiting, and if vomiting occurs, the parents should contact the health care provider. Options 1, 3, and 4 are all correct. Decreasing stimuli and providing rest decrease stress on the brain tissue. Checking for jaundice will assist in identifying the presence of liver dysfunction that occurs in Reye's syndrome.
Test-Taking Strategy: Use the process of elimination, noting the key words "indicate a need for further instruction." Options 1 and 3 can be eliminated first because they are similar. Next eliminate option 4, knowing that liver dysfunction is a concern in the child with Reye's syndrome. Review home care instructions for the child with Reye's syndrome if you had difficulty with this question.
Level of Cognitive Ability: Analysis
Client Needs: Health Promotion and Maintenance
Integrated Concept/Process: Teaching/Learning
Content Area: Child Health
Reference: Wong, D. (1999). *Whaley & Wong's nursing care of infants and children* (6th ed.). St. Louis: Mosby, p. 1806.
8. **1**
Rationale: Generalized tonic-clonic seizures cause rigidity of all body muscles, followed by intense jerking movements. Since airway obstruction and increased oral secretions can occur during and after the seizure, an airway and suctioning equipment are placed at the bedside. A tracheotomy is not performed during a seizure. An emergency cart would not be left at the bedside but would be available in the treatment room or nearby on the nursing unit.

Test-Taking Strategy: Use the process of elimination. Note the key words "need to be placed at the child's bedside." Remember that when an option contains two parts, both parts of the option must be correct in order for the option to be the correct one. Eliminate options 2 and 4 first, knowing that a tracheotomy is not performed. From the remaining options, focusing on the primary concern during seizure activity will direct you to option 1. If you had difficulty with this question, review the plan of care associated with seizure precautions.

Level of Cognitive Ability: Application
Client Needs: Safe, Effective Care Environment
Integrated Concept/Process: Communication and Documentation
Content Area: Child Health
Reference: Bowden, V., Dickey, S., & Greenberg, C. (1998). *Children and their families: The continuum of care.* Philadelphia: W.B. Saunders, p. 1352.

9. **1**
Rationale: Cerebral palsy is a chronic disability characterized by impaired movement and posture resulting from an abnormality in the extrapyramidal or pyramidal motor system. Meningitis is an infectious process of the central nervous system. Encephalitis is an inflammation of the brain that occurs as a result of viral illness or central nervous system infection. Down syndrome is an example of a congenital condition that results in moderate to severe retardation.
Test-Taking Strategy: Use the process of elimination. Eliminate options 2 and 3 first, noting that they are similar. Next, note the relationship between "palsy" in the question and "impaired muscle movement" in option 1. If you had difficulty with this question, review the characteristics associated with cerebral palsy.

Level of Cognitive Ability: Comprehension
Client Needs: Physiological Integrity
Integrated Concept/Process: Teaching/Learning
Content Area: Child Health
Reference: Wong, D. (1999). *Whaley & Wong's nursing care of infants and children* (6th ed.). St. Louis: Mosby, p. 1966.

10. **3**
Rationale: The goals of managing the child with cerebral palsy are early recognition and intervention to maximize the child's abilities. The cause of the disorder cannot be eliminated. It is best to minimize the occurrence of emotional disturbances if possible, but not to prevent them, because it is healthy for the child to express emotions. The disorder is not curable.
Test-Taking Strategy: Use the process of elimination. Eliminate options 1 and 4 first because they are similar. Next, eliminate option 2 because emotional disturbances cannot be prevented. Also, option 3 is the most global option. Review the therapeutic management of the child with cerebral palsy if you had difficulty with this question.

Level of Cognitive Ability: Application
Client Needs: Health Promotion and Maintenance
Integrated Concept/Process: Nursing Process/Planning
Content Area: Child Health
Reference: Wong, D. (1999). *Whaley & Wong's nursing care of infants and children* (6th ed.). St. Louis: Mosby, p. 1970.

11. **3**
Rationale: Down syndrome is a form of mental retardation. It is a congenital condition that results in moderate to severe mental retardation. A high percentage of cases are attributable to an extra chromosome (group G); hence the name trisomy 21. Options 1, 2, and 4 are incorrect characteristics of this syndrome.
Test-Taking Strategy: Use the process of elimination. Eliminate options 1 and 2 first because average or above average intelligence is not associated with this disorder. Eliminate option 4 because deficits in adaptive behavior do occur with Down syndrome. Knowing that Down syndrome is associated with an extra chromosome will assist in directing you to the correct option. If you had difficulty with this question, review the characteristics associated with Down syndrome.

Level of Cognitive Ability: Comprehension
Client Needs: Physiological Integrity
Integrated Concept/Process: Teaching/Learning
Content Area: Child Health
Reference: Wong, D. (1999). *Whaley & Wong's nursing care of infants and children* (6th ed.). St. Louis: Mosby, p. 1086.

12. **4**
Rationale: Nasotracheal suctioning is contraindicated in a child with a basilar skull fracture. Because of the nature of the injury, there is a high risk of secondary infection and the probability of the catheter entering the brain through the fracture. The child is either maintained on an NPO status or restricted to clear liquids until it is determined that vomiting will not occur. An IV line is maintained to administer fluids or medications if necessary. Fluid balance is closely monitored by daily weight, intake and output measurement, and serum osmolality to detect early signs of water retention, excessive dehydration, and states of hypertonicity or hypotonicity.
Test-Taking Strategy: Use the process of elimination. Eliminate options 1, 2, and 3 because they are similar in that they all address the issue of fluids. Remember that nasotracheal suctioning is contraindicated in a child with a skull fracture. If you had difficulty with this question, review the care of a child with this type of a skull fracture.

Level of Cognitive Ability: Analysis
Client Needs: Safe, Effective Care Environment
Integrated Concept/Process: Communication and Documentation
Content Area: Child Health
Reference: Wong, D. (1999). *Whaley & Wong's nursing care of infants and children* (6th ed.). St. Louis: Mosby, pp. 1793-1795.

13. **2**
Rationale: A diagnosis of meningitis is made by testing CSF obtained by lumbar puncture. In the case of bacterial meningitis, findings usually include an elevated pressure, turbid or cloudy CSF, elevated leukocytes, elevated protein, and decreased glucose levels.
Test-Taking Strategy: Use the process of elimination and knowledge regarding the diagnostic findings in meningitis. Eliminate options 3 and 4 first because clear CSF is not likely to be found if an infectious process such as meningitis. From this point, knowledge that an elevated protein level indicates a possible diagnosis of meningitis is helpful to answer the question. If you had difficulty with this question, review this diagnostic test.

Level of Cognitive Ability: Analysis
Client Needs: Physiological Integrity
Integrated Concept/Process: Nursing Process/Analysis

Content Area: Child Health
Reference: Bowden, V., Dickey, S., & Greenberg, C. (1998). *Children and their families: The continuum of care.* Philadelphia: W.B. Saunders, p. 1390.

14. 3

Rationale: A major priority of nursing care for a child suspected of having meningitis is to administer the prescribed antibiotic as soon as it is ordered. The child is also placed on respiratory isolation for at least 24 hours while culture results are obtained and the antibiotic is having an effect. Enteric precautions and neutropenic precautions are not associated with the mode of transmission of meningitis. Enteric precautions are instituted when the mode of transmission is through the gastrointestinal tract. Neutropenic precautions are instituted when a child has a low neutrophil count.

Test-Taking Strategy: Use the process of elimination and knowledge regarding the mode of transmission of meningitis. Eliminate options 2 and 4 first because both enteric and neutropenic precautions are unrelated to the mode of transmission. Knowledge that it takes approximately 24 hours for antibiotics to reach a therapeutic blood level will assist in directing you to option 3. If you had difficulty with this question, review the mode of transmission of meningitis.

Level of Cognitive Ability: Application
Client Needs: Safe, Effective Care Environment
Integrated Concept/Process: Nursing Process/Planning
Content Area: Child Health
Reference: Wong, D. (1999). *Whaley & Wong's nursing care of infants and children* (6th ed.). St. Louis: Mosby, p 1802.

15. 3

Rationale: Autistic disorder is a complex childhood disorder that involves abnormalities in behavior, social interactions, and communication. Autistic children are unable to relate to people or to respond to social and emotional cues. Characteristically, these children engage in repetitive behaviors, including head banging, twirling in circles, biting themselves, and flapping their hands or arms. Abnormal communication patterns include both verbal and nonverbal communication.

Test-Taking Strategy: Use the process of elimination. Note that options 1, 2, and 4 are similar in that they all address a normal response. If you had difficulty with this question, review the characteristics associated with autistic disorder.

Level of Cognitive Ability: Comprehension
Client Needs: Psychosocial Integrity
Integrated Concept/Process: Nursing Process/Assessment
Content Area: Child Health
Reference: Ball, J., & Bindler, R. (1999). *Pediatric nursing: Caring for children* (2nd ed.). Stamford, Conn.: Appleton & Lange, p. 958.

16. 4

Rationale: The most likely assessment findings in sexual abuse include difficulty walking or sitting; torn, stained, or bloody underclothing; pain, swelling, or itching of the genitals; and bruises, bleeding, or lacerations in the genital or anal area. Poor hygiene may be indicative of physical neglect. Bald spots on the scalp and fear of the parents are most likely associated with physical abuse.

Test-Taking Strategy: Use the process of elimination, noting the key words "sexually abused." The only option that specifically addresses an assessment finding related to sexual abuse is option 4. If you had difficulty with this question, review the assessment findings in a child suspected of being abused.

Level of Cognitive Ability: Analysis
Client Needs: Physiological Integrity
Integrated Concept/Process: Nursing Process/Assessment
Content Area: Child Health
Reference: Ball, J., & Bindler, R. (1999). *Pediatric nursing: Caring for children* (2nd ed.). Stamford, Conn.: Appleton & Lange, p. 996.

17. 2

Rationale: The primary legal nursing responsibility when child abuse is suspected is to report the case. All states and provinces in North America have laws for mandatory reporting of child maltreatment. Suspected child abuse is reported to the local authorities. Although documentation of assessment findings, assisting the family, and referring the family to appropriate resources and support groups are important, the primary legal responsibility is to report the suspected case.

Test-Taking Strategy: Use the process of elimination, noting the key words "primary" and "legal." In addition to the many implications associated with child abuse, abuse is a crime. With this in mind, option 2, reporting the case of abuse, is the primary responsibility. If you had difficulty with this question, review the responsibilities of the nurse when child abuse is suspected.

Level of Cognitive Ability: Application
Client Needs: Safe, Effective Care Environment
Integrated Concept/Process: Communication and Documentation
Content Area: Child Health
Reference: Wong, D. (1999). *Whaley & Wong's nursing care of infants and children* (6th ed.). St. Louis: Mosby, p. 765.

18. 4

Rationale: The newborn with spina bifida is at risk for infection before the closure of the sac. A sterile normal saline dressing is placed over the sac to maintain moisture of the sac and its contents. This prevents tearing or breakdown of the skin integrity at the site. Blood pressure may be difficult to assess during the newborn period and is not the best indicator of infection. Urine concentration is not well developed in the newborn stage of development. A thermometer will be needed to assess temperature, but in this newborn the priority is to maintain sterile normal saline dressings over the sac.

Test-Taking Strategy: Knowledge of the characteristics of spina bifida, the care involved, and the potential complications is needed to correctly answer this question. Eliminate options 1 and 3 first as unlikely needed items. Recalling that this newborn will have a sac and is at risk for infection will easily direct you to the correct option. Review care to the newborn with spina bifida if you had difficulty with this question.

Level of Cognitive Ability: Application
Client Needs: Physiological Integrity
Integrated Concept/Process: Nursing Process/Planning
Content Area: Child Health
Reference: Wong, D. (1999). *Whaley & Wong's nursing care of infants and children* (6th ed.). St. Louis: Mosby, p. 490.

19. 1

Rationale: Formerly called petit mal seizures, absence seizures are very brief episodes of altered awareness. There is no muscle activity except eyelid fluttering or twitching. The child has a blank facial expression. These seizures last only 5 to 10 seconds, but they may occur one after another several times a day. Myoclonic seizures are brief random contractions of a muscle group that can occur on one or both sides of the body. Simple partial seizures consist of twitching of an extremity, face, or neck, or the sensation of twitching or numbness in an extremity or face or neck.

Test-Taking Strategy: Knowledge of the characteristics of the various types of seizures is required to answer this question. Focusing on the type of seizure identified in the question, "absence" seizures, may assist in directing you to option 1. Review the characteristics of the various types of seizures if you had difficulty with this question.

Level of Cognitive Ability: Analysis
Client Needs: Health Promotion and Maintenance
Integrated Concept/Process: Nursing Process/Assessment
Content Area: Child Health
Reference: Wong, D. (1999). *Whaley & Wong's nursing care of infants and children* (6th ed.). St. Louis: Mosby, p. 1811.

20. **2**
Rationale: Decerebrate posturing is characterized by the rigid extension and pronation of the arms and legs. Option 1 describes decorticate posturing. Options 3 and 4 are incorrect.

Test-Taking Strategy: Knowledge of the clinical manifestations associated with decerebrate posturing is required to answer this question. Review the characteristics of posturing if you had difficulty with this question.

Level of Cognitive Ability: Analysis

Client Needs: Physiological Integrity
Integrated Concept/Process: Nursing Process/Assessment
Content Area: Child Health
Reference: Wong, D. (1999). *Whaley & Wong's nursing care of infants and children* (6th ed.). St. Louis: Mosby, p. 1817.

CRITICAL THINKING: FREE-TEXT ENTRY

Answer: Test the watery discharge for the presence of glucose
Rationale: Following a head injury, bleeding from the nose or ears needs further evaluation. A watery discharge from the nose (rhinorrhea) that is positive for glucose suggests leaking of cerebrospinal fluid (CSF) from a skull fracture. If the nurse noted watery discharge from the child's nose, the nurse would initially test the drainage for glucose using reagent strips such as Dextrostix. If the results of the test are positive, the nurse would then contact the physician.

Test-Taking Strategy: Focus on the key words "nurse's initial action." Recall that a concern following a head injury is the leakage of CSF. Also, recalling that CSF is clear and contains glucose will assist in answering the question. Review care to the child after a head injury if you had difficulty with this question.

Level of Cognitive Ability: Application
Client Needs: Physiological Integrity
Integrated Concept/Process: Nursing Process/Implementation
Content Area: Child Health
Reference: Wong, D. (1999). *Whaley & Wong's nursing care of infants and children* (6th ed.). St. Louis: Mosby, p. 1792.

REFERENCES

Ball, J., & Bindler, R. (1999). *Pediatric nursing: Caring for children* (2nd ed.). Stamford, Conn.: Appleton & Lange.

Bowden, V., Dickey, S, & Greenberg, C. (1998). *Children and their families: The continuum of care.* Philadelphia: W.B. Saunders.

Wong, D. (1999). *Whaley & Wong's nursing care of infants and children* (6th ed.). St. Louis: Mosby.

Eye, Ear, and Throat Disorders

I. STRABISMUS

A. Description
   1. Called "squint" or "lazy eye"
   2. A condition in which the eyes are not aligned because of lack of coordination of the extraocular muscles
   3. Most often results from muscle imbalance or paralysis of extraocular muscles, but may also result from conditions such as a brain tumor, myasthenia gravis, or infection
   4. Normal in the young infant but should not be present after about age 4 months

B. Assessment
   1. Amblyopia if not treated early
   2. Permanent loss of vision if not treated early
   3. Loss of binocular vision
   4. Impairment of depth perception
   5. Frequent headaches
   6. Squints or tilts head to see

C. Implementation
   1. Corrective lenses as indicated
   2. Instruct the parents regarding patching (occlusion therapy) of the "good" eye to strengthen the weak eye
   3. Prepare for botulinum toxin (Botox) injection into the eye muscle, which produces temporary paralysis and allows muscles opposite the paralyzed muscle to straighten the eye
   4. Inform the parents that the injection of botulinum toxin wears off in about 2 months, and if successful, correction will occur
   5. Prepare for surgery to realign the weak muscles as prescribed if nonsurgical interventions are unsuccessful
   6. Instruct the parents in the need for follow-up visits

II. CONJUNCTIVITIS

A. Description
   1. Also known as "pinkeye"
   2. Inflammation of the conjunctiva
   3. Usually caused by allergy, infection, or trauma
   4. Bacterial or viral conjunctivitis is extremely contagious
   5. Chlamydial conjunctivitis is rare in older children and if diagnosed in a child who is not sexually active, the child should be assessed for possible sexual **abuse**

B. Assessment
   1. Itching, burning, or scratchy eyelids
   2. Redness
   3. Edema
   4. Discharge

C. Implementation
   1. Instruct in infection control measures such as good handwashing and not sharing towels and washcloths
   2. Administer antibiotic or antiviral eye drops or ointment as prescribed if infection is present
   3. Administer antihistamines as prescribed if an allergy is present
   4. Instruct the child and parents in the administration of the prescribed medications
   5. Instruct the parents that the child should be kept home from school or day care until antibiotic eye drops have been administered for 24 hours
   6. Instruct in the use of cool compresses to lessen irritation, and in wearing dark glasses for photophobia
   7. Instruct the child to avoid rubbing the eye to prevent injury
   8. Instruct the child who is wearing contact lenses to discontinue wearing them and to obtain new lenses to eliminate the chance of reinfection

9. Instruct the adolescent that eye makeup should be discarded and replaced

III. OTITIS MEDIA
A. Description
   1. Infection of the middle ear occurring as a result of a blocked eustachian tube, which prevents normal drainage
   2. Otitis media is a common complication of an acute respiratory infection
   3. Infants and children are more prone to otitis media because their eustachian tubes are shorter, wider, and straighter
B. Assessment
   1. Fever
   2. Irritability and restlessness
   3. Loss of appetite
   4. Rolling of head from side to side
   5. Pulling on or rubbing the ear
   6. Earache or pain
   7. Signs of hearing loss
   8. Purulent ear drainage
   9. Red, opaque, bulging, or retracting tympanic membrane
C. Implementation
   1. Encourage fluids
   2. Teach the parents to feed infants in upright position
   3. Instruct the child to avoid chewing during the acute period because chewing increases pain
   4. Provide local heat and have the child lie with the affected ear down
   5. Instruct the parents in the appropriate procedure to clean drainage from the ear with sterile cotton swabs
   6. Instruct the parents in the administration of analgesics or antipyretics such as acetaminophen (Tylenol) to decrease fever and pain
   7. Instruct the parents in the administration of the prescribed antibiotics, emphasizing that the 10- to 14-day period is necessary to eradicate positive organisms
   8. Instruct the parents that screening for hearing loss may be necessary
   9. If ear drops are prescribed, instruct the parents that the auditory canal is straightened by pulling the pinna down and back in children younger than age 3, and by pulling the pinna up and back for a child older than 3 years
D. Myringotomy
   1. Description: insertion of tympanoplasty tubes into the middle ear to equalize pressure and keep the ear aerated
   2. Implementation postoperatively
      a. Instruct the parents and child to keep the ears dry

b. Earplugs should be worn during bathing, shampooing, and swimming
c. Diving and submerging under water are not allowed

IV. TONSILLECTOMY AND ADENOIDECTOMY
A. Description
   1. Tonsillitis refers to inflammation and infection of the tonsils
   2. Adenoiditis refers to inflammation and infection of the adenoids
B. Assessment
   1. Persistent or recurrent sore throat
   2. Enlarged bright red tonsils that may be covered with white exudate
   3. Difficulty in swallowing
   4. Mouth breathing and an unpleasant mouth odor
   5. Fever
   6. Cough
   7. Enlarged adenoids may cause nasal quality of speech, mouth breathing, hearing difficulty, snoring, or obstructive sleep apnea
C. Implementation preoperatively
   1. Assess for signs of active infection
   2. Assess bleeding and clotting studies because the throat is very vascular
   3. Prepare the child for a sore throat postoperatively, and inform the child that he or she will need to drink liquids
   4. Assess for any loose teeth to decrease the risk of aspiration during surgery
D. Implementation postoperatively
   1. Position prone or side-lying to facilitate drainage
   2. Have suction equipment available, but do not suction unless there is an airway obstruction
   3. Monitor for signs of hemorrhage; if hemorrhage occurs, turn the child to the side and notify the physician
   4. Discourage coughing or clearing the throat
   5. Provide clear, cool, noncitrus and noncarbonated fluids
   6. Avoid milk products initially because they will coat the throat
   7. Avoid red liquids, which will simulate the appearance of blood if the child vomits
   8. Do not give the child any straws, forks, or sharp objects that can be put in the mouth
   9. Administer acetaminophen (Tylenol) for sore throat as prescribed
   10. Instruct the parents to notify the physician if bleeding, persistent earache, or fever occurs
   11. Instruct the parents to keep the child away from crowds until healing has occurred

PRACTICE QUESTIONS

1. A day care nurse is observing a 2-year-old child. The nurse suspects that the child may have strabismus. Which of the following observations made by the nurse might be indicative of this condition?
   1. The child consistently tilts the head to see
   2. The child consistently turns the head to see
   3. The child does not respond when spoken to
   4. The child has difficulty hearing

2. A physician has told the mother of a newborn infant diagnosed with strabismus that surgery will be necessary to realign the weakened eye muscles. The mother asks the nurse when the surgery might be performed. The most appropriate response is to tell the mother that surgery will be performed:
   1. Immediately
   2. Shortly before the child starts school
   3. Before the child is 2 years old
   4. Before the child begins to read

3. The mother of a 6-year-old child arrives at a clinic because the child has been experiencing scratchy, red, and swollen eyes. The nurse notes a discharge from the eyes, and a culture is sent to the laboratory for analysis. Chlamydial conjunctivitis is diagnosed. On the basis of this diagnosis, the nurse determines that which of the following would require further investigation?
   1. The presence of an allergy
   2. Possible trauma
   3. Possible sexual abuse
   4. The presence of a respiratory infection

4. A nurse prepares a teaching plan for a mother of a child diagnosed with bacterial conjunctivitis. Which of the following, if stated by the mother, would indicate a need for further education?
   1. "I need to wash my hands frequently."
   2. "I need to clean the eye as prescribed."
   3. "I need to give the eye drops as prescribed."
   4. "It is OK to share towels and washcloths."

5. The mother of a child who had a myringotomy with insertion of tympanostomy tubes calls the nurse and tells the nurse that the tubes have fallen out. Which of the following is the most appropriate response to the mother?
   1. "Replace the tubes immediately so that the created opening does not close."
   2. "This is an emergency and requires immediate intervention. Bring the child to the emergency room."
   3. "This is not an emergency. I will speak to the physician and call you right back."
   4. "Place the tubes in hydrogen peroxide for 1 hour before replacing them in the child's ears."

6. Antibiotics are prescribed for a child after a myringotomy with insertion of tympanostomy tubes. The nurse provides discharge instructions to the parents regarding the administration of the antibiotics. Which of the following statements, if made by the parents, indicates that they understood the instructions?
   1. "Administer the antibiotics if the child has a fever."
   2. "Administer the antibiotics until the child feels better."
   3. "Administer the antibiotics until they are gone."
   4. "Begin to taper the antibiotics after 3 days of a full course."

7. The mother of a child who underwent a myringotomy with insertion of tympanostomy tubes calls a nurse and reports that the child is complaining of discomfort. Which of the following is the most appropriate response?
   1. "Give the child children's aspirin for the discomfort."
   2. "Give the child acetaminophen (Tylenol) for the discomfort."
   3. "You need to speak to the physician because the child should not be having any discomfort."
   4. "I will speak to the physician so that a narcotic can be prescribed."

8. A nurse provides discharge instructions to the mother of a child after a myringotomy with insertion of tympanostomy tubes. Which of the following is not included in the instructions?
   1. Be sure the child uses soft tissues to blow his nose
   2. Place earplugs with petroleum jelly in the ears during baths and showers
   3. Swimming in deep water is prohibited
   4. Swimming in lake water needs to be avoided

9. A nurse is reviewing the laboratory results for a child scheduled for tonsillectomy. The nurse determines that which of the following laboratory values is most significant to review?
   1. Prothrombin time (PT)
   2. Sedimentation rate
   3. Blood urea nitrogen (BUN)
   4. Creatinine

10. A child is scheduled for a tonsillectomy. A nurse plans care, knowing that which of the following would present the highest risk of aspiration during surgery?
    1. Difficulty in swallowing
    2. The presence of loose teeth
    3. Bleeding during surgery
    4. Exudate in the throat area

11. A nurse is preparing to care for a child after a tonsillectomy. The nurse documents on the plan of care to place the child in which most appropriate position?
    1. Supine
    2. Trendelenburg
    3. Side-lying
    4. High Fowler's

12. After a tonsillectomy, a nurse reviews the physician's postoperative orders. Which of the following physician's orders does the nurse question?
    1. Clear, cool liquids when awake
    2. No milk or milk products
    3. Monitor for bleeding
    4. Suction every 2 hours
13. A nurse is caring for a child after a tonsillectomy. The nurse monitors the child, knowing that which of the following may indicate that the child is bleeding?
    1. A decreased pulse rate
    2. An elevation in blood pressure (BP)
    3. Complaints of discomfort
    4. Frequent swallowing
14. After tonsillectomy, a child begins to vomit bright red blood. The most appropriate initial nursing action would be to:
    1. Administer the prescribed antiemetic
    2. Turn the child to the side
    3. Notify the physician
    4. Maintain a nothing-by-mouth (NPO) status

15. A child is scheduled for a tonsillectomy in a day stay surgical unit. On the day following surgery, the mother calls the surgical unit and expresses concern because the child has a very bad mouth odor. Which of the following responses is most appropriate?
    1. "The child probably has an infection."
    2. "You need to contact the physician immediately."
    3. "Bad mouth odor is normal and may be relieved by drinking more liquids."
    4. "Have the child gargle with mouthwash every 4 hours."

CRITICAL THINKING: FREE-TEXT ENTRY

A nurse is providing instructions to the mother of a 2-year-old-child regarding the correct procedure for administering ear drops. In order to straighten the auditory canal, the nurse tells the mother to pull on the pinna of the ear in which manner?

Answer: _____

ANSWERS

1. **1**
Rationale: The nurse may suspect strabismus in a child when the child complains of frequent headaches, squints, or tilts the head to see. Options 2, 3, and 4 are not indicative of this condition.
Test-Taking Strategy: Use the process of elimination. Eliminate options 3 and 4 first because they are similar. From the remaining options, recalling that the child may tilt the head to see will direct you to option 1. Review the signs of strabismus if you had difficulty with this question.
Level of Cognitive Ability: Analysis
Client Needs: Physiological Integrity
Integrated Concept/Process: Nursing Process/Assessment
Content Area: Child Health
Reference: Wong, D. (1999). *Whaley & Wong's nursing care of infants and children* (6th ed.). St. Louis: Mosby, p. 1100.
2. **3**
Rationale: In a child diagnosed with strabismus, surgery may be indicated to realign the weakened muscles. It is most often indicated when amblyopia (decreased vision in the deviated eye) is present. The surgery should be performed before the child is 2 years old. Options 1, 2, and 4 are incorrect.
Test-Taking Strategy: Use the process of elimination. Option 1 can be easily eliminated. Options 2 and 4 can be eliminated next because they address a similar time frame. If you had difficulty with this question, review the treatment for strabismus.
Level of Cognitive Ability: Application
Client Needs: Physiological Integrity

Integrated Concept/Process: Communication and Documentation
Content Area: Child Health
Reference: Ball, J., & Bindler, R. (1999). *Pediatric nursing: Caring for children* (2nd ed.). Stamford, Conn.: Appleton & Lange, p. 718.
3. **3**
Rationale: A diagnosis of chlamydial conjunctivitis in a child who is not sexually active should signal the health care provider to assess the child for possible sexual abuse. Allergy, infection, and trauma can cause conjunctivitis, but the causative organism is not likely to be chlamydia.
Test-Taking Strategy: Use the process of elimination. Note the age of the child and the organism that is identified in the question. This may assist in directing you to option 3. Options 1, 2, and 4 can be recognized as the common causes of conjunctivitis. These options are similar in that they all relate to a physiological problem. Review content related to chlamydial conjunctivitis if you had difficulty with this question.
Level of Cognitive Ability: Analysis
Client Needs: Psychosocial Integrity
Integrated Concept/Process: Nursing Process/Assessment
Content Area: Child Health
Reference: Ball, J., & Bindler, R. (1999). *Pediatric nursing: Caring for children* (2nd ed.). Stamford, Conn.: Appleton & Lange, p. 705.
4. **4**
Rationale: Bacterial conjunctivitis is highly contagious, and infection control measures should be taught. These include

good handwashing and not sharing towels and washcloths. Options 2 and 3 are correct treatment measures.

Test-Taking Strategy: Use the process of elimination. Note the key words "need for further education." Options 1, 2, and 3 can be easily eliminated by recalling that bacterial conjunctivitis is highly contagious. If you had difficulty with this question, review infection control measures for bacterial conjunctivitis.

Level of Cognitive Ability: Analysis
Client Needs: Safe, Effective Care Environment
Integrated Concept/Process: Teaching/Learning
Content Area: Child Health
Reference: Ball, J., & Bindler, R. (1999). *Pediatric nursing: Caring for children* (2nd ed.). Stamford, Conn.: Appleton & Lange, p. 715.

5. **3**

Rationale: The size and appearance of the tympanostomy tubes should be described to the parents after surgery. They should be reassured that if the tubes fall out, it is not an emergency, but that the physician should be notified.

Test-Taking Strategy: Use the process of elimination. Option 2 should be eliminated first because this will cause concern in the parent. Next, eliminate options 1 and 4 because they are similar and relate to replacing the tubes. Review parent instructions following this procedure, if you had difficulty with this question.

Level of Cognitive Ability: Application
Client Needs: Physiological Integrity
Integrated Concept/Process: Nursing Process/Implementation
Content Area: Child Health
Reference: Wong, D. (1999). *Whaley & Wong's nursing care of infants and children* (6th ed.). St. Louis: Mosby, p. 1473.

6. **3**

Rationale: It is important that parents are instructed regarding the administration of antibiotics. Antibiotics need to be taken as prescribed, and the full course needs to be completed. Options 1, 2, and 4 and incorrect. Antibiotics are not tapered but administered until they are completed.

Test-Taking Strategy: Use the process of elimination and recall that antibiotics must be taken for the full course, regardless of whether the child is feeling better. Note the key words "understood the instructions." Review concepts related to the administration of antibiotics if you had difficulty with this question.

Level of Cognitive Ability: Analysis
Client Needs: Health Promotion and Maintenance
Integrated Concept/Process: Teaching/Learning
Content Area: Child Health
Reference: Wong, D. (1999). *Whaley & Wong's nursing care of infants and children* (6th ed.). St. Louis: Mosby, p. 1473.

7. **2**

Rationale: After myringotomy with insertion of tympanostomy tubes, the child may experience some discomfort. Tylenol can be given to relieve the discomfort. A narcotic is not necessary, and aspirin should not be administered to a child.

Test-Taking Strategy: Use the process of elimination. Options 1 and 4 can be easily eliminated. It seems reasonable that the child may have some discomfort following this surgical procedure; therefore eliminate option 3. If you had difficulty

with this question, review postoperative care following this procedure.

Level of Cognitive Ability: Application
Client Needs: Health Promotion and Maintenance
Integrated Concept/Process: Teaching/Learning
Content Area: Child Health
Reference: Ball, J., & Bindler, R. (1999). *Pediatric nursing: Caring for children* (2nd ed.). Stamford, Conn.: Appleton & Lange, p. 733.

8. **1**

Rationale: Parents need to be instructed that the child should not blow his or her nose for 7 to 10 days. Bath and lake water are potential sources of bacterial contamination. Diving and swimming in deep water are prohibited. The child's ears need to be kept dry. Options 2, 3, and 4 are appropriate instructions.

Test-Taking Strategy: Use the process of elimination. Note the key word "not" in the stem of the question. Options 2, 3, and 4 are similar; all relate to the concept of keeping the ears dry. Option 1 may cause disruption of the surgical site. Review parent discharge instructions following this procedure if you had difficulty with this question.

Level of Cognitive Ability: Application
Client Needs: Health Promotion and Maintenance
Integrated Concept/Process: Teaching/Learning
Content Area: Child Health
Reference: Ball, J., & Bindler, R. (1999). *Pediatric nursing: Caring for children* (2nd ed.). Stamford, Conn.: Appleton & Lange, p. 733.

9. **1**

Rationale: Because the tonsillar area is so vascular, postoperative bleeding is a concern. The PT, partial thromboplastin time, platelet count, hemoglobin and hematocrit, white blood cell count, and urinalysis are performed preoperatively. The PT results would identify a potential for bleeding. The BUN, creatinine, and sedimentation rate would not determine the potential for bleeding.

Test-Taking Strategy: Focus on the issue of the question. The issue of the question relates to the potential for bleeding. Options 3 and 4 can be eliminated because they relate to kidney function. Similarly, option 2 can be eliminated because it is unrelated to the issue of the question. Review preoperative care to the child scheduled for tonsillectomy if you had difficulty with this question.

Level of Cognitive Ability: Analysis
Client Needs: Physiological Integrity
Integrated Concept/Process: Nursing Process/Assessment
Content Area: Child Health
Reference: Wong, D. (1999). *Whaley & Wong's nursing care of infants and children* (6th ed.). St. Louis: Mosby, p. 1466.

10. **2**

Rationale: In the preoperative period, the child should be observed for the presence of loose teeth to decrease the risk of aspiration during surgery. Options 1 and 4 are incorrect because these are characteristics that may indicate the need for the surgery. Bleeding during surgery will be controlled via packing and suction as needed.

Test-Taking Strategy: Use the process of elimination, noting that the child is scheduled for surgery. The issue of the

question relates to aspiration, and note the key words "highest risk" in the stem of the question. Options 1 and 4 can be easily eliminated because these are characteristics that may indicate the need for the surgery. Recall that the tonsillar area is vascular; anticipation of bleeding during surgery is expected and would be controlled. Therefore, eliminate option 3. Review preoperative assessment procedures related to tonsillectomy if you had difficulty with this question.
Level of Cognitive Ability: Analysis
Client Needs: Safe, Effective Care Environment
Integrated Concept/Process: Nursing Process/Planning
Content Area: Child Health
Reference: Wong, D. (1999). *Whaley & Wong's nursing care of infants and children* (6th ed.). St. Louis: Mosby, p. 1466.
11. **3**
Rationale: The child should be placed in a prone or side-lying position following tonsillectomy, to facilitate drainage. Options 1, 2, and 4 will not achieve this goal.
Test-Taking Strategy: Use the process of elimination. Visualize each of the positions described in the options. Keeping in mind that the goal is to facilitate drainage will easily direct you to option 3. Review positioning procedures following tonsillectomy if you had difficulty with this question.
Level of Cognitive Ability: Application
Client Needs: Safe, Effective Care Environment
Integrated Concept/Process: Communication and Documentation
Content Area: Child Health
Reference: Wong, D. (1999). *Whaley & Wong's nursing care of infants and children* (6th ed.). St. Louis: Mosby, p. 1466.
12. **4**
Rationale: After tonsillectomy, suction equipment should be available, but suctioning is not performed unless there is an airway obstruction, because of the risk of trauma to the oropharynx. Clear, cool liquids are encouraged. Milk and milk products are avoided initially because they coat the throat, cause the child to clear the throat, and increase the risk of bleeding. Option 3 is an important nursing intervention following any type of surgery.
Test-Taking Strategy: Use the process of elimination. Option 3 can be eliminated first because this is a nursing action, not a medical order. From the remaining options, consider the anatomical location of the surgery. This should easily direct you to option 4. Review postoperative care following tonsillectomy if you had difficulty with this question.
Level of Cognitive Ability: Analysis
Client Needs: Safe, Effective Care Environment
Integrated Concept/Process: Communication and Documentation
Content Area: Child Health
Reference: Wong, D. (1999). *Whaley & Wong's nursing care of infants and children* (6th ed.). St. Louis: Mosby, p. 1466.
13. **4**
Rationale: Frequent swallowing, restlessness, a fast and thready pulse, and vomiting bright red blood are signs of bleeding. An elevated BP and complaints of discomfort are not indications of bleeding.
Test-Taking Strategy: Use the concepts related to the signs of shock to assist in answering the question. These concepts

should assist in eliminating options 1 and 2. From the remaining options, knowing that discomfort does not indicate bleeding will direct you to option 4. Review the signs of bleeding after tonsillectomy if you had difficulty with this question.
Level of Cognitive Ability: Analysis
Client Needs: Physiological Integrity
Integrated Concept/Process: Nursing Process/Assessment
Content Area: Child Health
Reference: Wong, D. (1999). *Whaley & Wong's nursing care of infants and children* (6th ed.). St. Louis: Mosby, p. 1467.
14. **2**
Rationale: After tonsillectomy, if bleeding occurs, the child is turned to the side and then the physician is notified. An NPO status would be maintained, and an antiemetic may be prescribed; however, the initial nursing action would be to turn the child to the side.
Test-Taking Strategy: Use the process of elimination. Note the key word "initial" in the stem of the question. Although all of the options may be appropriate, to maintain physiological integrity, the initial action is to turn the child to the side. Review care of the postoperative child who vomits if you had difficulty with this question.
Level of Cognitive Ability: Application
Client Needs: Safe, Effective Care Environment
Integrated Concept/Process: Nursing Process/Implementation
Content Area: Child Health
Reference: Bowden, V., Dickey, S, & Greenberg, C. (1998). *Children and their families: The continuum of care.* Philadelphia: W.B. Saunders, p. 903.
15. **3**
Rationale: Bad mouth odor is normal following tonsillectomy and may be relieved by drinking more liquids. Options 1, 2, and 4 are incorrect. In addition, mouthwash gargles (option 4) will irritate the throat.
Test-Taking Strategy: Use the process of elimination. Eliminate option 4 first, knowing that mouthwash gargles will irritate the surgical site. Options 1 and 2 are similar and will cause additional concern in the mother. Review postoperative expectations following tonsillectomy if you had difficulty with this question.
Level of Cognitive Ability: Application
Client Needs: Health Promotion and Maintenance
Integrated Concept/Process: Teaching/Learning
Content Area: Child Health
Reference: Ball, J., & Bindler, R. (1999). *Pediatric nursing: Caring for children* (2nd ed.). Stamford, Conn.: Appleton & Lange, p. 746.

CRITICAL THINKING: FREE-TEXT ENTRY

Answer: In children younger than age 3, the parent is instructed that the auditory canal is straightened by pulling the pinna down and back.
Rationale: If ear drops are prescribed, instruct the parent that the auditory canal is straightened by pulling the pinna down and back in children younger than age 3, and by pulling the pinna up and back for a child older than 3 years.
Test-Taking Strategy: Focus on the age of the child and recall the anatomy of the ear and the principles related to th

administration of ear drops in a child to answer the question. Review these age-related principles if you had difficulty with this question.
Level of Cognitive Ability: Application
Client Needs: Health Promotion and Maintenance

Integrated Concept/Process: Teaching/Learning
Content Area: Child Health
Reference: Wong, D. (1999). *Whaley & Wong's nursing care of infants and children* (6th ed.). St. Louis: Mosby, p. 1270.

REFERENCES

Ball, J., & Bindler, R. (1999). *Pediatric nursing: Caring for children* (2nd ed.). Stamford, Conn.: Appleton & Lange.

Ball, J., & Bindler, R. (1999). *Quick reference to pediatric clinical skills.* Stamford, Conn.: Appleton & Lange.

Bowden, V., Dickey, S, & Greenberg, C. (1998). *Children and their families: The continuum of care.* Philadelphia: W.B. Saunders.

Wong, D. (1999). *Whaley & Wong's nursing care of infants and children* (6th ed.). St. Louis: Mosby.

35

Respiratory Disorders

I. EPIGLOTTITIS

A. Description
   1. A bacterial form of croup
   2. An inflammation of the epiglottis, which may be caused by *Haemophilus influenzae* type B or *Streptococcus pneumoniae*
   3. Occurs most frequently in age group 2 to 5
   4. The onset is abrupt, and the condition occurs most often in the winter
   5. Considered an emergency situation

B. Assessment
   1. High fever
   2. Sore, red, and inflamed throat
   3. Absence of spontaneous cough
   4. Drooling
   5. Difficulty in swallowing
   6. Muffled voice
   7. Inspiratory **stridor**
   8. Agitation
   9. Tripod positioning; while supporting the body with the hands, the child thrusts the chin forward and opens the mouth in an attempt to widen the airway

C. Implementation
   1. Maintain a patent airway
   2. Assess respiratory status and breath sounds, noting **nasal flaring,** the use of accessory muscles, and the presence of **stridor**
   3. Assess temperature by the axillary route, not the oral route
   4. To prevent spasm of epiglottis and airway occlusion, NO attempts should be made to visualize the posterior pharynx or to obtain a throat culture
   5. Prepare the child for lateral neck films to confirm the diagnosis
   6. Maintain NPO status
   7. Do not leave the child unattended
   8. Do not force the child to lie down
   9. Do not restrain the child
   10. Administer IV fluids and antibiotics as prescribed
   11. Administer analgesics and antipyretics (acetaminophen [Tylenol]) to reduce fever and throat pain as prescribed
   12. Provide cool-mist oxygen therapy as prescribed
   13. Provide high humidification to cool the airway and decrease swelling
   14. Have resuscitation equipment available, and prepare for enotracheal intubation or tracheotomy for severe respiratory distress
   15. Question the physician regarding the need for immunization (*Haemophilus* type B)

II. LARYNGOTRACHEOBRONCHITIS (LTB)

A. Description
   1. Inflammation of larynx, trachea, and bronchi
   2. Most common type of croup and may be viral or bacterial
   3. Has a gradual onset and may be preceded by an upper respiratory infection

B. Assessment
   1. Fever, low-grade to high
   2. Irritability and restlessness
   3. Hoarse voice
   4. Seal bark and brassy cough
   5. Inspiratory **stridor** and suprasternal **retractions**
   6. Use of accessory muscles for breathing
   7. Crackles and **wheezing** on lung auscultation
   8. Anorexia, nausea, and vomiting
   9. Signs of anoxia and carbon dioxide retention
   10. Cyanosis

C. Implementation
   1. Maintain a patent airway
   2. Assess respiratory status, monitoring for **nasal flaring,** sternal **retraction,** and inspiratory **stridor**

3. Monitor for pallor or cyanosis
4. Elevate the head of the bed and provide bed rest
5. Provide humidified oxygen via cool-mist tent for the hospitalized child
6. Instruct the parents to use a cool-air vaporizer or humidifier at home; other measures include having the child breathe in the cool night air or the air from an open freezer, or taking the child to a cool basement or garage
7. Provide and encourage fluid intake; IVs may be prescribed to maintain hydration status if the child is unable to take oral fluids
8. Administer acetaminophen (Tylenol) as prescribed to reduce fever
9. Avoid cough syrups and cold medicines, which may dry and thicken secretions
10. Administer bronchodilators if prescribed to relax smooth muscle and relieve **stridor**
11. Administer corticosteroids if prescribed for the antiinflammatory effect
12. Administer nebulized epinephrine (racemic epinephrine) as prescribed for children with severe disease, **stridor** at rest, **retractions,** or difficulty breathing
13. Administer antibiotics as prescribed, noting that they are not indicated unless a bacterial infection is present
14. Have resuscitation equipment available

III. BRONCHITIS
A. Description: Infection of the major bronchi that may be referred to as tracheobronchitis
B. Assessment
   1. Fever
   2. Dry, hacking, and nonproductive cough that is worse at night and becomes productive in 2 to 3 days
C. Implementation
   1. Monitor for respiratory distress
   2. Provide cool, humidified air
   3. Monitor for signs of dehydration, such as a sunken fontanel, poor skin turgor, and decreased and concentrated urinary output
   4. Increased fluid intake
   5. Administer acetaminophen (Tylenol) for fever as prescribed

IV. BRONCHIOLITIS/RESPIRATORY SYNCYTIAL VIRUS (RSV)
A. Description
   1. An inflammation of the bronchioles that causes a thick production of mucus that occludes bronchiole tubes and small bronchi
   2. RSV is a common cause of bronchiolitis
   3. RSV, although not airborne, is highly communicable and is usually transferred by the hands

B. Assessment
   1. Upper respiratory infection (URI) symptoms such as rhinorrhea and low-grade fever
   2. Lethargy, poor feeding, and irritability in infants
   3. Tachypnea
   4. Increased difficulty in breathing
   5. **Nasal flaring** and **retractions**
   6. Expiratory wheeze and grunt
   7. Diminished breath sounds
C. Implementation
   1. Maintain a patent airway
   2. Position the child at a 30- to 40-degree angle with the neck slightly extended to maintain an open airway and decrease pressure on the diaphragm
   3. Provide cool, humidified oxygen
   4. Encourage fluids; IV fluid may be necessary until the acute stage has passed
   5. Assess for signs of dehydration
D. The child with RSV
   1. Isolate in a single room or place in a room with another RSV child
   2. Maintain good handwashing procedures
   3. Ensure that nurses caring for these children do not care for other high-risk children
   4. Wear gowns when soiling of clothing may occur during care
   5. Administer ribavirin (Virazole), an antiviral respiratory medication, if prescribed
   6. Ribavirin is administered via aerosol by hood, tent, mask, or through ventilator tubing; pregnant health care providers should not care for a child receiving ribavirin
   7. The nurse wearing contact lenses should wear goggles when coming in contact with ribavirin, because the mist may dissolve soft lenses
   8. Prepare for the administration of respiratory syncytial virus immune globulin (RSV-IGIV or RespiGam)
      a. Used prophylactically to prevent RSV in high-risk infants
      b. RespiGam is an IV preparation of immunoglobulin G and is administered before the RSV epidemic season (November through April); subsequent doses are given every month to maintain protection
      c. Not administered to infants or children with congenital heart disease (CHD) or with cyanotic CHD

V. PNEUMONIA
A. Description
   1. Inflammation of the alveoli caused by a virus, mycoplasmal agents, bacteria, or the aspiration of foreign substances
   2. The causative agent is usually introduced into the lungs through inhalation or from the bloodstream

3. Viral pneumonia occurs more frequently than bacterial and is often associated with a viral upper respiratory infection (URI)
4. Primary atypical pneumonia (*Mycoplasma pneumoniae*) is the most common cause of pneumonia in children between the ages of 5 and 12 years; occurs primarily in the fall and winter months and is more prevalent in crowded living conditions
5. Bacterial pneumonia is often a serious infection; hospitalization is indicated when pleural effusion or empyema accompanies the disease, and is mandatory for children with staphylococcal pneumonia
6. Aspiration pneumonia occurs when food, secretions, liquids, or other materials enter the lung and cause inflammation and a chemical pneumonitis; classic symptoms include an increasing cough or fever with foul-smelling sputum, deteriorating results on chest x-rays, and other signs of airway involvement

B. Viral pneumonia
1. Assessment
   a. Mild fever, slight cough, and malaise, to high fever, severe cough, and prostration
   b. Nonproductive or productive cough of small amounts of whitish sputum
   c. Wheezes or fine crackles
2. Implementation
   a. Administer oxygen with cool mist as prescribed
   b. Increase fluid intake
   c. Administer antipyretics for fever as prescribed
   d. Administer chest physiotherapy and postural drainage as prescribed
   e. Antimicrobial therapy is reserved for children in whom the presence of infection is demonstrated by cultures

C. Primary atypical pneumonia
1. Assessment
   a. Fever, chills, anorexia, headache, malaise, and muscle pain
   b. Rhinitis, sore throat, and dry, hacking cough
   c. Cough is nonproductive initially; then produces seromucoid sputum that becomes mucopurulent or blood streaked
2. Implementation: Symptomatic

D. Bacterial pneumonia
1. Assessment
   a. Acute onset, fever, toxic appearance
   b. Infant: irritability, lethargy, poor feeding; abrupt fever (may be accompanied by seizures); respiratory distress (air hunger, tachypnea, and circumoral cyanosis)
   c. Older child: headache, chills, abdominal pain, chest pain, meningeal symptoms (meningism)

d. Hacking, nonproductive cough
e. Diminished breath sounds or scattered crackles
f. As the infection resolves, coarse crackles and **wheezing** are heard and the cough becomes productive with purulent sputum

2. Implementation
   a. Antimicrobial therapy is initiated as soon as the diagnosis is suspected
   b. Administer oxygen (via hood, mist tent, or nasal cannula) for respiratory distress as prescribed
   c. Place the child in a mist tent as prescribed; cool humidification moistens the airways and assists in temperature reduction
   d. Suction the infant to maintain a patent airway if the infant is unable to handle secretions
   e. Administer chest physiotherapy and postural drainage every 4 hours as prescribed
   f. Promote bed rest to conserve energy
   g. Encourage the child to lie on the affected side (if pneumonia is unilateral) to splint the chest and reduce the discomfort caused by pleural rubbing
   h. Provide liberal fluid intake (administer cautiously to prevent aspiration); IV fluids may be necessary
   i. Administer antipyretics for fever as prescribed; monitor temperature frequently because of the risk for febrile seizures
   j. Institute isolation precautions with pneumococcal or staphylococcal pneumonia (according to agency policy)
   k. Administer antitussives as prescribed before rest times and meals if the cough is disturbing
   l. Continuous closed chest drainage may be instituted if purulent fluid is present (usually noted in staphylococcus infections)
   m. Fluid accumulation in the pleural cavity may be removed by thoracentesis; thoracentesis also provides a means for obtaining fluid for culture and for instilling antibiotics directly into the pleural cavity

VI. TUBERCULOSIS (TB)
A. Description
   1. A contagious disease caused by *Mycobacterium tuberculosis*, an acid-fast bacillus
   2. Children are susceptible to the human *Mycobacterium tuberculosis* and to *Mycobacterium bovis*
   3. *Mycobacterium bovis* is common in parts of the world where TB is not controlled or pasteurization of milk is not practiced; the organism can be ingested via infected milk
   4. Multidrug-resistant strains of *Mycobacterium tuberculosis* occur because of client or family noncompliance with therapeutic regimens

5. The route of transmission of *Mycobacterium tuberculosis* is through inhalation of droplets from an individual with active TB
6. Most children are infected by a family member or by another individual with whom they have frequent contact, such as a baby-sitter

B. Assessment
1. May be asymptomatic or develop symptoms such as malaise, fever, cough, weight loss, anorexia, and lymphadenopathy
2. Specific symptoms related to the site of infection, such as the lungs, brain, or bone, may be present

C. Mantoux test
1. Will produce a positive reaction 2 to 10 weeks after the initial infection
2. Determines whether the child has been infected and has developed a sensitivity to the protein of the tubercle bacillus; a positive reaction does not confirm the presence of active disease
3. Once the child reacts positively, the child will always react positively; a positive reaction in a previously negative test indicates that the child has been infected since the last test
4. TB testing should not be done at the same time as measles immunization; viral interference from the measles vaccine may cause a false-negative reaction
5. Induration measuring 15 mm or greater is considered to be a positive reaction in children 4 years of age or older who do not have any risk factors
6. Induration measuring 10 mm or greater is considered to be a positive reaction in children younger than 4 years of age and in those with chronic illness or at high risk for exposure to TB
7. Induration measuring 5 mm or greater is considered to be positive for the highest risk groups, such as children with immunosuppressive conditions or human immunodeficiency virus (HIV)

D. Sputum culture
1. A definitive diagnosis is made by demonstrating the presence of mycobacteria in a culture
2. Because an infant or young child often swallows sputum rather than expectorates, gastric washings (aspiration of lavaged contents from the fasting stomach) may be done to obtain a specimen; specimen is obtained in the early morning before breakfast

E. Implementation
1. Medications
   a. Include isoniazid (INH), rifampin (Rifadin), and pyrazinamide
   b. A 9-month course of INH is prescribed to prevent a latent infection from progressing to clinically active TB and to prevent initial infection in children in high-risk situations; a

12-month course is prescribed for the HIV-infected child
   c. Recommendation for the child with clinically active TB: INH, rifampin, and pyrazinamide daily for 2 months; then, INH and rifampin twice weekly for 4 months
2. Place children with infectious disease on isolation precautions until medications have been initiated, sputum cultures demonstrate a diminished number of organisms, and cough is improving
3. Wear a mask if the child is coughing and does not reliably cover his or her mouth
4. Maintain airborne precautions with family members until they are demonstrated not to have infectious TB
5. Bacillus Calmette-Guérin (BCG) vaccine
   a. Produces limited immunity (definite although incomplete protection against TB)
   b. Positive tuberculin reactions develop after inoculation
   c. Not generally recommended; however, may be used for long-term protection of infants and children who are at high risk for continuing exposure to persons with infectious TB
6. Stress the importance of adequate rest and adequate diet
7. Instruct the child and family in measures to prevent transmission of TB

VII. ASTHMA
A. Description
1. Chronic inflammatory disease of the airways
2. Is commonly caused by physical and chemical irritants as foods, pollens, dust mites, cockroaches, smoke, animal dander, temperature changes, respiratory infection, activity, and stress
3. The allergic reaction in the airways can cause an immediate reaction, with obstruction occurring, and it can precipitate a late bronchial obstructive reaction several hours after the initial exposure
4. A common symptom is coughing in the absence of respiratory infection, especially at night
5. Status asthmaticus
   a. Child displays respiratory distress despite vigorous treatment measures
   b. A medical emergency that can result in respiratory failure and death if left untreated

B. Assessment
1. Episodes of **wheezing**, breathlessness, dyspnea, chest tightness, and cough, particularly at night and/or in the early morning
2. Itching localized at the front of the neck or over the upper part of the back
3. Exacerbations are episodes of progressively worsening shortness of breath, cough, **wheezing,**

chest tightness, decreases in expiratory airflow because of bronchospasm, mucosal edema, and mucus plugging; air is trapped behind occluded or narrow airways, and hypoxemia can occur

4. Asthmatic episode
   a. Begins with irritability, restlessness, headache, feeling tired, or chest tightness
   b. Respiratory symptoms include a hacking, irritable, nonproductive cough, caused by bronchial edema
   c. Accumulated secretions stimulate the cough, and the cough becomes rattling and productive of frothy, clear, gelatinous sputum
   d. Child may be pale or flushed, and the lips may have a deep, dark red color that may progress to cyanosis observed in the nailbeds and skin, especially around the mouth
   e. Restlessness, apprehension, and diaphoresis occur
   f. Younger children assume the tripod sitting position; older children sit upright with the shoulders in a hunched-over position, with the hands on the bed or a chair, and arms braced to facilitate the use of accessory muscles of breathing (child refuses to lie down)
   g. Child speaks in short, broken phrases
   h. **Retractions**
   i. Hyperresonance on percussion of the chest
   j. Breath sounds are coarse and loud, with crackles and coarse rhonchi and inspiratory and expiratory **wheezing;** expiration is prolonged
5. Exercise-induced bronchospasm (EIB): Cough, shortness of breath, chest pain or tightness, **wheezing,** and endurance problems during exercise
6. Severe spasm or obstruction: Breath sounds and crackles may become inaudible, and the cough is ineffective (represents a lack of air movement)
7. Ventilatory failure and asphyxia: Shortness of breath, with air movement in the chest restricted to the point of absent breath sounds accompanied by a sudden rise in the respiratory rate

C. Implementation: Acute episode
1. Assess airway patency
2. Administer humidified oxygen by nasal prongs or facemask as prescribed
3. Administer quick-relief (rescue) medications as prescribed
4. Continuously monitor respiratory status, pulse oximetry, and color; be alert to decreased **wheezing** or a silent chest, which may signal the inability to move air
5. Initiate an IV line, and prepare to correct dehydration, acidosis, or electrolyte imbalances

6. Prepare the child for a chest x-ray
7. Prepare to obtain arterial blood gases and serum electrolytes

D. Medications
1. Quick-relief (rescue medications)
   a. To treat symptoms and exacerbations
   b. Short-acting B_2-agonists: For acute exacerbations (albuterol [Proventil HFA, Ventolin], metaproterenol sulfate [Alupent], and terbutaline sulfate [Brethaire, Brethine, Bricanyl])
   c. Anticholinergics: For relief of acute bronchospasm (atropine sulfate, ipratropium bromide [Atrovent])
   d. Systemic corticosteroids: Antiinflammatory action to treat reversible airflow obstruction
2. Long-term control (preventer medications)
   a. Achieve and maintain control of inflammation
   b. Corticosteroids: Antiinflammatory action to reduce bronchial hyperactivity
   c. Cromolyn sodium (Intal): A nonsteroidal antiinflammatory (NSAID) that inhibits acute airway narrowing
   d. Nedocromil sodium (Tilade): An antiallergic and antiinflammatory used for maintenance therapy
   e. Long-acting B_2-agonists: For the prevention of EIB (albuterol [Proventil HFA, Ventolin], metaproterenol sulfate [Alupent], and terbutaline sulfate [Brethaire, Brethine, Bricanyl])
   f. Methylxanthines: For bronchodilation
   g. Leukotriene modifiers: To prevent bronchospasm and inflammatory cell infiltration (zafirlukast [Accolate] and zileuton [Zyflo]); used in children older than 12 years
   h. Long-acting bronchodilator: Used for long-term prevention of symptoms, especially nocturnal symptoms (salmeterol [Serevent])
3. Nebulizer, metered-dose inhaler (MDI), or peak expiratory flow meters (PEFMs)
   a. Used to deliver many of the medications used to treat asthma
   b. A non-chlorofluorocarbon (CFC) is available for albuterol (Proventil Hydrofluoroalkane [HFA])
   c. Turbuhaler (CFC-free MDI) delivers inhaled powder and eliminates the need for coordination of the device with inhalation and holding the breath
   d. If the child has difficulty using the MDI, medication can be administered by nebulization (medication is mixed with saline and then nebulized with compressed air by a machine)

E. Chest physiotherapy (CPT)
1. Includes breathing exercises and physical training
2. Not recommended during an acute exacerbation

▲ F. Allergen control
  1. Prevents and reduces exposure to airborne allergens
  2. Skin testing to identify allergens; immunotherapy is not recommended for allergens that can be eliminated effectively
  3. Dust mites: Maintain the humidity in the house under 50%
  4. Cockroaches: Exterminating, cleaning kitchen floors and cabinets, putting food away quickly after eating, taking the trash out in the evening

▲ G. Home care measures
  1. Instruct in measures to eliminate allergens
  2. Avoid extremes of environmental temperature; in cold temperatures, instruct the child to breathe through the nose, not the mouth, and to cover the nose and mouth with a scarf
  3. Avoid exposure to individuals with a viral respiratory infection
  4. Instruct the child in how to recognize early symptoms of an asthma attack
  5. Instruct the child in the administration of medications as prescribed
  6. Instruct the child in the use of a nebulizer, MDI, or PEFM
  7. Instruct the child in the cleaning of devices used for inhaled medications (oral candidiasis can occur with the use of aerosolized steroids)
  8. Encourage adequate rest, sleep, and a well-balanced diet
  9. Instruct the child in the importance of adequate fluid intake to liquefy secretions
  10. Assist in developing an exercise program
  11. Instruct the child in the procedure for respiratory treatments and exercises as prescribed
  12. Encourage the child to cough effectively
  13. Encourage the parents to keep immunizations up to date; annual influenza vaccinations are recommended
  14. Inform other health care providers and school personnel of the asthma condition
  15. Allow the child to take control of self-care measures on the basis of age appropriateness

VIII. CYSTIC FIBROSIS (CF)

A. Description
  1. A chronic multisystem disorder (autosomal recessive trait disorder) characterized by exocrine gland dysfunction
  2. The mucus produced by the exocrine glands is abnormally thick, causing obstruction of the small passageways of the affected organs
  3. The most common symptoms are pancreatic enzyme deficiency caused by duct blockage, progressive chronic lung disease associated with infection, and sweat gland dysfunction resulting in increased sodium and chloride sweat concentrations

  4. An increase in sodium and chloride in both sweat and saliva forms the basis for the most reliable diagnostic test, the sweat chloride test

B. Respiratory system
  1. Symptoms are produced by the stagnation of mucus in the airway, leading to bacterial colonization and destruction of lung tissue
  2. Emphysema and atelectasis occur as the airways become increasingly obstructed
  3. Chronic hypoxemia causes contraction and hypertrophy of the muscle fibers in pulmonary arteries and arterioles, leading to pulmonary hypertension and eventual cor pulmonale
  4. Pneumothorax from ruptured bullae and hemoptysis from erosion of the bronchial wall through an artery occur as the disease progresses
  5. **Wheezing** and dry nonproductive cough
  6. Dyspnea
  7. Cyanosis
  8. Clubbing of the fingers and toes
  9. Repeated episodes of bronchitis and pneumonia

C. Gastrointestinal system ▲
  1. Meconium ileus in the neonate
  2. Intestinal obstruction (distal intestinal obstructive syndrome) caused by thick intestinal secretions; signs include pain, abdominal distention, nausea, and vomiting
  3. Steatorrhea (frothy, foul-smelling stools)
  4. Deficiency of the fat-soluble vitamins A, D, E, and K, which causes easy bruising and anemia
  5. Malnutrition and failure to thrive; demonstrate hypoalbuminemia from diminished absorption of protein, resulting in generalized edema
  6. Rectal prolapse can occur as a result of the large, bulky stools, and lack of the supportive fat pads around the rectum

D. Integumentary system ▲
  1. Abnormally high concentrations of sodium and chloride in sweat
  2. Parents report that the infant tastes "salty" when kissed
  3. Dehydration and electrolyte imbalances, especially during hyperthermic conditions

E. Reproductive system
  1. Delayed **puberty** in females
  2. Fertility can be inhibited by highly viscous cervical secretions, which act as a plug and block sperm entry
  3. Males are usually sterile, caused by the blockage of the vas deferens by abnormal secretions or by failure of normal development of duct structures

F. Diagnostic tests ▲
  1. Quantitative sweat chloride test ▲
    a. The production of sweat is stimulated (pilocarpine iontophoresis), the sweat is collected, and the sweat electrolytes are measured (a minimum of 50 mg of sweat is needed)

b. Normally, sweat chloride concentration is less than 40 mEq/L

c. A chloride concentration greater than 60 mEq/L is a positive test result

d. Chloride concentrations of 40 to 60 mEq/L are highly suggestive of CF and require a repeat test

2. Chest x-ray: Reveals atelectasis and obstructive emphysema

3. Pulmonary function tests: Provide evidence of abnormal small airway function

4. Stool/fat and/or enzyme analysis: A 72-hour stool sample is collected to check the fat and/or enzyme (trypsin) content (food intake is recorded during the collection)

G. Implementation

1. Respiratory system

a. Goals of treatment include preventing and treating pulmonary infection by improving aeration, removing secretions, and administering antimicrobial medications

b. Chest physiotherapy (percussion and postural drainage) on awakening and in the evening (more frequently during pulmonary infection)

c. Chest physiotherapy should not be performed before or immediately after a meal

d. Bronchodilator medication by aerosol to open the bronchi for easier expectoration (administered before the CPT when the child has reactive airway disease or is **wheezing**)

e. Use of a Flutter Mucus Clearance Device (a small, hand-held plastic pipe with a stainless-steel ball on the inside) that facilitates removal of mucus); store away from small children because if the device separates, the steel ball poses a choking hazard

f. Use of a ThAIRapy vest device that provides high-frequency chest wall oscillation to help loosen secretions

g. Administration of recombinant human deoxyribonuclease (DNase), known generically as dornase alfa (Pulmozyme), which decreases the viscosity of mucus

h. Instruct the parents not to give cough suppressants, as they will inhibit expectoration of secretions and promote infection

i. Teach the child forced expiratory technique (huffing) to mobilize secretions

j. Develop a physical exercise program with the aim of establishing a good habitual breathing pattern

k. Administer antibiotics as prescribed, which may be prescribed prophylactically or when pulmonary symptoms develop

l. Aerosolized antibiotics may be prescribed and are administered after CPT is performed, or IV antibiotics may be prescribed and administered at home through a central venous access device

m. Administer oxygen as prescribed during acute episodes; monitor closely for oxygen narcosis

n. Monitor for hemoptysis; greater than 300 mL in 24 hours for the older child (less for a younger child) needs to be treated immediately

o. Hemoptysis may be controlled by bed rest, cough suppressants, antibiotics, and vitamin K; if hemoptysis persists, the site of bleeding may be cauterized or embolized

p. Lung transplantation is a final therapeutic option for the end-stage child

2. Gastrointestinal system

a. The goal of treatment for pancreatic insufficiency is to replace pancreatic enzymes; administered with meals and snacks (or within 30 minutes of eating meals and snacks) to ensure that digestive enzymes are mixed with food in the duodenum

b. The amount of pancreatic enzymes administered is adjusted to achieve normal **growth** and a decrease in the number of stools to two or three per day

c. Enteric-coated pancreatic enzymes should not be crushed or chewed

d. Pancreatic enzymes should not be given if the child is NPO

e. Encourage a well-balanced, high-protein, high-calorie diet; multivitamins and vitamins A, D, E, and K are also administered

f. Assess weight and monitor for failure to thrive

g. Monitor for constipation and intestinal obstruction

h. Supplement the child's diet with salt during extremely hot weather or if the child has a fever; include fluids such as Gatorade or Exceed, which provide an adequate supply of electrolytes

H. Home care

1. Instruct the parents about the prescribed treatment measures and their importance

2. Instruct the parents to be sure immunizations are up to date

3. Inform the parents that the child should be vaccinated yearly for pneumococcus and influenza

4. Inform the parents about the Cystic Fibrosis Foundation

IX. SUDDEN INFANT DEATH SYNDROME (SIDS)

A. Description

1. Unexpected death of an apparently healthy infant under age 1 year for which a thorough autopsy fails to demonstrate an adequate cause of deat'

2. The cause is not known

B. Characteristics
1. Maternal risk factors
   a. Maternal smoking
   b. Substance **abuse**
   c. Younger mothers
2. Birth risk factors
   a. Prematurity
   b. Low-birth-weight infants
   c. Multiple births
   d. Infants with central nervous system problems
3. Time of year: Most frequently during winter months
4. Time of death: Usually occurs during sleep
5. Age: Most frequently occurs from 2 months to 4 months of life
6. Sex and race
   a. Incidence higher in males
   b. Incidence higher in Native Americans and blacks
7. Sleep risk habits
   a. Prone position
   b. Use of soft bedding
   c. Overheating (thermal stress)
   d. Possibly: sleeping with an adult
C. Appearance when found
1. Apneic, blue, lifeless
2. Frothy blood-tinged fluid in the nose and mouth
3. May be found in any position but is typically found in a disheveled bed, with blankets over the head, and huddled in a corner
4. May be clutching bedding
5. Diaper is wet and full of stool
D. Prevention
1. Healthy infants should be placed in the supine position for sleep
2. Infants with gastroesophageal reflux or other airway anomalies that predispose to airway obstruction may be placed in a prone sleeping position
3. Soft moldable mattresses and bedding, such as pillows or quilts, should not be used under the infant for bedding
4. Stuffed animals should be removed from the crib while the infant is sleeping

PRACTICE QUESTIONS

1. A student nurse is caring for a 2-year-old child diagnosed with croup. A nursing instructor asks the student about the clinical manifestations associated with croup. Which statement by the student indicates a need for further research?
   1. "Symptoms usually worsen at night and are better during the day."
   "Symptoms usually worsen during the day and relieved during sleep."
   cough is harsh and brassy."

4. "Inspiratory stridor and a low-grade fever may be present."

2. A hospitalized 2-year-old child with croup is receiving corticosteroid therapy. The mother asks a nurse why the physician did not prescribe antibiotics. The most appropriate response is:
   1. "The child is too young to receive antibiotics."
   2. "The child still has the maternal antibodies from birth and does not need antibiotics."
   3. "Antibiotics are not indicated unless a bacterial infection is present."
   4. "The child may be allergic to antibiotics."

3. A child with croup is placed in a cool mist tent. The mother becomes concerned because the child is frightened, consistently crying, and trying to climb out of the tent. The most appropriate nursing action would be to:
   1. Call the physician and obtain an order for a mild sedative
   2. Tell the mother that the child must stay in the tent
   3. Place a toy in the tent to make the child feel more comfortable
   4. Let the mother hold the child and direct a cool mist over the child's face

4. A nurse caring for an infant with bronchiolitis is assessing for signs of dehydration. The nurse assesses which of the following, knowing that it is the most reliable method of determining fluid loss?
   1. Intake and output (I & O)
   2. Fontanels
   3. Mucous membranes
   4. Weight

5. An emergency room nurse is caring for a child diagnosed with epiglottitis. Assessing the child, the nurse monitors for which indication that the child may be experiencing airway obstruction?
   1. The child is leaning backward, supporting himself with the hands and arms
   2. A low-grade fever and complaints of a sore throat
   3. The child is leaning forward with the chin thrust out
   4. Nasal flaring and bradycardia

6. A nurse is caring for an infant with bronchiolitis. Diagnostic tests have confirmed respiratory syncytial virus (RSV). On the basis of this finding, which of the following would be the most appropriate nursing action?
   1. Move the infant to a room with another RSV child
   2. Leave the infant in the present room because RSV is not contagious
   3. Inform the staff that they must wear a mask when caring for the child
   4. Initiate strict enteric precautions

7. Ribavirin (Virazole) is prescribed for a hospitalized child with respiratory syncytial virus (RSV). The

nurse prepares to administer this medication via which of the following routes?
1. Subcutaneous
2. Intramuscular
3. Oxygen tent
4. Oral

8. A 10-year-old child with asthma is treated for acute exacerbation in the emergency room. A nurse reports which of the following, knowing that it is not an indication that the condition is improving?
1. Increased wheezing
2. Decreased wheezing
3. Warm, dry skin
4. A pulse rate of 90 beats per minute

9. The mother of an 8-year-old child being treated for right lower lobe pneumonia at home calls the clinic nurse. The mother tells the nurse that the child complains of discomfort on the right side and that the acetaminophen (Tylenol) is not very effective. The nurse most appropriately tells the mother to:
1. Increase the dose of the acetaminophen
2. Increase the frequency of the acetaminophen
3. Encourage the child to lie on the right side
4. Encourage the child to lie on the left side

10. The charge nurse of a newborn nursery is providing a teaching session to new employees regarding sudden infant death syndrome (SIDS). The charge nurse tells the new employees that SIDS usually occurs during sleep and:
1. Is more common in premature infants
2. Is more common in girls
3. Most frequently occurs between 8 and 10 months of age
4. Is more common in high-birth-weight infants

11. A new mother expresses concern to a nurse regarding sudden infant death syndrome (SIDS). She asks the nurse how to position her new infant for sleep. The nurse most appropriately tells the mother that the infant should be placed on his:
1. Back rather than on the stomach
2. Side or prone
3. Stomach with the face turned
4. Back or prone

12. A sweat test is performed on a child with a suspected diagnosis of cystic fibrosis (CF). The nurse reviews the test results and determines that which of the following is a positive result for CF?
1. Chloride level of 20 mEq/L
2. Chloride level of 30 mEq/L
3. Chloride level of 40 mEq/L
4. Chloride level of 70 mEq/L

13. A clinic nurse is providing instructions to a mother of a child with cystic fibrosis (CF) regarding the immunization schedule for the child. Which statement would the nurse make to the mother?
1. "The immunization schedule will need to be altered."
2. "The child will receive all of the immunizations except for the polio series."
3. "The child will receive the recommended basic series of immunizations along with a yearly pneumococcus and influenza vaccination."
4. "The child should not receive any hepatitis vaccines."

14. A clinic nurse reads the results of a Mantoux test on a 3-year-old child. The results indicate an area of induration measuring 10 mm. The nurse would interpret these results as:
1. Negative
2. Positive
3. Inconclusive
4. Definitive and requiring a repeat test

15. Isoniazid (INH) is prescribed for a 2-year-old child with a positive Mantoux test. The mother of the child asks the nurse how long the child will need to take the medication. The nurse tells the mother that the medication will need to be taken for:
1. Six months
2. Nine months
3. Twelve months
4. Eighteen months

CRITICAL THINKING: FREE-TEXT ENTRY

A mother arrives at an emergency room with her child, and a diagnosis of epiglottitis is documented. The nurse reviews the physician's orders and notes the following: obtain a throat culture, obtain axillary temperatures, administer humidified oxygen, administer acetaminophen (Tylenol) for fever. Which order written by the physician would the nurse question?

Answer: _____

ANSWERS

1. 2

Rationale: Croup often begins at night and may be preceded by several days of upper respiratory infection symptoms. It is characterized by a sudden onset of a harsh, brassy cough, sore throat, and inspiratory stridor. Symptoms usually worsen at night and are better in the day. It is usually accompanied by a low-grade fever, but occasionally the fever may be as high as 104° F.

Test-Taking Strategy: Use the process of elimination. Note the key words "need for further research." Eliminate option 4 first because of the word "may." Knowledge of the manifestations associated with this illness will assist in eliminating options 1 and 3. If you had difficulty with this question, review this disorder.

Level of Cognitive Ability: Analysis
Client Needs: Physiological Integrity
Integrated Concept/Process: Teaching/Learning
Content Area: Child Health
Reference: Ball, J., & Bindler, R. (1999). *Pediatric nursing: Caring for children* (2nd ed.). Stamford, Conn.: Appleton & Lange, p. 421.

2. 3

Rationale: Antibiotics are not indicated in the treatment of croup unless a bacterial infection is present. Options 1, 2, and 4 are correct. In addition, there are no supporting data in the question to indicate that the child may be allergic to antibiotics.

Test-Taking Strategy: Use the process of elimination. Eliminate option 4 because there are no supporting data in the question regarding the potential for allergies. Noting the age of the child will assist in eliminating both options 1 and 2. In addition, recalling the general principles related to the use of antibiotics will direct you to the correct option. Review the indications for the use of antibiotics if you had difficulty with this question.

Level of Cognitive Ability: Application
Client Needs: Health Promotion and Maintenance
Integrated Concept/Process: Teaching/Learning
Content Area: Child Health
Reference: Wong, D. (1999). *Whaley & Wong's nursing care of infants and children* (6th ed.). St. Louis: Mosby, p. 1476.

3. 4

Rationale: If the use of a tent or hood is causing distress, treatment may be more effective if the child is held by the parent and a cool mist is directed toward the child's face. A mild sedative would not be administered to the child. Crying will aggravate laryngospasm and increase hypoxia, which may cause airway obstruction. Options 2 and 3 will not alleviate the child's fear.

Test-Taking Strategy: Focus on the issue of the question. Options 1, 2, and 3 will not alleviate the child's fear and are similar in that they do not address the fear. Option 4 is the option that addresses the issue of the question. Review care to the child in a mist tent if you had difficulty with this question.

Level of Cognitive Ability: Application
Client Needs: Psychosocial Integrity
Integrated Concept/Process: Caring
Content Area: Child Health
Reference: Wong, D. (1999). *Whaley & Wong's nursing care of infants and children* (6th ed.). St. Louis: Mosby, p. 1478.

4. 4

Rationale: Weight is the most reliable method of measurement of body fluid loss or gain. One kilogram of weight change represents 1 liter of fluid loss or gain. Although options 1, 2, and 3 identify components of the assessment for dehydration, these are not the most reliable determinants.

Test-Taking Strategy: Use the process of elimination. Note the key words "most reliable." Options 2 and 3 can be easily eliminated first. From the remaining options, recall that it would be very difficult to obtain an accurate output on an infant. This concept should easily direct you toward option 4. Review assessment of dehydration if you had difficulty with this question.

Level of Cognitive Ability: Analysis
Client Needs: Physiological Integrity
Integrated Concept/Process: Nursing Process/Assessment
Content Area: Child Health
Reference: Ball, J., & Bindler, R. (1999). *Pediatric nursing: Caring for children* (2nd ed.). Stamford, Conn.: Appleton & Lange, p. 296.

5. 3

Rationale: Clinical manifestations suggestive of airway obstruction include tripod positioning (leaning forward while supported by arms, chin thrust out, mouth open), nasal flaring, tachycardia, a high fever, and a sore throat.

Test-Taking Strategy: Use the process of elimination. Eliminate option 4 first because tachycardia rather than bradycardia will occur in a child experiencing respiratory distress. Eliminate option 2 next, knowing that a high fever occurs with epiglottitis. From the remaining options, visualize the descriptions in each and determine which position would best assist a child experiencing respiratory distress. Review the indications of airway obstruction if you had difficulty with this question.

Level of Cognitive Ability: Analysis
Client Needs: Physiological Integrity
Integrated Concept/Process: Nursing Process/Assessment
Content Area: Child Health
Reference: Ball, J., & Bindler, R. (1999). *Pediatric nursing: Caring for children* (2nd ed.). Stamford, Conn.: Appleton & Lange, p. 425.

6. 1

Rationale: RSV is a highly communicable disorder. It is not transmitted via the airborne route. It is usually transferred by the hands, and meticulous handwashing is necessary to decrease the spread of organisms. The infant with RSV is isolated in a single room or placed in a room with another RSV child. Enteric precautions are not necessary; however, the nurse should wear a gown when soiling of clothing may occur.

Test-Taking Strategy: Use the process of elimination. Recall the method of the transmission and that the infant with RSV is isolated in a single room or placed in a room with another RSV child. Review the care of the infant with RSV, if you had difficulty with this question

Level of Cognitive Ability: Application
Client Needs: Safe, Effective Care Environment
Integrated Concept/Process: Nursing Process/Implementation
Content Area: Child Health
Reference: Ball, J., & Bindler, R. (1999). *Pediatric nursing: Caring for children* (2nd ed.). Stamford, Conn.: Appleton & Lange, p. 441.

7. 3

Rationale: Ribavirin (Virazole) is an antiviral respiratory medication that is used mainly in hospitalized children with severe RSV. Administration is via hood, face mask, or oxygen tent. It is not administered subcutaneously, intramuscularly, or orally.

Test-Taking Strategy: Use the process of administration. Recalling that this medication is aerosolized will direct you to option 3. If you are unfamiliar with this medication, review its method of administration.

Level of Cognitive Ability: Application
Client Needs: Physiological Integrity
Integrated Concept/Process: Nursing Process/Planning
Content Area: Child Health
Reference: Wong, D. (1999). *Whaley & Wong's nursing care of infants and children* (6th ed.). St. Louis: Mosby, p. 1480.

8. 2

Rationale: Decreased wheezing in a child with asthma may be incorrectly interpreted as a positive sign when, in fact, it may signal an inability to move air. A "silent chest" is an ominous sign during an asthma episode. With treatment, increased wheezing may actually signal that the child's condition is improving. The normal pulse rate in a 10-year-old is 70 to 110 beats per minute. Warm, dry skin indicates an improvement in condition, as the child is normally diaphoretic during exacerbation.

Test-Taking Strategy: Use the process of elimination. Note the key word "not" in the stem of the question. Options 3 and 4 can be easily eliminated. From the remaining options, recall that a "silent chest" is an ominous sign during an asthma episode. Review these clinical manifestations if you had difficulty with this question.

Level of Cognitive Ability: Analysis
Client Needs: Physiological Integrity
Integrated Concept/Process: Nursing Process/Assessment
Content Area: Child Health
Reference: Wong, D. (1999). *Whaley & Wong's nursing care of infants and children* (6th ed.). St. Louis: Mosby, p. 1510.

9. 3

Rationale: Splinting of the affected side by lying on that side may decrease discomfort. It is inappropriate to advise the mother to increase the dose or frequency of the acetaminophen. Lying on the left side will not be helpful in alleviating discomfort.

Test-Taking Strategy: Use the process of elimination. Options 1 and 2 can be easily eliminated. Recalling the principles related to splinting an incision in the postoperative client will assist in directing you to option 3 because these principles can be applied in this situation. Review care to the child with pneumonia if you had difficulty with this question.

Level of Cognitive Ability: Application
Client Needs: Physiological Integrity
Integrated Concept/Process: Teaching/Learning
Content Area: Child Health
Reference: Wong, D. (1999). *Whaley & Wong's nursing care of infants and children* (6th ed.). St. Louis: Mosby, p. 1484.

10. 1

Rationale: SIDS usually occurs during sleep. It most frequently occurs between the second and fourth months of life. It is more common in boys, low-birth-weight infants, and premature infants.

Test-Taking Strategy: Use the process of elimination and knowledge regarding the characteristics, etiology, and incidence of SIDS. Review this information if you are unfamiliar with it.

Level of Cognitive Ability: Application
Client Needs: Health Promotion and Maintenance
Integrated Concept/Process: Teaching/Learning
Content Area: Child Health
Reference: Ball, J., & Bindler, R. (1999). *Pediatric nursing: Caring for children* (2nd ed.). Stamford, Conn.: Appleton & Lange, p. 416.

11. 1

Rationale: Nurses should encourage parents to place healthy infants on their backs (supine) for sleep. The infant may have the ability to turn to a prone position from the side-lying position. Infants in the prone position (on the stomach) may be unable to move their heads to the side, thus increasing the risk of suffocation and lethal rebreathing.

Test-Taking Strategy: Use the process of elimination. Eliminate options 2, 3, and 4 because they are similar. Remember that the infant needs to be placed on his or her back. Review positioning of the healthy infant for sleep if you had difficulty with this question.

Level of Cognitive Ability: Application
Client Needs: Safe, Effective Care Environment
Integrated Concept/Process: Teaching/Learning
Content Area: Child Health
Reference: Wong, D. (1999). *Whaley & Wong's nursing care of infants and children* (6th ed.). St. Louis: Mosby, p. 653.

12. 4

Rationale: In a sweat test, sweating is stimulated on the child's forearm with pilocarpine, the sample is collected on absorbent material, and the amounts of sodium and chloride are measured. A sample of at least 50 mg of sweat is required for accurate results. A chloride level greater than 60 mEq/L is considered to be a positive test result. A chloride level of 40 mEq/L is suggestive of CF and requires a repeat test.

Test-Taking Strategy: Use the process of elimination. Note the key words "positive result." Use knowledge regarding this diagnostic test, and in this situation select the option that indicates the highest value. Review this diagnostic test if you are unfamiliar with it.

Level of Cognitive Ability: Analysis
Client Needs: Physiological Integrity
Integrated Concept/Process: Nursing Process/Analysis
Content Area: Child Health
Reference: Wong, D. (1999). *Whaley & Wong's nursing care of infants and children* (6th ed.). St. Louis: Mosby, p. 1521.

13. 3

Rationale: It is essential that children with CF be adequately protected from communicable diseases by immunization. It is recommended that in addition to the basic series of immunizations, children with CF should also receive yearly pneumococcus and influenza vaccines.

Test-Taking Strategy: Use the process of elimination. Eliminate options 1, 2, and 4 because they are similar. Recalling the importance of protection from communicable diseases, particularly in children with a disorder such as CF, will assist in directing you to option 3. Review the immunization schedule for the child with CF if you had difficulty with this question.

Level of Cognitive Ability: Application
Client Needs: Health Promotion and Maintenance
Integrated Concept/Process: Teaching/Learning
Content Area: Child Health
Reference: Wong, D. (1999). *Whaley & Wong's nursing care of infants and children* (6th ed.). St. Louis: Mosby, p. 1526.

14. **2**

Rationale: Induration measuring 10 mm or greater is considered to be a positive result in children younger that 4 years of age and in those with chronic illness or at high risk for environmental exposure to tuberculosis. A reaction of 5 mm or greater is considered to be a positive result for the highest risk groups, such as the child with an immunosuppressive condition or the child with human immunodeficiency virus. A reaction of 15 mm or greater is positive in children 4 years of age or older without any risk factors.

Test-Taking Strategy: Use the process of elimination. Options 3 and 4 are similar and can be eliminated first. From the remaining options, note the child's age to assist in directing you to option 2. If you had difficulty with this question, review the analysis of a Mantoux test in children.

Level of Cognitive Ability: Analysis
Client Needs: Physiological Integrity
Integrated Concept/Process: Nursing Process/Analysis
Content Area: Child Health
Reference: Wong, D. (1999). *Whaley & Wong's nursing care of infants and children* (6th ed.). St. Louis: Mosby, p. 1488.

15. **2**

Rationale: INH is given to prevent a latent TB infection from progressing to active disease. A chest x-ray film is obtained prior to initiation of preventive therapy. In infants and children, the recommended duration of INH therapy is 9 months. A minimum of 12 months of INH is recommended for children with human immunodeficiency virus.

Test-Taking Strategy: Knowledge regarding treatment with INH in a 2-year-old child is required to answer this question. Review the treatment plans for TB in children if you had difficulty with this question.

Level of Cognitive Ability: Application
Client Needs: Health Promotion and Maintenance
Integrated Concept/Process: Nursing Process/Implementation
Content Area: Child Health
Reference: Wong, D. (1999). *Whaley & Wong's nursing care of infants and children* (6th ed.). St. Louis: Mosby, p. 1488.

CRITICAL THINKING: FREE-TEXT ENTRY

Answer: Obtain a throat culture

Rationale: The throat of a child with suspected epiglottitis should not be examined or cultured because any stimulation with a tongue depressor or culture swab could cause laryngospasm and complete airway obstruction. Humidified oxygen and antipyretics are components of management. Axillary rather than oral temperatures should be taken.

Test-Taking Strategy: Recall that the high potential for laryngospasm and complete airway obstruction can occur from any throat stimulation in a child with epiglottitis. Review care to the child with epiglottitis if you had difficulty with this question.

Level of Cognitive Ability: Analysis
Client Needs: Safe, Effective Care Environment
Integrated Concept/Process: Nursing Process/Analysis
Content Area: Child Health
Reference: Ball, J., & Bindler, R. (1999). *Pediatric nursing: Caring for children* (2nd ed.). Stamford, Conn.: Appleton & Lange, p. 415.

REFERENCES

Altman, G., Buchsel, P., & Coxon, V. (2000). *Delmar's fundamental & advanced nursing skills.* Albany, N.Y.: Delmar.

Ball, J., & Bindler, R. (1999). *Pediatric nursing: Caring for children* (2nd ed.). Stamford, Conn.: Appleton & Lange.

Ball, J., & Bindler, R. (1999). *Quick reference to pediatric clinical skills.* Stamford, Conn.: Appleton & Lange.

Bowden, V., Dickey, S, & Greenberg, C. (1998). *Children and their families: The continuum of care.* Philadelphia: W.B. Saunders.

Clark, J., Queener, S., & Karb, V. (2000). *Pharmacologic basis of nursing practice* (6th ed.). St. Louis: Mosby.

Fischbach, F. (2000). *A manual of laboratory & diagnostic tests* (6th ed.). Philadelphia: Lippincott Williams & Wilkins.

Hodgson, B., & Kizior, R. (2001). *Saunders nursing drug handbook 2001.* Philadelphia: W.B. Saunders.

Web site (asthma): www.aafa.org and www.lungusa.org

Web site (CF): www.CFF.org

Web site (SIDS): www.sids.org

Wong, D. (1999). *Whaley & Wong's nursing care of infants and children* (6th ed.). St. Louis: Mosby.

Cardiovascular Disorders

▲ I. CONGESTIVE HEART FAILURE (CHF)

A. Description
1. Inability of the heart to pump sufficiently to meet the metabolic needs of the body
2. In infants and children, inadequate cardiac output is most commonly caused by congenital heart defects that produce an excessive volume or pressure load on the myocardium
3. In infants and children, a combination of both left-sided and right-sided heart failure is usually present
4. The goals of treatment are to improve cardiac function, remove accumulated fluid and sodium, decrease cardiac demands, improve tissue oxygenation, and decrease oxygen consumption

B. Assessment of early signs
1. Tachycardia, especially during rest and slight exertion
2. Tachypnea
3. Profuse scalp sweating, especially in infants
4. Fatigue and irritability
5. Sudden weight gain
6. Respiratory distress

C. Implementation
1. Monitor vital signs closely and for the early signs of CHF
2. Monitor for respiratory distress (count respirations for 1 full minute)
3. Monitor apical pulse (count pulse for 1 full minute) and monitor for dysrhythmias
4. Monitor temperature for hyperthermia and for other signs of infection, particularly respiratory infection
5. Monitor I & O; weigh diapers
6. Monitor daily weight to assess for fluid retention; a weight gain of 0.5 kg (1 pound) in 1 day is due to the accumulation of fluid
7. Monitor for facial or peripheral edema, auscultate lung sounds, and report abnormal findings
8. Elevate the head of the bed (semi-Fowler's position)
9. Maintain a neutral thermal environment to prevent cold stress in infants
10. Provide rest; decrease environmental stimuli
11. Administer cool, humidified oxygen as prescribed; use an oxygen hood for young infants and a nasal cannula or face tent for older infants and children
12. Organize nursing activities to allow for uninterrupted sleep
13. Maintain adequate nutritional status
14. Feed when hungry and soon after awakening (crying exhausts the limited energy supply), accommodating the infant's sleep and wake patterns; the infant should be well rested before feeding
15. Provide small, frequent feedings, which will be less tiring
16. Administer sedation as prescribed during the acute stage to promote rest
17. Administer digoxin (Lanoxin) as prescribed; monitor digoxin levels and for signs of digoxin toxicity, especially bradycardia and vomiting
18. Assess apical heart rate for 1 minute before administering digoxin
19. Check with physician regarding parameters for withholding digoxin; generally, digoxin is withheld if the pulse is below 90 to 110 beats per minute in infants and young children or below 70 beats per minute in older children
20. Note that infants rarely receive more than 1mL (50 µg, or 0.05 mg) of digoxin (Lanoxin) in one dose
21. Administer angiotensin-converting enzyme (ACE) inhibitors as prescribed; captopril (Capo-

---

BOX 36-1

Home Care Instructions for Administering Digoxin

Administer as prescribed
Administer 1 hour before or 2 hours after feedings
Use a calendar to mark off the dose administered
Do not mix the medication with foods or fluid
If a dose is missed and more than 4 hours has elapsed, withhold the dose and give the next dose at the scheduled time; if less than 4 hours has elapsed, administer the missed dose
If the child vomits, do not administer a second dose
If more than two consecutive doses have been missed, notify the physician; do not increase or double the dose for missed doses
If the child has teeth, give water after the medication; if possible, brush the teeth to prevent tooth decay from the sweetened liquid
If the child becomes ill, notify the physician
Keep the medication in a locked cabinet
Call the poison control center immediately if accidental overdose occurs

---

ten) or enalapril (Vasotec) is most commonly used

22. Monitor for hypotension, renal dysfunction, and cough when ACE inhibitors are administered
23. Administer diuretics as prescribed; monitor for hypokalemia with furosemide (Lasix) and with the thiazide diuretics
24. Administer potassium supplements and provide dietary sources of potassium as prescribed
25. Monitor serum electrolytes, particularly the potassium level
26. Restrict fluid as prescribed in the acute stage; monitor for dehydration
27. Check with the physician regarding sodium restriction; note that most infant formulas have slightly more sodium than does breast milk
▲ 28. Instruct the parents regarding the description of the diagnosis and administration of medications (Box 36-1)
29. Instruct the parents in cardiopulmonary resuscitation (CPR)

II. DEFECTS WITH INCREASED PULMONARY BLOOD FLOW (Box 36-2)

A. Description
   1. Intracardiac communications along the septum or an abnormal connection between the great arteries allows blood to flow from the high-pressure left side of the heart to the low-pressure right side of the heart
   2. The infant typically demonstrates signs and symptoms of CHF
B. Atrial septal defect (ASD)
   1. Abnormal opening between the atria that causes

BOX 36-2

Defects with Increased Pulmonary Blood Flow

Atrial septal defect (ASD)
Ventricular septal defect (VSD)
Atrioventricular canal (AVC) defect
Patent ductus arteriosus (PDA)

---

   an increased flow of oxygenated blood into the right side of the heart
   2. Right atrial and ventricular enlargement occurs
   3. Infant may be asymptomatic or may develop CHF
   4. Types
      a. ASD 1 (ostium primum): Opening is at the lower end of the septum
      b. ASD 2 (ostium secundum): Opening is near the center of the septum
      c. ASD 3 (sinus venosus defect): Opening is near the junction of the superior vena cava and the right atrium
   5. Nonsurgical treatment: ASD 2 may be closed by using devices during a cardiac catheterization
   6. Surgical treatment: Open repair with cardiopulmonary bypass is usually performed before school age
C. Ventricular septal defect (VSD)
   1. Abnormal opening between the right and left ventricles
   2. Many VSDs close spontaneously during the first year of life in children having small or moderate defects
   3. A characteristic murmur is present; CHF is common
   4. Nonsurgical treatment: Device closure during cardiac catheterization may be possible
   5. Surgical treatment: Open repair with cardiopulmonary bypass
D. Atrioventricular canal (AVC) defect
   1. Incomplete fusion of the endocardial cushions
   2. Most common cardiac defect in Down syndrome
   3. A characteristic murmur is present
   4. The infant usually has mild to moderate CHF; mild cyanosis increases with crying
   5. Surgical treatment: Can include either pulmonary artery banding for infants with severe symptoms (palliative) or complete repair via cardiopulmonary bypass
E. Patent ductus arteriosus (PDA)
   1. Failure of the fetal ductus arteriosus (artery connecting the aorta and the pulmonary artery) to close within the first weeks of life
   2. A characteristic machinery-like murmur is present; asymptomatic or may show signs of CHF
   3. A widened pulse pressure and bounding pulses are present

4. Medical management: indomethacin (prostaglandin inhibitor) may be administered to close a patent ductus in premature infants and some newborns
5. Nonsurgical management: Use of coils to occlude the PDA during cardiac catheterization
6. Surgical management: Surgical division or ligation of the patent vessel via a left thoracotomy; may be performed via assisted thoracoscopic surgery, which eliminates the need for thoracotomy

III. OBSTRUCTIVE DEFECTS (Box 36-3)
A. Description
   1. Blood exiting the heart meets an area of anatomic narrowing (**stenosis**) causing obstruction to blood flow
   2. The location of narrowing is usually near the valve of the obstructive defect
   3. Infants and children exhibit signs of CHF
   4. Children with mild obstruction may be asymptomatic
B. Coarctation of the aorta (COA)
   1. Localized narrowing near the insertion of the ductus arteriosus
   2. Collateral circulation develops during fetal life to maintain flow from the ascending to the descending aorta
   3. Signs of CHF in infants
   4. High blood pressure and bounding pulses in the arms, weak or absent femoral pulses, and cool lower extremities may be present
   5. Children may experience headaches, dizziness, fainting, and epistaxis resulting from hypertension
   6. Nonsurgical treatment: Balloon angioplasty in children; there is a high restenosis rate in neonates and infants with this procedure
   7. Surgical management
      a. Mechanical ventilation and inotropic support are often necessary before surgery
      b. Either resection of the coarcted portion with end-to-end anastomosis of the aorta or enlargement of the constricted section using a graft of prosthetic material or a portion of the left subclavian artery
      c. Because the defect is outside the heart, cardiopulmonary bypass is not required and a thoracotomy incision is used
C. Aortic **stenosis** (AS)
   1. Narrowing or stricture of the aortic valve, causing resistance to blood flow in the left ventricle, decreased cardiac output, left ventricular hypertrophy, and pulmonary vascular congestion
   2. Types
      a. Valvular **stenosis**: The most common type; is usually caused by malformed cusps, resulting in a bicuspid rather than a tricuspid valve, or fusion of the cusps

---

BOX 36-3

Obstructive Defects

Coarctation of the aorta (COA)
Aortic stenosis (AS)
Pulmonary stenosis (PS)

      b. Subvalvular **stenosis**: A stricture caused by a fibrous ring below a normal valve
      c. Supravalvular **Stenosis**: Occurs rarely
   3. A characteristic murmur is present
   4. Infants with severe defects demonstrate signs of decreased cardiac output with faint pulses, hypotension, tachycardia, and poor feeding
   5. Children show signs of exercise intolerance, chest pain, and dizziness when standing for long periods of time
   6. Nonsurgical treatment for valvular aortic **stenosis**: Balloon angioplasty during cardiac catheterization to dilate the narrowed valve
   7. Surgical treatment for valvular aortic **stenosis**: Aortic valvotomy under inflow occlusion (palliative); a valve replacement may be required at a second procedure
   8. Surgical treatment for subvalvular aortic **stenosis**: May involve incising a membrane if one exists or cutting the fibromuscular ring; a patch may be required
D. Pulmonary **stenosis** (PS)
   1. Narrowing at the entrance to the pulmonary artery
   2. Resistance to blood flow causes right ventricular hypertrophy and decreased pulmonary blood flow; the right ventricle may be hypoplastic
   3. Pulmonary **atresia** is the extreme form of PS in that there is total fusion of the commissures and no blood flows to the lungs
   4. A characteristic murmur is present
   5. May be asymptomatic; mild cyanosis or CHF occurs
   6. Newborns with severe narrowing will be cyanotic
   7. If PS is severe, CHF occurs
   8. Nonsurgical treatment: Balloon angioplasty during cardiac catheterization to dilate the narrowed valve
   9. Surgical treatment
      a. In infants, transventricular (closed) valvotomy procedure
      b. In children, pulmonary valvotomy with cardiopulmonary bypass

IV. DEFECTS WITH DECREASED PULMONARY BLOOD FLOW (Box 36-4)
A. Description
   1. Obstructed pulmonary blood flow and an anatomic defect (ASD or VSD) between the right and left sides of the heart

2. Pressure on the right side of the heart increases, exceeding left-sided pressure, which allows desaturated blood to **shunt** right to left, causing desaturation in the left side of the heart and in the systemic circulation
3. Typically hypoxemia and cyanosis appear

B. Tetralogy of Fallot (TOF)
   1. Includes four defects: VSD, PS, overriding aorta, and right ventricular hypertrophy
   2. If pulmonary vascular resistance is higher than systemic resistance, the **shunt** is from right to left; if systemic resistance is higher than pulmonary resistance, the **shunt** is left to right
   3. Infants
      a. May be acutely cyanotic at birth or may have mild cyanosis that progresses over the first year of life as the pulmonic **stenosis** worsens
      b. A characteristic murmur is present
      c. Acute episodes of cyanosis and hypoxia (hypercyanotic spells), called blue spells or tet spells, occur when the infant's oxygen requirements exceed the blood supply (usually during crying or after feeding)
   4. Children: With increasing cyanosis, there may be clubbing of the fingers, squatting, and poor **growth**
   5. Surgical treatment: Palliative **shunt**
      a. To increase pulmonary blood flow and increase oxygen saturation in infants who cannot undergo primary repair
      b. Blalock-Taussig or modified Blalock-Taussig **shunt** provides blood flow to the pulmonary arteries from the left or right subclavian artery
   6. Surgical treatment: Complete repair
      a. Usually performed in the first year of life
      b. Involves closure of the VSD and resection of the **stenosis,** with a pericardial patch to enlarge the right ventricular outflow tract
      c. Requires a median sternotomy and cardiopulmonary bypass

C. Tricuspid **atresia**
   1. Failure of the tricuspid valve to develop
   2. There is no communication from the right atrium to the right ventricle
   3. Blood flows through an ASD or a patent foramen ovale to the left side of the heart and through a VSD to the right ventricle and out to the lungs
   4. Often associated with pulmonic **stenosis** and transposition of the great arteries

5. Complete mixing of unoxygenated and oxygenated blood in the left side of the heart, resulting in systemic desaturation, pulmonary obstruction, and decreased pulmonary blood flow
6. Cyanosis, tachycardia, and dyspnea are seen in the newborn
7. Older children exhibit signs of chronic hypoxemia and clubbing
8. Surgical treatment
   a. For the neonate whose pulmonary blood flow depends on the patency of the ductus arteriosus, a continuous infusion of prostaglandin E_1 is initiated until surgery
   b. Placement of a **shunt** (pulmonary-to-systemic artery anastomosis) to increase blood flow to the lungs
   c. If the ASD is small, atrial septostomy is performed during cardiac catheterization
   d. Pulmonary artery banding may be performed to lessen the volume of blood to the lungs; a bidirectional Glenn **shunt** (cavopulmonary anastomosis) may be performed at age 6 to 9 months as a second stage
   e. Modified Fontan procedure: Systemic venous return is directed to the lungs, separating oxygenated and unoxygenated blood inside the heart and eliminating the excess volume load on the ventricle; does not restore normal anatomy or hemodynamics

V. **MIXED DEFECTS** (Box 36-5)
A. Description
   1. Fully saturated systemic blood flow mixes with the desaturated blood flow, causing a desaturation of the systemic blood flow
   2. Pulmonary congestion occurs and cardiac output decreases
   3. Signs of CHF; symptoms depend on the degree of desaturation
B. Transposition of the great arteries (TGA) or transposition of the great vessels (TGV)
   1. The pulmonary artery leaves the left ventricle, and the aorta exits from the right ventricle
   2. No communication between the systemic and pulmonary circulation
   3. Infants with minimal communication are severely cyanotic and depressed at birth
   4. Infants with large septal defects or a patent ductus arteriosus may be less severely cyanotic but may have symptoms of CHF
   5. Cardiomegaly is evident a few weeks after birth
   6. Nonsurgical treatment
      a. Prostaglandin E_1 may be initiated to temporarily increase blood mixing if systemic and pulmonary mixing is inadequate
      b. Balloon atrial septostomy during cardiac catheterization may be performed to increase

mixing and maintain cardiac output over a longer period

7. Surgical treatment
   a. Arterial switch procedure: Reestablishes normal circulation with the left ventricle acting as the systemic pump; involves transection and anastomosis of the great arteries, and the coronary arteries are switched from the proximal aorta to the proximal pulmonary artery, creating a new aorta
   b. Rastelli procedure: Creates physiologically normal circulation but requires multiple conduit replacements as the child grows; involves closure of the VSD and pulmonic valve and placement of a conduit from the right ventricle to the pulmonary artery

C. Total anomalous pulmonary venous connection (TAPVC)
   1. Failure of the pulmonary veins to join the left atrium
   2. Results in mixed blood being returned to the right atrium and shunted from the right to the left through an ASD
   3. The right side of the heart hypertrophies, whereas the left side of the heart may remain small
   4. CHF develops
   5. Cyanosis worsens with pulmonary vein obstruction; once obstruction occurs, the infant's condition deteriorates rapidly
   6. Surgical treatment
      a. Corrective repair performed in early infancy
      b. The pulmonary vein is anastomosed to the left atrium, the ASD is closed, and the anomalous pulmonary venous connection is ligated

D. Truncus arteriosus (TA)
   1. Failure of normal septation and division of the embryonic bulbar trunk into the pulmonary artery and the aorta, resulting in a single vessel that overrides both ventricles
   2. Blood from both ventricles mixes in the common great artery, causing desaturation and hypoxemia
   3. A characteristic murmur is present
   4. The infant exhibits moderate to severe CHF and variable cyanosis, poor **growth**, and activity intolerance
   5. Surgical treatment: Corrective repair via a modi-

fied Rastelli procedure performed in the first few months of life

E. Hypoplastic left heart syndrome (HLHS)
   1. Underdevelopment of the left side of the heart, resulting in a hypoplastic left ventricle and aortic **atresia**
   2. Mild cyanosis and signs of CHF occur until the ductus arteriosus closes; then, progressive deterioration with cyanosis and decreased cardiac output occurs, leading to cardiovascular collapse
   3. Fatal in the first few months of life without intervention
   4. Surgical treatment
      a. In the preoperative period, the neonate requires mechanical ventilation and a continuous infusion of prostaglandin E_1 to maintain ductal patency, ensuring adequate systemic blood flow
      b. Several-staged approach: Creation of a new aorta and a large atrial septal defect followed by a bidirectional Glenn **shunt**; the final repair is a modified Fontan repair
      c. Transplantation in the newborn period may be considered

VI. **IMPLEMENTATION: CARDIOVASCULAR DEFECTS**
A. Monitor for signs of a defect in the infant or child
B. Monitor vital signs closely
C. Monitor respiratory status for the presence of **nasal flaring** and use of accessory muscles, and notify the physician if any changes occur
D. Auscultate breath sounds for crackles, rhonchi, or rales
E. If respiratory effort is increased, place the child in reverse Trendelenburg position (elevate head and upper body) to decrease the work of breathing
F. Administer humidified oxygen as prescribed
G. Provide endotracheal tube and ventilator care if necessary and as prescribed, and restrain the hands of an intubated child
H. Monitor for hypercyanotic spells (Box 36-6)
I. Assess for signs of CHF, such as fluid retention in the eyes, hands, feet, and chest
J. Assess peripheral pulses
K. Monitor I & O and notify the physician if a decrease in urine output occurs
L. Assess urine output, weighing diapers as necessary
M. Obtain daily weight
N. Maintain fluid restriction if prescribed
O. Provide adequate nutrition (high calorie requirements) as prescribed
P. Administer medications as prescribed
Q. Keep child as stress free as possible; plan interventions to allow maximal rest for the child
R. Prepare parents and child, if appropriate, for surgery

BOX 36-6

Treatment for Hypercyanotic Spells

Place the infant in a knee-chest position
Administer 100% oxygen by face mask
Administer morphine sulfate as prescribed
Administer IV fluids as prescribed

S. Allow parents and child to verbalize feelings and concerns regarding disorder
T. Familiarize parents and child with hospital procedures and equipment

VII. CARDIAC SURGERY

A. Implementation postoperatively
   1. Monitor vital signs frequently
   2. Monitor temperature and notify the physician if a fever occurs
   3. Monitor for signs of sepsis, such as fever, chills, diaphoresis, lethargy, and altered levels of consciousness
   4. Maintain aseptic technique
   5. Monitor lines, tubes, or catheters that are in place and remove promptly as prescribed when no longer needed, to prevent infection
   6. Assess for signs of discomfort, such as irritability, changes in heart rate, respiratory rate, and blood pressure, and the inability to sleep
   7. Administer pain medications as prescribed, noting effectiveness
   8. Administer antibiotics and antipyretics as prescribed
   9. Encourage rest periods
   10. Facilitate parent-child contact as soon as possible
B. Postoperative home care (Box 36-7)

VIII. RHEUMATIC FEVER

A. Description
   1. An inflammatory autoimmune disease that affects the connective tissues of the heart, joints, subcutaneous tissues, and/or blood vessels of the central nervous system (CNS)
   2. The most serious complication is rheumatic heart disease, which affects the cardiac valves
   3. Presents 2 to 6 weeks following an untreated or partially treated group A beta-hemolytic streptococcal infection of the upper respiratory tract
   4. Jones criteria are utilized in determining the diagnosis
B. Assessment
   1. Aschoff bodies (lesions): found in the heart, blood vessels, brain, and serous surfaces of the joints and pleura
   2. Signs of carditis: shortness of breath, edema

BOX 36-7

Home Care After Cardiac Surgery

Omit play outside for several weeks
Avoid activities in which the child could fall, such as bike riding, for 2 to 4 weeks
Avoid crowds for 2 weeks after discharge
Follow a no-added-salt diet if prescribed
Do not add any new foods to the infant's eating schedule
Do not place creams, lotions, or powders on the incision until completely healed
The child may return to school the third week after discharge, starting with half-days
No physical education for 2 months
Instruct the parents to discipline the child normally
Instruct the parents about the importance of the 2-week follow-up
Avoid immunizations, invasive procedures, and dental visits for 2 months
Advise the parents regarding the importance of a dental visit every 6 months after age 3 and to inform the dentist of the cardiac problem so that antibiotics can be prescribed if necessary
Instruct the parents to call the physician when coughing, tachypnea, cyanosis, vomiting, diarrhea, anorexia, pain, fever, or any swelling, redness, or drainage occurs at the site of the incision

---

   of the face, abdomen or ankles, and precordial pain
   3. Signs of polyarthritis: edema, inflammation of large joints, and joint pain
   4. Erythema marginatum: erythematous macular rash on the trunk and extremities
   5. Subcutaneous nodules found in crops over the bony prominences
   6. Chorea: sudden, aimless, irregular movements of the extremities, involuntary facial grimaces, speech disturbances, emotional lability, and muscle weakness
   7. Fever: low-grade fever that spikes in the late afternoon
   8. Elevated antistreptolysin O titer
   9. Elevated sedimentation rate
   10. Elevated C-reactive protein
C. Implementation
   1. Assess vital signs
   2. Assess for the clinical manifestations
   3. Control joint pain and inflammation with massage and alternating hot and cold applications as prescribed
   4. Provide bed rest during acute febrile phase
   5. Limit physical exercise in the child with carditis
   6. Administer antibiotics (penicillin) as prescribed
   7. Administer salicylates and antiinflammatory agents as prescribed (should not be instituted

before the diagnosis is confirmed, because these medications mask the polyarthritis)

8. Initiate seizure precautions if the child is experiencing chorea
9. Instruct the parents about the importance of follow-up, and the need for antibiotic prophylaxis for dental work, infection, and invasive procedures
10. Advise the child to inform the parents if anyone in school develops a streptococcal throat infection

IX. KAWASAKI DISEASE
A. Description
   1. Known as mucocutaneous lymph node syndrome and is an acute systemic inflammatory illness
   2. The cause is unknown but may be associated with an infection from an organism or toxin
   3. Cardiac involvement is the most serious complication; aneurysms can develop
B. Assessment
   1. Acute stage
      a. Fever
      b. Conjunctival hyperemia
      c. Red throat
      d. Swollen hands, rash, and enlargement of the cervical lymph nodes
   2. Subacute stage
      a. Cracking lips and fissures
      b. Desquamation of the skin on the tips of the fingers and toes
      c. Joint pain
      d. Cardiac manifestations
      e. Thrombocytosis
   3. Convalescent stage: Child appears normal but signs of inflammation may be present
C. Implementation
   1. Monitor temperature frequently
   2. Assess heart sounds and rhythm
   3. Assess extremities for edema, redness, and desquamation
   4. Examine eyes for conjunctivitis
   5. Monitor mucous membranes for inflammation
   6. Monitor dietary and fluid intake (I & O)
   7. Administer soft foods and liquids that are neither too hot nor too cold
   8. Weigh daily
   9. Provide passive range-of-motion exercises to facilitate joint movement
   10. Administer acetylsalicylic acid (aspirin) as prescribed for its antipyretic and antiplatelet effect
   11. Administer IV immune globulin (IVIG) as prescribed; reduces the duration of fever and the incidence of coronary artery lesions and aneurysms
   12. Instruct the parents in the administration of

prescribed medications, the need to monitor for bleeding, and the need for follow-up to monitor for cardiac complications

PRACTICE QUESTIONS

1. A nurse caring for an infant with congenital heart disease is monitoring the infant closely for signs of congestive heart failure (CHF). The nurse assesses the infant closely for which early sign of CHF?
   1. Cough
   2. Tachycardia
   3. Slow and shallow breathing
   4. Pallor

2. A physician has prescribed oxygen PRN for an infant with congestive heart failure (CHF). In which situation would the nurse plan to administer the oxygen to the infant?
   1. During feeding
   2. When the mother is holding the infant
   3. When changing the infant's diapers
   4. When drawing blood for electrolyte values

3. An infant with congestive heart failure (CHF) is receiving diuretic therapy, and a nurse is closely monitoring the intake and output (I & O). The nurse uses which most appropriate method to assess the urine output?
   1. Inserting a Foley catheter
   2. Weighing the diapers
   3. Comparing intake with output
   4. Measuring the amount of water added to formula

4. A nurse is monitoring the daily weight of an infant with congestive heart failure (CHF). Which of the following alerts the nurse to suspect fluid accumulation and the need to call the physician?
   1. Bradypnea
   2. Diaphoresis
   3. Decreased blood pressure (BP)
   4. A weight gain of 1 pound in 1 day

5. A nurse provides home care instructions to the parents of a child with congestive heart failure (CHF) regarding the procedure for the administration of digoxin (Lanoxin). Which statement if made by a parent indicates the need for further education?
   1. "If the child vomits after medication administration, I will repeat the dose."
   2. "I will take the child's pulse before administering the medication."
   3. "I will not mix the medication with food."
   4. "If more than one dose is missed, I will call the physician."

6. A nurse is assigned to care for an infant with a diagnosis of tricuspid atresia. The nurse plans care, knowing that in this disorder:
   1. There is no communication between the systemic and pulmonary circulation

2. Frequent episodes of hypercyanotic spells occur
3. There is no communication from the right atrium to the right ventricle
4. A single vessel overrides both ventricles

7. Prostaglandin E$_1$ is prescribed for a child with transposition of the great arteries. The mother of the child is a registered nurse and asks the nurse why the child needs the medication. The most appropriate response would be to tell the mother that the medication:
   1. Maintains an adequate hormonal level
   2. Maintains the position of the great arteries
   3. Provides adequate oxygen saturation and maintains cardiac output
   4. Prevents tet spells

8. A clinic nurse reviews the record of a child just seen by a physician. The physician has documented a diagnosis of suspected aortic stenosis. The nurse expects to note documentation of which of the following clinical manifestations specifically found in this disorder?
   1. Hyperactivity
   2. Exercise intolerance
   3. Pallor
   4. Gastrointestinal disturbances

9. A nurse has provided home care instructions to the mother of a child who is being discharged following cardiac surgery. Which statement made by the mother indicates a need for further instructions?
   1. "Large crowds of people need to be avoided for at least 2 weeks following surgery."
   2. "I can apply lotion or powder to the incision if it is itchy."
   3. "A balance of rest and exercise is important."
   4. "Activities in which the child could fall need to be avoided for 2 to 4 weeks."

10. A nurse receives a telephone call from the admitting office and is told that a child with rheumatic fever (RF) will be arriving in the nursing unit for admission. On admission, the nurse prepares to ask the mother which question to elicit assessment information specific to the development of RF?
    1. "Did the child have a sore throat or an unexplained fever within the last 2 months?"
    2. "Has the child had any nausea or vomiting?"
    3. "Has the child complained of headaches?"
    4. "Has the child complained of back pain?"

11. Acetylsalicylic acid (aspirin) is prescribed for a child with rheumatic fever. A nurse would question this order if there were documented evidence that the child had which of the following?
    1. A viral infection
    2. Joint pain

3. Facial edema
4. Arthralgia

12. A nurse is caring for a child with a suspected diagnosis of rheumatic fever (RF). The nurse reviews the laboratory results, knowing that which laboratory study would assist in confirming the diagnosis of RF?
    1. White blood cell count
    2. Red blood cell count
    3. Immunoglobulin
    4. Antistreptolysin O titer

13. The nurse is caring for a child with a diagnosis of Kawasaki disease. The mother of the child asks the nurse about the disorder. The nurse tells the mother that:
    1. It is an acquired cell-mediated immunodeficiency disorder
    2. It is an inflammatory autoimmune disease that affects the connective tissue of the heart, joints, and subcutaneous tissues
    3. It is a chronic multisystem autoimmune disease characterized by the inflammation of connective tissue
    4. Is also called mucocutaneous lymph node syndrome and is a febrile generalized vasculitis of unknown etiology

14. A nurse is preparing for the admission of a child with a diagnosis of acute-stage Kawasaki disease. On assessment of the child, the nurse expects to note which clinical manifestation of the acute stage of the disease?
    1. Conjunctival hyperemia
    2. Cracked lips
    3. Desquamation of the skin
    4. A normal appearance

15. A nurse is reviewing the physician's orders for a child who was just admitted to the hospital with a diagnosis of Kawasaki disease. The nurse expects to note an order for which of the following as part of the treatment plan?
    1. Morphine sulfate
    2. Immune globulin
    3. Heparin infusion
    4. Digoxin (Lanoxin)

CRITICAL THINKING: FREE-TEXT ENTRY

A nurse is caring for an infant with a diagnosis of tetralogy of Fallot. The infant suddenly becomes cyanotic, and the nurse recognizes that the infant is experiencing a hypercyanotic spell. The nurse immediately places the infant in what position?

Answer: _____

ANSWERS

1. 2

Rationale: The early signs of CHF include tachycardia, tachypnea, profuse scalp sweating, fatigue and irritability, sudden weight gain, and respiratory distress. A cough may occur in CHF as a result of mucosal swelling and irritation, but it is not an early sign. Pallor may be noted in the infant with CHF, but is also not an early sign.

Test-Taking Strategy: Use the process of elimination and note the key word "early." Think about the physiology and the effects on the heart when fluid overload occurs. These concepts will assist in directing you to option 2. If you had difficulty with this question, review the early signs of CHF in an infant.

Level of Cognitive Ability: Analysis
Client Needs: Physiological Integrity
Integrated Concept/Process: Nursing Process/Assessment
Content Area: Child Health
Reference: Wong, D. (1999). *Whaley & Wong's nursing care of infants and children* (6th ed.). St. Louis: Mosby, p. 1600.

2. 4

Rationale: Crying exhausts the limited energy supply, increases the workload of the heart, and increases the oxygen demands. Oxygen administration may be prescribed for stressful periods, especially during bouts of crying or invasive procedures. Options 1, 2, and 3 are not likely to produce crying in the infant.

Test-Taking Strategy: Use the process of elimination. Recall the situations that would place stress and an increased workload on the heart. This concept should easily direct you to option 4. Drawing blood is an invasive procedure, which would likely cause the child to cry. Review care to the child with CHF if you had difficulty with this question.

Level of Cognitive Ability: Analysis
Client Needs: Physiological Integrity
Integrated Concept/Process: Nursing Process/Planning
Content Area: Child Health
Reference: Wong, D. (1999). *Whaley & Wong's nursing care of infants and children* (6th ed.). St. Louis: Mosby, p. 1601.

3. 2

Rationale: The most appropriate method for assessing urine output in an infant on diuretic therapy is to weigh the diapers. Comparing intake with output would not provide an accurate measure of urine output. Measuring the amount of water added to formula is unrelated to the amount of output. Although Foley catheter drainage is most accurate in determining output, it is not the most appropriate method in an infant, and places the infant at risk for infection.

Test-Taking Strategy: Use the process of elimination. Eliminate options 3 and 4 first because they will not provide an indication of urine output. From the remaining options, note the words "most appropriate" in the stem of the question. These words will direct you to option 2. Review care to the infant receiving diuretic therapy if you had difficulty with this question.

Level of Cognitive Ability: Analysis
Client Needs: Physiological Integrity
Integrated Concept/Process: Nursing Process/Assessment
Content Area: Child Health
Reference: Ball, J., & Bindler, R. (1999). *Pediatric nursing: Caring for children* (2nd ed.). Stamford, Conn.: Appleton & Lange, p. 302.

4. 4

Rationale: A weight gain of 0.5 kg (1 pound) in 1 day is due to the accumulation of fluid. The nurse should assess urine output, assess for evidence of facial or peripheral edema, auscultate lung sounds, and report the weight gain to the physician. Tachypnea and an increased BP would occur with fluid accumulation. Diaphoresis is a sign of CHF but is not specific to fluid accumulation, and usually occurs with exertional activities.

Test-Taking Strategy: Use the process of elimination and focus on the issue, fluid accumulation. Note the relationship between "fluid accumulation" in the question and "weight gain" in the correct option. Review the indications of fluid accumulation in an infant with CHF if you had difficulty with this question.

Level of Cognitive Ability: Analysis
Client Needs: Physiological Integrity
Integrated Concept/Process: Nursing Process/Analysis
Content Area: Child Health
Reference: Ball, J., & Bindler, R. (1999). *Pediatric nursing: Caring for children* (2nd ed.). Stamford, Conn.: Appleton & Lange, p. 301.

5. 1

Rationale: The parents need to be instructed that if the child vomits after the digoxin is administered, they are not to repeat the dose. Options 2, 3, and 4 are accurate instructions regarding the administration of this medication. In addition, the parents should be instructed that if a dose is missed and it is not identified until 4 hours later, the dose should not be administered.

Test-Taking Strategy: Use the process of elimination. Note the key words "need for further education." General knowledge regarding digoxin administration will assist in eliminating option 2. Principles related to administering medications to children will assist in eliminating option 3. From the remaining options, select option 1 over option 4 because if the child vomits, it would be difficult to determine if the medication was also vomited or was absorbed by the body. Review home care instructions regarding the administration of digoxin if you had difficulty with this question.

Level of Cognitive Ability: Analysis
Client Needs: Health Promotion and Maintenance
Integrated Concept/Process: Teaching/Learning
Content Area: Child Health
Reference: Wong, D. (1999). *Whaley & Wong's nursing care of infants and children* (6th ed.). St. Louis: Mosby, p. 1601.

6. 3

Rationale: In tricuspid atresia, there is no communication from the right atrium to the right ventricle. Option 1 describes transposition of the great arteries. Frequent episodes of hypercyanotic spells occur in tetralogy of Fallot. Option 4 describes truncus arteriosus.

Test-Taking Strategy: Use the process of elimination. Note the relationship between "tricuspid atresia" and the description in option 3. Recalling that the tricuspid valve is located between the right atrium and the right ventricle will direct you to this option. Review the characteristics of tricuspid atresia if you had difficulty with this question.

Level of Cognitive Ability: Comprehension
Client Needs: Physiological Integrity
Integrated Concept/Process: Nursing Process/Planning

Content Area: Child Health
Reference: Wong, D. (1999). *Whaley & Wong's nursing care of infants and children* (6th ed.). St. Louis: Mosby, p. 1615.

7. **3**

Rationale: A child with transposition of the great arteries may receive prostaglandin E₁ temporarily to increase blood mixing if systemic and pulmonary mixing is inadequate to provide an oxygen saturation of 75% or to maintain cardiac output. Options 1, 2, and 4 are incorrect. In addition, tet spells occur in tetralogy of Fallot.

Test-Taking Strategy: Use the ABCs—airway, breathing, and circulation—to answer the question. Option 3 addresses circulation. Review the purpose of this medication in this condition if you had difficulty with this question.
Level of Cognitive Ability: Application
Client Needs: Physiological Integrity
Integrated Concept/Process: Teaching/Learning
Content Area: Child Health
Reference: Wong, D. (1999). *Whaley & Wong's nursing care of infants and children* (6th ed.). St. Louis: Mosby, p. 1617.

8. **2**

Rationale: The child with aortic stenosis shows signs of exercise intolerance, chest pain, and dizziness when standing for long periods of time. Pallor may be noted, but is not specific to this type of disorder alone. Options 1 and 4 are not related to this disorder.

Test-Taking Strategy: Use the process of elimination, focusing on the disorder. Options 1 and 4 can be easily eliminated first because they are not associated with a cardiac disorder. From the remaining options, noting the word "specifically" in the stem of the question will direct you to option 2. Review the manifestations associated with aortic stenosis if you had difficulty with this question.
Level of Cognitive Ability: Analysis
Client Needs: Physiological Integrity
Integrated Concept/Process: Communication and Documentation
Content Area: Child Health
Reference: Wong, D. (1999). *Whaley & Wong's nursing care of infants and children* (6th ed.). St. Louis: Mosby, p. 1613.

9. **2**

Rationale: The mother should be instructed that lotions and powders should not be applied to the incision site. Options 1, 3, and 4 are accurate instructions regarding home care after cardiac surgery.

Test-Taking Strategy: Use the process of elimination. Note the key words "indicates a need for further instructions" in the stem of the question. Using general principles related to postoperative incisional site care will direct you to option 2. Review home care instructions following cardiac surgery if you had difficulty with this question.
Level of Cognitive Ability: Analysis
Client Needs: Health Promotion and Maintenance
Integrated Concept/Process: Teaching/Learning
Content Area: Child Health
Reference: Bowden, V., Dickey, S., & Greenberg, C. (1998). *Children and their families: The continuum of care.* Philadelphia: W.B. Saunders, p. 811.

10. **1**

Rationale: RF characteristically presents 2 to 6 weeks after an untreated or partially treated group A beta-hemolytic strepto-

coccal infection of the upper respiratory tract. Initially, the nurse determines if the child had a sore throat or an unexplained fever within the past 2 months. Options 2, 3, and 4 are unrelated to RF.

Test-Taking Strategy: Use the process of elimination. Note the similarity between rheumatic "fever" in the question and the word "fever" in the correct option. If you had difficulty with this question, review the etiology related to RF.
Level of Cognitive Ability: Analysis
Client Needs: Physiological Integrity
Integrated Concept/Process: Nursing Process/Assessment
Content Area: Child Health
Reference: Ball, J., & Bindler, R. (1999). *Pediatric nursing: Caring for children* (2nd ed.). Stamford, Conn.: Appleton & Lange, p. 496.

11. **1**

Rationale: Antiinflammatory agents including aspirin may be prescribed for the child with RF. Aspirin should not be given to a child who has chickenpox or other viral infections such as the flu. Options 2 and 4 are clinical manifestations of RF. Facial edema may be associated with the development of a cardiac complication.

Test-Taking Strategy: Use the process of elimination. Options 2 and 4 can be eliminated because they are similar. Knowledge that facial edema may indicate a cardiac complication will assist in eliminating this option. Review the contraindications related to the use of aspirin if you had difficulty with this question.
Level of Cognitive Ability: Analysis
Client Needs: Safe, Effective Care Environment
Integrated Concept/Process: Communication and Documentation
Content Area: Child Health
Reference: Hodgson, B., & Kizior, R. (2001). *Saunders nursing drug handbook 2001.* Philadelphia: W.B. Saunders, p. 76.

12. **4**

Rationale: A diagnosis of RF is confirmed by the presence of two major manifestations or one major and two minor manifestations from the Jones criteria. In addition, evidence of a recent streptococcal infection is confirmed by a positive antistreptolysin O titer, streptozyme assay, or an anti-DNase B assay. Options 1, 2, and 3 will not assist in confirming the diagnosis of RF.

Test-Taking Strategy: Use the process of elimination. Recalling that RF is characteristically associated with streptococcal infection will easily direct you to option 4. If you had difficulty with this question, review the Jones criteria.
Level of Cognitive Ability: Analysis
Client Needs: Physiological Integrity
Integrated Concept/Process: Nursing Process/Assessment
Content Area: Child Health
Reference: Ball, J., & Bindler, R. (1999). *Pediatric nursing: Caring for children* (2nd ed.). Stamford, Conn.: Appleton & Lange, p. 496.

13. **4**

Rationale: Kawasaki disease, also called mucocutaneous lymph node syndrome, is a febrile generalized vasculitis of unknown etiology. Option 1 describes human immunodeficiency virus (HIV) infection. Option 2 describes rheumatic fever. Option 3 describes systemic lupus erythematosus.

Test-Taking Strategy: Knowledge regarding the description of Kawasaki disease is required to answer this question. Review this disorder if you are unfamiliar with it.
Level of Cognitive Ability: Comprehension
Client Needs: Physiological Integrity
Integrated Concept/Process: Teaching/Learning
Content Area: Child Health
Reference: Wong, D. (1999). *Whaley & Wong's nursing care of infants and children* (6th ed.). St. Louis: Mosby, p. 1631.

14. **1**
Rationale: In the acute stage, the child presents with fever, conjunctival hyperemia, a red throat, swollen hands, a rash, and enlargement of the cervical lymph nodes. In the subacute stage, cracking lips and fissures, desquamation of the skin on the tips of the fingers and toes, joint pain, cardiac manifestations, and thrombocytosis occur. In the convalescent stage, the child appears normal but signs of inflammation may be present.
Test-Taking Strategy: Use the process of elimination. Noting the key words "acute stage" in the question will assist in directing you to option 1. Review the clinical manifestations associated with each stage of Kawasaki disease if you had difficulty with this question.
Level of Cognitive Ability: Analysis
Client Needs: Physiological Integrity
Integrated Concept/Process: Nursing Process/Assessment
Content Area: Child Health
Reference: Ball, J., & Bindler, R. (1999). *Pediatric nursing: Caring for children* (2nd ed.). Stamford, Conn.: Appleton & Lange, p. 500.

15. **2**
Rationale: Intravenous immune globulin (IVIG) is administered to the child with Kawasaki disease to decrease the incidence of coronary artery lesions and aneurysms and to decrease fever and inflammation. Options 1, 3, and 4 are not components of the treatment plan for this disease.
Test-Taking Strategy: Use the process of elimination. Remember that the pharmacological treatment for this disease is acetylsalicylic acid (aspirin) and IVIG. If you had difficulty with this question, review the treatment plan for the child with Kawasaki disease.
Level of Cognitive Ability: Analysis
Client Needs: Physiological Integrity
Integrated Concept/Process: Nursing Process/Analysis
Content Area: Child Health
Reference: Ball, J., & Bindler, R. (1999). *Pediatric nursing: Caring for children* (2nd ed.). Stamford, Conn.: Appleton & Lange, p. 500.

CRITICAL THINKING: FREE-TEXT ENTRY

Answer: The nurse places the infant in a knee-chest position
Rationale: If a hypercyanotic spell occurs, the nurse immediately places the infant in a knee-chest position. This position improves systemic arterial oxygen saturation.
Test-Taking Strategy: Focus on the issue of the question, a hypercyanotic spell. Think about the position that will improve oxygenation. Review the interventions if a hypercyanotic spell occurs in an infant, if you had difficulty with this question.
Level of Cognitive Ability: Application
Client Needs: Physiological Integrity
Integrated Concept/Process: Nursing Process/Implementation
Content Area: Child Health
Reference: Wong, D. (1999). *Whaley & Wong's nursing care of infants and children* (6th ed.). St. Louis: Mosby, p. 1607.

REFERENCES

Ball, J., & Bindler, R. (1999). *Pediatric nursing: Caring for children* (2nd ed.). Stamford, Conn.: Appleton & Lange.

Bowden, V., Dickey, S, & Greenberg, C. (1998). *Children and their families: The continuum of care.* Philadelphia: W.B. Saunders.

Hodgson, B., & Kizior, R. (2001). *Saunders nursing drug handbook 2001.* Philadelphia: W.B. Saunders.

Wong, D. (1999). *Whaley & Wong's nursing care of infants and children* (6th ed.). St. Louis: Mosby.

Gastrointestinal Disorders

I. VOMITING

A. Description
1. The major concerns when a child is vomiting are the risk of dehydration, the loss of fluid and electrolytes, and the development of metabolic alkalosis
2. Additional concerns include aspiration, atelectasis, and the development of pneumonia

B. Assessment
1. Signs of aspiration
2. Character of vomitus
3. Pain and abdominal cramping
4. Dehydration
5. Fluid and electrolyte imbalances
6. Metabolic alkalosis

C. Implementation
1. Maintain a patent airway
2. Position the child on side to prevent aspiration
3. Monitor vital signs
4. Monitor the character, amount, and frequency of vomiting
5. Assess the force of the vomiting, as projectile vomiting is indicative of pyloric **stenosis** or increased intracranial pressure
6. Monitor intake and output (I & 0) and for signs of dehydration
7. Monitor electrolyte levels
8. Provide oral rehydration therapy as tolerated and as prescribed; start feeding slowly, with small amounts of fluid at frequent intervals
9. Assess for diarrhea or abdominal pain
10. Advise the parents to inform the physician when signs of dehydration, blood in vomitus, forceful vomiting, or abdominal pain is present

II. DIARRHEA

A. Description: The major concerns when a child is having diarrhea are the risk of dehydration, the loss of fluid and electrolytes, and the development of metabolic acidosis

B. Assessment
1. Character of stools
2. Pain and abdominal cramping
3. Dehydration
4. Fluid and electrolyte imbalances
5. Metabolic acidosis

C. Implementation
1. Monitor vital signs
2. Monitor the character, amount, and frequency of diarrhea
3. Monitor skin integrity
4. Monitor I & O and for signs of dehydration
5. Monitor electrolyte levels
6. For mild to moderate dehydration, provide oral rehydration therapy; avoid carbonated beverages and those containing high amounts of sugar
7. For severe dehydration, maintain NPO status to place the bowel at rest and provide fluid and electrolyte replacement by IV as prescribed; if potassium is prescribed by IV, ensure that the child has voided prior to administering
8. Reintroduce a normal diet once rehydration is achieved
9. Provide enteric isolation as required
10. Instruct the parents in good handwashing technique

III. CLEFT LIP AND CLEFT PALATE

A. Description
1. A congenital anomaly that occurs as a result of failure of soft tissue or bony structure to fuse during embryonic development
2. Involves abnormal openings in the lip or palate that may occur unilaterally or bilaterally and are readily apparent at birth
3. Causes include genetic, **hereditary,** and environ-

mental factors; exposure to radiation or rubella virus; chromosome abnormalities; and teratogenic factors

4. Closure of cleft lip defect precedes that of the palate and is performed usually during the first weeks of life

5. Cleft palate repair is performed sometime between 12 and 18 months of age to allow for the palatal changes that take place with normal **growth;** a cleft palate is closed before the child develops faulty speech habits

B. Assessment

1. Cleft lip can range from a slight notch to a complete separation from the floor of the nose

2. Cleft palate can include nasal distortion, midline or bilateral cleft, and variable extension from the uvula and soft and hard palate

▲ C. Implementation

1. Assess the ability to suck, swallow, handle normal secretions, and breathe without distress

2. Assess fluid and calorie intake daily and monitor weight

3. Modify feeding techniques; plan to use specialized feeding techniques, obturators, and special nipples and feeders

▲ 4. Hold the child in an upright position and direct the formula to the side and back of the mouth to prevent aspiration; feed small amounts gradually and burp frequently

5. Position on side after feeding

6. Keep suction equipment and bulb syringe at bedside

7. Encourage breastfeeding if appropriate

8. Teach the parents special feeding or suctioning techniques

9. Teach the parents the ESSR (enlarge, stimulate sucking, swallow, rest) method of feeding (Box 37-1)

10. Encourage the parents to describe their feelings related to the deformity

D. Implementation postoperatively

1. Cleft lip repair

   a. A lip protector device may be taped securely to the cheeks to prevent trauma to the suture line

▲ b. Position the child on the side lateral to the repair or on the back; avoid the prone

position to prevent rubbing of the surgical site on the mattress

   c. After feeding, cleanse the suture line of formula or serosanguineous drainage with a cotton-tipped swab dipped in saline; apply antibiotic ointment if prescribed

2. Cleft palate repair

   a. Child is allowed to lie on the abdomen

   b. Feedings are resumed by bottle, breast, or cup

   c. Oral packing may be secured to the palate (removed in 2 to 3 days)

   d. Do not allow the child to brush his or her teeth

   e. Instruct the parents to avoid offering hard food items to the child, such as toast or cookies

3. Soft elbow or jacket restraints may be used ▲ (check agency policies and procedures) to keep the child from touching the repair site; remove restraints at least every 2 hours to assess skin integrity and allow for exercising the arms

4. Avoid contact with sharp objects near the ▲ surgical site

5. Avoid the use of oral suction or placing objects in the mouth such as tongue depressor, thermometer, straws, spoons, forks, or pacifiers

6. Provide analgesics for pain ▲

7. Instruct the parents in feeding techniques and in the care of the surgical site

8. Instruct the parents to monitor for signs of infection at the surgical site, such as redness, swelling, or drainage

9. Encourage the parents to hold the child

10. Initiate appropriate referrals for speech impairment or language-based **learning** difficulties

IV. ESOPHAGEAL ATRESIA AND TRACHEOESOPHAGEAL FISTULA

A. Description

1. The esophagus terminates before it reaches the stomach and/or a fistula is present that forms an unnatural connection with the trachea

2. The condition causes oral intake to enter the lungs or a large amount of air to enter the stomach, and choking, coughing, and severe abdominal distention can occur

3. Aspiration pneumonia and severe respiratory distress will develop, and death will occur without surgical intervention

4. Treatment includes maintenance of a patent airway, prevention of pneumonia, gastric or blind pouch decompression, supportive therapy, and surgical repair

B. Assessment

1. Frothy saliva in the mouth and nose, and drooling

BOX 37-1

ESSR Method of Feeding

ENLARGE the nipple
STIMULATE the suck reflex
SWALLOW
REST to allow the child to finish swallowing what has been placed in the mouth

2. Coughing and choking during feedings
3. Unexplained cyanosis
4. **Regurgitation** and vomiting
5. Abdominal distention
6. Inability to pass a small-gauge (no. 5 French) orogastric feeding tube via the mouth into the stomach

C. Implementation preoperatively
1. Infant may be placed in an incubator or radiant warmer and humidified oxygen is administered (intubation and mechanical ventilation may be necessary if respiratory distress occurs)
2. Maintain an NPO status
3. Maintain IV fluids as prescribed
4. Suction accumulated secretions from the mouth and pharynx
5. A double-lumen catheter is placed into the upper esophageal pouch and attached to intermittent or continuous low suction to keep the pouch empty of secretions; it is irrigated with normal saline as prescribed to prevent clogging
6. Maintain in an upright position to facilitate drainage and to prevent aspiration of gastric secretions
7. A gastrostomy tube may be placed and is left open so that air entering the stomach through the fistula can escape, minimizing the danger of **regurgitation**
8. Administer broad-spectrum antibiotics as prescribed, because of the high risk for aspiration pneumonia

D. Implementation postoperatively
1. Monitor respiratory status
2. Maintain IV fluids, antibiotics, and parenteral nutrition as prescribed
3. Monitor I & O and weight daily
4. Inspect surgical site
5. Provide care to the chest tube if in place
6. Assess for signs of pain
7. Assess for dehydration and possible fluid overload
8. Monitor for anastomotic leaks as evidenced by purulent chest drainage, increased temperature, and an increased white blood cell count
9. The double-lumen catheter is attached to low suction
10. If a gastrostomy tube is present, it is attached to gravity drainage until the infant can tolerate feedings (usually the 5th to 7th day postoperatively)
11. Before oral feedings and removal of the chest tube, a barium swallow is performed to verify the integrity of the esophageal anastomosis
12. Prior to feeding, the gastrostomy tube is elevated and secured above the level of the stomach to allow gastric secretions to pass to the duodenum and swallowed air to escape through the open gastrostomy tube

13. Feedings through the gastrostomy tube may be prescribed until the anastomosis is healed
14. Oral feedings are begun with sterile water, followed by frequent small feedings of formula
15. The gastrostomy tube may be removed prior to discharge or may be maintained for supplemental feedings at home
16. If the infant is awaiting esophageal replacement, a cervical esophagostomy may be performed
17. Assess cervical esophagostomy site for redness, breakdown, or exudate (continued discharge or saliva can cause skin breakdown); remove drainage frequently and apply a protective ointment, a barrier dressing, and/or a collection device
18. If the infant is awaiting esophageal replacement, nonnutritive sucking is provided by a pacifier; infants who remain NPO for extended periods and have not received oral stimulation frequently may have difficulty eating by mouth after surgery and develop oral hypersensitivity and food aversion
19. Instruct the parents in the techniques of suctioning, gastrostomy tube care and feedings, and skin site care as appropriate
20. Instruct parents to identify behaviors that indicate the need for suctioning, signs of respiratory distress, and signs of a constricted esophagus (poor feeding, dysphagia, drooling, or regurgitated undigested food)

V. GASTROESOPHAGEAL REFLUX (GER)

A. Description
1. Backflow of gastric contents into the esophagus as a result of relaxation or incompetence of the lower esophageal or cardiac sphincter
2. Complications include esophagitis, esophageal strictures, aspiration of gastric contents, and aspiration pneumonia
3. Most infants with GER have a mild problem that improves in about 1 year and requires only medical therapy
4. Treatment includes diet, positioning, medications, and surgery; however, surgery is performed only in children with severe complications from the GER

B. Assessment
1. Passive **regurgitation** or emesis
2. Poor weight gain
3. Hematemesis and melena
4. Irritability
5. Heartburn (in older children)
6. Anemia from blood loss

C. Implementation
1. Assess amount and characteristics of emesis
2. Assess the relation of vomiting to the times of feedings and infant activity
3. Monitor breath sounds before and after feedings
4. Place suction equipment at the bedside

5. Monitor I & O
6. Monitor for signs and symptoms of dehydration
7. Maintain IV fluids as prescribed

D. Positioning: Place in either the flat prone position or the head-elevated prone position following feedings and at night

E. Diet
1. Provide small, frequent feedings to decrease the amount of **regurgitation;** nasogastric tube feedings are indicated if severe **regurgitation** and poor **growth** are present
2. For infants, thicken formula by adding 1 tablespoon of rice cereal per 6 ounces of formula and crosscut the nipple; monitor for coughing during feeding
3. Breastfeeding may continue, and the mother may provide more frequent feeding times or express milk for thickening with rice cereal
4. Burp the infant frequently when feeding and handle the infant minimally after feedings
5. For toddlers, feed solids first, followed by liquids
6. The parents are instructed to avoid feeding the child fatty foods, chocolate, tomato products, carbonated liquids, fruit juices, citrus products, and spicy foods
7. Avoid vigorous play after feeding and avoid feeding just before bedtime

F. Medications
1. Administer antacids and histamine receptor antagonists as prescribed, to reduce the amount of acid present in gastric secretions and to prevent esophagitis
2. Administer prokinetic agents to accelerate gastric emptying and decrease reflux
3. Administer acetaminophen (Tylenol) as prescribed to relieve reflux pain

G. Surgery
1. If surgery is prescribed, it will require a procedure known as fundoplication, in which a wrap to the stomach fundus is made around the distal esophagus (restores the competence of the lower esophageal sphincter)
2. A gastrostomy may be performed at the same time as the fundoplication, for decompression of the stomach postoperatively
3. Fundoplication may be combined with pyloroplasty in children with GER who also have delayed gastric emptying
4. Postoperative care is similar to that for other types of abdominal surgery
5. Instruct parents in the potential postoperative problems, such as bloating symptoms or discomfort after consuming large, solid meals

VI. HYPERTROPHIC PYLORIC STENOSIS (HPS)
(Fig. 37-1)

A. Description
1. Hypertrophy of the circular muscles of the

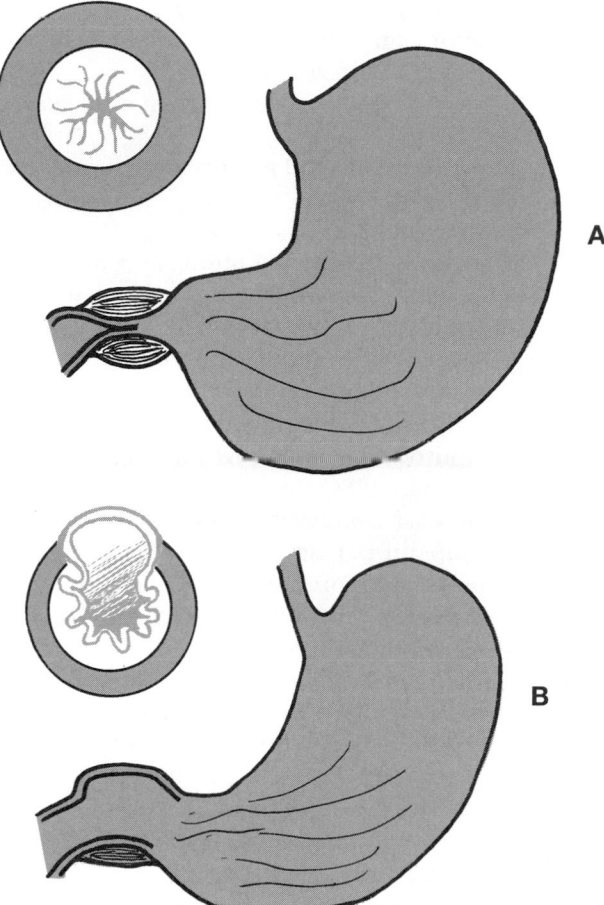

FIG. 37-1 Hypertrophic pyloric stenosis. **A,** Enlarged muscular tumor nearly obliterates pyloric channel. **B,** Longitudinal surgical division of muscle down to submucosa establishes adequate passageway. (From Wong DL et al: *Whaley & Wong's nursing care of infants and children,* ed 6, St Louis, 1999, Mosby.)

pylorus causes narrowing of the pyloric canal between the stomach and the duodenum
2. Usually develops in the first few weeks of life, causing projectile vomiting, dehydration, metabolic alkalosis, and failure to thrive

B. Assessment
1. Vomiting that progresses from mild **regurgitation** to forceful and projectile and usually occurs after a feeding
2. Vomitus contains gastric contents such as milk or formula; may contain mucus, may be blood tinged, and does not usually contain bile
3. Hunger and irritability
4. Peristaltic waves visible from left to right across the epigastrium during or immediately following a feeding
5. Olive-shaped mass in the epigastrium just right of the umbilicus
6. Dehydration and malnutrition
7. Electrolyte imbalances
8. Metabolic alkalosis

C. Implementation
1. Monitor vital signs
2. Monitor I & O and weight
3. Monitor for signs of dehydration and electrolyte imbalances
4. Prepare the child and parents for pyloromyotomy if prescribed

D. Pyloromyotomy
1. Description: An incision through the muscle fibers of the pylorus; may be performed by laparoscopy
2. Implementation preoperatively
   a. Monitor hydration status by daily weights, I & O, and urine for specific gravity
   b. Correct fluid and electrolyte imbalances; administer IV fluids as prescribed for rehydration
   c. Maintain NPO status
   d. Monitor the number and character of stools
   e. Maintain patency of the NG tube placed for stomach decompression
3. Implementation postoperatively
   a. Monitor I & O
   b. Maintain IV fluids until the infant is taking and retaining adequate amounts by mouth
   c. Begin small, frequent feedings of glucose, water, or electrolyte solution 4 to 6 hours postoperatively as prescribed; advance the diet to formula 24 hours postoperatively as prescribed
   d. Gradually increase amount and interval between feedings until a full feeding schedule is reinstated, usually by 48 hours postoperatively
   e. Feed the infant slowly, burping frequently; handle the infant minimally after feedings
   f. Monitor for abdominal distention
   g. Monitor the surgical wound and for signs of infection
   h. Instruct the parents about wound care and feeding

VII. LACTOSE INTOLERANCE

A. Description: Inability to tolerate lactose as a result of an absence or deficiency of lactase, an enzyme found in the secretions of the small intestine that is required for the digestion of lactose
B. Assessment
1. Symptoms occur after the ingestion of milk products
2. Diarrhea
3. Abdominal distention
4. Crampy, abdominal pain
5. Excessive flatus
C. Implementation
1. Eliminate the offending dairy product or administer an enzyme replacement
2. Provide information to parents about enzyme tablets (Lactaid, Lactrase, Dairy Ease) that predi-

gest the lactose in milk or supplement the body's own lactase
3. In infants, soy-based formulas can be substituted for cow's milk formula or human milk
4. Provide calcium and vitamin D supplements to prevent deficiency
5. Limit milk consumption to one glass at a time
6. If milk is consumed, drink with other foods rather than alone
7. Encourage consumption of hard cheese, cottage cheese, or yogurt (contains inactive lactase enzyme) instead of drinking milk
8. Encourage consumption of small amounts of dairy foods daily to help colonic bacteria adapt to ingested lactose
9. Instruct parents about the importance of calcium and vitamin D supplements
10. Instruct parents about the foods that contain lactose, including hidden sources

VIII. CELIAC DISEASE (GLUTEN-SENSITIVITY ENTEROPATHY)

A. Description
1. Intolerance to gluten, the protein component of wheat, barley, rye, and oats
2. It results in the accumulation of the amino acid glutamine, which is toxic to intestinal mucosal cells
3. Intestinal villi atrophy occurs, which affects absorption of ingested nutrients
4. Symptoms of the disorder occur most often between the ages of 1 and 5 years; there is usually an interval of several months between the introduction of gluten in the diet and the onset of symptoms
5. Strict dietary avoidance of gluten minimizes the risk of developing malignant lymphoma of the small intestine and other GI malignancies
B. Assessment
1. Acute or insidious diarrhea; stools are watery and pale with an offensive odor
2. Anorexia
3. Abdominal pain and distention
4. Muscle wasting, particularly in the buttocks and extremities
5. Vomiting
6. Anemia
7. Irritability
C. Celiac crisis
1. Precipitated by infection, fasting, and ingestion of gluten
2. Can lead to electrolyte imbalance, rapid dehydration, and severe acidosis
3. Causes profuse watery diarrhea and vomiting
D. Implementation
1. Gluten-free diet and substituting corn, rice, and millet as grain sources

---

BOX 37-2

Basics of a Gluten-Free Diet

FOODS ALLOWED
Meat such as beef, pork, and poultry, fish, eggs, milk and dairy products, vegetables, fruits, grains, rice, corn, gluten-free wheat flour, puffed rice, cornflakes, cornmeal, precooked gluten-free cereals

FOODS PROHIBITED
Commercially prepared ice cream; malted milk; prepared puddings; grains, including anything made from wheat, rye, oats, or barley, such as breads, rolls, cookies, cakes, crackers, cereal, spaghetti, macaroni noodles, beer, and ale

---

2. Lifelong elimination of gluten sources such as wheat, rye, oats, and barley
3. Mineral and vitamin supplements, including iron, folic acid, and fat-soluble supplements A, D, E, and K
4. Teach the parents about a gluten-free diet and to read food labels carefully for hidden sources of gluten (Box 37-2)
5. Instruct the parents in the measures to prevent celiac crisis
6. Inform the parents about the Celiac Sprue Association/United States of America

IX. APPENDICITIS

A. Description
1. Inflammation of the appendix
2. When the appendix becomes inflamed or infected, perforation may occur within a matter of hours, leading to peritonitis and sepsis
3. Treatment is surgical removal of the appendix before perforation occurs
B. Assessment
1. Pain in periumbilical area that descends to the right lower quadrant
2. Abdominal pain that is most intense at McBurney's point
3. Referred pain indicating the presence of peritoneal irritation
4. Rebound tenderness and abdominal rigidity
5. Elevated white blood cell (WBC) count
6. Side-lying position with abdominal guarding (legs flexed)
7. Difficulty walking and pain in the right hip
8. Low-grade fever
9. Anorexia, nausea, and vomiting after the pain develops
10. Diarrhea
C. Peritonitis (perforated appendix)
1. Assessment
a. Increased fever

b. Sudden relief of pain after the perforation; then, a subsequent increase in pain accompanied by right guarding of the abdomen occurs
c. Progressive abdominal distention
d. Tachycardia and tachypnea
e. Pallor
f. Chills
g. Restlessness and irritability
D. Appendectomy
1. Description: Surgical removal of the appendix
2. Implementation preoperatively
a. Maintain NPO status
b. Administer IV fluids and electrolytes as prescribed, to prevent dehydration and correct electrolyte imbalances
c. Monitor for signs of ruptured appendix and peritonitis
d. Administer antibiotics as prescribed
e. Monitor for changes in the level of pain
f. Monitor bowel sounds
g. Position in right side-lying or low to semi-Fowler's position to promote comfort
h. Apply ice packs to the abdomen for 20 to 30 minutes every hour if prescribed
i. Avoid the application of heat to the abdomen
j. Avoid laxatives or enemas
3. Implementation postoperatively
a. Monitor temperature for signs of infection
b. Maintain NPO status until bowel function has returned; advance diet gradually as tolerated and as prescribed when bowel sounds return
c. Assess incision for signs of infection, such as redness, swelling, drainage, and pain
d. If perforation of the appendix had occurred, expect a drain (Penrose drain) to be inserted or the incision may be left open to heal from the inside out
e. Expect that drainage from the drain may be profuse for the first 12 hours
f. Position the client in right side-lying or low to semi-Fowler's position with legs flexed to facilitate drainage
g. Change the dressing as prescribed, and record type and amount of drainage
h. Perform wound irrigations if prescribed
i. Maintain NG tube suction and patency of tube if present
j. Administer antibiotics and analgesics as prescribed

X. HIRSCHSPRUNG'S DISEASE (Fig. 37-2)

A. Description
1. A congenital anomaly also known as congenital aganglionosis or megacolon
2. Occurs as the result of an absence of ganglion cells in the rectum and upward in the colon

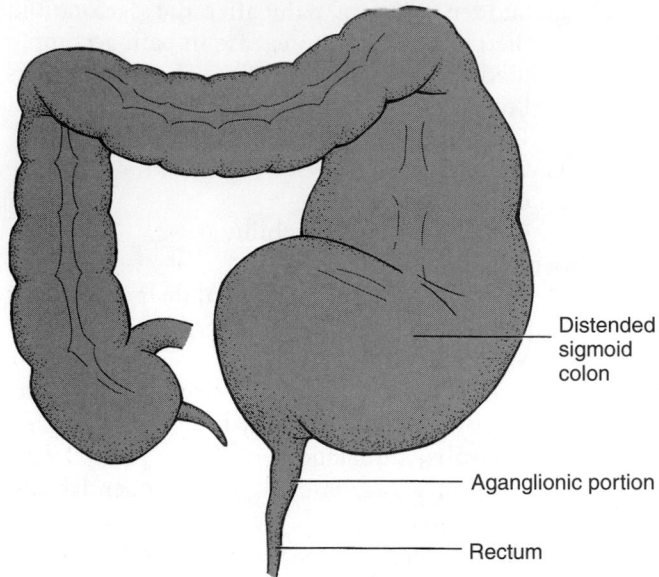

Distended sigmoid colon

Aganglionic portion

Rectum

FIG. 37-2 Hirschsprung's disease. (From Wong DL et al: *Whaley & Wong's nursing care of infants and children,* ed 6, St Louis, 1999, Mosby.)

3. Results in mechanical obstruction from inadequate motility in an intestinal segment
4. May be a familial congenital defect or may be associated with other anomalies, such as Down syndrome and genital urinary abnormalities
5. A rectal biopsy demonstrates histologic evidence of the absence of ganglionic cells
6. The most serious complication is enterocolitis; signs include fever, severe prostration, GI bleeding, and explosive watery diarrhea
7. Treatment for mild or moderate disease is based on relieving the chronic constipation with stool softeners and rectal irrigations; however, most children require surgery
8. Treatment for moderate to severe disease involves a two-step surgical procedure
9. Initially, in the neonatal period, the obstruction is relieved by a temporary colostomy to relieve obstruction and allow the normally innervated, dilated bowel to return to its normal size
10. A complete surgical repair is performed, when the child weighs approximately 9 kg (20 pounds), via a pull-through procedure to excise portions of the bowel; at this time, the colostomy is closed

B. Assessment
 1. Newborn infants
  a. Failure to pass meconium stool
  b. Refusal to suck
  c. Abdominal distention
  d. Bile-stained vomitus
 2. Children
  a. Failure to gain weight and delayed **growth**
  b. Abdominal distention

  c. Vomiting
  d. Constipation alternating with diarrhea
  e. Ribbon-like and foul-smelling stools
C. Implementation: Medical management
 1. Dietary management
 2. Stool softeners
 3. Daily rectal irrigations with normal saline to promote adequate elimination and prevent obstruction
D. Surgical management: Preoperative implementation
 1. Assess bowel function and administer bowel preparation as prescribed
 2. Maintain NPO status
 3. Monitor hydration and fluid and electrolyte status; provide IV fluids as prescribed for hydration
 4. Administer antibiotics as prescribed to clear the bowel of bacteria
 5. Monitor I & O and weight
 6. Measure abdominal girth
 7. Avoid rectal temperatures
 8. Monitor for respiratory distress associated with abdominal distention
E. Implementation postoperatively
 1. Monitor vital signs, avoiding rectal temperatures
 2. Measure abdominal girth
 3. Assess surgical site for redness, swelling, and drainage
 4. Assess the stoma for bleeding or skin breakdown
 5. Assess anal area for the presence of stool, redness, or discharge
 6. Maintain NPO status until bowel sounds return or flatus is passed; bowel sounds usually return within 48 to 72 hours
 7. Maintain the NG tube to allow intermittent suction until peristalsis returns
 8. Maintain the IV until the child tolerates appropriate oral intake; begin the diet with clear liquids, advancing to regular as tolerated and as prescribed
 9. Assess for dehydration and fluid overload
 10. Monitor I & O and weight
 11. Assess pain and provide comfort measures as required
 12. Provide the parents with instructions regarding colostomy care and skin care
 13. Teach the parents about the appropriate diet and the need for adequate fluid intake

XI. INTUSSUSCEPTION
A. Description
 1. Telescoping of one portion of the bowel into another portion
 2. Results in an obstruction to the passage of intestinal contents

B. Assessment
 1. Colicky abdominal pain that causes the child to scream and draw the knees to the abdomen
 2. Vomiting of gastric contents
 3. Bile-stained fecal emesis
 4. Currant jelly–like stools containing blood and mucus
 5. Hypoactive or hyperactive bowel sounds
 6. Tender distended abdomen, possibly with a palpable sausage-shaped mass in the upper right quadrant
C. Implementation
 1. Monitor for signs of perforation and shock as evidenced by fever, increased heart rate, changes in level of consciousness (LOC) or blood pressure, and respiratory distress, and report immediately
 2. Prepare for hydrostatic reduction if prescribed (not performed if signs of perforation or shock occur)
  a. Antibiotics, IV fluids, and NG decompression may be prescribed
  b. Monitor for the passage of normal, brown stool, which indicates that the intussusception has reduced itself
 3. After hydrostatic reduction:
  a. Monitor for the return of normal bowel signs, for the passage of barium, and the characteristics of stool
  b. Administer clear fluids and advance the diet gradually as prescribed
 4. If surgery is required, postoperative care is similar to that following any abdominal surgery

XII. ABDOMINAL WALL DEFECTS

A. Omphalocele
 1. Occurs when there is a herniation of the abdominal contents through the umbilical ring (hernia of the umbilical cord), usually with an intact peritoneal sac
 2. The protrusion is covered by a translucent sac that may contain bowel or other abdominal organs
 3. Rupture of the sac results in evisceration of the abdominal contents
 4. Immediately after birth, the sac is covered with sterile gauze soaked in normal saline to prevent drying of abdominal contents; a layer of plastic wrap is placed over the gauze to provide additional protection against heat and moisture loss
 5. Monitor vital signs every 2 to 4 hours, particularly temperature because the infant can lose heat through the sac
 6. Preoperatively: Maintain NPO status, administer IVs as prescribed to maintain hydration and electrolyte balance, monitor for signs of infection, and handle the infant carefully to prevent rupture of the sac
 7. Postoperatively: Control pain, prevent infection, maintain fluid and electrolyte balance, and ensure adequate nutrition
B. Gastroschisis
 1. Occurs when the herniation of the intestine is lateral to the umbilical ring
 2. There is no membrane covering the exposed bowel
 3. The exposed bowel is loosely covered in saline-soaked pads, and the abdomen is wrapped in a plastic drape; wrapping around the exposed bowel is contraindicated because if the exposed bowel expands, wrapping could cause pressure and necrosis
 4. Preoperatively: Care is similar to that for omphalocele; surgery is performed within several hours after birth because there is no membrane covering the sac
 5. Postoperatively: Most infants have a prolonged ileus and require mechanical ventilation and parenteral nutrition; otherwise, care is similar to that for omphalocele

XIII. UMBILICAL HERNIA, INGUINAL HERNIA, OR HYDROCELE

A. Description
 1. A hernia is a protrusion of the bowel through an abnormal opening in the abdominal wall
 2. In children, a hernia most commonly occurs at the umbilicus and through the inguinal canal
 3. A hydrocele is the presence of abdominal fluid in the scrotal sac
B. Assessment
 1. Umbilical hernia: soft swelling or protrusion around the umbilicus that is usually reducible with the finger
 2. Inguinal hernia
  a. Painless inguinal swelling that is reducible
  b. Swelling may disappear during periods of rest and is most noticeable when the infant cries or coughs
 3. Incarcerated hernia
  a. When the descended portion of bowel becomes tightly caught in the hernial sac, compromising blood supply
  b. A medical emergency requiring surgical repair
  c. Irritability
  d. Tenderness at site
  e. Anorexia
  f. Abdominal distention
  g. Difficulty defecating
  h. May lead to complete intestinal obstruction and gangrene
 4. Noncommunicating hydrocele
  a. Occurs when residual peritoneal fluid is trapped with no communication to the peritoneal cavity
  b. Usually disappears by age 1 year

5. Communicating hydrocele
   a. Associated with a hernia that remains open from the scrotum to the abdominal cavity
   b. Assessment includes a bulge in the inguinal area or the scrotum that increases with crying or straining and decreases when the child is at rest
C. Implementation postoperatively (hernia)
   1. Monitor vital signs
   2. Assess for wound infection
   3. Monitor for redness or drainage
   4. Monitor I & O and hydration status
   5. Advance the diet as tolerated
   6. Administer analgesics as prescribed
D. Implementation postoperatively (hydrocele)
   1. Provide ice bags and a scrotal support to relieve pain and swelling
   2. Instruct the child and parents to avoid tub bathing until the incision heals
   3. Instruct the child and parents to avoid strenuous physical activities

XIV. CONSTIPATION/ENCOPRESIS

A. Description
   1. Constipation is the infrequent and difficult passage of dry, hard stools
   2. **Encopresis** is fecal incontinence, and children often complain that soiling is involuntary and occurs without warning
   3. If the child does not have a neurological or anatomic disorder, **encopresis** is usually the result of fecal impaction and an enlarged rectum caused by chronic constipation
B. Assessment
   1. Constipation
      a. Abdominal pain and cramping without distention
      b. Palpable movable fecal masses
      c. Normal or decreased bowel sounds
      d. Malaise and headache
      e. Anorexia, nausea, and vomiting
   2. **Encopresis**
      a. Evidence of soiling of clothing
      b. Scratching or rubbing of anal area
      c. Fecal odor
      d. Social withdrawal
C. Implementation
   1. Simple constipation may resolve by using only dietary changes or methods to change the habit of retention
   2. Severe **encopresis** may require that interventions be continued over a period of 3 to 6 months
   3. Overcoming withholding
      a. Administer enemas as prescribed until the impaction is cleared
      b. Monitor for hypernatremia or hyperphosphatemia when administering repeated enemas
      c. Administer stool softener or laxative as prescribed
      d. Administer mineral oil, 30 to 75 mL bid, as prescribed; administer chilled or mixed with cold drinks to disguise the taste
   4. Dietary changes
      a. Increase water and fiber intake
      b. Decrease sugar and milk intake
      c. Administer fat-soluble vitamins during the use of mineral oil because the oil can interfere with vitamin absorption in the small intestine
   5. Changing the retention habit: have the child sit on the toilet for 5 to 10 minutes approximately 20 to 30 minutes after breakfast and dinner to assist with defecation

XV. IRRITABLE BOWEL SYNDROME

A. Description
   1. Occurs as a result of increased motility that can lead to spasm and pain
   2. The diagnosis is based on the elimination of pathology
   3. It is a self-limiting, intermittent problem with no definitive treatment
   4. Stress and emotional factors may contribute to its occurrence
B. Assessment
   1. Diffuse abdominal pain unrelated to meals or activity
   2. Alternating constipation and diarrhea with the presence of undigested food and mucus in the stool
C. Implementation
   1. Reassure that the problem is self-limiting and intermittent and will resolve
   2. Encourage the maintenance of a healthy, well-balanced, moderate-fiber diet
   3. Encourage health promotion activities such as exercise and school activities
   4. Inform the parents of psychosocial resources if required

XVI. IMPERFORATE ANUS

A. Description: Incomplete development or absence of the anus in its normal position in the perineum
B. Assessment
   1. Failure to pass meconium stool
   2. Absence or **stenosis** of the anal rectal canal
   3. Anal membrane
   4. External fistula to the peritoneum
C. Implementation
   1. Determine patency of the anus
   2. Monitor for the presence of stool in the urine and vagina and report immediately
D. Implementation postoperatively
   1. Monitor the skin for signs of infection
   2. Position side-lying with legs flexed or in a prone

position to keep the hips elevated to reduce edema and pressure on the surgical site

3. Keep the anal surgical incision clean and dry, and monitor for redness, swelling, or drainage
4. Maintain NPO status and NG tube if in place
5. Maintain IV fluids until gastrointestinal (GI) motility returns
6. Provide colostomy care if prescribed
7. A fresh colostomy stoma will be red and edematous, but this should decrease with time
8. Instruct the parents to perform anal dilatation if prescribed to achieve and maintain bowel patency
9. Instruct the parents to use only dilators supplied by the physician and a water-soluble lubricant and to insert the dilator no more than 1 to 2 cm into the anus to prevent damage to the mucosa

XVII. HEPATITIS

A. This section contains specific information regarding hepatitis as it relates to infants and children; refer to Chapters 25 and 53 for additional information on hepatitis
B. Description: An acute or chronic inflammation of the liver that may be caused by a virus, a medication reaction, or another disease process
C. Hepatitis A (HAV)
   1. Highest incidence occurs among preschool or school-aged children under 15 years of age
   2. Many affected children are asymptomatic, but mild nausea, vomiting, and diarrhea may occur
   3. Infected children who are asymptomatic can still spread HAV to others
D. Hepatitis B (HBV)
   1. Most HBV in children is acquired perinatally
   2. Newborn infants are at risk if the mother is infected with HBV or was a carrier of HBV during pregnancy
   3. Possible routes of maternal-fetal (infant) transmission include leakage of the virus across the placenta late in pregnancy or during labor; ingestion of amniotic fluid or maternal blood; and breastfeeding, especially if the mother has cracked nipples
   4. The severity in the infant varies from no liver disease to fulminant (severe, acute course) or chronic, active disease
   5. In children and adolescents, HBV occurs in specific high-risk groups, including children with hemophilia or other disorders who have received multiple blood transfusions, children or adolescents involved in drug abuse, institutionalized children, and preschool children in endemic areas, and if involvement with heterosexual activity or sexual activity with homosexual males occurs
   6. HBV infection can cause a carrier state and lead to

eventual cirrhosis or hepatocellular carcinoma in adulthood

E. Hepatitis C (HCV)
   1. Transmission is primarily by the parenteral route
   2. Some children may be asymptomatic, but HCV often becomes a chronic condition and can cause cirrhosis and hepatocellular carcinoma
F. Hepatitis D (HDV)
   1. Occurs in children already infected with HBV
   2. Both acute and chronic forms tend to be more severe than HBV and can lead to cirrhosis
G. Hepatitis E (HEV)
   1. Uncommon in children
   2. Is not a chronic condition, does not cause chronic liver disease, and has no carrier state
H. Hepatitis G
   1. Blood borne and is similar to HCV
   2. High-risk groups include transfusion recipients, IV drug users, and individuals infected with HCV
   3. Individuals are often asymptomatic, and most infections are chronic
I. Assessment
   1. Prodromal or anicteric phase
      a. Lasts 5 to 7 days
      b. Absence of jaundice
      c. Anorexia, malaise, lethargy, easy fatigability
      d. Fever (especially in adolescents)
      e. Nausea and vomiting
      f. Epigastric or right upper quadrant abdominal pain
      g. Arthralgia and skin rashes (more likely with HBV)
      h. Hepatomegaly
   2. Icteric phase
      a. Jaundice, which is best assessed in the sclera, nail beds, and mucous membranes
      b. Dark urine and pale stools
      c. Pruritus
J. Diagnostic evaluation: Refer to Chapter 10 for laboratory studies used to diagnose hepatitis
K. Prevention
   1. Proper handwashing and standard precautions can prevent the spread of viral hepatitis
   2. Prophylactic use of standard immune globulin (IG) to prevent HAV in situations of preexposure (such as anticipated travel to areas where HAV is prevalent) or within 2 weeks of exposure
   3. Hepatitis B immune globulin (HBIG) is effective in preventing infection following one-time exposures, such as accidental needle punctures or other contact of contaminated material with mucous membranes, and should be given to newborns whose mothers are HbsAg positive; should be given within 72 hours of exposure
   4. Hepatitis A vaccine is recommended for children 2 years and older who reside in communities

with high endemic rates and for preexposure prophylaxis

5. Hepatitis B vaccine: Refer to Chapter 45 for immunization schedule

L. Implementation
1. Strict handwashing
2. Hospitalization is required in the event of coagulopathy or fulminant hepatitis
3. Standard precautions are followed during hospitalization
4. Hospitalized child is not usually isolated in a separate room unless he or she is fecally incontinent and items are likely to become contaminated with feces
5. Children are discouraged from sharing toys
6. Instruct child and parents in good handwashing techniques
7. Instruct the parents to thoroughly disinfect diaper-changing surfaces with ¼ cup bleach to a gallon of water
8. Maintain comfort and provide adequate rest and sleep
9. Provide a low-fat, balanced diet
10. Provide enteric precautions for at least 1 week after the onset of jaundice with HAV
11. Inform the parents that because hepatitis A is not infectious within 1 week after the onset of jaundice, the child may return to school at that time if he or she feels well enough
12. Inform the parents that jaundice may get worse before it resolves
13. Caution parents about administering any medications to the child (liver is unable to detoxify and excrete medications)
14. Instruct the parents in the signs indicating a worsening of the child's condition, such as changes in the neurological status, bleeding, and fluid retention

XVIII. INGESTION OF POISONS

A. Lead poisoning
1. Description: Excessive accumulation of lead in the blood
2. Causes
   a. The pathway for exposure may be food, air, or water
   b. Dust and soil contaminated with lead may be a source of exposure
   c. Lead enters the child's body through ingestion or inhalation, or through placental transmission to an unborn child when the mother is exposed; the most common route is ingestion either from hand-to-mouth behavior from contaminated objects or from eating loose paint chips
   d. When lead enters the body, it affects the erythrocytes, bones and teeth, and organs

and tissues, including the brain and nervous system; the most serious consequences are the effects on the central nervous system

3. Universal screening
   a. Recommended in high-risk areas at the age of 1 to 2 years; children at high risk should be screened earlier
   b. Any child between the ages of 3 and 6 years who has not been screened should be tested
4. Targeted screening
   a. Acceptable in low-risk areas
   b. At the age of 1 to 2 years (or a child between the ages of 3 and 6 years who has not been screened) may be targeted for screening if determined to be at risk
5. Blood lead level (BLL) test
   a. Used for screening and diagnosis
   b. BLL less than 10 μg/dL: Reassess or rescreen in 1 year; sooner if exposure status changes
   c. BLL 10 to 14 μg/dL: Provide family lead education, follow-up testing, and social service referral if necessary
   d. BLL 15 to 19 μg/dL: Provide family lead education, follow-up testing, and social service referral if necessary; on follow-up testing, initiate actions for BLL of 20 to 44 μg/dL
   e. BLL 20 to 44 μg/dL: A BLL greater than 20 μg/dL is considered acute; provide coordination of care, clinical management, including treatment, environmental investigation, and lead-hazard control (the child must not remain in a lead-hazardous environment if resolution is necessary)
   f. BLL 70 μg/dL or greater: Medical treatment is immediately provided, including coordination of care, clinical management, environmental investigation, and lead-hazard control
6. Erythrocyte protoporphyrin (EP) test
   a. An indicator of anemia
   b. Normal value for a child is 35 μg/100 mL of whole blood or less
7. Chelation therapy
   a. Removing lead from the circulating blood and from some organs and tissues
   b. Does not counteract any effects of the lead
   c. Medications: dimercaprol (BAL in oil); calcium disodium edetate (CaNa₂EDTA); succimer (Chemet)
   d. Dimercaprol (BAL) is contraindicated in children with an allergy to peanuts because the medication is prepared in a peanut oil solution
   e. Ensure adequate urinary output before administering medications
   f. Provide adequate hydration and monitor

kidney function for nephrotoxicity when medication is given, because the medication is excreted via the kidneys

    g. Follow-up lead levels to monitor progress are essential

    h. Provide instructions to parents about safety from lead hazards, medication administration, and the need for follow-up

    i. Confirm that the child will be discharged to home without lead hazards

▲ B. Acetaminophen (Tylenol)
1. Description
    a. Seriousness of ingestion is determined by the amount ingested and the length of time before intervention
    b. Toxic dose is 150 mg/kg or greater in children
2. Assessment
    a. First 2 to 4 hours: malaise, nausea, vomiting, sweating, pallor, weakness
    b. Latent period: 24 to 36 hours; child improves
    c. Hepatic involvement: May last up to 7 days and be permanent; right upper quadrant pain, jaundice, confusion, stupor, elevated liver enzymes and bilirubin, prolonged prothrombin time (PT)

▲ 3. Implementation
    a. Administer antidote: *N*-acetylcysteine (NAC)
    b. Dilute antidote in juice or soda because of its offensive odor
    c. Loading dose is followed by maintenance doses

▲ C. Acetylsalicylic acid (aspirin, ASA)
1. Description
    a. May be caused by acute ingestion or chronic ingestion
    b. Acute: Severe toxicity occurs with 300 to 500 mg/kg
    c. Chronic: More than 100 mg/kg/day for 2 days or more; can be more serious than acute ingestion
2. Assessment
    a. GI effects: nausea, vomiting, and thirst from dehydration
    b. CNS effects: hyperpnea, confusion, tinnitus, convulsions, coma, respiratory failure, circulatory collapse
    c. Renal effects: oliguria
    d. Hematopoietic effects: bleeding tendencies
    e. Metabolic effects: diaphoresis, dehydration, fever, hyponatremia, hypokalemia, dehydration, hypoglycemia

▲ 3. Implementation
    a. Induce vomiting with syrup of Ipecac or perform gastric lavage
    b. Administer activated charcoal to decrease absorption of salicylate (important in early ASA toxicity)

    c. Administer IVs, sodium bicarbonate, electrolytes, or volume expanders as prescribed
    d. Administer vitamin K for bleeding tendencies as prescribed
    e. Administer glucose for hypoglycemia as prescribed
    f. Prepare the child for dialysis as prescribed if the child is unresponsive to the therapy

PRACTICE QUESTIONS

1. A 3-year-old child is hospitalized because of persistent vomiting. A nurse monitors the child closely for:
1. Diarrhea
2. Metabolic acidosis
3. Metabolic alkalosis
4. Hyperactive bowel sounds

2. A nurse is monitoring for signs of dehydration in a 1-year-old child who has been hospitalized for diarrhea. The nurse prepares to take the child's temperature and avoids which method of measurement?
1. Tympanic
2. Axillary
3. Rectal
4. Electronic

3. A home care nurse provides instructions to the mother of an infant with cleft palate regarding feeding. Which statement if made by the mother indicates a need for further instructions?
1. "I will use a nipple with a small hole to prevent choking."
2. "I will stimulate sucking by rubbing the nipple on the lower lip."
3. "I will allow the infant time to swallow."
4. "I will allow the infant to rest frequently to provide time for swallowing what has been placed in the mouth."

4. An infant has just returned to the nursing unit following a surgical repair of a cleft lip located on the right side of the lip. The nurse places the infant in which most appropriate position?
1. On the right side
2. On the left side
3. Prone
4. Supine

5. A clinic nurse reviews the record of an infant seen in the clinic. The nurse notes that a diagnosis of esophageal atresia with tracheoesophageal fistula (TEF) is suspected. The nurse expects to note which most likely sign of this condition documented in the record?
1. Severe projectile vomiting
2. Coughing at nighttime
3. Choking with feedings
4. Incessant crying

6. A nurse prepares a teaching plan for the parents of an infant with gastroesophageal reflux (GER) regarding proper positioning to manage reflux. The nurse documents that the infant should be maintained in which position following feedings and at night?
   1. 30-degree angle when supine
   2. 60-degree angle when supine
   3. Head-elevated prone position
   4. 20-degree angle when supine

7. A nurse provides feeding instructions to a mother of an infant diagnosed with gastroesophageal reflux (GER). To assist in reducing the episodes of emesis, the nurse tells the mother to:
   1. Thin the feedings by adding water to the formula
   2. Thicken the feedings by adding rice cereal to the formula
   3. Provide less frequent, larger feedings
   4. Burp the infant less frequently during feedings

8. A nurse admits a child to the hospital with a diagnosis of pyloric stenosis. On admission assessment, which data would the nurse expect to obtain when asking the mother about the child's symptoms?
   1. Vomiting large amounts of bile
   2. Watery diarrhea
   3. Increased urine output
   4. Projectile vomiting

9. A home care nurse instructs the mother about dietary measures for a 5-year-old child with lactose intolerance. The nurse tells the mother that is necessary to provide which dietary supplement in the child's diet?
   1. Zinc
   2. Protein
   3. Calcium
   4. Fats

10. A nurse provides home care instructions to the parents of a child with celiac disease. The nurse teaches the parents to include which of the following food items in the child's diet?
    1. Rice
    2. Rye toast
    3. Oatmeal
    4. Wheat bread

11. A clinic nurse reviews the record of a 3-week-old infant and notes that the physician has documented a diagnosis of suspected Hirschsprung's disease. The nurse reviews the assessment findings documented in the record, knowing that which symptom most likely led the mother to seek health care for the infant?
    1. Diarrhea
    2. Projectile vomiting
    3. Regurgitation of feedings
    4. Foul-smelling ribbon-like stools

12. A nurse is caring for a newborn infant with a suspected diagnosis of imperforate anus. The nurse monitors the infant, knowing that which of the following is not a clinical manifestation associated with this disorder?
    1. The presence of stool in the urine
    2. Failure to pass a rectal thermometer
    3. Failure to pass meconium in the first 24 hours after birth
    4. The passage of currant jelly–like stools

13. A nurse is preparing to care for a child with a diagnosis of intussusception. The nurse reviews the child's record and expects to note which symptom of this disorder documented?
    1. Bright red blood and mucus in the stools
    2. Profuse projectile vomiting
    3. Watery diarrhea
    4. Ribbon-like stools

14. A child is receiving succimer (Chemet) for the treatment of lead poisoning. A nurse monitors which of the following most important laboratory results?
    1. Potassium level
    2. Blood urea nitrogen (BUN)
    3. Red blood cell count
    4. White blood cell count

15. An emergency room nurse is caring for a child brought to the emergency room after the ingestion of approximately one-half bottle of acetylsalicylic acid (aspirin, ASA). The nurse anticipates that the most likely initial treatment will be:
    1. The administration of syrup of ipecac
    2. The administration of sodium bicarbonate
    3. The administration of vitamin K
    4. Dialysis

CRITICAL THINKING: FREE-TEXT ENTRY

A nurse is caring for a child who is scheduled for an appendectomy. The nurse reviews the physician's preoperative orders and notes the following: initiate an IV line, maintain an NPO status, administer a Fleet enema, and administer preoperative medication on call to the operating room. Which order written by the physician would the nurse question?

Answer: _____

ANSWERS

1. 3

Rationale: Vomiting will cause the loss of hydrochloric acid and subsequent metabolic alkalosis. Metabolic acidosis would occur in a child experiencing diarrhea, because of the loss of bicarbonate. Diarrhea may not accompany vomiting. Hyperactive bowel sounds are not necessarily associated with vomiting.

Test-Taking Strategy: Use the process of elimination. Recalling that gastric fluids are acidic in nature and that the loss of these fluids will lead to alkalosis will assist in answering the question. There are no data in the question to support options 1 and 4. Review the manifestations that occur with vomiting if you had difficulty with this question.

Level of Cognitive Ability: Analysis
Client Needs: Physiological Integrity
Integrated Concept/Process: Nursing Process: Assessment
Content Area: Child Health
Reference: Wong, D. (1999). *Whaley & Wong's nursing care of infants and children* (6th ed.). St. Louis: Mosby, p. 1296.

2. 3

Rationale: Rectal temperature measurements should be avoided if diarrhea is present. Use of a rectal thermometer can stimulate peristalsis and cause more diarrhea. Axillary and tympanic measurements of temperature would be acceptable. Most measurements are done via electronic devices.

Test-Taking Strategy: Use the process of elimination. Note the key word "avoids." Eliminate option 4 first because most methods of temperature measurement are done through an electronic device. Note the diagnosis stated in the question. This should easily direct you to option 3. Review care of the child with diarrhea if you had difficulty with this question.

Level of Cognitive Ability: Analysis
Client Needs: Physiological Integrity
Integrated Concept/Process: Nursing Process: Implementation
Content Area: Child Health
Reference: Bowden, V., Dickey, S, & Greenberg, C. (1998). *Children and their families: The continuum of care.* Philadelphia: W.B. Saunders, p. 351.

3. 1

Rationale: The mother is taught the ESSR method of feeding the child with a cleft palate: ENLARGE the nipple, STIMULATE the sucking reflex, SWALLOW, and REST to allow the infant to finish swallowing what has been placed in the mouth.

Test-Taking Strategy: Use the process of elimination. Note the key words "need for further instructions." Eliminate options 3 and 4 first because they are similar. Use basic principles regarding the methods to stimulate sucking to eliminate option 2. Review teaching guidelines for the child with cleft lip or palate if you had difficulty with this question.

Level of Cognitive Ability: Analysis
Client Needs: Health Promotion and Maintenance
Integrated Concept/Process: Teaching/Learning
Content Area: Child Health
Reference: Wong, D. (1999). *Whaley & Wong's nursing care of infants and children* (6th ed.). St. Louis: Mosby, p. 518.

4. 2

Rationale: After cleft lip repair, the infant should be positioned supine or on the side lateral to the repair to prevent the contact of the suture lines with the bed linens. It is best to place the infant on the left side rather than supine immediately after surgery, to prevent the risk of aspiration if the infant vomits.

Test-Taking Strategy: Use the process of elimination. Note the key words "just returned" and "most appropriate." Consider the anatomical location of the surgical site and the key words "right side" in the question. You should easily be directed to the correct option by using these concepts. Review postoperative positioning techniques if you had difficulty with this question.

Level of Cognitive Ability: Application
Client Needs: Safe, Effective Care Environment
Integrated Concept/Process: Nursing Process: Implementation
Content Area: Child Health
Reference: Wong, D. (1999). *Whaley & Wong's nursing care of infants and children* (6th ed.). St. Louis: Mosby, p. 519.

5. 3

Rationale: Any child who exhibits the "3 Cs," coughing and choking with feedings and unexplained cyanosis, should be suspected of TEF. Options 1, 2, and 4 are not specifically associated with TEF.

Test-Taking Strategy: Use the process of elimination, focusing on the diagnosis. Recalling the "3 Cs" associated with this disorder will assist in directing you to the correct option. Review the clinical manifestations associated with this disorder if you had difficulty with this question

Level of Cognitive Ability: Analysis
Client Needs: Physiological Integrity
Integrated Concept/Process: Communication and Documentation
Content Area: Child Health
Reference: Ball, J., & Bindler, R. (1999). *Pediatric nursing: Caring for children* (2nd ed.). Stamford, Conn.: Appleton & Lange, p. 604.

6. 3

Rationale: The infant should be placed in either the flat prone position or the head-elevated prone position following feedings and at night. The supine position is not recommended, since aspiration could occur if the infant vomits.

Test-Taking Strategy: Use the process of elimination. Visualize each of the positions, and think about the effect of the position in the infant with GER. Also note that options 1, 2, and 4 are similar. Review positioning for GER if you had difficulty with this question.

Level of Cognitive Ability: Application
Client Needs: Safe, Effective Care Environment
Integrated Concept/Process: Communication and Documentation
Content Area: Child Health
Reference: Wong, D. (1999). *Whaley & Wong's nursing care of infants and children* (6th ed.). St. Louis: Mosby, p. 1547.

7. 2

Rationale: Small, more frequent feedings with frequent burping are often prescribed in the treatment of GER. Feedings thickened with rice cereal may reduce episodes of emesis. If thickened formula is used, crosscutting of the nipple may be required.

Test-Taking Strategy: Use the process of elimination and basic principles related to feeding an infant to assist in eliminating options 3 and 4. Noting the key words "reducing the episodes of emesis" will assist in directing you to select option 2 over

option 1. Review therapeutic interventions associated with this disorder if you had difficulty with this question.
Level of Cognitive Ability: Application
Client Needs: Health Promotion and Maintenance
Integrated Concept/Process: Teaching/Learning
Content Area: Child Health
Reference: Ball, J., & Bindler, R. (1999). *Pediatric nursing: Caring for children* (2nd ed.). Stamford, Conn.: Appleton & Lange, pp. 609-610.

8. **4**
Rationale: Clinical manifestations of pyloric stenosis include projectile vomiting, irritability, hunger and crying, constipation, and signs of dehydration, including a decrease in urine output.
Test-Taking Strategy: Use the process of elimination. Considering the anatomical location of this disorder and its potential effects will assist in eliminating options 2 and 3. Recalling that a major clinical manifestation is projectile vomiting will assist in directing you to option 4. Review these clinical manifestations if you had difficulty with this question.
Level of Cognitive Ability: Analysis
Client Needs: Physiological Integrity
Integrated Concept/Process: Nursing Process/Assessment
Content Area: Child Health
Reference: Ball, J., & Bindler, R. (1999). *Pediatric nursing: Caring for children* (2nd ed.). Stamford, Conn.: Appleton & Lange, p. 607.

9. **3**
Rationale: Lactose intolerance is the inability to tolerate lactose, the sugar found in dairy products. Removing milk from the diet can provide adequate relief from symptoms. Additional dietary changes may be required to provide adequate sources of calcium and, in the infant, protein and calories.
Test-Taking Strategy: Use the process of elimination. Knowledge that lactose is the sugar found in dairy products will easily direct you to option 3, since dairy products contain high levels of calcium. Review the dietary management for lactose intolerance if you had difficulty with this question.
Level of Cognitive Ability: Application
Client Needs: Health Promotion and Maintenance
Integrated Concept/Process: Teaching/Learning
Content Area: Child Health
Reference: Ball, J., & Bindler, R. (1999). *Pediatric nursing: Caring for children* (2nd ed.). Stamford, Conn.: Appleton & Lange, p. 643.

10. **1**
Rationale: Dietary management is the mainstay of treatment in celiac disease. All wheat, rye, barley, and oats should be eliminated from the diet and replaced with corn, rice, or millet. Vitamin supplements, especially the fat-soluble vitamins, iron, and folic acid, may be needed in the early period of treatment to correct deficiencies. Dietary restrictions are likely to be lifelong, although small amounts of grains may be tolerated after ulcerations have healed.
Test-Taking Strategy: Use the process of elimination. Recalling that corn, rice, and millet are substitute food replacements in this disease will easily direct you to option 1. Review the dietary management in this disorder if you had difficulty with this question.
Level of Cognitive Ability: Application

Client Needs: Health Promotion and Maintenance
Integrated Concept/Process: Teaching/Learning
Content Area: Child Health
Reference: Ball, J., & Bindler, R. (1999). *Pediatric nursing: Caring for children* (2nd ed.). Stamford, Conn.: Appleton & Lange, p. 642.

11. **4**
Rationale: Chronic constipation beginning in the first month of life and resulting in pellet-like or ribbon stools that are foul smelling is a clinical manifestation of this disorder. Delayed passage or absence of meconium stool in the neonatal period is the cardinal sign. Bowel obstruction, especially in the neonatal period, abdominal pain and distension, and failure to thrive are also clinical manifestations. Options 1, 2, and 3 are not specifically associated with this disorder.
Test-Taking Strategy: Use the process of elimination and knowledge regarding the pathophysiology associated with Hirschsprung's disease to direct you to option 4. If you are unfamiliar with this disorder, review the assessment findings associated with it.
Level of Cognitive Ability: Analysis
Client Needs: Physiological Integrity
Integrated Concept/Process: Communication and Documentation
Content Area: Child Health
Reference: Ball, J., & Bindler, R. (1999). *Pediatric nursing: Caring for children* (2nd ed.). Stamford, Conn.: Appleton & Lange, p. 613.

12. **4**
Rationale: During the newborn assessment, this defect should be easily identified on site. However, a rectal thermometer or tube may be necessary to determine patency if meconium is not passed in the first 24 hours after birth. The presence of stool in the urine or the vagina or in a skin dimple should be reported immediately as an indication of abnormal anorectal development. Current jelly–like stools are not a clinical manifestation of this disorder.
Test-Taking Strategy: Note the key word "not" in the stem of the question. Use the process of elimination and the definition of the word "imperforate" to assist in answering this question. This should easily direct you to option 4. Review the important assessment data associated with this disorder if you had difficulty with this question.
Level of Cognitive Ability: Analysis
Client Needs: Physiological Integrity
Integrated Concept/Process: Nursing Process/Assessment
Content Area: Child Health
Reference: Ball, J., & Bindler, R. (1999). *Pediatric nursing: Caring for children* (2nd ed.). Stamford, Conn.: Appleton & Lange, p. 614.

13. **1**
Rationale: The child with intussusception classically presents with severe abdominal pain that is crampy and intermittent, causing the child to draw in the knees to the chest. Vomiting may be present but it is not projectile. Bright red blood and mucus are passed through the rectum and are commonly described as currant-jelly stools. Watery diarrhea and ribbon-like stools are not manifestations of this disorder.
Test-Taking Strategy: Use the process of elimination. Recalling that a classic manifestation is currant-jelly stools will assist in

directing you to option 1. Review this disorder if you had difficulty with this question.
Level of Cognitive Ability: Analysis
Client Needs: Physiological Integrity
Integrated Concept/Process: Communication and Documentation
Content Area: Child Health
Reference: Bowden, V., Dickey, S., & Greenberg, C. (1998). *Children and their families: The continuum of care.* Philadelphia: W.B. Saunders, p. 1073.

14. **2**
Rationale: Renal function is monitored closely during the administration of chelation therapy because the medications are excreted via the kidneys. Although it is important to monitor the red blood cell count for the presence of anemia in a child with lead poisoning, this laboratory result is not specific to chelation therapy. Options 1 and 4 are unrelated to the administration of chelation therapy.
Test-Taking Strategy: Use the process of elimination. Recalling that the medications used in chelation therapy are excreted via the kidneys will direct you to option 2. Review this treatment for lead poisoning if you had difficulty with this question.
Level of Cognitive Ability: Analysis
Client Needs: Physiological Integrity
Integrated Concept/Process: Nursing Process/Assessment
Content Area: Child Health
Reference: Ball, J., & Bindler, R. (1999). *Pediatric nursing: Caring for children* (2nd ed.). Stamford, Conn.: Appleton & Lange, p. 657.

15. **1**
Rationale: Initial treatment of salicylate overdose includes inducing vomiting with syrup of ipecac or gastric lavage. Activated charcoal may be administered to decrease absorption. IV fluids and sodium bicarbonate may be administered to enhance excretion but would not be the initial treatment.

Dialysis is used in extreme cases if the child is unresponsive to therapy. Vitamin K is the antidote for warfarin sodium (Coumadin) overdose.
Test-Taking Strategy: Use the process of elimination and knowledge regarding the treatment for aspirin overdose to answer this question. Note the key word "initial" in the stem of the question. This key word will assist in directing you to option 1. Review the treatment for this common overdose in children if you had difficulty with this question.
Level of Cognitive Ability: Analysis
Client Needs: Physiological Integrity
Integrated Concept/Process: Nursing Process/Planning
Content Area: Child Health
Reference: Wong, D. (1999). *Whaley & Wong's nursing care of infants and children* (6th ed.). St. Louis: Mosby, p. 742.

CRITICAL THINKING: FREE-TEXT ENTRY

Answer: Administer a Fleet enema
Rationale: In preoperative period, enemas or laxatives should not be administered. IV fluids would be started, and the child would be NPO. Prescribed preoperative medications most likely would be administered on call to the operating room.
Test-Taking Strategy: Consider the anatomical location and the concern of rupture in this disorder. Administering a Fleet enema would place the child at risk for a perforated appendix. Review preoperative care in the child with appendicitis if you had difficulty with this question.
Level of Cognitive Ability: Analysis
Client Needs: Safe, Effective Care Environment
Integrated Concept/Process: Nursing Process/Analysis
Content Area: Child Health
Reference: Ball, J., & Bindler, R. (1999). *Pediatric nursing: Caring for children* (2nd ed.). Stamford, Conn.: Appleton & Lange, p. 618.

REFERENCES

Ball, J., & Bindler, R. (1999). *Pediatric nursing: Caring for children* (2nd ed.). Stamford, Conn.: Appleton & Lange.
Bowden, V., Dickey, S., & Greenberg, C. (1998). *Children and their families: The continuum of care.* Philadelphia: W.B. Saunders.
Clark, J., Queener, S., & Karb, V. (2000). *Pharmacologic basis of nursing practice* (6th ed.). St. Louis: Mosby.

E-mail (Celiac Disease): Celiacusa@aol.com
Hodgson, B., & Kizior, R. (2001). *Saunders nursing drug handbook 2001.* Philadelphia: W.B. Saunders.
Wong, D. (1999). *Whaley & Wong's nursing care of infants and children* (6th ed.). St. Louis: Mosby.

Metabolic and Endocrine Disorders

I. FEVER

A. Description
1. An abnormal body temperature elevation
2. A child's temperature can vary depending on activity, emotional stress, the type of clothing the child is wearing, and the temperature of the environment
3. Assessment findings associated with the fever provide important indications of the seriousness of the fever

B. Assessment
1. Temperature elevation
2. Flushed skin
3. Diaphoresis
4. Chills
5. Restlessness or lethargy

C. Implementation
1. Monitor vital signs
2. Administer a sponge bath with lukewarm water for 20 to 30 minutes
3. Administer antipyretics such as acetaminophen (Tylenol) as prescribed
4. Do not administer aspirin (acetylsalicylic acid, ASA), because of the risk of Reye's syndrome
5. Retake the temperature 30 to 60 minutes after the antipyretic is administered
6. Provide adequate fluid intake as tolerated and as prescribed
7. Monitor for dehydration and fluid and electrolyte imbalance
8. Instruct the parents in how to take the temperature, how to safely medicate their child, and when it is necessary to call the physician

II. DEHYDRATION (Box 38-1)

A. Description
1. Dehydration is a common fluid and electrolyte imbalance in infants and children
2. Infants and children are more vulnerable to fluid volume deficit because a greater amount of their body water is in the extracellular fluid compartment
3. In infants and children, the organs that conserve water are immature, placing them at risk for fluid volume deficit
4. The causes can include decreased fluid intake, diaphoresis, vomiting, diarrhea, diabetic ketoacidosis, and extensive burns or other serious injuries

B. Assessment
1. Tachycardia
2. Dry skin and mucous membranes
3. Sunken eyeballs and fontanels
4. Decreased urine output and increased urine specific gravity
5. Changes in level of consciousness and responses to stimuli
6. Signs of circulatory failure, such as coolness and mottling of the extremities
7. Loss of skin elasticity and turgor
8. Delayed capillary filling time
9. Weight loss
10. Decreased blood pressure
11. Thirst
12. Absence of tears

C. Implementation
1. Monitor vital signs
2. Monitor for signs of dehydration
3. Monitor weight and monitor for changes, including fluid gains and losses
4. Monitor I & O and urine for specific gravity
5. Monitor level of consciousness
6. Monitor skin turgor and mucous membranes for dryness
7. Provide oral rehydration therapy with solutions, as prescribed, if the child is able to take fluids orally

BOX 38-1

Types of Dehydration

ISOTONIC DEHYDRATION
Electrolyte and water deficits occur in approximately balanced proportions

HYPERTONIC DEHYDRATION
Water loss exceeds electrolyte loss

HYPOTONIC DEHYDRATION
Electrolyte loss exceeds water loss

8. Administer IV fluids and electrolyte replacements, as prescribed, if the child is unable to take sufficient fluids orally
9. Introduce a regular diet as prescribed when the child is rehydrated
10. Provide instructions to the parents about the types and amounts of fluid to encourage, the signs of dehydration, and the indications of the need to notify the physician

III. PHENYLKETONURIA (PKU)

A. Description
   1. Genetic disorder that results in central nervous system (CNS) damage from toxic levels of phenylalanine in the blood
   2. An autosomal recessive disorder
   3. PKU is characterized by blood phenylalanine levels greater than 8 mg/dL (normal level is less than 2 mg/dL 2 to 5 days after birth)
   4. All 50 states require routine screening of all newborn infants for PKU

B. Assessment
   1. In all children
      a. Digestive problems and vomiting
      b. Seizures
      c. Musty or mousy odor of the urine
      d. Mental retardation
   2. In older children
      a. Eczema
      b. Hypertonia
      c. Hypopigmentation of the hair, skin, and irises
      d. Hyperactive behavior

C. Implementation
   1. Screening of newborn infants for PKU: the infant should have begun formula or breast milk feeding before specimen collection
   2. If initial screening is positive, a repeat test is performed and further diagnostic evaluation is required to verify the diagnosis
   3. Rescreen infants by 14 days of age if the initial screening was done before 48 hours of age
   4. If PKU is diagnosed:
      a. Restrict phenylalanine intake; high-protein foods (meats and dairy products) and aspartame are avoided because they contain large amounts of phenylalanine
      b. Monitor physical, neurological, and intellectual development
      c. Stress the importance of follow-up treatment
      d. Encourage the parents to express feelings about the diagnosis and the risk of PKU in future children

IV. TYPE 1 DIABETES MELLITUS (TYPE 1 DM)   ▲

A. Description
   1. Type 1 DM is also known as insulin-dependent diabetes mellitus (IDDM); the majority of children with diabetes mellitus have type 1
   2. Type 1 DM is caused by the partial or complete lack of secretory capacity of the beta cells of the pancreas, resulting in insulin deficiency
   3. Complete insulin deficiency requires the use of exogenous insulin to promote appropriate glucose use and to prevent complications related to elevated blood glucose levels, such as hyperglycemia, diabetic ketoacidosis, and death
   4. Diagnosis is based on the presence of classic symptoms and an elevated blood glucose level (normal blood glucose level is 80 to 120 mg/dL)

B. Assessment   ▲
   1. Polyuria, polydipsia, polyphagia
   2. Hyperglycemia
   3. Weight loss
   4. Unexplained fatigue or lethargy
   5. Headaches
   6. Stomachaches
   7. Occasional enuresis in a previously toilet-trained child
   8. Vaginitis in adolescent girls (caused by *Candida*, which thrives in hyperglycemic tissues)
   9. Fruity odor to breath
   10. Dehydration
   11. Blurred vision
   12. Slow wound healing
   13. Changes in level of consciousness (LOC)

C. Long-term effects
   1. Failure to grow at a normal rate
   2. Delayed maturation
   3. Recurrent infections
   4. Neuropathy
   5. Cardiovascular disease
   6. Retinal microvascular disease
   7. Renal microvascular disease

D. Complications
   1. Hypoglycemia
   2. Hyperglycemia
   3. Diabetic ketoacidosis
   4. Coma
   5. Hypokalemia
   6. Hyperkalemia

7. Microvascular changes
8. Cardiovascular changes
E. Diet
   1. Total number of calories is individualized on the basis of the child's age and **growth** expectations
   2. As prescribed by the physician, the child may be instructed to follow the food exchange from the American Diabetic Association diet or the dietary guidelines for Americans (Food Guide Pyramid) issued by the U.S. Departments of Agriculture and Health and Human Services
   3. Dietary intake should include three meals per day, eaten at consistent intervals, plus a midafternoon carbohydrate snack and a bedtime snack high in protein; a consistent intake of carbohydrates at each meal and snack is needed
   4. Instruct the child and the parents that the child should carry candy with him or her at all times
   5. Incorporate the diet into individual child's needs, likes and dislikes, lifestyle, and cultural and socioeconomic patterns
   6. Allow the child to participate in making food choices, to provide a sense of control
▲ F. Exercise
   1. Instruct the child in dietary adjustments when exercising
   2. Extra food needs to be consumed for increased activity, usually 10 to 15 g of carbohydrate for every 30 to 45 minutes of activity
   3. Instruct the child to monitor blood glucose prior to exercising
   4. Plan with the child an appropriate exercise regimen, incorporating the developmental stage
▲ G. Insulin
   1. Diluted insulin may be required for some infants to provide small enough doses to avoid hypoglycemia
   2. Diluted insulin should be clearly labeled to avoid dosage errors
   3. To prevent dosage errors, be certain that there is a match of the insulin concentration with the calibration of units on the insulin syringe
   4. A pen-shaped device that contains an insulin-filled cartridge may be prescribed for the adolescent
   5. Laboratory evaluation of glycosylated hemoglobin should be performed every 3 months
   6. Illness, infection, and stress increase the need for insulin, and insulin should not be withheld during illness, infection, or stress, because hyperglycemia and ketoacidosis can result
   7. When the child is NPO for a special procedure, verify with the physician the need to withhold the morning insulin, and when food, fluids, and insulin are to be given
   8. Instruct the child and parents in the administration of the insulin

9. Instruct the child and parents to recognize symptoms of hypoglycemia and hyperglycemia
10. Instruct the parents in the administration of intramuscular (IM) or subcutaneous (SC) glucagon if the child has a hypoglycemic reaction and is unable to consume sugar-containing items orally
11. Instruct the child and parents to always have a spare bottle of insulin available
12. Advise the parents to obtain a Medic-Alert bracelet indicating the type and daily insulin dosage prescribed for the child
H. Blood glucose monitoring
   1. Results provide information needed to maintain good glycemic control
   2. More accurate than urine testing
   3. Requires that the child prick himself or herself several times a day as prescribed
   4. Instruct the child and parents in the proper procedure for obtaining the blood glucose level
   5. Inform the child and parents that the procedure must be done precisely to obtain accurate results
   6. Stress the importance of handwashing before ▲ and after performing the procedure, to prevent infection
   7. Stress the importance of following the manufacturer's instructions for the blood glucose monitoring device
   8. Instruct the child and parents to calibrate the monitor as instructed by the manufacturer
   9. Instruct the child and parents to check the expiration date on the test strips used for the blood glucose monitoring
   10. Instruct the child and parents that if the blood glucose results do not seem reasonable, reread the instructions, reassess technique, check the expiration date of the test strips, and perform the procedure again to verify results
I. Urine testing
   1. Instruct the parents and child in the procedure for testing urine for ketones and glucose
   2. Teach the child that the second voided urine ▲ specimen is most accurate
   3. The presence of ketones may indicate impending ketoacidosis
   4. Urine glucose testing is not recommended as the only means of monitoring control in the child taking insulin, because it is a less reliable indicator as compared with blood glucose monitoring
J. Hypoglycemia ▲
   1. Description
      a. A blood glucose level below 60 mg/dL
      b. Occurs as a result of too much insulin, not enough food, or excessive activity
   2. Implementation (Box 38-2) ▲
      a. If able to, confirm with a blood glucose reading

BOX 38-2

Carbohydrates to Treat Hypoglycemia

½ cup (120 mL) of orange juice or a sugar-sweetened carbonated beverage
1 small box of raisins
3 to 4 hard candies
1 candy bar
2 or 3 glucose tablets

---

  b. Administer glucose immediately in the form of a carbohydrate-containing snack or drink, cake frosting, glucose tablets, or glucose paste
  c. Give an extra snack if the next meal is not planned for more than 30 minutes or if activity is planned
  d. If the child becomes unconscious, squeeze cake frosting or glucose paste onto the gums and retest the blood glucose level if the child does not improve within 15 to 20 minutes; if the reading remains low, administer additional sugar
  e. If the child remains unconscious, it may be necessary to administer glucagon
  f. In the hospital setting, prepare to administer IV dextrose
▲ K. Hyperglycemia
  1. Description: elevated blood glucose level over 200 mg/dL
▲ 2. Implementation: Instruct the parents to notify the physician when blood glucose results are greater than 200 mg/dL, when moderate or high ketonuria is present, when child is unable to take food or fluids, or when illness persists (Box 38-3)
▲ L. Diabetic ketoacidosis (DKA)
  1. Description
    a. A complication of diabetes mellitus that develops when a severe insulin deficiency occurs
    b. DKA is a life-threatening condition
    c. Hyperglycemia that progresses to metabolic acidosis occurs
    d. It develops over a period of several hours to days
    e. The blood glucose level is greater than 300 mg/dL and urine and serum ketones are positive
  2. Implementation
    a. Restore circulating volume and protect against cerebral, coronary, or renal hypoperfusion
    b. Correct dehydration with IV infusions of 0.9% or 0.45% saline as prescribed
    c. Correct hyperglycemia with IV Regular insulin administration as prescribed
    d. Monitor vital signs, urine output, and mental status closely

---

BOX 38-3

Sick Day Rules for the Diabetic Child

Always give insulin even if the child does not have an appetite, or contact the physician for specific instructions
Test blood glucose levels at least every 4 hours
Test for urinary ketones with each voiding
Notify the physician if moderate or large amounts of urinary ketones are present
Follow the child's usual meal plan
Encourage calorie-free liquids to aid in clearing ketones
Encourage rest, especially if urinary ketones are present
Notify the physician if vomiting, fruity odor to the breath, deep rapid respirations, decreasing level of consciousness, or persistent hyperglycemia occurs

---

    e. Correct acidosis and electrolyte imbalances
    f. Administer oxygen as prescribed
    g. Monitor blood glucose level frequently
    h. Monitor potassium level closely because when the child receives insulin to lower the blood glucose level, the serum potassium will decrease as the acidosis improves, and potassium replacement may be required
    i. Monitor the child closely for signs of fluid overload
    j. IV dextrose is added as prescribed when the blood glucose reaches an appropriate level
    k. Treat the cause of hyperglycemia

PRACTICE QUESTIONS

1. A nurse is gathering supplies in preparation to administer a tepid bath to a child with a fever. The nurse understands that which of the following items would not be needed for the bath?
   1. Washcloths and towels
   2. A bottle of alcohol
   3. Toys
   4. Lightweight pajamas
2. A nursing student is assigned to admit to the hospital a child who has been experiencing vomiting and diarrhea. A physician establishes a diagnosis of gastroenteritis and isotonic dehydration. A nursing instructor asks the student to describe isotonic dehydration. The nursing student responds accurately by telling the instructor that isotonic dehydration:
   1. Occurs when water and electrolytes are lost in approximately the same proportions as they exist in the body
   2. Occurs when the loss of electrolytes is greater than the loss of water
   3. Occurs when the loss of water is greater than the loss of electrolytes

4. Causes the serum sodium level to rise above 150 mEq/L

3. A clinic nurse is assessing a child for dehydration. The nurse determines that the child is moderately dehydrated if which symptom is noted on assessment?
1. Flat fontanels
2. Moist mucous membranes
3. Pale skin color
4. Oliguria

4. A physician orders IV potassium for a child with hypertonic dehydration. A nurse performs which of the following highest-priority assessments before administering the potassium?
1. Taking the temperature
2. Taking the blood pressure (BP)
3. Obtaining a weight
4. Checking the amount of urine output

5. A pediatric nurse educator provides a teaching session to the nursing staff regarding phenylketonuria (PKU). The nurse educator tells the nursing staff that:
1. PKU is an autosomal dominant disorder
2. Treatment includes dietary restriction of tyramine
3. All 50 states require routine screening of all newborn infants for PKU
4. PKU primarily affects the gastrointestional system

6. A mother brings her 3-week-old infant to a clinic for a phenylketonuria (PKU) rescreening blood test. The test indicates a serum phenylalanine level of 1 mg/dL. The nurse interprets this result as:
1. Inconclusive
2. Requiring rescreening at age 6 weeks
3. Positive
4. Negative

7. A school-aged child with type 1 diabetes mellitus has soccer practice three afternoons a week. The school nurse provides instructions regarding how to prevent hypoglycemia during practice. The school nurse tells the child to:
1. Take one half of the amount of prescribed insulin on practice days
2. Eat twice the amount normally eaten at lunchtime
3. Take the prescribed insulin at noontime rather than in the morning

4. Eat 6 graham crackers or drink a cup of orange juice prior to soccer practice

8. A home care nurse is teaching an adolescent with type 1 diabetes mellitus about insulin administration and rotation sites. Which of the following statements, if made by the adolescent, would indicate effective teaching?
1. "I need to use a location in one major site for the morning injection and another location in the same major site for the evening injection for 2 to 3 weeks before changing major sites."
2. "I need to use a different site for each insulin injection."
3. "I need to use the same site for 1 month before rotating to another site."
4. "I should use only my stomach and my thighs for injections."

9. The mother of a 6-year-old who has type 1 diabetes mellitus calls a clinic nurse and tells the nurse that the child has been sick. The mother reports that she checked the child's urine and it showed positive ketones. The nurse instructs the mother to:
1. Come to the clinic immediately
2. Hold the next dose of insulin
3. Administer an additional dose of Regular insulin
4. Encourage the child to drink calorie-free liquids

10. A child with type 1 diabetes mellitus is brought to an emergency room by the mother, who states that the child has been complaining of abdominal pain and has a fruity odor of the breath. Diabetic ketoacidosis (DKA) is diagnosed. Anticipating the plan of care, the nurse prepares to administer:
1. 5% dextrose IV infusion
2. Normal saline IV infusion
3. NPH insulin IV
4. Potassium IV

CRITICAL THINKING: FREE-TEXT ENTRY

An adolescent with type 1 diabetes mellitus is attending a dance in the school gym. The adolescent suddenly becomes flushed and complains of hunger and dizziness. The school nurse is at the dance. The nurse takes the child to the nurse's office and performs a blood glucose level that shows 60 mg/dL. What is the most appropriate nursing intervention?

Answer: _____

ANSWERS

1. 2
Rationale: Alcohol should not be used for bathing the child with a fever because it can cause rapid cooling, peripheral vasoconstriction, and chilling, thus elevating the temperature further. Washcloths can be used to squeeze water over the child's body. Towels are used to dry the child. Toys, especially water toys, can be used to provide distraction during the bath. Lightweight clothing should be placed on the child after the child is dried.

Test-Taking Strategy: Use the process of elimination, noting the key word "not." Options 1 and 4 can be easily eliminated. From the remaining options, recall the harmful effects of alcohol and the effect of potentially elevating the temperature with its use. Review the procedure for administering a tepid bath if you had difficulty with this question.
Level of Cognitive Ability: Application
Client Needs: Safe, Effective Care Environment
Integrated Concept/Process: Nursing Process/Planning
Content Area: Child Health
Reference: Wong, D. (1999). *Whaley & Wong's nursing care of infants and children* (6th ed.). St. Louis: Mosby, p. 1242.

2. 1
Rationale: Isotonic dehydration occurs when water and electrolytes are lost in approximately the same proportions as they exist in the body. In this type of dehydration, the serum sodium levels remain normal (135 to145 mEq/L). Option 2 describes hypotonic dehydration; in this type, the serum sodium level is less than 130 mEq/L. Options 3 and 4 describe hypertonic dehydration.
Test-Taking Strategy: Use the process of elimination. Thinking about the terms "hypotonic" and "hypertonic" and relating these terms to "losses" or "excesses" may assist in eliminating options 2, 3, and 4. Review these types of dehydration if you had difficulty with this question.
Level of Cognitive Ability: Analysis
Client Needs: Physiological Integrity
Integrated Concept/Process: Nursing Process/Analysis
Content Area: Child Health
Reference: Bowden, V., Dickey, S., & Greenberg, C. (1998). *Children and their families: The continuum of care.* Philadelphia: W.B. Saunders, p. 1000.

3. 4
Rationale: In moderate dehydration, the fontanels would be slightly sunken, the mucous membranes would be very dry, and the skin color would be dusky. In moderate dehydration, oliguria would be present.
Test-Taking Strategy: Use the process of elimination. Note the key words "moderately dehydrated." From the options presented, option 4 is the clinical manifestation of greatest concern. Review the manifestations related to mild, moderate, and severe dehydration if you had difficulty with this question.
Level of Cognitive Ability: Analysis
Client Needs: Physiological Integrity
Integrated Concept/Process: Nursing Process/Assessment
Content Area: Child Health
Reference: Ball, J., & Bindler, R. (1999). *Pediatric nursing: Caring for children* (2nd ed.). Stamford, Conn.: Appleton & Lange, p. 294.

4. 4
Rationale: The priority assessment before administering IV potassium would be to assess the status of the urine output. Potassium should never be administered in the presence of oliguria or anuria. If the urine output is less than 1 to 2 mL/kg/hr, it should not be administered. Although options 1, 2, and 3 are appropriate assessments for the child with dehydration, these assessments are not specifically related to the administration of IV potassium.
Test-Taking Strategy: Use the process of elimination. Recalling that the kidneys play a key role in the excretion and

reabsorption of potassium will easily direct you to option 4. Review this important medication if you had difficulty with this question.
Level of Cognitive Ability: Analysis
Client Needs: Physiological Integrity
Integrated Concept/Process: Nursing Process/Assessment
Content Area: Child Health
Reference: Wong, D. (1999). *Whaley & Wong's nursing care of infants and children* (6th ed.). St. Louis: Mosby, p. 1288.

5. 3
Rationale: PKU is an autosomal recessive disorder. Treatment includes dietary restriction of phenylalanine intake. PKU is a genetic disorder that results in central nervous system (CNS) damage from toxic levels of phenylalanine in the blood. Option 3 is accurate.
Test-Taking Strategy: Use the process of elimination. Recalling that PKU is a recessive disorder will assist in eliminating option 1. Reading option 2 carefully will direct you to eliminate this option because phenylalanine, not tyramine, is restricted. Recalling that PKU affects the CNS will direct you to option 3. Review the characteristics associated with this disorder if you had difficulty with this question.
Level of Cognitive Ability: Application
Client Needs: Physiological Integrity
Integrated Concept/Process: Teaching/Learning
Content Area: Child Health
Reference: Ball, J., & Bindler, R. (1999). *Pediatric nursing: Caring for children* (2nd ed.). Stamford, Conn.: Appleton & Lange, pp. 902-903.

6. 4
Rationale: PKU is characterized by blood phenylalanine levels greater than 8 mg/dL. A normal level is less than 2 mg/dL. A result of 1 mg/dL is a negative test result.
Test-Taking Strategy: Use the process of elimination. Eliminate options 1 and 2 first because they are similar. Note that the level identified in the question is a low level. This should assist in directing you to option 4. Review this important screening test if you had difficulty with this question.
Level of Cognitive Ability: Analysis
Client Needs: Physiological Integrity
Integrated Concept/Process: Nursing Process/Analysis
Content Area: Child Health
Reference: Ball, J., & Bindler, R. (1999). *Pediatric nursing: Caring for children* (2nd ed.). Stamford, Conn.: Appleton & Lange, p. 902.

7. 4
Rationale: An extra snack of 15 to 30 g of carbohydrate eaten before activities such as soccer practice will prevent hypoglycemia. Six graham crackers or a cup of orange juice will provide 15 to 30 g of carbohydrate. The child or parents should not be instructed to adjust the amount or time of insulin administration. Meal amounts should not be doubled.
Test-Taking Strategy: Use the process of elimination. Options 1 and 3 can be eliminated first because insulin doses and times should not be adjusted. From the remaining options, recalling the manifestations and treatment associated with hypoglycemia will direct you to option 4. Review treatment to prevent hypoglycemia if you had difficulty with this question.
Level of Cognitive Ability: Application
Client Needs: Health Promotion and Maintenance

Integrated Concept/Process: Self-Care
Content Area: Child Health
Reference: Wong, D. (1999). *Whaley & Wong's nursing care of infants and children* (6th ed.). St. Louis: Mosby, p. 1881.

8. 1

Rationale: To help decrease variations in absorption from day to day, the adolescent should use one major site for injections for 2 to 3 weeks before changing major sites. The injections are rotated to different locations within that major site. Options 2, 3, and 4 are incorrect,

Test-Taking Strategy: Use the process of elimination. Eliminate option 4 first because of the word "only." From the remaining options, recalling the physiology associated with absorption of insulin will direct you to option 1. If you had difficulty with this question, review insulin administration.

Level of Cognitive Ability: Analysis
Client Needs: Health Promotion and Maintenance
Integrated Concept/Process: Self-Care
Content Area: Child Health
Reference: Ball, J., & Bindler, R. (1999). *Pediatric nursing: Caring for children* (2nd ed.). Stamford, Conn.: Appleton & Lange, p. 893.

9. 4

Rationale: When the child is sick, the mother should test for urinary ketones with each voiding. If ketones are present, liquids are essential to aid in clearing the ketones. The child should be encouraged to drink calorie-free liquids. It is not necessary to bring the child to the clinic immediately. Insulin doses should not be adjusted or changed.

Test-Taking Strategy: Use the process of elimination. Eliminate options 2 and 3 first because insulin doses should not be adjusted or changed. From the remaining options, note the words "positive ketones." Recalling that liquids are essential to aid in clearing the ketones will direct you to the correct option. Review home care instructions for the sick diabetic child if you had difficulty with this question.

Level of Cognitive Ability: Application
Client Needs: Health Promotion and Maintenance
Integrated Concept/Process: Nursing Process/Implementation
Content Area: Child Health
Reference: Wong, D. (1999). *Whaley & Wong's nursing care of infants and children* (6th ed.). St. Louis: Mosby, p. 1877.

10. 2

Rationale: Rehydration is the initial step in resolving DKA. Normal saline is the initial IV rehydration fluid. NPH insulin is never administered by IV. Dextrose solutions are added to the treatment when the blood glucose level reaches an acceptable level. IV potassium may be required, depending on the potassium level, but would not be part of the initial treatment.

Test-Taking Strategy: Use the process of elimination. Eliminate option 1, knowing that dextrose would not be administered in a hyperglycemic state. Eliminate option 3 next, knowing that NPH insulin is never administered by IV. Knowledge that hydration is the initial treatment in DKA will easily direct you to option 2. Review the treatment for this important condition if you had difficulty with this question.

Level of Cognitive Ability: Analysis
Client Needs: Physiological Integrity
Integrated Concept/Process: Nursing Process/Planning
Content Area: Child Health
Reference: Wong, D. (1999). *Whaley & Wong's nursing care of infants and children* (6th ed.). St. Louis: Mosby, p. 1870.

CRITICAL THINKING: FREE-TEXT ENTRY

Answer: Give the child an oral source of glucose, such as 1/2 cup of a sugar-sweetened carbonated beverage

Rationale: A blood glucose below 70 mg/dL indicates hypoglycemia. The child is attending an activity that is different from the normal routine at school. Insulin requirements change with unfamiliar situations. When signs of hypoglycemia occur, the child needs an immediate source of glucose.

Test-Taking Strategy: Focus on the signs presented in the question to determine that the adolescent is experiencing hypoglycemia. Recall that when signs of hypoglycemia occur, the child needs an immediate source of glucose. If you had difficulty with this question, review the assessment data associated with hypoglycemia and the treatment if it occurs.

Level of Cognitive Ability: Analysis
Client Needs: Physiological Integrity
Integrated Concept/Process: Nursing Process/Implementation
Content Area: Child Health
Reference: Ball, J., & Bindler, R. (1999). *Pediatric nursing: Caring for children* (2nd ed.). Stamford, Conn.: Appleton & Lange, p. 889.

REFERENCES

Ball, J., & Bindler, R. (1999). *Pediatric nursing: Caring for children* (2nd ed.). Stamford, Conn.: Appleton & Lange.

Bowden, V., Dickey, S., & Greenberg, C. (1998). *Children and their families: The continuum of care.* Philadelphia: W.B. Saunders.

Hodgson, B., & Kizior, R. (2001). *Saunders nursing drug handbook 2001.* Philadelphia: W.B. Saunders.

Wong, D. (1999). *Whaley & Wong's nursing care of infants and children* (6th ed.). St. Louis: Mosby.

Renal and Urinary Disorders

I. GLOMERULONEPHRITIS

A. Description
1. A term that includes a variety of disorders, most of which are caused by an immunological reaction
2. It results in proliferative and inflammatory changes within the glomerular structure
3. Destruction, inflammation, and sclerosis of the glomeruli of both kidneys occur
4. Inflammation of the glomeruli results from an antigen-antibody reaction produced by an infection elsewhere in the body
5. Loss of kidney function develops

B. Causes
1. Immunological diseases
2. Autoimmune diseases
3. Streptococcal infection, group A beta-hemolytic
4. History of pharyngitis or tonsillitis 2 to 3 weeks prior to symptoms

C. Types
1. Acute: Occurs 2 to 3 weeks after a streptococcal infection
2. Chronic: Can occur after the acute phase or slowly over time

D. Complications
1. Renal failure
2. Hypertensive encephalopathy
3. Pulmonary edema
4. Heart failure

E. Assessment
1. Child is pale, irritable, and weak
2. Gross hematuria, or dark, smoky, cola-colored or red-brown urine
3. Proteinuria that produces a persistent and excessive foam in the urine
4. Oliguria or anuria
5. Urinary debris, moderate to high specific gravity, low urinary pH
6. Increased blood urea nitrogen (BUN) and creatinine
7. Azotemia
8. Abdominal or flank pain
9. Edema in the face and periorbital area, feet, or generalized
10. Hypertension
11. Increased antistreptolysin O titer (used to diagnose disorders caused by streptococcal infections)
12. Headache
13. Chills and fever
14. Anorexia, nausea, and vomiting

F. Implementation
1. Monitor vital signs, weight, intake and output (I & O), and the characteristics of urine
2. Limit activity; provide safety measures
3. Nutrition
   a. Restrictions depend on the stage and severity of the disease, especially the extent of the edema
   b. In uncomplicated cases, a regular diet is permitted but sodium is restricted to no added salt to foods
   c. Moderate sodium restriction is prescribed for the child with hypertension or edema
   d. Fluid and sodium intake is restricted as prescribed if edema is present and if urine output is significantly reduced
   e. Foods high in potassium are restricted during periods of oliguria
   f. Protein is restricted if the child has severe azotemia resulting from prolonged oliguria
4. Administer diuretics as prescribed if significant edema and fluid overload are present
5. Administer antihypertensives as prescribed for hypertension
6. Administer anticonvulsants as prescribed for seizures associated with hypertensive encephalopathy; initiate seizure precautions as indicated

433

7. Administer antibiotics as prescribed for the child with evidence of persistent streptococcal infections

8. Monitor for edema and fluid overload, ascites, pulmonary edema, and congestive heart failure (CHF)

9. Monitor for signs of renal failure, cardiac failure, and hypertensive encephalopathy

10. Instruct the parents to report signs of bloody urine, headache, or edema

11. Instruct the parents that the child needs to obtain treatment for infections, specifically sore throats and upper respiratory infections

II. NEPHROTIC SYNDROME

A. Description
1. A set of clinical manifestations arising from protein wasting secondary to diffuse glomerular damage
2. Defined as massive proteinuria, hypoalbuminemia, hyperlipemia, and edema
3. The primary objective of therapeutic management is to reduce the excretion of urinary protein and maintain protein-free urine

B. Assessment
1. Pale, irritable, and fatigued child
2. Child gains weight
3. Decreased urine output
4. Dark, frothy urine; hematuria may be present
5. Abdominal ascites
6. Waxy pallor of the skin
7. Hypertension
8. Anorexia
9. Anemia
10. Amenorrhea or abnormal menses

C. Implementation
1. Monitor vital signs
2. Monitor I & O and daily weights
3. Monitor urine for specific gravity and albumin
4. Monitor for edema
5. Monitor for signs of infection, particularly in the edematous child and in the child receiving corticosteroid therapy
6. Maintain bed rest if severe edema is present; activity is not restricted during remission
7. Nutrition
   a. A regular diet is prescribed if the child is in remission
   b. Sodium restriction is prescribed during periods of massive edema
   c. Normal protein intake is usually prescribed
8. Corticosteroid therapy
   a. Prescribed as soon as the diagnosis has been determined
   b. Continued until the urine is free from protein and remains normal for 10 days to 2 weeks; then it is tapered to discontinuation

c. If a tendency to relapse is demonstrated, a low-dose, every-other-day schedule of corticosteroid therapy may be prescribed and may continue for 6 months to a year

9. Administer immunosuppressant therapy as prescribed to reduce the relapse rate and induce long-term remission; may be administered in conjunction with the corticosteroid

10. Administer loop diuretic as prescribed (may be prescribed if edema interferes with respiration)

11. Administer plasma expanders such as salt-poor human albumin as prescribed to the severely edematous child

12. Administer antibiotics as prescribed for infection

13. Instruct the parents about testing the urine for albumin, medication administration, and general care of the child

14. Instruct the parents regarding the signs of infection and the need to avoid contact with other children who may be infectious

15. Instruct the parents about the side effects of corticosteroid therapy

III. ENURESIS

A. Description
1. Refers to a condition in which the child is unable to control bladder function even though the child has reached an age at which control of voiding is expected
2. By age 5, most children are aware of bladder fullness and are able to control voiding

B. Primary nocturnal enuresis
1. Bed-wetting in a child who has never been dry for extended periods
2. Common in children, and most children will eventually outgrow bed-wetting without therapeutic intervention
3. The child is not able to sense a full bladder and does not awaken to void
4. The child may have delayed maturation of the central nervous system (CNS)

C. Secondary or acquired enuresis
1. The onset of wetting after a period of established urinary continence
2. May occur during nighttime sleep (nocturnal), only during the waking hours (diurnal), or during both times of the day
3. The child may complain of dysuria, urgency, or frequency
4. The child should be assessed for urinary tract infections

D. Assessment
1. Normal voiding pattern
2. History of bed-wetting with no extended period of dryness in a child older than age 5 years

E. Implementation
1. Obtain urinalysis and urine culture as prescribed to rule out infection or existing disorder
2. Assist the family with identifying a treatment plan that will best fit their needs
3. Limit fluid intake at night, and encourage the child to void just before going to bed
4. Involve the child in caring for the wet sheets and changing the bed, to assist the child to take ownership of the problem
5. Provide reward systems as appropriate for the child
6. Incorporate behavioral conditioning techniques
7. Encourage follow-up to determine the effectiveness of the treatment

IV. CRYPTORCHIDISM
A. Description: Occurs when one or both testes fail to descend through the inguinal canal into the scrotal sac
B. Assessment: Testes not palpable or easily guided into the scrotum
C. Implementation
1. Monitor during the first 12 months of life to determine if spontaneous descent occurs
2. After age 1, medical or surgical treatment may be instituted
3. Human chorionic gonadotropin (hCG), a pituitary hormone administered by injection that stimulates the production of testosterone, and hormone therapy with luteinizing hormone–releasing hormone (nasal spray) may be prescribed
4. Surgical correction, if needed, is done by orchiopexy before the child's second birthday (preferably between 1 and 2 years of age) if the testes do not descend spontaneously
5. Monitor for bleeding and infection postoperatively
6. Instruct the parents in postoperative home care measures, including preventing infection, pain control, and activity restrictions
7. Provide an opportunity for parental counseling if the parents are concerned about the future fertility of the child

V. HYPOSPADIAS/EPISPADIAS
A. Description: Congenital defects involving abnormal placement of the urethral orifice of the penis
B. Assessment
1. Hypospadias: Urethral orifice located below the glans penis along the ventral surface
2. Epispadias: Urethral orifice located on the dorsal surface of the penis; often occurs with exstrophy of the bladder

C. Surgical implementation
1. Done before the age of toilet training, preferably between 16 and 18 months of age
2. The child should not be circumcised because the foreskin may be used in surgical reconstruction
D. Implementation postoperatively
1. The child will have a pressure dressing and may have some type of urinary diversion or a urinary stent (used to maintain patency of the urethral opening) while healing of the meatus occurs
2. Monitor vital signs
3. Encourage fluid intake to maintain adequate urine output and to maintain patency of the stent
4. Monitor I & O and the urine for cloudiness or a foul odor
5. Notify the physician if there is no urinary drainage for 1 hour, because this may indicate kinks in the system or obstruction by sediment
6. Provide pain medication (acetaminophen [Tylenol]) or medication to relieve bladder spasms (anticholinergic) as prescribed
7. Administer antibiotics as prescribed
8. Instruct the parents in the care of the urinary diversion or stent if present
9. Instruct the parents to avoid giving the child a tub bath until the stent, if present, is removed
10. Instruct the parents about fluid intake, medication administration, the signs and symptoms of infection, and the need for physician follow-up for dressing removal approximately 4 days after surgery

VI. BLADDER EXSTROPHY
A. Description
1. A congenital anomaly characterized by extrusion of the urinary bladder to the outside of the body through a defect in the lower abdominal wall
2. The cause is not known
3. Treatment requires surgical management and occurs in a series of staged reconstructions
4. Initial surgery for closure of the abdominal defect should occur within the first few days of life
5. The goal of subsequent operations is to reconstruct the bladder and genitalia and enable the child to achieve urinary continence
B. Assessment
1. Exposed bladder mucosa
2. Widened symphysis pubis
3. Defects of the external genitalia
C. Implementation
1. Monitor urinary output
2. Monitor for signs of urinary tract or wound infection
3. Maintain the integrity of the exposed bladder mucosa

4. Prevent the bladder tissue from drying, while allowing the drainage of urine, until surgical closure is performed
    a. The bladder is covered with sterile nonadherent clear plastic wrap or a sterile thin film dressing without adhesive
    b. Petroleum jelly is avoided because it tends to dry out, adhere to the bladder mucosa, and damage the delicate tissues when the dressing is removed
5. Monitor laboratory values and urinalysis to assess for renal function
6. Administer antibiotics as prescribed
7. Provide emotional support to the parents, and encourage verbalization of their fears and concerns

PRACTICE QUESTIONS

1. A nurse interviews the parents of a child recently diagnosed with glomerulonephritis. The nurse understands that which information collected during the assessment is most often associated with the diagnosis of glomerulonephritis?
    1. Streptococcal throat infection 2 weeks prior to diagnosis
    2. Child fell off a bike onto the handlebars
    3. Nausea and vomiting for the last 24 hours
    4. Urticaria and itching for 1 week prior to diagnosis
2. A nurse is assigned to care for a child suspected of having glomerulonephritis. The nurse reviews the child's record and notes that which finding is associated with the diagnosis of glomerulonephritis?
    1. Low blood urea nitrogen (BUN)
    2. Hypotension
    3. Low urinary specific gravity
    4. Red-brown urine
3. A nurse is developing a plan of care for a 7-year-old child diagnosed with acute glomerulonephritis. The nurse includes which priority intervention in the plan of care?
    1. Encourage limited activity and provide safety measures
    2. Catheterize the child to strictly monitor intake and output
    3. Force oral fluids to prevent hypovolemic shock
    4. Encourage classmates to visit and to keep the child informed of school events
4. A nurse is performing an admission assessment on a 2-year-old child who has been diagnosed with nephrotic syndrome. The nurse knows that the most common characteristic associated with nephrotic syndrome is:
    1. Generalized edema
    2. Frank bright red blood in the urine
    3. Increased urinary output
    4. Hypotension
5. A nurse is preparing a 2-year-old child with suspected nephrotic syndrome for diagnostic tests to confirm the diagnosis. The mother asks the nurse if the child will ever look thin again. The nurse most appropriately responds by telling the mother:
    1. "Wearing loose-fitting clothing should help conceal the extra weight."
    2. "In most cases, medication and diet will control the fluid retention."
    3. "Do you feel guilty because you didn't notice the weight gain?"
    4. "When children are little, it's expected they'll look a little chubby."
6. A 7-year-old child is seen in a clinic, and the primary health care provider documents a diagnosis of primary nocturnal enuresis. The mother asks a nurse about the diagnosis. The nurse plans to respond, knowing that primary nocturnal enuresis:
    1. Requires surgical intervention to improve the problem
    2. Is caused by a psychiatric problem
    3. Is common and most children will outgrow the problem without therapeutic intervention
    4. Does not respond to treatment
7. A child with cryptorchidism is being discharged following orchiopexy, which was performed on an outpatient basis. A nurse informs the parents that which care measure should take priority in the plan of care at home?
    1. Administering anticholinergics
    2. Measuring intake and output
    3. Applying cold, wet compresses to the surgical site
    4. Preventing infection at the surgical site
8. A nurse has provided discharge instructions to the mother of a 2-year-old child who has had an orchiopexy to correct cyptorchidism. Which of the following statements, if made by the mother of the child, indicates that further teaching is necessary?
    1. "I'll check his temperature."
    2. "I'll let him decide when to return to his play activities."
    3. "I'll give him medication so he'll be comfortable."
    4. "I'll check his voiding to be sure there's no problem."
9. A nurse collects a urine specimen preoperatively from a child with epispadias who is scheduled for surgical repair. When the nurse is analyzing the results of the urinalysis, which of the following would the nurse most likely expect to note?
    1. Hematuria
    2. Proteinuria
    3. Bacteriuria
    4. Glucosuria

10. A 1-year-old child with hypospadias is scheduled for surgery to correct this condition. The nurse prepares a nursing care plan for this child and understands that this surgery is taking place at a time when:
    1. Fears of separation are great
    2. Sibling rivalry will cause regression to occur
    3. Embarrassment about voiding irregularities is common
    4. Concern over size and function of the penis is present

11. An 18-month-old child is being discharged following surgical repair of hypospadias. Which postoperative nursing care measure should the nurse stress to the parents as they prepare to take this child home?
    1. Encourage toilet training to ensure that flow of urine is normal
    2. Restrict fluid intake to reduce urinary output for the first few days
    3. Avoid tub baths until the stent has been removed
    4. Leave the diapers off to allow the site to heal

12. A nurse is reviewing a treatment plan with the parents of a newborn infant with hypospadias. Which statement by the parents indicates their understanding of the plan?
    1. "Circumcision has been delayed to save tissue for surgical repair."
    2. "Catheterization will be necessary when the infant does not void."
    3. "Caution should be used when straddling the infant on a hip."
    4. "Vital signs should be taken daily to check for bladder infection."

13. The parents of a newborn infant have been told that their child was born with bladder exstrophy. The parents ask the nurse about this condition. The nurse plans to base the response on knowledge that this condition is:
    1. Caused by the use of medications taken by the mother during pregnancy

    2. A hereditary disorder that occurs in every other generation
    3. A condition in which the urinary bladder is abnormally located in the pelvic cavity
    4. An extrusion of the urinary bladder to the outside of the body through a defect in the lower abdominal wall

14. After performing an assessment of an infant with bladder exstrophy, a nurse prepares a plan of care. The nurse identifies which of the following nursing diagnoses as the priority for the infant?
    1. Alteration in elimination
    2. Impaired tissue integrity
    3. Parental knowledge deficit
    4. Potential for infection

15. A nurse is caring for an infant with a diagnosis of bladder exstrophy. To protect the exposed bladder tissue, the nurse plans to:
    1. Cover the bladder with petroleum jelly gauze
    2. Keep the bladder tissue dry by covering it with dry sterile gauze
    3. Cover the bladder with a nonadhering plastic wrap
    4. Apply sterile distilled water dressings over the bladder mucosa

CRITICAL THINKING: FREE-TEXT ENTRY

A nurse is performing an assessment on a child admitted to the hospital with a probable diagnosis of nephrotic syndrome. The nurse reviews the physician's orders and notes that the physician has ordered a urinalysis. The nurse obtains the specimen and would expect to observe what characteristics in the urine if nephrotic syndrome is present?

Answer: _____

ANSWERS

1. **1**

Rationale: Group A beta-hemolytic streptococcal infection is a cause of glomerulonephritis. Often the child becomes ill with streptococcal infection of the upper respiratory tract and then develops symptoms of acute poststreptococcal glomerulonephritis after an interval of 1 to 2 weeks. The assessment data in options 2, 3, and 4 are unrelated to a diagnosis of glomerulonephritis.

Test-Taking Strategy: Use the process of elimination. Option 2 relates to a kidney injury, not an infectious process. From the remaining options, recalling that a streptococcal infection 1 to 2 weeks prior to the development of glomerulonephritis is

the classic assessment finding will assist in directing you to option 1. If you had difficulty with this question, review the causes of glomerulonephritis.

Level of Cognitive Ability: Analysis
Client Needs: Physiological Integrity
Integrated Concept/Process: Nursing Process/Assessment
Content Area: Child Health
Reference: Ball, J., & Bindler, R. (1999). *Pediatric nursing: Caring for children* (2nd ed.). Stamford, Conn.: Appleton & Lange, p. 698.

2. **4**

Rationale: Gross hematuria, resulting in dark, smoky, cola-colored or red-brown urine, is a classic symptom of glomerulonephritis. Hypertension is also common. BUN levels may be elevated. A moderately elevated to high urinary specific gravity is associated with glomerulonephritis.

Test-Taking Strategy: Use the process of elimination. Eliminate options 2 and 3 first because hypertension and a high specific gravity are most likely to occur in this kidney disorder. Knowledge that BUN levels elevate will assist in directing you to option 4. If you had difficulty with this question, review the clinical manifestations associated with glomerulonephritis.

Level of Cognitive Ability: Analysis
Client Needs: Physiological Integrity
Integrated Concept/Process: Nursing Process/Analysis
Content Area: Child Health
Reference: Ball, J., & Bindler, R. (1999). *Pediatric nursing: Caring for children* (2nd ed.). Stamford, Conn.: Appleton & Lange, p. 698.

3. 1

Rationale: Activity is limited and most children, because of fatigue, voluntarily restrict their activities during the active phase of the disease. Catheterization may cause a risk of infection. Fluids should not be forced. Visitors should be limited to allow for adequate rest.

Test-Taking Strategy: Use the process of elimination. Eliminate option 4 because rest is the priority over socialization. Eliminate option 2 next. Although monitoring I & O is essential, the risk of infection could occur with catheterization. From the remaining options, eliminate option 3 because of the words "force oral fluids." Review the appropriate nursing interventions for the child with glomerulonephritis, if you had difficulty with this question.

Level of Cognitive Ability: Application
Client Needs: Physiological Integrity
Integrated Concept/Process: Nursing Process/Planning
Content Area: Child Health
Reference: Wong, D. (1999). *Whaley & Wong's nursing care of infants and children* (6th ed.). St. Louis: Mosby, p. 1383.

4. 1

Rationale: Nephrotic syndrome is defined as massive proteinuria, hypoalbuminemia, hyperlipemia, and edema. Urine is dark, foamy, and frothy, but microscopic hematuria is present; frank bright red blood in the urine does not occur. Urine output is decreased, and hypertension is likely to be present.

Test-Taking Strategy: Use the process of elimination. Eliminate options 3 and 4 first because urine output is most likely to be decreased in a renal disorder and hypertension is more likely to be present. Associate edema with nephrotic syndrome because this will be helpful to you if you encounter a similar question. If you had difficulty with this question, review the characteristics of nephrotic syndrome.

Level of Cognitive Ability: Analysis
Client Needs: Physiological Integrity
Integrated Concept/Process: Nursing Process/Assessment
Content Area: Child Health
Reference: Wong, D. (1999). *Whaley & Wong's nursing care of infants and children* (6th ed.). St. Louis: Mosby, p. 1385.

5. 2

Rationale: It is important to give the mother information that addresses the issue that is the parent's concern. Most children experience remission with treatment. Options 1 and 3 are nontherapeutic and may add to the mother's guilt. Option 4

does not acknowledge the concern and is a stereotypical response.

Test-Taking Strategy: Use therapeutic communication techniques, and focus on the mother's concern. Options 1, 3, and 4 do not address the mother's concern and are inappropriate and nontherapeutic responses. Remember, always address the mother's feelings and concerns.

Level of Cognitive Ability: Application
Client Needs: Physiological Integrity
Integrated Concept/Process: Communication and Documentation
Content Area: Child Health
Reference: Wong, D. (1999). *Whaley & Wong's nursing care of infants and children* (6th ed.). St. Louis: Mosby, p. 1385.

6. 3

Rationale: Primary nocturnal enuresis occurs in a child who has never been dry at night for extended periods. It is common in children, and most children will eventually outgrow bed-wetting without therapeutic intervention. The child is not able to sense a full bladder and does not awaken to void. The child may have delayed maturation of the central nervous system (CNS). The condition is not caused by a psychiatric problem.

Test-Taking Strategy: Use the process of elimination, noting the relationship between the words "enuresis" in the question and "bed-wetting" in the correct option. If you had difficulty with this question, review the characteristics associated with enuresis.

Level of Cognitive Ability: Application
Client Needs: Physiological Integrity
Integrated Concept/Process: Nursing Process/Planning
Content Area: Child Health
Reference: Wong, D. (1999). *Whaley & Wong's nursing care of infants and children* (6th ed.). St. Louis: Mosby, p. 867.

7. 4

Rationale: The most common complications associated with orchiopexy are bleeding and infection. The parents are instructed in postoperative home care measures, including preventing infection, pain control, and activity restrictions. Anticholinergics are prescribed for the relief of bladder spasms and are not necessary following orchiopexy. Measurement of intake and output is not required. Cold wet compresses are not prescribed. In addition, the moisture from a wet compress presents a potential for infection.

Test-Taking Strategy: Note the key word "priority" in the stem of the question. Use Maslow's Hierarchy of Needs theory to answer the question. Of the options presented, the potential for infection is the physiological priority. Review home care instructions following orchiopexy if you had difficulty with this question.

Level of Cognitive Ability: Application
Client Needs: Health Promotion and Maintenance
Integrated Concept/Process: Teaching/Learning
Content Area: Child Health
Reference: Wong, D. (1999). *Whaley & Wong's nursing care of infants and children* (6th ed.). St. Louis: Mosby, p. 540.

8. 2

Rationale: All vigorous activities should be restricted for 2 weeks following surgery to promote healing and prevent injury. This will prevent dislodging of the suture, which is internal. Normally, 2-year-olds will want to be very active; therefore, allowing the child to decide when to return to his play activities may prevent healing and cause injury. The parent should be taught to monitor the temperature, provide analgesics as needed, and monitor the urine output.

Test-Taking Strategy: Use the process of elimination. Note the key words "further teaching is necessary." Option 1 is an important action in order to recognize signs of infection. Option 3 is appropriate to keep pain to a minimum. Option 4 monitors voiding pattern, which is also important following this type of surgery. If you had difficulty with this question, review the discharge instructions following surgical correction of cryptorchidism.

Level of Cognitive Ability: Analysis
Client Needs: Health Promotion and Maintenance
Integrated Concept/Process: Teaching/Learning
Content Area: Child Health
Reference: Ball, J., & Bindler, R. (1999). *Pediatric nursing: Caring for children* (2nd ed.). Stamford, Conn.: Appleton & Lange, p. 702.

9. **3**

Rationale: Epispadias is a congenital defect involving abnormal placement of the urethral orifice of the penis. The urethral opening is located anywhere on the dorsum of the penis. This anatomical characteristic leads to the easy entry of bacteria into the urine. Options 1, 2, and 4 are not characteristically noted in this condition.

Test-Taking Strategy: Use knowledge regarding the anatomical characteristic of epispadias and the process of elimination to answer the question. Options 1, 2, and 4 do not relate to the potential for infection, which can be present in the condition of epispadias. If you had difficulty with this question, review the diagnostic findings associated with epispadias.

Level of Cognitive Ability: Analysis
Client Needs: Physiological Integrity
Integrated Concept/Process: Nursing Process/Assessment
Content Area: Child Health
Reference: Wong, D. (1999). *Whaley & Wong's nursing care of infants and children* (6th ed.). St. Louis: Mosby, p. 542.

10. **1**

Rationale: At the age of 1 year, a child's fears of separation are great, since the child is facing the developmental task of trusting others. Options 3 and 4 may be issues if the child was older. There are no data in the question to determine that siblings exist.

Test-Taking Strategy: Use the process of elimination and knowledge regarding the stages of growth and development to answer the question. Options 3 and 4 can be easily eliminated. Next, eliminate option 2 because there are no data in the question to determine that siblings exist. If you had difficulty with this question, review the stages of growth and development.

Level of Cognitive Ability: Analysis
Client Needs: Psychosocial Integrity
Integrated Concept/Process: Nursing Process/Planning
Content Area: Child Health
Reference: Wong, D. (1999). *Whaley & Wong's care of infants and children* (6th ed.). St. Louis: Mosby, pp. 581-582.

11. **3**

Rationale: After hypospadias repair, the parents are instructed to avoid giving the child a tub bath until the stent has been removed, to prevent infection. Diapers are placed on the child to prevent contamination of the surgical site. Fluids should be encouraged to maintain hydration. Toilet training should not be an issue during this stressful period.

Test-Taking Strategy: Use the process of elimination. Option 1 is eliminated first, since toilet training should not be initiated during times of stress, such as following surgery. Option 2 is inappropriate, since fluids should be encouraged rather than restricted. Eliminate option 4, since this action can cause contamination of the surgical site. If you had difficulty with this question, review the postoperative care following surgical repair of hypospadias.

Level of Cognitive Ability: Application
Client Needs: Health Promotion and Maintenance
Integrated Concept/Process: Teaching/Learning
Content Area: Child Health
Reference: Wong, D. (1999). *Whaley & Wong's nursing care of infants and children* (6th ed.). St. Louis: Mosby, p. 541.

12. **1**

Rationale: Hypospadias is a congenital defect involving abnormal placement of the urethral orifice of the penis. In hypospadias, the urethral orifice is located below the glans penis along the ventral surface. The infant should not be circumcised because the dorsal foreskin tissue will be used for surgical repair of the hypospadias. Options 2, 3, and 4 are unrelated to this disorder.

Test-Taking Strategy: Use the process of elimination. Note the key words "indicates their understanding." Recalling that hypospadias is a congenital defect involving abnormal placement of the urethral orifice of the penis will direct you to option 1. Review the treatment plan related to the repair of the hypospadias, if you had difficulty with this question.

Level of Cognitive Ability: Analysis
Client Needs: Health Promotion and Maintenance
Integrated Concept/Process: Teaching/Learning
Content Area: Child Health
Reference: Wong, D. (1999). *Whaley & Wong's nursing care of infants and children* (6th ed.). St. Louis: Mosby, p. 541.

13. **4**

Rationale: Bladder exstrophy is a congenital anomaly characterized by the extrusion of the urinary bladder to the outside of the body through a defect in the lower abdominal wall. The cause in not known, and a higher incidence occurs in the male. Options 1, 2, and 3 are not characteristics of this disorder.

Test Taking Strategy: Use the process of elimination. If you are unfamiliar with this condition, note the relationship of *exstrophy* in the name of the disorder to the word *extrusion* in the correct option. This should remind you that this condition is located external to the body. If you had difficulty with this question, review the characteristics of bladder exstrophy.

Level of Cognitive Ability: Analysis
Client Needs: Physiological Integrity
Integrated Concept/Process: Nursing Process/Planning
Content Area: Child Health
Reference: Wong, D. (1999). *Whaley & Wong's nursing care of infants and children* (6th ed.). St. Louis: Mosby, p. 542.

14. **2**

Rationale: In bladder exstrophy, the bladder is exposed and external to the body. The highest priority is impaired tissue integrity related to the exposed bladder mucosa. Although the infant needs to be monitored for elimination patterns and kidney function, this is not the priority concern for this condition. Parental knowledge deficit related to the diagnosis and treatment of the condition will need to be addressed, but again is not the priority. Although infection related to the anatomical location of the defect is an appropriate nursing diagnosis, it is a potential problem and not an actual one.

Test-Taking Strategy: Use the process of elimination. Eliminate option 4 first because this addresses a potential problem rather than an actual one. Eliminate option 3 next because physiological needs take precedence over psychosocial needs. From the remaining options, knowledge that the bladder mucosa is exposed in this condition should direct you to the correct option. Review this disorder if you had difficulty with this question.

Level of Cognitive Ability: Analysis
Client Needs: Physiological Integrity
Integrated Concept/Process: Nursing Process/Analysis
Content Area: Child Health
Reference: Wong, D. (1999). *Whaley & Wong's nursing care of infants and children* (6th ed.). St. Louis: Mosby, p. 543.

15. **3**

Rationale: In this disorder, care must be taken to protect the exposed bladder tissue from drying while allowing the drainage of urine. This is best accomplished by covering the bladder with a nonadhering plastic wrap. The use of petroleum jelly gauze should be avoided because this type of dressing can dry out, adhere to the mucosa, and damage the delicate tissue when removed. Dry sterile dressings and dressings soaked in solutions (that can dry out) also damage the mucosa when removed.

Test-Taking Strategy: Use the process of elimination. Also, note the key word "nonadhering" in the correct option. If you had difficulty with this question, review care of the infant with bladder exstrophy.

Level of Cognitive Ability: Application
Client Needs: Physiological Integrity
Integrated Concept/Process: Nursing Process/Planning
Content Area: Child Health
Reference: Wong, D. (1999). *Whaley & Wong's nursing care of infants and children* (6th ed.). St. Louis: Mosby, p. 543.

CRITICAL THINKING: FREE-TEXT ENTRY

Answer: Dark, frothy urine

Rationale: Nephrotic syndrome is defined as massive proteinuria, hypoalbuminemia, hyperlipemia, and edema. The urine volume is decreased, and the urine is dark and frothy in appearance. Hematuria may also be noted.

Test-Taking Strategy: Focus on the probable diagnosis of the child and think about the definition of nephrotic syndrome and its associated characteristics to answer the question. Review the clinical manifestations associated with nephrotic syndrome if you had difficulty with this question.

Level of Cognitive Ability: Analysis
Client Needs: Physiological Integrity
Integrated Concept/Process: Nursing Process/Assessment
Content Area: Child Health
Reference: Wong, D. (1999). *Whaley & Wong's nursing care of infants and children* (6th ed.). St. Louis: Mosby, p. 1386.

REFERENCES

Ball, J., & Bindler, R. (1999). *Pediatric nursing: Caring for children* (2nd ed.). Stamford, Conn.: Appleton & Lange.

Bowden, V., Dickey, S, & Greenberg, C. (1998). *Children and their families: The continuum of care.* Philadelphia: W.B. Saunders.

Wong, D. (1999). *Whaley & Wong's nursing care of infants and children* (6th ed.). St. Louis: Mosby.

Integumentary Disorders

I. ECZEMA (ATOPIC DERMATITIS)

A. Description
1. A superficial inflammatory process involving primarily the epidermis
2. The major goals of management are to relieve pruritus, hydrate the skin, reduce inflammation, and prevent or control secondary infections

B. Forms of eczema
1. Infantile: Usually begins at 2 to 6 months of age and generally undergoes spontaneous remission by 3 years of age
2. Childhood: May follow the infantile form and occurs at 2 to 3 years of age
3. Preadolescent and adolescent: Begins at about 12 years of age and may continue into the early adult years or indefinitely

C. Assessment
1. Redness
2. Itching
3. Minute papules and vesicles
4. Weeping, oozing, and crusting of lesions

D. Implementation
1. Avoid exposure to skin irritants such as soaps, detergents, fabric softeners, diaper wipes, and powder
2. Improve skin hydration
3. Apply cool, wet compresses to soothe the skin
4. Administer antihistamines and topical corticosteroids as prescribed; corticosteroids are applied in a thin layer and are rubbed into the area thoroughly
5. Prevent or minimize scratching; keep the nails short and clean, and place gloves or cotton socks over the hands
6. Eliminate conditions that increase itching, such as heat, woolen clothes or blankets, rough fabrics, or furry stuffed animals
7. Instruct the parents to wash clothing in a mild detergent and rinse thoroughly; putting the clothes through a second complete wash cycle without detergent will minimize the amount of residue remaining on the fabric
8. Instruct the parents in the measures to prevent skin infections
9. Instruct the parents to monitor the lesions for signs of infection (honey-colored crusts with surrounding erythema)

II. IMPETIGO

A. Description
1. A highly contagious, bacterial infection of the skin caused by beta-hemolytic streptococci or *Staphylococcus aureus* or both
2. The most common sites of infection are the face, around the mouth, the hands, the neck, and the extremities
3. The lesions begin as a vesicle or pustule that is surrounded by edema and redness, usually at a site that has been injured; this progresses to an exudative and crusting stage
4. After the crusting of the lesions, the initially serous vesicular fluid becomes cloudy, and the vesicle ruptures, leaving a honey-colored crust covering an ulcerated base

B. Assessment
1. Lesions
2. Pruritus
3. Burning
4. Secondary lymph node involvement

C. Implementation
1. Contact isolation; use standard (universal) precautions and implement agency-specific isolation procedures for the hospitalized child
2. Allow lesions to dry by air exposure
3. Assist the child with daily bathing with antibacterial soap, such as pHisoHex, as prescribed
4. Apply warm compresses to lesions 2 or 3 times

per day, as prescribed, to remove crusts and to allow for healing

5. Apply and instruct the parents in the use of antibiotic ointments; the infection is communicable for 48 hours after antibiotic ointment treatment is begun

6. Administer oral antibiotics, which may be prescribed if there is no response to topical antibiotic treatment

7. Apply and instruct the parents in the use of emollients, as prescribed, to prevent skin cracking

8. Instruct the parents in the methods to prevent the spread of the infection, especially careful handwashing

9. Inform the parents that the child needs to use separate towels, linens, and dishes

10. Inform the parents that all linens and clothing should be washed separately with detergent in hot water

III. PEDICULOSIS CAPITIS (LICE)

A. Description

1. An infestation of the hair and scalp with lice

2. The most common sites of involvement are the occipital area, behind the ears at the nape of the neck, and occasionally the eyebrows and eyelashes

3. The female louse lays her eggs (nits) on the hair shaft, close to the scalp; the incubation period is 8 to 10 days

4. Head lice live and reproduce only on humans and are transmitted by direct and indirect contact, such as sharing of brushes, hats, towels, and bedding

5. All contacts of the infested child should be examined

B. Assessment

1. Intense pruritis

2. Adult lice are difficult to see and appear as small gray specks, which may crawl very fast

3. Nits are visible and firmly attached to the hair shaft near the scalp; they are tiny silver or gray specks resembling dandruff

C. Implementation

1. Use of a pediculicide shampoo; the hair is towel dried, the nits are removed with a fine-toothed comb, and the treatment is repeated in 7 days

2. Use of permethrin (Nix) rinse
   a. Apply to washed and towel-dried hair, leave in place for 10 minutes, and then rinse
   b. After rinsing, towel dry the hair, and remove the nits with a fine-toothed comb

3. Instruct the parents in the use of shampoo and rinse as prescribed

4. Instruct the parents that bedding and clothing used by the child should be changed daily,

laundered in hot water with detergent, and dried in a hot dryer for 20 minutes

5. Instruct the parents that nonessential bedding and clothing can be stored in a tightly sealed bag for 10 days to 2 weeks and then washed

6. Instruct the parents to seal toys that cannot be washed or dry cleaned in a plastic bag for 2 weeks

7. Instruct the parents that hairbrushes or combs should be discarded or soaked in hot water (54.4° C [130° F])

8. Instruct the parents that furniture and carpets need to be vacuumed frequently

9. Teach the child not to share clothing, headwear, or brushes and combs

IV. SCABIES (Refer to Chapter 47 for additional information related to scabies)

A. Description

1. A parasitic skin disorder caused by an infestation of *Sarcoptes scabiei* (itch mite)

2. Is endemic among schoolchildren and institutionalized populations as a result of close personal contact

3. Incubation period
   a. Female mite burrows into epidermis, lays eggs, and dies in the burrow after 4 to 5 weeks
   b. The eggs hatch in 3 to 5 days, and larvae migrate to the skin to mature and complete their life cycle

4. Infectious period: During the course of the infestation

5. Transmission: By close personal contact with infected person

B. Assessment

1. Intense pruritis, especially at night

2. Burrows (fine grayish red lines that may be difficult to see) on the skin

C. Implementation

1. Topical application of a scabicide such as lindane cream (Kwell, Scabene), crotamiton (Eurax), or permethrin 5% (Elimite)

2. Lindane cream (Kwell, Scabene) should not be used in children younger than age 2 because of the risk of neurotoxicity and seizures

3. Instruct the parents in the application of the scabicide
   a. Application should be preceded by a warm soap-and-water bath
   b. Skin must be cool and dry before the application of the lotion
   c. Lotion is left in place for 8 to 14 hours before it is washed off

4. When permethrin 5% (Elimite) is used, the cream is thoroughly and gently massaged into all skin surfaces (not just the areas that have the rash) from the head to the soles of the feet; care should be taken to avoid contact with the eyes

A

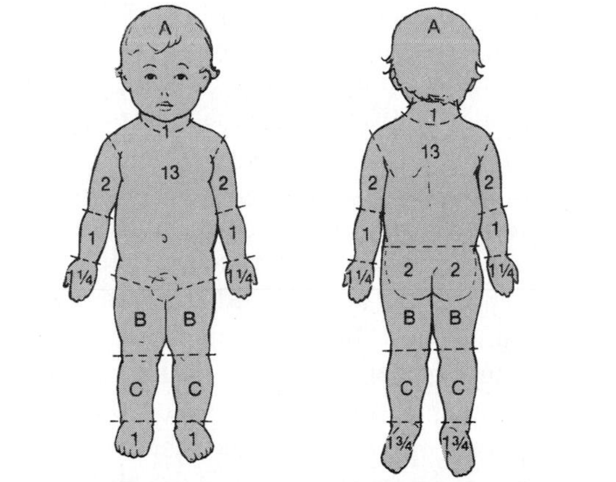

RELATIVE PERCENTAGES OF AREAS AFFECTED BY GROWTH

AREA	BIRTH	AGE 1 YR	AGE 5 YR
A = ½ of head	9½	8½	6½
B = ½ of one thigh	2¾	3¼	4
C = ½ of one leg	2½	2½	2¾

B

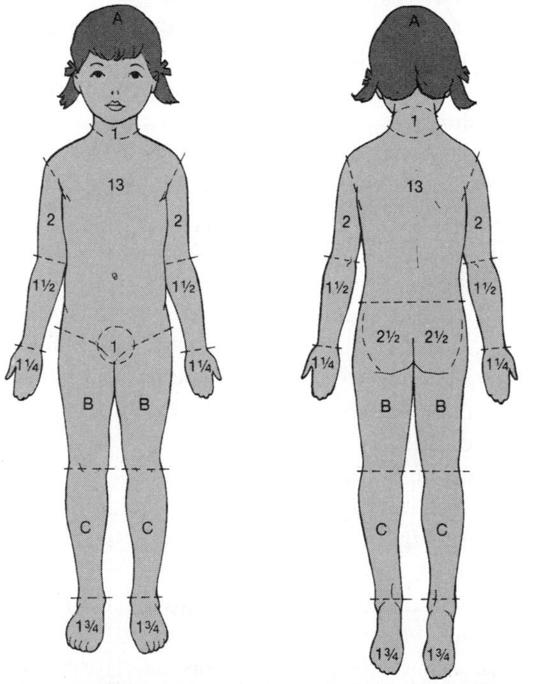

RELATIVE PERCENTAGES OF AREAS AFFECTED BY GROWTH

AREA	AGE 10 YR	AGE 15 YR	ADULT
A = ½ of head	5½	4½	3½
B = ½ of one thigh	4½	4½	4¾
C = ½ of one leg	3	3¼	3½

FIG. 40-1 Estimation of distribution of burns in children. **A,** Children from birth to age 5 years. **B,** Older children. (From Wong D: *Whaley & Wong's nursing care of infants and children,* ed. 6, St. Louis, 1999, Mosby.)

5. Household members and contacts of the infected child need to be treated at the same time
6. Instruct the parents about the importance of frequent handwashing
7. Instruct the parents that all clothing, bedding, and pillowcases used by the child need to be changed daily, washed in hot water with detergent, dried in a hot dryer, and ironed before reuse
8. Instruct the parents that nonwashable toys and other items should be sealed in plastic bags for 4 days

BOX 40-1

Parkland Formula for Fluid Resuscitation

4 mL Ringer's lactate solution × kg of body weight × % TBSA burned

One half of the total is administered in the first 8 hours postburn

One fourth of the total is administered in the second 8 hours postburn

One fourth of the total is administered in the third 8 hours postburn

Time is calculated from the time of injury, not the time of admission to the hospital

The criterion for successful burn, shock, and fluid resuscitation is a urine output of 1 mL/kg/ hr in children

V. **THE BURNED CHILD** (Refer to Chapter 47 for additional information related to burns)

A. Pediatric differences
   1. Very young children who have been severely burned have a higher mortality rate than older children and adults with comparable burns
   2. Lower burn temperatures and shorter exposure to heat can cause a more severe burn in a child than in an adult because a child's skin is thinner
   3. Severely burned children are at increased risk for fluid and heat loss, dehydration, and metabolic acidosis than an adult
   4. The higher proportion of body fluid to mass in children increases the risk of cardiovascular problems
   5. Burns involving more than 10% of total body surface area (TBSA) require some form of fluid resuscitation
   6. Infants and children are at increased risk for protein and calorie deficiency because they have smaller muscle mass and less body fat than adults
   7. Scarring is more severe in a child
   8. An immature immune system presents an increased risk of infection for infants and young children
   9. A delay in **growth** may occur following a burn

B. Extent of burn injury
   1. The rule of nines, used for an adult with a burn injury, gives an inaccurate estimate because of the differences in body proportion between children and adults

2. A modified rule of nines may be used for the pediatric population (Fig. 40-1)
C. Formulas of fluid resuscitation
   1. Several formulas are available that can be used to calculate the rate of fluid administration
   2. The Parkland formula for fluid resuscitation is commonly used (Box 40-1)

PRACTICE QUESTIONS

1. Corticream is prescribed by a physician for a child with atopic dermatitis (eczema). A nurse instructs the mother in how to appropriately apply the cream and tells the mother to:
   1. Avoid cleansing the area prior to application of the cream
   2. Apply the cream over the entire body
   3. Apply a thin layer of cream and rub into the area thoroughly
   4. Apply a thick layer of cream in affected areas only

2. A school nurse has provided an instructional session about impetigo to parents of the children attending the school. Which statement if made by a parent indicates a need for further instructions?
   1. "It is most common in humid weather."
   2. "It begins in an area of broken skin, such as an insect bite."
   3. "It is extremely contagious."
   4. "Lesions are most often located on the arms and chest."

3. A clinic nurse provides instructions to the mother of a child with impetigo regarding the application of antibiotic ointment. The mother asks the nurse when the child can return to school. The most appropriate response to the mother is:
   1. Twenty-four hours after using antibiotic ointment
   2. Forty-eight hours after using antibiotic ointment
   3. One week after using antibiotic ointment
   4. Ten days after using antibiotic ointment

4. A school nurse has provided instructions regarding the use of permethrin 1% (Nix) to the parents of children diagnosed with pediculosis capitis (head lice). Which statement if made by a parent indicates a need for further instructions?
   1. "The Nix can be obtained over-the-counter in a local pharmacy."
   2. "It is applied to the hair after shampooing and left on for 24 hours."
   3. "It is applied to the hair after shampooing, left on for 10 minutes, and then rinsed out."
   4. "The hair should not be shampooed for 24 hours following treatment."

5. A school nurse prepares a list of home care instructions for the parents of schoolchildren diagnosed with pediculosis capitis. Which of the following will the nurse include in the list?
   1. Use antilice sprays on all bedding and furniture
   2. Bring all bedding and linens to the cleaners to be dry cleaned
   3. Soak combs and brushes in warm water
   4. Vacuum floors, play areas, and furniture to remove any hairs that might carry live nits

6. A mother of a 3-year-old child arrives at a clinic and tells a nurse that the child has been continuously scratching the skin and has developed a rash. The nurse assesses the child and suspects the presence of scabies. The nurse bases this suspicion on which finding noted on assessment of the child's skin?
   1. Clusters of fluid-filled vesicles
   2. Fine thread-like lines
   3. Purple-colored lesions
   4. Thick, honey-colored crusts

7. Permethrin 5% (Elimite) is prescribed for a 4-year-old child with a diagnosis of scabies. A clinic nurse instructs the mother regarding the use of this treatment and tells the mother:
   1. That the lotion should be applied to areas of the rash only
   2. To apply the lotion and leave it on for 6 hours
   3. To apply the lotion to cool, dry skin at least one-half hour after bathing
   4. To avoid clothing the child while the lotion is in place

8. A 2-year-old child is admitted to a burn unit with partial- and full-thickness burns over 35% of the body. After admission assessment and review of the physician's orders, the priority nursing intervention focuses on:
   1. Sedating with morphine sulfate
   2. Restricting IV fluids
   3. Inserting a nasogastric tube
   4. Inserting a Foley catheter

9. A clinic nurse is reviewing the physician's orders for a child who has been diagnosed with scabies. Lindane (Kwell, Scabene) has been prescribed for the child. The nurse questions the order if which of the following is noted in the child's record?
   1. The child is 18 months old
   2. The child has a history of frequent respiratory infections
   3. A sibling is using lindane for the treatment of scabies
   4. The child is being bottle fed

10. A nurse is monitoring a burn child during the treatment for burn shock. The nurse understands that which of the following assessments provides the most accurate guide to determining the adequacy of fluid resuscitation?
    1. Skin turgor
    2. Level of edema at burn site

3. Adequacy of peripheral pulses
4. Neurological assessment

CRITICAL THINKING: FREE-TEXT ENTRY

A 10-kg child sustains a burn from a house fire, and the total body surface area (TBSA) of the burn is determined to be 50%. The Parkland formula for fluid resuscitation is used to determine the amount of fluid that this child requires. A nurse determines that the child will receive how many milliliters of fluid in the first 8 hours from the time of the injury?

Answer: _____

ANSWERS

1. **3**

Rationale: Corticream is a topical corticosteroid. It should be applied sparingly (thin layer) and rubbed into the area thoroughly. The affected area should be cleansed gently prior to application. Corticream should not be applied over extensive areas. Systemic absorption is more likely to occur with extensive application.

Test-Taking Strategy: Use the process of elimination. Eliminate option 1 first because it does not make sense not to cleanse an affected area. Eliminate option 2 because cream should be applied only to areas that are affected. Eliminate option 4 because of the word "thick." Review the procedure for the application of a topical corticosteroid if you had difficulty with this question.

Level of Cognitive Ability: Application
Client Needs: Health Promotion and Maintenance
Integrated Concept/Process: Teaching/Learning
Content Area: Child Health
Reference: Hodgson, B., & Kizior, R. (2001). *Saunders nursing drug handbook 2001.* Philadelphia: W.B. Saunders, pp. 498-500.

2. **4**

Rationale: Impetigo is most common during hot, humid summer months. It begins in an area of broken skin, such as an insect bite or atopic dermatitis. It may be caused by *Staphylococcus aureus,* group A beta-hemolytic streptococci, or a combination of these bacteria. It is extremely contagious. Lesions are usually located around the mouth and nose, but may be present on the extremities.

Test-Taking Strategy: Use the process of elimination, noting the key words "need for further instructions." Knowledge regarding the etiology and manifestations of impetigo will easily direct you to option 4. If you are unfamiliar with this disorder, review this content.

Level of Cognitive Ability: Analysis
Client Needs: Health Promotion and Maintenance
Integrated Concept/Process: Teaching/Learning
Content Area: Child Health
Reference: Ball, J., & Bindler, R. (1999). *Pediatric nursing: Caring for children* (2nd ed.). Stamford, Conn.: Appleton & Lange, p. 919.

3. **2**

Rationale: The child should not attend school for 24 to 48 hours after the initiation of systemic antibiotics or 48 hours after the use of antibiotic ointment. The school should be notified of the diagnosis. Options 1, 3, and 4 are incorrect time frames.

Test-Taking Strategy: Use general principles related to the administration of antibiotics to answer the question. Eliminate options 3 and 4 first because these time frames are closely related and rather lengthy. From the remaining options, noting the key word "ointment" in the question should assist in directing you to option 2. Review home care measures related to the administration of antibiotics if you had difficulty with this question.

Level of Cognitive Ability: Application
Client Needs: Safe, Effective Care Environment
Integrated Concept/Process: Teaching/Learning
Content Area: Child Health
Reference: Ball, J., & Bindler, R. (1999). *Pediatric nursing: Caring for children* (2nd ed.). Stamford, Conn.: Appleton & Lange, p. 921.

4. **2**

Rationale: Nix is an over-the-counter scabicide product that kills both lice and eggs with one application and has residual activity for 10 days. It is applied to the hair after shampooing and left for 10 minutes before rinsing out. The hair should not be shampooed for 24 hours after the treatment.

Test-Taking Strategy: Use the process of elimination, noting the key words "need for further instructions." Recalling the instructions for the use of this scabicide product will direct you to option 2. Review the procedure for using this product if you had difficulty with this question.

Level of Cognitive Ability: Analysis
Client Needs: Health Promotion and Maintenance
Integrated Concept/Process: Teaching/Learning
Content Area: Child Health
Reference: Ball, J., & Bindler, R. (1999). *Pediatric nursing: Caring for children* (2nd ed.). Stamford, Conn.: Appleton & Lange, p. 924.

5. **4**

Rationale: Thorough home cleaning is necessary to remove any remaining lice or nits. Antilice sprays are unnecessary. In addition, they should never be used on a child. Bedding and linens should be washed with hot water and dried on a hot setting. Items that cannot be washed should be dry cleaned or sealed in plastic bags in a warm place for 2 weeks. Combs and brushes should be soaked in the scabicide shampoo or hot water.

Test-Taking Strategy: Use the process of elimination. Eliminate option 1 first, knowing that antilice sprays should not be used. Eliminate option 2 next, knowing that bedding and linens can be washed. Also note the absolute term "all" in this option. From the remaining options, eliminate option 3 because of the words "warm water." If you had difficulty with this question, review these important home care instructions.

Level of Cognitive Ability: Application
Client Needs: Health Promotion and Maintenance
Integrated Concept/Process: Teaching/Learning
Content Area: Child Health
Reference: Ball, J., & Bindler, R. (1999). *Pediatric nursing: Caring for children* (2nd ed.). Stamford, Conn.: Appleton & Lange, p. 924.

6. 2
Rationale: Scabies appears as burrows or fine grayish thread-like lines. They may be difficult to see if they are obscured by excoriation and inflammation. Clusters of fluid-filled vesicles are seen in herpesvirus. Thick, honey-colored crusts are characteristic of impetigo. Purple-colored lesions may be indicative of various disorders, including systemic conditions.
Test-Taking Strategy: Use the process of elimination. Recalling that scabies infestation produces burrows will assist in directing you to option 2. If you are unfamiliar with the clinical manifestations associated with scabies, review this content
Level of Cognitive Ability: Analysis
Client Needs: Physiological Integrity
Integrated Concept/Process: Nursing Process/Assessment
Content Area: Child Health
Reference: Wong, D. (1999). *Whaley & Wong's nursing care of infants and children* (6th ed.). St. Louis: Mosby, pp. 839, 842.

7. 3
Rationale: Permethrin is thoroughly and gently massaged into all skin surfaces (not just the areas that have the rash), from the head to the soles of the feet. Care should be taken to avoid contact with the eyes. The lotion should be kept on for 8 to 14 hours, and then the child should be given a bath. The lotion should not be applied until at least one-half hour after bathing and should be applied only to cool, dry skin. The child should be clothed during treatment.
Test-Taking Strategy: Use the process of elimination. Options 1 and 4 can be easily eliminated. Also, note the absolute word "only" in option 1. Knowledge regarding the procedure for the application of this lotion will direct you to option 3. Review this treatment if you had difficulty with this question.
Level of Cognitive Ability: Application
Client Needs: Health Promotion and Maintenance
Integrated Concept/Process: Teaching/Learning
Content Area: Child Health
Reference: Wong, D. (1999). *Whaley & Wong's nursing care of infants and children* (6th ed.). St. Louis: Mosby, p. 842.

8. 4
Rationale: A Foley catheter is inserted into the child's bladder so that urine output can be accurately measured on an hourly basis. Although pain medication may be required, the child should not be sedated. IV fluids are not restricted and are administered at a rate sufficient to keep the child's urine output at 1 mL/kg of body weight per hour, thus reflecting adequate tissue perfusion. A nasogastric tube may or may not be required, but this is not the priority intervention.
Test-Taking Strategy: Use the process of elimination. Option 1 can be eliminated first because the child should not be sedated. Eliminate option 2 next, knowing that fluid resuscitation is an important component of therapy to prevent burn shock. From the remaining options, knowledge that urine output reflects adequate tissue perfusion will direct you to option 4. Review the treatment of burns if you had difficulty with this question.
Level of Cognitive Ability: Analysis
Client Needs: Physiological Integrity
Integrated Concept/Process: Nursing Process/Implementation
Content Area: Child Health
Reference: Bowden, V., Dickey, S., & Greenberg, C. (1998). *Children and their families: The continuum of care.* Philadelphia: W.B. Saunders, p. 1787.

9. 1
Rationale: Lindane is contraindicated for children younger than 2 years of age. These children have more permeable skin, and there may be high systemic absorption, placing the child at risk for central nervous system toxicity and seizures. Lindane is also used with caution in children between the ages of 2 and 10. Siblings and other household members should also be treated at the same time. Options 2 and 4 are unrelated to the use of lindane. Lindane is not recommended for use by a woman who is breast-feeding because the medication is secreted into breast milk.
Test-Taking Strategy: Use the process of elimination. Recall the concepts related to the body surface area of children and medication administration. These concepts will easily direct you to option 1. If you are unfamiliar with this medication, review the contraindications associated with its use.
Level of Cognitive Ability: Analysis
Client Needs: Safe, Effective Care Environment
Integrated Concept/Process: Analysis
Content Area: Child Health
Reference: Cleveland, L., Aschenbrenner, D., Venable, S., & Yensen, J. (1999). *Nursing management in drug therapy.* Philadelphia: Lippincott, p. 1005.

10. 4
Rationale: Sensorium is an accurate guide to determine the adequacy of fluid resuscitation. The burn injury itself does not affect the sensorium, so the child should be alert and oriented. Any alteration in sensorium should be evaluated further. A neurological assessment would determine the level of sensorium in the child. Options 1, 2, and 3 would not provide an accurate assessment of the adequacy of fluid resuscitation.
Test-Taking Strategy: Note the key words "most accurate" in the stem of the question. Although options 1, 2, and 3 may provide some information related to fluid volume, in a burn injury, from the options provided, neurological assessment is most accurate. Review assessments during fluid resuscitation and treatment for burn shock if you had difficulty with this question.
Level of Cognitive Ability: Analysis
Client Needs: Physiological Integrity
Integrated Concept/Process: Nursing Process/Assessment
Content Area: Child Health
Reference: Bowden, V., Dickey, S., & Greenberg, C. (1998). *Children and their families: The continuum of care.* Philadelphia: W.B. Saunders, p. 1787.

CRITICAL THINKING: FREE-TEXT ENTRY

Answer: 1000 mL
Rationale: The Parkland formula is calculated as 4 mL Ringer's lactate (RL) solution times kilograms of body weight times

percent TBSA burn. One half of the total is administered in the first 8 hours postburn. One fourth of the total is administered in the second 8 hours postburn. One fourth of the total is administered in the third 8 hours postburn. 4 mL × 10 kg × 50% TBSA burn = 2000 mL RL in 24 hours. The child would receive 1000 mL in the first 8 hours at 125 mL/ hour, 500 mL in the second 8 hours at 62 mL/ hour, and 500 mL in the third 8 hours at 62 mL/hour.

Test-Taking Strategy: Knowledge regarding the calculation of the amount of fluid required by the Parkland formula is required to answer this question. If you are unfamiliar with this method of calculation, review the formula.

Level of Cognitive Ability: Analysis
Client Needs: Physiological Integrity
Integrated Concept/Process: Nursing Process/Analysis
Content Area: Child Health
Reference: Bowden, V., Dickey, S., & Greenberg, C. (1998). *Children and their families: The continuum of care.* Philadelphia: W.B. Saunders, p. 1787.

REFERENCES

Ball, J., & Bindler, R. (1999). *Pediatric nursing: Caring for children* (2nd ed.). Stamford, Conn.: Appleton & Lange.

Bowden, V., Dickey, S., & Greenberg, C. (1998). *Children and their families: The continuum of care.* Philadelphia: W.B. Saunders.

Cleveland, L., Aschenbrenner, D., Venable, S., & Yensen, J. (1999). *Nursing management in drug therapy.* Philadelphia: Lippincott.

Hodgson, B., & Kizior, R. (2001). *Saunders nursing drug handbook 2001.* Philadelphia: W.B. Saunders.

Wong, D. (1999). *Whaley & Wong's nursing care of infants and children* (6th ed.). St. Louis: Mosby.

Musculoskeletal Disorders

I. DYSPLASIA OF THE HIP

A. Description
1. A condition in which the head of the femur is improperly seated in the acetabulum, or hip socket, of the pelvis
2. Can range from very mild to severely dislocated
3. Can be congenital or develop after birth

B. Assessment (Fig. 41-1)
1. Neonates: laxity of the ligaments around the hip, which allows the femoral head to be displaced from the acetabulum upon manipulation
2. Infants beyond the newborn period
   a. Asymmetry of the gluteal and thigh skinfolds when the child is placed prone and the legs are extended against the examining table
   b. Limited range of motion (ROM) in the affected hip
   c. Asymmetric abduction of the affected hip when the child is placed supine with the knees and hips flexed
   d. Apparent short femur on the affected side (Galeazzi sign, Allis sign)
3. The walking child: minimal to pronounced variations in gait with lurching toward the affected side; positive Trendelenburg sign
4. Positive Barlow or Ortolani's maneuver

C. Implementation
1. In the neonatal period, splinting of the hips with Pavlik harness to maintain flexion and abduction and external rotation
2. Following the neonatal period, traction and/or surgery to release muscles and tendons
3. Following surgery, positioning and immobilization in a spica cast until healing is achieved
4. Osteotomy following traction in profoundly affected children
5. Instruct parents regarding proper care of a Pavlik harness or spica cast (Fig. 41-2)

II. CONGENITAL CLUBFOOT

A. Description
1. A congenital malformation of the lower extremities
2. The defect may be unilateral or bilateral
3. Defects are rigid and cannot be manipulated into a neutral position
4. Long-term interval follow-up is required until the child reaches skeletal maturity

B. Assessment: the foot is plantar flexed with an inverted heel and adducted forefoot

C. Implementation
1. Treatment begins as soon after birth as possible
2. Serial manipulation and casting are performed weekly, and if correction is not achieved in 3 to 6 months, surgery is indicated
3. Monitor for pain
4. Monitor neurovascular status of the toes
5. Instruct parents in cast care and the signs of neurovascular impairment that requires physician notification

III. SCOLIOSIS

A. Description
1. A lateral curvature of the spine
2. Surgical and nonsurgical interventions are employed, and the type of treatment depends on the degree of curvature, the age of the child, and the amount of **growth** that is anticipated
3. Long-term monitoring is essential to detect any progression of the curve

B. Assessment
1. Visible curve fails to straighten when the child bends forward and hangs arms down toward feet

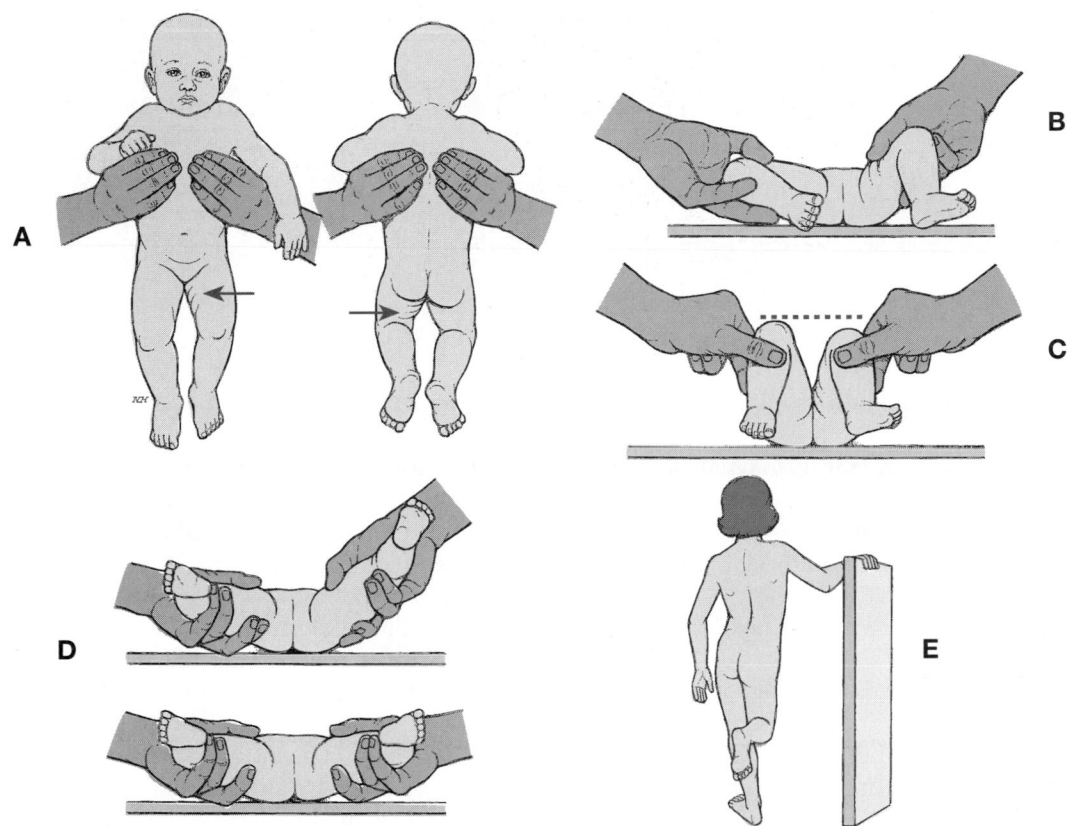

FIG. 41-1   Signs of developmental dysplasia of the hip. **A,** Assymetry of gluteal and thigh folds. **B,** Limited hip abduction, as seen in flexion. **C,** Apparent shortening of the femur, as indicated by the level of the knees in flexion. **D,** Ortolani click (in infant is under 4 weeks of age). **E,** Positive Trendelenburg sign or gait (if child is weight bearing). (From Wong D et al: *Whaley & Wong's nursing care of infants and children,* ed 6, St Louis, 1999, Mosby.)

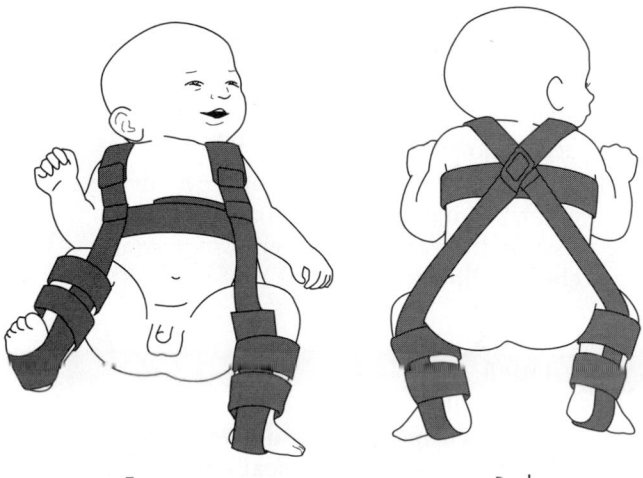

Front   Back

FIG. 41-2   Child in Pavlik harness. (From Ball JW: *Mosby's pediatric patient teaching guides,* St Louis, 1998, Mosby.)

2. Hips, ribs, and shoulders are asymmetrical
3. Apparent leg length discrepancy
C. Implementation
  1. Monitor progression of the curvature
  2. Prepare the child and parents for the use of a brace if prescribed

3. Prepare the child and parents for surgery (spinal fusion; placement of internal instrumentation rods) if prescribed
D. Braces
  1. Usually worn from 16 to 23 hours a day
  2. Inspect the skin for signs of redness or breakdown

TABLE 41-1

Assessment of JRA

Systemic JRA	Pauciarticular JRA	Polyarticular JRA
Fever	Mild joint pain and swelling	Morning joint stiffness
Salmon-pink rash	Affects large joints	Low-grade fever
Affects five or more joints	Affects no more than 4 joints	Affects weight-bearing joints
May also have anorexia, anemia, fatigue	Iridocyclitis	Affects five or more joints

3. Keep the skin clean and dry, avoiding lotions and powders
4. Advise the child to wear soft nonirritating clothing under the brace
5. Instruct in prescribed exercises
6. Encourage verbalization about body image

E. Implementation postoperatively
1. Maintain proper alignment; avoid twisting movements
2. Logroll the child when turning, to maintain alignment
3. Assess extremities for neurovascular status
4. Encourage coughing and deep breathing and use of incentive spirometry
5. Assess pain and administer prescribed analgesics
6. Monitor for incontinence
7. Monitor for superior mesenteric artery syndrome disorder, caused by mechanical changes in the position of the child's abdominal contents during surgery, and notify the physician if it occurs; symptoms include emesis and abdominal distention similar to that which occurs with intestinal obstruction or paralytic ileus
8. Instruct in activity restrictions
9. Instruct the child to roll from a side-lying position to a sitting position, and assist with ambulation
10. Prepare the child for the use of a molded plastic jacket to provide external stability of the spine when resuming activities

IV. JUVENILE RHEUMATOID ARTHRITIS (JRA)

A. Description
1. An autoimmune inflammatory disease affecting the joints; occurs most often in girls
2. The cause is unknown
3. Juvenile onset is diagnosed before 16 years of age
4. Iridocyclitis is a unique complication of JRA
5. Treatment of JRA is supportive and directed toward preserving joint function, controlling inflammation, minimizing deformity, and reducing the impact that the disease may have on the development of the child
6. Therapy includes medications, physical and occupational therapies, and child and family education
7. Surgical intervention may be implemented when the child has problems with joint contractures and unequal **growth** of extremities

B. Assessment (Table 41-1)

C. Implementation
1. Facilitate social and emotional development
2. Instruct the parents and child in the administration of medications as prescribed; these may include acetylsalicylic acid (aspirin, ASA), nonsteroidal antiinflammatory drugs (NSAIDs), slower-acting antirheumatic drugs (SAARDs), cytotoxic medications, or corticosteroids
3. Instruct the parent regarding the signs of aspirin toxicity; aspirin is stopped if signs of toxicity occur, and the physician is notified
4. Assist the child with ROM exercises and instruct in prescribed exercises
5. Encourage normal performance of activities of daily living (ADLs)
6. Instruct the parents and child in the use of hot or cold packs, splinting, and positioning the affected joint in a neutral position during painful episodes
7. Encourage and support prescribed physical and occupational therapy
8. Instruct in the importance of preventive eye care and reporting visual disturbances
9. Assess the child's perception regarding the chronic illness

V. FRACTURES

A. Description
1. A break in the continuity of the bone as a result of trauma, twisting, or bone decalcification
2. Fractures in children usually result from increased mobility and inadequate or immature motor and cognitive skills
3. Fractures in children may result from trauma or bone diseases
4. Fractures in infancy are generally rare and warrant further investigation to rule out the possibility of child **abuse**

5. The most frequently seen fracture in children is located in the forearm

▲ B. Assessment
1. Pain or tenderness over the involved area
2. Loss of function
3. Obvious deformity
4. Crepitation
5. Ecchymosis
6. Edema
7. Muscle spasm

▲ C. Initial care of a fracture
1. Assess the extent of injury and immobilize affected extremity
2. If a compound fracture exists, splint the extremity and cover the wound with a sterile dressing

D. Implementation
1. Reduction
   a. Restoring the bone to proper alignment
   b. Closed reduction: Accomplished by manual alignment of the fragments, followed by immobilization
   c. Open reduction: Requires the surgical insertion of internal fixation devices, such as rods, wires, or pins, that help maintain alignment while healing occurs
2. Retention: The application of traction or a cast to maintain alignment until healing occurs

E. Traction
1. Bryant's skin traction
   a. Used to stabilize a fractured femur or correct a congenital hip dislocation in children
   b. Position child flat with a 90-degree hip flexion
2. Russell's skin traction
   a. Used to stabilize a fractured femur before surgery
   b. Similar to Buck's traction but provides a double pull with the use of a knee sling
   c. Traction pulls at the knee and the foot
   d. Position the child with the foot of the bed slightly elevated
3. Balanced suspension
   a. Used with skin or skeletal traction
   b. Used to approximate fractures of the femur, tibia, or fibula
   c. Produced by a counterforce other than the child
   d. Types include Thomas splint with Pearson attachment, Steinmann pin, Kirschner wires
   e. Position child in low-Fowler's position, on either the side or the back
   f. Maintain a 20-degree angle from the thigh to the bed
   g. Protect the skin from breakdown
   h. Provide pin care if pins are used with the skeletal traction
   i. Clean pin site with normal saline and hydro-

gen peroxide or Betadine as prescribed and according to agency procedure

F. Casts ▲
1. Description
   a. Made of plaster or fiberglass to provide immobilization of bone and joints after a fracture or injury
   b. Fractures of the hip or the knee may require a spica cast
2. Implementation
   a. Examine the cast for pressure areas
   b. Monitor the extremity for circulatory impairment, such as pain, swelling, discoloration, tingling, numbness or coolness, or diminished pulse
   c. Notify the physician if circulatory impairment occurs
   d. Prepare for bivalving or cutting the cast if circulatory impairment occurs
   e. Instruct the child not to stick objects down ▲ the cast
   f. Teach the child to keep the cast clean and dry
   g. Instruct the child in isometric exercises to prevent muscle atrophy

PRACTICE QUESTIONS

1. A 1-month-old infant is seen in a clinic and is diagnosed with unilateral hip dysplasia. A nurse assesses the infant, knowing that which of the following findings would not be noted in this condition?
   1. An apparent short femur on the affected side
   2. Limited range of motion (ROM) in the affected hip
   3. Asymmetric adduction of the affected hip when the infant is placed supine with the knees and hips flexed
   4. Asymmetry of the gluteal skinfolds when the infant is placed prone and the legs are extended against the examining table

2. A nurse is assisting a physician during the examination of an infant with hip dysplasia. The physician performs Ortolani's maneuver. The nurse is aware that this maneuver is performed to:
   1. Push the unstable femoral head out of the acetabulum
   2. Reduce the dislocated femoral head back into the acetabulum
   3. Determine the extent of range of motion (ROM)
   4. Assess for asymmetry on the affected side

3. A clinic nurse provides instructions to the parents of an infant with hip dysplasia regarding care of the Pavlik harness. Which of the following does the nurse include in the instructions?
   1. The harness should be worn 12 hours a day

2. The harness needs be removed for diaper changes and for feeding
3. The harness should be removed only to check the skin and for bathing
4. The infant should not be moved when out of the harness

4. A mother brings her 2-week-old infant to a clinic for treatment following a diagnosis of clubfoot made at the time of birth. Which of the following statements, if made by the mother, indicates a need for further education regarding this disorder?
   1. "I need to bring my infant back to the clinic in 1 month for a new cast."
   2. "Treatment needs to be started as soon as possible."
   3. "I need to come to the clinic every week with my infant for the casting."
   4. "I realize my infant will require follow-up care until full grown."

5. A nurse is caring for a child after spinal fusion for the treatment of scoliosis. The child complains of abdominal discomfort and begins to have episodes of vomiting. On further assessment, the nurse notes abdominal distention. Which of the following nursing actions would be most appropriate?
   1. Administer an antiemetic
   2. Place the child in a Sims' position
   3. Notify the physician
   4. Increase the IV fluids

6. A nurse is providing instructions to the parents of a child with scoliosis regarding the use of a brace. Which of the following is not a component of the instructions given to the parents?
   1. Apply lotion under the brace to prevent skin breakdown
   2. Avoid the use of powder because it will cake under the brace
   3. Have the child wear soft-fabric clothing under the brace
   4. Encourage the child to perform prescribed exercises

7. A pediatric nurse educator provides a teaching session to the nursing staff regarding juvenile rheumatoid arthritis (JRA). Which of the following is not included in the teaching session?
   1. It most often occurs before the age of 16
   2. It is twice as likely to occur in boys than in girls
   3. A complication is iridocyclitis
   4. Clinical manifestations include morning stiffness and painful, stiff, swollen joints

8. The mother of a child with juvenile rheumatoid arthritis (JRA) calls the clinic nurse because the child is experiencing a painful exacerbation of the disease. The mother asks the nurse if the child should perform range-of-motion (ROM) exercises at this time. The most appropriate nursing response is:
   1. "The ROM exercises must be performed every day."
   2. "Avoid all exercise during painful periods."
   3. "Administer additional pain medication before performing ROM exercises."
   4. "Have the child perform simple isometric exercises during this time."

9. A 2-year-old child is placed in Bryant traction for treatment of a fractured femur. The nurse develops a plan of care for the child. Which of the following is not a component of the plan?
   1. Place the child in a supine position
   2. Place the child supine with the legs flexed slightly less than 90 degrees
   3. Ensure that the sacrum is resting on the mattress
   4. Ensure the use of a footplate to keep the traction straps away from the child's ankles

10. A 4-year-old child sustains a fall at home and is brought to the emergency room by the mother. After an x-ray, it has been determined that the child has a fractured arm and a plaster cast is applied. The nurse provides instructions to the mother regarding cast care for the child. Which of the following statements, if made by the mother, indicates a need for further education?
   1. "The cast may feel warm as the cast dries."
   2. "If the cast becomes wet, a blow drier set on the cool setting may be used to dry the cast."
   3. "A small amount of white shoe polish can touch up a soiled white cast."
   4. "I can use lotion or powder around the cast edges to relieve itching."

CRITICAL THINKING: FREE-TEXT ENTRY

A child is admitted to a hospital after application of a cast to the left arm to treat a fracture sustained from a fall. A nurse monitors the extremity for circulatory impairment and notes swelling, discoloration, coolness, and a diminished pulse. The child complains of pain and numbness in the affected extremity. On the basis of these assessment findings, what is the nurse's initial action?

Answer: _____

ANSWERS

1. 3

Rationale: Asymmetric abduction of the affected hip, when the child is placed supine with the knees and hips flexed, would be an assessment finding in hip dysplasia in infants beyond the newborn period. Options 1, 2, and 4 are accurate assessment findings in this disorder.

Test-Taking Strategy: Note the key word "not." Also note the age of the infant. Attempt to visualize each of the assessment findings described in the options. This will assist in directing you to option 3. If you had difficulty with this question, review the assessment findings is hip dysplasia.

Level of Cognitive Ability: Analysis
Client Needs: Physiological Integrity
Integrated Concept/Process: Nursing Process/Assessment
Content Area: Child Health
Reference: Ball, J., & Bindler, R. (1999). *Pediatric nursing: Caring for children* (2nd ed.). Stamford, Conn.: Appleton & Lange, p. 826.

2. 2

Rationale: In the Barlow maneuver, the examiner pushes the unstable femoral head out of the acetabulum. In the Ortolani maneuver, the examiner reduces the dislocated femoral head back into the acetabulum. A positive finding is a palpable clink upon entry or exit of the femoral head over the acetabular ring. Options 3 and 4 are done to assess for hip dysplasia.

Test-Taking Strategy: Use the process of elimination. Options 3 and 4 can be eliminated first because they are specific assessments performed to determine the presence of hip dysplasia. From the remaining options, it is necessary to know the purpose of Ortolani's maneuver. Review this maneuver if you had difficulty with this question.

Level of Cognitive Ability: Analysis
Client Needs: Physiological Integrity
Integrated Concept/Process: Nursing Process/Assessment
Content Area: Child Health
Reference: Ball, J., & Bindler, R. (1999). *Pediatric nursing: Caring for children* (2nd ed.). Stamford, Conn.: Appleton & Lange, p. 827.

3. 3

Rationale: The harness should be worn 16 to 23 hours a day and should be removed only to check the skin and for bathing. The infant can be moved when out of the harness, but the hips and buttocks should be supported carefully. The harness does not need to be removed for diaper changes or feedings.

Test-Taking Strategy: Use the process of elimination. Attempt to visualize this harness to assist in eliminating options 2 and 4. Select option 3 over option 1 because the time frame in option 1 is rather short. Review home care instruction regarding this harness if you had difficulty with this question.

Level of Cognitive Ability: Application
Client Needs: Health Promotion and Maintenance
Integrated Concept/Process: Teaching/Learning
Content Area: Child Health
Reference: Wong, D. (1999). *Whaley & Wong's nursing care of infants and children* (6th ed.). St. Louis: Mosby, p. 509.

4. 1

Rationale: Treatment for clubfoot is started as soon as possible after birth. Serial manipulation and casting are performed at least weekly. If sufficient correction is not achieved in 3 to 6 months, surgery is usually indicated. Because clubfoot can recur, all children with clubfoot require long-term interval follow-up until they reach skeletal maturity to ensure an optimal outcome.

Test-Taking Strategy: Use the process of elimination. Note the key words "indicates a need for further education." This will assist in eliminating options 2 and 4. Recalling that serial manipulations and casting are required weekly will assist in directing you to option 1. Review these treatment procedures if you had difficulty with this question,

Level of Cognitive Ability: Analysis
Client Needs: Health Promotion and Maintenance
Integrated Concept/Process: Teaching/Learning
Content Area: Child Health
Reference: Wong, D. (1999). *Whaley & Wong's nursing care of infants and children* (6th ed.). St. Louis: Mosby, p. 512.

5. 3

Rationale: A complication after surgical treatment of scoliosis is superior mesenteric artery syndrome. This disorder is caused by mechanical changes in the position of the child's abdominal contents, resulting from lengthening of the child's body. It results in a syndrome of emesis and abdominal distention similar to that which occurs with intestinal obstruction or paralytic ileus. Postoperative vomiting in children with body casts or those who have undergone spinal fusion warrants attention because of the possibility of superior mesenteric artery syndrome.

Test-Taking Strategy: Use the process of elimination. Eliminate option 4 first because it should not be implemented without a prescribed order. Eliminate option 2 next because this child requires logrolling, and Sims' position may cause injury following surgery. From the remaining options, note the assessment signs and symptoms in the question. These should alert you that physician notification is necessary. Review superior mesenteric artery syndrome if you had difficulty with this question.

Level of Cognitive Ability: Analysis
Client Needs: Physiological Integrity
Integrated Concept/Process: Nursing Process/Implementation
Content Area: Child Health
Reference: Wong, D. (1999). *Whaley & Wong's nursing care of infants and children* (6th ed.). St. Louis: Mosby, p. 1946.

6. 1

Rationale: The use of lotions or powders should be avoided because they can become sticky and cake under the brace, causing irritation. Options 2, 3, and 4 are appropriate instructions to the parents of a child with a brace.

Test-Taking Strategy: Use the process of elimination. Note the key word "not" in the stem of the question. Careful reading of the options will assist in directing you to option 1. Review home care instructions regarding the care of a child in a brace if you had difficulty with this question.

Level of Cognitive Ability: Application
Client Needs: Health Promotion and Maintenance
Integrated Concept/Process: Teaching/Learning
Content Area: Child Health
Reference: Ball, J., & Bindler, R. (1999). *Pediatric nursing: Caring for children* (2nd ed.). Stamford, Conn.: Appleton & Lange, p. 825.

7. 2

Rationale: JRA is twice as likely to occur in girls than in boys. Options 1, 3, and 4 are accurate regarding this disorder.

Test-Taking Strategy: Use the process of elimination. Note the key word "not" in the stem of the question. Simply recalling that JRA is twice as likely to occur in girls than in boys will direct you to option 2. Review this disorder if you are unfamiliar with it.

Level of Cognitive Ability: Application
Client Needs: Physiological Integrity
Integrated Concept/Process: Teaching/Learning
Content Area: Child Health
Reference: Ball, J., & Bindler, R. (1999). *Pediatric nursing: Caring for children* (2nd ed.). Stamford, Conn.: Appleton & Lange, p. 358.

8. 4

Rationale: During painful episodes, hot or cold packs and splinting and positioning the affected joint in a neutral position help reduce the pain. Although resting the extremity is appropriate, it is important to begin simple isometric or tensing exercises as soon as the child is able. These exercises do not involve joint movement.

Test-Taking Strategy: Use the process of elimination. Eliminate options 1, 2, and 3 because of the words "must," "all," and "additional" in these options. Review pain management and care during exacerbations if you had difficulty with this question.

Level of Cognitive Ability: Application
Client Needs: Health Promotion and Maintenance
Integrated Concept/Process: Teaching/Learning
Content Area: Child Health
Reference: Bowden, V., Dickey, S., & Greenberg, C. (1998). *Children and their families: The continuum of care.* Philadelphia: W.B. Saunders, pp. 1291-1292.

9. 3

Rationale: In Bryant's traction, the sacrum should be off the mattress. Options 1, 2, and 4 are accurate interventions in the use of this traction.

Test-Taking Strategy: Use the process of elimination. Note the key word "not" in the stem of the question. Attempt to visualize this type of traction in selecting the correct option. Review this type of traction and the associated nursing interventions if you had difficulty with this question.

Level of Cognitive Ability: Application

Client Needs: Physiological Integrity
Integrated Concept/Process: Nursing Process/Planning
Content Area: Child Health
Reference: Ball, J., & Bindler, R. (1999). *Pediatric nursing: Caring for children* (2nd ed.). Stamford, Conn.: Appleton & Lange, p. 857.

10. 4

Rationale: The mother needs to be instructed not to use lotion or powders on the skin around the cast edges or inside the cast. Lotions or powders can become sticky or caked and cause skin irritation. Options 1, 2, and 3 are appropriate instructions.

Test-Taking Strategy: Use the process of elimination. Note the key words "indicates a need for further education." Remember that lotions or powders can become sticky or caked and cause skin irritation. Review home care instructions regarding cast care if you had difficulty with this question.

Level of Cognitive Ability: Analysis
Client Needs: Health Promotion and Maintenance
Integrated Concept/Process: Teaching/Learning
Content Area: Child Health
Reference: Bowden, V., Dickey, S., & Greenberg, C. (1998). *Children and their families: The continuum of care.* Philadelphia: W.B. Saunders, pp. 1234-1235.

CRITICAL THINKING: FREE-TEXT ENTRY

Answer: Notify the physician immediately

Rationale: When circulatory impairment is evident, the nurse immediately contacts the physician. The physician will cut the cast in half to form a bivalve cast or make a large window in the cast to decrease the pressure. If the physician is not able to come and release the pressure, the nurse needs to be prepared to perform the procedure.

Test-Taking Strategy: Use the ABCs—airway, breathing, and circulation—to answer the question. Focus on the signs identified in the question to determine that circulatory impairment is evident. Review the nursing actions if circulatory impairment occurs after application of a cast, if you had difficulty with this question.

Level of Cognitive Ability: Analysis
Client Needs: Physiological Integrity
Integrated Concept/Process: Nursing Process/Implementation
Content Area: Child Health
Reference: Wong, D. (1999). *Whaley & Wong's nursing care of infants and children* (6th ed.). St. Louis: Mosby, p. 1925.

REFERENCES

Ball, J., & Bindler, R. (1999). *Pediatric nursing: Caring for children* (2nd ed.). Stamford, Conn.: Appleton & Lange.

Ball, J., & Bindler, R. (1999). *Quick reference to pediatric clinical skills.* Stamford, Conn.: Appleton & Lange.

Bowden, V., Dickey, S., & Greenberg, C. (1998). *Children and their families: The continuum of care.* Philadelphia: W.B. Saunders.

Wong, D. (1999). *Whaley & Wong's nursing care of infants and children* (6th ed.). St. Louis: Mosby.

Acquired Immunodeficiency Syndrome

I. ACQUIRED IMMUNODEFICIENCY SYNDROME (AIDS)

A. Description
1. A disorder caused by the human immunodeficiency virus (HIV) and characterized by generalized dysfunction of the immune system
2. Both cellular and humoral immunity are compromised
3. Horizontal transmission of HIV occurs through intimate sexual contact or parenteral exposure to blood or body fluids containing visible blood
4. Vertical (perinatal) transmission occurs when an HIV-infected pregnant woman passes the infection to her fetus
5. The most common opportunistic infection of children infected with HIV is *Pneumocystis carinii* pneumonia (PCP); it occurs most frequently between the ages of 3 and 6 months, when HIV status maybe indeterminate
6. The goals of therapy include slowing the growth of the virus, preventing and treating opportunistic infections, and providing nutritional support and symptomatic treatment

B. Assessment
1. During neonatal period
   a. Lymphadenopathy
   b. Hepatosplenomegaly
   c. *Pneumocystis carinii* pneumonia
   d. Progressive encephalopathy
   e. Microcephaly
2. Infants
   a. Failure to thrive
   b. Diarrhea
   c. Developmental delays
   d. Oral candidiasis
   e. Hepatosplenomegaly
   f. Chronic cough and lymphoid interstitial pneumonia (LIP)
   g. Chronic otitis media
3. Children/adolescents
   a. Malaise and fatigue
   b. Night sweats
   c. Weight loss
   d. Diarrhea
   e. Fever
   f. **Regression** of developmental milestones
   g. Generalized lymphadenopathy
   h. Nephropathy
   i. PCP and LIP
   j. Encephalopathy

C. Diagnostic tests
1. Enzyme-linked immunosorbent assay (ELISA)
   a. ELISA determines the response of antibodies to the HIV virus
   b. Useful in children older than 18 months
2. Western blot
   a. Confirms the presence of HIV antibodies
   b. Useful in children older than 18 months
   c. A positive HIV antibody test in children younger than 18 months indicates only that the mother is infected; other diagnostic tests will be employed, including the virus culture, polymerase chain reaction (PCR) for detection of proviral DNA, and p24 antigen detection, which is HIV specific
3. p24 antigen
   a. Used to detect HIV antigen in children younger than 18 months
   b. Test can be useful at any age
   c. Only a positive result is significant
   d. Two or more positive results are diagnostic for HIV infection
4. CD4+: Used to assess a child's immune status,

risk for disease progression, and the need for PCP prophylaxis after 1 year of age

II. CARE OF THE CHILD WITH HIV OR AIDS

A. Prophylaxis
  1. Provide prophylaxis as prescribed against PCP during the first year of life to the infant born to an HIV-infected woman; after 1 year of age, the need for prophylaxis is determined by the presence of severe immunosuppression or a history of PCP
  2. Provide continued prophylaxis through 12 months of age for children diagnosed with HIV
  3. For HIV-infected children older than 12 months, continued prophylaxis is based on CD4+ counts and whether PCP has previously occurred

B. Parent instructions regarding care to the child
  1. Frequent handwashing
  2. Assess for fever, malaise, fatigue, weight loss, vomiting and diarrhea, altered activity level, and oral lesions, and notify the physician if these occur
  3. The signs and symptoms of opportunistic infections
  4. The administration of antiretroviral medications as prescribed
  5. The child should avoid exposure to other illnesses
  6. Keep immunizations up to date
  7. Keep the child home when sick
  8. Do not kiss the child on the mouth
  9. Monitor weight
  10. Provide a high-calorie and high-protein diet
  11. Do not share eating utensils
  12. Wash eating utensils in the dishwasher
  13. Cover unused food and formula and refrigerate
  14. Discard unused refrigerated formula and food after 24 hours
  15. Wear gloves for care, especially when in contact with body fluids and changing diapers
  16. Change diapers frequently, away from food areas
  17. Fold soiled disposable diapers inward and tab, and dispose in a tightly covered plastic-lined container
  18. Dispose of trash daily
  19. Cover sandboxes when not in use to create a barrier to germs
  20. Clean up spills with bleach solution (10:1 ratio of water to bleach)

C. Immunizations
  1. Immunizations against common childhood illnesses are recommended for all children exposed to or infected with HIV
  2. The varicella (chickenpox) vaccine is avoided
  3. Oral poliovirus (OPV) is not recommended for routine vaccination for any child (refer to Chapter 45 for information on immunizations)

  4. Pneumococcal and influenza vaccines are recommended
  5. Measles, mumps, rubella (MMR) vaccine is administered if the child is not severely immunocompromised (the child receiving IV gamma globulin prophylaxis may not respond to the MMR vaccine)

PRACTICE QUESTIONS

1. A pediatric nurse educator provides a teaching session to the nursing staff regarding human immunodeficiency virus (HIV) and acquired immunodeficiency syndrome (AIDS). The nurse educator plans to include which information in the teaching session?
   1. Most newborn infants of HIV-positive women test positive for the HIV virus
   2. HIV primarily attacks the hematological system
   3. In AIDS, the B cells are depleted and cannot signal the T4 cells to form protective antibodies
   4. The virus attacks the immune system by destroying T lymphocytes

2. A newborn infant of a human immunodeficiency virus (HIV)–positive mother is tested for the presence of HIV antibodies. An enzyme-linked immunosorbent assay (ELISA) test is performed, and the results are positive. A nurse interprets these results as:
   1. Positive for HIV virus
   2. Indicating the presence of maternal infection
   3. Indicating the absence of maternal infection
   4. Negative for HIV virus

3. A physician prescribes laboratory studies for an infant of a human immunodeficiency virus (HIV)–positive woman to determine the presence of HIV antigen. The nurse anticipates that which laboratory study will be prescribed?
   1. Western blot
   2. Chest x-ray
   3. CD4+ count
   4. p24 antigen assay

4. A mother with human immunodeficiency virus (HIV) infection brings her 10-month-old infant to the clinic for a routine checkup. The physician has documented that the infant is asymptomatic for HIV infection. After the checkup, the mother tells the nurse that she is so pleased that the infant will not get HIV. The most appropriate nursing response to the mother is:
   1. "I am so pleased also that everything has turned out fine."
   2. "Everything looks great, but be sure that you return with your infant next month for the scheduled visit."
   3. "Most children infected with HIV develop symptoms within the first 9 months of life, and some become symptomatic sometime before age 3."

4. "Since symptoms have not developed, it is unlikely that the infant will develop HIV infection."

5. An infant with a human immunodeficiency virus (HIV)–infected mother is seen in the clinic on a monthly basis and is being monitored for symptoms indicative of HIV. The nurse assesses the infant, knowing that the most common opportunistic infection of children infected with HIV is:
   1. Gastroenteritis
   2. Meningitis
   3. *Pneumocystis carinii* pneumonia (PCP)
   4. Lymphoid interstitial pneumonia (LIP)

6. A clinic nurse is instructing the mother of a child with human immunodeficiency virus (HIV) regarding immunizations. The nurse tells the mother that:
   1. Household members need to avoid receiving the varicella vaccine
   2. Pneumococcal and influenza vaccines are recommended
   3. The hepatitis B vaccine will not to be given to the child
   4. A Western blot needs to be performed and the results evaluated prior to immunizations

7. A child with acquired immunodeficiency syndrome (AIDS) is hospitalized for the treatment of *Pneumocystis carinii* pneumonia (PCP). The child will be receiving nebulizer treatments at home when discharged. The nurse instructs the mother regarding the maintenance of the nebulizer equipment and tells the mother to:
   1. Clean the nebulizer pieces after each treatment with one-fourth strength bleach and water
   2. Clean the nebulizer pieces with warm water after each treatment and allow to air dry
   3. Boil the nebulizer pieces for 15 minutes after each treatment
   4. Clean the mouthpiece with alcohol after each use and soak in alcohol for 30 minutes at the end of each day

8. A child with human immunodeficiency virus (HIV) is receiving zidovudine (AZT, Retrovir). The nurse monitors which laboratory study to determine if the child is experiencing an adverse reaction from the medication?
   1. Sedimentation rate
   2. Complete blood count (CBC)
   3. Calcium level
   4. Potassium level

9. A nurse is caring for a 4-year-old child with a diagnosis of human immunodeficiency virus (HIV) infection. In planning care to address the psychosocial issues, the nurse would expect that this child:
   1. Is unable to grasp the concept of illness and death
   2. Begins to understand that something is wrong
   3. Begins to conceptualize the death process as involving physical harm
   4. Will express fear, withdrawal, and denial

10. A home care nurse provides instructions regarding basic infection control to the mother of a child with human immunodeficiency virus (HIV) infection. Which statement if made by the mother indicates the need for further instructions?
    1. "I will carefully wash all fresh fruits and vegetables."
    2. "I will wash baby bottles, nipples, and pacifiers in the dishwasher."
    3. "I will clean up any spills from the diaper with full-strength alcohol."
    4. "I will rub the inside of the nipple with salt and rinse well if it becomes slimy."

CRITICAL THINKING: FREE-TEXT ENTRY

The mother of an 18-month-old child with acquired immunodeficiency syndrome (AIDS) brings the child to the clinic for the scheduled immunizations. The child is up-to-date with immunizations, and at the last visit, when the child was 15 months of age, the child received a pneumococcal vaccine and an influenza vaccine. The nurse prepares to administer which scheduled immunization(s) for this child?

Answer: _____

ANSWERS

1. **4**

Rationale: The HIV virus attacks the immune system by destroying T lymphocytes. Infants born to HIV-positive women test positive for HIV antibody, not HIV virus. This is actually a measure of maternal antibody and not indicative of true infection in the infant. HIV attacks the immune system. T4 cells are depleted in number and cannot signal B cells to form protective antibodies to fight off the invading virus.

Test-Taking Strategy: Use the process of elimination. Eliminate option 2 first, knowing that HIV attacks the immune system. Eliminate option 1 next with the knowledge that newborn infants test positive for HIV antibody, but not the virus. Recalling that T4 cells are depleted will assist in eliminating option 3. Review the physiological occurrences in HIV and AIDS if you had difficulty with this question.
Level of Cognitive Ability: Application
Client Needs: Physiological Integrity
Integrated Concept/Process: Teaching/Learning

Content Area: Child Health
Reference: Bowden, V., Dickey, S., & Greenberg, C. (1998). *Children and their families: The continuum of care.* Philadelphia: W.B. Saunders, pp. 1645-1646.

2. 2
Rationale: A positive antibody test in a child younger than 18 months indicates only that the mother is infected, because maternal IgG antibodies persist in infants for 6 to 9 months and, in some cases, as long as 18 months. A positive ELISA is not indicative of true infection.
Test-Taking Strategy: Use the process of elimination. Noting the key words "newborn infant" in the question, and recalling that a positive antibody test in a child younger than 18 months indicates only that the mother is infected, will assist in directing you to the correct option. Review tests associated with HIV infection if you had difficulty with this question.
Level of Cognitive Ability: Analysis
Client Needs: Physiological Integrity
Integrated Concept/Process: Nursing Process/Analysis
Content Area: Child Health
Reference: Ball, J., & Bindler, R. (1999). *Pediatric nursing: Caring for children* (2nd ed.). Stamford, Conn.: Appleton & Lange, p. 348.

3. 4
Rationale: True infections in infants are confirmed by the detection of HIV by a p24 antigen assay, virus culture of HIV, or polymerase chain reaction (PCR). A Western blot confirms the presence of HIV antibodies. The CD4+ count indicates how well the immune system is working. A chest x-ray evaluates the presence of other manifestations associated HIV infection, such as pneumonia.
Test-Taking Strategy: Knowledge regarding the laboratory tests used to determine the presence of HIV infection is required to answer this question. If you are unfamiliar with these laboratory tests, review them. Specific laboratory tests to review include ELISA, Western blot, CD4+ counts, and p24 antigen assay.
Level of Cognitive Ability: Analysis
Client Needs: Physiological Integrity
Integrated Concept/Process: Nursing Process/Analysis
Content Area: Child Health
Reference: Bowden, V., Dickey, S., & Greenberg, C. (1998). *Children and their families: The continuum of care.* Philadelphia: W.B. Saunders, p. 1645.

4. 3
Rationale: Most children infected with HIV develop symptoms within the first 9 months of life. The remainder of these infected children become symptomatic sometime before age 3. Children, with their immature immune systems, have a much shorter incubation period than adults. Options 1, 2, and 4 are incorrect.
Test-Taking Strategy: Use the process of elimination. Eliminate options 1, 2, and 4 because they are similar in content. Option 3 is the only option that provides specific and accurate data regarding HIV infection in the infant. Review assessment findings associated with HIV infection if you had difficulty with this question.
Level of Cognitive Ability: Application
Client Needs: Psychosocial Integrity
Integrated Concept/Process: Teaching/Learning

Content Area: Child Health
Reference: Bowden, V., Dickey, S., & Greenberg, C. (1998). *Children and their families: The continuum of care.* Philadelphia: W.B. Saunders, p. 1646.

5. 3
Rationale: The most common opportunistic infection of children infected with HIV is PCP. It occurs most frequently between the ages of 3 and 6 months, when HIV status may be indeterminate. LIP is a form of chronic pneumonitis and is also characteristic of HIV infection; however, it is not the most common opportunistic infection. Although gastrointestinal disturbances and neurological abnormalities may occur in the child with HIV infection, options 1 and 2 are not specific opportunistic infections noted in the HIV-infected child.
Test-Taking Strategy: Use the process of elimination and note the key words "most common opportunistic infection." This focus will direct you to option 3. Review the common manifestations associated with HIV, if you had difficulty with this question.
Level of Cognitive Ability: Analysis
Client Needs: Physiological Integrity
Integrated Concept/Process: Nursing Process/Assessment
Content Area: Child Health
Reference: Wong, D. (1999). *Whaley & Wong's nursing care of infants and children* (6th ed.). St. Louis: Mosby, p. 1695.

6. 2
Rationale: Immunizations against common childhood illnesses are recommended for all children exposed to or infected with HIV. Pneumococcal and influenza vaccines are also recommended. The varicella (chickenpox) vaccine is avoided in the child who is HIV infected. The hepatitis B vaccine is administered according to the recommended immunization schedule. Option 4 is not necessary and is inaccurate.
Test-Taking Strategy: Use the process of elimination. Option 4 can be easily eliminated first. From the remaining options, recalling that *Pneumocystis carinii* is the most common opportunistic infection in the child infected with HIV will assist in directing you to option 2. Review immunizations in the immunodeficient child if you had difficulty with this question.
Level of Cognitive Ability: Application
Client Needs: Health Promotion and Maintenance
Integrated Concept/Process: Teaching/Learning
Content Area: Child Health
Reference: Wong, D. (1999). *Whaley & Wong's nursing care of infants and children* (6th ed.). St. Louis: Mosby, p. 1695.

7. 2
Rationale: Nebulizer pieces are cleaned with warm water after each treatment and allowed to air dry. They are soaked in white vinegar and water for 30 minutes at the end of each day. Options 1, 3, and 4 are inaccurate and would damage the nebulizer equipment.
Test-Taking Strategy: Use the process of elimination. Options 1, 3, and 4 are similar in that they will damage the equipment. Options 1 and 4 should be eliminated first because these cleaning agents are very strong and will damage the equipment. Next eliminate option 3 because the boiling process may also cause damage. Review home care instructions regarding respiratory treatments if you had difficulty with this question.

Level of Cognitive Ability: Application
Client Needs: Health Promotion and Maintenance
Integrated Concept/Process: Teaching/Learning
Content Area: Child Health
Reference: Altman, G., Buchsel, P., & Coxon, V. (2000). *Delmar's fundamental & advanced nursing skills.* Albany, N.Y.: Delmar, p. 542.

8. **2**

Rationale: Zidovudine effectively interferes with HIV replication but can cause bone marrow suppression. Anemia occurs most commonly after 4 to 6 weeks of therapy. Hematology studies need to be monitored for anemia and granulocytopenia. Renal and liver function tests should also be monitored. Options 1, 3, and 4 are not associated with the use of zidovudine.

Test-Taking Strategy: Use the process of elimination. Recalling that anemia is a concern with the administration of this medication will easily direct you to option 2. Review the adverse effects related to this medication if you had difficulty with this question.
Level of Cognitive Ability: Analysis
Client Needs: Physiological Integrity
Integrated Concept/Process: Nursing Process/Analysis
Content Area: Pharmacology
Reference: Hodgson, B., & Kizior, R. (2001). *Saunders nursing drug handbook 2001.* Philadelphia: W.B. Saunders, pp. 1067-1069.

9. **3**

Rationale: The preschool child will begin to conceptualize the death process as involving physical harm. A child from birth to 2 years of age will be unable to grasp the concept of illness and death. A school-aged child will begin to understand that something is wrong. An adolescent will express fear, withdrawal, and denial.

Test-Taking Strategy: Use concepts of growth and development and the related psychosocial issues to answer the question. Noting the age of the child will assist in directing you to the correct option. Review these concepts if you had difficulty with this question.
Level of Cognitive Ability: Analysis
Client Needs: Psychosocial Integrity
Integrated Concept/Process: Nursing Process/Analysis

Content Area: Child Health
Reference: Bowden, V., Dickey, S., & Greenberg, C. (1998). *Children and their families: The continuum of care.* Philadelphia: W.B. Saunders, p. 1652.

10. **3**

Rationale: The mother should be instructed to use a bleach solution for disinfecting contaminated objects or cleaning up spills from the child's diaper. Options 1, 2, and 4 are accurate instructions related to basic infection control.

Test-Taking Strategy: Use the process of elimination and note the key words "need for further instructions." Knowledge regarding basic infection control measures will easily direct you to option 3. Review these measures if you had difficulty with this question.
Level of Cognitive Ability: Analysis
Client Needs: Health Promotion and Maintenance
Integrated Concept/Process: Teaching/Learning
Content Area: Child Health
Reference: Ball, J., & Bindler, R. (1999). *Pediatric nursing: Caring for children* (2nd ed.). Stamford, Conn.: Appleton & Lange, p. 355.

CRITICAL THINKING: FREE-TEXT ENTRY

Answer: DTaP (diphtheria, tetanus, acellular pertussis)
Rationale: At the age of 12 to 18 months, the recommended immunizations include the DtaP and the varicella zoster vaccine. The varicella zoster vaccine is avoided in the child with AIDS.

Test-Taking Strategy: Focus on the issue, the immunization schedule for a child with AIDS. Note the age of the child and recall the immunization schedule. Remembering that the varicella zoster vaccine is avoided in the child with AIDS will assist in identifying the immunization to be administered in this child. Review the immunization schedule and the schedule for the child with AIDS if you had difficulty with this question.
Level of Cognitive Ability: Application
Client Needs: Health Promotion and Maintenance
Integrated Concept/Process: Nursing Process/Planning
Content Area: Child Health
Reference: Wong, D. (1999). *Whaley & Wong's nursing care of infants and children* (6th ed.). St. Louis: Mosby, p. 1695.

REFERENCES

Altman, G., Buchsel, P., & Coxon, V. (2000). *Delmar's fundamental & advanced nursing skills.* Albany, N.Y.: Delmar.

Ball, J., & Bindler, R. (1999). *Pediatric nursing: Caring for children* (2nd ed.). Stamford, Conn.: Appleton & Lange.

Bowden, V., Dickey, S., & Greenberg, C. (1998). *Children and their families: The continuum of care.* Philadelphia: W.B. Saunders.

Hodgson, B., & Kizior, R. (2001). *Saunders nursing drug handbook 2001.* Philadelphia: W.B. Saunders.

Wong, D. (1999). *Whaley & Wong's nursing care of infants and children* (6th ed.). St. Louis: Mosby.

Hematological Disorders

I. SICKLE CELL DISEASE (SCD)

A. Description
1. A group of diseases collectively termed hemo-globinopathies, in which hemoglobin (hemo-globin A [HgbA]) is partly or completely re-placed by abnormal sickle hemoglobin (HgbS)
2. Caused by the inheritance of a gene for a structurally abnormal portion of the hemoglo-bin (Hgb) chain
3. HgbS is sensitive to changes in the oxygen content of the red blood cell (RBC)
4. Insufficient oxygen causes the cells to assume a sickle shape, and the cells become rigid and clumped together, obstructing capillary blood flow
5. Situations that precipitate sickling include fever and emotional or physical stress; any condition that increases the body's need for oxygen or alters the transport of oxygen can result in sickle cell crisis
6. Risk factors include having parents heterozy-gous for HgbS or being African-American
7. The sickling response is reversible under condi-tions of adequate oxygenation and hydration; after repeated sickling, the cell becomes perma-nently sickled
8. The clinical manifestations are primarily the result of obstruction caused by sickled RBCs and increased RBC destruction
9. Sickle cell crises are acute exacerbations of the disease, which vary markedly in severity and frequency; these include vaso-occlusive crisis, splenic sequestration, and aplastic crisis
10. Care focuses on the prevention (preventing exposure to infection and maintaining nor-mal hydration) and treatment (oxygen, hy-dration, pain management, and bed rest) of the crisis

B. Assessment of the crisis
1. Vaso-occlusive crisis
   a. Most common type of crisis; caused by stasis of blood with clumping of the cells in the microcirculation, ischemia, and infarction
   b. Signs include fever, pain, and tissue en-gorgement
2. Splenic sequestration
   a. Life-threatening crisis caused by the pooling of blood in the spleen
   b. Signs include profound anemia, hypovole-mia, and shock
3. Aplastic crisis
   a. Caused by the diminished production and increased destruction of RBCs, triggered by viral infection or the depletion of folic acid
   b. Signs include profound anemia and pallor

C. Implementation
1. Administer oxygen and blood transfusions as prescribed to increase tissue perfusion
2. Administer analgesics as prescribed (around the clock); administration of meperidine (Demerol) is avoided because of the risk of normeperidine-induced seizures
3. Maintain adequate hydration and blood flow with intravenous (IV) normal saline as prescribed and with oral fluids
4. Assist the child to assume a comfortable position so that the child keeps the extremities extended to promote venous return; elevate the head of the bed no more than 30 degrees, avoid putting strain on painful joints, and do not raise the knee gatch of the bed
5. Encourage consumption of a high-calorie, high-protein diet with folic acid supplementation
6. Administer antibiotics as prescribed to prevent infection
7. Monitor for signs of increasing anemia and shock (mental status changes, pallor, vital sign changes)

8. Instruct the child and parents about the early signs and symptoms of crisis and the measures to prevent crisis

9. Inform the parents of the **hereditary** aspects of the disorder

II. IRON DEFICIENCY ANEMIA

A. Description
1. Iron stores are depleted, resulting in a decreased supply of iron for the manufacture of hemoglobin in RBCs
2. Commonly results from blood loss, increased metabolic demands, syndromes of gastrointestinal (GI) malabsorption, and dietary inadequacy

B. Assessment
1. Pallor
2. Weakness and fatigue
3. Irritability

C. Implementation
1. Increase the oral intake of iron
2. Instruct the child and parents in food choices that are high in iron (Box 43-1)
3. Administer iron supplements as prescribed
4. Teach the child and parents that liquid iron preparation stains the teeth and should be taken through a straw
5. Instruct the child and parents about the side effects of iron supplements (black stools, constipation, and foul aftertaste)

III. APLASTIC ANEMIA

A. Description
1. A deficiency of circulating erythrocytes resulting from the arrested development of RBCs within the bone marrow
2. There are several possible causes, including chronic exposure to myelotoxic agents, viruses, infection, autoimmune disorders, and allergic states
3. The definitive diagnosis is determined by bone marrow aspiration (demonstrates conversion of red bone marrow to fatty red bone marrow)
4. Therapeutic management includes blood transfusions, splenectomy, corticosteroids, immunosuppressive therapy, bone marrow transplant (treat-

---

BOX 43-1

Iron-Rich Foods

Liver
Meats
Egg yolks
Dark, green leafy vegetables
Breads and cereals
Kidney beans
Raisins

---

ment of choice if a suitable donor exists), and the administration of antilymphocyte globulin (ALG) or antithymocyte globulin (ATG) to suppress the autoimmune response

B. Assessment
1. Pancytopenia (a deficiency of erythrocytes, leukocytes, and thrombocytes)
2. Petechiae, purpura, bleeding, pallor, weakness, tachycardia, and fatigue

C. Implementation
1. Administer blood transfusions as prescribed and monitor for transfusion reactions; transfusions are discontinued as soon as the bone marrow begins to produce RBCs
2. Administer corticosteroids and immunosuppressive therapy as prescribed
3. Prepare the child for splenectomy; prescribed for the child with an enlarged spleen that is destroying normal RBCs or suppressing their development
4. Prepare the child for bone marrow transplant if planned
5. Administer ALG or ATG as prescribed and monitor for allergic reactions (fever, skin rash)
6. Advise the parents to obtain a Medic-Alert bracelet for the child

IV. HEMOPHILIA

A. Description
1. An X-linked recessive trait
2. Hemophilia A (classic hemophilia) results from a deficiency of factor VIII
3. Hemophilia B (Christmas disease) results from a deficiency of factor IX
4. Males inherit hemophilia from their mothers, and females inherit the carrier status from their fathers
5. Some females who are carriers have an increased tendency to bleed, and, although it is rare, females can have hemophilia if their fathers have the disorder and their mothers are carriers of the genetic disorder
6. The primary treatment is replacement of the missing clotting factor; products used are factor VIII concentrate and desmopressin acetate (DDAVP)

B. Assessment
1. Abnormal bleeding in response to trauma or surgery
2. Joint bleeding causing pain, tenderness, swelling, and limited range of motion
3. Tendency to bruise easily
4. Prolonged partial thromboplastin time (PTT)
5. Normal bleeding time, prothrombin time (PT), and platelet count

C. Implementation
1. Prepare to administer factor VIII concentrate or DDAVP

2. Monitor for bleeding and maintain bleeding precautions
3. Monitor for joint pain; immobilize the affected extremity if joint pain occurs
4. Assess neurological status (child is at risk for intracranial hemorrhage)
5. Monitor urine for hematuria
6. Control bleeding by immobilization, elevation, and the application of ice; in addition, apply pressure (15 minutes) for superficial bleeding
7. Instruct the child and parents about the signs of internal bleeding
8. Instruct the parents in how to control the bleeding
9. Instruct the parents regarding activities for the child, emphasizing the avoidance of contact sports
10. Instruct the parents to obtain a Medic-Alert bracelet for the child

V. β-THALASSEMIA MAJOR

A. Description
   1. An autosomal recessive disorder
   2. Also called Cooley's anemia and includes a group of disorders characterized by the reduced production of one of the globin chains in the synthesis of hemoglobin
   3. The incidence is highest in individuals of Mediterranean descent
   4. Treatment is supportive, and the goal of therapy is to maintain normal hemoglobin levels by the administration of blood transfusions
   5. Bone marrow transplantation may be offered as an alternative therapy
B. Assessment
   1. Severe anemia
   2. Pallor
   3. Failure to thrive
   4. Hepatosplenomegaly
   5. Microcytic, hypochromic RBCs
C. Implementation
   1. Instruct in the administration of folic acid (vitamin B_9) as prescribed, which stimulates the production of blood cells
   2. Administer blood transfusions as prescribed; monitor for transfusion reactions
   3. Monitor for iron overload and administer chelation therapy with deferoxamine (Desferal) as prescribed, to treat iron overload and to prevent organ damage from the elevated levels of iron caused by the multiple transfusion therapy
   4. Provide genetic counseling

PRACTICE QUESTIONS

1. A child suspected of having sickle cell disease (SCD) is seen in a clinic, and laboratory studies are performed. A nurse checks the laboratory results, knowing that which of the following would be increased in this disease?
   1. Platelet count
   2. Hematocrit level
   3. Reticulocyte count
   4. Hemoglobin level
2. A pediatric nursing instructor asks a nursing student to describe the cause of the clinical manifestations that occur in sickle cell disease. The student responds correctly by telling the instructor that:
   1. Sickled cells increase the blood flow through the body and cause a great deal of pain
   2. Sickled cells mix with the unsickled cells and cause the immune system to become depressed
   3. Bone marrow depression occurs because of the development of sickled cells
   4. Sickled cells are unable to flow easily through the microvasculature and their clumping obstructs blood flow
3. A clinic nurse instructs the mother of a child with sickle cell disease regarding the precipitating factors related to pain crisis. Which of the following, if identified by the mother as a precipitating factor, indicates the need for further instructions?
   1. Infection
   2. Trauma
   3. Fluid overload
   4. Stress
4. Laboratory studies are performed for a child suspected of having iron deficiency anemia (IDA). The nurse reviews the laboratory results, knowing that which of the following results would indicate this type of anemia?
   1. An elevated hemoglobin level
   2. A decreased reticulocyte count
   3. An elevated red blood cell (RBC) count
   4. RBCs that are microcytic and hypochromic
5. A home care nurse is instructing the parents of a child with iron deficiency anemia regarding the administration of a liquid oral iron supplement. The nurse tells the mother to:
   1. Administer the iron through a straw
   2. Administer the iron at mealtimes
   3. Add the iron to the formula for easy administration
   4. Mix the iron with cereal to administer
6. A pediatric nurse educator provides a teaching session to the nursing staff regarding hemophilia. Which of the following information regarding this disorder would the nurse plan to include in the discussion?
   1. Hemophilia is a Y-linked hereditary disorder
   2. Males inherit hemophilia from their fathers
   3. Females inherit hemophilia from their mothers
   4. Hemophilia A results from deficiency of factor VIII

7. A nurse analyzes the laboratory results of a child with hemophilia. The nurse understands that which of the following would most likely be abnormal in this child?
   1. Bleeding time
   2. Platelet count
   3. Prothrombin time (PT)
   4. Partial thromboplastin time (PTT)

8. A nurse is providing home care instructions to the mother of a 10-year-old child with hemophilia. Which of the following activities would the nurse suggest that the child could safely participate in with peers?
   1. Basketball
   2. Swimming
   3. Soccer
   4. Field hockey

9. A nursing student is presenting a clinical conference and discusses the etiology related to β-thalassemia. The nursing student informs the group that the child at greatest risk of developing this disorder is:
   1. A child whose intake of iron is extremely poor
   2. A breast-fed child of a mother with chronic anemia
   3. A child of Mediterranean descent
   4. A child of Mexican descent

10. A child with β-thalassemia is receiving long-term blood transfusion therapy for the treatment of this disorder. Chelation therapy is prescribed in order to prevent organ damage from the presence of too much iron in the body as a result of the transfusions. Which of the following medications would the nurse anticipate to be prescribed in chelation therapy?
    1. Dalteparin sodium (Fragmin)
    2. Meropenem (Merrem)
    3. Molindone HCl (Moban)
    4. Deferoxamine (Desferal)

CRITICAL THINKING: FREE-TEXT ENTRY

A nurse is reviewing a physician's orders for a child with sickle cell anemia who was admitted to the hospital for the treatment of vaso-occlusive crisis. The nurse notes that the physician has prescribed an increased fluid intake, intravenous (IV) fluids, oxygen, heat to the affected areas, and meperidine (Demerol) for pain. Which order documented by the physician will the nurse question?

Answer: _____

ANSWERS

1. 3

Rationale: A diagnosis is established on the basis of a complete blood count, examination for sickled red blood cells (RBCs) in the peripheral smear, and hemoglobin electrophoresis. Laboratory studies will show decreased hemoglobin and hematocrit levels and a decreased platelet count, an increased reticulocyte count, and the presence of nucleated red blood cells. Increased reticulocyte counts occur in children with SCD because the life span of their sickled RBCs is shortened.

Test-Taking Strategy: Use the process of elimination. Recalling that the life span of the sickled RBCs is shortened in SCD and noting the relationship between this concept and the reticulocytes will direct you to the correct option. Review the laboratory tests that are diagnostic for this disorder if you had difficulty with this question.

Level of Cognitive Ability: Analysis
Client Needs: Physiological Integrity
Integrated Concept/Process: Nursing Process/Assessment
Content Area: Child Health
References: Ball, J., & Bindler, R. (1999). *Pediatric nursing: Caring for children* (2nd ed.). Stamford, Conn.: Appleton & Lange, p. 524.
Bowden, V., Dickey, S., & Greenberg, C. (1998). *Children and their families: The continuum of care.* Philadelphia: W.B. Saunders, p. 1567.

2. 4

Rationale: All of the clinical manifestations of sickle cell disease (SCD) result from the sickled cells being unable to flow easily through the microvasculature, and their clumping obstructs blood flow. With reoxygenation, most of the sickled red blood cells resume their normal shape. Options 1, 2, and 3 are incorrect statements.

Test-Taking Strategy: Use the process of elimination. Recalling that sickled cells clump will direct you to the correct option. Review the pathophysiology associated with SCD if you had difficulty with this question.

Level of Cognitive Ability: Analysis
Client Needs: Physiological Integrity
Integrated Concept/Process: Teaching/Learning
Content Area: Child Health
Reference: Ball, J., & Bindler, R. (1999). *Pediatric nursing: Caring for children* (2nd ed.). Stamford, Conn.: Appleton & Lange, p. 523.

3. 3

Rationale: Pain crisis may be precipitated by infection, dehydration, hypoxia, trauma, or physical or emotional stress. The mother of a child with sickle cell disease should encourage fluid intake of one and one-half to two times the daily requirement to prevent dehydration.

Test-Taking Strategy: Use the process of elimination. Note the key words "the need for further instructions." Recalling that fluids are a main component of treatment in sickle cell disease to prevent pain crisis will direct you to option 3. Remember that fluids are required to prevent dehydration. Review the precipitating factors of pain crisis if you had difficulty with this question.

Level of Cognitive Ability: Analysis

Client Needs: Health Promotion and Maintenance
Integrated Concept/Process: Teaching/Learning
Content Area: Child Health
Reference: Ball, J., & Bindler, R. (1999). *Pediatric nursing: Caring for children* (2nd ed.). Stamford, Conn.: Appleton & Lange, p. 526.

4. **4**

Rationale: The results of a complete blood count (CBC) in children with IDA will show decreased hemoglobin levels and microcytic and hypochromic RBCs. The RBC count is decreased. The reticulocyte count is usually normal or slightly elevated.

Test-Taking Strategy: Use the process of elimination. Eliminate options 1 and 3 first, knowing that the hemoglobin and RBC counts would be decreased. From the remaining options, select option 4 over option 2 because of the relationship between anemia and RBCs. Review the laboratory findings in IDA if you had difficulty with this question.
Level of Cognitive Ability: Analysis
Client Needs: Physiological Integrity
Integrated Concept/Process: Nursing Process/Assessment
Content Area: Child Health
Reference: Wong, D. (1999). *Whaley & Wong's nursing care of infants and children* (6th ed.). St. Louis: Mosby, p. 1664.

5. **1**

Rationale: An oral iron supplement should be administered through a straw or medicine dropper placed at the back of the mouth because the iron will stain the teeth. The parents should be instructed to brush or wipe the teeth after administration. Iron is administered between meals because absorption is decreased if there is food in the stomach. Iron requires an acid environment to facilitate its absorption in the duodenum. It is not added to formula or mixed with cereal or other food items.

Test-Taking Strategy: Use the process of elimination. Eliminate options 3 and 4 first because they are similar and because medication should not be added to formula and food. Note the key word "liquid" in the question. This should assist you in recalling that liquid iron stains teeth. Review the teaching points related to this medication if you had difficulty with this question.
Level of Cognitive Ability: Application
Client Needs: Health Promotion and Maintenance
Integrated Concept/Process: Teaching/Learning
Content Area: Child Health
Reference: Wong, D. (1999). *Whaley & Wong's nursing care of infants and children* (6th ed.). St. Louis: Mosby, p. 1666.

6. **4**

Rationale: Males inherit hemophilia from their mothers, and females inherit the carrier status from their fathers. Hemophilia is inherited in a recessive manner via a genetic defect on the X chromosome. Hemophilia A results from a deficiency of factor VIII. Hemophilia B (Christmas Disease) is a deficiency of factor IX.

Test-Taking Strategy: Use the process of elimination. Read each option carefully, and use knowledge regarding hemophilia and its related etiology to answer the question. Review this important disorder if you had difficulty with this question.
Level of Cognitive Ability: Application
Client Needs: Physiological Integrity
Integrated Concept/Process: Teaching/Learning

Content Area: Child Health
Reference: Bowden, V., Dickey, S., & Greenberg, C. (1998). *Children and their families: The continuum of care*. Philadelphia: W.B. Saunders, p. 1535.

7. **4**

Rationale: Abnormal laboratory results in hemophilia indicate a prolonged partial thromboplastin time (PTT). The bleeding time, prothrombin time (PT), and platelet count are normal in hemophilia.

Test-Taking Strategy: Use the process of elimination and knowledge regarding the laboratory tests used to monitor hemophilia. Recalling the pathophysiology associated with this disorder will direct you to option 4. Review these laboratory tests if you had difficulty with this question.
Level of Cognitive Ability: Analysis
Client Needs: Physiological Integrity
Integrated Concept/Process: Nursing Process/Analysis
Content Area: Child Health
Reference: Bowden, V., Dickey, S., & Greenberg, C. (1998). *Children and their families: The continuum of care*. Philadelphia: W.B. Saunders, p. 1540.

8. **2**

Rationale: Children with hemophilia need to avoid contact sports and to take precautions, such as wearing elbow and knee pads and helmets with other sports. The safest activity for them is swimming.

Test-Taking Strategy: Use the process of elimination. Note the key word "safely" in the stem of the question. Recalling that bleeding is a major concern in this condition will assist in directing you to option 2. Eliminate options 1, 3, and 4 because these activities present the potential for injury. Review home care instructions for the child with hemophilia if you had difficulty with this question.
Level of Cognitive Ability: Application
Client Needs: Health Promotion and Maintenance
Integrated Concept/Process: Teaching/Learning
Content Area: Child Health
Reference: Wong, D. (1999). *Whaley & Wong's nursing care of infants and children* (6th ed.). St. Louis: Mosby, p. 1684.

9. **3**

Rationale: β-Thalassemia is inherited as an autosomal recessive pattern. This disorder is found primarily in individuals of Mediterranean descent. The disease has been reported in the Asian and African populations as well. Options 1, 2, and 4 are incorrect.

Test-Taking Strategy: Use the process of elimination. Recalling that this disorder occurs primarily in individuals of Mediterranean descent will direct you to the correct option. If you are unfamiliar with this disorder, review the information associated with its incidence and etiology.
Level of Cognitive Ability: Application
Client Needs: Physiological Integrity
Integrated Concept/Process: Teaching/Learning
Content Area: Child Health
Reference: Ball, J., & Bindler, R. (1999). *Pediatric nursing: Caring for children* (2nd ed.). Stamford, Conn.: Appleton & Lange, p. 529.

10. **4**

Rationale: The major complication of chronic transfusion therapy is hemosiderosis. In order to prevent organ damage from too much iron in the blood, chelation therapy with a medication called deferoxamine (Desferal) is used. Desferal is classified as an antidote for acute iron toxicity. Fragmin is an anticoagulant used as prophylaxis for postoperative deep vein thrombosis. Merrem is an antibiotic. Moban is an antipsychotic.

Test-Taking Strategy: Use the process of elimination and knowledge regarding the antidote for iron toxicity. If you had difficulty with this question, review these medications.

Level of Cognitive Ability: Analysis
Client Needs: Physiological Integrity
Integrated Concept/Process: Nursing Process/Analysis
Content Area: Child Health
References: Ball, J., & Bindler, R. (1999). *Pediatric nursing: Caring for children* (2nd ed.). Stamford, Conn.: Appleton & Lange, p. 531.
Hodgson, B., & Kizior, R. (2001). *Saunders nursing drug handbook 2001.* Philadelphia: W.B. Saunders, pp. 281, 289, 642, 700.

CRITICAL THINKING: FREE-TEXT ENTRY

Answer: Meperidine (Demerol) for pain
Rationale: Meperidine (Demerol) is not recommended for the child with sickle cell disease because of the risk for normeperidine-induced seizures. Normeperidine, a metabolite of meperidine, is a central nervous system stimulant that produces anxiety, tremors, myoclonus, and generalized seizures when it accumulates with repetitive dosing. The nurse would question the order for this pain control medication. Fluids, oxygen, and heat to affected areas are used to treat vaso-occlusive crisis.

Test-Taking Strategy: Focus on the pathophysiology that occurs in sickle cell disease to assist in identifying the order that needs to be questioned. Recalling the effects of meperidine will assist in identifying the answer. Review care of the child with sickle cell disease experiencing a crisis if you had difficulty with this question.

Level of Cognitive Ability: Analysis
Client Needs: Safe, Effective Care Environment
Integrated Concept/Process: Nursing Process/Analysis
Content Area: Child Health
Reference: Wong, D. (1999). *Whaley & Wong's nursing care of infants and children* (6th ed.). St. Louis: Mosby, p. 1672.

REFERENCES

Ball, J., & Bindler, R. (1999). *Pediatric nursing: Caring for children* (2nd ed.). Stamford, Conn.: Appleton & Lange.

Bowden, V., Dickey, S,, & Greenberg, C. (1998). *Children and their families: The continuum of care.* Philadelphia: W.B. Saunders.

Hodgson, B., & Kizior, R. (2001). *Saunders nursing drug handbook 2001.* Philadelphia: W.B. Saunders.

Wong, D. (1999). *Whaley & Wong's nursing care of infants and children* (6th ed.). St. Louis: Mosby.

Web site: www.thalassemia.org.

Web site: www.ahcpr.gov/

Oncological Disorders

I. LEUKEMIA (Table 44-1)

A. Description
1. Malignant exacerbation in the number of leukocytes, usually at an immature stage, in the bone marrow
2. Affects the bone marrow, causing anemia from decreased erythrocytes, infection from neutropenia, and bleeding from decreased platelet production
3. The cause is unknown and appears to involve gene damage of cells, leading to the transformation of cells from a normal state to a malignant state
4. Risk factors include genetic, viral, immunological, and environmental factors, and exposure to radiation, chemicals, and medications
5. Acute lymphocytic leukemia (ALL) is the most frequent type of cancer in children; peak onset is age 2 to 6 years
6. Is more common in boys than girls after age 1 year
7. Treatment involves the use of chemotherapeutic agents with or without cranial radiation
8. The phases of treatment include induction, which achieves a complete remission or disappearance of leukemic cells; intensification or consolidation therapy, which further decreases the tumor burden; central nervous system prophylactic therapy, which prevents leukemic cells from invading the central nervous system; and maintenance, which serves to maintain the remission phase
9. Bone marrow transplantation (BMT) may also be performed to treat some children with leukemia

B. Assessment
1. Infiltration of the bone marrow causes fever, pallor, fatigue, anorexia, hemorrhage (usually petechiae), and bone and joint pain; pathological fractures can occur as a result of bone marrow invasion with leukemic cells
2. Signs of infection as a result of neutropenia
3. Hepatosplenomegaly, lymphadenopathy
4. Normal, elevated, or low white blood cell (WBC) count
5. Decreased hemoglobin and hematocrit levels
6. Decreased platelet count
7. Positive bone marrow biopsy identifying leukemic blast (immature) phase cells
8. Signs of increased intracranial pressure, such as severe headache, vomiting, papilledema, irritability, lethargy, and eventually coma, as a result of central nervous system involvement
9. Signs of cranial nerve (cranial nerve VII, or the facial nerve, is most commonly affected) or spinal nerve involvement; clinical manifestations relate to the area involved
10. Clinical manifestations that indicate the invasion of leukemic cells to the kidneys, testes, prostate, ovaries, gastrointestinal (GI) tract, and lungs

C. Infection (Box 44-1)
1. A major cause of death in the immunosuppressed child
2. Can occur through autocontamination or cross-contamination

---

TABLE 44-1

Classification of Leukemia

Acute Lymphocytic Leukemia (ALL)	Acute Myelogenous Leukemia (AML)
Mostly lymphoblasts present in bone marrow	Mostly myeloblasts present in bone marrow
Age of onset is less than 15 years	Age of onset is between 15 and 39 years

3. Most common sites of infection are the skin (any break in the skin is a potential site of infection), respiratory tract, and GI tract
▲ D. Bleeding (Box 44-2)
   1. Children with platelet counts below 20,000/mm³ may need a platelet transfusion

---

2. For children with severe blood loss, packed red blood cells may be prescribed
E. Fatigue and nutrition ▲
   1. Assist the child in selecting a well-balanced diet
   2. Provide small meals that require little chewing
   3. Assist the child in self-care and mobility activities
   4. Allow adequate rest periods during care
   5. Do not perform activities unless they are essential
F. Chemotherapy
   1. Monitor for severe bone marrow suppression; ▲ during the period of greatest bone marrow suppression (the nadir), blood counts will be extremely low
   2. Monitor for infection and bleeding ▲
   3. Protect the child from life-threatening infec- ▲ tions
   4. Monitor for nausea, vomiting, and diarrhea
   5. Administer antiemetics as prescribed
   6. Monitor for signs of dehydration
   7. Monitor for signs of hemorrhagic cystitis
   8. Monitor for signs of peripheral neuropathy
   9. Assess oral mucous membranes for mucositis; administer frequent mouth rinses (normal saline with or without sodium bicarbonate solution) to promote healing if mucositis occurs

---

BOX 44-1

Protecting the Child from Infection

Initiate protective isolation procedures
Maintain the child in a private room and a room with high-efficiency particulate air (HEPA) filtration or laminar air flow system if possible
Be sure that the child's room is cleaned daily
Maintain frequent and thorough handwashing
Use strict aseptic technique for all nursing procedures
Limit the number of caregivers entering the child's room, and ensure that anyone entering the child's room is wearing a mask
Keep supplies for the child separate from supplies for other children
Reduce exposure to environmental organisms by eliminating raw fruits and vegetables and fresh flowers, and by not leaving standing water in the child's room
Assist the child with daily bathing, using antimicrobial soap
Assist the child to perform oral hygiene frequently
Assess for signs and symptoms of infection
Monitor temperature, pulse, and blood pressure
Change wound dressings daily and inspect wounds for redness, swelling, or drainage
Assess urine for color and cloudiness
Assess the skin and oral mucous membranes for signs of infection
Auscultate lung sounds
Encourage the child to cough and deep breathe
Monitor the WBC and the neutrophil count
Notify the physician if signs of infection are present, and prepare to obtain specimens for culture of open lesions, urine, and sputum
Initiate a bowel program to prevent constipation and rectal trauma
Avoid invasive procedures such as injections, rectal temperatures, and urinary catheterization
Administer antibiotic, antifungal, and antiviral medication as prescribed
Administer granulocyte colony-stimulating factor (GCSF) as prescribed
Instruct the parents to keep the child away from crowds and those with infections
Instruct the parents that the child should not receive immunization with a live virus
Keep any child with chickenpox or any child who has been exposed to the virus away from the child with leukemia
Instruct the parents to inform the teacher that they should be notified immediately if a case of chickenpox occurs in another child at school

---

BOX 44-2

Protecting the Child from Bleeding

Examine the child for signs and symptoms of bleeding
Handle the child gently
Measure abdominal girth, which can indicate internal hemorrhage
Instruct the child to use a soft toothbrush and to avoid dental floss
Provide soft foods that are cool to warm in temperature
Avoid injections if possible, to prevent trauma to the skin and bleeding
Apply firm and gentle pressure to a needle-stick site for at least 10 minutes
Pad side rails and sharp corners of the bed and furniture
Discourage the child from engaging in activities involving the use of sharp objects
Instruct the child to avoid constrictive or tight clothing
Use caution when taking the blood pressure, to prevent skin injury
Instruct the child to avoid blowing the nose
Avoid rectal suppositories, enemas, and rectal thermometers
Examine all body fluids and excrement for the presence of blood
Count the number of pads or tampons used if the female adolescent is menstruating
Instruct the child in the signs and symptoms of bleeding
Instruct the parents to avoid administering nonsteroidal antiinflammatory drugs (NSAIDs) and products that contain aspirin to the child

10. Instruct the parents in signs and symptoms to monitor after chemotherapy and when to notify the physician
11. Inform the parents that hair loss may occur from chemotherapy (hair will regrow in 3 to 6 months and may be a slightly different color or texture)
12. Instruct the parents about the care of a central venous access device as necessary
13. Listen to the child and family, and encourage them to verbalize their feelings and express their concerns
14. Introduce the family to other families of children with cancer
15. Consult social services and chaplains as necessary

II. HODGKIN'S DISEASE (Box 44-3)

A. Description
1. A malignancy of the lymph nodes that originates in a single lymph node or a single chain of nodes
2. It predictably metastasizes to nonnodal or extralymphatic sites, especially the spleen, liver, bone marrow, lungs, and mediastinum
3. Characterized by the presence of the Reed-Sternberg cell in the lymph nodes
4. Possible causes include viral infections and previous exposure to alkalating chemical agents
5. The prognosis is dependent on the stage of disease; the prognosis is excellent in children with localized disease
6. The primary treatment modalities are radiation and chemotherapy; each may be used alone or in combination, depending on the clinical staging of the disease

---

BOX 44-3

Staging of Hodgkin's Disease

STAGE I
Involvement of a single lymph node region or an extralymphatic organ or site

STAGE II
Involvement of two or more lymph node regions on the same side of the diaphragm or localized involvement of an extralymphatic organ or site

STAGE III
Involvement of lymph node regions on both sides of the diaphragm or localized involvement of an extralymphatic organ or site or spleen or both

STAGE IV
Diffuse or disseminated involvement of one or more extralymphatic organs with or without associated lymph node involvement

---

7. BMT may be a consideration in treating Hodgkin's disease

B. Assessment
1. Painless enlargement of lymph nodes
2. Enlarged, firm, nontender, movable nodes in the supraclavicular area; in children, the "sentinel" node located near the left clavicle may be the first enlarged node
3. Nonproductive cough as a result of mediastinal lymphadenopathy
4. Abdominal pain as a result of enlarged retroperitoneal nodes
5. Advanced lymph node and extralymphatic involvement may cause systemic symptoms such as low-grade and/or intermittent fever, anorexia, nausea, weight loss, night sweats, and pruritus
6. Positive biopsy of lymph node (presence of Reed-Sternberg cell) and positive bone marrow biopsy
7. Computed tomography (CT) scan of the liver, spleen, and bone marrow to detect metastasis

C. Implementation
1. For stages 1 and 2 without mediastinal node involvement, the treatment of choice is extensive external radiation of the involved lymph node regions
2. With more extensive disease, radiation along with multiagent chemotherapy is utilized
3. Monitor for drug-induced pancytopenia, which increases the risk for infection, bleeding, and anemia
4. Monitor for signs of infection and bleeding
5. Protect the child from infection
6. Provide a safe, hazard-free environment
7. Monitor for side effects related to chemotherapy or radiation; the most common complication of radiation to the neck area is hypothyroidism
8. Monitor for nausea and vomiting and administer antiemetics as prescribed
9. Monitor for skin irritation and breakdown as a result of radiation therapy

III. NEPHROBLASTOMA (WILMS' TUMOR)

A. Description
1. A tumor of the kidney that may present unilaterally and localized or bilaterally, sometimes with metastasis to other organs
2. The peak incidence is at 3 years of age
3. Its occurrence is associated with a genetic inheritance and with several congenital anomalies
4. Therapeutic management includes a combined treatment of surgery (partial to total nephrectomy) and chemotherapy with or without radiation, depending on the clinical stage and histologic pattern

B. Assessment
1. Swelling or mass within the abdomen (mass is

characteristically firm, nontender, confined to one side, and deep within the flank)
2. Abdominal pain
3. Urinary retention and/or hematuria
4. Anemia (secondary to hemorrhage within the tumor)
5. Pallor, anorexia, lethargy (occurs as a result of anemia)
6. Hypertension (caused by secretion of excess amounts of renin by the tumor)
7. Weight loss and fever
8. Symptoms of lung involvement, such as dyspnea, shortness of breath, and pain in the chest, if metastasis has occurred

C. Implementation preoperatively
1. Monitor vital signs, particularly blood pressure
2. Place a sign at the bedside: "Do Not Palpate Abdomen"
3. Avoid palpation of the abdomen
4. Measure abdominal girth

D. Implementation postoperatively
1. Monitor temperature and blood pressure closely
2. Monitor for signs of hemorrhage and infection
3. Maintain I & O and urine output closely
4. Monitor for abdominal distention, bowel sounds, and other signs of GI activity, because of the risk for intestinal obstruction

IV. NEUROBLASTOMA

A. Description
1. An embryonal tumor found in children that arises from the neural crest
2. The primary site is in the abdomen because the tumor arises from the adrenal gland or from the retroperitoneal sympathetic chain; other sites may be within the head, neck, chest, or pelvis
3. Most presenting signs are caused by the tumor compressing adjacent normal tissue and organs
4. Diagnostic evaluation is aimed at locating the primary site of the tumor
5. The prognosis is poor because of the frequency of invasiveness of the tumor and because in most cases, a diagnosis is not made until after metastasis has occurred
6. Therapeutic management
   a. Surgery to remove as much of the tumor as possible and to obtain biopsies; in stages I and II, complete surgical removal of the tumor is the treatment of choice
   b. Surgery is usually limited to biopsy in stages III and IV because of the extensive metastasis
   c. Radiation is commonly used with stage III disease and provides palliation for metastatic lesions in bones, lungs, liver, or brain
   d. Chemotherapy is the mainstay of treatment for extensive local or disseminated disease

B. Assessment
1. Firm, nontender, irregular mass in the abdomen that crosses the midline
2. Urinary frequency or retention from compression of the kidney, ureter, or bladder
3. Lymphadenopathy, especially in the cervical and supraclavicular area
4. Bone pain if skeletal involvement occurs
5. Supraorbital ecchymosis, periorbital edema, and exophthalmos as a result of invasion of retrobulbar soft tissue
6. Pallor, weakness, irritability, anorexia, weight loss
7. Signs of respiratory impairment (thoracic lesion)
8. Signs of neurological impairment (intracranial lesion)
9. Paralysis from compression of the spinal cord

C. Implementation preoperatively
1. Monitor for signs and symptoms related to the location of the tumor
2. Provide emotional support to the child and parents

D. Implementation postoperatively
1. Monitor for postoperative complications related to the location (organ) of the surgery
2. Monitor for complications related to chemotherapy or radiation if prescribed
3. Provide support to the parents and encourage them to express their feelings; many parents suffer from guilt for not having recognized signs in the child earlier
4. Refer the parents to appropriate community services

V. OSTEOGENIC SARCOMA

A. Description
1. The most common bone cancer in children
2. Usually found in the metaphysis of long bones, especially in the lower extremities, with most tumors occurring in the femur
3. Peak age of incidence is between 10 and 25 years
4. Symptoms in the earliest stage are almost always attributed to extremity injury or normal growing pains
5. Treatment may include surgical resection by limb salvage to remove affected tissue or amputation
6. Chemotherapy plays a vital role in treatment and may be employed both before and after surgery

B. Assessment
1. Localized pain at the affected site (may be severe or dull) that may be attributed to trauma or the vague complaint of "growing pains"; pain is often relieved by a flexed position
2. Palpable mass
3. Limping if weight-bearing limb is affected
4. Progressive limited range of motion and the child curtails physical activity

5. Child may be unable to hold heavy objects
6. Pathological fractures at the tumor site
C. Implementation
 1. Prepare the child and family for prescribed treatment modalities, which may include surgical resection by limb salvage to remove affected tissue, amputation, and chemotherapy
 2. Provide honesty and support for the child and family
 3. Prepare for prosthetic fitting as necessary
 4. Assist the child in dealing with problems of self-image

VI. BRAIN TUMORS
A. Description
 1. An infratentorial (below the tentorium cerebelli) tumor is located in the posterior third of the brain (primarily in the cerebellum or brainstem) and accounts for the frequency of symptoms resulting from increased intracranial pressure (ICP)
 2. A supratentorial tumor is located within the anterior two thirds of the brain, mainly the cerebrum
 3. The signs and symptoms of a brain tumor depend on its anatomical location and size and to some extent on the age of the child
 4. Therapeutic management includes surgery, radiation, and chemotherapy; the treatment of choice is total removal of the tumor without residual neurological damage
B. Assessment
 1. Headache that is worse on awakening and improves during the day
 2. Vomiting that is unrelated to feeding or eating
 3. Ataxia
 4. Seizures
 5. Behavioral changes
 6. Clumsiness; awkward gait or difficulty walking
 7. Diplopia
 8. Facial weakness
C. Implementation preoperatively
 1. Perform a neurological assessment
 2. Institute safety measures
 3. Assess weight loss and nutritional status
 4. Initiate seizure precautions
 5. The child's head will be shaved (provide a favorite cap or hat for the child)
 6. Prepare the child as much as possible; tell the child that he or she will wake up with a large head dressing
D. Implementation postoperatively
 1. Assess neurological and motor function and level of consciousness (LOC)
 2. Monitor temperature closely, which may be elevated because of hypothalamus or brainstem involvement during surgery; maintain a cooling blanket by the bedside

3. Monitor for signs of respiratory infection
4. Monitor for signs of meningitis (opisthotonos, Kernig and Brudzinski signs)
5. Monitor for signs of increased ICP or hemorrhage (check the back of the head dressing for posterior pooling of blood)
6. Assess pupillary response; sluggish, dilated, or unequal pupils are reported immediately because they may indicate increased ICP and potential brainstem herniation
7. Monitor for colorless drainage on the dressing or from the ears or nose, which indicates cerebrospinal fluid (CSF) and should be reported immediately
8. Assess the physician's order for positioning, including the degree of neck flexion
 a. If a large tumor was removed, the child is not placed on the operative side because the brain may suddenly shift to that cavity
 b. In an infratentorial procedure, the child is usually positioned flat and on either side
 c. In a supratentorial procedure, the head is usually elevated above the heart level to facilitate CSF drainage and to decrease excessive blood flow to the brain to prevent hemorrhage
 d. Never place the child in the Trendelenburg position because it increases ICP and the risk of hemorrhage
9. Monitor IV fluids carefully
10. Promote measures that prevent vomiting (vomiting increases ICP and the risk for incisional rupture)
11. Provide a quiet environment
12. Administer analgesics as prescribed
13. Provide emotional support to the child and parents, and promote maximum functioning in the child

PRACTICE QUESTIONS

1. A pediatric nurse clinician is discussing the pathophysiology related to childhood leukemia with a class of nursing students. Which statement made by a nursing student indicates a lack of understanding of the pathophysiology of this disease?
 1. Normal bone marrow is replaced by blast cells
 2. Red blood cell (RBC) production is affected
 3. The platelet count is decreased
 4. The presence of a Reed-Sternberg cell is found on biopsy

2. A 4-year-old child is admitted to the hospital for abdominal pain. The mother reports that the child has been pale and excessively tired and is bruising very easily. On physical examination, lymphadenopathy and hepatosplenomegaly are noted. Diagnostic studies are being performed on the child because acute lymphocytic leukemia (ALL) is sus-

pected. The nurse understands that which diagnostic study will confirm this diagnosis?
1. White blood cell (WBC) count
2. A lumbar puncture
3. Bone marrow biopsy
4. A platelet count

3. A nurse instructs the parents of a child with leukemia regarding measures related to monitoring for infection. Which statement if made by a parent indicates a need for further education?
1. "I will perform proper handwashing techniques."
2. "I will take a rectal temperature daily."
3. "I will inspect the skin daily for redness."
4. "I will inspect the mouth daily for lesions."

4. A 6-year-old child with leukemia is hospitalized and is receiving combination chemotherapy. Laboratory results indicate that the child is neutropenic, and protective isolation procedures are initiated. The grandmother of the child visits and brings a fresh bouquet of flowers picked from her garden and asks the nurse for a vase for the flowers. The nurse responds to the grandmother by telling her:
1. "I have a vase in the utility room and I will get it for you."
2. "The flowers from your garden are beautiful, but should not be placed in the child's room at this time."
3. "I will get the vase and wash it well before you put the flowers in it."
4. "When you bring the flowers into the room, place them on the bedside stand as far away from the child as possible."

5. A 9-year-old child with leukemia is in remission and has returned to school. The school nurse calls the mother of the child and tells the mother that a classmate has just been diagnosed with chickenpox. The mother immediately calls the clinic nurse because the leukemic child has never had chickenpox. The most appropriate response by the clinic nurse to the mother is:
1. "Monitor the child for an elevated temperature, and call the clinic if a temperature occurs."
2. "Keep the child out of school for a 2-week period."
3. "There is no need to be concerned."
4. "Bring the child into the clinic for a vaccine."

6. The nurse analyzes the laboratory values of a child with leukemia who is receiving chemotherapy. The nurse notes that the platelet count is 20,000/mm^3. On the basis of this laboratory result, which intervention will the nurse document in the plan of care?
1. Initiate protective isolation precautions
2. Monitor the temperature every 4 hours
3. Monitor closely for signs of infection
4. Use Toothettes for mouth care

7. A child with leukemia is complaining of nausea. A nurse suspects that the nausea is related to the chemotherapy. The nurse, concerned about the child's nutritional status, would most appropriately offer which of the following during this episode of nausea?
1. The child's favorite foods
2. Cool, clear liquids
3. Low-protein foods
4. Low-calorie foods

8. A 12-year-old child is seen in a clinic, and a diagnosis of Hodgkin's disease is suspected. Several diagnostic studies are performed to determine the presence of this disease. When evaluating the diagnostic results, a nurse would expect to note which of the following, if this child had Hodgkin's disease?
1. The presence of blast cells in the bone marrow
2. The presence of Reed-Sternberg cells in the lymph nodes
3. The presence of Epstein-Barr virus in the blood
4. Elevated vanillylmandelic acid (VMA) urinary levels

9. A nurse is performing an assessment on a 10-year-old child suspected of having Hodgkin's disease. The nurse understands that which data are most characteristic of this disease?
1. Painful, enlarged inguinal lymph nodes
2. Fever and malaise
3. Painless, firm, and movable adenopathy in the cervical area
4. Anorexia and weight loss

10. A pediatric nurse is assigned to care for a child with a diagnosis of Wilms' tumor. In planning care for the child, the nurse understands that this tumor is:
1. An abdominal tumor
2. A renal tumor
3. A brain tumor
4. A bone tumor

11. The mother of a 4-year-old child brings the child to a clinic and tells a pediatric nurse specialist that the child's abdomen seems to be very swollen. During further assessment of subjective data, the mother tells the nurse that the child is eating well and that the activity level of the child is unchanged. The nurse, suspecting the possibility of Wilms' tumor, would avoid which of the following during the physical assessment?
1. Palpating the abdomen for a mass
2. Assessing the urine for the presence of hematuria
3. Monitoring the temperature for the presence of fever
4. Monitoring the blood pressure for the presence of hypertension

12. A pediatric nurse specialist is providing a teaching session to the nursing staff regarding osteogenic sarcoma. Which of the following would not be a component of the information provided during this session?
1. The symptoms of the disease in the early stage

are almost always attributed to normal growing pains

2. The femur is the most common site of this sarcoma

3. Limping, if a weight-bearing limb is affected, is a clinical manifestation

4. The child does not experience pain at the primary tumor site

13. A nurse is caring for a child after surgical removal of a brain tumor. The nurse assesses the child for which of the following signs that would indicate that brainstem involvement occurred during the surgical procedure?

   1. Elevated temperature
   2. Orthostatic hypotension
   3. Inability to swallow
   4. Altered hearing ability

14. A nurse is monitoring a child for bleeding following surgery for removal of a brain tumor. The nurse checks the head dressing for the presence of blood and notes a colorless drainage on the back of the dressing. Which of the following would be the most appropriate nursing intervention?

   1. Circle the area of drainage and continue to monitor

   2. Reinforce the dressing
   3. Notify the physician
   4. Document the findings and continue to monitor

15. After surgical removal of a brain tumor, the physician writes an order to maintain the child in a flat position. In the postoperative period, a nurse is monitoring the child and notes that the child is restless, the pulse rate is elevated, and the blood pressure has dropped significantly from the baseline value. The nurse suspects that the child is in shock. Which of the following would be the most appropriate nursing action?

   1. Place the child in the Trendelenburg position
   2. Elevate the head of the bed
   3. Increase the IV fluids
   4. Notify the physician

CRITICAL THINKING: FREE-TEXT ENTRY

A pediatric nurse assists a physician in performing a lumbar puncture on a 3-year-old child with leukemia who is suspected of having central nervous system (CNS) metastasis. The nurse places the child in which position for this procedure?

Answer: _____

ANSWERS

1. **4**

Rationale: In leukemia, normal bone marrow is replaced by malignant blast cells. As the blast cells take over the bone marrow, eventually RBC and platelet production is affected and the child becomes anemic and thrombocytopenic. The Reed-Sternberg cell is found in Hodgkin's disease.

Test-Taking Strategy: Use the process of elimination. Note the key words "lack of understanding" in the stem of the question. Recalling that the Reed-Sternberg cell is found in Hodgkin's disease will easily direct you to option 4. Review the pathophysiology related to leukemia if you had difficulty with this question.

Level of Cognitive Ability: Analysis
Client Needs: Physiological Integrity
Integrated Concept/Process: Teaching/Learning
Content Area: Child Health
Reference: Ball, J., & Bindler, R. (1999). *Pediatric nursing: Caring for children* (2nd ed.). Stamford, Conn.: Appleton & Lange, p. 578.

2. **3**

Rationale: The confirmatory test for leukemia is microscopic examination of bone marrow obtained by bone marrow aspirate and biopsy. A lumbar puncture may be done to look for blast cells in the spinal fluid that are indicative of central nervous system disease. The WBC count may be normal, high, or low in leukemia. An altered platelet count occurs as a result of the disease, but may also occur as a result of chemotherapy, and does not confirm the diagnosis.

Test-Taking Strategy: Use the process of elimination. Note the key word "confirm" in the stem of the question. This key word and knowledge that the bone marrow is affected in leukemia will direct you to option 3. If you had difficulty with this question, review the significance of the bone marrow biopsy.

Level of Cognitive Ability: Analysis
Client Needs: Physiological Integrity
Integrated Concept/Process: Nursing Process/Assessment
Content Area: Child Health
Reference: Ball, J., & Bindler, R. (1999). *Pediatric nursing: Caring for children* (2nd ed.). Stamford, Conn.: Appleton & Lange, p. 578.

3. **2**

Rationale: The risk of injury to fragile mucous membranes is so great in the child with leukemia that only oral or axillary temperatures should be taken. Rectal abscesses can easily occur to damaged rectal tissue. No rectal temperatures should be taken. In addition, oral temperatures should be avoided if the child has oral ulcers. Options 1, 3, and 4 are appropriate measures to prevent infection.

Test-Taking Strategy: Use the process of elimination. Note the key words "a need for further education." Options 1 and 3 can be easily eliminated first. From the remaining options, note the word "rectal" in option 2. Recalling that rectal temperatures should be avoided will direct you to this option. Review home care instructions related to infection in the leukemic child if you had difficulty with this question.

Level of Cognitive Ability: Analysis
Client Needs: Health Promotion and Maintenance

Integrated Concept/Process: Teaching/Learning
Content Area: Child Health
Reference: Wong, D. (1999). *Whaley & Wong's nursing care of infants and children* (6th ed.). St. Louis: Mosby, p. 1730.

4. 2
Rationale: For the hospitalized neutropenic child, flowers or plants should not be kept in the room because standing water and damp soil harbor *Aspergillus* and *Pseudomonas*, to which these children are very susceptible. In addition, fruits and vegetables not peeled before being eaten harbor molds and should be avoided until the white blood cell count rises.
Test-Taking Strategy: Use the process of elimination. Note that options 1 and 3 are similar and should be eliminated first. From the remaining options, select option 2 over option 4 because this nursing response maintains the protective isolation procedures required. Review protective isolation procedures for the neutropenic child if you had difficulty with this question.
Level of Cognitive Ability: Application
Client Needs: Safe, Effective Care Environment
Integrated Concept/Process: Caring
Content Area: Child Health
Reference: Bowden, V., Dickey, S., & Greenberg, C. (1998). *Children and their families: The continuum of care.* Philadelphia: W.B. Saunders, p. 1602.

5. 4
Rationale: Immunocompromised children are unable to adequately fight varicella. Chickenpox can be deadly to the immunocompromised child. If an immunocompromised child who has not had chickenpox is exposed to someone with varicella, the child should receive varicella zoster immune globulin (VZIG) within 96 hours of exposure. Options 1, 2, and 3 are incorrect.
Test-Taking Strategy: Use the process of elimination. Note the key words "never had chickenpox" in the question. Recall that a child with leukemia is immunocompromised and is unable to fight infection. This should assist you in eliminating options 1, 2, and 3. Review protective procedures for the immunocompromised child if you had difficulty with this question.
Level of Cognitive Ability: Application
Client Needs: Health Promotion and Maintenance
Integrated Concept/Process: Nursing Process/Implementation
Content Area: Child Health
Reference: Wong, D. (1999). *Whaley & Wong's nursing care of infants and children* (6th ed.). St. Louis: Mosby, p. 731.

6. 4
Rationale: If a child is severely thrombocytopenic, and has a platelet count less than 20,000/mm^3, precautions need to be taken because of the increased risk of bleeding. The precautions include limiting activity that could result in head injury, using soft toothbrushes or Toothettes, checking urine and stools for blood, and administering stool softeners to prevent straining with constipation. In addition, suppositories and rectal temperatures are avoided. Options 1, 2, and 3 are related to the prevention of infection rather than bleeding.
Test-Taking Strategy: Use the process of elimination. Noting that the platelet count is low, and that a low platelet count places the child at risk for bleeding, will assist in directing you to option 4. In addition, note that options 1, 2, and 3 are

similar because they all relate to prevention of and monitoring for infection.
Level of Cognitive Ability: Analysis
Client Needs: Safe, Effective Care Environment
Integrated Concept/Process: Communication and Documentation
Content Area: Child Health
Reference: Wong, D. (1999). *Whaley & Wong's nursing care of infants and children* (6th ed.). St. Louis: Mosby, p. 1719.

7. 2
Rationale: When the child is nauseated, it is best to offer cool, clear liquids because they are soothing and better tolerated. It is best not to offer favorite foods when the child is nauseated because foods eaten during times of nausea will be associated with being sick. Supportive nutritional measures should also include oral supplements with high-protein and high-calorie foods.
Test-Taking Strategy: The issue of the question relates to the nutritional status in a child with nausea. Focusing on this issue will assist in eliminating options 3 and 4. From the remaining options, you may be tempted to select option 1. Remember that it is best not to offer favorite foods when the child is nauseated because foods eaten during times of nausea will be associated with being sick. Review these interventions related to nutrition if you had difficulty with this question.
Level of Cognitive Ability: Analysis
Client Needs: Physiological Integrity
Integrated Concept/Process: Nursing Process/Implementation
Content Area: Child Health
Reference: Wong, D. (1999). *Whaley & Wong's nursing care of infants and children* (6th ed.). St. Louis: Mosby, p. 1721.

8. 2
Rationale: Hodgkin's disease is a neoplasm of lymphatic tissue. The presence of giant, multinucleated cells (Reed-Sternberg cells) is the hallmark of this disease. The presence of blast cells in the bone marrow is indicative of leukemia. The Epstein-Barr virus is associated with infectious mononucleosis. Elevated VMA urinary levels may be found in children with neuroblastoma.
Test-Taking Strategy: Use the process of elimination. Recalling that the Reed-Sternberg cell is characteristic of Hodgkin's disease will easily direct you to option 2. Review the clinical manifestations associated with Hodgkin's disease if you had difficulty with this question.
Level of Cognitive Ability: Analysis
Client Needs: Physiological Integrity
Integrated Concept/Process: Nursing Process/Assessment
Content Area: Child Health
Reference: Wong, D. (1999). *Whaley & Wong's nursing care of infants and children* (6th ed.). St. Louis: Mosby, pp. 1737-1738.

9. 3
Rationale: Clinical manifestations specifically associated with Hodgkin's disease include painless, firm, and movable adenopathy in the cervical and supraclavicular area. Hepatosplenomegaly is also noted. Although fever, malaise, anorexia, and weight loss are associated with Hodgkin's disease, these manifestations are seen in many disorders.
Test-Taking Strategy: Use the process of elimination. Note the key words "most characteristic" in the stem of the question. Eliminate options 2 and 4 first because these symptoms are

general and vague. Recalling that painless adenopathy is associated with Hodgkin's disease will direct you to option 3. Review the clinical manifestations related to Hodgkin's disease if you had difficulty with this question.
Level of Cognitive Ability: Analysis
Client Needs: Physiological Integrity
Integrated Concept/Process: Nursing Process/Assessment
Content Area: Child Health
Reference: Wong, D. (1999). *Whaley & Wong's nursing care of infants and children* (6th ed.). St. Louis: Mosby, p. 1737.

10. 2
Rationale: Wilms' tumor, or nephroblastoma, is the most common renal tumor in children. Arising from the renal parenchyma of the kidney, this tumor grows very rapidly. It may be present unilaterally and localized or bilaterally, sometimes with metastasis to other organs. Options 1, 3, and 4 are incorrect.
Test-Taking Strategy: Knowledge regarding the location of Wilms' tumor is required to answer this question. If you are unfamiliar with this type of tumor, review this content
Level of Cognitive Ability: Application
Client Needs: Physiological Integrity
Integrated Concept/Process: Nursing Process/Planning
Content Area: Child Health
Reference: Ball, J., & Bindler, R. (1999). *Pediatric nursing: Caring for children* (2nd ed.). Stamford, Conn.: Appleton & Lange, p. 572.

11. 1
Rationale: If Wilms' tumor is suspected, the tumor mass should not be palpated by the nurse. Excessive manipulation can cause seeding of the tumor and spread of the cancerous cells. Fever, hematuria, and hypertension are clinical manifestations associated with Wilms' tumor.
Test-Taking Strategy: Use the process of elimination. Note the key word "avoid." Knowledge that this tumor is located in the kidney will assist in eliminating options 2, 3, and 4 because of the relationship of these options to renal function. Review the significant assessment procedures in the child with Wilms' tumor if you had difficulty with this question.
Level of Cognitive Ability: Application
Client Needs: Physiological Integrity
Integrated Concept/Process: Nursing Process/Assessment
Content Area: Child Health
Reference: Ball, J., & Bindler, R. (1999). *Pediatric nursing: Caring for children* (2nd ed.). Stamford, Conn.: Appleton & Lange, p. 574.

12. 4
Rationale: A clinical manifestation of osteogenic sarcoma is progressive, insidious, and intermittent pain at the tumor site. By the time these children receive medical attention, they may be in considerable pain from the tumor. Options 1, 2, and 3 are accurate regarding osteogenic sarcoma.
Test-Taking Strategy: Use the process of elimination. Note the key word "not" in the stem of the question. Knowledge that osteogenic sarcoma is a malignant tumor of the bone will easily direct you to option 4. Review the clinical manifestations associated with osteogenic sarcoma if you had difficulty with this question.
Level of Cognitive Ability: Application
Client Needs: Physiological Integrity

Integrated Concept/Process: Teaching/Learning
Content Area: Child Health
Reference: Ball, J., & Bindler, R. (1999). *Pediatric nursing: Caring for children* (2nd ed.). Stamford, Conn.: Appleton & Lange, p. 575.

13. 1
Rationale: Vital signs and neurological status are assessed frequently. Special attention is paid to the child's temperature, which may be elevated because of hypothalamus or brainstem involvement during surgery. A cooling blanket should either be in place on the bed or readily available if the child becomes hyperthermic. Options 3 and 4 are related to functional deficits following surgery. An elevated blood pressure and a widened pulse pressure may be associated with increased intracranial pressure.
Test-Taking Strategy: Use the process of elimination. Recalling the functions of the hypothalamus and the brainstem will easily direct you to option 1. If you had difficulty with this question, review the complications that can occur following surgical removal of a brain tumor.
Level of Cognitive Ability: Analysis
Client Needs: Physiological Integrity
Integrated Concept/Process: Nursing Process/Assessment
Content Area: Child Health
Reference: Wong, D. (1999). *Whaley & Wong's nursing care of infants and children* (6th ed.). St. Louis: Mosby, p. 1744.

14. 3
Rationale: Colorless drainage on the dressing would indicate the presence of cerebrospinal fluid and should be reported to the physician immediately. Options 1, 2, and 4 are inaccurate nursing interventions.
Test-Taking Strategy: Use the process of elimination. Eliminate options 1 and 4 first because they are similar. Note the key words "colorless drainage." This should quickly alert you to the possibility of the presence of cerebrospinal fluid and direct you to option 3. If you had difficulty with this question, review the significance of the presence of colorless drainage following cranial surgery.
Level of Cognitive Ability: Analysis
Client Needs: Physiological Integrity
Integrated Concept/Process: Nursing Process/Implementation
Content Area: Child Health
Reference: Wong, D. (1999). *Whaley & Wong's nursing care of infants and children* (6th ed.). St. Louis: Mosby, p. 1744.

15. 4
Rationale: The child is never placed in the Trendelenburg position because it increases intracranial pressure (ICP) and the risk of bleeding. In the event of shock, the physician is notified immediately before changing the child's position or increasing IV fluids. Increasing IV fluids can cause an increase in ICP.
Test-Taking Strategy: Recall the complications associated with cranial surgery to answer this question. Eliminate option 1 because this position increases ICP. Eliminate option 2 because this intervention will not assist in alleviating shock. In fact, this action could cause harm to the child. Eliminate option 3 because this action could increase ICP. In addition, the nurse should not increase IV fluids without a physician's order. Review care to the client after surgical removal of a brain tumor if you had difficulty with this question.

Level of Cognitive Ability: Application
Client Needs: Physiological Integrity
Integrated Concept/Process: Nursing Process/Implementation
Content Area: Child Health
Reference: Wong, D. (1999). *Whaley & Wong's nursing care of infants and children* (6th ed.). St. Louis: Mosby, p. 1744.

CRITICAL THINKING: FREE-TEXT ENTRY

Answer: Lateral recumbent with the knees flexed to the abdomen and the head bent with the chin resting on the chest
Rationale: This position separates the spinal processes and facilitates needle insertion into the subarachnoid space.

Test-Taking Strategy: Note the key word "lumbar" in the question. Visualize the position needed to access the subarachnoid space to obtain cerebrospinal fluid. Review this procedure if you are unfamiliar with it.
Level of Cognitive Ability: Application
Client Needs: Physiological Integrity
Integrated Concept/Process: Nursing Process/Implementation
Content Area: Child Health
Reference: Altman, G., Buchsel, P., & Coxon, V. (2000). *Delmar's fundamental & advanced nursing skills.* Albany, N.Y.: Delmar, p. 1345.

REFERENCES

Altman, G., Buchsel, P., & Coxon, V. (2000). *Delmar's fundamental & advanced nursing skills.* Albany, N.Y.: Delmar.

Ball, J., & Bindler, R. (1999). *Pediatric nursing: Caring for children* (2nd ed.). Stamford, Conn.: Appleton & Lange.

Bowden, V., Dickey, S., & Greenberg, C. (1998). *Children and their families: The continuum of care.* Philadelphia: W.B. Saunders.

Web site: www.braintumor.org.

Web site: www.cancer.org.

Wong, D. (1999). *Whaley & Wong's nursing care of infants and children* (6th ed.). St. Louis: Mosby.

Infectious and Communicable Diseases

I. RUBEOLA (MEASLES)
A. Description
1. Agent: Virus
2. Incubation period: 10 to 20 days
3. Communicable period: From 4 days before to 5 days after the rash appears; mainly during prodromal (catarrhal) stage
4. Source: Respiratory tract secretions, blood, or urine of infected person
5. Transmission: Airborne or direct contact with infectious droplets
B. Assessment
1. Fever
2. Malaise
3. Coryza and cough
4. Rash appears as red, discrete maculopapules that blanch easily with pressure and gradually turn a brownish color (lasts 6 to 7 days); rash begins behind the ears and spreads downward to the feet
5. Koplik spots: small, red spots with a bluish white center and a red base; located on the mucosa and last 3 days
C. Implementation
1. Respiratory precautions if the child is hospitalized
2. Restrict to quiet activities and bed rest
3. Use a cool mist vaporizer for cough and coryza
4. Dim lights if photophobia is present
5. Administer antipyretics for fever

II. ROSEOLA (EXANTHEMA SUBITUM)
A. Description
1. Agent: Human herpesvirus type 6 (HHV-6)
2. Incubation period: 5 to 15 days
3. Communicable period: Unknown but thought to extend from the febrile stage to the time the rash first appears
4. Source: Unknown
5. Transmission: Unknown
B. Assessment
1. Fever for 3 to 5 days followed by a rash (rose-pink maculas that blanch with pressure)
2. The rash appears 2 to 3 days after the onset of fever and lasts 1 to 2 days
C. Implementation: Supportive

III. RUBELLA (GERMAN MEASLES)
A. Description
1. Agent: Rubella virus
2. Incubation period: 14 to 21 days
3. Communicable period: 7 days before to approximately 5 days after the rash appears
4. Source: Nasopharyngeal secretions; virus is also present in blood, stool, and urine
5. Transmission
   a. Airborne or direct contact with infectious droplets
   b. Indirectly via articles freshly contaminated with nasopharyngeal secretions, feces, or urine
   c. Transplacental
B. Assessment
1. Low-grade fever
2. Malaise
3. Pinkish red maculopapular rash that begins on the face and spreads to the entire body
4. Petechial spots may occur on the soft palate
C. Implementation
1. Supportive treatment
2. Isolate the infected child from pregnant women

IV. MUMPS
A. Description
1. Agent: Paramyxovirus
2. Incubation period: 14 to 21 days

3. Communicable period: Immediately before and after the swelling begins
4. Source: Saliva of infected person and possibly urine
5. Transmission
   a. Direct contact with infected person
   b. Droplet spread from infected person
B. Assessment
   1. Fever
   2. Headache and malaise
   3. Anorexia
   4. Earache aggravated by chewing, followed by parotid glandular swelling
C. Implementation
   1. Respiratory precautions
   2. Bed rest until the parotid glandular swelling subsides
   3. Avoid foods that require chewing
   4. Apply hot or cold compresses as prescribed to the neck
   5. To relieve orchitis, apply warmth and local support with tight-fitting underpants

V. CHICKENPOX (VARICELLA)
A. Description
   1. Agent: Varicella zoster virus (VZV)
   2. Incubation period: 13 to 17 days
   3. Communicable period: 1 to 2 days before the onset of the rash to 6 days after the first crop of vesicles, when crusts have formed
   4. Source: Respiratory tract secretions of infected person; skin lesions
   5. Transmission: Direct contact, droplet (airborne) spread, and contaminated objects
B. Assessment
   1. Slight fever, malaise, and anorexia followed by a macular rash that first appears on the trunk and scalp and moves to the extremities
   2. Lesions become pustules, begin to dry, and develop a crust
   3. Lesions may appear on the mucous membranes of the mouth, the genital area, and the rectal area
C. Implementation
   1. In the hospital setting, strict isolation
   2. In the home setting, isolate the infected child until the vesicles have dried; isolate high-risk children from the infected child

VI. PERTUSSIS (WHOOPING COUGH)
A. Description
   1. Agent: *Bordetella pertussis*
   2. Incubation period: 5 to 21 days (usually 10 days)
   3. Communicable period: Greatest during the catarrhal stage
   4. Source: Discharge from the respiratory tract of the infected person
   5. Transmission: Direct contact or droplet spread

from infected person; indirect contact with freshly contaminated articles
B. Assessment: Symptoms of respiratory infection followed by increased severity of cough
C. Implementation
   1. Isolation during the catarrhal stage; if the child is hospitalized, institute respiratory precautions
   2. Administer antimicrobial therapy as prescribed
   3. Administer pertussis immune globulin as prescribed
   4. Reduce environmental factors that promote paroxysms of coughing, such as dust, smoke, and sudden changes in temperature
   5. Encourage fluid intake
   6. Provide high humidity with the use of a humidifier or tent

VII. DIPHTHERIA
A. Description
   1. Agent: *Corynebacterium diphtheriae*
   2. Incubation period: 2 to 5 days
   3. Communicable period: Variable; until virulent bacilli are no longer present (three negative cultures), usually 2 weeks but as long as 4 weeks
   4. Source: Discharge from the mucous membrane of the nose and nasopharynx, skin, and other lesions of the infected person
   5. Transmission: Direct contact with infected person, carrier, or contaminated articles
B. Assessment
   1. Low-grade fever, malaise, sore throat
   2. Foul-smelling, mucopurulent nasal discharge
   3. Gray membrane on the tonsils and pharynx
   4. Lymphadenitis (neck edema)
C. Implementation
   1. Strict isolation of the hospitalized child
   2. Administer antitoxin as prescribed (preceded by a skin or conjunctival test to rule out sensitivity to horse serum)
   3. Bed rest
   4. Administer antibiotics as prescribed

VIII. POLIOMYELITIS
A. Description
   1. Agent: Enteroviruses
   2. Incubation period: 7 to 14 days
   3. Communicable period: Not exactly known; the virus is present in the throat and feces shortly after infection and persists for approximately 1 week in the throat and 4 to 6 weeks in the feces
   4. Source: Oropharyngeal secretions and feces of the infected person
   5. Transmission: Direct contact with infected person; fecal-oral and oropharyngeal routes
B. Assessment
   1. Fever, malaise, anorexia, nausea, headache, sore throat

2. Abdominal pain followed by soreness and stiffness of the trunk, neck, and limbs that progresses to flaccid paralysis

C. Implementation
   1. Enteric precautions
   2. Supportive treatment
   3. Bed rest
   4. Monitor for respiratory paralysis
   5. Physical therapy

IX. SCARLET FEVER

A. Description
   1. Agent: Group A, beta-hemolytic streptococci
   2. Incubation period: 1 to 7 days
   3. Communicable period: During the incubation period and clinical illness, approximately 10 days; during the first 2 weeks of the carrier stage, although may persist for months
   4. Source: Nasopharyngeal secretions of infected person and carriers
   5. Transmission: Direct contact with infected person or droplet spread; indirectly by contact with contaminated articles, ingestion of contaminated milk, or other foods

B. Assessment
   1. Abrupt high fever, vomiting, headache, malaise, abdominal pain
   2. A red, fine papular rash in the axilla, groin, and neck that spreads to cover the entire body
   3. The rash blanches with pressure except in areas of deep creases and folds of the joints (Pastia's sign)
   4. The tongue is coated and papillae become red and swollen (white strawberry tongue); by the fourth to fifth day the white coat sloughs off, leaving prominent papillae (red strawberry tongue)
   5. Tonsils are edematous and covered with a gray-white exudate
   6. Pharynx is edematous and beefy red

C. Implementation
   1. Respiratory precautions until 24 hours after the initiation of treatment
   2. Supportive therapy
   3. Bed rest
   4. Encourage fluid intake
   5. Administer antibiotics as prescribed

X. ERYTHEMA INFECTIOSUM (FIFTH DISEASE)

A. Description
   1. Agent: Human parvovirus B19 (HPV)
   2. Incubation period: 4 to 14 days; may be as long as 20 days
   3. Communicable period: Uncertain but before the onset of symptoms in most children
   4. Source: Infected person
   5. Transmission: Unknown; possibly respiratory secretions and blood

B. Assessment
   1. Fever, myalgia, lethargy, nausea, vomiting, abdominal pain
   2. Stages of the rash
      a. Erythema of the face (slapped face appearance), chiefly on the cheeks; disappears by 1 to 4 days
      b. Approximately 1 day after the rash appears on the face, maculopapular red spots appear, symmetrically distributed in the extremities; rash progresses from proximal to distal surfaces and may last a week or more
      c. Rash subsides but may reappear if the skin becomes irritated or traumatized by such factors as the sun, heat, cold, or friction

C. Implementation
   1. Respiratory isolation of the hospitalized child
   2. Pregnant women should not be in contact with or care for the infected person
   3. Supportive
   4. Administer antipyretics, analgesics, and antiinflammatory medications as prescribed

XI. INFECTIOUS MONONUCLEOSIS

A. Description
   1. Agent: Epstein-Barr (EB) virus
   2. Incubation period: 4 to 6 weeks
   3. Communicable period: Unknown; the virus is shed before the onset of the disease until 6 months or longer after recovery
   4. Source: Oral secretions
   5. Transmission: Direct intimate contact, infected blood

B. Assessment
   1. Fever, sore throat, malaise, headache, fatigue, nausea, abdominal pain
   2. Lymphadenopathy and hepatosplenomegaly

C. Implementation
   1. Supportive
   2. Monitor for signs of splenic rupture, which include abdominal pain, left upper quadrant pain, or left shoulder pain

XII. ROCKY MOUNTAIN SPOTTED FEVER

A. Description
   1. Agent: *Rickettsia rickettsii*
   2. Incubation period: 2 to 14 days
   3. Source: Tick; mammal source: wild rodents, dogs
   4. Transmission: Bite of infected tick

B. Assessment
   1. Fever, malaise, anorexia, vomiting, headache, myalgia
   2. Maculopapular or petechial rash primarily on the extremities (ankles and wrists) but may spread to other areas, characteristically on the palms and soles

C. Implementation
   1. Vigorous supportive care

2. Administer antibiotics as prescribed
3. Teaching regarding protection from tick bites

XIII. ENTEROBIASIS (PINWORM)

A. Description
   1. Agent: *Enterobius vermicularis*
   2. Source
      a. Universally present in temperate climatic zones
      b. Eggs are ingested or inhaled (eggs float in the air), hatch in the upper intestine, mature in 2 to 8 weeks, and migrate to the cecal area; females then mate, migrate out the anus, and lay eggs
   3. Transmission
      a. Favored in crowded conditions
      b. Ingestion or inhalation of eggs
      c. Hands to mouth or fecal-oral route
      d. Contaminated items (pinworm eggs persist in the environment for 2 to 3 weeks)
B. Assessment: Intense perianal itching, irritability, restlessness, poor sleep, bed-wetting, distractibility, short attention span; in females, the worm may migrate to the vagina and urethra and cause infection
C. Implementation
   1. Identify the worms
      a. Use of a flashlight to inspect the anal area 2 to 3 hours after the child is asleep
      b. Tape test: Transparent, sticky tape is used to obtain a specimen from the child's perianal area; specimen is collected in the morning as soon as the child awakens and before a bowel movement or a bath
   2. Enteric precautions
   3. Anthelmintic medications (all household members are treated); course of medication is repeated in 2 weeks following the first course, to prevent reinfection
   4. Teach home care measures to prevent reinfection

XIV. IMMUNIZATIONS

A. Immunization schedule (Box 45-1)
▲ B. General contraindications to immunizations
   1. Severe febrile illness
   2. Live virus vaccines are generally not administered to anyone with an altered immune system
   3. Allergic reaction to a previously administered vaccine or a substance in the vaccine
C. Hepatitis B vaccine
   1. Protects against hepatitis B
   2. The first dose of hepatitis B is administered between the ages of birth and 2 months, the second dose is administered between the ages of 1 and 4 months, and the third dose is administered between the ages of 6 to 18 months
   3. All children from birth through 18 years of age

BOX 45-1	
Recommended Immunization Schedule for Healthy Infants and Children	
Birth	Hepatitis B
1 month	Hepatitis B
2 months	IPV, DTaP, Hib
4 months	DTaP, Hib, IPV
6 months	DTaP, Hib, hepatitis B, IPV
12-15 months	Hib, MMR
12-18 months	DtaP, varicella zoster
4-6 years	DTaP, IPV, MMR
11-12 years	MMR (if not administered at 4-6 years)
11-16 years	Td

need three doses of hepatitis B vaccine if they have not already received them
   4. Contraindication: Anaphylactic reaction to common baker's yeast
D. DTaP (diphtheria, tetanus, acellular pertussis) and Td
   1. Protects against diphtheria, tetanus, and pertussis
   2. DTaP is administered at 2 months, 4 months, 6 months, between 15 and 18 months of age, and between 4 and 6 years of age
   3. The fourth dose of DTaP can be given at 12 months of age if 6 months have elapsed since the previous dose and if the child might not return for follow-up by 18 months of age
   4. Td (tetanus, diphtheria booster) is given at 11 to 12 years of age if at least 5 years have passed since the last dose of DTaP/DTP (DTP = diphtheria, tetanus, pertussis)
   5. Contraindication: Encephalopathy within 7 days of administration of previous dose of DTP
E. Hib (*Haemophilus influenzae* type b) vaccine
   1. Protects against *Haemophilus influenzae* type b
   2. Hib is administered at 2 months, 4 months, 6 months, and between 12 and 15 months of age
   3. Depending on the brand of Hib vaccine used for the first and second doses, a dose at 6 months of age may not be needed
   4. Contraindication: None identified
F. IPV (inactivated poliovirus vaccine)
   1. Protects against polio
   2. IPV is administered at 2 months, 4 months, 6 months, and between 4 and 6 years of age
   3. The third dose of IPV is administered between 6 and 18 months of age
   4. Contraindication: Anaphylactic reaction to neomycin or streptomycin
G. MMR (measles, mumps, rubella)
   1. Protects against measles, mumps, and rubella (German measles)
   2. The first dose of MMR is administered between

12 and 15 months of age; the second dose is administered at 4 to 6 years of age (if the second dose was not given by 4 to 6 years of age, it should be given at the next visit)

3. MMR contains minute amounts of neomycin; measles and mumps vaccines, which are grown on chick embryo tissue cultures, are not believed to contain significant amounts of egg cross-reacting proteins
4. Contraindications
   a. Pregnancy
   b. Known altered immunodeficiency
   c. Allergy to contents of immunization (prior to the administration of MMR vaccine, assess for a known history of allergy to neomycin or related antibiotics)
   d. Presence of recently acquired passive immunity through blood transfusions, immunoglobulin, or maternal antibodies (MMR should be postponed for a minimum of 3 months after passive immunization with immunoglobulins or blood transfusions, except washed blood cells, which do not interfere with the immune response)

H. Varicella zoster vaccine
   1. Protects against chickenpox
   2. Varicella zoster vaccine is administered between 12 and 18 months of age
   3. Susceptible children 13 years of age and older (who have not had chickenpox or have not been previously vaccinated) need two doses given 4 to 8 weeks apart
   4. Contraindications
      a. Pregnancy
      b. Immunocompromised individuals
      c. Children receiving corticosteroids

I. OPV (oral poliovirus vaccine)
   1. No longer recommended for routine vaccination
   2. Not administered to anyone with an altered immune system or to any household contacts of an immunosuppressed child (the virus multiplies in the gastrointestinal tract and is excreted in the stool)

PRACTICE QUESTIONS

1. A child with rubeola (measles) is being admitted to the hospital. In preparing for the admission of the child, a nurse plans to place the child on which precautions?
   1. Contact
   2. Enteric
   3. Respiratory
   4. Protective

2. Several children have contracted rubeola (measles) in a local school. The school nurse conducts a teaching session for the mothers of the school children. Which statement made by a mother indicates a need for further teaching regarding this communicable disease?
   1. "Respiratory symptoms such as a profuse runny nose, cough, and fever occur prior to the development of a rash."
   2. "Small blue-white spots with a red base may appear in the mouth."
   3. "The rash usually begins behind the ears and spreads downward toward the feet."
   4. "The communicable period ranges from 10 days before the onset of symptoms to 15 days after the rash appears."

3. The mother of a 15-month-old child brings the child to a clinic and reports that the child has a fever and has developed a rash on the neck and trunk. Roseola is diagnosed. The mother is concerned that her other children will contract the disease. A nurse provides which of the following instructions to the mother regarding the prevention of transmission of the disease?
   1. The disease is transmitted through the urine and feces, so the other children should use a separate bathroom
   2. Disease transmission is unknown
   3. The disease is transmitted through the respiratory tract, so the child should be isolated from the other children as much as possible
   4. The disease is transmitted by contact with body fluids, so any items contaminated with body fluids need to discarded in a separate receptacle

4. A nurse provides instructions to the mother of a child with mumps regarding respiratory precautions. The mother asks the nurse about the length of time required for the respiratory precautions. The nurse most appropriately responds:
   1. "Respiratory isolation in not necessary."
   2. "Mumps is not transmitted by the respiratory system."
   3. "Respiratory precautions are indicated during the period of communicability."
   4. "Respiratory precautions are indicated for 18 days following the onset of parotid swelling."

5. A mother brings her 6-year-old child to the clinic because the child has developed a rash on the trunk and on the scalp. The mother reports that the child has had a low-grade temperature, has not felt like eating, and has been generally tired. The child is diagnosed with chickenpox. The mother inquires about the communicable period associated with chickenpox. A nurse plans to base the response on which of the following?
   1. The communicable period is unknown
   2. The communicable period is 1 to 2 days before the onset of the rash to 6 days after the first crop of vessicles, when crusts have formed
   3. The communicable period is 10 days before the onset of symptoms to 15 days after the rash appears

    4. The communicable period ranges from 2 weeks or less to several months

6. A nurse provides home care instructions to the parents of a child hospitalized with pertussis. The child is in the convalescent stage and is being prepared for discharge. Which of the following will not be included in the teaching plan?
   1. Maintain respiratory precautions and a quiet environment for at least 2 weeks
   2. Coughing spells may be triggered by dust or smoke
   3. Encourage fluid intake
   4. Good handwashing techniques must be instituted to prevent spreading the disease to others

7. A 6-month-old infant receives a DTaP (diphtheria, tetanus, and acellular pertussis) immunization at a well baby clinic. The mother returns home and calls the clinic to report that the infant has developed swelling and redness at the site of injection. The nurse tells the mother to:
   1. Apply a warm pack to the injection site
   2. Bring the infant back to the clinic
   3. Apply an ice pack to the injection site
   4. Monitor the infant for a fever

8. A child diagnosed with scarlet fever is being cared for at home. A home health nurse performs an assessment on the child, knowing that which of the following is not a clinical manifestation associated with this disease?
   1. Pastia's sign
   2. White strawberry tongue
   3. Edematous and beefy-red pharynx
   4. Koplik spots

9. A home health nurse visits a child with infectious mononucleosis and provides home care instructions to the parents about the care of the child. The nurse tells the parents to:
   1. Maintain the child on bed rest for 2 weeks
   2. Maintain respiratory precautions for 1 week
   3. Notify the physician if the child develops a fever
   4. Notify the physician if the child develops abdominal pain or left shoulder pain occurs

10. The mother of a preschooler who attends day care calls a clinic nurse and tells the nurse that the child is constantly itching the perianal area and that the area is irritated. The nurse suspects the possibility of pinworm infection (enterobiasis). The nurse instructs the mother to obtain a tape test rectal specimen. The nurse tells the mother to obtain the specimen:
    1. When the child is put to bed
    2. After toileting
    3. After bathing
    4. In the morning when the child awakens

11. A nursing student is assigned to administer immunizations to children in a clinic. The nursing instructor asks the student about the contraindications to receiving an immunization. The student responds correctly by telling the instructor that a contraindication to receiving an immunization is if a child has:
    1. A cold
    2. Otitis media
    3. Mild diarrhea
    4. A severe febrile illness

12. A mother brings her 4-month-old infant to a well baby clinic for immunizations. A nurse would prepare to administer which of the following immunizations to this infant?
    1. DTaP (diphtheria, tetanus, acellular pertussis), MMR (measles, mumps, rubella), IPV (inactivated poliovirus vaccine)
    2. MMR, Hib (*Haemophilus influenzae* type b), DTaP
    3. DTaP, Hib, IPV
    4. Varicella and hepatitis B vaccines

13. A clinic nurse prepares to administer an MMR (measles, mumps, rubella) vaccine to a 5-year-old child. The nurse administers this vaccine:
    1. Intramuscularly in the anterolateral aspect of the thigh
    2. Intramuscularly in the deltoid muscle
    3. Subcutaneously in the outer aspect of the upper arm
    4. Subcutaneously in the gluteal muscle

14. A child is scheduled to receive an MMR (measles, mumps, rubella) vaccine. The nurse preparing to administer the vaccine reviews the child's record and questions the order if which of the following is documented in the child's record?
    1. A local reaction at the site of injection of a previous MMR vaccine
    2. A history of an anaphylactic reaction to neomycin
    3. A history of frequent respiratory infections
    4. Recent recovery from a cold

15. A 15-year-old child is scheduled to receive a series of the hepatitis B vaccine. The child arrives at a clinic for the first dose. Before administering the vaccine, a nurse performs an assessment on the child and asks the child about a history of an allergy to:
    1. Baker's yeast
    2. Eggs
    3. Penicillin
    4. Sulfonamides

CRITICAL THINKING: FREE-TEXT ENTRY

A nurse is preparing to care for a child with rubella (German measles) and anticipates contact with infectious material during care. The nurse enters the supply closet where the masks, gloves, gowns, and goggles are kept. Which item(s) does the nurse obtain to care for this child?

Answer: _____

ANSWERS

1. 3

Rationale: Rubeola is transmitted via airborne particles or direct contact with infectious droplets. Respiratory precautions are required, and a mask is worn by those in contact with the child. Gowns and gloves are not indicated. Articles that are contaminated should be bagged and labeled. Options 1, 2, and 4 are not indicated in rubeola.

Test-Taking Strategy: Use the process of elimination. Recalling that rubeola is transmitted via the airborne route will easily direct you to option 3. Review the route of transmission and therapeutic management of rubeola if you had difficulty with this question.

Level of Cognitive Ability: Application
Client Needs: Safe, Effective Care Environment
Integrated Concept/Process: Nursing Process/Planning
Content Area: Child Health
Reference: Ball, J., & Bindler, R. (1999). *Pediatric nursing: Caring for children* (2nd ed.). Stamford, Conn.: Appleton & Lange, p. 388.

2. 4

Rationale: The communicable period for rubeola ranges from 4 days before to 5 days after the rash appears, mainly during the prodromal (catarrhal) stage. Options 1, 2, and 3 are accurate descriptions of rubeola. The small blue-white spots found in this communicable disease are called Koplik spots. Option 4, the incorrect option, describes the incubation period for rubella, not rubeola.

Test-Taking Strategy: Note the key words "need for further teaching" in the stem of the question. Recalling that the communicable period for rubeola ranges from 4 days before to 5 days after the rash appears will direct you to option 4. Review the clinical manifestations associated with rubeola if you had difficulty with this question.

Level of Cognitive Ability: Analysis
Client Needs: Health Promotion and Maintenance
Integrated Concept/Process: Teaching/Learning
Content Area: Child Health
Reference: Wong, D. (1999). *Whaley & Wong's nursing care of infants and children* (6th ed.). St. Louis: Mosby, p. 726.

3. 2

Rationale: The method of transmission of roseola is unknown. Options 1, 3, and 4 are not accurate transmission routes of roseola.

Test-Taking Strategy: Use the process of elimination. Eliminate options 1 and 4 first because they are similar. From the remaining options, recall that the method of transmission of roseola is unknown. Review the characteristics of roseola if you had difficulty with this question.

Level of Cognitive Ability: Application
Client Needs: Health Promotion and Maintenance
Integrated Concept/Process: Teaching/Learning
Content Area: Child Health
Reference: Ball, J., & Bindler, R. (1999). *Pediatric nursing: Caring for children* (2nd ed.). Stamford, Conn.: Appleton & Lange, p. 395.

4. 3

Rationale: Mumps is transmitted via direct contact with or droplet spread from an infected person and possibly by contact with the urine. Respiratory precautions are indicated during the period of communicability.

Test-Taking Strategy: Use the process of elimination. Options 1 and 2 can be eliminated first because they are similar. From the remaining options, select option 3 because it is the global option and addresses communicability. Also, the time frame indicated in option 4 seems rather lengthy. Review the infectious period related to mumps if you had difficulty with this question.

Level of Cognitive Ability: Application
Client Needs: Safe, Effective Care Environment
Integrated Concept/Process: Teaching/Learning
Content Area: Child Health
Reference: Ball, J., & Bindler, R. (1999). *Pediatric nursing: Caring for children* (2nd ed.). Stamford, Conn.: Appleton & Lange, p. 390.

5. 2

Rationale: The communicable period for chickenpox is 1 to 2 days before the onset of the rash to 6 days after the first crop of vessicles, when crusts have formed. In roseola, the communicable period is unknown. Option 3 describes rubella. Option 4 describes diphtheria.

Test-Taking Strategy: Use the process of elimination. Option 1 can be easily eliminated. Eliminate options 3 and 4 next because the time frames in these two options seem rather lengthy and are similar. If you had difficulty with this question, review the communicable period for chickenpox.

Level of Cognitive Ability: Analysis
Client Needs: Safe, Effective Care Environment
Integrated Concept/Process: Teaching/Learning
Content Area: Child Health
Reference: Wong, D. (1999). *Whaley & Wong's nursing care of infants and children* (6th ed.). St. Louis: Mosby, p. 722.

6. 1

Rationale: Pertussis is transmitted by direct contact or respiratory droplets from coughing. The communicable period occurs primarily during the catarrhal stage. Respiratory precautions are not required during the convalescent phase. Options 2, 3, and 4 are components of home care instructions.

Test-Taking Strategy: Use the process of elimination. Note the key words "convalescent" in the question and "not" in the stem of the question. Options 3 and 4 can be easily eliminated because they are general interventions associated with convalescence. Knowing that coughing spells are associated with pertussis will assist in directing you to option 1. In addition, 2 weeks of respiratory precautions is not required. If you had difficulty with this question, review home care instructions for the child with pertussis.

Level of Cognitive Ability: Application
Client Needs: Health Promotion and Maintenance
Integrated Concept/Process: Teaching/Learning
Content Area: Child Health
Reference: Ball, J., & Bindler, R. (1999). *Pediatric nursing: Caring for children* (2nd ed.). Stamford, Conn.: Appleton & Lange, p. 391.

7. 3

Rationale: Occasionally, tenderness, redness, or swelling may occur at the site of the injection. This can be relieved with ice packs for the first 24 hours, followed by warm compresses if the inflammation persists. It is not necessary to bring the infant back to the clinic. Option 4 may be an appropriate intervention but is not specific to the issue of the question.

Test-Taking Strategy: Use the process of elimination. Option 4 can be eliminated first because it does not relate specifically to the issue of the question. Eliminate option 2 next as an unnecessary intervention. From the remaining options, general principles related to the effects of heat and cold will easily direct you to option 3. Review interventions following immunizations and injections if you had difficulty with this question.
Level of Cognitive Ability: Application
Client Needs: Health Promotion and Maintenance
Integrated Concept/Process: Nursing Process/Implementation
Content Area: Child Health
Reference: Bowden, V., Dickey, S., & Greenberg, C. (1998). *Children and their families: The continuum of care.* Philadelphia: W.B. Saunders, p. 341.

8. 4
Rationale: Pastia's sign describes a rash seen in scarlet fever that will blanch with pressure except in areas of deep creases and the folds of joints. The tongue is initially coated with a white furry covering with red projecting papillae (white strawberry tongue). By the fourth to fifth day, the white strawberry tongue sloughs off, leaving a red swollen tongue (strawberry tongue). The pharynx is edematous and beefy red. Koplik spots are associated with rubeola.
Test-Taking Strategy: Use the process of elimination, noting the key word "not" in the stem of the question. Recalling that Koplik spots are associated with rubeola will assist in answering this question. Review the clinical manifestations associated with scarlet fever if you had difficulty with this question.
Level of Cognitive Ability: Analysis
Client Needs: Physiological Integrity
Integrated Concept/Process: Nursing Process/Assessment
Content Area: Child Health
Reference: Wong, D. (1999). *Whaley & Wong's nursing care of infants and children* (6th ed.). St. Louis: Mosby, p. 731.

9. 4
Rationale: The parents need to be instructed to notify the physician if abdominal pain, especially in the left upper quadrant, or left shoulder pain occurs because this may indicate splenic rupture. Children with enlarged spleens are also instructed to avoid contact sports until splenomegaly resolves. Bed rest is not necessary, and children usually self-limit their activity. Respiratory precautions are not required, although transmission can occur via direct intimate contact or contact with infected blood. Fever is treated with acetaminophen (Tylenol).
Test-Taking Strategy: Use the process of elimination and knowledge regarding the organs affected in mononucleosis. Options 1 and 2 can be eliminated first because they are unnecessary interventions in this disease. From the remaining options, knowledge that splenic rupture is a concern will direct you to option 4. Review the complications associated with mononucleosis if you had difficulty with this question.
Level of Cognitive Ability: Application
Client Needs: Health Promotion and Maintenance
Integrated Concept/Process: Teaching/Learning
Content Area: Child Health
Reference: Bowden, V., Dickey, S., & Greenberg, C. (1998). *Children and their families: The continuum of care.* Philadelphia: W.B. Saunders, p. 1662.

10. 4
Rationale: Diagnosis is confirmed by direct visualization of the worms. Parents can view the sleeping child's anus with a flashlight. The worm is white, thin, about $1/2$ inch long, and moves. A simple technique, the tape test, is used to capture worms and eggs. Transparent tape is lightly touched to the anus and then applied to a slide for examination. The best specimens are obtained as the child awakens, before toileting or bathing.
Test-Taking Strategy: Use the process of elimination. Thinking about the test and the purpose of the test (to obtain a specimen that contains worms and eggs) will easily direct you to option 4. Review the procedure for this test if you are unfamiliar with it.
Level of Cognitive Ability: Application
Client Needs: Physiological Integrity
Integrated Concept/Process: Nursing Process/Implementation
Content Area: Child Health
Reference: Bowden, V., Dickey, S., & Greenberg, C. (1998). *Children and their families: The continuum of care.* Philadelphia: W.B. Saunders, p. 1673.

11. 4
Rationale: A severe febrile illness is a reason to delay immunization, but only until the child has recovered from the acute stage of the illness. Minor illnesses such as a cold, otitis media, or mild diarrhea are not contraindications to immunization.
Test-Taking Strategy: Use the process of elimination, focusing on the issue of the question, a contraindication to receiving an immunization. Reviewing each option carefully will easily direct you to option 4. If you had difficulty with this question, review the contraindications associated with immunizations.
Level of Cognitive Ability: Analysis
Client Needs: Physiological Integrity
Integrated Concept/Process: Teaching/Learning
Content Area: Child Health
Reference: Wong, D. (1999). *Whaley & Wong's nursing care of infants and children* (6th ed.). St. Louis: Mosby, p. 603.

12. 3
Rationale: DTaP, Hib, and IPV are administered at 4 months of age. DTaP is administered at 2 months, 4 months, 6 months, between 15 and 18 months of age, and between 4 and 6 years of age. Hib is administered at 2 months, 4 months, 6 months, and between 12 and 15 months of age. IPV is administered at 2 months, 4 months, 6 months, and between 4 and 6 years of age. The first dose of MMR is administered between 12 and 15 months of age; the second dose is administered at 4 to 6 years of age (if the second dose was not given by 4 to 6 years of age, it should be given at the next visit). The first dose of hepatitis B is administered between the ages of birth and 2 months, the second dose is administered between the ages of 1 and 4 months, and the third dose is administered between the ages of 6 and 18 months. Varicella zoster vaccine is administered between 12 and 18 months of age.
Test-Taking Strategy: Knowledge regarding the immunization schedule for infants and children is required to answer this question. Noting the age of the infant in the question will assist in directing you to option 3. Learn the immunization schedule, if you are unfamiliar with it.
Level of Cognitive Ability: Application
Client Needs: Health Promotion and Maintenance

Integrated Concept/Process: Nursing Process/Implementation
Content Area: Child Health
References: Advisory Committee on Immunization Practices (2000). *When do children and teens need vaccinations?* St. Paul: Immunization Action Coalition, Item P4050.
Advisory Committee on Immunization Practices (2000). *Summary of rules for childhood immunization.* St. Paul: Immunization Action Coalition, Item P2010.
Web site: http://www2.cdc.gov/mmwr/.
Web site: http://www.immunize.org

13. 3
Rationale: MMR is administered subcutaneously in the outer aspect of the upper arm. The gluteal muscle is most often used for intramuscular injections. MMR is not administered by the intramuscular route.
Test-Taking Strategy: Use the process of elimination. Knowledge that MMR is administered subcutaneously will assist in eliminating options 1 and 2. From the remaining options, recalling that the gluteal muscle is most often used for intramuscular injections will assist in directing you to option 3. Review the procedures related to the administration of MMR if you had difficulty with this question.
Level of Cognitive Ability: Application
Client Needs: Physiological Integrity
Integrated Concept/Process: Nursing Process/Implementation
Content Area: Child Health
Reference: Wong, D. (1999). *Whaley & Wong's nursing care of infants and children* (6th ed.). St. Louis: Mosby, p. 595.

14. 2
Rationale: MMR contains minute amounts of neomycin. A history of an anaphylactic reaction to neomycin is considered a contraindication to the MMR vaccine. The general contraindication to all immunizations is a severe febrile illness. The presence of minor illnesses such as a common cold is not a contraindication. In addition, a history of frequent respiratory infections is not a contraindication to receiving a vaccine. A local reaction to an immunization is treated with ice packs for the first 24 hours after injection, followed by warm compresses if the inflammation persists.
Test-Taking Strategy: Use the process of elimination. Recalling that a general contraindication to all immunizations is a severe febrile illness will assist in eliminating options 3 and 4. From the remaining options, note that option 1 identifies a local reaction. This will direct you to option 2, the systemic reaction, and a potential life-threatening condition. Review the contraindications to receiving immunizations if you had difficulty with this question.

Level of Cognitive Ability: Analysis
Client Needs: Safe, Effective Care Environment
Integrated Concept/Process: Nursing Process/Analysis
Content Area: Child Health
Reference: Wong, D. (1999). *Whaley & Wong's nursing care of infants and children* (6th ed.). St. Louis: Mosby, p. 603.

15. 1
Rationale: A contraindication to receiving the hepatitis B vaccine is a previous anaphylactic reaction to common baker's yeast. An allergy to eggs, penicillin, and sulfonamides is unrelated to the contraindication to receiving this vaccine.
Test-Taking Strategy: Use the process of elimination and knowledge regarding the contraindications associated with the administration of vaccines. It is necessary to know that a contraindication to receiving the hepatitis B vaccine is an anaphylactic reaction to common baker's yeast. Review the contraindication to receiving the hepatitis B vaccine if you had difficulty with this question.
Level of Cognitive Ability: Analysis
Client Needs: Physiological Integrity
Integrated Concept/Process: Nursing Process/Assessment
Content Area: Child Health
Reference: Wong, D. (1999). *Whaley & Wong's nursing care of infants and children* (6th ed.). St. Louis: Mosby, p. 605.

CRITICAL THINKING: FREE-TEXT ENTRY

Answer: Mask, gown, and gloves
Rationale: The rubella virus is primarily present in nasopharyngeal secretions. The virus is also present in blood, stool, and urine. It is transmitted via the airborne route, by direct contact with infectious droplets, or indirectly via articles freshly contaminated with nasopharyngeal secretions, feces, or urine. Care for the child with rubella involves contact isolation. Contact isolation requires masks, gowns, and gloves if contact with infectious material is anticipated.
Test-Taking Strategy: Think about the source and route of transmission of the rubella virus. Recalling that contact precautions are required will assist in identifying the protective items needed in caring for this child. Review the modes of transmission of rubella if you had difficulty with this question.
Level of Cognitive Ability: Application
Client Needs: Safe, Effective Care Environment
Integrated Concept/Process: Nursing Process/Planning
Content Area: Child Health
Reference: Wong, D. (1999). *Whaley & Wong's nursing care of infants and children* (6th ed.). St. Louis: Mosby, p. 603.

REFERENCES

Advisory Committee on Immunization Practices (2000). *When do children and teens need vaccinations?* St. Paul: Immunization Action Coalition, Item P4050.
Advisory Committee on Immunization Practices (2000). *Summary of rules for childhood immunization.* St. Paul: Immunization Action Coalition, Item P2010.
Ball, J., & Bindler, R. (1999). *Pediatric nursing: Caring for children* (2nd ed.). Stamford, Conn.: Appleton & Lange.

Bowden, V., Dickey, S., & Greenberg, C. (1998). *Children and their families: The continuum of care.* Philadelphia: W.B. Saunders.
Web site: http://www2.cdc.gov/mmwr/.
Web site: http://www.immunize.org
Wong, D. (1999). *Whaley & Wong's nursing care of infants and children* (6th ed.). St. Louis: Mosby.

46

Pediatric Medications and Calculations

I. ORAL MEDICATIONS

A. Most oral pediatric medications are in liquid or suspension form, since children usually are not able to swallow a tablet

B. Solutions may be measured by using an oral syringe; if an oral syringe is not available, hypodermic syringes without the needle can be used for dosage measurement

C. When volumes are extremely small, oral liquids are measured by using a calibrated medication dropper

D. Medications in suspension settle to the bottom of the bottle between uses, and thorough mixing is required prior to pouring of the medication

E. Suspensions must be administered immediately after measurement, to prevent settling and administration of an incomplete dose

F. Administer oral medications with the child sitting in an upright position, and with the head elevated, to prevent aspiration if the child cries or resists

G. Never pinch the infant or child's nostrils when administering medication

H. Do not place medication in a baby's bottle

I. Draw the required dose of an unpleasant medication into a small syringe, and place the syringe into the side and toward the back of the infant's mouth; administer the medication slowly, allowing the infant to swallow

J. Place the small child sideways on the lap; the child's closest arm should be placed under the adult's arm and behind the adult's back; cradle the child's head and hold the child's hand, and administer the medication slowly with a plastic spoon or small plastic cup

K. Mix liquid medications with less than an ounce of fluid to disguise the taste if necessary

L. If a tablet or capsule has been administered, check the child's mouth to ensure that it has been swallowed; if swallowing is a problem, some tablets can be crushed and given in small amounts of pureed food or flavored syrup (enteric-coated tablets, timed-release tablets, and capsules cannot be crushed)

II. PARENTERAL MEDICATIONS

A. Subcutaneous (SC) and intramuscular (IM) medications

1. Medications most often given via the SC route are insulin and most immunizations

2. Any site with sufficient subcutaneous tissue may be used for SC injections; common sites include the central third of the lateral aspect of the upper arm, the abdomen, and the center third of the anterior thigh

3. The safe use of all injection sites is based on normal muscle development and the size of the child; the preferred site for IM injections in infants is the vastus lateralis

4. Usually not more than 0.5 mL (infant) to 2.0 mL (child) is injected per IM or SC site, and the site of injection is rotated if frequent injections are necessary

5. The usual needle length and gauge for pediatric clients are ½ to 1 inch and 22 to 25 gauge

6. Needle length can also be estimated by grasping the muscle for injection between the thumb and forefinger; half the resulting distance between thumb and forefinger would be the needle length

7. Pediatric dosages for SC and IM administration are calculated to the nearest hundredth and measured by using a tuberculin (TB) syringe

8. For the toddler or preschooler, place an adhesive bandage or decorated Band-Aid over the puncture site

B. Intravenous (IV) medications

1. IV medications are diluted for administration

2. When an infant or child is receiving an IV medication, the IV site needs to be assessed for

485

signs of infiltration and inflammation immediately before, during, and after completion of each medication

▲ 3. Signs of inflammation include redness, heat, swelling, and tenderness

▲ 4. Signs of infiltration include swelling, coolness, pain, and lack of blood return

▲ 5. If inflammation or infiltration occurs, the IV is discontinued and restarted at a new site

6. IV medication may be administered on a continuous basis by adding the medication to an IV solution bag and infusing it through a primary infusion line

7. IV medications may be administered on an intermittent basis, involving several doses within a 24-hour period

8. Medications for IV administration are diluted according to the directions accompanying the medication and according to the physician's orders and agency procedures

9. Infusion time for IV medications is determined on the basis of the directions accompanying the medication, the physician's orders, and agency procedures

▲ 10. Determine agency procedures related to the volume of flush for peripheral IV lines and for central lines

11. The flush volume (3 to 20 mL) must be included in the child's intake; the flush is started after the IV medication is completed and is infused at the same rate as the medication

C. Intermittent IV medication administration

1. Children receiving IV medications on an intermittent basis may or may not have a primary IV

2. If a primary IV exists, the medication may be administered by IV piggyback (IVPB) via a secondary line

3. If a primary line does not exist, an indwelling infusion catheter is used for medication administration

4. All intermittent medication administrations are preceded and followed by a flush to ensure that the medication has cleared the IV tubing and that the total dose has been administered

5. Electronic controllers and pumps are used to regulate and administer IVs and intermittent IV medications

D. Special IV administration sets

1. Special IV administration sets, referred to by their trade names (Burretrol, Soluset, Volutrol), may be used for medication preparation and administration

2. These special sets are all microdrip sets calibrated to deliver 60 drops (gtt) per mL

3. The total capacity of these special IV administration sets is between 100 and 150 mL, calibrated in 1-mL increments so that exact measurements of small volumes are possible

4. The medication is mixed with the appropriate amount of diluent and added to the special IV administration set, and the medication is allowed to infuse at the prescribed rate

5. Label the special IV administration set to identify the medication and fluid dosage added

6. Attach a label that states "medication infusing" during the medication infusion time

7. Attach a label that states "flush infusing" during the flush infusion time

E. Retrograde IV injection

1. The medication is mixed with the appropriate amount of diluent in a syringe

2. The IV tubing is clamped close to the child, the medication is injected through the port in the direction of the burette, the tubing is unclamped, the prescribed rate is set, and the medication is allowed to infuse over the prescribed time

F. Syringe pump for IV medication administration

1. A syringe containing the medication is fitted into a pump that is connected to the IV tubing through a Y-connector

2. The medication is administered over the prescribed time

III. CALCULATION OF MEDICATION DOSAGE BY BODY WEIGHT

A. Conversion of body weight

1. Pounds (lb) to kilograms (kg)
   a. 1 kg = 2.2 lb ▲
   b. To convert from pounds to kilograms, divide by 2.2
   c. Kilograms are expressed to the nearest tenth

2. Kilograms (kg) to pounds (lb)
   a. 1 kg = 2.2 lb ▲
   b. To convert from kilograms to pounds, multiply by 2.2
   c. Pounds are expressed to the nearest tenth

B. Calculating daily dosages

1. Dosages are expressed in terms of mg/kg/day, mg/lb/day, or mg/kg/dose

2. The total daily dosage is usually administered in divided (more than one) doses per day

3. Express the child's body weight in kilograms or pounds to correlate with the dosage specifications

4. Calculate the total daily dosage

5. Divide the total daily dosage by the number of doses to be administered in one day

IV. CALCULATION OF BODY SURFACE AREA (BSA)

A. The body surface area is determined by comparing body weight and height with averages or norms on a graph called a nomogram

B. Not all children are the same size at the same age; therefore, the nomogram chart is used to determine the BSA of a child

C. Look at the nomogram chart (Fig. 46-1), and note

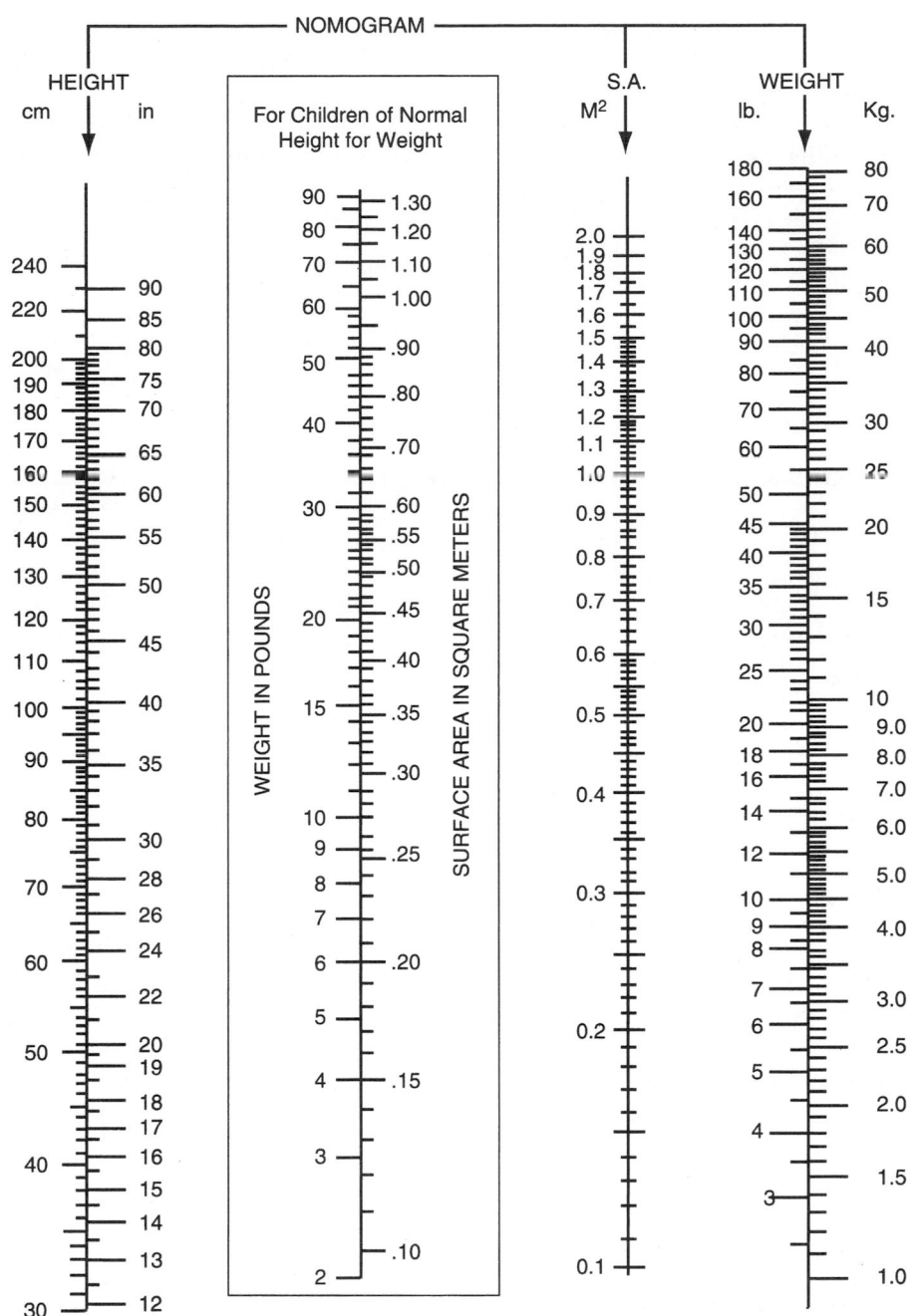

FIG. 46-1 West nomogram for infants and children. *Directions:* (1) find height; (2) find weight; (3) draw a straight line connecting the height and weight. Where the line intersects on the SA column is the body surface area (m²). (Modified from data of E. Boyd and C.D. West, in Behrman RE, Kliegman RM, Alvin AM: *Nelson textbook of pediatrics,* ed 15, Philadelphia, 1996, WB Saunders.)

that the height is on the left-hand side of the chart and the weight is on the right-hand side

D. Place a ruler on the chart

E. Line up the left side of the ruler on the height and the right side of the ruler on the weight; read the BSA at the point where the straight edge of the ruler intersects the surface area (SA) column

F. The estimated SA is given in square meters (m²)

EXAMPLE: Use the nomogram and calculate the

BSA for a child whose height is 58 inches and weight is 12 kg.

ANSWER: 0.66 m²

V. CALCULATION BASED ON BSA

A. When dosage recommendations for children specify mg, µg, or U per m², calculating the dosage is simple multiplication

EXAMPLE: The dosage recommendation is 4 mg

per m^2. The child has a BSA of 1.1 m^2. What is the dosage to be administered?

ANSWER: 1.1 × 4 mg = 4.4 mg

B. When dosages are specified only for adults, a formula is used to calculate a child's dosage from the adult dosage

EXAMPLE: A physician has prescribed an antibiotic for a child. The average adult dose is 250 mg. The child has a BSA of 0.41 m^2. What is the dose for the child?

ANSWER:

Formula:

$$\frac{\text{BSA of child (m}^2)}{1.73 \text{ m}^2} \times \text{Adult dose} = \text{Child's dose}$$

$$\frac{0.41}{1.73} \times 250 \text{ mg} = 59.24 \text{ mg}$$

PRACTICE QUESTIONS

1. Penicillin V (Veetids), 250 mg PO every 8 hours, is prescribed for a child with a respiratory infection. The child's weight is 45 pounds. The safe pediatric dosage is 25 to 50 mg/kg/day. The nurse determines that:
   1. The dose is too low
   2. The dose is too high
   3. The dose is within the safe dosage range
   4. There is not enough information to determine the safe dose

2. A physician has prescribed phenobarbital sodium (Luminal Sodium), 25 mg PO bid, for a child with febrile seizures. The medication label reads: phenobarbital sodium, 20 mg per 5 mL. A nurse has determined that the dosage prescribed is a safe for the child. The nurse prepares to administer how many milliliters per dose to the child?
   1. 2 mL
   2. 4.5 mL
   3. 6.25 mL
   4. 7.0 mL

3. Cloxacillin (Tegopen), 100 mg PO every 8 hours, is prescribed for a child with an elevated temperature who is suspected of having a respiratory tract infection. The child weighs 17 lb. The safe pediatric dosage is 50 mg/kg/day. The nurse determines that:
   1. The dose is too low
   2. The dose is too high
   3. The dose is safe
   4. There is not enough information to determine the safe dose

4. Sulfisoxazole (Gantrisin), 1.0 g PO qid, is prescribed for an adolescent with a urinary tract infection. The medication label reads: 500-mg tablets. A nurse has determined that the dosage prescribed is safe. The nurse administers how many tablets per dose to the adolescent?
   1. 0.5 tablet

   2. 1 tablet
   3. 2 tablets
   4. 3 tablets

5. Diphenhydramine hydrochloride (Benadryl), 25 mg PO every 6 hours, is prescribed for a child with an allergic reaction. The child weighs 25 kg. The safe pediatric dosage is 5 mg/kg/day. The nurse determines that:
   1. The dose is too low
   2. The dose is too high
   3. The dose is safe
   4. There is not enough information to determine the safe dose

6. Penicillin G procaine (Wycillin), 1,000,000 U IM, is prescribed for a child with an infection. The medication label reads: 1,200,000 U per 2 mL. A nurse has determined that the dose prescribed is safe. The nurse prepares to administer how many milliliters per dose to the child?
   1. 0.8 mL
   2. 1.2 mL
   3. 1.44 mL
   4. 1.66 mL

7. Morphine sulfate, 2.5 mg, IV piggyback, is prescribed for a child with cancer. The safe pediatric dose is 0.05 to 0.1 mg/kg/dose. The child weighs 50 kg. The nurse determines that:
   1. The dose is too low
   2. The dose is too high
   3. The dose is within the safe dosage range
   4. There is not enough information to determine the safe dosage range

8. Morphine sulfate, 2.5 mg, IV piggyback, in 10 mL of normal saline (NS), is prescribed for a child postoperatively. The medication label reads: 1/15 gr per mL. The nurse has determined that the dosage is safe. The nurse prepares to add how many milliliters of morphine sulfate to the 10 mL of NS solution?
   1. 0.62 mL
   2. 0.82 mL
   3. 1.35 mL
   4. 1.62 mL

9. A physician's order reads: ampicillin (Omnipen), 125 mg IV every 6 hours. The medication label reads: 1 g and reconstitute with 7.4 mL of bacteriostatic water. A nurse prepares to draw up how many milliliters to administer one dose?
   1. 0.54 mL
   2. 0.92 mL
   3. 1.1 mL
   4. 7.4 mL

10. A pediatric client with ventricular septal defect repair is placed on a maintenance dosage of digoxin (Lanoxin) elixir. The dosage is 0.07 mg/kg/day, and the client's weight is 7.2 kg. The physician orders the digoxin to be given bid. A nurse prepares how

much digoxin to administer to the client at each dose?

1. 0.25 mg
2. 0.37 mg
3. 0.50 mg
4. 2.50 mg

CRITICAL THINKING: FREE-TEXT ENTRY

Atropine sulfate, 0.2 mg IM, is prescribed for a child preoperatively. The medication label reads: 0.4 mg per mL. A nurse has determined that the dose prescribed is safe. The nurse prepares to administer how many milliliters to the child?

Answer: _____

ANSWERS

1. **3**

Rationale: Convert pounds to kilograms by dividing by 2.2.
Pounds to kilograms: 45 lb divided by 2.2 lb/kg = 20.45 kg
Dosage parameters: 25 mg/kg/day × 20.45 kg = 511.25 mg/day
50 mg/kg/day × 20.45 kg = 1022.50 mg/day
Dosage frequency: 250 mg × 3 doses (every 8 hours) = 750 mg/day
Dose is within the safe dosage range.
Test-Taking Strategy: Identify the key components of the question and what the question is asking. In this case, the question asks for the safe dosage range for medication. Change pounds to kilograms. Calculate the dosage parameters by using the safe dosage range identified in the question and the child's weight in kilograms. Remember to determine the total daily dosage prior to selecting an option.
Level of Cognitive Ability: Analysis
Client Needs: Safe, Effective Care Environment
Integrated Concept/Process: Nursing Process/Analysis
Content Area: Child Health
Reference: Kee, J., & Marshall, S. (2000). *Clinical calculations: With applications to general and specialty areas* (4th ed.). Philadelphia: W.B. Saunders, p. 219.

2. **3**

Rationale: Formula:
$$\frac{Desired}{Available} \times Volume = \frac{25\ mg}{20\ mg} \times 5\ mL = 6.25\ mL\ per\ dose$$
Test-Taking Strategy: Identify the key components of the question and what the question is asking. In this case, the question asks for the milliliters per dose. Use the formula to determine the correct dosage.
Level of Cognitive Ability: Application
Client Needs: Safe, Effective Care Environment
Integrated Concept/Process: Nursing Process/Planning
Content Area: Child Health
Reference: Kee, J., & Marshall, S. (2000). *Clinical calculations: With applications to general and specialty areas* (4th ed.). Philadelphia: W.B. Saunders, p. 78.

3. **3**

Rationale: Convert pounds to kilograms by dividing by 2.2.
Pounds to kilograms: 17 lb divided by 2.2 lb/kg = 7.72 kg
Dosage parameters: 50 mg/kg/day × 7.72 kg = 386 mg/day
Dosage frequency: 100 mg × 3 doses (every 8 hours) = 300 mg/day
The dose is safe.
Test-Taking Strategy: Identify the key components of the question and what the question is asking. In this case, the question asks for the safe dose of the medication. Change pounds to kilograms. Calculate the dose by using the safe dosage identified in the question and the child's weight in kilograms. Remember to determine the total daily dosage before selecting an option.
Level of Cognitive Ability: Analysis
Client Needs: Safe, Effective Care Environment
Integrated Concept/Process: Nursing Process/Analysis
Content Area: Child Health
Reference: Kee, J., & Marshall, S. (2000). *Clinical calculations: With applications to general and specialty areas* (4th ed.). Philadelphia: W.B. Saunders, p. 219.

4. **3**

Rationale: Change 1 g to milligrams, knowing that 1000 mg = 1 g. When converting from grams to milligrams (larger to smaller), move the decimal point 3 places to the right. Therefore, 1.0 g = 1000 mg.
Formula:
$$\frac{Desired}{Available} \times Tablet = \frac{1000\ mg}{500\ mg} \times 1\ Tablet = 2\ Tablets$$
Test-Taking Strategy: Identify the key components of the question and what the question is asking. In this case, the question asks for tablets per dose. Change grams to milligrams first. Then use the formula to determine the correct dose.
Level of Cognitive Ability: Application
Client Needs: Safe, Effective Care Environment
Integrated Concept/Process: Nursing Process/Implementation
Content Area: Child Health
Reference: Kee, J., & Marshall, S. (2000). *Clinical calculations: With applications to general and specialty areas* (4th ed.). Philadelphia: W.B. Saunders, p. 78.

5. **3**

Rationale:
Dosage parameters: 5 mg/kg/day × 25 kg = 125 mg/day
Dosage frequency: 25 mg × 4 doses (every 6 hours) = 100 mg/day
Dose is within the safe dosage range.
Test-Taking Strategy: Identify the key components of the question and what the question is asking. In this case, the question asks for the safe dose of the medication. Calculate the dosage parameters by using the safe dosage identified in the question and the child's weight in kilograms. Remember to determine the total daily dosage prior to selecting an option.
Level of Cognitive Ability: Analysis
Client Needs: Safe, Effective Care Environment
Integrated Concept/Process: Nursing Process/Analysis

Content Area: Child Health
Reference: Kee, J., & Marshall, S. (2000). *Clinical calculations: With applications to general and specialty areas* (4th ed.). Philadelphia: W.B. Saunders, p. 219.

6. 4
Rationale: Formula:
$$\frac{\text{Desired}}{\text{Available}} \times \text{Volume} = \frac{1,000,000}{1,200,000} \times 2 \text{ mL} = 1.66 \text{ mL per dose}$$
Test-Taking Strategy: Identify the key components of the question and what the question is asking. In this case, the question asks for the milliliters per dose. Use the formula to determine the correct dose.
Level of Cognitive Ability: Application
Client Needs: Safe, Effective Care Environment
Integrated Concept/Process: Nursing Process/Planning
Content Area: Child Health
Reference: Kee, J., & Marshall, S. (2000). *Clinical calculations: With applications to general and specialty areas* (4th ed.). Philadelphia: W.B. Saunders, p. 78.

7. 3
Rationale: Dosage parameters:
$$0.05 \text{ mg/kg/dose} \times 50 \text{ kg} = 2.5 \text{ mg/dose}$$
$$0.1 \text{ mg/kg/dose} \times 50 \text{ kg} = 5 \text{ mg/dose}$$
Dosage is within the safe dosage range.
Test-Taking Strategy: Identify the key components of the question and what the question is asking. In this case, the question asks for the safe dose of the medication. Calculate the dosage parameters, using the safe dosage range identified in the question and the child's weight in kilograms.
Level of Cognitive Ability: Analysis
Client Needs: Safe, Effective Care Environment
Integrated Concept/Process: Nursing Process/Analysis
Content Area: Child Health
Reference: Kee, J., & Marshall, S. (2000). *Clinical calculations: With applications to general and specialty areas* (4th ed.). Philadelphia: W.B. Saunders, p. 219.

8. 1
Rationale: Convert grains to milligrams
$$60 \text{ mg} = 1 \text{ gr}$$
$$1/15 \text{ gr} \times 60 \text{ mg} = 4 \text{ mg}$$
Formula:
$$\frac{\text{Desired}}{\text{Available}} \times \text{Volume} = \frac{2.5 \text{ mg}}{4 \text{ mg}} \times 1 \text{ mL} = 0.62 \text{ mL}$$
Test-Taking Strategy: Identify the key components of the question and what the question is asking. In this case, the question asks for the milliliters per dose. Begin by converting grains to milligrams. Then use the formula to determine the correct dose.
Level of Cognitive Ability: Application
Client Needs: Safe, Effective Care Environment
Integrated Concept/Process: Nursing Process/Planning
Content Area: Child Health
Reference: Kee, J., & Marshall, S. (2000). *Clinical calculations: With applications to general and specialty areas* (4th ed.). Philadelphia: W.B. Saunders, p. 78.

9. 2
Rationale: Convert 1 g to milligrams. In the metric system, to convert larger to smaller, multiply by 1000 or move the decimal point three places to the right.
$$1 \text{ g} = 1000 \text{ mg}$$
Formula:
$$\frac{\text{Desired}}{\text{Available}} \times \text{Volume} = \text{mL per dose}$$
$$\frac{125 \text{ mg}}{1000 \text{ mg}} \times 7.4 \text{ mL} = 0.925 \text{ mL} = 0.92 \text{ mL per dose}$$
Test-Taking Strategy: Identify the key components of the question and what the question is asking. In this case, the question asks for the milliliters per dose. Convert grams to milligrams first. Next, use the formula to determine the correct dose, knowing that 1000 mg = 7.4 mL.
Level of Cognitive Ability: Application
Client Needs: Safe, Effective Care Environment
Integrated Concept/Process: Nursing Process/Planning
Content Area: Fundamental Skills
Reference: Kee, J., & Marshall, S. (2000). *Clinical calculations: With applications to general and specialty areas* (4th ed.). Philadelphia: W.B. Saunders, p. 78.

10. 1
Rationale: Calculate the dosage by weight first:
$$0.07 \text{ mg/day} \times 7.2 \text{ kg} = 0.50 \text{ mg/day}$$
The physician orders digoxin bid; therefore, 2 doses in 24 hours will be administered.
$$0.50 \text{ mg/day divided by 2 doses} = 0.25 \text{ mg for each dose}$$
Test-Taking Strategy: Identify the key components of the question and what the question is asking. Read the question carefully, noting that the question states "bid" and "each dose." Calculate the dosage by weight first, and then determine the milligrams per each dose.
Level of Cognitive Ability: Application
Client Needs: Safe, Effective Care Environment
Integrated Concept/Process: Nursing Process/Planning
Content Area: Child Health
Reference: Kee, J., & Marshall, S. (2000). *Clinical calculations: With applications to general and specialty areas* (4th ed.). Philadelphia: W.B. Saunders, p. 78.

CRITICAL THINKING: FREE-TEXT ENTRY

Answer: 0.5 mL
Rationale: Formula:
$$\frac{\text{Desired}}{\text{Available}} \times \text{Volume} = \frac{0.2 \text{ mg}}{0.4 \text{ mg}} \times 1 \text{ mL} = 0.5 \text{ mL}$$
Test-Taking Strategy: Identify the key components of the question and what the question is asking. In this case, the question asks for the milliliters to be administered. Use the formula to determine the correct dose.
Level of Cognitive Ability: Application
Client Needs: Safe, Effective Care Environment
Integrated Concept/Process: Nursing Process/Planning
Content Area: Child Health
Reference: Kee, J., & Marshall, S. (2000). *Clinical calculations: With applications to general and specialty areas* (4th ed.). Philadelphia: W.B. Saunders, p. 78.

REFERENCES

Ball, J., & Bindler, R. (1999). *Pediatric nursing: Caring for children* (2nd ed.). Stamford, Conn.: Appleton & Lange.

Ball, J., & Bindler (1999). *Quick reference to pediatric clinical skills.* Stamford, Conn.: Appleton & Lange.

Bowden, V., Dickey, S, & Greenberg, C. (1998). *Children and their families: The continuum of care.* Philadelphia: W.B. Saunders.

Hodgson, B., & Kizior, R. (2001). *Saunders nursing drug handbook 2001.* Philadelphia: W.B. Saunders.

Kee, J., & Marshall, S. (2000). *Clinical calculations: With applications to general and specialty areas* (4th ed.). Philadelphia: W.B. Saunders.

Wong, D. (1999). *Whaley & Wong's nursing care of infants and children* (6th ed.). St. Louis: Mosby.

The Adult Client with an Integumentary Disorder

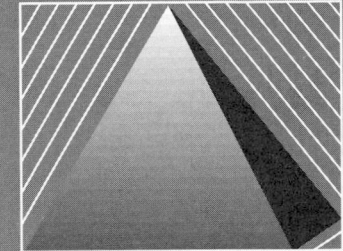

PYRAMID TERMS

burn Cell destruction of the layers of the skin and the resultant depletion of fluid and electrolytes.

carbon monoxide poisoning Carbon monoxide is a colorless, odorless, and tasteless gas that has an affinity for hemoglobin 200 times greater than that of oxygen. Oxygen molecules are displaced and carbon monoxide reversibly binds to hemoglobin to form carboxyhemoglobin. Tissue hypoxia occurs.

chemical burn Caused by tissue contact with strong acids, alkalis, or organic compounds. Systemic toxicity from cutaneous absorption can occur.

decubitus Localized area of skin breakdown that occurs as a result of poor circulation to the area; also called a pressure ulcer.

deep full-thickness burn Involves injury to the muscle and bone. Injured area appears black. Edema is absent.

electrical burn Caused by heat generated from electrical energy as it passes through the body. Results in internal tissue damage.

full-thickness burn Injured area appears deep red, black, white, or brown. Injured surface appears dry. Tissue disruption is noted, with fat exposed. Skin is edematous.

herpes zoster (shingles) An acute viral infection of the nerve structure caused by varicella-zoster virus. Herpes zoster is contagious to individuals who have not had chickenpox.

Kaposi's sarcoma Small, purplish brown lesions that are the most common malignancy associated with acquired immunodeficiency syndrome.

Lyme disease An infection acquired from a tick bite. Ticks live in wooded areas and survive by attaching to a host.

partial-thickness burn A mottled red base and broken epidermis with a wet shiny and weeping surface is present. Large blisters cover an extensive area. Skin is edematous and painful.

skin cancer A malignant lesion of the skin that may or may not metastasize. Causes include chronic friction and irritation to a skin area and exposure to ultraviolet rays. Diagnosis is confirmed by a skin biopsy that is positive for cancer cells.

smoke inhalation injury Results from the inhalation of superheated air, steam, toxic fumes, or smoke, and leads to respiratory insufficiency.

superficial-thickness burn Mild to severe erythema is noted, and the skin blanches with pressure.

thermal burn Caused by exposure to flames, hot liquids, steam, or hot objects.

PYRAMID TO SUCCESS

The Pyramid to Success focuses on the concept that the integumentary system provides the first line of defense against infections. Focus on the protective measures necessary to prevent infection. Pyramid points address the risk factors related to the development of integumentary disorders, the preventive measures related to skin cancer, and the content related to Kaposi's sarcoma and Lyme disease. Focus on the emergency measures related to a client with a burn, fluid resuscitation, monitoring for complications, and skin grafting. Psychosocial issues relate to the body image disturbances that can occur as a result of the integumentary disorder. The Integrated Concepts and Processes addressed in this unit include Nursing Process, Caring, Communication and Documentation, Cultural Awareness, Self-Care, and Teaching/Learning.

CLIENT NEEDS
Safe, Effective Care Environment

Confidentiality related to the disorder
Consultation with members of the health care team
Establishing priorities
Handling infectious materials
Informed consent for treatments and procedures
Medical and surgical asepsis
Referrals
Standard (universal) precautions

Health Promotion and Maintenance

Disease prevention measures
Health promotion programs
Health screening
Instructions to the client regarding care for integumentary disorder
Physical assessment of the integumentary system

Psychosocial Integrity

Coping mechanisms
End-of-life issues
Situational role changes
Unexpected body image changes
Use of support systems

Physiological Integrity

Adequate nutrition for healing
Alteration in body systems
Basic care and comfort
Comfort care
Expected effects of treatments

Fluid and electrolyte imbalances
Monitoring for complications
Monitoring laboratory values
Providing emergency care

REFERENCES

Craven, R., & Hirnle, C. (2000). *Fundamentals of nursing: Human health and function* (3rd ed.). Philadelphia: Lippincott.

Harkreader, H. (2000). *Fundamentals of nursing: Caring and clinical judgment.* Philadelphia: W.B. Saunders.

Ignatavicius, D., Workman, M., & Mishler, M. (1999). *Medical-surgical nursing across the health care continuum* (3rd ed.). Philadelphia: W.B. Saunders.

LeMone, P., & Burke, K. (2000). *Medical-surgical nursing: Critical thinking in client care* (2nd ed.). Upper Saddle River, N.J.: Prentice-Hall.

Lewis, S., Heitkemper, M., & Dirksen, S. (2000). *Medical-surgical nursing: Assessment and management of clinical problems* (5th ed.). St. Louis: Mosby.

National Council of State Boards of Nursing (eds.) (2000). *Test Plan for the National Council Licensure Examination for Registered Nurses.* Chicago: Author.

Potter, P., & Perry, A. (2001). *Fundamentals of nursing* (5th ed.). St. Louis: Mosby.

Smeltzer, S., & Bare, B. (2000). *Textbook of medical-surgical nursing* (9th ed). Philadelphia: Lippincott Williams & Wilkins.

Integumentary System

I. ANATOMY AND PHYSIOLOGY

A. The skin is the largest sensory organ of the body, with a surface area of 15 to 20 feet and a weight of about 9 pounds
B. Functions
   1. First line of defense against infections
   2. Protects underlying tissues and organs from injury
   3. Receives stimuli from the external environment; detects touch, pressure, pain, and temperature stimuli and relays that information to the nervous system
   4. Maintains normal body temperature
   5. Excretes salts, water, and organic wastes
   6. Protects the body from excessive water loss
   7. Synthesizes vitamin D_3, which converts to calcitriol, for normal calcium metabolism
   8. Stores nutrients
C. Layers
   1. Epidermis
   2. Dermis
   3. Hypodermis (subcutaneous fat)
D. Epidermal appendages
   1. Nails
   2. Hair
   3. Glands
      a. Sebaceous
      b. Sweat
E. Normal bacterial flora
   1. Types of normal bacterial flora
      a. Gram-positive and gram-negative staphylococci
      b. *Pseudomonas*
      c. *Streptococcus*
   2. Organisms are shed with normal exfoliation
   3. A pH of 4.2 to 5.6 halts the growth of bacteria

II. RISK FACTORS FOR INTEGUMENTARY DISORDERS

A. Exposure to chemical or environmental pollutants
B. Exposure to radiation
C. Exposure to the sun
D. Lack of personal hygiene habits
E. Use of cosmetics or harsh soaps
F. Medications, such as long-term corticosteroid and/or anticoagulant therapy
G. Nutritional deficiencies
H. Moderate to severe emotional stress
I. Infection, with injured areas as the potential entry points for infection
J. Changes associated with developmental stages and aging

III. PSYCHOSOCIAL IMPACT

A. Change in body image and decreased self-esteem
B. Social isolation and fear of rejection (from embarrassment about changes in skin appearance)
C. Restrictions in physical activity
D. Pain
E. Disruption or loss of employment
F. Cost of medications, hospitalizations, and follow-up care, including dressing supplies

IV. DIAGNOSTIC TESTS

A. Skin biopsy
   1. Description
      a. Obtaining a small piece of skin tissue for histopathologic study
      b. Methods include punch, excisional, incisional, and shave
   2. Implementation preprocedure
      a. Obtain informed consent
      b. Cleanse site as prescribed

3. Implementation postprocedure
   a. Place specimen, when obtained by physician, in the appropriate container and send to pathology laboratory for analysis
   b. Use surgically aseptic technique for biopsy site dressings
   c. Assess the biopsy site for bleeding and infection
   d. Instruct the client to keep dressing in place for at least 8 hours, and then to clean the site daily, as prescribed, and use antibiotic ointment as prescribed

B. Skin cultures
   1. Description
      a. Noninvasive procedure
      b. A small skin culture sample is obtained, using a sterile applicator and the appropriate type of culture tube (bacterial or viral)
      c. Viral culture is placed immediately on ice
      d. Sample is sent to laboratory to identify an existing organism
   2. Implementation: Obtain skin culture samples prior to instituting antibiotic therapy
   3. Implementation postprocedure: Send skin culture sample to the laboratory

C. Wood's light examination
   1. Description: Skin is viewed under ultraviolet light through a special glass (Wood's glass) to identify superficial infections of the skin
   2. Implementation preprocedure: Darken room prior to the examination
   3. Implementation postprocedure: Assist the client during adjustment from the darkened room

D. Skin testing
   1. Description
      a. The administration of an allergen to the skin's surface or into the dermis
      b. Administered by patch, scratch, or intradermal techniques
   2. Implementation preprocedure
      a. Discontinue systemic corticosteroids or antihistamine therapy for 48 hours prior to the test, as prescribed
      b. Obtain informed consent
      c. Have resuscitation equipment available if a scratch test is performed, as it may induce an anaphylactic reaction
   3. Implementation postprocedure
      a. Instruct the client to keep skin-testing patch area dry
      b. Instruct the client to avoid activities that may produce sweating if a patch test was performed
      c. Record the site, date, and time of the test
      d. Record the date and time for follow-up site reading

   e. Inspect the site for erythema, papules, vesicles, edema, and induration
   f. Provide the client with a list of potential allergens, if identified

V. SKIN DISORDERS

A. **Skin cancer**
   1. Description
      a. A malignant lesion of the skin, which may or may not metastasize
      b. Causes include chronic friction or irritation to a skin area and exposure to ultraviolet rays
      c. Diagnosis is confirmed by a skin biopsy that is positive for cancer cells
   2. Types
      a. Basal cell: The most common type, arising from the basal cells contained in the epidermis
      b. Squamous cell: The second most common type of **skin cancer** in whites; it is a tumor of the epidermal keratinocytes and can infiltrate surrounding structures, metastasize to lymph nodes, and be subsequently fatal
      c. Malignant melanoma: Cancer of the melanocytes that can metastasize to the brain, lungs, bone, liver, and skin and be ultimately fatal
   3. Assessment (Box 47-1)
      a. Change in color, size, or shape of preexisting lesion
      b. Pruritus
      c. Local soreness
   4. Implementation
      a. Instruct the client regarding preventive measures
      b. Instruct the client to monitor for lesions that do not heal or that change characteristics
      c. Instruct the client to have moles or lesions removed that are subject to chronic irritation
      d. Instruct the client to avoid contact with chemical irritants
      e. Instruct the client to wear layered clothing and use sun-screening lotions with an appropriate skin protection factor when outdoors
      f. Instruct the client to avoid sun exposure between 11:00 A.M. and 3:00 P.M.
      g. Assist with surgical excision of the lesion as prescribed

---

BOX 47-1

Appearance of Skin Cancer Lesions

A waxy nodule
An irregular, circular, bordered lesion with hues of tan, black, or blue
A small, red, nodular lesion
An oozing, bleeding, crusting lesion

B. Contact dermatitis
1. Description: An inflammatory response of the skin that produces skin changes after contact with a specific antigen
2. Assessment
   a. Pruritus and burning
   b. Edema
   c. Erythema at the point of contact
   d. Signs of infection
   e. Vesicles with drainage
3. Implementation
   a. Elevation of the extremity to reduce edema
   b. Application of cool, wet dressings and tepid baths as prescribed
   c. Maintain a cool environment
   d. Protect the affected area from trauma
   e. Prevent scratching and rubbing of the affected area
   f. Assist with skin testing, as prescribed, to determine allergen(s)
   g. Instruct the client to avoid contact with the allergen when determined
   h. Instruct the client to avoid harsh soaps
   i. Instruct the client to avoid using heating pads or blankets
   j. Administer antibiotic for infection, antipruritic or antihistamine for itching, and/or corticosteroids for inflammation, as prescribed

C. Poison ivy, poison oak, and poison sumac
1. Description: A dermatitis that develops from contact with urushiol from poison ivy, oak, or sumac plants
2. Assessment
   a. Papulovesicular lesions
   b. Severe itching
3. Implementation
   a. Cleanse the skin of the plant oils
   b. Apply cool, wet dressings with Burrow's solution, as prescribed, to relieve the itching
   c. Apply lotion or topical corticosteroids as prescribed

d. Administer oral corticosteroids, as prescribed, for severe reaction

D. **Lyme disease**
1. Description
   a. An infection caused by the spirochete *Borrelia burgdorferi*, acquired from a tick bite
   b. Ticks live in wooded areas and survive by attaching to a host
2. Assessment (Table 47-1)
3. Implementation
   a. Gently remove the tick with tweezers or fingers, wash the skin with antiseptic, and dispose of the tick by flushing it down the toilet
   b. Obtain a blood test 4 to 6 weeks after a bite to detect the presence of the disease (testing before this time is not reliable)
   c. Instruct the client in the administration of antibiotics, as prescribed, if the disease is confirmed
   d. Instruct the client to avoid areas that contain ticks, such as wooded grassy areas, especially in the summer months
   e. Instruct the client to wear long-sleeved tops, long pants, closed shoes, and hats while outside
   f. Instruct the client to spray the body with tick repellent before going outside
   g. Instruct the client to examine the body when returning inside

E. Erysipelas and cellulitis
1. Description
   a. Erysipelas is an acute, superficial, rapidly spreading inflammation of the dermis and lymphatics caused by beta-hemolytic streptococcus group A, which enters the tissue via an abrasion, bite, trauma, or wound
   b. Cellulitis is a skin infection into the deeper dermis and subcutaneous fat, and the causative organism is usually *Streptococcus pyogenes*

TABLE 47-1

Assessment and Stages of Lyme Disease

First Stage	Second Stage	Third Stage
Symptoms can occur several days to months following the bite	Occurs several weeks following the bite	Large joints become involved
A small red pimple develops that spreads into a ring-shaped rash	Joint pain	Arthritis progresses
Rash may be large or small or may not occur at all	Neurological complications	
Flulike symptoms occur, such as headaches, stiff neck, muscle aches, and fatigue	Cardiac complications	

2. Assessment
   a. Pain
   b. Itching
   c. Swelling
   d. Redness and warmth
3. Implementation
   a. Promote rest
   b. Apply warm compresses as prescribed (usually twice a day) to promote circulation and to decrease discomfort, erythema, and edema
   c. Administer antibiotics, as prescribed, for infection following a culture of the area
   d. Clean skin daily with an antibacterial type of soap as prescribed

F. Psoriasis
   1. Description
      a. A chronic, noninfectious skin inflammation involving keratin synthesis that results in psoriatic patches
      b. Various forms exist, with psoriasis vulgaris being the most common
      c. Possible causes of the disorder include stress, trauma, infection, and changes in climate
      d. The disorder may also be exacerbated by the use of certain medications
      e. Koebner's phenomenon is the development of psoriatic lesions at a site of injury, such as a scratched or sunburned area
   2. Assessment
      a. Pruritus
      b. Shedding, silvery, white scales on a raised, reddened, round plaque that usually affects the scalp, knees, elbows, extensor surfaces of arms and legs, and sacral regions
      c. A yellow discoloration, pitting, and a thickening of nails if they are affected
      d. Joint inflammation with psoriatic arthritis
   3. Implementation
      a. Administer and instruct the client regarding daily soaks and tepid, wet compresses, as prescribed, to the affected areas to remove scales; oils or coal tar preparations (Balnetar) are added to the bath water
      b. Assist the client to remove the scales during the soak, using a soft washcloth and gentle, circular motions; emollient creams or salicylic acid is applied to affected areas after the bath to continue to soften thick scales
   4. Topical pharmacological therapy
      a. Includes tar preparations, anthralin, salicylic acid, and corticosteroids; vitamin D preparation, calcipotriene (Dovonex), and a retinoid compound, tazarotene (Tazorac), suppress epidermopoiesis and cause sloughing of the rapidly growing epidermal cells
      b. Occlusive dressings may be applied following application of the corticosteroid, to increase its effectiveness
      c. Use plastic wrap or bags as the occlusive dressing, and use rubber gloves on the client's hands, plastic bags on the feet, and a shower cap on the head if affected; a plastic vinyl jogging suit may be used for the client being treated at home
   5. Intralesional therapy
      a. Involves the administration of injections into highly visible or isolated patches of psoriasis that are resistant to other forms of therapy
      b. Triamcinolone acetonide (Aristocort, Kenolog-10, Trymex) is injected, and care is taken so that normal skin is not injected with the medication
   6. Systemic therapy
      a. Systemic medications may be prescribed to treat extensive psoriasis that does not respond to other forms of therapy
      b. Prescribed medications may include methotrexate, hydroxyurea (Hydrea), and cyclosporine A (CyA)
   7. Photochemotherapy
      a. A combination of psoralens and ultraviolet-A (PUVA) light therapy (decreases cellular proliferation)
      b. The client takes a photosensitizing medication (8-methoxypsoralen) and is subsequently exposed to long-wave ultraviolet light
   8. Client education
      a. Instruct the client not to scratch the affected areas and to keep the skin lubricated to minimize itching
      b. Monitor for and instruct the client to recognize the signs and symptoms of infection
      c. Instruct the client to wear light cotton clothing over affected areas
      d. Instruct the client regarding prescribed treatments and medications and to avoid over-the-counter medications
      e. Assist the client to identify ways to reduce stress

G. **Kaposi's sarcoma**
   1. Description: Skin lesions that occur primarily in individuals with a compromised immune system
   2. Assessment
      a. Slow-growing tumors that appear as raised, oblong, purplish, reddish brown lesions; may be tender or nontender
      b. Organ involvement includes the lymph nodes, airways or lungs, or any part of gastrointestinal tract from the mouth to anus
   3. Implementation
      a. Maintain standard precautions
      b. Provide protective isolation if the immune system is depressed

c. Prepare the client for radiation therapy or chemotherapy as prescribed

d. Administer immunotherapy, as prescribed, to stabilize the immune system

H. **Herpes zoster (shingles)**

1. Description

a. An acute viral infection of the dorsal nerve root ganglion, caused by the varicella-zoster virus

b. Can be caused by the reactivation of the varicella-zoster virus or exposure to the virus, or can occur during any immunocompromised state

c. Diagnosis is determined by visual examination, skin cultures, and skin stains that identify the organism, and by an antinuclear antibody (ANA) blood test, which will produce a positive result

d. A culture provides the definitive diagnosis

e. **Herpes zoster** is contagious to individuals who have not had chickenpox

2. Assessment

a. Unilaterally clustered skin vesicles along peripheral sensory nerves on the trunk, thorax, or face

b. Fever

c. Burning and neuralgia

d. Pruritus

e. Paresthesia

3. Implementation

a. Isolate the client, because exudate from the lesions contains the virus

b. Maintain strict wound and skin precautions

c. Assess neurovascular status and seventh cranial nerve function

d. Assess for signs and symptoms of infection

e. Keep blisters intact if formed

f. Assist the client with acetic acid compresses, cool, wet compresses, and/or tepid baths, as prescribed

g. Prepare to assist the physician with a nerve block using lidocaine (Xylocaine) if prescribed

h. Administer antiviral agents, analgesics, antianxiety agents, antipruritics, and corticosteroids, as prescribed

i. Use an air mattress and a bed cradle on the client's bed, and keep environment cool; warmth and touch aggravate pain

j. Prevent the client from scratching or rubbing the affected area

k. Instruct the client to wear lightweight, loose cotton clothing and to avoid wool and synthetic clothing

I. Paronychia

1. Description: An infection of the tissue around the nail plate that most commonly occurs in middle-aged women and in clients with diabetes mellitus

2. Assessment

a. Redness and swelling around the nailbed

b. Soreness at the nailbed

3. Implementation

a. Monitor temperature

b. Monitor for infection around the nails

c. Monitor for cellulitis in the affected area

d. Assist the client with warm soaks as prescribed

e. Prepare to assist with incision and drainage of infected area if prescribed

f. Administer antibiotic or fungicidal ointments as prescribed

J. Impetigo: Refer to Chapter 40 for information on this disorder

K. Boils

1. Description

a. A deep bacterial inflammation of a hair follicle caused by staphylococcus

b. Commonly occur on the face, neck, arms, legs, and groin

2. Assessment

a. Redness on skin

b. Tender and painful furuncle

c. Skin swelling at the site

d. A yellow or white center at the furuncle

3. Implementation

a. Instruct the client in good handwashing technique to prevent the spread of infection

b. Apply hot moist compresses until drainage occurs

c. Assist the physician in incision and drainage, which relieves pain and allows the escape of purulent drainage

d. Instruct the client in daily cleanliness, the use of separate bath linens, and the administration of antibiotics if prescribed

L. Frostbite

1. Description

a. Damage to tissues and blood vessels as a result of prolonged exposure to cold

b. Fingers, toes, nose, and ears are often affected

2. Assessment

a. Numbness

b. Paresthesia

c. Pallor

d. Severe pain, swelling, erythema, and blistering occur once the client is in a warm environment

e. Necrosis and gangrene may develop in severe cases

3. Implementation

a. Handle the tissues gently

b. Rewarm the affected part rapidly and continuously with a warm water bath (90° to 107° F) for 15 to 20 minutes or until skin flushing occurs

   c. Avoid slow thawing, interrupted periods of warmth, or massage (may result in further tissue damage)

   d. Do not debride blisters

   e. Leave area exposed initially for continued assessment; then apply bulky dressings as prescribed, to permit drainage and provide protection

M. Scabies

  1. Description

   a. A parasitic skin disorder caused by an infestation of *Sarcoptes scabiei* (itch mite)

   b. Is endemic among schoolchildren and institutionalized populations because of close personal contact

   c. Risk factors include close personal contact with an infected person or a contaminated article

   d. There is a 1-month delay between the initial infestation and onset of pruritus in the host

  2. Assessment

   a. Erythematous papules and pustules

   b. Threadlike, brownish, linear burrows up to 1 cm long

   c. Secondary lesions consist of vesicles, crusts, reddish brown nodules, and excoriations

   d. Intense pruritus that worsens at night

  3. Implementation

   a. Administer antihistamines or topical steroids to relieve itching as prescribed

   b. Apply topical antiscabies creams or lotions such as lindane (Kwell, Scabene), crotamiton (Eurax), or permethrin 5% (Elimite) as prescribed

   c. Lindane (Kwell, Scabene) should not be used in children younger than age 2, because of the risk of neurotoxicity and seizures

   d. Instruct the client to apply the antiscabies preparation thinly to the entire skin from the neck down (face and scalp are not affected in scabies) and to leave on for 12 to 24 hours, as prescribed

   e. Instruct the client to apply antiscabies preparations to dry skin, because moist skin increases absorption and the potential for central nervous system side effects, such as seizures

   f. After treatment with antiscabies preparations, instruct the client to remove the medication by thoroughly washing with soap and water

   g. All family members and close contacts should be treated simultaneously

   h. Instruct the client that all bedding and clothing should be washed in very hot water and dried on the hot dryer cycle or dry cleaned (mites can survive up to 36 hours on linen)

N. Acne vulgaris

  1. Description

   a. A common, self-limiting, multifactorial disorder

   b. Requires active treatment for control until it spontaneously resolves

   c. The types of lesions include comedones (open and closed), pustules, papules, and nodules

   d. The exact cause is unknown, but may include androgenic influence on sebaceous glands, increased sebum production, and proliferation of *Propionibacterium acnes* (whose enzymes reduce lipids to irritating fatty acids)

   e. There is no evidence that chocolate, nuts, fatty foods, or cosmetics affect acne

   f. Exacerbations coincide with the menstrual cycle, as a result of hormonal activity

   g. Heat, humidity, and excessive perspiration have a role in increased acne

  2. Assessment

   a. Closed comedones: Whiteheads and noninflamed lesions that develop as a follicle, and enlarge with the retention of horny cells

   b. Open comedones: Blackheads that result from continuing accumulation of horny cells and sebum, which dilate the follicles

   c. Pustules and papules result as the inflammatory process progresses

   d. Nodules result from total disintegration of a comedone and subsequent collapse of the follicle

   e. Deep scarring can result from nodules

  3. Implementation

   a. Instruct the client in the administration (provide written instructions) of topical or oral antibiotics as prescribed

   b. Instruct the client in the use of isotretinoin (Accutane), if prescribed, to inhibit sebum production and reduce sebaceous gland size

   c. Instruct the client about the adverse effects of isotretinoin, which include cheilitis (lip inflammation), skin dryness, elevated triglycerides, and eye discomfort

   d. Instruct the client to stop taking vitamin A supplements during treatment with isotretinoin

   e. Inform the client that improvement may not be apparent for 4 to 6 weeks

   f. Instruct the client in appropriate skin-cleansing methods, with emphasis on not scrubbing the face and using only the agreed-upon topical agents

   g. Instruct the client not to squeeze, prick, or pick at lesions

   h. Instruct the client to use products labeled noncomedogenic and cosmetics that are water

TABLE 47-2

Stages of Decubiti

Stage 1	Stage 2	Stage 3	Stage 4
A reddened area that returns to normal skin color after 15 to 20 minutes of pressure relief, such as turning the client to another position The skin is intact Area is red and does not blanch with external pressure	Area in which the top layer is missing The ulcer usually is shallow with a pink to red base, and a white or yellow eschar may be present	Deep ulcers that extend into the dermis and subcutaneous tissues White, gray, or yellow eschar usually is present at the bottom of the ulcer, and the ulcer crater may have a lip or edge Purulent drainage is common	Deep ulcers that extend into muscle and bone Foul smelling Brown or black eschar Purulent drainage is common

based, and to avoid contact with excessively oil-based products

  i. Instruct the client on the importance of follow-up treatment

O. **Decubitus**
  1. Description
    a. An impairment of skin integrity
    b. Localized areas of necrosis of the skin and subcutaneous tissue as a result of pressure
    c. Prevention of skin breakdown is a major role of the nurse, particularly in caring for the bedridden or immobile client
  2. Risk factors
    a. Malnutrition
    b. Incontinence
    c. Immobility
    d. Skin shearing
    e. Decreased sensory perception
  3. Assessment (Table 47-2)
  4. Implementation
    a. Institute measures to prevent **decubitus**
    b. Assess the nutritional status of the client
    c. Provide adequate nutritional intake to promote tissue integrity
    d. Monitor for an alteration in skin integrity
    e. Relieve or remove pressure on the skin
    f. Turn and reposition the immobile client every 2 hours, or more frequently if necessary
    g. Ambulate the client
    h. Provide active and passive exercises every 8 hours
    i. Keep the skin clean and dry and the sheets wrinkle free
    j. Apply moisture barrier as prescribed to protect the skin
    k. Use assistive devices to prevent pressure, such as an air pressure mattress and/or sheepskin padding
    l. Apply medications or dressings to the wound as prescribed

VI. **BURN INJURIES**
  A. Description: Cell destruction of the layers of the skin and the resultant depletion of fluid and electrolytes
  B. **Burn** size
    1. Small **burns:** The body's response to injury is localized to the injured area
    2. Large or extensive **burns**
      a. Consist of 25% or more of the total body surface area (TBSA)
      b. The body's response to the injury is systemic
      c. Affect all of the major systems of the body
  C. Characteristics: Depth, extent, and location
    1. Minor **burns**
      a. **Partial-thickness burns** are no greater than 15% of the TBSA in the adult
      b. **Full-thickness burns** are less than 2% of the TBSA in the adult
      c. **Burn** areas do not involve the eyes, ears, hands, face, feet, or perineum
      d. There are no **electrical burns** or inhalation injuries
      e. The client is an adult younger than 60 years of age
      f. The client has no preexisting medical condition at the time of the **burn** injury
      g. No other injury occurred with the **burn**
    2. Moderate **burns**
      a. **Partial-thickness burns** are deep and are 15% to 25% of the TBSA in the adult
      b. **Full-thickness burns** are 2% to 10% of the TBSA in the adult
      c. **Burn** areas do not involve the eyes, ears, hands, face, feet, or perineum
      d. There are no **electrical burns** or inhalation injuries
      e. The client is an adult younger than 60 years of age
      f. The client has no chronic cardiac, pulmonary, or endocrine disorder at the time of the **burn** injury

TABLE 47-3

Methods to Estimate Extent of Burn Injury

Rule of Nines/Adult		Lund and Browder (Berkow) Method
Head and neck	9%	Modifies percentages for body segments according to age
Anterior trunk	18%	Provides a more accurate estimate of the burn size
Posterior trunk	18%	Uses a diagram of the body divided into sections, with the representative % of the TBSA*
Arms (9%)	18%	for ages throughout the life span
Legs (18%)	36%	Should be reevaluated after initial wound debridement
Perineum	1%	

*Total body surface area.

    g. No other complicated injury occurred with the **burn**

3. Major **burns**
    a. **Partial-thickness burns** are more than 25% of the TBSA in the adult
    b. **Full-thickness burns** are more than 10% of the TBSA
    c. **Burn** areas involve the eyes, ears, hands, face, feet, or perineum
    d. The **burn** injury was an electrical injury or inhalation injury
    e. The client is older than 60 years of age
    f. The client has a chronic cardiac, pulmonary, or metabolic disorder at the time of the **burn** injury
    g. **Burns** are accompanied by other injuries

▲ D. Estimating the extent of injury (Table 47-3)

E. **Burn** depth
  1. **Superficial thickness**
    a. Mild to severe erythema (pink to red), no blisters
    b. Skin blanches with pressure
    c. Painful, tingling
    d. Pain is eased by cooling
    e. Discomfort lasts about 48 hours; healing occurs in about 3 to 7 days
    f. Skin grafts are not required
  2. **Partial thickness**
    a. Large blisters covering an extensive area
    b. Edema
    c. Mottled red base and broken epidermis, with a wet, shiny, and weeping surface
    d. Painful
    e. Injured area is sensitive to cold air
    f. Superficial partial-thickness burn heals in 2 to 3 weeks
    g. Deep partial-thickness burn heals in 3 to 6 weeks
    h. Grafts may be used if the healing process is prolonged
  3. **Full thickness**
    a. Deep red, black, white, yellow, or brown area
    b. Injured surface appears dry

    c. Edema
    d. Tissue disruption with fat exposed
    e. Little or no pain
    f. Spontaneous healing will not occur
    g. Requires removal of eschar and split- or full-thickness skin grafting
    h. Scarring and wound contractures are likely to develop without preventive measures
    i. Healing takes weeks to months
  4. **Deep full thickness**
    a. Involves injury to the muscle and bone
    b. Injured area appears black
    c. Edema is usually absent
    d. Pain is absent
    e. No blisters
    f. Eschar is hard and inelastic
    g. Healing takes weeks to months
    h. Grafts are required

F. Age and general health
  1. Mortality rates are higher for children less than 4 years of age, particularly those less than 1 year old, and for clients over the age of 60 years
  2. Debilitating disorders, such as cardiac, respiratory, endocrine, and renal disorders, negatively influence the client's response to injury and treatment
  3. Mortality rate is higher when the client has a preexisting disorder at the time of the **burn** injury

G. **Burn** location
  1. **Burns** of the head, neck, and chest are associated with pulmonary complications
  2. **Burns** of the face are associated with corneal abrasion
  3. **Burns** of the ear are associated with auricular chondritis
  4. Hands and joints require intensive therapy to prevent disability
  5. The perineal area is prone to autocontamination by urine and feces
  6. Circumferential **burns** of the extremities can produce a tourniquet-like effect and lead to vascular compromise (compartment syndrome)
  7. Circumferential thoracic **burns** lead to inade-

quate chest wall expansion and pulmonary insufficiency

VII. TYPES OF BURNS

A. **Thermal burns:** Caused by exposure to flames, hot liquids, steam, or hot objects
B. **Chemical burns**
   1. Caused by tissue contact with strong acids, alkalis, or organic compounds
   2. Systemic toxicity from cutaneous absorption can occur
C. **Electrical burns**
   1. Caused by heat generated by electrical energy as it passes through the body
   2. Results in internal tissue damage
   3. Cutaneous burns cause muscle and soft tissue damage that may be extensive, particularly in high-voltage electrical injuries
   4. The voltage, type of current, contact site, and duration of contact are important to identify
   5. Alternating current is more dangerous than direct current because it is associated with cardiopulmonary arrest, ventricular fibrillation, tetanic muscle contractions, and long bone or vertebral fractures
D. **Radiation burns:** Caused by exposure to ultraviolet light, x-rays, or a radioactive source

VIII. INHALATION INJURIES

A. **Smoke inhalation injury**
   1. Description: Results from inhalation of superheated air, steam, toxic fumes, or smoke
   2. Assessment
      a. Facial **burns**
      b. Erythema
      c. Swelling of oropharynx and nasopharynx
      d. Singed nasal hairs
      e. Flaring nostrils
      f. Stridor, wheezing, and dyspnea
      g. Hoarse voice
      h. Sooty (carbonaceous) sputum and cough
      i. Agitation and anxiety
      j. Tachycardia
B. **Carbon monoxide poisoning**
   1. Description
      a. **Carbon monoxide** is a colorless, odorless, and tasteless gas that has an affinity for hemoglobin 200 times greater than that of oxygen
      b. Oxygen molecules are displaced, and **carbon monoxide** reversibly binds to hemoglobin to form carboxyhemoglobin
      c. Tissue hypoxia occurs
   2. Assessment (Table 47-4)
C. Smoke poisoning
   1. Description
      a. Caused by the inhalation of the by-products of combustion

TABLE 47-4

Carbon Monoxide Poisoning

Blood Level (%)	Clinical Manifestation
1-10	Impaired visual activity
11-20	Flushing
21-30	Nausea
	Impaired dexterity
31-40	Vomiting
	Dizziness
	Syncope
41-50	Tachypnea
	Tachycardia
Greater than 50	Coma and death

      b. A localized inflammatory reaction occurs, causing a decrease in bronchial ciliary action and a decrease in surfactant
   2. Assessment
      a. Mucosal edema in the airways
      b. Wheezing on auscultation
      c. After several hours, sloughing of the tracheobronchial epithelium may occur, and hemorrhagic bronchitis may develop
      d. Adult respiratory distress syndrome (ARDS) can result
D. Direct thermal heat injury
   1. Description
      a. Can occur to the lower airways by the inhalation of steam or explosive gases or the aspiration of scalding liquids
      b. Can occur to the upper airways, which appear erythematous and edematous, with mucosal blisters and ulcerations
      c. Mucosal edema can lead to upper airway obstruction, especially during the first 24 to 48 hours
      d. All clients with head or neck **burns** should be monitored closely for the development of airway obstruction and are immediately considered for endotracheal intubation if obstruction occurs
   2. Assessment
      a. Erythema and edema of the upper airways
      b. Mucosal blisters and ulcerations

IX. PATHOPHYSIOLOGY OF BURNS

A. Following the **burn,** vasoactive substances are released from the injured tissue, and these substances cause an increase in the capillary permeability, allowing the plasma to seep to the surrounding tissues
B. The direct injury to the vessels increases capillary permeability (capillary permeability decreases 18 to

26 hours postburn but does not normalize until 2 to 3 weeks following the injury)

C. Extensive **burns** result in generalized body edema and a decrease in circulating intravascular blood volume

D. The fluid losses result in a decrease in organ perfusion

E. The heart rate increases, cardiac output decreases, and the blood pressure drops

F. Initially hyponatremia and hyperkalemia occur

G. The hematocrit level increases as a result of plasma loss; this initial increase falls to below normal at the third to fourth day postburn as a result of the red blood cell (RBC) damage and loss at the time of injury

H. Initially, the body shunts blood from the kidneys, causing oliguria; then the body begins to reabsorb fluid, and diuresis of the excess fluid occurs over the next days to weeks

I. Blood flow to the gastrointestinal (GI) tract is diminished, leading to intestinal ileus and GI dysfunction

J. Immune system function is depressed, resulting in immunosuppression and thus increasing the risk of infection and sepsis

K. Pulmonary hypertension can develop, resulting in a decrease in the arterial oxygen tension and a decrease in lung compliance

L. Evaporative fluid losses through the **burn** wound are greater than normal, and the losses continue until complete wound closure occurs

M. If the intravascular space is not replenished with IV fluids, hypovolemic shock and ultimately death will occur

X. MANAGEMENT OF THE BURN INJURY (Box 47-2)

A. Emergent phase
   1. Description
      a. Begins at the time of injury and ends with the restoration of capillary permeability (fluid resuscitation), usually at 48 to 72 hours following the injury; includes prehospital and emergency room care
      b. The primary goal is to prevent hypovolemic shock and preserve vital organ functioning
   2. Prehospital care
      a. Begins at the scene of the accident and ends when emergency care is obtained
      b. Remove the victim from the source of the **burn**
      c. Remove the source of heat
      d. Assess airway, breathing, and circulation
      e. Assess for associated trauma
      f. Conserve body heat
      g. Cover **burns** with sterile or clean cloths
      h. Remove constricting jewelry and clothing
      i. Assess the need for intravenous fluids
      j. Transport

BOX 47-2

Phases of Management of the Burn Injury

EMERGENT PHASE
Begins at the time of injury and ends with the restoration of capillary permeability, usually at 48 to 72 hours after the injury
The primary goal is to prevent hypovolemic shock and preserve vital organ functioning
Includes prehospital care and emergency room care

RESUSCITATIVE PHASE
Begins with the initiation of fluids and ends when capillary integrity returns to near-normal levels and the large fluid shifts have decreased
The amount of fluid administered is based on the client's weight and the extent of injury
Most fluid replacement formulas are calculated from the time of injury and not from the time of arrival at the hospital
The goal is to prevent shock by maintaining adequate circulating blood volume and maintaining vital organ perfusion

ACUTE PHASE
Begins when the client is hemodynamically stable, capillary permeability is restored, and diuresis has begun
Usually begins 48 to 72 hours after the time of injury
Emphasis during this phase is placed on restorative therapy, and the phase continues until wound closure is achieved
The focus is on infection control, wound care, wound closure, nutritional support, pain management, and physical therapy

REHABILITATIVE PHASE
Final phase of burn care
Overlaps the acute care phase and goes well beyond hospitalization
Goals of this phase are designed so that the client can gain independence and achieve maximal function

---

   3. Emergency room care: Continuation of care administered at the scene of the injury
   4. Major **burns**
      a. Evaluate the degree and extent of the **burn** and treat life-threatening conditions
      b. Ensure a patent airway and administer 100% oxygen, as prescribed, if the **burn** occurred in an enclosed area
      c. Monitor for respiratory distress and assess the need for intubation
      d. Assess the oropharynx for blisters and erythema
      e. Monitor arterial blood gases (ABGs) and carboxyhemoglobin levels
      f. For an inhalation injury, administer 100% oxygen via a tight-fitting non-rebreather face mask, as prescribed, until carboxyhemoglobin levels fall below 15%

g. Initiate peripheral IV access to nonburned skin proximal to any extremity **burn**, or prepare for the insertion of a central venous pressure line, as prescribed

h. Assess for hypovolemia and prepare to administer IV fluids to maintain fluid balance

i. Monitor vital signs closely

j. Insert a Foley catheter as prescribed, and maintain urine output at 30 to 50 mL per hour

k. Maintain NPO status

l. Insert a nasogastric (NG) tube as prescribed, to prevent paralytic ileus, to prevent vomiting, and to reduce the risk of aspiration

m. Administer tetanus prophylaxis as prescribed

n. Administer pain medication, as prescribed, by the IV route

o. Prepare the client for an escharotomy or fasciotomy as prescribed

5. Minor **burns**

a. Administer small doses of morphine sulfate or meperidine (Demerol) as prescribed for pain

b. Instruct the client in the use of oral analgesics as prescribed

c. Administer tetanus prophylaxis as prescribed

d. Administer wound care as prescribed, which may include cleansing, debriding loose tissue, and removing any damaging agents, followed by the application of topical antimicrobial cream and a sterile dressing

e. Instruct the client in follow-up care, including active range-of-motion exercises and wound care treatments

▲ B. Resuscitative phase

1. Description

a. Begins with the initiation of fluids and ends when capillary integrity returns to near-normal levels and the large fluid shifts have decreased

b. The amount of fluid administered is based on client's weight and extent of injury

c. Most fluid replacement formulas are calculated from the time of injury and not from the time of arrival at the hospital

d. The goal is to prevent shock by maintaining adequate circulating blood volume and maintaining vital organ perfusion

2. Fluid resuscitation (Table 47-5)

a. The amount of fluid administered depends on how much intravenous fluid per hour is required to maintain a urinary output of 30 to 50 mL per hour

b. Successful fluid resuscitation is evidenced by stable vital signs, an adequate urine output, palpable peripheral pulses, and a clear sensorium

c. Urinary output is the most common and most sensitive assessment parameter for cardiac output and tissue perfusion

---

TABLE 47-5

Brooke and Parkland (Baxter) Fluid Resuscitation Formulas for First 24 Hours After a Burn Injury

Formula	Solution	Infusion Rate
BROOKE		
2 mL/kg/% BSA* burn	¾ crystalloid, ¼ colloid	½ in first 8 hours ½ in next 16 hours
+2000 mL/24 hr (maintenance)	D₅W maintenance	
PARKLAND (BAXTER)		
4 mL/kg/% BSA burn for 24-hr period	Crystalloid only (lactated Ringer's)	½ in first 8 hours ½ in next 16 hours

*Body surface area.

---

d. IV fluid replacement may be titrated (adjusted) on the basis of urinary output plus serum electrolyte levels to meet the perfusion needs of the **burn** client

e. If the hemoglobin and hematocrit levels decrease or if the urinary output exceeds 50 mL per hour, the rate of IV fluid administration may be decreased

3. Implementation

a. Monitor for tracheal or laryngeal edema, and administer respiratory treatments as prescribed

b. Monitor pulse oximetry and prepare for ABGs and carboxyhemoglobin (COHB) levels if inhalation injury is suspected

c. Elevate the head of the bed to 30 degrees or more for **burns** of the face and head

d. Initiate ECG monitoring

e. Monitor temperature and assess for infection

f. Initiate protective isolation techniques; maintain strict handwashing, use sterile sheets and linens when caring for the client, and use gloves, cap, masks, shoe covers, scrub clothes, and plastic aprons

g. Shave or cut body hair around wound margins

h. Monitor daily weights, expecting a weight gain of 15 to 20 pounds in the first 72 hours

i. Monitor gastric output and pH levels and for gastric discomfort and bleeding, indicating a stress ulcer

j. Administer antacids, H₂-receptor antagonists, and the antiulcer medication sucralfate (Carafate), as prescribed

k. Auscultate bowel sounds for ileus and monitor for abdominal distention and GI dysfunction

l. Monitor stools for occult blood

m. Obtain urine specimen for myoglobin and hemoglobin levels

n. Monitor IV fluids and hourly intake and output (I & O) to determine the adequacy of fluid replacement therapy; notify the physician if urine output is less than 30 or greater than 50 mL per hour

o. Elevate circumferential **burns** of the extremities on pillows above the level of heart to reduce dependent edema if no obvious fractures are present

p. Monitor pulses and capillary refill of the affected extremities, and assess perfusion of the distal extremity with a circumferential **burn**

q. Prepare for chest and other x-rays to rule out fractures or associated trauma

r. Keep the room temperature warm

s. Place the client on an air-fluidized bed and use a bed cradle to keep sheets off the client's skin

4. Pain management

a. Administer morphine sulfate or meperidine (Demerol), as prescribed, by the IV route

b. Avoid IM or SC routes because absorption through the soft tissue is unreliable when hypovolemia and large fluid shifts are occurring

c. Avoid administering medication by the oral route, because of the possibility of GI dysfunction

d. Medicate the client prior to painful procedures

5. Nutrition

a. Essential to promote wound healing and prevent infection

b. The basal metabolic rate (BMR) is 40 to 100 times higher than normal

c. Maintain nothing by mouth (NPO) status until the bowel sounds are heard; then advance to clear liquids as prescribed

d. Nutrition may be provided via enteral tube feeding, peripheral parenteral nutrition, or total parenteral nutrition

e. Provide a diet high in protein, carbohydrates, fats, and vitamins

f. Monitor calorie intake

6. Escharotomy

a. A lengthwise incision is made through the **burn** eschar to relieve constriction and pressure and to improve circulation

b. Performed for circulatory compromise resulting from circumferential **burns**

c. Performed at the bedside without anesthesia, because nerve endings have been destroyed by the **burn** injury

d. Escharotomy can be performed on the thorax to improve ventilation

e. After the escharotomy, assess pulses, color, movement, and sensation of affected extremity, and control any bleeding with pressure

f. Pack incision gently with fine-mesh gauze for 24 hours after escharotomy, as prescribed

g. Apply topical antimicrobial agents to the area, as prescribed, following the procedure

7. Fasciotomy

a. An incision is made, extending through the subcutaneous tissue and fascia

b. The procedure is performed if adequate tissue perfusion does not return after an escharotomy

c. Performed in the operating room with the client under general anesthesia

d. After the procedure, assess pulses, color, movement, and sensation of affected extremity, and control any bleeding with pressure

e. Apply topical antimicrobial agents and dressings to the area, as prescribed, after the procedure

C. Acute phase

1. Description

a. Begins when the client is hemodynamically stable, capillary permeability is restored, and diuresis has begun

b. Usually begins 48 to 72 hours after the time of injury

c. Emphasis during this phase is placed on restorative therapy, and the phase continues until wound closure is achieved

d. The focus is on infection control, wound care, wound closure, nutritional support, pain management, and physical therapy

2. Implementation

a. Continue with protective isolation techniques

b. Provide wound care as prescribed and prepare for wound closure

c. Provide pain management

d. Provide adequate nutrition as prescribed

e. Prepare client for rehabilitation

D. Wound care (Table 47-6)

1. Description: The cleansing, debridement, and dressing of the **burn** wounds

2. Hydrotherapy

a. Wounds are cleansed by immersion, showering, or spraying

b. Hydrotherapy occurs for 30 minutes or less, to prevent increased sodium loss through the **burn** wound, heat loss, pain, and stress

c. The client should be premedicated prior to the procedure

d. Hydrotherapy is generally not used for clients who are hemodynamically unstable or those with new skin grafts

e. Care is taken to minimize bleeding and maintain body temperature during the procedure

f. If hydrotherapy is not used, wounds are washed and rinsed in bed prior to the application of antimicrobial agents

TABLE 47-6

Open Method Versus Closed Method of Wound Care

Method	Advantages	Disadvantages
OPEN		
Antimicrobial cream applied, and wound is left open to the air without a dressing	Visualization of the wound	Increased change of hypothermia from exposure
Antimicrobial cream is applied every 12 hours	Easier mobility and joint range of motion	
	Simplicity in wound care	
CLOSED		
Gauze dressings are carefully wrapped from the distal to the proximal area of the extremity to ensure circulation is not compromised	Decreases evaporative fluid and heat loss	Mobility limitations
	Aids in debridement	Prevents effective range of motion exercises
No two burn surfaces should be allowed to touch, touching can promote webbing of digits, contractures, and poor cosmetic outcome		Wound assessment is limited
Dressings are changed every 8 to 12 hours		

TABLE 47-7

Debridement

Mechanical	Enzymatic	Surgical
Use of scissors and forceps to lift and trim away loose eschar	Application of prepared proteolytic and fibrinolytic topical enzymes that digest necrotic tissue, which facilitates eschar removal	Excision of eschar and coverage of wound
Wet to dry or wet to wet dressing changes		*Tangential:*
A painful procedure	Requires a moist environment to be effective; they are applied directly to the burn wound	Very thin layers of eschar are shaved until viable tissue is reached
		Fascial:
	Pain and bleeding are major problems	Used for very deep burns and removal of burn tissue and underlying fat down to the fascia

3. Debridement (Table 47-7)
   a. Removal of eschar to prevent bacterial proliferation under the eschar and to promote wound healing
   b. Debridement may be mechanical, enzymatic, or surgical
   c. Deep partial- or full-thickness burns: Wound is cleansed and debrided and topical antimicrobial agents are applied once or twice daily

E. Wound closure
   1. Description
      a. Prevents infection and loss of fluid
      b. Promotes healing
      c. Prevents contractures
      d. Performed on the 5th to 21st day, depending on the extent of the **burn**
   2. Temporary wound coverings (Box 47-3)
   3. Autografting (Box 47-4)
      a. Permanent wound coverage
      b. Surgical removal of a thin layer of the client's own unburned skin, which is then applied to the excised **burn** wound
      c. Performed in the operating room under anesthesia
      d. Monitor for bleeding following the graft, because bleeding beneath an autograft can prevent adherence
      e. Small amounts of blood or serum can be removed by gently rolling the fluid from the center of the graft to the periphery with a sterile gauze pad, where it can be absorbed
      f. For large accumulations of blood, the physician will aspirate the blood by using a small-gauge needle and syringe
      g. Autografts are immobilized after surgery for 3 to 7 days to allow time to adhere and attach to the wound bed
      h. Position for immobilization and elevation of the graft site to prevent movement, shearing of the graft, and edema

---

BOX 47-3

Temporary Wound Coverings

BIOLOGICAL
Amnion
Amniotic membranes from human placenta
Dressing is changed every 48 hours
Allograft (Homograft)
Donated human cadaver skin is harvested within 24 hours after death
Monitor for wound exudate and signs of infection
Rejection can occur within 24 hours
Xenograft (Heterograft)
Porcine skin is harvested after slaughter and preserved for storage
Rejection can occur within 24 to 72 hours
Xenograft over granulation tissue is replaced every 2 to 5 days until the wound heals naturally or until closure with autograft is complete

BIOSYNTHETIC AND SYNTHETIC
Visual inspection of wound is possible, as dressings are transparent or translucent
Monitor for wound exudate and signs of infection

BOX 47-4

Types of Skin Grafts

SPLIT THICKNESS
Graft of half of the epidermis; applied in sheets or postage stamp–like pieces

FULL THICKNESS
Graft consisting of epidermis and dermis; commonly used for reconstructive surgery months or years after the initial injury

PEDICLE FLAP
Commonly used for reconstructive surgery months or years after the initial injury

CULTURED EPITHELIUM
Use of the client's unburned skin
Keratinocytes are isolated and epithelial cells are cultured in a laboratory; these cells are then attached to the burn wound

---

4. Care of the graft site
   a. Elevate and immobilize graft site
   b. Keep site free from pressure
   c. Avoid weight bearing
   d. When the graft takes, roll a cotton-tipped applicator over the graft to remove exudate, because exudate can lead to infection and prevent graft adherence

   e. Monitor for foul-smelling drainage, increased temperature, increased white blood cell count, hematoma, or fluid accumulation
   f. Instruct the client to avoid using fabric softeners and harsh detergents in the laundry
   g. Instruct the client to lubricate healing skin with cocoa butter
   h. Instruct the client to protect the affected area from sunlight
   i. Instruct the client to use splints and support garments as prescribed

5. Care of the donor site
   a. Method of care will vary depending on physician's preference
   b. A moist gauze dressing is applied at the time of the surgery, to maintain pressure and stop any oozing
   c. The physician may prescribe site treatment with single-layer gauze impregnated with petrolatum or a biosynthetic dressing such as Biobrane
   d. Keep the donor site clean, dry, and free from pressure
   e. Prevent the client from scratching the donor site
   f. Apply lubricating lotions to soften the area and reduce the itching after the donor site is healed
   g. The donor site can be reused once healing has occurred (heals spontaneously within 7 to 14 days with proper care)

F. Physical therapy
   1. An individualized program of splinting, positioning, exercises, ambulation, and activities of daily living; implemented early in the acute phase of recovery to maximize functional and cosmetic outcomes
   2. Perform range-of-motion exercises as prescribed to reduce edema and maintain strength and joint function
   3. Ambulate the client as prescribed to maintain the strength of the lower extremities
   4. Apply splints as prescribed to maintain proper joint position and prevent contractures
      a. Static splints immobilize the joint and are applied for periods of immobilization, during sleeping, and for clients who cannot maintain proper positioning
      b. Dynamic splints exercise the affected joint
      c. Do not apply pressure to skin areas with splints, which could lead to further tissue and nerve damage
   5. Scarring is controlled by elastic wraps and bandages that apply continuous pressure to the healing skin during the period of time when the skin is vulnerable to shearing
   6. Antiburn scar support garments are worn 23

BOX 47-5

Surgical Options for Contractures and Scarring

Split-thickness and full-thickness skin grafts
Skin flaps
Z-plasties
Tissue expansion

hours a day until the **burn** scar tissue has matured, which takes 18 months to 2 years
G. Rehabilitative phase (Box 47-5)
 1. Description
  a. Final phase of **burn** care
  b. Overlaps the acute-care phase and goes well beyond hospitalization
  c. Goals of this phase are designed so that the client can gain independence and achieve maximal function
 2. Goals
  a. Promote wound healing
  b. Minimize deformities
  c. Increase strength and function
  d. Provide emotional support

PRACTICE QUESTIONS

1. A nurse is reviewing the health care records of clients scheduled to be seen at a health care clinic. The nurse determines that which of the following individuals is at the greatest risk for development of an integumentary disorder?
 1. An elderly female
 2. An adolescent
 3. An outdoor construction worker
 4. A physical education teacher
2. A client scheduled for a skin biopsy is concerned and asks a nurse how painful the procedure is. The most appropriate response by the nurse is:
 1. "There is no pain associated with this procedure."
 2. "There is some pain, but the physician will prescribe an analgesic following the procedure."
 3. "The local anesthetic may cause a burning or stinging sensation."
 4. "A preoperative medication will be given so you will be sleeping and will not feel any pain."
3. A nurse is reviewing the discharge instructions for a client who had a skin biopsy. Which of the following statements, if made by the client, would indicate a need for further instruction?
 1. "I will call the physician if I see any drainage from the wound."
 2. "I will return in 7 days to have the sutures removed."
 3. "I will use the antibiotic ointment as prescribed."

 4. "I will remove the dressing as soon as I get home and wash it with tap water."
4. A nurse prepares to assist a physician to examine a client's skin with a Wood's light. The nurse includes which of the following in the plan for this procedure?
 1. Obtain an informed consent
 2. Darken the room for the examination
 3. Shave the skin and scrub with Betadine solution
 4. Prepare a local anesthetic
5. A clinic nurse provides instructions to a client who is to return to the clinic in 1 week for a patch test. The patch test will be done to identify the allergen causing dermatitis. The nurse provides which instruction to the client?
 1. Remain NPO prior to the test
 2. Shower using an antibacterial soap on the morning of the test
 3. Discontinue the prescribed antihistamine 2 days before the test
 4. Consume only fluids on the day of the test
6. A nurse provides discharge instructions to a client after patch testing. Which statement if made by the client would indicate the need for further instruction?
 1. "I will return to the clinic in 2 days for the initial reading."
 2. "If the patch comes off, I need to reapply it."
 3. "I need to avoid activities that will cause me to sweat."
 4. "I need to keep the test sites dry at all times."
7. A clinic nurse implements a teaching plan for a client who has complained of chronic dry skin and episodes of pruritus. Which of the following if stated by the client would indicate a need for further teaching?
 1. "I should drink 8 to 10 glasses of water a day."
 2. "I need to avoid using astringents on my skin."
 3. "I should limit myself to one shower a day and apply emollient to my skin after the shower."
 4. "I should use a dehumidifier, especially during the winter months."
8. A camp nurse prepares to instruct a group of children about Lyme disease. Which of the following information would the nurse include in the instructions?
 1. It can be contagious by skin contact with an infected individual
 2. It can be caused by the inhalation of spores from bird droppings
 3. It is caused by contamination from cat feces
 4. It is caused by a tick carried by deer
9. A client is diagnosed with stage I of Lyme disease. A nurse assesses the client for which characteristic of this stage?
 1. Signs of neurological disorders
 2. Enlarged and inflamed joints

3. Arthralgias
4. Flulike symptoms

10. A female client arrives at a health care clinic and tells a nurse that she has just been bitten by a tick and would like to be tested for Lyme disease. The client tells the nurse that she removed the tick and flushed it down the toilet. Which of the following nursing actions is most appropriate?
    1. Refer the client for a blood test immediately
    2. Inform the client that there is not a test available for Lyme disease
    3. Instruct the client to return in 4 to 6 weeks to be tested, because testing before this time is not reliable
    4. Tell the client that testing is not necessary unless arthralgia develops

11. After diagnosis of Lyme disease, stage I, a nurse would anticipate that which of the following will be part of the treatment plan for the client?
    1. No treatment unless symptoms develop
    2. A 3-week course of oral antibiotic therapy
    3. Treatment with IV penicillin G
    4. Daily oatmeal baths for a period of 2 weeks

12. A cub scout leader who is a nurse is preparing a group of cub scouts for an overnight camping trip. The nurse provides the scouts with a list of methods to prevent Lyme disease. Which of the following would not be part of this list?
    1. Avoid the use of insect repellents, as they will attract the ticks
    2. Wear long-sleeved tops and long pants
    3. Bring a hat to wear during the trip
    4. Wear closed shoes and socks that can be pulled up over the pants

13. A male client calls an emergency room and tells a nurse that he has been cleaning a wooded area in the back yard and has discovered that he came directly in contact with poison ivy shrubs. The client tells the nurse that he cannot see anything on the skin and asks the nurse what to do. Which of the following is the most appropriate nursing response?
    1. "Come to the emergency room."
    2. "It is not necessary to do anything if you cannot see anything on your skin."
    3. "Take a shower immediately, lathering and rinsing several times."
    4. "Apply calamine lotion immediately to the exposed skin areas."

14. A client with acquired immunodeficiency syndrome (AIDS) is diagnosed with cutaneous Kaposi's sarcoma. A nurse understands that this diagnosis has been confirmed by which of the following?
    1. Appearance of reddish blue lesions on the skin
    2. Swelling in the lower extremities
    3. Punch biopsy of the cutaneous lesions
    4. Swelling in the genitalia area

15. Which of the following individuals is least likely to be at risk for the development of Kaposi's sarcoma?
    1. A male with a history of same-sex partners
    2. A renal transplant client
    3. A client receiving antineoplastic medications
    4. An individual working in an environment where exposure to asbestos exists

16. A nurse prepares to bathe and change the bed linens of a client with cutaneous Kaposi's sarcoma lesions. The lesions are open and draining a scant amount of serous fluid. Which of the following would the nurse most appropriately incorporate in the plan during the bathing of this client?
    1. Wearing a gown, gloves, and a mask
    2. Wearing a gown and gloves
    3. Wearing gloves
    4. Wearing a gown and gloves to change the bed linens and gloves only for the bath

17. A client is being admitted to the hospital for treatment of acute cellulitis of the lower left leg. The client asks the admitting nurse to explain what cellulitis means. The nurse bases the response on the understanding that the characteristics of cellulitis include:
    1. A skin infection into the dermis and subcutaneous tissue
    2. An acute superficial infection
    3. An inflammation of the epidermis
    4. An epidermal infection caused by *Staphylococcus*

18. A nurse prepares to care for a client with acute cellulitis of the lower leg. The nurse anticipates that which of the following will be prescribed for the client?
    1. Warm compresses to the affected area
    2. Cold compresses to the affected area
    3. Intermittent heat lamp treatments four times daily
    4. Alternating hot and cold compresses continuously

19. A clinic nurse assesses the skin of a Caucasian client with a diagnosis of psoriasis. The nurse understands that which characteristic is not associated with this skin disorder?
    1. Discoloration and pitting of the nails
    2. Silvery white, scaly patches on the scalp, elbows, knees, and sacral regions
    3. Complaints of pruritus
    4. Purple scaly lesions

20. Ultraviolet light (UVL) therapy is prescribed as a component of the treatment plan for a client with psoriasis. A nurse provides instructions to the client regarding the treatment. Which statement if made by the client indicates a need for further instructions?
    1. "Eye goggles need to be worn to prevent exposure to UVL."

2. "Treatments are limited to two or three times a week."

3. "The UVL treatments are given on consecutive days."

4. "Only the area requiring treatment should be exposed to the UVL."

21. A clinic nurse notes that the physician has documented a diagnosis of herpes zoster in a client's chart. On the basis of an understanding of the cause of this disorder, the nurse would determine that this definitive diagnosis was made following which diagnostic test?
    1. Skin biopsy
    2. Wood's light examination
    3. Culture of the lesion
    4. Patch test

22. A nurse is assigned to care for a client with herpes zoster. Which of the following characteristics would the nurse expect to note when assessing the lesions of this infection?
    1. A generalized body rash
    2. Small, blue-white spots with a red base
    3. A fiery red, edematous rash on the cheeks
    4. Clustered skin vesicles

23. A nurse manager is planning the clinical assignments for the day. The nurse manager avoids assigning which of the following staff members to a client with herpes zoster?
    1. A nurse who never had mumps
    2. An experienced registered nurse who never had chickenpox
    3. A nurse who never had roseola
    4. A nurse who never had German measles

24. A client returns to a clinic for follow-up treatment after a skin biopsy of a suspicious lesion that was performed 1 week ago. The biopsy report indicates that the lesion is a melanoma. The nurse understands that which of the following describes this type of lesion?
    1. Is highly metastatic
    2. Metastasis is rare
    3. Is characterized by local invasion
    4. Is encapsulated

25. When assessing a lesion diagnosed as malignant melanoma, a nurse would most likely expect to note which of the following?
    1. A small papule with a dry, rough scale
    2. A firm, nodular lesion topped with crust
    3. A pearly papule with a central crater and a waxy border
    4. An irregularly shaped lesion

26. A nurse prepares discharge instructions for a client after cryosurgery for the treatment of a malignant skin lesion. Which of the following would the nurse include in the plan of care?
    1. To clean the site with hydrogen peroxide to prevent infection

2. To apply ice to the site to prevent discomfort

3. To apply alcohol-soaked dressings twice a day

4. To avoid showering for 7 to 10 days

27. A health education nurse provides instructions to a group of clients regarding measures that will assist in preventing skin cancer. Which statement if made by a client indicates a need for further education?
    1. "I will use sunscreen when participating in outdoor activities."
    2. "I will examine my body monthly for any lesions that may be suspicious."
    3. "I will wear a hat, opaque clothing, and sunglasses when in the sun."
    4. "I will avoid sun exposure after 3:00 P.M."

28. A clinic nurse reviews a client's chart and notes that the physician has documented a diagnosis of paronychia. On the basis of this diagnosis, which of the following would the nurse expect to note during the assessment?
    1. Swelling of the skin near the parotid gland
    2. Red, shiny skin around the nailbed
    3. White, silvery patches on the elbows
    4. White, taut skin in the popliteal area

29. A nurse provides home care instructions to a client diagnosed with impetigo. Which of the following would not be a component of the teaching plan?
    1. Continue with the antibiotics as prescribed
    2. Wash the client's dishes separately from those of other household members
    3. It is not necessary to separate the client's linen and towels from those of other household members
    4. Wash hands thoroughly and frequently throughout the day

30. A client arriving at an emergency room has experienced frostbite of the right hand. Which of the following would a nurse note on assessment of the client's hand?
    1. Fiery red skin with edema in the nailbeds
    2. A pink, edematous hand
    3. Black fingertips surrounded by an erythematous rash
    4. A white color to the skin, which is insensitive to touch

31. A nurse prepares to treat a client with frostbite of the toes. Which of the following does the nurse anticipate to be prescribed for this condition?
    1. Rapid and continuous rewarming of the toes in a warm water bath until flushing of the skin occurs
    2. Rapid and continuous rewarming of the toes in hot water for 15 to 20 minutes
    3. Rapid and continuous rewarming of the toes after flushing returns
    4. Rapid and continuous rewarming of the toes in cold water for 45 minutes

32. An evening nurse reviews the nursing documentation in a client's chart and notes that the day nurse

has documented that the client has a stage II pressure ulcer (decubitus) in the sacral area. Which of the following would the nurse expect to note on assessment of the client's sacral area?

1. Skin is intact
2. Partial-thickness skin loss of the epidermis
3. A deep, crater-like appearance
4. The presence of sinus tracts

33. A nurse is assessing for the presence of cyanosis in a dark-skinned client. The nurse understands that which body area would provide the best assessment?

1. Backs of the hands
2. Earlobes
3. Palms of the hands
4. Sacrum

34. Which of the following individuals is least likely to be at risk for the development of psoriasis?

1. A 32-year-old African-American
2. A client with a family history of the disorder
3. An individual who has experienced a significant amount of emotional distress
4. A woman experiencing menopause

35. Which of the following clients would least likely be at risk for the development of skin breakdown?

1. A client who is unable to move about and is confined to bed
2. A client incontinent of urine and feces
3. A client with chronic nutritional deficiencies
4. A client with a lowered mental awareness status

36. A nurse is implementing a teaching plan for a group of adolescents regarding the causes of acne. Which of the following is the most appropriate nursing statement regarding the cause of this disorder?

1. "It is caused by eating chocolate, nuts, and fatty foods."
2. "It is caused by oily skin."
3. "The actual cause is not known."
4. "It is a result of exposure to heat and humidity."

37. Isotretinoin (Accutane) is prescribed for a client with severe cystic acne. A nurse provides instructions to the client regarding administration of the medication. Which of the following if stated by the client would indicate a need for further teaching regarding this medication?

1. "I need to continue to take my vitamin A supplements."
2. "I need to use emollients and lip balms for my dry skin and lips."
3. "The medication may cause dryness and burning in my eyes."
4. "I will need to return for a blood test to check my triglyceride level."

38. A clinic nurse inspects the skin of a client suspected of having scabies. Which of the following assess-

ment findings would the nurse note if this disorder were present?

1. The appearance of vesicles or pustules with a thick honey-colored crust
2. The presence of white patches scattered about the trunk
3. Multiple straight or wavy, threadlike lines beneath the skin
4. Patchy hair loss and round red macules with scales

39. A home health nurse visits a client suspected of having scabies. Which of the following precautions will the nurse institute during the assessment of the client?

1. Wear a mask and gloves
2. Wear gloves only
3. Wear a gown and gloves
4. Avoid touching client's home furnishings

40. A nurse inspects the oral cavity of a client with candidiasis (thrush). Which of the following would the nurse expect to note?

1. The presence of numerous small, red pinpoint lesions
2. The presence of blisters
3. The presence of white patches
4. The presence of purple-colored patches

41. A client was burned at 7:00 A.M. The client states that before the burn, the body weight was 198 pounds (90 kg). Using the Lund and Browder method, a physician has estimated that the total body surface area (TBSA) burned is 83%. Using the Parkland (Baxter) formula, a nurse determines that the total amount of intravenous lactated Ringer's solution that the client will receive by 3:00 P.M. of the same day that the burn occurred is which of the following?

1. 3735 mL
2. 7470 mL
3. 14,940 mL
4. 29,880 mL

42. A nurse is preparing to care for a burn client scheduled for an escharotomy procedure being performed for a third-degree circumferential arm burn. The nurse understands that the anticipated therapeutic outcome of the escharotomy is:

1. Brisk bleeding from the site
2. Formation of granulation tissue
3. Decreasing edema formation
4. Return of distal pulses

43. A client sustained a burn from cutaneous exposure to lye. At the site of injury, copious irrigation of the site was performed for 1 full hour. On the client's admission to the emergency department, the nurse assesses the burn site and determines that the presence of which of the following indicates that the chemical burn process is continuing?

1. Eschar

2. Liquefaction

3. Cherry-red, firm tissue

4. Intact blisters

44. A client is undergoing radiation therapy to treat lung cancer. After the treatment, the nurse notes erythema on the client's chest and neck, and the client is complaining of pain at the radiation site. The nurse interprets this assessment data as:

1. A superficial injury to tissue from the radiation

2. An allergic reaction to the radiation

3. A cutaneous reaction to products formed by the lysis of the neoplastic cells

4. An ischemic injury, much like decubitus formation, resulting from pressure from the linear accelerator

45. A nurse is caring for a client who sustained second- and third-degree burns on the anterior lower legs and anterior thorax. Which of the following does the nurse expect to note during the emergent phase of the burn injury?

1. Decreased heart rate

2. Increased blood pressure

3. Elevated hematocrit levels

4. Increased urinary output

46. A nurse is caring for a client who suffered an inhalation injury from a wood stove. The carbon monoxide blood report reveals a level of 12%. On the basis of this level, the nurse would anticipate which of the following signs in the client?

1. Flushing

2. Dizziness

3. Tachycardia

4. Coma

47. A client arrives at an emergency room after a burn injury that occurred in the basement at home. An inhalation injury is suspected. Which of the following would the nurse anticipate to be prescribed for the client?

1. 100% oxygen via a tight-fitting rebreather face mask

2. Oxygen via nasal cannula at 15 liters

3. 100% oxygen via a tight-fitting, non-rebreather face mask

4. Oxygen via nasal cannula at 10 liters

48. A nurse is administering IV fluids as prescribed to a client who sustained second- and third-degree burns of the back and legs. In evaluating the adequacy of fluid resuscitation, the nurse understands that which of the following would provide the most reliable indicator for determining the adequacy?

1. Vital signs

2. Urine output

3. Peripheral pulses

4. Mental status

49. A nurse is preparing to care for a burn client in protective isolation. The nurse plans care, knowing that which of the following is not a component of protective isolation techniques?

1. Using sterile sheets and linens

2. Strict handwashing

3. Wearing gloves and a gown only when giving direct care to the client

4. Wearing protective garb, including a mask, gloves, cap, shoe covers, scrub clothes, and plastic aprons

50. A nurse is caring for a client following an autograft to a burn wound on the right knee. Which of the following would the nurse anticipate to be prescribed for the client?

1. Immobilization of the affected leg

2. Out-of-bed activities

3. Placing the affected leg in a dependent position

4. Barhroom privileges

CRITICAL THINKING: FREE-TEXT ENTRY

An adult client was burned as a result of an explosion. The burn initially affected the client's entire face (anterior half of the head) and the upper half of the anterior torso, and there were circumferential burns to the lower half of both of the arms. The client's clothes caught on fire, and the client ran, causing subsequent burn injuries to the posterior surface of the head and the upper half of the posterior torso. According to the rule of nines, the extent of the burn injury would be which of the following?

Answer: _____

ANSWERS

1. **3**

Rationale: Prolonged exposure to the sun, unusual cold, or other conditions can damage the skin. The outdoor construction worker would fit into a high-risk category for the development of an integumentary disorder. Immobility and lack of nutrition would increase the elderly person's risk, but the elderly client is not at as high a risk as the outdoor construction worker. An adolescent may be prone to the development of acne, but this does not occur in all adolescents. The physical education teacher is at low or no risk of developing an integumentary problem.

Test-Taking Strategy: Use the process of elimination. Note the key words "greatest risk." Eliminate option 4 first. Eliminate

options 1 and 2 next because not all elderly persons or adolescents are at risk for the development of integumentary disorders. Noting the key word "outdoor" in option 3 should easily direct you to this option. If you had difficulty with this question, review the risk factors associated with integumentary disorders.
Level of Cognitive Ability: Analysis
Client Needs: Health Promotion and Maintenance
Integrated Concept/Process: Nursing Process/Assessment
Content Area: Adult Health/Integumentary
Reference: Lewis, S., Heitkemper, M., & Dirksen, S. (2000). *Medical-surgical nursing: Assessment and management of clinical problems* (5th ed.). St. Louis: Mosby, p. 493.

2. **3**
Rationale: Depending on the size and location of the lesion, a biopsy is usually a quick and almost painless procedure. The most common source of pain is the initial local anesthetic, which can produce a burning or stinging sensation. Preoperative medication is not necessary with this procedure.
Test-Taking Strategy: Use the process of elimination. Eliminate option 1 first because of the words "no pain." Eliminate option 2 because this option addresses care after the procedure, which is not the issue of the client's question to the nurse. Eliminate option 4 because a preoperative medication that puts the client to sleep is not a part of the procedure for a skin biopsy. If you had difficulty with this question, review the procedure related to a skin biopsy.
Level of Cognitive Ability: Application
Client Needs: Psychosocial Integrity
Integrated Concept/Process: Caring
Content Area: Adult Health/Integumentary
Reference: Ignatavicius, D., Workman, M., & Mishler, M. (1999). *Medical-surgical nursing across the health care continuum* (3rd ed.). Philadelphia: W.B. Saunders, p. 1709.

3. **4**
Rationale: After a skin biopsy, the nurse instructs the client to keep the dressing dry and in place for a minimum of 8 hours. After the dressing is removed, the site is cleaned once a day with tap water or saline to remove any dry blood or crusts. The physician may prescribe an antibiotic ointment to minimize local bacterial colonization. The nurse instructs the client to report any redness or excessive drainage at the site. Sutures are usually removed 7 to 10 days after biopsy.
Test-Taking Strategy: Use the process of elimination. Note the key words "indicate a need for further instruction." Eliminate option 3 first because of the words "as prescribed." Eliminate options 1 and 2 next. A client needs to report signs of drainage and needs to return to the physician for follow-up and suture removal. Consider the alteration in skin integrity that occurs with a skin biopsy. This should assist in directing you to option 4. Review care to the client following this procedure if you had difficulty with this question.
Level of Cognitive Ability: Analysis
Client Needs: Health Promotion and Maintenance
Integrated Concept/Process: Teaching/Learning
Content Area: Adult Health/Integumentary
Reference: Ignatavicius, D., Workman, M., & Mishler, M. (1999). *Medical-surgical nursing across the health care continuum* (3rd ed.). Philadelphia: W.B. Saunders, p. 1709.

4. **2**
Rationale: Examination of the skin under a Wood's light is always carried out in a darkened room. This is a noninvasive examination; therefore an informed consent is not required. A hand-held long wavelength ultraviolet light or a Wood's light is used. The skin does not need to be shaved, nor is a local anesthetic necessary. Areas of blue-green or red fluorescence are associated with certain skin infections. The procedure is painless.
Test-Taking Strategy: Use the process of elimination. Knowing that this is a noninvasive procedure will assist in eliminating options 1, 3, and 4. Review this procedure if you had difficulty answering this question.
Level of Cognitive Ability: Application
Client Needs: Physiological Integrity
Integrated Concept/Process: Nursing Process/Planning
Content Area: Adult Health/Integumentary
Reference: Ignatavicius, D., Workman, M., & Mishler, M. (1999). *Medical-surgical nursing across the health care continuum* (3rd ed.). Philadelphia: W.B. Saunders, p. 1709.

5. **3**
Rationale: Client preparation for a patch test includes instructing the client to discontinue the administration of systemic corticosteroids or antihistamines for at least 48 hours before the test. These medications must be discontinued to prevent suppression of the inflammatory response to the allergen. Topical steroid therapy may be continued, as long as the agent is not applied on the area to be tested. There is no need to restrict fluids or to remain NPO prior to the procedure. A patch test does not require a body shower with an antibacterial soap.
Test-Taking Strategy: Use the process of elimination. Eliminate options 1 and 4 first because these options are similar. From the remaining options, note the relationship between "allergen" in the question and "antihistamine" in the correct option. Review client preparation for a patch test if you had difficulty with this question.
Level of Cognitive Ability: Application
Client Needs: Physiological Integrity
Integrated Concept/Process: Teaching/Learning
Content Area: Adult Health/Integumentary
Reference: Ignatavicius, D., Workman, M., & Mishler, M. (1999). *Medical-surgical nursing across the health care continuum* (3rd ed.). Philadelphia: W.B. Saunders, p. 1709.

6. **2**
Rationale: If the client reapplies patches that come loose, this can interfere with an accurate interpretation of the allergic reactions. The nurse reinforces the necessity of removing loose or nonadherent test patches for reapplication at a later date. The initial reading is performed 2 days after application, and the final reading is performed 2 to 5 days later. The nurse instructs the client to keep the test sites dry at all times. The nurse also discourages physical activity that will result in sweating.
Test-Taking Strategy: Use the process of elimination. Note the key words "the need for further instruction." Eliminate options 3 and 4 first, since keeping the test site dry and avoiding sweating are similar. Knowledge that follow-up is important after any procedure should assist in directing you to

option 2. If you had difficulty with this question, review the client teaching points following a patch test.
Level of Cognitive Ability: Analysis
Client Needs: Health Promotion and Maintenance
Integrated Concept/Process: Teaching/Learning
Content Area: Adult Health/Integumentary
Reference: Ignatavicius, D., Workman, M., & Mishler, M. (1999). *Medical-surgical nursing across the health care continuum* (3rd ed.). Philadelphia: W.B. Saunders, p. 1709.

7. **4**
Rationale: The client should avoid using a dehumidifier because this will further dry room air. Instead, the client should use a room humidifier during the winter months or whenever the furnace is in use. The client should be taught to maintain a daily fluid intake of 3000 mL, unless contraindicated, and should avoid alcohol and caffeine ingestion. The client should avoid applying rubbing alcohol, astringents, or other drying agents to the skin. One bath or one shower per day for 15 to 20 minutes with warm water and a mild soap should be immediately followed by the application of an emollient to prevent evaporation of water from the hydrated epidermis.
Test-Taking Strategy: Use the process of elimination. Note the key words "a need for further teaching." Recalling that a dehumidifier is going to dry the air in the environment will assist in directing you to option 4. If you had difficulty with this question, review the client-teaching points related to dry skin and pruritus.
Level of Cognitive Ability: Analysis
Client Needs: Health Promotion and Maintenance
Integrated Concept/Process: Teaching/Learning
Content Area: Adult Health/Integumentary
Reference: Smeltzer, S., & Bare, B. (2000). *Brunner & Suddarth's textbook of medical-surgical nursing* (9th ed.). Philadelphia: Lippincott Williams & Wilkins, p. 1463.

8. **4**
Rationale: Lyme disease is a multisystem infection that results from a bite by a tick carried by several species of deer. Persons bitten by the *Ixodes* ticks are infected with the spirochete *Borrelia burgdorferi.* Lyme disease cannot be transmitted from one person to another. Histoplasmosis is caused by the inhalation of spores from bat or bird droppings. Toxoplasmosis is caused by the ingestion of cysts from contaminated cat feces.
Test-Taking Strategy: Use the process of elimination. Recalling that this disease is caused by a bite will assist in eliminating the incorrect options. If you had difficulty with this question, review the cause of Lyme disease.
Level of Cognitive Ability: Application
Client Needs: Health Promotion and Maintenance
Integrated Concept/Process: Teaching/Learning
Content Area: Adult Health/Integumentary
Reference: Smeltzer, S., & Bare, B. (2000). *Brunner & Suddarth's textbook of medical-surgical nursing* (9th ed.). Philadelphia: Lippincott Williams & Wilkins, p. 1884.

9. **4**
Rationale: The hallmark of stage I is the development of a skin rash within 2 to 30 days of infection, generally at the site of the tick bite. The rash develops into a concentric ring, giving it a

bull's eye appearance. The lesion enlarges up to 50 to 60 cm, and smaller lesions develop farther away from the original tick bite. In stage I, most infected persons develop flulike symptoms that last 7 to 10 days, and these symptoms may recur later. Neurological deficits occur in stage II. Arthralgias and joint enlargements are most likely to be noted in stage III.
Test-Taking Strategy: Use the process of elimination and eliminate options 2 and 3 first because they are similar. Next, note that the question asks for the characteristic of stage I. From the remaining two options, select the least serious, since the issue of the question relates to stage I. Expect neurological disorders to occur with progression of the disease. If you had difficulty with this question, review the stages of Lyme disease.
Level of Cognitive Ability: Analysis
Client Needs: Physiological Integrity
Integrated Concept/Process: Nursing Process/Assessment
Content Area: Adult Health/Integumentary
Reference: LeMone, P., & Burke, K. (2000). *Medical-surgical nursing: Critical thinking in client care* (2nd ed.). Upper Saddle River, N.J.: Prentice-Hall, p. 1669.

10. **3**
Rationale: A blood test is available to detect Lyme disease; however, it is not a reliable test if performed prior to 4 to 6 weeks following the tick bite. Antibody formation takes place in the following manner: IgM is detected 3 to 4 weeks after Lyme disease onset, peaks at 6 to 8 weeks, and then gradually disappears; IgG is detected 2 to 3 months after infection and may remain elevated for years. Options 1, 2, and 4 are incorrect.
Test-Taking Strategy: Use the process of elimination. Eliminate option 1 first. The word "immediately" should indicate that this is potentially an incorrect option. A blood test is available; therefore eliminate option 2. Eliminate option 4 because treatment should begin before the arthralgia develops. If you had difficulty with this question, review the method of diagnosing Lyme disease.
Level of Cognitive Ability: Application
Client Needs: Physiological Integrity
Integrated Concept/Process: Teaching/Learning
Content Area: Adult Health/Integumentary
Reference: LeMone, P., & Burke, K. (2000). *Medical-surgical nursing: Critical thinking in client care* (2nd ed.). Upper Saddle River, N.J.: Prentice-Hall, p. 1669.

11. **2**
Rationale: Prevention, public education, and early diagnosis are vital to the control and treatment of Lyme disease. A 3-week course of oral antibiotic therapy is recommended during stage I. Later stages of Lyme disease may require therapy with intravenous antibiotics, such as penicillin G. Options 1 and 4 are incorrect.
Test-Taking Strategy: Use the process of elimination. Note that the question addresses stage I. Eliminate option 3 because IV antibiotics will not be administered in this stage. Eliminate option 4, because although oatmeal baths may be helpful for pruritus, they would not be helpful for a systemic disorder. Waiting for symptoms to develop is an incorrect option. Review the treatment associated with Lyme disease if you had difficulty with this question.
Level of Cognitive Ability: Analysis

Client Needs: Physiological Integrity
Integrated Concept/Process: Nursing Process/Planning
Content Area: Adult Health/Integumentary
Reference: LeMone, P., & Burke, K. (2000). *Medical-surgical nursing: Critical thinking in client care* (2nd ed.). Upper Saddle River, N.J.: Prentice-Hall, p. 1669.

12. 1
Rationale: In the prevention of Lyme disease, individuals need to be instructed to use an insect repellent on the skin and clothes when they are in an area where ticks are likely to be found. Long-sleeve tops and long pants, closed shoes, and a hat or cap should be worn. If possible, heavily wooded areas or areas with thick underbrush should be avoided. Socks can be pulled up and over the pant legs to the prevent ticks from entering under clothing.
Test-Taking Strategy: Use the process of elimination. Note the key words "would not be part of this list." Note that option 1 uses the word "avoid." Reading carefully will assist in directing you to this option. If you had difficulty with this question, review the measures to prevent contact with ticks.
Level of Cognitive Ability: Application
Client Needs: Health Promotion and Maintenance
Integrated Concept/Process: Nursing Process/Implementation
Content Area: Adult Health/Integumentary
Reference: Lewis, S., Heitkemper, M., & Dirksen, S. (2000). *Medical-surgical nursing: Assessment and management of clinical problems* (5th ed.). St. Louis: Mosby, p. 493.

13. 3
Rationale: When an individual comes in contact with a poison ivy plant, the sap from the plant forms an invisible film upon the human skin. The client should be instructed to immediately shower and that the skin should be lathered several times and rinsed each time in running water. Calamine lotion is a treatment that is used if dermatitis develops. It is not necessary for the client to be seen in the emergency room at this time.
Test-Taking Strategy: Use the process of elimination. Recalling that dermatitis can develop from contact with an allergen and that contact with poison ivy results in an invisible film will assist in directing you to option 3. Review the immediate treatment for contact with poison ivy, if you had difficulty with this question.
Level of Cognitive Ability: Application
Client Needs: Health Promotion and Maintenance
Integrated Concept/Process: Nursing Process/Implementation
Content Area: Adult Health/Integumentary
Reference: Phipps, W., Sands, J., & Marek, J. (1999). *Medical-surgical nursing: Concepts & clinical practice* (6th ed.). St. Louis: Mosby, p. 2079.

14. 3
Rationale: Kaposi's sarcoma lesions begin as red, dark blue, or purple macules on the lower legs that change into plaques. These large plaques ulcerate or open and drain. The lesions spread by metastasis through the upper body and then to the face and oral mucosa. They can move to the lymphatic system, lungs, and gastrointestinal (GI) tract. Late disease results in swelling and pain in the lower extremities, penis, scrotum, or face. Diagnosis is made by punch biopsy of cutaneous lesions and biopsy of pulmonary and GI lesions.
Test-Taking Strategy: Use the process of elimination. Eliminate options 2 and 4 first because these symptoms occur late in the

development of Kaposi's sarcoma. From the remaining options, note the key word "confirmed." This key word will assist in directing you to the option that will confirm the diagnosis, the biopsy of the lesions. Review diagnostic measures for Kaposi's sarcoma if you had difficulty with this question.
Level of Cognitive Ability: Analysis
Client Needs: Physiological Integrity
Integrated Concept/Process: Nursing Process/Assessment
Content Area: Adult Health/Integumentary
Reference: Phipps, W., Sands, J., & Marek, J. (1999). *Medical-surgical nursing: Concepts & clinical practice* (6th ed.). St. Louis: Mosby, p. 2089.

15. 4
Rationale: Kaposi's sarcoma is a vascular malignancy that presents as a skin disorder. It is a common acquired immunodeficiency syndrome (AIDS) indicator. Malignancy is seen most frequently in men with a history of same-sex partners. Although the cause of Kaposi's sarcoma is not known, it is considered to be due to an alteration or failure in the immune system. The renal transplant client and the client receiving antineoplastic medications are at risk for immunosuppression. Exposure to asbestos is not related to the development of Kaposi's sarcoma.
Test-Taking Strategy: Use the process of elimination. Note the key words "least likely to be at risk." Option 1 can be easily eliminated. Note the similarity between options 2 and 3. These clients are at risk for immunosuppression. With this in mind, these options can be eliminated. If you had difficulty with this question, review the risk factors associated with Kaposi's sarcoma.
Level of Cognitive Ability: Analysis
Client Needs: Physiological Integrity
Integrated Concept/Process: Nursing Process/Assessment
Content Area: Adult Health/Integumentary
Reference: Phipps, W., Sands, J., & Marek, J. (1999). *Medical-surgical nursing: Concepts & clinical practice* (6th ed.). St. Louis: Mosby, p. 2089.

16. 2
Rationale: Gowns and gloves are required if the nurse anticipates contact with soiled items such as from wound drainage, or in caring for a client who is incontinent with diarrhea, or a client who has an ileostomy or a colostomy. Masks are not required unless droplet or airborne precautions are necessary. Regardless of the amount of wound drainage, a gown and gloves must be worn.
Test-Taking Strategy: Use the process of elimination and think about the method of transmission of infection when answering a question of this type. Read the question, noting the task that is presented; in this case, it is bathing and changing linens. Eliminate option 1 because the method of transmission is not respiratory in nature. Eliminate options 3 and 4 because neither provides adequate protection based on the method of transmission. If you had difficulty with this question, review standard and transmission-based precautions.
Level of Cognitive Ability: Application
Client Needs: Safe, Effective Care Environment
Integrated Concept/Process: Nursing Process/Planning
Content Area: Adult Health/Integumentary

Reference: Potter, P., & Perry, A. (2001). *Fundamentals of nursing* (5th ed.). St. Louis: Mosby, pp. 858-859.

17. 1

Rationale: Cellulitis is a skin infection into deeper dermis and subcutaneous tissue that results in a deep red erythema without sharp borders and spreads widely through tissue spaces. The skin is erythematous, edematous, tender, and sometimes nodular. Erysipelas is an acute, superficial, rapidly spreading inflammation of the dermis and lymphatics.

Test-Taking Strategy: Use the process of elimination. Eliminate options 2, 3, and 4 because they are similar. If you had difficulty with this question, review the characteristics of cellulitis and erysipelas.

Level of Cognitive Ability: Comprehension
Client Needs: Physiological Integrity
Integrated Concept/Process: Nursing Process/Planning
Content Area: Adult Health/Integumentary
Reference: LeMone, P., & Burke, K. (2000). *Medical-surgical nursing: Critical thinking in client care* (2nd ed.). Upper Saddle River, N.J.: Prentice-Hall, p. 576.

18. 1

Rationale: Warm compresses may be used to decrease the discomfort, erythema, and edema. After tissue and blood cultures are obtained, antibiotics will be initiated. The nurse should provide supportive care as prescribed to manage symptoms such as fatigue, fever, chills, headache, and myalgia. Heat lamps can cause more disruption to already inflamed tissue. Cold compresses and alternating cold and hot compresses are not the best measures.

Test-Taking Strategy: Use the process of elimination, noting that option 1 is different from the other options. The words "cold," "heat," and "hot" identify extremes in temperature. If you had difficulty with this question, review the treatment associated with cellulitis.

Level of Cognitive Ability: Analysis
Client Needs: Physiological Integrity
Integrated Concept/Process: Nursing Process/Planning
Content Area: Adult Health/Integumentary
Reference: Lewis, S., Heitkemper, M., & Dirksen, S. (2000). *Medical-surgical nursing: Assessment and management of clinical problems* (5th ed.). St. Louis: Mosby, p. 506.

19. 4

Rationale: Psoriatic patches are covered with silvery white scales. Affected areas include the scalp, elbows, knees, shins, sacral area, and trunk. Thickening, pitting, and discoloration of the nails occur. Pruritus may occur. The lesions in psoriasis are not purple scaly lesions.

Test-Taking Strategy: Use the process of elimination. Note the key word "not." Recalling that psoriasis is associated with the presence of silvery white, scaly patches will easily direct you to option 4. If you had difficulty with this question, review the manifestations associated with psoriasis.

Level of Cognitive Ability: Comprehension
Client Needs: Physiological Integrity
Integrated Concept/Process: Nursing Process/Assessment
Content Area: Adult Health/Integumentary
Reference: Ignatavicius, D., Workman, M., & Mishler, M. (1999). *Medical-surgical nursing across the health care continuum* (3rd ed.). Philadelphia: W.B. Saunders, p. 1739.

20. 3

Rationale: UVL treatments are limited to two or three times a week and are not given on consecutive days. Safety precautions are required during UVL therapy. It is best to expose to the UVL only those areas requiring treatment Protective wrap-around goggles prevent exposure of the eyes to UVL. The face should be shielded with a loosely applied pillow case if it is unaffected. Direct contact with the light bulbs of the treatment unit should be avoided to prevent burning of the skin.

Test-Taking Strategy: Use the process of elimination. Note the key words "indicates a need for further instructions." Recalling that safety precautions are necessary for this treatment and noting the words "given on consecutive days" will direct you to this option. If you had difficulty with this question, review client education for UVL treatments.

Level of Cognitive Ability: Analysis
Client Needs: Health Promotion and Maintenance
Integrated Concept/Process: Teaching/Learning
Content Area: Adult Health/Integumentary
Reference: Ignatavicius, D., Workman, M., & Mishler, M. (1999). *Medical-surgical nursing across the health care continuum* (3rd ed.). Philadelphia: W.B. Saunders, p. 1740.

21. 3

Rationale: With classic presentation of herpes zoster, the clinical examination is diagnostic. A viral culture of the lesion provides the definitive diagnosis. Herpes zoster is caused by a reactivation of the varicella-zoster virus, the cause of chickenpox. A biopsy would provide a cytological examination of tissue. In a Wood's light examination, the skin is viewed under ultraviolet light to identify superficial infections of the skin. A patch test is a skin test that involves the administration of an allergen to the skin's surface to identify specific allergies.

Test-Taking Strategy: Use the process of elimination. Recalling that herpes zoster is caused by a virus will assist in directing you to the correct option. Remember that a biopsy will determine tissue type, whereas a culture will identify an organism. Review the diagnostic measures for herpes zoster if you had difficulty with this question.

Level of Cognitive Ability: Comprehension
Client Needs: Physiological Integrity
Integrated Concept/Process: Nursing Process/Assessment
Content Area: Adult Health/Integumentary
Reference: Lewis, S., Heitkemper, M., & Dirksen, S. (2000). *Medical-surgical nursing: Assessment and management of clinical problems* (5th ed.). St. Louis: Mosby, p. 507.

22. 4

Rationale: The primary lesion of herpes zoster is a vesicle. The classic presentation is grouped vesicles on an erythematous base along a dermatome. Because they follow nerve pathways, the lesions do not cross the body's midline. Options 1, 2, and 3 are incorrect descriptions of herpes zoster.

Test-Taking Strategy: Use the process of elimination. Remembering that these lesions occur as grouped vesicles along a nerve pathway will assist in answering the question. If you had difficulty with this question, review the characteristics of herpes zoster lesions.

Level of Cognitive Ability: Analysis
Client Needs: Physiological Integrity
Integrated Concept/Process: Nursing Process/Assessment
Content Area: Adult Health/Integumentary

Reference: Lewis, S., Heitkemper, M., & Dirksen, S. (2000). *Medical-surgical nursing: Assessment and management of clinical problems* (5th ed.). St. Louis: Mosby, p. 507.

23. 2

Rationale: Herpes zoster is caused by a reactivation of the varicella-zoster virus, the causative virus for chickenpox. Individuals who have not been exposed to the varicella-zoster virus are susceptible to chickenpox. Health care workers who are unsure of their immune status should have varicella titers done before exposure to a person with herpes zoster. Options 1, 3, and 4 are unrelated to the herpes zoster virus.

Test-Taking Strategy: Use the process of elimination. Recalling that herpes zoster is caused by a reactivation of the varicella-zoster virus, the causative virus for chickenpox, will direct you to the correct option. Review the relationship between herpes zoster virus and chickenpox if you had difficulty with this question.

Level of Cognitive Ability: Analysis
Client Needs: Safe, Effective Care Environment
Integrated Concept/Process: Nursing Process/Planning
Content Area: Adult Health/Integumentary
Reference: Lewis, S., Heitkemper, M., & Dirksen, S. (2000). *Medical-surgical nursing: Assessment and management of clinical problems* (5th ed.). St. Louis: Mosby, p. 507.

24. 1

Rationale: Melanomas are pigmented, malignant lesions originating in the melanin-producing cells of the epidermis. This skin cancer is highly metastatic, and a person's survival depends on early diagnosis and treatment. Options 2, 3, and 4 are not characteristics of a melanoma.

Test-Taking Strategy: Use the process of elimination. Note the similarity between options 2, 3, and 4. Also, recalling that melanomas are highly metastatic will assist in directing you to the correct option. If you had difficulty with this question, review the characteristics of skin cancers.

Level of Cognitive Ability: Comprehension
Client Needs: Physiological Integrity
Integrated Concept/Process: Nursing Process/Assessment
Content Area: Adult Health/Integumentary
Reference: Ignatavicius, D., Workman, M., & Mishler, M. (1999). *Medical-surgical nursing across the health care continuum* (3rd ed.). Philadelphia: W.B. Saunders, p. 1745.

25. 4

Rationale: A melanoma is a irregularly shaped, pigmented papule or plaque with a red-, white-, or blue-toned color. Basal cell carcinoma appears as a pearly papule with a central crater and rolled waxy border. Squamous cell carcinoma is a firm, nodular lesion topped with a crust or a central area of ulceration. Actinic keratosis, a premalignant lesion, appears as a small macule or papule with a dry, rough, adherent yellow or brown scale.

Test-Taking Strategy: Use the process of elimination. Remembering that irregularly shaped lesions are a cause for concern will assist in directing you to option 4. If you had difficulty with this question, review the characteristics of malignant skin lesions.

Level of Cognitive Ability: Analysis
Client Needs: Physiological Integrity
Integrated Concept/Process: Nursing Process/Assessment
Content Area: Adult Health/Integumentary

Reference: Ignatavicius, D., Workman, M., & Mishler, M. (1999). *Medical-surgical nursing across the health care continuum* (3rd ed.). Philadelphia: W.B. Saunders, p. 1745.

26. 1

Rationale: Cryosurgery involves the local application of liquid nitrogen to isolated lesions and causes cell death and tissue destruction. The nurse prepares the client for swelling and increased tenderness of the treated area when the skin thaws. Tissue freezing is followed by hemorrhagic blister formation in 1 to 2 days. The nurse instructs the client to clean the treatment site with hydrogen peroxide to prevent secondary infection. A topical antibiotic may also be prescribed. Application of a warm, damp washcloth intermittently to the site will provide relief from any discomfort. Alcohol-soaked dressings will cause irritation. It is not necessary to avoid showering.

Test-Taking Strategy: Use the process of elimination. Eliminate option 4 first because there is no reason for the client to avoid showers. Eliminate option 3 next because alcohol-soaked dressings will cause irritation. From the remaining options, note that option 1 address the prevention of infection. Therefore, this is the best option to select. If you had difficulty with this question, review client education following cryosurgery.

Level of Cognitive Ability: Application
Client Needs: Health Promotion and Maintenance
Integrated Concept/Process: Teaching/Learning
Content Area: Adult Health/Integumentary
Reference: Ignatavicius, D., Workman, M., & Mishler, M. (1999). *Medical-surgical nursing across the health care continuum* (3rd ed.). Philadelphia: W.B. Saunders, p. 1745.

27. 4

Rationale: The client should be instructed to avoid sun exposure between the hours of 11:00 A.M. and 3:00 P.M. Sunscreen, a hat, opaque clothing, and sunglasses should be worn for outdoor activities. The client should be instructed to examine the body monthly for the appearance of any possible cancerous or precancerous lesions.

Test-Taking Strategy: Use the process of elimination. Note the key words "a need for further education." Note the key word "avoid" in option 4 to assist in directing you to this option. Review client education in the prevention of skin cancer if you had difficulty with this question.

Level of Cognitive Ability: Analysis
Client Needs: Health Promotion and Maintenance
Integrated Concept/Process: Teaching/Learning
Content Area: Adult Health/Integumentary
Reference: Ignatavicius, D., Workman, M., & Mishler, M. (1999). *Medical-surgical nursing across the health care continuum* (3rd ed.). Philadelphia: W.B. Saunders, p. 1745.

28. 2

Rationale: Paronychia, or infection around the nail, is characterized by red, shiny skin, often associated with painful swelling. These infections frequently result from trauma, picking at the nail, or disorders such as dermatitis. Often these become secondarily infected with bacteria or fungus, which later involves the nail. Warm soaks three or four times a day may reduce pain and pressure; however, incision and drainage of the inflamed site is frequently required. Options 1, 3, and 4 are incorrect.

Test-Taking Strategy: Use the process of elimination. Recalling that this disorder relates to an infection of the nail will easily direct you to the correct option. If you had difficulty with this question, review the definition of this disorder.
Level of Cognitive Ability: Analysis
Client Needs: Physiological Integrity
Integrated Concept/Process: Nursing Process/Assessment
Content Area: Adult Health/Integumentary
Reference: Phipps, W., Sands, J., & Marek, J. (1999). *Medical-surgical nursing: Concepts & clinical practice* (6th ed.). St. Louis: Mosby, p. 2062.

29. **3**
Rationale: The nurse would not tell a client that it is not necessary to separate his or her linen and towels from those of other household members. Thorough handwashing, separating linens and towels, and separate washing of the client's dishes are required because the infection is contagious as long as skin lesions are present. Antibiotics are administered and should be continued as prescribed.
Test-Taking Strategy: Use the process of elimination. Note the key word "not." Recalling that the infection is contagious as long as skin lesions are present will direct you to the correct option. If you had difficulty with this question, review client teaching related to home care and the prevention of transmission.
Level of Cognitive Ability: Application
Client Needs: Safe, Effective Care Environment
Integrated Concept/Process: Nursing Process/Planning
Content Area: Adult Health/Integumentary
Reference: LeMone, P., & Burke, K. (2000). *Medical-surgical nursing: Critical thinking in client care* (2nd ed.). Upper Saddle River, N.J.: Prentice-Hall, p. 579.

30. **4**
Rationale: Assessment findings in frostbite include a white or blue color, and the skin will be hard, cold, and insensitive to touch. As thawing occurs, flushing of the skin, the development of blisters or blebs, or tissue edema appears. Options 1, 2, and 3 are incorrect.
Test-Taking Strategy: Use the process of elimination. Noting the key words "insensitive to touch" in option 4 should direct you to this option. If you had difficulty with this question, review the characteristics associated with frostbite.
Level of Cognitive Ability: Analysis
Client Needs: Physiological Integrity
Integrated Concept/Process: Nursing Process/Assessment
Content Area: Adult Health/Integumentary
Reference: Lewis, S., Heitkemper, M., & Dirksen, S. (2000). *Medical-surgical nursing: Assessment and management of clinical problems* (5th ed.). St. Louis: Mosby, p. 1967.

31. **1**
Rationale: Acute frostbite is ideally treated with rapid and continuous rewarming of the tissue in a warm water bath for 15 to 20 minutes or until flushing of the skin occurs. Slow thawing or interrupted periods of warmth are avoided, because this can contribute to increased cellular damage. Cold or hot water is not used. Thawing can cause considerable pain, and the nurse administers analgesics as prescribed.
Test-Taking Strategy: Use the process of elimination. Eliminate options 2 and 4 because of the words "hot" and "cold." Eliminate option 3 because intervention would begin immedi-

ately. If you had difficulty with this question, review the interventions associated with frostbite.
Level of Cognitive Ability: Analysis
Client Needs: Physiological Integrity
Integrated Concept/Process: Nursing Process/Planning
Content Area: Adult Health/Integumentary
Reference: Lewis, S., Heitkemper, M., & Dirksen, S. (2000). *Medical-surgical nursing: Assessment and management of clinical problems* (5th ed.). St. Louis: Mosby, p. 1967.

32. **2**
Rationale: In a stage II pressure ulcer, the skin is not intact. There is partial-thickness skin loss of the epidermis or dermis. The ulcer is superficial and may be characterized as an abrasion, blister, or shallow crater. The skin is intact in stage I. A deep crater-like appearance occurs in stage III, and sinus tracts develop in stage IV.
Test-Taking Strategy: Use the process of elimination. Focus on the key words "stage II." If you had difficulty with this question, review the characteristics associated with each stage of pressure ulcers.
Level of Cognitive Ability: Analysis
Client Needs: Physiological Integrity
Integrated Concept/Process: Nursing Process/Assessment
Content Area: Adult Health/Integumentary
Reference: Phipps, W., Sands, J., & Marek, J. (1999). *Medical-surgical nursing: Concepts & clinical practice* (6th ed.). St. Louis: Mosby, p. 2048.

33. **3**
Rationale: In a dark-skinned client, the nurse examines the lips, tongue, nailbeds, conjunctiva, and palms of the hands and soles of the feet at regular intervals for subtle color changes. In a client with cyanosis, the lips and tongue are gray, and the palms, soles, conjunctiva, and nailbeds have a bluish tinge.
Test-Taking Strategy: Use the process of elimination, focusing on the issue, cyanosis in a dark-skinned client. Attempt to visualize assessment of the areas identified in each option to assist in directing you to option 3. Review this important assessment technique if you had difficulty with this question.
Level of Cognitive Ability: Comprehension
Client Needs: Physiological Integrity
Integrated Concept/Process: Nursing Process/Assessment
Content Area: Adult Health/Integumentary
Reference: Phipps, W., Sands, J., & Marek, J. (1999). *Medical-surgical nursing: Concepts & clinical practice* (6th ed.). St. Louis: Mosby, p. 2059.

34. **1**
Rationale: Psoriasis occurs equally among women and men, although the incidence is lower in darker-skinned races. A genetic predisposition has been recognized in some cases. Emotional distress, trauma, systemic illness, seasonal changes, and hormonal changes are linked to exacerbations.
Test-Taking Strategy: Note the key words "least likely." Use the process of elimination and knowledge regarding what psoriasis is and the etiology associated with the disorder to answer the question. If you had difficulty with the question, review the causes of the disorder and the factors that affect exacerbations.
Level of Cognitive Ability: Analysis
Client Needs: Health Promotion and Maintenance

Integrated Concept/Process: Nursing Process/Assessment
Content Area: Adult Health/Integumentary
Reference: Ignatavicius, D., Workman, M., & Mishler, M. (1999). *Medical-surgical nursing across the health care continuum* (3rd ed.). Philadelphia: W.B. Saunders, p. 1739.

35. 4
Rationale: Bed or chair confinement, inability to move, loss of bowel or bladder control, poor nutrition, absent or inconsistent care giving, and a lowered mental awareness can all contribute to the development of skin breakdown. The least likely risk, as presented in the options, is the lowered mental awareness status. Options 1, 2, and 3 identify physiological conditions, which are the risk priorities.
Test-Taking Strategy: Note the key words "least likely." Use Maslow's Hierarchy of Needs theory to answer the question. Remember that physiological needs are the priority. This will assist you in eliminating options 1, 2, and 3. Review the risk factors associated with skin breakdown if you had difficulty with this question.
Level of Cognitive Ability: Analysis
Client Needs: Physiological Integrity
Integrated Concept/Process: Nursing Process/Assessment
Content Area: Adult Health/Integumentary
Reference: Phipps, W., Sands, J., & Marek, J. (1999). *Medical-surgical nursing: Concepts & clinical practice* (6th ed.). St. Louis: Mosby. p. 2097.

36. 3
Rationale: The actual cause of acne is unknown. There is no evidence that oily skin or the consumption of foods such as chocolate, nuts, or fatty foods causes acne. Exacerbations that coincide with the menstrual cycle result from hormonal activity. Heat, humidity, and excessive perspiration may play a role in exacerbating acne but do not cause it.
Test-Taking Strategy: Use the process of elimination. Note that the question asks for the "cause" of acne. Options 1, 2, and 4 relate specifically to factors that exacerbate acne. Review the cause of and factors that exacerbate acne, if you had difficulty with this question.
Level of Cognitive Ability: Application
Client Needs: Health Promotion and Maintenance
Integrated Concept/Process: Nursing Process/Implementation
Content Area: Adult Health/Integumentary
Reference: LeMone, P., & Burke, K. (2000). *Medical-surgical nursing: Critical thinking in client care* (2nd ed.). Upper Saddle River, N.J.: Prentice-Hall, p. 592.

37. 1
Rationale: In severe cystic acne, isotretinoin (Accutane) is used to inhibit inflammation. Adverse effects include elevated triglycerides, skin dryness, eye discomfort such as dryness and burning, and cheilitis (lip inflammation). Close medical follow-up is required, and dry skin and cheilitis can be decreased by the use of emollients and lip balms. Vitamin A supplements are stopped during this treatment.
Test-Taking Strategy: Use the process of elimination. Note the key words "a need for further teaching." Recalling that vitamin A supplements need to be discontinued during this treatment will direct you to the correct option. If you had difficulty with this question, review the action, side effects, and adverse effects related to this medication.
Level of Cognitive Ability: Analysis

Client Needs: Health Promotion and Maintenance
Integrated Concept/Process: Teaching/Learning
Content Area: Pharmacology
Reference: LeMone, P., & Burke, K. (2000). *Medical-surgical nursing: Critical thinking in client care* (2nd ed.). Upper Saddle River, N.J.: Prentice-Hall, p. 594.

38. 3
Rationale: Scabies can be identified by the multiple straight or wavy, threadlike lines noted beneath the skin. The skin lesions are caused by the female, which burrows beneath the skin and lays its eggs. The eggs hatch in a few days, and the baby mites find their way to the skin surface, where they mate and complete the life cycle. Options 1, 2, and 4 are not characteristics of scabies.
Test-Taking Strategy: Use the process of elimination. Recalling that the scabies mite burrows beneath the skin surface will provide direction toward selection of the correct option. If you had difficulty with this question, review the characteristics associated with scabies.
Level of Cognitive Ability: Analysis
Client Needs: Physiological Integrity
Integrated Concept/Process: Nursing Process/Assessment
Content Area: Adult Health/Integumentary
Reference: Phipps, W., Sands, J., & Marek, J. (1999). *Medical-surgical nursing: Concepts & clinical practice* (6th ed.). St. Louis: Mosby, p. 2068.

39. 3
Rationale: The Centers for Disease Control and Prevention recommends the wearing of gowns and gloves for close contact with a person infested with scabies. Masks are not necessary. Transmission via clothing and other inanimate objects is uncommon. Scabies is usually transmitted from person to person by direct skin contact. All contacts that the client has had should be treated at the same time.
Test-Taking Strategy: Consider the mode of transmission of scabies and use the process of elimination. Since scabies is transmitted by direct skin contact, eliminate options 1, 2, and 4. If you had difficulty with this question, review standard precautions and the transmission mode of scabies.
Level of Cognitive Ability: Application
Client Needs: Safe, Effective Care Environment
Integrated Concept/Process: Nursing Process/Implementation
Content Area: Adult Health/Integumentary
Reference: Lewis, S., Heitkemper, M., & Dirksen, S. (2000). *Medical-surgical nursing: Assessment and management of clinical problems* (5th ed.). St. Louis: Mosby, p. 509.

40. 3
Rationale: Assessment of candidiasis (thrush) reveals white patches on the tongue, palate, and buccal mucosa. The lesions adhere firmly to the tissues and are difficult to remove. The lesions are often referred to as milk curds because of their appearance. Clients often describe the lesions as dry and hot. Options 1, 2, and 4 are not characteristics of thrush.
Test-Taking Strategy: Use the process of elimination. Recalling that candidiasis (thrush) presents as white patches will assist in answering the question. If you had difficulty with this question, review the characteristics associated with candidiasis (thrush).
Level of Cognitive Ability: Analysis
Client Needs: Physiological Integrity

Integrated Concept/Process: Nursing Process/Assessment
Content Area: Adult Health/Integumentary
Reference: Phipps, W., Sands, J., & Marek, J. (1999). *Medical-surgical nursing: Concepts & clinical practice* (6th ed.). St. Louis: Mosby, p. 2069.

41. 3
Rationale: The Parkland (Baxter) formula for estimating fluid requirements is 4 mL × kg × %TBSA. Half of this total is administered in the first 8 hours following the burn. Therefore, $4 \times 90 \times 83 = 29,880$ mL divided by $2 = 14,940$ mL.
Test-Taking Strategy: Knowledge regarding the Parkland (Baxter) formula is required to answer the question. Read the question carefully and remember that half of the total is administered in the first 8 hours following the burn. Review this formula, if you had difficulty with this question.
Level of Cognitive Ability: Analysis
Client Needs: Physiological Integrity
Integrated Concept/Process: Nursing Process/Analysis
Content Area: Adult Health/Integumentary
Reference: Lewis, S., Heitkemper, M., & Dirksen, S. (2000). *Medical-surgical nursing: Assessment and management of clinical problems* (5th ed.). St. Louis: Mosby, pp. 527; 537.

42. 4
Rationale: Escharotomies are performed to alleviate the compartment syndrome that can occur when edema forms under nondistensible eschar in a circumferential third-degree burn. Escharotomies are performed through avascular eschar to subcutaneous fat. Although bleeding may occur from the site, it is considered a complication rather that an anticipated therapeutic outcome. Usually, direct pressure with a bulky dressing and elevation will control the bleeding, but occasionally an artery is damaged that may require ligation. Formation of granulation tissue is not the intent of an escharotomy. Escharotomy will not affect the formation of edema.
Test-Taking Strategy: Use the ABCs—airway, breathing, and circulation—to answer the question. The only option that addresses circulation is option 4. If you had difficulty with this question, review the purpose of an escharotomy.
Level of Cognitive Ability: Analysis
Client Needs: Physiological Integrity
Integrated Concept/Process: Nursing Process/Evaluation
Content Area: Adult Health/Integumentary
Reference: Phipps, W., Sands, J., & Marek, J. (1999). *Medical-surgical nursing: Concepts & clinical practice* (6th ed.). St. Louis: Mosby, p. 2122.

43. 2
Rationale: Alkalis, such as lye, cause a liquefaction necrosis, and exposure to fat forms a soapy coagulum. Thick, leathery eschar forms with exposure to acids or heat. Cherry-red, firm tissue can occur as a result of thermal injury. Intact blisters indicate a partial-thickness thermal injury.
Test-Taking Strategy: Use the process of elimination, and focus on the issue of the question. Remembering that alkali burns cause a liquefaction necrosis and form a soapy coagulum will assist in answering the question. If you had difficulty with this question, review assessment findings in chemical burns.
Level of Cognitive Ability: Analysis
Client Needs: Physiological Integrity
Integrated Concept/Process: Nursing Process/Assessment
Content Area: Adult Health/Integumentary

Reference: Lewis, S., Heitkemper, M., & Dirksen, S. (2000). *Medical-surgical nursing: Assessment and management of clinical problems* (5th ed.). St. Louis: Mosby, p. 524.

44. 1
Rationale: Superficial injury from radiation can manifest with erythema (probably due to capillary damage), hyperpigmentation (from stimulation of melanocytes), dry desquamation (due to basal cell destruction), and/or moist desquamation (also due to basal cell destruction). Moist desquamation is comparable to a second-degree burn in histology, appearance, and sensation.
Test-Taking Strategy: Use the process of elimination, and note the relationship between "erythema" in the question and "superficial" in the correct option. If you had difficulty with this question, review the effects of radiation burns.
Level of Cognitive Ability: Analysis
Client Needs: Physiological Integrity
Integrated Concept/Process: Nursing Process/Assessment
Content Area: Adult Health/Integumentary
Reference: Lewis, S., Heitkemper, M., & Dirksen, S. (2000). *Medical-surgical nursing: Assessment and management of clinical problems* (5th ed.). St. Louis: Mosby, p. 527.

45. 3
Rationale: The emergent phase begins at the time of injury and ends with the restoration of capillary permeability, usually at 48 to 72 hours after the injury. During the emergent phase, the hematocrit increases to above normal because of hemoconcentration from the large fluid shifts. Hematocrit levels of 50% to 55% are expected during the first 24 hours after injury, with return to normal by 36 hours after injury. Initially, blood is shunted away from the kidneys, and renal perfusion and glomerular filtration are decreased, resulting in low urine output. Pulse rates are typically higher than normal and the blood pressure is decreased as a result of the large fluid shifts.
Test-Taking Strategy: Use the process of elimination, and think about how the body would react in such a traumatizing event. Eliminate options 1 and 4 first. Knowledge that the blood pressure would decrease as a result of the decrease in circulating blood volume will direct you to option 3. Review pathophysiology related to burn injuries if you had difficulty with this question.
Level of Cognitive Ability: Analysis
Client Needs: Physiological Integrity
Integrated Concept/Process: Nursing Process/Analysis
Content Area: Adult Health/Integumentary
Reference: Lewis, S., Heitkemper, M., & Dirksen, S. (2000). *Medical-surgical nursing: Assessment and management of clinical problems* (5th ed.). St. Louis: Mosby, p. 528.

46. 1
Rationale: Carbon monoxide levels between 1% and 10% result in impaired visual acuity; levels of 11% to 20% result in flushing and headache; levels of 21% to 30% result in nausea and impaired dexterity. Levels of 31% to 40% result in vomiting, dizziness, and syncope, levels of 41% to 50% result in tachypnea and tachycardia, and levels greater than 50% result in coma and death.
Test-Taking Strategy: Use the process of elimination, and focus on the carbon monoxide level presented in the question. If you had difficulty with this question, review these clinical manifestations.

Level of Cognitive Ability: Analysis
Client Needs: Physiological Integrity
Integrated Concept/Process: Nursing Process/Assessment
Content Area: Adult Health/Integumentary
Reference: Ignatavicius, D., Workman, M., & Mishler, M. (1999). *Medical-surgical nursing across the health care continuum* (3rd ed.). Philadelphia: W.B. Saunders, p. 1765.

47. **3**
Rationale: If an inhalation injury is suspected, administration of 100% oxygen via a tight-fitting non-rebreather face mask is prescribed until carboxyhemoglobin levels fall below 15%. In inhalation injuries, the oropharynx is inspected for evidence of erythema, blisters, or ulcerations. The need for endotracheal intubation is also assessed. Options 1, 2, and 4 are incorrect.
Test-Taking Strategy: Use the process of elimination. Recalling that 100% oxygen is required following an inhalation injury will assist in eliminating options 2 and 4. From the remaining options, recall that with a tight-fitting mask, a non-rebreather is preferred so that the client will not rebreath exhaled air. If you had difficulty with this question, review care of the client following an inhalation injury.
Level of Cognitive Ability: Analysis
Client Needs: Physiological Integrity
Integrated Concept/Process: Nursing Process/Analysis
Content Area: Adult Health/Integumentary
Reference: Lewis, S., Heitkemper, M., & Dirksen, S. (2000). *Medical-surgical nursing: Assessment and management of clinical problems* (5th ed.). St. Louis: Mosby, p. 533.

48. **2**
Rationale: Successful or adequate fluid resuscitation in the adult is signaled by stable vital signs, adequate urine output, palpable peripheral pulses, and clear sensorium. The most reliable indicator for determining adequacy of fluid resuscitation is the urine output. For an adult, the hourly urine volume should be 30 to 50 mL.
Test-Taking Strategy: Use the process of elimination. Note the key words "most reliable." Note the issue of the question, fluid resuscitation. Urine output is most similar to the issue of administering fluids. Review care to the burn client during fluid resuscitation if you had difficulty with this question.
Level of Cognitive Ability: Analysis
Client Needs: Physiological Integrity
Integrated Concept/Process: Nursing Process/Evaluation
Content Area: Adult Health/Integumentary
Reference: Lewis, S., Heitkemper, M., & Dirksen, S. (2000). *Medical-surgical nursing: Assessment and management of clinical problems* (5th ed.). St. Louis: Mosby, p. 537.

49. **3**
Rationale: Thorough handwashing should be done before and after each contact with the burn-injured client. Sterile sheets and linens are used. Protective garb, including gloves, cap, masks, shoe covers, scrub clothes, and plastic aprons, needs to be worn when the nurse is in the client's room or directly caring for the client.
Test-Taking Strategy: Use the process of elimination, noting the key word "not" in the stem of the question. Option 2 can

be easily eliminated. Note the absolute word "only" in option 3. Also, option 3 identifies the least thorough technique to prevent infection. If you had difficulty with this question, review protective isolation techniques when caring for a burn client.
Level of Cognitive Ability: Application
Client Needs: Safe, Effective Care Environment
Integrated Concept/Process: Nursing Process/Planning
Content Area: Adult Health/Integumentary
Reference: Lewis, S., Heitkemper, M., & Dirksen, S. (2000). *Medical-surgical nursing: Assessment and management of clinical problems* (5th ed.). St. Louis: Mosby, p. 538.

50. **1**
Rationale: Autografts placed over joints or on the lower extremities are often elevated and immobilized following surgery for 3 to 7 days. This period of immobilization allows the autograft time to adhere and attach to the wound bed. Options 2, 3, and 4 are incorrect.
Test-Taking Strategy: Use the process of elimination. Eliminate options 2 and 4 first because they are similar. From the remaining options, note that the autograft was placed over a joint. This should direct you to option 1. If you had difficulty with this question, review care of an autograft placed over a joint.
Level of Cognitive Ability: Analysis
Client Needs: Physiological Integrity
Integrated Concept/Process: Nursing Process/Analysis
Content Area: Adult Health/Integumentary
Reference: Phipps, W., Sands, J., & Marek, J. (1999). *Medical-surgical nursing: Concepts & clinical practice* (6th ed.). St. Louis: Mosby, p. 2127.

CRITICAL THINKING: FREE-TEXT ENTRY

Answer: 36%
Rationale: According to the rule of nines, with the initial burn, the anterior half of the head equals 4.5%, the upper half of the anterior torso equals 9%, and the lower half of both arms equals 9%. The subsequent burn included the posterior half of head, equaling 4.5%, and the upper half of the posterior torso, equaling 9%. This totals 36%.
Test-Taking Strategy: Knowledge regarding the rule of nines is required to answer this question. The entire head equals 9%, each entire arm equals 9% (both arms 18%), anterior or posterior torso each equals 18% (36% for entire torso), each entire leg equals 18% (both legs equal 36%), and the perineum equals 1%. Remember: 9 (head), 18 (arms), 36 (torso), 36 (legs), 1 (perineum), equaling 100. If you had difficulty with this question, learn the rule of nines.
Level of Cognitive Ability: Analysis
Client Needs: Physiological Integrity
Integrated Concept/Process: Nursing Process/Assessment
Content Area: Adult Health/Integumentary
Reference: Lewis, S., Heitkemper, M., & Dirksen, S. (2000). *Medical-surgical nursing: Assessment and management of clinical problems* (5th ed.). St. Louis: Mosby, p. 527.

REFERENCES

Ignatavicius, D., Workman, M., & Mishler, M. (1999). *Medical-surgical nursing across the health care continuum* (3rd ed.). Philadelphia: W.B. Saunders.

LeMone, P., & Burke, K. (2000). *Medical-surgical nursing: Critical thinking in client care* (2nd ed.). Upper Saddle River, N.J.: Prentice-Hall.

Lewis, S., Heitkemper, M., & Dirksen, S. (2000). *Medical-surgical nursing: Assessment and management of clinical problems* (5th ed.). St. Louis: Mosby.

Phipps, W., Sands, J., & Marek, J. (1999). *Medical-surgical nursing: Concepts & clinical practice* (6th ed.). St. Louis: Mosby.

Potter, P., & Perry, A. (2001). *Fundamentals of nursing* (5th ed.). St. Louis: Mosby.

Smeltzer, S., & Bare, B. (2000). *Brunner & Suddarth's textbook of medical-surgical nursing* (9th ed). Philadelphia: Lippincott Williams & Wilkins.

Integumentary Medications

I. EMOLLIENTS AND LOTIONS

A. Emollients (Box 48-1)
1. Oily or fatty substances that soften and soothe irritated skin by allowing the skin to retain water
2. Available as creams or ointments
3. Used for dry, scaly, itchy inflammatory conditions

B. Lotions (Box 48-2)
1. Liquid suspensions or dispersions
2. Require shaking before application
3. Although lotions are predominantly water, they have a drying effect on the skin when the water evaporates
4. Used as a wash for the skin, as soaks, or as wet dressings on ulcers or **burns**
5. Used for subacute inflammatory lesions after the severe exudate phase has ceased
6. Medicated lotions are often used as antiinflammatory agents because they provide a drying, protective, and cooling effect

II. RUBS AND LINIMENTS (Box 48-3)

A. Used for the temporary relief of muscular aches, rheumatism, arthritis, sprains, and neuralgia
B. Over-the-counter (OTC) products contain combinations of antiseptics, local anesthetics, analgesics, and counterirritants
C. Some products contain salicylates and, if used over a large area of the skin, may cause salicylate side effects such as tinnitus, nausea, or vomiting
D. A heating pad is not used with these products, as irritation or burning of the skin may occur

III. ANTIINFECTIVE AGENTS

A. Description
1. Include antiseptics and antibacterial, antifungal, antiviral, and antiparasitic medications
2. Topical antibiotics are safe and effective in certain conditions; extensive use may encourage the emergence of resistant bacteria

B. Antiseptics
1. Sodium hypochlorite (Dakin solution)
   a. A chloride solution that loosens, dissolves, and deodorizes necrotic tissue and blood clots
   b. It kills most common bacteria, including spores, amebas, fungi, protozoa, viruses, and yeast
   c. It is used for irrigating and cleaning necrotic or purulent wounds

---

BOX 48-1

Emollients

Cold cream
Glycerin
Lanolin
Petrolatum
Zinc ointment

BOX 48-2

Lotions

Aluminum acetate solution (Burrow's solution)
Calamine lotion (Caladryl lotion)
Potassium permanganate solution
Zinc stearate

BOX 48-3

Rubs and Liniments

Aspercreame
Ben-Gay
Deep-Down Rub
Hot cream/balm/stick
Myoflex

d. Loses its potency during storage, so fresh solution is prepared frequently

e. It should not be in contact with healing or normal tissue

2. Chlorhexidine gluconate (Hibiclens)
   a. Effective for cleaning wounds caused by staphylococci and other gram-positive bacteria
   b. Used for irrigating and cleansing wounds, but not for packing wounds because it may cause contact dermatitis

3. Acetic acid
   a. Effective for irrigating, cleansing, and packing wounds infected by *Pseudomonas aeruginosa*
   b. Healthy skin surrounding the wound must be protected with a petroleum barrier because it excoriates the skin

4. Hydrogen peroxide
   a. As a 3% solution, it has effervescent action that releases gas and breaks up necrotic tissue
   b. It is used to irrigate and clean necrotic tissue and pus from open wounds
   c. It is not used to pack wounds because it decomposes too rapidly
   d. When epithelial tissue begins to form, hydrogen peroxide is discontinued because it inhibits tissue formation

5. Hexachlorophene (pHisoHex, Septisol)
   a. A combination of hexachlorophene and alcohol
   b. Hexachlorophene is a bacteriostatic agent with activity against staphylococci and other gram-positive bacteria
   c. Hexachlorophene is heavily absorbed through broken skin and can cause neurotoxicity; it should not be used on wounds
   d. The alcohol component dries and irritates

tissue, is not a very effective germicide, and forms a film that can actually promote infection

e. All hexachlorophene products are well rinsed from the skin after their use to prevent systemic absorption

C. Antibacterials (Box 48-4)
   1. Description: Used for superficial skin infections
   2. Mupirocin (Bactroban)
      a. Topical antibacterial active against *Staphylococcus aureus*, beta-hemolytic streptococci, or *Streptococcus pyogenes*
      b. Applied three times daily; if improvement is not observed within 3 to 5 days, it is discontinued

D. Antifungals
   1. May cause erythema, stinging, blistering, peeling, pruritis, urticaria, and general skin irritation
   2. Client is reevaluated if no results are obtained after 4 weeks of treatment

E. Antiviral: Acyclovir (Zovirax)
   1. Inhibits DNA replication in the virus
   2. Used for herpes simplex types 1 and 2, varicella zoster, Epstein-Barr virus, and cytomegalovirus
   3. Can cause mild pain and transient burning and stinging
   4. Applied completely over the lesion every 3 hours six times daily for 1 week
   5. Rubber gloves are used to apply the ointment, to prevent the spread of infection

F. Antiparasitics
   1. Used to treat scabies (mites) and pediculosis (lice)
   2. May be harmful during pregnancy and in young children
   3. May irritate the skin, eyes, and mucous membranes
   4. May cause allergic reactions

IV. ANTIPRURITICS (Box 48-5)

A. Used to allay itching
B. Applied as wet dressings, pastes, lotions, creams, or ointments
C. Persons with dry skin should be instructed to bathe less frequently

V. KERATOLYTICS (Box 48-6)

A. Description
   1. Preparations that dissolve keratin

BOX 48-4

Antibacterials, Antifungals, Antiparasitics

ANTIBACTERIALS
Bacitracin
Mity-Mycin
Mupirocin (Bactroban)
Mycitracin Triple Antibiotic
Neomycin
Neo-Polycin ointment
Polymyxin B
Triple antibiotic

ANTIFUNGAL
Acyclovir (Zovirax)

ANTIPARASITICS
Crotamiton (Eurax)
Lindane (Kwell)
Permethrin 5% (Elimite)

BOX 48-5

Antipruritics

Calamine or phenol
Cornstarch or oatmeal baths
Solutions of potassium permanganate, aluminum subacetate, boric acid, or normal saline

---

BOX 48-6

Keratolytics

Cantharidin (Cantharone)
Masoprocol (Actinex)
Podophyllum resin (Pod-Ben 25)
Podofilox (Condylox)
Resorcinol (Fostex Medicated Bar, Meted-2, Sebulex)
Salicylic acid (Wart-Off, Freezone, Compound W)

BOX 48-7

Stimulants and Irritants

Coal tar
Compound benzoin tincture

BOX 48-8

Protectives

DuoDerm
Ensure-It (Deseret)
Mediskin and Silver
Op-Site
PolySkin
Tegaderm
Tegasorb
Uniflex
Vigilon
Zinc oxide paste (Unna's boot)

---

2. Soften scales and loosen the horny layer of the skin, resulting in minimal peeling or extensive desquamation
3. Used to treat superficial fungal infections, dermatitis, psoriasis, and localized dermatitis
B. Salicylic acid
   1. Used to treat seborrheic dermatitis, acne, and psoriasis, and to thin and remove calluses
   2. Can be absorbed systematically and can cause salicylism, characterized by dizziness and tinnitus; is not applied to large surface areas or open wounds
C. Podophyllum resin
   1. Used for various types of **skin cancer**
   2. Causes lesions to slough off, leaving a superficial ulcer and moderate dermatitis
   3. After the therapy is discontinued, the lesions are treated with a mild antiseptic ointment; healing usually occurs within a few days
D. Cantharidin (Cantharone)
   1. Used in treating warts
   2. Has an exfoliation effect only on the epidermal cells
   3. May cause tingling, itching, and burning
   4. Site may be very tender for a period of 2 to 6 days
E. Masoprocol (Actinex)
   1. Has antiproliferative activity against keratinocytes and is used to treat keratosis
   2. Occlusive dressings are not to be used
   3. Transient burning may be experienced after administration

VI. STIMULANTS AND IRRITANTS (Box 48-7)
A. Description: Produce a mild irritation to the surface of the skin, causing hyperemia and inflammation that promote the healing process
B. Coal tar
   1. Used in treating psoriasis, seborrheic dermatitis, and atopic dermatitis
   2. Has an unpleasant odor and frequently stains the skin and hair
   3. Can cause phototoxicity
C. Compound benzoin tincture
   1. Protects the skin when the client has bedsores, ulcers, cracked nipples, or fissures of any orifice

2. Causes a mild irritation that produces increased blood flow and healing

VII. PROTECTIVES (Box 48-8)
A. Description
   1. Preparations that provide a film on the skin to protect it from irritations such as light, moisture, air, and dust
   2. Promote natural healing without the usual formation of dry crust over the wound
   3. Allow exudate to collect beneath the dressing, forming an artificial blister
   4. Designed to be left in place for up to 7 days or until leakage occurs around the dressing
   5. Uniflex, PolySkin, and Ensure-It may be used to cover central and peripheral IV sites
   6. Op-Site, Tegasorb, Mediskin and Silver and Vigilon may be used for skin **burns**
B. Sunscreens
   1. Act by absorbing ultraviolet rays
   2. The best sunscreens contain PABA (para-aminobenzoic acid)
   3. Most effective when applied about 30 minutes to 1 hour before exposure to the sun; should be reapplied after swimming or sweating
   4. Can cause contact dermatitis and photosensitivity reactions
C. Nonadherent dressings
   1. Woven or nonwoven dressings that may be impregnated with saline, petrolatum, or antimicrobials
   2. Nonadherent dressings include Adaptic, Exu-Dry, Sofsorb, Telfa, Vaseline gauze, and Xeroform

VIII. GROWTH FACTORS

A. Description
   1. Used to promote wound healing
   2. Stimulate cells to divide and migrate, which results in wound healing, formation of granulation tissue, and new epidermis
B. Procuren solution
   1. Promotes healing by actively stimulating growth and granulation tissue, capillaries, and epithelium
   2. Applied to the wound and covered with petrolatum-impregnated gauze
   3. The material is left in place for 12 hours and then washed off; during the remaining 12 hours of the day, the wound is covered with sulfadiazine (Silvadene)

IX. ENZYMES

A. Description
   1. Used to promote healing of wounds and to debride skin ulcers
   2. Reduce inflammation resulting from trauma and infection
   3. Dissolve fibrin clots, which helps reduce the size of surface hematomas
   4. To be effective, must be in contact with affected tissue in adequate concentrations for a sufficient length of time
   5. Wound may need to be surgically debrided prior to application; if not administered to a clean, debrided wound, healing may be delayed
B. Enzymes that promote wound healing (Box 48-9)
   1. Papain (Panafil, Panafil White)
      a. Does not injure or affect healthy tissue or cells
      b. Enzyme must be in immediate contact with the purulent wound material
      c. Wounds are cleansed with prescribed irrigating solution between applications
      d. Hydrogen peroxide cannot be used to irrigate the wound, because it inactivates the papain
      e. Light dressings and cellophane wrap may be used over the wound to prevent soiling of clothing
      f. Dressings are changed frequently to prevent contamination and to remove necrotic debris
   2. Hyaluronidase (Wydase)
      a. Facilitates the absorption of fluid administered by subcutaneous hypodermoclysis
      b. Can be injected SC into an infiltrated IV site when a potent vasoconstrictor such as norepinephrine (Levophed) or metaraminol (Aramine) has infiltrated
      c. It reduces the sloughing of tissue that is likely to occur secondarily to infiltration
C. Enzymes to remove exudates (Box 48-10)
   1. Description
      a. Alter the thick, purulent drainage to a thin,

BOX 48-9

Enzymes That Promote Wound Healing

Hyaluronidase (Wydase)
Papain (Panafil, Panafil White)

BOX 48-10

Enzymes to Remove Exudates

Collagenase (Santyl)
Dextranomer (Debrisan)
Fibrinolysin and desoxyribonuclease (Elase)
Sutilains (Travase)

---

liquid material that can be easily wiped or irrigated off the wound
   b. Enzyme contact with the wound is necessary to promote wound healing
   c. Wound needs to be cleansed, and crosshatching of eschar on **burns** is performed prior to application
   2. Sutilains (Travase)
      a. Used to remove nonviable or necrotic tissue and purulent enzymes from **burns**, ulcers, traumatic injury, and peripheral vascular disease wounds
      b. Inactive on viable tissue
   3. Collagenase (Santyl)
      a. Used as a topical debriding agent
      b. Provides effective debridement of the collagen tissue at the wound edges where necrotic tissue is anchored
      c. Encourages the formation of granulation tissue at the wound edges and quicker epithelization of wounds
      d. Apply with a tongue depressor directly into deep wounds
      e. Prior to application, cleanse wound of debris by gently rubbing with a gauze pad with sterile water or Dakin solution, followed by sterile normal saline
      f. Remove all excess ointment each time dressing is changed
      g. Apply only to injured area; causes erythema in healthy tissues
      h. Protect healthy tissue by applying zinc oxide paste
      i. Discontinued when necrotic tissue is gone
   4. Fibrinolysin and desoxyribonuclease (Elase)
      a. Used to debride wounds, including **burns, decubitus** ulcers, and inflamed or infected lesions
      b. Clean wound with sterile water, pat dry; flush away necrotic debris with normal saline; then

apply a thin layer and cover with petrolatum gauze

▲ D. Dextranomer (Debrisan)
　　1. Not a debriding agent but is a cleansing agent that actually absorbs peptides and proteins
　　2. Effective in wet wounds only
　　3. It is not packed tightly into the wound because maceration of surrounding tissue may occur from contact with the agent

▲ X. **CORTICOSTEROIDS**
　A. Have antiinflammatory, antipruritic, and vasoconstrictive actions
　B. Contraindications
　　1. Clients demonstrating previous sensitivity to corticosteroids
　　2. Those with current systemic fungal, viral, or bacterial infections
　　3. Those with current complications related to corticosteroid therapy
　C. Local adverse effects
　　1. Hypopigmentation
　　2. Acneiform eruptions
　　3. Contact dermatitis
　　4. Burning, dryness, irritation, itching
　　5. Overgrowth of bacteria, fungi, and viruses
　　6. Skin atrophy
　D. Systemic adverse effects
　　1. Occur rarely
　　2. Adrenal suppression
　　3. Cushing's syndrome
　　4. Striae, skin atrophy
　　5. Ocular effects (glaucoma and cataracts)
　E. Topical steroids
　　1. Monitor plasma cortisol levels if prolonged therapy is necessary
　　2. Wash area just prior to application to increase medication penetration
　　3. Apply sparingly in a light film, rubbing gently
　　4. May apply to skin alone or with a dry occlusive dressing if prescribed by the physician
　　5. Instruct the client to report burning, irritation, or signs of infection to the physician

▲ XI. **ACNE PRODUCTS** (Box 48-11)
　A. Description
　　1. Mild acne can be treated with bar soaps, soap-free cakes, liquid cleansers, lotions, gels, and creams
　　2. For moderate acne, topical antiinflammatory medication such as benzoyl peroxide, tretinoin (Retin-A), isotretinoin (Accutane), azelaic acid (Azelex), and adapalene (Differin) may be prescribed; antibiotics may also be prescribed
　　3. Side effects can include excessive redness, extreme dryness of the skin leading to blistering and crusting, temporary pigmentation changes, and peeling of the skin

---

BOX 48-11

Acne Products

CLEANSERS
Acnomel
Brasivol
Clearasil Medicated Astringent
Fostex
pHisoDerm
Stri-Dex

DRYING AGENTS
Acnomel
Dry and Clear
Ionax
Listerex

MISCELLANEOUS
Adapalene (Differin)
Alpha-hydroxy acids
Antibiotics
Azelaic acid (Azelex)
Bensulfoid cream (benzoyl peroxide and sulfur)
Benzamycin gel (benzoyl peroxide and sulfur)
Benzoyl peroxide wash, gel
Isotretinoin (Accutane)
Rosorcinol (as an ingredient in other preparations)
Salicylic acid (as an ingredient in other preparations)
Trentinoin (Retin-A)

---

　　4. All products are kept away from the eyes, inside the nose, mucous membranes, and hair
　B. Benzoyl peroxide: A keratolytic agent that is bacteriostatic and may decrease the production of irritant free fatty acids in the follicle
　C. Tretinoin (Retin-A) and adapalene (Differin): Acids of vitamin A that are used to treat acne vulgaris; may also be used to treat **skin cancer** and aging of the skin
　D. Tretinoin (Retin-A)　　　　　　　　　　　　▲
　　1. Decreases cohesiveness of the epithelial cells, increasing cell mitosis and turnover; potentially irritating, particularly when used correctly
　　2. Within 48 hours of use, the skin generally becomes red and begins to peel
　　3. Temporary hyperpigmentation and hypopigmentation can occur
　　4. Client should avoid sun exposure because photosensitivity may occur
　　5. Applied liberally to the skin; the hands are washed thoroughly immediately after applying
　　6. Therapeutic results should be seen after 2 to 3 weeks but may not be optimal until after 6 weeks
　　7. Client may use cosmetics, but the skin needs to be cleaned thoroughly before applying the cosmetics
　E. Isotretinoin (Accutane)　　　　　　　　　　▲
　　1. A metabolite of vitamin A

2. Used to treat severe cystic acne, and its use is reserved for persons who have not responded to other therapies, including systemic antibiotics
3. Can cause xerosis and facial desquamation, palmoplantar desquamation, pruritus, brittle nails, and hair loss
4. Is administered with meals two times daily for a 15- to 20-week course; if another course of therapy is needed, an 8-week lapse of time should occur
5. Photosensitivity may occur, so the client needs to be instructed to decrease sun exposure
6. Alcohol consumption should be eliminated during therapy because alcohol may potentiate serum triglyceride elevation

F. Local antibiotics
1. Used to treat acne; include clindamycin (Cleocin T), erythromycin, tetracycline (Topicycline), and meclocycline (Meclan)
2. Therapeutic response generally requires 6 to 12 weeks of therapy
3. Side effects include acute contact dermatitis, transient stinging or burning, staining of the skin, erythema, and skin tenderness

XII. POISON IVY TREATMENT (See Box 48-12)

XIII. BURN PRODUCTS (Box 48-13)
A. Nitrofurazone (Furacin)
1. Applied topically to the **burn** as a solution, ointment, or cream
2. Has a broad spectrum of antibacterial activity
3. Used in **burns** when bacterial resistance to other agents is a problem
4. Topical: apply $^1/_{16}$ inch film directly to **burn**
5. Side effects: Contact dermatitis, rash
6. Less common side effects: Pruritus, local edema
B. Mafenide (Sulfamylon)
1. A water-soluble cream that is bacteriostatic for both gram-negative and gram-positive organisms
2. Is used to treat **burns** to reduce the bacteria present in avascular tissues
3. Diffuses through the devascularized areas of the skin; may precipitate metabolic acidosis (usually compensated by hyperventilation)
4. Apply $^1/_{16}$ inch film directly to the **burn**
5. Side effects can include local pain, rash
6. Systemic effects include bone marrow depression, hemolytic anemia, metabolic acidosis
7. Keep **burn** covered with mafenide at all times
8. Notify physician if hyperventilation occurs; if acidosis develops, mafenide is washed off the skin
C. Silver sulfadiazine (Flint SSD, Silvadene)
1. Has a broad spectrum of activity against gram-negative bacteria, gram-positive bacteria, and yeast

---

BOX 48-12
Poison Ivy Treatment Products

Calamine
Calomox
IV-Chex
Ivy-Rid
Rhuli cream/spray/gel

BOX 48-13
Burn Products

Mafenide (Sulfamylon)
Nitrofurazone (Furacin)
Silver nitrate
Silver sulfadiazine (Flint SSD, Silvadene)

---

2. Released slowly from the cream, which is selectively toxic to bacteria
3. Used primarily to prevent sepsis in clients with **burns**
4. Is not a carbonic anhydrase inhibitor and therefore does not cause acidosis
5. Rash and itching occur from topical application
6. Apply $^1/_{16}$ inch film (keep **burn** covered at all times with silver sulfadiazine)
7. Side effects include rash, itching
8. Systemic effects include leukopenia, interstitial nephritis
9. Monitor complete blood cell (CBC) count, particularly the white blood cells (WBC) frequently; if leukopenia develops, the medication is discontinued

D. Silver nitrate
1. An antiseptic solution active against gram-negative bacteria
2. Dressings are applied to the **burn,** which are then kept moist with silver nitrate, which stains anything that it comes in contact with; this discoloration is not usually permanent
3. Used on extensive **burns** that may precipitate fluid and electrolyte imbalances
4. Apply to dressing; do not apply to wounds, cuts, or broken skin

PRACTICE QUESTIONS

1. A physician has prescribed Myoflex topical cream for a client with a diagnosis of rheumatism who is complaining of muscular aches. Which of the following information does a nurse provide to the client regarding this medication?
   1. Apply a heating pad to the area after applying the medication

2. The medication acts by decreasing muscle spasms
3. The medication is prescribed to cause the skin to peel
4. The medication will act as a local anesthetic

2. An outbreak of pediculosis capitis has occurred at a local school. The school nurse is providing instructions to the mothers of the children attending the school regarding the application of permethrin 5% (Elimite). The nurse tells the mothers to:
   1. Apply at bedtime and rinse off in the morning
   2. Apply prior to washing the hair
   3. Avoid saturating the hair and scalp when applying
   4. Allow to remain on the hair 10 minutes and then rinse with water

3. A client is seen in a clinic for complaints of skin itchiness that has been persistent over the past several weeks. Following an assessment, it has been determined that the client has scabies. Lindane (Kwell) is prescribed, and a nurse provides instructions to the client regarding the use of the medication. The nurse tells the client to:
   1. Leave the cream on for 8 to 12 hours and then remove by washing
   2. Apply a thick layer of cream to the entire body
   3. Apply the cream for 2 days in a row
   4. Apply to the entire body and scalp, excluding the face

4. A topical corticosteroid is prescribed for a client with dermatitis. A nurse provides instructions to the client regarding the use of the medication. Which of the following, if stated by the client, would indicate a need for further instruction?
   1. "I need to apply the medication in a thin film."
   2. "I should gently rub the medication into the skin."
   3. "I should place a bandage over the site after applying the medication."
   4. "The medication will help to relieve the inflammation and itching."

5. A nurse is applying a topical corticosteroid to a client with eczema. The nurse would be concerned about the potential for systemic absorption of the medication if the medication was being applied to which of the following body areas?
   1. Back
   2. Axilla
   3. Palms of the hands
   4. Soles of the feet

6. Salicylic acid is prescribed for a client with a diagnosis of psoriasis. A nurse monitors the client, knowing that which of the following would indicate the presence of systemic toxicity from this medication?
   1. Decreased respirations

2. Diarrhea
3. Constipation
4. Tinnitus

7. A client is diagnosed with herpes simplex type 1. The physician prescribes a topical medication for treatment. A nurse anticipates that which of the following medications will be prescribed?
   1. Triple antibiotic
   2. Acyclovir (Zovirax)
   3. Mupirocin (Bactroban)
   4. Masoprocol (Actinex)

8. A physician has prescribed coal tar treatments for a client with psoriasis, and a nurse provides information to the client about the treatments. Which statement made by the client indicates a lack of understanding about the treatments?
   1. "The medication has an unpleasant odor."
   2. "The medication can stain the skin and hair."
   3. "The medication can cause systemic toxicity."
   4. "The medication can cause phototoxicity."

9. A camp nurse asks the children preparing to swim in a lake if they have applied sunscreen. The nurse reminds the children that chemical sunscreens are most effective when applied:
   1. One hour before exposure to the sun
   2. Immediately before exposure to the sun
   3. 15 minutes before exposure to the sun
   4. Immediately before swimming

10. Mafenide (Sulfamylon) is prescribed for a client with a burn injury. When applying the medication, the client complains of local discomfort and burning. Which of the following is the most appropriate nursing action?
    1. Discontinue the medication
    2. Notify the physician
    3. Apply a thinner film than prescribed to the burn site
    4. Inform the client that this is normal

11. A burn client is receiving treatments of topical mafenide (Sulfamylon) to the site of injury. A nurse monitors the client, knowing that which of the following indicates that a systemic effect has occurred?
    1. Local pain at the burn site
    2. Local rash at the burn site
    3. Hyperventilation
    4. Elevated blood pressure

12. Sodium hypochlorite (Dakin) solution is prescribed for a client with a leg wound that is draining purulent material. A home health nurse teaches a family member how to perform these treatments. Which statement if made by the family member indicates a need for further teaching?
    1. "The solution should not come in contact with normal skin tissue."

2. "I should rinse the solution off immediately following the irrigation."

3. "I will soak a sterile dressing with solution and pack it into the wound."

4. "I will prepare the solution prior to use."

13. A nurse has provided instructions to a client regarding the use of tretinoin (Retin-A). Which statement if made by the client indicates the need for further instructions?
    1. "I will wash my hands thoroughly after applying the medication."
    2. "Optimal results will be seen after 6 weeks."
    3. "I must apply a thin layer to the skin."
    4. "I will cleanse the skin thoroughly before applying the medication."

14. Isotretinoin (Accutane) is prescribed for a client with severe acne. Prior to the administration of this medication, a nurse would anticipate that which laboratory test will be prescribed?
    1. Complete blood count
    2. White blood cell count
    3. Triglyceride level
    4. Platelet count

15. A client with severe acne is seen in a clinic. A physician prescribes isotretinoin (Accutane). A nurse reviews the client's medication record and would contact the physician if the client were taking which medication?
    1. Digoxin (Lanoxin)
    2. Phenytoin (Dilantin)
    3. Vitamin A
    4. Furosemide (Lasix)

16. A registered nurse (RN) is observing a licensed practical nurse (LPN) perform a dressing change for a client with a leg ulcer. Sutilains (Travase) is being used to treat the ulcer. Which observation by the RN would indicate an inaccurate action by the LPN when performing the dressing change?
    1. The LPN cleans the wound with a sterile solution
    2. The LPN dries the wound and covers the Travase application with a dry sterile dressing
    3. The LPN moistens the wound with sterile normal saline and then applies the Travase
    4. The LPN places the Travase in the refrigerator following use

17. Dextranomer (Debrisan) is prescribed for a client with a decubitus ulcer. A nursing instructor asks the nursing student who is preparing to perform the treatment about the medication and the procedure.

Which statement if made by the student indicates a need for further research?
    1. "It is effective in wet wounds only."
    2. "It should be packed lightly into the wound."
    3. "Maceration of tissue surrounding the wound can occur from the medication."
    4. "The wound bed must be thoroughly dried prior to applying the medication."

18. Fibrinolysin and desoxyribonuclease (Elase) dry powder is prescribed to treat a skin ulcer. Which nursing intervention would not be a component of the plan of care regarding this treatment?
    1. Clean the wound with a sterile solution prior to applying Elase
    2. Prepare the solution just prior to use
    3. Apply a thick layer of medication and cover with a dry sterile dressing
    4. Apply a thin layer of medication and cover with a petrolatum gauze

19. A clinic nurse is performing an admission assessment on a client. The nurse notes that the client is taking azelaic acid (Azelex). Because of the medication prescription, the nurse would suspect that the client is being treated for:
    1. Herpes simplex
    2. Acne
    3. Eczema
    4. Hair loss

20. Minoxidil (Rogaine) is prescribed for a client to treat hair loss. The client asks a nurse if the hair will continue to grow when the medication is stopped. The most appropriate nursing response is:
    1. "The hair will continue to grow."
    2. "Newly gained hair is lost in 3 to 4 months."
    3. "It depends on how long you have been taking the Rogaine."
    4. "I'm not sure; you need to ask your physician."

CRITICAL THINKING: FREE-TEXT ENTRY

A home health care nurse makes a home visit to a client who has an ulcer on the medial aspect of the left ankle. The wound is being treated with Duoderm. The nurse removes the Duoderm, cleanses the wound as prescribed, and reapplies the Duoderm. The nurse schedules the next visit for wound care and for changing the Duoderm in how many days?

Answer: _____

ANSWERS

1. 4

Rationale: Myoflex is one of the many products used for the temporary relief of muscular aches, rheumatism, arthritis, sprains, and neuralgia. These types of products contain combinations of antiseptics, local anesthetics, analgesics, and counterirritants. A heating pad should not be applied because irritation or burning of the skin may occur. The medication does not act in a systemic manner (option 2). These types of products are not prescribed to cause the skin to peel, and if this sort of reaction occurs, the physician should be notified.

Test-Taking Strategy: Use the process of elimination. Noting the key words "topical cream" may assist in eliminating option 2. Eliminate option 3, knowing that this is not an expected therapeutic effect. Recalling the principles related to the application of heat will assist in eliminating option 1. Review this medication if you had difficulty with this question.

Level of Cognitive Ability: Application
Client Needs: Health Promotion and Maintenance
Integrated Concept/Process: Teaching/Learning
Content Area: Pharmacology
Reference: Gutierrez, K. (1999). *Pharmacotherapeutics: Clinical decision-making in nursing.* Philadelphia: W.B. Saunders, p. 1339.

2. 4

Rationale: The instructions for the use of Elimite include: wash, rinse, and towel dry hair; apply sufficient volume to saturate hair and scalp; allow to remain on hair 10 minutes and then rinse with water.

Test-Taking Strategy: Use the process of elimination. Note that both options 1 and 4 address a time frame for allowing the medication to remain on the hair. Recognizing this may provide you with the clue that one of these options is correct. Review this treatment if you are unfamiliar with it.

Level of Cognitive Ability: Application
Client Needs: Safe, Effective Care Environment
Integrated Concept/Process: Teaching/Learning
Content Area: Pharmacology
Reference: Kuhn, M. (1998). *Pharmacotherapeutics: A nursing process approach* (4th ed.). Philadelphia: F.A. Davis, p. 991.

3. 1

Rationale: Kwell is applied in a thin layer to the entire body below the head. No more than 30 g (1 ounce) should be used. The medication is removed by washing 8 to 12 hours later. In most cases, only one application is required.

Test-Taking Strategy: Use the process of elimination. Eliminate option 2 because of the word "thick." Eliminate option 4 because of the word "entire." From the remaining options, eliminate option 3, knowing that only one application is required. Review this medication if you are unfamiliar with it.

Level of Cognitive Ability: Application
Client Needs: Health Promotion and Maintenance
Integrated Concept/Process: Teaching/Learning
Content Area: Pharmacology
Reference: Gutierrez, K. (1999). *Pharmacotherapeutics: Clinical decision-making in nursing.* Philadelphia: W.B. Saunders, p. 579.

4. 3

Rationale: Clients should be advised not to use occlusive dressings (bandages or plastic wraps) to cover the affected site following the application of the topical corticosteroid, unless the physician has specifically prescribed wound coverage. Options 1, 2, and 4 are accurate statements related to the use of this medication.

Test-Taking Strategy: Use the process of elimination. Note the key words "need for further instruction." Eliminate option 4, knowing that this is the action of a corticosteroid. The words "thin" in option 1 and "gently" in option 2 should assist you in eliminating these options. If you had difficulty with this question, review this medication.

Level of Cognitive Ability: Analysis
Client Needs: Health Promotion and Maintenance
Integrated Concept/Process: Teaching/Learning
Content Area: Pharmacology
Reference: Lehne, R. (1998). *Pharmacology for nursing care* (3rd ed.). Philadelphia: W.B. Saunders, p. 1055.

5. 2

Rationale: Topical corticosteroids can be absorbed into the systemic circulation. Absorption is higher from regions where the skin is especially permeable (scalp, axilla, face, eyelids, neck, perineum, genitalia), and lower from regions where penetrability is poor (back, palms, soles).

Test-Taking Strategy: Use the process of elimination. Focus on the issue of the question, "permeability and the potential for systemic absorption." Eliminate options 3 and 4 because these body areas are similar in terms of skin substance. From the remaining options, think about permeability of the skin area. This should direct you to option 2. Review the principles related to the administration of topical corticosteroids if you had difficulty with this question.

Level of Cognitive Ability: Analysis
Client Needs: Physiological Integrity
Integrated Concept/Process: Nursing Process/Analysis
Content Area: Pharmacology
Reference: Salerno, E. (1999). *Pharmacology for health professionals.* St. Louis: Mosby, p. 752.

6. 4

Rationale: Salicylic acid is readily absorbed through the skin, and systemic toxicity (salicylism) can result. Symptoms include tinnitus, dizziness, hyperpnea, and psychological disturbances. Constipation and diarrhea are not associated with salicylism.

Test-Taking Strategy: Use the process of elimination. Noting the name of the medication will assist in directing you to the correct option if you can recall the toxic effects that occur with acetyl*salicylic* acid (Aspirin). Review the toxic effects of salicylic acid if you are unfamiliar with them.

Level of Cognitive Ability: Analysis
Client Needs: Physiological Integrity
Integrated Concept/Process: Nursing Process/Assessment
Content Area: Pharmacology
Reference: Hodgson, B., & Kizior, R. (2001). *Saunders nursing drug handbook 2001.* Philadelphia: W.B. Saunders, p. 76.

7. 2

Rationale: Acyclovir is a topical antiviral agent that inhibits DNA replication in the virus. It has activity against herpes simplex types 1 and 2, varicella-zoster virus, Epstein-Barr virus and cytomegalovirus. Triple antibiotic would not be effective in treating herpesvirus. Bactroban is a topical antibacterial active against *Staphylococcus aureus*, beta-hemolytic streptococci, or *Streptococcus pyogenes*. Actinex is a keratolytic.

Test-Taking Strategy: Use the process of elimination. Knowledge that herpes simplex is a virus will direct you to the option that identifies an antiviral medication. Review these medications if you are unfamiliar with them.

Level of Cognitive Ability: Analysis
Client Needs: Physiological Integrity
Integrated Concept/Process: Nursing Process/Analysis
Content Area: Pharmacology
Reference: Hodgson, B., & Kizior, R. (2001). *Saunders nursing drug handbook 2001.* Philadelphia: W.B. Saunders, p. 13.

8. **3**

Rationale: Coal tar is used to treat psoriasis and other chronic disorders of the skin. It suppresses DNA synthesis, mitotic activity, and cell proliferation. It has an unpleasant odor, can frequently stain the skin and hair, and can cause phototoxicity. Systemic toxicity does not occur.

Test-Taking Strategy: Use the process of elimination. Note the key words "lack of understanding" in the stem of the question. The name of the medication will assist in eliminating options 1 and 2. From the remaining options, it is necessary to know that the medication does not cause systemic toxicity. If you had difficulty with this question, review this treatment.

Level of Cognitive Ability: Analysis
Client Needs: Physiological Integrity
Integrated Concept/Process: Teaching/Learning
Content Area: Pharmacology
Reference: Lehne, R. (1998). *Pharmacology for nursing care* (3rd ed.). Philadelphia: W.B. Saunders, p. 1059.

9. **1**

Rationale: Sunscreens are most effective when applied about 30 minutes to 1 hour before exposure to the sun, so that they can penetrate the skin. All sunscreens should be reapplied after swimming or sweating.

Test-Taking Strategy: Use the process of elimination. Knowledge that sunscreens need to penetrate the skin will assist in eliminating options 2 and 3. Noting the key words "most effective" will assist in directing you to option 1. Review protective skin measures if you had difficulty with this question.

Level of Cognitive Ability: Application
Client Needs: Health Promotion and Maintenance
Integrated Concept/Process: Teaching/Learning
Content Area: Pharmacology
Reference: Kuhn, M. (1998). *Pharmacotherapeutics: A nursing process approach* (4th ed.). Philadelphia: F.A. Davis, p. 993.

10. **4**

Rationale: Mafenide is bacteriostatic for both gram-negative and gram-positive organisms and is used to treat burns to reduce bacteria present in avascular tissues. The client should be informed that the medication will cause local discomfort and burning.

Test-Taking Strategy: Use the process of elimination. Eliminate options 1 and 3 because it is not within the scope of nursing practice to alter or discontinue a medication therapy. Recalling that this is a normal, expected occurrence will easily direct you to option 4. If you had difficulty with this question, review the effects of this medication.

Level of Cognitive Ability: Application

Client Needs: Physiological Integrity
Integrated Concept/Process: Nursing Process/Implementation
Content Area: Pharmacology
Reference: Hodgson, B., & Kizior, R. (2001). *Saunders nursing drug handbook 2001.* Philadelphia: W.B. Saunders, p. 616.

11. **3**

Rationale: Sulfamylon is a carbonic anhydrase inhibitor and can suppress renal excretion of acid, thereby causing acidosis. Clients receiving this treatment should be monitored for acid-base imbalance. If acidosis becomes severe, the medication should be discontinued for 1 to 2 days. Options 1 and 2 describe local rather than systemic effects. An elevated blood pressure may be expected in the client with pain.

Test-Taking Strategy: Use the process of elimination. Note the key words "systemic effect." Options 1 and 2 can be eliminated because these are local rather than systemic effects. From the remaining options, recall that the client in pain would likely have an elevated blood pressure. This should direct you to option 3. Review the systemic effects of this medication if you had difficulty with this question.

Level of Cognitive Ability: Analysis
Client Needs: Physiological Integrity
Integrated Concept/Process: Nursing Process/Assessment
Content Area: Pharmacology
Reference: Hodgson, B., & Kizior, R. (2001). *Saunders nursing drug handbook 2001.* Philadelphia: W.B. Saunders, p. 616.

12. **3**

Rationale: Sodium hypochlorite is a chloride solution that is used for irrigating and cleaning necrotic or purulent wounds. Although it can be used for packing necrotic wounds, it cannot be used to pack purulent wounds, since the solution is inactivated by copious pus. It should not come in contact with healing or normal tissue, and it should be rinsed off immediately if used for irrigation. Solutions are unstable and must be prepared fresh for each use.

Test-Taking Strategy: Use the process of elimination. Note the key words "need for further teaching." Eliminate options 1 and 2 first because they are similar and indicate avoiding healthy tissue. It makes sense to prepare the solution prior to use; therefore eliminate option 4. If you are unfamiliar with the use of this solution, review these concepts.

Level of Cognitive Ability: Analysis
Client Needs: Health Promotion and Maintenance
Integrated Concept/Process: Teaching/Learning
Content Area: Pharmacology
Reference: Karch, A. (2000). *Focus on nursing pharmacology.* Philadelphia: Lippincott, p. 744.

13. **3**

Rationale: Tretinoin is applied liberally to the skin. The hands are washed thoroughly immediately after application. Therapeutic results should be seen after 2 to 3 weeks but may not be optimal until after 6 weeks. The skin needs to be cleansed thoroughly before the medication is applied.

Test-Taking Strategy: Use the process of elimination. Note the key words "need for further instructions." Eliminate options 1 and 4 first, using the principles of asepsis. Recalling that the medication is applied liberally to the skin and noting the absolute term "must" in option 3 will direct you to this option. Review this medication if you had difficulty with this question.

Level of Cognitive Ability: Analysis

Client Needs: Health Promotion and Maintenance
Integrated Concept/Process: Teaching/Learning
Content Area: Pharmacology
Reference: Kuhn, M. (1998). *Pharmacotherapeutics: A nursing process approach* (4th ed.). Philadelphia: F.A. Davis, p. 997.

14. 3
Rationale: Accutane can elevate triglyceride levels. Blood triglyceride content should be measured prior to treatment and periodically thereafter until the effect on the triglycerides has been evaluated. Options 1, 2, and 4 do not need to be specifically monitored during this treatment.
Test-Taking Strategy: Use the process of elimination. Eliminate options 1 and 2 first because a complete blood count will also measure the white blood cell count. From the remaining options, recall that the medication can affect the triglyceride level in the client. Review this medication if you had difficulty with this question
Level of Cognitive Ability: Analysis
Client Needs: Physiological Integrity
Integrated Concept/Process: Nursing Process/Analysis
Content Area: Pharmacology
Reference: Hodgson, B., & Kizior, R. (2001). *Saunders nursing drug handbook 2001.* Philadelphia: W.B. Saunders, p. 558.

15. 3
Rationale: Vitamin A, being a relative of isotretinoin, can produce generalized intensification of isotretinoin toxicity. Because of the potential for increased toxicity, vitamin A supplements should be discontinued prior to isotretinoin therapy. Options 1, 2, and 4 are not contraindicated with the use of isotretinoin.
Test-Taking Strategy: Use the process of elimination. Recalling that isotretinoin is a derivative of vitamin A will easily direct you to the correct option. If you are unfamiliar with this medication, review the contraindications associated with its use.
Level of Cognitive Ability: Analysis
Client Needs: Safe, Effective Care Environment
Integrated Concept/Process: Nursing Process/Analysis
Content Area: Pharmacology
Reference: Hodgson, B., & Kizior, R. (2001). *Saunders nursing drug handbook 2001.* Philadelphia: W.B. Saunders, p. 558.

16. 2
Rationale: The wound should be cleansed with a sterile solution prior to treatment. The nurse then thoroughly moistens the wound with normal saline or sterile water, applies a thin film of Travase extending ¼ to ½ inch beyond the area to be debrided, and then applies a loose thin dressing. The ointment should be refrigerated.
Test-Taking Strategy: Use the process of elimination. Note the key word "inaccurate" in the stem of the question. Recalling that the wound is moistened prior to application of the Travase will direct you to the correct option. Review the method of application of Travase if you had difficulty with this question.
Level of Cognitive Ability: Analysis
Client Needs: Physiological Integrity
Integrated Concept/Process: Nursing Process/Evaluation
Content Area: Pharmacology
Reference: Kuhn, M. (1998). *Pharmacotherapeutics: A nursing process approach* (4th ed.). Philadelphia: F.A. Davis, p. 1010.

17. 4
Rationale: Debrisan is a cleansing rather than a debriding agent. It is effective in wet wounds only. It is not packed tightly into the wound because maceration of surrounding tissue may result.
Test-Taking Strategy: Use the process of elimination. Note the key words "indicates a need for further research." Noting that option 1 indicates that the wound should be wet and option 4 indicates that the wound should be dry provides the clue that one of these options is correct. If you are unfamiliar with the use of Debrisan, review the procedure associated with its use.
Level of Cognitive Ability: Analysis
Client Needs: Physiological Integrity
Integrated Concept/Process: Nursing Process/Evaluation
Content Area: Pharmacology
Reference: Kuhn, M. (1998). *Pharmacotherapeutics: A nursing process approach* (4th ed.). Philadelphia: F.A. Davis, p. 1012.

18. 3
Rationale: The wound should be cleansed with a sterile solution and gently patted dry. A thin layer of Elase is applied and covered with a petrolatum gauze. If a dry powder is used, for best effects, the solution should be prepared just prior to use.
Test-Taking Strategy: Use the process of elimination. Note the word "not" in the stem of the question. Also, noting the key word "thick" in option 3 will direct you to this option. Review the method of application of Elase if you had difficulty with this question.
Level of Cognitive Ability: Application
Client Needs: Physiological Integrity
Integrated Concept/Process: Nursing Process/Planning
Content Area: Pharmacology
Reference: Kuhn, M. (1998). *Pharmacotherapeutics: A nursing process approach* (4th ed.). Philadelphia: F.A. Davis, p. 1010.

19. 2
Rationale: Azelex is a topical medication used to treat mild to moderate acne. It appears to work by suppressing growth of *Propionibacterium acnes* and by decreasing proliferation of keratinocytes. Options 1, 3, and 4 are incorrect.
Test-Taking Strategy: Use the process of elimination. It is necessary to know that Azelex is used to treat acne to answer this question correctly. Review this medication if you are unfamiliar with it.
Level of Cognitive Ability: Analysis
Client Needs: Physiological Integrity
Integrated Concept/Process: Nursing Process/Analysis
Content Area: Pharmacology
Reference: Karch, A. (2000). *Focus on nursing pharmacology.* Philadelphia: Lippincott, p. 747.

20. 2
Rationale: Hair regrowth with the use of Rogaine is most likely to occur when baldness has developed recently and has been limited to a small area. Upon discontinuation of the medication, newly gained hair is lost in 3 to 4 months, and the natural progression of hair loss resumes. Options 1 and 3 are incorrect. Option 4 places the client's question on hold and is inappropriate.
Test-Taking Strategy: Use the process of elimination. Option 4 can be easily eliminated because it places the client's question on hold. Knowledge regarding the clinical response and effects

of this medication is required to select the correct answer from the remaining options. If you are unfamiliar with this medication, review its effects.

Level of Cognitive Ability: Application
Client Needs: Psychosocial Integrity
Integrated Concept/Process: Nursing Process/Implementation
Content Area: Pharmacology
Reference: Hodgson, B., & Kizior, R. (2001). *Saunders nursing drug handbook 2001*. Philadelphia: W.B. Saunders, p. 690.

CRITICAL THINKING: FREE-TEXT ENTRY

Answer: Seven days
Rationale: The nurse would schedule the next home care visit in 7 days. Protective dressings such as Duoderm are designed

to be left in place for 7 days unless leakage occurs around the dressing.

Test-Taking Strategy: Note the key word "Duoderm." Recalling that these dressings are designed to be left in place for 7 days will easily assist in answering this question. Review the purpose and procedure for using protective dressings if you had difficulty with this question.

Level of Cognitive Ability: Application
Client Needs: Health Promotion and Maintenance
Integrated Concept/Process: Nursing Process/Planning
Content Area: Pharmacology
Reference: Lewis, S., Heitkemper, M., & Dirksen, S. (2000). *Medical-surgical nursing: Assessment and management of clinical problems* (5th ed.). St. Louis: Mosby, p. 205.

REFERENCES

Gutierrez, K. (1999). *Pharmacotherapeutics: Clinical decision-making in nursing*. Philadelphia: W.B. Saunders.

Hodgson, B., & Kizior, R. (2001). *Saunders nursing drug handbook 2001*. Philadelphia: W.B. Saunders.

Karch, A. (2000). *Focus on nursing pharmacology*. Philadelphia: Lippincott.

Kuhn, M. (1998). *Pharmacotherapeutics: A nursing process approach* (4th ed.). Philadelphia: F.A. Davis.

Lehne, R. (1998). *Pharmacology for nursing care* (3rd ed.). Philadelphia: W.B. Saunders.

Lewis, S., Heitkemper, M., & Dirksen, S. (2000). *Medical-surgical nursing: Assessment and management of clinical problems* (5th ed.). St. Louis: Mosby.

Salerno, E. (1999). *Pharmacology for health professionals*. St. Louis: Mosby.

The Adult Client with an Oncological Disorder

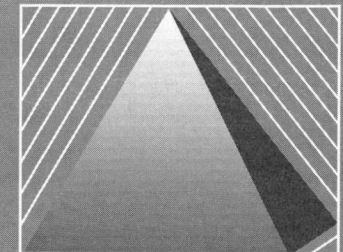

PYRAMID TERMS

benign Usually refers to growths that are encapsulated, remain localized, and are slow growing.

cancer A neoplastic disorder that can involve all body organs. Cells lose their normal growth-controlling mechanism, and the growth of cells is uncontrolled.

carcinogen A physical, chemical, or biological stressor that causes neoplastic changes in normal cells.

carcinoma in situ A lesion with all the histological characteristics of malignancies, except invasion.

carcinomas A new growth or malignant tumor that originates from epithelial cells, the skin, gastrointestinal (GI) tract, lungs, uterus, breast, and other organs.

hospice A concept of care for terminally ill clients that includes the idea of intensive caring rather than intensive care. The family and the client are the focus of nursing care, and the goal is to relieve pain and facilitate the optimal quality of life.

lymphomas Originate from lymphoid tissue.

leukemias or myelomas Originate from blood-forming organs.

malignant Refers to growths that are not encapsulated but metastasize and grow. These growths are cancerous lesions having the characteristics of disorderly, uncontrolled, and chaotic proliferation of cells.

metastasis The transfer of disease from one organ or part to another not directly connected with it. Secondary malignant lesions, originating from the primary tumor, are located in anatomically distant places.

nadir The period of time during which an antineoplastic medication has its most profound effects on the bone marrow.

neoplasm A new growth, which may be benign or malignant.

sarcomas Originate from muscle, bone, fat, the lymph system, or connective tissues.

staging A method of classifying malignancies based on the presence and extent of the tumor within the body.

tumor markers Specific bodily substances that seem to indicate tumor progression or regression.

undifferentiated cells Cells that have lost the capacity for specialized functions.

PYRAMID TO SUCCESS

Pyramid points focus on treatment modalities related to an oncological disorder, such as pain management, internal and external radiation, and chemotherapy, and on oncological disorders such as skin cancer, leukemia, breast cancer, and lung cancer. Specific focus relates to the nursing care related to these treatment modalities and disorders, and to client adaptation and the impact of the treatment or the disorder. Specifically, focus on the complications related to chemotherapy and the nursing measures required in monitoring for these complications, and in preventing life-threatening conditions such as infection and bleeding. Specific laboratory values include the white blood cell count and the platelet count. The Integrated Concepts and Processes addressed in this unit include Nursing Process, Caring, Communication and Documentation, Cultural Awareness, Self-Care, and Teaching/Learning.

CLIENT NEEDS
Safe, Effective Care Environment

Advance directives
Advocacy related to client's decisions
Client rights
Confidentiality regarding diagnosis
Establishing priorities
Ethical practice

Handling hazardous and infectious materials related to radiation and chemotherapy
Informed consent for treatments and procedures
Medical and surgical asepsis
Oncology-related consultations and referrals
Protective precautions
Standard (universal) precautions

Health Promotion and Maintenance

Client and family instructions regarding home care
Client lifestyle choices
Expected body image changes related to chemotherapy and treatments
Health screening measures for cancer
Health promotion programs regarding risks for cancer
Instructions regarding monthly breast or testicular self-examinations
Prevention of disease related to infection

Psychosocial Integrity

Ability to cope, adapt, and/or problem solve during illness or stressful events
Assisting the client and family to cope with the alteration in body image
End-of-life issues
Grief and loss related to death and the dying process
Mobilizing appropriate support and resource systems
Promoting a positive environment to maintain optimal quality of life
Religious and cultural preferences

Physiological Integrity

Administration of blood and blood products
Central venous access devices

Chemotherapy
Diagnostic tests and laboratory values such as white blood cell and platelet counts
Managing pain
Providing basic care and comfort
Monitoring for expected and unexpected responses to radiation and chemotherapy
Promoting nutrition
Protecting the client from the life-threatening side effects of treatments
Radiation therapy

REFERENCES

Craven, R., & Hirnle, C. (2000). *Fundamentals of nursing: Human health and function* (3rd ed.). Philadelphia: Lippincott.

Harkreader, H. (2000). *Fundamentals of nursing: Caring and clinical judgment*. Philadelphia: W.B. Saunders.

Ignatavicius, D., Workman, M., & Mishler, M. (1999). *Medical-surgical nursing across the health care continuum* (3rd ed.). Philadelphia: W.B. Saunders.

LeMone, P., & Burke, K. (2000). *Medical-surgical nursing: Critical thinking in client care* (2nd ed.). Upper Saddle River, N.J.: Prentice-Hall.

Lewis, S., Heitkemper, M., & Dirksen, S. (2000). *Medical-surgical nursing: Assessment and management of clinical problems* (5th ed.). St. Louis: Mosby.

National Council of State Boards of Nursing (eds.) (2000). *Test Plan for the National Council Licensure Examination for Registered Nurses*. Chicago: Author.

Potter, P., & Perry, A. (2001). *Fundamentals of nursing* (5th ed.). St. Louis: Mosby.

Smeltzer, S., & Bare, B. (2000) *Textbook of medical-surgical nursing* (9th ed). Philadelphia: Lippincott Williams & Wilkins.

49

Oncological Disorders

BOX 49-1
Common Sites of Metastasis

BREAST CANCER
Bone
Lung

LUNG CANCER
Brain

COLORECTAL CANCER
Liver

PROSTATE CANCER
Bone
Spine and legs

BRAIN TUMORS
Central nervous system

I. CANCER

A. Description
   1. A neoplastic disorder that can involve all body organs
   2. Cells lose their normal growth-controlling mechanism, and the growth of cells is uncontrolled
   3. **Cancer** produces serious health problems such as impaired immune and hematopoietic (blood-producing) function; altered gastrointestinal (GI) tract structure and function; motor and sensory deficits; and decreased respiratory function

B. **Metastasis** (Box 49-1)
   1. **Cancer** cells move from their original location to other sites
   2. Routes of **metastasis**
      a. Local seeding: Distribution of shed **cancer** cells in the local area of the primary tumor
      b. Blood-borne **metastasis:** Tumor cells enter the blood; most common cause of **cancer** spread
      c. Lymphatic spread: Primary sites rich in lymphatics are more susceptible to early metastatic spread

C. **Cancer** classification
   1. Solid tumors: Associated with the organs from which they develop, such as breast **cancer** or lung **cancer**
   2. Hematologic **cancers:** Originate from blood cell–forming tissues, such as the **leukemias** and the **lymphomas**

D. Grading and **staging**
   1. A method used to describe the tumor
   2. Includes the extent of the tumor, the extent to which malignancy has increased in size, the involvement of regional nodes, and metastatic development
   3. Grading a tumor classifies the cellular aspects of the **cancer**
   4. **Staging** classifies the clinical aspects of the **cancer**

E. Factors that influence **cancer** development
   1. Environmental factors
      a. Chemical **carcinogens:** Industrial chemicals, drugs, and tobacco
      b. Physical **carcinogens:** Ionizing radiation (diagnostic and therapeutic x-rays) and ultraviolet radiation (sun, tanning beds, and germicidal lights); chronic irritation and tissue trauma
      c. Viral **carcinogens:** Viruses capable of causing **cancer** are known as oncoviruses (Epstein-Barr virus, hepatitis B virus, human papillomavirus)
   2. Dietary factors: High-fat and low-fiber diets; high animal fat intake; preservatives, contaminants, additives; and nitrates
   3. Genetic predisposition: Inherited predisposition to specific **cancers,** inherited conditions associated with **cancer,** familial clustering, and chromosomal abberations

---

BOX 49-2

Warning Signs of Cancer

Change in bowel or bladder habits
Any sore that does not heal
Nagging cough or hoarseness
Unusual bleeding or discharge
Thickening or lump in breast or elsewhere
Indigestion
Obvious change in wart or mole

BOX 49 3

Diagnostic Tests

Cytology studies (Pap smear)
Chest x-ray
Complete blood count
Proctoscopic examination (including guaiac for occult blood)
Liver function studies
Radiographic studies (mammogram)
Radioisotope scans (liver, brain, bone, lung)
Magnetic resonance imaging (MRI)
Computed tomography (CT scan)
Presence of oncofetal antigens such as carcinoembryonic antigen (CEA) and alpha-fetoprotein AFP)
Bone marrow examination (if a hematolymphoid malignancy is suspected)
Biopsy

---

4. Age: Advancing age is a significant risk factor for the development of **cancer**
5. Immune function: Incidences of **cancer** are higher in immunosuppressed individuals, organ transplant recipients who are taking immunosuppressive medication, and individuals with acquired immunodeficiency syndrome (AIDS)

F. Prevention: Avoidance of known or potential **carcinogens** and avoidance or modification of the factors associated with the development of **cancer** cells

G. Early detection (Box 49-2)
   1. Mammography
   2. Papanicolaou ("Pap") test
   3. Stools for occult blood
   4. Sigmoidoscopy
   5. Breast self-examination
   6. Testicular self-examination
   7. Skin inspection

▲ **II. BREAST SELF-EXAMINATION (BSE)**
A. Performing BSE
   1. Perform 7 to 10 days after menses
   2. Postmenopausal clients or clients who have had a hysterectomy should select a specific day of the month and perform BSE monthly on that day
B. Procedure
   1. Before a mirror
      a. Inspect with arms at the side
      b. Raise arms overhead to inspect for changes in size or contour, dimpling, or changes in the nipple
      c. Inspect by resting the palms on the hips and pressing down firmly to flex the chest muscles
   2. Lying down
      a. Place a pillow under the right breast
      b. Use the pads of the middle three fingers of the left hand; press firmly on the right breast, and feel for lumps or changes by using a rubbing, circular pattern to cover all breast tissue
      c. Gently squeeze the nipple, looking for discharge
      d. Perform BSE on the left breast, using the same method

3. In the shower
   a. With fingers flat, move gently over every part of each breast
   b. Check for lumps or thickening

III. TESTICULAR SELF-EXAMINATION (TSE)   ▲
A. Select a day of the month and perform the examination on the same day each month
B. Perform after a warm bath or shower
C. Hold the scrotum in one hand
D. Examine each testicle separately by gently rolling it between the thumb and fingers of the other hand
E. Check for hard lumps or knots

IV. DIAGNOSTIC TESTS
A. Diagnostic tests to be performed will depend on the suspected primary or metastatic site(s) of the **cancer** (Box 49-3)
B. Biopsy   ▲
   1. Description
      a. Definitive means of diagnosing **cancer** and provides histologic proof of malignancy
      b. Involves the surgical incision of a small piece of tissue for microscopic examination
   2. Types
      a. Needle: Aspiration of cells
      b. Incisional: Wedge of suspected tissue is removed from a larger mass
      c. Excisional: Complete removal of the entire lesion
      d. **Staging:** Multiple needle or incisional biopsies in tissues where **metastasis** is suspected or likely
   3. Tissue examination
      a. Following excision, a frozen section or a permanent paraffin section is done in order to examine the specimen

b. The advantage of the frozen section is the speed with which the section can be prepared and the diagnosis made, as only minutes are required for this test

c. Permanent paraffin section takes about 24 hours; however, it provides clearer details than does the frozen section

4. Implementation

a. The procedure is usually performed in an outpatient surgical setting

b. Prepare the client for the diagnostic procedure, following the physician's instructions

c. Obtain an informed consent

▲ V. PAIN CONTROL

A. Causes of pain

1. Bone destruction
2. Obstruction of an organ
3. Compression of peripheral nerves
4. Infiltration/distention of tissue
5. Inflammation/necrosis
6. Psychological, such as fear or anxiety

▲ B. Implementation

1. Collaborate with other members of the health care team to develop a pain management program
2. Administer oral preparations if possible and if they provide adequate relief of pain
3. Mild or moderate pain may be treated with salicylates, acetaminophen (Tylenol), and nonsteroidal antiinflammatory drugs (NSAIDs)
4. Severe pain is treated with narcotics, such as codeine sulfate, meperidine (Demerol), morphine sulfate, and hydromorphone hydrochloride (Dilaudid)
5. Subcutaneous injections and continuous IV infusions of narcotics provide superior pain control
6. Monitor for side effects of medications
7. Monitor for effectiveness of medications
8. Provide nonpharmacological techniques of pain control, such as relaxation, guided imagery, biofeedback, and diversion
9. Do not undermedicate the **cancer** client who is in pain

VI. SURGERY

A. Description: Used to diagnose, stage, and treat **cancer**

B. Prophylactic surgery

1. Performed in clients with an existing premalignant condition or a known family history that strongly predisposes the person to the development of **cancer**
2. An attempt is made to remove the tissue or organ at risk and thus prevent the development of **cancer**

C. Curative surgery: All gross and microscopic tumor is either removed or destroyed

D. Control (cytoreductive) surgery

1. A "debulking" procedure that consists of removing part of the tumor
2. It decreases the number of **cancer** cells and increases the chance that other therapies will be successful

E. Palliative surgery

1. Performed to improve quality of life during the survival time
2. Performed to reduce pain, relieve airway obstruction, relieve obstructions in the GI or urinary tract, relieve pressure on the brain or spinal cord, prevent hemorrhage, remove infected or ulcerated tumors, or drain abscesses

F. Reconstructive or rehabilitative surgery: Performed to improve quality of life by restoring maximal function and appearance

G. Side effects of surgery

1. Loss or loss of function of a specific body part
2. Reduced function as a result of organ loss
3. Scarring or disfigurement
4. Grieving about altered body image or imposed change in lifestyle

VII. CHEMOTHERAPY ▲

A. Description

1. Kills or inhibits the reproduction of neoplastic cells
2. The effects are systemic; affects both healthy cells and cancerous cells
3. Normal cells most profoundly affected include those of the skin, hair, and lining of the GI tract, spermatocytes, and hematopoietic cells
4. Cell cycle phase–specific medications affect cells only during a certain phase of the reproductive cycle, and cell cycle phase–nonspecific medications affect cells in any phase of the reproductive cycle
5. Usually several medications are used in combination (combination therapy) to increase the therapeutic response
6. Combination chemotherapy is planned to avoid prescribing medications with **nadirs** (the time during which bone marrow activity and white blood cell counts are at their lowest) at or near the same time, to minimize immunosuppression
7. Antineoplastic therapy may be combined with other treatments, such as surgery and radiation
8. The preferred route of administration is by IV
9. Side effects include alopecia, nausea and vomiting, mucositis, skin changes, immunosuppression, anemia, and thrombocytopenia
10. Refer to Chapter 50 for information regarding the care of the client receiving chemotherapy

BOX 49-4

Teletherapy: Client Education

Wash area with water or mild soap and water, using the hand rather than a washcloth; rinse the soap thoroughly, and pat dry with a soft towel or cloth

Do not remove the radiation markings from the skin

Use no powders, ointments, lotions, or creams on the area unless prescribed

Wear soft clothing over the area, avoiding belts, buckles, straps, or any clothing that binds or rubs the skin

Avoid sun and heat exposure

Monitor for moist desquamation (weeping of the skin)

If moist desquamation occurs, cleanse the area with warm water and pat dry, apply antibiotic ointment or steroid cream as prescribed, and expose the site to air

BOX 49-5

Care of the Client with a Sealed Radiation Source

Place the client in a private room with a private bath

Place a caution sign on the client's door

Organize nursing tasks to minimize exposure to the radiation source

Nursing assignments to a client with a radiation implant should be rotated

Limit time to one-half hour per care provider per shift

Wear a dosimeter film badge to measure radiation exposure

Wear a lead shield to reduce the transmission of radiation

A nurse should never care for more than one client with a radiation implant at one time

Do not allow a pregnant nurse to care for the client

Do not allow children under the age of 16 or a pregnant woman to visit the client

Limit visitors to one-half hour per day; visitors should be at least 6 feet from the source

Save bed linens and dressings until the source is removed; then dispose of in the usual manner

Other equipment can be removed from the room at any time

VIII. RADIATION THERAPY

A. Description
1. Destroys **cancer** cells with minimal exposure of normal cells to the damaging effects of radiation; the cells damaged either die or become unable to divide
2. Effective on tissues directly within the path of the radiation beam
3. Side effects include skin changes and irritation, alopecia, fatigue, and altered taste sensation; also, the effects vary according to the site of treatment
4. Teletherapy and brachytherapy are the types of radiation therapy most commonly used to treat **cancer**

B. Teletherapy (Box 49-4)
1. Also called beam radiation; the actual radiation source is external to client
2. The client does not emit radiation and does not pose a hazard to anyone else

C. Brachytherapy
1. The radiation source comes into direct, continuous contact with tumor tissues for a specific time
2. The radiation source is within the client; for a period of time, the client emits radiation and can pose a hazard to others
3. Includes either an unsealed source or a sealed source of radiation
4. Unsealed radiation source
   a. Administered via the oral or IV route or by instillation into body cavities
   b. The source is not completely confined to one body area, and it enters body fluids and is eventually eliminated via various excreta, which are radioactive and harmful to others; most of the source is eliminated from the body within 48 hours; then neither the client nor the excreta are radioactive or harmful
5. Sealed radiation source (Boxes 49-5 and 49-6)
   a. A sealed, temporary or permanent radiation

BOX 49-6

A Dislodged Radiation Source

Do not touch a dislodged radiation source with bare hands

If the radiation source dislodges, use long-handled forceps to place the source in the lead container kept in the client's room, and call the physician

If unable to locate the radiation source, bar visitors and notify the physician

source (solid implant) implanted within the tumor target tissues
   b. The client emits radiation while the implant is in place, but the excreta are not radioactive
6. Removal of sealed radiation sources
   a. The client is no longer radioactive
   b. Inform the client that sexual partners cannot "catch" **cancer**
   c. Inform the female client that she may resume sexual intercourse after 7 to 10 days, if the implant was cervical or vaginal
   d. Provide a Betadine douche if prescribed, if the implant was placed in the cervix
   e. Administer a Fleets enema if prescribed
   f. Advise the client who had a cervical or vaginal implant to notify the physician if nausea, vomiting, diarrhea, frequent urination, vaginal or rectal bleeding, hematuria, foul-smelling vaginal discharge, abdominal pain or distention, or a fever occurs

IX. BONE MARROW TRANSPLANTATION

A. Description
1. Used in the treatment of **leukemia** for clients who have closely matched donors and who are experiencing temporary remission with chemotherapy
2. The goal of treatment is to rid the client of all leukemic or other **malignant** cells through treatment with high doses of chemotherapy and whole-body irradiation
3. Since these treatments are lethal to bone marrow, without the replacement of bone marrow function through transplantation, the client would die of infection or hemorrhage

B. Types of donor marrow
1. Allogeneic: Marrow donor is usually a sibling or parent with a similar tissue type
2. Syngeneic: Bone marrow from an identical twin
3. Autologous
   a. Most common type
   b. The marrow donor is also the recipient
   c. Marrow is harvested during disease remission and is stored frozen, to be reinfused later

C. Procedure
1. Harvest
   a. Marrow is harvested through multiple aspirations from the iliac crest to retrieve sufficient bone marrow for the transplant
   b. Approximately 500 to 1000 mL of marrow is aspirated
   c. Marrow is filtered for any residual **cancer** cells and to deplete cells that may cause graft-versus-host disease
   d. Allogeneic marrow is transfused immediately; autologous marrow is frozen for later use
   e. Harvest is obtained before the initiation of the conditioning regimen
2. Conditioning: Refers to an immunosuppression therapy regimen used to eradicate all **malignant** cells, provide a state of immunosuppression, and create space in the bone marrow for the engraftment of the new marrow
3. Transplantation
   a. Bone marrow is administered through the client's central line in a manner similar to a blood transfusion
   b. Marrow is infused over a 30-minute period or may be administered by IV push directly into the central line
4. Engraftment
   a. The transfused bone marrow cells move to the marrow-forming sites of the recipient's bones
   b. Engraftment occurs when the white blood cell, erythrocyte, and platelet counts begin to rise
   c. When successful, the engraftment process takes 2 to 5 weeks

D. Post-transplantation period
1. The client remains without any natural immunity until the donor marrow begins to proliferate and engraftment occurs
2. Infection and severe thrombocytopenia are major concerns until engraftment occurs

E. Complications
1. Failure to engraft: If the transplanted bone marrow fails to engraft, the client will die unless another transplantation is attempted and is successful
2. Graft-versus-host disease (GVHD)
   a. Although the recipient cannot recognize the donated bone marrow cells as foreign or nonself because of the total immunosuppression, the immune competent cells of the donated marrow recognize the client's cells as foreign and mount an immune offense against them
   b. The graft is actually trying to attack the host
   c. GVHD is managed with immunosuppressive agents, with caution to avoid suppressing the new immune system to the extent that the client becomes more susceptible to infection, or the transplanted cells stop engrafting
3. Veno-occlusive disease
   a. Involves occlusion of the hepatic venules by thrombosis or phlebitis
   b. Signs include right upper quadrant abdominal pain, jaundice, ascites, weight gain, and hepatomegaly
   c. Early detection is critical because there is no known way to open the hepatic vessels
   d. The client will be treated with fluids and supportive therapy

X. SKIN CANCER (Refer to Chapter 47)

XI. LEUKEMIA (Box 49-7)

A. Description
1. **Malignant** exacerbation in the number of leukocytes, usually at an immature stage, in the bone marrow
2. May be acute, with a sudden onset and short duration, or chronic, with a slow onset and persistent symptoms over a period of years
3. Affects the bone marrow, causing anemia, leukopenia, the production of immature cells, thrombocytopenia, and a decline in immunity
4. The cause is unknown and appears to involve gene damage of cells, leading to the transformation of cells from a normal state to a **malignant** state
5. Risk factors include genetic, viral, immunological, and environmental factors and exposure to radiation, chemicals, and medications

---

BOX 49-7

Classification of Leukemia

ACUTE LYMPHOCYTIC LEUKEMIA (ALL)
Mostly lymphoblasts present in bone marrow
Age of onset is less than 15 years

ACUTE MYELOGENOUS LEUKEMIA (AML)
Mostly myeloblasts present in bone marrow
Age of onset is between 15 and 39 years

CHRONIC MYELOGENOUS LEUKEMIA (CML)
Mostly granulocytes present in bone marrow
Age of onset is after 50 years

CHRONIC LYMPHOCYTIC LEUKEMIA (CLL)
Mostly lymphocytes present in bone marrow
Age of onset is after 50 years

BOX 49-8

Mouth Care for the Client with Mucositis

Inspect mouth daily
Offer complete mouth care before and after every meal
   and at bedtime
Brush teeth and tongue with a soft-bristled toothbrush
   or sponges
Provide mouth rinses every 12 hours (saline or sodium
   bicarbonate and water, as prescribed)
Administer topical anesthetic agents to the mouth sores
   as prescribed
Avoid the use of alcohol- or glycerin-based mouthwashes
   or swabs
Apply petrolatum jelly to the client's lips
Avoid foods that are hard or spicy

B. Assessment
   1. Anorexia, fatigue, weakness, weight loss
   2. Anemia
   3. Bleeding (nosebleeds, gum bleeding, rectal bleeding, hematuria, increased menstrual flow)
   4. Petechiae
   5. Prolonged bleeding after minor abrasions or lacerations
   6. Elevated temperature
   7. Lymphadenopathy and splenomegaly
   8. Palpitations, tachycardia, orthostatic hypotension
   9. Pallor and dyspnea on exertion
   10. Headache
   11. Bone pain and joint swelling
   12. Normal, elevated, or reduced WBC count
   13. Decreased hemoglobin and hematocrit levels
   14. Decreased platelet count
   15. Positive bone marrow biopsy identifying leukemic blast phase cells
C. Infection
   1. A major cause of death in the immunosuppressed client
   2. Can occur through autocontamination or cross-contamination
   3. Common sites of infection are the skin, respiratory tract, and GI tract
   4. Initiate protective isolation procedures
   5. Ensure frequent and thorough handwashing
   6. Ensure that anyone entering the client's room is wearing a mask
   7. Use strict aseptic technique for all procedures
   8. Keep supplies for the client separate from supplies for other clients; keep frequently used equipment in the room for the client's use only
   9. Limit the number of caregivers entering the client's room

   10. Maintain the client in a private room
   11. Place the client in a room with high-efficiency particulate air (HEPA) filtration or laminar air flow system if possible
   12. Reduce exposure to environmental organisms by eliminating raw fruits and vegetables (low-bacteria diet) from the diet and fresh flowers from the client's room and by not leaving standing water in the client's room
   13. Be sure that the client's room is cleaned daily
   14. Assist the client with daily bathing, using an antimicrobial soap
   15. Assist the client to perform oral hygiene frequently
   16. Initiate a bowel program to prevent constipation and prevent rectal trauma
   17. Avoid invasive procedures such as injections, rectal temperatures, and urinary catheterization
   18. Change wound dressings daily, and inspect the wounds for redness, swelling, or drainage
   19. Assess the urine for color and cloudiness
   20. Assess skin and oral mucous membranes for signs of infection (Box 49-8)
   21. Auscultate lung sounds, and encourage the client to cough and deep breathe
   22. Monitor temperature, pulse, and blood pressure
   23. Monitor WBC and neutrophil counts
   24. Notify the physician if signs of infection are present, and prepare to obtain specimens for culture of open lesions, urine, and sputum
   25. Administer prescribed antibiotic, antifungal, and antiviral medication
   26. Instruct the client to avoid crowds and those with infections
   27. Instruct the client about a low-bacteria diet (avoid salads, raw fruit and vegetables, undercooked meat, pepper, and paprika) and to avoid drinking water that has been standing for longer than 15 minutes

28. Instruct the client to avoid activities that expose the client to infection, such as changing a pet's litter box or working with houseplants or in the garden

29. Instruct clients that neither they nor their household contacts should receive immunization with a live virus

D. Bleeding

1. During the period of greatest bone marrow suppression (the **nadir**), the platelet count may be extremely low, less than $10,000/mm^3$

2. The client is at risk for bleeding when the platelet count falls below $50,000/mm^3$, and spontaneous bleeding frequently occurs when the platelet count is lower than $20,000/mm^3$

3. Clients with platelet counts below $20,000/mm^3$ may need a platelet transfusion

4. For clients with anemia and fatigue, packed red blood cells (RBCs) may be prescribed

5. Monitor laboratory values

6. Examine the client for signs and symptoms of bleeding; examine all body fluids and excrement for the presence of blood

7. Handle the client gently; use caution when taking blood pressures, to prevent skin injury

8. Measure abdominal girth, which can provide an indication of internal hemorrhage

9. Provide soft foods that are cool to warm

10. Avoid injections if possible, to prevent trauma to the skin and bleeding; apply firm and gentle pressure to a needle stick site for at least 10 minutes

11. Pad side rails and sharp corners of the bed and furniture

12. Avoid rectal suppositories, enemas, and thermometers

13. If the female client is menstruating, count the number of pads or tampons used

14. Administer blood products as prescribed

15. Instruct the client to use a soft toothbrush and avoid dental floss

16. Instruct the client to use only an electric razor for shaving

17. Instruct the client to avoid blowing the nose

18. Instruct the client to avoid constrictive or tight clothing or shoes

19. Discourage the client from engaging in activities involving the use of sharp objects

20. Instruct the client to avoid using NSAIDs and products that contain aspirin

E. Fatigue and nutrition

1. Assist the client in selecting a well-balanced diet

2. Provide small, frequent meals (high calorie, high protein, high carbohydrate) that require little chewing

3. Assist the client in self-care and mobility activities

4. Allow adequate rest periods during care

5. Do not perform activities unless they are essential

6. Administer blood products for anemia as prescribed

F. Implementation

1. Chemotherapy

a. Induction therapy: Aimed at achieving a rapid, complete remission of all manifestations of the disease

b. Consolidation therapy: Administered early in remission with the aim of cure

c. Maintenance therapy: May be prescribed for months or years following successful induction and consolidation therapy; the aim is to maintain remission

2. Administer antibiotic, antibacterial, antiviral, and antifungal medications as prescribed

3. Administer blood replacements as prescribed

4. Prepare the client for transplantation as prescribed

5. Administer colony-stimulating factors as prescribed

6. Maintain infection and bleeding precautions

7. Provide an adequate diet

8. Provide an activity schedule that will conserve energy

9. Instruct the client in appropriate home care measures

10. Provide psychosocial support and support services for home care

XII. HODGKIN'S DISEASE

A. Description

1. A malignancy of the lymph nodes that originates in a single lymph node or a single chain of nodes

2. **Metastasis** occurs to other, adjacent lymph structures and eventually invades nonlymphoid tissue

3. Usually involves lymph nodes, tonsils, spleen, and bone marrow and is characterized by the presence of the Reed-Sternberg cell in the nodes

4. Possible causes include viral infections and previous exposure to alkylating chemical agents

5. Prognosis is dependent on the stage of the disease (Box 49-9)

B. Assessment

1. Fever

2. Malaise, fatigue, and weakness

3. Night sweats

4. Loss of appetite and significant weight loss

5. Anemia and thrombocytopenia

6. Enlarged lymph nodes, spleen, and liver

7. Positive biopsy of lymph nodes, with cervical nodes most often affected first

8. Presence of Reed-Sternberg cell in nodes

9. Positive CT scan of the liver and spleen

C. Implementation

1. For stages I and II without mediastinal node involvement, the treatment of choice is extensive

---

BOX 49-9

Staging in Hodgkin's Disease

STAGE I
Involvement of a single lymph node region or an extra-lymphatic organ or site

STAGE II
Involvement of two or more lymph node regions on the same side of the diaphragm or localized involvement of an extralymphatic organ or site

STAGE III
Involvement of lymph node regions on both sides of the diaphragm

STAGE IV
Diffuse or disseminated involvement of one or more extralymphatic organs with or without associated lymph node involvement

---

external radiation of the involved lymph node regions
2. With more extensive disease, radiation along with multiagent chemotherapy is utilized
3. Monitor for side effects related to chemotherapy or radiation
4. Monitor for signs of infection and bleeding
5. Maintain infection and bleeding precautions
6. Discuss the possibility of sterility with the male client receiving radiation, and inform the client of options related to sperm banks

XIII. MULTIPLE MYELOMA

A. Description
   1. A **malignant** proliferation of plasma cells and tumors within the bone
   2. An excessive number of abnormal plasma cells invade the bone marrow, develop into tumors, and ultimately destroy bone; invasion of the lymph nodes, spleen, and liver occurs
   3. The abnormal plasma cells produce an abnormal antibody (**myeloma** protein or the Bence Jones protein) that is found in the blood and urine
   4. Causes decreased production of immunoglobulin and antibodies, and increased levels of uric acid and calcium, which can lead to renal failure
   5. The cause is unknown
B. Assessment
   1. Bone (skeletal) pain, especially in the pelvis, spine, and ribs
   2. Weakness and fatigue
   3. Recurrent infections
   4. Anemia

5. Bence Jones proteinuria and elevated total serum protein level
6. Osteoporosis (bone loss and the development of pathological fractures)
7. Thrombocytopenia and granulocytopenia
8. Elevated calcium and uric acid levels
9. Renal failure
10. Spinal cord compression and paraplegia

C. Implementation
   1. Administer chemotherapy as prescribed
   2. Provide supportive care to control symptoms and prevent complications, especially bone fractures, renal failure, and infections
   3. Maintain neutropenic and bleeding precautions as necessary
   4. Monitor for signs of bleeding, infection, and skeletal fractures
   5. Force fluids up to 3 to 4 liters a day, to offset potential problems associated with hypercalcemia, hyperuricemia, and proteinuria
   6. Monitor for signs of renal failure
   7. Encourage ambulation to prevent renal problems and to slow down bone resorption
   8. Provide skeletal support during moving, turning, and ambulating to prevent pathological fractures; provide a hazard-free environment
   9. Administer IVs and diuretics as prescribed to increase renal excretion of calcium
   10. Administer blood transfusions as prescribed for anemia
   11. Administer analgesics as prescribed to control pain
   12. Administer antibiotics as prescribed for infection
   13. Prepare the client for local radiation therapy if prescribed
   14. Instruct the client in home care measures and the signs and symptoms of infection

XIV. TESTICULAR CANCER

A. Description
   1. Arises from germinal epithelium from the sperm-producing germ cells or from nongerminal epithelium from other structures in the testicles (Box 49-10)
   2. Most often occurs between the ages of 15 and 40
   3. **Metastasis** occurs to the lung, liver, bone, and adrenal glands
B. Prevention: Routine testicular self-examination
C. Assessment
   1. Painless testicular swelling
   2. Dragging sensation in scrotum
   3. Palpable lymphadenopathy, abdominal masses, and gynecomastia may indicate **metastasis**
   4. Late signs include back or bone pain and respiratory symptoms

---

BOX 49-10

Types of Testicular Cancer

GERMINAL TUMORS
Seminomas
Nonseminomas

NONGERMINAL TUMORS
Interstitial cell tumors
Androblastoma

BOX 49-11

Preinvasive Cancers

CERVICAL INTRAEPITHELIAL NEOPLASIA (CIN)
CIN I: Mild dysplasia
CIN II: Moderate dysplasia
CIN III: Severe dysplasia to cancer in situ (CIS)

BOX 49-12

Treatment for Cervical Cancer

NONSURGICAL
External radiation
Internal radiation implants (intracavitary)
Chemotherapy
Laser therapy
Cryosurgery

SURGICAL
Conization
Hysterectomy
Pelvic exenteration

D. Implementation
1. Administer chemotherapy as prescribed
2. Prepare the client for radiation therapy as prescribed
3. Prepare the client for unilateral orchiectomy, if prescribed, for diagnosis and primary surgical management
4. Prepare the client for radical retroperitoneal lymph node dissection, if prescribed, to stage the disease and reduce tumor volume so that chemotherapy and radiation therapy are more effective
5. Discuss reproduction, sexuality, and fertility information and options with the client
6. Identify reproductive options such as sperm storage, donor insemination, and adoption
E. Postoperative implementation
1. Monitor for signs of bleeding and wound infection
2. Monitor intake and output (I & O)
3. Notify the physician if chills, fever, increasing pain or tenderness at the incision site, or drainage of the incision occurs
4. Instruct the client that he may resume normal activities within 1 week, except for lifting objects heavier that 20 pounds or stair climbing
5. Instruct the client to perform monthly TSE on the remaining testicle
6. Inform the client that sutures will be removed 7 to 10 days after surgery

XV. CERVICAL CANCER
A. Description
1. Preinvasive **cancer** in limited to the cervix (Box 49-11)
2. Invasive **cancer** is in the cervix and other pelvic structures
3. **Metastasis** is usually confined to the pelvis, but distant **metastasis** occurs through lymphatic spread
4. **Premalignant** changes are described on a continuum from dysplasia, which is the earliest premalignancy change, to **carcinoma in situ** (CIS), the most advanced **premalignant** change

B. Precipitating factors
1. Low socioeconomic groups
2. Early first marriage
3. Early and frequent intercourse
4. Multiple sex partners
5. High parity
6. Poor hygiene
C. Assessment
1. Painless vaginal bleeding postmenstrually and postcoitally
2. Foul-smelling or serosanguineous vaginal discharge
3. Pelvic, lower back, leg, or groin pain
4. Anorexia and weight loss
5. Leakage of urine and feces from the vagina
6. Dysuria
7. Hematuria
8. Cytological changes on Papanicolaou test
D. Implementation (Box 49-12)
E. Laser therapy
1. Used when all boundaries of the lesion are visible during colposcopic examination
2. Energy from the beam is absorbed by fluid in the tissues, causing them to vaporize
3. Minimal bleeding is associated with the procedure
4. Slight vaginal discharge is expected following the procedure, and healing occurs in 6 to 12 weeks
F. Cryosurgery
1. Freezing of the tissues by a probe with subsequent necrosis

2. No anesthesia is required, although cramping may occur during the procedure
3. A heavy, watery discharge will occur for several weeks following the procedure
4. Instruct the client to avoid intercourse and the use of tampons while the discharge is present

▲ G. Conization
   1. A cone-shaped area of the cervix is removed
   2. Performed in women who desire further childbearing
   3. Long-term follow-up care is needed, as new lesions can develop
   4. The risks of the procedure include hemorrhage, uterine perforation, incompetent cervix, cervical stenosis, and preterm labor in future pregnancies

H. Hysterectomy
   1. Description
      a. For microinvasive **cancer** if childbearing is not desired
      b. A vaginal approach is most commonly performed
      c. A radical hysterectomy and bilateral lymph node dissection may be performed for **cancer** that has spread beyond the cervix but not to the pelvic wall
   2. Postoperative implementation
      a. Monitor vital signs
   ▲ b. Assist with coughing and deep-breathing exercises
      c. Assist with range-of-motion (ROM) exercises and provide early ambulation
   ▲ d. Apply antiembolism stockings as prescribed
      e. Monitor I & O, Foley catheter drainage, and hydration status
   ▲ f. Monitor bowel sounds
      g. Monitor vaginal bleeding; more than one saturated pad per hour may indicate excessive bleeding
      h. Assess incision site for signs of infection
      i. Administer pain medication as prescribed
   ▲ j. Instruct the client to avoid stair climbing for 1 month and to avoid tub baths and sitting for long periods
   ▲ k. Avoid strenuous activity or lifting anything weighing more than 10 to 20 pounds
      l. Instruct the client to consume foods that aid in the healing
      m. Instruct the client to avoid sexual intercourse for 3 to 6 weeks as prescribed
      n. Instruct the client in the signs associated with complications

I. Pelvic exenteration (Box 49-13)
   1. Description
      a. A radical surgical procedure performed for recurrent **cancer** if there is no evidence of

tumor outside the pelvis and no lymph node involvement
      b. When the bladder is removed, an ileal conduit will be created and located on the right side of the abdomen to divert urine
      c. A colostomy may need to be created and will be located of the left side of the abdomen for the passage of feces
   2. Postoperative implementation
   ▲ a. Monitor for atelectasis and pneumonia
      b. Assist with coughing and deep-breathing exercises
   ▲ c. Monitor for hemorrhage, shock, and deep vein thrombosis
   ▲ d. Apply antiembolism stockings as prescribed
      e. Administer prophylactic heparin infusion as prescribed
   ▲ f. Monitor bowel sounds
      g. Monitor I & O and for signs of dehydration
      h. Monitor incision site for infection
      i. Administer perineal irrigations with half-strength normal saline (NS) and hydrogen peroxide as prescribed
      j. Provide sitz baths as prescribed
      k. Administer analgesics as prescribed for pain
      l. Instruct the client to avoid strenuous activity for 6 months
      m. Instruct the client that the perineal opening, if present, may drain for several months
      n. Instruct the client in the care of the ileal conduit and colostomy, if created
      o. Provide sexual counseling, as vaginal intercourse is not possible after anterior and total pelvic exenteration

XVI. OVARIAN CANCER
A. Description
   1. Grows rapidly, spreads fast, and is often bilateral
   2. **Metastasis** occurs by direct spread to the organs in the pelvis, by distal spread through lymphatic drainage, or by peritoneal seeding

---

BOX 49-13

Types of Pelvic Exenteration

ANTERIOR
Removal of the uterus, ovaries, fallopian tubes, vagina, bladder, urethra, and pelvic lymph nodes

POSTERIOR
Removal of the uterus, ovaries, fallopian tubes, descending colon, rectum, and anal canal

TOTAL
Combination of anterior and posterior

3. Prognosis is usually poor because the tumor is usually detected late
4. An exploratory laparotomy is performed to diagnose and stage the tumor

B. Assessment
1. Abdominal discomfort or swelling
2. GI disturbances
3. Dysfunctional vaginal bleeding
4. Abdominal mass

C. Implementation
1. External radiation is used if the tumor has invaded other organs
2. Chemotherapy is used postoperatively for all stages of ovarian **cancer**
3. Intraperitoneal chemotherapy, which involves the instillation of chemotherapy into the abdominal cavity
4. Immunotherapy, which alters the immunological response of the ovary and promotes tumor resistance
5. Total abdominal hysterectomy and bilateral salpingo-oophorectomy

XVII. ENDOMETRIAL CANCER

A. Description
1. A slow-growing tumor associated with the menopausal years
2. **Metastasis** occurs through the lymphatic system to the ovaries and pelvis, via the blood to the lungs, liver, and bone, or intraabdominally to the peritoneal cavity

B. Precipitating factors
1. History of uterine polyps
2. Nulliparity
3. Polycystic ovary disease
4. Estrogen stimulation
5. Late menopause
6. Family history

C. Assessment
1. Postmenopausal bleeding
2. Watery, serosanguineous discharge
3. Low back, pelvic, or abdominal pain
4. Enlarged uterus in advanced stages

D. Nonsurgical implementation
1. External radiation or internal radiation used alone or in combination with surgery, depending on the stage of **cancer**
2. Chemotherapy to treat advanced or recurrent disease
3. Progestational therapy with medroxyprogesterone (Depo-Provera) or megestrol acetate (Megace) for estrogen-dependent tumors
4. Tamoxifen (Nolvadex), an antiestrogen, may also be prescribed

E. Surgical implementation: Total abdominal hysterectomy and bilateral salpingo-oophorectomy

XVIII. BREAST CANCER

A. Description
1. Classified as invasive when it penetrates the tissue surrounding the mammary duct and grows in an irregular pattern
2. **Metastasis** occurs via lymph nodes
3. Common sites of **metastasis** are the bone, lungs, brain, and liver
4. Diagnosis is made by breast biopsy through a needle aspiration or by surgical removal of the tumor with microscopic examination for **malignant** cells

B. Precipitating factors
1. Family history
2. Early menarche and late menopause
3. Previous **cancer** of the breast, uterus, or ovaries
4. Nulliparity
5. Obesity
6. High-dose radiation exposure to chest

C. Assessment
1. Mass felt during BSE
2. Mass usually felt in the upper outer quadrant or beneath the nipple
3. A fixed, irregular nonencapsulated mass
4. A painless mass except in the very late stages
5. Nipple retraction or elevation
6. Asymmetry, with the affected breast being higher
7. Bloody or clear nipple discharge
8. Skin dimpling, retraction, or ulceration
9. Skin edema or peau d'orange skin
10. Axillary lymphadenopathy
11. Lymphedema of affected arm
12. Symptoms of bone or lung **metastasis**
13. Presence of the lesion on mammography

D. Prevention: Monthly BSE

E. Nonsurgical implementation
1. Chemotherapy
2. Radiation therapy
3. Hormonal manipulation via the use of estrogen in postmenopausal women or tamoxifen (Nolvadex) for estrogen receptor–positive tumors

F. Surgical implementation
1. Surgical breast procedures with possible breast reconstruction (Box 49-14)
2. Oophorectomy for estrogen receptor–positive tumors
3. Ablative therapy with adrenalectomy or chemical ablation, which blocks the production of cortisol, androstenedione, and aldosterone

G. Postoperative implementation
1. Monitor vital signs
2. Position in semi-Fowler's; turn from back or unaffected side, with the affected arm elevated above the level of the heart to promote drainage and prevent lymphedema

---

BOX 49-14

Surgical Breast Procedures

LUMPECTOMY
Excision and removal of the tumor
Lymph node dissection may also be performed

SIMPLE MASTECTOMY
Breast tissue and the nipple are removed
Lymph nodes are left intact

MODIFIED RADICAL MASTECTOMY
Breast tissue, nipple, and lymph nodes are removed
Muscles are left intact

HALSTED RADICAL MASTECTOMY
Breast tissue, nipple, underlying muscles, and lymph
nodes are removed

BOX 49-15

Client Instructions Following Mastectomy

Avoid overuse of the arm during the first few months
To prevent lymphedema, keep the affected arm elevated
Provide incision care with lanolin to soften and prevent
   wound contracture
Encourage use of Reach for Recovery volunteers
Encourage the client to perform BSE on the remaining
   breast
Protect the affected hand and arm
Avoid strong sunlight to the affected arm
Do not let the affected arm hang dependent
Do not carry a pocketbook or anything heavy over the
   affected arm
Avoid trauma, cuts, bruises, or burns to the affected side
Avoid wearing constricted clothing or jewelry on the
   affected side
Wear gloves when gardening
Use thick oven mitts when cooking
Use a thimble when sewing
Apply lanolin hand cream several times daily
Use cream cuticle remover
Call the physician if signs of inflammation occur in the
   affected arm
Wear a Medic-Alert bracelet stating lymphedema arm

---

3. Encourage coughing and deep breathing
4. If a drain (usually Jackson-Pratt) is in place, maintain suction and record the amount of drainage and drainage characteristics
5. Assess operative site for infection, swelling, or the presence of fluid collection under the skin flaps
6. Monitor incision site for restriction of dressing, impaired sensation, or color changes of the skin
7. If breast reconstruction was performed, the client will return from surgery with a surgical brassiere and the temporary prosthesis in place
8. Place a sign above the bed stating "No IVs, No IMs, No BPs, No Venipunctures in Affected Arm"
9. Provide the use of a pressure sleeve as prescribed if edema is severe
10. Administer diuretics and provide a low-salt diet as prescribed for severe lymphedema
11. Consult with the physician and the physical therapist regarding the appropriate exercise program
12. Assist with exercise as prescribed to decrease lymphedema and muscle weakness
13. Instruct the client about home care measures (Box 49-15)

XIX. GASTRIC CANCER
A. Description
   1. A **malignant** growth in the stomach
   2. Risk factors include a diet high in complex carbohydrates, grains, and salt, and low in fresh, green leafy vegetables and fresh fruit; smoking; alcohol; the use of nitrates; and a history of gastric ulcers
   3. Complications include hemorrhage, obstruction, **metastasis,** and dumping syndrome

4. The goal of treatment is to remove the tumor and provide a nutritional program
B. Assessment
   1. Fatigue
   2. Anorexia and weight loss
   3. Nausea and vomiting
   4. Indigestion and epigastric discomfort
   5. A sensation of pressure in the stomach
   6. Dysphagia
   7. Anemia
   8. Ascites
   9. Palpable mass
C. Implementation
   1. Monitor vital signs
   2. Monitor hemoglobin and hematocrit and administer blood transfusion as prescribed
   3. Monitor weight
   4. Assess nutritional status; encourage small, bland, easily digestible meals with vitamin and mineral supplements
   5. Administer pain medication as prescribed
   6. Prepare the client for chemotherapy or radiation therapy as prescribed
   7. Prepare the client for surgical resection of the tumor as prescribed (Box 49-16)
D. Postoperative implementation
   1. Monitor vital signs
   2. Place in Fowler's position for comfort
   3. Monitor I & O; administer fluids and electrolyte replacement by IV as prescribed

BOX 49-16

Surgical Implementation for Gastric Cancer

SUBTOTAL GASTRECTOMY

Billroth I

Also called gastroduodenostomy

Partial gastrectomy, and remaining segment is anastomosed to the duodenum

Billroth II

Also called gastrojejunostomy

Partial gastrectomy, with remaining segment anastomosed to the jejunum

TOTAL GASTRECTOMY

Also called esophagojejunostomy

Removal of the stomach with attachment of the esophagus to the jejunum or duodenum

4. Maintain NPO status as prescribed for 1 to 3 days until peristalsis returns
5. Monitor nasogastric (NG) suction
6. Do not irrigate or remove the NG tube; assist the physician with irrigation or removal
7. Assess for bowel sounds
8. Advance the diet from NPO to sips of clear water to six small bland meals a day, as prescribed
9. Monitor for complications of hemorrhage, dumping syndrome, diarrhea, hypoglycemia, and vitamin B_{12} deficiency

XX. INTESTINAL TUMORS

A. Description
  1. **Malignant** lesions that develop in the cells lining the bowel wall or develop as polyps in the colon or rectum
  2. Complications include bowel perforation with peritonitis, abscess and/or fistula formation, hemorrhage, and complete intestinal obstruction
  3. **Metastasis** occurs via the circulatory or lymphatic system, or by direct extension to other areas in the colon or other organs
B. Assessment
  1. Blood in stools
  2. Anorexia, vomiting, and weight loss
  3. Malaise
  4. Anemia
  5. Abnormal stools
    a. Ascending colon tumor: Diarrhea
    b. Descending colon tumor: Constipation or some diarrhea, or flat, ribbon-like stool resulting from a partial obstruction
    c. Rectal tumor: Alternating constipation and diarrhea
  6. Guarding or abdominal distention
  7. Abdominal mass (a late sign)
  8. Cachexia (a late sign)

C. Implementation
  1. Monitor for signs of complications, which include bowel perforation with peritonitis, abscess and/or fistula formation, hemorrhage, and complete intestinal obstruction
  2. Monitor for signs of intestinal perforation, which include low blood pressure (BP), rapid and weak pulse, distended abdomen, and elevated temperature
  3. Monitor for signs of intestinal obstruction, which include vomiting (may be fecal contents), pain, constipation, and abdominal distention
  4. Note that an early sign of intestinal obstruction is increased peristaltic activity, which produces an increase in bowel sounds; as the obstruction progresses, hypoactive sounds are heard
  5. Prepare for radiation preoperatively to facilitate surgical resection, and postoperatively to decrease the risk of recurrence or to reduce pain, hemorrhage, bowel obstruction, or **metastasis**
  6. Chemotherapy is used postoperatively to assist in the control of symptoms and the spread of the disease
D. Surgical implementation: Bowel resection and creation of colostomy or ileostomy
E. Colostomy/ileostomy
  1. Preoperative implementation
    a. Consult with the enterostomal therapist to assist in identifying optimal placement of ostomy
    b. Instruct the client to eat a low-residue diet for a day or two prior to surgery as prescribed
    c. Administer intestinal antiseptics and antibiotics, as prescribed, to decrease the bacterial content of the colon and to reduce the risk of infection from the surgical procedure
    d. Administer laxatives and enemas as prescribed
  2. Postoperative: colostomy
    a. Place a petroleum jelly gauze over the stoma to keep it moist, followed by a dry sterile dressing if a pouch system is not in place
    b. Place a pouch system on the stoma as soon as possible
    c. Monitor the stoma for size, unusual bleeding, or necrotic tissue
    d. Monitor for color changes in the stoma
    e. Note that the normal stoma color is red or pink, indicating high vascularity
    f. Note that a pale pink stoma indicates low hemoglobin and hematocrit levels, and a purple-black stoma indicates compromised circulation, requiring physician notification
    g. Monitor the pouch system for proper fit and signs of leakage
    h. Assess the functioning of the colostomy
    i. Expect that stool will be liquid postoperatively

but will become more solid, depending on the area of the colostomy

▲ j. Ascending colon colostomy: Expect liquid stool

▲ k. Transverse colon colostomy: Expect loose to semiformed stool

▲ l. Descending colon colostomy: Expect close to normal stool

m. Fecal matter should not be allowed to remain on the skin

n. Empty pouch when one-third full

o. Administer analgesics and antibiotics as prescribed

p. Irrigate perineal wound if present and if prescribed, and monitor for signs of infection

▲ q. Instruct the client to avoid foods that cause excessive gas formation and odor

r. Instruct the client in stoma care and irrigations as prescribed

s. Instruct the client that normal activities may be resumed when approved by the physician

3. Postoperative: ileostomy

▲ a. Healthy stoma is red; a color change to dark blue or black should be reported to the physician

▲ b. Postoperative drainage will be dark green and progress to yellow as the client begins to eat

▲ c. Stool is liquid

▲ d. Risk for dehydration and electrolyte imbalance exists

▲ e. Do not give suppositories through ileostomy

XXI. LUNG CANCER

A. Description
1. **Malignant** tumor of the lung that may be primary or metastatic
2. The lungs are a common target for **metastasis** from other organs
3. Bronchiogenic **carcinoma** spreads through direct extension and lymphatic dissemination
4. The four major types of lung **cancer** include small cell (oat cell), epidermal (squamous cell), adenocarcinoma, and large cell anaplastic **carcinoma**
5. Diagnosis is made by a chest x-ray, which will show a lesion or mass, and bronchoscopy and sputum studies, which will demonstrate a positive cytology for **cancer** cells

B. Causes
1. Cigarette smoking
2. Exposure to environmental pollutants
3. Exposure to occupational pollutants

C. Assessment
1. Cough
2. Dyspnea
3. Hoarseness
4. Hemoptysis
5. Chest pain

6. Anorexia and weight loss
7. Weakness

D. Implementation
1. Monitor vital signs
2. Monitor breathing patterns and breath sounds and for signs of respiratory impairment
3. Assess for tracheal deviation
4. Administer analgesics as prescribed for pain management
5. Place in Fowler's position for ease in breathing ▲
6. Administer oxygen as prescribed and humidification to moisten and loosen secretions ▲
7. Monitor pulse oximetry
8. Provide respiratory treatments as prescribed
9. Administer bronchodilators and corticosteroids as prescribed to decrease bronchospasm, inflammation, and edema
10. Provide a high-calorie, high-protein, high-vitamin diet
11. Provide activity as tolerated, rest periods, and active and passive ROM exercises
12. Monitor for bleeding, infection, and electrolyte imbalances

E. Nonsurgical implementation
1. Radiation therapy for localized intrathoracic lung **cancers** and for palliation of hemoptysis, obstructions, dysphagia, and pain
2. Chemotherapy
3. Immunotherapy directed at enhancing an effective immune response, which favorably affects the course of the disease

F. Surgical implementation
1. Laser therapy: To relieve endobronchial obstruction
2. Thoracentesis and pleurodesis: To remove pleural fluid and relieve hypoxia
3. Thoracotomy with pneumonectomy: Surgical removal of a lung
4. Thoracotomy with lobectomy: Surgical removal of one lobe of the lung for tumors confined to a single lobe
5. Thoracotomy with segmental resection: Surgical removal of a lobe segment for clients unable to tolerate lobectomy or pneumonectomy

G. Preoperative implementation
1. Explain the potential postoperative need for chest tubes
2. Note that closed chest drainage is not usually ▲ used for a pneumonectomy, and the serum fluid that accumulates in the empty thoracic cavity eventually consolidates, preventing shifts of the mediastinum, heart, and remaining lung

H. Postoperative implementation
1. Monitor vital signs
2. Assess cardiac and respiratory status; monitor ▲ for the absence and presence of lung sounds
3. Maintain chest tube drainage system, which will ▲

drain air and/or blood that accumulates in the pleural space

4. Assess chest tube insertion site for crepitus (subcutaneous air) and drainage
5. Administer oxygen as prescribed
6. Check physician's orders regarding client positioning; complete lateral turning is avoided
7. Monitor pulse oximetry
8. Provide activity as tolerated
9. Encourage active ROM exercises of the operative shoulder as prescribed
10. Refer to Chapter 20 for care of the client with a chest tube

XXII. LARYNGEAL CANCER

A. Description
1. A **malignant** tumor of the larynx
2. Laryngeal **cancer** presents as **malignant** ulcerations with underlying infiltration
3. **Metastasis** to the lung is common
4. Diagnosis is made by laryngoscopy and biopsy showing a positive cytology for **cancer** cells

B. Causes
1. Cigarette smoking
2. Exposure to environmental pollutants
3. Exposure to radiation
4. Voice strain

C. Assessment
1. Persistent hoarseness and sore throat
2. Painless neck mass
3. A feeling of a lump in the throat
4. Burning sensation in the throat
5. Dysphagia
6. Change in voice quality
7. Dyspnea
8. Weakness and weight loss
9. Hemoptysis
10. Foul breath odor

D. Implementation
1. Place in Fowler's position to promote optimal air exchange
2. Monitor respiratory status
3. Monitor for signs of aspiration of food and fluid
4. Administer oxygen as prescribed
5. Provide respiratory treatments as prescribed
6. Provide activity as tolerated
7. Provide a high-calorie, high-protein, high-vitamin diet
8. Provide nutritional support via total parenteral nutrition (TPN), NG tube feedings, or gastrostomy or jejunostomy tube, as prescribed
9. Administer analgesics as prescribed for pain

E. Nonsurgical implementation
1. Radiation therapy if the **cancer** is limited to a small area in one vocal cord
2. Chemotherapy, which may be done in combination with radiation and surgery

F. Surgical implementation
1. Depends on the tumor size and the amount of tissue to be resected
2. Types of resection include cordal stripping, cordectomy, partial laryngectomy, and total laryngectomy
3. A tracheostomy is performed with a total laryngectomy; this airway opening is always permanent and is referred to as a laryngectomy stoma

G. Preoperative implementation
1. Establish methods of communication for the client
2. Encourage the client to express feelings about changes in body image and loss of voice
3. Describe the rehabilitation program and information about the tracheostomy and suctioning

H. Postoperative implementation
1. Monitor vital signs
2. Monitor respiratory status; monitor airway patency and provide frequent suctioning to remove bloody secretions
3. Place the client in high Fowler's position
4. Maintain mechanical ventilator support or a tracheostomy collar with humidification, as prescribed
5. Monitor pulse oximetry
6. Maintain surgical drains in the neck area if present
7. Observe for hemorrhage and edema in the neck
8. Monitor IV fluids or TPN until nutrition is administered via NG, gastrostomy, or jejunostomy tube
9. Provide oral hygiene
10. Assess gag and cough reflexes and ability to swallow
11. Increase activity, as tolerated
12. Assess the color, amount, and consistency of sputum
13. Provide stoma and laryngectomy care (Box 49-17)
14. Provide consultation with speech and language pathologist as prescribed
15. Reinforce method of communication established preoperatively
16. Prepare the client for rehabilitation and speech therapy (Box 49-18)

XXIII. CANCER OF THE PROSTATE

A. Description
1. A slow-growing **cancer** of the prostate gland, which is usually a androgen-dependent type of adenocarcinoma
2. The risk increases in men with each decade after age 50
3. Prostate cancer can spread via direct invasion of surrounding tissues or by **metastasis,** through the

---

BOX 49-17

Stoma Care Following Laryngectomy

Teach the client clean suctioning technique

Instruct the client how to clean the incision and provide stoma care

Protect the neck from injury

Instruct the client to wear a stoma guard to shield the stoma

Avoid swimming, showering, and using aerosol sprays

Demonstrate ways to prevent debris from entering the stoma

Advise the client to wear loose-fitting, high-collar clothing to hide the stoma

Advise the client to increase humidity in the home

Instruct the client in ROM exercises for arms, shoulders, and neck as prescribed

Avoid exposure to people with infections

Alternate rest periods with activity

Increase fluid intake to 3000 mL/day as prescribed

Advise the client to obtain a Medic-Alert bracelet

BOX 49-18

Speech Rehabilitation Following Laryngectomy

ESOPHAGEAL SPEECH

Client produces esophageal speech by "burping" the air swallowed

Voice produced is monotone, cannot be raised or lowered, and carries no pitch

Client must have adequate hearing because the client uses the mouth to shape the words as they are heard

MECHANICAL DEVICES

Known as electrolarynges

Placed against the side of the neck; the air inside the neck and pharynx is vibrated, and the client articulates

A Cooper-Rand device consists of a plastic tube that is placed inside the client's mouth and vibrates on articulation

TRACHEOESOPHAGEAL FISTULA (TEF)

Surgical creation of a fistula between the trachea and the esophagus, with eventual placement of a prosthesis used to produce speech

The prosthesis provides the client with a means to divert the air from the lungs through the trachea, into the esophagus, and out of the mouth

Lip and tongue movement produces the speech

---

bloodstream and lymphatics, to the bony pelvis and spine

   4. Bone **metastasis** is a concern

B. Assessment

   1. Asymptomatic in early stages

   2. Hard, pea-sized nodule palpated on rectal examination

   3. Hematuria

   4. Late symptoms include weight loss, urinary obstruction, and pain radiating from the lumbosacral area down the leg

   5. Prostate-specific antigen (PSA) test does not necessarily indicate malignancy and is used routinely to monitor the client's response to therapy

   6. Elevated serum acid phosphatase indicates spread and **metastasis**

C. Nonsurgical implementation

   1. Prepare the client for hormone manipulation therapy as prescribed

   2. Administer luteinizing hormone, leuprolide acetate (Lupron), flutamide (Eulexin), or diethylstilbestrol (DES), as prescribed to slow the rate of growth of the tumor

   3. Goserelin acetate (Zoladex) may be prescribed for palliation in advanced prostatic **cancer** when orchiectomy or estrogen administration is neither acceptable nor indicated for the client

   4. Prepare the client for radiation (internal or external), which may be prescribed alone or in conjunction with surgery and may be prescribed preoperatively or postoperatively, to reduce the lesion and limit **metastasis**

   5. Prepare the client for the administration of chemotherapy in cases of hormone-resistant tumors

D. Surgical implementation

   1. Prepare the client for orchiectomy (palliative) if prescribed, which will limit the production of testosterone

   2. Prepare the client for transurethral resection of the prostate (TURP) or prostatectomy if prescribed

   3. Cyrosurgical ablation: A minimally invasive procedure that may be an alternative to radical prostatectomy; liquid nitrogen freezes the gland, and the dead cells are absorbed by the body

E. TURP

   1. Insertion of a scope into the urethra to excise prostatic tissue

   2. Bleeding is common following TURP, and monitoring for hemorrhage is an important nursing intervention

   3. Continuous bladder irrigation (CBI) will be prescribed postoperatively to maintain the urine at a pink color

   4. Bladder spasms are common following surgery, and antispasmodics may be prescribed

   5. Dribbling or incontinence may occur postoperatively, and it is important for the nurse to instruct the client to monitor for these occurrences

   6. Sterility may or may not occur following the surgical procedure

F. Suprapubic prostatectomy
  1. Removal of the prostate by an abdominal incision with a bladder incision
  2. The client will have an abdominal dressing that may drain copious amounts of urine, and the abdominal dressing will need to be changed frequently
  3. Severe hemorrhage is possible, and monitoring for blood loss is an important nursing intervention
  4. Bladder spasms are common, and antispasmodics may be prescribed
  5. CBI will be prescribed and administered to keep the urine pink
  6. A longer healing process is involved as compared with the TURP
  7. Sterility occurs with this procedure
G. Retropubic prostatectomy
  1. Removal of the prostate gland by a low abdominal incision without opening the bladder
  2. Less bleeding occurs with this procedure, as compared with suprapubic, and the client experiences fewer bladder spasms
  3. There is minimal abdominal drainage
  4. CBI may be used
  5. Sterility occurs with this procedure
H. Perineal prostatectomy
  1. The prostate gland is removed through an incision made between the scrotum and anus
  2. Minimal bleeding occurs with this procedure
  3. The client needs to be monitored closely for infection, because the risk of infection is increased with this type of prostatectomy
  4. Urinary incontinence is common
  5. The procedure causes sterility
  6. Teach the client how to perform perineal exercises
  7. Avoid inserting rectal tubes, taking the temperature rectally, or administering enemas
I. Postoperative implementation
  1. Monitor vital signs
  2. Monitor urinary output
  3. Monitor urine for hemorrhage and clots
  4. Increase fluids to 2400 to 3000 mL a day unless contraindicated
  5. Monitor for arterial bleeding as evidenced by bright red urine with numerous clots, and if it occurs, increase CBI and notify the physician immediately
  6. Monitor for venous bleeding as evidenced by burgundy-colored urine output; if it occurs, inform the physician, who may apply traction on the catheter
  7. Monitor hemoglobin and hematocrit levels
  8. Expect red to light pink urine for 24 hours, turning to amber in 3 days
  9. Ambulate the client as early as possible and as soon as urine begins to clear in color
  10. Inform the client that a continuous feeling of an urge to void is normal
  11. Instruct the client to avoid attempts to void around the catheter because this will cause bladder spasms
  12. Administer antibiotics, analgesics, stool softeners, and antispasmodics as prescribed
  13. Monitor three-way Foley catheter, which will have a 30- to 45-mL retention balloon
  14. Maintain CBI with sterile bladder irrigation solution as prescribed to keep the catheter free of obstruction and maintain the urine pink in color (Box 49-19)
J. Postoperative: suprapubic prostatectomy
  1. Monitor suprapubic and Foley catheter drainage
  2. Monitor CBI if prescribed
  3. Note that the Foley catheter will be removed 2 to 4 days postoperatively if the client has a suprapubic catheter
  4. If prescribed, clamp the suprapubic catheter after the Foley catheter is removed, and instruct client to attempt to void; after the client has voided, assess the residual urine in the bladder by unclamping the suprapubic catheter and measuring the output
  5. Prepare for removal of suprapubic catheter when client consistently empties bladder and residual urine is 75 mL or less
  6. Monitor suprapubic incision dressing, which may become saturated with urine, until the incision heals
K. Postoperative: retropubic prostatectomy
  1. Note that since the bladder is not entered, there is no urinary drainage on the abdominal dressing
  2. Assess for urinary or purulent drainage on the dressing; if this occurs, notify the physician
  3. Monitor for fever and increased pain, which may indicate an infection
L. Postoperative: perineal prostatectomy
  1. Note that the client will have an incision, which may or may not have a drain
  2. Avoid rectal thermometers, rectal tubes, and enemas, because they may cause trauma and bleeding

XXIV. BLADDER CANCER

A. Description
  1. Papillomatous growths in the bladder urothelium that undergo **malignant** changes and that may infiltrate the bladder wall
  2. Predisposing factors include cigarette smoking, exposure to industrial chemicals, and exposure to radiation
  3. Common sites of **metastasis** include the liver, bones, and lungs
  4. As the tumor progresses, it can extend into the rectum, vagina, other pelvic soft tissues, and retroperitoneal structures

---

BOX 49-19

Postoperative Care Following TURP

CONTINUOUS BLADDER IRRIGATION (CBI)
A three-way (lumen) irrigation to decrease bleeding and to keep the bladder free from clots:
One lumen for inflating the balloon (30 mL)
One lumen for instillation (inflow)
One lumen for outflow

IMPLEMENTATION
Maintain traction on the catheter if applied to prevent bleeding, by pulling the catheter taut and taping it to the abdomen or thigh
Instruct the client to keep the leg straight if traction is applied to the catheter and it is taped to the thigh
Catheter traction is not released without a physician's order; is usually released after any bright red drainage has diminished
Use NS or prescribed solution only, to prevent water intoxication
Run the solution at a rate, as prescribed, to keep the urine pink
Run the solution rapidly if bright red drainage or clots are present
Run the solution at about 40 gtt/minute when the bright red drainage clears
If the urinary catheter becomes obstructed, turn off the CBI and irrigate the catheter with 30 to 50 mL of normal saline if prescribed; notify physician if obstruction does not resolve

Monitor for TUR syndrome or severe hyponatremia (water intoxication) caused by the excessive absorption of bladder irrigation (altered mental status, bradycardia, increased blood pressure, and confusion)
Discontinue CBI and Foley catheter as prescribed, usually 24 to 48 hours after surgery
Monitor for continence and urinary retention when the catheter is removed
Inform the client that some burning, frequency, and dribbling may occur following catheter removal
Inform the client that he should be voiding 150 to 200 mL of clear yellow urine every 3 to 4 hours by 3 days after surgery
Inform the client that he may pass small clots and tissue debris for several days
Teach the client to avoid heavy lifting, stressful exercise, driving, Valsalva's maneuver, and sexual intercourse for 2 to 6 weeks to prevent strain, and to call the physician if bleeding occurs or there is a decrease in urinary stream
Instruct the client to drink 2400 to 3000 mL of fluid each day, preferably before 8 P.M.
Instruct the client to avoid alcohol, caffeinated beverages, and spicy foods, to avoid overstimulation of the bladder
Instruct the client that if the urine becomes bloody, to rest and increase fluid intake, and that if the bleeding does not subside, to notify the physician

---

B. Assessment
　1. Gross, painless hematuria
　2. Frequency, urgency, dysuria
　3. Clot-induced obstruction
　4. Bladder biopsy confirms diagnosis
C. Radiation
　1. Most bladder **cancers** are poorly radiosensitive and require high doses of radiation
　2. Radiation therapy is more acceptable for advanced disease that cannot be eradicated by surgery
　3. Palliative radiation may be used to relieve pain and bowel obstruction and control potential hemorrhage and leg edema secondary to venous or lymphatic obstruction
　4. Intracavitary radiation may be prescribed, which protects adjacent tissue
　5. External radiation combined with chemotherapy or surgery may be prescribed because the external radiation alone may be ineffective
　6. Complications of radiation
　　a. Abacterial cystitis
　　b. Proctitis
　　c. Fistula formation
　　d. Ileitis or colitis
　　e. Bladder ulceration and hemorrhage
D. Chemotherapy
　1. Intravesical instillation
　　a. An alkylating chemotherapeutic agent is instilled into the bladder
　　b. This method provides a concentrated topical treatment with little systemic absorption
　　c. Chemotherapeutic agents used are thiotepa, mitomycin (Mutamycin), doxorubicin (Adriamycin), cyclophosphamide (Cytoxan), and bacille Calmette-Guérin (BCG)
　　d. The medication is injected into a urethral catheter and retained for 2 hours
　　e. Following instillation, the client's position is rotated every 15 to 30 minutes, starting in the supine position to avoid lying on a full bladder
　　f. After 2 hours, the client voids in a sitting position and is instructed to increase fluids to flush the bladder
　　g. Treat the urine as biohazard and send to the radioisotope laboratory for monitoring
　　h. For 6 hours following intravesical chemotherapy, disinfect the toilet with household bleach after the client has voided
　2. Systemic chemotherapy
　　a. Used to treat inoperable or late tumors

b. Agents used include cisplatin (Platinol), doxorubicin (Adriamycin), cyclophosphamide (Cytoxan), methotrexate (Folex), and pyridoxine

3. Complications of chemotherapy
    a. Bladder irritation
    b. Hemorrhagic cystitis

E. Surgical implementation

1. TURP
    a. Local resection and fulguration (destruction of tissue by electrical current through electrodes placed in direct contact with the tissue)
    b. Performed for very early tumors for cure or for inoperable tumors for palliation

2. Partial cystectomy
    a. The removal of up to half of the bladder
    b. Done for early tumors and for clients who cannot tolerate a radical cystectomy
    c. During the initial postoperative period, bladder capacity is markedly reduced to about 60 mL; however, as the bladder tissue expands, the capacity increases to 200 to 400 mL
    d. Maintenance of a continuous output of urine following surgery is critical to prevent bladder distention and stress on the suture line
    e. A urethral catheter and a suprapubic catheter may be in place, and the suprapubic catheter may be left in place for 2 weeks until healing occurs

3. Cystectomy and urinary diversion
    a. Removal of the bladder and the urethra in women, and the bladder, the urethra, and usually the prostate and seminal vesicles in men
    b. When the bladder and urethra are removed, permanent urinary diversion is required
    c. The surgery may be performed in two stages if the tumor is extensive, with the creation of the urinary diversion first and the cystectomy several weeks later
    d. If a radical cystectomy is performed, lower extremity lymphedema may occur as a result of lymph node dissection, and impotence may occur in the male client

4. Ileal conduit
    a. Also called ureteroileostomy or Bricker's procedure
    b. Ureters are implanted into a segment of the ileum, with the formation of an abdominal stoma
    c. The urine flows into the conduit and is continually propelled out through the stoma by peristalsis
    d. The client is required to wear an appliance over the stoma to collect the urine
    e. Complications include obstruction, pyelonephritis, leakage at the anastomosis site, stenosis, hydronephrosis, calculi, skin irritation and ulceration, and stomal defects

5. Kock pouch
    a. A continent internal ileal reservoir created from a segment of the ileum and ascending colon
    b. The ureters are implanted into the side of the reservoir, and a special nipple valve is constructed to attach the reservoir to the skin
    c. Postoperatively, the client will have a 24 to 26 Foley catheter in place to drain urine continuously until the pouch has healed
    d. The catheter is irrigated gently with NS to prevent obstruction from mucus or clots
    e. Following removal of the catheter, the client is instructed in how to self-catheterize and to drain the reservoir at 4- to 6-hour intervals

6. Indiana pouch
    a. A continent reservoir is created from the ascending colon and terminal ileum, making a pouch larger than the Kock pouch
    b. Postoperatively, the client will have a 24 to 26 Foley catheter in place to drain urine continuously until the pouch has healed
    c. The Foley catheter is irrigated gently with NS to prevent obstruction from mucus or clots
    d. Following removal of the Foley catheter, the client is instructed in how to self-catheterize and to drain the reservoir at 4- to 6-hour intervals

7. Creation of a neobladder
    a. Similar to the creation of an internal reservoir, with the difference being that instead of emptying through an abdominal stoma, it empties through a pelvic outlet into the urethra
    b. The client empties the neobladder by relaxing the external sphincter and creating abdominal pressure or by intermittent self-catheterization

8. Percutaneous nephrostomy or pyelostomy
    a. Used when the **cancer** is inoperable, to prevent obstruction
    b. Involves a percutaneous or surgical insertion of a nephrostomy tube into the kidney for drainage
    c. Nursing implementation involves stabilizing the tube to prevent dislodgment and monitoring output

9. Ureterostomy
    a. May be performed as a palliative procedure if the ureters are obstructed by the tumor
    b. The ureters are attached to the surface of the abdomen, where the urine flows directly into a drainage appliance without a conduit
    c. Potential problems include infection, skin

irritation, and obstruction to urinary flow as a result of strictures at the opening
   10. Vesicostomy
       a. The bladder is sutured to the abdomen, and a stoma is created in the bladder wall
       b. The bladder empties through the stoma
   F. Preoperative implementation
   ▲ 1. Administer bowel preparation as prescribed, which may include a clear liquid diet, laxatives and enemas, and antibiotics to lower the bacterial count in the bowel
       2. Assist the surgeon and the enterostomal nurse in selecting an appropriate skin site for creation of the abdominal stoma
       3. Encourage the client to talk about his or her feelings related to the stoma creation
   G. Postoperative implementation
       1. Monitor vital signs
       2. Assess incision site
   ▲ 3. Assess stoma (should be red and moist) every hour for the first 24 hours (Box 49-20)
   ▲ 4. Monitor for edema in the stoma, which may be present in the immediate postoperative period
   ▲ 5. If the stoma appears dark and dusky, notify the physician immediately, as this indicates necrosis
       6. Monitor for prolapse or retraction of the stoma
       7. Assess for return of bowel function; monitor for peristalsis, which will return in 3 to 4 days
       8. Maintain NPO status as prescribed until bowel sounds return
   ▲ 9. Monitor urine flow, which is continuous (30 to 60 mL per hour) following surgery
   ▲ 10. Notify the physician if the urine output is less than 30 mL an hour or if there is no urine output for more than 15 minutes
   ▲ 11. Ureteral stents or catheters may be in place for 2 to 3 weeks or until healing occurs; maintain stability with catheters to prevent dislodgment
   ▲ 12. Following a continent diversion or creation of a neobladder, monitor urinary output closely and irrigate catheter gently to prevent obstruction, as prescribed, with 60 mL of NS (Box 49-21)
   ▲ 13. Monitor for hematuria
   ▲ 14. Monitor for signs of peritonitis
       15. Monitor for bladder distention following a partial cystectomy
       16. Monitor for shock, hemorrhage, thrombophlebitis, and lower extremity lymphedema following a radical cystectomy
       17. Monitor the urinary drainage pouch for leaks, and check skin integrity
       18. Monitor the pH of the urine (do not place the dipstick in the stoma), as strong alkali urine can cause skin irritation and facilitate crystal formation

---

BOX 49-20

Urinary Stoma Care

Instruct the client to change the appliance in the morning, when urinary production is slowest

Collect equipment, remove collection bag, use water or commercial solvent to loosen adhesive

Hold a rolled gauze pad against the stoma to collect and absorb urine during the procedure

Cleanse the skin around stoma and under the drainage bag with mild nonresidue soap and water

Inspect the skin for excoriation, and instruct the client to prevent urine from coming into contact with the skin

After the skin is dry, apply skin adhesive around the appliance

Instruct the client to cut the stoma opening of the skin barrier just large enough to fit over the stoma (no more that 3 mm larger than the stoma)

Instruct the client that the stoma will begin to shrink, requiring a smaller stoma opening on the skin barrier

Apply skin barrier before attaching the pouch or faceplate

Place the appliance over the stoma and secure in place

Encourage self-care; teach the client to use mirror

Instruct the client that the pouch may be drained by a bedside bag or leg bag, especially at night

Instruct the client to empty the urinary collection bag when it is one-third to one-half full, to prevent pulling of the appliance and leakage

Instruct the client to check the appliance seal if perspiring occurs

Instruct the client to leave the urinary pouch in place as long as it is not leaking, and change every 5 to 7 days

During appliance changes, leave the skin open to air as long as possible

Use a nonkaraya gum product because urine erodes karaya gum

To control odor, instruct the client to drink adequate fluids, to wash the appliance thoroughly with soap and lukewarm water, and to soak the collection pouch in dilute white vinegar for 20 to 30 minutes or place a special deodorant tablet into the pouch while it is being worn

Instruct the client who takes baths to keep the level of the water below the stoma and to avoid oily soaps

If the client plans to shower, instruct the client to direct the flow of water away from the stoma

---

   19. Instruct the client regarding the potential for urinary tract infection or the development of calculi
   20. Instruct the client to assess the skin for irritation ▲ and to monitor the urinary drainage pouch for any leakage
   21. Encourage the client to express feelings about changes in body image, embarrassment, and sexual dysfunction

---

BOX 49-21

Self-Irrigation and Catheterization of Stoma

IRRIGATION

Instruct the client to wash hands and use clean technique

Instruct the client to use a catheter and syringe and to instill 60 mL of NS or water into the reservoir and to gently aspirate or allow to drain

Instruct the client to irrigate until the drainage remains free of mucus but to be cautious not to overirrigate

CATHETERIZATION

Instruct the client to wash hands and use clean technique

Initially, the client is taught to insert a catheter every 2 to 3 hours to drain the reservoir; during each week thereafter, the interval is increased by 1 hour until the catheterization is done every 4 to 6 hours

Lubricate the catheter well with water-soluble lubricant, and instruct the client never to force the catheter into the reservoir

If resistance is met, instruct the client to pause, rotate the catheter, and apply gentle pressure to insert

Instruct the client to notify the physician if the client is unable to insert the catheter

When urine has stopped, instruct the client to take several deep breaths and move the catheter in and out 2 to 3 inches to ensure that the pouch is empty

Instruct the client to withdraw the catheter slowly, and to pinch the catheter when withdrawn so that it does not leak urine

Instruct the client to carry catheterization supplies with him or her

---

XXV. ONCOLOGICAL EMERGENCIES

A. Sepsis and disseminated intravascular coagulation (DIC)
1. Description: The client with an oncological disorder is at increased risk for infection; DIC is caused by sepsis
2. Implementation
   a. Maintain strict aseptic technique with the immunocompromised client and monitor closely for infection
   b. Administer IV antibiotics as prescribed
   c. Administer anticoagulants as prescribed during the early phase of DIC
   d. Administer cryoprecipitated clotting factors, as prescribed, when DIC progresses and hemorrhage is the primary problem
B. Syndrome of inappropriate antidiuretic hormone (SIADH)
1. Description
   a. Tumors can produce, secrete, or stimulate the brain to synthesize antidiuretic hormone (ADH)
   b. Mild symptoms include weakness, muscle cramps, loss of appetite, and fatigue; serum sodium levels range from 115 to 120 mEq/L
   c. More serious signs and symptoms relate to water intoxication and include weight gain, personality changes, confusion, and extreme muscle weakness
   d. As the serum sodium level approaches 110 mEq/L, seizures, coma, and eventually death will occur, unless the condition is rapidly treated
2. Implementation
   a. Initiate fluid restriction and increased sodium intake as prescribed
   b. Administer demeclocycline (Declomycin) as prescribed, an antagonist to ADH
   c. Monitor serum sodium levels
C. Spinal cord compression
1. Description
   a. Occurs when a tumor directly enters the spinal cord or when the vertebral column collapses from tumor entry
   b. Causes back pain, usually before neurological deficits occur
   c. Neurological deficits relate to the spinal level of compression and include numbness, tingling, loss of urethral, vaginal, and rectal sensation; and muscle weakness
2. Implementation
   a. Assess for back pain and neurological deficits
   b. Prepare the client for radiation and/or chemotherapy to reduce the size of the tumor and relieve compression
   c. Surgery may need to be performed to remove the tumor and relieve the pressure on the spinal cord
   d. Instruct the client in the use of neck or back braces if they are prescribed
D. Hypercalcemia
1. Description
   a. A late manifestation of extensive malignancy that occurs most often in clients with bone **metastasis**
   b. Decreased physical mobility contributes to or worsens hypercalcemia
   c. Early signs include fatigue, anorexia, nausea, vomiting, constipation, and polyuria
   d. More serious signs and symptoms include severe muscle weakness, diminished deep tendon reflexes, paralytic ileus, dehydration, and ECG changes
2. Implementation
   a. Monitor serum calcium level
   b. Administer oral or parenteral (normal saline) fluids as prescribed
   c. Administer medications to lower the calcium level as prescribed

d. Prepare the client for dialysis if the condition becomes life threatening or is accompanied by renal impairment

E. Superior vena cava (SVC) syndrome
  1. Description
    a. Occurs when the SVC is compressed or obstructed by tumor growth
    b. Signs and symptoms result from blockage of blood flow in the venous system of the head, neck, and upper trunk
    c. Early signs and symptoms generally occur in the morning and include edema of the face, especially around the eyes, and tightness of the shirt or blouse collar (Stokes' sign)
    d. As the condition worsens, edema in the arms and hands, dyspnea, erythema of the upper body, and epistaxis occur
    e. Life-threatening signs and symptoms include hemorrhage, cyanosis, mental status changes, decreased cardiac output, and hypotension
  2. Implementation
    a. Assess for signs and symptoms of SVC syndrome
    b. Prepare the client for radiation therapy to the mediastinal area

F. Tumor lysis syndrome (TLS)
  1. Description
    a. Occurs when large quantities of tumor cells are destroyed rapidly and are released into the bloodstream faster than the body's homeostatic mechanisms can handle them
    b. TLS is a positive sign that **cancer** treatment is effective; however, if left untreated, it can cause severe tissue damage and death
    c. Hyperkalemia and hyperuricemia occur; hyperuricemia can lead to acute renal failure
  2. Implementation
    a. Encourage oral hydration; IV hydration may be prescribed for the client experiencing nausea
    b. Instruct the client regarding the importance of fluid intake during chemotherapy
    c. Administer diuretics to increase the urine flow through the kidneys as prescribed
    d. Administer medications that increase the excretion of purines, such as allopurinol (Zyloprim), as prescribed
    e. Prepare to administer IV infusion of glucose and insulin to treat hyperkalemia
    f. Prepare the client for dialysis if hyperkalemia and hyperuricemia persist despite treatment

PRACTICE QUESTIONS

1. A nurse is instructing a client in how to perform a testicular self-examination (TSE). The nurse tells the client:
   1. To examine the testicles while lying down
   2. That the best time for the examination is after a shower
   3. To gently feel the testicle with one finger to feel for a growth
   4. That testicular exams should be done at least every 6 months

2. A community nurse is conducting a health promotion program at a local school and is discussing the risk factors associated with cancer. Which of the following, if identified by a student as a risk factor, indicates a need for further instructions?
   1. Viral factors
   2. Stress
   3. Low-fat and high-fiber diets
   4. Exposure to radiation

3. A client with cancer is receiving chemotherapy and develops thrombocytopenia. A nurse identifies which intervention as the highest priority in the nursing plan of care?
   1. Ambulation three times daily
   2. Monitoring temperature
   3. Monitoring the platelet count
   4. Monitoring for pathological fractures

4. A nurse is monitoring the laboratory results of a client preparing to receive chemotherapy. The nurse would determine that the white blood cell (WBC) count is normal if which of the following results were present?
   1. 3000 to 8000/mm^3
   2. 4000 to 10,000/mm^3
   3. 7000 to 15,000/mm^3
   4. 2000 to 5000/mm^3

5. A community health nurse is instructing a group of female clients about breast self-examination (BSE). The nurse would instruct the clients to perform the exam:
   1. At the onset on menstruation
   2. One week after menstruation begins
   3. Every month during ovulation
   4. Weekly at the same time of day

6. A nurse is caring for a client who has undergone a vaginal hysterectomy. The nurse avoids which of the following in the care of this client?
   1. Removal of antiembolism stockings twice daily
   2. Assisting with range-of-motion leg exercises
   3. Elevating the knee gatch on the bed
   4. Checking placement of pneumatic compression boots

7. A client suspected of having an ovarian tumor is scheduled for a pelvic ultrasound. A nurse provides which preprocedure instructions to the client?
   1. Maintain an NPO status prior to the procedure
   2. Eat a light breakfast only
   3. Drink six to eight glasses of water without voiding prior to the test
   4. Wear comfortable clothing and shoes for the procedure

8. A client is diagnosed as having a bowel tumor. Several diagnostic tests are prescribed. A nurse understands that which of the following tests will confirm the diagnosis of malignancy?
   1. Magnetic resonance imaging (MRI)
   2. Computerized tomography (CT) scan
   3. Abdominal ultrasound
   4. Biopsy of the tumor

9. A client is diagnosed with multiple myeloma. The client asks a nurse about the diagnosis. The nurse bases the response on which of the following descriptions of this disorder?
   1. Malignant exacerbation in the number of leukocytes
   2. Altered red blood cell production
   3. Altered production of lymph nodes
   4. Malignant proliferation of plasma cells and tumors within the bone

10. A nurse is reviewing the laboratory results of a client diagnosed with multiple myeloma. Which of the following would the nurse expect to specifically note in this disorder?
    1. Decreased number of plasma cells in the bone marrow
    2. Increased white blood cells
    3. Increased calcium level
    4. Decreased blood urea nitrogen (BUN)

11. A nurse is developing a plan of care for a client with multiple myeloma. The nurse includes which priority intervention in the plan of care?
    1. Coughing and deep breathing
    2. Forcing fluids
    3. Monitoring the red blood cell count
    4. Providing frequent oral care

12. An oncology nurse specialist is preparing an educational session about the characteristics of Hodgkin's disease. The nurse understands that which of the following is not a characteristic of this disease?
    1. Presence of Reed-Sternberg cells
    2. Involvement of lymph nodes, spleen, and liver
    3. Occurs most often in the elderly
    4. Prognosis depends on the stage of the disease

13. A community health nurse is conducting a health promotion program about testicular cancer for community members. The nurse understands that which of the following is not a sign of testicular cancer?
    1. Painless testicular swelling
    2. Heavy sensation in the scrotum
    3. Alopecia
    4. Back pain

14. A client is receiving external radiation to the neck for cancer of the larynx. The most likely side effect to be expected is:
    1. Constipation
    2. Dyspnea
    3. Sore throat
    4. Diarrhea

15. A nurse is caring for a client with an internal radiation implant. When caring for this client, the nurse should observe which of the following principles?
    1. Limit the time with the client to 1 hour per shift
    2. Do not allow pregnant women into the client's room
    3. Individuals younger than 16 years may be allowed to go in the room as long as they are 6 feet away from the client
    4. Remove dosimeter badge when entering the client's room

16. A cervical radiation implant is placed in a client for treatment of cervical cancer. A nurse initiates what most appropriate activity order for this client?
    1. Out of bed in a chair only
    2. Ambulate to the bathroom only
    3. Bed rest
    4. Out of bed ad lib

17. A client is hospitalized for insertion of an internal cervical radiation implant. While giving care, a nurse finds the radiation implant in the bed. The initial action by the nurse is to:
    1. Call the physician
    2. Pick up the implant with gloved hands and flush it down the toilet.
    3. Reinsert the implant into the vagina immediately
    4. Pick up the implant with long-handled forceps and place it in a lead container

18. A nurse is caring for a client experiencing hematologic toxicity as a result of chemotherapy. The nurse develops a plan of care for the client. The nurse plans to:
    1. Restrict all visitors
    2. Restrict fluid intake
    3. Insert an indwelling urinary catheter to prevent skin breakdown
    4. Restrict fresh fruits and vegetables in the diet

19. A nurse is reviewing the laboratory results of a client receiving chemotherapy. The platelet count is 10,000/mm^3. On the basis of this laboratory value, the priority nursing assessment is which of the following?
    1. Assess level of consciousness
    2. Assess temperature
    3. Assess bowel sounds
    4. Assess skin turgor

20. A home health care nurse is caring for a client with cancer. The client is complaining of acute pain. The most appropriate nursing assessment of the client's pain would include which of the following?
    1. The client's pain rating
    2. The nurse's impression of the client's pain
    3. Nonverbal cues from the client
    4. Pain relief after appropriate nursing intervention

21. A nurse is caring for a client 4 days after a pelvic

exenteration. The physician has changed the client's diet from NPO to clear liquids. The nurse makes which priority assessment before administering the diet?
1. Ability to ambulate
2. Urine specific gravity
3. Incision appearance
4. Bowel sounds

22. A client is admitted to a hospital with a diagnosis of suspected Hodgkin's disease. Which of the following assessment signs would a nurse expect to specifically note in the client?
1. Weakness
2. Fatigue
3. Weight gain
4. Enlarged lymph nodes

23. During the admission assessment of a client with advanced ovarian cancer, a nurse recognizes which symptom as typical of the disease?
1. Hypermenorrhea
2. Abdominal distention
3. Diarrhea
4. Abnormal bleeding

24. A nurse is reviewing the complications of conization with a client who has microinvasive cervical cancer. Which complication if identified by the client indicates a need for further teaching?
1. Infection
2. Infertility
3. Ovarian perforation
4. Hemorrhage

25. When assessing the laboratory results of the client with bladder cancer and bone metastasis, a nurse notes a calcium level of 12 mg/dL. The nurse recognizes that this is consistent with which oncological emergency?
1. Hyperkalemia
2. Spinal cord compression
3. Superior vena cava syndrome
4. Hypercalcemia

26. A client reports to a nurse that when performing testicular self-examination (TSE), he found a lump the size and shape of a pea. The most appropriate response to the client is which of the following?
1. "That's important to report even though it might not be serious."
2. "That could be cancer. I'll ask the doctor to examine you."
3. "Let me know if it gets bigger next month."
4. "Lumps like that are normal; don't worry."

27. A hospice nurse visits a client who is dying of ovarian cancer. During the visit, the client remarks, "If I can just live long enough to attend my daughter's graduation, I'll be ready to die." Which phase of coping is this client experiencing?
1. Denial

2. Bargaining
3. Depression
4. Anger

28. A nurse is caring for a client after a modified radical mastectomy. Which assessment finding would indicate that the client is experiencing a complication related to the surgery?
1. Sanguineous drainage in the Jackson-Pratt drain
2. Pain at the incisional site
3. Complaints of decreased sensation near the operative site
4. Arm edema on the operative side

29. A nurse is admitting a client with laryngeal cancer to a nursing unit. The nurse assesses for which most common risk factor for this type of cancer?
1. Use of chewing tobacco
2. Cigarette smoking
3. Urban living
4. Alcohol abuse

30. A female client who has been receiving radiation therapy for bladder cancer tells a nurse that it feels as if she is voiding through the vagina. The nurse interprets that the client may be experiencing:
1. Extreme stress resulting from the diagnosis of cancer
2. Altered perineal sensation as a side effect of radiation therapy
3. The development of a vesicovaginal fistula
4. Rupture of the bladder

31. A client with leukemia is receiving busulfan (Myleran). Allopurinol (Zyloprim) is prescribed for the client. The purpose of the allopurinol (Zyloprim) is to:
1. Prevent gouty arthritis
2. Prevent hyperuricemia
3. Prevent stomatitis
4. Prevent diarrhea

32. A client receiving chemotherapy is experiencing stomatitis. A nurse advises the client to use which of the following as the best substance to rinse the mouth?
1. Hydrogen peroxide mixture
2. Weak salt and bicarbonate mouth rinse
3. Lemon-flavored mouthwash
4. Alcohol-based mouthwash

33. A community nurse is conducting a health promotion program, and the topic of the discussion relates to the risk factors of gastric cancer. Which risk factor if identified by a client indicates a need for further discussion?
1. History of gastric polyps
2. History of pernicious anemia
3. A diet of smoked, highly salted, and spiced food
4. High meat and carbohydrate consumption

34. A gastrectomy is performed on a client with gastric cancer. In the immediate postoperative period, the

nurse notes bloody drainage from the nasogastric (NG) tube. Which of the following is the most appropriate nursing intervention?
1. Notify the physician
2. Continue to monitor the drainage
3. Measure abdominal girth
4. Irrigate the NG tube

35. A nurse is reviewing the medical history of a client admitted to a hospital with a diagnosis of colorectal cancer. The nurse understands that which of the following is not an associated risk factor for this type of cancer?
   1. A history of inflammatory bowel disease
   2. Family history of colon cancer
   3. A high-fiber diet
   4. A diet high in fats and carbohydrates

36. A nurse is performing an admission assessment on a client diagnosed with a right colon tumor. The nurse asks the client about which characteristic symptom of this type of a tumor?
   1. Diarrhea
   2. Flat ribbon-like stools
   3. Dull abdominal pain exacerbated by walking
   4. Crampy gas pains

37. A nurse is reviewing the preoperative orders for a client with a colon tumor who is scheduled for abdominal perineal resection. The nurse notes that the physician has prescribed neomycin for the client. The nurse determines that this medication has been prescribed:
   1. Because the client has an infection
   2. To prevent an infection
   3. To decrease the bacteria in the bowel
   4. Because the client is allergic to penicillin

38. A nurse is assessing the perineal wound in a client who has returned from the operating room following an abdominal perineal resection. The nurse notes serosanguineous drainage from the wound. Which of the following nursing interventions is most appropriate?
   1. Notify the physician
   2. Change the dressing as prescribed
   3. Clamp the Penrose drain
   4. Remove and replace the perineal packing

39. A nurse is assessing the colostomy of a client who had an abdominal perineal resection for a bowel tumor. Which of the following assessment findings indicates that the colostomy is beginning to function?
   1. Bloody drainage from the colostomy
   2. The client's ability to tolerate food
   3. Absent bowel sounds
   4. The passage of flatus

40. A nurse is caring for a client following a radical neck dissection and creation of a tracheostomy performed for laryngeal cancer. The nurse is providing discharge instructions to the client. Which statement if made by the client indicates a need for further instructions?
   1. "I need to apply a thin layer of petrolatum to the skin around the stoma to prevent cracking."
   2. "I will protect the stoma from water."
   3. "I need to use an air conditioner to provide cool air to assist in breathing."
   4. "I need to keep powders and sprays away from the stoma site."

41. A nurse is caring for a client with a suspected diagnosis of cancer of the prostate. The nurse analyzes the laboratory values and notes that the serum acid phosphatase level is elevated. The nurse knows that this laboratory test is most often useful in determining:
   1. The diagnosis of prostate cancer
   2. Complications associated with cancer
   3. The progression or regression of the cancer
   4. The likelihood of associated bone cancer

42. Hormone therapy is prescribed as the mode of treatment for a client with prostatic cancer. A nurse understands that the goal of this form of treatment is to:
   1. Limit the levels of circulating androgens
   2. Increase the levels of circulating androgens
   3. Increase testosterone levels
   4. Increase prostaglandin levels

43. A nurse is caring for a client with cancer of the prostate after a prostatectomy. The nurse provides discharge instructions to the client and tells the client to:
   1. Notify the physician if small blood clots are noticed during urination
   2. Avoid driving the car for 1 week
   3. Restrict fluid intake to prevent incontinence
   4. Avoid lifting objects heavier than 20 pounds for at least 6 weeks

44. An oncology nurse is providing a teaching session to a group of nursing students regarding the risks and causes of bladder cancer. Which statement if made by a student indicates a need for further teaching?
   1. "It most often occurs in women."
   2. "It is generally seen in clients older than age 40."
   3. "Environmental health hazards have been attributed as a cause."
   4. "Using cigarettes, artificial sweeteners, and coffee drinking can increase the risk."

45. A nurse is reviewing the history of a client with bladder cancer. The nurse expects to note documentation of which most common symptom of this type of cancer?
   1. Frequency of urination
   2. Urgency on urination
   3. Hematuria
   4. Dysuria

46. A nurse is caring for a client following intravesical instillation of an alkylating chemotherapeutic agent into the bladder for the treatment of bladder cancer. After the instillation, the nurse would most appropriately instruct the client to:
    1. Urinate immediately
    2. Maintain strict bed rest
    3. Retain the instillation fluid for 30 minutes
    4. Change position every 15 minutes

47. A nurse is assessing the stoma of a client after a ureterostomy. Which of the following would the nurse expect to note?
    1. A pale stoma
    2. A red and moist stoma
    3. A dry stoma
    4. A dark-colored stoma

48. A nurse is caring for a client after a radical mastectomy. Which of the following nursing interventions would assist in preventing lymphedema of the affected arm?
    1. Placing cool compresses on the affected arm
    2. Elevating the affected arm on a pillow above heart level
    3. Maintaining an IV site below the antecubital area on the affected side
    4. Avoiding arm exercises in the immediate postoperative period

49. A nurse is preparing a client for mammography. The nurse tells the client:
    1. That mammography takes about 1 hour
    2. To avoid the use of deodorants, powders, or creams on the day of the test
    3. That there is no discomfort associated with the procedure
    4. To maintain an NPO status on the day of the test

50. A nurse is monitoring a client for signs and symptoms related to vena cava syndrome. Which of the following is an early sign of this oncological emergency?
    1. Periorbital edema
    2. Arm edema
    3. Mental status changes
    4. Cyanosis

CRITICAL THINKING: FREE-TEXT ENTRY

A nurse is caring for a client with metastatic breast cancer. The client develops a new and sudden sharp pain in the back. On the basis of this assessment finding, what is the most appropriate nursing intervention?

Answer: _____

ANSWERS

1. **2**

Rationale: The TSE is recommended monthly after a warm bath or shower, when the scrotal skin is relaxed. The client should stand to examine the testicles. Using both hands, with fingers under the scrotum and thumbs on top, the client should gently roll the testicles, feeling for any lumps.
Test-Taking Strategy: Use the process of elimination. Eliminate option 4 first because of the words "6 months." Next eliminate option 3 because of the word "one." From the remaining options, eliminate option 1 by trying to visualize the process of the self-examination. If you had difficulty with this question, review the procedure for this self-examination.
Level of Cognitive Ability: Application
Client Needs: Health Promotion and Maintenance
Integrated Concept/Process: Self-Care
Content Area: Adult Health/Oncology
Reference: Potter, P., & Perry, A. (2001). *Fundamentals of nursing* (5th ed.). St. Louis: Mosby, pp. 811-813.

2. **3**

Rationale: Viruses may be one of multiple agents acting to initiate carcinogenesis and have been associated with several types of cancer. Increased stress has been associated with causing the growth and proliferation of cancer cells. Two forms of radiation, ultraviolet and ionizing, can lead to cancer. A diet high in fat may be a factor in the development of breast, colon, and prostate cancers. High-fiber diets may reduce the risk of colon cancer.

Test-Taking Strategy: Use the process of elimination. Note the key words "indicates a need for further instructions" in the stem of the question. Read each option carefully, utilizing the process of elimination. Familiarity with the risk factors related to cancer will easily direct you to option 3. Review these risk factors if you had difficulty with this question.
Level of Cognitive Ability: Application
Client Needs: Health Promotion and Maintenance
Integrated Concept/Process: Teaching/Learning
Content Area: Adult Health/Oncology
Reference: Ignatavicius, D., Workman, M., & Mishler, M. (1999). *Medical-surgical nursing across the health care continuum* (3rd ed.). Philadelphia: W.B. Saunders, p. 487.

3. **3**

Rationale: Thrombocytopenia indicates a decrease in the number of platelets in the circulating blood. A major concern is monitoring for and preventing bleeding. Option 2 relates to monitoring for infection, particularly if leukopenia is present. Options 1 and 4, although important in the plan of care, are not directly related to thrombocytopenia.
Test-Taking Strategy: Use the process of elimination. Note the key word "thrombocytopenia" in the question. Recalling that this condition places the client at risk for bleeding will assist in eliminating options 1, 2, and 4. Review the nursing interventions related to this disorder if you had difficulty with this question.
Level of Cognitive Ability: Application

Client Needs: Physiological Integrity
Integrated Concept/Process: Nursing Process/Implementation
Content Area: Adult Health/Oncology
Reference: Lewis, S., Heitkemper, M., & Dirksen, S. (2000). *Medical-surgical nursing: Assessment and management of clinical problems* (5th ed.). St. Louis: Mosby, pp. 754-757.

4. 2
Rationale: The normal WBC count ranges from 4000 to 10,000/mm³. Option 1 indicates a low range. Options 3 and 4 indicate elevated ranges.
Test-Taking Strategy: Use the process of elimination. Knowledge regarding the normal WBC count is required to answer this question. Learn this value if you are unfamiliar with it.
Level of Cognitive Ability: Comprehension
Client Needs: Physiological Integrity
Integrated Concept/Process: Nursing Process/Assessment
Content Area: Adult Health/Oncology
Reference: LeMone, P., & Burke, K. (2000). *Medical-surgical nursing: Critical thinking in client care* (2nd ed.). Upper Saddle River, N.J.: Prentice-Hall, p. 241.

5. 2
Rationale: The BSE should be performed monthly several days after the menstrual period. It is not recommended to perform the examination weekly. At the onset of menstruation and during ovulation, hormonal changes occur that may alter breast tissue.
Test-Taking Strategy: Use the process of elimination. Option 4 can be easily eliminated because of the word "weekly." Eliminate options 1 and 3 next because of the similarity that exists in regard to the hormonal changes that occur during these times. Review the procedure for performing BSE if you had difficulty with this question.
Level of Cognitive Ability: Application
Client Needs: Health Promotion and Maintenance
Integrated Concept/Process: Self-Care
Content Area: Adult Health/Oncology
Reference: Leahy, J., & Kizilay, P. (1998). *Foundations of nursing practice: A nursing process approach.* Philadelphia: W.B. Saunders, pp. 332-333.

6. 3
Rationale: The client is at risk for deep vein thrombosis or thrombophlebitis after this surgery, as for any other major surgery. For this reason, the nurse implements measures that will prevent this complication. Range-of-motion exercises, antiembolism stockings, and pneumatic compression boots are all helpful. The nurse should avoid using the knee gatch in the bed, which inhibits venous return, thus placing the client more at risk for deep vein thrombosis or thrombophlebitis.
Test-Taking Strategy: Use the process of elimination. Note the key word "avoids." This tells you that the correct option is an incorrect nursing action. Review postoperative nursing interventions following vaginal hysterectomy if you had difficulty with this question.
Level of Cognitive Ability: Application
Client Needs: Physiological Integrity
Integrated Concept/Process: Nursing Process/Implementation
Content Area: Adult Health/Oncology
Reference: Beare, P., & Myers, J. (1998). *Adult health nursing* (3rd ed.). St. Louis: Mosby, p. 1669.

7. 3
Rationale: A pelvic ultrasound requires the ingestion of large volumes of water just prior to the procedure. A full bladder is necessary so that this organ will be visualized as such and not mistaken for a possible pelvic growth. An abdominal ultrasound may require that the client abstain from food or fluid for several hours before the procedure. Option 4 is unrelated to this specific procedure.
Test-Taking Strategy: Use the process of elimination. Noting the key word "pelvic" will assist in eliminating option 4. From the remaining options, focusing on the key word will assist in directing you to option 3. Review preparation for a pelvic ultrasound if you had difficulty with this question.
Level of Cognitive Ability: Application
Client Needs: Physiological Integrity
Integrated Concept/Process: Nursing Process/Planning
Content Area: Adult Health/Oncology
Reference: Leahy, J., & Kizilay, P. (1998). *Foundations of nursing practice: A nursing process approach.* Philadelphia: W.B. Saunders, p. 151.

8. 4
Rationale: A biopsy is done to determine whether a tumor is malignant or benign. MRI, CT scan, and ultrasound will visualize the presence of a mass but will not confirm a diagnosis of malignancy.
Test-Taking Strategy: Use the process of elimination. Note the key word "confirm." This key word should easily direct you to option 4. Review the purpose of the tests identified in the options, if you had difficulty with this question.
Level of Cognitive Ability: Analysis
Client Needs: Physiological Integrity
Integrated Concept/Process: Nursing Process/Analysis
Content Area: Adult Health/Oncology
Reference: Smeltzer, S., & Bare, B. (2000) *Brunner & Suddarth's textbook of medical-surgical nursing* (9th ed.). Philadelphia: Lippincott Williams & Wilkins, p. 272.

9. 4
Rationale: Multiple myeloma is a B cell neoplastic condition characterized by abnormal malignant proliferation of plasma cells and the accumulation of abnomal plasma cells in the bone marrow. Option 1 describes the leukemic process. Options 2 and 3 are not characteristics of multiple myeloma.
Test-Taking Strategy: Use the process of elimination. Focus on the name of the disorder, multiple myeloma, to direct you to option 4. Review this information if you are unfamiliar with this oncological disorder.
Level of Cognitive Ability: Analysis
Client Needs: Physiological Integrity
Integrated Concept/Process: Teaching/Learning
Content Area: Adult Health/Oncology
Reference: Lewis, S., Heitkemper, M., & Dirksen, S. (2000). *Medical-surgical nursing: Assessment and management of clinical problems* (5th ed.). St. Louis: Mosby, pp. 780-781.

10. 3
Rationale: Findings indicative of multiple myeloma are an increased number of plasma cells in the bone marrow, anemia, hypercalcemia resulting from the release of calcium from the deteriorating bone tissue, and an elevated BUN. An increased white blood cell count may or may not be present and is not specifically related to multiple myeloma.

Test-Taking Strategy: Use the process of elimination. Noting the name of the disorder will direct you to option 3. Review this information if you are unfamiliar with this oncological disorder.
Level of Cognitive Ability: Analysis
Client Needs: Physiological Integrity
Integrated Concept/Process: Nursing Process/Assessment
Content Area: Adult Health/Oncology
Reference: Lewis, S., Heitkemper, M., & Dirksen, S. (2000). *Medical-surgical nursing: Assessment and management of clinical problems* (5th ed.). St. Louis: Mosby, pp. 780-781.

11. 2
Rationale: Hypercalcemia secondary to bone destruction is a priority concern in the client with multiple myeloma. The nurse should administer fluids in adequate amounts to maintain an output of 1.5 to 2.0 L/day. Clients require about 3 L of fluid per day. The fluid is needed not only to dilute the calcium overload but also to prevent protein from precipitating in the renal tubules. Options 1, 3, and 4 may be components of the plan of care, but are not the priority in this client.
Test-Taking Strategy: Use the process of elimination. Recalling the pathophysiology of this disorder and that forcing fluids is specific to the care of a client with this disorder will direct you to option 2. Review the specific manifestations of this disorder if you had difficulty with this question.
Level of Cognitive Ability: Analysis
Client Needs: Physiological Integrity
Integrated Concept/Process: Nursing Process/Planning
Content Area: Adult Health/Oncology
Reference: Lewis, S., Heitkemper, M., & Dirksen, S. (2000). *Medical-surgical nursing: Assessment and management of clinical problems* (5th ed.). St. Louis: Mosby, p. 781.

12. 3
Rationale: Hodgkin's disease is a disorder of young adults. Options 1, 2, and 4 are characteristics of this disease.
Test-Taking Strategy: Use the process of elimination. Note the key word "not" in the stem of the question. Recalling that Hodgkin's occurs in the young adult will easily direct you to option 3. Review the characteristics of this disorder if you had difficulty with this question.
Level of Cognitive Ability: Analysis
Client Needs: Physiological Integrity
Integrated Concept/Process: Nursing Process/Planning
Content Area: Adult Health/Oncology
Reference: LeMone, P., & Burke, K. (2000). *Medical-surgical nursing: Critical thinking in client care* (2nd ed.). Upper Saddle River, N.J.: Prentice-Hall, p. 1317.

13. 3
Rationale: Alopecia is not an assessment finding in testicular cancer. It may, however, occur as a result of radiation or chemotherapy. Options 1, 2, and 4 are assessment findings in testicular cancer. Back pain may indicate metastasis to the retroperitoneal lymph nodes.
Test-Taking Strategy: Note the key word "not" in the stem of the question. Use the process of elimination, remembering that alopecia occurs as a result of chemotherapy rather than from the disease. Review the manifestations associated with testicular cancer if you had difficulty with this question.
Level of Cognitive Ability: Application

Client Needs: Health Promotion and Maintenance
Integrated Concept/Process: Teaching/Learning
Content Area: Adult Health/Oncology
Reference: Smeltzer, S., & Bare, B. (2000) *Brunner & Suddarth's textbook of medical-surgical nursing* (9th ed). Philadelphia: Lippincott Williams & Wilkins, p. 1319.

14. 3
Rationale: In general, only the area in the treatment field is affected by the radiation. Skin reactions, fatigue, nausea, and anorexia may occur with radiation to any site, whereas other side effects occur only when specific areas are involved in treatment. A client receiving radiation to the larynx is most likely to experience a sore throat. Options 1 and 4 may occur with radiation to the gastrointestinal (GI) tract. Dyspnea may occur with lung involvement.
Test-Taking Strategy: Use the process of elimination. Eliminate options 1 and 4 first because they are similar and GI related. Consider the anatomical location of the radiation therapy to assist you in selecting option 3. Review the effects of radiation therapy if you had difficulty with this question.
Level of Cognitive Ability: Analysis
Client Needs: Physiological Integrity
Integrated Concept/Process: Nursing Process/Assessment
Content Area: Adult Health/Oncology
Reference: Ignatavicius, D., Workman, M., & Mishler, M. (1999). *Medical-surgical nursing across the health care continuum* (3rd ed.). Philadelphia: W.B. Saunders, p. 596.

15. 2
Rationale: The time that the nurse spends in a room of a client with an internal radiation implant is 30 minutes per 8-hour shift. The dosimeter badge must be worn when in the client's room. Children younger than 16 years and pregnant women are not allowed in the client's room.
Test-Taking Strategy: Use the process of elimination. Option 4 can be eliminated first. Knowledge of the time frame related to exposure to the client will assist in eliminating option 1. From the remaining options, select option 2 because of the possible risks associated with exposure to the mother and fetus. Review these principles if you had difficulty with this question.
Level of Cognitive Ability: Application
Client Needs: Safe, Effective Care Environment
Integrated Concept/Process: Nursing Process/Implementation
Content Area: Adult Health/Oncology
Reference: Monahan, F., & Neighbors, M. (1998). *Medical-surgical nursing: Foundations for clinical practice* (2nd ed.). Philadelphia: W. B. Saunders, p. 1519.

16. 3
Rationale: The client with a cervical radiation implant should be maintained on bed rest in the dorsal position to prevent movement of the radiation source. The head of the bed is elevated to a maximum of 10 to 15 degrees for comfort. The nurse avoids turning the client on the side. If turning is absolutely necessary, a pillow is placed between the knees and, with the body in straight alignment, the client is logrolled.
Test-Taking Strategy: Use the process of elimination. Consider the anatomical location of the implant and the risk of dislodgment to answer the question. In addition, note that options 1, 2, and 4 are similar. If you had difficulty with this question, review care to the client with a radiation implant.
Level of Cognitive Ability: Application

Client Needs: Safe, Effective Care Environment
Integrated Concept/Process: Nursing Process/Implementation
Content Area: Adult Health/Oncology
Reference: Monahan, F., & Neighbors, M. (1998). *Medical-surgical nursing: Foundations for clinical practice* (2nd ed.). Philadelphia: W. B. Saunders, p. 1835.

17. 4
Rationale: A lead container and long-handled forceps should be kept in the client's room at all times during internal radiation therapy. If the implant becomes dislodged, the nurse should pick up the implant with long-handled forceps and place it in the lead container. Options 1, 2, and 3 are inaccurate interventions.
Test-Taking Strategy: Use the process of elimination. Note the key word "initial" in the stem of the question. Option 3 is not an appropriate action. Eliminate option 2 next because the implant would not be discarded. Although the physician would be notified, the initial action is option 4. Review the initial measures related to a dislodged implant if you had difficulty with this question.
Level of Cognitive Ability: Application
Client Needs: Safe, Effective Care Environment
Integrated Concept/Process: Nursing Process/Implementation
Content Area: Adult Health/Oncology
Reference: Monahan, F., & Neighbors, M. (1998). *Medical-surgical nursing: Foundations for clinical practice* (2nd ed.). Philadelphia: W. B. Saunders, p. 1519.

18. 4
Rationale: In the immunocompromised client, a low-bacteria diet is implemented. This includes avoiding fresh fruits and vegetables and thorough cooking of all foods. Not all visitors are restricted, but the client is protected from people with known infections. Fluids should be encouraged. Invasive measures such as an indwelling urinary catheter should be avoided to prevent infections.
Test-Taking Strategy: Use the process of elimination. Eliminate option 1 because of the word "all." Next eliminate option 2 because it is not reasonable to eliminate fluids in a client receiving chemotherapy, who is at risk for fluid and electrolyte imbalances. Eliminate option 3 because of the risk of infection that exists with this measure. Review interventions for the client with hematologic toxicity if you had difficulty with this question.
Level of Cognitive Ability: Application
Client Needs: Safe, Effective Care Environment
Integrated Concept/Process: Nursing Process/Planning
Content Area: Adult Health/Oncology
Reference: Monahan, F., & Neighbors, M. (1998). *Medical-surgical nursing: Foundations for clinical practice* (2nd ed.). Philadelphia: W.B. Saunders, pp. 1536-1537.

19. 1
Rationale: A high risk for hemorrhage exists when the platelet count is less than 20,000/mm³. Fatal central nervous system hemorrhage or massive gastrointestinal hemorrhage can occur when the platelet count is less than 10,000/mm³. The client should be assessed for changes in level of consciousness, which may be an early indication of an intracranial hemorrhage. Option 2 is a priority nursing assessment when the white blood cell count is low and the client is at risk for an infection. Although options 3 and 4

are important to assess, they are not the priority in this situation.
Test-Taking Strategy: Use the process of elimination. Note the key word "priority" in the stem of the question. Recalling the normal platelet count and determining that a low count places the client at risk for bleeding will assist in eliminating options 2, 3, and 4 as assessment measures for bleeding. Review the normal platelet count and the nursing interventions for a client with a low count if you had difficulty with this question.
Level of Cognitive Ability: Analysis
Client Needs: Physiological Integrity
Integrated Concept/Process: Nursing Process/Assessment
Content Area: Adult Health/Oncology
Reference: Lewis, S., Heitkemper, M., & Dirksen, S. (2000). *Medical-surgical nursing: Assessment and management of clinical problems* (5th ed.). St. Louis: Mosby, p. 756.

20. 1
Rationale: The client's self-report is a critical component of pain assessment. The nurse should ask the client about the description of the pain and listen carefully to the client's words used to describe the pain. The nurse's impression of the client's pain is not appropriate in determining the client's level of pain. Nonverbal cues from the client are important but are not the most appropriate pain assessment measure. Assessing pain relief is an important measure, but this option is not related to the issue of the question.
Test-Taking Strategy: Use the process of elimination. Noting the issue of the question will assist in eliminating option 4. Eliminate option 2 because the nurse is not the client of the question. From the remaining two options, the subjective data from the client will provide the most accurate description of the pain.
Level of Cognitive Ability: Analysis
Client Needs: Physiological Integrity
Integrated Concept/Process: Caring
Content Area: Adult Health/Oncology
Reference: Monahan, F., & Neighbors, M. (1998). *Medical-surgical nursing: Foundations for clinical practice* (2nd ed.). Philadelphia: W.B. Saunders, p. 1556.

21. 4
Rationale: The client is kept NPO until peristalsis returns, usually in 4 to 6 days. When signs of bowel function return, clear fluids are given to the client. If no distention occurs, the diet is advanced as tolerated. The most important assessment is to assess bowel sounds prior to feeding the client. Options 1, 2, and 3 are unrelated to the issue of the question.
Test-Taking Strategy: Use the process of elimination. Note the key word "priority" and the key words "NPO to clear liquids" in the stem of the question. Knowledge regarding general postoperative care measures will assist in selecting the correct option. Option 4 is the only option that relates to gastrointestinal function, which is the issue of the question.
Level of Cognitive Ability: Analysis
Client Needs: Physiological Integrity
Integrated Concept/Process: Nursing Process/Assessment
Content Area: Adult Health/Oncology
Reference: Monahan, F., & Neighbors, M. (1998). *Medical-surgical nursing: Foundations for clinical practice* (2nd ed.). Philadelphia: W.B. Saunders, p. 1832

22. **4**

Rationale: Hodgkin's disease is a chronic progressive neoplastic disorder of lymphoid tissue characterized by the painless enlargement of lymph nodes with progression to extralymphatic sites such as the spleen and liver. Weight loss is most likely to be noted. Fatigue and weakness may occur, but are not significantly related to the disease.

Test-Taking Strategy: Use the process of elimination. Knowledge that Hodgkin's disease affects the lymph nodes will easily direct you to option 4. Option 3 can be easily eliminated first because in such a disorder, weight loss is most likely to occur. Options 1 and 2 are similar and rather vague symptoms that can occur in many disorders. Review the manifestations associated with Hodgkin's disease if you had difficulty with this question.

Level of Cognitive Ability: Analysis
Client Needs: Physiological Integrity
Integrated Concept/Process: Nursing Process/Assessment
Content Area: Adult Health/Oncology
Reference: Smeltzer, S., & Bare, B. (2000) *Brunner & Suddarth's textbook of medical-surgical nursing* (9th ed.). Philadelphia: Lippincott Williams & Wilkins, pp. 763-764.

23. **2**

Rationale: Clinical manifestations of ovarian cancer include abdominal distention, urinary frequency and urgency, pleural effusion, malnutrition, pain from pressure caused by the growing tumor and the effects of urinary or bowel obstruction, constipation, ascites with dyspnea, and ultimately general severe pain. Abnormal bleeding, often resulting in hypermenorrhea, is associated with uterine cancer.

Test-Taking Strategy: Use the process of elimination. Eliminate options 1 and 4 first because they are similar. From the remaining options, consider the anatomical location of the cancer. This will assist in directing you to option 2. Review the manifestations associated with ovarian cancer if you had difficulty with this question.

Level of Cognitive Ability: Analysis
Client Needs: Physiological Integrity
Integrated Concept/Process: Nursing Process/Assessment
Content Area: Adult Health/Oncology
Reference: LeMone, P., & Burke, K. (2000). *Medical-surgical nursing: Critical thinking in client care* (2nd ed.). Upper Saddle River, N.J.: Prentice-Hall, p. 2036.

24. **3**

Rationale: Conization is generally not performed on women who desire to bear children because it can lead to incompetence of the cervix or infertility. Complications of the procedure include hemorrhage, infection, and, less frequently, cervical stenosis.

Test-Taking Strategy: Use the process of elimination. Note the key words "need for further teaching" and the words "cervical cancer" in the question. Select option 3 because this option addresses an "ovarian" condition, not a cervical one. Review the complications associated with this procedure if you had difficulty with this question.

Level of Cognitive Ability: Analysis
Client Needs: Health Promotion and Maintenance
Integrated Concept/Process: Teaching/Learning
Content Area: Adult Health/Oncology

Reference: Monahan, F., & Neighbors, M. (1998). *Medical-surgical nursing: Foundations for clinical practice* (2nd ed.). Philadelphia: W.B. Saunders, p. 1784.

25. **4**

Rationale: Hypercalcemia is a serum calcium level greater than 10 mg/dL. It most often occurs in clients who have bone metastasis, and is a late manifestation of extensive malignancy. The presence of cancer in the bone causes the bone to release calcium into the bloodstream.

Test-Taking Strategy: Use the process of elimination. Knowledge regarding the normal calcium level will easily direct you to option 4. Note the relationship between "calcium level" in the question and "hypercalcemia" in the correct option. Review oncological emergencies if you had difficulty with this question.

Level of Cognitive Ability: Analysis
Client Needs: Physiological Integrity
Integrated Concept/Process: Nursing Process/Assessment
Content Area: Adult Health/Oncology
Reference: Ignatavicius, D., Workman, M., & Mishler, M. (1999). *Medical-surgical nursing across the health care continuum* (3rd ed.). Philadelphia: W.B. Saunders, p. 258.

26. **1**

Rationale: Testicular cancer almost always occurs in only one testicle and is usually a pea-sized, painless lump. It is highly curable when found early. The finding should be reported to the physician.

Test-Taking Strategy: Use the process of elimination. Eliminate option 4 because it does not address the client's concern and is a block to communication. Option 3 places the client's concern on hold and is an inappropriate and inaccurate response. Option 2 is nontherapeutic and may cause concern in the client. Review TSE and therapeutic communication techniques if you had difficulty with this question.

Level of Cognitive Ability: Application
Client Needs: Psychosocial Integrity
Integrated Concept/Process: Caring
Content Area: Adult Health/Oncology
Reference: Monahan, F., & Neighbors, M. (1998). *Medical-surgical nursing: Foundations for clinical practice* (2nd ed.). Philadelphia: W.B. Saunders, p. 334.

27. **2**

Rationale: Denial, bargaining, anger, depression, and acceptance are recognized stages that a person facing a life-threatening illness experiences. Bargaining identifies a behavior in which the individual is willing to do anything to avoid loss or change the prognosis or fate. Denial is expressed as shock and disbelief and may be the first response to hearing bad news. Depression may be manifested by hopelessness, weeping openly, or remaining quiet or withdrawn. Anger may also be a first response to upsetting news, and the predominant theme is "Why me?" or the blaming of others.

Test-Taking Strategy: Use the process of elimination. Focus on the client's statement as identified in the question to assist in selecting the correct option. From this point, you should easily be able to eliminate options 1, 3, and 4. Review these stages if you had difficulty with this question.

Level of Cognitive Ability: Analysis
Client Needs: Psychosocial Integrity

Integrated Concept/Process: Nursing Process/Analysis
Content Area: Adult Health/Oncology
Reference: Potter, P., & Perry, A. (2001). *Fundamentals of nursing* (5th ed.). St. Louis: Mosby, p. 633.

28. **4**

Rationale: Arm edema on the operative side (lymphedema) is a complication following mastectomy and can occur immediately postoperatively or may occur months or even years after surgery. Options 1, 2, and 3 are expected occurrences following mastectomy and are not indicative of a complication.

Test-Taking Strategy: Use the process of elimination, considering the normal, expected occurrences following a mastectomy. You should easily be able to eliminate options 1, 2, and 3. If you had difficulty with this question, review the complications following mastectomy.

Level of Cognitive Ability: Analysis
Client Needs: Physiological Integrity
Integrated Concept/Process: Nursing Process/Assessment
Content Area: Adult Health/Oncology
Reference: LeMone, P., & Burke, K. (2000). *Medical-surgical nursing: Critical thinking in client care* (2nd ed.). Upper Saddle River, N.J.: Prentice-Hall, p. 2068.

29. **2**

Rationale: The most common risk factor associated with laryngeal cancer is cigarette smoking. Approximately three quarters of those diagnosed with this form of cancer smoke currently or have done so in the past. Alcohol abuse seems to have a synergistic effect with cigarette smoking. Air pollution is also a contributing cause, as well as chronic laryngitis and voice abuse.

Test-Taking Strategy: Use the process of elimination. Note the key words "most common" in the question. Begin to answer this question by eliminating options 3 and 4. Since cancer of the upper and lower airway is most often related to tobacco, these are the options that are most likely correct. To discriminate between the last two options, knowing that cigarettes are the most harmful guides you to choose this option over the chewing tobacco.

Level of Cognitive Ability: Application
Client Needs: Health Promotion and Maintenance
Integrated Concept/Process: Nursing Process/Assessment
Content Area: Adult Health/Oncology
Reference: Phipps, W., Sands, J., & Marek, J. (1999). *Medical-surgical nursing: Concepts & clinical practice* (6th ed.). St. Louis: Mosby, p. 889.

30. **3**

Rationale: A vesicovaginal fistula is a genital fistula that occurs between the bladder and the vagina. The fistula is an abnormal opening between these two body parts, and if this occurs, the client may experience drainage of urine through the vagina. The client's complaint is not associated with options 1, 2, and 4.

Test-Taking Strategy: Use the process of elimination. Noting the key words "voiding through the vagina" should easily direct you to option 3. Review the symptoms associated with vesicovaginal fistula if you had difficulty with this question.

Level of Cognitive Ability: Analysis
Client Needs: Physiological Integrity
Integrated Concept/Process: Nursing Process/Analysis

Content Area: Adult Health/Oncology
Reference: Monahan, F., & Neighbors, M. (1998). *Medical-surgical nursing: Foundations for clinical practice* (2nd ed.). Philadelphia: W.B. Saunders, p. 1821.

31. **2**

Rationale: Allopurinol decreases uric acid production and reduces uric acid concentrations in both serum and urine. In the client receiving chemotherapy, uric acid levels elevate as a result of the massive cell destruction that occurs from the chemotherapy. This medication prevents or treats hyperuricemia secondary to chemotherapy. Although the medication is used to treat gout, it is not the purpose in this client situation. This medication is not used to prevent stomatitis or diarrhea.

Test-Taking Strategy: Use the process of elimination. Recalling that hyperuricemia occurs as a result of chemotherapy will assist in directing you to option 2. If you had difficulty with this question or are unfamiliar with this medication, review its action in the client receiving chemotherapy.

Level of Cognitive Ability: Analysis
Client Needs: Physiological Integrity
Integrated Concept/Process: Nursing Process/Analysis
Content Area: Adult Health/Oncology
Reference: Hodgson, B., & Kizior, R. (2001). *Saunders nursing drug handbook 2001.* Philadelphia: W.B. Saunders, pp. 24-25.

32. **2**

Rationale: An acidic environment in the mouth is favorable for bacterial growth, particularly in an area already compromised by chemotherapy. Therefore, the client is advised to rinse the mouth before every meal and at bedtime with a weak salt and sodium bicarbonate mouth rinse. This lessens the growth of bacteria and limits plaque formation. The other substances are irritating to oral tissue. If hydrogen peroxide must be used because of severe plaque, it should be a very weak solution, because it dries the mucous membranes.

Test-Taking Strategy: Use the process of elimination. Options 3 and 4 can be eliminated first because of the irritating effects of these solutions. From the remaining options, note the word "weak" in the correct option. Review the treatment measures for stomatitis if you had difficulty with this question.

Level of Cognitive Ability: Application
Client Needs: Health Promotion and Maintenance
Integrated Concept/Process: Self-Care
Content Area: Adult Health/Oncology
Reference: Monahan, F., & Neighbors, M. (1998). *Medical-surgical nursing: Foundations for clinical practice* (2nd ed.). Philadelphia: W.B. Saunders, pp. 1529-1530.

33. **4**

Rationale: High meat and carbohydrate consumption plays a role in the development of cancer of the pancreas. Options 1, 2, and 3 are risk factors related to gastric cancer. In addition, an increased risk exists in the male population in clients 50 years of age and older and in clients with a history of precancerous lesions and chronic gastritis.

Test-Taking Strategy: Use the process of elimination. Note that the question asks about the risk factors associated with gastric cancer. Note the key words "indicate a need for further discussion." Eliminate options 1 and 2 because they are directly related to gastric disorders. Eliminate option 3, knowing that spicy foods cause gastric irritation. Review the risk factors associated with gastric cancer if you had difficulty with this question.

Level of Cognitive Ability: Application
Client Needs: Health Promotion and Maintenance
Integrated Concept/Process: Teaching/Learning
Content Area: Adult Health/Oncology
Reference: Monahan, F., & Neighbors, M. (1998). *Medical-surgical nursing: Foundations for clinical practice* (2nd ed.). Philadelphia: W.B. Saunders, pp. 1058, 1126.

34. 2
Rationale: After gastrectomy, drainage from the NG tube is normally bloody for 24 hours postoperatively and then changes to brown tinged and then to yellow or clear. Since bloody drainage is expected in the immediate postoperative period, the nurse should continue to monitor the drainage. There is no need to notify the physician at this time. Measuring abdominal girth is performed to detect the development of distention. Following gastrectomy, an NG tube should not be irrigated unless there are specific physician's orders to do so.
Test-Taking Strategy: Use the process of elimination. Note the key word "immediate" and the words "most appropriate" in the question. These key items should easily direct you to option 2. If you had difficulty with this question, review the expected postoperative findings after gastrectomy.
Level of Cognitive Ability: Application
Client Needs: Physiological Integrity
Integrated Concept/Process: Nursing Process/Implementation
Content Area: Adult Health/Oncology
Reference: Monahan, F., & Neighbors, M. (1998). *Medical-surgical nursing: Foundations for clinical practice* (2nd ed.). Philadelphia: W.B. Saunders, p. 999.

35. 3
Rationale: Colorectal cancer most often occurs in populations with diets low in fiber and high in refined carbohydrates, fats, and meats. Other risk factors include a family history of the disease, rectal polyps, and active inflammatory disease of at least 10 years' duration.
Test-Taking Strategy: Use the process of elimination. Note the key word "not" in the stem of the question. Eliminate options 1 and 2 because they are similar and directly related to the issue of colorectal cancer. Knowledge that a high-fiber diet is recommended as a preventive measure will assist in selecting the correct option. Review the risk factors associated with colorectal cancer if you had difficulty with this question.
Level of Cognitive Ability: Comprehension
Client Needs: Health Promotion and Maintenance
Integrated Concept/Process: Nursing Process/Assessment
Content Area: Adult Health/Oncology
Reference: Monahan, F., & Neighbors, M. (1998). *Medical-surgical nursing: Foundations for clinical practice* (2nd ed.). Philadelphia: W.B. Saunders, p. 1100.

36. 3
Rationale: Characteristic symptoms of right colon tumors include vague, dull abdominal pain exacerbated by walking and dark red or mahogany blood mixed in the stool. Options 1, 2, and 4 are symptoms associated with left colon tumors.
Test-Taking Strategy: Use the process of elimination. Note the key words "right colon tumor." Knowledge regarding the signs of right and left colon tumors is required to answer this

question. If you are not familiar with the differences, review these types of tumors.
Level of Cognitive Ability: Analysis
Client Needs: Physiological Integrity
Integrated Concept/Process: Nursing Process/Assessment
Content Area: Adult Health/Oncology
Reference: Monahan, F., & Neighbors, M. (1998). *Medical-surgical nursing: Foundations for clinical practice* (2nd ed.). Philadelphia: W.B. Saunders, p. 1100.

37. 3
Rationale: To reduce the risk of contamination at the time of surgery, the bowel is emptied and cleansed. Laxatives and enemas are given to empty the bowel. Intestinal antiinfectives such as neomycin or kanamycin are administered to decrease the bacteria in the bowel.
Test-Taking Strategy: Use the process of elimination. Eliminate options 1 and 4 first because there is no reference made to this information in the question. Recalling the concepts related to the flora of the intestinal tract will assist in directing you to option 3 as the primary purpose of this medication. Review this important preoperative intervention if you had difficulty with this question.
Level of Cognitive Ability: Analysis
Client Needs: Physiological Integrity
Integrated Concept/Process: Nursing Process/Analysis
Content Area: Adult Health/Oncology
Reference: Monahan, F., & Neighbors, M. (1998). *Medical-surgical nursing: Foundations for clinical practice* (2nd ed.). Philadelphia: W.B. Saunders, p. 1101.

38. 2
Rationale: Immediately after surgery, profuse serosanguineous drainage from the perineal wound is expected. There is no need to notify the physician at this time. A Penrose drain should not be clamped because this action will cause the accumulation of drainage within the tissue. Both Penrose drains and packing are removed gradually over a period of 5 to 7 days, as prescribed. The nurse should not remove the perineal packing.
Test-Taking Strategy: Use the process of elimination. Note the key words "most appropriate." Eliminate options 3 and 4, knowing that these are inappropriate interventions. Knowledge of the normal expectations following this type of surgery will assist in directing you to option 2 as the most appropriate action. Review postoperative expectations following abdominal perineal resection if you had difficulty with this question.
Level of Cognitive Ability: Application
Client Needs: Physiological Integrity
Integrated Concept/Process: Nursing Process/Implementation
Content Area: Adult Health/Oncology
Reference: Monahan, F., & Neighbors, M. (1998). *Medical-surgical nursing: Foundations for clinical practice* (2nd ed.). Philadelphia: W. B. Saunders, pp. 1101-1102.

39. 4
Rationale: After abdominal perineal resection, the nurse would expect the colostomy to begin to function within 72 hours after surgery, although it may take up to 5 days. The nurse should assess for a return of peristalsis and listen for bowel sounds and check for the passage of flatus. Absent

bowel sounds would not indicate the return of peristalsis. The client would remain NPO until bowel sounds return and the colostomy is functioning. Bloody drainage is not expected from a colostomy.

Test-Taking Strategy: Use the process of elimination. Note the key words "beginning to function." These key words should assist in eliminating option 3. Knowledge of general postoperative measures will assist in eliminating option 2. Focus on the issue of the question to assist in eliminating option 1 as a correct option. Review postoperative care of a client following abdominal perineal resection if you had difficulty with this question.

Level of Cognitive Ability: Analysis
Client Needs: Physiological Integrity
Integrated Concept/Process: Nursing Process/Assessment
Content Area: Adult Health/Oncology
Reference: Monahan, F., & Neighbors, M. (1998). *Medical-surgical nursing: Foundations for clinical practice* (2nd ed.). Philadelphia: W.B. Saunders, p. 1103.

40. 3
Rationale: Air conditioners need to be avoided to protect from excessive coldness. A humidifier in the home should be used if excessive dryness is a problem. Options 1, 2, and 4 are appropriate interventions regarding stoma care following radical neck dissection and creation of a tracheostomy.

Test-Taking Strategy: Use the process of elimination. Note the key words "need for further instructions." You should easily be able to eliminate options 2 and 4. From the remaining options, recalling that a humidifier rather than an air conditioner is recommended will assist you in selecting the correct option. If you had difficulty with this question, review discharge instructions following radical neck dissection.

Level of Cognitive Ability: Analysis
Client Needs: Health Promotion and Maintenance
Integrated Concept/Process: Teaching/Learning
Content Area: Adult Health/Oncology
Reference: Monahan, F., & Neighbors, M. (1998). *Medical-surgical nursing: Foundations for clinical practice* (2nd ed.). Philadelphia: W.B. Saunders, p. 631.

41. 3
Rationale: Serum acid phosphatase levels are elevated in clients with prostatic cancer because acid phosphatase, which is produced by the acinar cells, is absorbed into the circulation rather than secreted into the seminal fluid and kept in the prostate. This makes measurement of serum acid phosphatase a useful biochemical test for monitoring the progression or regression of prostatic cancer.

Test-Taking Strategy: Use the process of elimination. Eliminate option 1 first, knowing that biopsy is necessary to confirm the diagnosis of cancer. From the remaining options, select option 3 because it is the most global response. Review this serum test if you had difficulty with this question.

Level of Cognitive Ability: Analysis
Client Needs: Physiological Integrity
Integrated Concept/Process: Nursing Process/Analysis
Content Area: Adult Health/Oncology
Reference: Monahan, F., & Neighbors, M. (1998). *Medical-surgical nursing: Foundations for clinical practice* (2nd ed.). Philadelphia: W.B. Saunders, p. 1757.

42. 1
Rationale: Hormone therapy (androgen deprivation) is a mode of treatment for prostatic cancer. The goal is to limit the amounts of circulating androgens because prostate cells depend on androgen for cellular maintenance. Deprivation of androgen can often lead to regression of disease and improvement of symptoms.

Test-Taking Strategy: Use the process of elimination. Note that options 2, 3, and 4 all indicate an increase. Review the goal of this form of therapy if you had difficulty with this question.

Level of Cognitive Ability: Analysis
Client Needs: Physiological Integrity
Integrated Concept/Process: Nursing Process/Analysis
Content Area: Adult Health/Oncology
Reference: Monahan, F., & Neighbors, M. (1998). *Medical-surgical nursing: Foundations for clinical practice* (2nd ed.). Philadelphia: W.B. Saunders, p. 1759.

43. 4
Rationale: Small pieces of tissue or blood clots can be passed during urination for up to 2 weeks after surgery. Driving a car and sitting for long periods of time are restricted for at least 3 weeks. A high daily fluid intake should be maintained to limit clot formation and prevent infection. Option 4 is an accurate discharge instruction following prostatectomy.

Test-Taking Strategy: Use the process of elimination. Option 3 can be easily eliminated first. Eliminate option 2 next, because 1 week is a rather short time period. Recalling that blood clots are expected following this type of surgery will assist in directing you to option 4. Review client teaching points following prostatectomy if you had difficulty with this question.

Level of Cognitive Ability: Application
Client Needs: Health Promotion and Maintenance
Integrated Concept/Process: Teaching/Learning
Content Area: Adult Health/Oncology
Reference: Monahan, F., & Neighbors, M. (1998). *Medical-surgical nursing: Foundations for clinical practice* (2nd ed.). Philadelphia: W.B. Saunders, p. 1720.

44. 1
Rationale: The incidence of bladder cancer is three times greater in men than in women and affects the Caucasian population twice as often as African-Americans. Options 2, 3, and 4 are associated with the incidence of bladder cancer.

Test-Taking Strategy: Use the process of elimination. Note the key words "need for further teaching." Basic information regarding the risks associated with cancer will assist in eliminating options 2, 3, and 4. If you had difficulty with this question, review these risks.

Level of Cognitive Ability: Analysis
Client Needs: Health Promotion and Maintenance
Integrated Concept/Process: Teaching/Learning
Content Area: Adult Health/Oncology
Reference: Monahan, F., & Neighbors, M. (1998). *Medical-surgical nursing: Foundations for clinical practice* (2nd ed.). Philadelphia: W.B. Saunders, p. 1419.

45. 3
Rationale: The most common symptom in clients with cancer of the bladder is hematuria. The client may also experience irritative voiding symptoms such as frequency, urgency, and

dysuria, and these symptoms are often associated with cancer in situ.

Test-Taking Strategy: Use the process of elimination. Note the key words "most common" in the stem of the question. Options 1, 2, and 4 are symptoms that are most often associated with bladder infection. Review the clinical manifestations associated with bladder cancer if you had difficulty with this question.

Level of Cognitive Ability: Analysis
Client Needs: Physiological Integrity
Integrated Concept/Process: Communication and Documentation
Content Area: Adult Health/Oncology
Reference: Monahan, F., & Neighbors, M. (1998). *Medical-surgical nursing: Foundations for clinical practice* (2nd ed.). Philadelphia: W.B. Saunders, p. 1419.

46. 4
Rationale: Normally the medication is injected into the bladder through a urethral catheter, the catheter is clamped or removed, and the client is asked to retain the fluid for 2 hours. The client is to change position every 15 to 30 minutes from side to side, and from supine to prone, or to resume all activity immediately. The client then voids and is instructed to drink water to flush the bladder.

Test-Taking Strategy: Use the process of elimination. Note the key words "intravesical instillation" and think about the purpose of this treatment to direct you to option 4. If you are unfamiliar with this treatment measure, review the nursing interventions.

Level of Cognitive Ability: Application
Client Needs: Physiological Integrity
Integrated Concept/Process: Nursing Process/Implementation
Content Area: Adult Health/Oncology
Reference: Lewis, S., Heitkemper, M., & Dirksen, S. (2000). *Medical-surgical nursing: Assessment and management of clinical problems* (5th ed.). St. Louis: Mosby, p. 1284.

47. 2
Rationale: Following ureterostomy, the stoma should be red and moist. A pale stoma may indicate an inadequate vascular supply. A dry stoma may indicate a body fluid deficit. Any sign of darkness or duskiness in the stoma may indicate a loss of vascular supply and must be reported immediately or necrosis can occur.

Test-Taking Strategy: Use the process of elimination. You should easily be able to eliminate options 1 and 4. From the remaining options, note the key word "moist" in option 2. This should indicate that this is an expected and positive assessment. If you had difficulty with this question, review expected and unexpected findings following ureterostomy.

Level of Cognitive Ability: Analysis
Client Needs: Physiological Integrity
Integrated Concept/Process: Nursing Process/Assessment
Content Area: Adult Health/Oncology
Reference: Ignatavicius, D., Workman, M., & Mishler, M. (1999). *Medical-surgical nursing across the health care continuum* (3rd ed.). Philadelphia: W.B. Saunders, p. 1848.

48. 2
Rationale: Following mastectomy, the arm should be elevated above the level of the heart. Simple arm exercises should be encouraged. No BP readings, injections, IV lines, or blood

draws should be performed on the affected arm. Cool compresses are not a suggested measure to prevent lymphedema from occurring.

Test-Taking Strategy: Use the process of elimination. Note the key words "assist in preventing." Use the process of elimination, and note the relationship between the words "lymphedema" in the question and "elevating" in the correct option. Review these important measures if you had difficulty with this question.

Level of Cognitive Ability: Application
Client Needs: Physiological Integrity
Integrated Concept/Process: Nursing Process/Implementation
Content Area: Adult Health/Oncology
Reference: Ignatavicius, D., Workman, M., & Mishler, M. (1999). *Medical-surgical nursing across the health care continuum* (3rd ed.). Philadelphia: W.B. Saunders, p. 1976.

49. 2
Rationale: Mammography takes about 15 to 30 minutes to complete. Some discomfort may be experienced because of the breast compression required to obtain a clear image. There is no reason to maintain an NPO status prior to the procedure. Option 2 is an accurate instruction.

Test-Taking Strategy: Use the process of elimination. Eliminate options 3 and 4 first. Attempt to visualize the procedure to assist in selecting the correct option. If you are unfamiliar with this screening test, review this information.

Level of Cognitive Ability: Application
Client Needs: Physiological Integrity
Integrated Concept/Process: Nursing Process/Implementation
Content Area: Adult Health/Oncology
Reference: Ignatavicius, D., Workman, M., & Mishler, M. (1999). *Medical-surgical nursing across the health care continuum* (3rd ed.). Philadelphia: W.B. Saunders, pp. 1948-1949.

50. 1
Rationale: Vena cava syndrome occurs when the superior vena cava is compressed or obstructed by tumor growth. Early signs and symptoms generally occur in the morning and include edema of the face, especially around the eyes, and client complaints of tightness of a shirt or blouse collar. As the compression worsens, the client experiences edema of the hands and arms. Mental status changes and cyanosis are late signs.

Test-Taking Strategy: Use the process of elimination. Note the key word "early" in the stem of the question. This key word should assist in eliminating options 2, 3, and 4. If you are unfamiliar with vena cava syndrome, review this oncological emergency.

Level of Cognitive Ability: Analysis
Client Needs: Physiological Integrity
Integrated Concept/Process: Nursing Process/Assessment
Content Area: Adult Health/Oncology
Reference: Ignatavicius, D., Workman, M., & Mishler, M. (1999). *Medical-surgical nursing across the health care continuum* (3rd ed.). Philadelphia: W.B. Saunders, p. 515.

CRITICAL THINKING: FREE-TEXT ENTRY

Answer: Notify the physician
Rationale: Spinal cord compression should be suspected in a client with metastatic disease, particularly when a new and sudden onset of back pain occurs. Spinal cord compression

causes back pain before neurological changes occur. Spinal cord compression is an oncological emergency, and the physician should be notified.

Test-Taking Strategy: Noting the key words "new and sudden sharp pain in the back" will assist in identifying the appropriate nursing intervention. If you had difficulty with this question or are unfamiliar with spinal cord compression, review this oncological emergency.

Level of Cognitive Ability: Application
Client Needs: Physiological Integrity
Integrated Concept/Process: Nursing Process/Implementation
Content Area: Adult Health/Oncology
Reference: Ignatavicius, D., Workman, M., & Mishler, M. (1999). *Medical-surgical nursing across the health care continuum* (3rd ed.). Philadelphia: W.B. Saunders, p. 514.

REFERENCES

Beare, P., & Myers, J. (1998). *Adult health nursing* (3rd ed.). St. Louis: Mosby.

Hodgson, B., & Kizior, R. (2001). *Saunders nursing drug handbook 2001.* Philadelphia: W.B. Saunders.

Ignatavicius, D., Workman, M., & Mishler, M. (1999). *Medical-surgical nursing across the health care continuum* (3rd ed.). Philadelphia: W.B. Saunders.

Leahy, J., & Kizilay, P. (1998). *Foundations of nursing practice: A nursing process approach.* Philadelphia: W.B. Saunders.

LeMone, P., & Burke, K. (2000). *Medical-surgical nursing: Critical thinking in client care* (2nd ed.). Upper Saddle River, N.J.: Prentice-Hall.

Lewis, S., Heitkemper, M., & Dirksen, S. (2000). *Medical-surgical nursing: Assessment and management of clinical problems* (5th ed.). St. Louis: Mosby.

Monahan, F., & Neighbors, M. (1998). *Medical-surgical nursing: Foundations for clinical practice* (2nd ed.). Philadelphia: W.B. Saunders.

Phipps, W., Sands, J., & Marek, J. (1999). *Medical-surgical nursing: Concepts & clinical practice* (6th ed.). St. Louis: Mosby.

Potter, P., & Perry, A. (2001). *Fundamentals of nursing* (5th ed.). St. Louis: Mosby.

Smeltzer, S., & Bare, B. (2000). *Brunner & Suddarth's textbook of medical-surgical nursing* (9th ed). Philadelphia: Lippincott Williams & Wilkins.

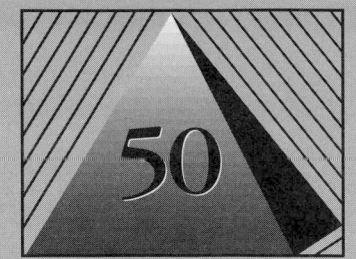

50

Antineoplastic Medications

I. GENERAL CONSIDERATIONS

A. Description
1. Kill or inhibit the reproduction of neoplastic cells
2. The effect of antineoplastic medications may not be limited to neoplastic cells; normal cells are also affected by the medication
3. Cell cycle phase–specific medications affect cells only during a certain phase of the reproductive cycle
4. Cell cycle phase–nonspecific medications affect cells in any phase of the reproductive cycle
5. Usually several medications are used in combination to increase the therapeutic response
6. Antineoplastic medications may be combined with other treatments, such as surgery and radiation
7. The routes of antineoplastic medication administration can vary; the IV route is the preferred route
8. Side effects result from the effects of the antineoplastic medication on normal cells

B. Side effects
1. Mucositis
2. Alopecia
3. Anorexia, nausea, and vomiting
4. Diarrhea
5. Anemia
6. Low white blood cell (WBC) count (neutropenia)
7. Thrombocytopenia
8. Infertility

C. Implementation
1. Physiological integrity
   a. Monitor complete blood count (CBC), WBC count, platelet count, and electrolytes
   b. Initiate bleeding precautions if thrombocytopenia occurs
   c. When the platelet count is less than 50,000 cells/uL, any small trauma can lead to episodes of prolonged bleeding; when the platelet count is less than 20,000 cells/uL, spontaneous and uncontrollable bleeding can occur
   d. Monitor for petechiae, ecchymosis, bleeding of the gums, and nosebleeds because the decreased platelet count can precipitate bleeding tendencies
   e. Avoid IM injections and venipunctures as much as possible to prevent bleeding
   f. Initiate neutropenic precautions if the WBC count decreases
   g. Monitor for fever, sore throat, unusual bleeding, or signs and symptoms of infection
   h. Inform the client that loss of appetite may also be due to a bitter taste in the mouth from the medications
   i. Monitor for nausea and vomiting and provide a high-calorie diet with protein supplements
   j. Administer antiemetics several hours before chemotherapy and for 12 to 48 hours afterward, as prescribed, because antineoplastic medications stimulate the vomiting centers
   k. Encourage hydration; IV fluids will be administered before and during therapy
   l. Promote a fluid intake of at least 2000 mL a day to maintain adequate renal function
   m. Administer allopurinol (Zyloprim) as prescribed to reduce the serum uric acid that occurs from the rapid destruction of cells by the antineoplastic medication
2. Safe, effective care environment
   a. Prepare IV chemotherapy in an air-vented space
   b. Prepare to administer the antineoplastic medication in short, high-dose, intermittent courses, as prescribed, to maximize antineoplastic effects while allowing normal cells to recover
   c. Wear gloves, a gown, and a mask when handling IV medications

d. Monitor for phlebitis with IV administration, as these medications irritate the veins

e. Monitor for extravasation (leakage of medication into surrounding skin and subcutaneous tissue), which causes tissue necrosis, and notify the physician if this occurs; heat or ice is applied, depending on the medication, and an antidote may be injected into the site

f. Discard IV equipment in designated containers

3. Psychosocial integrity

a. Instruct the client in the potential for hair loss and that varying degrees of hair loss may occur after the first or second treatment

b. Discuss the purchase of a wig before treatment starts

c. Inform the client that new hair growth will occur several months after the final treatment

d. Instruct the client about the need for contraception, as these medications have teratogenic effects

e. Discuss the potential effect of infertility, which may be irreversible

f. Encourage pretreatment counseling

4. Health promotion and maintenance

a. Instruct the client that if diarrhea is a problem, to avoid hot foods and high-fiber foods, which increase peristalsis

b. Instruct the client to inspect the oral mucosa for erythema and ulcers, to rinse the mouth after meals, and to provide good oral hygiene

c. Instruct the client to use saline or sodium bicarbonate mouth rinses for mouth sores

d. Instruct the client in the use of antifungal medications for mouth sores, if prescribed for the development of a superinfection

e. Instruct the client to avoid crowds and persons with infections and to report signs of infection such as fever, chills, or sore throat

f. Instruct individuals with colds or infections to wear a mask when visiting or to avoid visiting the client

g. Instruct the client to use a soft toothbrush and an electric razor to minimize the risk of bleeding

h. Instruct the client to avoid aspirin-containing products to minimize the risk of bleeding

i. Instruct the client to avoid alcohol to minimize the risk of toxicity

j. Instruct the client to consult the physician before receiving vaccinations

D. Anaphylactic reactions

1. Precautions

a. Obtain an allergy history

b. Administer a test dose when prescribed by the physician

c. Stay with the client during the administration of medication

d. Monitor vital signs

e. Have emergency equipment and medications readily available

f. Provide an IV line for the administration of emergency medications if needed

2. Signs of anaphylactic reaction

a. Dyspnea

b. Chest tightness or pain

c. Pruritis/urticaria

d. Tachycardia

e. Dizziness

f. Anxiety/agitation

g. Flushed appearance

h. Inability to speak

i. Nausea and abdominal pain

j. Hypotension

k. Decreased sensorium

l. Cyanosis

3. Implementation for anaphylactic reaction

a. Stop medication

b. Maintain airway

c. Notify physician

d. Maintain IV access with 0.9 % normal saline

e. Place client in supine position with legs elevated if not contraindicated

f. Monitor vital signs

g. Administer prescribed emergency medications

II. ALKYLATING MEDICATIONS (Box 50-1)

A. Description

1. Affects the synthesis of DNA by causing crosslinking of DNA to inhibit cell reproduction

2. Cell cycle phase–nonspecific medications

B. Side effects

1. Anorexia, nausea, and vomiting

2. Stomatitis

3. Skin rash

4. Pain during IV administration

5. Busulfan (Myleran) may cause hyperuricemia

6. Chlorambucil (Leukeran) and mechlorethamine HCl (Mustargen) may cause gonadal suppression and hyperuricemia

7. Cisplatin (Platinol) may cause ototoxicity, tinnitus, hypokalemia, hypocalcemia, hypomagnesemia, and nephrotoxicity

8. Cyclophosphamide (Cytoxan) may cause alopecia, gonadal suppression, hemorrhagic cystitis, and hematuria

C. Implementation

1. Assess vital signs and the temperature for signs of infection

2. Monitor CBC, WBC, platelet, uric acid, and electrolyte counts

3. Withhold medication if the platelet count is less than 75,000 cells/uL or the WBC count is less than 4000 cells/uL, and notify the physician

4. Assess results of pulmonary function tests

BOX 50-1

Alkylating Medications

NITROGEN MUSTARDS
Chlorambucil (Leukeran)
Cyclophosphamide (Cytoxan)
Estramustine phosphate sodium (Emcyt)
Ifosfamide (Ifex)
Mechlorethamine HCl (Mustargen)
Melphalan (Alkeran)

NITROSOUREAS
Busulfan (Myleran)
Carmustine (BCNU)
Chlorozotozin (DCNU)
Lomustine (CCNU)
Semustine (Methyl CCNU)
Streptozocin (Zanosar)

ALKYLATING-LIKE MEDICATIONS
Altretamine (Hexalen)
Carboplatin (Paraplatin)
Cisplatin (Platinol)
Dacarbazine (DTIC)
Thiotepa

BOX 50-2

Antitumor Antibiotic Medications

Bleomycin sulfate (Blenoxane)
Dactinomycin (Actinomycin D)
Daunorubicin (Cerubidine)
Doxorubicin (Adriamycin)
Idarubicin (Idamycin)
Mitomycin (Mutamycin)
Mitoxantrone (Novantrone)
Plicamycin (Mithracin)

---

5. Assess results of chest radiographs and renal and liver function studies
6. Hydrate the client with IV and/or oral fluids before administering the antineoplastic medication, as prescribed
7. Administer antiemetic 30 to 60 minutes before the antineoplastic medication, as prescribed
8. As prescribed, reduce IV site pain by altering IV rates, diluting the medication, or warming the injection site to distend vein and increase blood flow
9. Monitor IV site for irritation and phlebitis
10. When administering cisplatin (Platinol), assess the client for dizziness, tinnitus, hearing loss, incoordination, and numbness or tingling of extremities
11. Monitor for signs of hemorrhagic cystitis, such as hematuria or dysuria, during cyclophosphamide (Cytoxan) or ifosfamide (Ifex) therapy, and encourage the client to drink increased fluids (2 to 3 liters per day)
12. Instruct the client that cyclophosphamide (Cytoxan), when prescribed orally, is administered without food
13. Instruct the client to follow a diet low in purines to alkalize urine and lower uric acid blood levels
14. Instruct the client in how to avoid infection
15. Instruct the client to report signs of infection or bleeding
16. Instruct the client about good oral hygiene and use of a soft toothbrush

III. ANTITUMOR ANTIBIOTIC MEDICATIONS
(Box 50-2)
A. Description
1. Interfere with DNA and ribonucleic acid synthesis
2. Cell cycle phase–nonspecific medications
B. Side effects
1. Nausea and vomiting
2. Fever
3. Bone marrow depression
4. Skin rash
5. Alopecia
6. Stomatitis
7. Gonadal suppression
8. Hyperuricemia
9. Vesication (blistering of tissue at IV site) ▲
10. Plicamycin (Mithracin) affects bleeding time
11. Daunorubicin (Cerubidine) may cause congestive heart failure (CHF) and dysrhythmias
12. Doxorubicin (Adriamycin) and idarubicin (Idamycin) may cause cardiotoxicity, cardiomyopathy, and ECG changes ▲
13. Pulmonary toxicity can occur with bleomycin sulfate (Blenoxane) ▲
C. Implementation ▲
1. Assess vital signs and temperature for signs of infection
2. Monitor CBC, WBC, platelet, uric acid, bleeding time, and electrolyte counts
3. Withhold medication if the platelets are less than 75,000 cells/uL or the WBC count is less than 4000 cells/uL, and notify the physician
4. Assess results of pulmonary function tests
5. Monitor for ECG changes
6. Assess lung sounds for rales
7. Assess for signs of CHF, including dyspnea, crackles, peripheral edema, and weight gain
8. Assess results of chest radiographs and renal and liver function studies
9. Hydrate the client with IV and/or oral fluids before the antineoplastic medication
10. Administer antiemetic 30 to 60 minutes before the antineoplastic medication
11. As prescribed, reduce IV site pain by altering

IV rates, diluting the medication, or warming injection site to distend vein and increase blood flow

12. Monitor IV site for irritation, phlebitis, and vesication

▲ 13. Assess for myocardial toxicity, dyspnea, dysrhythmias, hypotension, and weight gain when administering doxorubicin (Adriamycin) or idarubicin (Idamycin)

▲ 14. Monitor pulmonary status when administering bleomycin (Blenoxane)

15. Avoid the use of aspirin, anticoagulants, and thrombolytic agents with plicamycin (Mithracin)

IV. ANTIMETABOLITE MEDICATIONS (Box 50-3)

A. Description
1. Halt the synthesis of cell protein
2. Replace normal proteins required for DNA synthesis
3. Cell cycle phase–specific and affect the S phase

B. Side effects
1. Anorexia, nausea, and vomiting
2. Diarrhea
3. Alopecia
4. Stomatitis
5. Depression of bone marrow
6. Cytarabine HCl (ara-C, Cytosar-U) may cause alopecia, stomatitis, hyperuricemia, and hepatotoxicity

▲ 7. 5-Fluorouracil (5-FU; Adrucil) may cause alopecia, stomatitis, diarrhea, phototoxicity reactions, and cerebellar dysfunction

8. 6-Mercaptopurine (Purinethol) may cause hyperuricemia and hepatotoxicity

▲ 9. Methotrexate (Folex) may cause alopecia, stomatitis, hyperuricemia, photosensitivity, hepatotoxicity, and hematological, GI, and skin toxicity

▲ C. Implementation
1. Monitor vital signs and temperature for signs of infection
2. Assess CBC, WBC, uric acid, and platelet count
3. Hold medication if the WBC count is less than 4000 cells/uL or the platelet count is less than 75,000 cells/uL, and notify the physician
4. Monitor renal function studies
5. Monitor for cerebellar dysfunction
6. Assess for photosensitivity
7. Administer antiemetics 30 to 60 minutes before the antineoplastic medication, as prescribed
8. Monitor IV site for extravasation
9. Encourage fluid intake of 2 to 3 liters a day
10. Encourage good oral hygiene
11. Instruct the client in how to avoid infections and bleeding

▲ 12. When administering 5-fluorouracil (5-FU; Adrucil), assess for signs of cerebellar dysfunc-

---

BOX 50-3

Antimetabolite Medications

FOLIC ACID ANTAGONIST
Methotrexate (Folex)

PYRIMIDINE ANALOGS
Cytarabine HCl (Ara-C, Cytosar-U)
Floxuridine (FUDR)
5-Fluorouracil (5-FU, Adrucil)
Procarbazine HCl (Matulane)

PURINE ANALOGS
6-Mercaptopurine (Purinethol)
Thioguanine

MISCELLANEOUS RIBONUCLEOTIDE REDUCTASE INHIBITORS
Hydroxyurea (Hydrea)
Trimetrexate glucuronate (Neutrexine)

ANTIMICROTUBULE
Pentostatin (Nipent)

OTHER ANTIMETABOLITE MEDICATIONS
5-Azacytidine
Cladribine (Leustatin)
Fludarabine (Fludara)
Hexamethylmelamine
Vidarabune (Vira-A)

---

tion, such as dizziness, weakness, and ataxia, and assess for stomatitis and diarrhea, which may necessitate medication discontinuation

13. When administering methotrexate (Folex) in ▲ large doses, prepare to administer leucovorin (folinic acid or citrovorum factor) as prescribed to prevent fatal toxicity (known as leucovorin rescue)

14. When administering 5-fluorouracil (5-FU; Adru- ▲ cil) or methotrexate (Folex), instruct the client to use sunscreen and to wear protective clothing to prevent photosensitivity reactions

V. VINCA (PLANT) ALKALOIDS (Box 50-4)

A. Description
1. Prevent mitosis, causing cell death
2. Mitotic inhibitor that prevents cell division
3. Cell cycle phase–specific and act on the M phase

B. Side effects
1. Leukopenia
2. Neurotoxicity with vincristine sulfate (On- ▲ covin), manifested as numbness and tingling in the fingers and toes
3. Ptosis
4. Hoarseness
5. Motor instability
6. Anorexia, nausea, and vomiting
7. Constipation

BOX 50-4

Plant (Vinca) Alkaloids

Etoposide (VePesid)
Paclitaxel (Taxol)
Taxotere (Docetaxel)
Teniposide (Vumon)
Vinblastine sulfate (Velban)
Vincristine sulfate (Oncovin)
Vindesine (Eldisine)
Vinorelbine (Navelbine)

BOX 50-5

Hormonal Medications and Enzymes

ANDROGENS
Progesterone (Gesterol 50)
Testolactone (Teslac)
Fluoxymesterone (Halotestin)

HORMONAL ANTAGONISTS, ENZYMES
Aminoglutethimide (Cytadren)
Asparaginase (Elspar)
Diethylstilbestrol (DES, Stilphostrol)
Flutamide (Eulexin)
Goserelin acetate (Zoladex)
Leuprolide acetate (Lupron)
Megestrol acetate (Megace)
Mitotane (Lysodren)
Tamoxifen citrate (Nolvadex)
Leuprolide acetate (Lupron)

---

8. Peripheral neuropathy
9. Alopecia
10. Stomatitis
11. Hyperuricemia
12. Phlebitis at IV site

▲ C. Implementation
  1. Monitor vital signs
  2. Monitor WBC, CBC, uric acid, and platelet counts
  3. Monitor for hoarseness
  4. Assess eyes for ptosis
  5. Assess motor stability and initiate safety precautions as necessary
▲ 6. Monitor for neurotoxicity with vincristine sulfate (Oncovin), manifested as numbness and tingling in the fingers and toes

VI. HORMONAL MEDICATIONS AND ENZYMES
  (Box 50-5)
A. Description
  1. Suppress the immune system and block normal hormones in hormone-sensitive tumors
  2. Change the hormonal balance and slow the growth rates of certain tumors
B. Side effects
  1. Anorexia, nausea, and vomiting
  2. Leukopenia
  3. Impaired pancreatic function with asparaginase (Elspar)
  4. Gynecomastia
  5. Breast swelling
  6. Hot flashes
  7. Weight gain
  8. Hemorrhagic cystitis, hypouricemia, and hypercholesterolemia, with mitotane (Lysodren)
  9. Hypertension
  10. Thromboembolitic disorders
  11. Edema
  12. Sex characteristic alterations
  13. Electrolyte imbalances
  14. Tamoxifen citrate (Nolvadex) may cause edema, hypercalcemia, and elevated cholesterol and triglyceride levels
▲ 15. Tamoxifen citrate (Nolvadex) decreases the effects of estrogen

16. Diethylstilbestrol (DES, Stilphostrol) may cause impotence and gynecomastia in men
17. Diethylstilbestrol (DES, Stilphostrol) may alter effects of insulin, oral anticoagulants, and oral hypoglycemic agents
C. Implementation   ▲
  1. Monitor vital signs
  2. Assess medications that the client is currently taking
  3. Monitor serum calcium levels with androgens
  4. Monitor for signs of alterations in sexual characteristics
  5. Monitor pancreatic function with asparaginase (Elspar)
  6. Encourage oral intake of 2 to 3 liters of fluids per day
  7. Monitor uric acid and cholesterol levels
  8. Monitor for signs of hemorrhagic cystitis

VII. IMMUNOTHERAPY: BIOLOGICAL RESPONSE MODIFIERS
A. Description
  1. Stimulate the immune system to recognize **cancer** cells and take action to eliminate or destroy them
  2. Interleukins: Help different immune system cells to recognize and destroy abnormal body cells
  3. Interferons: Slow down tumor cell division, stimulate proliferation and activation of natural killer cells, and help **cancer** cells resume a more normal appearance and revert to their previous characteristics
B. Colony-stimulating factors (CSF): Induce more rapid bone marrow recovery after suppression by chemotherapy (Box 50-6)

BOX 50-6

Colony-Stimulating Factors (CSF)

Granulocyte/Macrophage Colony-Stimulating Factor (GM-CSF)
Sargramostim (Leukine, Prokine)
Granulocyte Colony-Stimulating Factor (G-CSF)
Filgrastim (Neupogen)
Erythropoietin (EPO)
Epoetin alfa (Epogen)

PRACTICE QUESTIONS

1. A client with breast cancer is being treated with cyclophosphamide (Cytoxan). A nurse understands that this medication is:
   1. Cell cycle phase–specific, affecting cells only during a certain phase of the cell reproductive cycle
   2. Cell cycle phase–nonspecific, affecting cells in any phase of the reproductive cell cycle
   3. Cell cycle phase–specific, affecting the S phase of the reproductive cell cycle
   4. Cell cycle phase–specific, affecting the M phase of the reproductive cell cycle

2. A client with bladder cancer is receiving cisplatin (Platinol) and vincristine (Oncovin). A nurse understands that the purpose of administering both of these medications is to:
   1. Prevent gastrointestinal (GI) side effects
   2. Prevent alopecia
   3. Decrease the destruction of cells
   4. Increase the therapeutic response

3. A nurse is monitoring the laboratory results for a client receiving an antineoplastic medication by the intravenous (IV) route. The nurse prepares to initiate bleeding precautions if which laboratory result is noted?
   1. A white blood cell (WBC) count of 5000 cells/μL
   2. A platelet count of 50,000 cells/μL
   3. A clotting time of 10 minutes
   4. An ammonia level of 20 μg/dL

4. A nurse is analyzing the laboratory results of a client with leukemia who received a regimen of chemotherapy. Which of the following laboratory values would the nurse specifically note as a result of the massive cell destruction that occurred from the chemotherapy?
   1. Anemia
   2. Decreased platelets
   3. Decreased leukocyte count
   4. Increased uric acid level

5. A client with leukemia is receiving busulfan (Myleran). The physician prescribes allopurinol (Zyloprim) for the client. A nurse prepares to administer the medication and understands that the purpose of the allopurinol is to prevent:
   1. Gouty arthritis
   2. Hyperuricemia
   3. Alopecia
   4. Diarrhea

6. A nurse is providing medication instructions to a client with breast cancer who is receiving cyclophosphamide (Cytoxan). The nurse tells the client to:
   1. Take the medication with food
   2. Increase fluid intake to 2000 to 3000 mL daily
   3. Decrease sodium intake while taking the medication
   4. Increase potassium intake while taking the medication

7. A client with non-Hodgkin's lymphoma is receiving daunorubicin (Cerubidine). Which of the following would indicate to the nurse that the client is experiencing a toxic effect related to the medication?
   1. Complaints of nausea and vomiting
   2. Fever
   3. Rales on auscultation of the lungs
   4. Diarrhea

8. A nurse is assigned to care for a client with testicular cancer who is receiving plicamycin (Mithracin). The nurse reviews the client's record and would question which prescribed medication if noted in the physician's orders?
   1. Warfarin (Coumadin)
   2. Allopurinol (Zyloprim)
   3. Acetaminophen (Tylenol)
   4. Ondansetron (Zofran)

9. A client with squamous cell carcinoma of the larynx is receiving bleomycin sulfate (Blenoxane) by IV. The nurse caring for the client anticipates that which diagnostic study will be prescribed?
   1. Pulmonary function studies
   2. Electrocardiogram
   3. Cervical x-rays
   4. Echocardiogram

10. Cytarabine (Cytosar) is prescribed for a client with acute lymphocytic leukemia. A nurse understands that this medication is classified as an antimetabolite and is a:
    1. Cell cycle phase–nonspecific medication
    2. Cell cycle phase–specific medication affecting the M phase
    3. Cell cycle phase–specific medication affecting the S phase
    4. Medication that affects cells in any phase of the reproductive cell cycle

11. A clinic nurse prepares a teaching plan for a client receiving an antineoplastic medication. When implementing the plan, the nurse tells the client to:
    1. Take aspirin (acetylsalicylic acid, ASA) as needed for headache
    2. Drink beverages containing alcohol in moderate amounts

3. Consult with the physician before receiving immunizations
4. Be sure to receive flu and pneumonia vaccines

12. A client with lung cancer is receiving a high dose of methotrexate (Folex). Leucovorin (citrovorum factor, folic acid) is also prescribed. A nurse understands that the purpose of administering the leucovorin is to:
    1. Preserve normal cells
    2. Promote DNA synthesis
    3. Promote medication excretion
    4. Promote the synthesis of nucleic acids

13. A client with ovarian cancer is being treated with vincristine (Oncovin). A nurse monitors the client, knowing that which of the following is a side effect specific to this medication?
    1. Diarrhea
    2. Numbness and tingling in the fingers and toes
    3. Chest pain
    4. Hair loss

14. A nurse is reviewing the history and physical of a client who will be receiving asparaginase (Elspar), an antineoplastic agent. The nurse contacts the physician prior to administering the medication if which of the following is documented in the client's history?
    1. Myocardial infarction
    2. Chronic obstructive pulmonary disease
    3. Diabetes mellitus
    4. Pancreatitis

15. Tamoxifen (Nolvadex) is prescribed for a client with metastatic breast carcinoma. The nurse administering the medication understands that the primary action of this medication is to:
    1. Increase DNA and RNA synthesis
    2. Compete with estradiol for binding to estrogen in tissues containing high concentrations of receptors
    3. Increase estrogen concentration and estrogen response
    4. Promote the biosynthesis of nucleic acids

16. A client with metastatic breast cancer is receiving Tamoxifen (Nolvadex). A nurse specifically monitors which of the following laboratory values while the client is taking this medication?
    1. Potassium level
    2. Glucose level
    3. Calcium level
    4. Prothrombin time

17. Megestrol acetate (Megace), an antineoplastic medication, is prescribed for a client with metastatic endometrial carcinoma. A nurse reviews the client's history and contacts the physician if which of the following is documented in the client's history?
    1. Asthma
    2. Myocardial infarction
    3. Thrombophlebitis
    4. Gout

18. A female client with carcinoma of the breast is admitted to a hospital for treatment with IV vincristine (Oncovin). The client tells a nurse that she has been told by her friends that she is going to lose all of her hair. The most appropriate nursing response is which of the following?
    1. "You will not lose your hair."
    2. "Your friends are correct."
    3. "Hair loss may occur, but it will grow back just as it is now."
    4. "Hair loss may occur, and it will grow back, but it may have a different color or texture."

19. A clinic nurse prepares instructions for a client who developed stomatitis following the administration of a course of antineoplastic medications. The nurse tells the client to:
    1. Rinse the mouth with baking soda or saline
    2. Avoid foods and fluids for the next 24 hours
    3. Swab the mouth daily with lemon and glycerin pads
    4. Brush the teeth and use waxed dental floss three times a day

20. A client with acute myelocytic leukemia is being treated with busulfan (Myleran). Which of the following laboratory values would a nurse specifically monitor during treatment with this medication?
    1. Blood glucose
    2. Uric acid level
    3. Potassium level
    4. Clotting time

CRITICAL THINKING: FREE-TEXT ENTRY

A nurse is monitoring the intravenous (IV) infusion of an antineoplastic medication. During the infusion, the client complains of pain at the insertion site. On inspection of the site, the nurse notes redness and swelling, and that the infusion of the medication has slowed. On the basis of these assessment data, what is the nurse's initial action?

Answer: _____

ANSWERS

1. 2

Rationale: Cyclophosphamide (Cytoxan) is an antineoplastic medication of the alkylating classification. Medications in this classification affect any phase of the reproductive cell cycle. Cell phase–specific medications affect cells only during a certain phase of the reproductive cycle. Antimetabolite medications are cell cycle phase–specific and affect the S phase. Vinca alkaloids are cell cycle phase–specific and act on the M phase.

Test-Taking Strategy: Use the process of elimination. Note that option 2 is the option that is different. Option 2 addresses the action as cell cycle phase–nonspecific, whereas options 1, 3, and 4 address a cell cycle phase–specific action. If you had difficulty with this question, review the action of alkylating medications.

Level of Cognitive Ability: Analysis
Client Needs: Physiological Integrity
Integrated Concept/Process: Nursing Process/Analysis
Content Area: Pharmacology
Reference: Clark, J., Queener, S., & Karb, V. (2000). *Pharmacologic basis of nursing practice* (6th ed.). St. Louis: Mosby, p. 617.

2. 4

Rationale: Cisplatin (Platinol) is an alkylating-like medication, and vincristine (Oncovin) is a vinca (plant) alkaloid. Alkylating medications are cell cycle phase–nonspecific. Vinca alkaloids are cell cycle phase–specific and act on the M phase. Combinations of medications are used to enhance tumoricidal effects and increase the therapeutic response.

Test-Taking Strategy: Use the process of elimination. Option 3 can be easily eliminated first. Eliminate options 1 and 2 next. It may be possible, with some specific interventions, to reduce GI effects and alopecia, but it is unlikely that these occurrences can be prevented. Review the purpose of combination medication therapy if you had difficulty with this question.

Level of Cognitive Ability: Analysis
Client Needs: Physiological Integrity
Integrated Concept/Process: Nursing Process/Analysis
Content Area: Pharmacology
Reference: Karch, A. (2000). *Focus on nursing pharmacology.* Philadelphia: Lippincott, p. 140.

3. 2

Rationale: Bleeding precautions need to be initiated when the platelet count decreases. The normal platelet count is 150,000 to 450,000 cells/μL. When the platelets are less than 50,000 cells/μL, any small trauma can lead to episodes of prolonged bleeding. The normal WBC count is 5000 to 10,000/μL. When the WBC count drops, neutropenic precautions need to be implemented. The normal clotting time is 8 to 15 minutes. The normal ammonia value is 15 to 45 μg/dL.

Test-Taking Strategy: Use the process of elimination and knowledge regarding normal laboratory values. Options 1, 3, and 4 identify normal laboratory values. Remember, correlate a low platelet count with the need for bleeding precautions, and a low WBC count with the need for neutropenic precautions. Review the indications to implement bleeding precautions in a client receiving chemotherapy, if you had difficulty with this question.

Level of Cognitive Ability: Analysis
Client Needs: Safe, Effective Care Environment

Integrated Concept/Process: Nursing Process/Planning
Content Area: Pharmacology
Reference: Ignatavicius, D., Workman, M., & Mishler, M. (1999). *Medical-surgical nursing across the health care continuum* (3rd ed.). Philadelphia: W.B. Saunders, p. 509.

4. 4

Rationale: Hyperuricemia is especially common following treatment for leukemias and lymphomas, since chemotherapy results in massive cell kill. Although options 1, 2, and 3 may also be noted, an increased uric acid level is specifically related to cell destruction.

Test-Taking Strategy: Note the key words "massive cell destruction" in the question. Recalling the cell response to destruction will assist in directing you to option 4. Review this concept if you had difficulty with this question.

Level of Cognitive Ability: Analysis
Client Needs: Physiological Integrity
Integrated Concept/Process: Nursing Process/Assessment
Content Area: Pharmacology
Reference: Clark, J., Queener, S., & Karb, V. (2000). *Pharmacologic basis of nursing practice* (6th ed.). St. Louis: Mosby, pp. 620-623.

5. 2

Rationale: Busulfan (Myleran) is as alkylating medication used in the treatment of acute myelocytic leukemia and in the palliative treatment of chronic myelogenous leukemia. Hyperuricemia can result from the use of this medication. Allopurinol (Zyloprim), an antigout medication, is used with chemotherapy to prevent or treat hyperuricemia that occurs from the rapid destruction of cells by the antineoplastic medication. Allopurinol is not used to prevent alopecia and diarrhea.

Test-Taking Strategy: Use the process of elimination, recalling that hyperuricemia occurs from the rapid destruction of cells by the antineoplastic medication. This knowledge will easily direct you to option 2. Review the purpose of administering allopurinol to a client receiving chemotherapy if you had difficulty with this question.

Level of Cognitive Ability: Analysis
Client Needs: Physiological Integrity
Integrated Concept/Process: Nursing Process/Analysis
Content Area: Pharmacology
Reference: Hodgson, B., & Kizior, R. (2001). *Saunders nursing drug handbook 2001.* Philadelphia: W.B. Saunders, pp. 24, 134.

6. 2

Rationale: Hemorrhagic cystitis is a toxic effect that can occur with the use of cyclophosphamide (Cytoxan). The client needs to be instructed to drink copious amounts of fluid during the administration of this medication. Clients should also monitor urine output for hematuria. The medication should be taken on an empty stomach, unless gastrointestinal upset occurs. Hyperkalemia can result from the use of the medication; therefore, the client would not be told to increase potassium intake. The client would not be instructed to alter the sodium intake.

Test-Taking Strategy: Use the process of elimination. Recalling that cyclophosphamide can cause hemorrhagic cystitis will easily direct you to option 2. If you had difficulty with this question, review the toxic effects associated with this medication.

Level of Cognitive Ability: Application
Client Needs: Health Promotion and Maintenance
Integrated Concept/Process: Teaching/Learning
Content Area: Pharmacology
Reference: Hodgson, B., & Kizior, R. (2001). *Saunders nursing drug handbook 2001.* Philadelphia: W.B. Saunders, pp. 270-272.

7. **3**

Rationale: Cardiotoxicity noted by abnormal ECG findings and/or cardiomyopathy manifested as congestive heart failure is a toxic effect of daunorubicin. Bone marrow depression is also a toxic effect. Nausea and vomiting are a frequent side effect associated with the medication; they begin a few hours after administration and last 24 to 48 hours. Fever is a frequent side effect, and diarrhea can occur occasionally. Options 1, 2, and 4, however, are not toxic effects.

Test-Taking Strategy: Use the process of elimination, keeping in mind that the question is asking about a toxic effect. Use of the ABCs—airway, breathing, and circulation—will easily direct you to option 3. If you had difficulty with this question, review the toxic effects associated with daunorubicin.

Level of Cognitive Ability: Analysis
Client Needs: Physiological Integrity
Integrated Concept/Process: Nursing Process/Analysis
Content Area: Pharmacology
Reference: Hodgson, B., & Kizior, R. (2001). *Saunders nursing drug handbook 2001.* Philadelphia: W.B. Saunders, pp. 286-289.

8. **1**

Rationale: Plicamycin (Mithracin) is an antitumor antibiotic chemotherapeutic agent. Because plicamycin affects bleeding time, the use of aspirin, anticoagulants, and thrombolytic agents should be avoided. Warfarin (Coumadin) is an anticoagulant, and the risk of hemorrhage is increased if this medication is administered during plicamycin (Mithracin) therapy. Allopurinol (Zyloprim), an antigout medication, may be used with chemotherapy to prevent or treat hyperuricemia secondary to cell destruction caused by cancer chemotherapy. Acetaminophen (Tylenol) may be used to treat mild discomfort. Ondansetron (Zofran) is an antiemetic used to prevent or treat nausea and vomiting during chemotherapy.

Test-Taking Strategy: Use the process of elimination, recalling the classifications of the medications identified in the options. Recalling that plicamycin affects bleeding time will direct you to option 1. If you are unfamiliar with these medications, review their classifications and purposes. In addition, review the medication interactions associated with plicamycin.

Level of Cognitive Ability: Analysis
Client Needs: Safe, Effective Care Environment
Integrated Concept/Process: Communication and Documentation
Content Area: Pharmacology
Reference: Hodgson, B., & Kizior, R. (2001). *Saunders nursing drug handbook 2001.* Philadelphia: W.B. Saunders, p. 772.

9. **1**

Rationale: Bleomycin sulfate (Blenoxane) is an antineoplastic medication that can cause interstitial pneumonitis that can progress to pulmonary fibrosis. Pulmonary function studies along with hematologic, hepatic, and renal function tests need to be monitored. The nurse needs to monitor lung sounds for dyspnea and rales that indicate pulmonary toxicity. The

medication needs to be discontinued immediately if pulmonary toxicity occurs. Options 2, 3, and 4 are unrelated to the specific use of this medication.

Test-Taking Strategy: Use the process of elimination. Eliminate options 2 and 4 first because they are both cardiac related and are therefore similar. From the remaining options, use the ABCs—airway, breathing, and circulation—to direct you to option 1. If you had difficulty with this question, review the toxic effects of this medication.

Level of Cognitive Ability: Analysis
Client Needs: Physiological Integrity
Integrated Concept/Process: Nursing Process/Analysis
Content Area: Pharmacology
Reference: Hodgson, B., & Kizior, R. (2001). *Saunders nursing drug handbook 2001.* Philadelphia: W.B. Saunders, pp. 120-122.

10. **3**

Rationale: Cytarabine (Cytosar) is an antimetabolite. Antimetabolites are classified as cell cycle phase–specific and affect the S phase (DNA synthesis and metabolism) of the reproductive cell cycle. Alkylating medications affect any phase of the cell reproductive cycle. Vinca alkaloids are cell cycle phase–specific and act on the M phase of the cell reproductive cycle.

Test-Taking Strategy: Use the process of elimination. Eliminate options 1 and 4 first because they are similar. From this point, knowledge regarding the action of an antimetabolite is required to answer the question. Review the specific action of an antimetabolite if you had difficulty with this question.

Level of Cognitive Ability: Analysis
Client Needs: Physiological Integrity
Integrated Concept/Process: Nursing Process/Analysis
Content Area: Pharmacology
Reference: Clark, J., Queener, S., & Karb, V. (2000). *Pharmacologic basis of nursing practice* (6th ed.). St. Louis: Mosby, pp. 632-633.

11. **3**

Rationale: Since antineoplastic medications lower the body's resistance, clients must be instructed not to receive immunizations without a physician's approval. Clients also need to avoid contact with individuals who may have recently received the oral polio vaccine. Aspirin and aspirin-containing products need to be avoided to minimize the risk of bleeding. Alcohol needs to be avoided to minimize the risk of toxicity.

Test-Taking Strategy: Use the process of elimination. Remember that antineoplastic medications lower the body's resistance. Review the client teaching points regarding these medications, if you had difficulty with this question.

Level of Cognitive Ability: Application
Client Needs: Health Promotion and Maintenance
Integrated Concept/Process: Teaching/Learning
Content Area: Pharmacology
Reference: Clark, J., Queener, S., & Karb, V. (2000). *Pharmacologic basis of nursing practice* (6th ed.). St. Louis: Mosby, p. 632.

12. **1**

Rationale: High concentrations of methotrexate (Folex) cause harm and damage to normal cells. To save normal cells, leucovorin is given. This is known as leucovorin rescue. Leucovorin bypasses the metabolic block caused by methotrexate, thereby permitting normal cells to synthesize. It should be noted that leucovorin rescue is potentially hazardous. Failure to administer leucovorin in the right dose at the right time can be fatal.

Test-Taking Strategy: Use the process of elimination. Eliminate options 2 and 4 first because they are similar. Nucleic acids include RNA and DNA. Eliminate option 3 because increased fluids and diuretics are normally administered to promote medication excretion. This leaves option 1 as the correct answer. If you had difficulty with this question, review the purpose of leucovorin rescue.

Level of Cognitive Ability: Analysis
Client Needs: Physiological Integrity
Integrated Concept/Process: Nursing Process/Analysis
Content Area: Pharmacology
Reference: Clark, J., Queener, S., & Karb, V. (2000). *Pharmacologic basis of nursing practice* (6th ed.). St. Louis: Mosby, p. 636.

13. 2

Rationale: A side effect specific to vincristine (Oncovin) is peripheral neuropathy, which occurs in nearly every client. This can be manifested as numbness and tingling in the fingers and toes. Depression of the Achilles tendon reflex may be the first clinical sign indicating peripheral neuropathy. Constipation rather than diarrhea is most likely to occur with this medication, although diarrhea may occur occasionally. Hair loss occurs with nearly all of the antineoplastic medications. Chest pain is unrelated to this medication.

Test-Taking Strategy: Use the process of elimination. Eliminate options 1 and 4 first because these side effects are associated with many of the antineoplastic agents. Note that the question asks for the side effect "specific" to this medication. Correlate peripheral neuropathy with vincristine (Oncovin).

Level of Cognitive Ability: Analysis
Client Needs: Physiological Integrity
Integrated Concept/Process: Nursing Process/Assessment
Content Area: Pharmacology
Reference: Hodgson, B., & Kizior, R. (2001). *Saunders nursing drug handbook 2001.* Philadelphia: W.B. Saunders, pp. 1053-1054.

14. 4

Rationale: Asparaginase (Elspar) is contraindicated if hypersensitivity exists, in pancreatitis, or if the client has a history of pancreatitis. The medication impairs pancreatic function, and pancreatic function tests should be performed before therapy begins, and when a week or more has elapsed between the administration of the doses. The client needs to be monitored for signs of pancreatitis, which include nausea, vomiting, and abdominal pain.

Test-Taking Strategy: Use the process of elimination. Recalling that this medication affects pancreatic function will direct you to option 4. Review this medication if you had difficulty answering this question.

Level of Cognitive Ability: Analysis
Client Needs: Physiological Integrity
Integrated Concept/Process: Nursing Process/Assessment
Content Area: Pharmacology
Reference: Hodgson, B., & Kizior, R. (2001). *Saunders nursing drug handbook 2001.* Philadelphia: W.B. Saunders, pp. 72-74.

15. 2

Rationale: Tamoxifen (Nolvadex) is an antineoplastic medication that competes with estradiol for binding to estrogen in tissues containing high concentrations of receptors. It is used

in the treatment of metastatic breast carcinoma in women and men. It is also effective in delaying the recurrence of cancer following mastectomy. It reduces DNA synthesis and estrogen response.

Test-Taking Strategy: Use the process of elimination. Eliminate options 1 and 4 first because they are similar. Nucleic acids include DNA and RNA. From this point, select option 2, because it is unlikely that treatment of metastatic breast carcinoma would focus on increasing estrogen concentration and estrogen response. If you had difficulty with this question, review the action of this medication.

Level of Cognitive Ability: Analysis
Client Needs: Physiological Integrity
Integrated Concept/Process: Nursing Process/Assessment
Content Area: Pharmacology
Reference: Hodgson, B., & Kizior, R. (2001). *Saunders nursing drug handbook 2001.* Philadelphia: W.B. Saunders, p. 961.

16. 3

Rationale: Tamoxifen (Nolvadex) may increase calcium, cholesterol, and triglyceride levels. Prior to the initiation of therapy, a CBC, a platelet count, and serum calcium levels should be assessed. These blood levels, along with the cholesterol and triglyceride levels, should be monitored periodically during therapy. The nurse should assess for hypercalcemia while the client is taking this medication. Signs of hypercalcemia include increased urine volume, excessive thirst, nausea, vomiting, constipation, hypotonicity of muscles, and deep bone or flank pain.

Test-Taking Strategy: Use the process of elimination. Recalling that this medication causes hypercalcemia will direct you to option 3. Review this medication if you had difficulty answering this question.

Level of Cognitive Ability: Analysis
Client Needs: Physiological Integrity
Integrated Concept/Process: Nursing Process/Assessment
Content Area: Pharmacology
Reference: Hodgson, B., & Kizior, R. (2001). *Saunders nursing drug handbook 2001.* Philadelphia: W.B. Saunders, p. 962.

17. 3

Rationale: Megestrol acetate (Megace) suppresses the release of luteinizing hormone from the anterior pituitary by inhibiting pituitary function and reducing tumor size. It is used with caution if the client has a history of thrombophlebitis.

Test-Taking Strategy: Use the process of elimination. Recalling that megestrol acetate (Megace) is a hormonal antagonist enzyme and that a side effect is thrombolytic disorders will direct you to option 3. Review this medication if you had difficulty answering this question.

Level of Cognitive Ability: Analysis
Client Needs: Physiological Integrity
Integrated Concept/Process: Communication and Documentation
Content Area: Pharmacology
Reference: Hodgson, B., & Kizior, R. (2001). *Saunders nursing drug handbook 2001.* Philadelphia: W.B. Saunders, p. 634.

18. 4

Rationale: Alopecia (hair loss) can occur following the administration of many antineoplastic medications. Alopecia is reversible, but new hair growth may have a different color and texture.

Test-Taking Strategy: Use the process of elimination. Eliminate option 2 because it is a nontherapeutic response. Next, eliminate options 1 and 3 because they are incorrect. Review content related to hair loss and antineoplastic medications, if you had difficulty with this question.
Level of Cognitive Ability: Application
Client Needs: Psychosocial Integrity
Integrated Concept/Process: Caring
Content Area: Pharmacology
Reference: Hodgson, B., & Kizior, R. (2001). *Saunders nursing drug handbook 2001*. Philadelphia: W.B. Saunders, p. 1054.

19. **1**
Rationale: Stomatitis (ulceration in the mouth) can occur as a result of the administration of antineoplastic medications. The client should be instructed to examine the mouth daily and to report any signs of ulceration. If stomatitis occurs, the client should be instructed to rinse the mouth with baking soda or saline. Food and fluid are important and should not be restricted. If chewing and swallowing are painful, the client may switch to a liquid diet that includes milkshakes and ice cream. Instruct the client to avoid spicy foods and foods with hard crusts or edges. The client should avoid toothbrushing and flossing when stomatitis is severe. Lemon and glycerin swabs may cause pain and further irritation.
Test-Taking Strategy: Knowing that stomatitis involves ulcerations in the mucous membrane of the mouth will assist you in the process of eliminating the incorrect options. Eliminate option 2 first because foods and fluids would not be restricted in a client who received antineoplastic medication. Eliminate option 3 because lemon can be irritating to ulcerated lesions. Eliminate option 4 because a toothbrush and floss will also irritate ulcerations and may cause bleeding. If you had difficulty with this question, review the client teaching points related to stomatitis.
Level of Cognitive Ability: Application
Client Needs: Physiological Integrity

Integrated Concept/Process: Teaching/Learning
Content Area: Pharmacology
Reference: Clark, J., Queener, S., & Karb, V. (2000). *Pharmacologic basis of nursing practice* (6th ed.). St. Louis: Mosby, p. 619.

20. **2**
Rationale: Busulfan (Myleran) can cause an increase in the uric acid level. Hyperuricemia can produce uric acid nephropathy, renal stones, and acute renal failure. Options 1, 3, and 4 are not specifically related to this medication.
Test-Taking Strategy: Use the process of elimination. Recall that busulfan (Myleran) increases uric acid levels. If you had difficulty with this question, review the effects of busulfan (Myleran).
Level of Cognitive Ability: Analysis
Client Needs: Physiological Integrity
Integrated Concept/Process: Nursing Process/Assessment
Content Area: Pharmacology
Reference: Hodgson, B., & Kizior, R. (2001). *Saunders nursing drug handbook 2001*. Philadelphia: W.B. Saunders, pp. 133-134.

CRITICAL THINKING: FREE-TEXT ENTRY

Answer: Stop the infusion and notify the physician
Rationale: Redness and swelling and a slowed infusion are signs of extravasation. If extravasation occurs during the administration of an IV antineoplastic medication, the infusion is stopped and the physician is notified.
Test-Taking Strategy: Focus on the assessment signs in the question. Attempt to visualize the situation to identify the initial nursing action. Review nursing actions if extravasation occurs, if you had difficulty with this question.
Level of Cognitive Ability: Application
Client Needs: Safe, Effective Care Environment
Integrated Concept/Process: Nursing Process/Implementation
Content Area: Pharmacology
Reference: Ignatavicius, D., Workman, M., & Mishler, M. (1999). *Medical-surgical nursing across the health care continuum* (3rd ed.). Philadelphia: W.B. Saunders, p. 504.

REFERENCES

Clark, J., Queener, S., & Karb, V. (2000). *Pharmacologic basis of nursing practice* (6th ed.). St. Louis: Mosby.

Hodgson, B., & Kizior, R. (2001). *Saunders nursing drug handbook 2001*. Philadelphia: W.B. Saunders.

Ignatavicius, D., Workman, M., & Mishler, M. (1999). *Medical-surgical nursing across the health care continuum* (3rd ed.). Philadelphia: W.B. Saunders.

Karch, A. (2000). *Focus on nursing pharmacology*. Philadelphia: Lippincott.

The Adult Client with an Endocrine Disorder

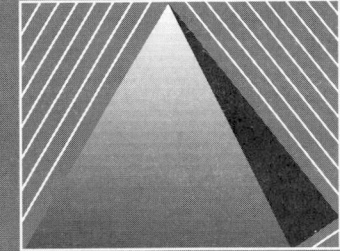

PYRAMID TERMS

addisonian crisis A life-threatening disorder caused by adrenal hormone insufficiency. It is precipitated by infection, trauma, stress, or surgery. Death can occur from shock, vascular collapse, or hyperkalemia.

Addison's disease Hyposecretion of adrenal cortex hormones (glucocorticoids and mineralocorticoids) from the adrenal gland, resulting in deficiency of the steroid hormones. The condition is fatal if left untreated.

adrenalectomy The surgical removal of an adrenal gland. Lifelong steroid replacement is necessary with a bilateral adrenalectomy. Temporary steroid replacement, up to 2 years, is necessary for a unilateral adrenalectomy.

Chvostek's sign A spasm of the facial muscles elicited by tapping the facial nerve in the region of the parotid gland. It is noted in hypocalcemia.

Cushing's syndrome A condition resulting from the hypersecretion of glucocorticoids from the adrenal cortex.

dawn phenomenon Results from a nocturnal release of growth hormone, which may cause blood glucose elevations about 3 A.M. Treatment includes administering an evening dose of intermediate-acting insulin at 10 P.M.

diabetic ketoacidosis (DKA) A complication of diabetes mellitus that develops when a severe insulin deficiency occurs. DKA is a life-threatening condition. Hyperglycemia that progresses to ketoacidosis occurs. Seen in clients with type 1 diabetes mellitus, undiagnosed diabetics, and persons who stop prescribed treatment for diabetes. It develops over a period of several hours to days.

diabetes insipidus The hyposecretion of antidiuretic hormone (ADH) and a deficiency of vasopressin. Results in failure of tubular reabsorption of water in the kidneys.

diabetes mellitus A chronic and potentially disabling disease characterized by elevated blood glucose levels. A chronic disorder of glucose intolerance and impaired carbohydrate, protein, and lipid metabolism caused by a deficiency of insulin. A deficiency of insulin results in hyperglycemia.

Graves' disease (hyperthyroidism) Known as thyrotoxicosis. A hyperthyroid state resulting from hypersecretion of thyroid hormone.

hyperglycemia Elevated blood glucose level.

hyperglycemic hyperosmolar nonketotic syndrome (HHNS) Extreme hyperglycemia without acidosis. Usually occurs in type 2 diabetes mellitus when diabetes is uncontrolled or undiagnosed, or during stress or infection. The major difference between HHNS and DKA is the lack of ketone production with HHNS. Onset is usually slow, taking from hours to days.

hypoglycemia (insulin reaction) Described as a blood glucose level below 50 to 60 mg/dL. Occurs as a result of too much insulin, not enough food, or excessive activity.

hypophysectomy The removal of the pituitary gland.

insulin waning A progressive rise in the blood glucose level from bedtime to morning. Treatment includes increasing the evening (predinner or bedtime) dose of intermediate- or long-acting insulin, or instituting a dose of insulin before the evening meal if one is not already prescribed.

myxedema (hypothyroidism) A hypothyroid state resulting from a hyposecretion of thyroid hormone. The condition occurs in adulthood.

myxedema coma A rare but serious disorder that results from persistently low thyroid production. It can be precipitated by acute illness, rapid withdrawal of thyroid medication, anesthesia and surgery, hypothermia, and the use of sedatives and narcotics.

Somogyi's phenomenon A rebound phenomenon that occurs during the initial period of serum glucose control. It develops at peak insulin times and during the night. Normal or elevated blood glucose levels are present at bedtime, a decrease occurs at about 2 to 3 A.M. to hypoglycemic levels, and a subsequent increase occurs as a result of the production of counterregulatory hormones. Treatment includes decreasing the evening (predinner or bedtime) dose of intermediate-acting insulin, or increasing the bedtime snack.

thyroidectomy Removal of the thyroid gland. Performed in conditions in which persistent hyperthryoidism exists.

thyroid storm An acute and fatal thyroid condition that occurs as a result of manipulation of the thyroid gland during surgery and the release of thyroid hormone into the bloodstream. It can also occur as a result of severe infection and stress.

Trousseau's sign A sign found in hypocalcemia. Carpal spasm can be elicited by compressing the upper arm and causing ischemia to the nerves distally.

▲ PYRAMID TO SUCCESS

The endocrine system is made up of organs or glands that secrete hormones and release them directly into the circulation. The endocrine system can be easily understood if you remember that basically one of two situations can occur: either hypersecretion or hyposecretion of hormones from the organ or gland. When an excess of the hormone occurs, treatment is aimed at blocking the hormone release through medication or surgery. When a deficit of the hormone exists, treatment is aimed at replacement therapy. Pyramid points focus on diabetes mellitus, including the prevention and treatment of complications, insulin therapy, hypoglycemic and hyperglycemic reactions, and diabetic ketoacidosis; Addison's disease and addisonian crisis; Cushing's syndrome; thyroid disorders; thyroid storm; and care of the client after thyroidectomy or adrenalectomy. The Integrated Concepts and Processes addressed in this unit include Nursing Process, Caring, Communication and Documentation, Cultural Awareness, Self-Care, and Teaching/Learning.

▲ CLIENT NEEDS
Safe, Effective Care Environment

Accident prevention in the client with altered mental status
Advocacy related to client's decisions
Confidentiality related to client's condition
Consultation with members of the health care team
Handling hazardous and infectious materials
Informed consent related to diagnostic tests and procedures
Medical and surgical asepsis

Health Promotion and Maintenance

Addressing lifestyle choices
Describing expected body image changes
Disease prevention related to potential complications
Instructions regarding the prescribed treatment plan

Instructions regarding the effect of diet therapy, exercise, and the administration of insulin to the client with diabetes mellitus
Health screening related to diabetes mellitus
Human sexuality

Psychosocial Integrity

Coping mechanisms related to the endocrine disturbance
Grief and loss related to loss of a body part
Role changes and support systems
Sensory or perceptual alterations related to the disorder
Unexpected body image disturbances

Physiological Integrity

Alterations in body systems
Basic care and comfort measures
Expected effects of medication administration
Fluid and electrolyte imbalances
Identifying potential complications
Laboratory values for diagnostic tests
Promoting nutrition
Protecting the client from the life-threatening side effects of treatments
Providing care in emergencies

REFERENCES

Craven, R., & Hirnle, C. (2000). *Fundamentals of nursing: Human health and function* (3rd ed.). Philadelphia: Lippincott.

Harkreader, H. (2000). *Fundamentals of nursing: Caring and clinical judgment.* Philadelphia: W.B. Saunders.

Ignatavicius, D., Workman, M., & Mishler, M. (1999). *Medical-surgical nursing: Across the health care continuum* (3rd ed.). Philadelphia: W.B. Saunders.

LeMone, P., & Burke, K. (2000). *Medical-surgical nursing: Critical thinking in client care* (2nd ed.). Upper Saddle River, N.J.: Prentice-Hall.

Lewis, S., Heitkemper, M., & Dirksen, S. (2000). *Medical-surgical nursing: Assessment and management of clinical problems* (5th ed.). St. Louis: Mosby.

National Council of State Boards of Nursing (eds.) (2000). *Test Plan for the National Council Licensure Examination for Registered Nurses.* Chicago: Author.

Potter, P., & Perry, A. (2001). *Fundamentals of nursing* (5th ed.). St. Louis: Mosby.

Smeltzer, S., & Bare, B. (2000) *Textbook of medical-surgical nursing* (9th ed). Philadelphia: Lippincott Williams & Wilkins.

51

Endocrine System

I. ANATOMY AND PHYSIOLOGY OF ENDOCRINE GLANDS (Box 51-1)

A. Functions (Box 51-2)
   1. Maintenance and regulation of vital functions
   2. Response to stress and injury
   3. Growth and development
   4. Energy metabolism
   5. Reproduction
   6. Fluid, electrolyte, and acid-base balance

B. Pituitary gland (Box 51-3)
   1. The master gland
   2. Located at the base of the brain
   3. Influenced by the hypothalamus
   4. Directly affects the function of the other endocrine glands
   5. Promotes growth of body tissue
   6. Influences water absorption by the kidney
   7. Controls sexual development and function

C. Adrenal gland
   1. Rest upon each kidney
   2. Regulates sodium and electrolyte balance
   3. Affects carbohydrate, fat, and protein metabolism
   4. Influences the development of sexual characteristics
   5. Sustains the "flight or fight" response
   6. Adrenal cortex
      a. The outer shell of the adrenal gland
      b. Synthesizes glucocorticoids and mineralocorticoids and secretes small amounts of sex hormones (androgens, estrogens) (Box 51-4)
   7. Adrenal medulla
      a. The inner core of the adrenal gland
      b. Works as part of the sympathetic nervous system
      c. Produces epinephrine and norepinephrine

D. Thyroid gland
   1. Located in the anterior part of the neck

2. Controls the rate of body metabolism and growth
   3. Produces thyroxine (T_4), triiodothyronine (T_3), and thyrocalcitonin

E. Parathyroid gland
   1. Located near the thyroid
   2. Controls calcium and phosphorus metabolism
   3. Produces parathyroid hormone (PTH)

F. Pancreas
   1. Located posterior to the liver
   2. Influences carbohydrate metabolism
   3. Indirectly influences fat and protein metabolism
   4. Produces insulin and glucagon

G. Ovaries and testes
   1. Ovaries
      a. Located in the pelvic cavity
      b. Produce estrogen and progesterone

BOX 51-1

Endocrine Glands

Pituitary
Adrenal
Thyroid
Parathyroid
Pancreas
Ovaries
Testes

BOX 51-2

Risk Factors for Endocrine Disorders

Hereditary
Congenital
Trauma
Environmental
Secondary to other disorders

BOX 51-3

Pituitary Gland

ANTERIOR LOBE PRODUCTION
ACTH (adrenocorticotropic hormone)
TSH (thyroid-stimulating hormone)
STH (somatotropic growth-stimulating hormone)
FSH (follicle-stimulating hormone)
LH (luteinizing hormone)
PRL (prolactin)
GH (growth hormone)
MSH (melanocyte-stimulating hormone)

POSTERIOR LOBE PRODUCTION
ADH (vasopressin, antidiuretic hormone)
Oxytocin

BOX 51-4

Adrenal Cortex

GLUCOCORTICOIDS
Cortisol, Cortisone, Corticosterone
Responsible for glucose metabolism, protein metabolism, fluid and electrolyte balance, suppression of the inflammatory response to injury, the protective immune response to invasion by infectious agents, and resistance to stress

MINERALOCORTICOIDS
Aldosterone
Regulates electrolyte balance by promoting sodium retention and potassium excretion

---

2. Testes
   a. Located in the scrotum
   b. Control the development of the secondary sex characteristics
   c. Produce testosterone

II. DIAGNOSTIC TESTS

A. Stimulation/suppression tests
   1. Stimulation testing
      a. In the client with suspected underactivity of an endocrine gland, a stimulus may be provided to determine whether the gland is capable of normal hormone production
      b. Measured amounts of selected hormones are administered to stimulate the target gland to maximal production
      c. Hormone levels are measured
      d. Failure of the hormone to rise with stimulation indicates hypofunction
   2. Suppression tests
      a. Used when hormone levels are high or in the upper range of normal
      b. Failure of hormone production to be suppressed during standardized testing indicates hyperfunction

B. Radioactive iodine (RAI) uptake
   1. A thyroid function test that measures the absorption of the iodine isotope to determine how the thyroid gland is functioning
   2. The amount of radioactivity is measured 2, 6, and 24 hours after ingestion of the capsule
   3. Normal value is 5% to 35% in 24 hours
   4. Elevated values are indicative of **hyperthyroidism, thyrotoxicosis,** decreased iodine intake, or increased iodine excretion
   5. Decreased values indicate a low T_4, the use of antithyroid medications, thyroiditis, **myxedema,** or **hypothyroidism**

C. T_3 and T_4 resin uptake test
   1. Blood tests for the diagnosis of thyroid disorders
   2. T_3 and T_4 regulate thyroid-stimulating hormone
   3. Normal values
      a. T_3: 80 to 230 ng/dL
      b. T_4: 5.0 to 12.0 μg/dL
      c. Thyroxine, free (FT_4): 0.8 to 2.4 ng/dL
   4. The T_3 is elevated in **hyperthyroidism,** decreases with the aging process, and may be decreased in **hypothyroidism**
   5. The T_4 is elevated in **hyperthyroidism** and decreased in **hypothyroidism**

D. Thyroid-stimulating hormone (TSH)
   1. Blood test used to differentiate the diagnosis of primary **hypothyroidism**
   2. Normal value is: 0.2 to 5.4 μU/mL
   3. Elevated values indicate primary **hypothyroidism**
   4. Decreased values indicate **hyperthyroidism** or secondary **hypothyroidism**

E. Thyroid scan
   1. Performed to identify nodules or growths in the thyroid gland
   2. A radioisotope of iodine or technetium is administered prior to the scanning of the thyroid gland
   3. Reassure the client that the level of radioactive medication is not dangerous to self or others
   4. Determine whether the client has received radiographic contrast agents within the past 3 months, because these may invalidate scan
   5. Check with the physician regarding discontinuing medications containing iodine for 14 days prior to the test and the need to discontinue thyroid medication 4 to 6 weeks before the test
   6. Instruct the client to maintain an NPO status after midnight on the day prior to the test; if iodine is used, the client will fast for an additional 45 minutes after ingestion of the oral isotope and the scan will be performed in 24 hours

7. If technetium is used, it is administered by the IV route 30 minutes before the scan

F. Needle aspiration of thyroid tissue
1. Aspiration of thyroid tissue for cytological examination
2. No client preparation is necessary
3. Light pressure is applied to the aspiration site after the procedure

G. Glucose tolerance test (GTT)
1. Aids in the diagnosis of **diabetes mellitus**
2. If the glucose levels peak at higher than normal at 1 and 2 hours after injection or ingestion of glucose, and are slower than normal to return to fasting levels, then **diabetes mellitus is confirmed**
3. Client preparation
   a. Eat a high-carbohydrate (200- to 300-g) diet for 3 days before the test
   b. Avoid alcohol, coffee, and smoking for 36 hours before testing
   c. Fast for 10 to 16 hours prior to the test
   d. Avoid strenuous exercise for 8 hours before and after the test
   e. Withhold morning insulin or oral hypo-glycemic medication (client with **diabetes mellitus**)
   f. The test will take 3 to 5 hours, requires intravenous or oral administration of glucose, and multiple blood samples

H. Glycosylated hemoglobin
1. Description
   a. Glycosylated hemoglobin is blood glucose bound to hemoglobin
   b. HbA_{1c} (glycosylated hemoglobin A) is a reflection of how well blood glucose levels have been controlled for up to the prior 4 months
   c. **Hyperglycemia** in a client with **diabetes mellitus** is usually a cause of an increase in HbA_{1c}
2. Values
   a. Values are expressed as a percentage of total hemoglobin
   b. Diabetic with good control: 7.5% or less
   c. Diabetic with fair control: 7.6% to 8.9%
   d. Diabetic with poor control: 9% or greater
3. Nursing consideration: fasting is not required

III. DISORDERS OF PITUITARY GLAND (Box 51-5)

A. Hypopituitarism
1. Description: The hyposecretion of growth hor-mone (GH) by the anterior pituitary gland
2. Assessment
   a. Retarded physical growth
   b. Premature aging
   c. Low intellectual development

BOX 51-5

Disorders of the Pituitary Gland

ANTERIOR PITUITARY
Hypopituitarism
Hyperpituitarism

POSTERIOR PITUITARY
Diabetes insipidus
SIADH (syndrome of inappropriate antidiuretic hormone)

---

   d. Poor development of secondary sex charac-teristics
3. Implementation
   a. Provide emotional support to client and family
   b. Encourage client and family to express feelings related to altered body image
   c. Prepare to administer human growth hor-mone (hGH)

B. Hyperpituitarism
1. Description
   a. The hypersecretion of GH by the anterior pituitary gland, which results in giantism or acromegaly
   b. Giantism occurs in childhood before the closure of the epiphyses of the long bones
   c. Acromegaly occurs in middle age, after the closure of the epiphyses of the long bones
2. Assessment
   a. Large hands and feet
   b. Thickening and protrusion of the jaw
   c. Arthritic changes
   d. Visual disturbances
   e. Diaphoresis
   f. Oily, rough skin
   g. Organomegaly
   h. Hypertension
   i. Dysphagia
   j. Deepening of the voice
3. Implementation
   a. Provide emotional support to client and family, and encourage client and family to express feelings related to altered body image
   b. Provide frequent skin care
   c. Provide pharmacological and nonpharmaco-logical interventions for joint pain
   d. Prepare the client for radiation of the pituitary gland if prescribed
   e. Prepare the client for **hypophysectomy** if planned

C. **Hypophysectomy**
1. Description
   a. The removal of the pituitary gland

b. Complications include increased intracranial pressure (ICP), bleeding, and meningitis

2. Postoperative implementation
   a. Initiate postoperative care similar to craniotomy care
   b. Monitor vital signs, neurological status, and level of consciousness (LOC)
   c. Elevate the head of the bed
   d. Monitor for increased ICP
   e. Monitor for bleeding
   f. Monitor for any postnasal drip, which might indicate leakage of cerebrospinal fluid (CSF)
   g. Instruct the client to avoid sneezing, coughing, and blowing the nose
   h. Monitor electrolyte values and for temporary **diabetes insipidus** resulting from antidiuretic hormone (ADH) disturbances
   i. Monitor intake and output (I & O) and avoid water intoxication
   j. Administer glucocorticoids, if prescribed, on time
   k. Administer antibiotics, analgesics, and antipyretics as prescribed
   l. Instruct the client in the administration of prescribed medications, which may include hormones and glucocorticoids if the entire gland was removed

D. **Diabetes insipidus**
   1. Description
      a. A hyposecretion of ADH and a deficiency of vasopressin
      b. Results in failure of tubular reabsorption of water in the kidneys
   2. Assessment
      a. Polyuria of 4 to 24 L per day
      b. Polydipsia
      c. Dehydration
      d. Decreased skin turgor, dry mucous membranes
      e. Inability to concentrate urine
      f. A low urinary specific gravity: 1.006 or less
      g. Fatigue
      h. Muscle pain and weakness
      i. Headache
      j. Postural hypotension
      k. Tachycardia
   3. Implementation
      a. Monitor vital signs and neurological and cardiovascular status
      b. Provide a safe environment, particularly in the client with a change in LOC or mental status
      c. Monitor electrolyte values and for signs of dehydration
      d. Monitor I & O, weights, specific gravity of urine
      e. Maintain the intake of adequate fluids

f. Instruct the client to avoid foods or liquids with a diuretic type action
g. Administer chlorpropamide (Diabenese) or clofibrate (Atromid-S) if prescribed; these medications augment that action of ADH and are used if only a partial deficit of ADH exists
h. Administer vasopressin tannate (Pitressin Tannate), desmopressin acetate (DDAVP, Stimate), or lypressin (Diapid) as prescribed; used when the ADH deficiency is severe
i. Instruct the client in the administration of medications as prescribed
j. Instruct the client to wear a Medic-Alert bracelet

E. Syndrome of inappropriate antidiuretic hormone (SIADH)
   1. Description
      a. A disorder in which a continued release of ADH occurs
      b. Results in water intoxication
   2. Assessment
      a. Signs of fluid volume overload
      b. Changes in LOC and mental status changes
      c. Weight gain
      d. Hypertension
      e. Tachycardia
      f. Anorexia, nausea, and vomiting
      g. Hyponatremia
   3. Implementation
      a. Monitor vital signs and cardiac and neurological status
      b. Provide a safe environment, particularly for the client with changes in LOC or mental status
      c. Monitor I & O and obtain daily weights
      d. Monitor fluid and electrolyte balance
      e. Restrict fluid intake as prescribed
      f. Administer diuretics and IV fluids as prescribed; monitor IV fluids carefully because of the risk for water intoxication
      g. Administer demeclocycline (Declomycin) as prescribed (inhibits ADH-induced water reabsorption and produces water diuresis)

IV. **DISORDERS OF ADRENAL GLANDS** (Box 51-6)
A. **Addison's disease**
   1. Description
      a. Hyposecretion of adrenal cortex hormones (glucocorticoids and mineralocorticoids)
      b. The condition is fatal if left untreated
   2. Assessment
      a. Lethargy, fatigue, and muscle weakness
      b. Gastrointestinal (GI) disturbances
      c. Weight loss
      d. Menstrual changes in women; impotence in men

e. **Hypoglycemia**
f. Hyperkalemia
g. Postural hypotension
h. Dehydration
i. Emotional disturbances
3. Implementation
   a. Monitor vital signs, particularly BP, weight, and I & O
   b. Monitor blood glucose and potassium levels
   c. Administer glucocorticoid or mineralocorticoid medications as prescribed
   d. Observe for **addisonian crisis** secondary to stress, infection, trauma, or surgery
4. Client education
   a. Avoid individuals with an infection
   b. Avoid stress
   c. Avoid strenuous exercise
   d. Need for lifelong glucocorticoid therapy
   e. Avoid over-the-counter medications
   f. Wear a Medic-Alert bracelet

▲ B. **Addisonian crisis**
1. Description
   a. A life-threatening disorder caused by acute adrenal insufficiency
   b. It is precipitated by stress, infection, trauma, or surgery
   c. Can cause hyponatremia, hyperkalemia, **hypoglycemia**, and shock
2. Assessment
   a. Severe headache
   b. Severe abdominal, leg, and lower back pain
   c. Generalized weakness
   d. Irritability and confusion
   e. Severe hypotension
   f. Shock
3. Implementation
   a. Prepare to administer IV glucocorticoids as prescribed; hydrocortisone sodium succinate (Solu-Cortef) is usually prescribed initially
   b. Following resolution of the crisis, administer oral glucocorticoid and mineralocorticoid as prescribed
   c. Monitor vital signs, particularly BP

   d. Monitor neurological status, noting irritability and confusion
   e. Monitor I & O
   f. Monitor laboratory values, particularly the sodium, potassium, and blood glucose
   g. Administer IV fluids as prescribed to restore electrolyte balance
   h. Protect the client from infection
   i. Maintain bed rest and provide a quiet environment

C. **Cushing's syndrome** ◀
1. Description
   a. A condition resulting from the hypersecretion of glucocorticoids from the adrenal cortex
   b. Can be caused by an increased pituitary secretion of adrenocorticotropic hormone (ACTH), a pituitary adenoma, or an adrenal adenoma
2. Assessment
   a. Truncal obesity with thin extremities
   b. Moonface
   c. Buffalo hump
   d. Supraclavicular fat pads
   e. Generalized muscle wasting and weakness
   f. Fragile skin that easily bruises
   g. Reddish-purple striae on the abdomen and upper thighs
   h. Hirsutism (masculine characteristics in female)
   i. Hypertension
   j. Elevated blood glucose, sodium, and white blood cell (WBC) counts
   k. Decreased calcium and potassium levels
3. Implementation
   a. Monitor vital signs, particularly blood pressure (BP)
   b. Monitor I & O and weight
   c. Monitory laboratory values, particularly the blood glucose, WBC, sodium, potassium, and calcium levels
   d. Provide good skin care
   e. Allow the client to discuss feelings related to body appearance
   f. Administer aminoglutethimide (Elipten, Cytadren), an adrenal enzyme inhibitor, as prescribed
   g. Administer chemotherapeutic agents as prescribed for inoperable adrenal tumors
   h. Prepare the client for radiation as prescribed if the condition results from a pituitary adenoma
   i. Prepare the client for **hypophysectomy** if the condition results from increased pituitary secretion of ACTH
   j. Prepare the client for **adrenalectomy** if the condition results from an adrenal adenoma;

glucorticoid replacement may be required following **adrenalectomy**

D. Hyperaldosteronism (Conn's syndrome)
1. Description
   a. A hypersecretion of aldosterone from the adrenal cortex of the adrenal gland
   b. Most commonly caused by an adenoma
2. Assessment
   a. Symptoms relate to the hypokalemia and hypertension that occur
   b. Headache, fatigue, muscle weakness, nocturia
   c. Polydipsia and polyuria
   d. Paresthesias
   e. Visual changes
   f. Hypernatremia
   g. Low urine specific gravity and increased urinary aldosterone
3. Implementation
   a. Monitor vital signs, particularly BP
   b. Monitor for signs of hypokalemia
   c. Monitor I & O and urine for specific gravity
   d. Administer spironolactone (Aldactone) as prescribed to promote fluid balance; medication is a potassium-sparing diuretic and aldosterone antagonist
   e. Administer potassium supplements as prescribed
   f. Administer antihypertensives as prescribed
   g. Prepare the client for **adrenalectomy**
   h. Maintain sodium restriction, if prescribed, preoperatively
   i. Administer glucocorticoids preoperatively, as prescribed, to prevent adrenal hypofunction
   j. Instruct the client regarding the need for glucocorticoids following **adrenalectomy**
   k. Instruct the client about the need to wear a Medic-Alert bracelet
E. Pheochromocytoma
1. Description
   a. A catecholamine-producing tumor usually found in the adrenal gland but also may be found in the abdomen
   b. It causes hypersecretion of the hormones of adrenal medulla and secretion of excessive amounts of epinephrine and norepinephrine
   c. It is typically a benign tumor but can be malignant
   d. Surgical excision of adrenal gland is the primary treatment
   e. Symptomatic treatment is initiated if surgical excision is not possible
   f. The complications associated with pheochromocytoma include hypertensive retinopathy and nephropathy, myocarditis, congestive heart failure (CHF), increased platelet aggregation, and cerebrovascular accident (CVA)
   g. Death can occur from shock, CVA, renal failure, dysrhythmias, or dissecting aortic aneurysm
2. Assessment
   a. Hypertension
   b. Severe headaches
   c. Palpitations
   d. Profuse diaphoresis
   e. Flushing
   f. Pain in the chest or abdomen with nausea and vomiting
   g. Heat intolerance
   h. Weight loss
   i. Tremors
   j. **Hyperglycemia** and glycosuria
3. Implementation
   a. Monitor vital signs, particularly the BP
   b. Monitor for hypertensive crisis; be alert to stimuli that can precipitate a hypertensive crisis, such as increased abdominal pressure, micturition, and vigorous abdominal palpation
   c. Avoid stimuli that can precipitate a hypertensive crisis
   d. Instruct the client not to smoke, drink caffeine-containing beverages, or change position suddenly
   e. Keep phentolamine (Regitine) at the bedside for hypertensive crisis
   f. Prepare to administer an alpha-adrenergic blocking agent, phenoxybenzamine (Dibenzyline), as prescribed, to control blood pressure
   g. Monitor blood glucose and urine for glucose and acetone
   h. Promote rest and a nonstressful environment
   i. Provide a diet high in calories, vitamins, and minerals
   j. Prepare the client for **adrenalectomy**
F. **Adrenalectomy**
1. Description
   a. The surgical removal of an adrenal gland
   b. Lifelong glucocorticoid replacement is necessary with a bilateral **adrenalectomy**
   c. Temporary glucocorticoid replacement, up to 2 years, is necessary for a unilateral **adrenalectomy**
   d. Catecholamine levels drop as a result of surgery, which can result in cardiovascular collapse, hypotension, and shock, and the client needs to be monitored closely
   e. Hemorrhage can also occur owing to the high vascularity of the adrenal glands
2. Preoperative implementation
   a. Monitor electrolytes and correct electrolyte imbalances
   b. Assess for dysrhythmias
   c. Monitor for **hyperglycemia**

d. Protect the client from infections

e. Administer glucocorticoids as prescribed

3. Postoperative implementation

a. Monitor vital signs

b. Monitor I & O, and if the urinary output is less that 30 mL per hour, notify the physician, because this may be indicative of renal failure and impending shock

c. Monitor daily weights

d. Monitor electrolytes

e. Monitor for signs of shock and hemorrhage, particularly during first 24 to 48 hours

f. Assess the dressing for drainage

g. Monitor for paralytic ileus, as manifested by abdominal distention and pain, nausea, vomiting, and diminished or absent bowel sounds, because paralytic ileus can develop from internal bleeding

h. Administer IV fluids, as prescribed, to maintain blood volume

i. Administer glucocorticoids as prescribed

j. Administer pain medication as prescribed, remembering that meperidine (Demerol) can cause hypotension

k. Instruct the client in the importance of glucocorticoid therapy following surgery

l. Instruct the client regarding the need to wear a Medic-Alert bracelet

V. DISORDERS OF THE THYROID GLAND
(Box 51-7)

A. **Hypothyroidism (myxedema)**

1. Description

a. A hypothyroid state resulting from a hyposecretion of thyroid hormone

b. Characterized by a decreased rate of body metabolism

2. Assessment

a. Lethargy and fatigue

b. Weakness, muscle aches, paresthesias

c. Intolerance to cold

d. Weight gain

e. Dry skin and hair

f. Loss of body hair

g. Bradycardia

h. Constipation

i. Generalized puffiness and edema around the eyes and face

j. Forgetfulness and loss of memory

k. Menstrual disturbances

l. Cardiac disorders

3. Implementation

a. Monitor vital signs, including heart rate and rhythm

b. Administer thyroid replacement; levothyroxine sodium (Synthroid) is most commonly prescribed

---

c. Instruct the client about thyroid replacement therapy

d. Instruct the client in low-calorie, low-cholesterol, low-saturated-fat diet

e. Assess the client for constipation; provide roughage and fluids to prevent constipation

f. Provide a warm environment for the client

g. Avoid sedatives and narcotics because of increased sensitivity to these medications

h. Monitor for overdose of thyroid medications, characterized by tachycardia, restlessness, nervousness, and insomnia

i. Instruct the client to report episodes of chest pain immediately

B. **Myxedema coma**

1. Description

a. A rare but serious disorder that results from persistently low thyroid production

b. It can be precipitated by acute illness, rapid withdrawal of thyroid medication, anesthesia and surgery, hypothermia, or the use of sedatives and narcotics

2. Assessment

a. Hypotension

b. Bradycardia

c. Hypothermia

d. Hyponatremia

e. **Hypoglycemia**

f. Respiratory failure

g. Coma

3. Implementation

a. Maintain a patent airway

b. Administer IV fluids as prescribed

c. Administer levothyroxine sodium (Synthroid) IV as prescribed

d. Administer IV glucose as prescribed

e. Administer corticosteroids as prescribed

f. Assess client's temperature frequently

g. Monitor blood pressure

h. Keep client warm

i. Monitor for changes in mental status

j. Monitor electrolytes and glucose level

C. **Hyperthyroidism (Graves' disease)**

1. Description

a. A hyperthyroid state resulting from hypersecretion of thyroid hormone

b. Characterized by an increased rate of body metabolism

c. Thyrotoxicosis refers to the signs and symptoms

that appear when body tissues are stimulated by increased thyroid hormones

2. Assessment
   a. Enlarged thyroid gland (goiter)
   b. Cardiac dysrhythmias, such as tachycardia and palpitations
   c. Protruding eyeballs (exophthalmos)
   d. Hypertension
   e. Heat intolerance
   f. Diaphoresis
   g. Weight loss
   h. Diarrhea
   i. Smooth, soft skin and hair
   j. Nervousness and fine tremors of hands
   k. Personality changes
   l. Irritability and agitation
   m. Mood swings

3. Implementation
   a. Provide adequate rest
   b. Administer sedatives as prescribed
   c. Provide a cool and quiet environment
   d. Obtain daily weights
   e. Provide a high-calorie diet
   f. Avoid the administration of stimulants
   g. Administer antithyroid medications that block thyroid synthesis, as prescribed
   h. Administer iodine preparations that inhibit the release of thyroid hormone, as prescribed
   i. Administer propranolol (Inderal) for tachycardia as prescribed
   j. Prepare the client for radioactive iodine therapy as prescribed, to destroy thyroid cells
   k. Prepare the client for **thyroidectomy** if prescribed

D. **Thyroid storm**
   1. Description
      a. An acute and life-threatening condition that occurs in a client with uncontrollable **hyperthyroidism**
      b. It can occur from manipulation of the thyroid gland during surgery and the release of thyroid hormone into the bloodstream
      c. Antithyroid medications, beta-blockers, glucocorticoids, and iodides are administered to the client prior to thyroid surgery, to prevent its occurrence
      d. It can also occur from severe infection and stress
   2. Assessment
      a. Fever
      b. Tachycardia
      c. Systolic hypertension
      d. Nausea, vomiting, and diarrhea
      e. Agitation, tremors, anxiety
      f. Irritability, agitation, restlessness, confusion, and seizures as the condition progresses
      g. Delirium and coma

3. Implementation
   a. Maintain a patent airway and adequate ventilation
   b. Administer antithyroid medications, sodium iodide solution, propranolol (Inderal), and glucocorticoids as prescribed
   c. Monitor vital signs
   d. Monitor continually for cardiac dysrhythmias
   e. Administer nonsalicylate antipyretics as prescribed (salicylates increase free thyroid hormone levels)
   f. Use a cooling blanket to decrease temperature as prescribed

E. **Thyroidectomy**
   1. Description
      a. Removal of the thyroid gland
      b. Performed when persistent hyperthryoidism exists
   2. Preoperative implementation
      a. Obtain vital signs and weight
      b. Assess electrolyte levels
      c. Assess for **hyperglycemia** and glycosuria
      d. Instruct the client in how to perform coughing and deep-breathing exercises and how to support the neck in the postoperative period when coughing and moving
      e. Administer antithyroid medications, sodium iodide solution, propranolol (Inderal), and glucocorticoids, as prescribed, to prevent the occurrence of **thyroid storm**
   3. Postoperative implementation
      a. Monitor for respiratory distress
      b. Have a tracheotomy set, oxygen, and suction at the bedside
      c. Maintain semi-Fowler's position
      d. Monitor surgical site for edema and for signs of bleeding; check dressing anteriorly and at the back of the neck
      e. Limit client talking, and assess level of hoarseness
      f. Monitor for laryngeal nerve damage, as evidenced by respiratory obstruction, dysphonia, high-pitched voice, stridor, dysphagia, and restlessness
      g. Monitor for signs of hypocalcemia and tetany, which can be due to trauma to the parathyroid gland (Box 51-8)
      h. Prepare to administer calcium gluconate or calcium chloride as prescribed for tetany
      i. Monitor for **thyroid storm**

VI. DISORDERS OF THE PARATHYROID GLAND

A. Hypoparathyroidism
   1. Description
      a. A condition caused by hyposecretion of parathyroid hormone by the parathyroid gland

---

BOX 51-8

Signs of Tetany

Positive Chvostek's sign
Positive Trousseau's sign
Wheezing and dyspnea (bronchospasm, laryngospasm)
Dysphagia
Numbness and tingling of the face and extremities
Carpopedal spasm
Visual disturbances (photophobia)
Muscle and abdominal cramps
Cardiac dysrhythmias
Seizures

---

   b. Can occur following **thyroidectomy** because of removal of parathyroid tissue
 2. Assessment
   a. Hypocalcemia and hyperphosphatemia
   b. Numbness and tingling in the face
   c. Muscle cramps and cramps in the abdomen or in the extremities
    d. Positive **Trousseau's sign** or **Chvostek's sign**
   e. Signs of overt tetany, such as bronchospasm, laryngospasm, carpopedal spasm, dysphagia, photophobia, cardiac dysrhythmias, seizures
   f. Hypotension
   g. Anxiety, irritability, depression
 3. Implementation
   a. Monitor vital signs
    b. Monitor for signs of hypocalcemia and tetany
   c. Initiate seizure precautions
   d. Place a tracheotomy set, oxygen, and suctioning at the bedside
   e. Prepare to administer IV calcium gluconate or calcium chloride for hypocalcemia
   f. Provide a high-calcium and low-phosphorus diet
   g. Instruct the client in the administration of calcium supplements as prescribed
   h. Instruct the client in the administration of vitamin D supplements as prescribed; vitamin D enhances the absorption of calcium from the GI tract
   i. Instruct the client in the administration of phosphate binders, as prescribed, to promote the excretion of phosphate through the GI tract
   j. Instruct the client to wear a Medic-Alert bracelet
B. Hyperparathyroidism
 1. Description: A condition caused by hypersecretion of parathyroid hormone by the parathyroid gland
 2. Assessment
   a. Hypercalcemia and hypophosphatemia
   b. Fatigue and muscle weakness

   c. Skeletal pain and tenderness
   d. Bone deformities that result in pathological fractures
   e. Anorexia, nausea, vomiting, epigastric pain
   f. Weight loss
   g. Constipation
   h. Hypertension
   i. Cardiac dysrhythmias
   j. Renal stones
 3. Implementation
   a. Monitor vital signs, particularly the BP
   b. Monitor for cardiac dysrhythmias
   c. Monitor I & O and for signs of renal stones
   d. Monitor for skeletal pain; move client slowly and carefully
   e. Encourage fluids
   f. Administer furosemide (Lasix) as prescribed to lower calcium levels
   g. Administer IV normal saline as prescribed to lower calcium levels
   h. Administer phosphates as prescribed, which interfere with calcium absorption
   i. Administer calcitonin (Calcimar) as prescribed, to decrease skeletal calcium release and increase renal clearance of calcium
   j. Administer calcium chelators as prescribed to lower calcium levels
   k. Monitor calcium and phosphorus levels
   l. Notify the physician immediately if a precipitous drop in the calcium level occurs; assess for tingling and numbness in the muscles and signs of hypocalcemia
   m. Prepare the client for parathyroidectomy as prescribed
C. Parathyroidectomy
 1. Description: Removal of one or more of the parathyroid glands
 2. Preoperative implementation
   a. Monitor electrolytes, calcium, phosphate, and magnesium levels
   b. Ensure that calcium levels are decreased to near normal
   c. Inform the client that talking may be painful for the first day or two after surgery
 3. Postoperative implementation
   a. Monitor for respiratory distress
   b. Place a tracheotomy set, oxygen, and suctioning at the bedside
   c. Monitor vital signs
   d. Position the client in semi-Fowler's
   e. Assess neck dressing for bleeding; 1 to 5 mL of serosanguineous drainage is expected
   f. Monitor for hypocalcemic crisis, as evidenced by tingling and twitching in the extremities and face
   g. Assess for positive **Trousseau's** or **Chvostek's sign,** which signals the potential for tetany

h. Monitor for changes in voice pattern and hoarseness

i. Monitor for laryngeal nerve damage

j. Instruct the client in the administration of calcium and vitamin D supplements as prescribed

VII. DISORDERS OF THE PANCREAS

A. **A. Diabetes mellitus** (Table 51-1)

1. Description
   a. A chronic disorder of impaired glucose intolerance and carbohydrate, protein, and lipid metabolism; caused by a deficiency of insulin
   b. A deficiency of insulin results in **hyperglycemia**
   c. Macrovascular complications include coronary disease, cardiomyopathy, hypertension, cerebrovascular disease, peripheral vascular disease, and infection
   d. Microvascular complications include retinopathy, nephropathy, and neuropathy

2. Assessment
   a. Polyuria
   b. Polydipsia
   c. Polyphagia
   d. **Hyperglycemia**
   e. Weight loss
   f. Blurred vision
   g. Slow wound healing
   h. Vaginal infections
   i. Weakness and paresthesias
   j. Signs of inadequate circulation to the feet

3. Diet
   a. The total number of calories is individualized on the basis of the client's current or desired weight and the presence of other existing health problems
   b. As prescribed by the physician, the client may be advised to follow the food exchange from the American Diabetic Association diet or the dietary guidelines for Americans (Food Guide Pyramid) issued by the U.S. Departments of Agriculture and Health and Human Services
   c. Incorporate diet into individual client needs, lifestyle, and cultural and socioeconomic patterns

4. Exercise
   a. Lowers blood glucose level
   b. Reduces cardiovascular risks
   c. Improves circulation and muscle tone
   d. Decreases total cholesterol and triglyceride levels
   e. Encourages weight loss
   f. Instruct the client in dietary adjustments when exercising; dietary adjustments are individualized
   g. Instruct the client to monitor blood glucose prior to exercising; if the client plans to participate in extended periods of exercise, blood glucose levels should be checked before, during, and after the exercise period
   h. Initially, the client who requires insulin should be instructed to eat a 15-g carbohydrate snack (a fruit exchange) or a snack of complex carbohydrate with a protein before engaging in moderate exercise, to prevent **hypoglycemia**
   i. If the client requires extra food during exercise to prevent **hypoglycemia,** it need not be deducted from the regular meal plan
   j. If the blood glucose level is greater than 250 mg/dL and urinary ketones are present, the client is instructed not to exercise until the blood glucose is closer to normal and urinary ketones are negative

5. Oral hypoglycemic medications
   a. Prescribed for clients with **diabetes mellitus** type 2
   b. Assess the client's knowledge of **diabetes mellitus** and the use of oral hypoglycemic agents
   c. Assess vital signs and blood glucose levels
   d. Assess the medications that the client is currently taking
   e. Aspirin, alcohol, sulfonamides, oral contraceptives, and monoamine oxidase inhibitors (MAOIs) increase the hypoglycemic effect
   f. Glucocorticoids, thiazide diuretics, and estrogen increase blood glucose levels
   g. Instruct the client in how to recognize symptoms of **hypoglycemia** and **hyperglycemia**
   h. Instruct the client to avoid over-the-counter medications unless prescribed by the physician
   i. Instruct the client not to ingest alcohol with sulfonylureas
   j. Inform the client that insulin may be needed during stress, surgery, or infection
   k. Instruct the client in the necessity of compliance with the prescribed medication
   l. Advise the client to obtain a Medic-Alert bracelet

6. Insulin
   a. Used in the treatment of type 1 **diabetes mellitus** and in type 2 **diabetes mellitus** when diet and weight control therapy have failed to maintain satisfactory blood glucose levels

TABLE 51-1

Major Types of Diabetes Mellitus

Type 1: insulin-dependent diabetes mellitus
Type 2: non–insulin-dependent diabetes mellitus

b. Regular insulin is used in the emergency treatment of **diabetic ketoacidosis**

c. Aspirin, alcohol, oral anticoagulants, oral hypoglycemics, beta-blockers, tricyclic antidepressants, tetracycline, and MAOIs increase the hypoglycemic effect of insulin

d. Glucocorticoids, thiazide diuretics, thyroid agents, oral contraceptives, and estrogen increase blood glucose levels

e. Illness, infection, and stress increase the need for insulin, and insulin should not be withheld during illness, infection, or stress, because **hyperglycemia** and ketoacidosis can result

f. Instruct the client to recognize symptoms of **hypoglycemia** and **hyperglycemia**

g. The peak action time of insulin is very important because of the possibility of hypoglycemic reactions occurring during that time

B. Complications of insulin therapy

1. Local allergic reactions

a. Redness, swelling, tenderness, and induration or a wheal at the site of injection 1 to 2 hours after administration

b. Usually occurs during the early stages of insulin therapy

c. Instruct the client to avoid the use of alcohol to cleanse the skin prior to injection

d. The physician may prescribe an antihistamine to be taken 1 hour prior to injection

2. Insulin lipodystrophy

a. Lipoatrophy is loss of subcutaneous fat and appears as slight dimpling or more serious pitting of subcutaneous fat; the use of human insulin helps to prevent this complication

b. Liperhypertrophy is the development of fibro-fatty masses at the injection site and is caused by repeated use of an injection site

c. Instruct the client to avoid injecting insulin into affected sites

d. Instruct the client about the importance of rotating insulin injection sites

3. Insulin resistance

a. The client taking insulin develops immune antibodies that bind the insulin, thereby decreasing the insulin available for use in the body

b. Treatment consists of administering a purer insulin preparation; occasionally prednisone is prescribed to block the production of antibodies

4. **Dawn phenomenon**

a. Results from a nocturnal release of growth hormone, which may cause the blood glucose to begin to rise at about 3:00 A.M.

b. Treatment includes administering an evening dose of intermediate-acting insulin at 10:00 P.M.

5. **Somogyi's phenomenon**

a. A rebound phenomenon that occurs during the initial period of blood glucose control; develops at peak insulin times and during the night

b. Normal or elevated blood glucose levels are present at bedtime, a decrease occurs at about 2:00 A.M. to 3:00 A.M. to hypoglycemic levels, and a subsequent increase occurs as a result of the production of counterregulatory hormones

c. Treatment includes decreasing the evening (predinner or bedtime) dose of intermediate-acting insulin, or increasing the bedtime snack

6. **Insulin waning**

a. A progressive rise in the blood glucose level from bedtime to morning

b. Treatment includes increasing the evening (predinner or bedtime) dose of intermediate- or long-acting insulin, or instituting a dose of insulin before the evening meal if one is not already prescribed

C. Insulin administration

1. Subcutaneous injections and mixing insulin: Refer to Chapter 52

2. Insulin pens

a. A device that uses a small, prefilled insulin cartridge that is loaded into a penlike holder; a disposable needle is attached to the device for injection

b. The client inserts the needle for injection, and the insulin is delivered by dialing in a dose or pushing a button for every 1- to 2-unit increment administered

3. Jet injectors

a. A device that delivers insulin through the skin under pressure in an extremely fine stream

b. Insulin administered by this device usually absorbs faster

c. Can cause bruising at the site of insulin delivery

4. Insulin pumps

a. Continuous subcutaneous insulin infusion is administered by an externally worn device that contains a syringe attached to a long, thin, narrow-lumened tube with a needle or Teflon catheter attached to the end

b. The client inserts the needle or Teflon catheter into the subcutaneous tissue (usually on the abdomen) and secures it with tape or a transparent dressing; the pump is worn either on a belt or in a pocket; the needle or Teflon catheter is changed at least every 3 days

c. A continuous basal rate of insulin infuses, and on the basis of the blood glucose level, the anticipated food intake, and the activity level, the client delivers a bolus of insulin before each meal

d. The pump uses Regular insulin (buffered to prevent the precipitation of insulin crystals within the catheter); some physicians may prescribe the use of Lispro insulin

5. Implantable insulin delivery
   a. An insulin pump is implanted in the peritoneal cavity, where insulin can be absorbed in a more physiological manner
   b. Not widely used because mechanical problems associated with the pump, the catheter, and the insulin delivery exist

6. Inhalant insulin delivery
   a. Regular insulin is administered in an inhaler during inspiration
   b. A less effective method of administration; absorption across the nasal mucosa is rapid; however, only a small amount of insulin is actually absorbed

7. Pancreas transplants
   a. The goal of pancreatic transplantation is to halt or reverse the complications of **diabetes mellitus**
   b. The pancreas is transplanted into the peritoneal cavity; the exocrine secretions drain into the urinary bladder
   c. Performed on a limited number of clients (mostly clients receiving kidney transplantations simultaneously)
   d. Immunosuppressive therapy is prescribed to prevent and treat rejection

D. Self-monitoring of blood glucose
   1. Provides the client with the current blood glucose level and information to maintain good glycemic control
   2. Requires a finger prick to obtain a drop of blood for testing
   3. Must be used with caution in clients with diabetic retinopathy and neuropathy
   4. Instruct the client in the proper procedure for obtaining the blood glucose level
   5. Inform the client that the procedure must be done precisely to obtain accurate results
   6. Stress the importance of following the manufacturer's instructions
   7. Stress the importance of handwashing before and after performing the procedure, to prevent infection
   8. Instruct the client to calibrate the monitor as instructed by the manufacturer
   9. Instruct the client to check the expiration date on the test strips
   10. Instruct the client that if the blood glucose results do not seem reasonable, to reread the instructions, reassess technique, check the expiration date of the test strips, and perform the procedure again to verify results

E. Urine testing
   1. A less reliable indicator as compared with blood glucose monitoring
   2. Instruct the client in the procedure for testing urine for glucose and ketones
   3. Teach the client that the second voided urine specimen is most accurate
   4. The presence of ketones may indicate impending **ketoacidosis**
   5. Urine ketone testing should be performed during illness and whenever the client with type 1 **diabetes mellitus** has glycosuria or persistently elevated blood glucose levels (greater than 240 mg/dL for two consecutive testing periods)

VIII. ACUTE COMPLICATIONS OF DIABETES MELLITUS

A. **Hypoglycemia**
   1. Description
      a. Occurs when the blood glucose level falls to less than 50 to 60 mg/dL
      b. Caused by too much insulin or oral hypoglycemic agents, too little food, or excessive activity
   2. Assessment (Table 51-2)
      a. Mild **hypoglycemia**: A capillary blood glucose level of 40 to 60 mg/dL
      b. Moderate **hypoglycemia**: A capillary blood glucose level of 20 to 40 mg/dL
      c. Severe **hypoglycemia**: The client is unconscious or experiencing seizures
   3. Implementation
      a. Give 10 to 15 g of a fast-acting simple carbohydrate (Box 51-9)

TABLE 51-2

Assessment of Hypoglycemia

Mild	Moderate	Severe
Sweating	Inability to concentrate	Disoriented behavior
Tremor		Difficulty arousing from sleep
Tachycardia	Headache	
Palpitations	Lightheadedness	Loss of consciousness
Nervousness	Confusion	Seizures
Hunger	Memory lapses	
	Numbness of the lips and tongue	
	Slurred speech	
	Impaired coordination	
	Emotional changes	
	Irrational or combative behavior	
	Double vision	
	Drowsiness	

b. Retest the blood glucose level in 15 minutes, and retreat if it is less than 70 to 75 mg/dL

c. If symptoms persist for more than 15 minutes after the initial treatment, the treatment is repeated even if testing of blood glucose is not possible

d. Once symptoms resolve, a snack containing protein and carbohydrate, such as milk or cheese and crackers, is recommended unless the client plans to eat a regular meal or snack within 30 to 60 minutes

4. Implementation for severe **hypoglycemia**

a. If the client is unconscious and cannot swallow, an injection of glucagon is administered either subcutaneously or intramuscularly

b. After the injection of glucagon, it may take up to 20 minutes for the client to regain consciousness

c. A simple carbohydrate followed by a snack should be given to prevent recurrence of **hypoglycemia**

d. In the hospital or emergency department, the client may be treated with an IV injection of 25 to 50 mL of 50% dextrose in water

e. The client needs to be instructed to always carry some form of fast-acting simple carbohydrate with him or her

f. If the client has a hypoglycemic reaction and does not have any of the recommended emergency foods available, any available food should be eaten; high-fat foods slow the absorption of glucose, and the hypoglycemic symptoms may not resolve quickly

g. Family members need to be instructed in the administration of glucagon

h. The client is instructed that if a severe hypoglycemic reaction occurs, the physician needs to be notified

B. **Diabetic ketoacidosis (DKA)**

1. Description

a. A life-threatening complication of **diabetes mellitus** that develops when a severe insulin deficiency occurs

b. The main clinical manifestations include **hyperglycemia,** dehydration and electrolyte loss, and acidosis

c. The major causes include a decreased or missed dose of insulin, illness or infection, and undiagnosed and untreated **diabetes mellitus**

d. It develops over a period over several hours to days

2. Assessment (Box 51-10)

a. Blood glucose levels may vary from 300 to 800 mg/dL

b. Low serum bicarbonate and a low pH

c. Sodium and potassium levels may be low, normal, or high, depending on the amount of water loss and dehydration status

3. Implementation

a. Restore circulating volume and protect against cerebral, coronary, or renal hypoperfusion

b. Treat dehydration with rapid IV infusions of 0.9% or 0.45% saline as prescribed; dextrose is added to IV fluids, such as D_5NS or 5% dextrose in 0.45% saline, when the blood glucose level reaches 250 to 300 mg/dL

c. Treat **hyperglycemia** with IV Regular insulin administration as prescribed

d. Correct electrolyte imbalance (potassium level may be elevated as a result of dehydration and acidosis)

e. Monitor potassium level closely because when the client receives treatment for the dehydration and acidosis, the serum potassium will decrease and potassium replacement may be required

4. Insulin IV administration

a. Use Regular insulin only

b. b. A dose of 5 to 10 units of Regular insulin by IV bolus may be prescribed before a continuous infusion is begun

c. Mix the prescribed IV dose of Regular insulin for continuous infusion in 0.9% or 0.45% saline as prescribed

d. Flush the insulin solution through the entire intravenous infusion set and discard the first 50 mL of solution prior to connecting and

---

BOX 51-9

Simple Carbohydrates to Treat Hypoglycemia

Three or four commercially prepared glucose tablets
4 to 6 ounces of fruit juice or regular soda
6 to 10 Life Savers or hard candy
2 to 3 teaspoons of sugar or honey

BOX 51-10

Assessment of Diabetic Ketoacidosis

Polyuria
Polydipsia
Blurred vision
Weakness
Headache
Hypotension
Weak, rapid pulse
Anorexia, nausea, vomiting, and abdominal pain
Acetone breath (a fruity odor)
Kussmaul respirations
Mental status changes

administering to the client; insulin molecules adhere to the glass and plastic of IV infusion sets

e. Always place the insulin infusion on an IV infusion controller

f. Insulin is infused continuously until subcutaneous administration resumes

g. Monitor vital signs and for signs of fluid overload

h. Monitor potassium levels, glucose levels, and urinary output, and for signs of increased intracranial pressure

i. If the blood glucose level falls too far, too fast before the brain has time to equilibrate, water is pulled from the blood to the cerebrospinal fluid and the brain, causing cerebral edema and increased intracranial pressure

j. The potassium level will fall rapidly within the first hour of treatment as the dehydration and the acidosis are treated

k. Potassium is administered IV as prescribed when the potassium reaches normal level, to prevent hypokalemia; ensure adequate renal function before administering potassium

5. Client education (Box 51-11)

C. **Hyperglycemic hyperosmolar nonketotic syndrome (HHNS)**

1. Description
   a. Extreme **hyperglycemia** without ketosis and acidosis
   b. Occurs most often in individuals with type 2 **diabetes mellitus**
   c. The major difference between **HHNS** and **DKA** is that ketosis and acidosis do not occur with **HHNS**
   d. Onset is usually slow and takes hours to days to develop

2. Assessment
   a. Blood glucose level is from 600 to 1200 mg/dL
   b. Hypotension
   c. Dehydration
   d. Tachycardia
   e. Mental status changes
   f. Neurological deficits
   g. Seizures

3. Implementation
   a. Similar to the treatment for **DKA**
   b. Includes fluid replacement, correction of electrolyte imbalances, and insulin administration
   c. Insulin plays a less critical role in the treatment of **HHNS** than it does for the treatment of **DKA** because insulin is not needed for reversal of acidosis in **HHNS**

BOX 51-11

Client Education: Guidelines During Illness

Take insulin or oral antidiabetic medications as prescribed

Test blood glucose and test the urine for ketones every 3 to 4 hours

If the usual meal plan cannot be followed, substitute soft foods six to eight times a day

If vomiting, diarrhea, or fever occurs, consume liquids every ½ to 1 hour to prevent dehydration and to provide calories

Notify the physician if vomiting, diarrhea, or fever persists, if blood glucose levels are greater than 250 to 300 mg/dL, when ketonuria is present for more than 24 hours, when unable to take food or fluids for a period of 4 hours, or when illness persists for more than 2 days

---

IX. **CHRONIC COMPLICATIONS OF DIABETES MELLITUS**

A. Diabetic retinopathy
   1. Description
      a. A chronic and progressive noninflammatory impairment of the retinal circulation that eventually causes hemorrhage
      b. Permanent vision changes and blindness can occur
      c. The client has difficulty with carrying out the daily tasks of blood glucose testing and insulin injections
   2. Assessment
      a. A change in vision due to ruptured vessels
      b. Blurred vision resulting from macular edema
      c. Sudden loss of vision as a result of retinal detachment
      d. Cataracts resulting from lens opacity
   3. Implementation
      a. Maintain safety
      b. Early prevention by the control of hypertension and blood glucose levels
      c. Photocoagulation (laser therapy) to remove hemorrhagic tissue to decrease scarring
      d. Vitrectomy to remove vitreous hemorrhages and thus decrease tension on the retina, preventing detachment
      e. Cataract removal with lens implant

B. Diabetic nephropathy
   1. Description: a progressive decrease in kidney function
   2. Assessment
      a. Microalbuminuria
      b. Thirst
      c. Fatigue
      d. Anemia

e. Weight loss

f. Signs of malnutrition

g. Frequent urinary tract infections

h. Signs of a neurogenic bladder

3. Implementation

a. Early prevention by the control of hypertension and blood glucose levels

b. Assess vital signs

c. Monitor I & O

d. Monitor BUN and creatinine levels, and for albuminuria

e. Restrict dietary protein, sodium, and potassium as prescribed

f. Avoid nephrotoxic medications

g. Prepare the client for dialysis procedures as prescribed

h. Prepare the client for kidney transplants as prescribed

i. Prepare the client for pancreas transplants as prescribed

C. Diabetic neuropathy

1. Description

a. General deterioration of the nervous system

b. Complications include foot injuries resulting from trauma and the development of ulcers, frequently requiring amputation

2. Assessment

a. Paresthesias

b. Decreased or absent reflexes

c. Decreased sensation to vibration or light touch

d. Pain, aching, and burning in the lower extremities

e. Poor peripheral pulses

f. Skin breakdown and signs of infection

g. Weakness or loss of sensation in cranial nerves III, IV, V, or VI

h. Dizziness and postural hypotension

i. Nausea and vomiting

j. Diarrhea or constipation

k. Incontinence

l. Dyspareunia

m. Impotence

n. Hypoglycemic unawareness

3. Implementation

a. Early prevention by the control of hypertension and blood glucose levels

b. Careful foot care to prevent trauma (Box 51-12)

c. Apply topical capsaicin (Axsain, Zostrix) for temporary relief of neuralgia, if prescribed

d. Administer medications as prescribed for pain relief

e. Initiate bladder-training programs

f. Instruct in the use of estrogen-containing lubricants for women with dyspareunia

---

BOX 51-12

Preventive Foot Care Instructions

Meticulous skin care and proper foot care

Inspect feet daily and monitor feet for redness, swelling, or break in skin integrity

Notify the physician if redness or a break in the skin occurs

Avoid thermal injuries from hot water, heating pads, and baths

Wash feet with warm (not hot) water and dry thoroughly (avoid foot soaks)

Do not soak feet

Do not treat corns, blisters, or ingrown toenails

Do not cross legs or wear tight garments that may constrict blood flow

Apply moisturizing lotion to the feet but not between the toes

Prevent moisture from accumulating between the toes

Wear loose socks and well-fitting (not tight) shoes, and instruct the client not to go barefoot

Change into clean cotton socks daily

Wear socks to keep feet warm

Do not wear the same pair of shoes 2 days in a row

Do not wear open-toed shoes or shoes with a strap that goes between the toes

Check shoes for cracks or tears in the lining and for foreign objects before putting them on

Break in new shoes gradually

Cut toenails straight across and smooth nails with an emery board

Do not smoke

---

g. Prepare the male client with impotence for penile injections or implantable devices as prescribed

h. Prepare for surgical decompression for compression lesions related to the cranial nerves as prescribed

X. OPERATIVE CARE FOR THE DIABETIC CLIENT

A. Preoperative care

1. Check with physician regarding withholding oral hypoglycemic medications or insulin

2. Some long-acting oral antidiabetic medications are discontinued 24 to 48 hours prior to surgery

3. Insulin dose may be adjusted or may be withheld if IV insulin administration during surgery is planned

4. Monitor blood glucose level

5. Administer IV fluids as prescribed

B. Postoperative care

1. Administer IV glucose and insulin infusions as prescribed until the client can tolerate oral feedings

2. Administer supplemental short-acting insulin as prescribed, on the basis of blood glucose results

3. Monitor blood glucose levels frequently if the client is receiving total parenteral nutrition
4. When the client is tolerating food, ensure that the client receives an adequate amount of carbohydrates daily to prevent **hypoglycemia** and ketosis

PRACTICE QUESTIONS

1. After hypophysectomy, a client complains of being very thirsty and having to urinate frequently. The initial nursing action is to:
   1. Document the complaints
   2. Increase fluid intake
   3. Assess urine specific gravity
   4. Assess for urinary glucose

2. A nurse is caring for a client after hypophysectomy. The nurse notices clear nasal drainage from the client's nostril. The initial nursing action would be to:
   1. Continue to observe the drainage
   2. Test the drainage for glucose
   3. Lower the head of the bed
   4. Obtain a culture of the drainage

3. After several diagnostic tests, a client is diagnosed with diabetes insipidus. A nurse performs an assessment on the client, knowing that which symptom is indicative of this disorder?
   1. Diarrhea
   2. Polydipsia
   3. Weight gain
   4. Fatigue

4. A nurse develops a plan of care for a client with Graves' disease and includes which of the following in the plan?
   1. Provide small meals
   2. Provide extra blankets
   3. Provide a high-fiber diet
   4. Provide a restful environment

5. A nurse is performing an assessment on a client following a thyroidectomy. The nurse notes that the client has developed hoarseness and a weak voice. Which nursing action is most appropriate?
   1. Notify the physician immediately
   2. Reassure the client that this is usually a temporary condition
   3. Check for signs of bleeding
   4. Administer calcium gluconate

6. A client is admitted to an emergency room, and a diagnosis of myxedema coma is made. Which action would the nurse prepare to carry out initially?
   1. Warm the client
   2. Administer fluid replacement
   3. Maintain an airway
   4. Administer thyroid hormone

7. A client is taking NPH insulin daily every morning. The nurse instructs the client that the most likely time for a hypoglycemic reaction to occur is:
   1. 2 to 4 hours after administration
   2. 4 to 12 hours after administration
   3. 12 to 16 hours after administration
   4. 18 to 24 hours after administration

8. A nurse is preparing a teaching plan for a client with diabetes mellitus regarding proper foot care. Which instruction is included in the plan?
   1. Soak feet in hot water
   2. Apply a moisturizing lotion to dry feet but not between the toes
   3. Always have a podiatrist cut your toenails; never cut them yourself
   4. Avoid using a mild soap on the feet

9. A client is brought to the emergency room in an unresponsive state, and a diagnosis of hyperglycemic hyperosmolar nonketotic syndrome (HHNS) is made. The nurse would prepare to immediately initiate which of the following anticipated physician's orders?
   1. 100 units of NPH insulin
   2. Endotracheal intubation
   3. IV replacement of sodium bicarbonate
   4. IV infusion of normal saline

10. An external insulin pump is prescribed for a client with diabetes mellitus. The client asks the nurse about the functioning of the pump. The nurse bases the response on the information that the pump:
    1. Gives a small continuous dose of Regular insulin subcutaneously, and the client can self-bolus with an additional dosage from the pump prior to each meal
    2. Is timed to release programmed doses of Regular or NPH insulin into the bloodstream at specific intervals
    3. Is surgically attached to the pancreas and infuses Regular insulin into the pancreas, which in turn releases the insulin into the bloodstream
    4. Continuously infuses small amounts of NPH insulin into the bloodstream while regularly monitoring blood glucose levels

11. A client newly diagnosed with diabetes mellitus has been stabilized with insulin injections daily. A nurse prepares a discharge teaching plan regarding the insulin. The teaching plan should reinforce which of the following concepts?
    1. Increase the amount of insulin prior to unusual exercise
    2. Acetone in the urine will signify a need for less insulin
    3. Always keep insulin vials refrigerated
    4. Systematically rotate insulin injection sites

12. A client with a diagnosis of diabetic ketoacidosis

(DKA) is being treated in an emergency room. Which finding would a nurse expect to note as confirming this diagnosis?
1. Elevated blood glucose level and a low plasma bicarbonate
2. Decreased urine output
3. Increased respirations and an increase in pH
4. Comatose state

13. A nurse teaches a client with diabetes mellitus about differentiating between hypoglycemia and ketoacidosis. The client demonstrates an understanding of the teaching by stating that glucose will be taken if which of the following symptoms develops?
    1. Fruity breath odor
    2. Shakiness
    3. Blurred vision
    4. Polyuria

14. A client with diabetes mellitus demonstrates acute anxiety when first admitted for the treatment of hyperglycemia. The most appropriate intervention to decrease the client's anxiety would be to:
    1. Administer a sedative
    2. Make sure the client knows all the correct medical terms to understand what is happening
    3. Ignore the signs and symptoms of anxiety so that they will soon disappear
    4. Convey empathy, trust, and respect toward the client

15. A nurse provides instructions to a client newly diagnosed with type 1 diabetes mellitus. The nurse recognizes accurate understanding of measures to prevent diabetic ketoacidosis (DKA) when the client states:
    1. "I will stop taking my insulin if I'm too sick to eat."
    2. "I will decrease my insulin dose during times of illness."
    3. "I will notify my physician if my blood glucose level is greater than 250 mg/dL."
    4. "I will adjust my insulin dose according to the level of glucose in my urine."

16. A client is admitted to a hospital with a diagnosis of diabetic ketoacidosis (DKA). The initial blood glucose level was 950 mg/dL. A continuous IV infusion of Regular insulin is initiated along with rehydration with IV normal saline. The serum glucose level is now 240 mg/dL. The nurse would next prepare to administer which of the following?
    1. IV fluids containing 5% dextrose
    2. NPH insulin subcutaneously
    3. An ampule of 50% dextrose
    4. Phenytoin (Dilantin) for the prevention of seizures

17. A physician has prescribed propylthiouracil (PTU)

for a client with hyperthyroidism. A nurse develops a plan of care for the client. A priority nursing assessment to be included in the plan regarding this medication is to assess for:
1. Signs and symptoms of hypothyroidism
2. Signs and symptoms of hyperglycemia
3. Relief of pain
4. Signs of renal toxicity

18. A nurse develops a plan of care for a client with hyperparathyroidism who is receiving calcitonin salmon (Calcimar). Which of he following outcome criteria has the highest priority regarding this medication?
    1. Absence of side effects
    2. Achievement of normal serum calcium levels
    3. Relief of pain
    4. Verbalization of appropriate medication knowledge

19. A physician prescribes levothyroxine sodium (Synthroid), 0.15 mg PO daily, for a client with hypothyroidism. A nurse will prepare to administer this medication:
    1. Three times a day in equal doses of 0.5 mg each to ensure consistent serum drug levels
    2. In the morning to prevent sleeplessness
    3. Only when the client complains of fatigue and cold intolerance
    4. At various times during the day to prevent tolerance from occurring

20. A nurse is monitoring a client receiving chlorpropamide (Diabenese). The nurse knows that which of the following is not a therapeutic outcome for this client?
    1. A decrease in polyuria
    2. A fasting blood glucose of 110 mg/dL
    3. A decrease in polyphagia
    4. A glycosylated hemoglobin of 10%

21. A nurse is monitoring a client with diabetes insipidus. Desmopressin (DDAVP, Stimate) has been prescribed for the client. Which of the following outcomes reflects a therapeutic effect of this medication?
    1. Serum osmolality greater than 320 mOsm/kg
    2. Increased blood pressure
    3. Decreased urine output
    4. Urine osmolality less than 100 mOsm/kg

22. A nurse is monitoring a client newly diagnosed with diabetes mellitus for signs of complications. Which of the following, if exhibited in the client, would indicate hyperglycemia and warrant physician notification?
    1. Hypertension
    2. Diaphoresis
    3. Polyuria
    4. Increased pulse rate

23. A nurse is preparing a plan of care for a client with

diabetes mellitus who has hyperglycemia. The priority nursing diagnosis would be:
1. High risk for fluid volume deficit
2. Knowledge deficit: disease process and treatment
3. Altered nutrition: less than body requirements
4. Ineffective family coping: compromised

24. A home health nurse visits a client with a diagnosis of type 1 diabetes mellitus. The client relates a history of vomiting and diarrhea and tells the nurse that no food or medication has been consumed for 36 hours. Which additional statement by the client indicates a need for further teaching?
1. "I need to stop my insulin."
2. "I need to increase my fluid intake."
3. "I need to call the physician because of these symptoms."
4. "I need to monitor my blood glucose every 3 to 4 hours."

25. A nurse is assisting a client with diabetes mellitus who is recovering from diabetic ketoacidosis (DKA) to develop a plan to prevent a recurrence. Which of the following is most important to include in the plan of care?
1. Eat six small meals per day
2. Receive appropriate follow-up health care
3. Monitor blood glucose levels frequently
4. Test urine for ketone levels

26. A nurse is caring for a client admitted to the emergency room with diabetic ketoacidosis (DKA). In the acute phase, the priority nursing action is to prepare to:
1. Administer IV Regular insulin
2. Administer IV 5% dextrose
3. Correct the acidosis
4. Apply an ECG monitor

27. A client with type 2 diabetes mellitus diabetes mellitus has a blood glucose over 600 mg/dL and is complaining of polydipsia, polyuria, weight loss, and weakness. A nurse reviews the physician's documentation and would expect to note which of the following diagnoses?
1. Diabetic ketoacidosis (DKA)
2. Hypoglycemia
3. Hyperglycemic hyperosmolar nonketotic syndrome (HHNS)
4. Pheochromocytoma

28. The family of a bedridden client with type 2 diabetes mellitus calls a nurse to report the following symptoms: blood glucose of 400 mg/dL (by fingerstick), polydipsia, and increased lethargy. To determine a possible diagnosis, the nurse asks the family which most important question?
1. "Has there been any change in the dietary intake?"
2. "Have there been any ketones in the urine?"
3. "Has there been any fever?"

4. "Have you increased the amount of fluids provided?"

29. A nurse performs a physical assessment on a client with type 2 diabetes mellitus. Findings include a fasting blood glucose of 120 mg/dL, temperature of 101° F, pulse of 88, respirations of 22, and blood pressure of 140/84 mm Hg. Which finding would be of most concern to the nurse?
1. Pulse
2. Blood pressure
3. Respiration
4. Temperature

30. A nurse is interviewing a client with type 2 diabetes mellitus. Which statement by the client indicates an understanding of the treatment for this disorder?
1. "I am taking oral insulin instead of shots."
2. "The medications I'm taking help release the insulin I already make."
3. "By taking these medications I am able to eat more."
4. "When I become ill, I need to increase the number of pills I take."

31. A nurse is providing discharge instructions to a client who has Cushing's syndrome. Which statement by the client indicates that instructions related to dietary management were understood?
1. "I am fortunate that I do not need to follow any special diet."
2. "I will need to limit the amount of protein in my diet."
3. "I am fortunate that I can eat all the salty foods I enjoy."
4. "I can eat foods that have a lot of potassium in them."

32. A client with type 1 diabetes mellitus calls the nurse to report recurrent episodes of hypoglycemia with exercising. Which statement by the client indicates an inadequate understanding of the peak action of NPH insulin and exercise?
1. "The best time for me to exercise is every afternoon."
2. "The best time for me to exercise is after I eat."
3. "The best time for me to exercise is after breakfast."
4. "The best time for me to exercise is before bedtime."

33. A nurse is completing an assessment on an elderly client who is being admitted for a diagnostic workup for primary hyperparathyroidism. Which client complaint would be characteristic of this disorder?
1. Diarrhea
2. Polyuria
3. Polyphagia
4. Weight gain

34. A nurse is caring for a postoperative parathyroidectomy client. Which client complaint would indicate

that a serious, life-threatening complication may be developing, requiring immediate notification of the physician?

1. Difficulty in voiding
2. Abdominal cramps
3. Laryngeal stridor
4. Mild to moderate incisional pain

35. A nurse notes that a client with type 1 diabetes mellitus has lipodystrophy on both upper thighs. The nurse would appropriately inquire if the client:

1. Cleanses the skin with alcohol before each injection
2. Rotates sites for injection
3. Aspirates for blood prior to injection into the subcutaneous tissue
4. Administers the insulin at a 45-degree angle

36. A nurse is caring for a client with type 1 diabetes mellitus. Which client complaint would alert the nurse to the presence of a possible hypoglycemic reaction?

1. Hot, dry skin
2. Muscle cramps
3. Anorexia
4. Tremors

37. A nurse needs to maintain food and fluid intake to minimize the risk of dehydration in a frail, elderly, client with diabetes mellitus who has gastroenteritis. The most appropriate nursing intervention is to:

1. Offer water only, until the client is able to tolerate solid foods
2. Withhold all fluids until vomiting has ceased for at least 4 hours
3. Encourage the client to take 8 to 12 ounces of fluid every hour while awake
4. Maintain a clear liquid diet for at least 5 days before advancing to solids, to allow inflammation of the bowel to dissipate

38. A client who is currently taking levothyroxine sodium (Synthroid) complains of cold intolerance, constipation, dry skin, weight gain, and puffy eyes. On the basis of these findings, the nurse would anticipate which of the following prescriptions?

1. Increase levothyroxine sodium dosage after checking the T_4 level
2. Decrease levothyroxine sodium dosage after checking the T_4 level
3. Discontinue levothyroxine sodium, since the client is having an adverse reaction
4. No change in medication, since these are common side effects that will diminish with time

39. A client with diabetes mellitus visits a health care clinic. The client's diabetes mellitus had previously been well controlled with glyburide (DiaBeta), 5 mg PO qd, but recently the fasting blood glucose has been running 180 to 200 mg/dL. Which

medication, if added to the client's regimen, may have contributed to the hyperglycemia?

1. Prednisone (Deltasone)
2. Atenolol (Tenormin)
3. Phenelzine (Nardil)
4. Allopurinol (Zyloprim)

40. A nurse is caring for a client with diabetes insipidus who is receiving vasopressin (Pitressin). The nurse monitors the client, knowing that which of the following is not a therapeutic effect of this medication?

1. Increased gastrointestinal tract smooth muscle tone and contractions
2. Decreased urine output
3. Increased reabsorption of water by the renal tubules
4. Vasodilation of vascular vessels

41. A client is diagnosed with pheochromocytoma. A nurse prepares a plan of care for the client, and in the planning the nurse understands that pheochromocytoma is a condition that:

1. Causes profound hypotension
2. Causes the release of excessive amounts of catecholamines
3. Is not curable and is treated symptomatically
4. Is manifested by severe hypoglycemia

42. A nurse is performing an admission assessment on a client admitted with a diagnosis of pheochromocytoma. The nurse assesses for the major symptom associated with pheochromocytoma when the nurse:

1. Tests the client's urine for glucose
2. Obtains the client's weight
3. Palpates the skin for its temperature
4. Takes the client's blood pressure

43. A nurse collects urine specimens for catecholamine testing from a client with suspected pheochromocytoma. The results of the catecholamine test are reported as 20 µg/100 mL urine. The nurse analyzes these results as:

1. Normal
2. Lower than normal, ruling out pheochromocytoma
3. Higher than normal, indicating pheochromocytoma
4. Insignificant and unrelated to pheochromocytoma

44. A nurse is caring for a client with pheochromocytoma. The client is scheduled for adrenalectomy. In the preoperative period, the priority nursing action would be to monitor:

1. Vital signs
2. Urine for glucose and acetone
3. Intake and output
4. Blood urea nitrogen (BUN) results

45. A nurse is caring for a client with pheochromocytoma. As part of the nursing care plan, the nurse

monitors for hypertensive crisis. In the event that hypertensive crisis occurs, the nurse would anticipate that the most likely medication to be prescribed would be:

1. Propranolol (Inderal)
2. Phentolamine mesylate (Regitine)
3. Phenoxybenzamine hydrochloride (Dibenzyline)
4. Prazosin hydrochloride (Minipress)

46. A nurse is caring for a client with pheochromocytoma. The client asks for a snack and something warm to drink. The most appropriate choice for this client to meet nutritional needs would be which of the following?

1. Graham crackers and warm milk
2. Toast with peanut butter and cocoa
3. Crackers with cheese and tea
4. Vanilla wafers and coffee with cream and sugar

47. A nurse is performing an assessment on a client with pheochromocytoma. Which of the following assessment data would indicate a potential complication associated with this disorder?

1. A urinary output of 50 mL per hour
2. An irregular heart rate
3. A blood urea nitrogen (BUN) of 20 mg/dL
4. A coagulation time of 5 minutes

48. A community health nurse visits a client at home. Prednisone (Deltasone), 10 mg PO daily, has been prescribed for the client. The nurse teaches the client about the medication. Which statement, if made by the client, indicates that further teaching is necessary?

1. "I need to take the medication every day at the same time."
2. "I can take aspirin or my antihistamine if I need it."

3. "If I gain more than 5 pounds a week, I will call my doctor."
4. "I need to avoid coffee, tea, cola, and chocolate in my diet."

49. A nurse is preparing to provide instructions to a client with Addison's disease regarding diet therapy. The nurse knows that which of the following diets would most likely be prescribed for this client?

1. Low sodium
2. High sodium
3. Low protein
4. Low carbohydrate

50. A nursing instructor asks a student to describe the pathophysiology that occurs in Cushing's disease. Which statement by the student indicates an accurate understanding of this disorder?

1. "It is characterized by an oversecretion of glucocorticoid hormones."
2. "It is characterized by an undersecretion of glucocorticoid hormones."
3. "It is characterized by an oversecretion of insulin."
4. "It is characterized by an undersecretion of corticotropic hormones."

CRITICAL THINKING: FREE-TEXT ENTRY

A nurse is reviewing a physician's orders for a client with hypothyroidism. The physician has prescribed the following medications: docusate sodium (Colace), morphine sulfate, and levothyroxine sodium (Synthroid). Which medication order would the nurse question and verify?

Answer: _____

ANSWERS

1. **3**

Rationale: After hypophysectomy, diabetes insipidus can occur temporarily because of antidiuretic hormone (ADH) deficiency. This deficiency is related to surgical manipulation. The nurse should assess specific gravity and notify the physician if the results are less than 1.006.

Test-Taking Strategy: Use the process of elimination. Recalling that diabetes insipidus is a complication of this type of surgery will assist in eliminating option 4. Note the key word "initial." Knowledge of the nursing assessment measures in diabetes insipidus will easily direct you to option 3. Review the complications of hypophysectomy if you had difficulty with this question.

Level of Cognitive Ability: Application
Client Needs: Physiological Integrity
Integrated Concept/Process: Nursing Process/Implementation

Content Area: Adult Health/Endocrine
Reference: Smeltzer, S., & Bare, B. (2000). *Brunner & Suddarth's textbook of medical-surgical nursing* (9th ed.). Philadelphia: Lippincott Williams & Wilkins, p. 1033.

2. **2**

Rationale: After hypophysectomy, the client should be monitored for rhinorrhea, which could indicate a cerebrospinal fluid (CSF) leak. If this occurs, the drainage should be collected and tested for the presence of CSF. The head of the bed should not be lowered, to prevent increased intracranial pressure. Clear nasal drainage would not indicate the need for a culture. Continuing to observe the drainage without taking action could result in a serious complication.

Test-Taking Strategy: Use the process of elimination. Note the key word "initial." This indicates that an action is required. Option 3 can be easily eliminated. Option 4 can be easily eliminated because the drainage is clear. Because an action is

required, eliminate option 1. Review the complications following hypophysectomy if you had difficulty with this question.
Level of Cognitive Ability: Application
Client Needs: Physiological Integrity
Integrated Concept/Process: Nursing Process/Implementation
Content Area: Adult Health/Endocrine
Reference: Phipps, W., Sands, J., & Marek, J. (1999). *Medical-surgical nursing: Concepts & clinical practice* (6th ed.). St. Louis: Mosby, p. 1062.

3. 2
Rationale: Polydipsia and polyuria are classic symptoms of diabetes insipidus. The urine is pale, and the specific gravity is low. Anorexia and weight loss occur. Options 1 and 4 are not specific to this disorder.
Test-Taking Strategy: Use the process of elimination. Eliminate option 4 first because this symptom is rather vague and occurs in many conditions. Knowledge of the manifestations of diabetes insipidus will assist in eliminating options 1 and 3. If you had difficulty with this question, review the clinical manifestations associated with diabetes insipidus.
Level of Cognitive Ability: Analysis
Client Needs: Physiological Integrity
Integrated Concept/Process: Nursing Process/Assessment
Content Area: Adult Health/Endocrine
Reference: Smeltzer, S., & Bare, B. (2000). *Brunner & Suddarth's textbook of medical-surgical nursing* (9th ed.). Philadelphia: Lippincott Williams & Wilkins, p. 1033.

4. 4
Rationale: Because of the hypermetabolic state, the client with Graves' disease needs to be provided with an environment that is restful both physically and mentally. Six full meals a day that are well balanced and high in calories are required because of the accelerated metabolic rate. Foods that increase peristalsis, such as high-fiber foods, need to be avoided. These clients suffer from heat intolerance and require a cool environment.
Test-Taking Strategy: Use the process of elimination. The key concept to bear in mind when answering this question is that clients with Graves' disease experience an accelerated metabolic rate. This concept should assist you in eliminating options 1, 2, and 3. Review the plan of care for the client with Graves' disease if you had difficulty with this question.
Level of Cognitive Ability: Application
Client Needs: Physiological Integrity
Integrated Concept/Process: Nursing Process/Planning
Content Area: Adult Health/Endocrine
Reference: Phipps, W., Sands, J., & Marek, J. (1999). *Medical-surgical nursing: Concepts & clinical practice* (6th ed.). St. Louis: Mosby, p. 1078.

5. 2
Rationale: Weakness and hoarseness of the voice can occur as a result of trauma from the surgery. If this develops, the client should be reassured that the problem will subside in a few days. Unnecessary talking should be discouraged. It is not necessary to notify the physician immediately. These signs do not indicate bleeding or the need to administer calcium gluconate.
Test-Taking Strategy: Use the process of elimination. Options 3 and 4 can easily be eliminated because they are unrelated to the signs presented in the question. There are no data

presented requiring immediate physician notification. Review care of the client following thyroidectomy if you had difficulty with this question.
Level of Cognitive Ability: Analysis
Client Needs: Physiological Integrity
Integrated Concept/Process: Nursing Process/Implementation
Content Area: Adult Health/Endocrine
Reference: Black, J., & Matassarin-Jacobs, E. (1997). *Medical-surgical nursing: Clinical management for continuity of care* (5th ed.). Philadelphia: W.B. Saunders. p. 2023.

6. 3
Rationale: The initial nursing action would be to maintain a patent airway. Oxygen would be administered, followed by fluid replacement, keeping the client warm, monitoring vital signs, and administering thyroid hormones by the IV route.
Test-Taking Strategy: Use the process of elimination. Note the key word "initially." All of the options are appropriate interventions, but use the ABCs—airway, breathing, and circulation—in selecting the correct option. Review the initial interventions for myxedema coma if you had difficulty with this question.
Level of Cognitive Ability: Application
Client Needs: Physiological Integrity
Integrated Concept/Process: Nursing Process/Implementation
Content Area: Adult Health/Endocrine
Reference: Smeltzer, S., & Bare, B. (2000). *Brunner & Suddarth's textbook of medical-surgical nursing* (9th ed.). Philadelphia: Lippincott Williams & Wilkins, p. 1039.

7. 2
Rationale: NPH is an intermediate-acting insulin. The onset of action is 3 to 4 hours, it peaks in 4 to 12 hours, and its duration of action is 16 to 20 hours. Hypoglycemic reactions most likely occur during peak time.
Test-Taking Strategy: Use the process of elimination and knowledge regarding the onset, peak, and duration of action for NPH insulin. If you had difficulty with this question, review the characteristics of NPH insulin.
Level of Cognitive Ability: Application
Client Needs: Health Promotion and Maintenance
Integrated Concept/Process: Teaching/Learning
Content Area: Adult Health/Endocrine
Reference: Smeltzer, S., & Bare, B. (2000). *Brunner & Suddarth's textbook of medical-surgical nursing* (9th ed.). Philadelphia: Lippincott Williams & Wilkins, p. 987.

8. 2
Rationale: The client is instructed to use a moisturizing lotion on the feet and to avoid applying the lotion between the toes. The client should be instructed not to soak the feet and should avoid hot water to prevent burns. The client may cut the toenails straight across and even with the toe itself, and would consult a podiatrist if the toenails were thick or hard to cut or if vision was poor. The client should be instructed to wash the feet daily with a mild soap.
Test-Taking Strategy: Use the process of elimination. Eliminate option 3 because of the word "always" and option 1 because of the word "hot." Eliminate option 4 next because of the words "avoid" and "mild." Review diabetic foot care instructions if you had difficulty with this question.
Level of Cognitive Ability: Application
Client Needs: Health Promotion and Maintenance

Integrated Concept/Process: Self-Care
Content Area: Adult Health/Endocrine
Reference: Monahan, F., & Neighbors, M. (1998). *Medical-surgical nursing: Foundations for clinical practice* (2nd ed.). Philadelphia: W.B. Saunders, p. 1252.

9. **4**

Rationale: The primary goal of treatment in HHNS is to rehydrate the client to restore fluid volume and to correct electrolyte deficiency. IV fluid replacement is similar to that administered in diabetic ketoacidosis (DKA) and begins with IV infusion of normal saline. Regular, not NPH, insulin would be administered. The use of sodium bicarbonate to correct acidosis is avoided because it can precipitate a further drop in serum potassium levels. Intubation and mechanical ventilation are not required to treat HHNS.

Test-Taking Strategy: Use the process of elimination. If you can recall the treatment for DKA, you will easily be able to answer this question. Treatment for HHNS is similar to the treatment for DKA. Review the treatment for HHNS if you had difficulty with this question.
Level of Cognitive Ability: Application
Client Needs: Physiological Integrity
Integrated Concept/Process: Nursing Process/Planning
Content Area: Adult Health/Endocrine
Reference: Monahan, F., & Neighbors, M. (1998). *Medical-surgical nursing: Foundations for clinical practice* (2nd ed.). Philadelphia: W.B. Saunders, pp. 1249-1250.

10. **1**

Rationale: An insulin pump provides a small continuous dose of Regular insulin subcutaneously throughout the day and night, and the client can self-bolus with additional dosage from the pump prior to each meal as needed. Regular insulin is used in an insulin pump. An external pump is not surgically attached to the pancreas.

Test-Taking Strategy: Use the process of elimination. Knowledge that Regular insulin is used in an insulin pump will assist in eliminating options 2 and 4. Noting the word "external" in the question will assist in eliminating option 3. Review the use of the insulin pump if you are unfamiliar with it.
Level of Cognitive Ability: Analysis
Client Needs: Health Promotion and Maintenance
Integrated Concept/Process: Teaching/Learning
Content Area: Adult Health/Endocrine
Reference: Monahan, F., & Neighbors, M. (1998). *Medical-surgical nursing: Foundations for clinical practice* (2nd ed.). Philadelphia: W.B. Saunders, pp. 1238-1239.

11. **4**

Rationale: Insulin dosages should not be adjusted and should not be increased prior to unusual exercise. If acetone is found in the urine, it may possibly indicate the need for additional insulin. To minimize the discomfort associated with insulin injections, insulin should be administered at room temperature. Injection sites should be systematically rotated from one area to another.

Test-Taking Strategy: Use the process of elimination. Eliminate option 3 first because of the word "always." Knowledge regarding insulin administration and the significance of acetone in the urine will assist in eliminating options 1 and 2. If you had difficulty with this question, review the components of insulin management.

Level of Cognitive Ability: Application
Client Needs: Health Promotion and Maintenance
Integrated Concept/Process: Teaching/Learning
Content Area: Adult Health/Endocrine
Reference: Smeltzer, S., & Bare, B. (2000). *Brunner & Suddarth's textbook of medical-surgical nursing* (9th ed.). Philadelphia: Lippincott Williams & Wilkins, p. 1001.

12. **1**

Rationale: In DKA, the arterial pH is less than 7.35, plasma bicarbonate is less than 15 mEq/L, the blood glucose level is higher than 250 mg/dL, and ketones are present in the blood and urine. The client would be experiencing polyuria, and Kussmaul's respirations would be present. A comatose state may occur if DKA is not treated, but coma would not confirm the diagnosis.

Test-Taking Strategy: Use the process of elimination. Note the key word "confirming" in the stem of the question. Eliminate option 4 because a comatose state can exist is many conditions. Eliminate option 3 because in acidosis the pH would be low. Remember that polyuria exists in DKA. Review the clinical manifestations of DKA if you had difficulty with this question.
Level of Cognitive Ability: Analysis
Client Needs: Physiological Integrity
Integrated Concept/Process: Nursing Process/Assessment
Content Area: Adult Health/Endocrine
Reference: Monahan, F., & Neighbors, M. (1998). *Medical-surgical nursing: Foundations for clinical practice* (2nd ed.). Philadelphia: W.B. Saunders, pp. 1249, 1251.

13. **2**

Rationale: Shakiness is a sign of hypoglycemia and would indicate the need for food or glucose. A fruity breath odor, blurred vision, and polyuria are signs of hyperglycemia.

Test-Taking Strategy: Focus on the issue of the question, the treatment of hypoglycemia. Recalling the signs of hypoglycemia will direct you to option 2. Review these signs if you had difficulty with this question.
Level of Cognitive Ability: Analysis
Client Needs: Health Promotion and Maintenance
Integrated Concept/Process: Nursing Process/Evaluation
Content Area: Adult Health/Endocrine
Reference: Monahan, F., & Neighbors, M. (1998). *Medical-surgical nursing: Foundations for clinical practice* (2nd ed.). Philadelphia: W.B. Saunders, p. 1251.

14. **4**

Rationale: The most appropriate intervention is to address the client's feelings related to the anxiety. Administering a sedative is not the most appropriate intervention. The nurse should not ignore the client's anxious feelings. A client will not relate to medical terms, particularly when anxiety exists.

Test-Taking Strategy: Use therapeutic communication techniques to answer the question. Remember that the client's feelings come first. Keeping this in mind will easily direct you to option 4. Review therapeutic communication techniques if you had difficulty with this question.
Level of Cognitive Ability: Application
Client Needs: Psychosocial Integrity
Integrated Concept/Process: Caring
Content Area: Adult Health/Endocrine

Reference: Leahy, J., & Kizilay, P. (1998). *Foundations of nursing practice: a nursing process approach.* Philadelphia: W.B. Saunders, p. 223.

15. 3

Rationale: During illness, the client should monitor blood glucose levels and should notify the physician if the level is over 250 mg/dL. Insulin should never be stopped. In fact, insulin may need to be increased during times of illness. Doses should not be adjusted without the physician's advice to do so.

Test-Taking Strategy: Use the process of elimination. Note that options 1, 2, and 4 are similar and all relate to adjustment of insulin doses. Review diabetic management during illness if you had difficulty with this question.

Level of Cognitive Ability: Analysis
Client Needs: Health Promotion and Maintenance
Integrated Concept/Process: Nursing Process/Evaluation
Content Area: Adult Health/Endocrine
Reference: Monahan, F., & Neighbors, M. (1998). *Medical-surgical nursing: Foundations for clinical practice* (2nd ed.). Philadelphia: W.B. Saunders, pp. 1240-1241.

16. 1

Rationale: During management of DKA, when the blood glucose level falls to 250 to 300 mg/dL, the infusion rate is reduced and 5% dextrose is added to maintain a blood glucose level of about 250 mg/dL, or until the client recovers from ketosis. NPH insulin is not used to treat DKA. Fifty percent dextrose is used to treat hypoglycemia. Dilantin is not a usual treatment measure for DKA.

Test-Taking Strategy: Use the process of elimination. Eliminate option 2 first, knowing that Regular insulin is used in the management of DKA. Eliminate option 3 next, knowing that this is the treatment for hypoglycemia. Note the key words "the serum glucose level is now 240 mg/dL." This should indicate that the IV solution of 5% dextrose is the next step in management of care. Review care of the client with DKA if you had difficulty with this question.

Level of Cognitive Ability: Analysis
Client Needs: Physiological Integrity
Integrated Concept/Process: Nursing Process/Planning
Content Area: Adult Health/Endocrine
Reference: Monahan, F., & Neighbors, M. (1998). *Medical-surgical nursing: Foundations for clinical practice* (2nd ed.). Philadelphia: W.B. Saunders, p. 1249-1250.

17. 1

Rationale: Excessive dosing with PTU may convert the client from a hyperthyroid state to a hypothyroid state. If this occurs, the dosage should be reduced. Temporary administration of thyroid hormone may be required. PTU is not used for pain and does not cause hyperglycemia or renal toxicity.

Test-Taking Strategy: Read the question carefully, noting the client's diagnosis. Noting that PTU is used to treat hyperthyroidism should easily direct you to option 1. If you had difficulty with this question, review the side effects and adverse effects of this medication.

Level of Cognitive Ability: Application
Client Needs: Physiological Integrity
Integrated Concept/Process: Nursing Process/Assessment
Content Area: Adult Health/Endocrine
Reference: Hodgson, B., & Kizior, R. (2001). *Saunders nursing drug handbook 2001.* Philadelphia: W.B. Saunders, pp. 880-881.

18. 2

Rationale: Calcitonin can lower plasma calcium levels in clients with hypercalcemia secondary to hyperparathyroidism. The therapeutic effect in this client situation would be a reduction in serum calcium levels. Options 1, 3, and 4 are incorrect outcome criteria.

Test-Taking Strategy: Use the process of elimination. Reading the question carefully, noting the client's diagnosis, will assist in directing you to option 2. In addition, note the relationship between the name of the medication and the word "calcium" in option 2. Review the action of this medication if you are unfamiliar with it.

Level of Cognitive Ability: Analysis
Client Needs: Health Promotion and Maintenance
Integrated Concept/Process: Nursing Process/Evaluation
Content Area: Adult Health/Endocrine
Reference: Hodgson, B., & Kizior, R. (2001). *Saunders nursing drug handbook 2001.* Philadelphia: W.B. Saunders, pp. 137-138.

19. 2

Rationale: Synthroid is a synthetic thyroid hormone that increases cellular metabolism. It should be given in the morning in a single dose to prevent sleeplessness. It should be given at the same time each day to maintain an adequate drug level.

Test-Taking Strategy: Use the process of elimination. Focus on the key word "daily" in the question to direct you to option 2. Review the administration of this medication if you had difficulty with this question.

Level of Cognitive Ability: Application
Client Needs: Physiological Integrity
Integrated Concept/Process: Nursing Process/Planning
Content Area: Adult Health/Endocrine
Reference: Hodgson, B., & Kizior, R. (2001). *Saunders nursing drug handbook 2001.* Philadelphia: W.B. Saunders, pp. 589-590.

20. 4

Rationale: Diabenese is an oral hypoglycemic agent given to reduce the serum glucose level and the signs and symptoms of hyperglycemia. Therefore, a decrease in both polyuria and polyphagia, and symptoms of hyperglycemia, would denote a beneficial response to Diabenese. Laboratory values are also used to assess the client's response to treatment. A fasting blood glucose level of 110 mg/dL is within normal limits. However, a glycosylated hemoglobin of 10% denotes poor glycemic control.

Test-Taking Strategy: Use the process of elimination. Note the key word "not" in the stem of the question. Knowledge that Diabenese is an oral hypoglycemic agent tells you to look for an option that would denote hyperglycemia (lack of response to medication). Options 1 and 3 are similar and can be eliminated first. Knowledge of the normal blood glucose level will assist in eliminating option 2. Review the action and expected therapeutic outcome of Diabenese if you had difficulty with this question.

Level of Cognitive Ability: Analysis
Client Needs: Physiological Integrity
Integrated Concept/Process: Nursing Process/Evaluation
Content Area: Adult Health/Endocrine
Reference: Hodgson, B., & Kizior, R. (2001). *Saunders nursing drug handbook 2001.* Philadelphia: W.B. Saunders, pp. 1104-1106.

21. **3**

Rationale: Desmopressin is a synthetic form of antidiuretic hormone. It causes increased reabsorption of water with a resultant decrease in urine output. The therapeutic response to DDAVP or Stimate would demonstrate a decrease in serum osmolality, because more fluid is retained, and an increase in urine osmolality, because less fluid is excreted. Increased blood pressure is a side effect rather than a therapeutic effect of DDAVP or Stimate.

Test-Taking Strategy: Use the process of elimination and note the client's diagnosis. Focus on the issue, therapeutic effect. Knowledge of the therapeutic effects of the medication will direct you to the correct option. Review these therapeutic effects if you had difficulty with this question.

Level of Cognitive Ability: Analysis
Client Needs: Physiological Integrity
Integrated Concept/Process: Nursing Process/Evaluation
Content Area: Adult Health/Endocrine
Reference: Hodgson, B., & Kizior, R. (2001). *Saunders nursing drug handbook 2001.* Philadelphia: W.B. Saunders, pp. 293-295.

22. **3**

Rationale: Classic symptoms of hyperglycemia include polydipsia, polyuria, and polyphagia. Options 1, 2, and 4 are not signs of hyperglycemia.

Test-Taking Strategy: Use the process of elimination. Remember the 3 Ps: polyuria, polydipsia, polyphagia. Learn the signs of hyperglycemia if you had difficulty with this question.

Level of Cognitive Ability: Analysis
Client Needs: Physiological Integrity
Integrated Concept/Process: Nursing Process/Assessment
Content Area: Adult Health/Endocrine
Reference: Monahan, F., & Neighbors, M. (1998). *Medical-surgical nursing: Foundations for clinical practice* (2nd ed.). Philadelphia: W.B. Saunders, p. 1251.

23. **1**

Rationale: Increased blood glucose will cause the kidneys to excrete the glucose in the urine. This glucose is accompanied by fluids and electrolytes, causing an osmotic diuresis leading to dehydration. This fluid loss must be replaced when it becomes severe. Options 2, 3, and 4 are not specifically related to the issue of the question.

Test-Taking Strategy: Use Maslow's Hierarchy of Needs to answer this question. Option 1 indicates a physiological need and is the priority. Options 2, 3, and 4 are nursing diagnoses that may need to be addressed after providing for the high-priority physiological needs.

Level of Cognitive Ability: Analysis
Client Needs: Physiological Integrity
Integrated Concept/Process: Nursing Process/Analysis
Content Area: Adult Health/Endocrine
Reference: Monahan, F., & Neighbors, M. (1998). *Medical-surgical nursing: Foundations for clinical practice* (2nd ed.). Philadelphia: W.B. Saunders, pp. 1250-1251.

24. **1**

Rationale: When a client with diabetes mellitus is unable to eat normally because of illness, the client should still take the prescribed insulin or oral medication. Additional fluids should be consumed, and the physician is notified. The client should monitor the blood glucose level every 3 to 4 hours.

Test-Taking Strategy: Use the process of elimination and knowledge regarding the guidelines related to illness in the diabetic client to answer this question. Remembering that the client needs to take insulin will easily direct you to option 1. Review these guidelines if you had difficulty with this question.

Level of Cognitive Ability: Analysis
Client Needs: Health Promotion and Maintenance
Integrated Concept/Process: Nursing Process/Evaluation
Content Area: Adult Health/Endocrine
Reference: Smeltzer, S., & Bare, B. (2000). *Brunner & Suddarth's textbook of medical-surgical nursing* (9th ed.). Philadelphia: Lippincott Williams & Wilkins, p. 1006.

25. **3**

Rationale: Client education following DKA should emphasize the need for home glucose monitoring two to four times per day. It is also important to instruct the client to notify the health care provider when illness occurs. The presence of urine ketones indicates that DKA has already occurred. The client should eat well-balanced meals with snacks as prescribed.

Test-Taking Strategy: Use the process of elimination and focus on the issue "prevent a reccurrence." Option 1 is not an accurate component of the dietary measures for a client with diabetes mellitus. Option 2 will not prevent DKA, and option 4 does not prevent DKA but actually confirms the diagnosis. Review the measures to prevent DKA if you had difficulty with this question.

Level of Cognitive Ability: Application
Client Needs: Health Promotion and Maintenance
Integrated Concept/Process: Self-Care
Content Area: Adult Health/Endocrine
Reference: Monahan, F., & Neighbors, M. (1998). *Medical-surgical nursing: Foundations for clinical practice* (2nd ed.). Philadelphia: W.B. Saunders, pp. 1242-1243.

26. **1**

Rationale: Lack (absolute or relative) of insulin is the primary cause of DKA. Treatment consists of insulin administration (Regular insulin), IV fluids (normal saline initially), and potassium replacement, followed by correcting acidosis. Applying an ECG monitor is not a priority action.

Test-Taking Strategy: Use the process of elimination and focus on the client's diagnosis. Note the key word "priority." Remember that in DKA, the initial treatment is Regular insulin. Normal saline is administered initially; therefore option 2 is incorrect. Options 3 and 4 may be components of the treatment plan, but are not the priority. Review the initial treatment for DKA if you had difficulty with this question.

Level of Cognitive Ability: Application
Client Needs: Physiological Integrity
Integrated Concept/Process: Nursing Process/Implementation
Content Area: Adult Health/Endocrine
Reference: Phipps, W., Sands, J., & Marek, J. (1999). *Medical-surgical nursing: Concepts & clinical practice* (6th ed.). St. Louis: Mosby, pp. 1170-1172.

27. **3**

Rationale: HHNS is seen in clients with type 2 diabetes mellitus. The onset of symptoms may be gradual. The symptoms may include polyuria, polydipsia, dehydration, mental status alterations, weight loss, and weakness. Options 1, 2, and 4 are incorrect interpretations of the client's symptoms.

Test-Taking Strategy: Use the process of elimination and note the key words "with a blood glucose over 600 mg/dL." This will assist in eliminating options 2 and 4. Recalling that HHNS most commonly occurs in type 2 diabetes mellitus will easily direct you to option 3. Review the clinical manifestations of HHNS if you had difficulty with this question.
Level of Cognitive Ability: Analysis
Client Needs: Physiological Integrity
Integrated Concept/Process: Nursing Process/Analysis
Content Area: Adult Health/Endocrine
Reference: Smeltzer, S., & Bare, B. (2000). *Brunner & Suddarth's textbook of medical-surgical nursing* (9th ed.). Philadelphia: Lippincott Williams & Wilkins, pp. 1007-1008.

28. 2
Rationale: Hyperglycemic hyperosmolar nonketotic syndrome (HHNS) is differentiated from diabetic ketoacidosis (DKA) by the absence of ketones in the urine. Options 1, 3, and 4 will not assist in determining a potential diagnosis.
Test-Taking Strategy: Use the process of elimination and note the signs and symptoms presented in the question. Eliminate options 1 and 4 first because they are similar. From the remaining options, option 2 is most specifically related to a client with diabetes mellitus. Review the differences between DKA and HHNS if you had difficulty with this question.
Level of Cognitive Ability: Analysis
Client Needs: Health Promotion and Maintenance
Integrated Concept/Process: Nursing Process/Assessment
Content Area: Adult Health/Endocrine
Reference: Smeltzer, S., & Bare, B. (2000). *Brunner & Suddarth's textbook of medical-surgical nursing* (9th ed.). Philadelphia: Lippincott Williams & Wilkins, p. 1007.

29. 4
Rationale: An elevated temperature may be indicative of infection. Infection is a leading cause of hyperglycemic hyperosmolar nonketotic syndrome (HHNS) or diabetic ketoacidosis (DKA). The other findings noted in the question are within normal limits.
Test-Taking Strategy: Use the process of elimination and knowledge of the normal values of vital signs to direct you to option 4. The client's temperature is the only abnormal value. Remember that an elevated temperature can indicate an infectious process that can lead to complications in the client with diabetes mellitus. Review normal and abnormal findings in the client with diabetes mellitus if you had difficulty with this question.
Level of Cognitive Ability: Analysis
Client Needs: Physiological Integrity
Integrated Concept/Process: Nursing Process/Analysis
Content Area: Adult Health/Endocrine
Reference: Smeltzer, S., & Bare, B. (2000). *Brunner & Suddarth's textbook of medical-surgical nursing* (9th ed.). Philadelphia: Lippincott Williams & Wilkins, p. 1005.

30. 2
Rationale: Clients with type 2 diabetes mellitus have decreased or impaired insulin secretion. Oral hypoglycemic agents are given to these clients to facilitate glucose utilization. Insulin injections may be given during times of stress-induced hyperglycemia. Oral insulin is not available because of the breakdown of the insulin by digestion. Options 1, 3, and 4 are incorrect.

Test-Taking Strategy: Use the process of elimination, focusing on the issue, type 2 diabetes mellitus. Eliminate option 1 because "oral insulin" is not available. Treatment with medication does not mean that the client can eat more; therefore eliminate option 3. Recalling that during times of illness insulin may be required will eliminate option 4. Review treatment measures for type 2 diabetes mellitus if you had difficulty with this question.
Level of Cognitive Ability: Analysis
Client Needs: Physiological Integrity
Integrated Concept/Process: Nursing Process/Evaluation
Content Area: Adult Health/Endocrine
Reference: Lewis, S., Heitkemper, M., & Dirksen, S. (2000). *Medical-surgical nursing: Assessment and management of clinical problems* (5th ed.). St. Louis: Mosby, pp. 1371-1372.

31. 4
Rationale: A diet low in carbohydrates and sodium but ample in protein and potassium is encouraged for a client with Cushing's syndrome. Such a diet promotes weight loss, reduction of edema and hypertension, control of hypokalemia, and rebuilding of wasted tissue.
Test-Taking Strategy: Use the process of elimination. Eliminate option 1 because it reflects that no dietary change is necessary. Eliminate option 2 next because protein is most likely limited in liver or renal disorders. From the remaining options, eliminate option 3 because excess sodium is not normally healthy. Review dietary management in Cushing's syndrome if you had difficulty with this question.
Level of Cognitive Ability: Analysis
Client Needs: Health Promotion and Maintenance
Integrated Concept/Process: Nursing Process/Evaluation
Content Area: Adult Health/Endocrine
Reference: Smeltzer, S., & Bare, B. (2000). *Brunner & Suddarth's textbook of medical-surgical nursing* (9th ed.). Philadelphia: Lippincott Williams & Wilkins, pp. 1061-1062.

32. 1
Rationale: A hypoglycemic reaction may occur in response to increased exercise. Clients should avoid exercise during the peak time of insulin. NPH insulin peaks at 4 to 12 hours; therefore afternoon exercise will occur during the peak of the medication. Options 2, 3, and 4 do not address peak action times.
Test-Taking Strategy: Use the process of elimination and note the key words "inadequate understanding." Focus on the issue, "peak action of the NPH." Recalling that NPH peaks at 4 to 12 hours will direct you to option 1. Review the peak action time of NPH if you had difficulty with this question.
Level of Cognitive Ability: Analysis
Client Needs: Physiological Integrity
Integrated Concept/Process: Nursing Process/Evaluation
Content Area: Adult Health/Endocrine
Reference: Smeltzer, S., & Bare, B. (2000). *Brunner & Suddarth's textbook of medical-surgical nursing* (9th ed.). Philadelphia: Lippincott Williams & Wilkins, p. 987.

33. 2
Rationale: Hypercalcemia is the hallmark of hyperparathyroidism. Elevated serum calcium levels produce osmotic diuresis and thus polyuria. This diuresis leads to dehydration (weight loss rather than weight gain). Both options 1 and 3 are gastrointestinal (GI) symptoms and are not associated with

the common GI symptoms typical of hyperparathyroidism (nausea, vomiting, anorexia, constipation).

Test-Taking Strategy: Use the process of elimination. Note that options 1, 3, and 4 are all GI symptoms and are similar. Review the clinical manifestations of hyperparathyroidism if you had difficulty with this question.

Level of Cognitive Ability: Analysis
Client Needs: Physiological Integrity
Integrated Concept/Process: Nursing Process/Assessment
Content Area: Adult Health/Endocrine
Reference: LeMone, P., & Burke, K. (2000). *Medical-surgical nursing: Critical thinking in client care* (2nd ed.). Upper Saddle River, N.J.: Prentice-Hall, p. 700.

34. **3**
Rationale: During the postoperative period, the nurse carefully observes the client for signs of hemorrhage, which causes swelling and compression of adjacent tissue. Laryngeal stridor is a harsh, high-pitched sound heard on inspiration and expiration; it is caused by compression of the trachea, leading to respiratory distress. It is an acute emergency situation that requires immediate attention to avoid complete obstruction of the airway. Options 1, 2, and 4 do not identify signs of a life-threatening complication.

Test-Taking Strategy: Consider the anatomical location of the surgical procedure and use the ABCs—airway, breathing, and circulation—to select the correct option. Options 1, 2, and 4 are usual postoperative findings that are not life threatening. Option 3 addresses airway. Review postoperative care of the parathyroidectomy client if you had difficulty with this question.

Level of Cognitive Ability: Analysis
Client Needs: Physiological Integrity
Integrated Concept/Process: Nursing Process/Assessment
Content Area: Adult Health/Endocrine
Reference: Phipps, W., Sands, J., & Marek, J. (1999). *Medical-surgical nursing: Concepts & clinical practice* (6th ed.). St. Louis: Mosby, p. 1099.

35. **2**
Rationale: Lipodystrophy (hypertrophy of subcutaneous tissue at the injection site) occurs in some clients with diabetes mellitus when injection sites are used for a prolonged period of time. Thus, clients are instructed to adhere to a rotating injection site plan to avoid tissue changes. Cleansing with alcohol, aspiration, and angle of insulin administration do not produce this complication.

Test-Taking Strategy: Use the process of elimination and knowledge of the definition of lipodystrophy to answer this question. This will easily direct you to option 2. Review this complication of insulin therapy if you had difficulty with this question.

Level of Cognitive Ability: Analysis
Client Needs: Physiological Integrity
Integrated Concept/Process: Nursing Process/Assessment
Content Area: Adult Health/Endocrine
Reference: Ignatavicius, D., Workman, M., & Mishler, M. (1999). *Medical-surgical nursing across the health care continuum* (3rd ed.). Philadelphia: W.B. Saunders, p. 1659.

36. **4**
Rationale: Decreased blood glucose levels produce autonomic nervous system symptoms, which are classically manifested as

nervousness, irritability, and tremors. Option 1 is more likely to occur with hyperglycemia. Options 2 and 3 are unrelated to the signs of hypoglycemia.

Test-Taking Strategy: Use the process of elimination and focus on the issue, hypoglycemic reaction. Recalling the signs of this type of reaction will easily direct you to option 4. Review the signs of hypoglycemia if you had difficulty with this question.

Level of Cognitive Ability: Analysis
Client Needs: Physiological Integrity
Integrated Concept/Process: Nursing Process/Assessment
Content Area: Adult Health/Endocrine
Reference: Smeltzer, S., & Bare, B. (2000). *Brunner & Suddarth's textbook of medical-surgical nursing* (9th ed.). Philadelphia: Lippincott Williams & Wilkins, pp. 1002-1003.

37. **3**
Rationale: Small amounts of fluid may be tolerated even when vomiting is present. The nurse should encourage liquids containing both glucose and electrolytes every hour. Options 1, 2, and 4 will not provide the adequate intake needed by the client with diabetes mellitus.

Test-Taking Strategy: Use the process of elimination. Eliminate options 1 and 2 because of the words "only" and "all." The time frame in option 4 (5 days) is unreasonable; therefore select option 3. Review care of the client with diabetes mellitus during times of illness if you had difficulty with this question.

Level of Cognitive Ability: Application
Client Needs: Physiological Integrity
Integrated Concept/Process: Nursing Process/Implementation
Content Area: Adult Health/Endocrine
Reference: Ignatavicius, D., Workman, M., & Mishler, M. (1999). *Medical-surgical nursing across the health care continuum* (3rd ed.). Philadelphia: W.B. Saunders, p. 1678.

38. **1**
Rationale: Manifestations of hypothyroidism include cold intolerance, constipation, loss of initiative, thick dry skin, weight gain, a notably puffy appearance of the skin around the eyes, slowed intellectual function, including retarded speech and apathy, and low metabolic rate. Synthroid is used to correct hypothyroidism. This dosage is not therapeutic and needs to be increased.

Test-Taking Strategy: Use the process of elimination. Note the key words "currently taking." Knowledge that the signs presented in the question relate to the manifestations associated with hypothyroidism will easily direct you to option 1. The dosage needs to be increased. Review the expected therapeutic effect of Synthroid if you had difficulty with this question.

Level of Cognitive Ability: Analysis
Client Needs: Physiological Integrity
Integrated Concept/Process: Nursing Process/Analysis
Content Area: Adult Health/Endocrine
Reference: Hodgson, B., & Kizior, R. (2001). *Saunders nursing drug handbook 2001.* Philadelphia: W.B. Saunders, pp. 589-590.

39. **1**
Rationale: Prednisone may decrease the effect of oral hypoglycemics, insulin, diuretics, and potassium supplements. Options 2, a beta blocker, and 3, an MAO inhibitor, have their own intrinsic hypoglycemic activity. Option 4 decreases urinary excretion of sulfonylurea agents, causing increased levels of the oral agents, which can lead to hypoglycemia.

Test-Taking Strategy: Use the process of elimination and recall that prednisone decreases the effects of hypoglycemia. Review medication interactions with hypoglycemics if you had difficulty with this question.
Level of Cognitive Ability: Analysis
Client Needs: Physiological Integrity
Integrated Concept/Process: Nursing Process/Analysis
Content Area: Adult Health/Endocrine
Reference: Hodgson, B., & Kizior, R. (2001). *Saunders nursing drug handbook 2001*. Philadelphia: W.B. Saunders, pp. 855-857.

40. **4**
Rationale: Vasopressin, an antidiuretic hormone, causes vasoconstriction with reduced blood flow in coronary, peripheral, cerebral, and pulmonary vessels. Options 1, 2, and 4 are therapeutic effects of the medication.
Test-Taking Strategy: Use the process of elimination. Note the key word "not" in the stem of the question. Eliminate options 2 and 3 because they are similar. Noting the name of the medication, "vasopressin," will direct you to option 4. If you had difficulty with this question, review the effect of this medication.
Level of Cognitive Ability: Analysis
Client Needs: Physiological Integrity
Integrated Concept/Process: Nursing Process/Evaluation
Content Area: Adult Health/Endocrine
Reference: Hodgson, B., & Kizior, R. (2001). *Saunders nursing drug handbook 2001*. Philadelphia: W.B. Saunders, pp. 1043-1045.

41. **2**
Rationale: Pheochromocytoma is a catecholamine-producing tumor and causes secretion of excessive amounts of epinephrine and norepinephrine. Hypertension is the principal manifestation, and the client has episodes of a high blood pressure accompanied by pounding headaches. The excessive release of catecholamine also results in excessive conversion of glycogen into glucose in the liver. Consequently, hyperglycemia and glucosuria occur during attacks. Pheochromocytoma is curable. The primary treatment is surgical removal of one or both of the adrenal glands, depending on whether the tumor is unilateral or bilateral.
Test-Taking Strategy: Use the process of elimination and knowledge of the manifestations of pheochromocytoma to answer this question. If you are unfamiliar with this disorder, review this content.
Level of Cognitive Ability: Comprehension
Client Needs: Physiological Integrity
Integrated Concept/Process: Nursing Process/Planning
Content Area: Adult Health/Endocrine
Reference: Smeltzer, S., & Bare, B. (2000). *Brunner & Suddarth's textbook of medical-surgical nursing* (9th ed.). Philadelphia: Lippincott Williams & Wilkins, pp. 1056-1057.

42. **4**
Rationale: Hypertension is the major symptom associated with pheochromocytoma. Taking the client's blood pressure would assess the blood pressure status. Glycosuria, weight loss, and diaphoresis are also clinical manifestations of pheochromocytoma, yet hypertension is the major symptom.
Test-Taking Strategy: Use the process of elimination, noting the key words "major symptom." Use the ABCs—airway, breathing, and circulation. A method of assessing circulation is

to take the blood pressure. Review the clinical manifestations of pheochromocytoma if you had difficulty with this question.
Level of Cognitive Ability: Analysis
Client Needs: Physiological Integrity
Integrated Concept/Process: Nursing Process/Assessment
Content Area: Adult Health/Endocrine
Reference: Smeltzer, S., & Bare, B. (2000). *Brunner & Suddarth's textbook of medical-surgical nursing* (9th ed.). Philadelphia: Lippincott Williams & Wilkins, pp. 1056-1057.

43. **3**
Rationale: Assays of catecholamines are performed on single-voided urine specimens, 2- to 4-hour specimens, and 24-hour urine specimens. The normal range of urinary catecholamines is up to 14 μg/100 mL of urine, with higher levels occurring in pheochromocytoma.
Test-Taking Strategy: Recall that pheochromocytoma is a catecholamine-producing tumor. Since the question addresses urine specimens for catecholamine testing, expect the results to indicate higher than normal amounts of catecholamine. In addition, the question addresses that the client is suspected of having pheochromocytoma, so if you need to select an answer and you are not quite sure, select the option that has similarity to a thought in the question. In this case, suspected pheochromocytoma is similar to "indicating pheochromocytoma" in option 3. Review diagnostic tests for pheochromocytoma if you had difficulty with this question.
Level of Cognitive Ability: Analysis
Client Needs: Physiological Integrity
Integrated Concept/Process: Nursing Process/Analysis
Content Area: Adult Health/Endocrine
Reference: Smeltzer, S., & Bare, B. (2000). *Brunner & Suddarth's textbook of medical-surgical nursing* (9th ed.). Philadelphia: Lippincott Williams & Wilkins, p. 1057.

44. **1**
Rationale: Hypertension is the hallmark of pheochromocytoma. Severe hypertension can precipitate a cerebrovascular accident or sudden blindness. Although all of the options are accurate nursing interventions for the client with pheochromocytoma, the priority nursing action is to monitor the vital signs, particularly the blood pressure.
Test-Taking Strategy: Use the process of elimination. Note the key words "priority nursing action." Use the ABCs—airway, breathing, and circulation. Monitoring vital signs is the nursing action that would assess airway, breathing, and circulation. Also, options 2, 3, and 4 all refer to the assessment of the renal system, whereas option 1 does not. Review preoperative care of the client with pheochromocytoma if you had difficulty with this question.
Level of Cognitive Ability: Application
Client Needs: Physiological Integrity
Integrated Concept/Process: Nursing Process/Implementation
Content Area: Adult Health/Endocrine
Reference: Ignatavicius, D., Workman, M., & Mishler, M. (1999). *Medical-surgical nursing across the health care continuum* (3rd ed.). Philadelphia: W.B. Saunders, p. 1611.

45. **2**
Rationale: The most likely medication to be prescribed in hypertensive crisis is phentolamine mesylate (Regitine). This medication is a short-acting alpha-adrenergic blocker and would be given by IV bolus or drip for hypertensive crisis.

Phenoxybenzamine hydrochloride (Dibenzyline) is an oral medication and produces long-acting alpha-adrenergic blockade. It is used in the management of pheochromocytoma and is most suitable for preoperative management of hypertension and prevention of hypertensive crisis. Prazosin hydrochloride (Minipress), an alpha blocker, is used less frequently for the preoperative pheochromocytoma client because of its shorter duration of action. The physician would not prescribe beta-receptor blocking agents in clients with suspected or confirmed pheochromocytoma until after alpha-adrenergic blockade has been initiated, because these medications may cause the blood pressure to rise. After alpha-adrenergic blockade, low doses of propranolol (Inderal) may be used to treat tachycardia and dysrhythmias.
Test-Taking Strategy: Use the process of elimination. Note that the question asks about hypertensive crisis, and such a situation requires immediate intervention. Recalling that phentolamine mesylate (Regitine) is a short-acting medication will direct you to this option. Review medications to treat hypertensive crisis if you had difficulty with this question.
Level of Cognitive Ability: Analysis
Client Needs: Physiological Integrity
Integrated Concept/Process: Nursing Process/Analysis
Content Area: Adult Health/Endocrine
Reference: Ignatavicius, D., Workman, M., & Mishler, M. (1999). *Medical-surgical nursing across the health care continuum* (3rd ed.). Philadelphia: W.B. Saunders, p. 1611.

46. 1
Rationale: The client with pheochromocytoma needs to be provided with a diet high in vitamins, minerals, and calories. Of particular importance are the foods or beverages that contain caffeine, such as cocoa, coffee, tea, or colas. These foods are prohibited because they can precipitate a hypertensive crisis.
Test-Taking Strategy: Use the process of elimination. Note that options 2, 3, and 4 are similar in that they all include a drink that contains caffeine. This strategy represents selection of the option that is different. Review dietary measures for the client with pheochromocytoma if you had difficulty with this question.
Level of Cognitive Ability: Application
Client Needs: Physiological Integrity
Integrated Concept/Process: Nursing Process/Implementation
Content Area: Adult Health/Endocrine
Reference: Ignatavicius, D., Workman, M., & Mishler, M. (1999). *Medical-surgical nursing across the health care continuum* (3rd ed.). Philadelphia: W.B. Saunders. p. 1611.

47. 2
Rationale: The complications associated with pheochromocytoma include hypertensive retinopathy and nephropathy, myocarditis, increased platelet aggregation, and cerebrovascular accident (CVA). Death can occur from shock, CVA, renal failure, dysrhythmias, or dissecting aortic aneurysm. An irregular heart rate indicates the presence of a dysrhythmia. A urinary output of 50 mL per hour is an adequate output. A BUN of 20 mg/dL is a normal finding. A coagulation time of 5 minutes is normal.
Test-Taking Strategy: Use the process of elimination and the ABCs—airway, breathing, and circulation. An irregular heart rate is associated with circulation. In addition, if you knew the normal hourly expectations associated with urinary output and the normal laboratory values for coagulation time and BUN, you would easily be directed to option 2. Review the complications associated with pheochromocytoma if you had difficulty with this question.
Level of Cognitive Ability: Analysis
Client Needs: Physiological Integrity
Integrated Concept/Process: Nursing Process/Assessment
Content Area: Adult Health/Endocrine
Reference: Smeltzer, S., & Bare, B. (2000). *Brunner & Suddarth's textbook of medical-surgical nursing* (9th ed). Philadelphia: Lippincott Williams & Wilkins, p. 1056.

48. 2
Rationale: Aspirin and other over-the-counter medications should not be taken unless the client consults with the physician. The client needs to take the medication at the same time every day and should be instructed not to stop the medication. A slight weight gain as a result of an improved appetite is expected, but after the dosage is stabilized, a weight gain of 5 pounds or more weekly should be reported to the physician. Caffeine-containing foods and fluids need to be avoided because they may contribute to steroid-ulcer development.
Test-Taking Strategy: Use the process of elimination, noting the key words "further teaching is necessary." Remember that a client should not take other medications, especially over-the-counter medications, without first consulting with his or her physician. Review teaching points for the client taking prednisone if you had difficulty with this question.
Level of Cognitive Ability: Analysis
Client Needs: Health Promotion and Maintenance
Integrated Concept/Process: Nursing Process/Evaluation
Content Area: Adult Health/Endocrine
Reference: Hodgson, B., & Kizior, R. (2001). *Saunders nursing drug handbook 2001.* Philadelphia: W.B. Saunders, p. 857.

49. 2
Rationale: A high-sodium, high-complex-carbohydrate, and high-protein diet will be prescribed for the client with Addison's disease. To prevent excess fluid and sodium loss, the client is instructed to maintain an adequate salt intake daily and to increase salt intake during hot weather, before strenuous exercise, and in response to fever, vomiting, or diarrhea.
Test-Taking Strategy: Use the process of elimination and knowledge regarding the pathophysiology associated with Addison's disease to answer this question. If you are unfamiliar with this disorder, review the pathophysiology and dietary measures associated with Addison's disease.
Level of Cognitive Ability: Analysis
Client Needs: Health Promotion and Maintenance
Integrated Concept/Process: Nursing Process/Planning
Content Area: Adult Health/Endocrine
Reference: Monahan, F., & Neighbors, M. (1998). *Medical-surgical nursing: Foundations for clinical practice* (2nd ed.). Philadelphia: W.B. Saunders, p. 1284.

50. 1
Rationale: Cushing's syndrome is characterized by an oversecretion of glucocorticoid hormones. Addison's disease is characterized by the failure of the adrenal cortex to produce and secrete adrenocorticol hormones. Options 3 and 4 are inaccurate regarding Cushing's syndrome.

Test-Taking Strategy: Use the process of elimination. Option 3 can be easily eliminated if you remember that in Cushing's (up) syndrome there is an oversecretion and in Addison's (down) diseae there is an undersecretion. This may assist in answering questions similar to this one. Review the pathophysiology associated with Cushing's syndrome if you had difficulty with this question.
Level of Cognitive Ability: Analysis
Client Needs: Physiological Integrity
Integrated Concept/Process: Teaching/Learning
Content Area: Adult Health/Endocrine
Reference: Monahan, F., & Neighbors, M. (1998). *Medical-surgical nursing: Foundations for clinical practice* (2nd ed.). Philadelphia: W.B. Saunders. p. 1285.

CRITICAL THINKING: FREE-TEXT ENTRY

Answer: Morphine sulfate
Rationale: Medications are administered very cautiously to the client with hypothyroidism because of altered metabolism and excretion and depressed metabolic rate and respiratory status. Morphine sulfate would further depress bodily functions. Levothyroxine sodium (Synthroid), a thyroid hormone, is a component of therapy. Stool softeners, such as docusate sodium (Colace), are prescribed to prevent constipation.
Test-Taking Strategy: Keeping in mind that a depressed metabolic rate occurs in the client with hypothyroidism will assist in identifying the medication order that requires verification. Review the pathophysiology associated with hypothyroidism if you had difficulty with this question.
Level of Cognitive Ability: Analysis
Client Needs: Safe, Effective Care Environment
Integrated Concept/Process: Nursing Process/Analysis
Content Area: Adult Health/Endocrine
Reference: Smeltzer, S., & Bare, B. (2000). *Brunner & Suddarth's textbook of medical-surgical nursing* (9th ed.). Philadelphia: Lippincott Williams & Wilkins, p. 1040.

REFERENCES

Hodgson, B., & Kizior, R. (2001). *Saunders nursing drug handbook 2001.* Philadelphia: W.B. Saunders.

Ignatavicius, D., Workman, M., & Mishler, M. (1999). *Medical-surgical nursing: Across the health care continuum* (3rd ed.). Philadelphia: W.B. Saunders.

Leahy, J., & Kizilay, P. (1998). *Foundations of nursing practice: A nursing process approach.* Philadelphia: W.B. Saunders.

Lehne, R. (1998). *Pharmacology for nursing care* (3rd ed.). Philadelphia: W.B. Saunders.

LeMone, P., & Burke, K. (2000). *Medical-surgical nursing: Critical thinking in client care* (2nd ed.). Upper Saddle River, N.J.: Prentice-Hall.

Lewis, S., Heitkemper, M., & Dirksen, S. (2000). *Medical-surgical nursing: Assessment and management of clinical problems* (5th ed.). St. Louis: Mosby.

Monahan, F., & Neighbors, M. (1998). *Medical-surgical nursing: Foundations for clinical practice* (2nd ed.). Philadelphia: W. B. Saunders.

Phipps, W., Sands, J., & Marek, J. (1999). *Medical-surgical nursing: Concepts & clinical practice* (6th ed.). St. Louis: Mosby.

Potter, P., & Perry, A. (2001). *Fundamentals of nursing* (5th ed.). St. Louis: Mosby.

Smeltzer, S., & Bare, B. (2000). *Brunner & Suddarth's textbook of medical-surgical nursing* (9th ed.). Philadelphia: Lippincott Williams & Wilkins.

Endocrine Medications

I. PITUITARY MEDICATIONS

A. Description
1. Anterior pituitary gland: Secretes growth hormone (GH), thyroid-stimulating hormone (TSH), adrenocorticotropic hormone (ACTH), and gonadotropins (follicle-stimulating hormone, or FSH, and luteinizing hormone, or LH)
2. Posterior pituitary gland: Secretes antidiuretic hormones (ADH, vasopressin) and oxytocin

B. Growth hormones and related medications
1. Uses and side effects (Table 52-1)
2. Implementation
   a. Assess child's physical growth and compare growth with standards
   b. Recommend annual bone age determinations for children receiving growth hormones
   c. Monitor blood and urine glucose levels
   d. Teach the client and family about the importance of follow-up regarding blood and urine glucose testing

II. ANTIDIURETIC HORMONES (Box 52-1)

A. Description
1. Enhance reabsorption of water in the kidneys, promoting an antidiuretic effect and regulating fluid balance
2. Used in **diabetes insipidus**

B. Side effects
1. Flushing
2. Headache
3. Nausea and abdominal cramps
4. Water intoxication
5. Hypertension with water intoxication
6. Nasal congestion with nasal administration

BOX 52-1

Antidiuretic Hormones

Desmopressin acetate (DDAVP, Stimate)
Lypressin (Diapid)
Vasopressin (Pitressin)

TABLE 52-1

Growth Hormones and Related Medications

Medication(s)	Use	Side Effects
Somatrem (Protropin)	Growth failure	Development of antibodies to GH
Somatropin (Humatrope)	Growth failure	Headache, muscle pain, weakness,
		Mild hyperglycemia, allergic reaction (rash, swelling), pain at injection site
Sermorelin (Geref)	Growth failure	Pain, swelling, redness at injection site; facial flushing, nausea,
	Diagnose pituitary function	vomiting, headache, altered taste, chest tightness
Bromocriptine (Parlodel)	Acromegaly	Nausea, headache, dizziness
Octreotide (Sandostatin)	Acromegaly	Diarrhea, nausea, abdominal discomfort, increased glucose

▲ C. Implementation
1. Monitor weight
2. Monitor intake and output (I & O) and urine osmolality
3. Monitor electrolytes
4. Restrict fluid intake as prescribed to prevent water intoxication
5. Monitor for signs of water intoxication, such as drowsiness, listlessness, and headache
6. Instruct the client in how to use the intranasal medication
7. Instruct the client to report signs of water intoxication or symptoms of headache or shortness of breath

▲ III. THYROID HORMONES (Box 52-2)
A. Description
1. Control the metabolic rate of tissues and accelerate heat production and oxygen consumption
2. To replace hormonal deficit in the treatment of **hypothyroidism, myxedema,** or cretinism
3. Enhance the action of oral anticoagulants, sympathomimetics, and antidepressants, and decrease the action of insulin, oral hypoglycemics, and digitalis preparations
4. Phenytoin (Dilantin) and aspirin can enhance the action of thyroid hormone

▲ B. Side effects
1. Nausea and vomiting
2. Cramps and diarrhea
3. Weight loss
4. Nervousness and tremors
5. Headache
6. Hypertension
7. Tachycardia and dysrhythmias
8. Sweating and heat intolerance
9. Insomnia
10. Toxicity: **Hyperthyroidism**

▲ C. Implementation
1. Assess client for history of medications currently being taken
2. Monitor vital signs
3. Monitor weight
4. Monitor triiodothyronine (T_3), thyroxine (T_4), and thyroid-stimulating hormone (TSH) levels
▲ 5. Instruct the client to take the medication at the same time each day, preferably in the morning without food
6. Instruct the client in how to monitor pulse rate ▲
7. Advise the client to report symptoms of **hyper-** ▲ **thyroidism,** such as tachycardia, chest pain, palpitations, and excessive sweating
8. Instruct the client to avoid foods that can inhibit thyroid secretion, such as strawberries, peaches, pears, cabbage, turnips, spinach, kale, Brussels sprouts, cauliflower, radishes, and peas
9. Advise the client to avoid over-the-counter-medications
10. Instruct the client to wear a Medic-Alert bracelet

IV. ANTITHYROID MEDICATIONS (Box 52-3) ▲
A. Description
1. Inhibit the synthesis of thyroid hormone ▲
2. Used for **hyperthyroidism,** or **Graves' disease**
B. Side effects
1. Nausea and vomiting
2. Diarrhea
3. Hypersensitivity
4. Agranulocytosis ▲
5. Toxicity: **Hypothyroidism**
6. Iodism: Characterized by vomiting, abdominal pain, metallic taste in the mouth, rash, and sore salivary glands
C. Implementation ▲
1. Monitor vital signs
2. Monitor T_3, T_4, and TSH levels
3. Monitor weight
4. Instruct the client to take medication with meals ▲ to avoid gastrointestinal (GI) upset
5. Instruct the client in how to monitor the ▲ pulse rate
6. Inform the client of side effects and when to notify the physician
7. Advise the client to contact the physician if a fever or sore throat develops
8. Instruct the client in the signs of **hypothyroidism**
9. Instruct the client regarding the importance of medication compliance and that abruptly stopping the medication could cause thyroid crisis **(thyroid storm)**
10. Instruct the client to monitor for signs and ▲ symptoms of thyroid crisis (fever, flushed skin,

---

BOX 52-2

Thyroid Hormones

Levothyroxine (Synthroid, Levothroid, Levoxyl)
Liothyronine (Cytomel)
Liotrix (Thyrolar)
Thyroglobulin (Proloid)
Thyroid (Thyrar)

BOX 52-3

Antithyroid Medications

Iodine solution (Lugol solution, potassium iodide solution)
Methimazole (Tapazole)
Propylthiouracil (PTU)

confusion and behavioral changes, tachycardia, dysrhythmias, and signs of heart failure)
11. Instruct the client to monitor for signs of iodism
12. Advise the client to consult physician before eating iodized salt and iodine-rich foods
13. Instruct the client to avoid acetylsalicylic acid (aspirin) and medications containing iodine

V. PARATHYROID MEDICATIONS (Box 52-4)
A. Description
1. Parathyroid hormone regulates serum calcium levels
2. Low serum levels of calcium stimulate parathyroid hormone release
3. Hyperparathyroidism results in a high serum calcium level and bone demineralization, and medication is used to lower the serum calcium level
4. Hypoparathyroidism results in a low serum calcium level, which increases neuromuscular excitability, and the treatment includes calcium and vitamin D supplements
5. Parathyroid and antihypercalcemic agents may cause hypermagnesemia

6. Calcium salts administered with digoxin (Lanoxin) increases the risk of digoxin toxicity
7. Oral calcium salts reduce the absorption of tetracycline hydrochloride
B. Implementation
1. Monitor electrolyte and calcium levels
2. Assess for signs and symptoms of hypocalcemia and hypercalcemia
3. Assess for symptoms of tetany in the client with hypocalcemia
4. Instruct the client in the signs and symptoms of hypercalcemia and hypocalcemia
5. Instruct the client to check over-the-counter medication labels for the possibility of calcium content
6. Instruct the client receiving oral calcium to maintain an adequate intake of vitamin D, because vitamin D enhances absorption of calcium

VI. ADRENOCORTICOTROPIC HORMONES (Box 52-5)
A. Description
1. Stimulate the adrenal cortex to secrete cortisol
2. Produce an antiinflammatory effect
3. Used to diagnose adrenocortical disorders (Box 52-6)
4. Used to treat acute multiple sclerosis
B. Side effects
1. Nausea and vomiting
2. Increased appetite
3. Mood swings
4. Petechiae

BOX 52-4

Medications to Treat Calcium Disorders

CALCIUM SUPPLEMENTS
Calcium carbonate (BioCal, Caltrate 600, Rolaids, Tums)
Calcium carbonate, oyster-shell derived (OsCal 500, Oysco, Oyst-Cal)
Calcium citrate (Citracal)
Calcium glubionate (Calcionate, Neo-Calglucon)
Calcium gluconate
Calcium lactate
Dibasic calcium phosphate
Tribasic calcium phosphate (Posture)

VITAMIN D SUPPLEMENTS
Calcifediol (Calderol)
Calcitriol (Calcijex, Rocaltrol)
Dihydrotachysterol (DHT, Hytakerol)
Ergocalciferol (Calciferol, Drisdol)

CALCIUM REGULATORS
Alendronate (Fosamax)
Calcitonin human (Cibacalcin)
Calcitonin salmon (Calcimar, Miacalcin)
Etidronate (Didronel)
Pamidronate (Aredia)
Risedronate (Actonel)
Tiludronate (Skelid)

ANTIHYPERCALCEMICS
Edetate disodium (Disotate. Endrate)
Gallium nitrate (Ganite)

BOX 52-5

Medications for Adrenal Replacement Therapy

Betamethasone (Celestone)
Cortisone (Cortone)
Fludrocortisone (Florinef)
Hydrocortisone (Cortef)
Triamcinolone (Aristocort, Kenacort)
Dexamethasone (Decadron)
Methylprednisolone (Depo-Medrol, Solu-Medrol)
Prednisolone (Delta-Cortef, Prelone)
Prednisone (Orasone, Deltasone, Meticorten)

BOX 52-6

Medications Used in Diagnosing Adrenal Gland Dysfunction

Corticotropin (Acthar)
Corticotropin repository (Acthar gel)
Cosyntropin (Cortrosyn)

5. Water and sodium retention
6. Hypokalemia
7. Hypocalcemia

C. Implementation
1. Monitor vital signs
2. Monitor I & O, weight, and for edema
3. Monitor for signs of infection
4. Monitor electrolyte and calcium levels
5. Avoid administering to the client with adrenocortical hyperfunction
6. Instruct the client to decrease salt intake
7. Instruct the client to report side effects such as muscle weakness, edema, petechiae, ecchymosis, decrease in growth, decreased wound healing, and menstrual irregularities
8. Monitor for adverse effects when the medication is discontinued; dose should be tapered and not stopped abruptly, because adrenal hypofunction may result
9. Advise the client to wear Medic-Alert bracelet

VII. CORTICOSTEROIDS (GLUCOCORTICOIDS)
(Box 52-5)

A. Description
1. Produce metabolic effects
2. Alter the normal immune response and suppress inflammation
3. Promote sodium and water retention and potassium excretion
4. Produce antiinflammatory, antiallergic, and anti-stress effects
5. May be used as a replacement for adrenocortical insufficiency

B. Side effects
1. **Hyperglycemia**
2. Hypokalemia
3. Sodium and water retention
4. Edema
5. Cause muscle wasting, osteoporosis, growth retardation in children, peptic ulcer, increased serum glucose levels, hypertension, convulsions, mood swings, cataracts, glaucoma, fragile skin, hirsutism, altered fat distribution
6. Mask the signs and symptoms of infection

C. Contraindications and cautions
1. Contraindicated in hypersensitivity, psychosis, and fungal infections
2. Use with caution in **diabetes mellitus**
3. Dexamethasone (Decadron) decreases the effects of oral anticoagulants and oral antidiabetic agents
4. Increase the potency of medications taken concurrently, such as aspirin, and nonsteroidal antiinflammatory drugs (NSAIDs), thus increasing the risk of GI bleeding and ulceration
5. Use of potassium-wasting diuretics increases potassium loss, resulting in hypokalemia

6. Barbiturates, phenytoin (Dilantin), and rifampin (Rifadin) decrease the effect of prednisone
7. The action of dexamethasone (Decadron) is decreased by the use of phenytoin (Dilantin), theophylline, rifampin (Rifadin), barbiturates, and antacids
8. NSAIDs, aspirin, and estrogen increase the effect of dexamethasone (Decadron)
9. Should be used with extreme caution in clients with infections because they mask the signs and symptoms of an infection
10. Advise the client to wear Medic-Alert bracelet

D. Implementation
1. Monitor vital signs
2. Monitor serum electrolytes and blood glucose level
3. Monitor for hypokalemia and **hyperglycemia**
4. Monitor I & O, weight, and for edema
5. Monitor for hypertension
6. Assess medical history for glaucoma, cataracts, peptic ulcer, mental health disorders, or **diabetes mellitus**
7. Monitor the older client for signs and symptoms of increased osteoporosis
8. Assess for changes in muscle strength
9. Prepare a schedule for the client on short-term, tapered doses
10. Instruct the client to take at mealtime or with food
11. Advise the client to eat foods high in potassium
12. Instruct the client to avoid individuals with respiratory infections
13. Advise the client to inform all health care providers of taking the medication
14. Instruct the client to report signs and symptoms of a medication overdose or **Cushing's syndrome**, including a moon face, puffy eyelids, edema in the feet, increased bruising, dizziness, bleeding, and menstrual irregularities
15. Note that the client may need additional doses during periods of stress, such as surgery
16. Instruct the client not to stop medication abruptly, as abrupt withdrawal can result in severe adrenal insufficiency
17. Advise the client to consult with the physician before receiving vaccinations
18. Advise the client to wear Medic-Alert bracelet

E. Mineralocorticoids
1. Description
   a. Steroid hormones that enhance the reabsorption of sodium and chloride and promote the excretion of potassium and hydrogen from the renal tubules, thereby helping to maintain fluid and electrolyte balance
   b. Used for replacement therapy in primary and secondary adrenal insufficiency in **Addison's disease**

2. Medication: Fludrocortisone (Florinef)
3. Side effects
   a. Sodium and water retention
   b. Hypokalemia
   c. Hypocalcemia
   d. Increased susceptibility to infection
   e. Delayed wound healing
   f. GI distress
   g. Diarrhea or constipation
   h. Increased appetite
   i. Weight gain
   j. Insomnia
   k. Mood swings
   l. Abdominal distention
4. Implementation
   a. Monitor vital signs
   b. Monitor weight
   c. Monitor electrolytes and calcium level
   d. Instruct the client to take medication with food or milk
   e. Instruct the client to consume a high-potassium diet
   f. Instruct the client not to stop the medication abruptly
   g. Instruct the client to notify the physician if signs of infection, muscle aches, sudden weight gain, or headaches occur
   h. Instruct the client to avoid exposure to disease or trauma
   i. Instruct the client not to take aspirin or any other medication without consulting the physician
   j. Instruct the client to wear a Medic-Alert bracelet

VIII. ANDROGENS (Box 52-7)

A. Description
   1. Used either to replace deficient hormones or to treat hormone-sensitive disorders
   2. Can cause bleeding if the client is taking oral anticoagulants (increase the effect of anticoagulants)
   3. Cause decreased serum glucose concentration, thereby reducing insulin requirements in the client with **diabetes mellitus**
   4. Hepatotoxic medications are avoided with the use of androgens because of the risk of additive damage to the liver
   5. Usually avoided in men with known prostatic or breast carcinoma because androgens often stimulate growth of these tumors
B. Side effects
   1. Masculine secondary sexual characteristics (body hair growth, lowered voice, muscle growth)
   2. Bladder irritation and urinary tract infections
   3. Breast tenderness
   4. Gynecomastia
   5. Priapism

BOX 52-7

Androgens

Fluoxymesterone (Android-F, Halotestin)
Methyltestosterone (Android, Testred, Virilon)
Testosterone (Andro, Histerone, Testaqua)
Testosterone (Androderm, Testoderm)
Testosterone (Testopel pellets)
Testosterone cypionate (Andronate, Depotest, Virilon-IM)
Testosterone enanthate (Delatest, Delatestryl, Everone)
Testosterone propionate (Testex)

---

   6. Menstrual irregularities
   7. Virilism
   8. Edema
   9. Nausea, vomiting, or diarrhea
   10. Acne
   11. Changes in libido
   12. Hepatotoxicity
C. Implementation
   1. Monitor vital signs
   2. Monitor for edema, weight gain, and skin changes
   3. Assess mental status and neurological function
   4. Assess for signs of liver dysfunction, including right upper quadrant abdominal pain, malaise, fever, jaundice, pruritus
   5. Assess for the development of secondary sexual characteristics
   6. Instruct the client to take with meals or a snack
   7. Instruct the client to notify the physician if priapism develops
   8. Instruct the client to notify the physician if fluid retention occurs
   9. Instruct women to use a nonhormonal contraceptive while on therapy

IX. ESTROGENS AND PROGESTINS

A. Description
   1. Estrogens are steroids that stimulate female reproductive tissue
   2. Progestins are steroids that specifically stimulate the uterine lining
   3. Estrogen and progestin preparations may be used to stimulate the endogenous hormones to restore hormonal balance or to treat hormone-sensitive tumors (suppress tumor growth) (Boxes 52-8 and 52-9)
B. Contraindications and cautions
   1. Estrogens
      a. Contraindicated in clients with breast cancer, endometrial hyperplasia, or endometrial cancer
      b. Increase the risk of toxicity when used with hepatotoxic medications
   2. Progestins: Contraindicated in clients with

BOX 52-8

Estrogens

Chlorotrianisene (Tace)
Dienestrol (Dienestrol)
Diethylstibesterol (DES)
Estradiol (Estrace, Climara, Estraderm, FemPatch, Vivelle)
Estradiol cypionate (Depo-Estradiol)
Estradiol valerate (Delestrogen)
Estrogens, conjugated (Premarin)
Estrogens, esterified (Estratab)
Estrone (Aquest, Estragyn 5)
Estropipate (Ogen Ortho-Est)
Ethinyl Estradiol (Estinyl)

BOX 52-9

Progestins

Hydroxyprogesterone (Hylutin)
Levonorgestrel (Norplant)
Medroxyprogesterone (Cycrin, Provera)
Medroxyprogesterone (Depo-Provera)
Medroxyprogesterone and conjugated estrogens
  (Premphase, Prempro)
Megestrol (Megace)
Norethindrone acetate (Aygestin)
Progesterone (Prometrium)
Progesterone (Gesterol, Crinone, Progestasert)

---

thromboembolitic disorders, and avoided in clients with breast tumors or hepatic disease

C. Side effects
1. Breast tenderness
2. Nausea, vomiting, and diarrhea
3. Malaise, depression, excessive irritability
4. Weight gain
5. Edema and fluid retention
6. Atherosclerosis
7. Hypertension
8. Migraine headaches and vomiting (estrogen)

▲ D. Implementation
1. Monitor vital signs
2. Monitor for hypertension
3. Assess for edema and weight gain
4. Advise the client not to smoke
5. Advise the client to undergo routine breast and pelvic examinations

X. ORAL CONTRACEPTIVES

A. Description
1. These medications contain a combination of estrogen and a progestin or a progestin alone
2. Estrogen-progestin combinations suppress ovulation and change the cervical mucus, making it difficult for sperm to enter

3. Medications that contain only progestins are less effective than the combined medications
4. Usually taken for 21 consecutive days and stopped for 7 days; then the administration cycle is repeated
5. Provide reversible prevention of pregnancy
6. Useful in controlling irregular or excessive menstrual cycles
7. Risk factors associated with the development of ▲ complications related to the use of oral contraceptives include smoking, obesity, and hypertension
8. Contraindicated in women with hypertension ▲ or thrombolytic disease
9. Avoided with the use of hepatotoxic medi- ▲ cations
10. Interfere with the activity of bromocriptine (Parlodel) and anticoagulants and increase the toxicity of tricyclic antidepressants
11. May alter blood glucose levels

B. Side effects
1. Breakthrough bleeding
2. Excessive cervical mucus formation
3. Breast tenderness

C. Implementation ▲
1. Monitor vital signs and weight
2. Instruct the client in the administration of the medication (it may take up to 1 week for full contraceptive effect to occur when the medication is begun)
3. Instruct the client with **diabetes mellitus** to monitor blood glucose levels carefully
4. Instruct the client to report signs of thromboembolitic complications
5. Instruct the client to notify the physician if vaginal bleeding or menstrual irregularities occur or if pregnancy is suspected
6. Inform the client that many medications interfere with the effectiveness of birth control pills
7. Instruct the client to perform breast self-examination monthly and about the importance of yearly physical examinations
8. If the client decides to discontinue the oral contraceptive to become pregnant, recommend that the client use an alternative form of birth control for 2 months after discontinuation to ensure more complete excretion of hormonal agents before conception

XI. FERTILITY MEDICATIONS (Box 52-10)

A. Description
1. Act to stimulate follicle development and ovulation in functioning ovaries and are combined with human chorionic gonadotropin (HCG) to maintain the follicles once ovulation has occurred
2. Contraindicated in the presence of primary ovarian function, thyroid or adrenal dysfunction,

---

BOX 52-10

Fertility Medications

Bromocriptine (Parlodel)
Chorionic gonadotropin (A.P.L., Profasi)
Clomiphene (Clomid)
Follitropin alfa (Gonal-F)
Follitropin beta (Follistin)
Menotropins (Humegon, Pergonal)
Urofollitropin (Metrodin, Fertinex)

---

ovarian cysts, pregnancy, or idiopathic uterine bleeding

3. Used with caution in clients with thromboembolitic or respiratory diseases

B. Side effects
1. Risk of multiple births and birth defects
2. Ovarian overstimulation (abdominal pain, distention, ascites, pleural effusion)
3. Headache
4. Fluid retention and bloating
5. Nausea
6. Uterine bleeding
7. Ovarian enlargement
8. Gynecomastia
9. Febrile reactions

C. Implementation
1. Instruct the client regarding administration of the medication
2. Provide a calendar of treatment days and instructions on when intercourse should occur, to increase therapeutic effectiveness of the medication
3. Provide information about the risks and hazards of multiple births
4. Instruct the client to notify the physician if signs of ovarian stimulation occur
5. Inform the client about the need for regular follow-up for evaluation

XII. MEDICATIONS FOR PENILE ERECTION DYSFUNCTION

A. Description
1. Alprostadil (Caverject, MUSE) is a prostaglandin that relaxes smooth muscle and promotes blood flow into the corpus cavernosum
2. Sildenafil (Viagara) may be classified as a cardiovascular agent and selectively inhibits receptors and increases nitrous oxide levels, allowing blood flow into the corpus cavernosum
3. Contraindicated in the presence of any anatomical obstruction or condition that might predispose to priapism and in clients with penile implants
4. Caution should be used in clients with bleeding disorders

5. Sildenafil (Viagara) is used cautiously in clients with coronary artery disease, active peptic ulcer, or retinitis pigmentosa
6. Sildenafil (Viagara) cannot be administered to clients taking any organic nitrates

B. Side effects
1. Alprostadil (Caverject, MUSE): Pain at the injection site, infection, priapism, fibrosis, rash
2. Sildenafil (Viagara); Headache, flushing, dyspepsia, urinary tract infection, diarrhea, dizziness, rash

C. Implementation
1. Perform a thorough assessment of health and medication history
2. Instruct the client regarding administration of the medication; alprostadil (Caverject, MUSE) is injected, and sildenafil (Viagara) is taken orally
3. Inform the client of the side effects necessitating the need to notify the physician

XIII. MEDICATIONS FOR DIABETES MELLITUS

A. Insulin and oral hypoglycemic medications
1. Description
   a. Insulin increases glucose transport into cells and promotes conversion of glucose to glycogen, decreasing serum glucose levels
   b. Oral hypoglycemic agents stimulate the pancreas to produce more insulin and increase the sensitivity of peripheral receptors to insulin, thereby decreasing serum glucose levels
2. Contraindications and concerns
   a. Insulin is contraindicated in clients with hypersensitivity
   b. Oral hypoglycemic agents are contraindicated in type 1 **diabetes mellitus** and in individuals allergic to sulfonylureas
   c. Sulfonylureas can affect cardiac function and oxygen consumption and lead to cardiac dysrhythmias
   d. Use of hypoglycemic medications with beta-adrenergic blocking agents masks signs and symptoms of **hypoglycemia**
   e. Anticoagulants, chloramphenicol (Chloromycetin), clofibrate (Atromid-S), salicylates, propranolol (Inderal), monoamine oxidase inhibitors (MAOIs), pentamidine (Pentam-300), and sulfonamides may cause **hypoglycemia**
   f. Corticosteroids, sympathomimetics, thiazide diuretics, phenytoin (Dilantin), thyroid preparations, oral contraceptives, and estrogen compounds may cause **hyperglycemia**
   g. Side effects of the sulfonylureas include gastrointestinal symptoms and dermatological reactions; **hypoglycemia** can occur when an excessive dose is administered or when meals are omitted or delayed, food intake is decreased, or activity is increased

h. Chlorpropamide (Diabenese) can cause a disulfiram (Antabuse) type of reaction when alcohol is ingested
B. Oral hypoglycemic medications
1. Prescribed for clients with type 2 **diabetes mellitus**
2. Sulfonylureas
a. Classified as first- or second-generation sulfonylureas (Box 52-11)
b. Stimulate the beta cells to produce more insulin
3. Nonsulfonylureas (Box 52-11)
a. Affect the hepatic and gastrointestinal production of glucose
b. May be used in combination with a sulfonylurea
4. Implementation
a. Assess the client's knowledge of **diabetes mellitus** and the use of oral antidiabetic agents
b. Obtain a medication history regarding the medications that the client is currently taking
c. Assess vital signs and blood glucose levels
d. Instruct the client to recognize symptoms of **hypoglycemia** and **hyperglycemia**
e. Instruct the client to avoid over-the-counter medications unless prescribed by the physician
f. Instruct the client not to ingest alcohol with sulfonylureas
g. Inform the client that insulin may be needed during stress, surgery, or infection
h. Instruct the client in the necessity of compliance with prescribed medication
i. Advise the client to obtain a Medic-Alert bracelet

C. Insulin (Table 52-2)
1. Primarily acts in the liver, muscle, and adipose tissue by attaching to receptors on cellular membranes and facilitating the passage of glucose, potassium, and magnesium

---

BOX 52-11

First- and Second-Generation Sulfonylureas and Nonsulfonylureas

FIRST-GENERATION SULFONYLUREAS
Short Acting
Tolbutamide (Orinase)
Intermediate Acting
Acetohexamide (Dymelor)
Tolazamide (Tolinase)
Long Acting
Chlorpropamide (Diabenese)

SECOND-GENERATION SULFONYLUREAS
Glipizide (Glucotrol, Glucotrol XL)
Glyburide (DiaBeta, Micronase, Glynase)
Glimepiride (Amaryl)

NONSULFONYLUREAS
Biguanide
Metformin (Glucophage)
Alpha Glucosidase Inhibitor
Acarbose (Precose)
Miglitol (Glyset)
Thiozolidinediones
Troglitazone (Rezulin)
Pioglitazone (Actos)
Rosiglitazone (Avandia)
Meglitinide
Rapaglinide (Prandin)

TABLE 52-2

Common Types of Insulin

Type	Onset	Peak	Duration
RAPID-ACTING INSULIN			
Lispro (Humalog)	10-15 minutes	1 hour	3 hours
SHORT-ACTING INSULIN			
Humulin Regular	0.5-1 hour	2-3 hours	4-6 hours
INTERMEDIATE-ACTING INSULIN			
Humulin NPH	3-4 hours	4-12 hours	16-20 hours
Humulin Lente	3-4 hours	4-12 hours	16-20 hours
LONG-ACTING INSULIN			
Humulin Ultralente	6-8 hours	12-16 hours	20-30 hours
PREMIXED INSULIN			
70% NPH and 30% Regular	0.5-1 hour	2-12 hours	18-24 hours

2. Prescribed for clients with type 1 **diabetes mellitus**
3. Storing insulin
   a. Exposure to extremes in temperature is avoided; insulin should not be frozen or kept in direct sunlight or a hot car
   b. Before injection, insulin should be at room temperature
   c. If a vial of insulin will be used up in a month, it may be kept at room temperature; otherwise, the vial should be refrigerated
4. Insulin injection sites
   a. The main areas for injections are the abdomen, arms (posterior surface), thighs (anterior surface), and hips
   b. Insulin injected into the abdomen may absorb more evenly and rapidly than at other sites
   c. Systematic rotation within one anatomical area is recommended to prevent lipodystrophy; client should be instructed not to use the same site more than once in a 2- to 3-week period
   d. Injections should be 1.5 inches apart within the anatomical area
   e. Heat, massage, and exercise of the injected area can increase absorption rates and may result in **hypoglycemia**
   f. Injection into scar tissue may delay absorption of insulin
5. Administering insulin
   a. To prevent dosage errors, be certain that there is a match of the insulin concentration noted on the vial with the calibration of units on the insulin syringe; the usual concentration of insulin is U 100 (100 units per mL)
   b. Most insulin syringes have a 27- to 29-gauge needle that is approximately 0.5 inch long
   c. Before use, roll, not shake (to avoid bubbles) the insulin bottle to ensure that the insulin and ingredients are mixed well; otherwise an inaccurate dose will be drawn.
   d. Premixed insulins (NPH to Regular insulin) are available as 70/30 (most commonly used), 80/20, 60/40, 50/50
   e. A 3-week supply of insulin may be prepared and kept in the refrigerator; prefilled syringes should be kept flat or with the needle in an upright position to avoid clogging of the needle
   f. Inject air into the insulin bottle (a vacuum makes it difficult to draw up the insulin)
   g. It is recommended to draw up the Regular (shorter-acting) insulin first
   h. Regular Insulin may be mixed with any other type of insulin
   i. Insulin zinc suspensions may be mixed only with each other and Regular insulin, not with other types of insulin
   j. Administer a mixed dose of insulin within 5 to 15 minutes of preparation; after this time the Regular insulin binds with the NPH insulin and its action is reduced
   k. Aspiration is generally not recommended with self-injection of insulin
   l. Administer insulin at a 45- to 90-degree angle and at a 45- to 60-degree angle in thin persons
   m. REMEMBER: Regular insulin is the only type of insulin that can be administered by IV

D. Glucagon
   1. A hormone secreted by the alpha cells of the islets of Langerhans in the pancreas
   2. Increases blood glucose by stimulating glycogenolysis in the liver
   3. Can be administered by SC, IM, or IV routes
   4. Used to treat insulin-induced **hypoglycemia** when the client is semiconscious or unconscious and is unable to ingest liquids
   5. The blood glucose level begins to increase within 5 to 20 minutes after administration
   6. Instruct the family in the procedure for administration
   7. Refer to Chapter 51 for additional information regarding implementation for severe **hypoglycemia**

E. Diazoxide (Proglycem)
   1. Increases blood glucose by inhibiting insulin release from the beta cells and stimulating the release of epinephrine from the adrenal medulla
   2. Used to treat chronic **hypoglycemia** caused by hyperinsulinism resulting from islet cell cancer or hyperplasia
   3. It is not used for **hypoglycemic** reactions from insulin

PRACTICE QUESTIONS

1. Somatren (Protropin) is administered to a client with pituitary dwarfism. A nurse monitors the client, knowing that the expected therapeutic effect of this medication is to:
   1. Promote weight gain
   2. Stimulate linear growth
   3. Increase bone density
   4. Decrease the mobilization of fats
2. Desmopressin acetate (DDAVP, Stimate) is prescribed for the treatment of diabetes insipidus. The nurse administering the medication monitors the client, knowing that the primary action of the medication is to:
   1. Decrease permeability in the kidneys to water
   2. Decrease water reabsorption
   3. Increase renal excretion of water
   4. Promote renal conservation of water
3. A nurse is monitoring a client receiving desmopressin acetate (DDAVP, Stimate) for adverse reac-

tions to the medication. Which of the following indicates the presence of an adverse reaction?
1. Increased urination
2. Weight loss
3. Drowsiness
4. Insomnia

4. Vasopressin (Pitressin) is prescribed for a client with diabetes insipidus. A nurse is particularly cautious in monitoring the client receiving this medication if the client has which of the following preexisting conditions?
1. Depression
2. Endometriosis
3. Coronary artery disease
4. Pheochromocytoma

5. A nurse provides instructions to a client who is taking levothyroxine (Synthroid). The nurse tells the client to take the medication:
1. With food
2. On an empty stomach
3. At bedtime with a snack
4. At lunchtime

6. A nurse provides medication instructions to a client who is taking levothyroxine (Synthroid). The nurse instructs the client to notify the physician if which of the following occurs?
1. Cold intolerance
2. Tremors
3. Excessively dry skin
4. Fatigue

7. A nurse performs an admission assessment on a client who visits a health care clinic for the first time. The client tells the nurse that propylthiouracil (PTU) is taken daily. The nurse continues to collect data from the client, suspecting that the client has a history of:
1. Cushing's syndrome
2. Addison's disease
3. Myxedema
4. Graves' disease

8. A nurse is instructing a client regarding the administration of lypressin (Diapid). The nurse instructs the client that the medication will be taken by which of the following routes?
1. Oral
2. Subcutaneous
3. Intranasal
4. Intramuscular

9. A client is receiving somatropin (Humatrope). The nurse monitors which most significant laboratory study during therapy with this medication?
1. Amylase
2. Lipase
3. Blood urea nitrogen (BUN)
4. Thyroid-stimulating hormone (TSH)

10. A client is scheduled for a subtotal thyroidectomy. Iodine solution (Lugol solution, potassium iodide solution) is prescribed. A nurse prepares to administer the medication, knowing that the therapeutic effect of this medication is to:
1. Increase thyroid hormone production
2. Suppress thyroid hormone production
3. Replace thyroid hormone
4. Prevent the oxidation of iodide

11. Iodine solution (Lugol solution, potassium iodide solution) is prescribed for a client with thyrotoxic crisis. The client calls a clinic nurse and complains of a brassy taste and burning sensations in the mouth. The most appropriate instruction to the client is which of the following?
1. Continue with the medication
2. Take half of the prescribed dose for the next 24 hours
3. Stop the medication for the next 24 hours and then continue as prescribed
4. Stop the medication and notify the physician

12. A nurse provides instructions to a client taking fludrocortisone (Florinef). The nurse instructs the client to notify the physician if which of the following occurs?
1. Weight loss
2. Nausea
3. Swelling of the feet
4. Fatigue

13. Calcium carbonate (OsCal) is prescribed for a client with hypocalcemia. A nurse instructs the client to take the medication:
1. With meals
2. One hour after meals
3. Just before meals
4. Every 4 hours

14. Calcitriol (Rocaltrol) is prescribed for a client with hypocalcemia. A nurse provides dietary instructions to the client. Which of the following food items would the nurse instruct the client to avoid while taking this medication?
1. Dark green leafy vegetables
2. Milk
3. Whole grain cereals
4. Sardines

15. A daily dose of prednisone (Deltasone) is prescribed for a client. A nurse provides instructions to the client regarding administration of the medication. The nurse instructs the client that the best time to take this medication is:
1. At bedtime
2. At noon
3. Early morning
4. Anytime, at the same time, each day

16. Prednisone (Deltasone) is prescribed for a client with diabetes mellitus who is taking NPH insulin daily. Which of the following prescriptions does the nurse anticipate during therapy with the prednisone?
1. A decreased amount of daily NPH insulin
2. An increased amount of daily NPH insulin

3. An additional dose of prednisone daily
4. The addition of an oral hypoglycemic medication daily

17. A nurse is teaching a client how to mix Regular insulin and NPH insulin in the same syringe. Which of the following actions, if performed by the client, indicates the need for further teaching?
   1. Injects air into NPH insulin vial first
   2. Injects an amount of air equal to the desired dose of insulin into the vial
   3. Withdraws the NPH insulin first
   4. Withdraws the Regular insulin first

18. A home care nurse visits a client recently diagnosed with diabetes mellitus. The client is taking NPH insulin daily. The client asks the nurse how to store the unopened vials of insulin. The nurse tells the client to:
   1. Freeze the insulin
   2. Refrigerate the insulin
   3. Keep the insulin at room temperature
   4. Store the insulin in a dark, dry place

19. Tolbutamide (Orinase) is prescribed for a client with diabetes mellitus. A nurse instructs the client to avoid which of the following while taking this medication?
   1. Carbonated beverages

2. Organ meats
3. Alcohol
4. Whole grain cereals

20. Sildenafil citrate (Viagra) is prescribed to treat a client with erectile dysfunction. A nurse reviews the client's medical record and would question the prescription if which of the following is noted in the client's history?
   1. Neuralgia
   2. Use of nitroglycerin
   3. Use of multivitamins
   4. Insomnia

CRITICAL THINKING: FREE-TEXT ENTRY

A home care nurse prefills syringes containing NPH and Regular insulin for a client with diabetes mellitus who has difficulty with seeing and accurately preparing dosages. The client can administer the injection. Considering the stability of insulin, how many prefilled syringes will the nurse prepare for the client for self-administration?

Answer: _____

ANSWERS

1. **2**
Rationale: Protropin is a growth stimulator used in the long-term treatment of growth failure resulting from endogenous growth hormone deficiency. It stimulates linear growth and increases the number and size of muscle cells and red cell mass. It affects carbohydrate metabolism by antagonizing the action of insulin, increases mobilization of fats, and increases cellular protein synthesis. Options 1, 3, and 4 are not actions of this medication.
Test-Taking Strategy: Focus on the client's diagnosis to assist in the process of elimination. Note the relationship between "dwarfism" in the question and "growth" in the correct option. Review the action of this medication if you had difficulty with this question.
Level of Cognitive Ability: Analysis
Client Needs: Physiological Integrity
Integrated Concept/Process: Nursing Process/Evaluation
Content Area: Pharmacology
Reference: Hodgson, B., & Kizior, R. (2001). *Saunders nursing drug handbook 2001.* Philadelphia: W.B. Saunders, p. 938.

2. **4**
Rationale: DDAVP promotes renal conservation of water. The hormone accomplishes this by acting on the collecting ducts of the kidney to increase their permeability to water, which results in increased water reabsorption.
Test-Taking Strategy: Use the process of elimination. Focus on the diagnosis in the question to assist in answering the question. Recalling the manifestations related to the loss of large volumes of urine in this disorder will assist in directing you to option 4. Review diabetes insipidus and the action of DDAVP if you had difficulty with this question.
Level of Cognitive Ability: Analysis
Client Needs: Physiological Integrity
Integrated Concept/Process: Nursing Process/Analysis
Content Area: Pharmacology
Reference: Hodgson, B., & Kizior, R. (2001). *Saunders nursing drug handbook 2001.* Philadelphia: W.B. Saunders, p. 294.

3. **3**
Rationale: Water intoxication (overhydration) or hyponatremia is an adverse reaction to DDAVP. Early signs include drowsiness, listlessness, and headache. Decreased urination, rapid weight gain, confusion, seizures, and coma may also occur in overhydration.
Test-Taking Strategy: Use the process of elimination. Knowledge that this medication is used in the treatment of diabetes insipidus will assist in eliminating options 1 and 2. Recalling the action of the medication will assist in determining that water intoxication is an adverse reaction. This thought process will direct you to option 3. Review the adverse reactions related to this medication if you had difficulty with this question.
Level of Cognitive Ability: Analysis
Client Needs: Physiological Integrity
Integrated Concept/Process: Nursing Process/Assessment
Content Area: Pharmacology

Reference: Hodgson, B., & Kizior, R. (2001). *Saunders nursing drug handbook 2001.* Philadelphia: W.B. Saunders, p. 295.

4. 3

Rationale: Because of its powerful vasoconstrictor actions, vasopressin can cause adverse cardiovascular effects. By constricting arteries of the heart, vasopressin can cause angina pectoris and even myocardial infarction, especially if administered to clients with coronary artery disease. In addition, vasopressin may cause gangrene by decreasing blood flow in the periphery. Options 1, 2, and 4 are incorrect.

Test-Taking Strategy: Use the process of elimination. Attempt to make a relationship between the name of the medication, *vaso*pressin, and coronary artery disease, the correct option. Review the cautions associated with the administration of this medication if you had difficulty with this question.

Level of Cognitive Ability: Analysis
Client Needs: Physiological Integrity
Integrated Concept/Process: Nursing Process/Analysis
Content Area: Pharmacology
Reference: Salerno, E. (1999). *Pharmacology for health professionals.* St. Louis: Mosby, p. 544.

5. 2

Rationale: Oral doses of Synthroid should be taken on an empty stomach to enhance absorption. Dosing is usually done in the morning before breakfast.

Test-Taking Strategy: Use the process of elimination. Note the similarity between options 1, 3, and 4 in that these options all address administering the medication with food. Review client teaching points regarding the administration of Synthroid if you had difficulty with this question.

Level of Cognitive Ability: Application
Client Needs: Health Promotion and Maintenance
Integrated Concept/Process: Teaching/Learning
Content Area: Pharmacology
Reference: Hodgson, B., & Kizior, R. (2001). *Saunders nursing drug handbook 2001.* Philadelphia: W.B. Saunders, p. 589.

6. 2

Rationale: Excessive doses of Synthroid can produce signs and symptoms of hyperthyroidism. These include tachycardia, angina, tremors, nervousness, insomnia, hyperthermia, heat intolerance, and sweating. The client should be instructed to notify the physician if these occur. Options 1, 3, and 4 are signs of hypothyroidism.

Test-Taking Strategy: Use the process of elimination, recalling the symptoms associated with hypothyroidism, the purpose of administering Synthroid, and the effects of the medication. Options 1, 3, and 4 are symptoms related to hypothyroidism. Review the adverse effects of this medication if you are unfamiliar with them.

Level of Cognitive Ability: Application
Client Needs: Health Promotion and Maintenance
Integrated Concept/Process: Teaching/Learning
Content Area: Pharmacology
Reference: Cleveland, L., Aschenbrenner, D., Venable, S., & Yensen, J. (1999). *Nursing management in drug therapy.* Philadelphia: Lippincott, p. 633.

7. 4

Rationale: PTU inhibits thyroid hormone synthesis and is used to treat hyperthyroidism, or Graves' disease. Myxedema indicates hypothyroidism. Cushing's syndrome and Addison's disease are disorders related to adrenal function.

Test-Taking Strategy: Use the process of elimination and knowledge regarding the action of the medication and the treatment measures for Graves' disease to answer the question. Review this medication and Graves' disease if you had difficulty with this question.

Level of Cognitive Ability: Analysis
Client Needs: Physiological Integrity
Integrated Concept/Process: Nursing Process/Assessment
Content Area: Pharmacology
Reference: Hodgson, B., & Kizior, R. (2001). *Saunders nursing drug handbook 2001.* Philadelphia: W.B. Saunders, p. 880.

8. 3

Rationale: Lypressin is administered by the intranasal route. It is used to treat diabetes insipidus. The usual adult dosage is 1 to 2 sprays into each nostril four times daily. Options 1, 2, and 4 are incorrect routes of administration.

Test-Taking Strategy: Use the process of elimination and knowledge that lypressin is administered by the intranasal route. Review this medication if you are unfamiliar with it.

Level of Cognitive Ability: Application
Client Needs: Health Promotion and Maintenance
Integrated Concept/Process: Teaching/Learning
Content Area: Pharmacology
Reference: Clark, J., Queener, S., & Karb, V. (2000). *Pharmacologic basis of nursing practice* (6th ed.). St. Louis: Mosby, p. 762.

9. 4

Rationale: An adverse reaction to Humatrope is hypothyroidism. Thyroid function is monitored throughout therapy. Options 1 and 2 would evaluate pancreatic function, and option 3 evaluates renal function.

Test-Taking Strategy: Use the process of elimination. Eliminate options 1 and 2 first because both evaluate pancreatic function and therefore are similar. Next, eliminate option 3 because it evaluates renal function. Recalling that Humatrope is a growth hormone will assist in directing you to option 4. If you had difficulty with this question, review interventions associated with the administration of Humatrope.

Level of Cognitive Ability: Analysis
Client Needs: Physiological Integrity
Integrated Concept/Process: Nursing Process/Assessment
Content Area: Pharmacology
Reference: Wilson, B., Shannon, M., & Stang, C. (2000). *Nurses drug guide 2000.* Stamford, Conn.: Appleton & Lange, p. 1287.

10. 2

Rationale: Lugol solution is administered to hyperthyroid individuals in preparation for thyroidectomy to suppress thyroid function. Initial effects develop within 24 hours; peak effects develop in 10 to 15 days. In most cases, plasma levels of thyroid hormone are reduced with propythiouracil (PTU) before Lugol solution therapy is initiated. Then Lugol solution along with PTU is administered for the last 10 days prior to surgery.

Test-Taking Strategy: Use the process of elimination. Eliminate options 1 and 3 first because they are similar. From the remaining options, select option 2 because of its relationship to the issue of the question. If you had difficulty with this question, review the purpose of this medication for the client scheduled for subtotal thyroidectomy.

Level of Cognitive Ability: Analysis
Client Needs: Physiological Integrity
Integrated Concept/Process: Nursing Process/Planning
Content Area: Pharmacology
Reference: Cleveland, L., Aschenbrenner, D., Venable, S., & Yensen, J. (1999). *Nursing management in drug therapy.* Philadelphia: Lippincott, p. 640.

11. **4**
Rationale: Chronic ingestion of iodine can produce iodism. The client needs to be instructed about the symptoms of iodism, which includes a brassy taste, burning sensations in the mouth, soreness of gums and teeth, frontal headache, coryza, salivation, and skin eruptions. The client needs to be instructed to notify the physician if these symptoms occur.
Test-Taking Strategy: Use the process of elimination. Eliminate options 2 and 3 first because the nurse cannot legally alter medication prescriptions without a physician's order. Consider the client symptoms presented in the question, and eliminate option 1 as a reasonable choice. Review the adverse effects of iodine solution if you had difficulty with this question.
Level of Cognitive Ability: Application
Client Needs: Physiological Integrity
Integrated Concept/Process: Nursing Process/Implementation
Content Area: Pharmacology
Reference: Cleveland, L., Aschenbrenner, D., Venable, S., & Yensen, J. (1999). *Nursing management in drug therapy.* Philadelphia: Lippincott, p. 640.

12. **3**
Rationale: Excessive doses of Florinef cause retention of sodium and water and excessive excretion of potassium, resulting in expansion of blood volume, hypertension, cardiac enlargement, edema, and hypokalemia. The client needs to be informed about the signs of sodium and water retention, such as unusual weight gain or swelling of the feet or lower legs. If these signs occur, the physician needs to be notified.
Test-Taking Strategy: Use the process of elimination. Recalling that Florinef can cause water retention will easily direct you to option 3. Review client teaching points related to this medication if you had difficulty with this question.
Level of Cognitive Ability: Application
Client Needs: Health Promotion and Maintenance
Integrated Concept/Process: Teaching/Learning
Content Area: Pharmacology
Reference: Salerno, E. (1999). *Pharmacology for health professionals.* St. Louis: Mosby, p. 561.

13. **2**
Rationale: The client should be instructed to take the medication exactly as prescribed. When used as a calcium supplement, it should be taken 1 to 1.5 hours after meals. The client should take the tablets with a full glass of water; however, it can be taken with milk.
Test-Taking Strategy: Use the process of elimination. Option 4 can be easily eliminated first. From the remaining options, eliminate options 1 and 3 because they are similar. If you are unfamiliar with the administration of calcium supplements, review this information.
Level of Cognitive Ability: Application
Client Needs: Health Promotion and Maintenance
Integrated Concept/Process: Self-Care

Content Area: Pharmacology
Reference: Wilson, B., Shannon, M., & Stang, C. (2000). *Nurses drug guide 2000.* Stamford, Conn.: Appleton & Lange, p. 200.

14. **3**
Rationale: The client who is taking an antihypocalcemic medication should be instructed to avoid eating too much spinach, rhubarb, bran, or whole grain cereals because they decrease calcium absorption. Good dietary sources of calcium are milk products, dark green leafy vegetables (although spinach needs to be avoided), clams, oysters, sardines, and orange juice fortified with calcium.
Test-Taking Strategy: Note that the client diagnosis is "hypocalcemia." Note the key word "avoid" in the stem of the question. Use the process of elimination and knowledge regarding food items high in calcium to assist in selecting the correct option. This should assist in eliminating options 1, 2, and 4. Review this medication and food sources high in calcium if you had difficulty with this question.
Level of Cognitive Ability: Application
Client Needs: Health Promotion and Maintenance
Integrated Concept/Process: Self-Care
Content Area: Pharmacology
Reference: Kuhn, M. (1998). *Pharmacotherapeutics: A nursing process approach* (4th ed.). Philadelphia: F.A. Davis, p. 684.

15. **3**
Rationale: Glucocorticoids should be administered before 9 A.M. Administration at this time helps minimize adrenal insufficiency and mimics the burst of glucocorticoids released naturally by the adrenals each morning. Options 1, 2, and 4 are incorrect.
Test-Taking Strategy: Use the process of elimination. Recalling that this medication is a glucocorticoid will direct you to option 3. If you had difficulty with this question, review the administration of glucocorticoids.
Level of Cognitive Ability: Application
Client Needs: Health Promotion and Maintenance
Integrated Concept/Process: Self-Care
Content Area: Pharmacology
Reference: Lehne, R. (1998). *Pharmacology for nursing care* (3rd ed.). Philadelphia: W.B. Saunders, p. 717.

16. **2**
Rationale: Glucocorticoids can elevate blood glucose levels. Clients with diabetes mellitus may need their dosages of insulin or oral hypoglycemic medications increased during glucocorticoid therapy.
Test-Taking Strategy: Use the process of elimination. Recalling that glucocorticoids can increase blood glucose levels will easily direct you to option 2. Review the effects of glucocorticoids if you had difficulty with this question.
Level of Cognitive Ability: Analysis
Client Needs: Physiological Integrity
Integrated Concept/Process: Nursing Process/Analysis
Content Area: Pharmacology
Reference: Clark, J., Queener, S., & Karb, V. (2000). *Pharmacologic basis of nursing practice* (6th ed.). St. Louis: Mosby, p. 471.

17. **3**
Rationale: When preparing a mixture of Regular insulin with another insulin preparation, draw the Regular insulin into the syringe first. This sequence will avoid contaminating the vial of Regular insulin with insulin of another type. Options 1, 2,

and 4 identify the correct actions for preparing NPH and Regular insulin.
Test-Taking Strategy: Use the process of elimination, noting the key words "need for further teaching." Remember "RN"; draw up the Regular insulin before the NPH insulin. Review the procedure for preparing NPH and Regular insulin if you had difficulty with this question.
Level of Cognitive Ability: Analysis
Client Needs: Health Promotion and Maintenance
Integrated Concept/Process: Nursing Process/Evaluation
Content Area: Pharmacology
Reference: Hodgson, B., & Kizior, R. (2001). *Saunders nursing drug handbook 2001.* Philadelphia: W.B. Saunders, p. 531.
18. **2**
Rationale: Insulin in unopened vials should be stored under refrigeration until needed. Vials should not be frozen. When stored unopened under refrigeration, insulin can be used up to the expiration date on the vial.
Test-Taking Strategy: Use the process of elimination. Note the key words "store the unopened vials" in the question. Remembering that insulin should not be frozen will assist in eliminating option 1. Options 3 and 4 are similar and should be eliminated. Review client teaching points related to insulin if you had difficulty with this question.
Level of Cognitive Ability: Application
Client Needs: Health Promotion and Maintenance
Integrated Concept/Process: Self-Care
Content Area: Pharmacology
Reference: Lehne, R. (1998). *Pharmacology for nursing care* (3rd ed.). Philadelphia: W.B. Saunders, p. 583.
19. **3**
Rationale: When alcohol is combined with tolbutamide, a disulfiram-like reaction may occur. This syndrome includes flushing, palpitations, and nausea. Alcohol can potentiate the hypoglycemic effects of tolbutamide. Clients need to be instructed to avoid alcohol consumption while taking this medication.
Test-Taking Strategy: Use the process of elimination. Eliminate options 1, 2, and 4 because these food items are allowed in a diabetic diet. Remembering that alcohol can affect the action of many medications will assist in directing you to option 3. Review this medication if you had difficulty with this question.
Level of Cognitive Ability: Application

Client Needs: Health Promotion and Maintenance
Integrated Concept/Process: Self-Care
Content Area: Pharmacology
Reference: Wilson, B., Shannon, M., & Stang, C. (2000). *Nurses drug guide 2000.* Stamford, Conn.: Appleton & Lange, p. 1386.
20. **2**
Rationale: Sildenafil citrate (Viagra) enhances the vasodilation effect of nitric oxide in the corpus cavernosus of the penis, thus sustaining an erection. Because of the effect of the medication, it is contraindicated with concurrent use of organic nitrates and nitroglycerin. It is not contraindicated with the use of vitamins. Neuralgia and insomnia are side effects of the medication.
Test-Taking Strategy: Use the process of elimination, noting the key words "would question the prescription." Recalling the action of the medication will easily direct you to option 2. If you had difficulty with this question, review the contraindications associated with the use of this medication.
Level of Cognitive Ability: Analysis
Client Needs: Safe, Effective Care Environment
Integrated Concept/Process: Nursing Process/Analysis
Content Area: Pharmacology
Reference: Wilson, B., Shannon, M., & Stang, C. (2000). *Nurses drug guide 2000.* Stamford, Conn.: Appleton & Lange, p. 1271.

CRITICAL THINKING: FREE-TEXT ENTRY

Answer: Seven prefilled syringes
Rationale: Mixtures of insulin in prefilled syringes should be stored in a refrigerator, where they will be stable for 1 week. The syringe should be stored vertically with the needle pointing up to avoid clogging the needle. Prior to administration, the syringe should be agitated gently to resuspend the insulin.
Test-Taking Strategy: It is necessary to know the concepts related to insulin stability and storage to answer this question. Review these concepts if you are unfamiliar with the principles related to prefilling insulin syringes.
Level of Cognitive Ability: Application
Client Needs: Health Promotion and Maintenance
Integrated Concept/Process: Self-Care
Content Area: Pharmacology
Reference: Hodgson, B., & Kizior, R. (2001). *Saunders nursing drug handbook 2001.* Philadelphia: W.B. Saunders, p. 531.

REFERENCES

Cleveland, L., Aschenbrenner, D., Venable, S., & Yensen, J. (1999). *Nursing management in drug therapy.* Philadelphia: Lippincott.

Clark, J., Queener, S., & Karb, V. (2000). *Pharmacologic basis of nursing practice* (6th ed.). St. Louis: Mosby.

Hodgson, B., & Kizior, R. (2001). *Saunders nursing drug handbook 2001.* Philadelphia: W.B. Saunders.

Kuhn, M. (1998). *Pharmacotherapeutics: A nursing process approach* (4th ed.). Philadelphia: F.A. Davis.

Lehne, R. (1998). *Pharmacology for nursing care* (3rd ed.). Philadelphia: W.B. Saunders.

Salerno, E. (1999). *Pharmacology for health professionals.* St. Louis: Mosby.

Wilson, B., Shannon, M., & Stang, C. (2000). *Nurses drug guide 2000.* Stamford, Conn.: Appleton & Lange.

The Adult Client with a Gastrointestinal Disorder

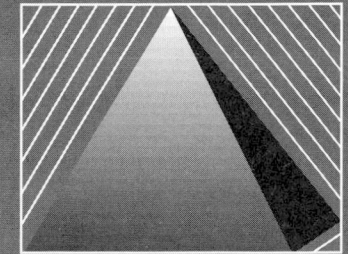

PYRAMID TERMS

ascites The accumulation of fluid within the peritoneal cavity that results in venous congestion of the hepatic capillaries. This leads to plasma leaking directly from the liver surface and portal vein.

asterixis Also termed liver flap. A coarse tremor characterized by rapid, nonrhythmic extensions and flexions in the wrist and fingers.

Billroth I Also called gastroduodenostomy; partial gastrectomy and remaining segment is anastomosed to duodenum.

Billroth II Also called gastrojejunostomy; partial gastrectomy with remaining segment anastomosed to the jejunum.

cholecystectomy Removal of the gallbladder.

cholecystitis An inflammation of the gallbladder, which may occur as an acute or a chronic process. Acute inflammation is associated with gallstones (cholelithiasis). Chronic cholecystitis results when inefficient bile emptying and gallbladder muscle wall disease cause a fibrotic and contracted gallbladder.

choledochotomy Incision into the common bile duct to remove the stone.

cirrhosis A chronic, progressive disease of the liver characterized by diffuse damage to cells, with fibrosis and nodular regeneration. Repeated destruction of hepatic cells causes the formation of scar tissue.

Crohn's disease An inflammatory disease that can occur anywhere in the gastrointestinal (GI) tract but most often affects the terminal ileum and leads to thickening and scarring, a narrowed lumen, fistulas, ulcerations, and abscesses. It is characterized by remissions and exacerbations.

Cullen's sign Bluish discoloration of the abdomen and periumbilical area, seen in acute hemorrhagic pancreatitis.

diverticulitis Inflammation of one or more diverticuli. Results when a diverticulum perforates, with local abscess formation. A perforated diverticulum can progress to intraabdominal perforation with generalized peritonitis.

diverticulosis Outpouching or herniations of the intestinal mucosa. They can occur in any part of the intestine but are most common in the sigmoid colon.

dumping syndrome Rapid emptying of the gastric contents into the small intestine. Occurs following gastric resection.

esophageal varices Dilated and tortuous veins in the submucosa of the esophagus. They are caused by portal hypertension, are often associated with liver cirrhosis, and are at high risk for rupture if portal circulation pressure rises.

fetor hepaticus The fruity, musty breath odor associated with chronic liver disease.

gastrectomy Also called esophagojejunostomy. Removal of the stomach with attachment of the esophagus to the jejunum or duodenum.

gastric resection Also called antrectomy. Involves removal of the lower half of the stomach and usually includes a vagotomy.

hiatal hernia Also known as esophageal or diaphragmatic hernia. A portion of the stomach herniates through the diaphragm and into the thorax. It results from weakening of the muscles of the diaphragm and is aggravated by factors that increase abdominal pressure, such as pregnancy, ascites, obesity, tumors, and heavy lifting.

Kock ileostomy (continent ileostomy) An intraabdominal pouch is constructed from the terminal ileum. The pouch is connected to the stoma with a nipple-like valve constructed from a portion of the ileum. The stoma is flush with the skin.

Murphy's sign A sign of gallbladder disease, consisting of pain on taking a deep breath when the examiner's fingers are on the approximate location of the gallbladder.

pancreatitis An acute or chronic inflammation of the pancreas, with associated escape of pancreatic enzymes into surrounding tissue. Acute pancreatitis occurs suddenly as one attack or can be recurrent but resolves. Chronic pancreatitis is a continual inflammation and destruction of the pancreas, with scar tissue replacing pancreatic tissue.

peristalsis Wavelike rhythmic contractions that propel material through the GI tract.

portal hypertension A persistent increase in pressure within the portal vein that develops as a result of obstruction to flow.

pyloroplasty Enlarging the pylorus to prevent or decrease pyloric obstruction, thereby enhancing gastric emptying.

Turner's sign A gray-blue discoloration of the flanks, seen in acute hemorrhagic pancreatitis.

Ulcerative colitis Ulcerative and inflammatory disease of the bowel that results in poor absorption of nutrients. Acute ulcerative colitis results in vascular congestion, hemorrhage, edema, and ulceration of the bowel mucosa. Chronic ulcerative colitis causes muscular hypertrophy, fat deposits, and fibrous tissue, with bowel thickening, shortening, and narrowing.

vagotomy Surgical division of the vagus nerve to eliminate the vagal impulses that stimulate hydrochloric acid secretion in the stomach.

▲ PYRAMID TO SUCCESS

Pyramid points focus on diagnostic tests, nursing care related to the various gastric or intestinal tubes, gastric surgery, cirrhosis, hepatitis, pancreatitis, and colostomy care. Focus on preprocedure and postprocedure care of the client undergoing a gastrointestinal diagnostic test. Remember that informed consent is required for any invasive procedure. Focus on diet restrictions before and after the diagnostic test, and remember that the gag reflex or bowel sounds must return before a client is allowed to consume food or fluids. Pyramid points include instructions to the client and family regarding the prevention of gastrointestinal disorders and the complications associated with the disorders. Focus on teaching the client and family about diet and nutrition specific to a disorder, tube and wound care, preventing the transmission of infection, and care of a colostomy or an ileostomy. Remember that body image disturbances can occur in clients with a GI disorder. Specific focus relates to the client with a diversion, such as an ileostomy or a colostomy, and to the social isolation issues that can occur, and coping strategies. The Integrated Concepts and Processes addressed in this unit include Nursing Process, Caring, Communication and Documentation, Cultural Awareness, Self-Care, and Teaching/Learning.

▲ CLIENT NEEDS

Safe, Effective Care Environment

Confidentiality issues related to the GI disorder
Consultation related to nutritional status
Establishing priorities
Handling infectious drainage and secretions
Informed consent for treatments and surgical procedures
Preventing the transmission of disease
Referrals to home care and community services
Standard precautions

Health Promotion and Maintenance

Health screening related to GI disorders
Health promotion programs related to GI disorders
Physical assessment techniques of the GI system
Teaching related to prescribed dietary and other treatment measures
Teaching related to colostomy or ileostomy care
Teaching related to preventing the transmission of disease

Psychosocial Integrity

Coping mechanisms
End-of-life issues
Grief and loss
Support systems
Unexpected body image changes related to colostomy or ileostomy

Physiological Integrity

Care of GI tubes
Diagnostic tests related to the GI system
Elimination
Fluid and electrolyte imbalances
Infectious diseases of the GI tract
Medication therapy specific to the GI disorder
Monitoring for complications related to tests, procedures, and surgical interventions
Nonpharmacological and pharmacological comfort measures
Nutrition and oral hydration
Personal hygiene
Parenteral fluids
Total parenteral nutrition

REFERENCES

Craven, R., & Hirnle, C. (2000). *Fundamentals of nursing: Human health and function* (3rd ed.). Philadelphia: Lippincott.

Harkreader, H. (2000). *Fundamentals of nursing: Caring and clinical judgment.* Philadelphia: W.B. Saunders.

Ignatavicius, D., Workman, M., & Mishler, M. (1999). *Medical-surgical nursing: Across the health care continuum* (3rd ed.). Philadelphia: W.B. Saunders.

LeMone, P., & Burke, K. (2000). *Medical-surgical nursing: Critical thinking in client care* (2nd ed.). Upper Saddle River, N.J.: Prentice-Hall.

Lewis, S., Heitkemper, M., & Dirksen, S. (2000). *Medical-surgical nursing: Assessment and management of clinical problems* (5th ed.). St. Louis: Mosby.

National Council of State Boards of Nursing (eds.) (2000). *Test Plan for the National Council Licensure Examination for Registered Nurses.* Chicago: Author.

Potter, P., & Perry, A. (2001). *Fundamentals of nursing* (5th ed.). St. Louis: Mosby.

Smeltzer, S., & Bare, B. (2000). *Textbook of medical-surgical nursing* (9th ed.). Philadelphia: Lippincott Williams & Wilkins.

Gastrointestinal System

I. ANATOMY AND PHYSIOLOGY

A. Functions of the gastrointestinal (GI) system
1. Process food substances
2. Absorb the products of digestion into the blood
3. Excrete unabsorbed materials
4. Provide an environment for microorganisms to synthesize nutrients, such as vitamin K
5. For risk factors associated with the GI system, see Box 53-1

B. Mouth
1. Contains the lips, cheeks, palate, tongue, teeth, salivary glands, muscles, and maxillary bones
2. Saliva contains the amylase enzyme (ptyalin) that aids in digestion

C. Esophagus
1. A collapsible muscular tube, about 10 inches long
2. Carries food from the pharynx to the stomach

D. Stomach: Contains the cardia, the fundus, the body, and the pylorus
1. Mucous glands
   a. Located in mucosa
   b. Prevent autodigestion by providing an alkaline protective covering
2. Lower esophageal (cardiac) sphincter: Prevents reflux of gastric contents into the esophagus
3. Pyloric sphincter: Regulates the rate of stomach emptying into the small intestine
4. Hydrochloric acid: Kills microorganisms, breaks food into small particles, and provides a chemical environment that is required by the gastric enzymes
5. Pepsin: The chief coenzyme of gastric juice, which converts proteins into proteases and peptones
6. Intrinsic factor: Necessary for the absorption of vitamin B_{12}
7. Gastrin: Controls gastric acidity

E. Small intestine
1. Duodenum: Contains the openings of the bile and pancreatic ducts
2. Jejunum: Approximately 8 feet long
3. Ileum: Approximately 12 feet long
4. The small intestine terminates into the cecum

F. Pancreatic intestinal juice enzymes
1. Amylase digests starch to maltose
2. Maltase reduces maltose to monosaccharide glucose
3. Lactase splits lactose into galactose and glucose
4. Sucrase reduces sucrose to fructose and glucose
5. Nucleoses split nucleic acids to nucleotides
6. Enterokinase activates trypsinogen to trypsin

BOX 53-1

Risk Factors Associated with the GI System

Family history of GI disorders
Chronic laxative use
Tobacco use
Chronic alcohol use
Chronic high stress levels
Allergic reactions to food or medications
Chronic use of aspirin or nonsteroidal antiinflammatory drugs (NSAIDs)
Long-term GI conditions such as ulcerative colitis may predispose to colorectal cancer
Previous abdominal surgery or trauma may lead to adhesions
Neurological disorders can impair movement, particularly with chewing and swallowing
Cardiac, respiratory, and endocrine disorders may lead to constipation
Diabetes mellitus may predispose to oral candidal infections

G. Large intestine
  1. Approximately 5 feet long
  2. Absorbs water and eliminates wastes
  3. Manufacture of vitamins, including some B vitamins and vitamin K
  4. Colon
      a. Ascending
      b. Transverse
      c. Descending
      d. Sigmoid
      e. Rectum
  5. Ileocecal valve: Prevents contents of large intestine from entering ileum
  6. Anal sphincters: Guard the anal canal
H. Peritoneum
  1. Lines the abdominal cavity
  2. Forms the mesentery that supports the intestines and blood supply
I. Liver
  1. The largest gland in the body, weighing 3 to 4 pounds
  2. Contains Kupffer's cells, which remove bacteria in the portal venous blood
  3. Removes excess glucose and amino acids from the portal blood
  4. Synthesizes glucose, amino acids, and fats
  5. Aids in the digestion of fats, carbohydrates, and proteins
  6. Stores and filters blood (200 to 400 mL of blood stored)
  7. Stores vitamins A, D, and B$_{12}$ and iron
  8. Secretes bile to emulsify fats (500 to 1000 mL of bile a day)
  9. Hepatic ducts
      a. Deliver bile to the gallbladder via the cystic duct and to the duodenum via the common bile duct
      b. The common bile duct opens into the duodenum, with the pancreatic duct at the ampulla of Vater
      c. The sphincter prevents the reflux of intestinal contents into the common bile duct and pancreatic duct
J. Gallbladder
  1. Stores and concentrates bile
  2. Contracts to force bile into the duodenum during the digestion of fats
  3. The cystic duct joins the hepatic duct to form the common bile duct
  4. The sphincter of Oddi guards the entrance into the duodenum
  5. The presence of fatty materials in the duodenum stimulates the liberation of cholecystokinin, which causes contraction of the gallbladder and relaxation of the sphincter of Oddi
K. Pancreas
  1. Exocrine gland
      a. Secretes sodium bicarbonate to neutralize the acidity of the stomach contents as they enter the duodenum
      b. Pancreatic juices contain enzymes for digesting carbohydrates, fats, and proteins
  2. Endocrine gland
      a. Insulin secretion is produced by the islets of Langerhans
      b. Insulin is secreted into the bloodstream and is important for carbohydrate metabolism
      c. Secretes glucagon to raise blood glucose levels
      d. Secretes somatostatin to exert a hypoglycemic effect

II. DIAGNOSTIC PROCEDURES

A. Upper GI tract study (barium swallow)
  1. Description: An examination of the upper GI tract under fluoroscopy after the client drinks barium sulfate
  2. Preprocedure: NPO after midnight prior to the day of the test
  3. Postprocedure
      a. A laxative may be prescribed
      b. Instruct the client to drink increased oral fluids to help pass the barium
      c. Monitor stools for the passage of barium (stools will appear chalky white) because barium can cause a bowel obstruction
B. Lower GI tract study (barium enema)
  1. Description
      a. A fluoroscopic and radiographic examination of the large intestine after rectal instillation of barium sulfate
      b. May be done with or without air
  2. Preprocedure
      a. A low-residue diet for 1 to 2 days prior to the test
      b. A clear liquid diet and a laxative the evening before the test
      c. NPO after midnight prior to the day of the test
      d. Cleansing enemas on the morning of the test
  3. Postprocedure
      a. Instruct the client to drink increased oral fluids to help pass the barium
      b. Administer a mild laxative as prescribed to facilitate emptying of the barium
      c. Monitor stools for the passage of barium
      d. Notify the physician if a bowel movement does not occur within 2 days
C. Gastric analysis
  1. Description
      a. The passage of a nasogastric (NG) tube into the stomach to aspirate gastric contents for the analysis of acidity (pH), appearance, and volume; the entire gastric contents are aspirated, and then specimens are collected every 15 minutes for 1 hour
      b. Histamine or pentagastrin may be adminis-

tered subcutaneously to stimulate gastric secretions; may produce a flushed feeling
c. Esophageal reflux of gastric acid may be performed by ambulatory pH monitoring; a probe is placed just above the lower esophageal sphincter, is connected to an external recording device, and provides a computer analysis and graphic display of results
2. Preprocedure
a. Fasting for 8 to 12 hours prior to the test
b. Avoid tobacco and chewing gum for 6 hours prior to the test
c. Medications that stimulate gastric secretions are withheld for 24 to 48 hours
3. Postprocedure
a. May resume normal activities
b. Refrigerate gastric samples if not tested within 4 hours
D. Upper GI fiberoscopy
1. Description
a. Also known as esophagogastroduodenoscopy (EGD)
b. Following sedation, an endoscope is passed down the esophagus to view the gastric wall, sphincters, and duodenum; tissue specimens can be obtained
2. Preprocedure
a. NPO for 6 to 12 hours prior to the test
b. A local anesthetic (spray or gargle) is administered along with midazolam (Versed) IV (provides conscious sedation and relieves anxiety) just before the scope is inserted
c. Atropine may be administered to reduce secretions, and glucagon may be administered to relax smooth muscle
d. Client is positioned on the left side to facilitate saliva drainage and to provide easy access of the endoscope
e. Airway patency is monitored during the test, and pulse oximetry is used to monitor oxygen saturation; emergency equipment should be readily available
3. Postprocedure
a. NPO until the gag reflex returns (1 to 2 hours)
b. Monitor for signs of perforation (pain, bleeding, unusual difficulty in swallowing, elevated temperature)
c. Maintain bed rest for the sedated client until alert
d. Lozenges, saline gargles, or oral analgesics can relieve minor sore throat, after the gag reflex returns
E. Anoscopy, proctoscopy, and sigmoidoscopy
1. Description
a. Anoscopy: Use of a rigid scope to examine the anal canal; client is placed in the knee-chest position with the back inclined at a 45-degree angle

b. Proctoscopy and sigmoidoscopy: Use of a flexible scope to examine the rectum and sigmoid colon; client is placed on the left side with the right leg bent and placed anteriorly
c. Biopsies and polypectomies can be performed
2. Preprocedure: Enemas until the returns are clear
3. Postprocedure: Monitor for rectal bleeding and signs of perforation
F. Fiberoptic colonoscopy
1. Description
a. A fiberoptic endoscopy study in which the lining of the large intestine is visually examined; biopsies and polypectomies can be performed
b. Cardiac and respiratory function is monitored continuously during the test
c. Performed with the client lying on the left side with the knees drawn up to the chest; position may be changed during the test to facilitate passing of the scope
2. Preprocedure
a. Adequate cleansing of the colon is necessary, as prescribed by the physician
b. A clear liquid diet is started at noon on the day before the test
c. Consult with the physician regarding medications that must be withheld prior to the test
d. Client is NPO after midnight on the day before the test
e. Midazolam (Versed) IV is administered to provide sedation
f. Glucagon may be administered to relax smooth muscle
3. Postprocedure
a. Provide bed rest until alert
b. Monitor for signs of perforation
c. Instruct the client to report any bleeding to the physician
G. Laparoscopy (peritoneoscopy): Performed with a fiberoscopic laparoscope that allows direct visualization of organs and structures within the abdomen; biopsies may be obtained
H. Cholecystography
1. Description: Performed to detect gallstones and to assess the ability of the gallbladder to fill, concentrate its contents, contract, and empty
2. Preprocedure
a. Assess allergies to iodine or seafood
b. Contrast agents such as iopanoic acid (Telepaque), iodipamide meglumine (Cholografin), and sodium ipodate (Oragrafin) are administered 10 to 12 hours (evening before) before the test
c. Client is NPO after the contrast agent is administered
d. Instruct the client that if a rash, itching, hives, or difficulty in breathing occurs after taking the contrast agent, to report to the emergency room

3. Postprocedure
   a. Inform the client that dysuria is common because the contrast agent is excreted in the urine
   b. A normal diet may be resumed (a fatty meal may enhance excretion of the contrast agent)

I. Endoscopic retrograde cholangiopancreatography (ERCP)
  1. Description
    a. Examination of the hepatobiliary system via a flexible endoscope inserted into the esophagus to the descending duodenum; multiple positions are required during the procedure to pass the endoscope
    b. If medication is administered prior to the procedure, the client is monitored closely for signs of respiratory and central nervous system depression, hypotension, oversedation, and vomiting
  2. Preprocedure
    a. Client is NPO for several hours prior to the procedure
    b. Sedation is administered prior to the procedure
  3. Postprocedure
    a. Monitor vital signs
    b. Monitor for the return of the gag reflex
    c. Monitor for signs of perforation or infection

J. Percutaneous transhepatic cholangiography
  1. Description
    a. Involves the injection of dye directly into the biliary tree
    b. The hepatic ducts within the liver, the entire length of the common bile duct, the cystic duct, and the gallbladder are clearly outlined
  2. Preprocedure
    a. Client is NPO
    b. Sedating medication is administered
  3. Postprocedure
    a. Monitor vital signs
    b. Monitor for signs of bleeding, peritonitis, and septicemia; report the presence of pain immediately
    c. Administer antibiotics as prescribed to reduce the risk of sepsis

K. Paracentesis
  1. Description: Transabdominal removal of fluid from the peritoneal cavity for analysis
  2. Preprocedure
    a. Obtain informed consent
    b. Void prior to the start of procedure to empty bladder and to move bladder out of the way of the paracentesis needle
    c. Measure abdominal girth, weight, and baseline vital signs
    d. Note that the client is positioned upright on the edge of the bed with the back supported and the feet resting on a stool (Fowler's position is used for the client confined to bed)
  3. Postprocedure
    a. Monitor vital signs
    b. Measure fluid collected, describe, and record
    c. Label fluid samples and send to the laboratory for analysis
    d. Apply a dry sterile dressing to the insertion site; monitor site for bleeding
    e. Measure abdominal girth and weight
    f. Monitor for hypovolemia, electrolyte loss, mental status changes, or encephalopathy
    g. Monitor for hematuria resulting from bladder trauma
    h. Instruct the client to notify the physician if the urine becomes bloody, pink, or red

L. Liver biopsy
  1. Description: A needle is inserted through the abdominal wall to the liver to obtain a tissue sample for biopsy and microscopic examination
  2. Preprocedure
    a. Obtained informed consent
    b. Assess results of coagulation tests (prothrombin time, partial thromboplastin time, platelet count)
    c. Administer a sedative as prescribed
    d. Note that the client is placed in the supine or left lateral position during the procedure to expose the right side of the upper abdomen
  3. Postprocedure
    a. Assess vital signs
    b. Assess biopsy site for bleeding
    c. Monitor for peritonitis
    d. Maintain bed rest for several hours
    e. Place client on the right side with a pillow under the costal margin to decrease the risk of hemorrhage, and instruct the client to avoid coughing and straining
    f. Instruct the client to avoid heavy lifting and strenuous exercise for 1 week

M. GI motility studies
  1. Radionuclide Testing: Assesses gastric emptying and colonic emptying time; a capsule containing radioactive material is administered to the client, and the time it takes for the radioactive material to move through the colon indicates colonic motility
  2. Esophageal manometry: Detects motility disorders of the esophagus and lower esophageal sphincter; client is NPO for 8 to 12 hours before the test, and medications that affect GI motility are withheld
  3. Gastrointestinal, small intestinal, and colonic manometry: Evaluates delayed gastric emptying and gastric and intestinal motility disorders; often is an ambulatory outpatient procedure that lasts 24 to 72 hours

4. Anorectal manometry: Measures the resting tone and contractibility of the anal sphincters to evaluate the client with chronic constipation or fecal incontinence; phosphosoda or a cleansing enema is administered 1 hour prior to the test
5. Electrogastrography: Used to detect motor or neurological dysfunction in the stomach; records gastric electrical activity
6. Rectal sensory function test: Evaluates rectal sensory function and neuropathy to evaluate the client with chronic constipation, diarrhea, or incontinence

N. Defecography
1. Measures anorectal function
2. Thick barium is instilled into the rectum, fluoroscopy is performed, and the function of the rectum and anal sphincter is visualized while the client attempts to pass the barium
3. Digital subtraction methods may be used for more rapid imaging and mapping of rectal evacuation
4. No preparation is required

O. Stool specimens
1. Includes inspecting the specimen for consistency and color and testing for occult blood
2. Tests for fecal urobilinogen, fat, nitrogen, parasites, pathogens, food substances, and other substances; these tests require that the specimen be sent to the laboratory
3. Random specimens are promptly sent to the laboratory
4. Quantitative 24- to 72- hour collections must be kept refrigerated until they are taken to the laboratory
5. Some specimens require that a certain diet be followed or that certain medications be withheld; check agency guidelines regarding specific procedures

P. Hydrogen breath test
1. Evaluates carbohydrate absorption by determining the amount of hydrogen expelled in the breath after it is produced in the colon and absorbed in the blood
2. Used to aid in the diagnosis of bacterial overgrowth in the intestine

Q. Urea breath test
1. Detects the presence of *Helicobacter pylori,* the bacterium that causes peptic ulcer disease
2. The client consumes a capsule of carbon-labeled urea and provides a breath sample 10 to 20 minutes later
3. The client is instructed to avoid antibiotics or loperamide (Pepto-Bismal) for 1 month before the test; sucralfate (Carafate) and omeprazole (Prilosec) for 1 week before the test; and cimetidine (Tagamet), famotidine (Pepcid), ranitidine (Zantac), and nizatidine (Axid) for 24 hours before breath testing
4. *Helicobacter pylori* can also be detected by assessing serum antibody levels

R. Liver and pancreas laboratory studies (refer to Chapter 10)
1. Alkaline phosphatase: Released during liver damage or biliary obstruction
2. Prothrombin time (PT): Prolonged with liver damage
3. Serum ammonia: Assesses the ability of the liver to deaminate protein by-products
4. Liver enzymes (transaminase studies): Elevated with liver damage
5. Cholesterol: Increase indicates **pancreatitis** or biliary obstruction
6. Bilirubin: Increase indicates liver damage or biliary obstruction
7. Amylase and lipase: Elevations indicate **pancreatitis**

III. ASSESSMENT
A. Abdominal assessment
1. Inspect skin for color, abnormalities, contour, and tautness, and the abdomen for distention
2. Auscultate for bowel sounds
3. Percuss for air or solids
4. Palpate for tenderness

B. Bowel sounds
1. Auscultate bowel sounds before percussion and palpation
2. Normal bowel sounds occur 5 to 30 times a minute or every 5 to 15 seconds
3. Auscultate in all abdominal quadrants
4. Listen at least 5 minutes in each quadrant before assuming sounds are absent

IV. GASTROINTESTINAL TUBES
(Refer to Chapter 20)

V. GASTROESOPHAGEAL REFLUX (GER)
A. Description
1. The back-flow of gastric and duodenal contents into the esophagus
2. Caused by an incompetent lower esophageal sphincter, pyloric stenosis, or a motility disorder
3. Symptoms may mimic those of a heart attack

B. Assessment
1. Pyrosis
2. Dyspepsia
3. Regurgitation
4. Pain and difficulty with swallowing
5. Hypersalivation

C. Implementation
1. Instruct the client to avoid factors that decrease lower esophageal sphincter pressure or cause esophageal irritation

2. Instruct the client to eat a low-fat, high-fiber diet; to avoid caffeine, tobacco, and carbonated beverages; to avoid eating and drinking 2 hours before bedtime; to avoid wearing tight clothes; and to elevate the head of the bed on 6- to 8- inch blocks
3. Avoid the use of anticholinergics, which delay stomach emptying
4. Instruct the client regarding prescribed medications, such as antacids, histamine H_2-receptor antagonists, or gastric acid pump inhibitors
5. Instruct the client regarding the administration of prokinetic medications, if prescribed, which accelerate gastric emptying
6. If medical management is unsuccessful, surgery may be required and involves a fundoplication (wrapping a portion of the gastric fundus around the sphincter area of the esophagus); may be performed by laparoscopy

VI. HIATAL HERNIA

A. Description
1. Also known as esophageal or diaphragmatic hernia
2. A portion of the stomach herniates through the diaphragm and into the thorax
3. It results from weakening of the muscles of the diaphragm and is aggravated by factors that increase abdominal pressure, such as pregnancy, **ascites,** obesity, tumors, and heavy lifting
4. Complications include ulceration, hemorrhage, regurgitation and aspiration of stomach contents, strangulation, and incarceration of the stomach in the chest with possible necrosis, peritonitis, and mediastinitis

B. Assessment
1. Heartburn
2. Regurgitation or vomiting
3. Dysphagia
4. Feeling of fullness

C. Implementation
1. Medical and surgical management is similar to that for GER
2. Provide small, frequent meals and minimize the amount of liquids
3. Advise the client not to recline for 1 hour after eating
4. Avoid anticholinergics, which delay stomach emptying

VII. GASTRITIS

A. Description
1. Inflammation of the stomach or gastric mucosa
2. Acute: Caused by the ingestion of food contaminated with disease-causing microorganisms or food that is irritating or too highly seasoned, the overuse of aspirin or other nonsteroidal antiin-

flammatory drugs (NSAIDs), excessive alcohol intake, bile reflux, or radiation therapy
3. Chronic: Caused by benign or malignant ulcers, or by the bacteria *Helicobacter pylori*; may also be caused by autoimmune diseases, dietary factors, medications, alcohol, smoking, or reflux

B. Assessment
1. Acute
   a. Abdominal discomfort
   b. Headache
   c. Anorexia, nausea, and vomiting
   d. Hiccuping
2. Chronic
   a. Anorexia, nausea, and vomiting
   b. Heartburn after eating
   c. Belching
   d. Sour taste in the mouth
   e. Vitamin B_{12} deficiency

C. Implementation
1. Acute: Food and fluids may be withheld until symptoms subside; then, ice chips, followed by clear liquids, and then solid food is introduced
2. Monitor for signs of hemorrhagic gastritis such as hematemesis, tachycardia, and hypotension, and notify the physician if these signs occur
3. Instruct the client to avoid irritating foods, fluids, and other substances such as spicy and highly seasoned foods, caffeine, alcohol, and nicotine
4. Instruct the client in the use of prescribed medications, such as antibiotics and bismuth salts (Pepto-Bismol)
5. Provide the client with information about the importance of vitamin B_{12} injections, if a deficiency is present

VIII. PEPTIC ULCER DISEASE

A. Description
1. An ulceration in the mucosal wall of the stomach, pylorus, duodenum, or esophagus, in portions that are accessible to gastric secretions; erosion may extend through the muscle
2. May be referred to as gastric, duodenal, or esophageal ulcers, depending on location
3. The most common peptic ulcers are gastric ulcers and duodenal ulcers

B. Gastric ulcers
1. Description
   a. Involve ulceration of the mucosal lining that extends to the submucosal layer of the stomach
   b. Predisposing factors include stress, smoking, the use of corticosteroids, NSAIDs, alcohol, a history of gastritis, a family history of gastric ulcers, or infection with *Helicobacter pylori*
   c. Complications include hemorrhage, perforation, and pyloric obstruction

2. Assessment
   a. Gnawing, sharp pain in or left of the midepigastric region 1 to 2 hours after eating
   b. Nausea and vomiting
   c. Hematemesis
3. Implementation
   a. Monitor vital signs and for signs of bleeding
   b. Administer small, frequent bland feedings during the active phase
   c. Administer histamine H_2-receptor antagonists as prescribed to decrease the secretion of gastric acid
   d. Administer antacids as prescribed to neutralize gastric secretions
   e. Administer anticholinergics as prescribed to reduce gastric motility
   f. Administer mucosal barrier protectants as prescribed 1 hour before each meal
   g. Administer prostaglandins as prescribed for their protective and antisecretory actions
4. Client education
   a. Avoid consuming alcohol and substances that contain caffeine or chocolate
   b. Avoid smoking
   c. Avoid aspirin or NSAIDs
   d. Obtain adequate rest and reduce stress
5. Implementation during active bleeding
   a. Monitor vital signs closely
   b. Assess for signs of dehydration, hypovolemic shock, sepsis, and respiratory insufficiency
   c. Maintain NPO status and administer IV fluid replacement as prescribed; monitor I & O
   d. Monitor hemoglobin and hematocrit
   e. Administer blood transfusions as prescribed
   f. Assist with the insertion of an NG tube for decompression and for lavage access
   g. Assist with normal saline or tap water lavage at room temperature to reduce active bleeding
   h. Prepare to assist with administering vasopressin (Pitressin) by IV, as prescribed, to induce vasoconstriction and reduce bleeding
6. Surgical implementation
   a. Total **gastrectomy:** Also called esophagojejunostomy; removal of the stomach with attachment of the esophagus to the jejunum or duodenum
   b. **Vagotomy:** Surgical division of the vagus nerve to eliminate the vagal impulses that stimulate hydrochloric acid secretion in the stomach
   c. **Gastric resection:** Also called antrectomy; involves removal of the lower half of the stomach and usually includes a **vagotomy**
   d. **Billroth I:** Also called gastroduodenostomy; partial **gastrectomy,** with remaining segment anastomosed to duodenum
   e. **Billroth II:** Also called gastrojejunostomy; partial **gastrectomy,** with remaining segment anastomosed to jejunum
   f. **Pyloroplasty:** Enlarges the pylorus to prevent or decrease pyloric obstruction, thereby enhancing gastric emptying
7. Postoperative Implementation
   a. Monitor vital signs
   b. Position in Fowler's for comfort and to promote drainage
   c. Administer fluids and electrolyte replacements IV as prescribed; monitor I & O
   d. Assess bowel sounds
   e. Monitor NG suction as prescribed
   f. Do not irrigate or remove the NG tube
   g. Assist the physician with NG irrigation or removal of the NG tube
   h. Maintain NPO status as prescribed for 1 to 3 days until **peristalsis** returns
   i. Progress the diet from NPO to sips of clear water to six small bland meals a day as prescribed, when bowel sounds return
   j. Monitor for postoperative complications of hemorrhage, **dumping syndrome,** diarrhea, hypoglycemia, and vitamin B_{12} deficiency

C. Duodenal ulcers
   1. Description
      a. A break in the mucosa of the duodenum
      b. Risk factors and causes include alcohol intake, smoking, stress, caffeine, the use of aspirin, corticosteroids, and NSAIDs, and infection with *Helicobacter pylori*
      c. Complications include bleeding, perforation, gastric outlet obstruction, and intractable disease
   2. Assessment
      a. Burning pain in the midepigastric area 2 to 4 hours after eating and during the night
      b. Pain that is often relieved by eating
      c. Melena
   3. Implementation
      a. Monitor vital signs
      b. Perform abdominal assessment
      c. Instruct the client in a bland diet with small, frequent meals
      d. Provide for adequate rest
      e. Encourage the cessation of smoking
      f. Instruct the client to avoid alcohol intake, caffeine, and the use of aspirin, corticosteroids, and NSAIDs
      g. Administer antacids as prescribed to neutralize acid secretions
      h. Administer histamine H_2-receptor antagonists as prescribed to block the secretion of acid
   4. Surgical implementation: Surgery is performed only if the ulcer is unresponsive to medications

---

BOX 53-2

Foods Rich in Vitamin B$_{12}$

Brewer's yeast
Citrus fruits
Dried beans
Green leafy vegetables
Liver
Nuts
Organ meats

---

or if hemorrhage, obstruction, or perforation occurs

D. **Dumping syndrome**
　1. Description
　　a. Rapid emptying of the gastric contents into the small intestine
　　b. Occurs following **gastric resection**
　2. Assessment
　　a. Symptoms occurring 30 minutes after eating
　　b. Nausea and vomiting
　　c. Feelings of abdominal fullness and abdominal cramping
　　d. Diarrhea
　　e. Palpitations and tachycardia
　　f. Perspiration
　　g. Weakness and dizziness
　　h. Borborygmi
　3. Client education
　　a. Eat a high-protein, high-fat, low-carbohydrate diet
　　b. Eat small meals and avoid consuming fluids with meals
　　c. Avoid sugar and salt
　　d. Lie down after meals
　　e. Take antispasmodic medications as prescribed to delay gastric emptying

IX. VITAMIN B$_{12}$ DEFICIENCY

A. Description
　1. Results from either an inadequate intake of vitamin B$_{12}$ or a lack of absorption of ingested vitamin B$_{12}$ from the intestinal tract
　2. Pernicious anemia results from a deficiency of intrinsic factor, which is necessary for intestinal absorption of vitamin B$_{12}$
B. Assessment
　1. Severe pallor
　2. Fatigue
　3. Weight loss
　4. Smooth, beefy-red tongue
　5. Slight jaundice
　6. Paresthesias of the hands and feet
　7. Disturbances with gait and balance
C. Implementation
　1. Increase dietary intake of foods rich in vitamin

B$_{12}$ if the anemia is the result of a dietary deficiency (Box 53-2)
　2. Administer vitamin B$_{12}$ injections, as prescribed, on a weekly basis initially, and then monthly for maintenance (lifelong) if the anemia is the result of a deficiency of the intrinsic factor

X. GASTRIC CANCER (Refer to Chapter 49)

XI. ESOPHAGEAL VARICES

A. Description
　1. Dilated and tortuous veins in the submucosa of the esophagus
　2. Caused by **portal hypertension,** are often associated with liver **cirrhosis,** and are at high risk for rupture if portal circulation pressure rises
　3. Bleeding varices are an emergency
　4. The goal of treatment is to control bleeding, prevent complications, and prevent the reoccurrence of bleeding
B. Assessment
　1. Hematemesis
　2. Melena
　3. Tarry stools
　4. **Ascites**
　5. Jaundice
　6. Hepatomegaly and splenomegaly
　7. Dilated abdominal veins
　8. Hemorrhoids
　9. Signs of shock
C. Implementation
　1. Monitor vital signs
　2. Elevate the head of the bed
　3. Monitor for orthostatic hypotension
　4. Monitor lung sounds and for the presence of respiratory distress
　5. Administer oxygen as prescribed to prevent tissue hypoxia
　6. Monitor level of consciousness (LOC)
　7. Maintain NPO status
　8. Administer IV fluids as prescribed to restore fluid volume and correct electrolyte imbalances; monitor I & O
　9. Monitor hemoglobin, hematocrit, and coagulation factors
　10. Administer blood transfusions or clotting factors as prescribed
　11. Assist in inserting an NG tube or a balloon tamponade as prescribed
　12. Assist with the administration of iced saline irrigations to achieve vasoconstriction of the varices
　13. Prepare to assist with administering vasopressin (Pitressin) by IV or intraarterial infusion, as prescribed, to induce vasoconstriction and reduce bleeding
　14. Prepare to assist with administering nitroglyc-

erin (Tridil) with the vasopressin (Pitressin) to prevent vasoconstriction of the coronary arteries

15. Instruct the client to avoid activities that will initiate vasovagal responses
16. Prepare the client for endoscopic procedures or surgical procedures as prescribed

D. Endoscopic injection (Sclerotherapy)
   1. Injection of a sclerosing agent into and around bleeding varices
   2. Complications include chest pain, pleural effusion, aspiration pneumonia, esophageal stricture, and perforation of the esophagus

E. Endoscopic variceal ligation
   1. Ligation of the varices with an elastic rubber band
   2. Sloughing, followed by superficial ulceration, occurs in the area of ligation within 3 to 7 days

F. Surgical shunt procedures
   1. Splenorenal: Involves splenectomy, with anastomosis of the splenic vein to the left renal vein
   2. Portacaval: Shunting of the blood from the portal vein to the inferior vena cava
   3. Mesocaval: Involves a side anastomosis of the superior mesenteric vein to the proximal end of the inferior vena cava
   4. Transjugular intrahepatic portal/systemic
      a. Uses the normal vascular anatomy of the liver to create a shunt with the use of a metallic stent
      b. The shunt is between the portal and systemic venous system within the liver and is aimed at relieving **portal hypertension**

XII. ULCERATIVE COLITIS

A. Description
   1. Ulcerative and inflammatory disease of the bowel that results in poor absorption of nutrients
   2. Commonly begins in the rectum and spreads upward toward the cecum
   3. The colon becomes edematous and may develop bleeding lesions and ulcers; the ulcers may lead to perforation
   4. Scar tissue develops and causes loss of elasticity and loss of ability to absorb nutrients
   5. Characterized by various periods of remissions and exacerbations
   6. Acute **ulcerative colitis** results in vascular congestion, hemorrhage, edema, and ulceration of the bowel mucosa
   7. Chronic **ulcerative colitis** causes muscular hypertrophy, fat deposits, and fibrous tissue with bowel thickening, shortening, and narrowing
   8. Surgical intervention involves creation of an ostomy; the ostomy can be created within the ileum or at various sites within the large bowel
   9. An ileostomy is the surgical creation of an opening into the ileum or small intestine that

allows for drainage of fecal matter from the ileum to the outside of the body
   10. A colostomy is the surgical creation of an opening into the colon that allows for drainage of fecal matter from the colon to the outside of the body

B. Assessment
   1. Anorexia
   2. Weight loss
   3. Malaise
   4. Abdominal tenderness and cramping
   5. Severe diarrhea that may contain blood and mucus
   6. Dehydration and electrolyte imbalances
   7. Anemia
   8. Vitamin K deficiency

C. Implementation
   1. Acute phase: Maintain NPO status, administer IVs and electrolytes, or total parenteral nutrition (TPN), as prescribed
   2. Restrict the client's activity, to reduce intestinal activity
   3. Monitor bowel sounds and for abdominal tenderness and cramping
   4. Monitor stools, noting color, consistency, and the presence or absence of blood
   5. Monitor for perforation, peritonitis, and hemorrhage
   6. Following the acute phase, the diet progresses from clear liquids to low residue as tolerated
   7. Instruct the client to consume a low-residue, high-protein diet; vitamins and iron supplements may be prescribed
   8. Instruct the client to avoid gas-forming foods and milk products, and foods such as whole wheat grains, nuts, raw fruits and vegetables, pepper, alcohol, and caffeine-containing products
   9. Instruct the client to avoid smoking
   10. Administer bulk-forming agents such as bran, psyllium, or methylcellulose, to decrease diarrhea and relieve symptoms
   11. Administer antimicrobial, corticosteroids, and immunosuppressants as prescribed to prevent infection and reduce inflammation

D. Surgical implementation
   1. Total proctocolectomy with permanent ileostomy
      a. Curative and involves the removal of the entire colon (colon, rectum, and anus with anal closure)
      b. The end of the terminal ileum forms the stoma, which is located in the right lower quadrant
   2. **Kock ileostomy** (continent ileostomy)
      a. An intraabdominal pouch (that stores the feces) is constructed from the terminal ileum

b. The pouch is connected to the stoma with a nipple-like valve constructed from a portion of the ileum; the stoma is flush with the skin

c. A catheter is used to empty the pouch, and a small dressing or adhesive bandage is worn over the stoma between emptyings

3. Ileoanal reservoir

   a. A two-stage procedure that involves the excision of the rectal mucosa, an abdominal colectomy, construction of a reservoir to the anal canal, and a temporary loop ileostomy

   b. The ileostomy is closed in approximately 3 to 4 months after the capacity of the reservoir is increased

4. Ileoanal anastomosis (ileorectostomy)

   a. Does not require an ileostomy

   b. A 12- to 15-cm rectal stump is left after the colon is removed, and the small intestine is inserted into this rectal sleeve and anastomosed

   c. Requires a large, compliant rectum

5. Preoperative colostomy/ileostomy

   a. Consult with enterostomal therapist to assist in identifying optimal placement of the ostomy

   b. Instruct the client to eat a low-residue diet for a day or two prior to surgery, as prescribed

   c. Administer intestinal antiseptics and antibiotics, as prescribed, to cleanse the bowel and to decrease the bacterial content of the colon

   d. Administer laxatives and enemas as prescribed

6. Postoperative colostomy

   a. Place a petrolatum gauze over the stoma as prescribed to keep it moist, followed by a dry sterile dressing if a pouch (external) system is not in place

   b. Place a pouch system on the stoma as soon as possible

   c. Monitor the stoma for size, unusual bleeding, or necrotic tissue

   d. Monitor for color changes in the stoma

   e. Note that the normal stoma color is pink to bright red and shiny, indicating high vascularity

   f. Note that a pale pink stoma indicates low hemoglobin and hematocrit levels and a purple-black stoma indicates compromised circulation, requiring physician notification

   g. Assess the functioning of the colostomy

   h. Expect that stool is liquid in the immediate postoperative period, but becomes more solid depending on the area of the colostomy: ascending colon, liquid; transverse colon, loose to semiformed; descending colon, close to normal

   i. Monitor the pouch system for proper fit and signs of leakage

---

BOX 53-3

Colostomy Irrigation

PURPOSE

An enema given through the stoma to stimulate bowel emptying

DESCRIPTION

Instilling 500 to 1000 mL of lukewarm tap water through the stoma and allowing the water and stool to drain into a collection bag

PROCEDURE

If ambulatory, position the client sitting on toilet

If on bed rest, position the client on the side

Hang the irrigation bag so that the bottom of the bag is at the level of the client's shoulder, or slightly higher

Insert the irrigation tube carefully, without force

Begin the flow of irrigation

Clamp tubing if cramping occurs; release tubing as cramping subsides

Avoid frequent irrigations with water, which can lead to loss of fluids and electrolytes

Perform irrigation around the same time each day

Perform irrigation preferably 1 hour after a meal

---

j. Empty the pouch when it is one-third full

k. Fecal matter should not be allowed to remain on the skin

l. Administer analgesics and antibiotics as prescribed

m. Irrigate the perineal wound (if present) as prescribed and monitor for signs of infection

n. Instruct the client to avoid foods that cause excess gas formation and odor

o. Instruct the client about stoma care and irrigations as prescribed (Box 53-3)

p. Instruct the client that normal activities may be resumed when approved by the physician

7. Postoperative ileostomy

   a. Note that normal stool is liquid

   b. Monitor for dehydration and electrolyte imbalance

   c. Do not give suppositories through an ileostomy

XIII. CROHN'S DISEASE (REGIONAL ENTERITIS)

A. Description

1. An inflammatory disease that can occur anywhere in the GI tract but most often affects the terminal ileum and leads to thickening and scarring, a narrowed lumen, fistulas, ulcerations, and abscesses

2. It is characterized by remissions and exacerbations

B. Assessment

1. Fever

2. Cramplike and colicky pain after meals
3. Diarrhea (semisolid); may contain mucus and pus
4. Abdominal distention
5. Anorexia, nausea, and vomiting
6. Weight loss
7. Anemia
8. Dehydration
9. Electrolyte imbalances

C. Implementation: Care is similar to that for the client with **ulcerative colitis;** however, surgery is avoided as much as possible because recurrence of the disease process in the same region is likely to occur

XIV. INTESTINAL TUMORS AND BOWEL OBSTRUCTIONS (Refer to Chapter 49)

XV. DIVERTICULOSIS AND DIVERTICULITIS

A. Description
1. **Diverticulosis**
   a. Outpouching or herniations of the intestinal mucosa
   b. They can occur in any part of the intestine but are most common in the sigmoid colon
2. **Diverticulitis**
   a. Inflammation of one or more diverticuli that results when a diverticulum perforates
   b. A perforated diverticulum can progress to intraabdominal perforation with generalized peritonitis

B. Assessment
1. Left lower quadrant abdominal pain that increases with coughing, straining, or lifting
2. Elevated temperature
3. Nausea and vomiting
4. Flatulence
5. Cramplike pain
6. Abdominal distention and tenderness
7. Palpable, tender rectal mass
8. Blood in the stools

C. Implementation
1. Provide bed rest during the acute phase
2. Maintain NPO status or provide clear liquids during the acute phase as prescribed
3. Introduce a fiber-containing diet gradually, when the inflammation is resolved
4. Administer antibiotics, analgesics, and anticholinergics to reduce bowel spasms as prescribed
5. Instruct the client to refrain from lifting, straining, coughing, or bending, to avoid increased intraabdominal pressure
6. Monitor for perforation, hemorrhage, fistulas, abscesses
7. Instruct the client to increase fluid intake to 2500 to 3000 mL daily, unless contraindicated
8. Instruct the client to eat soft high-fiber foods such as whole grains
9. Instruct the client to avoid gas-forming foods or foods containing indigestible roughage, seeds, or nuts because these food substances become trapped in diverticula and cause inflammation
10. Instruct the client to consume a small amount of bran daily and to take bulk-forming laxatives as prescribed to increase stool mass
11. Instruct the client to avoid high-fiber foods when inflammation occurs because these foods will further irritate the mucosa

D. Surgical implementation
1. Colon resection with primary anastomosis
2. Temporary or permanent colostomy may be required for increased bowel inflammation

XVI. HEMORRHOIDS

A. Description
1. Dilated varicose veins of the anal canal
2. May be internal, external, or prolapsed
3. Internal hemorrhoids lie above the anal sphincter and cannot be seen upon inspection of the perianal area
4. External hemorrhoids lie below the anal sphincter and can be seen on inspection
5. Prolapsed hemorrhoids can become thrombosed or inflamed
6. Hemorrhoids are caused by **portal hypertension,** straining, irritation, or increased venous or abdominal pressure

B. Assessment
1. Bright red bleeding with defecation
2. Rectal pain
3. Rectal itching

C. Implementation
1. Apply cold packs to the anal/rectal area followed by sitz baths as prescribed
2. Apply witch hazel soaks and topical anesthetics as prescribed
3. Encourage a high-fiber diet and fluids to promote bowel movements without straining
4. Administer stool softeners as prescribed

D. Endoscopic procedures
1. Sclerotherapy
2. Endoscopic ligation

E. Surgical procedures
1. Cryosurgery
2. Hemorrhoidectomy

F. Postoperative implementation
1. Assist the client to a prone or side-lying position to prevent bleeding
2. Maintain ice packs over the dressing as prescribed until the packing is removed by the physician
3. Monitor for urinary retention
4. Administer stool softeners as prescribed
5. Instruct the client to increase fluids and high-fiber foods

6. Instruct the client to limit sitting to short periods of time
7. Instruct the client in the use of sitz baths three or four times a day as prescribed

XVII. APPENDICITIS

A. Description
   1. Inflammation of the appendix
   2. When the appendix becomes inflamed or infected, rupture may occur within a matter of hours, leading to peritonitis and sepsis
B. Assessment
   1. Pain in the periumbilical area that descends to the right lower quadrant
   2. Abdominal pain that is most intense at McBurney's point
   3. Rebound tenderness and abdominal rigidity
   4. Low-grade fever
   5. Elevated white blood cell (WBC) count
   6. Anorexia, nausea, and vomiting
   7. Client in side-lying position, with abdominal guarding and legs flexed
   8. Constipation or diarrhea
C. Peritonitis: Inflammation of the peritoneum
   1. Increased fever and chills
   2. Progressive abdominal distention and abdominal pain
   3. Right guarding of the abdomen
   4. Tachycardia and tachypnea
   5. Pallor
   6. Restlessness
D. Appendectomy: Surgical removal of the appendix
   1. Preoperative implementation
      a. Maintain NPO status
      b. Administer IV fluids to prevent dehydration
      c. Monitor for changes in level of pain
      d. Monitor for signs of ruptured appendix and peritonitis
      e. Position in right side-lying or low to semi-Fowler's position to promote comfort
      f. Monitor bowel sounds
      g. Apply ice packs to the abdomen for 20 to 30 minutes every hour as prescribed
      h. Administer antibiotics as prescribed
      i. Avoid the application of heat to the abdomen
      j. Avoid laxatives or enemas
   2. Postoperative implementation
      a. Monitor temperature for signs of infection
      b. Assess incision for signs of infection, such as redness, swelling, and pain
      c. Maintain NPO status until bowel function has returned
      d. Advance diet gradually as tolerated and as prescribed, when bowel sounds return
      e. If rupture of the appendix occurred, expect a Penrose drain to be inserted, or the incision may be left open to heal from the inside out

f. Expect that drainage from the Penrose drain may be profuse for the first 12 hours
g. Position the client in right side-lying or low to semi-Fowler's position, with legs flexed, to facilitate drainage
h. Change the dressing as prescribed and record the type and amount of drainage
i. Perform wound irrigations if prescribed
j. Maintain NG suction and patency of NG tube if present
k. Administer antibiotics and analgesics as prescribed

XVIII. CIRRHOSIS (Box 53-4)

A. Description
   1. A chronic, progressive disease of the liver, characterized by diffuse damage to cells with fibrosis and nodular regeneration
   2. Repeated destruction of hepatic cells causes the formation of scar tissue
B. Complications
   1. **Portal hypertension:** A persistent increase in pressure within the portal vein that develops as a result of obstruction to flow
   2. **Ascites**
      a. The accumulation of fluid within the peritoneal cavity that results in venous congestion of the hepatic capillaries
      b. This leads to plasma leaking directly from the liver surface and portal vein
   3. Bleeding **esophageal varices:** Fragile, thin-

BOX 53-4

Types of Cirrhosis

LAENNEC'S CIRRHOSIS
Alcohol-induced, nutritional, or portal cirrhosis
Cellular necrosis causes eventual widespread scar tissue, with fibrotic infiltration of the liver

POSTNECROTIC CIRRHOSIS
Occurs after massive liver necrosis
Results as a complication of acute viral hepatitis or exposure to hepatotoxins
Scar tissue causes destruction of liver lobules and entire lobes

BILIARY CIRRHOSIS
Develops from chronic biliary obstruction, bile stasis, and inflammation, resulting in severe obstructive jaundice

CARDIAC CIRRHOSIS
Associated with severe, right-sided congestive heart failure (CHF) and results in an enlarged, edematous, congested liver
The liver becomes anoxic, resulting in liver cell necrosis and fibrosis

walled, distended esophageal veins that become irritated and rupture

4. Coagulation defects
   a. Decreased synthesis of bile fats in the liver prevent the absorption of fat-soluble vitamins
   b. Without vitamin K and clotting factors II, VII, IX, and X, the client is prone to bleeding
5. Jaundice: Occurs because the liver is unable to metabolize bilirubin and because the edema, fibrosis, and scarring of the hepatic bile ducts interfere with normal bile and bilirubin secretion
6. Portal systemic encephalopathy: End-stage hepatic failure and **cirrhosis,** characterized by altered LOC, neurological symptoms, impaired thinking, and neuromuscular disturbances
7. Hepatorenal syndrome
   a. Progressive renal failure associated with hepatic failure
   b. Characterized by a sudden decrease in urinary output, elevated BUN and creatinine, decreased urine sodium excretion, and increased urine osmolarity

C. Assessment
   1. Anorexia and weight loss
   2. Early morning nausea and vomiting (presence of blood in vomitus)
   3. Dyspepsia
   4. Flatulence and changes in bowel habits
   5. Emaciation
   6. Fatigue
   7. Jaundice
   8. Abdominal pain or tenderness
   9. **Ascites**
   10. Peripheral edema
   11. Dry skin and rashes
   12. Petechiae or ecchymosis
   13. Spider angiomas on the nose, cheeks, upper thorax, and shoulders
   14. Hepatomegaly
   15. Protruding umbilicus
   16. Dilated abdominal veins
   17. **Fetor hepaticus,** the fruity, musty breath odor of chronic liver disease
   18. **Asterixis** (liver flap): A coarse tremor characterized by rapid, nonrhythmic extension and flexions in the wrist and fingers
   19. Delirium

D. Implementation
   1. Elevate the head of the bed to minimize shortness of breath
   2. If **ascites** and edema are absent and the client does not exhibit signs of impending coma, a high-protein diet supplemented with vitamins is prescribed
   3. Provide supplemental vitamins (B complex, vitamin A, C, and K, folic acid, and thiamine) as prescribed
   4. Restrict sodium intake and fluid intake as prescribed
   5. Initiate enteral feedings or TPN as prescribed
   6. Administer diuretics as prescribed
   7. Monitor I & O and electrolyte balance
   8. Weigh client and measure abdominal girth daily
   9. Monitor LOC; assess for precoma state (tremors, delirium)
   10. Monitor for **asterixis**
   11. Maintain gastric intubation to assess bleeding and/or esophagogastric balloon tamponade to control bleeding varices, if prescribed
   12. Administer blood products as prescribed
   13. Monitor coagulation laboratory results; administer vitamin K if prescribed
   14. Administer low-sodium antacids as prescribed
   15. Administer lactulose (Chronulac), which decreases the pH of the bowel, decreases production of ammonia by bacteria in the bowel, and facilitates the excretion of ammonia
   16. Administer neomycin (Mycifradin) as prescribed to inhibit protein synthesis in bacteria and decrease the production of ammonia
   17. Avoid medications such as narcotics, sedatives, and barbiturates, and any hepatotoxic medications or substances
   18. Instruct the client about the restriction of alcohol intake
   19. Prepare the client for paracentesis to remove abdominal fluid
   20. Prepare the client for surgical shunting procedures if prescribed

XIX. CHOLECYSTITIS

A. Description
   1. An inflammation of the gallbladder that may occur as an acute or chronic process
   2. Acute inflammation is associated with gallstones (cholelithiasis)
   3. Chronic **cholecystitis** results when inefficient bile emptying and gallbladder muscle wall disease cause a fibrotic and contracted gallbladder
   4. A calculus **cholecystitis** occurs in the absence of gallstones and is due to bacterial invasion via the lymphatic or vascular systems

B. Assessment
   1. Nausea and vomiting
   2. Indigestion
   3. Belching
   4. Flatulence
   5. Epigastric pain that radiates to the scapula 2 to 4 hours after eating fatty foods and may persist for 4 to 6 hours
   6. Pain localized in right upper quadrant
   7. Guarding, rigidity, and rebound tenderness
   8. Mass palpated in the right upper quadrant
   9. **Murphy's sign** (cannot take a deep breath when

the examiner's fingers are passed below the hepatic margin)
   10. Elevated temperature
   11. Tachycardia
   12. Signs of dehydration
▲ C. Biliary obstruction
   1. Jaundice
   2. Dark orange and foamy urine
   3. Steatorrhea and clay-colored feces
   4. Pruritus
  D. Implementation
▲   1. Maintain NPO status during nausea and vomiting episodes
   2. Maintain nasogastric decompression as prescribed for severe vomiting
   3. Administer antiemetics as prescribed for nausea and vomiting
▲   4. Administer analgesics as prescribed to relieve pain and reduce spasm (note: morphine sulfate or codeine sulfate may cause spasm of the sphincter of Oddi and increase pain)
   5. Administer antispasmodics (anticholinergics) as prescribed to relax smooth muscle
▲   6. Instruct the client with chronic **cholecystitis** to eat low-fat meals more frequently in small amounts
▲   7. Instruct the client to avoid gas-forming foods
   8. Prepare the client for nonsurgical and surgical procedures as prescribed
  E. Nonsurgical implementation
   1. Dissolution therapy
     a. To remove cholesterol stones
     b. Chenodeoxycholic acid (Chenodiol) or ursodiol (Actigall) is administered PO to decrease the size of the stones or to dissolve small stones
     c. Direct contact with repeated injections and aspirations of a dissolution agent via percutaneous catheter may be performed
   2. Extracorporeal shock wave lithotripsy
     a. Shock waves are administered that disintegrate stones in the biliary system
     b. Oral dissolution follows
  F. Surgical implementation
   1. **Cholecystectomy:** Removal of the gallbladder
   2. **Choledochotomy:** Incision into the common bile duct to remove the stone
   3. Surgical procedures may be performed by laparoscopy
  G. Postoperative implementation
▲   1. Monitor for respiratory complications secondary to pain at the incisional site
▲   2. Encourage coughing and deep breathing
   3. Encourage early ambulation
   4. Instruct the client about splinting the abdomen to prevent discomfort during coughing

---

BOX 53-5

Care of a T Tube

PURPOSE AND DESCRIPTION
A tube that is placed after surgical exploration of the common bile duct. It preserves the patency of the duct and ensures drainage of bile until edema resolves and bile is effectively draining into the duodenum. A gravity drainage bag is attached to the T tube to collect the drainage.

IMPLEMENTATION
Position client in semi-Fowler's to facilitate drainage
Monitor the amount, color, consistency, and odor of drainage
Report sudden increases in bile output to the physician
Monitor for inflammation and protect the skin from irritation
Keep the drainage system below the level of the gallbladder
Monitor for foul odor and purulent drainage and report to the physician
Avoid irrigation, aspiration, or clamping of the T tube without a physician's order
As prescribed, clamp the tube before eating, and observe for abdominal discomfort and distention, nausea, chills, or fever; unclamp the tube if nausea or vomiting occurs

---

   5. Administer antiemetics as prescribed for nausea and vomiting
   6. Administer analgesics as prescribed for pain relief
▲   7. Maintain NPO status and NG tube suction as prescribed
   8. Advance diet from clear liquids to solids when prescribed and as tolerated by the client
   9. Maintain and monitor drainage from the T tube, if present (Box 53-5)

XX. PANCREATITIS
  A. Description
   1. An acute or chronic inflammation of the pancreas with associated escape of pancreatic enzymes into surrounding tissue
   2. Acute **pancreatitis** occurs suddenly as one attack or can be recurrent, but resolves
   3. Chronic **pancreatitis** is a continual inflammation and destruction of the pancreas, with scar tissue replacing pancreatic tissue
   4. Precipitating factors include trauma, the use of alcohol, biliary tract disease, viral or bacterial disease, hyperlipedemia, hypercalcemia, cholelithiasis, hyperparathyroidism, ischemic vascular disease, and peptic ulcer disease
  B. Acute
   1. Assessment
     a. Abdominal pain, including a sudden onset at ▲

the midepigastric or left upper quadrant location with radiation to the back

b. Pain that is aggravated by a fatty meal, alcohol, or lying in a recumbent position

c. Abdominal tenderness and guarding

d. Nausea and vomiting

e. Weight loss

f. **Cullen's sign** (discoloration of the abdomen and periumbilical area)

g. **Turner's sign** (bluish discoloration of the flanks)

h. Absent or decreased bowel sounds

i. Elevated WBC, glucose, bilirubin, alkaline phosphatase, urinary amylase

j. Elevated lipase and amylase

2. Implementation

a. Maintain NPO status and maintain hydration with IV fluids as prescribed

b. Administer TPN for severe nutritional depletion

c. Administer supplemental preparations and vitamins and minerals to increase caloric intake if prescribed

d. Maintain NG tube to decrease gastric distention and suppress pancreatic secretion

e. Administer meperidine hydrochloride (Demerol) as prescribed for pain because it causes less incidence of smooth muscle spasm of the pancreatic ducts and sphincter of Oddi (note: avoid morphine sulfate or codeine sulfate, which may cause spasms)

f. Administer antacids as prescribed to neutralize gastric secretions

g. Administer histamine H_2-receptor antagonists as prescribed to decrease hydrochloric acid production and prevent activation of pancreatic enzymes

h. Administer anticholinergics as prescribed to decrease vagal stimulation, decrease GI motility, and inhibit pancreatic enzyme secretion

i. Instruct the client in the importance of avoiding alcohol

j. Instruct the client in the importance of follow-up visits with the physician

k. Instruct the client to notify the physician if acute abdominal pain, jaundice, clay-colored stools, or dark urine develops

C. Chronic

1. Assessment

a. Abdominal pain and tenderness

b. Left upper quadrant mass

c. Steatorrhea and foul-smelling stools that may increase in volume as pancreatic insufficiency increases

d. Weight loss

e. Muscle wasting

f. Jaundice

g. Signs and symptoms of diabetes mellitus

2. Implementation

a. Instruct the client in the prescribed dietary measures (fat and/or protein intake may be limited)

b. Instruct the client to avoid heavy meals

c. Instruct the client about the importance of avoiding alcohol

d. Provide supplemental preparations and vitamins and minerals to increase caloric intake

e. Administer pancreatic enzymes as prescribed to aid in the digestion and absorption of fat and protein

f. Administer insulin or oral hypoglycemic medications as prescribed to control diabetes mellitus, if present

g. Instruct the client in the use of pancreatic enzyme medications

h. Instruct the client in the treatment plan for glucose management

i. Instruct the client to notify the physician if increased steatorrhea occurs or if abdominal distention or cramping and skin breakdown develop

j. Instruct the client in the importance of follow-up visits

XXI. HEPATITIS

A. Description

1. An inflammation of the liver caused by a virus, bacteria, or exposure to medications or

2. hepatotoxins

3. The goals of treatment include resting the inflamed liver to reduce metabolic demands and increasing the blood supply, thus promoting cellular regeneration and preventing complications

B. Types of viral hepatitis

1. Hepatitis A (HAV), infectious hepatitis

2. Hepatitis B (HBV), serum hepatitis

3. Hepatitis C (HCV), non-A, non-B hepatitis or posttransfusion hepatitis

4. Hepatitis D (HDV), delta agent hepatitis

5. Hepatitis E (HEV), enterically transmitted or epidemic non-A, non-B hepatitis

6. Hepatitis G (HGV), non-A, non-B, non-C hepatitis

C. Stages of viral hepatitis (Box 53-6)

D. Assessment

1. Preicteric stage

a. Flulike symptoms: malaise, fatigue

b. Anorexia, nausea, vomiting, diarrhea

c. Pain: headache, muscle aches, polyarthritis

d. Serum bilirubin and enzyme levels are elevated

BOX 53-6

Stages of Viral Hepatitis

PREICTERIC STAGE
The first stage of hepatitis preceding the appearance of jaundice

ICTERIC STAGE
The second stage of hepatitis, which includes the appearance of jaundice and associated symptoms such as elevated bilirubin levels, dark or tea-colored urine, and clay-colored stools

POSTICTERIC STAGE
The convalescent stage, in which the jaundice decreases and the color of the urine and the color of the stool return to normal

  2. Icteric stage
    a. Jaundice
    b. Pruritus
    c. Brown-colored urine
    d. Lighter-colored stools
    e. Decrease in preicteric phase symptoms
  3. Posticteric stage
    a. Energy levels increase
    b. Pain subsides
    c. GI symptoms are minimal to absent
    d. Serum bilirubin and enzyme levels return to normal
E. Laboratory assessment
  1. Alanine aminotransferase (ALT)
    a. Elevated to more than 1000 mU/mL and may rise to as high as 4000 mU/mL
    b. Normal adult blood value: 6 to 24 U/L
  2. Aspartate aminotransferase (AST)
    a. May rise to 1000 to 2000 mU/mL
    b. Normal adult blood value: 8 to 26 U/L
  3. Alkaline phosphatase levels
    a. May be normal or mildly elevated
    b. Normal adult blood value: 4.5 to 13 King-Armstrong units/dL
  4. Serum total bilirubin levels
    a. Elevated to greater than 2.5 mg/dL
    b. Normal: less than 1.5 mg/dL
    c. Elevated levels of bilirubin in the urine

XXII. HEPATITIS A (HAV)
A. Description
  1. Formerly known as infectious hepatitis
  2. Commonly seen during the fall and early winter
B. Increased-risk individuals
  1. Commonly seen in young children
  2. Individuals in institutionalized settings
  3. Health care personnel
▲ C. Transmission
  1. Fecal-oral route

  2. Person-to-person contact
  3. Parenteral
  4. Contaminated fruits, vegetables, or uncooked shellfish
  5. Contaminated water or milk
  6. Poorly washed utensils
D. Incubation period
  1. Incubation period is 2 to 6 weeks
  2. Infectious period is 2 to 3 weeks prior to, and 1 week after, developing jaundice
E. Testing
  1. Infection is established by the presence of hepatitis A virus (HAV) antibodies (anti-HAV) in the blood
  2. IgM and IgG are normally present in the blood, and increased levels indicate infection and inflammation
  3. Ongoing inflammation of the liver is evidenced by the presence of elevated immunoglobulin M (IgM) antibodies, which persist in the blood for 4 to 6 weeks
  4. Previous infection is indicated by the presence of elevated immunoglobulin G (IgG) antibodies
F. Complication: Fulminant hepatitis
G. Prevention
  1. Strict handwashing
  2. Stool and needle precautions
  3. Treatment of municipal water supplies
  4. Serologic screening of food handlers
  5. Hepatitis A vaccine (Havrix)
  6. Immune globulin (IG): For individuals exposed to HAV who have never received the hepatitis A vaccine; administer during the period of incubation and within 2 weeks of exposure
  7. IG is recommended for household members and sexual contacts of individuals with hepatitis A
  8. Preexposure prophylaxis with IG is recommended for individuals traveling to countries with poor or uncertain sanitation conditions

XXIII. HEPATITIS B (HBV)
A. Description
  1. Is nonseasonal in nature
  2. All age groups are affected
B. Increased-risk individuals
  1. Drug addicts
  2. Clients undergoing long-term hemodialysis
  3. Health care personnel
C. Transmission
  1. Blood or body fluid contact
  2. Infected blood products
  3. Infected saliva or semen
  4. Contaminated needles
  5. Sexual contact
  6. Parenteral
  7. Perinatal period
  8. Blood or body fluids contact at birth

D. Incubation period: 6 to 24 weeks
E. Testing
   1. Infection is established by the presence of hepatitis B antigen-antibody systems in the blood
   2. Presence of hepatitis B surface antigens (HBsAG) is the serologic marker to establish the diagnosis of hepatitis B
   3. The client is considered infectious if these antigens are present in the blood
   4. If the serologic marker (HBsAG) is present after 6 months, it indicates a carrier state or chronic hepatitis
   5. Normally the serologic marker (HBsAG) level declines and disappears after the acute hepatitis B episode
   6. The presence of antibodies to HBsAG (anti-HBS) indicates recovery and immunity to hepatitis B
   7. Hepatitis B early antigen (HBeAG) is detected in the blood about 1 week after the appearance of HbsAG, and its presence determines the infective state of the client
F. Complications
   1. Fulminant hepatitis
   2. Chronic liver disease
   3. **Cirrhosis**
   4. Primary hepatocellular carcinoma
G. Prevention
   1. Strict handwashing
   2. Screening blood donors
   3. Testing of all pregnant women
   4. Needle precautions
   5. Avoiding intimate sexual contact if hepatitis B surface antigen (HBsAG) is positive
   6. Hepatitis B vaccine: Engerix-B, Recombivax HB
   7. Hepatitis B immune globulin (HBIG): For individuals exposed to HBV either through sexual contact or through the percutaneous or transmucosal route, who have never had hepatitis B and have never received hepatitis B vaccine

XXIV. HEPATITIS C (HCV)
A. Description
   1. Occurs year round
   2. Can occur in any age group
   3. Is common among drug abusers and is the major cause of posttransfusion hepatitis
   4. Risk factors are similar as HBV, since hepatitis C is also parenterally transmitted
B. Increased-risk individuals
   1. Parenteral drug users
   2. Clients receiving frequent transfusions
   3. Health care personnel
C. Transmission: Same as HBV; primarily through blood
D. Incubation period: 5 to 10 weeks
E. Testing: Anti-HCV is the antibody to HCV and is most accurate in detecting chronic states of hepatitis C

F. Complications
   1. Chronic liver disease
   2. **Cirrhosis**
   3. Primary hepatocellular carcinoma
G. Prevention
   1. Strict handwashing
   2. Needle precautions
   3. Screening of blood donors

XXV. HEPATITIS D (HDV)
A. Description
   1. Common in the Mediterranean and Middle Eastern areas
   2. Seen with hepatitis B and may cause infection only in the presence of active HBV infection
   3. Coinfection with the delta agent intensifies the acute symptoms of hepatitis B
   4. Transmission and risk of infection are the same as for HBV, via contact with blood and blood products
   5. Prevention of HBV infection with vaccine also prevents HDV infection, since HDV is dependent on HBV for replication
B. High-risk individuals
   1. Drug users
   2. Clients receiving hemodialysis
   3. Clients receiving frequent blood transfusions
C. Transmission: Same as HBV
D. Incubation period: 7 to 8 weeks
E. Testing: Serologic hepatitis delta virus (HDV) determination is made by detection of the hepatitis D antigen (HDAg) early in the course of the infection and by detection of anti-HDV antibody in the later disease stages
F. Complications
   1. Chronic liver disease
   2. Fulminant hepatitis
G. Prevention: Because hepatitis D must coexist with hepatitis B, the precautions that help prevent hepatitis B are also useful in preventing delta hepatitis

XXVI. HEPATITIS E (HEV)
A. Description
   1. A waterborne virus
   2. Prevalent in areas where sewage disposal is inadequate or where communal bathing in contaminated rivers is practiced
   3. Risk of infection is the same as HAV
   4. Presents as a mild disease except in infected women in the third trimester of pregnancy, in whom the mortality rate is high
B. Increased-risk individuals
   1. Travelers to countries that have a high incidence of hepatitis E, such as India, Burma (Myanmar), Afghanistan, Algeria, and Mexico
   2. Eating or drinking food or water contaminated with the virus

⬥ C. Transmission: Same as HAV
D. Incubation period: 2 to 9 weeks
E. Testing: Specific serologic tests for hepatitis E virus (HEV) include detection of IgM and IgG antibodies to hepatitis E (anti-HEV)
F. Complications
1. High mortality rate in pregnant women
2. Fetal demise
⬥ G. Prevention
1. Strict handwashing
2. Treatment of water supplies and sanitation measures

XXVII. HEPATITIS G (HGV)

A. Non-A, non-B, non-C hepatitis
B. Autoantibodies are absent
C. Risk factors are similar to those for hepatitis C
D. Hepatitis G (HGV) has been found in some blood donors, IV drug users, hemodialysis clients, and clients with hemophilia; however, HGV does not appear to cause significant liver disease

⬥ **XXVIII. INSTRUCTIONS FOR HOME CARE FOR THE CLIENT AND FAMILY** (Box 53-7)

BOX 53-7

Client and Family Education for Hepatitis

Strict and frequent handwashing
Do not share bathrooms unless the client strictly adheres to personal hygiene measures
Individual washcloths, towels, and drinking and eating utensils, as well as toothbrushes and razors, must be labeled and identified
The client must not prepare food for other family members
The client should avoid alcohol and over-the-counter medications, particularly acetaminophen (Tylenol) and sedatives, because these medications are hepatotoxic
The client should increase activity gradually to prevent fatigue
The client should consume small, frequent meals of high-carbohydrate, low-fat foods
The client is not to donate blood
The client may maintain normal contact with people as long as proper personal hygiene is maintained
Close personal contact such as kissing should be discouraged until HbsAg test results are negative
The client is to avoid sexual activity until hepatitis B surface antigen (HBsAg) results are negative
The client needs to carry a Medic-Alert card noting the date of hepatitis onset
The client needs to inform other health professionals, such as medical or dental personnel, of the onset of hepatitis
The client needs to keep follow-up appointments with the health care provider

---

PRACTICE QUESTIONS

1. A nurse is participating in a health screening clinic and is preparing teaching materials about colorectal cancer. The nurse plans to include which of the following in a list of risk factors for colorectal cancer?
   1. Age over 30 years
   2. High-fiber, low-fat diet
   3. Distant relative with colorectal cancer
   4. Personal history of ulcerative colitis or gastrointestinal (GI) polyps

2. A hospitalized client with gastroesophageal reflux disease (GERD) is complaining of chest discomfort that feels like heartburn following a meal. After administering an ordered antacid, a nurse encourages the client to lie in which of the following positions?
   1. Supine with the head of bed flat
   2. On the stomach with the head flat
   3. On the left side with the head of bed elevated 30 degrees
   4. On the right side with the head of bed elevated 30 degrees

3. A nurse is planning to teach a client with gastroesophageal reflux disease (GERD) about substances that will increase the lower esophageal sphincter (LES) pressure. Which of the following items would the nurse include in this list?
   1. Fatty foods
   2. Nonfat milk
   3. Chocolate
   4. Coffee

4. A client has undergone esophagogastroduodenoscopy (EGD). A nurse places highest priority on which of the following items as part of the client's care plan?
   1. Assessing for the return of the gag reflex
   2. Giving warm gargles for a sore throat
   3. Monitoring the temperature
   4. Monitoring complaints of heartburn

5. A nurse has taught a client about an upcoming endoscopic retrograde cholangiopancreatography (ERCP) procedure. The nurse determines that the client has not fully understood the information if the client makes which of the following statements?
   1. "I know I must sign the consent form."
   2. "I'm glad I don't have to lie still for this procedure."
   3. "I'm glad some IV medication will be given to relax me."
   4. "I hope the throat spray keeps me from gagging."

6. A client being seen in a physician's office has just been scheduled for a barium swallow the next day. A nurse writes down which of the following instructions for the client to follow before the test?
   1. Remove all metal and jewelry before the test
   2. Eat a regular supper and breakfast

3. Continue to take all oral medications as scheduled
4. Monitor own bowel movement (BM) pattern for constipation

7. A nurse has given postprocedure instructions to a client who underwent colonoscopy. The nurse would conclude that the client did not fully understand the directions if the client stated that:
   1. Intake should be light at first, then progress to regular intake
   2. It is normal to feel gassy or bloated after the procedure
   3. The abdominal muscles may be tender from the procedure
   4. It is all right to drive once the client has been home for an hour or so

8. A nurse is performing an abdominal assessment. The initial assessment would be which of the following?
   1. Auscultation
   2. Inspection
   3. Palpation
   4. Percussion

9. Polyethylene glycol electrolyte solution (GoLYTELY) is prescribed for a client scheduled for a colonoscopy. The client begins to experience diarrhea following administration of the solution. What action by the nurse is most appropriate?
   1. Cancel the diagnostic test
   2. Start an IV
   3. Administer an enema
   4. Explain that diarrhea is expected

10. A nurse is caring for a client with a diagnosis of chronic gastritis. The nurse monitors the client, knowing that this client is at risk for which of the following vitamin deficiencies?
    1. Vitamin A
    2. Vitamin B_{12}
    3. Vitamin C
    4. Vitamin E

11. A nurse is reviewing the medication record of a client with acute gastritis. Which medication, if noted on the client's record, would the nurse question?
    1. Digoxin (Lanoxin)
    2. Indomethacin (Indocin)
    3. Furosemide (Lasix)
    4. Propranolol hydrochloride (Inderal)

12. A nurse is assessing a client 24 hours following a cholecystectomy. The nurse notes that the T tube has drained 750 mL of green-brown drainage. Which nursing intervention is most appropriate?
    1. Notify the physician
    2. Document the findings
    3. Irrigate the T tube
    4. Clamp the T tube

13. A nurse is monitoring a client with a diagnosis of

peptic ulcer. Which assessment finding would most likely indicate perforation of the ulcer?
   1. Bradycardia
   2. Numbness in the legs
   3. Nausea and vomiting
   4. A rigid boardlike abdomen

14. A nurse provides medication instructions to a client with peptic ulcer disease. Which statement, if made by the client, indicates the best understanding of the medication therapy?
    1. "The cimetidine (Tagamet) will cause me to produce less stomach acid."
    2. "Sucralfate (Carafate) will change the fluid in my stomach."
    3. "Antacids will coat my stomach."
    4. "Omeprazole (Prilosec) will coat the ulcer and help it heal."

15. A client with peptic ulcer disease is scheduled for a pyloroplasty. The client asks a nurse about the procedure. The nurse plans to respond, knowing that a pyloroplasty involves:
    1. Cutting the vagus nerve
    2. Removing the distal portion of the stomach
    3. Removal of the ulcer and a large portion of the cells that produce hydrochloric acid
    4. An incision and resuturing of the pylorus to relax the muscle and enlarge the opening from the stomach to the duodenum

16. A client with a peptic ulcer is scheduled for a vagotomy. The client asks the nurse about the purpose of this procedure. The nurse tells the client that the procedure:
    1. Decreases food absorption in the stomach
    2. Heals the gastric mucosa
    3. Halts stress reactions
    4. Reduces the stimulus to acid secretions

17. A nurse is caring for a client following a Billroth II procedure. On review of the postoperative orders, which of the following, if prescribed, would the nurse question and verify?
    1. Irrigating the nasogastric (NG) tube
    2. Coughing and deep breathing exercises
    3. Leg exercises
    4. Early ambulation

18. A nurse is providing discharge instructions to a client following gastrectomy. Which measure will the nurse instruct the client to follow to assist in preventing dumping syndrome?
    1. Eat high-carbohydrate foods
    2. Limit the fluids taken with meals
    3. Ambulate following a meal
    4. Sit in a high-Fowler's position during meals

19. A nurse is monitoring a client for the early signs and symptoms of dumping syndrome. Which of the following symptoms indicate this occurrence?
    1. Abdominal cramping and pain
    2. Bradycardia and indigestion

3. Sweating and pallor
4. Double vision and chest pain

20. A nurse is preparing a discharge teaching plan for a client who had a herniorrhaphy. Which of the following would the nurse include in the plan?
    1. Restricting pain medication
    2. Maintaining bed rest
    3. Avoiding coughing
    4. Irrigating the drain

21. A nurse is instructing a client who had a herniorrhaphy in how to reduce postoperative swelling following the procedure. The nurse tells the client to:
    1. Apply heat to the abdomen
    2. Elevate the scrotum
    3. Limit oral fluids
    4. Remain on a low-fiber diet

22. A nurse is caring for a hospitalized client with a diagnosis of ulcerative colitis. Which finding, if noted on assessment of the client, would the nurse report to the physician?
    1. Bloody diarrhea
    2. Hypotension
    3. A hemoglobin level of 12 mg/dL
    4. Rebound tenderness

23. A nurse is caring for a client postoperatively following creation of a colostomy. Which of the following nursing diagnoses would the nurse include in the plan of care?
    1. Altered nutrition: more than body requirements
    2. Body image disturbance
    3. Fear related to poor prognosis
    4. Sexual dysfunction

24. A nurse is reviewing the record of a client with Crohn's disease. Which of the following stool characteristics would the nurse expect to be documented in the client's record?
    1. Chronic constipation
    2. Diarrhea
    3. Constipation alternating with diarrhea
    4. Stool constantly oozing from the rectum

25. A nurse is performing a colostomy irrigation on a client. During the irrigation, the client begins to complain of abdominal cramps. Which of the following is the most appropriate nursing action?
    1. Notify the physician
    2. Increase the height of the irrigation
    3. Stop the irrigation temporarily
    4. Medicate for pain and resume the irrigation

26. A nurse is teaching a client how to perform a colostomy irrigation. To enhance the effectiveness of the irrigation, what measure should the nurse instruct the client to do?
    1. Increase fluid intake
    2. Reduce the amount of irrigation solution
    3. Massage the abdomen gently
    4. Place heat on the abdomen

27. A nurse is reviewing the record of a client with a diagnosis of cirrhosis and notes that there is documentation of the presence of asterixis. To assess for the presence of this sign, the nurse would do which of the following?
    1. Ask the client to extend the arms
    2. Assess for the presence of Homans' sign
    3. Instruct the client to lean forward
    4. Measure the abdominal girth

28. A client with ascites is scheduled for a paracentesis. A nurse is assisting the physician in performing the procedure. Which of the following positions will the nurse assist the client to assume for this procedure?
    1. Supine
    2. Left side-lying
    3. Right side-lying
    4. Upright position

29. A nurse is reviewing the laboratory results for a client with cirrhosis and notes that the ammonia level is elevated. Which of the following diets would the nurse anticipate would most likely be prescribed for this client?
    1. High carbohydrate
    2. Moderate fat
    3. High protein
    4. Low protein

30. A client is admitted to the hospital for treatment of acute hepatitis B. Which activity order would the nurse expect to be prescribed?
    1. Bed rest
    2. Encourage ambulation
    3. Out of bed in a chair
    4. No activity restrictions

31. It has been determined that a client with hepatitis contracted the infection from contaminated food. A nurse understands that this client is most likely experiencing what type of hepatitis?
    1. Hepatitis A
    2. Hepatitis B
    3. Hepatitis C
    4. Hepatitis D

32. A client is suspected of having hepatitis. Which diagnostic test results will assist in confirming this diagnosis?
    1. Decreased erythrocyte sedimentation rate
    2. Elevated serum bilirubin
    3. Elevated hemoglobin
    4. Elevated blood urea nitrogen (BUN)

33. A nurse is reviewing a physician's orders for a client admitted with acute pancreatitis. Which physician's order would the nurse question if noted on the client's chart?
    1. NPO status
    2. Insert a nasogastric tube
    3. An anticholinergic medication
    4. Morphine sulfate for pain

34. A nurse is doing an admission assessment on a client with a history of duodenal ulcer. To determine whether the problem is currently active, the nurse would assess the client for which of the following most frequent symptoms of duodenal ulcer?
    1. Pain that is relieved by food intake
    2. Pain that radiates down the right arm
    3. Nausea and vomiting
    4. Weight loss

35. A client with peptic ulcer disease (PUD) needs dietary modification to reduce episodes of epigastric pain. A nurse would plan to teach the client that which of the following items does not need to be limited or eliminated with this disease?
    1. Wine
    2. Baked chicken
    3. Coffee
    4. Fresh fruit

36. The medication history of a client with peptic ulcer disease (PUD) reveals intermittent use of several medications. A nurse would teach the client to avoid which of these medications because of the irritating effects on the lining of the gastrointestinal (GI) tract?
    1. Omeprazole (Prilosec)
    2. Ibuprofen (Motrin)
    3. Sucralfate (Carafate)
    4. Nizatidine (Axid)

37. A nurse instructs an ileostomy client to do which of the following as part of essential care of the stoma?
    1. Cleanse the peristomal skin meticulously
    2. Take in high-fiber foods such as nuts
    3. Massage the area below the stoma
    4. Limit fluid intake to prevent diarrhea

38. A client with hiatal hernia chronically experiences heartburn following meals. The nurse would plan to teach the client to avoid which of the following, which is contraindicated with a hiatal hernia?
    1. Taking in small, frequent, bland meals
    2. Lying recumbent following meals
    3. Raising the head of bed on 6-inch blocks
    4. Taking histamine H_2-receptor antagonist medication

39. A client who has undergone creation of a colostomy has a nursing diagnosis of body image disturbance. A nurse would conclude that the client is making the most significant progress toward identified goals if the client:
    1. Watches the nurse empty the ostomy bag
    2. Looks at the ostomy site
    3. Reads the ostomy product literature
    4. Practices cutting the ostomy appliance

40. A nurse is assessing for stoma prolapse in a client with a colostomy. The nurse would observe which of the following if stoma prolapse occurred?
    1. Sunken and hidden stoma
    2. Dark and bluish-colored stoma
    3. Narrowed and flattened stoma
    4. Protruding and swollen stoma

41. A client has a new colostomy, created 2 days earlier. The client is beginning to pass malodorous flatus from the stoma. The nurse interprets that:
    1. This indicates inadequate preoperative bowel preparation
    2. This is a normal, expected event
    3. The client is experiencing early signs of ischemic bowel
    4. The client should not have the nasogastric tube removed

42. A client with a new colostomy is concerned about the odor from stool in the ostomy drainage bag. The nurse teaches the client to include which of the following foods in the diet to reduce odor?
    1. Yogurt
    2. Broccoli
    3. Cucumbers
    4. Eggs

43. A nurse has given instructions to a client with an ileostomy about foods to eat to thicken the stool. The nurse would conclude that the client did not fully understand the instructions if the client stated that eating which of the following foods makes the stool less watery?
    1. Pasta
    2. Boiled rice
    3. Bran
    4. Low-fat cheese

44. A client has just had surgery to create an ileostomy. A nurse assesses the client in the immediate postoperative period for which of the following most frequent complications of this type of surgery?
    1. Intestinal obstruction
    2. Fluid and electrolyte imbalance
    3. Malabsorption of fat
    4. Folate deficiency

45. A nurse is doing preoperative teaching with a client who is about to undergo creation of a Kock pouch. The nurse interprets that the client has the best understanding of the nature of the surgery if the client makes which of the following statements?
    1. "I will need to drain the pouch regularly with a catheter."
    2. "I will need to wear a drainage bag for the rest of my life."
    3. "The drainage from this type of ostomy will be formed."
    4. "I will be able to pass stool by the rectum eventually."

46. A client with a newly created Kock pouch has an order to discontinue the continuous suction to the catheter placed in the pouch during surgery. The nurse anticipates that which of the follow-

ing solutions will be ordered for periodic catheter irrigation once the suction has been removed?
1. 10 to 20 mL normal saline
2. 50 to 60 mL tap water
3. 30 to 40 mL sterile water
4. 120 mL normal saline

47. A nurse is monitoring a client admitted to the hospital with a diagnosis of appendicitis. The client is scheduled for surgery in 2 hours. The client begins to complain of increased abdominal pain and begins to vomit. On assessment, the nurse notes that the abdomen is distended and bowel sounds are diminished. Which of the following is the most appropriate nursing intervention?
1. Administer the prescribed pain medication
2. Notify the physician
3. Call and ask the operating room team to perform the surgery as soon as possible
4. Reposition the client and apply a heating pad on warm setting to the client's abdomen

48. A client has been admitted with a diagnosis of acute pancreatitis. A nurse would assess this client for pain that is:
1. Severe and unrelenting, located in the epigastric area and radiating to the back
2. Severe and unrelenting, located in the left lower quadrant and radiating to the groin
3. Burning and aching, located in the epigastric area and radiating to the umbilicus
4. Burning and aching, located in the left lower quadrant and radiating to the hip

49. A client with chronic pancreatitis needs information on dietary modification to manage the health problem. A nurse should plan as priority instruction to teach the client to limit which of the following items in the diet?
1. Carbohydrate
2. Protein
3. Fat
4. Water-soluble vitamins

50. A nurse has taught a client with chronic pancreatitis about risk factor modification to reduce the incidence of recurrences. The nurse concludes that the client has understood the information if the client states that it will be necessary to control which of the following?
1. Diabetes mellitus
2. Alcohol intake
3. Duodenal ulcer
4. Crohn's disease

51. A nurse is evaluating the effect of dietary counseling on a client with cholecystitis. The nurse would conclude that the client understands the instructions given if the client states that which of the following food items is acceptable in the diet?
1. Baked scrod
2. Sauces and gravies
3. Fried chicken
4. Fresh whipped cream

52. A nurse would assess a client experiencing an acute episode of cholecystitis for pain that is located in the right:
1. Upper quadrant and radiates to the left scapula and shoulder
2. Upper quadrant and radiates to the right scapula and shoulder
3. Lower quadrant and radiates to the umbilicus
4. Lower quadrant and radiates to the back

53. A client with cirrhosis is beginning to show signs of hepatic encephalopathy. A nurse would plan a dietary consult to limit the amount of which of the following ingredients in the client's diet?
1. Fat
2. Carbohydrate
3. Protein
4. Minerals

54. A client with cirrhosis complicated by ascites is admitted to a hospital. The client has stated that a 10-pound weight gain occurred over the last week and a half. The client has edema of both feet and ankles. The abdomen is distended, taut, and shiny with striae. The nurse would select which of the following as the most appropriate nursing diagnosis for this client?
1. Altered Nutrition: More Than Body Requirements
2. Impaired Gas Exchange
3. Risk for Impaired Skin Integrity
4. Fluid Volume Excess

55. A client with Crohn's disease has a nursing diagnosis of Pain. A nurse would teach the client to avoid which of the following in managing this problem?
1. Lying supine with the legs straight
2. Applying heat to the abdomen
3. Using antispasmodic medication
4. Using relaxation techniques

56. A client with Crohn's disease has an order to begin taking antispasmodic medication. A nurse should time the medication so that each dose is taken:
1. 30 minutes before meals
2. During meals
3. 60 minutes after meals
4. Upon arising and at bedtime

57. A client with cirrhosis is scheduled for a liver biopsy. Which of these nursing measures would be included in the plan of care to assess for the possible development of bile peritonitis following a liver biopsy?
1. Monitoring for bloody diarrhea
2. Assessing for rebound tenderness
3. Assessing for increased flatulence
4. Monitoring for abdominal pain

58. A client is admitted to a hospital with viral hepatitis, complaining of "no appetite" and "losing

my taste for food." In order to provide adequate nutrition, the nurse would instruct the client to:

1. Eat a good supper when anorexia is not as severe
2. Eat less often, preferably only three large meals daily
3. Drink a lot of fluids, especially carbonated beverages
4. Select foods high in fat

59. A client has developed hepatitis A after eating contaminated oysters. A nurse assesses the client for which of the following?
   1. Dark stools
   2. Left upper quadrant discomfort
   3. Malaise
   4. Weight gain

60. A nurse is caring for an African-American who has a diagnosis of acute viral hepatitis. Which of the following specific areas should the nurse assess for jaundice in this client?
   1. Flexor surfaces of the extremities
   2. Hard palate of the mouth
   3. Nailbeds
   4. Skin

CRITICAL THINKING: FREE-TEXT ENTRY

A nurse assists a physician in performing a liver biopsy. After the procedure, the nurse places the client in which position?

Answer: _____

ANSWERS

1. 4

Rationale: Common risk factors for colorectal cancer include age over 40, first-degree relative with colorectal cancer, high-fat, low-fiber diet, and history of bowel problems, such as ulcerative colitis or familial polyposis.

Test-Taking Strategy: Use the process of elimination, reading each option carefully. Eliminate option 1 because of the age. Eliminate option 2 because this diet is healthy. Eliminate option 3 because of the word "distant." Review risk factors for colorectal cancer if you had difficulty with this question.

Level of Cognitive Ability: Application

Client Needs: Health Promotion and Maintenance

Integrated Concept/Process: Teaching/Learning

Content Area: Adult Health/Gastrointestinal

Reference: Monahan, F., & Neighbors, M. (1998). *Medical-surgical nursing: Foundations for clinical practice* (2nd ed.). Philadelphia: W.B. Saunders, p. 969.

2. 3

Rationale: The discomfort of reflux is aggravated by positions that compress the abdomen and the stomach. These include lying flat on either the back or the stomach after a meal, or lying on the right side. The left side-lying position with the head of the bed elevated is most likely to give relief to the client.

Test-Taking Strategy: Use the process of elimination. To answer this question correctly, evaluate each of the positions described in terms of their ability to put pressure on the stomach and cause reflux. Using knowledge of anatomy and these basic nursing positions, you should be able to eliminate each of the incorrect options. Review care of the client with GERD if you had difficulty with this question.

Level of Cognitive Ability: Application

Client Needs: Physiological Integrity

Integrated Concept/Process: Nursing Process/Implementation

Content Area: Adult Health/Gastrointestinal

Reference: Beare, P., & Myers, J. (1998). *Adult health nursing* (3rd ed.). St. Louis: Mosby, p. 1485.

3. 2

Rationale: Foods that increase the LES pressure will decrease reflux and lessen the symptoms of GERD. The food substance that will increase the LES pressure is nonfat milk. The other substances listed decrease the LES pressure, thus increasing reflux symptoms. Aggravating substances include chocolate, coffee, fatty foods, and alcohol.

Test-Taking Strategy: Use the process of elimination. It is necessary to understand the effect of various food substances on LES pressure and GERD. However, if you were unsure, select the option that identifies the healthiest food item. Review the dietary regimen for a client with GERD if you had difficulty with this question.

Level of Cognitive Ability: Application

Client Needs: Health Promotion and Maintenance

Integrated Concept/Process: Teaching/Learning

Content Area: Adult Health/Gastrointestinal

Reference: Beare, P., & Myers, J. (1998). *Adult health nursing* (3rd ed.). St. Louis: Mosby, p. 1484.

4. 1

Rationale: The nurse places highest priority on assessing for return of the gag reflex. This assessment addresses the client's airway. The client's vital signs are monitored also, and a sudden sharp increase in temperature could indicate perforation of the GI tract. This complication would be accompanied by other signs as well, such as pain. Monitoring for sore throat and heartburn are also important; however, the client's airway is the priority.

Test-Taking Strategy: Use the ABCs: airway, breathing, and circulation. Note the key words "highest priority." Option 1 addresses airway. Review care to the client following EGD if you had difficulty with this question.

Level of Cognitive Ability: Analysis

Client Needs: Safe, Effective Care Environment

Integrated Concept/Process: Nursing Process/Planning

Content Area: Adult Health/Gastrointestinal

Reference: Beare, P., & Myers, J. (1998). *Adult health nursing* (3rd ed.). St. Louis: Mosby, p. 1465.

5. 2

Rationale: The client does have to lie still for ERCP, which takes about an hour to perform. The client also has to sign a consent form. IV sedation is given to relax the client, and an anesthetic spray is used to help keep the client from gagging as the endoscope is passed.

Test-Taking Strategy: Use the process of elimination. Note the key words "has not fully understood." Invasive procedures require consent, so option 1 can be eliminated. Noting the name of the procedure and considering the anatomical location will assist in eliminating options 3 and 4. Review this procedure if you had difficulty with this question.

Level of Cognitive Ability: Analysis

Client Needs: Physiological Integrity

Integrated Concept/Process: Nursing Process/Evaluation

Content Area: Adult Health/Gastrointestinal

Reference: Beare, P., & Myers, J. (1998). *Adult health nursing* (3rd ed.). St. Louis: Mosby, p. 1472.

6. 1

Rationale: A barium swallow is an x-ray that uses a substance called barium for contrast to highlight abnormalities in the gastrointestinal (GI) tract. The client is told to remove all jewelry before the test, so it will not interfere with x-ray visualization of the field. The client should fast for 8 to 12 hours before the test, depending on the physician's instructions. Most oral medications are also withheld before the test. It is important after the procedure to monitor for constipation, which can occur as a result of the presence of barium in the GI tract.

Test-Taking Strategy: Note the key words "barium swallow" and "before." They tell you that the correct option is an item that the client needs to comply with before the test is done. Eliminate option 4 first, since it is a part of aftercare. Knowing that the procedure is a type of x-ray that involves barium for contrast allows you to eliminate options 2 and 3. Review preprocedure client instructions for this test if you had difficulty with this question.

Level of Cognitive Ability: Application

Client Needs: Physiological Integrity

Integrated Concept/Process: Communication and Documentation

Content Area: Adult Health/Gastrointestinal

Reference: Beare, P., & Myers, J. (1998). *Adult health nursing* (3rd ed.). St. Louis: Mosby, p. 1465.

7. 4

Rationale: The client should not drive for several hours after discharge because the client would have received sedative medications during the procedure. Important decisions should also be delayed for at least 24 hours for the same reason. The client should resume intake slowly, and progress as tolerated. The client may experience gas or abdominal tenderness for a short while after the procedure, and this is normal.

Test-Taking Strategy: Use the process of elimination. Note the key words "did not fully understand." Recalling that sedating medications are administered will direct you to option 4. Review postprocedure instructions following colonoscopy if you had difficulty with this question.

Level of Cognitive Ability: Analysis

Client Needs: Physiological Integrity

Integrated Concept/Process: Self-Care

Content Area: Adult Health/Gastrointestinal

Reference: Monahan, F., & Neighbors, M. (1998). *Medical-surgical nursing: Foundations for clinical practice* (2nd ed.). Philadelphia: W.B. Saunders, p. 976.

8. 2

Rationale: The appropriate sequence for abdominal examination is inspection, auscultation, percussion, and palpation. Auscultation is performed after inspection to ensure that the motility of the bowel and bowel sounds are not altered by percussion or palpation.

Test-Taking Strategy: Use the process of elimination and visualize this procedure. Remember that the sequence for abdominal assessment is different from the usual systematic approach. Review this technique if you had difficulty with this question.

Level of Cognitive Ability: Application

Client Needs: Health Promotion and Maintenance

Integrated Concept/Process: Nursing Process/Assessment

Content Area: Adult Health/Gastrointestinal

Reference: Potter, P., & Perry, A. (2001). *Fundamentals of nursing* (5th ed.). St. Louis: Mosby, p. 800.

9. 4

Rationale: The solution GoLYTELY is a bowel evacuant used to cleanse the bowel in preparation for a colonoscopy. It is expected to cause a mild diarrhea and will clear the bowel in 4 to 5 hours. Options 1, 2, and 3 are inappropriate actions.

Test-Taking Strategy: Use the process of elimination. Knowledge regarding the purpose of this medication will assist in eliminating option 3 and easily direct you to option 4. Options 1 and 2 are not within the scope of nursing practice and should be eliminated. Review the action and purpose of this medication if you had difficulty with this question.

Level of Cognitive Ability: Application

Client Needs: Physiological Integrity

Integrated Concept/Process: Nursing Process/Implementation

Content Area: Adult Health/Gastrointestinal

Reference: Hodgson, B., & Kizior, R. (2001). *Saunders nursing drug handbook 2001*. Philadelphia: W.B. Saunders, p. 841.

10. 2

Rationale: Chronic gastritis causes deterioration and atrophy of the lining of the stomach, leading to the loss of the function of the parietal cells. The source of the intrinsic factor is lost, which results in the inability to absorb vitamin B_{12}. This leads to the development of pernicious anemia.

Test-Taking Strategy: Recalling the pathophysiology related to pernicious anemia and vitamin B_{12} deficiency will direct you to option 2. If you are unfamiliar with vitamin B_{12} deficiency and its relationship to gastric disorders, review this content.

Level of Cognitive Ability: Analysis

Client Needs: Physiological Integrity

Integrated Concept/Process: Nursing Process/Assessment

Content Area: Adult Health/Gastrointestinal

Reference: Smeltzer, S., & Bare, B. (2000). *Brunner & Suddarth's textbook of medical-surgical nursing* (9th ed.). Philadelphia: Lippincott Williams & Wilkins, pp. 858-860.

11. 2

Rationale: Indocin is a nonsteroidal antiinflammatory drug and can cause ulceration of the esophagus, stomach, duodenum, or small intestine. It is contraindicated in a client with GI disorders. Lasix is a loop diuretic. Digoxin is an antidysrhythmic. Inderal is a beta-adrenergic blocker. Lasix, digoxin, and Inderal are not contraindicated in clients with gastric disorders.

Test-Taking Strategy: Identify the classification of each of the medications listed. Use the process of elimination, selecting option 2 since this medication is the one that would affect the GI tract. Review these medications if you are unfamiliar with them.

Level of Cognitive Ability: Analysis
Client Needs: Safe, Effective Care Environment
Integrated Concept/Process: Nursing Process/Analysis
Content Area: Adult Health/Gastrointestinal
Reference: Hodgson, B., & Kizior, R. (2001). *Saunders nursing drug handbook 2001.* Philadelphia: W.B. Saunders, pp. 324-326, 452-454, 528-530, 877-880.

12. **2**
Rationale: Following cholecystectomy, drainage from the T tube is initially bloody and then turns to green-brown. The drainage is measured as output. The amount of expected drainage will range from 500 to 1000 mL per day. The nurse would document the output.

Test-Taking Strategy: Use the process of elimination. Options 3 and 4 can be eliminated because a T tube is not irrigated and would not be clamped with this amount of drainage. From the remaining options, it is necessary to know normal expected findings following this surgical procedure. Review postoperative assessment findings following cholecystectomy if you had difficulty with this question.

Level of Cognitive Ability: Analysis
Client Needs: Physiological Integrity
Integrated Concept/Process: Nursing Process/Implementation
Content Area: Adult Health/Gastrointestinal
Reference: Monahan, F., & Neighbors, M. (1998). *Medical-surgical nursing: Foundations for clinical practice* (2nd ed.). Philadelphia: W.B. Saunders, p. 1114.

13. **4**
Rationale: Perforation is a surgical emergency. It is characterized by sudden, sharp, intolerable severe pain beginning in the midepigastric area and spreading over the abdomen, which becomes rigid and boardlike. Nausea and vomiting may occur. Tachycardia may occur as hypovolemic shock develops. Numbness in the legs is not an associated finding.

Test-Taking Strategy: Use the process of elimination. Note the key words "most likely." Option 2 can be easily eliminated. Eliminate option 1 next because tachycardia rather that bradycardia would develop if the client is bleeding. From the remaining two options, focusing on the key words will assist in directing you to option 4. Review the signs of a perforated ulcer if you had difficulty with this question.

Level of Cognitive Ability: Analysis
Client Needs: Physiological Integrity
Integrated Concept/Process: Nursing Process/Assessment
Content Area: Adult Health/Gastrointestinal
Reference: Monahan, F., & Neighbors, M. (1998). *Medical-surgical nursing: Foundations for clinical practice* (2nd ed.). Philadelphia: W.B. Saunders, p. 1029.

14. **1**
Rationale: Tagamet, a histamine H_2-receptor antagonist, will decrease the secretion of gastric acid. Carafate promotes

healing by coating the ulcer. Antacids neutralize acid in the stomach. Prilosec inhibits gastric acid secretion.

Test-Taking Strategy: Use the process of elimination and knowledge regarding the actions of the medications identified in the options. If you are unfamiliar with these medications or their actions, review this content.

Level of Cognitive Ability: Analysis
Client Needs: Health Promotion and Maintenance
Integrated Concept/Process: Teaching/Learning
Content Area: Adult Health/Gastrointestinal
Reference: Monahan, F., & Neighbors, M. (1998). *Medical-surgical nursing: Foundations for clinical practice* (2nd ed.). Philadelphia: W.B. Saunders, pp. 1027-1028.

15. **4**
Rationale: Option 4 describes the procedure for a pyloroplasty. A vagotomy involves cutting the vagus nerve. A subtotal gastrectomy involves removing the distal portion of the stomach. A Billroth II procedure involves removal of the ulcer and a large portion of the cells that produce hydrochloric acid.

Test-Taking Strategy: Use the process of elimination. Note the relationship between the words "pyloroplasty" and "pylorus" in the correct option. Review this procedure if you had difficulty with this question.

Level of Cognitive Ability: Comprehension
Client Needs: Physiological Integrity
Integrated Concept/Process: Nursing Process/Planning
Content Area: Adult Health/Gastrointestinal
Reference: Monahan, F., & Neighbors, M. (1998). *Medical-surgical nursing: Foundations for clinical practice* (2nd ed.). Philadelphia: W.B. Saunders, p. 1028.

16. **4**
Rationale: A vagotomy, or cutting of the vagus nerve, is done to eliminate parasympathetic stimulation of gastric secretion. Options 1, 2, and 3 are incorrect descriptions of a vagotomy.

Test-Taking Strategy: Knowledge regarding the purpose of a vagotomy is required to answer this question. If you are unfamiliar with this procedure, review this content.

Level of Cognitive Ability: Comprehension
Client Needs: Physiological Integrity
Integrated Concept/Process: Teaching/Learning
Content Area: Adult Health/Gastrointestinal
Reference: Monahan, F., & Neighbors, M. (1998). *Medical-surgical nursing: Foundations for clinical practice* (2nd ed.). Philadelphia: W.B. Saunders, p. 1028.

17. **1**
Rationale: In a Billroth II resection, the proximal remnant of the stomach is anastamosed to the proximal jejunum. Patency of the NG tube is critical for preventing the retention of gastric secretions. The nurse should never irrigate or reposition the gastric tube after gastric surgery, unless specifically ordered by the physician. In this situation, the nurse should clarify the order. Options 2, 3, and 4 are appropriate postoperative interventions.

Test-Taking Strategy: Use the process of elimination. Eliminate options 2, 3, and 4 because they are general postoperative measures. Consider the anatomical location of the surgical procedure to assist in directing you to option 1. Review postoperative measures following a Billroth II, if you had difficulty with this question.

Level of Cognitive Ability: Analysis

Client Needs: Safe, Effective Care Environment
Integrated Concept/Process: Communication and Documentation
Content Area: Adult Health/Gastrointestinal
Reference: Ignatavicius, D., Workman, M., & Mishler, M. (1999). *Medical-surgical nursing across the health care continuum* (3rd ed.). Philadelphia: W.B. Saunders, pp. 1392-1393.

18. 2
Rationale: The client should be instructed to decrease the amount of fluid taken at meals. The client should also be instructed to avoid high-carbohydrate foods including fluids, such as fruit nectars; to assume a low-Fowler's position during meals; to lie down for 30 minutes after eating to delay gastric emptying; and to take antispasmotics as prescribed.
Test-Taking Strategy: Use the process of elimination. Eliminate options 3 and 4 first because these measures will promote gastric emptying. From the remaining options, select option 2 because this measure will delay gastric emptying. If you are unfamiliar with this syndrome, review the important client teaching points.
Level of Cognitive Ability: Application
Client Needs: Health Promotion and Maintenance
Integrated Concept/Process: Self-Care
Content Area: Adult Health/Gastrointestinal
Reference: Monahan, F., & Neighbors, M. (1998). *Medical-surgical nursing: Foundations for clinical practice* (2nd ed.). Philadelphia: W.B. Saunders, p. 1000.

19. 3
Rationale: Early manifestations of dumping syndrome occur 5 to 30 minutes after eating. Symptoms include vertigo, tachycardia, syncope, sweating, pallor, palpitations, and the desire to lie down.
Test-Taking Strategy: Use the process of elimination. Focus on the key word "early" to direct you to option 3. Review the early manifestations of this syndrome if you had difficulty with this question.
Level of Cognitive Ability: Analysis
Client Needs: Physiological Integrity
Integrated Concept/Process: Nursing Process/Assessment
Content Area: Adult Health/Gastrointestinal
Reference: Ignatavicius, D., Workman, M., & Mishler, M. (1999). *Medical-surgical nursing across the health care continuum* (3rd ed.). Philadelphia: W.B. Saunders, p. 1396.

20. 3
Rationale: Bedrest is not required following this surgical procedure. The client should take analgesics as needed and as prescribed to control pain. A drain is not used in this surgical procedure, although the client may be instructed in simple dressing changes. Coughing is avoided to prevent disruption of the tissue integrity, which can occur because of the location of this surgical procedure.
Test-Taking Strategy: Use the process of elimination. General postoperative measures will assist in eliminating options 1 and 2. From the remaining options, consider the anatomical location of the surgery and the surgical procedure to assist in selecting option 3. Review postoperative measures following this surgical procedure, if you had difficulty with this question.
Level of Cognitive Ability: Application
Client Needs: Health Promotion and Maintenance
Integrated Concept/Process: Nursing Process/Planning

Content Area: Adult Health/Gastrointestinal
Reference: Monahan, F., & Neighbors, M. (1998). *Medical-surgical nursing: Foundations for clinical practice* (2nd ed.). Philadelphia: W.B. Saunders, p. 1096.

21. 2
Rationale: After herniorrhaphy, the client should be instructed to elevate of the scrotum and apply ice packs while in bed to decrease pain and swelling. The client is also instructed to apply a scrotal support when out of bed. Heat will increase swelling.
Test-Taking Strategy: Focus on the issue, to reduce swelling. Basic knowledge regarding the effects of heat and cold will assist in eliminating option 1. Options 3 and 4 can be eliminated next because they are similar and these actions will cause constipation. Limiting oral fluids and consuming a low-fiber diet can also cause constipation. Straining with a bowel movement needs to be avoided. Review postoperative care following herniorrhaphy, if you had difficulty with this question.
Level of Cognitive Ability: Application
Client Needs: Health Promotion and Maintenance
Integrated Concept/Process: Self-Care
Content Area: Adult Health/Gastrointestinal
Reference: Monahan, F., & Neighbors, M. (1998). *Medical-surgical nursing: Foundations for clinical practice* (2nd ed.). Philadelphia: W.B. Saunders, p. 1096.

22. 4
Rationale: Rebound tenderness may be indicative of peritonitis. Bloody diarrhea is expected to occur in ulcerative colitis. Because of the blood loss, the client may be hypotensive and the hemoglobin level may be lower than normal. Signs of peritonitis must be reported to the physician.
Test-Taking Strategy: Use the process of elimination. Consider the expected manifestations that would occur in ulcerative colitis. This will assist in eliminating option 1. Recalling that bleeding would cause a lowered hemoglobin and hypotension will assist in eliminating options 2 and 3. Review the normal assessment findings in ulcerative colitis, if you had difficulty with this question.
Level of Cognitive Ability: Analysis
Client Needs: Physiological Integrity
Integrated Concept/Process: Nursing Process/Analysis
Content Area: Adult Health/Gastrointestinal
Reference: Ignatavicius, D., Workman, M., & Mishler, M. (1999). *Medical-surgical nursing across the health care continuum* (3rd ed.). Philadelphia: W.B. Saunders, pp. 1422, 1434.

23. 2
Rationale: Risk for body image disturbance relates to loss of bowel control, the presence of a stoma, the release of fecal material onto the abdomen, the passage of flatus, odor, and the need for an appliance (external pouch). There are no data in the question to support options 3 and 4. A risk for Altered Nutrition: Less Than Body Requirements is the more likely nursing diagnosis.
Test-Taking Strategy: Use the process of elimination. Use the data presented in the question to assist in selecting the correct option. There are no data in the question to support options 3 and 4. Reading option 1 carefully will assist in eliminating this option. Review care to the client following a colostomy if you had difficulty with this question.

Level of Cognitive Ability: Analysis
Client Needs: Psychosocial Integrity
Integrated Concept/Process: Caring
Content Area: Adult Health/Gastrointestinal
Reference: Monahan, F., & Neighbors, M. (1998). *Medical-surgical nursing: Foundations for clinical practice* (2nd ed.). Philadelphia: W.B. Saunders, p. 1007

24. **2**
Rationale: Crohn's disease is characterized by nonbloody diarrhea of usually not more than four or five stools daily. Over time, the diarrhea episodes do increase in frequency, duration, and severity. Options 1, 3, and 4 are not characteristics of Crohn's disease.
Test-Taking Strategy: Use the process of elimination. Eliminate option 4 first as the most unlikely occurrence. From the remaining options, it is necessary to be familiar with the characteristics of Crohn's disease. If you are unfamiliar with this disorder, review this content.
Level of Cognitive Ability: Analysis
Client Needs: Physiological Integrity
Integrated Concept/Process: Nursing Process/Assessment
Content Area: Adult Health/Gastrointestinal
Reference: Monahan, F., & Neighbors, M. (1998). *Medical-surgical nursing: Foundations for clinical practice* (2nd ed.). Philadelphia: W.B. Saunders, p. 1067.

25. **3**
Rationale: If cramping occurs during a colostomy irrigation, the irrigation flow is stopped temporarily and the client is allowed to rest. Cramping may occur from an infusion that is too rapid or is causing too much pressure. Increasing the height of the irrigation will cause further discomfort. The physician does not need to be notified. Medicating the client for pain is not the most appropriate action.
Test-Taking Strategy: Focus on the issue, abdominal cramping during irrigation. This will assist in eliminating options 1, 2, and 4. If you had difficulty answering this question, review the procedure for colostomy irrigation.
Level of Cognitive Ability: Application
Client Needs: Physiological Integrity
Integrated Concept/Process: Nursing Process/Implementation
Content Area: Adult Health/Gastrointestinal
Reference: Potter, P., & Perry, A. (2001). *Fundamentals of nursing* (5th ed.). St. Louis: Mosby, p. 1472.

26. **3**
Rationale: To enhance effectiveness of the irrigation, the client is instructed to change position, ambulate, massage the abdomen gently, and drink something warm. Options 1, 2, and 4 will not enhance the effectiveness of this procedure.
Test-Taking Strategy: Focus on the issue of the question, which is the measure that will enhance the effectiveness of the irrigation. This focus will assist in eliminating options 1, 2, and 4. If you are unfamiliar with this procedure, review this content.
Level of Cognitive Ability: Application
Client Needs: Health Promotion and Maintenance
Integrated Concept/Process: Teaching/Learning
Content Area: Adult Health/Gastrointestinal
Reference: Ignatavicius, D., Workman, M., & Mishler, M. (1999). *Medical-surgical nursing across the health care continuum* (3rd ed.). Philadelphia: W.B. Saunders, p. 1419.

27. **1**
Rationale: Asterixis is irregular flapping movements of the fingers and wrists when the hands and arms are outstretched, with the palms down, wrists bent up, and fingers spread. It is the most common and reliable sign that hepatic encephalopathy is developing. Options 2, 3, and 4 are incorrect.
Test-Taking Strategy: Use the process of elimination and knowledge regarding the procedure for this assessment to answer this question. Review this assessment procedure if you had difficulty with this question.
Level of Cognitive Ability: Application
Client Needs: Health Promotion and Maintenance
Integrated Concept/Process: Nursing Process/Assessment
Content Area: Adult Health/Gastrointestinal
Reference: Monahan, F., & Neighbors, M. (1998). *Medical-surgical nursing: Foundations for clinical practice* (2nd ed.). Philadelphia: W.B. Saunders, p. 1150.

28. **4**
Rationale: An upright position allows the intestine to float posteriorly and helps prevent intestinal laceration during catheter insertion. Options 1, 2, and 3 are incorrect positions.
Test-Taking Strategy: Attempt to visualize this procedure in selecting the correct option. Knowing that fluid will be aspirated from the abdominal cavity will assist in directing you to option 4. If you had difficulty with this question, review this procedure.
Level of Cognitive Ability: Application
Client Needs: Physiological Integrity
Integrated Concept/Process: Nursing Process/Implementation
Content Area: Adult Health/Gastrointestinal
Reference: Ignatavicius, D., Workman, M., & Mishler, M. (1999). *Medical-surgical nursing across the health care continuum* (3rd ed.). Philadelphia: W.B. Saunders, p. 1471.

29. **4**
Rationale: Most of the ammonia in the body is found in the gastrointestinal tract. Protein provided by the diet is transported to the liver by the portal vein. The liver breaks down protein, and this results in the formation of ammonia. A low-protein diet would be prescribed.
Test-Taking Strategy: Recall the physiology of the liver in answering this question. Note the key words "most likely." You should be easily directed to option 4. Also note that options 3 and 4 are opposite, which should provide you with the clue that one of these options is correct. Review dietary measures for the client with a high ammonia level if you had difficulty with this question.
Level of Cognitive Ability: Analysis
Client Needs: Physiological Integrity
Integrated Concept/Process: Nursing Process/Analysis
Content Area: Adult Health/Gastrointestinal
Reference: Ignatavicius, D., Workman, M., & Mishler, M. (1999). *Medical-surgical nursing across the health care continuum* (3rd ed.). Philadelphia: W.B. Saunders, pp. 1476-1477.

30. **1**
Rationale: Fatigue is a normal response to hepatic cellular damage. During the acute stage, rest is an essential intervention to reduce the liver's metabolic demands and increase its blood supply. Options 2, 3, and 4 are incorrect.
Test-Taking Strategy: Use the process of elimination. Note the key word "acute" in the question. Knowing that the liver will

need to rest in order to heal will easily assist you to option 1. If you are unfamiliar with the care of a client with hepatitis, review this content.
Level of Cognitive Ability: Analysis
Client Needs: Physiological Integrity
Integrated Concept/Process: Nursing Process/Analysis
Content Area: Adult Health/Gastrointestinal
Reference: Monahan, F., & Neighbors, M. (1998). *Medical-surgical nursing: Foundations for clinical practice* (2nd ed.). Philadelphia: W.B. Saunders, p. 1177.

31. **1**
Rationale: Hepatitis A is transmitted by the fecal-oral route via contaminated food or infected food handlers. Hepatitis B, C, and D are most commonly transmitted via infected blood or body fluids.
Test-Taking Strategy: Knowledge regarding the modes of transmission of the various types of hepatitis is required to answer this question. Review this content if you are unfamiliar with it.
Level of Cognitive Ability: Comprehension
Client Needs: Safe, Effective Care Environment
Integrated Concept/Process: Nursing Process/Assessment
Content Area: Adult Health/Gastrointestinal
Reference: Monahan, F., & Neighbors, M. (1998). *Medical-surgical nursing: Foundations for clinical practice* (2nd ed.). Philadelphia: W.B. Saunders, p. 1170.

32. **2**
Rationale: Laboratory indicators of hepatitis include elevated liver enzyme levels, elevated serum bilirubin levels, elevated erythrocyte sedimentation rates, and leukopenia. An elevated BUN may indicate renal dysfunction. A hemoglobin level is unrelated to this diagnosis.
Test-Taking Strategy: Use the process of elimination. Eliminate option 4 because a BUN identifies renal rather than hepatic dysfunction. Thinking about the organ that is involved in hepatitis should assist in directing you to option 2, the liver function test. Review diagnostic tests for hepatitis if you had difficulty with this question.
Level of Cognitive Ability: Analysis
Client Needs: Physiological Integrity
Integrated Concept/Process: Nursing Process/Assessment
Content Area: Adult Health/Gastrointestinal
Reference: Monahan, F., & Neighbors, M. (1998). *Medical-surgical nursing: Foundations for clinical practice* (2nd ed.). Philadelphia: W.B. Saunders, p. 1172.

33. **4**
Rationale: Meperidine (Demerol) rather than morphine sulfate is the medication of choice because morphine sulfate can cause spasms in the sphincter of Oddi. Options 1, 2, and 3 are appropriate interventions for the client with acute pancreatitis.
Test-Taking Strategy: Note the key word "acute" in the question. Recalling the pathophysiology associated with this disorder will direct you to option 4. Review the treatment for acute pancreatitis if you had difficulty with this question.
Level of Cognitive Ability: Analysis
Client Needs: Safe, Effective Care Environment
Integrated Concept/Process: Nursing Process/Analysis
Content Area: Adult Health/Gastrointestinal

Reference: Monahan, F., & Neighbors, M. (1998). *Medical-surgical nursing: Foundations for clinical practice* (2nd ed.). Philadelphia: W.B. Saunders, p. 1118.

34. **1**
Rationale: The most frequent symptom of duodenal ulcer is pain that is relieved by food intake. These clients generally describe the pain as a burning, heavy, sharp, or "hungry" pain that often localizes in the midepigastric area. The client with duodenal ulcer does not usually experience weight loss or nausea and vomiting. These symptoms are more typical in the client with a gastric ulcer.
Test-Taking Strategy: Use the process of elimination. To answer this question accurately, it is necessary to be able to discriminate between symptoms of duodenal and gastric ulcer. This will allow you to eliminate options 3 and 4 first. Choose option 1 over option 2, knowing that the pain does not radiate down the right arm, or by knowing that there is a pattern of pain-food-relief with duodenal ulcer. Review the clinical manifestations of a duodenal ulcer if you had difficulty with this question.
Level of Cognitive Ability: Application
Client Needs: Physiological Integrity
Integrated Concept/Process: Nursing Process/Assessment
Content Area: Adult Health/Gastrointestinal
Reference: Monahan, F., & Neighbors, M. (1998). *Medical-surgical nursing: Foundations for clinical practice* (2nd ed.). Philadelphia: W.B. Saunders, p. 1026.

35. **2**
Rationale: Dietary modification for the client with PUD includes eliminating foods that are irritating to the client. Items that are generally eliminated or avoided are highly spiced foods, alcohol, caffeine, chocolate, and fresh fruits. Other foods may be taken according to the client's tolerance of that specific food.
Test-Taking Strategy: Use the process of elimination, noting the key words "does not need to be limited." Recalling which types of foods and beverages are irritating to the gastrointestinal mucosa will direct you to option 2. If this question was difficult, review this content.
Level of Cognitive Ability: Application
Client Needs: Health Promotion and Maintenance
Integrated Concept/Process: Teaching/Learning
Content Area: Adult Health/Gastrointestinal
Reference: Monahan, F., & Neighbors, M. (1998). *Medical-surgical nursing: Foundations for clinical practice* (2nd ed.). Philadelphia: W.B. Saunders, p. 1027.

36. **2**
Rationale: Ibuprofen is a nonsteroidal antiinflammatory drug (NSAID), which is typically irritating to the lining of the GI tract, and should be avoided by clients with a history of peptic ulcer disease. The other medications listed are frequently used in the treatment of PUD. Omeprazole is a proton-pump inhibitor, which blocks transport of hydrogen ions into the lumen of the GI tract. Sucralfate coats the surface of an ulcer to promote healing. Nizatidine is a histamine H_2-receptor antagonist, which reduces the secretion of gastric acid.
Test-Taking Strategy: Use the process of elimination. Recalling the types of medications that are irritating to the GI tract or knowing which medications are used in the treatment of PUD will direct you to option 2. Review the pharmacological

treatment measures for PUD if you had difficulty with this question.
Level of Cognitive Ability: Application
Client Needs: Health Promotion and Maintenance
Integrated Concept/Process: Teaching/Learning
Content Area: Adult Health/Gastrointestinal
Reference: Monahan, F., & Neighbors, M. (1998). *Medical-surgical nursing: Foundations for clinical practice* (2nd ed.). Philadelphia: W.B. Saunders, p. 1028.

37. 1
Rationale: The peristomal skin must receive meticulous cleansing because the ileostomy drainage has more enzymes and is more caustic to the skin than colostomy drainage. Foods such as nuts, and those with seeds, will pass through the ileostomy. The client should be taught that these foods will remain undigested. The area below the ileostomy may be massaged if needed if the ileostomy becomes blocked by high-fiber foods. Fluid intake should be at least 6 to 8 glasses of water per day to prevent dehydration.
Test-Taking Strategy: Use the process of elimination and focus on the issue. Note the key words "essential care" and "stoma." They tell you that the correct answer will be the option that deals with the stoma directly. Review client instructions regarding ileostomy care if you had difficulty with this question.
Level of Cognitive Ability: Application
Client Needs: Health Promotion and Maintenance
Integrated Concept/Process: Teaching/Learning
Content Area: Adult Health/Gastrointestinal
Reference: Monahan, F., & Neighbors, M. (1998). *Medical-surgical nursing: Foundations for clinical practice* (2nd ed.). Philadelphia: W.B. Saunders, p. 1014.

38. 2
Rationale: Hiatal hernia is due to a protrusion of a portion of the stomach above the diaphragm, where the esophagus usually is positioned. The client usually experiences pain as a result of reflux with ingestion of irritating foods, lying flat following meals or at night, or with ingestion of large or fatty meals. Relief is obtained with intake of small, frequent, and bland meals; with use of histamine H_2-antagonists and antacids; and with elevation of the thorax following meals and during sleep.
Test-Taking Strategy: Use the process of elimination, noting the key word "contraindicated." Thinking about the pathophysiology that occurs in hiatal hernia will direct you to option 2. Review this pathophysiology if you had difficulty with this question.
Level of Cognitive Ability: Application
Client Needs: Health Promotion and Maintenance
Integrated Concept/Process: Teaching/Learning
Content Area: Adult Health/Gastrointestinal
Reference: Monahan, F., & Neighbors, M. (1998). *Medical-surgical nursing: Foundations for clinical practice* (2nd ed.). Philadelphia: W.B. Saunders, p. 1044.

39. 4
Rationale: The client is expected to have a body image disturbance after colostomy. The client progresses through normal grieving stages to adjust to this change. The client demonstrates the greatest deal of acceptance when the client participates in the actual colostomy care. Each of the incorrect

options represents an interest in colostomy care but is a passive activity. The correct option shows the client participating in self-care.
Test-Taking Strategy: Use the process of elimination. Note the key words "colostomy" and "most significant progress." Eliminate options 1, 2, and 3 because they are similar and indicate passive activities. Review psychosocial adjustment in a client with colostomy if you had difficulty with this question.
Level of Cognitive Ability: Analysis
Client Needs: Psychosocial Integrity
Integrated Concept/Process: Self-Care
Content Area: Adult Health/Gastrointestinal
Reference: Monahan, F., & Neighbors, M. (1998). *Medical-surgical nursing: Foundations for clinical practice* (2nd ed.). Philadelphia: W.B. Saunders, p. 1010.

40. 4
Rationale: A prolapsed stoma is one in which the bowel protrudes through the stoma, with an elongated and swollen appearance. A stoma retraction is characterized by sinking of the stoma. Ischemia of the stoma would be associated with dusky or bluish color. A stoma with a narrowed opening at the level of either the skin or the fascia is said to be stenosed.
Test-Taking Strategy: Use the process of elimination. Focus on the key word "prolapse" to direct you to option 4. If this question was difficult, review the complications associated with a colostomy stoma.
Level of Cognitive Ability: Analysis
Client Needs: Physiological Integrity
Integrated Concept/Process: Nursing Process/Assessment
Content Area: Adult Health/Gastrointestinal
Reference: Monahan, F., & Neighbors, M. (1998). *Medical-surgical nursing: Foundations for clinical practice* (2nd ed.). Philadelphia: W.B. Saunders, p. 1005.

41. 2
Rationale: As peristalsis returns after creation of a colostomy, the client begins to pass malodorous flatus. This indicates returning bowel function, and is an expected event. Within 72 hours of surgery, the client should begin passing stool via the colostomy. Options 1, 3, and 4 are incorrect.
Test-Taking Strategy: Use the process of elimination. Recalling the normal progression of bowel activity following ostomy formation will direct you to option 2. Review the expected findings following a creation of a colostomy if you had difficulty with this question.
Level of Cognitive Ability: Analysis
Client Needs: Physiological Integrity
Integrated Concept/Process: Nursing Process/Analysis
Content Area: Adult Health/Gastrointestinal
Reference: Monahan, F., & Neighbors, M. (1998). *Medical-surgical nursing: Foundations for clinical practice* (2nd ed.). Philadelphia: W.B. Saunders, pp. 1004-1005.

42. 1
Rationale: The client should be taught to include deodorizing foods in the diet, such as beet greens, parsley, buttermilk, and yogurt. Spinach also reduces odor, but is a gas-forming food as well. Broccoli, cucumbers, and eggs are gas-forming foods.
Test-Taking Strategy: Use the process of elimination. Recalling the effect of various foods on the gastrointestinal tract of the client with an ostomy will direct you to option 1. If this

question was difficult, review which foods cause odor or gas, and those that have a deodorizing effect.
Level of Cognitive Ability: Application
Client Needs: Health Promotion and Maintenance
Integrated Concept/Process: Teaching/Learning
Content Area: Adult Health/Gastrointestinal
Reference: Monahan, F., & Neighbors, M. (1998). *Medical-surgical nursing: Foundations for clinical practice* (2nd ed.). Philadelphia: W.B. Saunders, p. 1009.

43. **3**
Rationale: Foods that help to thicken the stool of the client with an ileostomy include pasta, boiled rice, and low-fat cheese. Bran is high in dietary fiber, and thus will increase output of watery stool by increasing propulsion through the bowel. Ileostomy output is liquid by nature. Addition or elimination of various foods can help to thicken or loosen this liquid drainage.
Test-Taking Strategy: Use the process of elimination, noting the key words "did not fully understand." Recalling that high-fiber foods such as bran can cause watery stools will direct you to the correct option. Review dietary measures for the client with an ileostomy if you had difficulty with this question.
Level of Cognitive Ability: Analysis
Client Needs: Health Promotion and Maintenance
Integrated Concept/Process: Nursing Process/Evaluation
Content Area: Adult Health/Gastrointestinal
Reference: Monahan, F., & Neighbors, M. (1998). *Medical-surgical nursing: Foundations for clinical practice* (2nd ed.). Philadelphia: W.B. Saunders, p. 1014.

44. **2**
Rationale: A major complication that occurs most frequently after ileostomy is fluid and electrolyte imbalance. The client requires constant monitoring of intake and output to prevent this from occurring. Losses require replacement by IV until the client can tolerate a diet orally. Intestinal obstruction is a less frequent complication. Fat malabsorption and folate deficiency are complications that could occur later in the postoperative period.
Test-Taking Strategy: Use the process of elimination. Note the key words "ileostomy," "complications," and "immediate postoperative period." They tell you that the correct option is one that occurs early in the postoperative course, and that occurs with relative frequency. If you had difficulty with this question, review the postoperative complications following this surgical procedure.
Level of Cognitive Ability: Application
Client Needs: Physiological Integrity
Integrated Concept/Process: Nursing Process/Assessment
Content Area: Adult Health/Gastrointestinal
Reference: Monahan, F., & Neighbors, M. (1998). *Medical-surgical nursing: Foundations for clinical practice* (2nd ed.). Philadelphia: W.B. Saunders, p. 1013.

45. **1**
Rationale: A Kock pouch is a continent ileostomy. As the ileostomy begins to function, the client drains it every 3 to 4 hours, and then decreases to about three times a day or as needed when full. The client does not need to wear a drainage bag, but should wear an absorbent dressing to absorb mucous drainage from the stoma. Ileostomy drainage is liquid in nature. The client would be able to pass stool from the rectum

only if an ileal-anal pouch or anastamosis was created. This type of operation is a two-stage procedure.
Test-Taking Strategy: Use the process of elimination. Focusing on the key word "pouch" will assist in directing you to option 1. If this question was difficult, review this content.
Level of Cognitive Ability: Analysis
Client Needs: Physiological Integrity
Integrated Concept/Process: Teaching/Learning
Content Area: Adult Health/Gastrointestinal
Reference: Monahan, F., & Neighbors, M. (1998). *Medical-surgical nursing: Foundations for clinical practice* (2nd ed.). Philadelphia: W.B. Saunders, pp. 1012-1013.

46. **1**
Rationale: To maintain catheter patency and drainage, the catheter is irrigated with 10 to 20 mL of normal saline. This prevents the pouch from overfilling, causing tension on the new suture lines. Water is not used because it is hypotonic. Small amounts are used to prevent rupture of the suture lines in the newly created pouch.
Test-Taking Strategy: Use the process of elimination. Begin to answer this question by eliminating options 2 and 4 first. These amounts are large and could cause harm to the suture lines. Choose option 1 over option 3 because it is a smaller volume, and because it is an isotonic solution. Review postoperative care following this surgical procedure if you had difficulty with this question.
Level of Cognitive Ability: Analysis
Client Needs: Physiological Integrity
Integrated Concept/Process: Nursing Process/Analysis
Content Area: Adult Health/Gastrointestinal
Reference: Monahan, F., & Neighbors, M. (1998). *Medical-surgical nursing: Foundations for clinical practice* (2nd ed.). Philadelphia: W.B. Saunders, p. 1013.

47. **2**
Rationale: On the basis of the signs and symptoms presented in the question, the nurse should suspect peritonitis and the physician should be notified. Administering pain medication is not an appropriate intervention. Heat should never be applied to the abdomen of a client with suspected appendicitis. It is not within the scope of nursing practice to schedule the surgical time, although the physician would probably perform the surgery earlier than the prescheduled time.
Test-Taking Strategy: Use the process of elimination. Focus on the signs and symptoms in the question and consider the complications that can occur with appendicitis. Options 3 and 4 can be easily eliminated. Noting that the signs presented in the question indicate a complication will assist in directing you to option 2. Review care to the client with appendicitis if you had difficulty with this question.
Level of Cognitive Ability: Analysis
Client Needs: Physiological Integrity
Integrated Concept/Process: Nursing Process/Implementation
Content Area: Adult Health/Gastrointestinal
Reference: Ignatavicius, D., Workman, M., & Mishler, M. (1999). *Medical-surgical nursing across the health care continuum* (3rd ed.). Philadelphia: W.B. Saunders, pp. 1434-1435.

48. **1**
Rationale: The pain associated with acute pancreatitis is often severe and unrelenting, is located in the epigastric region, and radiates to the back. The other options are incorrect.

Test-Taking Strategy: Use the process of elimination. Noting the key word "acute" will assist in eliminating options 3 and 4. From the remaining options, recalling the anatomical location of the pancreas will direct you to option 1. Review the manifestations in acute pancreatitis if you had difficulty with this question.
Level of Cognitive Ability: Analysis
Client Needs: Physiological Integrity
Integrated Concept/Process: Nursing Process/Assessment
Content Area: Adult Health/Gastrointestinal
Reference: Ignatavicius, D., Workman, M., & Mishler, M. (1999). *Medical-surgical nursing across the health care continuum* (3rd ed.). Philadelphia: W.B. Saunders, p. 1507.

49. **3**
Rationale: The client should limit fat in the diet. The client should also take small meals. This will also reduce the amount of carbohydrate and protein that the client must digest at any one time. The client does not need to limit water-soluble vitamins in the diet.
Test-Taking Strategy: Use the process of elimination. Note the key words "priority instruction." Recalling the function of the pancreas will easily direct you to option 3. Review dietary measures for the client with pancreatitis if you had difficulty with this question.
Level of Cognitive Ability: Application
Client Needs: Health Promotion and Maintenance
Integrated Concept/Process: Teaching/Learning
Content Area: Adult Health/Gastrointestinal
Reference: Ignatavicius, D., Workman, M., & Mishler, M. (1999). *Medical-surgical nursing across the health care continuum* (3rd ed.). Philadelphia: W.B. Saunders, p. 1513.

50. **2**
Rationale: Chronic pancreatitis is aggravated by continued alcohol intake. Each of the other options are not associated with pancreatitis.
Test-Taking Strategy: Use the process of elimination. Remember that options that are similar are not likely to be correct. In this instance, two of the incorrect options (3 and 4) represent other disorders of the digestive system. Choose option 2 over option 1 by recalling that diabetes mellitus is an endocrine disorder of the pancreas, while pancreatitis is an exocrine disorder. Review the factors that contribute to a recurrence of pancreatitis if you had difficulty with this question.
Level of Cognitive Ability: Analysis
Client Needs: Physiological Integrity
Integrated Concept/Process: Nursing Process/Evaluation
Content Area: Adult Health/Gastrointestinal
Reference: Phipps, W., Sands, J., & Marek, J. (1999). *Medical-surgical nursing: Concepts & clinical practice* (6th ed.). St. Louis: Mosby, p. 1385.

51. **1**
Rationale: The client with cholecystitis should decrease overall intake of dietary fat. Foods that should be avoided to achieve this end include sauces and gravies, fatty meats, fried foods, products made with cream, and heavy desserts. The correct option is baked scrod, which is low in fat.
Test-Taking Strategy: Use the process of elimination. Recalling the function of the gallbladder and knowledge of the foods that are low in fat will direct you to option 1. Review dietary measures for the client with cholecystitis if you had difficulty with this question.

Level of Cognitive Ability: Analysis
Client Needs: Health Promotion and Maintenance
Integrated Concept/Process: Nursing Process/Evaluation
Content Area: Adult Health/Gastrointestinal
Reference: Monahan, F., & Neighbors, M. (1998). *Medical-surgical nursing: Foundations for clinical practice* (2nd ed.). Philadelphia: W.B. Saunders, p. 1111.

52. **2**
Rationale: During an acute "gallbladder attack," the client may complain of severe right upper quadrant pain that radiates to the right scapula and shoulder. This is governed by the pattern on dermatomes in the body. The other options are incorrect.
Test-Taking Strategy: Use the process of elimination. Knowledge of the anatomical location of the gallbladder will direct you to option 2. Review the characteristics of the pain associated with cholecystitis if you had difficulty with this question.
Level of Cognitive Ability: Application
Client Needs: Physiological Integrity
Integrated Concept/Process: Nursing Process/Assessment
Content Area: Adult Health/Gastrointestinal
Reference: Monahan, F., & Neighbors, M. (1998). *Medical-surgical nursing: Foundations for clinical practice* (2nd ed.). Philadelphia: W.B. Saunders, p. 1109.

53. **3**
Rationale: Ammonia is yielded as a product of protein metabolism. Clients with hepatic encephalopathy have high serum ammonia levels, which are responsible for the encephalopathy symptoms. Limiting protein intake will curb the elevation in serum ammonia, and prevent further deterioration of the client's mental status.
Test-Taking Strategy: Recalling the function of the liver and the pathophysiology associated with cirrhosis will direct you to option 3. Review this content if you had difficulty with this question.
Level of Cognitive Ability: Application
Client Needs: Health Promotion and Maintenance
Integrated Concept/Process: Nursing Process/Planning
Content Area: Adult Health/Gastrointestinal
Reference: Monahan, F., & Neighbors, M. (1998). *Medical-surgical nursing: Foundations for clinical practice* (2nd ed.). Philadelphia: W.B. Saunders, p. 1183.

54. **4**
Rationale: The client with weight gain who also has cirrhosis complicated by ascites is most often retaining fluid. This is especially true when the client has not demonstrated an appreciable increase in food intake, or when the weight gain is massive in relation to the time frame given. This makes Fluid Volume Excess the most appropriate nursing diagnosis. The client does not have Altered Nutrition: More Than Body Requirements; in fact, this client is most likely malnourished as part of the overall clinical picture. No data are given to support Impaired Gas Exchange, although in some clients, upward pressure on the diaphragm from ascites does impair respiration. Risk for Impaired Skin Integrity assumes a lower priority than diagnoses that are actual.
Test-Taking Strategy: Focus on the data provided in the question. Note the key words "most appropriate." Begin to answer this question by eliminating option 3, since it is not an actual nursing diagnosis. Eliminate option 2 next because there are no supportive data. Choose correctly between the

remaining options, knowing that the weight gain is due to fluid retention. Review the complications associated with cirrhosis if you had difficulty with this question.
Level of Cognitive Ability: Analysis
Client Needs: Physiological Integrity
Integrated Concept/Process: Nursing Process/Analysis
Content Area: Adult Health/Gastrointestinal
Reference: Monahan, F., & Neighbors, M. (1998). *Medical-surgical nursing: Foundations for clinical practice* (2nd ed.). Philadelphia: W.B. Saunders, p. 1155.

55. 1
Rationale: Pain associated with Crohn's disease is alleviated by the use of analgesics and antispasmodics. It is also reduced by having the client practice relaxation techniques, applying local heat to the abdomen, and lying with the legs flexed. Lying with the legs extended is not useful because it increases the muscle tension in the abdomen, which could aggravate inflamed intestinal tissues as the abdominal muscles are stretched.
Test-Taking Strategy: Use the process of elimination and use general knowledge of pain management strategies, application of heat, and client positioning to answer this question. Note the key word "avoid." If this question was difficult, review pain management techniques for the client with Crohn's disease.
Level of Cognitive Ability: Application
Client Needs: Physiological Integrity
Integrated Concept/Process: Teaching/Learning
Content Area: Adult Health/Gastrointestinal
Reference: Monahan, F., & Neighbors, M. (1998). *Medical-surgical nursing: Foundations for clinical practice* (2nd ed.). Philadelphia: W.B. Saunders, p. 1069.

56. 1
Rationale: In order to be effective in decreasing bowel motility, antispasmodic medications should be administered 30 minutes before mealtimes. The other options are incorrect.
Test-Taking Strategy: Use concepts related to medication action to anticipate when the doses should be timed. Because antispasmodics slow down gut motility, it can be reasoned that they should be taken before meals, an activity that normally stimulates increased gastrointestinal motility. Review the administration of antispasmodics if you had difficulty with this question.
Level of Cognitive Ability: Application
Client Needs: Physiological Integrity
Integrated Concept/Process: Nursing Process/Implementation
Content Area: Adult Health/Gastrointestinal
Reference: Monahan, F., & Neighbors, M. (1998). *Medical-surgical nursing: Foundations for clinical practice* (2nd ed.). Philadelphia: W.B. Saunders, p. 1069.

57. 4
Rationale: Abdominal pain is the most common symptom of peritonitis. Although tenderness over the involved area is a universal sign, rebound tenderness is associated with appendicitis. Bloody diarrhea is a major symptom of ulcerative colitis. Increased flatulence commonly occurs with irritable bowel syndrome.
Test-Taking Strategy: Use the process of elimination and focus on the issue, an assessment finding that indicates peritonitis. Recalling the signs associated with peritonitis will direct you to option 4. Review the assessment findings associated with peritonitis, if you had difficulty with this question.

Level of Cognitive Ability: Analysis
Client Needs: Physiological Integrity
Integrated Concept/Process: Nursing Process/Assessment
Content Area: Adult Health/Gastrointestinal
Reference: Lewis, S., Heitkemper, M., & Dirksen, S. (2000). *Medical-surgical nursing: Assessment and management of clinical problems* (5th ed.). St. Louis: Mosby, p. 1151.

58. 3
Rationale: Although no special diet is required in the treatment of viral hepatitis, it is generally recommended that clients consume a diet with low fat content, since fat may be poorly tolerated because of decreased bile production. Small, frequent meals are preferable and may even prevent nausea. Frequently, appetite is better in the morning, so it is easier to eat a good breakfast. Carbonated beverages are used to counteract anorexia. An adequate fluid intake of 2500 to 3000 mL per day is also important.
Test-Taking Strategy: Use the process of elimination. Knowledge regarding the nutritional problems associated with hepatitis will assist in directing you to the correct option. Review measures to provide adequate nutrition for the client with hepatitis if you had difficulty with this question.
Level of Cognitive Ability: Application
Client Needs: Physiological Integrity
Integrated Concept/Process: Teaching/Learning
Content Area: Adult Health/Gastrointestinal
Reference: Lewis, S., Heitkemper, M., & Dirksen, S. (2000). *Medical-surgical nursing: Assessment and management of clinical problems* (5th ed.). St. Louis: Mosby, pp. 1199, 1201.

59. 3
Rationale: Hepatitis causes gastrointestinal symptoms such as anorexia, nausea, right upper quadrant discomfort, and weight loss. Fatigue and malaise are common. Stools will be light or clay colored if conjugated bilirubin is unable to flow out of the liver because of inflammation or obstruction of the bile ducts.
Test-Taking Strategy: Use the process of elimination. Recalling the function of the liver will easily direct you to option 3. If you had difficulty with this question, review the signs and symptoms of hepatitis.
Level of Cognitive Ability: Application
Client Needs: Physiological Integrity
Integrated Concept/Process: Nursing Process/Assessment
Content Area: Adult Health/Gastrointestinal
Reference: Lewis, S., Heitkemper, M., & Dirksen, S. (2000). *Medical-surgical nursing: Assessment and management of clinical problems* (5th ed.). St. Louis: Mosby, p. 1199.

60. 2
Rationale: Jaundice occurs in the skin and mucous membranes. In light-skinned persons, it is first seen in the sclera of the eyes and later in the skin. In dark-skinned persons, jaundice is observed in the inner canthus of the eyes and hard palate of the mouth. Pallor is detected in the nailbeds, and flushing associated with increased body temperature is best noted in the flexor surfaces of the extremities.
Test-Taking Strategy: Use the process of elimination. Recalling that jaundice is not observed in a dark-skinned client will assist in eliminating options 1 and 4. Knowing that pallor is assessed in the nailbeds will direct you to option 2. Review assessment techniques if you had difficulty with this question.
Level of Cognitive Ability: Analysis

Client Needs: Physiological Integrity
Integrated Concept/Process: Cultural Awareness
Content Area: Adult Health/Gastrointestinal
Reference: Lewis, S., Heitkemper, M., & Dirksen, S. (2000). *Medical-surgical nursing: Assessment and management of clinical problems* (5th ed.). St. Louis: Mosby, p. 1199.

CRITICAL THINKING: FREE-TEXT ENTRY

Answer: After the liver biopsy, the client is placed on the right side
Rationale: In order to splint and provide pressure at the puncture site, the client is kept on the right side for a minimum of 2 hours.

Test-Taking Strategy: Recalling the anatomical location of the liver will assist in answering this question. Review postprocedure care following a liver biopsy if you had difficulty with this question.
Level of Cognitive Ability: Application
Client Needs: Physiological Integrity
Integrated Concept/Process: Nursing Process/Implementation
Content Area: Adult Health/Gastrointestinal
Reference: Lewis, S., Heitkemper, M., & Dirksen, S. (2000). *Medical-surgical nursing: Assessment and management of clinical problems* (5th ed.). St. Louis: Mosby, p. 1032.

REFERENCES

Altman, G., Buchsel, P., & Coxon, V. (2000). *Delmar's fundamental & advanced nursing skills.* Albany, N.Y.: Delmar.

Beare, P., & Myers, J. (1998). *Adult health nursing* (3rd ed.). St. Louis: Mosby.

Cleveland, L., Aschenbrenner, D., Venable, S., & Yensen, J. (1999). *Nursing management in drug therapy.* Philadelphia: Lippincott.

Corbett, J. (2000). *Laboratory tests and diagnostic procedures* (5th ed.). Upper Saddle River: N.J.: Prentice-Hall.

Craven, R., & Hirnle, C. (2000). *Fundamentals of nursing: Human health and function* (3rd ed.). Philadelphia: Lippincott.

Elkin, M., Perry, A., & Potter, P. (2000). *Nursing interventions and clinical skills* (2nd ed.). St. Louis: Mosby.

Grodner, M., Anderson, S., & DeYoung, S. (2000). *Foundations and clinical applications of nutrition: A nursing approach.* St. Louis: Mosby.

Gutierrez, K. (1999). *Pharmacotherapeutics; Clinical decision-making in nursing.* Philadelphia: W.B. Saunders.

Hodgson, B., & Kizior, R. (2001). *Saunders nursing drug handbook 2001.* Philadelphia: W.B. Saunders.

Ignatavicius, D., Workman, M., & Mishler, M. (1999). *Medical-surgical nursing across the health care continuum* (3rd ed.). Philadelphia: W.B. Saunders.

LeMone, P., & Burke, K. (2000). *Medical-surgical nursing: Critical thinking in client care* (2nd ed.). Upper Saddle River, N.J.: Prentice-Hall.

Lewis, S., Heitkemper, M., & Dirksen, S. (2000). *Medical-surgical nursing: Assessment and management of clinical problems* (5th ed.). St. Louis: Mosby.

Monahan, F., & Neighbors, M. (1998). *Medical-surgical nursing: Foundations for clinical practice* (2nd ed.). Philadelphia: W.B. Saunders.

Phipps, W., Sands, J., & Marek, J. (1999). *Medical-surgical nursing: Concepts & clinical practice* (6th ed.). St. Louis: Mosby.

Potter, P., & Perry, A. (2001). *Fundamentals of nursing* (5th ed.). St. Louis: Mosby.

Salerno, E. (1999). *Pharmacology for health professionals.* St. Louis: Mosby.

Smeltzer, S., & Bare, B. (2000). *Brunner & Suddarth's textbook of medical-surgical nursing* (9th ed.). Philadelphia: Lippincott Williams & Wilkins.

Wilson, B., Shannon, M., & Stang, C. (2000). *Nurses drug guide 2000.* Stamford, Conn.: Appleton & Lange.

Gastrointestinal Medications

I. ANTACIDS AND MUCOSAL PROTECTIVE MEDICATIONS (Box 54-1)

A. Description
1. React with gastric acid to produce neutral salts or salts of low acidity
2. Inactivate pepsin and enhance mucosal protection but do not coat the ulcer crater to protect it from the acid and pepsin
3. Used for peptic ulcer disease and gastroesophageal reflux disease (GRD)
4. Should be taken on a regular schedule
5. Are usually administered seven times a day, 1 and 3 hours after each meal and at bedtime
6. To provide maximum benefit, treatment should elevate the gastric pH above 5
7. Antacid tablets should be chewed thoroughly and followed with a glass of water or milk
8. Liquid preparations should be shaken before dispensing
9. Interactions with other medications can be minimized by allowing 1 hour between antacid administration and the administration of other medications
10. Can interfere with the action of sucralfate (Carafate), and to minimize this interaction, the medications should be administered 1 hour apart from each other

B. Sucralfate (Carafate)
1. Creates a protective barrier against acid and pepsin
2. Administered orally; should be taken on an empty stomach
3. Administer at least 30 minutes apart from an antacid
4. May cause constipation
5. May impede absorption of warfarin sodium (Coumadin), phenytoin (Dilantin), theophylline, digoxin (Lanoxin), and some antibiotics and should be administered at least 2 hours apart from these medications

C. Misoprostol (Cytotec)
1. Used to prevent gastric ulcers caused by long-term therapy with nonsteroidal antiinflammatory drugs (NSAIDs)
2. Suppresses secretion of gastric acid
3. Promotes secretion of bicarbonate and cytoprotective mucus
4. Maintains submucosal blood flow by promoting vasodilation
5. Administered with meals
6. Causes diarrhea and abdominal pain
7. Contraindicated for use in pregnancy

D. Magnesium hydroxide
1. Rapid acting
2. Also referred to as milk of magnesia
3. Most prominent side effect is diarrhea
4. Usually administered in combination with aluminum hydroxide, an antacid that assists in preventing diarrhea
5. Contraindicated in clients with intestinal obstruction, appendicitis, or undiagnosed abdominal pain
6. In clients with renal impairment, magnesium can accumulate to high levels, causing signs of toxicity

E. Aluminum hydroxide (Amphojel, Alu-Cap, Dialume)
1. Slow acting
2. Contains significant amounts of sodium
3. Used with caution in clients with hypertension or heart failure
4. Most common side effect is constipation
5. Can reduce the effects of tetracyclines, warfarin sodium (Coumadin), and digoxin (Lanoxin)
6. Can reduce phosphate absorption and thereby cause hypophosphatemia

---

BOX 54-1

Antacids and Mucosal Protective Medications

Aluminum hydroxide gel (Amphogel, AlternaGEL)
Aluminum carbonate gel (Basaljel)
Bismuth subsalicylate (Pepto-Bismol)
Calcium carbonate (Tums)
Magnesium hydroxide (Milk of Magnesia, MOM)
Misoprostol (Cytotec)
Sulcralfate (Carafate)

BOX 54-2

Histamine H₂ Receptor Antagonists

Cimetidine (Tagamet)
Famotidine (Pepcid)
Nizatidine (Axid)
Ranitidine (Zantac)
Ranitidine bismuth citrate (Tritec)

BOX 54-3

Antimicrobials Effective Against *Helicobacter pylori*

Amoxicillin (Amoxil)
Clarithromycin (Biaxin)
Metronidazole (Flagyl)
Tetracycline (Achromycin)

BOX 54-4

Proton Pump Inhibitors

Omeprazole (Prilosec)
lansoprazole (Prevacid)

F. Calcium carbonate (Tums)
  1. Rapid acting
  2. Common side effect is constipation
G. Sodium bicarbonate
  1. Rapid onset
  2. Liberates carbon dioxide, increases intraabdominal pressure, and promotes flatulence
  3. Used with caution in clients with hypertension or heart failure
  4. Can cause systemic alkalosis in clients with renal impairment
  5. Is useful for treating acidosis and elevating urinary pH to promote excretion of acidic medications following overdose

II. HISTAMINE H₂ RECEPTOR ANTAGONISTS (Box 54-2)

A. Description
  1. Suppress secretion of gastric acid
  2. Alleviate symptoms of heartburn and assist in preventing complications of peptic ulcer disease
  3. Prevent stress ulcers and reduce the recurrence of all ulcers
  4. Promote healing in GRD
  5. Contraindicated in hypersensitivity
  6. Used with caution in clients with impaired renal or hepatic function
B. Cimetidine (Tagamet)
  1. Can be administered orally, intramuscularly, or IV
  2. Food reduces the rate of absorption; if taken with meals, absorption will be slowed
  3. By the IV route, a 300-mg dose can be diluted in a total volume of 20 mL and injected slowly over not less than 2 minutes, or it may diluted in 100 mL and infused over 15 to 20 minutes
  4. Antacids can decrease the absorption of cimetidine
  5. Cimetidine and antacids should be administered at least 1 hour apart from each other
  6. Passes the blood-brain barrier, and central nervous system (CNS) side effects can occur
  7. May cause mental confusion, agitation, psychosis, depression, anxiety, and disorientation
  8. Dosage should be reduced in clients with renal impairment
  9. IV administration can cause hypotension and dysrhythmias
  10. If administered with warfarin sodium (Coumadin), phenytoin (Dilantin), theophylline or lidocaine, the dosages of these medications should be reduced
C. Ranitidine (Zantac)
  1. Can be administered orally, IM, or IV
  2. Side effects are uncommon
  3. It does not penetrate the blood brain-barrier as cimetidine does
  4. Zantac is not affected by food
  5. For IV injection, it should be diluted with a volume of 20 mL and administered slowly over 5 minutes or more, or diluted in 100 mL and administered over 15 to 20 minutes
D. Famotidine (Pepcid) and nizatidine (Axid)
  1. Similar to Zantac and Tagamet
  2. Do not need to be administered with food
E. Ranitidine bismuth citrate (Tritec)
  1. Used to treat active duodenal ulcers associated with *Helicobacter pylori*
  2. Administered with the antibiotic clarithromycin (Biaxin) (Box 54-3)

III. PROTON PUMP INHIBITORS (Box 54-4)

A. Suppress gastric acid secretion
B. Used with active ulcer disease, erosive esophagitis, and pathological hypersecretory conditions

---

BOX 54-5

Gastrointestinal Stimulants

Bethanechol chloride (Urecholine, Duvoid)
Cisapride (Propulsid)
Metoclopramide (Reglan)
Neostigmine methylsulfate (Prostigmin)

C. Contraindicated in hypersensitivity
D. Common side effects include headache, diarrhea, abdominal pain, and nausea

IV. GASTROINTESTINAL STIMULANTS (Box 54-5)

A. Stimulate motility of the upper GI tract and increase rate of gastric emptying without stimulating gastric, biliary, or pancreatic secretions
B. Used for gastroesophageal reflux
C. May cause restlessness, drowsiness, extrapyramidal reactions, dizziness, insomnia, headache
D. Contraindicated in clients with sensitivity
▲ E. Contraindicated in clients with mechanical obstruction, perforation, or GI hemorrhage
▲ F. Can precipitate hypertensive crisis in clients with pheochromocytoma
G. Safety in pregnancy is not established
H. Reglan can cause Parkinson-like reactions; if they occur, the medication is discontinued
I. Propulsid may increase the absorption of cimetidine (Tagamet) and ranitidine (Zantac) when administered concurrently
J. Anticholinergics and narcotic analgesics antagonize the effects of metoclopramide (Reglan)
K. Alcohol, sedatives, cyclosporine (Sandimmune), and tranquilizers produce an additive effect

V. BILE ACID SEQUESTRANTS (Box 54-6)

A. Description
1. Used to treat pruritis associated with biliary disease
2. Act by absorbing and combining with intestinal bile salts, which are then secreted in the feces, preventing intestinal reabsorption
3. May be used in the treatment of hypercholesterolemia in adults
▲ 4. Used cautiously in clients with bowel obstruction or severe constipation, because of the adverse GI effects
5. Taste and palatability are often reasons for noncompliance and can be improved by the use of flavored products or mixing the medication with various juices
6. Stool softeners and other sources of fiber can be used to abate the GI side effects
B. Side effects
1. Constipation
2. Bloating

BOX 54-6

Bile Acid Sequestrants

Cholestyramine (Questran, Prevalite)
Colestipol (Colestid)

BOX 54-7

Medications for Cholelithiasis

Chenodiol (Chenix)
Monoctanoin (Moctanin)
Ursodiol (Actigall)

---

3. Flatulence
4. Nausea
5. Fecal impaction and intestinal obstruction
6. Exacerbation of hemorrhoids
7. Hypoprothrombinemia
8. Decreased vitamin absorption

VI. MEDICATIONS FOR CHOLELITHIASIS (Box 54-7)

A. Chenodiol (Chenix)
1. Decreases cholesterol production, lowering content of bile, and thus facilitates dissolution of gallstones
2. Can cause diarrhea and possible hepatotoxicity
3. Baseline liver function studies should be performed
4. Client should be instructed to contact the physician if abdominal pain, sudden right upper quadrant pain, nausea, or vomiting occurs ▲
5. Administer with food or milk
6. Avoid aluminum-containing antacids
B. Ursodiol (Actigall)
1. A naturally occurring bile salt
2. Suppresses hepatic synthesis and secretion of cholesterol and inhibits intestinal absorption of cholesterol
3. Requires months of therapy for dissolution of gallstone to occur
4. Ultrasound images are obtained within 6 months to determine effectiveness of therapy
5. Clients should be instructed to report nausea, vomiting, diarrhea, or rash to the physician
6. Administer with food or milk
7. Avoid aluminum-containing antacids
C. Monoctanoin (Moctanin)
1. Used when stones made of calcium are resistant to dissolution by oral chenodiol
2. Administered through a T tube, nasal biliary catheter, or percutaneous transhepatic catheter
3. Effective only when in contact with the stone
4. Major side effects include diarrhea, nausea, and abdominal pain

BOX 54-8

Medications to Treat Hepatic Encephalopathy

Lactulose (Cephulac)
Neomycin (Mycifradin)

BOX 54-9

Pancreatic Enzyme Replacements

Pancreatin (Creon)
Pancrelipase (Cotazym, Pancrease, Viokase)

BOX 54-10

Commonly Administered Antiemetics

Diphenidol hydrochloride (Vontrol)
Dolesetron (Anzemet)
Dronabinol (Marinol)
Granisetron (Kytril)
Hydroxyzine hydrochloride (Atarax)
Hydroxyzine pamoate (Vistaril)
Meclizine hydrochloride (Antivert)
Metoclopramide (Reglan)
Ondansetron (Zofran)
Prochlorperazine (Compazine)
Promethazine hydrochloride (Phenergan)
Thiethylperazine malate (Torecon)
Trimethobenzamide hydrochloride (Tigan)

BOX 54-11

Laxatives

BULK-FORMING LAXATIVES
Methylcellulose (Citrucel)
Calcium polycarbophil (Fibercon)
Psyllium hydrophilic mucilloid (Metamucil, Fiberall, Konsyl, Serutan, Modane Bulk)

STIMULANT CATHARTICS
Bisacodyl (Dulcolax)
Cascara sagrada
Castor oil, emulsified (Neoloid)
Phenolphthalein (Ex-Lax)
Senna concentrate (Senexon, Senna-Gen)

OSMOTIC (SALINE) CATHARTICS
Glycerin suppositories (Senokot)
Lactulose (Chronulac)
Magnesium citrate (Citroma)
Magnesium hydroxide (Milk of Magnesia, MOM)
Magnesium sulfate (Epsom salts)
Potassium bitartrate and sodium bicarbonate (Coe-Two)
Sodium phosphates (Fleet Phospho-Soda)

STOOL SOFTENERS
Docusate calcium (Surfak)
Docusate sodium (Colace)
Docusate with casanthranol (Peri-Colace)

LUBRICANT
Mineral oil

VII. MEDICATIONS TO TREAT HEPATIC ENCEPHALOPATHY (Box 54-8)

A. Lactulose (Cephulac)
  1. Reduces ammonia levels
  2. Improves protein tolerance in clients with advanced hepatic **cirrhosis**
  3. Lowers the colonic pH from 7 to 5; this acidification pulls ammonia into the bowel to be excreted in the feces, thus lowering the ammonia level
  4. Administered orally in the form of a syrup
B. Neomycin (Mycifradin)
  1. Reduces the number of colonic bacteria that normally convert urea and amino acids into ammonia
  2. Administered orally or via nasogastric (NG) tube
  3. Used with caution in clients with kidney impairment

VIII. PANCREATIC ENZYME REPLACEMENTS (Box 54-9)

A. Used to supplement or replace pancreatic enzymes
B. Taken with meals or a snack (food helps to buffer the stomach acid)
C. A high-fiber diet may increase the efficacy of the medication
D. Side effects include abdominal cramps or pain, nausea, and diarrhea
E. Products that contain calcium carbonate or magnesium hydroxide interfere with the action of the medication

IX. ANTIEMETICS (Box 54-10)

A. Medications used to control vomiting
B. The choice of the antiemetic is determined by the cause of the nausea and vomiting
C. Monitor for drowsiness and protect the client from injury
D. Monitor vital signs and I & O
E. Limit odors in the client's room when the client is nauseated and/or vomiting
F. Limit oral intake to clear liquids when the client is nauseated and/or vomiting

X. LAXATIVES (Box 54-11)

A. Bulk-forming laxatives
  1. Description
    a. Absorb water into the feces and increase bulk to produce large and soft stools

b. For short-term use
c. Contraindicated in bowel obstruction
2. Side effects
   a. GI disturbances
   b. Dehydration
   c. Electrolyte imbalance
   d. Dependency with chronic use
B. Stimulant cathartics
   1. Description: Stimulate motility of large intestine
   2. Biscodyl (Dulcolax): Do not administer within 60 minutes of an antacid or milk
   3. Cascara (castor oil): Administer with juice; produces results in 2 to 6 hours
C. Saline cathartics
   1. Attract water into the large intestine to produce bulk
   2. Stimulate **peristalsis**
   3. Achieve results in 2 to 6 hours
D. Stool softeners
   1. Inhibit absorption of water so fecal mass remains large and soft
   2. Used to avoid straining
E. Lubricants
   1. Act to soften the feces
   2. Ease the strain of passing stool
   3. Lessen irritation to hemorrhoids
   4. Mineral oil
      a. Can cause lipid pneumonia if accidentally aspirated
      b. Interferes with absorption of fat-soluble vitamins A, D, E, and K

XI. MEDICATIONS TO CONTROL DIARRHEA
(Box 54-12)
A. Opioids
   1. Decrease intestinal motility and **peristalsis**
   2. When poisons, infections, or bacterial toxins are the cause of the diarrhea, opioids worsen the condition by delaying the elimination of toxins
   3. Tincture of opium has an unpleasant taste and can be diluted with 15 to 30 mL of water for administration
B. Other antidiarrheals: Refer to Box 54-12

XII. ANTISPASMODICS (Box 54-13)
A. Description: Relax smooth muscle of the GI tract
B. Side effects
   1. Constipation or diarrhea
   2. Rash
   3. Euphoria
   4. Dizziness
   5. Drowsiness
   6. Headache
   7. Nausea
   8. Weakness

BOX 54-12

Medications to Control Diarrhea

OPIOIDS AND RELATED MEDICATIONS
Codeine phosphate; codeine sulfate
Difenoxin with atropine (Motofen)
Diphenoxylate hydrochloride with atropine (Lomotil)
Loperamide hydrochloride (Imodium)
Tincture of opium

ABSORBENT ANTIDIARRHEALS
Bismuth subsalicylate (Pepto-Bismol)
Kaolin and pectin (Kao-Spen, Kapectolin)
Somatostatin Analog
Octreotide (Sandostatin)

BOX 54-13

Antispasmodics

Dicyclomine hydrochloride (Antispas)
Dicyclomine hydrochloride (Bentyl)

PRACTICE QUESTIONS

1. A client is receiving propantheline bromide (Pro-Banthine) as adjunctive treatment for peptic ulcer disease. A nurse should administer this medication:
   1. With meals
   2. Just after meals
   3. 30 minutes before meals
   4. With antacids

2. A client is taking docusate sodium (Colace). A nurse monitors for which of the following to determine whether the client is having a therapeutic effect from this medication?
   1. Absence of abdominal pain
   2. Hematest-negative stools
   3. Reduction in steatorrhea
   4. Regular bowel movements

3. A client is taking cascara sagrada and develops abdominal cramps. A nurse interprets that the client is most likely experiencing:
   1. A common side effect of this medication
   2. Partial bowel obstruction
   3. A case of influenza
   4. Peptic ulcer disease

4. A client taking bisacodyl (Dulcolax) wants to achieve rapid effect from the medication. A nurse then tells the client to take the medication:
   1. With a large meal
   2. On an empty stomach
   3. At bedtime
   4. With two glasses of juice

5. A client who is advised to take senna (Senokot) for

the treatment of constipation asks a nurse how this medication works. The nurse would incorporate which of the following when formulating a response?

1. It coats the bowel wall and makes it slippery
2. It adds fiber and bulk to the stool
3. It accumulates water and increases peristalsis
4. It stimulates the vagus nerve to improve bowel tone

6. A client has a PRN order for loperamide (Imodium). A nurse should plan to administer this medication if the client has:
   1. Hematest-positive nasogastric tube drainage
   2. Abdominal pain
   3. Constipation
   4. An episode of diarrhea

7. A nurse has given instructions to a client who just received a prescription for diphenoxylate with atropine (Lomotil). The nurse concludes that the client understands the use of the medication and its properties if the client states to:
   1. Stay within the prescribed dose because it can be habit forming
   2. Take the medication with a bulk-forming laxative
   3. Expect increased salivation while taking the medication
   4. Anticipate side effects of nervous system excitability

8. A client has been started on psyllium (Metamucil). A nurse would teach this client to take this medication with:
   1. Gelatin, applesauce, or pudding
   2. A full glass of liquid, followed by a second
   3. A multivitamin and mineral supplement
   4. A dose of an antacid

9. A nurse teaches a client taking metoclopramide (Reglan) to discontinue the medication immediately and call the physician if which of the following side effects occurs with long-term use?
   1. Anxiety or irritability
   2. Dry mouth not minimized by the use of sugar-free hard candy
   3. Excessive drowsiness or excitability
   4. Uncontrolled rhythmic movements of the face or limbs

10. A client has just taken a dose of trimethobenzamide (Tigan). A nurse plans to monitor this client for relief of:
    1. Nausea and vomiting
    2. Abdominal pain
    3. Heartburn
    4. Constipation

11. A client has a PRN order for ondansetron (Zofran). A nurse would administer this medication to the postoperative client for relief of:
    1. Urinary retention
    2. Incisional pain
    3. Nausea and vomiting
    4. Paralytic ileus

12. A client has an order to take magnesium citrate to prevent constipation following a barium study of the upper gastrointestinal (GI) tract. A nurse plans to administer this medication:
    1. With a full glass of water
    2. With fruit juice only
    3. On ice
    4. At room temperature

13. A nurse is administering a dose of prochlorperazine (Compazine) to a client for nausea and vomiting. The nurse would assess the client for which of the following frequent side effects of this medication?
    1. Diarrhea
    2. Drooling
    3. Excessive lacrimation
    4. Blurred vision

14. A client has begun medication therapy with pancrelipase (Pancrease). A nurse would conclude that the medication is having the optimal intended benefit if which of the following effects is observed?
    1. Reduction of steatorrhea
    2. Absence of abdominal pain
    3. Relief of heartburn
    4. Weight loss

15. A client asks a nurse why the medication cisapride (Propulsid) has been prescribed. The nurse would incorporate which of the following into a reply?
    1. It is being used to relieve nighttime heartburn from gastroesophageal reflux
    2. It is used to prevent nausea and vomiting
    3. It can help to heal gastrointestinal (GI) hemorrhage sites more quickly
    4. It may reverse a bowel obstruction, thus avoiding surgery

16. A nurse is giving a client directions for proper use of aluminum hydroxide tablets (Alu-Caps). The nurse tells the client to:
    1. Chew the tablets thoroughly and follow with 4 ounces of water
    2. Swallow the tablets whole with a full glass of water
    3. Take the tablets at the same time as other medications
    4. Take each dose with a laxative to prevent constipation

17. A client with a history of duodenal ulcer is taking calcium carbonate chewable tablets. A nurse would conclude that the client is experiencing optimal effects of the medication if:
    1. Muscle twitching stops
    2. Heartburn is relieved
    3. Serum calcium levels rise
    4. Serum phosphorus levels decrease

18. A hospitalized client asks a nurse for sodium bicarbonate to relieve heartburn following a meal. The nurse interprets that this client could not receive this medication if the client were currently being treated for which of the following conditions?
    1. Urinary calculi
    2. Chronic bronchitis
    3. Metabolic alkalosis
    4. Respiratory acidosis

19. A client is complaining of gas pains following surgery and requests medication. A nurse selects which of the following medications from the PRN medication list to give to the client?
    1. Magnesium hydroxide (Milk of Magnesia)
    2. Droperidol (Inapsine)
    3. Acetaminophen (Tylenol)
    4. Simethicone (Mylicon)

20. An elderly client has recently been started on cimetidine (Tagamet). A nurse would plan to monitor the client for which of the following most frequent central nervous system (CNS) side effects of this medication?
    1. Confusion
    2. Dizziness
    3. Tremors
    4. Hallucinations

21. A client with a gastric ulcer has an order for sucralfate (Carafate), 1 g by mouth qid. A nurse would schedule the medication for which of the following times?
    1. With meals and at bedtime
    2. One hour before meals and at bedtime
    3. Every 6 hours around the clock
    4. One hour after meals and at bedtime

22. A client who chronically uses nonsteroidal antiinflammatory drugs (NSAIDs) has been taking misoprostol (Cytotec). A nurse would conclude that the medication was having the intended therapeutic effect if the client did not experience which of the following symptoms?
    1. Decreased platelet count
    2. Decreased white blood cell count
    3. Epigastric pain
    4. Diarrhea

23. A physician has written an order for ranitidine (Zantac), 300 mg once daily. A nurse would schedule the medication for which of the following times?
    1. Before breakfast
    2. After lunch
    3. With supper
    4. At bedtime

24. A client is taking lansoprazole (Prevacid) for long-term chronic management of Zollinger-Ellison syndrome. A nurse advises the client to take which of the following products if needed for headache?
    1. Acetaminophen (Tylenol)
    2. Ibuprofen (Motrin)
    3. Naproxen (Aleve)
    4. Acetylsalicylic acid (Aspirin)

25. A client has been taking omeprazole (Prilosec) for 4 weeks. An ambulatory care nurse would conclude that the client is receiving the optimal intended effect of the medication if the client reports absence of which of the following symptoms?
    1. Constipation
    2. Heartburn
    3. Diarrhea
    4. Flatulence

CRITICAL THINKING: FREE-TEXT ENTRY

A client with esophageal reflux has been given a prescription for metoclopramide (Reglan) four times a day. A nurse teaches the client to take the medication at which times during the day?

Answer: _____

ANSWERS

1. **3**

Rationale: Propantheline bromide is an antimuscarinic anticholinergic medication that decreases gastrointestinal (GI) secretions. It should be administered 30 minutes prior to meals. The other options are incorrect.

Test-Taking Strategy: Use the process of elimination. Option 4 could be eliminated first, since most medications cannot be administered with antacids because of interactive effects. Next, eliminate options 1 and 2 because they are similar. Review this medication if you had difficulty with this question.

Level of Cognitive Ability: Application
Client Needs: Physiological Integrity

Integrated Concept/Process: Nursing Process/Implementation
Content Area: Pharmacology
Reference: Wilson, B., Shannon, M., & Stang, C. (2000). *Nurses drug guide 2000.* Stamford, Conn.: Appleton & Lange, p. 1189.

2. **4**

Rationale: Docusate sodium is a stool softener that promotes absorption of water into the stool, producing a softer consistency of stool. The intended effect is relief or prevention of constipation. The medication does not relieve abdominal pain, stop gastrointestinal (GI) bleeding, or decrease the amount of fat in the stools.

Test-Taking Strategy: Use the process of elimination. Recalling that docusate sodium is used to soften the stool will direct you to option 4. Review the expected effects of this medication if you had difficulty with this question.

Level of Cognitive Ability: Application
Client Needs: Health Promotion and Maintenance
Integrated Concept/Process: Nursing Process/Evaluation
Content Area: Pharmacology
Reference: Hodgson, B., & Kizior, R. (2001). *Saunders nursing drug handbook 2001.* Philadelphia: W.B. Saunders, pp. 344-345.

3. 1
Rationale: Cascara sagrada is a laxative that causes nausea and abdominal cramps as the most frequent side effects. Other health problems (options 2, 3, and 4) are not determined on the basis of a single symptom.

Test-Taking Strategy: Use the process of elimination. Remember that options that are similar are not likely to be correct. This will allow you to eliminate the two gastrointestinal disorders (options 2 and 4). From the remaining options, choose option 1 over option 3, knowing that laxatives can cause abdominal cramping. Review the effects of this medication if you had difficulty with this question.

Level of Cognitive Ability: Analysis
Client Needs: Physiological Integrity
Integrated Concept/Process: Nursing Process/Analysis
Content Area: Pharmacology
Reference: Hodgson, B., & Kizior, R. (2001). *Saunders nursing drug handbook 2001.* Philadelphia: W.B. Saunders, pp. 157-158.

4. 2
Rationale: Most rapid results from bisacodyl occur when it is taken on an empty stomach. It will not have a rapid effect if taken with a large meal. If it is taken at bedtime, the client will have a bowel movement in the morning. Taking the medication with two glasses of juice will not add to its effect.

Test-Taking Strategy: Use the process of elimination, noting the key words "rapid effects." Review the administration of this medication if you had difficulty with this question.

Level of Cognitive Ability: Application
Client Needs: Health Promotion and Maintenance
Integrated Concept/Process: Nursing Process/Implementation
Content Area: Pharmacology
Reference: Wilson, B., Shannon, M., & Stang, C. (2000). *Nurses drug guide 2000.* Stamford, Conn.: Appleton & Lange, p. 158.

5. 3
Rationale: Senna works by changing the transport of water and electrolytes in the large intestine, which causes accumulation of water in the mass of stool and increased peristalsis. The other options are incorrect.

Test-Taking Strategy: Knowledge regarding the action of this medication is required to answer this question. If you are unfamiliar with this medication, review its action.

Level of Cognitive Ability: Comprehension
Client Needs: Health Promotion and Maintenance
Integrated Concept/Process: Teaching/Learning
Content Area: Pharmacology
Reference: Wilson, B., Shannon, M., & Stang, C. (2000). *Nurses drug guide 2000.* Stamford, Conn.: Appleton & Lange, p. 1267.

6. 4
Rationale: Loperamide is an antidiarrheal agent. It is commonly administered after loose stools. It is used in the management of acute diarrhea, and also in chronic diarrhea such as with inflammatory bowel disease. It can also be used to reduce the volume of drainage from an ileostomy.

Test-Taking Strategy: Recalling that this medication is an antidiarrheal agent will direct you to option 4. Review the action of this medication if you had difficulty with this question.

Level of Cognitive Ability: Application
Client Needs: Physiological Integrity
Integrated Concept/Process: Nursing Process/Planning
Content Area: Pharmacology
Reference: Cleveland, L., Aschenbrenner, D., Venable, S., & Yensen, J. (1999). *Nursing management in drug therapy.* Philadelphia: Lippincott, p. 603.

7. 1
Rationale: The client should not exceed the recommended dose because the medication may be habit forming. The medication is an antidiarrheal and therefore should not be taken with a laxative. Side effects of the medication include dry mouth and drowsiness.

Test-Taking Strategy: Use the process of elimination. Noting the key word "atropine" will assist in eliminating options 3 and 4. Recalling that the medication is an antidiarrheal will assist in eliminating option 2. Review the properties of this medication if you had difficulty with this question.

Level of Cognitive Ability: Analysis
Client Needs: Physiological Integrity
Integrated Concept/Process: Nursing Process/Evaluation
Content Area: Pharmacology
Reference: Hodgson, B., & Kizior, R. (2001). *Saunders nursing drug handbook 2001.* Philadelphia: W.B. Saunders, p. 334.

8. 2
Rationale: Metamucil is a bulk-forming laxative. It should be taken with a full glass of water or juice, followed by another glass of liquid. This will help prevent impaction of the medication in the stomach or small intestine. The other options are incorrect.

Test-Taking Strategy: Use the process of elimination. Option 4 should be eliminated first because most medications are not taken with antacids. Eliminate options 1 and 3 next because they have no physiological benefit for medication effect. Review client teaching points related to this medication if you had difficulty with this question.

Level of Cognitive Ability: Application
Client Needs: Physiological Integrity
Integrated Concept/Process: Teaching/Learning
Content Area: Pharmacology
Reference: Hodgson, B., & Kizior, R. (2001). *Saunders nursing drug handbook 2001.* Philadelphia: W.B. Saunders, p. 886.

9. 4
Rationale: If the client experiences tardive dyskinesia (rhythmic movements of the face or limbs), the client should stop the medication and call the physician. These side effects may be irreversible. Excitability is not a side effect of this medication. Anxiety, irritability, and dry mouth are side effects that are not so harmful to the client.

Test-Taking Strategy: Use the process of elimination, focusing on the key words "discontinue the medication immediately." Select option 4 because these side effects are most harmful to the client. Review the side effects of this medication if you had difficulty with this question.

Level of Cognitive Ability: Application
Client Needs: Health Promotion and Maintenance
Integrated Concept/Process: Teaching/Learning
Content Area: Pharmacology
Reference: Hodgson, B., & Kizior, R. (2001). *Saunders nursing drug handbook 2001.* Philadelphia: W.B. Saunders, p. 672.

10. **1**
Rationale: Tigan is an antiemetic agent that is used in the treatment of nausea and vomiting. The other options are incorrect.
Test-Taking Strategy: Use the process of elimination. Recalling that this medication is an antiemetic will direct you to option 1. Review this medication if you had difficulty with this question.
Level of Cognitive Ability: Application
Client Needs: Physiological Integrity
Integrated Concept/Process: Nursing Process/Evaluation
Content Area: Pharmacology
Reference: Clark, J., Queener, S., & Karb, V. (2000). *Pharmacologic basis of nursing practice* (6th ed.). St. Louis: Mosby, p. 311.

11. **3**
Rationale: Ondansetron is an antiemetic that is used in the treatment of postoperative nausea and vomiting, as well as nausea and vomiting associated with chemotherapy. The other options are incorrect.
Test-Taking Strategy: Use the process of elimination. Recalling that this medication is an antiemetic will direct you to option 3. Review this medication if you had difficulty with this question.
Level of Cognitive Ability: Application
Client Needs: Physiological Integrity
Integrated Concept/Process: Nursing Process/Implementation
Content Area: Pharmacology
Reference: Clark, J., Queener, S., & Karb, V. (2000). *Pharmacologic basis of nursing practice* (6th ed.). St. Louis: Mosby, pp. 310-311.

12. **3**
Rationale: Magnesium citrate is available as an oral solution. It is used commonly as a laxative in preparation for or following certain studies of the GI tract. It should be served on ice, and should not be allowed to stand for prolonged periods. This would reduce the carbonation and make the solution even less palatable. Options 1, 2, and 4 are incorrect.
Test-Taking Strategy: Use the process of elimination. Eliminate options 1 and 2 first, knowing that magnesium citrate is itself a liquid. From the remaining options, it is necessary to know that it should be given cold to enhance palatability. Review this medication if you had difficulty with this question.
Level of Cognitive Ability: Application
Client Needs: Physiological Integrity
Integrated Concept/Process: Nursing Process/Planning
Content Area: Pharmacology
Reference: Clark, J., Queener, S., & Karb, V. (2000). *Pharmacologic basis of nursing practice* (6th ed.). St. Louis: Mosby, p. 296.

13. **4**
Rationale: The nurse would assess the client for blurred vision as a frequent side effect of prochlorperazine. Other frequent side effects of this phenothiazine-type antiemetic and antipsychotic are dry eyes, dry mouth, and constipation.
Test-Taking Strategy: Use the process of elimination. Recalling that this medication is a phenothiazine-type antiemetic and

knowing the side effects of these medications will direct you to option 4. Review this medication if you had difficulty with this question.
Level of Cognitive Ability: Application
Client Needs: Physiological Integrity
Integrated Concept/Process: Nursing Process/Assessment
Content Area: Pharmacology
Reference: Hodgson, B., & Kizior, R. (2001). *Saunders nursing drug handbook 2001.* Philadelphia: W.B. Saunders, p. 867.

14. **1**
Rationale: Pancrease is a pancreatic enzyme used as a digestive aid in clients with pancreatitis. The medication should reduce the amount of fatty stools (steatorrhea). Another intended effect could be improved nutritional status. It is not used to treat abdominal pain or heartburn. It could result in weight gain, but should not result in weight loss if it is aiding in digestion.
Test-Taking Strategy: Use the process of elimination and focus on the name of the medication. Use knowledge of physiology of the pancreas to assist in directing you to the correct option. Review this medication if you had difficulty with this question.
Level of Cognitive Ability: Analysis
Client Needs: Physiological Integrity
Integrated Concept/Process: Nursing Process/Evaluation
Content Area: Pharmacology
Reference: Hodgson, B., & Kizior, R. (2001). *Saunders nursing drug handbook 2001.* Philadelphia: W.B. Saunders, pp. 786-787.

15. **1**
Rationale: Cisapride is a GI prokinetic agent that is often given to treat nighttime heartburn that is associated with gastroesophageal reflux disease. It is not used as an antiemetic. It is contraindicated in conditions in which increased GI motility could cause harm, such as with GI hemorrhage, bowel perforation, or mechanical bowel obstruction.
Test-Taking Strategy: Use the process of elimination. Focusing on the name of the medication, Propulsid, may assist in directing you to option 1. Review the action of this medication if you had difficulty with this question.
Level of Cognitive Ability: Application
Client Needs: Physiological Integrity
Integrated Concept/Process: Teaching/Learning
Content Area: Pharmacology
Reference: Hodgson, B., & Kizior, R. (2001). *Saunders nursing drug handbook 2001.* Philadelphia: W.B. Saunders, pp. 225-226.

16. **1**
Rationale: Aluminum hydroxide tablets should be chewed thoroughly before they are swallowed. This prevents them from entering the small intestine undissolved. They should not be swallowed whole. Antacids should be taken at least 2 hours apart from other medications to prevent interactive effects. Constipation is a side effect of the use of aluminum products, but it is not correct for the client to take a laxative with each dose. This promotes laxative abuse; the client should first try other means to prevent constipation.
Test-Taking Strategy: Use the process of elimination. Eliminate option 4 first, since this action does not promote healthy bowel function. Next eliminate option 3 by using general knowledge of antacid interactive effects. From the remaining options, use principles of digestion and medication use to

direct you to option 1. Review this medication if you had difficulty with this question.

Level of Cognitive Ability: Application
Client Needs: Physiological Integrity
Integrated Concept/Process: Teaching/Learning
Content Area: Pharmacology
Reference: Hodgson, B., & Kizior, R. (2001). *Saunders nursing drug handbook 2001.* Philadelphia: W.B. Saunders, pp. 34-35.

17. 2

Rationale: Calcium carbonate can be used as an antacid for the relief of heartburn and indigestion. It can also be used as a calcium supplement (option 3), or to bind phosphorus in the gastrointestinal tract with renal failure (option 4). Option 1 is incorrect, although adequate calcium levels are needed for proper neurological function.

Test-Taking Strategy: Use the process of elimination. Focusing on the client's diagnosis will direct you to option 2. Review this medication if you had difficulty with this question.

Level of Cognitive Ability: Analysis
Client Needs: Health Promotion and Maintenance
Integrated Concept/Process: Nursing Process/Evaluation
Content Area: Pharmacology
Reference: Wilson, B., Shannon, M., & Stang, C. (2000). *Nurses drug guide 2000.* Stamford, Conn.: Appleton & Lange, p. 198.

18. 3

Rationale: Sodium bicarbonate is an electrolyte modifier and antacid. It would further aggravate metabolic alkalosis, which is a difficult acid-base imbalance to correct. The other options are incorrect.

Test-Taking Strategy: Use the process of elimination. Focusing on the name of the medication, "sodium bicarbonate," will direct you to option 3, "metabolic alkalosis." Review the contraindications associated with the use of sodium bicarbonate if you had difficulty with this question.

Level of Cognitive Ability: Analysis
Client Needs: Physiological Integrity
Integrated Concept/Process: Nursing Process/Analysis
Content Area: Pharmacology
Reference: Hodgson, B., & Kizior, R. (2001). *Saunders nursing drug handbook 2001.* Philadelphia: W.B. Saunders, p. 932.

19. 4

Rationale: Simethicone is an antiflatulent used in the relief of pain resulting from excessive gas in the gastrointestinal tract. MOM is an antacid and laxative. Droperidol is used to treat postoperative nausea and vomiting. Acetaminophen is a nonnarcotic analgesic.

Test-Taking Strategy: Use the process of elimination and focus on the key words "gas pains." Recalling the classifications of the medications in each of the options will direct you to option 4. Review the actions of Mylicon if you had difficulty with this question.

Level of Cognitive Ability: Analysis
Client Needs: Physiological Integrity
Integrated Concept/Process: Nursing Process/Implementation
Content Area: Pharmacology
Reference: Wilson, B., Shannon, M., & Stang, C. (2000). *Nurses drug guide 2000.* Stamford, Conn.: Appleton & Lange, p. 1273.

20. 1

Rationale: Elderly clients are especially susceptible to CNS side effects of cimetidine. The most frequent of these is confusion.

Less common CNS side effects include headache, dizziness, drowsiness, and hallucinations.

Test-Taking Strategy: Use the process of elimination and note the key words "most frequent." Use knowledge of the elderly and medication effects to direct you to option 1. Review the side effects of cimetidine if you had difficulty with this question.

Level of Cognitive Ability: Application
Client Needs: Physiological Integrity
Integrated Concept/Process: Nursing Process/Planning
Content Area: Pharmacology
Reference: Clark, J., Queener, S., & Karb, V. (2000). *Pharmacologic basis of nursing practice* (6th ed.). St. Louis: Mosby, p. 318.

21. 2

Rationale: The medication should be scheduled for administration 1 hour before meals and at bedtime. The medication is timed to allow it to form a protective coating over the ulcer before food intake stimulates gastric acid production and mechanical irritation. The other options are incorrect.

Test-Taking Strategy: Use the process of elimination. Focus on the diagnosis of the client to assist in directing you to option 2. Review the administration of this medication if you had difficulty with this question.

Level of Cognitive Ability: Application
Client Needs: Physiological Integrity
Integrated Concept/Process: Nursing Process/Implementation
Content Area: Pharmacology
Reference: Hodgson, B., & Kizior, R. (2001). *Saunders nursing drug handbook 2001.* Philadelphia: W.B. Saunders, p. 951.

22. 3

Rationale: The client who chronically uses NSAIDs is prone to gastric mucosal injury. Misoprostol is specifically given to prevent this occurrence. Diarrhea can be a side effect of the medication, but is not an intended effect. Options 1 and 2 are incorrect.

Test-Taking Strategy: The key words in this question are "intended therapeutic effect" and "did not experience." They tell you that the medication is being given to prevent the occurrence of specific symptoms. Recalling that NSAIDs can cause gastric mucosal injury will direct you to option 3. Review this medication and the side effects of NSAIDs if you had difficulty with this question.

Level of Cognitive Ability: Analysis
Client Needs: Health Promotion and Maintenance
Integrated Concept/Process: Nursing Process/Evaluation
Content Area: Pharmacology
Reference: Hodgson, B., & Kizior, R. (2001). *Saunders nursing drug handbook 2001.* Philadelphia: W.B. Saunders, p. 693.

23. 4

Rationale: A single daily dose of ranitidine is scheduled to be given at bedtime. This allows for a prolonged effect, and for the greatest protection of the gastric mucosa. The other options are incorrect.

Test-Taking Strategy: Use the process of elimination. Recalling the action of the medication and focusing on the key words "once daily" will direct you to option 4. Review this medication if you had difficulty with this question.

Level of Cognitive Ability: Application
Client Needs: Physiological Integrity
Integrated Concept/Process: Nursing Process/Implementation
Content Area: Pharmacology

Reference: Hodgson, B., & Kizior, R. (2001). *Saunders nursing drug handbook 2001.* Philadelphia: W.B. Saunders, p. 901.

24. **1**

Rationale: Zollinger-Ellison syndrome is a hypersecretory condition of the stomach. The client should avoid taking medications that are irritating to the stomach lining. Irritants would include aspirin and nonsteroidal antiinflammatory drugs (NSAIDs). The client should be advised to take Tylenol for a headache.

Test-Taking Strategy: Use the process of elimination. Remember that options that are similar are not likely to be correct. With this in mind, eliminate options 2 and 3 first because both of these medications are NSAIDs. Choose Tylenol over aspirin because it is least irritating to the stomach. Review this condition and this medication if you had difficulty with this question.

Level of Cognitive Ability: Application
Client Needs: Physiological Integrity
Integrated Concept/Process: Teaching/Learning
Content Area: Pharmacology
Reference: Hodgson, B., & Kizior, R. (2001). *Saunders nursing drug handbook 2001.* Philadelphia: W.B. Saunders, pp. 577-579.

25. **2**

Rationale: Omeprazole is a gastric pump inhibitor and is classified as an antiulcer agent. The intended effect of the medication is relief of pain from gastric irritation, often referred to as heartburn by clients. It is not used to treat the conditions identified in options 1, 3, and 4.

Test-Taking Strategy: Use the process of elimination. Recalling the classification of this medication will direct you to option 2. Review the action of this medication if you had difficulty with this question.

Level of Cognitive Ability: Analysis
Client Needs: Health Promotion and Maintenance
Integrated Concept/Process: Nursing Process/Evaluation
Content Area: Pharmacology
Reference: Hodgson, B., & Kizior, R. (2001). *Saunders nursing drug handbook 2001.* Philadelphia: W.B. Saunders, pp. 771-772.

CRITICAL THINKING: FREE-TEXT ENTRY

Answer: 30 minutes before meals and at bedtime

Rationale: The client should be taught to take this medication 30 minutes before meals and at bedtime. This allows the medication time to begin working before the client takes in food, which requires digestion and movement.

Test-Taking Strategy: Focusing on the client's diagnosis will assist in answering this question. Review administration of this medication if you had difficulty with this question.

Level of Cognitive Ability: Application
Client Needs: Physiological Integrity
Integrated Concept/Process: Teaching/Learning
Content Area: Pharmacology
Reference: Hodgson, B., & Kizior, R. (2001). *Saunders nursing drug handbook 2001.* Philadelphia: W.B. Saunders, p. 617.

REFERENCES

Clark, J., Queener, S., & Karb, V. (2000). *Pharmacologic basis of nursing practice* (6th ed.). St. Louis: Mosby.

Cleveland, L., Aschenbrenner, D., Venable, S., & Yensen, J. (1999). *Nursing management in drug therapy.* Philadelphia: Lippincott.

Gutierrez, K. (1999). *Pharmacotherapeutics: Clinical decision-making in nursing.* Philadelphia: W.B. Saunders.

Hodgson, B., & Kizior, R. (2001). *Saunders nursing drug handbook 2001.* Philadelphia: W.B. Saunders.

Ignatavicius, D., Workman, M., & Mishler, M. (1999). *Medical-surgical nursing across the health care continuum* (3rd ed.). Philadelphia: W.B. Saunders.

Salerno, E. (1999). *Pharmacology for health professionals.* St. Louis: Mosby.

Smeltzer, S., & Bare, B. (2000). *Brunner & Suddarth's textbook of medical-surgical nursing* (9th ed.). Philadelphia: Lippincott Williams & Wilkins.

Wilson, B., Shannon, M., & Stang, C. (2000). *Nurses drug guide 2000.* Stamford, Conn.: Appleton & Lange.

The Adult Client with a Respiratory Disorder

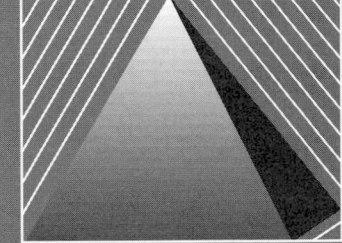

PYRAMID TERMS

bacille Calmette-Guérin (BCG) vaccine A vaccine containing attenuated tubercle bacilli that may be given to people in foreign countries or to those traveling to foreign countries, to produce increased resistance to tuberculosis (TB).

chronic airflow limitation, chronic obstructive lung disease (COLD), chronic obstructive pulmonary disease (COPD) A group of diseases that includes emphysema, asthma, bronchiectasis, and bronchitis. Characterized by progressive airflow limitations into and out of the lungs, elevated airway resistance, irreversible lung distention, and arterial blood gas imbalance. Can lead to pulmonary insufficiency, pulmonary hypertension, and cor pulmonale. In emphysema, the stimulus to breathe is a low Po_2 instead of an increased Pco_2.

emphysema A chronic pulmonary disease marked by a narrowing of the small airways and the trapping of air, with destructive changes in their walls. Also known as chronic obstructive pulmonary disease (COPD).

Mantoux test The most reliable determinant of infection with tuberculosis (TB). A small amount (0.1 mL) of intermediate-strength purified protein derivative (PPD) containing 5 tuberculin units is given intradermally in the forearm. An area of induration measuring 10 mm or more in diameter, 48 to 72 hours after injection, indicates that the individual has been exposed to TB.

mechanical ventilation The use of a ventilator if a client is unable to ventilate enough on his or her own to maintain proper levels of oxygen and carbon dioxide in the blood. Types of ventilators include negative-pressure and positive-pressure ventilators. Various ventilator modes are adjusted to the client's individual needs.

multidrug-resistant strain (MDR-TB) A multidrug-resistant strain of TB can occur as a result of improper or noncompliant use of treatment programs and the development of mutations in the tubercle bacilli.

Mycobacterium tuberculosis The causative organism (bacillus) of tuberculosis. An aerobic bacterium that is a nonmotile, nonsporulating, acid-fast rod that secrets niacin.

pneumothorax The accumulation of atmospheric air in the pleural space, which results in a rise in intrathoracic pressure and reduced vital capacity. The loss of negative intrapleural pressure results in collapse of the lung. Diagnosis of pneumothorax is made by chest x-ray.

suctioning A sterile procedure that involves the removal of respiratory secretions that accumulate in the tracheobronchial airway when the client is unable to expectorate secretions. Performed to maintain a patent airway.

tuberculosis (TB) A highly communicable disease caused by *Mycobacterium tuberculosis*. It is transmitted by the airborne route via droplet infection.

PYRAMID TO SUCCESS

The Pyramid to Success focuses on respiratory acid-base imbalances and reading arterial blood gas results; infectious diseases, particularly tuberculosis; and respiratory care in relation to oxygen delivery systems and mechanical ventilation. Pyramid points focus on the client with pneumonia, respiratory failure, chronic obstructive pulmonary disease, or pneumothorax. The Pyramid to Success includes the care of the client with tuberculosis, especially with regard to the importance of the medication regimen, providing adequate nutrition and adequate rest to promote the healing process, and the prevention of the progression of the disease. Focus on assisting the client to cope with the social isolation issues that exist during the period of illness and on teaching the client and family the critical measures of screening and of preventing respiratory disease and the transmission of disease. The Integrated Concepts and Processes addressed in this unit include Nursing Process, Caring, Communication and Documentation, Cultural Awareness, Self-Care, and Teaching/Learning.

CLIENT NEEDS
Safe, Effective Care Environment

Asepsis when caring for wounds or tracheostomy sites and during mechanical ventilation or suctioning
Client rights

Confidentiality related to the respiratory disorder

Consultations and referrals related to the respiratory disorder

Establishing priorities

Handling infectious materials such as sputum or body fluids

Informed consent related to diagnostic and surgical procedures

Respiratory precautions

Standard (universal) precautions

Health Promotion and Maintenance

Education related to the prevention of transmission of infection

Education related to medication administration

Education related to breathing exercises and respiratory therapy and care

Education related to adequate fluid and nutritional intake

Education related to the need for follow-up care

Health promotion programs

Health screening related to risks for respiratory disorders

Respiratory assessment techniques

Prevention of respiratory disorders and infectious diseases

Psychosocial Integrity

Body image changes related to tracheostomy if performed

Coping mechanisms

Community resources

Grief and loss

End-of-life issues

Religious and spiritual influences

Situational role changes

Support systems

Physiological Integrity

Alterations in body systems

Acid-base imbalances

Comfort interventions

Infectious diseases

Mechanical ventilation

Medical emergencies

Nutrition and oral hygiene

Oxygen delivery systems

Personal hygiene and rest and sleep

Pharmacological therapy

Reading arterial blood gas results

Respiratory care

REFERENCES

Craven, R., & Hirnle, C. (2000). *Fundamentals of nursing: Human health and function* (3rd ed.). Philadelphia: Lippincott.

Harkreader, H. (2000). *Fundamentals of nursing: Caring and clinical judgment.* Philadelphia: W.B. Saunders.

Ignatavicius, D., Workman, M., & Mishler, M. (1999). *Medical-surgical nursing across the health care continuum* (3rd ed.). Philadelphia: W.B. Saunders.

LeMone, P., & Burke, K. (2000). *Medical-surgical nursing: Critical thinking in client care* (2nd ed.). Upper Saddle River, N.J.: Prentice-Hall.

Lewis, S., Heitkemper, M., & Dirksen, S. (2000). *Medical-surgical nursing: Assessment and management of clinical problems* (5th ed.). St. Louis: Mosby.

National Council of State Boards of Nursing (eds.) (2000). *Test Plan for the National Council Licensure Examination for Registered Nurses.* Chicago: Author.

Potter, P;, & Perry, A. (2001). *Fundamentals of nursing* (5th ed.). St. Louis: Mosby.

Smeltzer, S., & Bare, B. (2000). *Textbook of medical-surgical nursing* (9th ed.). Philadelphia: Lippincott Williams & Wilkins.

The Respiratory System

I. ANATOMY AND PHYSIOLOGY

A. Primary functions
1. Provides oxygen for metabolism in the tissues
2. Removes carbon dioxide, the waste product of metabolism

B. Secondary functions
1. Facilitates sense of smell
2. Produces speech
3. Maintains acid-base balance
4. Maintains body water levels
5. Maintains heat balance

C. Upper respiratory tract
1. Nose: Humidifies, warms, and filters inspired air
2. Sinuses
   a. Air-filled cavities within the hollow bones that surround the nasal passages
   b. Provide resonance during speech
3. Pharynx
   a. Located behind the oral and nasal cavities
   b. Divided into the nasopharynx, oropharynx, and laryngopharynx
   c. Passageway for both the respiratory and digestive tracts
4. Larynx
   a. Located above the trachea and just below the pharynx at the root of the tongue
   b. Commonly called the voice box
   c. Contains two pairs of vocal cords, the false and true cords
   d. The opening between the true vocal cords is the glottis
   e. The glottis plays an important role in coughing, which is the most fundamental defense mechanism of the lungs
5. Epiglottis
   a. Leaf-shaped elastic structure that is attached along one end to the top of the larynx
   b. It prevents food from entering the tracheobronchial tree by closing over the glottis during swallowing

D. Lower respiratory tract
1. Trachea
   a. Located in front of the esophagus
   b. Branches into the right and left mainstem bronchi at the carina
2. Mainstem bronchi
   a. Begin at the carina
   b. The right bronchus is slightly wider, shorter, and more vertical than the left bronchus
   c. The mainstem bronchi divide into five secondary or lobar bronchi that enter each of the five lobes of the lung
   d. The bronchi are lined with cilia, which propel mucus up and away from the lower airway to the trachea, where it can be expectorated or swallowed
3. Bronchioles
   a. Branch from the secondary bronchi and subdivide into the small terminal and respiratory bronchioles
   b. They contain no cartilage and depend on the elastic recoil of the lung for patency
   c. The terminal bronchioles contain no cilia and do not participate in gas exchange
4. Alveolar ducts and alveoli
   a. Acinus (pl: acini) is a term used to indicate all structures distal to the terminal bronchiole
   b. Alveolar ducts branch from the respiratory bronchioles
   c. Alveolar sacs, which arise from the ducts, contain clusters of alveoli, which are the basic units of gas exchange
   d. Cells in the walls of the alveoli secrete surfactant, a phospholipid protein that reduces the surface tension in the alveoli; without surfactant, the alveoli would collapse

5. Lungs
   a. Located in the pleural cavity in the thorax
   b. Extend from just above the clavicles to the diaphragm, the major muscle of inspiration
   c. The right lung, which is larger than the left, is divided into three lobes, the upper, middle, and lower lobes
   d. The left lung, which is somewhat narrower than the right lung to accommodate the heart, is divided into two lobes
   e. Innervation of the respiratory structures is accomplished by the phrenic nerve, the vagus nerve, and the thoracic nerves
   f. The parietal pleura lines the inside of the thoracic cavity, including the upper surface of the diaphragm
   g. The visceral pleura covers the pulmonary surfaces
   h. A thin fluid layer, which is produced by the cells lining the pleura, lubricates the visceral pleura and the parietal pleura, allowing them to glide smoothly and painlessly during respiration
   i. Blood flow through the lungs occurs via the pulmonary system and the bronchial system
6. Accessory muscles of respiration: Include the scalene muscles, which elevate the first two ribs; the sternocleidomastoid muscles, which raise the sternum; and the trapezius and pectoralis muscles, which fix the shoulders
7. The respiratory process
   a. The diaphragm descends into the abdominal cavity during inspiration, causing negative pressure in the lungs
   b. The negative pressure draws air from the area of greater pressure, the atmosphere, into the area of lesser pressure, the lungs
   c. In the lungs, air passes through the terminal bronchioles into the alveoli to oxygenate the body tissues
   d. At the end of inspiration, the diaphragm and intercostal muscles relax and the lungs recoil
   e. As the lungs recoil, pressure within the lungs becomes greater than atmospheric pressure, causing the air, which now contains the cellular waste products of carbon dioxide and water, to move from the alveoli in the lungs to the atmosphere
   f. Expiration is a passive process (Box 55-1)

II. DIAGNOSTIC TESTS

A. Chest x-ray (CXR) film (radiograph)
   1. Description: Provides information regarding the anatomic location and appearance of the lungs
   2. Preprocedure
      a. Remove all jewelry and other metal objects from the chest area

---

BOX 55-1

Risk Factors For Respiratory Disease

Smoking
Use of chewing tobacco
Allergies
Frequent respiratory illnesses
Chest injury
Surgery
Exposure to chemicals and environmental pollutants
Crowded living conditions
Family history of infectious disease
Geographic residence and travel to foreign countries

BOX 55-2

Suctioning Procedure

Aseptic technique
Hyperoxygenate by a resuscitation bag, increasing the oxygen flow rate, or by asking the client to take deep breaths
Lubricate the catheter with sterile water
Tracheal suctioning: insert catheter 4 inches
Nasotracheal suctioning: insert catheter to induce cough reflex
Do not apply suction while inserting the catheter
Apply suction intermittently for 10 to 15 seconds; rotate the catheter and withdraw
Hyperoxygenate the client and encourage deep breaths

---

   b. Assess the client's ability to inhale and hold breath
   c. Question females regarding pregnancy or the possibility of pregnancy ▲
   3. Postprocedure: Assist the client to dress
B. Sputum specimen
   1. Description: A specimen obtained by expectoration or tracheal **suctioning** to assist in the identification of organisms or abnormal cells (Box 55-2)
   2. Preprocedure
      a. Determine specific purpose of collection and check with institutional policy for appropriate collection of specimen
      b. Obtain an early morning sterile specimen ▲ from **suctioning** or expectoration after a respiratory treatment, if a treatment is prescribed
      c. Obtain 15 mL of sputum
      d. Instruct the client to rinse the mouth with water prior to collection
      e. Instruct the client to take several deep breaths and then cough deeply to obtain sputum
      f. Always collect the specimen before starting antibiotics

3. Postprocedure
   a. If a culture of sputum is prescribed, transport specimen to laboratory immediately
   b. Assist the client with mouth care
C. Bronchoscopy
   1. Description: Direct visual examination of the larynx, trachea, and bronchi with a fiberoptic bronchoscope
   2. Preprocedure
      a. Obtain informed consent
      b. NPO from midnight prior to the procedure
      c. Obtain vital signs
      d. Assess the results of coagulation studies
      e. Remove dentures or eyeglasses
      f. Prepare suction equipment
      g. Administer medication for sedation as prescribed
      h. Have emergency resuscitation equipment readily available
   3. Postprocedure
      a. Monitor vital signs
      b. Maintain semi-Fowler's position
      c. Assess for the return of the gag reflex
      d. Maintain NPO status until gag reflex returns
      e. Have an emesis basin readily available for client to expectorate sputum
      f. Monitor for bloody sputum
      g. Monitor respiratory status, particularly if sedation was administered
      h. Monitor for complications, such as bronchospasm, bronchial perforation indicated by facial or neck crepitus, dysrhythmias, fever, bacteremia, hemorrhage, hypoxemia, and **pneumothorax**
      i. Notify the physician if fever, difficulty in breathing, or other signs of complications occur following the procedure
D. Pulmonary angiography
   1. Description
      a. An invasive fluoroscopic procedure in which a catheter is inserted through the antecubital or femoral vein into the pulmonary artery or one of its branches
      b. Involves an injection of iodine or radiopaque or contrast material
   2. Preprocedure
      a. Obtain informed consent
      b. Assess for allergies to iodine, seafood, or other radiopaque dyes
      c. Maintain NPO status for 8 hours prior to the procedure
      d. Monitor vital signs
      e. Assess results of coagulation studies
      f. Establish an IV access
      g. Administer sedation as prescribed
      h. Instruct the client that he or she must lie still during the procedure
      i. Instruct the client that he or she may feel an urge to cough, flushing, nausea, or a salty taste following injection of the dye
      j. Have emergency resuscitation equipment available
   3. Postprocedure
      a. Monitor vital signs
      b. Avoid taking blood pressures for 24 hours in the extremity used for the injection
      c. Monitor peripheral neurovascular status
      d. Assess insertion site for bleeding
      e. Monitor for delayed reaction to the dye
E. Thoracentesis
   1. Description: Removal of fluid or air from the pleural space via a transthoracic aspiration
   2. Preprocedure
      a. Obtain consent
      b. Obtain vital signs
      c. Prepare the client for ultrasound or chest radiograph, if prescribed, prior to procedure
      d. Assess results of coagulation studies
      e. Note that the client is positioned sitting upright, with the arms and head supported by a table at the bedside during the procedure
      f. If the client cannot sit up, the client is placed lying in bed on the unaffected side with the head of the bed elevated 45 degrees
      g. Instruct the client not to cough, breath deeply, or move during the procedure
   3. Postprocedure
      a. Monitor vital signs
      b. Monitor respiratory status
      c. Apply a pressure dressing, and assess the puncture site for bleeding and crepitus
      d. Monitor for signs of **pneumothorax,** air embolism, and pulmonary edema
F. Pulmonary function test (PFTs)
   1. Description: Include a number of different tests used to evaluate lung mechanics, gas exchange, and acid-base disturbance through spirometric measurements, lung volumes, and arterial blood gases
   2. Preprocedure
      a. Determine if an analgesic that may depress the respiratory function is being administered
      b. Consult with the physician regarding holding bronchodilators prior to testing
      c. Instruct the client to void prior to procedure and to wear loose clothing
      d. Remove dentures
      e. Instruct the client to refrain from smoking or eating a heavy meal for 4 to 6 hours prior to the test
   3. Postprocedure: Resume normal diet and any bronchodilators and respiratory treatments that were held prior to the procedure

G. Lung biopsy
   1. Description
      a. A percutaneous lung biopsy is performed to obtain tissue for analysis by culture or cytologic examination
      b. A needle biopsy is done to identify pulmonary lesions, changes in lung tissue, and the cause of pleural effusion
   2. Preprocedure
      a. Obtain informed consent
      b. Maintain NPO status prior to the procedure
      c. Inform the client that a local anesthetic will be used but that a sensation of pressure during needle insertion and aspiration may be felt
      d. Administer analgesics and sedatives as prescribed
   3. Postprocedure
      a. Monitor vital signs
      b. Apply a dressing to the biopsy site and monitor for drainage or bleeding
      c. Monitor for signs of respiratory distress, and notify the physician if they occur
      d. Monitor for signs of **pneumothorax** and air emboli, and notify the physician if they occur
      e. Prepare the client for chest x-ray film if prescribed

H. Ventilation perfusion lung scan
   1. Description
      a. In the perfusion scan, blood flow to the lungs is evaluated
      b. The ventilation scan determines the patency of the pulmonary airways and detects abnormalities in ventilation
      c. A radionuclide may be injected for the procedure
   2. Preprocedure
      a. Obtain informed consent
      b. Assess for allergies to dye, iodine, or seafood
      c. Remove jewelry around the chest area
      d. Review breathing methods that may be required during testing
      e. Establish an IV access
      f. Administer sedation if prescribed
      g. Have emergency resuscitation equipment available
   3. Postprocedure
      a. Monitor client for reaction to the radionuclide
      b. For 24 hours following the procedure, rubber gloves worn when urine is being discarded should be washed with soap and water before removing; then the hands should be washed after the gloves are removed
      c. Instruct client to wash hands carefully with soap and water for 24 hours following the procedure

I. Skin tests
   1. Description: An intradermal injection used to assist in diagnosing various infectious diseases

---

BOX 55-3

Normal ABG Values

pH: 7.35 to 7.45
Pco_2: 35 to 45 mm Hg
HCO_3: 22 to 27 mEq/L
Po_2: 80 to 100 mm Hg
O_2 saturation: 96% to 100%
Oxyhemoglobin dissociation curve: no shift

---

   2. Preprocedure: Determine hypersensitivity or previous reactions to skin tests
   3. Procedure
      a. Use a test site that is free of excessive body hair, dermatitis, and blemishes
      b. Apply at the upper one third of inner surface of left arm
      c. Circle and mark the injection test site
      d. Document the date, time, and test site
   4. Postprocedure
      a. Advise the client not to scratch the test site, to prevent infection and abscess formation
      b. Instruct the client to avoid washing the test site
      c. Interpret the reaction at the injection site 24 to 72 hours after administration of the test antigen
      d. Assess the test site for the amount of induration (hard swelling) in millimeters and the presence of erythema and vesiculation (small blister-like elevations)

J. Arterial blood gases (ABGs)
   1. Description: Measure the dissolved oxygen and carbon dioxide in the arterial blood and reveal the acid-base state and how well the oxygen is being carried to the body (Box 55-3)
   2. Preprocedure
      a. Perform Allen's test prior to drawing radial artery specimens
      b. Have the client rest for 30 minutes prior to specimen collection
      c. Avoid **suctioning** prior to drawing ABGs
      d. Do not turn off oxygen unless the ABGs are ordered to be drawn at room air
   3. Postprocedure
      a. Place the specimen on ice
      b. Note the client's temperature on laboratory form
      c. Note the oxygen and type of ventilation that the client is receiving on the laboratory form
      d. Apply pressure to the puncture site for 5 to 10 minutes and longer if the client is on anticoagulant therapy or has a bleeding disorder
      e. Transport the specimen to the laboratory within 15 minutes
      f. Refer to Chapter 9 for discussion of the analysis of ABG results

K. Pulse oximetry

1. Description
   a. A noninvasive test that registers the oxygen saturation of the client's hemoglobin
   b. This arterial oxygen saturation (SaO_2) is recorded as a percentage
   c. The normal value is 95% to 100%
   d. After a hypoxic client uses up the readily available oxygen (measured as the arterial oxygen pressure, PaO_2, on arterial blood gas testing), the reserve oxygen, that oxygen attached to the hemoglobin (SaO_2), is drawn on to provide oxygen to the tissues
   e. A pulse oximeter reading can alert the nurse to hypoxemia before clinical signs occur

2. Procedure
   a. A sensor is placed on the client's finger, toe, nose, earlobe, or forehead to measure oxygen saturation, which is then displayed on a monitor
   b. Maintain the transducer at heart level
   c. Do not select an extremity with an impediment to blood flow
   d. Results lower than 91% necessitate immediate treatment
   e. If the SaO_2 is below 85%, the body's tissues have a difficult time becoming oxygenated; an SaO_2 of less than 70% is life threatening

III. **RESPIRATORY TREATMENTS**

A. Chest physiotherapy (CPT)
   1. Description: Percussion and vibration over the thorax to loosen secretions in the affected area of the lungs
   2. Implementation
      a. A layer of material (gown or pajamas) is placed between the hands and the client's skin
      b. Best time to perform is in the morning upon rising, 1 hour before meals, or 2 to 3 hours after meals
      c. Stop CPT if pain occurs
      d. Dispose of sputum properly
      e. Provide mouth care after procedure
   3. Contraindications
      a. When bronchospasm is increased by its use
      b. History of pathological fractures
      c. Rib fractures
      d. Chest incisions

B. Postural drainage
   1. Description
      a. Use of gravity to drain secretions from segments of the lungs
      b. May be combined with CPT
   2. Implementation
      a. Position the client properly (lung segment to be drained is uppermost)
      b. Best time for the procedure is in the morning

upon arising, 1 hour before meals, or 2 to 3 hours after meals
   c. Stop postural drainage if cyanosis or exhaustion occurs
   d. Maintain position 5 to 20 minutes after procedure
   e. Dispose of sputum properly
   f. Provide mouth care after the procedure
   3. Contraindications
      a. Unstable vital signs
      b. Increased intracranial pressure

C. Incentive spirometry (Box 55-4)

IV. **OXYGEN**

A. Implementation
   1. Assess color and vital signs prior to and during treatment
   2. Place an OXYGEN IN USE sign at the client's bedside
   3. Assess for the presence of chronic lung problems
   4. Humidify the oxygen

B. Nasal cannula (nasal prongs) (Box 55-5)
   1. Description
      a. Used at flow rates of 1 to 6 L/min, providing approximate oxygen concentrations of 24% (at 1 L/min) to 44% (at 6 L/min)
      b. Flow rates higher than 6 L/min do not significantly increase oxygenation, because the anatomic reserve or dead space (oral and nasal cavities) is full
      c. Used for the client with chronic airflow limitation (**CAL**) and for long-term oxygen use; however, the **CAL** client who retains carbon dioxide should never receive oxygen at a rate higher than 2 to 3 L/min unless on a

---

BOX 55-4

Client Instructions for Incentive Spirometry

Use the lips to form seal around mouthpiece
Inspire deeply
Hold inspiration for a few seconds
Forcefully exhale
Avoid the use of spirometry at mealtimes because it may produce nausea

---

BOX 55-5

F_{IO_2} Delivered via Nasal Cannula

24% at 1 L/min
28% at 2 L/min
32% at 3 L/min
36% at 4 L/min
40% at 5 L/min
44% at 6 L/min

BOX 55-6

F$_{IO_2}$ Delivered via Simple Face Mask

40% at 5 L/min
45% to 50% at 6 L/min
55% to 60% at 8 L/min
Pyramid Point: Flow rate must be set to at least 5 L/min
to flush the mask of carbon dioxide

BOX 55-7

F$_{IO_2}$ Delivered via Partial Rebreather Mask

70% to 90% F$_{IO_2}$ is delivered at 6-15 L/min
Pyramid Point: A flow rate high enough to maintain the
bag two-thirds full during inspiration is needed

---

mechanical ventilator, because of the potential for apnea or respiratory arrest
  d. Effective oxygen concentration can be delivered to both nose breathers and mouth breathers with the use of a nasal cannula
2. Implementation
  a. Place the nasal prongs in the nostrils, with the openings facing the client
  b. Add humidification as prescribed when a flow rate higher than 2 L/min is prescribed
  c. Check the water level and change the humidifier as needed
  d. Assess the client for changes in respiratory rate or depth
  e. Assess the mucosa because high flow rates have a drying effect and increase mucosal irritation
  f. Assess skin integrity, because the oxygen tubing can irritate the skin
  g. Provide water-soluble jelly to the nares PRN
C. Simple face mask (Box 55-6)
1. Description
  a. A face mask used to deliver oxygen concentrations of 40% to 60% for short-term oxygen therapy or to deliver oxygen in an emergency
  b. A minimal flow rate of 5 L/min is needed to prevent the rebreathing of exhaled air
2. Implementation
  a. Be sure the mask fits securely over the nose and mouth because a poorly fitting mask reduces the F$_{IO_2}$ delivered
  b. Assess skin and provide skin care to the area covered by the mask, because pressure and moisture under the mask may cause skin breakdown
  c. Monitor the client closely for risk of aspiration, because the mask limits the client's ability to clear the mouth, especially if vomiting occurs
  d. Provide emotional support to decrease anxiety in the client who feels claustrophobic
  e. Consult with the physician regarding switching the client from a mask to a nasal cannula during eating
D. Partial rebreather mask (Box 55-7)
1. Description
  a. A partial rebreather mask consists of a mask

with a reservoir bag that provides an oxygen concentration of 70% to 90%, with flow rates of 6 to 15 L/min
  b. The client rebreathes one third of the exhaled tidal volume, which is high in oxygen, thus providing a high fraction of inspired oxygen (F$_{IO_2}$)
2. Implementation
  a. Make sure that the reservoir does not twist or kink, which results in a deflated bag
  b. Adjust the flow rate to keep the reservoir bag inflated two-thirds full during inspiration, because deflation results in decreased oxygen delivered and rebreathing of exhaled air
E. Nonrebreather mask
1. Description
  a. A nonrebreather mask provides the highest concentration of the low-flow systems and can deliver an F$_{IO_2}$ greater than 90%, depending on the client's ventilatory pattern
  b. It is most frequently used in the client with deteriorating respiratory status who might require intubation
  c. The nonrebreather mask has a one-way valve between the mask and the reservoir and two flaps over the exhalation ports
  d. The valve allows the client to draw the entire quantity of oxygen from the reservoir bag
  e. The flaps prevent room air from entering through the exhalation ports
  f. During exhalation, air leaves through these exhalation ports while the one-way valve prevents exhaled air from reentering the reservoir bag
2. F$_{IO_2}$ delivered: 60% to 100% F$_{IO_2}$ at a liter flow that maintains the bag two-thirds full
3. Implementation
  a. Remove mucus or saliva from the mask
  b. Assess the client closely
  c. Ensure that the valve and flaps are intact and functional during each breath
  d. Valves should open during expiration and close during inhalation
  e. Suffocation can occur if the reservoir bag kinks or if the oxygen source disconnects
F. High-flow oxygen delivery systems
1. A high-flow system provides oxygen concentrations of 24% to 100% at 8 to 15 L/min

2. High-flow systems include the Venturi mask, aerosol mask, face tent, tracheostomy collar, and T piece
3. These devices, when properly fitted, deliver a consistent and accurate oxygen concentration that meets the client's inspiratory effort

▲ G. Venturi mask
1. Description
▲   a. The Venturi mask delivers the most accurate oxygen concentration
   b. Its operation is based on a mechanism that pulls in a specific proportional amount of room air for each liter flow of oxygen
   c. An adapter is located between the bottom of the mask and the oxygen source; the adapter contains holes of different sizes that allow only specific amounts of air to mix with the oxygen
   d. The adapter allows selection of the amount of oxygen desired
2. FIO_2 delivered: 24% to 55% FIO_2 with flow rates of 4 to 10 L/min
3. Implementation
   a. Monitor closely to ensure an accurate flow rate for specific FIO_2
   b. Keep the orifice for the Venturi adapter open and uncovered to ensure adequate oxygen delivery.
   c. Ensure that the mask fits snugly and that tubing is free of kinks because the FIO_2 is altered if kinking occurs or if the mask fits poorly
   d. Assess the client for dry mucous membranes; humidity or aerosol can be added to the system

H. Face tent, aerosol mask, tracheostomy collar, and T piece
1. Face tent
   a. Fits over the client's chin, with the top extending halfway across the face
   b. The oxygen concentration varies, but the face tent is useful instead of a tight-fitting mask for the client who has facial trauma or burns
2. Aerosol mask: Used for the client who requires high humidity after extubation or upper air-way surgery, or for the client who has thick secretions
3. Tracheostomy collar and T piece
   a. The tracheostomy collar can be used to deliver high humidity and the desired oxygen to the client with a tracheostomy.
   b. A special adapter, called the T piece, can be used to deliver any desired FIO_2 to the client with a tracheostomy, laryngectomy, or endotracheal tube
   c. Refer to Chapter 20 for information on endotracheal and tracheostomy tubes
4. FIO_2 delivered: 24% to 100% FIO_2 with flow rates of at least 10 L/min

5. Implementation
   a. Change delivery system to a nasal cannula during mealtimes
   b. Assess that the aerosol mist escapes from the vents of the delivery system during inspiration and expiration
   c. Empty condensation from the tubing to prevent the client from being lavaged with water and to promote an adequate flow rate
   d. Ensure that there is sufficient water in the canister, and change the aerosol water container as needed
   e. Keep the exhalation port on the T piece open ▲ and uncovered (if the port is occluded, the client can suffocate)
   f. Position the T piece so that it does not pull on the tracheostomy or endotracheal tube and cause erosion of skin at the tracheostomy insertion site
   g. Make sure the humidifier creates enough mist; a mist should be seen during inspiration and expiration

V. MECHANICAL VENTILATION
A. Types
1. Pressure-cycled ventilator
   a. Pushes air into the lungs until an airway pressure is reached
   b. Used for short periods, as in the postanesthesia care unit and for respiratory therapy
2. Time-cycled ventilator
   a. Pushes air into the lungs until a preset time has elapsed
   b. Primarily used in the pediatric or neonatal client
3. Volume-cycled ventilator
   a. Pushes air into the lungs until a preset volume is delivered
   b. A constant tidal volume is delivered regardless of the changing compliance of the lungs and chest wall or the airway resistance in the client or ventilator
4. Microprocessor ventilator
   a. A computer or microprocessor is built into the ventilator to allow continuous monitoring of ventilatory functions, alarms, and client parameters
   b. Is more responsive to clients who have severe lung disease or require prolonged weaning

B. Modes of ventilation
1. Controlled
   a. The client receives a set tidal volume at a set rate
   b. Used for clients who cannot initiate respiratory effort
   c. The least used mode; if the client attempts to

initiate a breath, the efforts are blocked by the ventilator

2. Assist-control (AC)
   a. Most commonly used mode
   b. Tidal volume and ventilatory rate are preset on the ventilator
   c. The ventilator takes over the work of breathing for the client
   d. The ventilator is programmed to respond to the client's inspiratory effort if the client does initiate a breath
   e. The ventilator delivers the preset tidal volume when the client initiates a breath, while allowing the client to control the rate of breathing
   f. If the client's spontaneous ventilatory rate increases, the ventilator continues to deliver a preset tidal volume with each breath, which may cause hyperventilation and respiratory alkalosis

3. Synchronized intermittent mandatory ventilation (SIMV)
   a. Similar to AC in that the tidal volume and ventilatory rate are preset on the ventilator;
   b. SIMV allows the client to breath spontaneously at his or her own rate and tidal volume between the ventilator breaths
   c. Can be used as a primary ventilatory mode or as a weaning mode
   d. When SIMV is used as a weaning mode, the number of SIMV breaths is gradually decreased and the client gradually resumes spontaneous breathing

C. Ventilator controls and settings
   1. Tidal volume: The volume of air that the client receives with each breath
   2. Rate: Number of ventilator breaths delivered per minute
   3. Fraction of inspired oxygen (FIO_2): The oxygen concentration delivered to the client, which is determined by the client's condition and the arterial blood gases
   4. Sighs
      a. Volumes of air that are 1.5 to 2 times the set tidal volume, delivered 6 to 10 times per hour
      b. May be used to prevent atelectasis
   5. Peak airway inspiratory pressure (PIP)
      a. Pressure needed by the ventilator to deliver a set tidal volume at a given compliance
      b. Monitoring PIP reflects changes in compliance of the lungs and resistance in the ventilator or client
   6. Continuous positive airway pressure (CPAP)
      a. Application of positive airway pressure throughout the entire respiratory cycle for spontaneously breathing clients

   b. Keeps the alveoli open during inspiration and prevents alveolar collapse
   c. Used primarily as a weaning modality
   d. During CPAP, no ventilator breaths are delivered, but the ventilator delivers oxygen and provides monitoring and an alarm system
   e. The respiratory pattern is determined by the client's efforts

7. Positive end-expiratory pressure (PEEP)
   a. Positive pressure exerted during the expiratory phase of ventilation
   b. Improves oxygenation by enhancing gas exchange and preventing atelectasis
   c. The need for PEEP indicates a severe gas exchange disturbance

8. Implementation
   a. Assess the client first and the ventilator second
   b. Assess vital signs, lung sounds, respiratory status, and breathing patterns
   c. Monitor skin color, particularly in the lips and nailbeds
   d. Monitor chest for bilateral expansion
   e. Obtain pulse oximetry readings
   f. Monitor ABG results
   g. Assess the need for **suctioning** and observe the type, color, and amount of secretions
   h. Assess ventilator settings
   i. Assess level of water in humidifier and temperature of the humidification system because extremes in temperature can cause damage to the mucosa airway
   j. Ensure that the alarms are set
   k. If a cause for an alarm cannot be determined, ventilate the client manually with a resuscitation bag until the problem is corrected
   l. Empty the ventilator tubing when moisture collects
   m. Turn the client at least every 2 hours or get the client out of bed, as prescribed, to prevent complications of immobility
   n. Have resuscitation equipment available at the bedside

D. Causes of alarms
   1. High-pressure alarm
      a. Increased secretions in the airway
      b. Wheezing or bronchospasm causing decreased airway size
      c. Displacement of the endotracheal tube
      d. Obstructed endotracheal tube as a result of water or a kink in the tubing
      e. Client coughs, gags, or bites on the oral endotracheal tube
      f. Client is anxious or fights the ventilator
   2. Low-pressure alarm
      a. Disconnection or leak in the ventilator or in the client's airway cuff
      b. The client stops spontaneous breathing

E. Complications
1. Hypotension caused by the application of positive pressure, which increases intrathoracic pressure and inhibits blood return to the heart
2. Respiratory complications such as **pneumothorax** or subcutaneous **emphysema** as a result of positive pressure
3. Gastrointestinal alterations such as stress ulcers
4. Malnutrition if nutrition is not maintained
5. Infections
6. Muscular deconditioning
7. Ventilator dependence or inability to wean
F. Weaning: The process of going from ventilator dependence to spontaneous breathing
1. SIMV
   a. The client breathes between the ventilator's preset breaths per minute rate
   b. The SIMV rate is gradually decreased until the client is breathing on his or her own without the use of the ventilator
2. T piece
   a. The client is taken off the ventilator, and the ventilator is replaced with a T piece or CPAP, which delivers humidified oxygen
   b. The client is taken off the ventilator for short periods initially and allowed to breathe spontaneously
   c. Weaning progresses as the client is able to tolerate progressively longer periods off the ventilator
3. Pressure support (PS)
   a. A predetermined pressure on the ventilator assists the client in his or her respiratory effort
   b. As weaning continues, the amount of pressure is gradually decreased
   c. With PS, pressure may be maintained while the ventilator's preset breaths per minute are gradually decreased

VI. CHEST INJURIES

A. Rib fracture
1. Description
   a. Results from direct blunt chest trauma and causes a potential for intrathoracic injury, such as **pneumothorax** or pulmonary contusion
   b. Pain with movement and chest splinting result in impaired ventilation and inadequate clearance of secretions
2. Assessment
   a. Pain at injury site that increases with inspiration
   b. Tenderness at site
   c. Shallow respirations
   d. Client splints chest
   e. Fractures noted on chest x-ray film
3. Implementation
   a. Note that ribs usually unite spontaneously

   b. Position the client in high Fowler's position
   c. Administer pain medication as prescribed to maintain adequate ventilatory status
   d. Monitor for increased respiratory distress
   e. Instruct the client to self-splint with hands and arms
   f. Prepare the client for an intercostal nerve block as prescribed if the pain is severe
B. Flail chest
1. Description
   a. A blunt chest trauma associated with accidents, which may result in hemothorax and rib fractures
   b. The loose segment of the chest wall becomes paradoxical to the expansion and contraction of the rest of the chest wall
2. Assessment
   a. Paradoxical respirations (inward movement of a segment of the thorax during inspiration with outward movement during expiration)
   b. Severe pain in chest
   c. Dyspnea
   d. Cyanosis
   e. Tachycardia
   f. Hypotension
   g. Tachypnea, shallow respirations
   h. Diminished breath sounds
3. Implementation
   a. Position the client in high Fowler's
   b. Administer humidified oxygen as prescribed
   c. Monitor for increased respiratory distress
   d. Encourage coughing and deep breathing
   e. Administer pain medication as prescribed
   f. Maintain bed rest and limit activity to reduce oxygen demands
   g. Prepare for intubation with **mechanical ventilation,** with positive end-expiratory pressure for severe flail chest associated with respiratory failure and shock
C. Pulmonary contusion
1. Description
   a. Characterized by interstitial hemorrhage associated with intraalveolar hemorrhage, resulting in decreased pulmonary compliance
   b. The major complication is adult respiratory distress syndrome (ARDS)
2. Assessment
   a. Dyspnea
   b. Hypoxemia
   c. Increased bronchial secretions
   d. Hemoptysis
   e. Restlessness
   f. Decreased breath sounds
   g. Rales and wheezes
3. Implementation
   a. Maintain airway and ventilation
   b. Position the client in high Fowler's

c. Administer oxygen as prescribed

d. Monitor for increased respiratory distress

e. Maintain bed rest and limit activity to reduce oxygen demands

f. Prepare for **mechanical ventilation** with positive end-expiratory pressure if required

D. Pneumothorax

1. Description

a. The accumulation of atmospheric air in the pleural space, which results in a rise in intrathoracic pressure and reduced vital capacity

b. The loss of negative intrapleural pressure results in collapse of the lung

c. A spontaneous **pneumothorax** occurs with the rupture of a bleb

d. An open **pneumothorax** occurs when an opening through the chest wall allows the entrance of positive atmospheric pressure into the pleural space

e. A tension **pneumothorax** occurs from a blunt chest injury or from **mechanical ventilation** with positive end-expiratory pressure when there is a buildup of positive pressure in the pleural space

f. Diagnosis of **pneumothorax** is made by chest x-ray film

2. Assessment

a. Dyspnea

b. Tachycardia

c. Tachypnea

d. Sharp chest pain

e. Absent breath sounds on affected side

f. Decreased chest expansion unilaterally

g. Cyanosis

h. Hypotension

i. Subcutaneous **emphysema**

j. Sucking sound with open chest wound

k. Tracheal deviation to the unaffected side with tension **pneumothorax**

3. Implementation

a. Apply a dressing over an open chest wound

b. Administer oxygen as prescribed

c. Position the client in high Fowler's

d. Prepare for chest tube placement until the lung has fully expanded

e. Monitor chest tube drainage system

f. Monitor for subcutaneous **emphysema**

g. Refer to Chapter 20 for information on chest tubes

VII. RESPIRATORY FAILURE

A. Description

1. Occurs when the client cannot eliminate carbon dioxide from the alveoli

2. The carbon dioxide retention results in hypoxemia

3. Oxygen reaches the alveoli but cannot be absorbed or used properly

4. The lungs can move air sufficiently but cannot oxygenate the pulmonary blood properly

5. Respiratory failure occurs as a result of a mechanical abnormality of the lungs or chest wall, a defect in the respiratory control center in the brain, or an impairment in the function of the respiratory muscles

6. The $Paco_2$ level is greater than 45 mm Hg

B. Assessment

1. Dyspnea

2. Headache

3. Restlessness

4. Confusion

5. Tachycardia

6. Cyanosis

7. Dysrhythmias

8. Decreased level of consciousness

9. Alterations in respirations and breath sounds

C. Implementation

1. Identify and treat the cause of respiratory failure

2. Administer oxygen to maintain the Pao_2 level above 60 to 70 mm Hg

3. Position the client in high Fowler's

4. Encourage deep breathing

5. Administer bronchodilators as prescribed

6. Prepare the client for **mechanical ventilation** if supplemental oxygen cannot maintain acceptable Pao_2 levels

VIII. ADULT RESPIRATORY DISTRESS SYNDROME (ARDS)

A. Description

1. A form of acute respiratory failure caused by a diffuse lung injury, leading to extravascular lung fluid

2. The major site of injury is the alveolar capillary membrane

3. The interstitial edema causes compression and obliteration of the terminal airways and leads to reduced lung volume and compliance

4. The ABGs identify respiratory acidosis and hypoxemia that does not respond to an increased percentage of oxygen

5. The chest x-ray film shows interstitial edema

6. Some of the causes include sepsis, fluid overload, shock, trauma, neurological injuries, burns, disseminated intravascular coagulation (DIC), drug ingestion, and the inhalation of toxic substances

B. Assessment

1. Tachypnea

2. Dyspnea

3. Decreased breath sounds

4. Deteriorating blood gas levels

5. Hypoxemia despite high concentrations of delivered oxygen

6. Decreased pulmonary compliance

7. Pulmonary infiltrates

C. Implementation
1. Identify and treat cause of the ARDS
2. Administer oxygen as prescribed
3. Position client in high Fowler's
4. Restrict fluid intake as prescribed
5. Provide respiratory treatments as prescribed
6. Administer diuretics, anticoagulants, or corticosteroids as prescribed
7. Prepare the client for intubation and **mechanical ventilation,** using positive end-expiratory pressure (PEEP)

IX. CHRONIC OBSTRUCTIVE PULMONARY DISEASE (COPD)

A. Description
1. Also known as **chronic obstructive lung disease (COLD)** and **chronic airflow limitation (CAL)**
2. A group of diseases that includes **emphysema,** asthma, bronchiectasis, and bronchitis
3. Characterized by progressive airflow limitations into and out of the lungs, elevated airway resistance, irreversible lung distention, and arterial blood gas imbalance
4. **COPD** leads to pulmonary insufficiency, pulmonary hypertension, and cor pulmonale
5. In **emphysema,** the stimulus to breathe is a low Po_2 instead of an increased Pco_2

B. Assessment
1. Cough
2. Exertional dyspnea
3. Wheezing and crackles
4. Sputum production
5. Weight loss
6. Barrel chest (**emphysema**)
7. Use of accessory muscles for breathing
8. Cyanosis
9. Clubbing of fingers
10. Orthopnea
11. Cardiac dysrhythmias
12. Congestion and hyperinflation on chest x-ray film
13. ABGs indicate respiratory acidosis and hypoxemia
14. PFTs demonstrate decreased vital capacity

C. Implementation
1. Monitor vital signs
2. Administer a low concentration of oxygen (2 to 3 L/min) as prescribed; the stimulus to breathe is a low Po_2 instead of an increased Pco_2
3. Monitor pulse oximetry
4. Provide respiratory treatments and chest physiotherapy
5. Instruct the client in diaphragmatic or abdominal and pursed-lip breathing techniques
6. Record the color, amount, and consistency of sputum
7. Suction the client, if necessary, to clear airway and prevent infection
8. Monitor weight
9. Encourage small, frequent meals to prevent dyspnea
10. Provide a high-calorie, high-protein diet with supplements
11. Encourage fluids up to 3000 mL/day to keep secretions thin, unless contraindicated
12. Position in high Fowler's and leaning forward to aid in breathing
13. Allow activity as tolerated
14. Administer bronchodilators as prescribed, and instruct the client in the use of both oral and inhalant medications
15. Administer corticosteroids as prescribed to reduce inflammation
16. Administer mucolytics as prescribed to thin secretions
17. Administer antibiotics for infection if prescribed

D. Client education
1. Stop smoking
2. Recognize the signs and symptoms of respiratory infection and hypoxia
3. Adhere to activity limitations, alternating rest periods with activity
4. Avoid exposure to individuals with infections and avoid crowds
5. Demonstrate pursed-lip and diaphragmatic or abdominal breathing
6. Instruct the client in the use of medications and inhalers
7. Instruct the client in the use in oxygen therapy
8. Instruct the client in nutritional requirements
9. Avoid eating gas-producing foods, spicy foods, and extremely hot or cold foods
10. Instruct in the importance of receiving immunizations as recommended
11. When dusting, use a wet cloth
12. Avoid powerful odors
13. Avoid extremes in temperature
14. Avoid fireplaces, pets, and feather pillows

X. PNEUMONIA

A. Description
1. An infection of the pulmonary tissue, including the interstitial spaces, the alveoli, and the bronchioles
2. The edema associated with inflammation stiffens the lung, decreases lung compliance and vital capacity, and causes hypoxemia
3. Can be community acquired or hospital acquired
4. The chest x-ray presents as diffuse patches throughout the lungs or consolidation in a lobe
5. A sputum culture identifies the organism
6. The white blood cells (WBCs) and the erythrocyte sedimentation rate (ESR) are elevated

B. Assessment
1. Chills
2. Elevated temperature

3. Pleuritic pain
4. Rales, rhonchi, and wheezes ▲
5. Use of accessory muscles for breathing
6. Cyanosis
7. Mental status changes
8. Sputum production ▲
C. Implementation
   1. Administer oxygen as prescribed
   2. Monitor respiratory status
   3. Monitor for labored respirations, cyanosis, cold and clammy skin
   4. Encourage coughing and deep breathing and use of incentive spirometer ▲
   5. Position in semi-Fowler's to facilitate breathing and lung expansion ▲
   6. Change position frequently and ambulate as tolerated to mobilize secretions ▲
   7. Provide chest physiotherapy
   8. Perform nasotracheal **suctioning** if the client is unable to clear secretions
   9. Monitor pulse oximetry
   10. Monitor and record color, consistency, and amount of sputum
   11. Provide a high-calorie, high-protein diet with small frequent meals
   12. Encourage fluids up to 3 liters a day to thin secretions unless contraindicated ▲
   13. Provide a balance of rest and activity, increasing activity gradually
   14. Administer antibiotics as prescribed
   15. Administer antipyretics, bronchodilators, cough suppressants, mucolytic agents, and expectorants as prescribed
   16. Prevent the spread of infection by handwashing and the proper disposal of secretions
D. Client education ▲
   1. The importance of rest, proper nutrition, and adequate fluid intake
   2. Avoid chilling and exposure to individuals with respiratory infections or viruses
   3. Instruct the client regarding medications and the use of inhalants as prescribed
   4. Instruct the client to notify physician if chills, fever, dyspnea, hemoptysis, or increased fatigue occurs
   5. Instruct the client in the importance of receiving immunizations as recommended ▲

XI. PLEURAL EFFUSION

A. Description
   1. The collection of fluid in the pleural space
   2. Any condition that interferes with either secretion or drainage of this fluid will lead to pleural effusion
B. Assessment
   1. Pleuritic pain that is sharp and increases with inspiration ▲

2. Dyspnea on exertion
3. Dry nonproductive cough caused by bronchial irritation or mediastinal shift ▲
4. Tachycardia
5. Elevated temperature
6. Decreased breath sounds
7. Chest x-ray shows pleural effusion and a mediastinal shift away from the fluid ▲
C. Implementation
   1. Identify and treat underlying cause ▲
   2. Monitor breath sounds
   3. Position the client in high Fowler's ▲
   4. Encourage coughing and deep breathing ▲
   5. Prepare the client for thoracentesis
   6. If pleural effusion is recurrent, prepare the client for pleurectomy or pleurodesis
D. Pleurectomy
   1. Consists of surgically stripping the parietal pleura away from the visceral pleura
   2. This produces an intense inflammatory reaction that promotes adhesion formation between the two layers during healing
E. Pleurodesis
   1. Involves the instillation of a sclerosing substance into the pleural space via a thoracotomy tube
   2. This creates an inflammatory response that scleroses tissues together

XII. EMPYEMA

A. Description
   1. The collection of pus within the pleural cavity
   2. The fluid is thick, opaque, and foul smelling
   3. The most common cause is pulmonary infection and lung abscess caused by thoracic surgery or chest trauma, in which bacteria are introduced directly into the pleural space
   4. Treatment focuses on emptying the empyema cavity, reexpanding the lung, and controlling the infection
B. Assessment
   1. Recent febrile illnesses or trauma
   2. Chest pain
   3. Cough
   4. Dyspnea
   5. Anorexia and weight loss
   6. Malaise
   7. Elevated temperature and chills
   8. Night sweats
   9. Diminished chest wall movement on the affected side ▲
   10. Pleural exudate on chest x-ray ▲
C. Implementation
   1. Monitor breath sounds
   2. Position client in semi-Fowler's or high Fowler's ▲
   3. Encourage coughing and deep breathing
   4. Administer antibiotics as prescribed
   5. Instruct the client to splint chest as necessary

6. Assist with chest tube insertion to promote drainage and lung expansion
7. If marked pleural thickening occurs, prepare the client for decortication, if prescribed; this is a surgical procedure that involves removal of the restrictive mass of fibrin and inflammatory cells

XIII. PLEURISY
A. Description
  1. Inflammation of the visceral and parietal membranes
  2. These membranes rub together during respiration and cause pain
  3. May be caused by pulmonary infarction or pneumonia
  4. It usually occurs on one side of the chest, usually in the lower lateral portions in the chest wall
B. Assessment
  1. Knife-like pain that is aggravated on deep breathing and coughing
  2. Dyspnea
  3. Pleural friction rub heard on auscultation
  4. Apprehension
C. Implementation
  1. Identify and treat cause
  2. Monitor lung sounds
  3. Administer analgesics as prescribed
  4. Apply hot or cold applications as prescribed
  5. Encourage coughing and deep breathing
  6. Instruct the client to lie on affected side to splint chest

XIV. PULMONARY EMBOLISM
A. Description
  1. Occurs when a thrombus that forms in a deep vein detaches and travels to the right side of the heart and then lodges in a branch of the pulmonary artery
  2. Clients prone to pulmonary embolism are those at risk for deep vein thrombosis, including those with prolonged immobilization, surgery, obesity, pregnancy, congestive heart failure (CHF), advanced age, or prior history of thromboembolism
  3. Fat emboli can occur as a complication following a fracture of a flat long bone
  4. Treatment is aimed at preventing venous status and includes range-of-motion exercises and early ambulation following surgery, the use of antiembolism or pneumatic compression stockings, and preventing pressure under the popliteal space
B. Assessment
  1. Dyspnea accompanied by anginal and pleuritic pain, exacerbated by inspiration
  2. Chest pain
  3. Tachypnea and tachycardia
  4. Hypotension
  5. Shallow respirations

6. Rales on auscultation
7. Cough
8. Blood-tinged sputum
9. Distended neck veins
10. Cyanosis
C. Implementation
  1. Administer oxygen as prescribed
  2. Position client in high Fowler's
  3. Monitor lung sounds
  4. Maintain bed rest and active and passive range-of-motion exercises as prescribed
  5. Encourage use of incentive spirometry as prescribed
  6. Monitor pulse oximetry
  7. **Prepare** for intubation and **mechanical ventilation** for severe hypoxemia
  8. Administer anticoagulation with IV heparin (bolus), followed by continuous infusion during the acute phase
  9. Administer warfarin (Coumadin) orally, as prescribed, when heparin infusion is discontinued
  10. Monitor prothrombin time (PT) and partial thromboplastin time (PTT) closely
  11. Prepare the client for embolectomy, vein ligation, or insertion of an umbrella filter, as prescribed

XV. LUNG CANCER AND LARYNGEAL CANCER
(Refer to Chapter 49)

XVI. CARBON MONOXIDE POISONING
A. Description
  1. Carbon monoxide is a colorless, odorless, and tasteless gas that has an affinity for hemoglobin 200 times greater than that of oxygen
  2. Oxygen molecules are displaced and carbon monoxide reversibly binds to hemoglobin to form carboxyhemoglobin; tissue hypoxia occurs
B. Assessment (Table 55-1)
C. Implementation
  1. Remove victim from exposure
  2. Administer oxygen
  3. Assess need for basic life support

TABLE 55-1

Assessment: Levels of Carbon Monoxide

Level	Assessment Finding
5% to 10%	Impaired visual acuity
11% to 20%	Flushing
21% to 30%	Nausea and impaired dexterity
31% to 40%	Vomiting, dizziness, and syncope
41% to 50%	Tachypnea and tachycardia
Greater than 50%	Coma and death

4. Monitor vital signs
5. Monitor carbon monoxide levels

XVII. HISTOPLASMOSIS
A. Description
    1. A pulmonary fungal infection caused by spores of *Histoplasma capsulatum*
    2. Transmission occurs by the inhalation of spores, which are commonly located in contaminated soil
    3. Spores are also usually found in bird droppings
B. Assessment
    1. Dyspnea
    2. Chills
    3. Elevated temperature
    4. Chest pain
    5. Pulmonary infiltrates on chest x-ray
    6. Elevated WBC count
    7. Positive skin test for histoplasmosis
    8. Positive agglutination test
    9. Splenomegaly, hepatomegaly
C. Implementation
    1. Administer oxygen as prescribed
    2. Monitor breath sounds
    3. Administer antiemetics, antihistamines, antipyretics, and corticosteroids as prescribed
    4. Administer fungicidal medications as prescribed
    5. Encourage coughing and deep breathing
    6. Position client in semi-Fowler's
    7. Monitor vital signs
    8. Monitor for nephrotoxicity from fungicidal medications
    9. Instruct the client to spray area with water before sweeping barn and chicken coups

XVIII. SARCOIDOSIS
A. Description
    1. Epitheloid cell tubercles in lung
    2. Cause is unknown
    3. High titer of Epstein-Barr virus may be identified
    4. Virus incidence is highest in blacks and young adults
B. Assessment
    1. Night sweats
    2. Fever
    3. Weight loss
    4. Cough
    5. Skin nodules
    6. Polyarthritis
    7. Kveim test: Sarcoid node antigen is injected intradermally and causes local nodular lesion in approximately 1 month
C. Implementation
    1. Administer corticosteroids to control symptoms
    2. Monitor temperature
    3. Increase fluid intake

4. Provide frequent periods of rest
5. Encourage small, nutritious meals

XIX. OCCUPATIONAL LUNG DISEASE: SILICOSIS
A. Description
    1. Known as asbestosis and coal workers' pneumoconiosis
    2. Fibrotic disease of the lungs caused by the inhalation of inorganic dusts over long periods of time
    3. Common in miners and sandblasters
    4. **Tuberculosis (TB)** is a frequent complication
B. Assessment
    1. Frequent respiratory infections
    2. Blood-streaked sputum
    3. Cough
    4. Chest x-ray: Nodular lesions of lungs
C. Implementation
    1. Administer antitussive for cough
    2. Administer medication for **TB** as prescribed
    3. Eliminate the toxic substances
    4. Administer oxygen as prescribed
    5. Encourage coughing and deep breathing

XX. TUBERCULOSIS
A. Description
    1. A highly communicable disease caused by *Mycobacterium tuberculosis*
    2. *Mycobacterium tuberculosis* is a nonmotile, nonsporulating, acid-fast rod that secrets niacin, and when the bacillus reaches a susceptible site, it multiplies freely
    3. Because *Mycobacterium tuberculosis* is an aerobic bacterium, it primarily affects the pulmonary system, especially the upper lobes, where the oxygen content is greatest, but can also affect other areas of the body, such as the brain, intestines, peritoneum, kidney, joints, and liver
    4. An exudative-type response causes a nonspecific pneumonitis and the development of granulomas in the lung tissue
    5. **Tuberculosis (TB)** has an insidious onset, and many clients are not aware of symptoms until the disease is well advanced
    6. A **multidrug-resistant strain (MDR-TB)** of TB can exist as a result of improper or noncompliant use of treatment programs and the development of mutations in the tubercle bacilli
    7. The goal of treatment is to prevent transmission, control symptoms, and prevent progression of the disease
B. Risk factors
    1. Alcoholism
    2. Intravenous drug use
    3. Malnutrition
    4. Infection

5. The elderly
6. The homeless
7. Refugees
8. Minority groups
9. Individuals from a lower socioeconomic group
10. Children younger than 5 years of age
11. Individuals living in crowded areas, such as long-term care facilities, prisons, and mental health facilities
12. Individuals in constant, frequent contact with an untreated or undiagnosed individual
13. Individuals with immune dysfunction or human immunodeficiency virus (HIV) infection or individuals who are immunosuppressed as a result of medication therapy
14. Drinking unpasteurized milk if the cow is infected with bovine **TB**

C. Transmission
1. Via airborne route by droplet infection
2. When an infected individual coughs, laughs, sneezes, or sings, droplet nuclei containing **TB** bacteria enter the air and may be inhaled by others
3. Identification of those individuals in close contact with the infected individual is important so that they can be tested and treated as necessary
4. When contacts have been identified, these people are assessed with a tuberculin test and chest x-ray to determine infection with **TB**
5. After the infected individual has received **TB** medication for 2 to 3 weeks, the risk of transmission is greatly reduced

D. Disease progression
1. Droplets enter the lungs, and the bacteria form a tubercle lesion
2. The body's defense systems encapsulate the tubercle, leaving a scar
3. If encapsulation does not occur, bacteria may enter the lymph system, travel to the lymph nodes, and cause an inflammatory response called granulomatous inflammation
4. Primary lesions form; the primary lesions may become dormant, but can be reactivated and become a secondary infection when reexposed to the bacterium
5. In an active phase, **TB** can cause necrosis and cavitation in the lesions, leading to rupture and the spread of necrotic tissue, and damage to various parts of the body

E. Client history
1. Past exposure to **TB**
2. Client's country of origin and travel to foreign countries in which there is a high incidence of **TB**
3. Recent history of influenza, pneumonia, febrile illness, cough, or foul-smelling sputum production

4. Previous tests for **TB** and what the results were
5. Recent **bacille Calmette-Guérin (BCG) vaccine** (a vaccine containing attenuated tubercle bacilli that may be given to people in foreign countries or to persons traveling to foreign countries, to produce increased resistance to **TB**)
6. An individual who has received **BCG** will have a positive skin test and should be evaluated for **TB** with a chest x-ray

F. Clinical manifestations
1. May be asymptomatic in primary infection
2. Fatigue
3. Lethargy
4. Anorexia
5. Weight loss
6. Low-grade fever
7. Chills
8. Night sweats
9. Persistent cough and the production of mucoid and mucopurulent sputum, which is occasionally streaked with blood
10. Chest tightness and a dull, aching chest pain may accompany the cough

G. Chest assessment
1. A physical examination of the chest does not provide conclusive evidence of **TB**
2. Chest x-ray is not definitive, but the presence of multinodular infiltrates with calcification in the upper lobes suggests **TB**
3. If the disease is active, caseation and inflammation may be seen on the chest x-ray
4. Advanced disease
   a. Dullness with percussion over involved parenchymal areas, bronchial breath sounds, rhonchi and/or crackles
   b. Partial obstruction of a bronchus, caused by endobronchial disease or compression by lymph nodes, may produce localized wheezing and dyspnea

H. Sputum cultures
1. Sputum specimens are obtained for an acid-fast smear
2. A sputum culture identifying *Mycobacterium tuberculosis* confirms the diagnosis
3. After medications are started, sputum samples are obtained again to determine the effectiveness of therapy
4. Most clients have negative cultures after 3 months of compliance with medication therapy

I. **Mantoux test**
1. The most reliable determinant of infection with **TB**
2. A positive reaction does not mean that active disease is present but indicates exposure to **TB** or the presence of inactive (dormant) disease
3. Once the test result is positive, it will be positive in any future tests

4. A small amount (0.1 mL) of intermediate-strength purified protein derivative (PPD) containing 5 tuberculin units is administered intradermally in the forearm

5. An area of induration measuring 10 mm or more in diameter, 48 to 72 hours after injection, indicates that the individual has been exposed to **TB**

6. For individuals with HIV infection or who are immunosuppressed, a reaction of 5 mm or greater is considered positive

7. Once an individual's skin test is positive, a chest x-ray is necessary to rule out active **TB** or to detect old, healed lesions

J. The hospitalized client
1. The client with active **TB** is placed in respiratory isolation precautions in a well-ventilated room
2. The room should have at least six exchanges of fresh air per hour and should be ventilated to the outside environment if possible
3. The nurse wears a particulate respirator (a special individually fitted mask) when caring for the client and a gown when there is a possibility of contamination of clothing
4. Hands are always thoroughly washed before and after caring for the client
5. If the client needs to leave the room for a test or procedure, the client is required to wear a mask
6. Isolation is discontinued when the client is no longer considered infectious
7. After the infected individual has received **TB** medication for 2 to 3 weeks, the risk of transmission is greatly reduced
8. When the results of two sputum cultures are negative, the client is no longer considered infectious

K. The client at home
1. Provide the client and family with information about **TB** and allay concerns about the contagious aspect of the infection
2. Instruct the client to follow the medication regimen exactly as prescribed and always to have a supply of the medication on hand
3. Advise the client of the side effects of the medication and ways of minimizing them to ensure compliance
4. Reassure the client that after 2 to 3 weeks of medication therapy, it is unlikely that the client will infect anyone
5. Inform the client that activities should be resumed gradually
6. Instruct the client about the need for adequate nutrition and a well-balanced diet to promote healing and to prevent recurrence of infection
7. Instruct the client to increase foods rich in iron, protein, and vitamin C
8. Inform the client and family that respiratory isolation is not necessary because family members have already been exposed

9. Instruct the client to cover the mouth and nose when coughing or sneezing and to confine used tissues to plastic bags

10. Instruct the client and family about thorough handwashing

11. Inform the client that a sputum culture is needed every 2 to 4 weeks once medication therapy is initiated

12. Inform the client that when the results of two sputum cultures are negative, the client is no longer considered infectious and can usually return to his or her former employment

13. Advise the client to avoid excessive exposure to silicone or dust because these substances can cause further lung damage

14. Instruct the client regarding the importance of compliance with treatment, follow-up care, and sputum cultures, as prescribed

L. Medications (Refer to Chapter 56)

PRACTICE QUESTIONS

1. A nurse is preparing to obtain a sputum specimen from a client. Which of the following nursing actions will facilitate obtaining the specimen?
   1. Limiting fluids
   2. Having the client take three deep breaths
   3. Asking the client to spit into the collection container
   4. Asking the client to obtain the specimen after eating

2. A nurse is caring for a client after a bronchoscopy and biopsy. Which of the following signs if noted in the client should be reported immediately to the physician?
   1. Blood-streaked sputum
   2. Dry cough
   3. Hematuria
   4. Stridor

3. A nurse is suctioning a client via a tracheostomy tube. When suctioning, the nurse must limit the suctioning to a maximum of:
   1. 5 seconds
   2. 15 seconds
   3. 30 seconds
   4. 1 minute

4. A nurse is suctioning a client through an endotracheal tube. During the suctioning procedure the nurse notes cardiac irregularities on the monitor. Which of the following is the most appropriate nursing intervention?
   1. Continue to suction
   2. Ensure that the suction is limited to 15 seconds
   3. Stop the procedure and reoxygenate the client
   4. Notify the physician immediately

5. An unconscious client is admitted to an emergency room. Arterial blood gas measurements reveal a pH of 7.30, a low bicarbonate level, a normal carbon dioxide level, and a normal oxygen level. An elevated potassium level is also present. These results indicate the presence of:
   1. Metabolic acidosis
   2. Respiratory acidosis
   3. Combined respiratory and metabolic acidosis
   4. Overcompensated respiratory acidosis

6. An emergency room nurse is assessing a client who sustained a blunt injury to the chest wall. Which of these signs would indicate the presence of a pneumothorax?
   1. A sucking sound at the site of injury
   2. Diminished breath sounds
   3. A low respiratory rate
   4. The presence of a barrel chest

7. A nurse is caring for a client hospitalized with acute exacerbation of chronic obstructive pulmonary disease (COPD). Which of the following would the nurse expect to note in evaluating this client?
   1. Increased oxygen saturation with exercise
   2. Hypocapnia
   3. A hyperinflated chest on x-ray
   4. A widened diaphragm noted on chest x-ray

8. An oxygen delivery system is prescribed for a client with chronic airflow limitation (CAL) in order to deliver a precise oxygen concentration. Which of the following types of oxygen delivery systems would the nurse anticipate to be prescribed?
   1. Venturi mask
   2. Aerosol mask
   3. Face tent
   4. Tracheostomy collar

9. Theophylline (Theo-Dur) tablets are prescribed for a client with chronic airflow limitation (CAL). A nurse instructs the client about the medication. Which of the following nursing statements would not be a component of the teaching plan?
   1. "Take the medication on an empty stomach."
   2. "Take the medication with food."
   3. "Continue to take the medication even if you are feeling better."
   4. "Periodic blood levels will need to be obtained."

10. A nurse is instructing a hospitalized client with a diagnosis of emphysema about measures that will enhance the effectiveness of breathing during dyspneic periods. Which of the following positions will the nurse instruct the client to assume?
    1. Side-lying in bed
    2. Sitting in a recliner chair
    3. Sitting up in bed
    4. Sitting on the side of the bed and leaning on an overbed table

11. A community nurse is conducting an educational session with community members regarding tuberculosis (TB). The nurse tells the group that the first symptom associated with TB is:
    1. Bloody, productive cough
    2. A morning cough with the expectoration of mucoid sputum
    3. Chest pain
    4. Dyspnea

12. A nurse performs an admission assessment on a client with a diagnosis of tuberculosis (TB). The nurse reviews the results of which diagnostic test that will confirm this diagnosis?
    1. Bronchoscopy
    2. Chest x-ray
    3. Sputum culture
    4. Tuberculin skin test

13. A nursing instructor asks a nursing student to describe the route of transmission of tuberculosis. The nursing instructor concludes that the student understands this route of transmission if the student states that TB is transmitted by:
    1. The airborne route
    2. Blood and body fluids
    3. The fecal-oral route
    4. Hand to mouth

14. A nurse is caring for a client with emphysema. The client is receiving oxygen. The nurse assesses the oxygen flow rate to ensure that it does not exceed:
    1. 1 liter per minute
    2. 2 liters per minute
    3. 6 liters per minute
    4. 10 liters per minute

15. Which of the following arterial blood gas results indicates metabolic alkalosis?
    1. pH of 7.34, P_{CO_2} of 50, HCO_3 of 32, P_{O_2} of 70
    2. pH of 7.46, P_{CO_2} of 30, HCO_3 of 26, P_{O_2} of 80
    3. pH of 7.38, P_{CO_2} of 45, HCO_3 of 22, P_{O_2} of 50
    4. pH of 7.47, P_{CO_2} of 40, HCO_3 of 36, P_{O_2} of 78

16. A nurse reviews the arterial blood gas values of a client. The results indicate respiratory acidosis. Which of the following values would indicate that this acid-base imbalance exists?
    1. pH of 7.48
    2. P_{CO_2} of 32
    3. pH of 7.30
    4. HCO_3 of 20

17. A nurse instructs a client to use the pursed-lip method of breathing. The client asks the nurse about the purpose of this type of breathing. The nurse responds, knowing that the primary purpose of pursed-lip breathing is to:
    1. Promote oxygen intake
    2. Strengthen the diaphragm
    3. Strengthen the intercostal muscles
    4. Promote carbon dioxide elimination

18. The low-pressure alarm sounds on a ventilator. A nurse assesses the client and then attempts to determine the cause of the alarm. The nurse is

unsuccessful in determining the cause of the alarm and takes what initial action?
1. Checks the client's vital signs
2. Ventilates the client manually
3. Administers oxygen
4. Starts cardiopulmonary resuscitation (CPR)

19. A nurse reviews the arterial blood gas values and notes a pH of 7.50, a Pco_2 of 30 mm Hg, and an HCO_3 of 25 mm Hg. The nurse interprets these values as indicating:
1. Respiratory acidosis uncompensated
2. Respiratory alkalosis uncompensated
3. Metabolic acidosis uncompensated
4. Metabolic acidosis partially compensated

20. Aminophylline (theophylline) is administered to a client with acute bronchitis. A nurse administers the medication, knowing that the primary action of this medication is to:
1. Promote expectoration
2. Suppress the cough
3. Relax smooth muscles of the bronchial airway
4. Prevent infection

21. A nurse evaluates the blood theophylline level of a client receiving aminophylline (theophylline) by IV. The nurse would determine that a therapeutic blood level exists if which of the following were noted in the laboratory report?
1. 5 µg/mL
2. 15 µg/mL
3. 25 µg/mL
4. 30 µg/mL

22. A nurse is caring for a client with adult respiratory distress syndrome (ARDS). Which of the following would the nurse expect to note in the client?
1. Decreased respiratory rate
2. Pallor
3. Low arterial Pao_2
4. An elevated arterial Pao_2

23. A client is receiving isoetharine hydrochloride (Bronkosol) via a nebulizer. The nurse monitors the client for which side effect of this medication?
1. Constipation
2. Diarrhea
3. Bradycardia
4. Tachycardia

24. Isoniazid (INH) and rifampin (Rifadin) have been prescribed for a client with tuberculosis. A nurse reviews the medical record of the client. Which of the following, if noted in the client's history, would require physician notification?
1. Heart disease
2. Allergy to penicillin
3. Hepatitis B
4. Rheumatic fever

25. A client with tuberculosis is being treated with isoniazid (INH) and rifampin (Rifadin). A nurse is preparing instructions for the client regarding these

medications. Which of the following statements would be included in the plan of care?
1. "You must discontinue the medication if gastrointestinal (GI) irritation occurs."
2. "You must take the medication with meals."
3. "The entire year-long course of the medication needs to be completed."
4. "Fluids must be increased while taking this medication, to prevent renal failure."

26. A client exposed to tuberculosis (TB) is taking isoniazid (INH) and develops signs and symptoms of the disease. The client is instructed to add rifampin (Rifadin) to the medication regimen. A nurse explains to the client that the purpose of adding this second medication is:
1. That rifampin offsets the side effects of INH
2. To be certain that resistant organisms are eliminated
3. That these medications potentiate each other
4. That INH offsets the side effects of rifampin

27. A client is suspected of having a pulmonary embolus (PE). A nurse assesses the client, knowing that which of the following is not a common clinical manifestation of PE?
1. Decreased respirations
2. Tachypnea
3. Dyspnea
4. Chest pain

28. A nurse is teaching a client about the use of a respiratory inhaler. Which of the following would not be a component of the teaching plan?
1. Remove the cap and shake the inhaler well before use
2. Press the canister down with your finger as you breathe in
3. Inhale the mist and quickly exhale
4. Wait 1 minute between puffs if more than one puff has been prescribed

29. A female client is scheduled to have a chest x-ray. Which of the following questions is of most importance to the nurse assessing this client?
1. "Is there any possibility that you could be pregnant?"
2. "Are you wearing any metal chains or jewelry?"
3. "Can you hold your breath easily?"
4. "Are you able to hold your arms above your head?"

30. A client has just returned to a nursing unit following bronchoscopy. A nurse would implement which of the following nursing interventions for this client?
1. Forcing fluids for the next 24 hours
2. Ensuring the return of the gag reflex before offering food or fluids
3. Administering atropine intravenously
4. Administering small doses of midazolam (Versed)

31. A client has an order to have radial arterial blood gases drawn. Prior to drawing the sample, a nurse occludes the:
    1. Brachial and radial arteries, and then releases them and observes the circulation to the hand
    2. Radial and ulnar arteries, releases one, evaluates the color of the hand, and repeats the process with the other artery
    3. Radial artery and observes for color changes in the affected hand
    4. Ulnar artery and observes for color changes in the affected hand

32. A nurse is assessing the respiratory status of a client who has suffered a fractured rib. Which observation, if made by the nurse, would not be related to the rib fracture?
    1. Pain, especially with inspiration
    2. Slow, deep respirations
    3. Splinting or guarding the chest
    4. Bruising over the fracture area

33. A client with chest injury has suffered flail chest. A nurse assesses the client for which most distinctive sign of flail chest?
    1. Cyanosis
    2. Hypotension
    3. Dyspnea, especially on exhalation
    4. Paradoxical chest movement

34. A client has been admitted with chest trauma after a motor vehicle accident and has undergone subsequent intubation. A nurse checks the client when the ventilator's high-pressure alarm sounds, and notes that the client has absence of breath sounds in the right upper lobe of the lung. The nurse immediately assesses for other signs of:
    1. Displaced endotracheal tube
    2. Adult respiratory distress syndrome (ARDS)
    3. Pulmonary embolism
    4. Right pneumothorax

35. A client with no history of respiratory disease is admitted with respiratory failure. A nurse assesses the arterial blood gas report for which of the following results that are consistent with this disorder?
    1. Pao_2 58 mm Hg, $Paco_2$ 32 mm Hg
    2. Pao_2 60 mm Hg, $Paco_2$ 45 mm Hg
    3. Pao_2 49 mm Hg, $Paco_2$ 52 mm Hg
    4. Pao_2 73 mm Hg, $Paco_2$ 62 mm Hg

36. A nurse is teaching a client with chronic respiratory failure how to use a metered-dose inhaler correctly. The nurse instructs the client to:
    1. Inhale through the nose
    2. Inhale quickly
    3. Take two inhalations during one breath
    4. Hold the breath after inhalation

37. A nurse is assessing a client with multiple trauma who is at risk for developing adult respiratory distress syndrome (ARDS). The nurse assesses for which earliest sign of ARDS?
    1. Inspiratory crackles
    2. Bilateral wheezing
    3. Intercostal retractions
    4. Increased respiratory rate

38. A nurse is taking pulmonary artery catheter measurements of a client with adult respiratory distress syndrome (ARDS). The pulmonary capillary wedge pressure (PCWP) reading is 12 mm Hg. The nurse interprets that this reading is:
    1. High and expected
    2. Low and unexpected
    3. Normal and expected
    4. Uncertain and unexpected

39. A nurse is assessing a client with chronic airflow limitation (CAL) and notes that the client has a "barrel chest." The nurse interprets that this client has which of the following forms of CAL?
    1. Chronic obstructive bronchitis
    2. Emphysema
    3. Bronchial asthma
    4. Both bronchial asthma and bronchitis

40. A client diagnosed with pleurisy is being started on medication therapy with indomethacin (Indocin). A nurse teaches the client that this medication is a:
    1. Topical anesthetic that alleviates surface pain
    2. Mild narcotic analgesic to allow the client to deep breathe
    3. Corticosteroid to decrease the inflammatory response at the site
    4. Nonsteroidal antiinflammatory drug (NSAID) to enhance coughing and deep breathing

41. A client has experienced pulmonary embolism. A nurse assesses for which symptom, which is most commonly reported?
    1. Dyspnea when deep breaths are taken
    2. Hot, flushed feeling
    3. Chest pain that occurs suddenly
    4. Sudden chills and fever

42. A client experiencing confusion and tremors is admitted to a nursing unit An initial arterial blood gas report indicates that the $Paco_2$ level is 72 mm Hg, while the Pao_2 level is 64 mm Hg. A nurse interprets that the client is most likely experiencing:
    1. Carbon monoxide poisoning
    2. Carbon dioxide narcosis
    3. Respiratory alkalosis
    4. Metabolic acidosis

43. A client with carbon dioxide narcosis has a potassium level of 6.2 mEq/L. A nurse interprets that this result is:
    1. Unexpected, and indicates a concurrent history of renal insufficiency
    2. Unexpected, and indicates a deficit of hydrogen ions in the bloodstream

3. Expected, and indicates the result of massive hemolysis

4. Expected, and indicates that acidosis has driven hydrogen ions into the cell, forcing potassium out

44. A client is admitted with carbon dioxide narcosis. In addition to respiratory failure, a nurse plans to monitor the client for which complication of this disorder?
    1. Paralytic ileus
    2. Hypernatremia
    3. Increased intracranial pressure
    4. Hyperglycemia

45. A nurse is evaluating the respiratory status of a client with carbon dioxide narcosis who is being mechanically ventilated. Upon evaluation of a set of arterial blood gases, the nurse notes that the client's carbon dioxide level has dropped significantly. The nurse then evaluates the client for which adverse effect of this rapid change?
    1. Tachypnea
    2. Hyponatremia
    3. Seizure activity
    4. Confusion

46. A client with acquired immunodeficiency syndrome (AIDS) has histoplasmosis. A nurse assesses the client for which of the following signs and symptoms?
    1. Weight gain
    2. Dyspnea
    3. Hypothermia
    4. Headache

47. A client has been admitted to a nursing unit with pulmonary sarcoidosis. A nurse assesses the client for which of the following signs indicating a complication of the disorder?
    1. Bilateral lung crackles
    2. Flat neck veins
    3. Elevated central venous pressure (CVP)
    4. Shrunken liver

48. A nurse is caring for a client with exacerbation of sarcoidosis. A nurse teaches the client about adverse effects of medication therapy, which would include:
    1. Weight loss
    2. Hyperglycemia
    3. Hyperkalemia
    4. Pruritis

49. A nurse is giving discharge instructions to a client with pulmonary sarcoidosis. The nurse concludes that the client understands the information if the client reports which of the following early signs of exacerbation?
    1. Fever
    2. Weight loss
    3. Fatigue
    4. Shortness of breath

50. A nurse is taking the nursing history of a client with silicosis. The nurse assesses whether the client wears which of the following items during periods of exposure to silica particles?
    1. Mask
    2. Gown
    3. Gloves
    4. Eye protection

51. A client tells a nurse that a physician has stated a diagnosis of uncomplicated or simple silicosis. The client asks the nurse exactly what this means. In formulating a response, the nurse incorporates the knowledge that:
    1. There is evidence of silica in the bloodstream but no clinical symptoms
    2. The client has normal pulmonary function studies (PFTs) but has shortness of breath
    3. The client has mild ventilation restriction and has fibrosis on chest x-ray
    4. There is massive pulmonary fibrosis on chest x-ray but no extrapulmonary symptoms

52. A client has been taking benzonatate (Tessalon Perles) as prescribed. A nurse concludes that the medication is having the intended effect if the client experiences:
    1. Decreased anxiety level
    2. Increased comfort level
    3. Reduction in nausea and vomiting
    4. Decreased frequency and intensity of cough

53. A client has been taking pyrazinamide (PMS Pyrazinamide) for 1 month. The client asks a nurse if the therapy is due to be terminated soon. The nurse evaluates that the medication probably will be continued on the basis of a positive finding in which of the following reports?
    1. Blood culture
    2. Sputum culture
    3. Urine culture
    4. Wound culture

54. A nurse working on a medical respiratory nursing unit is caring for several clients with respiratory disorders. The nurse would determine that which of the following clients on the nursing unit is at the least risk for infection with tuberculosis?
    1. A newly immigrated woman from Korea
    2. An uninsured man who is homeless
    3. An elderly woman admitted from a long-term care facility
    4. A man who is an inspector for the U. S. Postal Service

55. A client has an order to receive purified protein derivative (PPD), 0.1 mL, intradermally. A nurse administers the medication by using a tuberculin syringe with a:
    1. 26-gauge, 5/8 inch needle inserted almost parallel to the skin with the bevel side up

2. 26-gauge, 5/8 inch needle inserted at a 45-degree angle with the bevel side down

3. 20-gauge, 1-inch needle inserted almost parallel to the skin with the bevel side up

4. 20-gauge, 1-inch needle inserted at a 30-degree angle with the bevel side down

56. A nurse is reading a Mantoux skin test for a client with no documented health problems. The site has no induration and a 1 mm area of ecchymosis. The nurse interprets that the result is:

1. Positive
2. Negative
3. Uncertain
4. Borderline

57. A nurse is caring for a client diagnosed with tuberculosis (TB). Which assessment, if made by the nurse, would not be consistent with the usual clinical presentation of tuberculosis?

1. Nonproductive or productive cough
2. Anorexia and weight loss
3. Chills and night sweats
4. High-grade fever

58. A nurse is teaching a client with tuberculosis (TB) about dietary elements that should be increased in the diet. The nurse suggests that the client increase intake of:

1. Meats and citrus fruits
2. Grains and broccoli
3. Eggs and spinach
4. Potatoes and fish

59. A nurse has conducted discharge teaching with a client who was diagnosed with tuberculosis (TB). The client has been on medication for a week and a half. The nurse evaluates that the client has understood the information if the client makes which of the following statements?

1. "I need to continue drug therapy for 2 months."
2. "I should not be contagious after 2 to 3 weeks of medication therapy."
3. "I can't shop at the mall for the next 6 months."
4. "I can return to work if a sputum culture comes back negative."

60. A nurse is preparing to give a bed bath to an immobilized client with tuberculosis (TB). The nurse should plan to wear which of the following items when performing this care?

1. Particulate respirator, gown, and gloves
2. Particulate respirator and protective eyewear
3. Surgical mask and gloves
4. Surgical mask, gown, and protective eyewear

CRITICAL THINKING: FREE-TEXT ENTRY

A client who is human immunodeficiency virus (HIV)–positive has had a Mantoux skin test. The nurse notes a 7-mm area of induration at the site of the skin test. The nurse interprets the results and documents what interpretation on the client's record?

Answer: _____

ANSWERS

1. 2
Rationale: To obtain a sputum specimen, the client should rinse the mouth to reduce contamination, breathe deeply, and then cough into a sputum specimen container. The client should be encouraged to cough and not spit, so as to obtain sputum. Sputum can be thinned by fluids or by a respiratory treatment such as inhalation of nebulized saline or water. The optimal time to obtain a specimen is upon arising in the morning.
Test-Taking Strategy: Use the process of elimination. Option 1 can be eliminated first because general principles indicate that fluids assist in loosening or thinning secretions. Eliminate option 3 because of the word "spit." Spit is very different from sputum. Next eliminate option 4 because of the words "after eating." Review this procedure if you had difficulty with this question.
Level of Cognitive Ability: Application
Client Needs: Physiological Integrity
Integrated Concept/Process: Nursing Process/Implementation
Content Area: Adult Health/Respiratory
Reference: Smeltzer, S., & Bare, B. (2000). *Brunner & Suddarth's textbook of medical-surgical nursing* (9th ed.). Philadelphia: Lippincott Williams & Wilkins, p. 432.

2. 4
Rationale: If a biopsy was performed during a broncoscopy, blood-streaked sputum is expected for several hours. Frank blood is indicative of hemorrhage. A dry cough may be expected. The client should be assessed for signs of complications, which would include cyanosis, dyspnea, stridor, hemoptysis, hypotension, tachycardia, and dysrhythmias. Hematuria is unrelated to this procedure.
Test-Taking Strategy: Use the process of elimination. Eliminate option 3 first because it is unrelated to the procedure. Next eliminate option 2 because a dry cough may be expected. Noting that a biopsy has been performed will assist in eliminating option 1, as pink-tinged sputum would be expected. Note that option 4, the correct option, relates to airway. If you had difficulty with this question, review postprocedure care following broncoscopy with biopsy.
Level of Cognitive Ability: Analysis
Client Needs: Physiological Integrity
Integrated Concept/Process: Nursing Process/Analysis
Content Area: Adult Health/Respiratory
Reference: Monahan, F., & Neighbors, M. (1998). *Medical-surgical nursing: Foundations for clinical practice* (2nd ed.). Philadelphia: W.B. Saunders, p. 549.

3. **2**

Rationale: Hypoxemia can be caused by prolonged suctioning, which stimulates the pacemaker cells within the heart. A vasovagal response may occur, causing bradycardia. It is important to limit the suctioning pass to 15 seconds and to preoxygenate the client prior to suctioning.

Test-Taking Strategy: Use the process of elimination. Recall that during suctioning, the client's airway is blocked; therefore you should be able to eliminate options 3 and 4 readily easily. From the remaining options, eliminate option 1 because of the very short time frame. It does not seem reasonable that 5 seconds would achieve removal of secretions. Review the procedure for suctioning, if you had difficulty with this question

Level of Cognitive Ability: Application

Client Needs: Physiological Integrity

Integrated Concept/Process: Nursing Process/Implementation

Content Area: Adult Health/Respiratory

Reference: Ignatavicius, D., Workman, M., & Mishler, M. (1999). *Medical-surgical nursing across the health care continuum* (3rd ed.). Philadelphia: W.B. Saunders, p. 580.

4. **3**

Rationale: During suctioning, the nurse should monitor the client closely for side effects, including hypoxemia, cardiac irregularities resulting from vagal stimulation, mucosal trauma, hypotension, and paroxysmal coughing. If side effects develop, especially cardiac irregularities, the procedure is stopped and the client is reoxygenated.

Test-Taking Strategy: Use the process of elimination, recalling that suctioning can cause cardiac irregularities. This principle should easily direct you to option 3. If you had difficulty with this question, review the complications and interventions associated with suctioning procedure.

Level of Cognitive Ability: Application

Client Needs: Physiological Integrity

Integrated Concept/Process: Nursing Process/Implementation

Content Area: Adult Health/Respiratory

Reference: Smith, S., Duell, D., & Martin, B. (2000). *Clinical nursing skills: Basic to advanced skills* (5th ed.). Upper Saddle River, N.J.: Prentice Hall Health, p. 771.

5. **1**

Rationale: In an acidotic condition, the pH would be low, indicating the acidosis. In addition, a low bicarbonate level along with the low pH would indicate a metabolic state.

Test-Taking Strategy: Use the Pyramid Steps for evaluating the results of a blood gas. Remember to look at the pH first. This pH of 7.30 would indicate an acidosis. Next look at the CO_2 level, which in this situation is normal; therefore a respiratory condition does not exist. This will assist in eliminating options 2, 3, and 4. Noting that the bicarbonate level is low, as is the pH, should assist in directing you to option 1, a metabolic condition. Review blood gas analysis if you had difficulty with this question.

Level of Cognitive Ability: Analysis

Client Needs: Physiological Integrity

Integrated Concept/Process: Nursing Process/Analysis

Content Area: Adult Health/Respiratory

Reference: Monahan, F., & Neighbors, M. (1998). *Medical-surgical nursing: Foundations for clinical practice* (2nd ed.). Philadelphia: W.B. Saunders, p. 544.

6. **2**

Rationale: This client has sustained a blunt or a closed chest injury. Basic symptoms of a closed pneumothorax are shortness of breath and chest pain. A larger pneumothorax may present with tachypnea, cyanosis, diminished breath sounds, and subcutaneous emphysema. There may also be hyperresonance on the affected side.

Test-Taking Strategy: Use the process of elimination. Note the key word "blunt" in the question. This will assist in eliminating option 1, sucking chest wound injury. Knowing that in a respiratory injury increased respirations will occur will assist in eliminating option 3. Option 4 can be eliminated because a barrel chest is a characteristic finding in a client with chronic obstructive pulmonary disease. Review the signs of pneumothorax if you had difficulty with this question.

Level of Cognitive Ability: Analysis

Client Needs: Physiological Integrity

Integrated Concept/Process: Nursing Process/Analysis

Content Area: Adult Health/Respiratory

Reference: Monahan, F., & Neighbors, M. (1998). *Medical-surgical nursing: Foundations for clinical practice* (2nd ed.). Philadelphia: W.B. Saunders, pp. 692-693.

7. **3**

Rationale: Clinical manifestations of COPD include hypoxemia, hypercapnia, dyspnea on exertion and at rest, oxygen desaturation with exercise, and the use of accessory muscles of respiration. Chest x-ray will reveal a hyperinflated chest and a flattened diaphragm if the disease is advanced.

Test-Taking Strategy: Use the process of elimination. Eliminate option 1 because oxygen desaturation rather than saturation would occur. Next eliminate option 2 because in the client with COPD, hypercapnia would be noted. From the remaining options, reading carefully will assist in directing you to option 3. If you are unfamiliar with the manifestations associated with COPD, review this content.

Level of Cognitive Ability: Analysis

Client Needs: Physiological Integrity

Integrated Concept/Process: Nursing Process/Assessment

Content Area: Adult Health/Respiratory

Reference: Monahan, F., & Neighbors, M. (1998). *Medical-surgical nursing: Foundations for clinical practice* (2nd ed.). Philadelphia: W.B. Saunders, p. 668.

8. **1**

Rationale: The Venturi mask delivers the most accurate oxygen concentration. It is the best oxygen delivery system for the client with CAL because it delivers a precise oxygen concentration. The face tent, the aerosol mask, and the tracheostomy collar are also high-flow oxygen delivery systems but are most often used to administer high humidity.

Test-Taking Strategy: Use the process of elimination. Note the key words "precise oxygen concentration." Eliminate options 2, 3, and 4 because they are similar in that they are used to provide high humidity. Review the various types of oxygen delivery systems if you had difficulty with this question.

Level of Cognitive Ability: Analysis

Client Needs: Physiological Integrity

Integrated Concept/Process: Nursing Process/Analysis

Content Area: Adult Health/Respiratory

Reference: Ignatavicius, D., Workman, M., & Mishler, M. (1999). *Medical-surgical nursing across the health care continuum* (3rd ed.). Philadelphia: W.B. Saunders, p. 570.

9. 1

Rationale: The medication should be administered with food such as milk and crackers to prevent gastrointestinal (GI) irritation. Options 2, 3, and 4 are appropriate instructions regarding the use of this medication.

Test-Taking Strategy: Use the process of elimination, noting the key word "not." Noting that options 1 and 2 are opposite in terms of administering the medication should alert you that one of these options is the correct answer. Recalling that the client with CAL experiences GI upset will easily direct you to option 1. If you are unfamiliar with this medication, review this content.

Level of Cognitive Ability: Application

Client Needs: Health Promotion and Maintenance

Integrated Concept/Process: Teaching/Learning

Content Area: Pharmacology

Reference: Ignatavicius, D., Workman, M., & Mishler, M. (1999). *Medical-surgical nursing across the health care continuum* (3rd ed.). Philadelphia: W.B. Saunders, p. 625.

10. 4

Rationale: Positions that will assist the client with breathing include sitting up and leaning on an overbed table, sitting up and resting the elbows on the knees, and standing and leaning against the wall.

Test-Taking Strategy: Use the process of elimination. Eliminate options 2 and 3 first because they are similar. Next eliminate option 1 because this position will not enhance breathing. If you had difficulty with this question, review the positions that will decrease the work of breathing in a client with emphysema.

Level of Cognitive Ability: Application

Client Needs: Physiological Integrity

Integrated Concept/Process: Teaching /Learning

Content Area: Adult Health/Respiratory

Reference: Ignatavicius, D., Workman, M., & Mishler, M. (1999). *Medical-surgical nursing across the health care continuum* (3rd ed.). Philadelphia: W.B. Saunders, p. 622.

11. 2

Rationale: The first pulmonary symptom includes a slight morning cough with the expectoration of mucoid sputum. Options 1, 3, and 4 are late symptoms and signify cavitation and extensive lung involvement.

Test-Taking Strategy: Use the process of elimination. Note the key word "first" in the stem of the question. This should easily direct you to option 2. If you are unfamiliar with the signs associated with TB, review this content.

Level of Cognitive Ability: Application

Client Needs: Health Promotion and Maintenance

Integrated Concept/Process: Teaching/Learning

Content Area: Adult Health/Respiratory

Reference: Monahan, F., & Neighbors, M. (1998). *Medical-surgical nursing: Foundations for clinical practice* (2nd ed.). Philadelphia: W.B. Saunders, p. 651.

12. 3

Rationale: Definitive diagnosis of TB is confirmed through culture and isolation of *Mycobacterium tuberculosis*. A presumptive diagnosis is made on the basis of a tuberculin skin test, a sputum smear that is positive for acid-fast bacteria, a chest x-ray, and histologic evidence of graunulomatous disease on biopsy.

Test-Taking Strategy: Note the key word "confirm" in the stem of the question. Confirmation is made by identifying *Mycobacterium tuberculosis*. If you had difficulty with this question, review the diagnostic procedures related to TB.

Level of Cognitive Ability: Analysis

Client Needs: Physiological Integrity

Integrated Concept/Process: Nursing Process/Assessment

Content Area: Adult Health/Respiratory

Reference: Monahan, F., & Neighbors, M. (1998). *Medical-surgical nursing: Foundations for clinical practice* (2nd ed.). Philadelphia: W.B. Saunders, p. 652.

13. 1

Rationale: Tuberculosis is an infectious disease caused by the bacillus *Mycobacterium tuberculosis* and is spread primarily by the airborne route. Options 2, 3, and 4 are incorrect.

Test-Taking Strategy: Recalling that TB is a respiratory disease will easily direct you to option 1. If you had difficulty with this question, review the transmission of this disease.

Level of Cognitive Ability: Analysis

Client Needs: Safe, Effective Care Environment

Integrated Concept/Process: Teaching/Learning

Content Area: Adult Health/Respiratory

Reference: Monahan, F., & Neighbors, M. (1998). *Medical-surgical nursing: Foundations for clinical practice* (2nd ed.). Philadelphia: W.B. Saunders, p. 650.

14. 2

Rationale: One to three liters of oxygen by nasal cannula may be required to raise the Pao2 to 60 to 80 mm Hg. However, oxygen is used cautiously and should not exceed 2 L. Because of the long-standing hypercapnia, the respiratory drive is triggered by low oxygen levels rather than increased carbon dioxide levels, as is the case in a normal respiratory system.

Test-Taking Strategy: Use the process of elimination, focusing on the client's diagnosis. Recalling that in the client with emphysema, respiratory drive is triggered by low oxygen levels will direct you to option 2. If you are unfamiliar with this important concept, review this content.

Level of Cognitive Ability: Analysis

Client Needs: Physiological Integrity

Integrated Concept/Process: Nursing Process/Analysis

Content Area: Adult Health/Respiratory

Reference: Smeltzer, S., & Bare, B. (2000). *Brunner & Suddarth's textbook of medical-surgical nursing* (9th ed.). Philadelphia: Lippincott Williams & Wilkins, p. 455.

15. 4

Rationale: In a metabolic alkalosis, the pH is elevated along with the bicarbonate level. Option 4 is the only option that reflects these values.

Test-Taking Strategy: Remember that when an alkalotic condition exists, the pH will be elevated. This will assist in eliminating options 1 and 3. Next, recall that in a metabolic condition, the HCO_3 will move in the same direction as the pH. The only option that represents these conditions is option 4. Review the process of blood gas analysis, if you had difficulty with this question.

Level of Cognitive Ability: Analysis

Client Needs: Physiological Integrity

Integrated Concept/Process: Nursing Process/Analysis
Content Area: Adult Health/Respiratory
Reference: Monahan, F., & Neighbors, M. (1998). *Medical-surgical nursing: Foundations for clinical practice* (2nd ed.). Philadelphia: W.B. Saunders, p. 544.

16. **3**
Rationale: In respiratory acidosis, the pH will be lower than normal and the P_{CO_2} will be elevated. The normal pH is 7.35 to 7.45. The normal P_{CO_2} is 35 to 45 mm Hg. The only option that reflects these conditions is option 3.
Test-Taking Strategy: Remember that when an acidotic condition exists, the pH will be low. Next, recall that in a respiratory acidotic condition, the P_{CO_2} will move in the opposite direction from the pH. The only option that represents these conditions is option 3. Review the process of blood gas analysis, if you had difficulty with this question.
Level of Cognitive Ability: Analysis
Client Needs: Physiological Integrity
Integrated Concept/Process: Nursing Process/Analysis
Content Area: Adult Health/Respiratory
Reference: Monahan, F., & Neighbors, M. (1998). *Medical-surgical nursing: Foundations for clinical practice* (2nd ed.). Philadelphia: W.B. Saunders, p. 544.

17. **4**
Rationale: Pursed-lip breathing facilitates maximal expiration for clients with obstructive lung disease. This type of breathing allows better expiration by increasing airway pressure that keeps air passages open during exhalation. Options 1, 2, and 3 are not the purposes of this type of breathing.
Test-Taking Strategy: Attempt to visualize the use of this procedure to assist you in answering correctly. Knowledge regarding the respiratory conditions in which this type of breathing is helpful will also assist in directing you to option 4. Review the purpose of this breathing technique, if you had difficulty with this question.
Level of Cognitive Ability: Analysis
Client Needs: Physiological Integrity
Integrated Concept/Process: Teaching/Learning
Content Area: Adult Health/Respiratory
Reference: Phipps, W., Sands, J., & Marek, J. (1999). *Medical-surgical nursing: Concepts & clinical practice* (6th ed.). St. Louis: Mosby, p. 991.

18. **2**
Rationale: If at any time an alarm is sounding and the nurse cannot quickly ascertain the problem, the client is disconnected from the ventilator and manual resuscitation is used to support respirations until the problem can be corrected. There is no reason to begin CPR. Checking vital signs is not the initial action. Although oxygen is helpful, it will not provide ventilation to the client.
Test-Taking Strategy: Use the process of elimination. Read the question carefully, and note that the issue relates to adequate ventilation of the client. Focusing on this issue will easily direct you to option 2. If you are unfamiliar with management of ventilators and alarms, review this content.
Level of Cognitive Ability: Application
Client Needs: Physiological Integrity
Integrated Concept/Process: Nursing Process/Implementation
Content Area: Adult Health/Respiratory

Reference: Smeltzer, S., & Bare, B. (2000). *Brunner & Suddarth's textbook of medical-surgical nursing* (9th ed.). Philadelphia: Lippincott Williams & Wilkins, p. 507.

19. **2**
Rationale: In respiratory alkalosis, the pH will be higher than normal and the P_{CO_2} will be low. The normal pH is 7.35 to 7.45. The normal P_{CO_2} is 35 to 45 mm Hg. The only option that reflects these conditions is option 2.
Test-Taking Strategy: Remember that when an alkalotic condition exists, the pH will be high. Next, recall that in a respiratory alkalotic condition, the P_{CO_2} will move in the opposite direction from the pH. The only option that represents these conditions is option 2. Compensation can be identified if the pH is within normal limits. Review the process of blood gas analysis, if you had difficulty with this question.
Level of Cognitive Ability: Analysis
Client Needs: Physiological Integrity
Integrated Concept/Process: Nursing Process/Analysis
Content Area: Adult Health/Respiratory
Reference: Monahan, F., & Neighbors, M. (1998). *Medical-surgical nursing: Foundations for clinical practice* (2nd ed.). Philadelphia: W.B. Saunders, p. 544.

20. **3**
Rationale: Aminophylline is a bronchodilator that directly relaxes the smooth muscles of the bronchial airway. Options 1, 2, and 4 are not direct actions of this medication.
Test-Taking Strategy: Use the process of elimination. Recalling that this medication is a bronchodilator will direct you to option 3. Review this medication if you had difficulty with this question.
Level of Cognitive Ability: Analysis
Client Needs: Physiological Integrity
Integrated Concept/Process: Nursing Process/Implementation
Content Area: Pharmacology
Reference: Hodgson, B., & Kizior, R. (2001). *Saunders nursing drug handbook 2001*. Philadelphia: W.B. Saunders, pp. 44-47.

21. **2**
Rationale: Safe and effective therapy requires periodic measurement of theophylline blood levels. A level of 15 µg/mL is appropriate. Adverse effects occur at levels above 20 µg/mL. Options 3 and 4 represent toxic levels. Option 1 indicates that the client may require an increased dose of medication.
Test-Taking Strategy: Note the issue of the question, a therapeutic blood level. Recalling that this level is 10 to 20 µg/mL will direct you to option 2. Review this therapeutic level if you had difficulty with this question.
Level of Cognitive Ability: Analysis
Client Needs: Physiological Integrity
Integrated Concept/Process: Nursing Process/Analysis
Content Area: Pharmacology
Reference: Hodgson, B., & Kizior, R. (2001). *Saunders nursing drug handbook 2001*. Philadelphia: W.B. Saunders, pp. 44-47.

22. **3**
Rationale: The earliest clinical sign of ARDS if an increased respiratory rate. Breathing becomes labored, and the client may exhibit air hunger, retractions, and cyanosis. Arterial blood gas analysis reveals increasing hypoxemia, with a Pao_2 of less than 60 mm Hg.

Test-Taking Strategy: Use the process of elimination. Note that options 3 and 4 relate to the same issue but present opposite conditions. This may provide you with the clue that one of these options is the correct one. Considering the diagnosis of the client, the best choice is option 3. Review the clinical manifestations associated with ARDS if you had difficulty with this question.
Level of Cognitive Ability: Analysis
Client Needs: Physiological Integrity
Integrated Concept/Process: Nursing Process/Assessment
Content Area: Adult Health/Respiratory
Reference: Ignatavicius, D., Workman, M., & Mishler, M. (1999). *Medical-surgical nursing across the health care continuum* (3rd ed.). Philadelphia: W.B. Saunders, p. 693.

23. **4**
Rationale: Side effects that can occur from the use of this medication include tremors, nausea, nervousness, palpitations, tachycardia, peripheral vasodilation, and dryness of the mouth or throat.
Test-Taking Strategy: Recalling that this medication causes sympathomimetic stimulation will easily direct you to option 4. If you are unfamiliar with the side effects related to this medication, review this content.
Level of Cognitive Ability: Analysis
Client Needs: Physiological Integrity
Integrated Concept/Process: Nursing Process/Assessment
Content Area: Pharmacology
Reference: Hodgson, B., & Kizior, R. (2001). *Saunders nursing drug handbook 2001.* Philadelphia: W.B. Saunders, pp. 548-550.

24. **3**
Rationale: Both isoniazid and rifampin are contraindicated in clients with acute liver disease or a history of hepatic injury. Option 3 is the only option that addresses hepatic dysfunction.
Test-Taking Strategy: Use the process of elimination. Eliminate options 1 and 4 first because they both relate to cardiac disorders. From the remaining options, it is necessary to know that these medications may cause hepatotoxicity. Review the contraindications associated with the use of these medications if you had difficulty with this question.
Level of Cognitive Ability: Analysis
Client Needs: Physiological Integrity
Integrated Concept/Process: Nursing Process/Assessment
Content Area: Pharmacology
Reference: Hodgson, B., & Kizior, R. (2001). *Saunders nursing drug handbook 2001.* Philadelphia: W.B. Saunders, pp. 550-552, 906-908.

25. **3**
Rationale: The client needs to be instructed that the entire year-long course of the medication needs to be completed. It is preferable to take the medication 1 hour before or 2 hours after meals. If GI irritation occurs, the medication should not be discontinued, and in this situation a small amount of food may be taken to reduce the irritation. It is not necessary to increase fluids during this medication therapy.
Test-Taking Strategy: Use the process of elimination. Note that options 1, 2, and 4 contain the absolute word "must." Review

the client teaching points related to these medications, if you had difficulty with this question.
Level of Cognitive Ability: Application
Client Needs: Health Promotion and Maintenance
Integrated Concept/Process: Teaching/Learning
Content Area: Pharmacology
Reference: Hodgson, B., & Kizior, R. (2001). *Saunders nursing drug handbook 2001.* Philadelphia: W.B. Saunders, pp. 550-552, 906-908.

26. **2**
Rationale: Clients diagnosed with active TB are usually started on more than one medication, to be certain that the resistant organisms are eliminated. The dosages of some medications may initially be large because the bacilli are difficult to kill. Options 1, 3, and 4 are inaccurate.
Test-Taking Strategy: Use the process of elimination. Recalling the concern related to multidrug-resistant therapy will direct you to option 2. If you are unfamiliar with this therapy, review this content.
Level of Cognitive Ability: Application
Client Needs: Health Promotion and Maintenance
Integrated Concept/Process: Teaching/Learning
Content Area: Pharmacology
Reference: Ignatavicius, D., Workman, M., & Mishler, M. (1999). *Medical-surgical nursing across the health care continuum* (3rd ed.). Philadelphia: W.B. Saunders, p. 677.

27. **1**
Rationale: The most common clinical manifestations of PE are tachypnea, dyspnea, and chest pain.
Test-Taking Strategy: Use the process of elimination. Note the key word "not." Also, note that options 1 and 2 address a similar issue but opposite effects. This may provide you with the clue that one of these options is the correct one. You would expect an increased respiratory rate in PE; therefore, select option 1. Review the clinical manifestations of PE if you had difficulty with this question.
Level of Cognitive Ability: Analysis
Client Needs: Physiological Integrity
Integrated Concept/Process: Nursing Process/Assessment
Content Area: Adult Health/Respiratory
Reference: Ignatavicius, D., Workman, M., & Mishler, M. (1999). *Medical-surgical nursing across the health care continuum* (3rd ed.). Philadelphia: W.B. Saunders. p. 684.

28. **3**
Rationale: The client should be instructed to hold his or her breath at least 5 to 10 seconds before exhaling the mist. Options 1, 2, and 4 are accurate instructions regarding the use of the inhaler.
Test-Taking Strategy: Use the process of elimination, noting the key word "not." Attempt to visualize this procedure to answer the question. If you are unfamiliar with the client teaching points related to the use of an inhaler, review this procedure.
Level of Cognitive Ability: Application
Client Needs: Health Promotion and Maintenance
Integrated Concept/Process: Teaching/Learning
Content Area: Adult Health/Respiratory
Reference: Altman, G., Buchsel, P., & Coxon, V. (2000). *Delmar's fundamental & advanced nursing skills.* Albany, N.Y.: Delmar, p. 542.

29. 1

Rationale: The most important item to ask about is the client's pregnancy status, because pregnant women should not be exposed to radiation. Clients are also asked to remove any chains or metal objects that could interfere with obtaining an adequate film. A chest x-ray is most often done at full inspiration, which gives optimal lung expansion. If a lateral view of the chest is ordered, the client is asked to raise the arms above the head. Most films are done in posterior-anterior (PA) view.

Test-Taking Strategy: Note the key words "most important." Eliminate options 3 and 4 first, because they can be determined by the radiological technologist. Option 1 is a higher priority than option 2, because of potential negative teratogenic consequences to the fetus. Review client preparation for a chest x-ray if you had difficulty with this question.

Level of Cognitive Ability: Application

Client Needs: Physiological Integrity

Integrated Concept/Process: Nursing Process/Assessment

Content Area: Adult Health/Respiratory

Reference: Potter, P., & Perry, A. (2001). *Fundamentals of nursing* (5th ed.). St. Louis: Mosby, p. 1674.

30. 2

Rationale: After bronchoscopy, the nurse keeps the client on NPO status until the gag reflex returns. This is because the preoperative sedation and the local anesthesia impair swallowing and the protective laryngeal reflexes for a number of hours. Forcing fluids is unnecessary, since there is no use of contrast dye that would need flushing from the system. Atropine and midazolam would be administered before the procedure, not after.

Test-Taking Strategy: Use the process of elimination. Recall that the client has lost the protective cough, gag, and swallow reflexes during this procedure. Knowledge of this implication helps you to choose option 2 as the only possible answer. Review nursing care measures following a bronchoscopy, if you had difficulty with this question.

Level of Cognitive Ability: Application

Client Needs: Physiological Integrity

Integrated Concept/Process: Nursing Process/Implementation

Content Area: Adult Health/Respiratory

Reference: Smeltzer, S., & Bare, B. (2000). *Brunner & Suddarth's textbook of medical-surgical nursing* (9th ed.). Philadelphia: Lippincott Williams & Wilkins, p. 397.

31. 2

Rationale: Prior to drawing an arterial blood gas, the nurse assesses the collateral circulation to the hand with the Allen test. This involves compressing both the radial and ulnar arteries and asking the client to close and open the fist. This should cause the hand to become pale. The nurse then releases pressure on one artery and observes if circulation is quickly restored. The process is then repeated, releasing the other artery. The blood sample may be safely taken if there is adequate collateral circulation.

Test-Taking Strategy: Use the process of elimination, recalling that collateral circulation to the hand must be ensured before arterial blood gases are drawn. Consider the anatomy of the blood vessels that lead to the hand to direct you to option 2. If you are unfamiliar with the Allen test, review this procedure.

Level of Cognitive Ability: Application

Client Needs: Physiological Integrity

Integrated Concept/Process: Nursing Process/Implementation

Content Area: Adult Health/Respiratory

Reference: Potter, P., & Perry, A. (2001). *Fundamentals of nursing* (5th ed.). St. Louis: Mosby, p. 790.

32. 2

Rationale: Rib fractures are a common injury, especially in the elderly, and result from a blunt injury or a fall. Typical signs and symptoms include pain and tenderness that is localized at the fracture site and is exacerbated by inspiration and palpation; shallow respirations; splinting or guarding the chest protectively to minimize chest movement; and possible bruising at the fracture site.

Test-Taking Strategy: Use the process of elimination, noting the key word "not." Knowing that fractured ribs can cause pain and bruising helps to eliminate options 1 and 4 first. To discriminate between options 2 and 3, knowing that pain causes shallow, guarded respirations helps you to choose option 2 as the unrelated finding. Review the assessment findings in rib fractures, if you had difficulty with this question.

Level of Cognitive Ability: Analysis

Client Needs: Physiological Integrity

Integrated Concept/Process: Nursing Process/Assessment

Content Area: Adult Health/Respiratory

Reference: Smeltzer, S., & Bare, B. (2000). *Brunner & Suddarth's textbook of medical-surgical nursing* (9th ed.). Philadelphia: Lippincott Williams & Wilkins, p. 1857.

33. 4

Rationale: Flail chest results from fracture of two or more ribs in at least two places each. This results in a "floating" section of ribs. Because this section is unattached to the rest of the bony rib cage, this segment results in paradoxical chest movement. This means that the force of inspiration pulls the fractured segment inward, while the rest of the chest expands. Likewise, during exhalation the segment balloons outward, while the rest of the chest moves inward. This is a telltale sign of flail chest.

Test-Taking Strategy: Use the process of elimination, focusing on the key words "most distinctive." Cyanosis and hypotension occur with many different disorders, and are therefore eliminated first. From the remaining options, choose paradoxical chest movement over dyspnea on exhalation by remembering that a flail chest has broken rib segments that move independently of the rest of the rib cage. Review the assessment findings in flail chest if you had difficulty with this question.

Level of Cognitive Ability: Application

Client Needs: Physiological Integrity

Integrated Concept/Process: Nursing Process/Assessment

Content Area: Adult Health/Respiratory

Reference: Smeltzer, S., & Bare, B. (2000). *Brunner & Suddarth's textbook of medical-surgical nursing* (9th ed.). Philadelphia: Lippincott Williams & Wilkins, p. 482.

34. 4

Rationale: Pneumothorax is characterized by restlessness, tachycardia, dyspnea, pain with respiration, asymmetrical chest expansion, and diminished or absent breath sounds on the affected side. Pneumothorax can cause increased airway pressure because of resistance to lung inflation. ARDS and pulmonary embolism are not characterized by absent breath sounds. An endotracheal tube that is inserted too far can cause absent breath sounds, but the lack of breath sounds would most likely be on the left side, because of the degree of curvature of the right and left mainstem bronchi.

Test-Taking Strategy: Use the process of elimination. Focus on the symptoms presented in the question. Note the relationship between "right" upper lobe and "right" pneumothorax in option 4. Review the manifestations associated with pneumothorax, if you had difficulty with this question.
Level of Cognitive Ability: Analysis
Client Needs: Physiological Integrity
Integrated Concept/Process: Nursing Process/Assessment
Content Area: Adult Health/Respiratory
Reference: Lewis, S., Heitkemper, M., & Dirksen, S. (2000). *Medical-surgical nursing: Assessment and management of clinical problems* (5th ed.). St. Louis: Mosby, p. 643.

35. 3
Rationale: Respiratory failure is described as a Pao_2 of 50 mm Hg or less and a $Paco_2$ of 50 mm Hg or greater in a client with no history of respiratory disease. In a client with a history of a respiratory disorder with hypercapnia, elevations of 5 mm or more from the client's baseline are considered diagnostic.
Test-Taking Strategy: Use the process of elimination. Focusing on the client's diagnosis will direct you to option 3, the option with the lowest Pao_2 level. Review the blood gas findings in a client with respiratory failure, if you had difficulty with this question.
Level of Cognitive Ability: Analysis
Client Needs: Physiological Integrity
Integrated Concept/Process: Nursing Process/Analysis
Content Area: Adult Health/Respiratory
Reference: Ignatavicius, D., Workman, M., & Mishler, M. (1999). *Medical-surgical nursing across the health care continuum* (3rd ed.). Philadelphia: W.B. Saunders, p. 690.

36. 4
Rationale: Instructions for using a metered-dose inhaler include to shake the canister; hold it right side up; inhale slowly and evenly through the mouth; deliver one spray per breath; and hold the breath after inhalation.
Test-Taking Strategy: This question tests a fundamental concept of medication administration using inhalers. Visualize the procedure and use the process of elimination. If you selected the incorrect option, review the key principles of this medication therapy.
Level of Cognitive Ability: Application
Client Needs: Health Promotion and Maintenance
Integrated Concept/Process: Teaching/Learning
Content Area: Adult Health/Respiratory
Reference: Ignatavicius, D., Workman, M., & Mishler, M. (1999). *Medical-surgical nursing across the health care continuum* (3rd ed.). Philadelphia: W.B. Saunders, p. 628.

37. 4
Rationale: The earliest detectable sign of ARDS is an increased respiratory rate, which can begin anywhere from 1 to 96 hours after the initial insult to the body. This is followed by increasing dyspnea, air hunger, retraction of accessory muscles, and cyanosis. Breath sounds may be clear or may consist of fine inspiratory crackles or diffuse coarse crackles.

Test-Taking Strategy: Use the process of elimination, noting the key word "earliest." Eliminate option 3 first, since intercostal retraction is a later sign of respiratory distress. Of the remaining options, recall that adventitious breath sounds (options 1 and 2) would occur later than an increased respiratory rate. Review the early signs of ARDS if you had difficulty with this question.
Level of Cognitive Ability: Application
Client Needs: Physiological Integrity
Integrated Concept/Process: Nursing Process/Assessment
Content Area: Adult Health/Respiratory
Reference: Ignatavicius, D., Workman, M., & Mishler, M. (1999). *Medical-surgical nursing across the health care continuum* (3rd ed.). Philadelphia: W.B. Saunders, p. 692.

38. 3
Rationale: The normal PCWP is 8 to 13 mm Hg, and the client is considered to have high readings if they exceed 18 to 20 mm Hg. The client with ARDS has a normal PCWP, which is an expected finding, since the edema is in the interstitium of the lung and is noncardiac in origin.
Test-Taking Strategy: To answer this question correctly, it is necessary to know that the PCWP is normal. This makes sense if you know that in ARDS fluid accumulates in the interstitium of the lung, and not in the vascular bed. Learn the normal PCWP reading, if you are unfamiliar with it.
Level of Cognitive Ability: Analysis
Client Needs: Physiological Integrity
Integrated Concept/Process: Nursing Process/Analysis
Content Area: Adult Health/Respiratory
Reference: Ignatavicius, D., Workman, M., & Mishler, M. (1999). *Medical-surgical nursing across the health care continuum* (3rd ed.). Philadelphia: W.B. Saunders, p. 693.

39. 2
Rationale: The client with emphysema has hyperinflation of the alveoli and flattening of the diaphragm. These lead to increased anteroposterior diameter, which is referred to as "barrel chest." The client also has dyspnea with prolonged expiration and has hyperresonant lungs to percussion.
Test-Taking Strategy: Use the process of elimination. Recall that the "barrel chest" is a result of long-term hyperinflation of the lungs and air trapping. By knowing that emphysema is the only type of CAL in which this occurs, you are able to eliminate each of the other, incorrect options. Review the characteristics of emphysema if you had difficulty with this question.
Level of Cognitive Ability: Analysis
Client Needs: Physiological Integrity
Integrated Concept/Process: Nursing Process/Assessment
Content Area: Adult Health/Respiratory
Reference: Ignatavicius, D., Workman, M., & Mishler, M. (1999). *Medical-surgical nursing across the health care continuum* (3rd ed.). Philadelphia: W.B. Saunders, pp. 615-616.

40. 4
Rationale: Indomethacin is an NSAID, which has an analgesic effect and allows the client to cough and deep breathe more effectively. Options 1, 2, and 3 are incorrect.
Test-Taking Strategy: Recalling that the medication needed to treat this condition would be an antiinflammatory helps you to eliminate options 1 and 2. From the remaining options, remember that indomethacin is an NSAID. This medication is

also used to treat inflammation of the epicardium in the pericardial sac, which is called pericarditis. If you are unfamiliar with this medication, review its uses and actions.
Level of Cognitive Ability: Application
Client Needs: Health Promotion and Maintenance
Integrated Concept/Process: Teaching/Learning
Content Area: Pharmacology
Reference: Smeltzer, S., & Bare, B. (2000). *Brunner & Suddarth's textbook of medical-surgical nursing* (9th ed.). Philadelphia: Lippincott Williams & Wilkins, p. 444.

41. 3
Rationale: The most common initial symptom in pulmonary embolism is chest pain that is sudden in onset. The next most commonly reported symptom is dyspnea, which is accompanied by an increased respiratory rate. Other typical symptoms of pulmonary embolism include tachycardia, fever, diaphoresis, cough, anxiety, and possibly syncope.
Test-Taking Strategy: Use the process of elimination. Since pulmonary embolism does not result from either an infectious process or an allergic reaction, options 2 and 4 are eliminated first. To discriminate between options 1 and 3, look at them closely. Option 1 states dyspnea when deep breaths are taken. Although dyspnea commonly occurs with pulmonary embolism, dyspnea is not associated only with deep breathing. Therefore, option 1 is eliminated. Review the signs of pulmonary embolism if you had difficulty with this question.
Level of Cognitive Ability: Application
Client Needs: Physiological Integrity
Integrated Concept/Process: Nursing Process/Assessment
Content Area: Adult Health/Respiratory
Reference: Smeltzer, S., & Bare, B. (2000). *Brunner & Suddarth's textbook of medical-surgical nursing* (9th ed.). Philadelphia: Lippincott Williams & Wilkins, p. 472.

42. 2
Rationale: Carbon dioxide narcosis is a condition that results from extreme hypercapnia, with carbon dioxide levels in excess of 70 mm Hg. The client experiences symptoms such as confusion and tremors, which may progress to convulsions and possibly coma.
Test-Taking Strategy: Use the process of elimination, focusing on the data in the question. Noting that the CO_2 level is elevated will easily direct you to the correct option, CO_2 narcosis. Review the clinical manifestations associated with CO_2 narcosis if you had difficulty with this question.
Level of Cognitive Ability: Analysis
Client Needs: Physiological Integrity
Integrated Concept/Process: Nursing Process/Analysis
Content Area: Adult Health/Respiratory
Reference: Smeltzer, S., & Bare, B. (2000). *Brunner & Suddarth's textbook of medical-surgical nursing* (9th ed.). Philadelphia: Lippincott Williams & Wilkins, p. 231.

43. 4
Rationale: With the severe respiratory acidosis that occurs in carbon dioxide narcosis, compensatory mechanisms fail. As hydrogen ion concentrations continue to rise, hydrogen ions are driven into the cell, forcing intracellular potassium out. This is an expected finding in this situation.
Test-Taking Strategy: Use the process of elimination and knowledge regarding the effects of acidosis on the body. Eliminate options 1 and 2, knowing that hyperkalemia is an

expected finding. Eliminate option 3 next because this condition is unrelated to hemolysis. Review the manifestations of this disorder if you had difficulty with this question.
Level of Cognitive Ability: Analysis
Client Needs: Physiological Integrity
Integrated Concept/Process: Nursing Process/Analysis
Content Area: Adult Health/Respiratory
Reference: Smeltzer, S., & Bare, B. (2000). *Brunner & Suddarth's textbook of medical-surgical nursing* (9th ed.). Philadelphia: Lippincott Williams & Wilkins, p. 231.

44. 3
Rationale: Carbon dioxide acts as a vasodilator to cerebral blood vessels. With sufficient rise in carbon dioxide, the client may suffer increased intracranial pressure, which is initially reflected as papilledema and dilated conjunctival blood vessels. Options 1, 2, and 4 are unrelated to this disorder.
Test-Taking Strategy: Use the process of elimination. Knowing that carbon dioxide dilates the cerebral blood vessels will direct you to option 3, since the cerebral circulation is one of the three components that contribute to the net intracranial pressure. Review the complications associated with carbon dioxide narcosis, if you had difficulty with this question.
Level of Cognitive Ability: Application
Client Needs: Physiological Integrity
Integrated Concept/Process: Nursing Process/Assessment
Content Area: Adult Health/Respiratory
Reference: Smeltzer, S., & Bare, B. (2000). *Brunner & Suddarth's textbook of medical-surgical nursing* (9th ed.). Philadelphia: Lippincott Williams & Wilkins, p. 231.

45. 3
Rationale: With a rapid drop in carbon dioxide levels, the kidneys are unable to excrete bicarbonate ions at the same pace. The client can experience rebound metabolic alkalosis, with resulting seizure activity. The nurse evaluates the client's status carefully during this period.
Test-Taking Strategy: Use the process of elimination and knowledge regarding how the body maintains acid-base balance. Because a rapid decline in carbon dioxide often results in metabolic alkalosis, the client is at risk for seizure activity. Review the basic acid-base abnormalities and their manifestations if you had difficulty with this question.
Level of Cognitive Ability: Analysis
Client Needs: Physiological Integrity
Integrated Concept/Process: Nursing Process/Analysis
Content Area: Adult Health/Respiratory
Reference: Smeltzer, S., & Bare, B. (2000). *Brunner & Suddarth's textbook of medical-surgical nursing* (9th ed.). Philadelphia: Lippincott Williams & Wilkins, p. 231.

46. 2
Rationale: Histoplasmosis is an opportunistic fungal infection that can occur in the client with AIDS. The infection begins as a respiratory infection, and can progress to disseminated infection. Typical signs and symptoms include fever, dyspnea, cough, and weight loss. There may be enlargement of the client's lymph nodes, liver, and spleen as well.
Test-Taking Strategy: Use the process of elimination. Recalling that histoplasmosis is an infectious process helps you to eliminate option 3. Since the client has AIDS as well as another infection, weight gain is an unlikely symptom, and can be eliminated next. Knowing that histoplasmosis begins as a

respiratory infection helps you to choose dyspnea over headache as the correct option. Review the signs of histoplasmosis, if you had difficulty with this question.

Level of Cognitive Ability: Application
Client Needs: Physiological Integrity
Integrated Concept/Process: Nursing Process/Assessment
Content Area: Adult Health/Respiratory
Reference: Ignatavicius, D., Workman, M., & Mishler, M. (1999). *Medical-surgical nursing across the health care continuum* (3rd ed.). Philadelphia: W.B. Saunders, 446.

47. **3**

Rationale: Pulmonary sarcoidosis can lead to cor pulmonale (or right-sided heart failure), which is characterized by distended neck veins, elevated CVP, engorged liver, and peripheral edema. Bilateral crackles would indicate left-sided heart failure, not right-sided heart failure.

Test-Taking Strategy: Recall that sarcoidosis is a restrictive lung disease. A complication of restrictive lung disease is cor pulmonale, since the right side of the heart has to work hard on a continuous basis to overcome pulmonary resistance. Knowing this, you would eliminate options 2 and 4, because they are the opposite of the symptoms expected with right-sided heart failure. Choose option 3 over option 1 by knowing how to discriminate between left- and right-sided heart failure. Review the complications of pulmonary sarcoidosis and the signs of right- and left-sided heart failure, if you had difficulty with this question.

Level of Cognitive Ability: Application
Client Needs: Physiological Integrity
Integrated Concept/Process: Nursing Process/Assessment
Content Area: Adult Health/Respiratory
Reference: Ignatavicius, D., Workman, M., & Mishler, M. (1999). *Medical-surgical nursing across the health care continuum* (3rd ed.). Philadelphia: W.B. Saunders, p. 637

48. **2**

Rationale: The usual treatment for exacerbations of sarcoidosis includes systemic corticosteroids. Side effects of this therapy include weight gain, changes in mood, and hyperglycemia. Hyperkalemia and pruritis are unrelated findings.

Test-Taking Strategy: Recall that sarcoidosis is a restrictive lung disease, and that exacerbations are treated with corticosteroids. Knowing that corticosteroids cause hyperglycemia will direct you to the correct option. Review the medication therapy used in the treatment of sarcoidosis, if you had difficulty with this question.

Level of Cognitive Ability: Analysis
Client Needs: Physiological Integrity
Integrated Concept/Process: Teaching/Learning
Content Area: Adult Health/Respiratory
Reference: Ignatavicius, D., Workman, M., & Mishler, M. (1999). *Medical-surgical nursing across the health care continuum* (3rd ed.). Philadelphia: W.B. Saunders, p. 637.

49. **4**

Rationale: Dry cough and dyspnea are typical signs and symptoms of pulmonary sarcoidosis. Others include chest pain, hemoptysis, and pneumothorax. Systemic signs and symptoms include weakness and fatigue, malaise, fever, and weight loss.

Test-Taking Strategy: Use the process of elimination. Note the key word "early." Since sarcoidosis is a pulmonary problem,

eliminate options 1 and 2 first. Select option 4 over option 3, since the shortness of breath (and impaired ventilation) appears first, and would cause the fatigue as a secondary symptom. Review the early signs of exacerbation in sarcoidosis if you had difficulty with this question.

Level of Cognitive Ability: Analysis
Client Needs: Health Promotion and Maintenance
Integrated Concept/Process: Teaching/Learning
Content Area: Adult Health/Respiratory
Reference: Smeltzer, S., & Bare, B. (2000). *Brunner & Suddarth's textbook of medical-surgical nursing* (9th ed.). Philadelphia: Lippincott Williams & Wilkins, p. 476.

50. **1**

Rationale: Silicosis results from chronic, excessive inhalation of particles of free crystalline silica dust. The client should wear a mask to limit inhalation of this substance, which can cause restrictive lung disease after years of exposure. Options 2, 3, and 4 are not necessary.

Test-Taking Strategy: Use the process of elimination. Recalling that exposure to silica dust causes the illness and that the dust is inhaled into the respiratory tract will direct you to option 1. If you had difficulty with this question, review the protective measures associated with silicosis.

Level of Cognitive Ability: Analysis
Client Needs: Physiological Integrity
Integrated Concept/Process: Nursing Process/Assessment
Content Area: Adult Health/Respiratory
Reference: Ignatavicius, D., Workman, M., & Mishler, M. (1999). *Medical-surgical nursing across the health care continuum* (3rd ed.). Philadelphia: W.B. Saunders, p. 640.

51. **3**

Rationale: The client with simple silicosis may be asymptomatic or have mild ventilatory restriction, and has evidence of fibrosis on chest x-ray. Pulmonary function studies reveal some decreases in vital capacity and total lung volume. There is no evidence of massive fibrosis at this stage. This disease is restricted to the respiratory system only.

Test-Taking Strategy: Use the process of elimination. Option 4 has the least amount of "fit" with a disorder that is described as simple or uncomplicated, and therefore is eliminated first. Since silicosis is a pulmonary disease, option 1 is eliminated. Option 2 is incongruent; it would be difficult for one to have shortness of breath and have normal PFTs. Review the pathophysiology associated with simple silicosis, if you had difficulty with this question.

Level of Cognitive Ability: Analysis
Client Needs: Physiological Integrity
Integrated Concept/Process: Nursing Process/Analysis
Content Area: Adult Health/Respiratory
Reference: Ignatavicius, D., Workman, M., & Mishler, M. (1999). *Medical-surgical nursing across the health care continuum* (3rd ed.). Philadelphia: W.B. Saunders, pp. 639-640.

52. **4**

Rationale: Benzonatate is a locally acting antitussive. Its effectiveness is measured by the degree to which it decreases the intensity and frequency of cough, without eliminating the cough reflex. Options 1, 2, and 3 are not effects of this medication.

Test-Taking Strategy: Recalling that the medication is an antitussive will direct you to option 4. Review this medication if you are unfamiliar with it.

Level of Cognitive Ability: Analysis
Client Needs: Physiological Integrity
Integrated Concept/Process: Nursing Process/Evaluation
Content Area: Pharmacology
Reference: Hodgson, B., & Kizior, R. (2001). *Saunders nursing drug handbook 2001.* Philadelphia: W.B. Saunders, pp. 101-102.

53. **2**
Rationale: Pyrazinamide is an antitubercular medication that is given in conjunction with other antitubercular medications. Its use might not be discontinued if sputum cultures continue to be positive. Options 1, 3, and 4 are not directly related to the use of this medication.
Test-Taking Strategy: Recalling that this medication is an antitubercular medication will direct you to option 2. If this question was difficult, review this medication.
Level of Cognitive Ability: Analysis
Client Needs: Physiological Integrity
Integrated Concept/Process: Nursing Process/Evaluation
Content Area: Pharmacology
Reference: Hodgson, B., & Kizior, R. (2001). *Saunders nursing drug handbook 2001.* Philadelphia: W.B. Saunders, pp. 887-888.

54. **4**
Rationale: People at high risk for acquiring tuberculosis include immigrants from Asia, Africa, Latin America, and Oceania; medically underserved populations (ethnic minorities, homeless); those with human immunodeficiency virus or other immunosuppressive disorders; residents in group settings (long-term care, correctional facilities); and health care workers.
Test-Taking Strategy: Use the process of elimination, noting the key words "least risk." Begin to answer this question by eliminating options 1 and 2, since immigrants and the medically underserved are more frequently affected by the disease. From the remaining options, the postal inspector may or may not come into contact with many people, depending on the job description. The client from the long-term care facility, however, lives in a group setting, where a large number of people share a common environment 24 hours a day. Review the risk factors associated with TB if you had difficulty with this question.
Level of Cognitive Ability: Analysis
Client Needs: Physiological Integrity
Integrated Concept/Process: Nursing Process/Assessment
Content Area: Adult Health/Respiratory
Reference: Smeltzer, S., & Bare, B. (2000). *Brunner & Suddarth's textbook of medical-surgical nursing* (9th ed.). Philadelphia: Lippincott Williams & Wilkins, p. 437.

55. **1**
Rationale: A Mantoux skin test is administered by giving 0.1 mL of purified protein derivative (PPD) intradermally. This involves drawing the medication into a tuberculin syringe with a 25- to 27-gauge, 5/8 inch needle. The injection is given by inserting the needle as close as possible to a parallel position with the skin, and with the needle bevel facing up. This results in formation of a wheal, when the PPD is administered correctly.
Test-Taking Strategy: Remember that a tuberculin syringe is small and measures small amounts of medication dosages. Use the process of elimination, eliminating options 3 and 4 first because these options indicate the use of larger syringes

and needles. Remembering that the bevel side is up during administration of PPD will assist in directing you to the correct option from the remaining choices. If this question was difficult, review the basics of this injection technique.
Level of Cognitive Ability: Application
Client Needs: Physiological Integrity
Integrated Concept/Process: Nursing Process/Implementation
Content Area: Adult Health/Respiratory
Reference: Smeltzer, S., & Bare, B. (2000). *Brunner & Suddarth's textbook of medical-surgical nursing* (9th ed.). Philadelphia: Lippincott Williams & Wilkins, p. 438.

56. **2**
Rationale: A positive reading has an induration measuring 10 mm or more, and is considered abnormal. A small area of ecchymosis is insignificant, and is probably related to injection technique.
Test-Taking Strategy: Recall that induration is necessary for a positive response. Since the client in this question has no induration, the result can only be negative. Review Mantoux skin testing results, if you had difficulty with this question.
Level of Cognitive Ability: Analysis
Client Needs: Physiological Integrity
Integrated Concept/Process: Nursing Process/Analysis
Content Area: Adult Health/Respiratory
Reference: Smeltzer, S., & Bare, B. (2000). *Brunner & Suddarth's textbook of medical-surgical nursing* (9th ed.). Philadelphia: Lippincott Williams & Wilkins, p. 439.

57. **4**
Rationale: The client with tuberculosis usually experiences cough (either productive or nonproductive), fatigue, anorexia, weight loss, dyspnea, hemoptysis, chest discomfort or pain, chills and sweats (which may occur at night), and a low-grade fever.
Test-Taking Strategy: Use the process of elimination. Options 1 and 2 may be eliminated first, since they are symptoms that are common in the client with TB. From the remaining options, you need to know either that the client may get night sweats or that the fever is low grade. Review the clinical manifestations associated with TB, if you had difficulty with this question.
Level of Cognitive Ability: Analysis
Client Needs: Physiological Integrity
Integrated Concept/Process: Nursing Process/Assessment
Content Area: Adult Health/Respiratory
Reference: Smeltzer, S., & Bare, B. (2000). *Brunner & Suddarth's textbook of medical-surgical nursing* (9th ed.). Philadelphia: Lippincott Williams & Wilkins, p. 440-441.

58. **1**
Rationale: The nurse teaches the client with TB to increase intake of protein, iron, and vitamin C. Foods rich in vitamin C include citrus fruits, berries, melons, pineapple, broccoli, cabbage, green peppers, tomatoes, potatoes, chard, kale, asparagus, and turnip greens. Food sources that are rich in iron include liver and other meats. Less than 10% of iron is absorbed from eggs, and less than 5 % is absorbed from grains and vegetables.
Test-Taking Strategy: Use the process of elimination. Recall that the diet in tuberculosis should be high in protein, vitamin C, and iron. Knowing which types of foods contain these various nutrients will direct you to option 1. If you

had difficulty with this question, review these nutritional concepts.

Level of Cognitive Ability: Application
Client Needs: Health Promotion and Maintenance
Integrated Concept/Process: Teaching/Learning
Content Area: Adult Health/Respiratory
Reference: Ignatavicius, D., Workman, M., & Mishler, M. (1999). *Medical-surgical nursing across the health care continuum* (3rd ed.). Philadelphia: W.B. Saunders, p. 677.

59. **2**
Rationale: The client is continued on medication therapy for 6 to 12 months, depending on the situation. The client is generally considered to be not contagious after 2 to 3 weeks of medication therapy. The client is instructed to wear a mask if there will be exposure to crowds, until the medication is effective in preventing transmission. The client is allowed to return to work when the results of two sputum cultures are negative.
Test-Taking Strategy: Use the process of elimination. Knowing that the medication therapy lasts for at least 6 months helps you to eliminate option 1 first. Knowing that two sputum cultures must be negative helps you to eliminate option 4 next. From the remaining options, recalling that the client is not contagious after 2 to 3 weeks of therapy will direct you to option 2. If you had difficulty with this question, review the infectious period of TB.
Level of Cognitive Ability: Analysis
Client Needs: Physiological Integrity
Integrated Concept/Process: Teaching/Learning
Content Area: Adult Health/Respiratory
Reference: Ignatavicius, D., Workman, M., & Mishler, M. (1999). *Medical-surgical nursing across the health care continuum* (3rd ed.). Philadelphia: W.B. Saunders, p. 677.

60. **1**
Rationale: The nurse who is in contact with a client with TB should wear an individually fitted particulate respirator. The nurse would also wear gloves as per universal precautions. The nurse wears a gown when there is a possibility that the

clothing could become contaminated, such as when giving a bed bath.
Test-Taking Strategy: Use the process of elimination. Knowing that the nurse should wear a particulate respirator eliminates options 3 and 4. Knowledge of basic universal precautions directs you to option 1. Review precautions related to the care of a client with TB if you had difficulty with this question.
Level of Cognitive Ability: Application
Client Needs: Safe, Effective Care Environment
Integrated Concept/Process: Nursing Process/Implementation
Content Area: Adult Health/Respiratory
Reference: Ignatavicius, D., Workman, M., & Mishler, M. (1999). *Medical-surgical nursing across the health care continuum* (3rd ed.). Philadelphia: W.B. Saunders, p. 677.

CRITICAL THINKING: FREE-TEXT ENTRY

Answer: Positive skin test
Rationale: The client with HIV is considered to have positive results on Mantoux skin testing with an area of 5 mm of induration or greater. The client without HIV is positive with induration greater than 10 mm. The client with HIV is immunosuppressed, making a smaller area of induration positive for this type of client. It is also possible for the client infected with HIV to have false-negative readings because of the immunosuppression factor.
Test-Taking Strategy: Remembering that the client with HIV is immunosuppressed will assist in determining the interpretation of the area of induration. Review results of TB skin testing in an immunosuppressed client if you had difficulty with this question.
Level of Cognitive Ability: Analysis
Client Needs: Physiological Integrity
Integrated Concept/Process: Nursing Process/Analysis
Content Area: Adult Health/Respiratory
Reference: Ignatavicius, D., Workman, M., & Mishler, M. (1999). *Medical-surgical nursing across the health care continuum* (3rd ed.). Philadelphia: W.B. Saunders, p. 677.

REFERENCES

Altman, G., Buchsel, P., & Coxon, V. (2000). *Delmar's fundamental & advanced nursing skills.* Albany, N.Y.: Delmar.

Hodgson, B., & Kizior, R. (2001). *Saunders nursing drug handbook 2001.* Philadelphia: W.B. Saunders.

Ignatavicius, D., Workman, M., & Mishler, M. (1999). *Medical-surgical nursing across the health care continuum* (3rd ed.). Philadelphia: W.B. Saunders.

LeMone, P., & Burke, K. (2000). *Medical-surgical nursing: Critical thinking in client care* (2nd ed.). Upper Saddle River, N.J.: Prentice-Hall.

Lewis, S., Heitkemper, M., & Dirksen, S. (2000). *Medical-surgical nursing: Assessment and management of clinical problems* (5th ed.). St. Louis: Mosby.

Monahan, F., & Neighbors, M. (1998). *Medical-surgical nursing: Foundations for clinical practice* (2nd ed.). Philadelphia: W.B. Saunders.

Phipps, W., Sands, J., & Marek, J. (1999). *Medical-surgical nursing: Concepts & clinical practice* (6th ed.). St. Louis: Mosby.

Potter, P., & Perry, A. (2001). *Fundamentals of nursing* (5th ed.). St. Louis: Mosby.

Smeltzer, S., & Bare, B. (2000). *Brunner & Suddarth's textbook of medical-surgical nursing* (9th ed.). Philadelphia: Lippincott Williams & Wilkins.

Smith, S., Duell, D., & Martin, B. (2000). *Clinical nursing skills: Basic to advanced skills* (5th ed.). Upper Saddle River, N.J.: Prentice-Hall Health.

Respiratory Medications

I. BRONCHODILATORS

A. Description

1. Sympathomimetic bronchodilators dilate the airways of the respiratory tree, making air exchange and respiration easier for the client, and relax the smooth muscle of the bronchi (Box 56-1)
2. Xanthine bronchodilators stimulate the central nervous system and respiration, dilate coronary and pulmonary vessels, cause diuresis, and relax smooth muscle (Box 56-2)
3. Used to treat allergic rhinitis and sinusitis, acute bronchospasm, acute and chronic asthma, bronchitis, **chronic obstructive pulmonary disease, and emphysema**
4. Contraindicated in individuals with hypersensitivity, peptic ulcer disease, severe cardiac disease and cardiac dysrhythmias, hyperthyroidism, or uncontrolled seizure disorders
5. Used with caution in clients with hypertension, diabetes mellitus, or narrow-angle glaucoma
6. Theophylline increases the risk of digitalis toxicity and decreases the effects of lithium and phenytoin (Dilantin)
7. If theophylline and a beta-adrenergic agonist are administered together, cardiac dysrhythmias may result
8. Beta blockers, cimetidine (Tagamet), and erythromycin increase the effects of theophylline
9. Barbiturate and carbamazepine (Tegretol) decrease the effects of theophylline

B. Side effects
1. Palpitations and tachycardia
2. Dysrhythmias
3. Restlessness, nervousness, tremors
4. Anorexia, nausea, and vomiting
5. Headaches and dizziness
6. Hyperglycemia
7. Decreased clotting time

8. Mouth dryness and throat irritation with inhalers
9. Tolerance and paradoxic bronchoconstriction with inhalers

C. Implementation
1. Assess vital signs
2. Monitor for cardiac dysrhythmias
3. Assess for cough, wheezing, decreased breath sounds, and sputum production
4. Monitor for restlessness and confusion
5. Provide adequate hydration
6. Administer the medication at regular intervals around the clock to maintain a sustained therapeutic level

---

Bronchodilators: Xanthines

Aminophylline (generic, Truphylline, Phyllocontin)
Theophylline
Theophylline (Aerolate, Slo-Phyllin, Theolair)
Theophylline (Theo-Dur, Slo-Bid, Theo-24, Uni-Dur, Uniphyl)
Oxtriphylline (Choledyl, Choledyl-SA)

Glucocorticoids (Corticosteroids)

Beclomethasone dipropionate (Vanceril, Beclovent)
Triamcinolone (Azmacort)
Fluticasone (Flonase, Flovent)
Flunisolide (AeroBid)

Inhaled Nonsteroidal Antiallergy Agents

MAST-CELL STABLIZERS
Cromolyn sodium (Intal)
Nedocromil (Tilade)

---

7. Administer oral medications with or after meals to decrease gastrointestinal (GI) irritation
8. Instruct the client not to crush enteric-coated or sustained-release tablets or capsules
9. Instruct the client to avoid caffeine products, such as coffee, tea, cola, and chocolate
10. Instruct the client in the side effects of bronchodilators
11. Instruct the client in how to monitor the pulse and to report any abnormalities to the physician
12. Instruct the client in how to use an inhaler or nebulizer and how to monitor the amount of medication remaining in an inhaler canister
13. Instruct the client to avoid over-the-counter medications
14. Instruct the client to stop smoking and provide information regarding support resources
15. Instruct the client with diabetes mellitus to monitor blood glucose levels
16. Instruct the client with asthma to wear a Medic-Alert bracelet
17. Monitor for a therapeutic serum theophylline level of 10 to 20 μg/mL
18. Note that toxicity is likely to occur when the serum level is greater than 20 μg/mL
19. IV aminophylline or theophylline preparations should be administered slowly and always via an infusion pump

II. GLUCOCORTICOIDS (CORTICOSTEROIDS) (Box 56-3)
A. Act as antiinflammatory agents and reduce edema of the airways
B. Refer to Chapter 52 for information on glucocorticoids

III. INHALED NONSTEROIDAL ANTIALLERGY AGENTS (Box 56-4)
A. Description
  1. Antiasthmatic, antiallergic, and mast cell stabilizers that inhibit mast cell release after exposure to antigens
  2. Used for the treatment of allergic rhinitis, bronchial asthma, and exercised-induced bronchospasm

  3. Contraindicated in clients with known hypersensitivity
  4. Oral cromolyn sodium is used with caution in clients with impaired hepatic or renal function
B. Side effects
  1. Cough or bronchospasm following inhalation
  2. Nasal sting or sneezing following inhalation
  3. Unpleasant taste in the mouth
C. Implementation
  1. Monitor vital signs
  2. Monitor respirations and assess lung sounds for rhonchi, wheezing, and rales
  3. Instruct the client to drink a few sips of water before and after inhalation to prevent cough and unpleasant taste in the mouth
  4. Administer oral capsules (cromolyn sodium) at least 30 minutes before meals
  5. Instruct the client not to discontinue the medication abruptly because a rebound asthmatic attack can occur

IV. LEUKOTRIENE MODIFIERS (Box 56-5)
A. Description
  1. Used in the prophylaxis and treatment of chronic bronchial asthma
  2. Not used for acute asthma episodes
  3. Inhibit bronchoconstriction caused by specific antigens
  4. Reduce airway edema and smooth muscle constriction
  5. Contraindicated with hypersensitivity and in breast-feeding mothers
  6. Used with caution in clients with impaired hepatic function
  7. Coadministration of inhaled glucocorticoids increases the risk of upper respiratory infection
B. Side effects
  1. Headache
  2. Nausea and vomiting
  3. Dyspepsia

BOX 56-5

Leukotriene Modifiers

Montelukast (Singulair)
Zafirlukast (Accolate)
Zileuton (Zyflo)

BOX 56-6

Antihistamines

Astemizole (Hismanal)
Azatadine maleate (Optimine)
Azelastine hydrochloride (Astelin)
Brompheniramine maleate (Dimetane)
Cetirizine hydrochloride (Zyrtec)
Chlorpheniramine maleate (Aller-Chlor, Chlor-Trimeton)
Clemastine fumarate (Tavist)
Cyproheptadine hydrochloride (Periactin)
Dexchlorpheniramine maleate (Polaramine)
Diphenhydramine (Benadryl)
Doxylamine succinate (Unisom)
Fexofenadine (Allegra)
Loratadine (Claritin)
Methdilazine hydrochloride (Tacaryl)
Phenindamine tartrate (Nolahist)
Pyrilamine maleate (Nisaval)
Trimeprazine tartrate (Temaril)
Tripelennamine citrate or hydrochloride (PBZ-SR)
Triprolidine hydrochloride (Myidil)

4. Diarrhea
5. Generalized pain, myalgia
6. Fever
7. Dizziness
C. Implementation
1. Monitor vital signs
2. Assess lung sounds for rhonchi, wheezing, and rales
3. Assess liver function laboratory values
4. Monitor for cyanosis
5. Instruct the client to take medication 1 hour before or 2 hours after meals
6. Instruct the client to increase fluid intake
7. Instruct the client not to discontinue medication and to take as prescribed even during symptom-free periods

V. ANTIHISTAMINES (Box 56-6)
A. Description
1. Called histamine antagonists or H_1 blockers; these medications compete with histamine for receptor sites, thus preventing a histamine response
2. When the H_1 receptor is stimulated, the extravascular smooth muscles, including those lining the nasal cavity, are constricted
3. Decrease nasopharyngeal secretions by blocking the H_1 receptor and decrease nasal itching that causes sneezing
4. Used for the common cold, rhinitis, nausea and vomiting, motion sickness, urticaria, and as a sleep aid
5. Can cause central nervous system (CNS) depression if taken with alcohol, narcotics, hypnotics, or barbiturates
6. Used with caution in clients with **chronic obstructive pulmonary disease (COPD)** because of their drying effect
 7. Diphenhydramine (Benadryl) has an anticholinergic effect and should be avoided in clients with narrow-angle glaucoma
B. Side effects
1. Drowsiness and fatigue
2. Dizziness
3. Urinary retention
4. Blurred vision
5. Wheezing
6. Constipation
7. Dry mouth

8. GI Irritation
9. Hypotension
10. Hearing disturbances
11. Photosensitivity
12. Nervousness and irritability
13. Confusion
14. Nightmares
C. Implementation
1. Monitor vital signs
2. Monitor for signs of urinary dysfunction
3. Administer with food or milk
4. Avoid subcutaneous (SC) injection and administer intramuscular (IM) injection in a large muscle if the IM route is prescribed
5. Instruct the client to avoid hazardous activities, ▲ alcohol, and other CNS depressants
6. Instruct the client taking medication for motion ▲ sickness to take the medication 30 minutes before the event, and then before meals and at bedtime during the event
7. Instruct the client to suck on hard candy or ice chips for dry mouth

VI. NASAL DECONGESTANTS (Box 56-7)
A. Description
1. Stimulate the alpha-adrenergic receptors, thus producing vasoconstriction of the capillaries within the nasal mucosa
2. Shrink nasal mucosal membranes and reduce fluid secretion
3. Used for allergic rhinitis, hay fever, and acute coryza (profuse nasal discharge)
4. Contraindicated or used with extreme caution in ▲

BOX 56-7

Nasal Decongestants

Oxymetazoline hydrochloride (Afrin)
Phenylephrine hydrochloride (Neo-Synephrine)
Phenylpropanolamine hydrochloride (Dimetapp)
Pseudoephedrine hydrochloride (Sudafed)
Xylometazoline hydrochloride (Otrivin)

BOX 56-8

Expectorants and Mucolytic Agents

EXPECTORANTS
Guaifenesin (glycerylguaiacolate) (Anti-Tuss, Glycotuss,
   Humibid, Robitussin)

MUCOLYTIC
Acetylcysteine (Mucomyst)

BOX 56-9

Antitussives

NARCOTICS
Codeine, codeine phosphate, codeine sulfate
Hydrocodone bitartrate (Hycodan)

NONNARCOTICS
Dextromethorphan hydrochloride (Benylin,
   Robitussin DM)
Diphenhydramine hydrochloride (Benylin Cough Syrup,
   Benadryl)

---

clients with hypertension, cardiac disease, hyperthyroidism, or diabetes mellitus

5. Nasal decongestants can cause tolerance and
   rebound nasal congestion (vasodilation), caused
   by irritation of the nasal mucosa, and should not
   be used for more than 48 hours

B. Side effects
   1. Frequent use of decongestants, especially nasal
      sprays or drops, can result in tolerance and
      rebound nasal congestion (vasodilation), caused
      by irritation of the nasal mucosa
   2. Nervousness
   3. Restlessness
   4. Hypertension
   5. Hyperglycemia

C. Implementation
   1. Assess the client for existing medical disorders
   2. Monitor for cardiac dysrhythmias
   3. Monitor blood glucose levels
   4. Instruct the client to avoid caffeine in large
      amounts because it can increase restlessness and
      palpitations
   5. Instruct the client in the importance of limiting
      the use of nasal sprays and drops

VII. EXPECTORANTS AND MUCOLYTIC AGENTS
   (Box 56-8)
A. Description
   1. Loosen bronchial secretions so that they can be
      eliminated with coughing
   2. Used for dry, unproductive cough and to stimu-
      late bronchial secretions
   3. Mucolytic agents with dextromethorphan should
      not be used by clients with **COPD** because they
      suppress the cough
   4. Acetylcysteine (Mucomyst) can increase airway
      resistance and should not be used in clients with
      asthma

B. Side effects
   1. GI irritation
   2. Skin rash
   3. Oropharyngeal irritation

C. Implementation
   1. Instruct the client to take medication with a full
      glass of water to loosen mucus
   2. Instruct the client to maintain an adequate fluid
      intake

3. Encourage the client to cough and deep breathe
4. Acetylcysteine (Mucomyst), administered by nebulization, should not be mixed with another
   medication
5. If acetylcysteine (Mucomyst), is administered
   with a bronchodilator, the bronchodilator
   should be administered 5 minutes before the
   acetylcysteine
6. Monitor for side effects of acetylcysteine (Mucomyst), such as nausea and vomiting, stomatitis,
   and runny nose

VIII. ANTITUSSIVES (Box 56-9)
A. Description
   1. Act on the cough control center in the medulla to
      suppress the cough reflex
   2. Used for a cough that is nonproductive and
      irritating
B. Side effects
   1. Dizziness, drowsiness, sedation
   2. GI irritation, nausea
   3. Dry mouth
   4. Constipation
   5. Respiratory depression
C. Implementation
   1. Instruct the client that if the cough lasts longer
      than 1 week and a fever or rash occurs, the
      physician should be notified
   2. Encourage the client to take adequate fluids with
      the medication
   3. Encourage the client to sleep with the head of the
      bed elevated
   4. Instruct the client to avoid hazardous activities

5. Note that drug dependency can occur
6. Avoid administration to the client with a head injury or postoperative cranial surgery
7. Avoid administration to the client using narcotics, sedative hypnotics, barbiturates, or antidepressants, because CNS depression can occur
8. Instruct the client to avoid the use of alcohol

▲ **IX. NARCOTIC ANTAGONIST** (Box 56-10)
   A. Description
      1. Reverses respiratory depression in narcotic overdose
      2. Avoid use in nonnarcotic respiratory depression
   B. Side effects
      1. CNS depression
      2. Nausea, vomiting
      3. Tremors
      4. Sweating
      5. Increased blood pressure
      6. Tachycardia
   C. Implementation
      1. Assess vital signs, especially respirations

BOX 56-10

Narcotic Antagonist

Naloxone hydrochloride (Narcan)

---

2. Have oxygen and resuscitative equipment available during administration

X. USE OF AN INHALER   ▲
   A. Client instructions (Fig. 56-1)
   B. If two different inhaled medications are prescribed, and one of the medications contains a glucocorticoid (corticosteroid), administer the bronchodilator first and the corticosteroid second
   C. Wait 5 minutes following the bronchodilator before inhaling the corticosteroid

XI. TUBERCULOSIS (TB) MEDICATIONS
   A. Description
      1. The most effective method for treating the disease and preventing transmission
      2. Treatment of identified lesions depends on whether the individual has active disease or has been exposed to the disease
      3. Treatment is difficult because the bacterium has a waxy substance on the capsule, which makes penetration and destruction difficult
      4. The use of a multiple-medication regimen destroys organisms as quickly as possible and minimizes the emergence of medication-resistant organisms   ▲
      5. Active **TB** is treated with a combination of medications to which the organism is susceptible

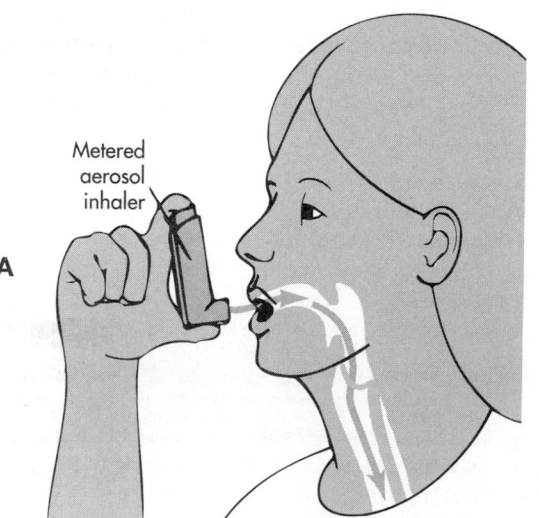
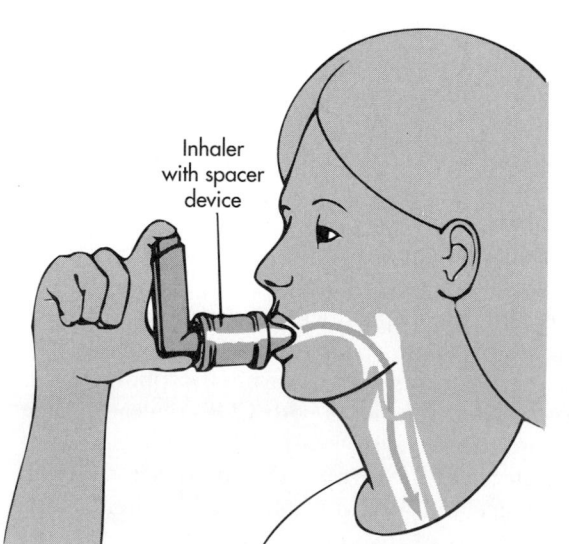

FIG. 56-1 Inhaled drugs commonly used in asthma treatment include beta-adrenergic bronchodilators, cromolyn sodium, and aerosol glucocorticoids. Metered-dose inhaler **(A)** should not be put in mouth but held about two fingerwidths (1½ inch) in front of mouth. Alternatively, inhaler with spacer device **(B)** can be used. Patients should breathe deeply once before activating the inhaler and then continue breathing in for about 5 seconds. Patients should then hold the breath for 10 to 15 seconds before breathing out slowly. If second dose is needed, patients should wait 1 to 2 minutes before taking another dose. (From Clark JF, Queener S, Karb VB: *Pharmacologic basis of nursing practice*, ed 6, St Louis, 2000, Mosby.)

6. Individuals with active **TB** are treated for 6 to 9 months; however, clients with human immunodeficiency virus (HIV) infection will be treated for a longer period of time

7. After the infected individual has received medication for 2 to 3 weeks, the risk of transmission is greatly reduced

8. Most clients have negative sputum cultures after 3 months of compliance with medication therapy

9. Individuals who have been exposed to active **TB** are treated with preventive isoniazid (INH) for 9 to 12 months

B. First-line or second-line medications
1. First-line medications provide the most effective antituberculosis activity
2. Second-line medications are used in combination with first-line medications, but are more toxic
3. Current infecting organisms are proving resistant to standard first-line medications, and the resistant organisms develop because individuals with the disease fail to complete the course of treatment; surviving bacteria adapt to the medication and become resistant
4. Multidrug therapies are instituted because of the resistant organisms

C. **Multidrug-resistant tuberculosis (MDR-TB)**
1. Occurs when a client receiving two medications (first-line and second-line medications) discontinues one of the medications without the physician's knowledge
2. The client briefly experiences some response from the single medication, but then large numbers of resistant organisms begin to grow
3. The client, infectious again, transmits the drug-resistant organism to other individuals
4. As this event is repeated, an organism develops that is resistant to many of the first-line **tuberculosis** medications

XII. FIRST-LINE MEDICATIONS FOR TB (Table 56-1)

A. Isoniazid (INH) (Laniazid, Nydrazid)
1. Description
   a. Bactericidal
   b. Inhibits synthesis of mycolic acids and acts to kill actively growing organisms in the extracellular environment
   c. Inhibits growth of dormant organisms in the macrophages and caseating granulomas
   d. Active only during cell division
   e. Used in combination with other antitubercular medications
2. Contraindications and cautions
   a. Contraindicated in clients with hypersensitivity or with acute liver disease
   b. Use with caution in clients with chronic liver disease, alcoholism, or renal impairment

c. Use with caution in clients taking niacin, nicotinic acid (Nicobid)
d. Use with caution in clients taking hepatotoxic medications because the risk for hepatotoxicity increases
e. Alcohol increases the risk of hepatotoxicity
f. Isoniazid (INH) may increase the risk of toxicity of carbamazepine (Tegretol) and phenytoin (Dilantin)
g. Isoniazid (INH) may decrease ketoconazole (Nizoral) concentrations

3. Side effects
   a. Hypersensitivity reactions
   b. Peripheral neuritis
   c. Neurotoxicity
   d. Hepatotoxicity
   e. Pyridoxine (vitamin B_6) deficiency
   f. Irritation at injection site with IM administration
   g. Nausea and vomiting
   h. Dry mouth
   i. Dizziness
   j. Hyperglycemia
   k. Increased liver function tests
   l. Hepatitis

4. Implementation
   a. Assess for hypersensitivity
   b. Assess for hepatic dysfunction
   c. Assess for sensitivity to niacin, nicotinic acid (Nicobid)
   d. Monitor liver function tests
   e. Monitor for signs of hepatitis, such as anorexia, nausea, vomiting, weakness, fatigue, dark urine, or jaundice, and if these symptoms occur, withhold the medication and notify the physician
   f. Monitor for tingling, numbness or burning of the extremities
   g. Assess mental status

TABLE 56-1

First-Line and Second-Line Medications for Tuberculosis

First Line	Second Line
Isoniazid (INH) (Laniazid, Nydrazid)	Capreomycin (Capastat)
Rifampin (Rifadin)	Ethionamide (Trecator-SC)
Ethambutol (Myambutol)	Aminosalicylate sodium (Tubasal)
Streptomycin	Cycloserine (Seromycin)
Pyrazinamide (Pyrazinamide)	Kanamycin (Kantrex)

OTHER MEDICATIONS

Rifampin and isoniazid (Rifamate): Treatment of tuberculosis after dosage of separate medications has been established

Rifampin, isoniazid, and pyrazinamide: Short-course treatment of tuberculosis

h. Monitor for visual changes, and notify the physician if they occur

i. Assess for dizziness and initiate safety precautions

j. Monitor complete blood cell (CBC) count and blood glucose levels

k. Administer 1 hour before or 2 hours after a meal because food may delay absorption

l. Administer at least 1 hour before antacids, especially those antacids that contain aluminum

5. Client education

a. Instruct the client not to skip doses and to take medication for the full length of the prescribed therapy

b. Instruct the client not to take any other medication without consulting the physician

c. Advise the client of the importance of follow-up physician visits, vision testing, and laboratory tests

d. Instruct the client to avoid alcohol

e. Advise the client to take medication on an empty stomach with 8 ounces of water 1 hour before or 2 hours after meals and to avoid taking antacids with the medication

f. Instruct the client to avoid tyramine-containing foods because they may cause a reaction such as red and itching skin, a pounding heartbeat, lightheadedness, a hot or clammy feeling, or a headache, and if this does occur, to notify the physician

g. Instruct the client in the signs of neurotoxicity, hepatitis, and hepatotoxicity

h. Instruct the client to notify the physician if signs of neurotoxicity, hepatitis and hepatotoxicity, or visual changes occur

B. Rifampin (Rifadin)

1. Description

a. Inhibits bacterial RNA synthesis

b. Binds to DNA-dependent RNA polymerase and blocks RNA transcription

c. Used in conjunction with at least one other antitubercular medication

2. Contraindications and cautions

a. Contraindicated in clients with hypersensitivity

b. Use with caution in clients with hepatic dysfunction or alcoholism

c. Use of alcohol or hepatotoxic medications may increase the risk of hepatotoxicity

d. Decreases the effects of several medications, including oral anticoagulants, oral hypoglycemics, chloramphenicol (Chloromycetin), digoxin (Lanoxin), disopyramide phosphate (Norpace), mexiletine (Mexitil), quinidine polygalacturonate (Cardioquin), tocainide hydrochloride (Tonocard), fluconazole (Diflu-

can), methadone hydrochloride (Dolophine), phenytoin (Dilantin), and verapamil hydrochloride (Calan)

3. Side effects

a. Hypersensitivity reaction including fever, chills, shivering, headache, muscle and bone pain, and dyspnea

b. Heartburn

c. Nausea, vomiting, diarrhea

d. Increased liver function tests

e. Hepatotoxicity and hepatitis

f. Increased uric acid levels

g. Blood dyscrasias

h. Colitis

4. Implementation

a. Assess for hypersensitivity

b. Evaluate CBC, uric acid, and liver function tests

c. Assess for signs of hepatitis, and if they occur, withhold the medication and notify the physician

d. Monitor stools for signs of colitis

e. Monitor mental status

f. Assess for visual changes

5. Client education

a. Instruct the client not to skip doses and to take medication for the full length of the prescribed therapy

b. Instruct the client not to take any other medication without consulting the physician

c. Advise the client of the importance of follow-up physician visits and laboratory tests

d. Instruct the client to avoid alcohol

e. Advise the client to take medication on an empty stomach with 8 ounces of water 1 hour before or 2 hours after meals and to avoid taking antacids with the medication

f. Instruct the client that urine, feces, sweat, and tears will be red-orange in color and that soft contact lens can become permanently discolored

g. Instruct the client to notify the physician if jaundice (yellow eyes or skin) develops or if weakness, fatigue, nausea, vomiting, sore throat, fever, or unusual bleeding occurs

C. Ethambutol (Myambutol)

1. Description

a. Bacteriostatic

b. Interferes with cell metabolism and multiplication by inhibiting one or more metabolites in susceptible organism

c. Inhibits bacterial RNA synthesis

d. Active only during cell division

e. Is slow acting and must be used in combination with other bactericidal agents

2. Contraindications and cautions

a. Contraindicated in clients with hypersensitivity or optic neuritis and in children under 13 years of age

b. Use with caution in clients with renal dysfunction, gout, ocular defects, diabetic retinopathy, cataracts, or ocular inflammatory conditions

c. Use with caution in clients taking neurotoxic medications, as the risk for neurotoxicity increases

3. Side effects
   a. Hypersensitivity reactions
   b. Anorexia, nausea, vomiting
   c. Dizziness
   d. Malaise
   e. Mental confusion
   f. Joint pain
   g. Dermatitis
   h. Optic neuritis
   i. Peripheral neuritis
   j. Thrombocytopenia
   k. Increased uric acid levels
   l. Anaphylactoid reaction

4. Implementation
   a. Assess for hypersensitivity
   b. Evaluate results of CBC, uric acid, and renal and liver function tests
   c. Obtain baseline visual acuity and color discrimination, especially to the color green
   d. Monitor for visual changes such as altered color perception and decreased visual acuity, and if changes occur, withhold the medication and notify the physician
   e. Administer once every 24 hours and administer with food to decrease gastrointestinal (GI) upset
   f. Monitor uric acid concentrations and assess for painful or swollen joints or signs of gout
   g. Monitor I & O and for adequate renal function
   h. Assess mental status
   i. Monitor for dizziness and initiate safety precautions
   j. Assess for peripheral neuritis (numbness, tingling or burning of the extremities), and if it occurs, notify the physician

5. Client education
   a. Inform the client that he or she can prevent nausea related to the medication by taking the daily dose at bedtime, or to take prescribed antinausea medications
   b. Instruct the client not to skip doses and to take the medication for the full length of the prescribed therapy
   c. Instruct the client not to take any other medication without consulting the physician
   d. Advise the client of the importance of follow-up physician visits, vision testing, and laboratory tests

e. Instruct the client to notify the physician immediately if any visual problems occur, or a rash, swelling and pain in the joints, or numbness, tingling, or burning in the hands or feet

D. Streptomycin
1. Description
   a. An aminoglycoside antibiotic that is used in conjunction with at least one other antitubercular medication
   b. Bactericidal, because of receptor-binding action, interfering with protein synthesis in susceptible organisms

2. Contraindications and cautions
   a. Contraindicated in clients with hypersensitivity, myasthenia gravis, parkinsonism, or eighth cranial nerve damage
   b. Use with caution in the elderly, in neonates because of renal insufficiency and immaturity, and in young infants because the medication may cause CNS depression
   c. The risk of toxicity increases when taken with other aminoglycosides, or nephrotoxicity- or ototoxicity-producing medications

3. Side effects (Box 56-11)
   a. Hypersensitivity
   b. Visual changes
   c. Increased liver and renal function tests
   d. Peripheral neuritis such as burning of the face or mouth

4. Implementation
   a. Assess for hypersensitivity
   b. Monitor liver and renal function tests
   c. Monitor for ototoxic, neurotoxic, and nephrotoxic reactions
   d. Obtain baseline audiometric test and repeat every 1 to 2 months because the medication impairs the eighth cranial nerve
   e. Assess hearing acuity
   f. Monitor for visual changes
   g. Assess hydration status and maintain adequate hydration during therapy

BOX 56-11

Side Effects of Streptomycin

NEPHROTOXICITY	NEUROTOXICITY
Changes in urine output	Muscle numbness
Increased thirst	Tingling
Decreased appetite	Twitching
Nausea, vomiting	Seizures

VESTIBULAR OTOTOXICITY	AUDITORY OTOTOXICITY
Dizziness	Ringing in the ears
Clumsiness	Loss of hearing
Unsteadiness	A full feeling in the ears

h. Monitor I & O

i. Assess urinalysis

j. Monitor for signs of peripheral neuritis

5. Client education

a. Instruct the client not to skip doses and to take medication for the full length of the prescribed therapy

b. Instruct the client not to take any other medication without consulting the physician

c. Advise the client of the importance of follow-up physician visits and laboratory tests

d. Instruct the client to notify the physician if hearing loss, changes in vision, or urinary problems occur

E. Pyrazinamide

1. Description

a. Exact mechanism of action is unknown

b. May be bacteriostatic or bactericidal, depending on its concentration at the infection site and susceptibility of infecting organism

c. Used in conjunction with at least one other antitubercular medication after failure or ineffectiveness of the primary medications occurs

2. Contraindications and cautions

a. Contraindicated in clients with hypersensitivity

b. Use with caution in clients with diabetes mellitus, renal impairment, or gout, and in children

c. May decrease the effects of allopurinol (Zyloprim), colchicine, probenecid (Benemid), sulfinpyrazone (Anturane)

d. Cross-sensitivity is possible with isoniazid (INH), ethionamide (Trecator-SC) or niacin, nicotinic acid (Nicobid)

3. Side effects

a. Increases liver function and uric acid levels

b. Arthralgia, myalgia

c. Photosensitivity

d. Hepatotoxicity

e. Thrombocytopenia

4. Implementation

a. Assess for hypersensitivity

b. Evaluate CBC, liver function tests, and uric acid levels

c. Observe for hepatotoxic effects, and if they occur, withhold the medication and notify the physician

d. Assess for painful or swollen joints

e. Evaluate blood glucose levels because diabetes mellitus may be difficult to control while on medication

5. Client education

a. Instruct the client to take the medication with food to reduce GI distress

b. Instruct the client to avoid sunlight or ultraviolet light until photosensitivity is determined

c. Instruct the client to notify the physician if any side effects occur

d. Instruct the client not to skip doses and to take the medication for the full length of the prescribed therapy

e. Instruct the client not to take any other medication without consulting the physician

f. Advise the client of the importance of follow-up physician visits and laboratory tests

XIII. SECOND-LINE MEDICATIONS FOR TB

A. Capreomycin sulfate (Capastat Sulfate)

1. Description

a. Mechanism of action is unknown

b. Used to treat **MDR-TB** when significant resistance to other medications is expected

c. Must be given by the IM route

2. Contraindications and cautions

a. The risk of nephrotoxicity, ototoxicity, and neuromuscular blockade is increased with the use of aminoglycosides or loop diuretics

b. Use with caution in clients with renal insufficiency, acoustic nerve impairment, hepatic disorder, myasthenia gravis, or parkinsonism

c. Do not administer to clients receiving streptomycin

3. Side effects

a. Nephrotoxicity

b. Ototoxicity

c. Neuromuscular blockade

4. Implementation

a. Perform baseline audiometric testing

b. Assess renal, hepatic, and electrolyte levels before administration

c. Monitor I & O

d. Reconstituted medication may be stored for 48 hours at room temperature

e. Administer deep IM in a large muscle mass

f. Rotate injection sites

g. Observe injection site for redness, excessive bleeding, and inflammation

5. Client education

a. Instruct the client not to perform tasks that require mental alertness

b. Instruct the client to report any hearing loss, balance disturbances, respiratory difficulty, weakness, or signs of hypersensitivity reactions

B. Kanamycin (Kantrex)

1. Description

a. An aminoglycoside antibiotic that is used in conjunction with at least one other antitubercular medication

b. Bactericidal, because of receptor-binding action, interfering with protein synthesis in susceptible microorganisms

2. Contraindications and cautions
   a. Contraindicated in clients with hypersensitivity, neuromuscular disorders, or eighth cranial nerve damage
   b. Use with caution in the elderly, in neonates because of renal insufficiency and immaturity, and in young infants because it may cause CNS depression
   c. The risk of toxicity increases when taken with other aminoglycosides, or nephrotoxicity- or ototoxicity-producing medications
3. Side effects
   a. Hypersensitivity
   b. Pain and irritation at the injection site
   c. Nephrotoxicity as evidenced by increased blood urea nitrogen (BUN) and serum creatinine
   d. Ototoxicity as evidenced by tinnitus, dizziness, ringing/roaring in the ears, and reduced hearing
   e. Neurotoxicity as evidenced by headache, dizziness, lethargy, tremors, and visual disturbances
   f. Superinfections
4. Implementation
   a. Assess for hypersensitivity
   b. Monitor for ototoxic, neurotoxic, and nephrotoxic reactions
   c. Monitor liver and renal function tests
   d. Obtain baseline audiometric test and repeat every 1 to 2 months because the medication impairs the eighth cranial nerve
   e. Assess hearing acuity
   f. Monitor for visual changes
   g. Assess hydration status and maintain adequate hydration during therapy
   h. Monitor I & O
   i. Assess urinalysis
   j. Monitor for superinfection
5. Client education
   a. Instruct the client not to skip doses and to take medication for the full length of the prescribed therapy
   b. Instruct the client not to take any other medication without consulting the physician
   c. Advise the client of the importance of follow-up physician visits and laboratory tests
   d. Instruct the client to notify the physician if hearing loss, changes in vision, or urinary problems occur

C. Ethionamide (Trecator-SC)
   1. Description
      a. Mechanism of action is unknown
      b. Used to treat **MDR-TB** when significant resistance to other medications is expected
   2. Contraindications and cautions
      a. Contraindicated in clients with hypersensitivity
      b. Use with caution in clients with diabetes mellitus or renal dysfunction
   3. Side effects
      a. Anorexia, nausea, vomiting
      b. Metallic taste in the mouth
      c. Orthostatic hypotension
      d. Jaundice
      e. Mental changes
      f. Peripheral neuritis
      g. Rash
   4. Implementation
      a. Assess liver and renal function tests
      b. Monitor glucose levels in the client with diabetes mellitus
      c. Administer pyridoxine as prescribed to reduce the risk of neurotoxicity
   5. Client education
      a. Instruct the client to take medication with food or meals to minimize GI irritation
      b. Instruct the client to change positions slowly
      c. Instruct the client to report signs of a rash, which can progress to exfoliative dermatitis if the medication is not discontinued
      d. Instruct the client to avoid alcohol
      e. Instruct the client to report signs of jaundice and other side effects of the medication if they occur

D. Aminosalicylate sodium (Tubasal)
   1. Description
      a. Inhibits folic acid metabolism in mycobacteria
      b. Used to treat **MDR-TB** when significant resistance to other medications is expected
   2. Contraindications and cautions
      a. Contraindicated with hypersensitivity to aminosalicylates, salicylates, or compounds containing para-aminophenyl group
      b. Aminobenzoates block the absorption of aminosalicylate sodium
   3. Side effects
      a. Hypersensitivity
      b. Bitter taste in the mouth
      c. GI tract irritation
      d. Exfoliative dermatitis
      e. Blood dyscrasias
      f. Crystalluria
      g. Changes in thyroid function
   4. Implementation
      a. Assess for hypersensitivity
      b. Offer clear water to rinse the mouth and chewing gum or hard candy to alleviate the bitter taste
      c. Encourage fluid intake to prevent crystalluria
      d. Monitor I & O
   5. Client education
      a. Instruct the client to discard the medication if a purplish brown discoloration occurs

    b. Instruct the client to take the medication with food or antacid

    c. Inform the client that urine may turn red on contact with hypochlorite bleach if bleach was used to clean a toilet

    d. Instruct the client not to take aspirin or over-the-counter medications without the physician's approval

    e. Inform the client with diabetes mellitus that a false-positive result can occur in glucose monitoring

    f. Instruct the client to report signs of a blood dyscrasia, such as sore throat or mouth, malaise, fatigue, bruising, or bleeding

  E. Cycloserine (Seromycin)

    1. Description

      a. Interferes with cell wall biosynthesis

      b. Used to treat **MDR-TB** when significant resistance to other medications is expected

    2. Contraindications and cautions

      a. Use of alcohol or ethionamide (Trecator-SC) increases the risk of seizures

      b. Use with caution in clients with epilepsy, depression, severe anxiety, psychosis, or renal insufficiency, or the client who uses alcohol

    3. Side effects

      a. Hypersensitivity

      b. CNS reactions

      c. Neurotoxicity

      d. Seizures

      e. Congestive heart failure (CHF)

      f. Headache

      g. Vertigo

      h. Altered level of consciousness (LOC)

      i. Irritability, nervousness, anxiety

      j. Confusion

      k. Mood changes, depression, thoughts of suicide

    4. Implementation

      a. Monitor LOC

      b. Monitor for changes in mental status and thought processes

      c. Monitor renal and hepatic function tests

      d. Monitor serum drug level to avoid the risk of neurotoxicity; peak concentrations, measured 2 hours after dosing, should be 25 to 35 μg/mL

    5. Client education

      a. Instruct the client to take the medication after meals to prevent GI upset

      b. Instruct the client to avoid alcohol

      c. Instruct the client to report signs of a rash or signs of CNS toxicity

      d. Instruct the client to avoid driving or performing tasks that require alertness until the reaction to the medication has been determined

    e. Advise the client of the need for serum drug levels weekly, as prescribed

PRACTICE QUESTIONS

1. A nurse is preparing to administer albuterol (Proventil) to a client. The nurse assesses which of the following parameters before and during therapy?
   1. Urine output and blood urea nitrogen (BUN)
   2. Nausea and vomiting
   3. Lung sounds and presence of dyspnea
   4. Headache and level of consciousness

2. A home care nurse has observed a client self-administer a dose of metaproterenol sulfate (Alupent) via metered-dose inhaler. Within a short time, the client begins to wheeze loudly. The nurse interprets that this is due to:
   1. Insufficient dosage of the medication, which needs to be increased
   2. Probable interaction of this medication with an over-the-counter cold remedy
   3. Tolerance to the medication, indicating a need for a stronger type of bronchodilator
   4. Paradoxical bronchospasm, which must be reported to the physician

3. A nurse has an order to give a client metaproterenol sulfate (Alupent), two puffs, and beclamethasone (Vanceril), two puffs, by metered-dose inhaler. The nurse administers the medication by giving the:
   1. Beclomethasone first and then the metaproterenol
   2. Metaproterenol first and then the beclomethasone
   3. Alternating a single puff of each, beginning with the beclomethasone
   4. Alternating a single puff of each, beginning with the metaproterenol

4. A client receiving theophylline is due to have a theophylline level drawn. A nurse questions the client to ensure that the client has not ingested which of the following substances prior to the sample being drawn?
   1. Sedatives
   2. Narcotics
   3. Glucose
   4. Caffeine

5. A client has begun therapy with oxtriphylline (Choledyl). A nurse plans to teach the client to limit the intake of which of the following while taking this medication?
   1. Oysters, lobster, and shrimp
   2. Coffee, cola, and chocolate
   3. Cottage cheese, cream cheese, and dairy creamers
   4. Grapefruit, oranges, and pineapple

6. A nurse has administered a dose of salmeterol (Serevent) to a client. The client develops a generalized rash and urticaria, and the eyelids begin to swell. The nurse should:
   1. Call the physician immediately
   2. Encourage the client to quickly drink oral fluids
   3. Apply a lanolin-based cream to the rash
   4. Assess the client's vision with a Snellen chart

7. A client is receiving acetylcystine (Mucomyst) by nebulizer. A nurse should have which of the following items available for possible use after giving this medication?
   1. Suction equipment
   2. Nasogastric tube
   3. Intubation tray
   4. Ambu bag

8. A client has an order to take guaifenesin (Humibid LA). A nurse concludes that the client understands the most effective use of this medication if the client states to:
   1. Take the tablet with a full glass of water
   2. Take an extra dose if the cough is accompanied by fever
   3. Watch for irritability as a side effect
   4. Crush the sustained-release tablet if immediate relief is needed

9. A nurse is preparing to administer a dose of naloxone HCl (Narcan) intravenously to a client with an intravenous narcotic overdose. The nurse plans to have which of the following available as supportive equipment in case it is needed?
   1. Nasogastric tube
   2. Paracentesis tray
   3. Central line insertion tray
   4. Resuscitation equipment

10. A nurse is teaching a client about the effects of diphenhydramine hydrochloride (Benadryl), which has been ordered as a cough suppressant. The nurse would not include which of the following items in the list of instructions?
    1. Avoid driving or other activities requiring mental alertness while taking this medication
    2. Use sugarless gum, candy, or oral rinses to decrease dry mouth
    3. Avoid using alcohol while taking this medication
    4. Administer on an empty stomach

11. A client has been prescribed a cough formula containing codeine sulfate. A nurse has given the client instructions for its use. The nurse concludes that the client understands the instructions if the client verbalizes to self-assess for:
    1. Excitability
    2. Constipation
    3. Rapid pulse
    4. Excessive urination

12. A cromolyn sodium (Intal) inhaler is prescribed for a client with allergic asthma. A nurse provides instructions regarding the side effects of this medication. Which of the following undesirable side effects is associated with this medication?
    1. Constipation
    2. Hypotension
    3. Insomnia
    4. Bronchospasm

13. Terbutaline sulfate (Brethine) is prescribed for a client with bronchitis. A nurse understands that this medication should be used with caution if which of the following existing medical conditions is present in the client?
    1. Hypothyroidism
    2. Polycystic disease
    3. Osteoarthritis
    4. Diabetes mellitus

14. Zafirlukast (Accolate) is prescribed for a client with bronchial asthma. Which of the following laboratory tests does a nurse expect to be prescribed prior to the administration of this medication?
    1. Platelet count
    2. Complete blood cell count
    3. Liver function tests
    4. Neutrophil count

15. A client has been taking isoniazid (INH) for a month and a half. The client complains to a nurse about numbness, paresthesias, and tingling in the extremities. The nurse interprets that the client is experiencing:
    1. Small blood vessel spasm
    2. Impaired peripheral circulation
    3. Hypercalcemia
    4. Peripheral neuritis

16. A client is to begin a 6-month course of therapy with isoniazid (INH). A nurse plans to teach the client to:
    1. Use alcohol in small amounts only
    2. Report yellow eyes or skin immediately
    3. Increase intake of Swiss or aged cheeses
    4. Avoid vitamin supplements during therapy

17. A client has been started on long-term therapy with rifampin (Rifadin). A nurse teaches the client that the medication:
    1. Should be double dosed if one dose is forgotten
    2. May be discontinued independently if symptoms are gone in 3 months
    3. Causes orange discoloration of sweat, tears, urine, and feces
    4. Should always be taken with food or antacids

18. A nurse has given a client taking ethambutol (Myambutol) information about the medication. The nurse evaluates that the client understands the instructions if the client states to immediately report:
    1. Gastrointestinal (GI) side effects

2. Impaired sense of hearing
3. Orange-red discoloration of body secretions
4. Difficulty in discriminating the color red from green

19. Cycloserine (Seromycin) is added to the medication regimen for a client with tuberculosis. Which of the following would a clinic nurse include in the client teaching plan regarding this medication?
   1. To take the medication prior to meals
   2. To return to the clinic weekly for serum drug levels
   3. It is not necessary to call the physician if a skin rash occurs
   4. It is not necessary to restrict alcohol intake with this medication

20. A client with tuberculosis is being started on antituberculosis therapy with isoniazid (INH).

Before giving the client the first dose, a nurse assesses that which of the following baseline studies has been completed?
   1. Coagulation times
   2. Electrolytes
   3. Serum creatinine
   4. Liver enzymes

CRITICAL THINKING: FREE-TEXT ENTRY

A nurse receives a report of the serum theophylline level of a client receiving theophylline by continuous intravenous infusion. The result is 18 µg/mL. The nurse documents what interpretation regarding this result?

Answer: _____

ANSWERS

1. **3**
Rationale: Albuterol is a bronchodilator of the adrenergic type. The nurse assesses respiratory pattern, lung sounds, pulse, and blood pressure prior to and during therapy. The color, character, and amount of sputum are also noted.
Test-Taking Strategy: Use the process of elimination. Knowing that this medication is a bronchodilator allows you to eliminate each of the incorrect options. Use the ABCs—airway, breathing, and circulation—to answer the question. Option 3 is the only option that addresses airway. Review this medication if you had difficulty with this question.
Level of Cognitive Ability: Application
Client Needs: Physiological Integrity
Integrated Concept/Process: Nursing Process/Assessment
Content Area: Pharmacology
Reference: Hodgson, B., & Kizior, R. (2001). *Saunders nursing drug handbook 2001.* Philadelphia: W.B. Saunders, p. 20.

2. **4**
Rationale: The client taking adrenergic bronchodilators may experience paradoxical bronchospasm, which is evidenced by the client's wheezing. This can occur with excessive use of inhalers. Further medication should be withheld, and the physician should be notified. Options 1, 2, and 3 are incorrect interpretations.
Test-Taking Strategy: Use the process of elimination. Eliminate option 1 first, since the client began wheezing after the medication was administered, and not before. Option 3 may be eliminated next, since tolerance does not generally occur. From the remaining options, knowing that wheezing is associated with broncho-spasm will direct you to option 4. Review the side effects associated with the use of inhaled broncodilators if you had difficulty with this question.
Level of Cognitive Ability: Analysis
Client Needs: Physiological Integrity
Integrated Concept/Process: Nursing Process/Analysis
Content Area: Pharmacology

Reference: Hodgson, B., & Kizior, R. (2001). *Saunders nursing drug handbook 2001.* Philadelphia: W.B. Saunders, pp. 648-650.

3. **2**
Rationale: Metaproterenol sulfate is an adrenergic type of bronchodilator. Beclomethasone is a glucocorticoid. Bronchodilators are always administered before glucocorticoids, when both are to be given on the same time schedule. This allows for widening of the air passages by the bronchodilator, which then makes the glucocorticoid more effective.
Test-Taking Strategy: Use the process of elimination. To answer this question correctly, it is necessary to know two different things. First you must know that a bronchodilator is always given before a glucocorticoid. This would allow you to eliminate options 3 and 4, since you would not alternate the medications. To discriminate between options 1 and 2, it is necessary to know that metaproterenol is a bronchodilator, while beclomethasone is a glucocorticoid. Review these medications if you had difficulty with this question.
Level of Cognitive Ability: Application
Client Needs: Physiological Integrity
Integrated Concept/Process: Nursing Process/Implementation
Content Area: Pharmacology
Reference: Hodgson, B., & Kizior, R. (2001). *Saunders nursing drug handbook 2001.* Philadelphia: W.B. Saunders, p. 99.

4. **4**
Rationale: Theophylline is a xanthine bronchodilator. Prior to the drawing of a serum level of the medication, the client should avoid taking in foods or beverages that contain xanthine, such as colas, coffee, or chocolate. Thus, the client is told to avoid caffeine intake before the test.
Test-Taking Strategy: Use the process of elimination. Recalling that this medication is a xanthine bronchodilator will direct you to option 4. Review client teaching points related to this medication if you had difficulty with this question.
Level of Cognitive Ability: Application
Client Needs: Physiological Integrity

Integrated Concept/Process: Nursing Process/Assessment
Content Area: Pharmacology
Reference: Wilson, B., Shannon, M., & Stang, C. (2000). *Nurses drug guide 2000.* Stamford, Conn.: Appleton & Lange, p. 52.

5. 2
Rationale: Oxtriphylline (Choledyl) is a xanthine bronchodilator. The nurse teaches the client to limit the intake of xanthine-containing foods while taking this medication. These include coffee, cola, and chocolate.
Test-Taking Strategy: Use the process of elimination. It is necessary to understand that oxtriphylline is a xanthine bronchodilator and to know that intake of excessive amounts of foods naturally high in xanthines should be curtailed. Review the foods naturally high in xanthines, if you had difficulty with this question.
Level of Cognitive Ability: Application
Client Needs: Health Promotion and Maintenance
Integrated Concept/Process: Teaching/Learning
Content Area: Pharmacology
Reference: Salerno, E. (1999). *Pharmacology for health professionals.* St. Louis: Mosby, p. 462.

6. 1
Rationale: Hypersensitivity reaction can occur in clients taking ephedrine, epinephrine, isoproterenol, or salmeterol. Signs and symptoms include rash, urticaria, and swelling of the face, lips, or eyelids. The nurse should call the physician immediately if any of these occur. The other options are incorrect.
Test-Taking Strategy: Use the process of elimination. Recognizing that the signs and symptoms listed in the question are typical of a hypersensitivity reaction allows you to eliminate options 3 and 4 first. From the remaining options, recall that the client needs treatment with an antihistamine or epinephrine, not oral fluids.
Level of Cognitive Ability: Application
Client Needs: Physiological Integrity
Integrated Concept/Process: Nursing Process/Implementation
Content Area: Pharmacology
Reference: Hodgson, B., & Kizior, R. (2001). *Saunders nursing drug handbook 2001.* Philadelphia: W.B. Saunders, p. 917.

7. 1
Rationale: Acetylcystine can be given orally or by a nasogastric tube to treat acetaminophen overdose, or it may be given by inhalation for use as a mucolytic. The nurse administering this medication as a mucolytic should have suction equipment available, in case the client cannot manage to clear the increased volume of liquefied secretions.
Test-Taking Strategy: Use the process of elimination. Note the key word "nebulizer." This will assist in directing you to option 1. If you had difficulty with this question, review the purpose of this medication and the related nursing interventions.
Level of Cognitive Ability: Application
Client Needs: Physiological Integrity
Integrated Concept/Process: Nursing Process/Planning
Content Area: Pharmacology
Reference: Deglin, J., & Vallerand, A. (2001). *Davis's drug guide for nurses* (7th ed.). Philadelphia: F.A. Davis, pp. 7-9.

8. 1
Rationale: Guaifenesin (Humibid LA) is an expectorant. It should be taken with a full glass of water to decrease viscosity of secretions. Sustained-release preparations should not be broken open, crushed, or chewed. The medication may occasionally cause dizziness, headache, or drowsiness as side effects. The client should contact the physician if the cough lasts longer than 1 week, or is accompanied by fever, rash, sore throat, or persistent headache.
Test-Taking Strategy: Use the process of elimination. Begin to answer this question by eliminating option 4 first. Sustained-relief preparations are not crushed or broken. Option 2 is eliminated next because fever indicates infection, and an "extra dose" of an expectorant is not helpful in treating infection. From the remaining options, knowing that increased fluids helps to liquefy secretions for more effective coughing directs you to option 1 as correct. If you had difficulty with this question, review this medication.
Level of Cognitive Ability: Analysis
Client Needs: Health Promotion and Maintenance
Integrated Concept/Process: Nursing Process/Evaluation
Content Area: Pharmacology
Reference: Hodgson, B., & Kizior, R. (2001). *Saunders nursing drug handbook 2001.* Philadelphia: W.B. Saunders, p. 482.

9. 4
Rationale: The nurse administering naloxone for suspected narcotic overdose should have resuscitation equipment readily available to support naloxone therapy if it is needed. Other adjuncts that may be needed include oxygen, mechanical ventilator, and vasopressors.
Test-Taking Strategy: Use the process of elimination. Note the key words "intravenous narcotic overdose." Recalling the effects of these medications will direct you to option 4. Option 4 is also the most global response. Review this medication if you had difficulty with this question.
Level of Cognitive Ability: Application
Client Needs: Physiological Integrity
Integrated Concept/Process: Nursing Process/Planning
Content Area: Pharmacology
Reference: Deglin, J., & Vallerand, A. (2001). *Davis's drug guide for nurses* (7th ed.). Philadelphia: F.A. Davis, p. 841.

10. 4
Rationale: Diphenhydramine (Benadryl) has several uses, including antihistamine, antitussive, antidyskinetic, and sedative/hypnotic. Instructions for use include to take with food or milk to decrease gastrointestinal upset and to use oral rinses or sugarless gum or hard candy to minimize dry mouth. Since the medication causes drowsiness, the client should avoid use of alcohol or central nervous system depressants, operating a car, or engaging in other activities requiring mental acuity during use.
Test-Taking Strategy: Use the process of elimination, noting the key word "not." Knowing that the medication has a sedative effect helps you to eliminate options 1 and 3 first. Recalling that the medication causes a dry mouth helps you choose option 4 as the answer to the question, according to the way the question is stated. If you had difficulty with this question, review client education related to this medication.
Level of Cognitive Ability: Application
Client Needs: Health Promotion and Maintenance
Integrated Concept/Process: Teaching/Learning
Content Area: Pharmacology

Reference: Deglin, J., & Vallerand, A. (2001). *Davis's drug guide for nurses* (7th ed.). Philadelphia: F.A. Davis, p. 383.

11. 2

Rationale: The client is taught about side effects that could occur with the use of codeine sulfate. The most common side effects include drowsiness, confusion, hypotension, nausea and vomiting, and constipation. Others include bradycardia, respiratory depression, and urinary retention.

Test-Taking Strategy: Use the process of elimination. Remember that codeine sulfate causes constipation. Review the side effects of this medication if you had difficulty with this question.

Level of Cognitive Ability: Analysis
Client Needs: Health Promotion and Maintenance
Integrated Concept/Process: Nursing Process/Evaluation
Content Area: Pharmacology
Reference: Hodgson, B., & Kizior, R. (2001). *Saunders nursing drug handbook 2001*. Philadelphia: W.B. Saunders, pp. 1179-1180.

12. 4

Rationale: The most common undesired side effects associated with inhalation therapy of cromolyn sodium (Intal) are bronchospasm, cough, nasal congestion, throat irritation, and wheezing. Clients receiving this medication orally may experience pruritis, nausea, diarrhea, and myalgia.

Test-Taking Strategy: Use the process of elimination. Note the key words "undesirable side effects." This should assist in directing you to option 4. In addition, use the ABCs—airway, breathing, and circulation—to select the correct option. Option 4 addresses airway. Review the undesirable side effects of this medication if you had difficulty with this question.

Level of Cognitive Ability: Analysis
Client Needs: Physiological Integrity
Integrated Concept/Process: Teaching/Learning
Content Area: Pharmacology
Reference: Salerno, E. (1999). *Pharmacology for health professionals.* St. Louis: Mosby, p. 464.

13. 4

Rationale: Terbutaline sulfate (Brethine) is contraindicated in clients with hypersensitivity to sympathomimetics. It should be used with caution in clients with impaired cardiac function, diabetes mellitus, hypertension, or hyperthyroidism, and clients with a history of seizures. The medication may increase blood glucose levels.

Test-Taking Strategy: This is a difficult question, and knowledge regarding this medication is required to answer correctly. Review the contraindications associated with this medication, if you are unfamiliar with them.

Level of Cognitive Ability: Analysis
Client Needs: Physiological Integrity
Integrated Concept/Process: Nursing Process/Analysis
Content Area: Pharmacology
Reference: Hodgson, B., & Kizior, R. (2001). *Saunders nursing drug handbook 2001*. Philadelphia: W.B. Saunders, pp. 969-970.

14. 3

Rationale: Zafirlukast (Accolate) is a leukotriene receptor antagonist that is used in the prophylaxis and long-term treatment of bronchial asthma. It is used with caution in clients with impaired hepatic function. Liver function labora-tory tests should be performed to obtain a baseline, and the levels should be monitored during administration of the medication.

Test-Taking Strategy: Use the process of elimination, eliminating options 2 and 4 first because a complete blood count would include a neutrophil count. From the remaining options, you would need to know that this medication would affect hepatic function. If you had difficulty with this question, review this medication.

Level of Cognitive Ability: Analysis
Client Needs: Physiological Integrity
Integrated Concept/Process: Nursing Process/Analysis
Content Area: Pharmacology
Reference: Hodgson, B., & Kizior, R. (2001). *Saunders nursing drug handbook 2001*. Philadelphia: W.B. Saunders, pp. 1064-1065.

15. 4

Rationale: A common side effect of INH is peripheral neuritis. This is manifested by numbness, tingling, and paresthesias in the extremities. This side effect can be minimized with pyridoxine (vitamin B_6) intake. Options 1, 2, and 3 are incorrect.

Test-Taking Strategy: Use the process of elimination. Options 1 and 2 would not cause the symptoms presented in the question, but instead would cause pallor and coolness. From the remaining options, you should know either that peripheral neuritis is a side effect of the medication or that these signs and symptoms do not correlate with hypercalcemia. Review the side effects associated with INH, if you had difficulty with this question.

Level of Cognitive Ability: Analysis
Client Needs: Physiological Integrity
Integrated Concept/Process: Nursing Process/Analysis
Content Area: Pharmacology
Reference: Hodgson, B., & Kizior, R. (2001). *Saunders nursing drug handbook 2001*. Philadelphia: W.B. Saunders, p. 551.

16. 2

Rationale: INH is hepatotoxic, and therefore the client is taught to report signs and symptoms of hepatitis immediately (which include yellow skin and sclera). For the same reason, alcohol should be avoided during therapy. The client should avoid intake of Swiss cheese, fish such as tuna, and foods containing tyramine because they may cause a reaction characterized by redness and itching of the skin, flushing, sweating, tachycardia, headache, or lightheadedness. The client can avoid developing peripheral neuritis by increasing the intake of pyridoxine (vitamin B_6) during the course of INH therapy.

Test-Taking Strategy: Use the process of elimination. Since alcohol intake is prohibited with the use of many medications, option 1 should be eliminated first. Since the client receiving this medication typically is supplemented with vitamin B_6, option 4 is incorrect and is eliminated next. Recalling that the medication is hepatotoxic will direct you to option 2. If you had difficulty with this question, review this medication.

Level of Cognitive Ability: Application
Client Needs: Health Promotion and Maintenance
Integrated Concept/Process: Teaching/Learning
Content Area: Pharmacology

Reference: Deglin, J., & Vallerand, A. (2001). *Davis's drug guide for nurses* (7th ed.). Philadelphia: F.A. Davis, p. 537.

17. **3**

Rationale: Rifampin should be taken exactly as directed. Doses should not be doubled or skipped. The client should not stop therapy until directed to do so by a physician. The medication should be administered on an empty stomach unless it causes gastrointestinal upset, and then it may be taken with food. Antacids, if prescribed, should be taken at least 1 hour prior to the medication. Rifampin causes orange-red discoloration of body secretions, and will permanently stain soft contact lenses.

Test-Taking Strategy: Use the process of elimination. Options 1 and 2 are examples of poor medication advice in general, and are eliminated first. Eliminate option 4 next because of the absolute word "always." If you had difficulty with this question, review the side effects associated with this medication.

Level of Cognitive Ability: Application
Client Needs: Physiological Integrity
Integrated Concept/Process: Teaching/Learning
Content Area: Pharmacology
Reference: Deglin, J., & Vallerand, A. (2001). *Davis's drug guide for nurses* (7th ed.). Philadelphia: F.A. Davis, p. 888.

18. **4**

Rationale: Ethambutol causes optic neuritis, which decreases visual acuity and the ability to discriminate between the colors red and green. This poses a potential safety hazard when a client is driving a motor vehicle. The client is taught to report this symptom immediately. The client is also taught to take the medication with food if GI upset occurs. Impaired hearing results from antitubercular therapy with streptomycin. Orange-red discoloration of secretions occurs with rifampin (Rifadin).

Test-Taking Strategy: Use the process of elimination. Option 1 is the least likely symptom to report; rather, it should be managed by taking the medication with food. To discriminate among the other options, it is necessary to know that this medication causes optic neuritis, resulting in difficulty with red-green discrimination. If this question was difficult, review antitubercular medications, since the incorrect options for this question are typical side effects of other antitubercular medications.

Level of Cognitive Ability: Analysis
Client Needs: Health Promotion and Maintenance
Integrated Concept/Process: Teaching/Learning
Content Area: Pharmacology
Reference: Deglin, J., & Vallerand, A. (2001). *Davis's drug guide for nurses* (7th ed.). Philadelphia: F.A. Davis, p. 375.

19. **2**

Rationale: Cycloserine (Seromycin) is an antitubercular medication that requires weekly serum drug level determinations to monitor for the potential of neurotoxicity. Serum drug levels less than 30 mg/mL reduce the incidence of neurotoxicity. The medication needs to be taken after meals to prevent gastrointestinal irritation. The client needs to be instructed to notify the physician if a skin rash or early signs of central nervous system toxicity are noted. Alcohol needs to be avoided because it increases the risk of seizure activity.

Test-Taking Strategy: Use the process of elimination. Eliminate options 3 and 4 first because they are the least likely correct options. From this point, knowing that the medication level needs to be monitored will assist in selecting the correct option. If you had difficulty with this question, review this medication.

Level of Cognitive Ability: Application
Client Needs: Health Promotion and Maintenance
Integrated Concept/Process: Teaching/Learning
Content Area: Pharmacology
Reference: Clark, J., Queener, S., & Karb, V. (2000). *Pharmacologic basis of nursing practice* (6th ed.). St. Louis: Mosby, p. 555.

20. **4**

Rationale: INH therapy can cause an elevation of hepatic enzymes and hepatitis. Therefore, liver enzymes are monitored when therapy is initiated, and during the first 3 months of therapy. They may be monitored longer in the client who is over age 50 or abuses alcohol.

Test-Taking Strategy: Use the process of elimination. In order to answer this question correctly, it is necessary to know that this medication can be toxic to the liver. Review the adverse effects of the various anti-TB medications, if this is an area that is unfamiliar to you.

Level of Cognitive Ability: Application
Client Needs: Physiological Integrity
Integrated Concept/Process: Nursing Process/Assessment
Content Area: Pharmacology
Reference: Hodgson, B., & Kizior, R. (2001). *Saunders nursing drug handbook 2001*. Philadelphia: W.B. Saunders, p. 551.

CRITICAL THINKING: FREE-TEXT ENTRY

Answer: The theophylline blood level is within the therapeutic range.

Rationale: The normal therapeutic range for a theophylline level is 10 to 20 µg/mL. A level above 20 µg/mL is considered toxic. The value of 18 µg/mL places the client within the therapeutic range.

Test-Taking Strategy: It is necessary to know the therapeutic theophylline level to interpret this result. Review this therapeutic range if you had difficulty with this question.

Level of Cognitive Ability: Analysis
Client Needs: Physiological Integrity
Integrated Concept/Process: Nursing Process/Analysis
Content Area: Pharmacology
Reference: Salerno, E. (1999). *Pharmacology for health professionals*. St. Louis: Mosby, pp. 462-463.

REFERENCES

Clark, J., Queener, S., & Karb, V. (2000). *Pharmacologic basis of nursing practice* (6th ed.). St. Louis: Mosby.

Deglin, J., & Vallerand, A. (2001). *Davis's drug guide for nurses* (7th ed.). Philadelphia: F.A. Davis.

Gutierrez, K. (1999). *Pharmacotherapeutics: Clinical decision-making in nursing.* Philadelphia: W.B. Saunders.

Hodgson, B., & Kizior, R. (2001). *Saunders nursing drug handbook 2001.* Philadelphia: W.B. Saunders.

Salerno, E. (1999). *Pharmacology for health professionals.* St. Louis: Mosby.

Smeltzer, S., & Bare, B. (2000). *Brunner & Suddarth's textbook of medical-surgical nursing* (9th ed.). Philadelphia: Lippincott Williams & Wilkins.

Wilson, B., Shannon, M., & Stang, C. (2000). *Nurses drug guide 2000.* Stamford, Conn.: Appleton & Lange.

The Adult Client with a Cardiovascular Disorder

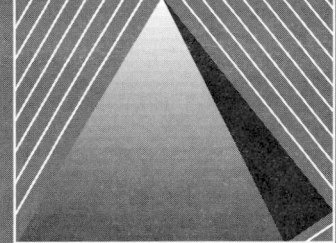

PYRAMID TERMS

afterload The force against which the heart has to pump to eject blood from the ventricle. Factors and conditions that would impede blood flow increase left ventricular afterload.

arterial anastomoses Ensure that when one of the blood-supplying arteries is damaged, flow is maintained from the other arteries. Blood flow to the hands, feet, brain, and other organs is protected by arterial anastomoses.

arterial pressure The pressure of the blood against the arterial walls. It can be measured indirectly by sphygmomanometer or directly by arterial catheter. Readings are expressed as systolic over diastolic. Arterial pressure increases when the cardiac output (CO), peripheral resistance, or blood volume increases.

automaticity The ability of cardiac cells to initiate an impulse spontaneously and repetitively without external neurohormonal control. The pacemaker cells have the highest rate of automaticity of all cardiac cells.

baroreceptors Also called pressoreceptors and are located in the walls of the aortic arch and carotid sinuses. Baroreceptors are specialized nerve endings that are affected by changes in the arterial blood pressure. Increases in arterial pressure stimulate baroreceptors, and the heart rate and arterial pressure decrease. Decreases in arterial pressure lead to a lessened stimulation of the baroreceptors, and vasoconstriction occurs, as does an increase in heart rate.

blood pressure (BP) The force exerted by the blood against the walls of the blood vessels. If the BP falls too low, blood flow to the tissues, heart, brain, and other organs becomes inadequate. If the BP becomes too high, the risk of vessel rupture and damage increases.

capillary pressure or hydrostatic pressure The pressure exerted by the blood against the capillary wall. Normal capillary pressure is 25 to 30 mm Hg at the arterial end of the capillaries and 10 to15 mm Hg at the venous end.

cardiac output The total volume of blood pumped through the heart in 1 minute. The normal cardiac output is 4 to 8 liters per minute. Cardiac output = stroke volume × heart rate.

chemoreceptors Located in the aortic arch and carotid bodies. Hypoxemia stimulates chemoreceptors, which then transmit impulses to the central nervous system.

conductivity The ability of the heart muscle fibers to propagate electrical impulses along and across cell membranes.

contractility Refers to the inherent ability of the myocardium to alter contractile force and velocity. Sympathetic stimulation increases myocardial contractility and thus increases stroke volume. Conditions that decrease myocardial contractility reduce stroke volume.

diastole The phase of the cardiac cycle in which the heart relaxes between contractions. It represents the period of time when the two ventricles are dilated by the blood flowing into them.

diastolic pressure The force of the blood exerted against the artery walls when the heart relaxes or fills. Normal diastolic pressure is 60 to 90 mm Hg.

excitability The ability of cardiac muscle cells to depolarize in response to a stimulus. Excitability is influenced by hormones, electrolytes, nutrition, oxygen supply, medication, infections, and nerve characteristics.

Frank-Starling law States that the more the heart fills within reasonable limits during diastole, the greater the force of contraction during systole and the greater the stroke volume. The exception to the law is during heart failure, when increasing blood volume into the ventricle decreases stroke volume. If the left ventricle fills to such an extent that it overdistends the myocardium, cardiac output begins to decrease and the heart begins to fail.

hepatojugular reflex Position the client with the head of the bed elevated 45 degrees, and locate the internal jugular vein. Compress the upper right abdomen for 30 to 40 seconds. Sudden distention of the neck veins after abdominal compression is usually indicative of right-sided heart failure.

mean arterial pressure (MAP) Is equivalent to one third of the pulse pressure plus the diastolic blood pressure. MAP is used in hemodynamic monitoring.

paradoxical blood pressure An exaggerated decrease in systolic pressure, by more than 10 mm Hg, during the inspiratory phase of the respiratory cycle. Normal decrease is 3 to 10 mm Hg.

postural (orthostatic) hypotension A blood pressure decrease of more than 20 mm Hg in the systolic pressure or a decrease of more than 10 mm Hg in the diastolic pressure and a 10% to 20% increase in heart rate. Occurs when the client's blood pressure is not adequately maintained while he or she is moving from a lying to a sitting or standing position.

preload The volume of blood stretching the left ventricle at the end of diastole. Preload is determined by the total circulating blood volume and is increased by an increase in venous return to the heart.

pulse pressure The difference between the systolic and diastolic pressures. Normal pulse pressure is 30 to 40 mm Hg.

refractoriness The heart's inability to respond to a new stimulus while still in a state of contraction from an earlier stimulus. Refractoriness prevents uncontrolled rapid cardiac contractions and helps to preserve the heart rhythm.

stretch receptors Located in the vena cava and the right atrium. Respond to pressure changes that affect circulatory blood volume. When the blood pressure decreases because of hypovolemia, a sympathetic response occurs, causing an increased heart rate and blood vessel constriction. When the blood pressure increases because of hypervolemia, an opposite effect occurs.

stroke volume The amount of blood ejected from the left ventricle with each contraction. The normal stroke volume is 70 to 130 mL per heart beat. The stroke volume can be affected by preload, afterload, contractility, and the Frank-Starling law.

systole The phase of contraction of the heart, especially of the ventricles, during which blood is forced into the aorta and the pulmonary artery.

systolic pressure The maximum pressure of blood exerted against the artery walls when the heart contracts. Normal systolic pressure is 100 to 140 mm Hg.

venous pressure The force exerted by the blood against the vein walls. Normal venous pressures are highest in the extremities (5 to 14 cm H_2O in the arm) and lowest closest to the heart (6 to 8 cm H_2O in the inferior vena cava).

▲ PYRAMID TO SUCCESS

Pyramid points focus on assessment data related to cardiovascular risks, health screening and promotion, complications of the various cardiovascular disorders, emergency implementation measures, and client education. Focus on the assessment findings in angina, myocardial infarction (MI), congestive heart failure (CHF) and pulmonary edema, pericarditis, dysrhythmias, pacemakers, aneurysms, hypertension, and arterial and vascular disorders. It is necessary to be able to identify the most common dysrhythmias and determine the appropriate interventions for these dysrhythmias. Focus also on the care of the client following diagnostic treatments and surgical procedures. Note appropriate and therapeutic client positions, particularly with arterial and venous disorders of the extremities. Focus on treatments and medications prescribed for the various cardiovascular disorders and client teaching related to prescribed treatment plans. Be familiar with the components related to cardiac rehabilitation. The Integrated Concepts and Processes addressed in this unit include Nursing Process, Caring, Communication and Documentation, Cultural Awareness, Self-Care, and Teaching/Learning.

CLIENT NEEDS
Safe, Effective Care Environment

Cardiovascular consultations and referrals
Client rights
Consultation with members of the health care team
Establishing priorities
Informed consent related to treatments and procedures
Medical and surgical asepsis
Standard (universal) precautions

Health Promotion and Maintenance

Alterations in lifestyle
Cardiac rehabilitation
Cardiovascular assessment techniques
Health screening and health promotion programs
Mobilization of appropriate community resources
Prevention of cardiovascular disease
Teaching related to diet therapy, exercise, and medications

Psychosocial Integrity

Accepting lifestyle changes
Coping mechanisms
Fear, anxiety, and denial
Grief and loss
End of life
Religious, spiritual, and cultural influences on health
Situational role changes
Support systems
Unexpected body image changes

Physiological Integrity

Assisting with basic care measures
Administration of IV medications
Activity limitations and rest and sleep
Hemodynamics
Interventions required in emergencies
Medical emergencies
Monitoring cardiac enzymes, troponin levels, and laboratory values related to the cardiovascular system
Monitoring for complications related to cardiovascular disorders
Monitoring for therapeutic effects of medications
Nonpharmacological and pharmacological comfort interventions

REFERENCES

Clark, J., Queener, S., & Karb, V. (2000). *Pharmacologic basis of nursing practice* (6th ed.). St. Louis: Mosby.

Fischbach, F. (2000). *A manual of laboratory & diagnostic tests* (6th ed.). Philadelphia: Lippincott Williams & Wilkins.

Gutierrez, K. (1999). *Pharmacotherapeutics: Clinical decision-making in nursing*. Philadelphia: W.B. Saunders,

Ignatavicius, D., Workman, M., & Mishler, M. (1999). *Medical-surgical nursing across the health care continuum* (3rd ed.). Philadelphia: W.B. Saunders.

Lewis, S., Heitkemper, M., & Dirksen, S. (2000). *Medical-surgical nursing: Assessment and management of clinical problems* (5th ed.). St. Louis: Mosby.

National Council of State Boards of Nursing (eds.) (2000). *Test Plan for the National Council Licensure Examination for Registered Nurses.* Chicago: Author.

Smeltzer, S., & Bare, B. (2000). *Brunner & Suddarth's textbook of medical-surgical nursing* (9th ed.). Philadelphia: Lippincott Williams & Wilkins.

Cardiovascular Disorders

I. ANATOMY AND PHYSIOLOGY

A. Heart and heart layers
   1. The heart is located in the left side of the mediastinum
   2. The epicardium covers the outer surface of the heart
   3. The myocardium is the middle layer and is the actual contracting muscle of the heart
   4. The endocardium is the innermost layer and lines the inner chambers and heart valves

B. Pericardium
   1. The pericardium encases and protects the heart from trauma and infection
   2. The parietal pericardium is the tough, fibrous outer membrane that attaches anteriorly to the lower half of the sternum, posteriorly to the thoracic vertebrae, and inferiorly to the diaphragm
   3. The visceral pericardium is the thin, inner layer that closely adheres to the heart
   4. The pericardial space is between the parietal and visceral layers; it holds 5 to 20 mL of pericardial fluid, which lubricates the pericardial surfaces and cushions the heart

C. Heart chambers
   1. The right atrium receives deoxygenated blood from the body via the superior and inferior vena cava
   2. The right ventricle receives blood from the right atrium and pumps it to the lungs via the pulmonary artery
   3. The left atrium receives oxygenated blood from the lungs via four pulmonary veins
   4. The left ventricle is the largest and most muscular chamber; it receives oxygenated blood from the lungs via the left atrium and pumps blood into the systemic circulation via the aorta

D. Heart valves
   1. The atrioventricular (AV) valves lie between the atria and the ventricles
   2. The AV valves close at the beginning of ventricular contraction and prevent blood from flowing back into the atria from the ventricles; these valves open when the ventricle relaxes
   3. The bicuspid or mitral valve is located on the left side of the heart
   4. The tricuspid valve is located on the right side of the heart
   5. The pulmonic semilunar valve lies between the right ventricle and the pulmonary artery
   6. The aortic semilunar valve lies between the left ventricle and the aorta
   7. The semilunar valves prevent blood from flowing back into the ventricles during relaxation; they open during ventricular contraction and close when the ventricles begin to relax.

E. Atrioventricular (AV) node
   1. The AV node is located in the lower aspect of the atrial septum
   2. The AV node receives electrical impulses from the sinoatrial (SA) node

F. The bundle of His (AV bundle)
   1. The bundle of His fuses with the AV node to form another pacemaker site
   2. It branches into the right bundle branch (RBB), which extends down the right side of the interventricular septum, and the left bundle branch (LBB), which extends into the left ventricle
   3. The right and left bundle branches terminate into Purkinje fibers
   4. If the SA node fails, the bundle of His can initiate and sustain a heart rate at 40 to 60 beats per minute

G. Purkinje fibers
   1. Purkinje fibers are a diffuse network of conduct-

ing strands located beneath the ventricular endocardium

2. These fibers spread the wave of depolarization through the ventricles

▶ H. Coronary arteries
1. The coronary arteries supply the capillaries of the myocardium with blood
2. The right coronary artery (RCA) supplies the right atrium and ventricle, the inferior portion of the left ventricle, the posterior septal wall, and the SA and AV nodes
3. The left coronary artery (LCA) consists of two major branches, the left anterior descending (LAD) and the circumflex arteries
4. The LAD artery supplies blood to the anterior wall of the left ventricle, the anterior ventricular septum, and the apex of the left ventricle
5. The circumflex artery supplies blood to the left atrium and the lateral and posterior surfaces of the left ventricle

I. Sinoatrial (SA) node
1. The SA node or pacemaker initiates each heart beat
2. It is located at the junction of the superior vena cava and the right atrium
3. It generates electrical impulses at approximately 60 to 100 times per minute and is controlled by the sympathetic and parasympathetic systems

J. Heart sounds
1. The first heart sound (S_1) is heard as the AV valves close
2. The second heart sound (S_2) is heard when the semilunar valves close
3. A third heart sound (S_3) may be heard if ventricular wall compliance is decreased and structures in the ventricular wall vibrate; this can occur in conditions such as congestive heart failure or valvular regurgitation; however, an S_3 heart sound may be normal in individuals younger than 30 years of age
4. A fourth heart sound (S_4) may be heard on atrial **systole** if resistance to ventricular filling is present; this is an abnormal finding, and the causes include cardiac hypertrophy, disease, or injury to the ventricular wall

K. Heart rate
1. The faster the heart rate, the less time the heart has for filling, and the **cardiac output** decreases
2. An increase in heart rate increases oxygen consumption
3. The normal heart rate is 60 to 100 beats per minute
4. Sinus tachycardia is a rate greater than 100 beats per minute
5. Sinus bradycardia is a rate less than 60 beats per minute

L. Autonomic nervous system
1. Stimulation of sympathetic nerve fibers releases

the neurotransmitter norepinephrine, producing an increased heart rate, increased conduction speed through the AV node, increased atrial and ventricular **contractility,** and peripheral vasoconstriction; stimulation occurs when a decrease in pressure is detected

2. Stimulation of the parasympathetic nerve fibers releases the neurotransmitter acetylcholine, which decreases the heart rate and lessens atrial and ventricular **contractility** and **conductivity;** stimulation occurs when an increase in pressure is detected

M. **Blood pressure** control
1. **Baroreceptors,** also called pressoreceptors, are located in the walls of the aortic arch **and** carotid sinuses
2. **Baroreceptors** are specialized nerve endings that are affected by changes in the arterial **blood pressure**
3. Increases in **arterial pressure** stimulate **baroreceptors,** and the heart rate and **arterial pressure** decrease
4. Decreases in **arterial pressure** reduce stimulation of the **baroreceptors,** and vasoconstriction occurs, as does an increase in heart rate
5. **Stretch receptors,** located in the vena cava and the right atrium, respond to pressure changes that affect circulatory blood volume
6. When the **blood pressure** decreases as a result of hypovolemia, a sympathetic response occurs, causing an increased heart rate and blood vessel constriction; when the **blood pressure** increases as a result of hypervolemia, an opposite effect occurs
7. The antidiuretic hormone (ADH) influences **blood pressure** indirectly by regulating vascular volume
8. Increases in blood volume result in decreased ADH release, increasing diuresis, and decreasing blood volume and thus **blood pressure**
9. Decreases in blood volume result in increased ADH release; this promotes an increase in blood volume and thus **blood pressure**
10. Renin, a potent vasoconstrictor, causes the **blood pressure** to increase
11. Renin converts angiotensinogen to angiotensin I; angiotensin I is then converted to angiotensin II in the lungs
12. Angiotensin II stimulates the release of aldosterone, which promotes water and sodium retention by the kidneys; this action increases blood volume and **blood pressure**

N. The vascular system
1. Arteries are vessels through which the blood passes away from the heart to various parts of the body; they convey highly oxygenated blood from the left side of heart to the tissues

2. Arterioles control the blood flow into the capillaries
3. Capillaries allow the exchange of fluid and nutrients between the blood and the interstitial spaces
4. Venules receive blood from the capillary bed and move blood into the veins
5. Veins transport deoxygenated blood from the tissues back to the heart and lungs for oxygenation
6. Valves help return blood to the heart against the force of gravity
7. The lymphatics drain the tissues and return the tissue fluid to the blood

II. DIAGNOSTIC TESTS AND PROCEDURES
A. Cardiac enzymes
   1. CK-MB (creatine kinase, myocardial muscle)
      a. An elevation in value indicates myocardial damage
      b. An elevation occurs within 4 to 6 hours and peaks 18 to 24 hours following an acute ischemic attack
      c. Normal value in conventional units is 0 to 7 U/L
   2. Lactic dehydrogenase (LDH)
      a. Elevations in LDH occur 24 hours following myocardial infarction and peak in 48 to 72 hours
      b. When the serum concentration of LDH_1 is higher than that for LDH_2, the pattern is indicated as "flipped," signifying myocardial necrosis
      c. Normal value in conventional units is 70 to 200 IU/L.
   3. Troponin
      a. Composed of three proteins: cardiac troponin, troponin I, and troponin T
      b. Troponin I, especially, has a high affinity for myocardial injury; it rises within 3 hours and persists for up to 7 days
      c. Normal values are quite low, with troponin T normally ranging from 0.0 to 0.2 ng/mL, and troponin I being less than 0.6 ng/mL; thus any rise can indicate myocardial cell damage
   4. Myoglobin
      a. An oxygen-binding protein found in cardiac and skeletal muscle
      b. Level rises within 1 hour after cell death, peaks in 4 to 6 hours, and returns to normal within 24 to 36 hours (and in some clients even faster)
B. Complete blood cell (CBC) count
   1. The red blood cell (RBC) count decreases in rheumatic heart disease and infective endocarditis and increases in conditions characterized by inadequate tissue oxygenation

2. The white blood cell (WBC) count increases in infectious and inflammatory diseases of the heart and after myocardial infarction (MI) because large numbers of WBCs are needed to dispose of the necrotic tissue resulting from the infarction
3. An elevated hematocrit can result from vascular volume depletion
4. Decreases in hematocrit and hemoglobin can indicate anemia
C. Blood coagulation factors: An increase in coagulation factors can occur during and after MI, which places the client at greater risk of thrombophlebitis and extension of clots in the coronary artery
D. Serum lipids
   1. The lipid profile measures serum cholesterol, triglycerides, and lipoprotein levels
   2. The lipid profile is used to assess the risk of developing coronary artery disease
   3. The desirable range for serum cholesterol is less than 200 mg/dL, with the LDH cholesterol less than 130 mg/dL and the HDL cholesterol at 30 to 70 mg/dL
E. Electrolytes
   1. Potassium
      a. Hypokalemia causes increased cardiac electrical instability, ventricular dysrhythmias, and increased risk of digitalis toxicity
      b. In hypokalemia, the electrocardiogram would show flattening and inversion of the T wave, the appearance of a U wave, and sagging of the ST segment
      c. Hyperkalemia causes asystole and ventricular dysrhythmias
   2. Sodium
      a. The serum sodium level decreases with the use of diuretics
      b. The serum sodium level decreases in heart failure, indicating water excess
F. Calcium
   1. Hypocalcemia can cause ventricular dysrhythmias, prolonged QT interval, and cardiac arrest
   2. Hypercalcemia can cause a shortened QT interval, AV block, tachycardia or bradycardia, digitalis hypersensitivity, and cardiac arrest
G. Phosphorus level: Phosphorus levels should be interpreted with calcium levels because the kidneys retain or excrete one electrolyte in an inverse relationship to the other
H. Magnesium
   1. A low magnesium level can cause ventricular tachycardia and fibrillation
   2. A high magnesium level can cause muscle weakness, hypotension, bradycardia, and a prolonged PR interval and wide QRS complex
I. Blood urea nitrogen (BUN): The BUN is elevated in heart disorders that adversely affect renal circulation, such as heart failure and cardiogenic shock

J. Blood glucose: An acute cardiac episode can elevate the blood glucose

K. Chest x-ray film
1. Description
   a. Done to determine the size, silhouette, and position of the heart
   b. Specific pathological changes are difficult to determine via x-ray, but anatomical changes can be seen
2. Implementation
   a. Prepare the client for x-ray film, explaining the purpose and procedure
   b. Remove jewelry

▲ L. Electrocardiogram (ECG) (Box 57-1)
1. Description: a common noninvasive diagnostic test that evaluates the heart's function by recording electrical activity
2. Implementation
   a. Determine the client's ability to lie still, and advise the client to lie still, breathe normally, and refrain from talking during the test
   b. Reassure the client that an electrical shock will not occur
   c. Document any cardiac medications the client is taking

M. Holter monitoring
1. Description
   a. A noninvasive test in which the client wears a Holter monitor and an ECG tracing is recorded continuously over a period of 24 hours or more
   b. It identifies dysrhythmias if they occur and evaluates the effectiveness of antidysrhythmics or pacemaker therapy

▲ 2. Implementation: Instruct the client to resume normal daily activities and to maintain a diary documenting activities and any symptoms that may develop

N. Echocardiogram
1. Description
   a. A noninvasive procedure based on the principles of ultrasound
   b. It evaluates structural and functional changes in the heart
2. Implementation: Determine the client's ability to lie still, and advise the client to lie still, breathe normally, and refrain from talking during the test

O. Exercise testing (stress test)
1. Description
   a. A noninvasive test that studies the heart during activity and detects and evaluates coronary artery disease
   b. Treadmill testing is the most commonly used mode of stress testing
   c. Stress testing may be used in conjunction with myocardial radionuclide testing, at which

---

BOX 57-1

Electrocardiogram (ECG) Basics

An ECG reflects the electrical activity of cardiac cells and records electrical activity at a speed of 25 mm/sec

An ECG strip consists of horizontal squares representing seconds and vertical squares representing voltage

Each small square represents 0.04 second

Each large square represents 0.20 second

The P wave represents atrial depolarization

The PR interval represents the time it takes an impulse to travel from the atria through the AV node, bundle of His, and bundle branches to the Purkinje fibers

Normal PR interval duration ranges from 0.12 to 0.2 second

The PR interval is measured from the beginning of the P wave to the end of the PR segment

The QRS complex represents ventricular depolarization

Normal QRS complex duration ranges from 0.04 to 0.1 second

The Q wave appears as the first negative deflection in the QRS complex and reflects initial ventricular septal depolarization

The R wave is the first positive deflection in the QRS complex

The S wave appears as the second negative deflection in the QRS complex

The J point marks the end of the QRS complex and the beginning of the ST segment

The QRS duration is measured from the end of the PR segment to the J point

The ST segment represents part of ventricular repolarization

The T wave represents ventricular repolarization and ventricular diastole

The U wave may follow the T wave

A prominent U wave may indicate an electrolyte abnormality such as hypokalemia

The QT interval represents ventricular refractory time, or the total time required for ventricular depolarization and repolarization

The QT interval is measured from the beginning of the QRS complex to the end of the T wave

The QT interval normally lasts 0.32 to 0.4 second but varies with the client's heart rate, age, and sex

---

point the procedure becomes invasive because a radionuclide must be injected
   d. A consent form is required if a radionuclide is injected
2. Preprocedure implementation
   a. Obtain consent if required
   b. Provide adequate rest the night before the procedure
   c. Instruct the client to eat a light meal 1 to 2 hours before the procedure
   d. Instruct the client to avoid smoking, alcohol, and caffeine prior to the procedure

c. Ask the physician about taking prescribed medication on the day of the procedure

f. Instruct the client to wear nonconstrictive, comfortable clothing and supportive shoes

3. Postprocedure implementation

a. Instruct the client to notify the physician if any chest pain, dizziness, or shortness of breath occurs

b. Instruct the client to avoid taking a hot bath or shower for at least 1 to 2 hours

P. Digital subtraction angiography

1. Description

a. Combines x-ray techniques and a computerized subtraction technique with fluoroscopy for visualization of the cardiovascular system

b. A contrast medium (dye) is injected

2. Preprocedure implementation

a. Assess the client for allergy to contrast medium (dye), iodine, or seafood

b. Obtain consent

3. Postprocedure implementation

a. Monitor vital signs (VS)

b. Assess injection site for bleeding or discomfort

Q. Nuclear cardiology

1. Description

a. The use of radionuclide techniques and scanning in cardiovascular assessment

b. The most common tests include technetium pyrophosphate scanning, thallium imaging, and multigated cardiac blood pool imaging (MUGA)

2. Preprocedure implementation

a. Obtain consent

b. Inform the client that a small amount of radioisotope will be injected, and that the radiation exposure and risks are minimal

3. Postprocedure implementation

a. Assess vital signs (VS)

b. Assess injection site for bleeding or discomfort

c. Inform the client that fatigue may be experienced

R. Cardiac catheterization

1. Description

a. Involves insertion of a catheter into the heart and surrounding vessels

b. Obtains information about the structure and performance of the heart valves and circulatory system

2. Preprocedure implementation

a. Obtain a consent form

b. Assess for allergies to seafood, iodine, or radiopaque dyes

c. Withhold solid food for 6 to 8 hours and liquids for 4 hours to prevent vomiting and aspiration during the procedure

d. Document the client's height and weight, because these data will be needed to determine the amount of dye to be administered

e. Document baseline vital signs, and note the quality and presence of peripheral pulses for postprocedure comparison

f. Inform the client that a local anesthetic will be administered prior to catheter insertion

g. Inform the client that he or she may feel fatigued because of the need to lie still and quiet on a relatively hard table for up to 2 hours

h. Inform the client that he or she may feel a fluttery feeling as the catheter passes through the heart, a flushed, warm feeling when the dye is injected, a desire to cough, and palpitations caused by heart irritability

i. Prepare insertion site by shaving and cleaning with an antiseptic solution if prescribed

j. Administer preprocedure medications if prescribed

k. Insert an IV if prescribed

3. Postprocedure implementation

a. Monitor VS and cardiac rhythm for dysrhythmias at least every 30 minutes for 2 hours initially

b. Assess for chest pain, and if dysrhythmias or chest pain occurs, notify the physician

c. Monitor peripheral pulses and the color, warmth, and sensation of the extremity distal to insertion site at least every 30 minutes for 2 hours initially

d. Notify the physician if the client complains of numbness and tingling, if the extremity becomes cool, pale, or cyanotic, or if loss of the peripheral pulses occurs

e. Monitor the pressure dressing for bleeding or hematoma formation

f. Apply a sandbag to the insertion site to provide additional pressure if required

g. Monitor for bleeding, and if bleeding occurs, apply pressure immediately and notify the physician

h. Monitor for hematoma, and if a hematoma develops, notify the physician

i. Keep extremity extended for 4 to 6 hours, keeping the leg straight to prevent arterial occlusion

j. Maintain strict bed rest for 6 to 12 hours; however, the client may turn from side to side; do not elevate the head of the bed more than 15 degrees

k. If the antecubital vessel was used, immobilize the arm with an armboard

l. Encourage fluids, if not contraindicated, to promote renal excretion of the dye

m. Monitor for nausea, vomiting, rash, or other signs of hypersensitivity to the dye

S. Central venous pressure (CVP)

1. Description

a. The CVP is the pressure within the superior

vena cava and reflects the pressure under which blood is returned to the superior vena cava and right atrium

b. CVP is measured with a central venous line in the superior vena cava or by a balloon flotation catheter in the pulmonary artery

c. Normal CVP pressure is 5 to 10 mm Hg

d. An elevated CVP measurement indicates an increase in blood volume as a result of sodium and water retention, excessive IV fluids, alterations in fluid balance, or renal failure

e. A decreased CVP measurement indicates a decrease in circulating blood volume, and may be due to hemorrhage or severe vasodilation with pooling of blood in the extremities that limits venous return, and fluid imbalances

2. Measuring CVP

a. The right atrium is located at the midaxillary line at the fourth intercostal space, and the zero point on the transducer needs to be at the level of the right atrium

b. The client needs to be supine, with the head of the bed at 45 degrees

c. The client needs to be relaxed; note that activity that increases intrathoracic pressure, such as coughing or straining, will cause false increases in the readings

d. If the client is on a ventilator, the reading should be taken at the point of end-expiration

e. To maintain patency of the line, a constant, small amount of fluid is delivered under pressure

III. THERAPEUTIC MANAGEMENT

A. Percutaneous transluminal coronary angioplasty (PTCA)

1. Description

a. One or more arteries are dilated with a balloon catheter to open the vessel lumen and improve arterial blood flow

b. The client can experience reocclusion after the procedure, thus the procedure may need to be repeated

c. Complications can include arterial dissection or rupture, immobilization of plaque fragments, spasm, and acute MI

d. Firm commitment is needed on the client's part to stop smoking, lose weight, alter exercise pattern, and stop any behaviors that lead to progression of artery occlusion

2. Preprocedure implementation

a. Maintain NPO status after midnight

b. Prepare the groin area with antiseptic soap and shave per institutional procedure and as prescribed

c. Assess baseline VS and peripheral pulses

3. Postprocedure implementation

a. Monitor VS closely

b. Assess distal pulses in both extremities

c. Maintain bed rest as prescribed, keeping the limb straight for 6 to 8 hours

d. Administer anticoagulants and antiplatelet agents as prescribed to prevent thrombus formation

e. Monitor IV nitroglycerin that may be prescribed to prevent coronary artery spasm

f. Instruct the client in the administration of nitrates, calcium channel blockers, antiplatelet agents, and anticoagulants as prescribed

g. Instruct the client to take daily aspirin permanently if prescribed

h. Assist the client with planning lifestyle modifications

B. Laser-assisted angioplasty

1. Description

a. A laser probe is advanced through a cannula similar to that used for PTCA

b. Used also for clients with small occlusions in the distal superficial femoral, proximal popliteal, and common iliac arteries

c. Heat from the laser vaporizes the plaque to open the occluded artery

2. Preprocedure and postprocedure care

a. Similar to that for the PTCA

b. Monitor for complications of coronary dissection, acute occlusion, perforation, embolism, and MI

C. Coronary artery stents

1. Description

a. Used instead of PTCA to eliminate the risk of acute coronary vessel closure and to improve long-term patency of the vessel

b. A balloon catheter bearing the stent is inserted into the coronary artery and positioned at the site of occlusion

c. When placed in the coronary artery, the stent reopens the blocked artery

2. Postprocedure implementation

a. Acute thrombosis is a major concern following the procedure, and the client is placed on antiplatelet and anticoagulation therapy for several months following the procedure

b. Monitor for complications of the procedure, such as stent migration or occlusion, coronary artery dissection, and bleeding resulting from anticoagulation

D. Atherectomy

1. Description

a. Removes plaque from an artery by the use of a cutting chamber on the inserted catheter or a rotating blade that pulverizes the plaque

b. Used to improve blood flow to ischemic limbs in individuals with peripheral arterial disease

2. Postprocedure implementation: monitor for complications of perforation, embolus, and reocclusion

E. Transmyocardial revascularization
1. Used for clients with widespread atherosclerosis involving vessels that are too small and numerous for replacement or balloon catheterization
2. Uses a high-powered laser that creates 15 to 30 holes (channels) in the heart
3. Blood enters these small channels, providing the affected region of the heart with oxygenated blood
4. Performed through a small chest incision
5. The opening on the heart's surface heals over; however, the main channels remain and perfuse the myocardium

F. Arterial revascularization
1. Description
   a. Performed to increase arterial blood flow to the affected limb
   b. Inflow procedures involve bypassing the arterial occlusion above the superficial femoral arteries
   c. Outflow procedures involve bypassing the arterial occlusions at or below the superficial femoral arteries
   d. Graft material is sutured above and below the occlusion to facilitate blood flow around the occlusion
2. Preoperative implementation
   a. Assess baseline VS and peripheral pulses
   b. Insert IV and urinary catheter as prescribed
   c. Maintain central venous catheter and/or arterial line if inserted
3. Postoperative implementation
   a. Assess VS
   b. Monitor the **blood pressure** and notify the physician if changes occur
   c. Monitor for hypotension, which may indicate hypovolemia
   d. Monitor for hypertension, which may place stress on the graft and facilitate clot formation
   e. Maintain bed rest for 24 hours as prescribed
   f. Instruct the client to keep affected extremity straight, limit movement, and avoid bending the knee and hip
   g. Monitor for warmth, redness, and edema, which are often expected outcomes because of increased blood flow
   h. Monitor for graft occlusion, which often occurs within the first 24 hours
   i. Assess peripheral pulses and for adverse changes in color and temperature of the extremity
   j. Monitor for a sharp increase in pain, since pain is frequently the first indicator of postoperative graft occlusion

k. If signs of graft occlusion occur, notify the physician immediately
l. Encourage coughing and deep breathing and the use of incentive spirometry
m. Maintain NPO status, with progression to clear liquids as prescribed
n. Use strict aseptic technique when in contact with the incision
o. Assess the incision for drainage, warmth, or swelling
p. Monitor for excessive bleeding (a small amount of bloody drainage is expected)
q. Monitor the area over the graft for hardness, tenderness, and warmth, which may indicate infection; if this occurs, notify the physician immediately
r. Instruct the client about proper foot care and measures to prevent ulcer formation
s. Instruct the client to take medications as prescribed
t. Instruct the client in how to care for incision
u. Assist the client in modifying lifestyle to prevent further plaque formation

G. Coronary artery bypass graft (CABG)
1. Description
   a. The occluded coronary arteries are bypassed with the client's own venous or arterial blood vessels
   b. The saphenous vein, radial artery, or internal mammary artery is used to bypass lesions in the coronary arteries
   c. Performed when the client does not respond to medical management of coronary artery disease (CAD) or when disease progression is evident
2. Preoperative implementation
   a. Familiarize the client and family with the cardiac surgical critical care unit
   b. Instruct the client in how to splint the chest incision, cough and deep breathe, and perform arm and leg exercises
   c. Instruct the client to inform the nurse of any postoperative pain, as pain medication will be available
   d. Inform the client to expect a sternal incision, possible arm or leg incision(s), one or two chest tubes, a Foley catheter, and several IV fluid catheters
   e. Inform the client that an endotracheal (ET) tube will be in place and connected to a ventilator for 6 to 24 hours
   f. Advise the client to breathe with the ventilator and not fight it
   g. Inform the family that the client will not be able to talk while the ET tube is in place
   h. Encourage the client and family to discuss anxieties and fears related to surgery

i. Note that prescribed medications are to be discontinued preoperatively (diuretics 2 to 3 days prior to surgery, digitalis 12 hours prior to surgery, and aspirin and anticoagulants 1 week prior to surgery)

j. Administer medications as prescribed, which may include potassium chloride, antihypertensives, antidysrhythmics, and antibiotics

3. Cardiac surgical unit
   a. Maintain mechanical ventilation for 6 to 24 hours as prescribed
   b. Monitor heart rate and rhythm, pulmonary artery and **arterial pressures,** and neurological status
   c. Monitor mediastinal and pericardial tubes and water seal drainage system, and report drainage exceeding 100 to 150 mL per hour
   d. Ground epicardial pacer wires
   e. Assess fluid and electrolyte balance
   f. Restrict fluids, as prescribed, to 1500 to 2000 mL because the client usually has edema
   g. Monitor for hypotension, which can cause collapse of a vein graft
   h. Monitor for hypertension because increased pressure promotes leakage from the suture line and may cause bleeding
   i. Monitor the temperature and initiate rewarming procedures using warm or thermal blankets if the temperature drops below 96.8° F; rewarm the client no faster than 1.8° F per hour to prevent shivering, and discontinue when the temperature approaches 98.6° F
   j. Administer potassium IV, as prescribed, to maintain the potassium level between 4 and 5 mEq/L to prevent dysrhythmias
   k. Monitor for signs of cardiac tamponade, which will include sudden cessation of previously heavy mediastinal drainage, jugular vein distention with clear lung sounds, and pulsus paradoxus
   l. Monitor pain, differentiating sternotomy pain from anginal pain, which would indicate graft failure

4. Transfer from the cardiac surgical unit
   a. Monitor VS, level of consciousness (LOC), and peripheral perfusion
   b. Monitor for dysrhythmias
   c. Auscultate lungs and assess respiratory status
   d. Encourage the client to splint the incision, cough, deep breathe, and use incentive spirometer to raise secretions and prevent atelectasis
   e. Monitor temperature and WBC count, which if elevated after 3 to 4 days indicate infection
   f. Provide adequate fluids and hydration as prescribed to liquefy secretions
   g. Assess suture line and chest tube insertion sites for redness, purulent discharge, and signs of infection
   h. Assess sternal suture line for instability, which may indicate an infection
   i. Guide the client to gradually resume activity
   j. Assess the client for tachycardia, **orthostatic hypotension,** and fatigue before, during, and after activity
   k. Discontinue activities if the **BP** drops more than 10 to 20 mm Hg or if the pulse increases more than 10 beats per minute
   l. Monitor episodes of pain closely
   m. See Box 57-2 for home care instructions

H. Heart transplant
   1. A donor heart from an individual with a comparable body weight and ABO compatibility is transplanted into a recipient within less than 6 hours of procurement
   2. The surgeon removes the diseased heart, leaving the posterior portion of the atria to serve as an anchor for the new heart
   3. Because a remnant of the client's atria remains, two unrelated P waves are noted on the ECG
   4. The transplanted heart is denervated and unresponsive to vagal stimulation; because the heart is denervated, clients do not experience angina
   5. Symptoms of heart rejection include hypotension, dysrhythmias, weakness, fatigue, and dizziness
   6. Endomyocardial biopsies are performed at regular scheduled intervals and whenever rejection is suspected
   7. Clients require lifetime immunosuppressive therapy
   8. The heart rate approximates 100 beats per minute, and responds slowly to exercise or stress

---

BOX 57-2

Home Care Instructions Following Cardiac Surgery

Progression with activities at home

Limit pushing or pulling activities for 6 weeks following discharge

Incisional care and record signs of redness, swelling, or drainage

Sternotomy incision heals in about 6 to 8 weeks

Avoid crossing legs, wear elastic hose as prescribed until edema subsides, and elevate surgical limb when sitting in a chair

Use of prescribed medications

Dietary measures, including the avoidance of saturated fats and cholesterol and the use of salt

Sexual intercourse can be resumed on the advice of the physician after exercise tolerance is assessed; if the client can walk one block or climb two flights of stairs without symptoms, he or she can safely resume sexual activity with regard to increases in heart rate, **contractility**, and **cardiac output**

IV. CARDIAC DYSRHYTHMIAS

A. Normal sinus rhythm (Fig. 57-1)
1. Rhythm originates from the SA node
2. Atrial and ventricular rhythms are regular
3. Atrial and ventricular rates are 60 to 100 beats per minute (Fig. 57-2; Box 57-3)

B. Sinus bradycardia
1. Description
   a. Atrial and ventricular rates are below 60 beats per minute
   b. Treatment may be necessary if the client is symptomatic
   c. Note that a low heart rate may be normal for some individuals
2. Implementation
   a. Attempt to determine cause, and if a medication is suspected of causing the bradycardia, hold the medication and notify the physician
   b. Administer oxygen as prescribed
   c. Administer atropine sulfate as prescribed to increase the heart rate to 60 beats per minute
   d. Be prepared to apply a noninvasive pacemaker initially as prescribed, if the atropine sulfate does not increase the heart rate sufficiently

e. Avoid additional doses of atropine sulfate because they will induce tachycardia
f. Monitor for hypotension and administer IV fluids as prescribed
g. Depending on the cause of the bradycardia, the client may need a permanent pacemaker

C. Sinus tachycardia
1. Description: atrial and ventricular rates are 100 to180 beats per minute
2. Implementation
   a. Identify the cause of the tachycardia

BOX 57-3

Six-Second Strip Method to Determine Heart Rate

Can be used to determine heart rate for both regular and irregular rhythms

To determine atrial rate, count the number of PP intervals in 6 seconds and multiply by 10 to obtain a full minute rate

To determine ventricular rate, count the number of RR intervals in 6 seconds and multiply by 10 to obtain a full minute rate

For accuracy, timing should begin on the P wave or the QRS complex and end exactly at 30 large blocks later

---

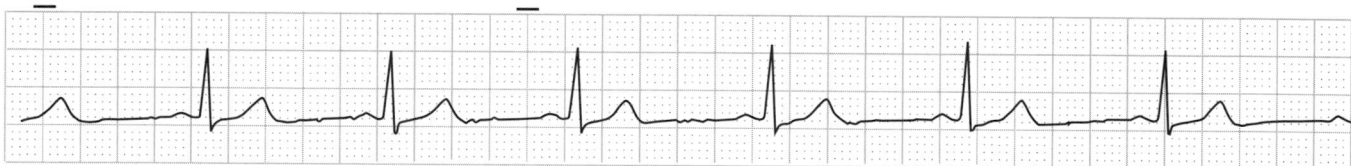

FIG. 57-1   Normal sinus rhythm. (From Paul S, Hebra JD: *The nurse's guide to cardiac rhythm interpretation*, Philadelphia, 1998, WB Saunders.)

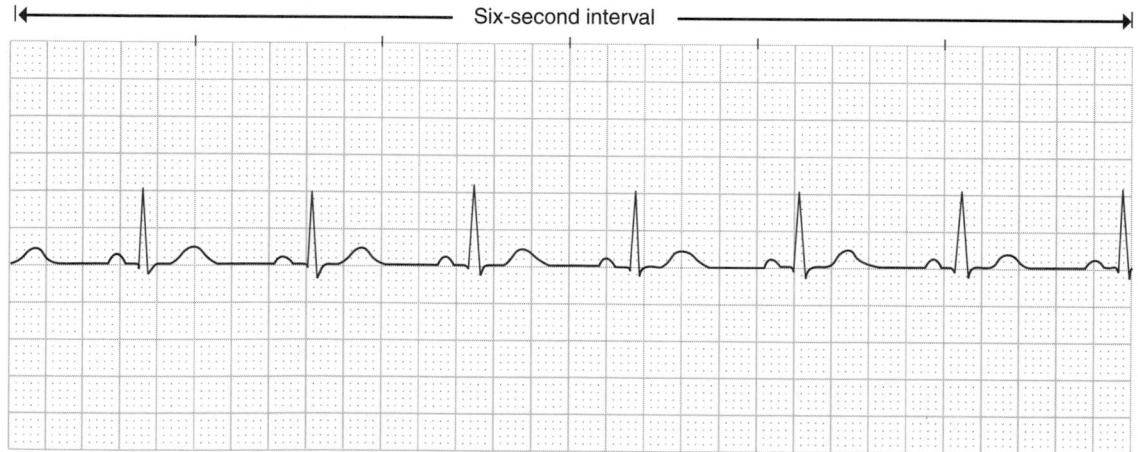

FIG. 57-2   Six-second method for calculating heart rate: seven QRS complexes in a six-second interval is equal to a heart rate of 70 beats per minute. (From Paul S, Hebra JD: *The nurse's guide to cardiac rhythm interpretation*, Philadelphia, 1998, WB Saunders.)

b. Decrease the heart rate to normal by treating the cause

D. Atrial fibrillation (Fig. 57-3)
1. Description
    a. Multiple rapid impulses from many foci depolarize in the atria in a totally disorganized manner at a rate of 350 to 600 times per minute
    b. The atria quiver, which can lead to the formation of thrombi
    c. P wave is absent
2. Implementation
    a. Administer oxygen
    b. Administer anticoagulants as prescribed because of the risk of emboli
    c. Administer cardiac medications as prescribed to control the ventricular rhythm and assist in the maintenance of **cardiac output**
    d. Prepare the client for cardioversion as prescribed
    e. Instruct the client in the use of medications as prescribed to control the dysrhythmia

E. Premature ventricular contractions (PVCs) (Box 57-4)
1. Description
    a. Early ventricular complexes result from increased irritability of the ventricles
    b. PVCs frequently occur in repetitive rhythms, such as bigeminy, trigeminy, and quadrigeminy

---

BOX 57-4

Premature Ventricular Contractions (PVCs)

Bigeminy: PVC every other heart beat
Trigeminy: PVC every third heart beat
Quadrigeminy: PVC every fourth heartbeat
Couplet or pair: Two sequential PVCs
Unifocal: Uniform upward or downward deflection, arising from the same ectopic foci
Multifocal: Different shapes, with the impulse generation from different sites
R-on-T phenomenon: PVC falls on preceding beat's T wave, which is considered a vulnerable period; may precipitate ventricular fibrillation

---

c. The QRS complexes may be unifocal or multifocal
2. Implementation
    a. Notify the physician if PVCs are noted
    b. Identify the cause and treat based on the cause
    c. Evaluate electrolytes, particularly the potassium level, since hypokalemia can cause PVCs
    d. Administer oxygen as prescribed
    e. Administer lidocaine as prescribed
    f. Notify the physician if the client complains of chest pain or if PVCs increase in frequency, are multifocal, occur on the T wave (R on T), or occur in runs of ventricular tachycardia

F. Ventricular tachycardia (VT) (Fig. 57-4)
1. Description
    a. Occurs when there is a repetitive firing of an irritable ventricular ectopic focus at a rate of 140 to 250 beats per minute or more
    b. May present as a paroxysm of three self-limiting beats or more, or may be a sustained rhythm
    c. Can cause cardiac arrest
2. Stable client with sustained VT
    a. Administer oxygen as prescribed
    b. Administer antidysrhythmics as prescribed
3. Unstable client with VT
    a. Administer oxygen and antidysrhythmic therapy as prescribed
    b. Prepare for synchronized cardioversion if client is unstable
    c. Attempt cough cardiopulmonary resuscitation (CPR) by asking the client to cough hard every 1 to 3 seconds
4. Pulseless client: defibrillation and cardiopulmonary resuscitation (CPR)

G. Ventricular fibrillation (Fig. 57-5)
1. Description
    a. Impulses from many irritable foci fire in a totally disorganized manner
    b. Chaotic rapid rhythm in which the ventricles quiver
    c. Rapidly fatal if not successfully terminated within 3 to 5 minutes
    d. Client lacks a pulse, **blood pressure,** respirations, and heart sounds

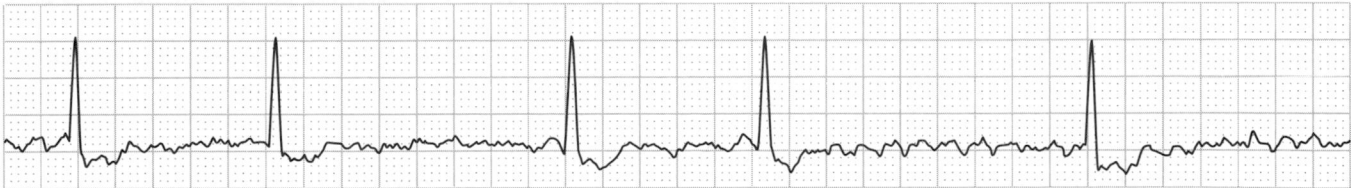

FIG. 57-3 Atrial fibrillation. Note the chaotic undulations of the atria and irregular response of the ventricles. (From Paul S, Hebra JD: *The nurse's guide to cardiac rhythm interpretation,* Philadelphia, 1998, WB Saunders.)

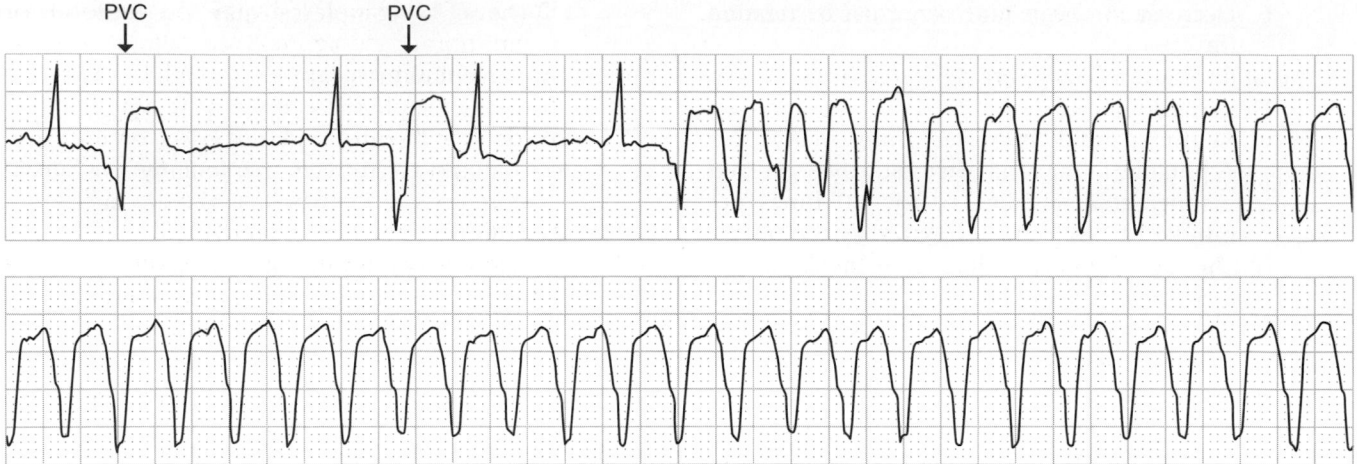

FIG. 57-4   Ventricular tachycardia. Note the PVCs prior to the onset of the tachycardia (second and fourth beats on the strip). The PVC that initiates the tachycardia has the identical morphology (shape) of the first PVC. (From Paul S, Hebra JD: *The nurse's guide to cardiac rhythm interpretation,* Philadelphia, 1998, WB Saunders.)

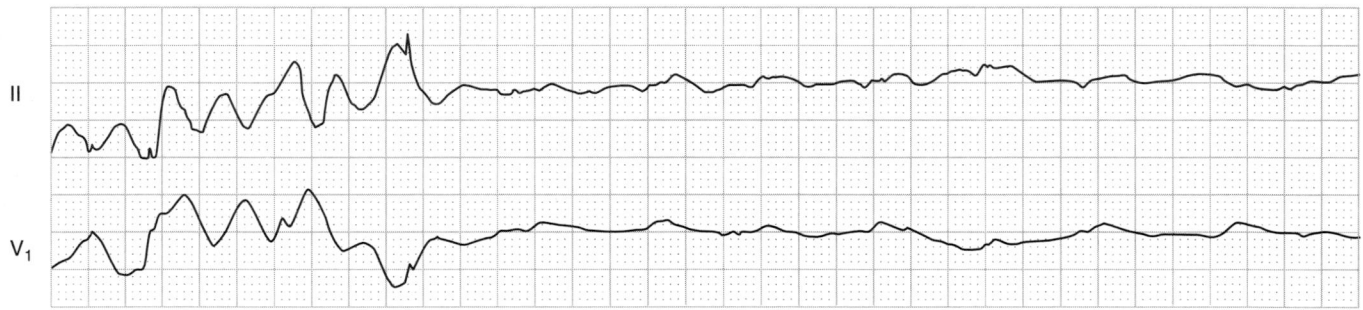

FIG. 57-5   Coarse ventricular fibrillation degenerating into fine ventricular fibrillation. (From Paul S, Hebra JD: *The nurse's guide to cardiac rhythm interpretation,* Philadelphia, 1998, WB Saunders.)

2. Implementation
   a. Defibrillate immediately, up to three times consecutively at 200, 300, and 360 joules
   b. Initiate CPR
   c. Administer oxygen as prescribed
   d. Administer epinephrine (Adrenalin) and antidysrhythmic therapy with lidocaine as prescribed
   e. Prepare to administer additional prescribed antidysrhythmics

V. MANAGEMENT OF DYSRHYTHMIAS
A. Vagal maneuvers
   1. Description: Induce vagal stimulation of the cardiac conduction system; used to terminate supraventricular tachydysrhythmias
   2. Carotid sinus massage
      a. The physician instructs the client to turn the head away from the side to be massaged
      b. The physician massages over the carotid artery

for 6 to 8 seconds until there is a change in cardiac rhythm
   c. Observe the cardiac monitor for a change in rhythm
   d. Record an ECG rhythm strip before, during, and after the procedure
   e. Have a defibrillator and resuscitative equipment available
   f. Monitor VS, cardiac rhythm, and level of consciousness (LOC) following the procedure
3. Valsalva maneuvers
   a. The physician instructs the client to bear down or induces a gag reflex in the client, both of which stimulate a vagal reflex
   b. Monitor the heart rate, rhythm, and **BP**
   c. Observe the cardiac monitor for a change in rhythm
   d. Record an ECG rhythm strip before, during, and after the procedure
   e. Provide an emesis basin if the gag reflex is

stimulated, and initiate precautions to prevent aspiration

    f. Have a defibrillator and resuscitative equipment available

B. Cardioversion

  1. Description

    a. Synchronized countershock to convert an undesirable rhythm to a stable rhythm

    b. An elective procedure performed by the physician

    c. A lower amount of energy is used than with defibrillation

    d. Defibrillator is synchronized to the client's R wave to avoid discharging the shock during the vulnerable period (T wave)

    e. If the defibrillator were not synchronized, it would discharge on the T wave and cause VF

  2. Preprocedure implementation

    a. Obtain consent

    b. Administer sedation as prescribed

    c. Hold digoxin (Lanoxin) 48 hours preprocedure as prescribed to prevent postcardioversion ventricular irritability

  3. During the procedure

    a. Ensure that the skin is clean and dry in the area where the electrode paddles will be placed

    b. Stop the oxygen during the procedure to avoid the hazard of fire

    c. Be sure that no one is touching the bed or the client when delivering the countershock

  4. Postprocedure implementation

    a. Maintain airway patency

    b. Administer oxygen as prescribed

    c. Assess VS

    d. Assess LOC

    e. Monitor cardiac rhythm

    f. Monitor for indications of successful response, such as conversion to sinus rhythm, strong peripheral pulses, and an adequate **BP**

C. Defibrillation

  1. Description

    a. An asynchronous countershock used to terminate pulseless VT or VF

    b. Three rapid consecutive shocks are delivered, with the first at an energy of 200 joules

    c. If unsuccessful, the shock is repeated at 200 to 300 joules

    d. The third and subsequent shock will be at 360 joules

  2. During the procedure

    a. Stop the oxygen during the procedure to avoid the hazard of fire

    b. Be sure that no one is touching the bed or the client when delivering the countershock

D. Use of paddle electrodes

  1. Apply conductive pads

  2. One paddle is placed at the third intercostal space to the right of the sternum; the other is placed at the fifth intercostal space on the left midaxillary line

  3. Apply firm pressure with the paddles

  4. Be sure that no one is touching the bed or the client when delivering the countershock

E. Automatic external defibrillator (AED)

  1. Used by laypersons and emergency medical technicians for prehospital cardiac arrest

  2. Place the client on a firm dry surface

  3. Stop CPR

  4. Ensure that no one is touching the client, to avoid motion artifact during rhythm analysis

  5. Place the electrode paddles in the correct position on the client's chest

  6. Press the analyzer button to identify the rhythm, which may take 30 seconds; the machine will advise whether a shock is necessary

  7. Shocks are recommended for pulseless VF only

  8. If shock is recommended, the shock is initially delivered at an energy of 200 joules

  9. If unsuccessful, the shock is repeated at 200 to 300 joules

  10. The third and subsequent shock will be at 360 joules

  11. If unsuccessful, CPR is continued for 1 minute, and then another series of three shocks is delivered, each at 360 joules of energy

F. Implantable cardioverter defibrillator (ICD)

  1. Description

    a. Monitors cardiac rhythm and detects and terminates episodes of VT and VF

    b. It senses VT or VF and delivers 25 to 30 joules up to four times if necessary

    c. Used in clients with episodes of spontaneous sustained VT or VF unrelated to an MI or in clients whose medication therapy has been unsuccessful in controlling life-threatening dysrhythmias

    d. Electrodes are placed in the right atrium and ventricle and apical pericardium

    e. The generator is implanted in the abdomen

  2. Client education

    a. Basic functioning of the ICD

    b. How to perform cough CPR

    c. How to take the pulse; the pulse is taken daily and a diary of pulse rates is maintained

    d. Wear loose-fitting clothing

    e. Avoid contact sports and strenuous activities

    f. Report any fever, redness, swelling, or drainage from the insertion site

    g. Report symptoms of fainting, nausea, weakness, blackouts, and rapid pulse rates to the physician

    h. During shock discharge, the client may feel faint or short of breath

i. Instruct the client to sit or lie down if he or she feels a shock and to notify the physician

j. Instruct the client and family in how to access emergency medical system

k. Encourage the family to learn CPR

l. Advise the client to maintain a diary of any shocks that are delivered, including the date, preceding activity, the number of shocks, and if the shocks were successful

m. Instruct the client to avoid electromagnetic fields directly over the ICD because they can inactivate the device

n. Instruct the client to move away from the magnetic field immediately if beeping tones are heard, and notify the physician

o. Keep a pacemaker ID in the wallet, and obtain and wear a Medic-Alert bracelet

p. Inform all health care providers that an ICD has been inserted

VI. PACEMAKERS

A. Description: a temporary or permanent device that provides electrical stimulation and maintains the heart rate when the client's intrinsic pacemaker fails to provide a perfusing rhythm

B. Settings

1. Synchronous or demand pacemaker: Senses the client's rhythm and paces only if the client's intrinsic rate falls below the set pacemaker rate

2. Asynchronous or fixed rate: Paces at a preset rate regardless of the client's intrinsic rhythm

3. Overdrive pacing: To suppress the underlying rhythm in tachydysrhythmias so that the sinus node will regain control of the heart

▲ C. Spikes

1. When a pacing stimulus is delivered to the heart, a spike (straight vertical line) is seen on the monitor or ECG strip

2. The spike should be followed by a P wave indicating atrial depolarization, or a QRS complex indicating ventricular depolarization; this pattern is referred to as "capture," indicating that the pacemaker successfully depolarized, or captured, the chamber

3. If the electrode is in the ventricle, the spike is in front of the QRS complex; if the electrode is in the atrium, the spike is before the P wave

4. If the electrode is in both the atrium and the ventricle, the spike is before both the P wave and the QRS complex

D. Temporary pacemakers

1. Noninvasive temporary pacing (NTP)

a. Used as an emergency measure or when a client is being transported and the risk of bradydysrhythmia exists

b. A large electrode patch is placed on the chest and back

c. Wash the skin with soap and water prior to applying electrodes

d. Do not shave the hair or apply alcohol or tinctures to the skin

e. Place the posterior electrode between the spine and left scapula behind the heart, avoiding placement over bone

f. Place the anterior electrode between V_2 and V_5 positions over the heart

g. Do not place the anterior electrode over female breast tissue; rather, displace breast tissue and place under the breast

h. Do not take the pulse or **BP** on the left side; the results will not be accurate because of the muscle twitching and electrical current

i. Ensure that electrodes are in good contact with the skin

j. If loss of "capture" occurs, assess the skin contact of the electrodes and increase the current until "capture" is regained

2. Transvenous invasive temporary pacing

a. Pacing lead wire is placed through antecubital, femoral, jugular, or subclavian vein into the right atrium for atrial pacing, or through the right ventricle, and positioned in contact with the endocardium

b. Monitor cardiac rhythm continuously

c. Monitor vital signs

d. Monitor pacemaker insertion site

e. Restrict client movement to prevent lead wire displacement

3. Epicardial invasive temporary pacing: applied by using a transthoracic approach; the lead wires are loosely threaded on the epicardial surface of the heart after cardiac surgery

4. Reducing the risk of microshock ▲

a. Use only inspected and approved equipment

b. Insulate the exposed portion of wires with plastic or rubber material (fingers of rubber gloves) when wires are not attached to the pulse generator, and cover with nonconductive tape

c. Ground all electrical equipment, using a three-pronged plug

d. Wear gloves when handling exposed wires

e. Keep dressings dry

E. Permanent pacemakers

1. Pulse generator is internal and surgically implanted in a subcutaneous pocket under the clavicle or abdominal wall

2. The leads are passed transvenously via the cephalic or subclavian vein to the endocardium on the right side of the heart

3. May be single chambered, in which the lead wire is placed in the chamber to be paced, or may be dual chambered, with lead wires placed in the atrium and right ventricle

BOX 57-5

Pacemakers: Client Education

Instruct the client about the pacemaker, including the programmed rate

Instruct the client in the signs of battery failure and when to notify the physician

Instruct the client to report any fever, redness, swelling, or drainage from the insertion site

Report signs of dizziness, weakness or fatigue, swelling of the ankles or legs, chest pain, or shortness of breath

Keep a pacemaker identification card in the wallet and obtain and wear a Medic-Alert bracelet

Instruct the client in how to take the pulse, to take the pulse daily, and to maintain a diary of pulse rates

Wear loose-fitting clothing

Avoid contact sports

Inform all health care providers that a pacemaker has been inserted

Instruct the client to inform airport security that he or she has a pacemaker, because the pacemaker may set off the security detector

Instruct the client that most electrical appliances can be used without any interference with the functioning of the pacemaker; however, advise the client not to operate electrical appliances directly over the pacemaker site

Avoid transmitter towers and antitheft devices in stores

Instruct the client that if any unusual feelings occur when near any electrical devices, to move 5 to 10 feet away and check the pulse

Emphasize the importance of follow-up with the physician

4. It is programmed when inserted and can be reprogrammed if necessary by noninvasive transmission from an external programmer to the implanted generator
5. Pacemakers are powered by a lithium battery that has an average life span of 10 years, are nuclear powered with a life span of 20 years or longer, or are designed to be recharged externally
6. Provide client teaching as per Box 57-5

VII. CORONARY ARTERY DISEASE (CAD)

A. Description
   1. A narrowing or obstruction of one or more coronary arteries as a result of atherosclerosis, an accumulation of lipid-containing plaque in the arteries
   2. Causes decreased perfusion of myocardial tissue and inadequate myocardial oxygen supply
   3. Leads to hypertension, angina, dysrhythmias, myocardial infarction, heart failure, and death
   4. Collateral circulation, more than one artery supplying a muscle with blood, is normally present in the coronary arteries, especially in older persons

5. The development of collateral circulation takes time and develops when chronic ischemia occurs, to meet the metabolic demands; therefore, an occlusion of a coronary artery in a younger individual is more likely to be lethal than in an older individual
6. Symptoms occur when the coronary artery is occluded to the point that inadequate blood supply to the muscle occurs, causing ischemia
7. Coronary artery narrowing is significant if the lumen diameter of the left main artery is reduced at least 50%, or if any major branch is reduced at least 75%
8. The goal of treatment is to alter the atherosclerotic progression

B. Assessment
   1. Findings may be normal during asymptomatic periods
   2. Chest pain
   3. Palpitations
   4. Dyspnea
   5. Syncope
   6. Cough or hemoptysis
   7. Excessive fatigue

C. Diagnostic studies
   1. ECG
      a. When blood flow is reduced and ischemia occurs, ST segment depression or T wave inversion is noted; the ST segment returns to normal when the blood flow returns
      b. With infarction, cell injury results in ST segment elevation, followed by T wave inversion
   2. Cardiac catheterization
      a. Provides the most definitive source for diagnosis
      b. Shows the presence of atherosclerotic lesions
   3. Blood lipid levels
      a. May be elevated
      b. Cholesterol-lowering medications may be prescribed to reduce the development of atherosclerotic plaques

D. Implementation
   1. Instruct the client regarding the purpose of diagnostic medical and surgical procedures and the expected preprocedure and postprocedure expectations
   2. Assist the client to identify risk factors that can be modified
   3. Assist the client to set goals to promote lifestyle changes that will reduce the impact of risk factors
   4. Assist the client to identify barriers to compliance with the therapeutic plan and to identify methods to overcome barriers
   5. Instruct the client regarding a low-calorie, low-sodium, low-cholesterol, and low-fat diet, with an increase in dietary fiber

6. Stress to the client that dietary changes are not temporary and must be maintained for life; instruct the client regarding prescribed medications
7. Provide community resources to the client regarding exercise, smoking reduction, and stress reduction

E. Surgical procedures
1. PTCA to compress the plaque against the walls of the artery and dilate the vessel
2. Laser angioplasty to vaporize the plaque
3. Atherectomy to remove the plaque from the artery
4. Vascular stent to prevent the artery from closing and to prevent restenosis
5. Coronary artery bypass graft to improve blood flow to the myocardial tissue that is at risk for ischemia or infarction because of the occluded artery

F. Medications
1. Nitrates to dilate the coronary arteries and to decrease **preload** and **afterload**
2. Calcium channel blockers to dilate coronary arteries and reduce vasospasm
3. Cholesterol-lowering medications to reduce the development of atherosclerotic plaques
4. Beta-blockers to reduce **blood pressure** in individuals who are hypertensive

▲ **VIII. ANGINA**
A. Description
1. Chest pain resulting from myocardial ischemia caused by inadequate myocardial blood and oxygen supply
2. Caused by an imbalance between oxygen supply and demand
3. Causes include obstruction of coronary blood flow because of atherosclerosis, coronary artery spasm, and conditions increasing myocardial oxygen consumption
4. The goal of treatment is to provide relief of an acute attack, correct the imbalance between myocardial oxygen supply and demand, and prevent the progression of the disease and further attacks to reduce the risk of MI

B. Patterns of angina
1. Stable angina
a. Also called exertional angina
b. Occurs with activities that involve exertion or emotional stress, and is relieved with rest or nitroglycerin
c. It usually has a stable pattern of onset, duration, severity, and relieving factors
2. Unstable angina
a. Also called preinfarction angina
b. Occurs with an unpredictable degree of exertion or emotion and increases in occurrence, duration, and severity over time
c. Pain may not be relieved with nitroglycerin

3. Variant angina
a. Also called Prinzmetal's or vasospastic angina
b. Results from coronary artery spasm, is similar to classic angina, but lasts longer
c. May occur at rest
d. Attacks may be associated with ST segment elevation noted on the ECG
4. Intractable angina: A chronic, incapacitating angina that is unresponsive to interventions
5. Preinfarction angina
a. Associated with acute coronary insufficiency
b. Lasts longer than 15 minutes
c. A symptom of worsening cardiac ischemia
6. Postinfarction angina: Occurs after an MI, when residual ischemia may cause episodes of angina

C. Assessment
1. Pain
a. Can develop slowly or quickly
b. Usually described as mild or moderate pain
c. Substernal, crushing, squeezing pain
d. May radiate to the shoulders, arms, jaw, neck, back
e. Usually lasts less than 5 minutes; however, can last up to 15 to 20 minutes
f. Relieved by nitroglycerin or rest
2. Dyspnea
3. Pallor
4. Sweating
5. Palpitations and tachycardia
6. Dizziness and faintness
7. Hypertension
8. Digestive disturbances

D. Diagnostic studies
1. ECG: Normal during rest, with ST depression or elevation and/or T wave inversion during an episode of pain
2. Stress test: Chest pain or changes in the ECG or vital signs during testing may indicate ischemia
3. Cardiac enzymes: Normal findings in angina
4. Cardiac Catheterization: Provides a definitive diagnosis by providing information about the patency of the coronary arteries

E. Implementation   ▲
1. Immediate management
a. Assess pain
b. Provide bed rest
c. Administer oxygen at 3 L by nasal cannula as prescribed
d. Administer nitroglycerin as prescribed to dilate the coronary arteries, reduce the oxygen requirements of the myocardium, and relieve the chest pain
e. Obtain a 12-lead ECG
f. Provide continuous cardiac monitoring
2. Following acute episode   ▲
a. Instruct the client regarding the purpose of diagnostic medical and surgical procedures

and the preprocedure and postprocedure expectations

b. Assist the client to identify angina-precipitating events

c. Instruct the client to stop activity and rest if chest pain occurs and to take nitroglycerin as prescribed

d. Instruct the client to seek medical attention if pain persists

e. Instruct the client regarding prescribed medications

f. Provide diet instructions to the client, stressing that dietary changes are not temporary and must be maintained for life

g. Assist the client to identify risk factors that can be modified

h. Assist the client to set goals that will promote changes in lifestyle to reduce the impact of risk factors

i. Assist the client to identify barriers to compliance with therapeutic plan and to identify methods to overcome barriers

j. Provide community resources to the client regarding exercise, smoking reduction, and stress reduction

F. Surgical procedures: Refer to CAD

G. Medications
   1. Refer to medications to treat CAD
   2. Antiplatelet therapy to inhibit platelet aggregation and reduce the risk of developing an acute MI

▲ IX. MYOCARDIAL INFARCTION (MI)

A. Description
   1. Occurs when myocardial tissue is abruptly and severely deprived of oxygen
   2. Ischemia can lead to necrosis of myocardial tissue if blood flow is not restored
   3. Infarction does not occur instantly but evolves over several hours
   4. Obvious physical changes do not occur in the heart until 6 hours after the infarction, when the infarcted area appears blue and swollen
   5. After 48 hours, the infarct turns gray with yellow streaks as neutrophils invade the tissue
   6. By 8 to 10 days after infarction, granulation tissue forms
   7. Over 2 to 3 months, the necrotic area develops into a scar; scar tissue permanently changes the size and shape of the entire left ventricle

B. Location of MI
   1. Obstruction of the left anterior descending (LAD) artery results in anterior or septal MI or both
   2. Obstruction of the circumflex artery results in posterior wall MI or lateral wall MI
   3. Obstruction of the right coronary artery results in inferior wall MI

C. Risk factors
   1. Atherosclerosis
   2. CAD
   3. Elevated cholesterol levels
   4. Smoking
   5. Hypertension
   6. Obesity
   7. Physical inactivity
   8. Impaired glucose tolerance
   9. Stress

D. Diagnostic studies
   1. Total CK levels
      a. Rise within 3 hours after the onset of chest pain
      b. Peak within 24 hours after damage and death of cardiac tissue
   2. CK-MB isoenzyme
      a. Peak elevation occurs 12 to 24 hours after the onset of chest pain
      b. Levels return to normal 48 to 72 hours later
   3. Troponin levels
      a. Rise within 3 hours
      b. Remain elevated for up to 7 days
   4. Myoglobin: Rises within 1 hour after cell death, peaks in 4 to 6 hours, and returns to normal within 24 to 36 hours or less
   5. LDH levels
      a. Rise within 12 to 24 hours after MI
      b. Peak between 40 and 72 hours and fall to normal in 7 days
      c. Serum levels of LDH_1 isoenzyme rise higher than serum levels of LDH_2
   6. WBC count: an elevated white blood cell count of 10,000 to 20,000 cells/mm^3 appears on the second day following the MI and lasts up to a week
   7. ECG
      a. ST segment elevation, T wave inversion, abnormal Q wave
      b. Hours to days after the MI, ST and T wave changes will return to normal but the Q wave usually remains permanently
   8. Diagnostic tests following the acute stage
      a. Exercise tolerance test or stress test may be prescribed to assess for ECG changes and ischemia and to evaluate for medical therapy or identify clients who may need invasive therapy
      b. Thallium scans may be prescribed to assess for ischemia or necrotic muscle tissue
      c. MUGA scans: May be used to evaluate left ventricular function
      d. Cardiac catheterization: Performed to determine the extent and location of obstructions of the coronary arteries

E. Assessment
   1. Pain
      a. Crushing substernal pain

b. May radiate to the jaw, back, and left arm

c. Occurs without cause, primarily early in the morning

d. Is unrelieved by rest or nitroglycerin, and relieved only by opioids

e. Lasts 30 minutes or longer

2. Nausea and vomiting

3. Diaphoresis

4. Dyspnea

5. Dysrhythmias

6. Feelings of fear and anxiety

7. Pallor, cyanosis, coolness of extremities

F. Complications of MI

1. Dysrhythmias

2. Heart failure

3. Pulmonary edema

4. Cardiogenic shock

5. Thrombophlebitis

6. Pericarditis

7. Mitral valve insufficiency

8. Postinfarction angina

9. Ventricular rupture

10. Dressler's syndrome (a combination of pericarditis, pericardial effusion, and pleural effusion, which can occur several weeks to months following an MI)

G. Implementation, acute stage

1. Obtain a description of the chest discomfort

2. Assess vital signs

3. Assess cardiovascular status and maintain cardiac monitoring

4. Obtain a 12-lead ECG

5. Administer nitroglycerin as prescribed

6. Administer morphine sulfate as prescribed to relieve chest discomfort that is unresponsive to nitroglycerin

7. Administer oxygen at 2 to 4 liters by nasal cannula as prescribed

8. Place the client in semi-Fowler's position to enhance comfort and tissue oxygenation

9. Establish an IV access route

10. Administer IV nitroglycerin and antidysrhythmics as prescribed

11. Monitor thrombolytic therapy, which may be prescribed within the first 6 hours of the coronary event

12. Monitor for signs of bleeding if the client is receiving thrombolytics

13. Monitor laboratory values as prescribed

14. Administer beta-blockers to slow the heart rate and increase myocardial perfusion, while reducing the force of myocardial contraction, as prescribed

15. Monitor for complications related to the MI

16. Monitor for cardiac dysrhythmias, since tachycardia and PVCs frequently occur in the first few hours after MI

17. Assess distal peripheral pulses and skin temperature, since poor **cardiac output** may be identified by cool diaphoretic skin and diminished or absent pulses

18. Monitor I & O

19. Assess respiratory rate and breath sounds for signs of heart failure, as indicated by the presence of crackles or wheezes or dependent edema

20. Monitor the **BP** closely after the administration of medications; if the **BP** is less than 100 systolic or 25 mm Hg lower than the previous reading, lower the head of the bed and notify the physician

21. Provide reassurance to the client and family

H. Implementation following acute episode

1. Maintain bed rest for the first 24 to 36 hours

2. Allow the client to stand to void or use a bedside commode if prescribed

3. Provide range-of-motion exercises to prevent thrombus formation and maintain muscle strength

4. Progress to dangling at the side of the bed or out of bed to the chair for 30 minutes three times a day as prescribed

5. Progress to ambulation in the client's room and to the bathroom, and then in the hallway, three times a day

6. Monitor for complications

7. Encourage the client to verbalize feelings regarding the MI

I. Cardiac rehabilitation: Process of actively assisting the client with cardiac disease to achieve and maintain a vital and productive life within the limitations of the heart disease

X. HEART FAILURE

A. Description

1. The inability of the heart to maintain adequate circulation to meet the metabolic needs of the body, because of an impaired pumping capability

2. **Cardiac output** is diminished, and peripheral tissue is not adequately perfused

3. Congestion of the lungs and periphery may occur

B. Classification

1. Acute: Occurs suddenly

2. Chronic: Develops over time; however, a client with chronic heart failure can develop an acute episode

C. Types of heart failure

1. Right-sided heart failure/left-sided heart failure

a. Because the two ventricles of the heart represent two separate pumping systems, it is possible for one to fail alone for a short period

b. Most heart failure begins with left ventricular failure and progresses to failure of both ventricles

c. Acute pulmonary edema, a medical emergency, results from left ventricular failure

d. If pulmonary edema is not treated, death will occur from suffocation as the client literally drowns in own fluids

2. Forward failure/backward failure

a. In forward failure, an inadequate output of the affected ventricle causes decreased perfusion to vital organs

b. In backward failure, blood backs up behind the affected ventricle, causing increased pressure in the atrium behind the affected ventricle

3. Low output/high output

a. In low-output failure, not enough **cardiac output** is available to meet the demands of the body

b. High-output failure occurs when a condition causes the heart to work harder to meet the demands of the body

4. Systolic failure/diastolic failure

a. Systolic failure leads to problems with contraction and the ejection of blood

b. Diastolic failure leads to problems with the heart relaxing and filling with blood

D. Compensatory mechanisms

1. Act to restore **cardiac output** to near-normal levels

2. Initially these mechanisms increase **cardiac output;** however, they eventually have a damaging effect on pump action

3. Contribute to an increase in myocardial oxygen consumption, and when this occurs, myocardial reserve is exhausted and clinical manifestations of heart failure develop

4. Include increased heart rate, improved **stroke volume,** arterial vasoconstriction, sodium and water retention, and myocardial hypertrophy

E. Assessment

1. Right-sided heart failure

a. Signs of right-sided failure will be evident in the systemic circulation

b. Pitting, dependent edema in the feet, legs, sacrum, back, buttocks

c. Ascites from portal hypertension

d. Tenderness of right upper quadrant, organomegaly

e. Distended neck veins

f. Pulsus alternans (regular alteration of weak and strong beats noted in the pulse)

g. Abdominal pain, bloating

h. Anorexia, nausea

i. Fatigue

j. Weight gain

k. Nocturnal diuresis

2. Left-sided heart failure

a. Signs of left-sided failure will be evident in the pulmonary system

b. Cough, which may become productive with frothy sputum

c. Dyspnea upon exertion

d. Orthopnea

e. Paroxysmal nocturnal dyspnea

f. Presence of rales or crackles on auscultation

g. Tachycardia

h. Pulsus alternans

i. Fatigue

j. Pallor

k. Cyanosis

l. Confusion and disorientation

m. Signs of cerebral anoxia

3. Acute pulmonary edema

a. Severe dyspnea and orthopnea

b. Pallor

c. Tachycardia

d. Expectoration of large amounts of blood-tinged, frothy sputum

e. Wheezing and rales

f. Bubbling respirations

g. Acute anxiety, apprehension, restlessness

h. Profuse sweating

i. Cold, clammy skin

j. Cyanosis

k. Nasal flaring

l. Use of accessory breathing muscles

m. Tachypnea

n. Hypocapnia, evidenced by muscle cramps, weakness, dizziness, and paresthesias

F. Immediate management

1. Place the client in high Fowler's position, with the legs in a dependent position, to reduce pulmonary congestion and relieve edema

2. Administer oxygen in high concentrations by mask or cannula, as prescribed, to improve gas exchange and pulmonary function

3. Prepare for intubation and ventilator support if required; monitor lung sounds for rales and decreased breath sounds

4. Suction as needed to maintain a patent airway

5. Assess level of consciousness

6. Provide reassurance to the client

7. Monitor vital signs closely, noting tachycardia or pulsus alternans

8. Monitor for hypotension resulting from decreased tissue perfusion, or hypertension resulting from anxiety or history of hypertension

9. Monitor heart rate and dysrhythmias by using a cardiac monitor

10. Assess for edema in dependent areas and in the sacral, lumbar, and posterior thigh region in the client on bed rest

11. Insert a Foley catheter as prescribed and monitor urine output closely following administration of a diuretic

12. Monitor I & O

13. Avoid the administration of unnecessary IV fluids
14. Administer morphine sulfate as prescribed to provide sedation and vasodilation, and monitor for respiratory depression or hypotension after administration
15. Administer diuretics as prescribed to reduce **preload,** enhance renal excretion of sodium and water, reduce circulating blood volume, and reduce pulmonary congestion
16. Administer digitalis as prescribed to increase ventricular **contractility** and improve **cardiac output**
17. Administer bronchodilators as prescribed for severe bronchospasm or bronchoconstriction
18. Administer additional inotropic medications, such as dopamine (Intropin) or dobutamine (Dobutrex), as prescribed, to facilitate myocardial **contractility** and enhance **stroke volume**
19. Administer vasodilators as prescribed to reduce **afterload,** increase the capacity of the systemic venous bed, and decrease venous return to the heart
20. Monitor weight to determine a response to treatment
21. Assess for hepatomegaly and ascites, and measure and record abdominal girth
22. Monitor peripheral pulses
23. Analyze arterial blood gas results, and evaluate electrolyte values for imbalances
24. Monitor potassium level closely, which may decrease as a result of diuretic therapy, and administer potassium supplements as prescribed to prevent digitalis toxicity

G. Following the acute episode
   1. Encourage the client to verbalize feelings about the lifestyle changes required as a result of the heart failure
   2. Assist the client to identify precipitating risk factors of heart failure and methods of eliminating these risk factors
   3. Instruct the client in the prescribed medication regimen, which may include digoxin (Lanoxin), a diuretic, and vasodilators
   4. Advise the client to notify the physician if side effects occur from the medications
   5. Advise the client to avoid over-the-counter medications
   6. Instruct the client to contact the physician if he or she is unable to take medications because of illness
   7. Instruct the client to avoid large amounts of caffeine, found in coffee, tea, cocoa, chocolate, and some carbonated beverages
   8. Instruct the client about the prescribed low-sodium, low-fat, and low-cholesterol diet
   9. Provide the client with a list of potassium-rich foods, since diuretics will cause hypokalemia (except for potassium-sparing diuretics)
   10. Instruct the client regarding fluid restriction, if prescribed, advising the client to spread the fluid out during the day, and to suck on hard candy to reduce thirst
   11. Instruct the client to space periods of activity and rest
   12. Advise the client to avoid isometric activities, which increase pressure in the heart
   13. Instruct the client to monitor daily weight
   14. Instruct the client to report signs of fluid retention, such as edema or weight gain

XI. CARDIOGENIC SHOCK

A. Description
   1. Failure of the heart to pump adequately, thereby reducing **cardiac output** and compromising tissue perfusion
   2. Necrosis of more than 40% of the left ventricle occurs, usually as a result of occlusion of major coronary vessels
   3. The goal of treatment is to maintain tissue oxygenation and perfusion and improve the pumping ability of the heart

B. Assessment
   1. Hypotension: **BP** less than 90 mm Hg systolic or 30 mm Hg less than the client's baseline
   2. Urine output of less than 30 mL/hr
   3. Cold, clammy skin
   4. Poor peripheral pulses
   5. Tachycardia
   6. Pulmonary congestion
   7. Tachypnea
   8. Disorientation, restlessness, and confusion
   9. Continuing chest discomfort

C. Implementation
   1. Administer IV morphine sulfate as prescribed to decrease pulmonary congestion and relieve pain
   2. Administer oxygen as prescribed
   3. Prepare for intubation and mechanical ventilation
   4. Administer diuretics and nitrates as prescribed while monitoring **blood pressure** constantly
   5. Administer vasopressors and positive inotropics as prescribed to maintain organ perfusion
   6. Prepare the client for insertion of an intraaortic balloon pump (IABP), if prescribed, to facilitate emptying of the left ventricle and improve **cardiac output**
   7. Prepare the client for immediate reperfusion procedures such as PTCA or CABG
   8. Monitor arterial blood gas levels and prepare to treat imbalances
   9. Monitor urinary output
   10. Assist with the insertion of Swan-Ganz catheter to assess heart failure

11. Monitor distal pulses and maintain the transducer at the level of the right atrium if the client has Swan-Ganz catheter

XII. INFLAMMATORY DISEASES OF THE HEART

A. Pericarditis
   1. Description
      a. An acute or chronic inflammation of the pericardium
      b. Chronic pericarditis, a chronic inflammatory thickening of the pericardium, constricts the heart, causing compression
      c. The pericardial sac becomes inflamed
      d. Can result in loss of pericardial elasticity or an accumulation of fluid within the sac
      e. Heart failure or cardiac tamponade may result
   2. Assessment
      a. Precordial pain in the anterior chest that radiates to the left side of the neck, shoulder, or back
      b. Pain that is aggravated by breathing (particularly inspiration), coughing, and swallowing
      c. Pain is worse when in the supine position and may be relieved by leaning forward
      d. Pericardial friction rub (scratchy, high-pitched sound) heard on auscultation; produced by the rubbing of the inflamed pericardial layers
      e. Fever and chills
      f. Fatigue and malaise
      g. Elevated WBC count
      h. ECG changes
      i. Signs of right-sided heart failure in clients with chronic constrictive pericarditis
   3. Implementation
      a. Assess the nature of the pain
      b. Position the client side-lying, high Fowler's, or upright and leaning forward
      c. Administer analgesics, nonsteroidal antiinflammatory drugs (NSAIDs), or corticosteroids for pain as prescribed
      d. Avoid the administration of aspirin and anticoagulants because they increase the risk of tamponade
      e. Auscultate for a pericardial friction rub
      f. Evaluate the blood culture report
      g. Administer antibiotics for bacterial infection as prescribed
      h. Administer diuretics and digoxin (Lanoxin) as prescribed to the client with chronic constrictive pericarditis
      i. Monitor for signs of cardiac tamponade, including pulsus paradoxus, jugular vein distention with clear lung sounds, muffled heart sounds, narrowed **pulse pressure**, tachycardia, and decreased **cardiac output**
      j. Notify the physician if signs of cardiac tamponade occur

B. Myocarditis
   1. Description: an acute or chronic inflammation of the myocardium as a result of pericarditis, systemic infection, or allergic response
   2. Assessment
      a. Fever
      b. Pericardial friction rub
      c. A gallop rhythm
      d. A murmur that sounds like fluid passing an obstruction
      e. Pulsus alternans
      f. Signs of heart failure
      g. Fatigue
      h. Dyspnea
      i. Tachycardia
      j. Chest pain
   3. Implementation
      a. Assist the client to a position of comfort, such as sitting up and leaning forward
      b. Administer analgesics, salicylates, NSAIDs as prescribed, to reduce fever and pain
      c. Administer oxygen as prescribed
      d. Provide adequate rest periods
      e. Limit activities to avoid overexertion and to decrease the workload of the heart
      f. Administer digoxin (Lanoxin) as prescribed, and monitor for signs of digoxin toxicity
      g. Administer antidysrhythmics as prescribed
      h. Administer antibiotics as prescribed to treat the causative organism
      i. Monitor for complications, which can include thrombus, heart failure, or cardiomyopathy

C. **Endocarditis**
   1. Description
      a. An inflammation of the inner lining of the heart and valves
      b. Occurs primarily in clients who are IV drug abusers, have had valve replacements, or have mitral valve prolapse or other structural defects
      c. Ports of entry for the infecting organism include the oral cavity (especially if the client had a dental procedure in the previous 3 to 6 months), cutaneous invasion, infections, or invasive procedures or surgery
   2. Assessment
      a. Fever
      b. Anorexia
      c. Weight loss
      d. Fatigue
      e. Cardiac murmurs
      f. Heart failure
      g. Embolic complications from vegetation fragments traveling through the circulation
      h. Petechiae
      i. Splinter hemorrhages in the nailbeds
      j. Osler's nodes (reddish tender lesions) on the pads of the fingers, hands, and toes

k. Janeway's lesions (nontender hemorrhagic lesions) on the fingers, toes, nose, or earlobes
l. Splenomegaly
m. Clubbing of the fingers
3. Implementation
   a. Provide adequate rest balanced with activity to prevent thrombus formation
   b. Maintain antiembolism stockings
   c. Monitor cardiovascular status
   d. Monitor for signs of heart failure
   e. Monitor for signs of emboli
   f. Monitor for splenic emboli, as evidenced by sudden abdominal pain radiating to the left shoulder, and the presence of rebound abdominal tenderness on palpation
   g. Monitor for renal emboli, as evidenced by flank pain radiating to the groin, hematuria, and pyuria
   h. Monitor for confusion, aphasia, or dysphagia, which may be indicative of CNS emboli
   i. Monitor for pulmonary emboli as evidenced by pleuritic chest pain, dyspnea, and cough
   j. Assess skin, mucous membranes, and conjunctiva for petechiae
   k. Assess nailbeds for splinter hemorrhages
   l. Assess for Osler's nodes on the pads of the fingers, hands, and toes
   m. Assess for Janeway's lesions on the fingers, toes, nose, or earlobes
   n. Assess for clubbing of the fingers
   o. Evaluate blood culture results
   p. Administer IV antibiotic as prescribed
   q. Plan and arrange for discharge, providing resources required for the continued administration of IV antibiotics
4. Client education
   a. Instruct the client about the signs and symptoms of complications and to notify the physician if they occur
   b. Inform the client about the importance of good oral hygiene
   c. Instruct the client to brush teeth twice daily with a soft toothbrush, followed by oral rinses
   d. Instruct the client to avoid irrigation devices, electric toothbrushes, and flossing, because these activities can cause the gums to bleed, allowing bacteria to enter the mucous membranes and bloodstream
   e. Advise the client of the importance of prophylactic antibiotics prior to any invasive procedure and the importance of informing all health care professionals of his or her disease history

▲ **XIII. CARDIAC TAMPONADE**
A. Description
   1. A pericardial effusion occurs when the space between the parietal and visceral layers of the pericardium fill with fluid
   2. Pericardial effusion places the client at risk for cardiac tamponade, an accumulation of fluid in the pericardial cavity
   3. Tamponade restricts ventricular filling, and **cardiac output** drops
   4. Acute tamponade occurs when small volumes (20 to 50 mL) of fluid accumulate in the pericardium
B. Assessment
   1. Pulsus paradoxus
   2. Increased CVP
   3. Jugular venous distention with clear lungs
   4. Distant, muffled heart sounds
   5. Decreased **cardiac output**
C. Implementation
   1. The client needs to be placed in a critical care unit for hemodynamic monitoring
   2. Administer IV fluids as prescribed to manage decreased **cardiac output**
   3. Prepare the client for chest x-ray film or echocardiogram
   4. Prepare the client for pericardiocentesis to withdraw pericardial fluid if prescribed
   5. Monitor for recurrence of tamponade following pericardiocentesis
   6. If the client experiences recurrent tamponade or recurrent effusions, or develops adhesions from chronic pericarditis, a portion (pericardial window) or all of the pericardium (pericardiectomy) may be removed to allow adequate ventricular filling and contraction

XIV. VALVULAR HEART DISEASE
A. Description
   1. Occurs when the heart valves cannot fully open (stenosis) or close completely (insufficiency or regurgitation)
   2. Prevents efficient blood flow through the heart
B. Types
   1. Mitral stenosis: Valvular tissue thickens and narrows the valve opening
   2. Mitral insufficiency/regurgitation: Valve is incompetent, preventing complete valve closure
   3. Mitral valve prolapse: Valve leaflets protrude into the left atrium during **systole**
   4. Aortic stenosis: Valvular tissue thickens and narrows the valve opening
   5. Aortic insufficiency: Valve is incompetent, preventing complete valve closure
C. Repair procedures
   1. Balloon valvuloplasty
      a. An invasive, nonsurgical procedure
      b. The passage of a balloon catheter from the femoral vein through the atrial septum to the mitral valve, or through the femoral artery to the aortic valve

c. The balloon is inflated to enlarge the orifice

d. Institute precautions for arterial puncture if appropriate

e. Monitor for bleeding from the catheter insertion site

f. Monitor for signs of systemic emboli

g. Monitor for signs of a regurgitant valve by monitoring cardiac rhythm, heart sounds, and **cardiac output**

2. Mitral annuloplasty: tightening and suturing the malfunctioning valve annulus to eliminate or markedly reduce regurgitation

3. Commissurotomy/valvotomy

a. Accomplished with cardiopulmonary bypass during open heart surgery

b. The valve is visualized, thrombi are removed from the atria, fused leaflets are incised, and calcium is debrided from the leaflets, thus widening the orifice

D. Valve replacement procedures

1. Mechanical prosthetic valves

a. Prosthetic valves are very durable but can fail

b. Thromboembolism is a problem following the valve replacement, and lifetime anticoagulant therapy is required

2. Bioprosthetic valves

a. Biological grafts are xenografts (valves from other species): porcine valves (pig), bovine valves (cow); or homografts (human cadavers)

b. There is little risk of clot formation; therefore, long-term anticoagulation is not indicated

3. Preoperative implementation: Consult with the physician regarding discontinuing anticoagulants 72 hours prior to surgery

4. Postoperative implementation

a. Monitor closely for signs of bleeding

b. Monitor **cardiac output** and for signs of heart failure

c. Administer digoxin (Lanoxin) as prescribed to maintain **cardiac output** and prevent atrial fibrillation

d. Provide client teaching (Box 57-6)

E. Mitral stenosis

1. Assessment

a. Asymptomatic initially

b. Symptoms occur when the orifice is reduced by 50%

c. Dyspnea

d. Orthopnea

e. Paroxysmal nocturnal dyspnea

f. Dry cough

g. Rumbling apical diastolic murmur

h. Right-sided heart failure

i. Hepatomegaly

j. Neck vein distention

k. Pitting peripheral edema

BOX 57-6

Client Instructions Following Valve Replacement

Adequate rest is important and fatigue is usual

Need for anticoagulant therapy if a mechanical prosthetic valve was inserted

Hazards related to anticoagulant therapy and to notify the physician if bleeding or excessive bruising occurs

Importance of good oral hygiene to reduce the risk of infective endocarditis

Brush teeth twice daily with a soft toothbrush, followed by oral rinses

Avoid irrigation devices, electric toothbrushes, and flossing, because these activities can cause the gums to bleed, allowing bacteria to enter the mucous membranes and bloodstream

Monitor incision and report any drainage or redness

Avoid any dental procedures for 6 months

Heavy lifting (greater than 10 pounds) is to be avoided, and exercise caution when in an automobile to prevent injury to the sternal incision

If a prosthetic valve was inserted, a soft audible clicking sound may be heard

Importance of prophylactic antibiotics prior to any invasive procedure and the importance of informing all health care professionals of the valvular disease history

Obtain and wear a Medic-Alert bracelet

---

l. Hemoptysis and pulmonary edema as pulmonary hypertension and congestion progress

m. Development of atrial fibrillation, indicating that the client may decompensate (notify physician immediately)

2. Implementation

a. Administer prescribed treatment for heart failure

b. Administer oxygen as prescribed

c. Provide a low-sodium diet

d. Administer diuretics and digoxin (Lanoxin) as prescribed

e. Administer antibiotics as prescribed if infective endocarditis is present

f. Administer antidysrhythmics and anticoagulants for atrial fibrillation, as prescribed

g. Prepare the client for commissurotomy or valve replacement as indicated

F. Mitral valve prolapse

1. Assessment

a. Fatigue

b. Atypical chest pain

c. Palpitations

d. Dizziness and syncope

e. Tachycardia

f. Systolic click

2. Implementation

a. Administer propranolol (Inderal) for dyspnea and chest pain as prescribed

b. Administer prophylactic antibiotics as prescribed

G. Mitral insufficiency
1. Assessment
   a. Dyspnea
   b. Orthopnea
   c. Fatigue
   d. Dizziness
   e. Palpitations
   f. Signs of right-sided heart failure
   g. Atrial fibrillation
   h. Neck vein distention
   i. Pitting peripheral edema
   j. High-pitched systolic murmur
2. Implementation
   a. Administer prescribed treatment for heart failure
   b. Administer oxygen as prescribed
   c. Provide a low-sodium diet
   d. Administer diuretics and digoxin (Lanoxin) as prescribed
   e. Administer antibiotics as prescribed if infective endocarditis is present
   f. Administer antidysrhythmics and anticoagulants for atrial fibrillation, as prescribed
   g. Prepare the client for commissurotomy or valve replacement as indicated

H. Aortic stenosis
1. Assessment
   a. Dyspnea on exertion
   b. Angina
   c. Syncope on exertion
   d. Fatigue
   e. Orthopnea
   f. Paroxysmal nocturnal dyspnea
   g. Harsh systolic crescendo-decrescendo murmur
2. Implementation
   a. Administer prescribed treatment for heart failure
   b. Administer oxygen as prescribed
   c. Provide a low-sodium diet
   d. Administer diuretics and digoxin (Lanoxin) as prescribed
   e. Administer antibiotics as prescribed if infective endocarditis is present
   f. Prepare the client for valve replacement, as indicated

I. Aortic insufficiency
1. Assessment
   a. Dyspnea
   b. Orthopnea
   c. Paroxysmal nocturnal dyspnea
   d. Fatigue
   e. Angina
   f. Tachycardia
   g. Blowing decresendo diastolic murmur

2. Implementation
   a. Administer prescribed treatment for heart failure
   b. Administer oxygen as prescribed
   c. Provide a low-sodium diet
   d. Administer diuretics and digoxin (Lanoxin) as prescribed
   e. Administer antibiotics as prescribed if infective endocarditis is present
   f. Prepare the client for valve replacement, as indicated

J. Tricuspid stenosis
1. Assessment
   a. Easily fatigued
   b. Effort intolerance
   c. Complaint of fluttering sensations in the neck (obstructed venous flow)
   d. Cyanosis
   e. Signs of right-sided heart failure
   f. Symptoms of decreased **cardiac output**
   g. Ascites
   h. Hepatomegaly
   i. Peripheral edema
   j. Rumbling diastolic murmur
   k. Jugular vein distention with clear lung fields
2. Implementation
   a. Administer prescribed treatment for heart failure
   b. Administer oxygen as prescribed
   c. Provide a low-sodium diet
   d. Administer diuretics and digoxin (Lanoxin) as prescribed
   e. Administer antibiotics as prescribed if infective endocarditis is present
   f. Prepare the client for valve replacement, as indicated

K. Tricuspid insufficiency
1. Assessment
   a. Asymptomatic in mild situations
   b. Signs of right-sided heart failure
   c. Ascites
   d. Hepatomegaly
   e. Pleural effusion
   f. Peripheral edema
   g. Systolic murmur heard at the left sternal border, fourth intercostal space
2. Implementation
   a. Administer prescribed treatment for heart failure
   b. Administer oxygen as prescribed
   c. Provide a low-sodium diet
   d. Administer diuretics and digoxin (Lanoxin) as prescribed
   e. Administer antibiotics as prescribed if infective endocarditis is present
   f. Prepare the client for valve replacement, as indicated

L. Pulmonary stenosis
   1. Assessment
      a. Asymptomatic in a mild condition
      b. Dyspnea
      c. Fatigue
      d. Syncope
      e. Signs of right-sided heart failure
      f. Ascites
      g. Hepatomegaly
      h. Peripheral edema
      i. Systolic thrill heard at left sternal border
   2. Implementation
      a. Administer prescribed treatment for heart failure
      b. Administer oxygen as prescribed
      c. Provide a low-sodium diet
      d. Administer diuretics and digoxin (Lanoxin) as prescribed
      e. Administer antibiotics as prescribed if infective endocarditis is present
      f. Prepare the client for pulmonary valve commissurotomy, as indicated
M. Pulmonary insufficiency
   1. Assessment
      a. Asymptomatic in mild condition
      b. Dyspnea
      c. Fatigue
      d. Syncope
      e. Signs of right-sided heart failure
      f. Ascites
      g. Hepatomegaly
      h. Peripheral edema
      i. Systolic thrill heard at the left sternal border
   2. Implementation
      a. Administer prescribed treatment for heart failure
      b. Administer oxygen as prescribed
      c. Provide a low-sodium diet
      d. Administer diuretics and digoxin (Lanoxin) as prescribed
      e. Administer antibiotics as prescribed if infective endocarditis is present
      f. Prepare the client for valve replacement, as indicated

XV. CARDIOMYOPATHY
A. Description
   1. A subacute or chronic disorder of the heart muscle
   2. Treatment is palliative, not curative, and the client needs to deal with numerous lifestyle changes and a shortened life span
B. Dilated cardiomyopathy (DCM)
   1. Description
      a. Most common type
      b. Heart ejects less than 40% of the blood in the left ventricle (normal is 70%), and reduced **cardiac output** leads to heart failure
   2. Assessment
      a. Symptoms of left ventricular heart failure
      b. Weakness and fatigue
      c. Activity intolerance
      d. Chest pain
      e. Dysrhythmias
      f. Eventually signs of right-sided heart failure
   3. Implementation
      a. Symptomatic treatment of heart failure
      b. Diuretics, cardiac glycosides, and vasodilators to increase **cardiac output**
      c. Antidysrhythmics to control dysrhythmias
      d. Instruct the client to report any signs of dizziness or fainting, which may indicate a dysrhythmia
      e. Instruct the client to avoid ingestion of alcohol because of its cardiac depressant effect
      f. Heart transplant
C. Hypertropic cardiomyopathy (HCM)
   1. Description
      a. Characterized by massive ventricular hypertrophy, leading to hypercontraction of the left ventricle and rigid ventricle walls
      b. Causes obstruction of the left ventricular outflow
   2. Assessment
      a. Exertional dyspnea
      b. Syncope
      c. Chest pain that occurs at rest, is prolonged, is unrelated to exertion, and is not relieved by nitrates
      d. Dysrhythmias
   3. Implementation
      a. Symptomatic treatment, similar to the care of a client with MI
      b. Conversion of atrial fibrillation if it occurs
      c. Instruct the client to report any signs of dizziness or fainting, which may indicate a dysrhythmia
      d. Instruct the client to avoid ingestion of alcohol because of its cardiac depressant effect
      e. Beta-blockers and calcium antagonists to decrease the outflow obstruction and decrease the heart rate
      f. Vasodilators and cardiac glycosides are contraindicated because vasodilator and positive inotropic effects augment the obstruction
      g. Ventriculomyotomy or muscle resection with mitral valve replacement
D. Restrictive cardiomyopathy
   1. Description: Characterized by restriction of filling of the ventricles
   2. Assessment
      a. Exertional dyspnea
      b. Weakness
   3. Implementation
      a. Symptomatic treatment of heart failure

b. Exercise restriction

c. Diuretics, cardiac glycosides, and vasodilators to increase **cardiac output**

d. Antidysrhythmics to control dysrhythmias

e. Instruct the client to report any signs of dizziness or fainting, which may indicate a dysrhythmia

f. Instruct the client to avoid ingestion of alcohol because of its cardiac depressant effect

XVI. VASCULAR DISORDERS

A. Venous thrombosis
 1. Description
  a. Thrombus can be associated with an inflammatory process
  b. When a thrombus develops, inflammation occurs, thickening the vein wall and leading to embolization
 2. Types
  a. Thrombophlebitis: A thrombus associated with inflammation
  b. Phlebothrombus: A thrombus without inflammation
  c. Phlebitis: Vein inflammation associated with invasive procedures such as IVs
  d. Deep vein thrombophlebitis (DVT): More serious than a superficial thrombophlebitis because of the risk for pulmonary embolism
 3. Risks factors for thrombus formation
  a. Venous stasis from varicose veins, heart failure, immobility
  b. Hypercoagulability disorders
  c. Injury to the venous wall from IV injections, fractures, trauma
  d. Following surgery, particularly hip surgery and open prostate surgery
  e. Pregnancy
  f. Ulcerative colitis
  g. Use of oral contraceptives
▲ B. Phlebitis
▲ 1. Assessment
  a. Red, warm area radiating up an extremity
  b. Pain and soreness
  c. Swelling
 2. Implementation
  a. Apply warm moist soaks as prescribed to dilate the vein and promote circulation
  b. Assess temperature of soak prior to applying
  c. Assess for signs of complications, such as tissue necrosis, infection, or pulmonary embolus
▲ C. Deep vein thrombophlebitis (DVT)
▲ 1. Assessment
  a. Calf or groin tenderness or pain with or without swelling
  b. Positive Homans' sign
  c. Warm skin that is tender to touch

2. Implementation
 a. Provide bed rest
 b. Elevate the affected extremity above the level ▲ of the heart as prescribed
 c. Avoid using the knee gatch or a pillow under ▲ the knees
 d. Do not massage the extremity ▲
 e. Provide thigh-high compression or antiembolism stockings as prescribed to reduce venous stasis and to assist in the venous return of blood to the heart
 f. Administer intermittent or continuous warm, moist compresses as prescribed
 g. Palpate the site gently, monitoring for warmth and edema
 h. Measure and record the circumferences of the thighs and calves
 i. Monitor for shortness of breath and chest pain, which can indicate pulmonary emboli
 j. Administer thrombolytic therapy (t-PA, tissue plasminogen activator) if prescribed, which must be initiated within 5 days after the onset of symptoms
 k. Administer heparin therapy as prescribed to prevent enlargement of the existing clot and prevent the formation of new clots
 l. Monitor APTT during heparin therapy
 m. Administer warfarin (Coumadin) as prescribed when the symptoms of DVT have resolved
 n. Monitor PT and INR during warfarin (Coumadin) therapy
 o. Monitor for the hazards and side effects associated with anticoagulant therapy
 p. Administer analgesics as prescribed to reduce pain
 q. Administer diuretics as prescribed to reduce lower extremity edema
 r. Provide client teaching (Box 57-7)
D. Venous insufficiency
 1. Description
  a. Results from prolonged venous hypertension, which stretches the veins and damages the valves
  b. The resultant edema and venous stasis cause venous stasis ulcers, swelling, and cellulitis
  c. Treatment focuses on decreasing edema and promoting venous return from the affected extremity
  d. Treatment for venous stasis ulcers focuses on healing the ulcer and preventing stasis and ulcer recurrence
 2. Assessment
  a. Stasis dermatitis or discoloration along the ankles and extending up to the calf
  b. Edema
  c. The presence of ulcer formation

Instructions for the Client with DVT

Hazards of anticoagulation therapy
Recognize the signs and symptoms of bleeding
Avoid prolonged sitting or standing, constrictive clothing, or crossing legs when seated
Elevate the legs for 10 to 20 minutes every few hours each day
Plan a progressive walking program
Inspect the legs for edema, and measure the circumference of the legs
Antiembolism stockings as prescribed
Avoid smoking
Avoid any medications unless prescribed by the physician
Importance of follow-up physician visits and laboratory studies
Obtain and wear a Medic-Alert bracelet

3. Implementation
   a. Instruct the client to wear elastic or compression stockings during the day and evening as prescribed
   b. Instruct the client to put elastic stockings on upon awakening before getting out of bed
   c. Advise the client to put a clean pair of elastic stockings on each day and that it will probably be necessary to wear the stockings for the remainder of life
   d. Instruct the client to avoid prolonged sitting or standing, constrictive clothing, or crossing legs when seated
   e. Instruct the client to elevate the legs for 10 to 20 minutes every few hours each day
   f. Instruct the client to elevate legs above the level of the heart when in bed
   g. Instruct the client in the use of an intermittent sequential pneumatic compression system, if prescribed; instruct the client to apply the compression system twice daily for 1 hour in the morning and evening
   h. Advise the client with an open ulcer that the compression system is applied over a dressing
4. Wound care
   a. Provide care to the wound as prescribed by the physician
   b. Assess the client's ability to care for the wound, and initiate home care resources as necessary
   c. If an Unna boot (a dressing constructed of gauze moistened with zinc oxide) is prescribed, it will be changed by the physician weekly
   d. The wound is cleansed with normal saline prior to application of the Unna boot; providone-iodine (Betadine) or hydrogen per-

oxide is not used because they destroy granulation tissue
   e. The Unna boot is covered with an elastic wrap that hardens, to promote venous return and prevent stasis
   f. Monitor for signs of arterial occlusion from an Unna boot that may be too tight
   g. Keep tape off of the client's skin
5. Medications
   a. Apply topical agents to wound as prescribed to debride the ulcer, eliminate necrotic tissue, and promote healing
   b. When applying topical agents, apply an oil-based agent such as petroleum jelly (Vaseline) on surrounding skin, because debriding agents can injure healthy tissue
   c. Administer antibiotics as prescribed if infection or cellulitis occurs
E. Varicose veins
   1. Description
      a. Distended protruding veins that appear darkened and tortuous
      b. Vein walls weaken and dilate, and valves become incompetent
   2. Assessment
      a. Pain in the legs with dull aching after standing
      b. A feeling of fullness in the legs
      c. Ankle edema
   3. Trendelenburg test
      a. Place the client in a supine position with the legs elevated
      b. When the client sits up, if varicosities are present, veins fill from the proximal end; veins normally fill from the distal end
   4. Implementation
      a. Assist with the Trendelenburg test
      b. Emphasize the importance of antiembolism stockings as prescribed
      c. Instruct the client to elevate the legs as much as possible
      d. Instruct the client to avoid constrictive clothing and pressure on the legs
      e. Prepare the client for sclerotherapy or vein stripping, as prescribed
   5. Sclerotherapy
      a. A solution is injected into the vein, followed by the application of a pressure dressing
      b. An incision and drainage of the trapped blood in the sclerosed vein are performed 14 to 21 days after the injection, followed by the application of a pressure dressing for 12 to 18 hours
   6. Vein stripping
      a. Varicose veins are removed if they are larger than 4 mm in diameter or if they are in clusters
      b. Preoperatively assist the physician with vein marking

c. Evaluate pulses as a baseline for comparison postoperatively

d. Maintain elastic (Ace) bandages on the client's legs postoperatively

e. Monitor the groin and leg for bleeding through the elastic bandages

f. Monitor the extremity for edema, warmth, color, and pulses

g. Elevate the legs above the level of the heart postoperatively

h. Encourage range-of-motion exercises of the legs

i. Instruct the client to avoid leg dangling or chair sitting

j. Instruct the client to elevate the legs when sitting

k. Emphasize the importance of wearing elastic stockings after bandage removal

XVII. ARTERIAL DISORDERS

A. Peripheral arterial disease (PAD)
   1. Description
      a. A chronic disorder in which partial or total arterial occlusion deprives the lower extremities of oxygen and nutrients
      b. Tissue damage occurs below the level of the arterial occlusion
      c. Atherosclerosis is the most common cause of PAD
   2. Assessment
      a. Intermittent claudication (pain in the muscles resulting from an inadequate blood supply)
      b. Rest pain, characterized by numbness, burning, or aching in the distal portion of the lower extremities, which awakens the client at night and is relieved by placing the extremity in a dependent position
      c. Lower back or buttock discomfort
      d. Loss of hair and dry scaly skin on the lower extremities
      e. Thickened toenails
      f. Cold and gray-blue color of skin in the lower extremities
      g. Elevational pallor and dependent rubor in the lower extremities
      h. Decreased or absent peripheral pulses
      i. Signs of arterial ulcer formation occurring on or between the toes, or on the upper aspect of the foot, that are characterized as painful
      j. **Blood pressure** measurements at the thigh, calf, and ankle are lower than the brachial pressure (normally **BP** readings in the thigh and calf are higher than those in the upper extremities)
   3. Implementation
      a. Assess pain

b. Monitor the extremities for color, motion and sensation, and pulses

c. Obtain **BP** measurements

d. Assess for signs of ulcer formation or signs of gangrene

e. Assist in developing an individualized exercise program, which is initiated gradually and slowly increased

f. Encourage prescribed exercise, which will improve arterial flow through the development of collateral circulation

g. Instruct the client to walk to the point of claudication, stop and rest, and then walk a little further

h. As swelling in the extremities prevents arterial blood flow, instruct the client to elevate the feet at rest, but to refrain from elevating them above the level of the heart, because extreme elevation slows arterial blood flow to the feet

i. In severe cases of PAD, clients with edema may sleep with the affected limb hanging from the bed or they may sit upright in a chair for comfort

j. Instruct the client with PAD to avoid crossing the legs, which interferes with blood flow

k. Instruct the client to avoid exposure to cold (causes vasoconstriction) to the extremities and to wear socks or insulated shoes for warmth at all times

l. Instruct the client never to apply direct heat to the limb, such as with a heating pad or hot water, because the decreased sensitivity in the limb will cause burning

m. Instruct the client to inspect the skin on the extremities daily and to report any signs of skin breakdown

n. Instruct the client to avoid tobacco and caffeine because of their vasoconstrictive effects

o. Instruct the client in the use of hemorrheologic and antiplatelet medications as prescribed

p. Inform the client of the importance of taking all medications prescribed by the physician

   4. Procedures to improve arterial blood flow
      a. Percutaneous transluminal angioplasty
      b. Laser-assisted angioplasty
      c. Atherectomy
      d. Bypass surgery (aortofemoral or femoral-popliteal)

B. Raynaud's disease
   1. Description
      a. Vasospasms of the arterioles and arteries of the upper and lower extremities
      b. Vasospasm causes constriction of the cutaneous vessels

c. Attacks are intermittent and occur with exposure to cold or stress

d. Affects primarily fingers, toes, ears, and cheeks

2. Assessment

a. Blanching of the extremity, followed by cyanosis during vasoconstriction

b. Reddened tissue when the vasospasm is relieved

c. Numbness, tingling, swelling, and a cold temperature at the affected body part

3. Implementation

a. Monitor pulses

b. Administer vasodilators as prescribed

c. Instruct the client regarding medication therapy

d. Assist the client to identify and avoid precipitating factors such as cold and stress

e. Instruct the client to avoid smoking

f. Instruct the client to wear warm clothing, socks, and gloves in cold weather

g. Advise the client to avoid injuries to fingers and hands

▲ C. Buerger's disease (thromboangiitis obliterans)

1. Description

a. An occlusive disease of the median and small arteries and veins

b. The distal upper and lower limbs are most commonly affected

2. Assessment

a. Intermittent claudication

b. Ischemic pain occurring in the digits while at rest

c. Aching pain that is more severe at night

d. Cool, numb, or tingling sensation

e. Diminished pulses in the distal extremities

f. Extremities are cool and red in the dependent position

g. Development of ulcerations in the extremities

3. Implementation

a. Instruct the client to stop smoking

b. Monitor pulses

c. Instruct the client to avoid injury to the upper and lower extremities

d. Administer vasodilators as prescribed

e. Instruct the client regarding medication therapy

▲ **XVIII. AORTIC ANEURYSMS**

A. Description

1. Abnormal dilation of the arterial wall, caused by localized weakness and stretching in the medial layer or wall of an artery

2. The aneurysm can be located anywhere along the abdominal aorta

3. The goal of treatment is to limit the progression of the disease by modifying risk factors, controlling the **BP** to prevent strain on the aneurysm, recognizing symptoms early, and preventing rupture

B. Types

1. Fusiform: Diffuse dilation that involves the entire circumference of the arterial segment

2. Saccular: Distinct localized outpouching of the artery wall

3. Dissecting: Created when blood separates the layers of the artery wall, forming a cavity between them

4. False (pseudoaneurysm)

a. Occurs when the clot and connective tissue are outside the arterial wall

b. Formed after complete rupture and subsequent formation of a scar sac

C. Assessment

1. Thoracic

a. Pain extending to neck, shoulders, lower back, or abdomen

b. Syncope

c. Dyspnea

d. Increased pulse

e. Cyanosis

f. Weakness

2. Abdominal

a. Prominent, pulsating mass in abdomen, at or above the umbilicus

b. Systolic bruit over the aorta

c. Tenderness on deep palpation

d. Abdominal or lower back pain

3. Rupturing aneurysm

a. Severe abdominal or back pain

b. Lumbar pain radiating to the flank and groin

c. Hypotension

d. Increased pulse rate

e. Signs of shock

4. Diagnostic tests

a. Done to confirm the presence, size, and location of the aneurysm

b. Includes abdominal ultrasound, CT scan, and arteriography

5. Implementation

a. Monitor vital signs

b. Assess risk factors for the arterial disease process

c. Obtain information regarding back or abdominal pain

d. Question the client regarding the sensation of palpation in the abdomen

e. Inspect the skin for the presence of vascular disease or breakdown

f. Check peripheral circulation, including pulses, temperature, and color

g. Observe for signs of rupture

h. Note any tenderness over the abdomen

i. Monitor for abdominal distention

6. Nonsurgical implementation
   a. Modify risk factors
   b. Instruct the client regarding the procedure for monitoring **BP**
   c. Instruct the client on the importance of regular physician visits to follow the size of the aneurysm
   d. Instruct the client that if severe back or abdominal pain or fullness, soreness over the umbilicus, sudden development of discoloration in the extremities, or a persistent elevation of **BP** occurs, to notify the physician immediately
   e. Instruct the client with a thoracic aneurysm to immediately report the occurrence of chest or back pain, shortness of breath, difficulty swallowing, or hoarseness

D. Pharmacological implementation
   1. Administer antihypertensives to maintain the **BP** within normal limits and to prevent strain on the aneurysm
   2. Instruct the client in the purpose of the medications
   3. Instruct the client about the side effects and schedule of the medication

▲ E. Abdominal aneurysm resection
   1. Description: Surgical resection or excision of the aneurysm; the excised section is replaced with a graft that is sewn end-to-end
   2. Preoperative implementation
      a. Assess all peripheral pulses as a baseline for postoperative comparison
      b. Instruct the client on coughing and deep breathing exercises
      c. Administer bowel preparation as prescribed
   3. Postoperative implementation
      a. Monitor vital signs
      b. Monitor peripheral pulses distal to the graft site
      c. Monitor for signs of graft occlusion, including changes in pulses, cool to cold extremities below the graft, white or blue extremities or flanks, severe pain, or abdominal distention
      d. Limit elevation of the head of the bed to 45 degrees to prevent flexion of the graft
      e. Monitor for hypovolemia and renal failure resulting from significant blood loss during surgery
      f. Monitor urine output hourly, and notify the physician if it is less than 50 mL per hour
      g. Monitor serum creatinine and BUN daily
      h. Monitor respiratory status and auscultate breath sounds to identify respiratory complications
      i. Encourage turning, coughing and deep breathing, and splinting the incision
      j. Ambulate as prescribed

   k. Maintain nasogastric tube to low suction until bowel sounds return
   l. Assess for bowel sounds and report their return to the physician
   m. Monitor for pain and administer medication as prescribed
   n. Assess incision site for bleeding or signs of infection
   o. Prepare the client for discharge by providing instructions regarding pain management, wound care, and activity restrictions
   p. Instruct the client not to lift objects heavier than 15 to 20 pounds for 6 to 12 weeks
   q. Advise the client to avoid activities requiring pushing, pulling, or straining
   r. Instruct the client not to drive a vehicle until approved by the physician

F. Thoracic aneurysm repair ▲
   1. Description
      a. A thoracotomy or median sternotomy approach is used to enter the thoracic cavity
      b. The aneurysm is exposed and excised, and a graft or prosthesis is sewn onto the aorta
      c. Total cardiopulmonary bypass is necessary for excision of aneurysms in the ascending aorta
      d. Partial cardiopulmonary bypass is used for clients with an aneurysm in the descending aorta
   2. Postoperative implementation
      a. Monitor vital signs
      b. Monitor for signs of hemorrhage, such as a drop in **BP** and increased pulse rate and respirations, and report to the physician immediately
      c. Monitor chest tubes for an increase in chest drainage, which may indicate bleeding or separation at the graft site
      d. Assess sensation and motion of all extremities and notify the physician if deficits occur, which can be due to a lack of blood supply during surgery
      e. Monitor respiratory status and auscultate breath sounds to identify respiratory complications
      f. Encourage turning, coughing and deep breathing, splinting the incision
      g. Monitor cardiac status for dysrhythmias
      h. Monitor for pain and administer medication as prescribed
      i. Assess the incision site for bleeding or signs of infection
      j. Prepare the client for discharge by providing instructions regarding pain management, wound care, and activity restrictions
      k. Instruct the client not to lift objects heavier than 15 to 20 pounds for 6 to 12 weeks
      l. Advise the client to avoid activities requiring pushing, pulling, or straining

m. Instruct the client not to drive a vehicle until approved by the physician

XIX. EMBOLECTOMY

A. Description
   1. Removal of an embolus from an artery, using a catheter
   2. A patch graft may be required to close the artery
B. Preoperative implementation
   1. Obtain a baseline vascular assessment
   2. Administer anticoagulants as prescribed
   3. Administer thrombolytics as prescribed
   4. Place a bed cradle on the bed
   5. Avoid bumping or jarring the bed
   6. Maintain the extremity in slightly dependent position
C. Postoperative implementation
   1. Assess cardiac, respiratory, and neurological status
   2. Monitor affected extremity for color, temperature, and pulse
   3. Assess sensory and motor function of the affected extremity
   4. Monitor for signs and symptoms of new thrombi or emboli
   5. Administer oxygen as prescribed
   6. Monitor pulse oximetry
   7. Monitor for complications caused by reperfusion of the artery, such as spasms and swelling of the skeletal muscles
   8. Monitor for signs of swollen skeletal muscles, such as edema, pain on passive movement, poor capillary refill, numbness, and muscle tenseness
   9. Maintain bed rest initially, with the client in semi-Fowler's position
   10. Place a bed cradle on the bed
   11. Check the incision site for bleeding or hematoma
   12. Administer anticoagulants as prescribed
   13. Monitor laboratory values related to anticoagulant therapy
   14. Instruct the client to recognize the signs and symptoms of infection and edema
   15. Instruct the client to avoid prolonged sitting or crossing the legs when sitting
   16. Instruct the client to elevate the legs when sitting
   17. Instruct the client to wear antiembolism stockings as prescribed and how to remove and reapply the stockings
   18. Instruct the client to ambulate daily
   19. Instruct the client about anticoagulant therapy and the hazards associated with anticoagulants

XX. VENA CAVAL FILTER AND LIGATION OF INFERIOR VENA CAVA

A. Vena caval filter: Insertion of an intracaval filter (umbrella) that partially occludes the inferior vena cava and traps emboli to prevent pulmonary emboli
B. Ligation: Suturing or placing clips on the inferior vena cava to prevent pulmonary emboli
C. Preoperative implementation: If the client has been taking an anticoagulant, consult with the physician regarding discontinuation of the medication to prevent hemorrhage
D. Postoperative implementation
   1. Monitor vital signs
   2. Assess cardiac and respiratory status
   3. Administer oxygen as prescribed
   4. Monitor pulse oximetry
   5. Maintain semi-Fowler's position
   6. Avoid hip flexion
   7. Provide activity as prescribed
   8. Check the insertion site for bleeding and hematoma
   9. Assess for peripheral edema
   10. Maintain antiembolism stockings as prescribed
   11. Monitor laboratory values related to anticoagulant therapy
   12. Instruct the client to recognize the signs and symptoms of infection and edema
   13. Instruct the client to avoid prolonged sitting or crossing legs when sitting
   14. Instruct the client to elevate the legs when sitting
   15. Instruct the client to wear antiembolism stockings as prescribed and how to remove and reapply the stockings
   16. Instruct the client to ambulate daily
   17. Instruct the client about anticoagulant therapy and the hazards associated with anticoagulants

XXI. HYPERTENSION

A. Description
   1. Persistent elevation of the **systolic blood pressure** above 140 mm Hg and the **diastolic blood pressure** above 90 mm Hg
   2. Most significant predictor of developing coronary artery disease
   3. Major risk factor for coronary, cerebral, renal, and peripheral vascular disease
   4. The disease is initially asymptomatic
   5. The goals of treatment include to reduce the **blood pressure** and to prevent or lessen the extent of organ damage (Table 57-1)

TABLE 57-1

Hypertension

Organ Involvement	Complications
Eyes	Visual changes
Brain	Cerebrovascular accident (CVA)
Cardiovascular system	CHF, hypertensive crisis
Kidneys	Renal failure

6. Nonpharmacological approaches, such as lifestyle changes, may be initially prescribed, and if the **BP** cannot be decreased after a reasonable time period (1 to 3 months), then the client may require pharmacological treatment

B. Primary or essential hypertension
   1. No known etiology
   2. Risk factors
      a. Aging
      b. Family history
      c. Black race, with higher prevalence in males
      d. Obesity
      e. Smoking
      f. Stress

C. Secondary hypertension
   1. Treatment depends on the cause and the organs involved
   2. Occurs as a result of other disorders or conditions
   3. Precipitating disorders or conditions
      a. Cardiovascular disorders
      b. Renal disorders
      c. Endocrine system disorders
      d. Pregnancy
      e. Medications

D. Assessment
   1. May be asymptomatic
   2. Headache
   3. Visual disturbances
   4. Dizziness
   5. Chest pain
   6. Tinnitus
   7. Flushed face
   8. Epistaxis

E. Implementation
   1. Goals
      a. To reduce the **blood pressure**
      b. To prevent or lessen the extent of organ damage
   2. Question the client regarding the signs and symptoms indicative of hypertension
   3. Obtain the **blood pressure (BP)** two or more times on both arms with the client supine and standing
   4. Compare the **blood pressure** with prior documentation
   5. Determine family history of hypertension
   6. Identify current medication therapy
   7. Obtain weight
   8. Evaluate dietary patterns and sodium intake
   9. Assess for visual changes or retinal damage
   10. Assess for cardiovascular changes, such as distended neck veins, increased heart rate, dysrhythmias
   11. Evaluate chest x-ray for heart enlargement
   12. Assess neurological system
   13. Evaluate renal function
   14. Evaluate results of diagnostic and laboratory studies

F. Nonpharmacological implementation
   1. Weight reduction, if necessary, or maintenance of ideal weight
   2. Dietary sodium restriction to 2 g daily as prescribed
   3. Moderate intake of alcohol and caffeine-containing products
   4. Initiation of a regular exercise program
   5. Avoidance of smoking
   6. Relaxation techniques and biofeedback therapy
   7. Elimination of unnecessary medications that may contribute to the hypertension

G. Stepped-care approach
   1. Description
      a. If a pharmacological approach to treating hypertension is required, a single medication is prescribed and monitored for its effectiveness
      b. Medications are added to the treatment regimen until the **BP** is controlled
      c. Refer to Chapter 58 for medications to treat hypertension
   2. Step 1: a single medication is prescribed, which may be a diuretic, beta-blocker, calcium channel blocker, or angiotensin-converting enzyme (ACE) inhibitor
   3. Step 2
      a. Step 1 therapy is evaluated after 1 to 3 months
      b. If the response is not adequate, compliance is evaluated
      c. The medication may be increased or a new medication is prescribed, or a second medication is added the treatment plan
   4. Step 3
      a. Compliance is evaluated
      b. Further evaluation of Step 2
      c. If a therapeutic response is not adequate, a second medication is substituted or a third medication is added to the treatment plan
   5. Step 4
      a. Compliance is evaluated
      b. Careful assessment of factors limiting the antihypertensive response is done
      c. A third or fourth medication may be added to the treatment plan

H. See Box 57-8 for client education

XXII. HYPERTENSIVE CRISIS

A. Description
   1. Any clinical condition requiring immediate reduction in **blood pressure**
   2. An acute and life-threatening condition
   3. The accelerated hypertension requires emergency treatment, since target organ damage (brain, heart, kidneys, retina of the eye) can occur quickly

BOX 57-8

Client Education for Hypertension

Describe the importance of compliance with the treatment plan

Describe the disease process, explaining that symptoms usually do not develop until organs have suffered damage

Initiate and assist the client in planning a regular exercise program, avoiding heavy weight lifting and isometric exercises

Emphasize the importance of beginning the exercise program gradually

Encourage the client to express feelings about daily stress

Assist the client to identify ways to reduce stress

Teach relaxation techniques

Instruct the client in how to incorporate relaxation techniques into the daily living pattern

Instruct the client and family in the technique for monitoring blood pressure

Instruct the client to maintain a diary of blood pressure readings

Emphasize the importance of lifelong medication and the need for follow-up treatment

Instruct the client and family about the dietary restrictions, which may include sodium, fat, calories, and cholesterol

Instruct the client in how to shop for and prepare low-sodium meals

Provide a list of products that contain sodium

Instruct the client to read labels of products to determine sodium content, focusing on substances listed as sodium, NaCl, or MSG

Instruct the client to bake, roast, or boil foods, avoid salt in preparation of foods, and avoid using salt at the table

Instruct the client that fresh foods are best to consume and to avoid canned foods

Instruct the client about the actions, side effects, and scheduling of medications

Advise the client that if uncomfortable side effects occur, to contact the physician and not to stop the medication

Instruct the client to avoid over-the-counter medications

Stress the importance of follow-up care

---

4. Death can be caused by stroke, renal failure, or cardiac disease

B. Assessment
   1. A **diastolic pressure** above 120 mm Hg
   2. Headache
   3. Drowsiness
   4. Confusion
   5. Changes in neurological status
   6. Tachycardia and tachypnea
   7. Dyspnea

8. Cyanosis
9. Seizures

C. Implementation
   1. Maintain a patent airway
   2. Administer IV antihypertensive medications as prescribed, which may include nitroprusside (Nipride), diazoxide (Hyperstat), or trimethaphan camsylate (Arfonad)
   3. Monitor vital signs, assessing BP every 5 minutes
   4. Assess for hypotension during the administration of antihypertensives
   5. Place the client in a supine position if hypotension occurs
   6. Have emergency medications and resuscitation equipment readily available
   7. Maintain bed rest, with the head of the bed elevated at 45 degrees
   8. Monitor IV therapy, assessing for fluid overload
   9. Monitor I & O
   10. Insert Foley catheter as prescribed
   11. Monitor urinary output, and if oliguria or anuria occurs, notify the physician

PRACTICE QUESTIONS

1. A client with angina pectoris has a 12-lead ECG taken during an episode of chest pain. A nurse examines the tracing for which ECG change caused by myocardial ischemia?
   1. Prolonged PR interval
   2. Widened QRS complex
   3. ST segment elevation or depression
   4. Tall, peaked T waves

2. A client is scheduled for a cardiac catheterization using a radiopaque dye. Which of the following assessments is most critical before the procedure?
   1. Intake and output
   2. Baseline peripheral pulse rates
   3. Height and weight
   4. Allergy to iodine or shellfish

3. A client is scheduled for a dipyridamole (Persantine) thallium 201 scan. A nurse would assess to make sure that the client avoided which of the following prior to the procedure?
   1. Milk products
   2. Caffeine
   3. Excess sugar
   4. Fatty meal

4. A client with no history of cardiovascular disease presents to the ambulatory clinic with flulike symptoms. The client suddenly complains of chest pain. Which of the following questions would best help a nurse to discriminate pain caused by a noncardiac problem?
   1. "Have you ever had this pain before?"

2. "Can you describe the pain to me?"

3. "Does the pain get worse when you breathe in?"

4. "Can you rate the pain on a scale of 1 to 10, with 10 being the worst?"

5. A client is admitted to an emergency room with chest pain and is being ruled out for myocardial infarction (MI). Vital signs are as follows: at 11:00 A.M., pulse (P) 92, respiratory rate (RR) 24, blood pressure (BP) 140/88 mm Hg; 11:15 A.M., P 96, RR 26, BP 128/82 mm Hg; 11:30 A.M., P 104, RR 28, BP 104/68 mm Hg; 11:45 A.M., P 118, RR 32, BP 88/58 mm Hg. A nurse alerts the physician because these changes are most consistent with:

1. Cardiogenic shock

2. Cardiac tamponade

3. Pulmonary embolism

4. Dissecting thoracic aortic aneurysm

6. A client with myocardial infarction (MI) has been transferred from a coronary care unit (CCU) to a general medical unit with cardiac monitoring via telemetry. A nurse plans to allow for which of the following client activities?

1. Strict bed rest for 24 hours after transfer

2. Bathroom privileges and self-care activities

3. Unsupervised hallway ambulation with distances under 200 feet

4. Ad lib activities since the client is monitored

7. A nurse notes bilateral 2+ edema in the lower extremities of a client with myocardial infarction (MI) who was admitted 2 days ago. The nurse would plan to do which of the following next?

1. Review the intake and output records for the last 2 days

2. Change the time of diuretic administration from morning to evening

3. Request a sodium restriction of 1 g/day from the physician

4. Order daily weights starting on the following morning

8. A nurse is conducting a health history with a client with a primary diagnosis of heart failure. Which of the following disorders reported by the client does not play a role in exacerbating the heart failure?

1. Recent upper respiratory infection

2. Nutritional anemia

3. Peptic ulcer disease

4. Atrial fibrillation

9. A nurse is preparing for the admission of a client with heart failure who is being sent directly to the hospital from the physician's office. The nurse would plan on having which of the following medications readily available for use?

1. Diltiazem (Cardizem)

2. Digoxin (Lanoxin)

3. Propranolol (Inderal)

4. Metoprolol (Lopressor)

10. A client with myocardial infarction suddenly becomes tachycardic, shows signs of air hunger, and begins coughing frothy pink-tinged sputum. A nurse listens to breath sounds, expecting to hear bilateral:

1. Rhonchi

2. Crackles in bases

3. Rales to apices

4. Wheezes

11. A nurse caring for a client in one room is told by another nurse that a second client has developed severe pulmonary edema. Upon entering the second client's room, the nurse would expect the client to be:

1. Slightly anxious

2. Mildly anxious

3. Moderately anxious

4. Extremely anxious

12. A client with pulmonary edema has been on diuretic therapy. The client has an order for additional furosemide (Lasix) in the amount of 40 mg IV push. Knowing that the client will also be started on digoxin (Lanoxin), a nurse checks the client's most recent:

1. Digoxin level

2. Sodium level

3. Potassium level

4. Creatinine level

13. A client with myocardial infarction is going into cardiogenic shock. Because of myocardial ischemia, a nurse would carefully assess the client for:

1. Ventricular dysrhythmias

2. Bradycardia

3. Rising diastolic blood pressure

4. Falling central venous pressure (CVP)

14. A client in cardiogenic shock has a multilumen pulmonary artery catheter placed. The nurse would interpret that the client is most unstable if which of the following cardiac output (CO) and pulmonary capillary wedge pressure (PCWP) readings were obtained?

1. CO 5 L/min, PCWP low

2. CO 4 L/min, PCWP high

3. CO 3 L/min, PCWP high

4. CO 2 L/min, PCWP low

15. A client in cardiogenic shock had insertion of an intraaortic balloon pump (IABP) 24 hours ago via the left femoral approach. A nurse notes that the left foot is cool and mottled and the left pedal pulse is weak. The nurse would:

1. Document the data, as this is expected because of the catheter size

2. Reevaluate the neurovascular status in another hour

3. Increase the rate of intravenous nitroglycerin that is infusing

4. Call the physician immediately

16. A nurse assesses the sternotomy incision of a client on the third day after cardiac surgery. The incision shows some slight "puffiness" along the edges and is nonreddened, with no apparent drainage. Temperature is 99° F orally. The white blood cell (WBC) count is 7500/mm³. The nurse interprets that the incision line:
    1. Is slightly edematous but shows no active signs of infection
    2. Shows no sign of infection, although the WBC count is elevated
    3. Shows early signs of infection, although the temperature is near normal
    4. Shows early signs of infection, supported by an elevated WBC count

17. A client who had cardiac surgery 24 hours ago has a urine output averaging 20 mL/hr for 2 hours. The client received a single bolus of 500 mL of intravenous fluid. Urine output for the subsequent hour was 25 mL. Daily laboratory results indicate that the blood urea nitrogen (BUN) is 45 mg/dL and the serum creatinine is 2.2 mg/dL. A nurse interprets that the client is at risk for:
    1. Hypovolemia
    2. Urinary tract infection (UTI)
    3. Glomerulonephritis
    4. Acute renal failure

18. A nurse is preparing to ambulate a client on the third day after cardiac surgery. The nurse would plan to do which of the following to enable the client to best tolerate the ambulation?
    1. Encourage the client to cough and deep breathe
    2. Premedicate the client with an analgesic
    3. Provide the client with a walker
    4. Remove telemetry equipment

19. A nurse is assessing an ECG rhythm strip. The P waves and QRS complexes are regular. The PR interval is 0.16 second, and QRS complexes measure 0.06 second. The overall heart rate is 64 beats per minute. The nurse assesses the cardiac rhythm as:
    1. Normal sinus rhythm
    2. Sinus bradycardia
    3. Sick sinus syndrome
    4. First-degree heart block

20. A client is wearing a continuous cardiac monitor, which begins to sound its alarm. A nurse sees no ECG complexes on the screen. The first action of the nurse is to:
    1. Check the client status and lead placement
    2. Press the recorder button on the ECG console
    3. Call the physician
    4. Call a code blue

21. A client's ECG strip shows atrial and ventricular rates of 80 complexes per minute. The PR interval is 0.14 second, the QRS complex measures 0.08 second, and the PP interval is slightly irregular. The nurse interprets that this rhythm is:
    1. Normal sinus rhythm
    2. Sinus bradycardia
    3. Sinus tachycardia
    4. Sinus dysrhythmia

22. A nurse notices frequent artifact on the ECG monitor for a client whose leads are connected by cable to a console at the bedside. The nurse examines the client to determine the cause. Which of the following items would not be responsible for the artifact?
    1. Frequent movement of the client
    2. Tightly secured cable connections
    3. Leads applied over hairy areas
    4. Leads applied to the limbs

23. A nurse is watching the cardiac monitor and notices that the rhythm suddenly changes. There are no P waves, the QRS complexes are wide, and the ventricular rate is regular but over 100. The nurse determines that the client is experiencing:
    1. Premature ventricular contractions (PVCs)
    2. Ventricular tachycardia (VT)
    3. Ventricular fibrillation (VF)
    4. Sinus tachycardia

24. A client has frequent bursts of ventricular tachycardia (VT) on the cardiac monitor. A nurse is most concerned with this dysrhythmia because:
    1. It is uncomfortable for the client, giving a sense of impending doom
    2. It produces a low cardiac output that quickly leads to cerebral and myocardial ischemia
    3. It is almost impossible to convert to a normal rhythm
    4. It can develop into ventricular fibrillation at any time

25. A nurse is viewing the cardiac monitor in a client's room and notes that the client has just gone into ventricular tachycardia (VT). The client is awake and alert and has good skin color. The nurse would prepare to do which of the following?
    1. Immediately defibrillate
    2. Prepare for pacemaker insertion
    3. Administer lidocaine hydrochloride (Xylocaine) intravenously
    4. Administer epinephrine (Adrenalin) intravenously

26. A nurse is caring for a client with unstable ventricular tachycardia (VT). The nurse instructs the client to do which of the following, if prescribed, during an episode of VT?
    1. Breathe deeply, regularly, and easily
    2. Inhale deeply and cough forcefully every 1 to 3 seconds
    3. Lie down flat in bed
    4. Remove any metal jewelry

27. A client is having frequent premature ventricular contractions (PVCs). A nurse would place priority on assessment of which of the following items?
    1. Blood pressure and peripheral perfusion
    2. Sensation of palpitations
    3. Causative factors such as caffeine
    4. Precipitating factors such as infection

28. A client has developed atrial fibrillation, with a ventricular rate of 150 beats per minute. A nurse assesses the client for:
    1. Hypotension and dizziness
    2. Nausea and vomiting
    3. Hypertension and headache
    4. Flat neck veins

29. A nurse is watching the cardiac monitor, and a client's rhythm suddenly changes. There are no P waves; instead there are wavy lines. The QRS complexes measure 0.08 second, but they are very irregular, with a rate of 120 beats per minute. The nurse interprets that this rhythm is:
    1. Sinus tachycardia
    2. Atrial fibrillation
    3. Ventricular tachycardia
    4. Ventricular fibrillation

30. A client with rapid-rate atrial fibrillation asks a nurse why the physician is going to perform carotid massage. The nurse responds that this procedure may stimulate the:
    1. Vagus nerve to slow the heart rate
    2. Vagus nerve to increase the heart rate, overdriving the rhythm
    3. Diaphragmatic nerve to slow the heart rate
    4. Diaphragmatic nerve to overdrive the rhythm

31. A nurse notes that a client with sinus rhythm has a premature ventricular contraction (PVC) that falls on the T wave of the preceding beat. The client's rhythm suddenly changes to one with no P waves or definable QRS complexes. Instead there are coarse wavy lines of varying amplitude. The nurse assesses this rhythm to be:
    1. Ventricular tachycardia
    2. Ventricular fibrillation
    3. Atrial fibrillation
    4. Asystole

32. A nurse is preparing to defibrillate a client in ventricular fibrillation (VF). The nurse places the paddles on the client's chest and, before defibrillating the client, assesses that:
    1. The client has received lidocaine hydrochloride (Xylocaine)
    2. The rhythm is actually VF
    3. The machine has been set to the "synchronize" mode
    4. The client has been intubated

33. A client in ventricular fibrillation is about to be defibrillated. A nurse knows that in order to effectively convert this rhythm, the machine should be set at which of the following energy levels for the first delivery?
    1. 50 joules
    2. 100 joules
    3. 200 joules
    4. 360 joules

34. A nurse would evaluate that defibrillation of a client was most successful if which of the following observations was made?
    1. Nonarousable, sinus rhythm, blood pressure (BP) 88/60 mm Hg
    2. Arousable, sinus rhythm, BP 116/72 mm Hg
    3. Nonarousable, supraventricular tachycardia, BP 122/ 60 mm Hg
    4. Arousable, marked bradycardia, BP 86/54 mm Hg

35. A nurse is evaluating a client's response to cardioversion. Which of the following observations would be of highest priority to the nurse?
    1. Oxygen flow rate
    2. Status of airway
    3. Blood pressure
    4. Level of consciousness

36. A nurse is performing cardiopulmonary resuscitation (CPR) on a client who had a cardiac arrest. An automatic external defibrillator (AED) is available to treat the client. The nurse uses the AED and assesses the cardiac rhythm by:
    1. Applying standard ECG monitoring leads to the client and observing the rhythm
    2. Holding the defibrillator paddles firmly against the chest
    3. Applying the adhesive patch electrodes to the chest and moving away from the client
    4. Connecting standard ECG electrodes to a trans-telephonic monitoring device

37. A nurse employed in a cardiac unit determines that which of the following clients is the least likely to have implantation of an internal automatic cardioverter-defibrillator (AICD)?
    1. A client with three episodes of cardiac arrest unrelated to myocardial infarction
    2. A client with ventricular dysrhythmias despite medication therapy
    3. A client with an episode of cardiac arrest related to myocardial infarction
    4. A client with syncopal episodes related to ventricular tachycardia

38. A nurse is caring for a client who has just had implantation of an automatic internal cardioverter-defibrillator (AICD). The nurse would immediately determine which of the following items, based on priority?
    1. Activation status of the device, heart rate cutoff, and number of shocks it is programmed to deliver

2. Presence of a Medic-Alert card for the client to carry
3. Anxiety level of the client and family
4. Knowledge of restrictions of postdischarge physical activity

39. A nurse is caring for a client immediately after insertion of a permanent demand pacemaker via the right subclavian vein. The nurse takes care not to dislodge the pacing catheter by:
    1. Limiting movement and abduction of the right arm
    2. Limiting movement and abduction of the left arm
    3. Assisting the client to get out of bed and ambulate with a walker
    4. Having the physical therapist do active range of motion to the right arm

40. A client diagnosed with thrombophlebitis 1 day ago suddenly complains of chest pain and shortness of breath and is visibly anxious. A nurse immediately assesses the client for other signs and symptoms of:
    1. Myocardial infarction
    2. Pneumonia
    3. Pulmonary embolism
    4. Pulmonary edema

41. A client seeks treatment in a physician's office for unsightly varicose veins, and sclerotherapy is recommended. Before leaving the examining room, the client says to the nurse, "Can you tell me again how this sclerotherapy is done?" In formulating a response, the nurse incorporates the knowledge that sclerotherapy consists of:
    1. Injecting an agent into the vein to damage the vein wall and close the vein off
    2. Tying off the vein at the upper end to prevent stasis from occurring
    3. Tying off the vein at the lower end to prevent stasis from occurring
    4. Surgical removal of the varicosity

42. A client is having a follow-up physician office visit after vein ligation and stripping. The client describes a sensation of "pins and needles" in the affected leg. On the basis of evaluation of this comment, the nurse:
    1. Reassures the client that this is only temporary
    2. Advises the client to take acetaminophen (Tylenol) until it is gone
    3. States that warm packs should help
    4. Reports the complaint to the physician

43. A 24-year-old male seeks medical attention for complaints of claudication in the arch of the foot. A nurse also notes superficial thrombophlebitis of the lower leg. The nurse would next assess the client for:
    1. Familial tendency toward peripheral vascular disease

2. Smoking history
3. Recent exposure to allergens
4. History of recent insect bites

44. A nurse has given instructions to the client with Raynaud's disease about self-management of the disease process. The nurse would evaluate that the client needs further reinforcement if the client states that:
    1. Smoking cessation is very important
    2. Sources of caffeine should be eliminated from the diet
    3. Taking nifedipine (Procardia) as prescribed will decrease vessel spasm
    4. Moving to a warmer climate is needed

45. A nurse is caring for a client who had a percutaneous insertion of an inferior vena cava (IVC) filter, and was on heparin therapy prior to surgery. The nurse would inspect the surgical site most closely for signs of:
    1. Thrombosis and infection
    2. Bleeding and infection
    3. Bleeding and wound dehiscence
    4. Wound dehiscence and evisceration

46. A nurse is assessing the blood pressure of a client diagnosed with primary hypertension. The nurse ensures accurate measurement by avoiding which of the following?
    1. Seating the client with arm bared, supported, and at heart level.
    2. Measuring the blood pressure after the client has been seated quietly for 5 minutes.
    3. Using a cuff with a rubber bladder that encircles at least 80% of the limb.
    4. Taking the blood pressure within 30 minutes after nicotine or caffeine ingestion.

47. Intravenous heparin therapy is ordered for a client. While implementing this order, a nurse ensures that which of the following medications is available on the nursing unit?
    1. Vitamin K (AquaMEPHYTON)
    2. Aminocaproic acid (Amicar)
    3. Potassium chloride (KCl)
    4. Protamine sulfate (protamine sulfate)

48. A client is at risk for pulmonary embolism and is on anticoagulant therapy with warfarin sodium (Coumadin). The client's prothrombin time is 20 seconds, with a control of 11 seconds. The nurse assesses that this result is:
    1. The same as the client's own baseline level
    2. Lower than the needed therapeutic level
    3. Within the therapeutic range
    4. Higher than the therapeutic range

49. A client who has been receiving heparin therapy is also started on warfarin sodium (Coumadin). The client asks a nurse why both medications are being administered. In formulating a response, the

nurse incorporates the understanding that warfarin sodium:

1. Stimulates breakdown of specific clotting factors by the liver, and it takes 2 to 3 days for this to exert an anticoagulant effect
2. Inhibits synthesis of specific clotting factors in the liver, and it takes 3 to 4 days for this medication to exert an anticoagulant effect
3. Stimulates production of the body's own thrombolytic substances, but it takes 2 to 4 days for this to begin
4. Has the same mechanism of action as heparin, and the cross-over time is needed for the serum level of warfarin sodium to be therapeutic

50. A nurse has an order to begin administering warfarin sodium (Coumadin) to a client. While implementing this order, the nurse ensures that which of the following medications is available on the nursing unit as the antidote for Coumadin?
   1. Vitamin K (AquaMEPHYTON)
   2. Aminocaproic acid (Amicar)
   3. Potassium chloride (KCl)
   4. Protamine sulfate (protamine sulfate)

51. A client is admitted to a hospital with acute myocardial infarction and is started on tissue plasminogen activator (t-PA, Activase) by infusion. Of the following parameters, which one would a nurse determine requires the least frequent assessment to detect complications with this therapy?
   1. Oxygen saturation
   2. Neurological signs
   3. Blood pressure and pulse
   4. Complaints of abdominal and back pain

52. A client is admitted with pulmonary thromboembolism and is to be treated with streptokinase (Streptase). A nurse would report which of the following assessments to the physician before this therapy is initiated?
   1. Adventitious breath sounds
   2. Respiratory rate of 28 breaths per minute
   3. Temperature of 99.4° F orally
   4. Blood pressure (BP) of 198/110 mm Hg

53. A client is receiving thrombolytic therapy with a continuous infusion of streptokinase (Streptase). The client suddenly becomes extremely anxious and complains of itching. A nurse hears stridor, and upon examination of the client, notes generalized urticaria and hypotension. The nurse should:
   1. Administer oxygen and protamine sulfate
   2. Cut the infusion rate in half and sit the client up in bed
   3. Stop the infusion and call the physician
   4. Administer diphenhydramine (Benadryl) and continue the infusion

54. A nurse is assessing the neurovascular status of a client who returned to the surgical nursing unit 4 hours ago after undergoing aortoiliac bypass graft. The affected leg is warm, and the nurse notes redness and edema. The pedal pulse is palpable and unchanged from admission. The nurse interprets that the neurovascular status is:
   1. Normal, because of increased blood flow through the leg
   2. Slightly deteriorating and should be monitored for another hour
   3. Moderately impaired, and the surgeon should be called
   4. Adequate from an arterial approach, but venous complications are arising

55. A nurse is evaluating the condition of a client after pericardiocentesis for cardiac tamponade. Which of the following observations would indicate that the procedure was unsuccessful?
   1. Rising central venous pressure (CVP)
   2. Rising blood pressure (BP)
   3. Client expressions of relief
   4. Clearly audible heart sounds

56. A nurse is assessing a client with an abdominal aortic aneurysm (AAA). Which of the following assessment findings by the nurse is probably unrelated to the AAA?
   1. Pulsatile abdominal mass
   2. Hyperactive bowel sounds in the area
   3. Systolic bruit over the area of the mass
   4. Subjective sensation of "heart beating" in the abdomen

57. A nurse is caring for a client who had a resection of an abdominal aortic aneurysm (AAA) yesterday. The client has an IV with a rate of 150 mL/hr, unchanged for the last 10 hours. The client's urine output for the last 3 hours was 90 mL, 50 mL, and 28 mL (28 mL most recent). The client's blood urea nitrogen (BUN) is 35 mg/dL, and serum creatinine is 1.8 mg/dL, drawn this morning. Which of the following actions should the nurse take next?
   1. Put the IV on a pump so that the infusion rate is sure to stay stable
   2. Check to see if the client had a serum albumin level drawn
   3. Check the urine specific gravity
   4. Call the physician

58. A client is admitted with a venous stasis leg ulcer. A nurse assesses the ulcer, expecting to note that the ulcer:
   1. Has a pale-colored base
   2. Is deep, with even edges
   3. Has little granulation tissue
   4. Has brown pigmentation surrounding it

59. A home care nurse is making a routine visit to a client receiving digoxin (Lanoxin) in the treatment of heart failure. The nurse would particularly assess the client for:
   1. Thrombocytopenia and weight gain
   2. Anorexia, nausea, and visual disturbances

3. Diarrhea and hypotension
4. Fatigue and muscle twitching

60. A client with angina complains that the anginal pain is prolonged and severe and occurs at the same time each day, most often in the morning. On further assessment, a nurse notes that that the pain occurs in the absence of precipitating factors. This type of anginal pain is best described as:
1. Stable angina
2. Unstable angina
3. Variant angina
4. Nonanginal pain

CRITICAL THINKING: FREE-TEXT ENTRY

A nurse is caring for a client in a room at the end of the hallway. The client is attached to a cardiac monitor, and the nurse notes that the client suddenly has a short burst of ventricular tachycardia followed by ventricular fibrillation (VF). The client immediately loses consciousness. What is the nurse's initial nursing action?

Answer: _____

ANSWERS

1. 3
Rationale: An ECG taken with pain captures ischemic changes, which include ST segment elevation or depression. A prolonged PR interval indicates first-degree heart block. A widened QRS complex indicates delay in intraventricular conduction, such as bundle branch block. Tall, peaked T waves may indicate hyperkalemia.
Test-Taking Strategy: Use the process of elimination. Recalling that myocardial ischemia causes cellular derangements that alter the processes of depolarization will direct you to option 3. Review the ECG changes that occur with myocardial ischemia if you had difficulty with this question.
Level of Cognitive Ability: Analysis
Client Needs: Physiological Integrity
Integrated Concept/Process: Nursing Process/Analysis
Content Area: Adult Health/Cardiovascular
Reference: Ignatavicius, D., Workman, M., & Mishler, M. (1999). *Medical-surgical nursing across the health care continuum* (3rd ed.). Philadelphia: W.B. Saunders, p. 907.

2. 4
Rationale: This procedure requires a consent, because it involves injection of a radiopaque dye into the blood vessel. The risk of allergic reaction and possible anaphylaxis is serious, and must be assessed before the procedure. Although options 1, 2, and 3 are accurate, they are not the most critical preprocedure assessments.
Test-Taking Strategy: Use the process of elimination. Note the key words "most critical." Recalling the concern related to allergy to the dye and the risk of anaphylaxis makes option 4 correct. Review preprocedure interventions for a cardiac catheterization, if you had difficulty with this question.
Level of Cognitive Ability: Application
Client Needs: Physiological Integrity
Integrated Concept/Process: Nursing Process/Assessment
Content Area: Adult Health/Cardiovascular
Reference: Ignatavicius, D., Workman, M., & Mishler, M. (1999). *Medical-surgical nursing across the health care continuum* (3rd ed.). Philadelphia: W.B. Saunders, p. 740.

3. 2
Rationale: This test is an alternative to the exercise thallium 201 scan. The dipyridamole (Persantine) dilates the coronary arteries as exercise would. Before the procedure, any form of caffeine should be withheld, as well as aminophylline or

theophylline. Aminophylline is the antagonist to dipyridamole. It is not necessary to avoid the items identified in options 1, 3, and 4.
Test-Taking Strategy: Use the process of elimination, noting the key word "avoided." Factors that put a strain on the heart, such as nicotine and caffeine, can interfere with cardiac diagnostic test results. Look for items such as these in similarly worded questions. Review preprocedure client instructions for this test if you had difficulty with this question.
Level of Cognitive Ability: Analysis
Client Needs: Physiological Integrity
Integrated Concept/Process: Nursing Process/Assessment
Content Area: Adult Health/Cardiovascular
Reference: Phipps, W., Sands, J., & Marek, J. (1999). *Medical-surgical nursing: Concepts & clinical practice* (6th ed.). St. Louis: Mosby, p. 629.

4. 3
Rationale: Chest pain is assessed by using the standard pain assessment parameters (e.g., characteristics, location, intensity, duration, precipitating and alleviating factors, and associated symptoms). Options 1, 2, and 4 may or may not help discriminate the origin of pain. Pain of pleuropulmonary origin usually worsens on inspiration.
Test-Taking Strategy: Use the process of elimination, focusing on the issue, pain resulting from a noncardiac problem. The three incorrect options, although appropriate to use in practice, are general assessment questions only. Option 3 will discriminate between a cardiac and noncardiac cause of pain. Review pain assessment measures for the client with a cardiovascular problem if you had difficulty with this question.
Level of Cognitive Ability: Analysis
Client Needs: Physiological Integrity
Integrated Concept/Process: Nursing Process/Assessment
Content Area: Adult Health/Cardiovascular
Reference: Ignatavicius, D., Workman, M., & Mishler, M. (1999). *Medical-surgical nursing across the health care continuum* (3rd ed.). Philadelphia: W.B. Saunders, pp. 726-727.

5. 1
Rationale: Cardiogenic shock occurs with severe damage (greater than 40%) to the left ventricle. Classic signs include hypotension, rapid pulse that becomes weaker, decreased urine output, and cool, clammy skin. Respiratory rate increases as the body develops metabolic acidosis from shock.

Cardiac tamponade is accompanied by distant, muffled heart sounds and prominent neck vessels. Pulmonary embolism presents suddenly with severe dyspnea accompanying the chest pain. Dissecting aortic aneurysms are usually accompanied by back pain.

Test-Taking Strategy: Use the process of elimination. Recalling that the early serious complications of MI include dysrhythmias, cardiogenic shock, and sudden death will direct you to option 1. There is no information in the question that would guide you to another option. Review the complications of MI if you had difficulty with this question.

Level of Cognitive Ability: Analysis
Client Needs: Physiological Integrity
Integrated Concept/Process: Nursing Process/Analysis
Content Area: Adult Health/Cardiovascular
Reference: Phipps, W., Sands, J., & Marek, J. (1999). *Medical-surgical nursing: Concepts & clinical practice* (6th ed.). St. Louis: Mosby, p. 443.

6. **2**
Rationale: Upon transfer from the CCU, the client is allowed self-care activities and bathroom privileges. Supervised ambulation in the hall for brief distances is encouraged, with distances gradually increased (50, 100, 200 feet).

Test-Taking Strategy: Use the process of elimination. Eliminate options 3 and 4 first, since they are excessive, given that the client has just transferred from the CCU. Option 1 is not appropriate, since the client would be doing less activity than in the CCU prior to transfer. Review activity prescriptions for the client with an MI, if you had difficulty with this question.

Level of Cognitive Ability: Application
Client Needs: Physiological Integrity
Integrated Concept/Process: Nursing Process/Planning
Content Area: Adult Health/Cardiovascular
Reference: Smeltzer, S., & Bare, B. (2000). *Brunner & Suddarth's textbook of medical-surgical nursing* (9th ed.). Philadelphia: Lippincott Williams & Wilkins, p. 631.

7. **1**
Rationale: Edema, the accumulation of excess fluid in the interstitial spaces, can be measured by intake greater than output, and by a sudden increase in weight. Diuretics should be given in the morning whenever possible, to avoid nocturia. Strict sodium restrictions are reserved for clients with severe symptoms.

Test-Taking Strategy: Use the process of elimination, noting the key word "next." Use the steps of the nursing process to prioritize. Option 1 is the only option that addresses assessment of data. Review care to the client with MI if you had difficulty with this question.

Level of Cognitive Ability: Application
Client Needs: Physiological Integrity
Integrated Concept/Process: Nursing Process/Assessment
Content Area: Adult Health/Cardiovascular
Reference: Ignatavicius, D., Workman, M., & Mishler, M. (1999). *Medical-surgical nursing across the health care continuum* (3rd ed.). Philadelphia: W.B. Saunders, p. 728.

8. **3**
Rationale: Heart failure is precipitated or exacerbated by physical or emotional stress, dysrhythmias, infections, anemia, thyroid disorders, pregnancy, Paget's disease, nutritional deficiencies (thiamine, alcoholism), pulmonary disease, and hypervolemia.

Test-Taking Strategy: Use the process of elimination. Note the key word "not." Remembering that heart failure is exacerbated by factors that increase the workload of the heart will assist in eliminating options 1, 2, and 4. Review the precipitating factors associated with heart failure, if you had difficulty with this question.

Level of Cognitive Ability: Analysis
Client Needs: Physiological Integrity
Integrated Concept/Process: Nursing Process/Assessment
Content Area: Adult Health/Cardiovascular
Reference: Smeltzer, S., & Bare, B. (2000). *Brunner & Suddarth's textbook of medical-surgical nursing* (9th ed.). Philadelphia: Lippincott Williams & Wilkins, pp. 662-663.

9. **2**
Rationale: Digoxin exerts a positive inotropic effect on the heart, while slowing the overall rate through a variety of mechanisms. It is the medication of choice to treat heart failure. Diltiazem (calcium channel blocker) and propranolol and metoprolol (beta-adrenergic blockers) have a negative inotropic effect, and would worsen the failing heart.

Test-Taking Strategy: Use the process of elimination. Options 3 and 4 can be eliminated first because they are both beta-blockers. From the remaining options, use knowledge of the classification and actions of these medications to direct you to option 2. Review these medications if you had difficulty with this question.

Level of Cognitive Ability: Application
Client Needs: Physiological Integrity
Integrated Concept/Process: Nursing Process/Planning
Content Area: Adult Health/Cardiovascular
Reference: Ignatavicius, D., Workman, M., & Mishler, M. (1999). *Medical-surgical nursing across the health care continuum* (3rd ed.). Philadelphia: W.B. Saunders, p. 817.

10. **3**
Rationale: Pulmonary edema is characterized by extreme breathlessness, dyspnea, air hunger, and production of frothy pink-tinged sputum. Auscultation of the lungs reveals rales to the apices. Wheezes, rhonchi, and crackles in the bases are not associated with pulmonary edema.

Test-Taking Strategy: Use the process of elimination. Recall that fluid produces sounds that are called rales or crackles, which eliminates options 1 or 4. From the remaining options, think about the physiology of pulmonary edema. Crackles in bases would not produce such extreme symptoms as are noted in pulmonary edema. If you had difficulty with this question, review the manifestations found in pulmonary edema.

Level of Cognitive Ability: Analysis
Client Needs: Physiological Integrity
Integrated Concept/Process: Nursing Process/Assessment
Content Area: Adult Health/Cardiovascular
Reference: Smeltzer, S., & Bare, B. (2000). *Brunner & Suddarth's textbook of medical-surgical nursing* (9th ed.). Philadelphia: Lippincott Williams & Wilkins, pp. 657-658.

11. **4**
Rationale: Pulmonary edema causes the client to be extremely agitated and anxious. The client may complain of a sense of drowning, suffocation, or smothering.

Test-Taking Strategy: Use the process of elimination. Noting the key word "severe" will direct you to option 4. Review the clinical manifestations associated with severe pulmonary edema if you had difficulty with this question.

Level of Cognitive Ability: Analysis
Client Needs: Psychosocial Integrity
Integrated Concept/Process: Nursing Process/Assessment
Content Area: Adult Health/Cardiovascular
Reference: Smeltzer, S., & Bare, B. (2000). *Brunner & Suddarth's textbook of medical-surgical nursing* (9th ed.). Philadelphia: Lippincott Williams & Wilkins, pp. 657-658.

12. **3**
Rationale: The serum potassium level is measured in the client receiving both digoxin and furosemide. Heightened digitalis effect leading to digoxin toxicity can occur in the client with hypokalemia. Hypokalemia also predisposes the cardiac client to ventricular dysrhythmias.
Test-Taking Strategy: Use the process of elimination. Eliminate option 1 because the client will just be beginning digoxin therapy. There are no data to indicate the presence of renal insufficiency; therefore eliminate option 4. Furosemide therapy can cause both hyponatremia and hypokalemia, but remember that the risk of hypokalemia has more severe consequences in this situation. Review the nursing considerations related to administering furosemide if you had difficulty with this question.
Level of Cognitive Ability: Analysis
Client Needs: Physiological Integrity
Integrated Concept/Process: Nursing Process/Assessment
Content Area: Adult Health/Cardiovascular
Reference: Smeltzer, S., & Bare, B. (2000). *Brunner & Suddarth's textbook of medical-surgical nursing* (9th ed.). Philadelphia: Lippincott Williams & Wilkins, pp. 666-667.

13. **1**
Rationale: Classic signs of cardiogenic shock as they relate to this question include low blood pressure and tachycardia. The CVP would rise as the backward effects of the left ventricular failure became apparent. Dysrhythmias commonly occur as a result of decreased oxygenation to the myocardium.
Test-Taking Strategy: Use the process of elimination. Focus on the key words "myocardial ischemia." Recall that ischemia makes the myocardium irritable, producing dysrhythmias. Also, knowledge of the classic signs of shock helps you to eliminate the incorrect options. Review the clinical manifestations associated with cardiogenic shock, if you had difficulty with this question.
Level of Cognitive Ability: Analysis
Client Needs: Physiological Integrity
Integrated Concept/Process: Nursing Process/Assessment
Content Area: Adult Health/Cardiovascular
Reference: Smeltzer, S., & Bare, B. (2000). *Brunner & Suddarth's textbook of medical-surgical nursing* (9th ed.). Philadelphia: Lippincott Williams & Wilkins, p. 673.

14. **3**
Rationale: The normal CO is 4 to 8 liters per minute. With cardiogenic shock, the cardiac output falls below normal, because of failure of the heart as a pump. The PCWP, on the other hand, rises, because it is a reflection of the left ventricular end-diastolic pressure (LVEDP), which rises with pump failure.
Test-Taking Strategy: Use the process of elimination. Knowing that the normal cardiac output is 4 to 8 L/min helps you eliminate options 1 and 2. From the remaining options, think about what the pressure would do in the lungs behind a failing heart to direct you to option 3. Review these concepts, if you had difficulty with this question.

Level of Cognitive Ability: Analysis
Client Needs: Physiological Integrity
Integrated Concept/Process: Nursing Process/Assessment
Content Area: Adult Health/Cardiovascular
Reference: Phipps, W., Sands, J., & Marek, J. (1999). *Medical-surgical nursing: Concepts & clinical practice* (6th ed.). St. Louis: Mosby, p. 634.

15. **4**
Rationale: The nursing interventions for the client with an intraaortic balloon pump are the same as for any cardiovascular surgery client. The peripheral circulation to the affected limb is monitored for signs of occlusion, such as coolness, mottling, pain, tingling, and decreased or absent distal pulse. Adverse changes are reported immediately.
Test-Taking Strategy: Focus on the data provided in this question. From these data, use the ABCs—airway, breathing, and circulation. Since these data indicate a circulatory problem, select option 4. Review nursing care for a client with an IABP if you had difficulty with this question.
Level of Cognitive Ability: Application
Client Needs: Physiological Integrity
Integrated Concept/Process: Nursing Process/Implementation
Content Area: Adult Health/Cardiovascular
Reference: Smeltzer, S., & Bare, B. (2000). *Brunner & Suddarth's textbook of medical-surgical nursing* (9th ed.). Philadelphia: Lippincott Williams & Wilkins, p. 674.

16. **1**
Rationale: Sternotomy incision sites are assessed for signs and symptoms of infection, such as redness, swelling, induration, and drainage. Elevated temperature and WBC count after 3 to 4 days postoperatively usually indicate infection.
Test-Taking Strategy: Use the process of elimination. Eliminate options 2 and 4 because the WBC count is within normal range. From the remaining options, focus on the data in the question. A nonreddened incision with no apparent drainage indicates no signs of infection. Review the signs of infection if you had difficulty with this question.
Level of Cognitive Ability: Analysis
Client Needs: Physiological Integrity
Integrated Concept/Process: Nursing Process/Analysis
Content Area: Adult Health/Cardiovascular
Reference: Ignatavicius, D., Workman, M., & Mishler, M. (1999). *Medical-surgical nursing across the health care continuum* (3rd ed.). Philadelphia: W.B. Saunders, p. 926.

17. **4**
Rationale: The client who undergoes cardiac surgery is at risk for renal injury from poor perfusion, hemolysis, low cardiac output, or vasopressor medication therapy. Renal insult is signaled by decreased urine output, and increased BUN and creatinine. The client may need medications such as dopamine (Intropin) to increase renal perfusion, and could possibly need peritoneal dialysis or hemodialysis. There are no data in the question to indicate the presence of hypovolemia, UTI, or glomerulonephritis.
Test-Taking Strategy: Use the process of elimination. Eliminate options 2 and 3 first because there are no data to indicate infection or inflammation. Noting that the urine output is inadequate will assist in eliminating option 1. Review the complications associated with cardiac surgery if you had difficulty with this question.
Level of Cognitive Ability: Analysis

Client Needs: Physiological Integrity
Integrated Concept/Process: Nursing Process/Analysis
Content Area: Adult Health/Cardiovascular
Reference: Smeltzer, S., & Bare, B. (2000). *Brunner & Suddarth's textbook of medical-surgical nursing* (9th ed.). Philadelphia: Lippincott Williams & Wilkins, pp. 617-618.

18. **2**
Rationale: The nurse should encourage regular use of pain medication for the first 48 to 72 hours after cardiac surgery, because analgesia will promote rest, decrease myocardial oxygen consumption resulting from pain, and allow better participation in activities such as coughing, deep breathing, and ambulation. Options 1 and 3 will not help in tolerating ambulation. Removal of telemetry equipment is contraindicated unless prescribed.
Test Taking Strategy: Use the process of elimination. Focus on the issue, how to best tolerate the ambulation. Coughing and deep breathing will not actively help endurance, so eliminate option 1. Removal of telemetry equipment is contraindicated unless ordered. From the remaining options, focusing on the issue will direct you to option 2. Review comfort measures for the client following cardiac surgery if you had difficulty with this question.
Level of Cognitive Ability: Application
Client Needs: Physiological Integrity
Integrated Concept/Process: Nursing Process/Planning
Content Area: Adult Health/Cardiovascular
Reference: Smeltzer, S., & Bare, B. (2000). *Brunner & Suddarth's textbook of medical-surgical nursing* (9th ed.). Philadelphia: Lippincott Williams & Wilkins, p. 617.

19. **1**
Rationale: Normal sinus rhythm is defined as a regular rhythm with an overall rate of 60 to 100 beats per minute. The PR and QRS measurements are normal, measuring 0.12 to 0.20 second and 0.04 to 0.10 second, respectively.
Test-Taking Strategy: A baseline knowledge of normal ECG measurements is needed to answer this question. Review this content if you are unfamiliar with it.
Level of Cognitive Ability: Analysis
Client Needs: Physiological Integrity
Integrated Concept/Process: Nursing Process/Assessment
Content Area: Adult Health/Cardiovascular
Reference: Smeltzer, S., & Bare, B. (2000). *Brunner & Suddarth's textbook of medical-surgical nursing* (9th ed.). Philadelphia: Lippincott Williams & Wilkins, p. 568.

20. **1**
Rationale: Sudden loss of ECG complexes indicates either ventricular asystole or possibly electrode displacement. Accurate assessment of the client and equipment is necessary to determine the cause and identify the appropriate intervention.
Test-Taking Strategy: Use the steps of the nursing process. Option 1 is the only option that addresses assessment. Review care to the client on a cardiac monitor if you had difficulty with this question. Remember, always assess the client directly before taking any action.
Level of Cognitive Ability: Application
Client Needs: Physiological Integrity
Integrated Concept/Process: Nursing Process/Implementation
Content Area: Adult Health/Cardiovascular

Reference: Ignatavicius, D., Workman, M., & Mishler, M. (1999). *Medical-surgical nursing across the health care continuum* (3rd ed.). Philadelphia: W.B. Saunders, p. 783.

21. **4**
Rationale: Sinus dysrhythmia has all the characteristics of normal sinus rhythm, except there is an irregular PP interval. This is due to phasic changes in the rate of firing of the sinoatrial (SA) node, and may occur with vagal tone and with respiration. It does not affect the cardiac output. Options 1, 2, and 3 identify rhythms that are regular.
Test-Taking Strategy: Use the process of elimination. Eliminate options 1, 2, and 3 because they are similar in that the rhythm of each of these is regular. Review the characteristics of sinus dysrhythmia if you had difficulty with this question.
Level of Cognitive Ability: Analysis
Client Needs: Physiological Integrity
Integrated Concept/Process: Nursing Process/Analysis
Content Area: Adult Health/Cardiovascular
Reference: Smeltzer, S., & Bare, B. (2000). *Brunner & Suddarth's textbook of medical-surgical nursing* (9th ed.). Philadelphia: Lippincott Williams & Wilkins, p. 569.

22. **2**
Rationale: Motion artifact, or "noise," can be caused by frequent client movement, electrode placement on limbs, and insufficient adhesion to the skin, such as placing electrodes over hairy areas of the skin. Electrode placement over bony prominences should also be avoided. Signal interference can also occur with electrode removal and cable disconnection.
Test-Taking Strategy: Use the process of elimination, focusing on the issue, artifact. Note the key word "not." Recalling the causes of artifact will direct you to option 2. Review these causes if you had difficulty with this question.
Level of Cognitive Ability: Analysis
Client Needs: Physiological Integrity
Integrated Concept/Process: Nursing Process/Assessment
Content Area: Adult Health/Cardiovascular
Reference: Ignatavicius, D., Workman, M., & Mishler, M. (1999). *Medical-surgical nursing across the health care continuum* (3rd ed.). Philadelphia: W.B. Saunders, p. 758.

23. **2**
Rationale: VT is characterized by the absence of P waves, wide QRS complexes (usually greater than 0.14 second), and a rate between 100 and 250 impulses per minute. The rhythm is usually fairly regular.
Test-Taking Strategy: Use the process of elimination. Eliminate option 4 first, since there are no P waves. PVCs are isolated ectopic beats superimposed on an underlying rhythm, so option 1 is eliminated next. Recalling that there are no true QRS complexes with VF will direct you to option 2. Review the characteristics of VT if you are unfamiliar with it.
Level of Cognitive Ability: Analysis
Client Needs: Physiological Integrity
Integrated Concept/Process: Nursing Process/Assessment
Content Area: Adult Health/Cardiovascular
Reference: Ignatavicius, D., Workman, M., & Mishler, M. (1999). *Medical-surgical nursing across the health care continuum* (3rd ed.). Philadelphia: W.B. Saunders. pp. 761-762.

24. **4**

Rationale: VT is a life-threatening dysrhythmia that results from an irritable ectopic focus that takes over as pacemaker for the heart. The low cardiac output that results can quickly lead to cerebral and myocardial ischemia. Clients frequently experience a feeling of impending death. VT is treated with antidysrhythmic medications or magnesium sulfate, cardioversion (client awake), or defibrillation (loss of consciousness). VT can deteriorate into ventricular fibrillation at any time.

Test-Taking Strategy: Use the process of elimination. Note the key words "most concerned." Option 3 is incorrect and is eliminated first. From the remaining options, focusing on the key words will direct you to option 4 because this option identifies the life-threatening condition. Review the concerns associated with VT if you had difficulty with this question.

Level of Cognitive Ability: Analysis
Client Needs: Physiological Integrity
Integrated Concept/Process: Nursing Process/Analysis
Content Area: Adult Health/Cardiovascular
Reference: Smeltzer, S., & Bare, B. (2000). *Brunner & Suddarth's textbook of medical-surgical nursing* (9th ed.). Philadelphia: Lippincott Williams & Wilkins, p. 575.

25. **3**

Rationale: First-line treatment of ventricular tachycardia in a client who is hemodynamically stable is the use of antidysrhythmics, such as lidocaine (Xylocaine), procainamide (Pronestyl), and bretylium (Bretylol). Cardioversion may also be needed to correct the rhythm. Defibrillation is used only when there is loss of consciousness. Epinephrine would stimulate an already excitable ventricle, and is contraindicated.

Test-Taking Strategy: Use the process of elimination. Eliminate option 2, recalling that pacemakers are used most often to treat bradycardias and heart block. Knowing that epinephrine is a sympathomimetic eliminates option 4. From the remaining options, noting that the client is awake and alert will direct you to option 3. Review treatment for VT if you had difficulty with this question.

Level of Cognitive Ability: Application
Client Needs: Physiological Integrity
Integrated Concept/Process: Nursing Process/Planning
Content Area: Adult Health/Cardiovascular
Reference: Smeltzer, S., & Bare, B. (2000). *Brunner & Suddarth's textbook of medical-surgical nursing* (9th ed.). Philadelphia: Lippincott Williams & Wilkins, p. 575.

26. **2**

Rationale: Cough CPR is sometimes used in the client with unstable VT. The nurse tells the client to use cough CPR, if prescribed, by inhaling deeply and coughing forcefully every 1 to 3 seconds. It may either terminate the dysrhythmia or sustain the cerebral and coronary circulation for a short time until other measures can be implemented. Options 1, 3, and 4 will not assist in terminating the dysrhythmia.

Test-Taking Strategy: To answer this question, it is necessary to be familiar with the treatment for unstable VT. Review the concept of cough CPR if you are not familiar with it.

Level of Cognitive Ability: Application
Client Needs: Physiological Integrity
Integrated Concept/Process: Teaching/Learning
Content Area: Adult Health/Cardiovascular
Reference: Ignatavicius, D., Workman, M., & Mishler, M. (1999). *Medical-surgical nursing across the health care continuum* (3rd ed.). Philadelphia: W.B. Saunders, p. 781.

27. **1**

Rationale: PVCs can cause hemodynamic compromise. The shortened ventricular filling time with the ectopic beat leads to decreased stroke volume and, if frequent enough, to decreased cardiac output. The client may be asymptomatic or may feel palpitations. They can be caused by cardiac disorders, or by any number of physiological stressors, such as infection, illness, surgery, or trauma, as well as intake of caffeine, nicotine, or alcohol.

Test-Taking Strategy: Note the key words "priority on assessment." Use the ABCs—airway, breathing, and circulation—to direct you to option 1. Review the effects of PVCs if you had difficulty with this question.

Level of Cognitive Ability: Analysis
Client Needs: Physiological Integrity
Integrated Concept/Process: Nursing Process/Assessment
Content Area: Adult Health/Cardiovascular
Reference: Ignatavicius, D., Workman, M., & Mishler, M. (1999). *Medical-surgical nursing across the health care continuum* (3rd ed.). Philadelphia: W.B. Saunders, p. 906.

28. **1**

Rationale: The client with uncontrolled atrial fibrillation with a ventricular rate over 100 beats per minute is at risk for low cardiac output because of loss of atrial kick. The nurse assesses the client for palpitations, chest pain or discomfort, hypotension, pulse deficit, fatigue, weakness, dizziness, syncope, shortness of breath, and distended neck veins.

Test-Taking Strategy: Use the process of elimination. Flat neck veins are normal or indicate hypovolemia, so option 4 is eliminated. Nausea and vomiting (option 2) is associated with vagus nerve activity, and does not correlate with a tachycardic state. From the remaining options, think of the consequences of falling cardiac output to direct you to option 1. Review the effects of atrial fibrillation if you had difficulty with this question.

Level of Cognitive Ability: Analysis
Client Needs: Physiological Integrity
Integrated Concept/Process: Nursing Process/Assessment
Content Area: Adult Health/Cardiovascular
Reference: Ignatavicius, D., Workman, M., & Mishler, M. (1999). *Medical-surgical nursing across the health care continuum* (3rd ed.). Philadelphia: W.B. Saunders, pp. 777-778.

29. **2**

Rationale: Atrial fibrillation is characterized by a loss of P waves; an undulating, wavy baseline; QRS duration that is often within normal limits; and a very irregular ventricular rate, which can range from 60 to 100 beats per minute (when controlled with medications) to a rate of 100 to 160 (when uncontrolled).

Test-Taking Strategy: Use the process of elimination. Noting the key words "there are no P waves" should direct you to option 2. Loss of P waves is characteristic of this dysrhythmia. Review the characteristics of atrial fibrillation if you had difficulty with this question.

Level of Cognitive Ability: Analysis
Client Needs: Physiological Integrity

Integrated Concept/Process: Nursing Process/Assessment
Content Area: Adult Health/Cardiovascular
Reference: Ignatavicius, D., Workman, M., & Mishler, M. (1999). *Medical-surgical nursing across the health care continuum* (3rd ed.). Philadelphia: W.B. Saunders, p. 777.

30. **1**

Rationale: Carotid sinus massage is one of maneuvers used for vagal stimulation to decrease a rapid heart rate and possibly terminate a tachydysrhythmia. The others include inducing the gag reflex and asking the client to strain or bear down. Medication therapy is often needed as an adjunct to keep the rate down, or maintain the normal rhythm. Options 2, 3, and 4 are incorrect descriptions of this procedure.

Test-Taking Strategy: Knowledge of anatomy and physiology alone may be sufficient to answer this question. Eliminate options 2 and 4, since a rapid-rate dysrhythmia would need to be slowed. Recalling the functions of the vagus nerve and the diaphragmatic nerve will direct you to option 1. The vagus nerve affects heart rate. The diaphragmatic nerve affects respiration. If you are unfamiliar with the functions of these nerves, review this content.

Level of Cognitive Ability: Application
Client Needs: Physiological Integrity
Integrated Concept/Process: Teaching/Learning
Content Area: Adult Health/Cardiovascular
Reference: Ignatavicius, D., Workman, M., & Mishler, M. (1999). *Medical-surgical nursing across the health care continuum* (3rd ed.). Philadelphia: W.B. Saunders, pp. 789-790.

31. **2**

Rationale: Ventricular fibrillation is characterized by irregular, chaotic undulations of varying amplitudes. There is no measurable rate, and no visible P waves or QRS complexes. It results from electrical chaos in the ventricles.

Test-Taking Strategy: Use the process of elimination and knowledge regarding the characteristics of ventricular fibrillation. The lack of visible QRS complexes eliminates atrial fibrillation and ventricular tachycardia. Recalling that asystole is lack of any electrical activity of the heart will direct you to option 2. Review the characteristics of ventricular fibrillation if you had difficulty with this question.

Level of Cognitive Ability: Analysis
Client Needs: Physiological Integrity
Integrated Concept/Process: Nursing Process/Assessment
Content Area: Adult Health/Cardiovascular
Reference: Ignatavicius, D., Workman, M., & Mishler, M. (1999). *Medical-surgical nursing across the health care continuum* (3rd ed.). Philadelphia: W.B. Saunders, pp. 782-783.

32. **2**

Rationale: Until the defibrillator is attached and charged, the client is resuscitated by using cardiopulmonary resuscitation. Once the defibrillator has been attached, the ECG is checked to verify that the rhythm is VF or pulseless ventricular tachycardia. Leads are also checked for any loose connections. A nitroglycerin patch, if present, is removed. The client does not have to be intubated in order to be defibrillated. Lidocaine may be given subsequently, but is not required before defibrillation. The machine is not set to the synchronous mode, because there is no underlying rhythm to synchronize with.

Test-Taking Strategy: Use the process of elimination, focusing on the issue, VF. Note that option 2 directly addresses this

issue and also addresses assessment of the client. Review the procedure for defibrillation if you had difficulty with this question.

Level of Cognitive Ability: Analysis
Client Needs: Physiological Integrity
Integrated Concept/Process: Nursing Process/Assessment
Content Area: Adult Health/Cardiovascular
Reference: Smeltzer, S., & Bare, B. (2000). *Brunner & Suddarth's textbook of medical-surgical nursing* (9th ed.). Philadelphia: Lippincott Williams & Wilkins, pp. 582-583.

33. **3**

Rationale: The client may be defibrillated up to three times in succession. The energy levels used are 200, 300, and 360 joules for the first, second, and third attempts, respectively.

Test-Taking Strategy: This is a difficult question to answer unless you are familiar with the defibrillation procedure. As a general rule, though, remember that lower levels of energy are used for cardioversion. Higher levels are used in defibrillation. Review this procedure if you had difficulty with this question.

Level of Cognitive Ability: Analysis
Client Needs: Physiological Integrity
Integrated Concept/Process: Nursing Process/Analysis
Content Area: Adult Health/Cardiovascular
Reference: Ignatavicius, D., Workman, M., & Mishler, M. (1999). *Medical-surgical nursing across the health care continuum* (3rd ed.). Philadelphia: W.B. Saunders, p. 798.

34. **2**

Rationale: After defibrillation, the client requires continuous monitoring of ECG rhythm, hemodynamic status, and neurological status. Respiratory and metabolic acidosis develops during ventricular fibrillation because of lack of respiration and cardiac output. These can cause cerebral as well as cardiopulmonary complications. Arousable status, adequate BP, and a sinus rhythm indicate successful response to defibrillation.

Test-Taking Strategy: Use the process of elimination. Note the key words "most successful." Eliminate options 1 and 3 first, since the client is nonarousable. From the remaining options, select option 2 because a sinus rhythm is a more successful response as compared with marked bradycardia. Review the expected effects of defibrillation if you had difficulty with this question.

Level of Cognitive Ability: Analysis
Client Needs: Physiological Integrity
Integrated Concept/Process: Nursing Process/Evaluation
Content Area: Adult Health/Cardiovascular
Reference: Ignatavicius, D., Workman, M., & Mishler, M. (1999). *Medical-surgical nursing across the health care continuum* (3rd ed.). Philadelphia: W.B. Saunders, p. 792.

35. **2**

Rationale: Nursing responsibilities after cardioversion include maintenance of a patent airway, oxygen administration, assessment of vital signs and level of consciousness, and dysrhythmia detection.

Test Taking Strategy: Use the process of elimination, noting the key words "highest priority." Use the ABCs—airway, breathing, and circulation—to direct you to option 2. Review care of the client following cardioversion if you had difficulty with this question.

Level of Cognitive Ability: Analysis
Client Needs: Physiological Integrity

Integrated Concept/Process: Nursing Process/Assessment
Content Area: Adult Health/Cardiovascular
Reference: Ignatavicius, D., Workman, M., & Mishler, M. (1999). *Medical-surgical nursing across the health care continuum* (3rd ed.). Philadelphia: W.B. Saunders, p. 797.

36. 3

Rationale: The nurse or rescuer puts two large adhesive patch electrodes on the client's chest in the usual defibrillator positions. The nurse stops CPR and orders anyone near the client to move away and not touch the client. The defibrillator then analyzes the rhythm, which may take up to 30 seconds. The machine then indicates if it is necessary to defibrillate.

Test-Taking Strategy: Use the process of elimination. If you are not familiar with this piece of equipment, look first at the word "automatic" in the name. This implies that a person is not as involved in the process as with a conventional defibrillator and will help to eliminate option 2. Since standard ECG monitoring leads do not play an active role once resuscitation is underway (options 1 and 4), you can eliminate these similar options. Review the procedure related to the use of an AED if you had difficulty with this question.
Level of Cognitive Ability: Application
Client Needs: Physiological Integrity
Integrated Concept/Process: Nursing Process/Implementation
Content Area: Adult Health/Cardiovascular
Reference: Ignatavicius, D., Workman, M., & Mishler, M. (1999). *Medical-surgical nursing across the health care continuum* (3rd ed.). Philadelphia: W.B. Saunders, p. 798.

37. 3

Rationale: An AICD detects and delivers an electric shock to terminate life-threatening episodes of ventricular tachycardia and ventricular fibrillation. These devices are implanted in clients who are considered high risk, including those who have survived sudden cardiac death unrelated to myocardial infarction, those who are refractive to medication therapy, and those who have syncopal episodes related to ventricular tachycardia.

Test-Taking Strategy: Use the process of elimination. Note the key words "least likely." Ventricular dysrhythmias that induce syncope or occur while the client is on medication are likely to be true indications for the AICD, so eliminate options 2 and 4 first. From the remaining options, the main difference is whether or not the cardiac arrest was related to myocardial infarction (MI). Of these two, the one most likely to be responsive to AICD would be the client without MI, since those dysrhythmias are spontaneous. Review the indications for the use of an AICD, if you had difficulty with this question.
Level of Cognitive Ability: Analysis
Client Needs: Physiological Integrity
Integrated Concept/Process: Nursing Process/Analysis
Content Area: Adult Health/Cardiovascular
Reference: Ignatavicius, D., Workman, M., & Mishler, M. (1999). *Medical-surgical nursing across the health care continuum* (3rd ed.). Philadelphia: W.B. Saunders, p. 800.

38. 1

Rationale: The nurse who is caring for the client after insertion of an AICD needs to determine device settings, similar to after insertion of a permanent pacemaker. Specifically, the nurse needs to know if it is activated, the heart rate cutoff above which it will fire, and the number of shocks it is programmed to deliver. Options 2, 3, and 4 are also nursing interventions but are not the priority.

Test-Taking Strategy: Use Maslow's Hierarchy of Needs theory. Option 1 is the option that identifies the physiological need. Review care to the client following insertion of an AICD if you had difficulty with this question.
Level of Cognitive Ability: Application
Client Needs: Physiological Integrity
Integrated Concept/Process: Nursing Process/Assessment
Content Area: Adult Health/Cardiovascular
Reference: Ignatavicius, D., Workman, M., & Mishler, M. (1999). *Medical-surgical nursing across the health care continuum* (3rd ed.). Philadelphia: W.B. Saunders, p. 800.

39. 1

Rationale: In the first several hours after insertion of either a permanent or a temporary pacemaker, the most common complication is pacing electrode dislodgment. The nurse helps prevent this complication by limiting the client's activities.

Test-Taking Strategy: Use the process of elimination. Note that the pacemaker was inserted on the right side. Therefore, to prevent pacing electrode dislodgment, motion must be limited on that side. Options 3 and 4 involve movement of the right arm and are eliminated first. Limiting the movement of the left arm (option 2) is of no benefit to the client. Thus, option 1 is the correct option. Review care to the client following insertion of a pacemaker if you had difficulty with this question.
Level of Cognitive Ability: Application
Client Needs: Physiological Integrity
Integrated Concept/Process: Nursing Process/Implementation
Content Area: Adult Health/Cardiovascular
Reference: Smeltzer, S., & Bare, B. (2000). *Brunner & Suddarth's textbook of medical-surgical nursing* (9th ed.). Philadelphia: Lippincott Williams & Wilkins, p. 585.

40. 3

Rationale: Pulmonary embolism is a life-threatening complication of deep vein thrombosis and thrombophlebitis. Chest pain is the most common symptom, which is sudden in onset, and may be aggravated by breathing. Other signs and symptoms include dyspnea, cough, diaphoresis, and apprehension.

Test-Taking Strategy: Focus on the client's diagnosis to answer the question. Recalling the complications related to thrombophlebitis will direct you to option 3. Review these complications and the associated signs and symptoms if you had difficulty with this question.
Level of Cognitive Ability: Analysis
Client Needs: Physiological Integrity
Integrated Concept/Process: Nursing Process/Assessment
Content Area: Adult Health/Cardiovascular
Reference: Smeltzer, S., & Bare, B. (2000). *Brunner & Suddarth's textbook of medical-surgical nursing* (9th ed.). Philadelphia: Lippincott Williams & Wilkins, pp. 471-472.

41. 1

Rationale: Sclerotherapy is the injection of a sclerosing agent into a varicosity. The agent damages the vessel and causes aseptic thrombosis, which results in vein closure. With no blood flow through the vessel, there is no distention. The surgical procedure for varicose veins is vein ligation and stripping. This procedure involves tying off the varicose vein and large tributaries, and then removal of the vein with the use of hook and wires via multiple small incisions in the leg.

Test-Taking Strategy: Use the process of elimination. Note the name of the procedure, "sclerotherapy." A vessel that is sclerosed is blocked. This will direct you to option 1. Review this procedure, if you had difficulty with this question.

Level of Cognitive Ability: Comprehension
Client Needs: Physiological Integrity
Integrated Concept/Process: Teaching/Learning
Content Area: Adult Health/Cardiovascular
Reference: Lemone, P., & Burke, K. (2000). *Medical-surgical nursing: Critical thinking in client care* (2nd ed.). Upper Saddle River, N.J.: Prentice-Hall, p. 1252.

42. **4**
Rationale: Hypersensitivity or a sensation of "pins and needles" in the surgical limb may indicate temporary or permanent nerve injury following surgery. The saphenous vein and the saphenous nerve run close together in the distal third of the leg. Since complications from this surgery are relatively rare, this symptom should be reported.

Test-Taking Strategy: Use the process of elimination. Pins and needles sensations usually indicate nerve irritation or damage. If you know this, options 2 and 3 can be eliminated. Reassuring the client about something being "only temporary" is not often an appropriate action, unless this is known to be absolutely true. Review the complications associated with vein ligation and stripping if you had difficulty with this question.

Level of Cognitive Ability: Analysis
Client Needs: Physiological Integrity
Integrated Concept/Process: Nursing Process/Implementation
Content Area: Adult Health/Cardiovascular
Reference: Lemone, P., & Burke, K. (2000). *Medical-surgical nursing: Critical thinking in client care* (2nd ed.). Upper Saddle River, N.J.: Prentice-Hall, p. 1254.

43. **2**
Rationale: The mixture of arterial and venous manifestations (claudication and phlebitis, respectively) in the young male client suggests thromboangiitis obliterans (Buerger's disease). This is a relatively uncommon disorder that is characterized by inflammation and thrombosis of smaller arteries and veins. This disorder is typically found in young adult males who smoke. The cause is not precisely known, but is suspected to have an autoimmune component.

Test-Taking Strategy: Use the process of elimination and knowledge of this disorder to answer the question. Eliminate options 3 and 4 because they would most likely cause local skin reactions. From the remaining options, focus on the key words "next assess." It is often better to assess a modifiable factor before a nonmodifiable one. Review this disorder if you had difficulty with this question.

Level of Cognitive Ability: Analysis
Client Needs: Physiological Integrity
Integrated Concept/Process: Nursing Process/Assessment
Content Area: Adult Health/Cardiovascular
Reference: Lemone, P., & Burke, K. (2000). *Medical-surgical nursing: Critical thinking in client care* (2nd ed.). Upper Saddle River, N.J.: Prentice-Hall, p. 1223.

44. **4**
Rationale: Raynaud's disease responds favorably to eliminating caffeine from the diet and by the cessation of smoking.

Medications may inhibit vessel spasm and prevent symptoms. Avoiding exposure to cold through a variety of means is very important. However, moving to a warmer climate may not necessarily be beneficial because the symptoms could still occur with the use of air conditioning, and during periods of cooler weather.

Test-Taking Strategy: Use the process of elimination. Note the key words "needs further reinforcement." Think about the measures used to treat the disease to direct you to option 4. Also, relocation is the least favorable of all the options, from the viewpoints of practicality and encountering new environmental concerns.

Level of Cognitive Ability: Analysis
Client Needs: Physiological Integrity
Integrated Concept/Process: Teaching/Learning
Content Area: Adult Health/Cardiovascular
Reference: Lemone, P., & Burke, K. (2000). *Medical-surgical nursing: Critical thinking in client care* (2nd ed.). Upper Saddle River, N.J.: Prentice-Hall, p. 1226-1227.

45. **2**
Rationale: After IVC filter insertion, the nurse inspects the surgical site for bleeding and signs and symptoms of infection. Otherwise, care is the same as for any other postoperative client.

Test-Taking Strategy: Use the process of elimination. Since these devices are inserted percutaneously through a deep vein, options 3 and 4 are eliminated because there is no abdominal incision. From the remaining options, noting that the client has been on anticoagulant therapy before surgery because of the high risk of pulmonary embolism will direct you to option 2. Review care of the client following insertion of an IVC filter if you had difficulty with this question.

Level of Cognitive Ability: Analysis
Client Needs: Physiological Integrity
Integrated Concept/Process: Nursing Process/Assessment
Content Area: Adult Health/Cardiovascular
Reference: Smeltzer, S., & Bare, B. (2000). *Brunner & Suddarth's textbook of medical-surgical nursing* (9th ed.). Philadelphia: Lippincott Williams & Wilkins, p. 475.

46. **4**
Rationale: Blood pressure should be taken with the client seated with the arm bared, positioned with support and at heart level. The client should sit with the legs on the floor, feet uncrossed, and not speak during the recording. The client should not have smoked tobacco or taken in caffeine in the 30 minutes preceding the measurement. The client should rest quietly for 5 minutes before the reading is taken. The cuff bladder should encircle at least 80% of the limb being measured. Gauges other than a mercury sphygmomanometer should be calibrated every 6 months to ensure accuracy. Finally, two or more readings should be averaged.

Test-Taking Strategy: Use the process of elimination, noting the key word "avoiding." Looking for the option that identifies variables that interfere with accuracy (caffeine and nicotine) will direct you to option 4. Review this skill and procedure if you had difficulty with this question.

Level of Cognitive Ability: Application
Client Needs: Physiological Integrity
Integrated Concept/Process: Nursing Process/Assessment
Content Area: Adult Health/Cardiovascular

Reference: Lemone, P., & Burke, K. (2000). *Medical-surgical nursing: Critical thinking in client care* (2nd ed.). Upper Saddle River, N.J.: Prentice-Hall, p. 1198.

47. 4

Rationale: The antidote to heparin is protamine sulfate, and should be readily available for use if excessive bleeding or hemorrhage should occur. Vitamin K is an antidote for warfarin sodium. Aminocaproic acid is the antidote for thrombolytic therapy. KCl is administered for a potassium deficit.

Test-Taking Strategy: Knowledge regarding the various antidotes is needed to answer this question. Learn these antidotes if you had difficulty with this question.

Level of Cognitive Ability: Application
Client Needs: Physiological Integrity
Integrated Concept/Process: Nursing Process/Implementation
Content Area: Adult Health/Cardiovascular
Reference: Hodgson, B., & Kizior, R. (2001). *Saunders nursing drug handbook 2001.* Philadelphia: W.B. Saunders, p. 1098.

48. 3

Rationale: The therapeutic range for prothrombin time (PT) is 1.5 to 2 times the control for clients at high risk for thrombus. Based on the client's control value, the therapeutic range for this individual would be 16.5 to 22 seconds. Therefore, the result is within the therapeutic range.

Test Taking Strategy: Use the process of elimination. Look at the control value. Remembering that the purpose of anticoagulant therapy is to prolong clotting times will assist in eliminating options 1 and 2. Since the PT value identified in the question is not even double the control, select option 3 from the remaining options. Review the therapeutic PT level for a client at risk for pulmonary embolism if you had difficulty with this question.

Level of Cognitive Ability: Analysis
Client Needs: Physiological Integrity
Integrated Concept/Process: Nursing Process/Assessment
Content Area: Adult Health/Cardiovascular
Reference: Hodgson, B., & Kizior, R. (2001). *Saunders nursing drug handbook 2001.* Philadelphia: W.B. Saunders, pp. 1062-1064.

49. 2

Rationale: Warfarin sodium works in the liver. It inhibits synthesis of four vitamin K–dependent clotting factors (X, IX, VII, and II), but it takes 3 to 4 days before the therapeutic effect of warfarin is exhibited.

Test-Taking Strategy: Use the process of elimination. Heparin and warfarin sodium do not act in the same way, so eliminate option 4 first. Warfarin is an anticoagulant, not a thrombolytic, so option 3 is eliminated next. From the remaining options, recalling that the liver synthesizes clotting factors will direct you to option 2. Review the action of warfarin sodium if you had difficulty with this question.

Level of Cognitive Ability: Application
Client Needs: Physiological Integrity
Integrated Concept/Process: Teaching/Learning
Content Area: Adult Health/Cardiovascular
Reference: Ignatavicius, D., Workman, M., & Mishler, M. (1999). *Medical-surgical nursing across the health care continuum* (3rd ed.). Philadelphia: W.B. Saunders, pp. 874-875.

50. 1

Rationale: The antidote to warfarin (Coumadin) is vitamin K, and should be readily available for use if excessive bleeding or hemorrhage should occur. Aminocaproic acid is the antidote for thrombolytic agents. Protamine sulfate is the antidote for heparin. KCl is administered to treat potassium deficit.

Test-Taking Strategy: Knowledge regarding the various antidotes is needed to answer this question. Review these antidotes if you had difficulty with this question.

Level of Cognitive Ability: Application
Client Needs: Physiological Integrity
Integrated Concept/Process: Nursing Process/Implementation
Content Area: Adult Health/Cardiovascular
Reference: Hodgson, B., & Kizior, R. (2001). *Saunders nursing drug handbook 2001.* Philadelphia: W.B. Saunders, pp. 1062-1064.

51. 1

Rationale: Thrombolytic agents dissolve existing clots, and bleeding can occur anywhere in the body. The nurse monitors for any obvious signs of bleeding and also for occult signs of bleeding, which would include hemoglobin and hematocrit, blood pressure and pulse, neurological signs, assessment of abdominal and back pain, and the presence of blood in the urine or stool.

Test-Taking Strategy: Remember that bleeding is the primary complication of thrombolytic therapy. Note the key words "least frequent measurement." Therefore, look for the option that is not related to bleeding. A change in neurological signs could indicate cerebral bleeding; abdominal and back pain could indicate abdominal bleeding; change in blood pressure and pulse could be general indicators of hemorrhage. Oxygen saturation is not an indicator of bleeding in the respiratory tract; more likely, hemoptysis would be noted. Review nursing considerations for the client receiving t-PA, if you had difficulty with this question.

Level of Cognitive Ability: Analysis
Client Needs: Physiological Integrity
Integrated Concept/Process: Nursing Process/Assessment
Content Area: Adult Health/Cardiovascular
Reference: Ignatavicius, D., Workman, M., & Mishler, M. (1999). *Medical-surgical nursing across the health care continuum* (3rd ed.). Philadelphia: W.B. Saunders, p. 875.

52. 4

Rationale: Thrombolytic therapy is contraindicated in a number of preexisting conditions in which there is a risk of uncontrolled bleeding, similar to the case in anticoagulant therapy. It is also contraindicated in severe uncontrolled hypertension because of the risk of cerebral hemorrhage. Therefore, the nurse would report the results of the BP to the physician before initiating therapy.

Test-Taking Strategy: Use the process of elimination and focus on the client's diagnosis. Options 1, 2, and 3 may be present in the client with pulmonary thromboembolism, and are not necessarily signs that warrants reporting before this therapy is initiated. Review the contraindications associated with the administration of this medication if you had difficulty with this question.

Level of Cognitive Ability: Analysis
Client Needs: Safe, Effective Care Environment
Integrated Concept/Process: Nursing Process/Analysis

Content Area: Adult Health/Cardiovascular
Reference: Hodgson, B., & Kizior, R. (2001). *Saunders nursing drug handbook 2001.* Philadelphia: W.B. Saunders, pp. 946-948.

53. 3
Rationale: The client is experiencing an anaphylactic reaction to streptokinase, which is allergenic. The infusion should be discontinued, the physician is notified, and the client should receive treatment with epinephrine, antihistamines, and corticosteroids.
Test-Taking Strategy: Recall that allergic reaction and possible anaphylaxis are risks associated with streptokinase therapy. Also, focusing on the signs and symptoms in the question will assist in answering the question. When a severe allergic reaction occurs, the offending substance should be stopped, and lifesaving treatment should begin. Review the adverse effects of this medication if you had difficulty with this question.
Level of Cognitive Ability: Analysis
Client Needs: Physiological Integrity
Integrated Concept/Process: Nursing Process/Analysis
Content Area: Adult Health/Cardiovascular
Reference: Smeltzer, S., & Bare, B. (2000). *Brunner & Suddarth's textbook of medical-surgical nursing* (9th ed.). Philadelphia: Lippincott Williams & Wilkins, p. 1391.

54. 1
Rationale: An expected outcome of surgery is warmth, redness, and edema in the surgical extremity, because of increased blood flow. Options 2, 3, and 4 are incorrect interpretations.
Test-Taking Strategy: Use the process of elimination. Option 3 can be eliminated because the pedal pulse is unchanged from admission. Venous complications from immobilization resulting from surgery would not be apparent within 4 hours, so option 4 is eliminated. From the remaining options, think about the effects of sudden reperfusion in an ischemic limb. There would be redness from new blood flow, and edema from the sudden change in pressure in the blood vessels. Review the expected assessment findings following this surgical procedure if you had difficulty with this question.
Level of Cognitive Ability: Analysis
Client Needs: Physiological Integrity
Integrated Concept/Process: Nursing Process/Assessment
Content Area: Adult Health/Cardiovascular
Reference: Ignatavicius, D., Workman, M., & Mishler, M. (1999). *Medical-surgical nursing across the health care continuum* (3rd ed.). Philadelphia: W.B. Saunders, p. 858.

55. 1
Rationale: Following pericardiocentesis, a rise in blood pressure and a fall in CVP are expected. The client usually expresses immediate relief. Heart sounds are no longer muffled or distant.
Test-Taking Strategy: Use the process of elimination. Note the key word "unsuccessful." Successful therapy is measured by the disappearance of the original signs and symptoms of cardiac tamponade. Therefore, look for the option that identifies a sign consistent with continued tamponade. Review signs of cardiac tamponade and the expected effects of pericardiocentesis if you had difficulty with this question.
Level of Cognitive Ability: Analysis
Client Needs: Physiological Integrity
Integrated Concept/Process: Nursing Process/Evaluation

Content Area: Adult Health/Cardiovascular
Reference: Lemone, P., & Burke, K. (2000). *Medical-surgical nursing: Critical thinking in client care* (2nd ed.). Upper Saddle River, N.J.: Prentice-Hall, p. 1168.

56. 2
Rationale: Not all clients with AAA exhibit symptoms. Those who do may describe a feeling of the "heart beating" in the abdomen when supine, or being able to feel the mass throbbing. A pulsatile mass may be palpated in the middle and upper abdomen. A systolic bruit may be auscultated over the mass. Hyperactive bowel sounds are not specifically related to an AAA.
Test-Taking Strategy: Use the process of elimination. Note the key word "unrelated." Note that options 1, 3, and 4 are similar in that they identify a circulatory component. Review the signs of AAA if you had difficulty with this question.
Level of Cognitive Ability: Analysis
Client Needs: Physiological Integrity
Integrated Concept/Process: Nursing Process/Assessment
Content Area: Adult Health/Cardiovascular
Reference: Lemone, P., & Burke, K. (2000). *Medical-surgical nursing: Critical thinking in client care* (2nd ed.). Upper Saddle River, N.J.: Prentice-Hall, p. 1231.

57. 4
Rationale: Following AAA resection or repair, the nurse monitors the client for signs of renal failure. This can occur because there is often much blood loss during the surgery, and depending on the aneurysm location, the renal arteries may be hypoperfused for a short period during surgery. The nurse monitors hourly intake and output, and notes the results of daily BUN and creatinine levels. Urine output less than 50 mL/hr is reported to the physician.
Test-Taking Strategy: Focus on the information in the question and the abnormal assessment data. In this question, there are elevations in BUN and creatinine levels, as well as a significant drop in hourly urine output. These assessment findings should direct you to option 4. Review the complications associated with this surgical procedure if you had difficulty with this question.
Level of Cognitive Ability: Analysis
Client Needs: Physiological Integrity
Integrated Concept/Process: Nursing Process/Implementation
Content Area: Adult Health/Cardiovascular
Reference: Lemone, P., & Burke, K. (2000). *Medical-surgical nursing: Critical thinking in client care* (2nd ed.). Upper Saddle River, N.J.: Prentice-Hall, p. 1234-1235.

58. 4
Rationale: Venous leg ulcers, also called stasis ulcers, tend to be more superficial than arterial ulcers, and the ulcer bed is pink. The edges of the ulcer are uneven, and there is evidence of granulation tissue. There is a brown pigmentation to the skin, from accumulation of metabolic waste products resulting from venous stasis. The client also exhibits peripheral edema.
Test-Taking Strategy: Use the process of elimination. It is necessary to discriminate between the signs and symptoms of arterial and venous leg ulcers. Knowing that the information in options 1, 2, and 3 is due to tissue malnutrition (and thus an arterial problem), will direct you to option 4. Review the assessment findings in arterial and venous conditions if you had difficulty with this question.
Level of Cognitive Ability: Analysis

Client Needs: Physiological Integrity
Integrated Concept/Process: Nursing Process/Assessment
Content Area: Adult Health/Cardiovascular
Reference: Lemone, P., & Burke, K. (2000). *Medical-surgical nursing: Critical thinking in client care* (2nd ed.). Upper Saddle River, N.J.: Prentice-Hall, p. 1257.

59. 2
Rationale: The first signs and symptoms of digitalis toxicity in adults include abdominal pain, nausea, vomiting, visual disturbances (blurred, yellow, or green vision, halos around lights), bradycardia, and other dysrhythmias. Options 1, 3, and 4 are unrelated to digoxin therapy.
Test Taking Strategy: Use the process of elimination, noting that the client is receiving digoxin. Recalling the signs of digoxin toxicity will direct you to option 2. Review these signs if you had difficulty with this question.
Level of Cognitive Ability: Application
Client Needs: Physiological Integrity
Integrated Concept/Process: Nursing Process/Assessment
Content Area: Adult Health/Cardiovascular
Reference: Hodgson, B., & Kizior, R. (2001). *Saunders nursing drug handbook 2001.* Philadelphia: W.B. Saunders, pp. 324-326.

60. 3
Rationale: Stable angina is induced by exercise and relieved by rest or nitroglycerin tablets. Unstable angina occurs at lower and lower levels of activity, or at rest, is less predictable and is often a precursor of myocardial infarction. Variant angina, or Prinzmetal's angina, is prolonged and severe, and occurs at the same time each day, most often in the morning.

Test-Taking Strategy: Use the process of elimination, focusing on the data in the question. Noting the key words "occurs at the same time each day" will direct you to option 1. If you had difficulty with this question, review the characteristics of the various types of angina.
Level of Cognitive Ability: Comprehension
Client Needs: Physiological Integrity
Integrated Concept/Process: Nursing Process/Assessment
Content Area: Adult Health/Cardiovascular
Reference: Monahan, F., & Neighbors, M. (1998). *Medical-surgical nursing: Foundations for clinical practice* (2nd ed.). Philadelphia: W.B. Saunders, p. 286.

CRITICAL THINKING: FREE-TEXT ENTRY

Answer: Calls for help and initiates cardiopulmonary resuscitation (CPR)
Rationale: When ventricular fibrillation (VF) occurs, the nurse calls for help, remains with the client, and initiates cardiopulmonary resuscitation (CPR).
Test-Taking Strategy: Use the ABCs—airway, breathing, and circulation—to answer the question. CPR needs to be initiated. Review interventions for the client with VF if you had difficulty with this question.
Level of Cognitive Ability: Application
Client Needs: Physiological Integrity
Integrated Concept/Process: Nursing Process/Implementation
Content Area: Adult Health/Cardiovascular
Reference: Ignatavicius, D., Workman, M., & Mishler, M. (1999). *Medical-surgical nursing across the health care continuum* (3rd ed.). Philadelphia: W.B. Saunders, p. 783.

REFERENCES

Hodgson, B., & Kizior, R. (2001). *Saunders nursing drug handbook 2001.* Philadelphia: W.B. Saunders.

Ignatavicius, D., Workman, M., & Mishler, M. (1999). *Medical-surgical nursing across the health care continuum* (3rd ed.). Philadelphia: W.B. Saunders.

Jarvis, C. (2000). *Physical examination and health assessment* (3rd ed.). Philadelphia: W.B. Saunders.

LeMone, P., & Burke, K. (2000). *Medical-surgical nursing: Critical thinking in client care* (2nd ed.). Upper Saddle River, N.J.: Prentice-Hall.

Monahan, F., & Neighbors, M. (1998). *Medical-surgical nursing: Foundations for clinical practice* (2nd ed.). Philadelphia: W.B. Saunders.

Phipps, W., Sands, J., & Marek, J. (1999). *Medical-surgical nursing: Concepts & clinical practice* (6th ed.). St. Louis: Mosby.

Smeltzer, S., & Bare, B. (2000). *Brunner & Suddarth's textbook of medical-surgical nursing* (9th ed.). Philadelphia: Lippincott Williams & Wilkins.

Cardiovascular Medications

I. ANTICOAGULANTS (Box 58-1)

A. Description
1. Prevent the extension and formation of clots by inhibiting factors in the clotting cascade and decreasing blood coagulability
2. Used for thrombosis, pulmonary embolism, and myocardial infarction (MI)
3. Contraindicated with active bleeding, except for disseminated intravascular coagulation (DIC), bleeding disorders or blood dyscrasias, ulcers, liver and kidney disease, and spinal cord or brain injuries

B. Side effects (Box 58-2)
1. Hemorrhage
2. Hematuria
3. Epistaxis
4. Ecchymosis
5. Bleeding gums
6. Thrombocytopenia
7. Hypotension

C. Heparin sodium (Liquaemin Sodium)
1. Description
   a. Prevents thrombin from converting fibrinogen to fibrin
   b. Prevents thromboembolism
   c. The therapeutic dose does not dissolve clots, but prevents new thrombus formation
2. Blood levels
   a. Normal activated partial thromboplastin time (APTT) is 20 to 36 seconds
   b. Maintain APTT at 1.5 to 2.5 times normal
   c. At therapeutic levels, heparin will increase the APTT by a factor of 1.5 to 2
   d. APTT therapy should be measured every 4 to 6 hours during initial therapy, and then on a daily basis
   e. If the APTT is too long, greater than 80 seconds, the dosage should be lowered
   f. If APTT is too short, less than 60 seconds, the dosage should be increased
   g. Normal clotting time is 8 to 15 minutes; maintain the clotting time at 15 to 20 minutes
3. Implementation
   a. Monitor clotting time and APTT
   b. Monitor platelet count
   c. Observe for bleeding gums, bruises, nosebleeds, hematuria, hematemesis, occult blood in the stool, and petechiae
   d. When administering heparin subcutaneously, inject into the abdomen with a small needle (25- to 28 gauge) at a 90-degree angle and do not aspirate or rub the injection site
   e. Instruct the client regarding measures to prevent bleeding
   f. Antidote: protamine sulfate

D. Warfarin sodium (Coumadin)
1. Description
   a. Decreases prothrombin activity and prevents the use of vitamin K by the liver
   b. Used for long-term anticoagulation
   c. Prolongs clotting time and is monitored by the prothrombin time (PT)
   d. Used mainly to prevent thromboembolitic conditions such as thrombophlebitis, pulmonary embolism, and embolism formation caused by atrial fibrillation, thrombosis, myocardial infarction (MI), or heart valve damage
   e. Usually given for 2 to 3 months after an MI to decrease the incidence of deep vein thrombosis and thromboembolism
2. Blood levels
   a. Average PT is 9.6 to 11.8 seconds
   b. Warfarin sodium prolongs the PT
3. International normalized ratio (INR)
   a. The normal INR is 1.3 to 2.0
   b. The INR is determined by multiplying the observed PT ratio (the ratio of the client's PT

BOX 58-1

Anticoagulants

ORAL
Anisindione (Miradon)
Warfarin sodium (Coumadin)

PARENTERAL
Ardeparin (Normiflo)
Dalteparin (Fragmin)
Danaparoid (Orgaran)
Enoxaprin (Lovenox)
Heparin sodium (Liquaemin)

BOX 58-2

Substances to Avoid with Anticoagulants

Green leafy vegetables and foods high in vitamin K
Allopurinol (Zyloprim)
Cimetadine (Tagamet)
Corticosteroids
Nonsteroidal antiinflammatory drugs (NSAIDs)
Oral hypoglycemic agents
Phenytoin (Dilantin)
Salicylates
Sulfonamides

---

to a control PT) by a correction factor specific to a particular thromboplastin preparation used in the testing

   c. The treatment goal is to raise the INR to an appropriate value

   d. An INR of 2 to 3 is appropriate for most clients, although for some clients, the target INR is 3.0 to 4.5

   e. If the INR is below the recommended range, warfarin sodium should be increased

   f. If the INR is above the recommended range, warfarin sodium should be reduced

  4. Implementation

   a. Monitor PT and INR

   b. Observe for bleeding gums, bruises, nosebleeds, hematuria, hematemesis, occult blood in the stool, and petechiae

   c. Instruct the client regarding measures to prevent bleeding

   d. Antidote: Vitamin K, phytonadione (Aqua-MEPHYTON)

II. THROMBOLYTIC MEDICATIONS (Box 58-3)

A. Description

  1. Activate plasminogen; plasminogen generates plasmin (the enzyme that dissolves clots)

  2. Used early in the course of myocardial infarct (within 4 to 6 hours of the onset of the infarct) to restore blood flow, limit myocardial damage,

---

BOX 58-3

Thrombolytic Medications

Alteplase (Activase, t-PA, tissue plasminogen activator)
Anistreplase (APSAC) (Eminase)
Reteplase (Retavase)
Streptokinase (Kabikinase, Streptase)
Urokinase (Abbokinase)

---

preserve left ventricular function, and prevent death

B. Contraindications

  1. Active internal bleeding

  2. History of cerebrovascular accident (CVA)

  3. Intracranial problems

  4. Intracranial surgery or trauma within the previous 2 months

  5. History of thoracic, pelvic, or abdominal surgery in the previous 10 days

  6. History of hepatic or renal disease

  7. Uncontrolled hypertension

  8. Recently required, prolonged cardiopulmonary resuscitation (CPR)

C. Side effects

  1. Bleeding

  2. Dysrhythmias

  3. Fever

  4. Allergic reactions

D. Implementation

  1. Obtain APTT, PT, fibrinogen level, hematocrit, and platelet count

  2. Monitor vital signs

  3. Assess pulses

  4. Monitor for bleeding

  5. Monitor all excretions for occult blood

  6. Monitor for neurological changes such as slurred speech, lethargy, confusion, and hemiparesis

  7. Monitor for hypotension and tachycardia

  8. Avoid injections if possible

  9. Apply direct pressure over a puncture site for 20 to 30 minutes

  10. Handle the client as little as possible when moving

  11. Instruct the client to use electric razor for shaving and to brush teeth gently

  12. Discontinue the medication if bleeding develops, and notify the physician

  13. Antidote

   a. Aminocaproic acid (Amicar)

   b. Used only in acute, life-threatening conditions

III. ANTIPLATELET MEDICATIONS (Box 58-4)

A. Description

  1. Inhibit the aggregation of platelets in the clotting process, thereby prolonging the bleeding time

BOX 58-4

Antiplatelet Medications

Abciximab (ReoPro)
Aspirin (acetylsalicylic acid, ASA)
Clopidolgrel bisulfate (Plavix)
Dipyridamole (Persantine)
Eptifibatide (Integril)
Ticlopidine hydrochloride (Ticlid)

BOX 58-5

Positive Inotropic/Cardiotonic Medications

AMRINONE (INOCOR)
Used for short-term management of congestive heart failure in those who have not responded adequately to cardiac glycosides, diuretics, and vasodilators

MILRINONE (PRIMACOR)
Used for short-term management of congestive heart failure or may be given prior to heart transplantation

2. May be used in conjunction with anticoagulants
3. Used in the prophylaxis of long-term complications following MI, coronary revascularization, and CVAs
4. Contraindicated in bleeding disorders and known sensitivity

B. Side effects
1. Gastrointestinal (GI) bleeding
2. Bruising
3. Hematuria
4. Tarry stools

C. Implementation
1. Determine sensitivity prior to administration
2. Monitor vital signs
3. Instruct the client to take medication with food if GI upset occurs
4. Monitor bleeding time
5. Monitor for side effects related to bleeding
6. Instruct the client in the use of the medication
7. Instruct the client to monitor for side effects related to bleeding and in the measures to prevent bleeding

IV. **POSITIVE INOTROPIC/CARDIOTONIC MEDICATIONS** (Box 58-5)
A. Description
1. Stimulate myocardial **contractility** and produce a positive inotropic effect
2. The increase in myocardial **contractility** increases cardiac, peripheral, and kidney function by increasing **cardiac output,** decreasing **preload,** improving blood flow to the periphery and kidneys, decreasing edema, and increasing fluid excretion; as a result, fluid retention in the lungs and extremities is decreased

B. Side effects
1. Dysrhythmias
2. Hypotension
3. Thrombocytopenia

C. Toxic/adverse reactions
1. Hepatotoxicity manifested by elevated liver enzyme levels
2. Hypersensitivity manifested by wheezing, shortness of breath, pruritis, urticaria, clammy skin, and flushing

D. Implementation
1. For intravenous (IV) administration
   a. Do not dilute with dextrose-containing solutions
   b. For continuous IV, administer with an infusion pump
   c. Stop infusion if the client's **blood pressure (BP)** drops or dysrhythmias occur
2. Monitor apical pulse and **BP**
3. Monitor for hypersensitivity
4. Assess lung sounds for wheezing and rales
5. Monitor for edema
6. Monitor for relief of congestive heart failure (CHF) as noted by reduction in edema, lessening of dyspnea, orthopnea, and fatigue
7. Monitor electrolytes, liver enzymes, platelet count, and renal function studies; may decrease potassium and increase liver enzymes

E. Milrinone (Primacor)
1. Side effects
   a. Headache
   b. Hypotension
   c. Angina
2. Toxic/adverse reactions: dysrhythmias
3. Implementation
   a. For IV injection of loading dose, administer slowly over 10 minutes
   b. For continuous IV, administer with an infusion pump
   c. Monitor apical pulse and **BP**
   d. Stop infusion if the client's **BP** drops or dysrhythmias occur
   e. Assess lung sounds for wheezing and rales
   f. Monitor for edema
   g. Monitor for relief of CHF as noted by reduction in edema, lessening of dyspnea, orthopnea, and fatigue

V. **CARDIAC GLYCOSIDES** (Box 58-6)
A. Description
1. Inhibit sodium-potassium pump, thus increasing intracellular calcium, which causes the heart muscle fibers to contract more efficiently

BOX 58-6

Cardiac Glycosides

Digoxin (Lanoxicaps, Lanoxin)
Digitoxin (Crystodigin)

2. Produce a positive inotropic action, which increases the force of myocardial contractions
3. Produce a negative chronotropic action, which depresses the sinoatrial (SA) node, reduces conduction of the impulse through the atrioventricular (AV) node, and slows the heart rate
4. Produce a negative dromotropic action that decreases the conduction of the heart cells
5. The increase in myocardial **contractility** increases cardiac, peripheral, and kidney function by increasing **cardiac output**, decreasing **preload**, improving blood flow to the periphery and kidneys, decreasing edema, and increasing fluid excretion; as a result, fluid retention in the lungs and extremities is decreased
6. Used for CHF, atrial tachycardia, atrial fibrillation, and atrial flutter
7. Contraindicated in ventricular dysrhythmias and second- or third-degree heart block
8. Used with caution in clients with renal disease, hypothyroidism, and hypokalemia

B. Side effects
   1. Anorexia, nausea, vomiting
   2. Headache
   3. Visual disturbances: diplopia, blurred vision, yellow-green halos
   4. Photophobia
   5. Drowsiness
   6. Bradycardia
   7. Fatigue, weakness

C. Implementation
   1. Monitor for toxicity as evidenced by anorexia, nausea, vomiting, visual disturbances, confusion, bradycardia, heart block, premature ventricular contractions (PVCs), and tachydysrhythmias
   2. Monitor serum digoxin level, electrolyte levels, and renal function tests
   3. Therapeutic digoxin range is 0.5 to 2.0 ng/mL, and levels above 2.0 ng/mL are toxic
   4. An increased risk of toxicity exists in clients with hypercalcemia, hypokalemia, hypomagnesemia, or hypothyroidism
   5. Monitor potassium level, and if hypokalemia occurs (potassium below 3.5 mEq/L), notify the physician
   6. Instruct the client to avoid over-the-counter medications
   7. Monitor the client taking a potassium-wasting diuretic or corticosteroids closely for hypokalemia, because the hypokalemia can cause digoxin toxicity
   8. Note that elderly clients are more sensitive to toxicity
   9. Advise the client to eat foods high in potassium, such as fresh and dried fruits, fruit juices, vegetables, and potatoes
   10. Monitor the apical pulse
   11. If the apical pulse rate is below 60, the medication should be held and the physician notified
   12. Teach the client how to measure pulse
   13. Teach the client to notify physician if the pulse rate is below 60 or above 100
   14. Teach the client the signs and symptoms of toxicity
   15. Antidote: digoxin immune FAB (Digibind) is used in extreme toxicity

VI. ANTIHYPERTENSIVE MEDICATIONS (Box 58-7)

A. Thiazide diuretics (Box 58-8)
   1. Description
      a. Increase sodium and water excretion by inhibiting sodium reabsorption in the distal tubule of the kidney
      b. Used for hypertension and peripheral edema
      c. Used in clients with normal renal function
      d. Not effective for immediate diuresis
      e. Contraindicated in renal failure
      f. Used with caution in the client taking lithium, because lithium toxicity can occur
      g. Used with caution in the client taking digoxin, corticosteroids, or antidiabetic medications
   2. Side effects
      a. Hypercalcemia, hyperglycemia, hyperuricemia
      b. Hypokalemia, hyponatremia
      c. Hypovolemia
      d. Hypotension
      e. Headaches
      f. Nausea, vomiting
      g. Constipation
      h. Rashes
      i. Photosensitivity
      j. Blood dyscrasias
   3. Implementation
      a. Monitor vital signs
      b. Monitor weight
      c. Monitor urine output
      d. Monitor electrolytes, glucose, calcium, and uric acid levels
      e. Check peripheral extremities for edema
      f. Instruct the client to take the medication in the morning to avoid nocturia and sleep interruption
      g. Instruct the client in how to record the **BP**
      h. Instruct the client to eat foods rich in potassium

BOX 58-7

Classifications of Diuretics

Thiazide diuretics
Loop diuretics
Osmotic diuretics
Potassium-sparing diuretics
Carbonic anhydrase inhibitors

BOX 58-8

Thiazide and Thiazide-like Diuretics

THIAZIDE DIURETICS
Bendroflumethiazide (Naturetin)
Benzthiazide (Exna)
Chlorothiazide (Diuril)
Hydrochlorothiazide (Esidrix, Oretic, HydroDIURIL)
Hydroflumethiazide (Saluron, Diucardin)
Methyclothiazide (Aquatensen, Enduron)
Polythiazide (Renese)
Thichlormethiazide (Metahydrin, Naqua, Trichlorex)

THIAZIDE-LIKE DIURETICS
Chlorthalidone (Hygroton, Thalitone)
Indapamide (Lozol)
Metolazone (Zaroxolyn)
Quinethazone (Hydromox, Mykrox)

---

i. Instruct the client in how to take potassium supplements if prescribed
j. Instruct the client to take medication with food to avoid GI upset
k. Instruct the client to change positions slowly to prevent **orthostatic hypotension**
l. Instruct the client to use sunscreen when in direct sunlight
m. Instruct the client with diabetes mellitus to have the blood glucose checked periodically

B. Loop diuretics (Box 58-9)
  1. Description
    a. Inhibit sodium and chloride reabsorption from the loop of Henle and the distal tubule
    b. They have little effect on the blood glucose; however, they cause marked depletion of water and electrolytes, increased uric acid levels, and the excretion of calcium
    c. Are more potent than the thiazide diuretics, causing rapid diuresis, thus decreasing vascular fluid volume, **cardiac output,** and **blood pressure**
    d. Used for hypertension, edema associated with CHF, hypercalcemia, and renal disease
    e. Use with caution in the client taking digoxin or lithium

---

BOX 58-9

Loop Diuretics

Furosemide (Lasix)
Bumetanide (Bumex)
Ethacrynic acid (Edecrin)
Torsemide (Demadex)

---

    f. Use with caution in the client on aminoglycosides, anticoagulants, corticosteroids, or amphotericin B
  2. Side effects
    a. Hypokalemia, hyponatremia, hypocalcemia, hypomagnesemia
    b. Hypochloremia
    c. Thrombocytopenia
    d. Hyperuricemia
    e. **Orthostatic hypotension**
    f. Skin disturbances
    g. Ototoxicity and deafness
    h. Thiamine deficiency
    i. Dehydration
  3. Implementation
    a. Monitor vital signs
    b. Monitor weight
    c. Monitor urine output
    d. Monitor electrolytes, calcium, magnesium, and uric acid levels
    e. Check the peripheral extremities for edema
    f. Monitor for signs of digitalis or lithium toxicity if the client is on these medications
    g. Instruct the client to take the medication in the morning to avoid nocturia and sleep interruption
    h. Instruct the client in how to record the **BP**
    i. Instruct the client to eat foods rich in potassium
    j. Instruct the client in how to take potassium supplements if prescribed
    k. Instruct the client to take medication with food to avoid GI upset
    l. Instruct the client to change positions slowly to prevent **orthostatic hypotension**
    m. Administer IV furosemide (Lasix) slowly, because hearing loss can occur if injected rapidly

C. Osmotic diuretics
  1. Refer to Chapter 64 for information regarding osmotic diuretics
  2. Refer to Box 58-10 for a list of these medications

D. Carbonic anhydrase inhibitors (Box 58-11)
  1. Description
    a. Block the action of the enzyme carbonic anhydrase, needed to maintain acid-base balance

b. Inhibition of this enzyme, carbonic anhydrase, causes increased sodium, potassium, and bicarbonate excretion
c. Metabolic acidosis can occur with prolonged use
d. Used to decrease intraocular pressure in open-angle (chronic) glaucoma, and to produce diuresis, manage epilepsy, and treat high-altitude sickness
e. Used to treat metabolic alkalosis
f. Contraindicated in narrow-angle or acute glaucoma
2. Side effects
   a. Hyperglycemia, hyperuricemia, hypercalcemia
   b. Hypokalemia
   c. Anorexia, nausea, vomiting
   d. **Orthostatic hypotension**
   e. Renal calculi
   f. Hemolytic anemia
3. Implementation
   a. Monitor vital signs
   b. Monitor weight
   c. Monitor urine output
   d. Monitor electrolytes, glucose, calcium, and uric acid levels
   e. Monitor mental status
   f. Instruct the client to monitor for signs of renal calculi
E. Potassium-sparing diuretics (Box 58-12)
   1. Description
      a. Act on the distal tubule to promote sodium and water excretion and potassium retention
      b. Used for edema and hypertension, to increase urine output, to treat fluid retention and overload associated with CHF, hepatic cirrhosis, or nephrotic syndrome, and for diuretic-induced hypokalemia
      c. Contraindicated in severe kidney or hepatic disease or in severe hyperkalemia
      d. Used with caution in the client with diabetes
      e. Used with caution in the client taking antihypertensives or lithium
      f. Used with caution in the client taking angiotensin converting enzyme (ACE) inhibitors, because hyperkalemia can result
      g. Used with caution in the client taking potassium supplements
   2. Side effects
      a. Hyperkalemia
      b. Nausea, vomiting, diarrhea
      c. Rash
      d. Dizziness, weakness
      e. Headache
      f. Dry mouth
      g. Photosensitivity
      h. Anemia
      i. Thrombocytopenia
   3. Implementation
      a. Monitor vital signs
      b. Monitor urine output
      c. Monitor for signs and symptoms of hyperkalemia, such as nausea, diarrhea, abdominal cramps, tachycardia followed by bradycardia, peaked narrow T wave on the electrocardiogram (ECG), or oliguria
      d. Monitor for a potassium level greater than 5.3 mEq/L, which indicates hyperkalemia
      e. Instruct the client to avoid foods high in potassium
      f. Instruct the client to avoid exposure to direct sunlight
      g. Instruct the client to monitor for signs of hyperkalemia
      h. Instruct the client to avoid salt substitutes because they contain potassium
      i. Instruct the client to take with or after meals to decrease GI irritation

VII. PERIPHERALLY ACTING ALPHA-ADRENERGIC BLOCKERS (Box 58-13)
A. Description
   1. Decrease sympathetic vasoconstriction by reducing the effects of norepinephrine at peripheral nerve endings, resulting in vasodilation and decreased **BP**

BOX 58-13

Peripherally Acting Alpha-Adrenergic Blockers

Doxazosin mesylate (Cardura)
Prazosin (Minipress)
Terazosin (Hytrin)
Guanadrel (Hylorel)
Guanethidine (Ismelin)
Reserpine (Serpasil)
Phenoxybenzamine (Dibenzyline)
Phentolamine (Regitine)
Tolazoline (Priscoline)

---

2. Used to maintain renal blood flow
3. Used to treat hypertension

B. Side effects
1. **Orthostatic hypotension**
2. Reflex tachycardia
3. Sodium and water retention
4. GI disturbances
5. Nausea
6. Drowsiness
7. Nasal congestion
8. Edema
9. Weight gain
10. Reserpine (Serpasil) can cause depression, GI irritation, and impotence

C. Implementation
1. Monitor vital signs
2. Monitor for fluid retention and edema
3. Instruct the client to change positions slowly to prevent **orthostatic hypotension**
4. Instruct the client in how to monitor the **BP**
5. Instruct the client to monitor for edema
6. Instruct the client to decrease salt intake
7. Instruct the client to avoid over-the-counter medications

VIII. CENTRALLY ACTING SYMPATHOLYTICS (ADRENERGIC BLOCKERS) (Box 58-14)

A. Description
1. Stimulate alpha-receptors in the central nervous system (CNS) to inhibit vasoconstriction, thus reducing peripheral resistance
2. Used to treat hypertension
3. Contraindicated in impaired liver function

B. Side effects
1. Sodium and water retention
2. Drowsiness, dizziness
3. Dry mouth
4. Bradycardia
5. Edema
6. Impotence
7. Hypotension
8. Depression

BOX 58-14

Centrally Acting Sympatholytics

Clonidine (Catapres)
Methyldopa (Aldomet)
Guanabenz (Wytensin)

C. Implementation
1. Monitor vital signs
2. Instruct the client not to discontinue medication, because abrupt withdrawal can cause severe rebound hypertension
3. Monitor liver function tests

IX. ANGIOTENSIN-CONVERTING ENZYME (ACE) INHIBITORS (Box 58-15)

A. Description
1. Prevent peripheral vasoconstriction by blocking conversion of angiotensin I to angiotensin II
2. Used to treat hypertension
3. Avoid use with potassium supplements and potassium-sparing diuretics

B. Side effects
1. Nausea, vomiting, diarrhea
2. Persistent cough
3. Hypotension
4. Hyperkalemia
5. Tachycardia
6. Headache
7. Dizziness, fatigue
8. Insomnia
9. Hypoglycemic reaction in the client with diabetes mellitus
10. Bruising, petechiae, bleeding
11. Diminished taste

C. Implementation
1. Monitor vital signs
2. Monitor protein, albumin, blood urea nitrogen (BUN), creatinine, white blood cells (WBC), potassium levels
3. Monitor for hypoglycemic reactions in the client with diabetes mellitus
4. Instruct the client to take captopril (Capoten) 20 minutes to 1 hour before a meal
5. Monitor for bruising, petechiae, or bleeding with captopril
6. Instruct the client not to discontinue medications because rebound hypertension can occur
7. Instruct the client not to take over-the-counter medications
8. Instruct the client in how to take the **BP**
9. Instruct the client that if dizziness occurs and persists, to notify the physician
10. Inform the client that the taste of food may be diminished during the first month of therapy

---

BOX 58-15

ACE Inhibitors

Benazepril (Lotensin)
Captopril (Capoten)
Enalapril (Vasotec)
Fosinopril (Monopril)
Lisinopril (Prinivil, Zestril)
Moexipril (Univasc)
Quinapril (Accupril)
Ramipril (Altrace)
Trandolapril (Mavik)

BOX 58-16

Antianginal Medications

Erythrityl tetranitrate (Cardilate)
Isosorbide mononitrate (Imdur, Monoket)
Isosorbide dinitrate (Iso-Bid, Isordil, Isotrate, Sorbitrate)
Nitroglycerin (Nitrostat, Nitrolingual, Klavikordal, Nitrogard, Nitrong, Nitronet)
Nitroglycerin ointment 2% (Nitro-Bid, Nitrol, Nitrong, Nitrodisc, Nitro-Dur, Transderm-Nitro)
Pentaerythritol tetranitrate (Pentylan Duotrate, Peritrate)

X. ANTIANGINAL MEDICATIONS (Box 58-16)

A. Nitrates
  1. Description
     a. Produce vasodilation
     b. Decrease **preload** and **afterload** and reduce myocardial oxygen consumption
     c. Contraindicated in the client with marked hypotension, increased intracranial pressure (ICP), or severe anemia
     d. Used with caution with severe renal or hepatic disease
     e. Avoid abrupt withdrawal of long-acting preparations to prevent the rebound effect of severe pain from myocardial ischemia
  2. Side effects
     a. Headache
     b. **Orthostatic hypotension**
     c. Dizziness, weakness
     d. Faintness
     e. Nausea, vomiting
     f. Flushing or pallor
     g. Confusion
     h. Rash
     i. Dry mouth
     j. Reflex tachycardia
     k. Paradoxical bradycardia
  3. Sublingual medications
     a. Monitor vital signs
     b. Offer sips of water before giving, because dryness may inhibit medication absorption
     c. Instruct the client to place under the tongue and leave until fully dissolved
     d. Instruct the client not to swallow the medication
     e. Instruct the client to take 1 tablet for pain, and repeat every 5 minutes for a total of three doses
     f. Instruct the client to seek medical help immediately if pain is not relieved in 15 minutes, following the three doses
     g. Inform the client that a stinging or biting sensation may indicate that the tablet is fresh

     h. Instruct the client to store medication in a dark, tightly closed bottle
     i. Instruct the client to check the expiration date on the medication bottle, because expiration may occur within 6 months of obtaining medication
     j. Instruct the client to take acetaminophen (Tylenol) for a headache
  4. Translingual medications
     a. Instruct the client to direct spray against the oral mucosa
     b. Instruct the client to avoid inhaling the spray
  5. Sustained-released medications: instruct the client to swallow and not to chew or crush the medication
  6. Transmucosal-buccal medications
     a. Instruct the client to place between the upper lip and gum or in the buccal area between the cheek and gum
     b. Inform the client that the medication will adhere to the oral mucosa and slowly dissolve
  7. Transdermal patch
     a. Instruct the client to apply the patch to a hairless area, using a new patch and a different site each day
     b. As prescribed, instruct the client to remove the patch after 12 to 14 hours, allowing 10 to 12 "patch-free" hours each day to prevent tolerance
     c. Do not apply the patch on the chest in the area of defibrillator-cardioverter paddle placement, because skin burns can result
  8. Topical ointments
     a. Instruct the client to remove the ointment on the skin from the previous dose
     b. Instruct the client to squeeze a ribbon of ointment of the prescribed length onto the applicator paper
     c. Instruct the client to spread the ointment over a 6 × 6 inch area, using the chest, back, abdomen, upper arm, or anterior thigh (avoiding hairy areas), and cover with a plastic wrap

    d. Instruct the client to rotate sites and to avoid touching the ointment when applying

    e. Do not apply the ointment on the chest in the area of defibrillator-cardioverter paddle placement, because skin burns can result

XI. BETA-ADRENERGIC BLOCKERS (Box 58-17)

A. Description
1. Inhibit response to beta-adrenergic stimulation, thus decreasing **cardiac output**
2. Block the release of the catecholamines, epinephrine, and norepinephrine, thus decreasing the heart rate and **blood pressure**
3. Decrease the workload of the heart and decrease oxygen demands
4. Used for angina, dysrhythmias, hypertension, migraine headaches, prevention of MI, and glaucoma
5. Contraindicated in the client with asthma, bradycardia, CHF, severe renal or hepatic disease, hyperthyroidism, or CVA
6. Used with caution in the client with diabetes mellitus, because it may mask symptoms of hypoglycemia
7. Used with caution in the client on antihypertensives

B. Side effects
1. Bradycardia
2. Bronchospasm
3. Hypotension
4. Weakness, fatigue
5. Nausea, vomiting
6. Dizziness
7. Hyperglycemia
8. Agranulocytosis
9. Behavioral or psychotic response
10. Depression
11. Nightmares

C. Implementation
1. Monitor vital signs
2. Hold the medication if the pulse or **BP** is not within the prescribed parameters
3. Monitor for signs of CHF
4. Assess for respiratory distress and for signs of wheezing and dyspnea
5. Instruct the client to report dizziness, lightheadedness, or nasal congestion
6. Instruct the client not to stop the medication, because rebound hypertension, rebound tachycardia, or an anginal attack can occur
7. Advise the client on insulin that early signs of hypoglycemia, such as tachycardia and nervousness, can be masked by the beta-blocker
8. Instruct the client on insulin to monitor the blood glucose level
9. Instruct the client in how to take pulse and **BP**
10. Instruct the client to change positions slowly to prevent **orthostatic hypotension**
11. Instruct the client to avoid over-the-counter cold medications and nasal decongestants

XII. CALCIUM CHANNEL BLOCKERS (Box 58-18)

A. Description
1. Decrease cardiac **contractility** (negative inotropic effect by relaxing smooth muscle) and the workload of the heart, thus decreasing the need for oxygen
2. Promote vasodilatation of the coronary and peripheral vessels
3. Used for angina, dysrhythmias, or hypertension
4. Used with caution in the client with CHF, bradycardia, or AV block

B. Side effects
1. Bradycardia
2. Hypotension
3. Reflex tachycardia as a result of hypotension
4. Headache
5. Dizziness, lightheadedness
6. Fatigue

BOX 58-17

Beta-Adrenergic Blockers

Acebutolol (Sectral)
Atenolol (Tenormin)
Betaxolol (Betoptic)
Bisoprolol fumarate (Zebeta)
Carteolol (Cartrol)
Carvedilol (Coreg)
Esmolol (Brevibloc)
Labetalol (Normodyne, Trandate, Vescal)
Levbunolol (Betagan)
Metipranolol (Opti-Pranolol)
Metoprolol (Lopressor, Toprol-XL)
Nadolol (Corgard)
Penbutolol (Levotol)
Pindolol (Visken)
Propranolol (Inderal)
Sotalol (Betapace)
Timolol (Blocadren, Timoptic)

BOX 58-18

Calcium Channel Blockers

Amlodipine (Norvasc)
Bepridal (Bepadin, Vascor)
Diltiazem (Cardizem, Cardizem SR)
Felodipine (Plendil)
Isradipine (DynaCirc)
Nicardipine (Cardene)
Nifedipine (Procardia, Procardia XL, Adalat CC)
Nisoldipine (Sular)
Verapamil (Calan, Isoptin)

7. Peripheral edema
8. Constipation
9. Flushing of the skin
10. Changes in liver and kidney function

C. Implementation
1. Monitor vital signs
2. Monitor for signs of CHF
3. Monitor liver enzyme levels
4. Monitor kidney function tests
5. Instruct the client not to discontinue the medication
6. Instruct the client in how to take a pulse
7. Instruct the client to notify the physician if dizziness or fainting occurs
8. Instruct the client not to crush or chew sustained-released tablets

XIII. PERIPHERAL VASODILATORS (Box 58-19)

A. Description
1. Decrease peripheral resistance by exerting a direct action on the arteries or on both the arteries and the veins
2. Increase blood flow to the extremities
3. Used in peripheral vascular disorders of venous and arterial vessels
4. Most effective for disorders resulting from vasospasm (Raynaud's disease)
5. These medications may decrease some of the symptoms of cerebral vascular insufficiency

B. Side effects
1. Lightheadedness, dizziness

BOX 58-19

Peripheral Vasodilators

ALPHA-ADRENERGIC BLOCKER
Tolazoline (Priscoline)

BETA-ADRENERGIC AGONISTS
Isoxsuprine (Vasodilan)
Nylidrin (Arlidin)

DIRECT-ACTING PERIPHERAL VASODILATOR
Ergoloid mesylates (Hydergine)

ALPHA BLOCKERS
Doxazosin mesylate (Cardura)
Prazosin hydrochloride (Minipress)
Terazosin hydrochloride (Hytrin)

CALCIUM CHANNEL BLOCKERS
Nifedipine (Procardia)
Nimodipine (Nimotop)

HEMORRHEOLOGIC
Pentoxifylline (Trental)
Increases microcirculation and tissue perfusion

---

2. **Postural hypotension**
3. Tachycardia
4. Palpitations
5. Flushing
6. GI distress

C. Implementation
1. Monitor vital signs, especially the **BP** and the heart rate
2. Monitor for **orthostatic hypotension** and tachycardia
3. Monitor for signs of inadequate blood flow to the extremities, such as pallor, coldness of the extremities, and pain
4. Instruct the client that it may take up to 3 months for a desired therapeutic response
5. Advise the client not to smoke because smoking increases vasospasm
6. Instruct the client to avoid aspirin or aspirin-like compounds unless approved by the physician
7. Instruct the client to take the medication with meals if GI disturbances occur
8. Instruct the client to avoid alcohol because it may cause a hypotensive reaction
9. Encourage the client to change positions slowly to avoid **orthostatic hypotension**

XIV. DIRECT-ACTING ARTERIOLAR VASODILATORS (Box 58-20)

A. Description
1. Relax the smooth muscles of the blood vessels, mainly the arteries, causing vasodilation
2. Promote an increase in blood flow to the brain and kidneys
3. With vasodilation, the **blood pressure** drops and sodium and water are retained, resulting in peripheral edema
4. Diuretics may be given to decrease the edema
5. Used in the client with moderate to severe hypertension
6. Used during acute hypertensive emergencies

B. Side effects
1. Hypotension
2. Reflex tachycardia caused by vasodilatation and the drop in **BP**
3. Palpitations

BOX 58-20

Direct-Acting Vasodilators

Diazoxide (Hyperstat)
Fenoldopam (Corlopam)
Hydralazine (Apresoline)
Minoxidil (Loniten)
Nitroglycerin (Nitro-Bid, Nitrol, Nitrostat, Tridil)
Sodium nitroprusside (Nipride, Nitropress)
Trimethaphan camsylate (Arfonad)

4. Edema
5. Dizziness
6. Headaches
7. Nasal congestion
8. GI bleeding
9. Neurological symptoms
10. Confusion
11. Excess hair growth with minoxidil (Loniten)
12. With sodium nitroprusside (Nipride), cyanide toxicity and thiocyanate toxicity can occur

C. Implementation
   1. Monitor vital signs
   2. Sodium nitroprusside
      a. Monitor cyanide and thiocyanate levels
      b. Protect from light because the medication decomposes
      c. When administering, solution must be wrapped in aluminum foil and is stable for 24 hours
      d. Discard if the medication is red or blue

XV. ANTIDYSRHYTHMIC MEDICATIONS

A. Description: suppress dysrhythmias by inhibiting abnormal pathways of electrical conduction through the heart

B. Class 1A Antidysrhythmics
   1. Disopyramide phosphate (Norpace)
   2. Procainamide hydrochloride (Pronestyl)
   3. Quinidine sulfate (Quinidine)

C. Class 1B antidysrhythmics
   1. Lidocaine (Xylocaine)
   2. Mexiletine hydrochloride (Mexitil)
   3. Tocainide hydrochloride (Tonocard)

D. Class 1C antidysrhythmics
   1. Flecainide acetate (Tambocor)
   2. Moricizine hydrochloride (Ethmozine)
   3. Propafenone hydrochloride (Rythmol)
   4. Side effects
      a. Hypotension
      b. Heart failure
      c. Worsened or new dysrhythmias
      d. Nausea, vomiting, or diarrhea

E. Class II Antidysrhythmics
   1. Acebutolol hydrochloride (Sectral)
   2. Esmolol hydrochloride (Brevibloc)
   3. Propranolol hydrochloride (Inderal)
   4. Sotalol hydrochloride (Betapace)
   5. Side effects
      a. Dizziness
      b. Fatigue
      c. Hypotension
      d. Bradycardia
      e. Heart failure
      f. Dysrhythmias
      g. Heart block
      h. Bronchospasms
      i. GI distress

F. Class III Antidysrhythmics
   1. Amiodarone hydrochloride (Cordarone)
   2. Bretylium tosylate (Bretylol)
   3. Ibutilide fumarate (Covert)
   4. Side effects
      a. Hypotension
      b. Bradycardia
      c. Nausea, vomiting
      d. Amiodarone hydrochloride may cause pulmonary fibrosis, photosensitivity, bluish skin discoloration, corneal deposits, peripheral neuropathy, tremor, poor coordination, abnormal gait, hypothyroidism
      e. Bretylium tosylate may cause vertigo, syncope, dizziness

G. Class IV antidysrhythmics
   1. Verapamil hydrochloride (Calan)
   2. Diltiazem hydrochloride (Cardizem)
   3. Side effects
      a. Dizziness
      b. Hypotension
      c. Bradycardia
      d. Edema
      e. Constipation

H. Other antidysrhythmics
   1. Adenosine (Adenocard)
   2. Atropine sulfate
   3. Digoxin (Lanoxin)
   4. Magnesium sulfate
   5. Phenytoin (Dilantin)
   6. Adenosine can cause dysrhythmias, dyspnea, facial flushing
   7. Atropine is used to treat sinus bradycardia and is contraindicated in glaucoma, urinary retention, and ileus
   8. Side effects: atropine can cause hallucinations, tachycardia, dry mouth, and constipation

I. Implementation for antidysrhythmics
   1. Monitor heart rate, respiratory rate, and **BP**
   2. Monitor ECG
   3. Provide cardiac monitoring
   4. Maintain therapeutic serum drug levels
   5. Before administering lidocaine, always check the vial label to prevent administering a form that contains epinephrine or preservatives, because these solutions are used for local anesthesia only
   6. Do not administer with food because food may affect absorption
   7. Mexiletine or tocainide may be administered with food or antacids to reduce GI distress
   8. Always administer IV antidysrhythmics via an infusion pump
   9. Monitor for signs of fluid retention, such as weight gain, peripheral edema, or shortness of breath
   10. Advise the client to limit fluid and salt intake to minimize fluid retention

11. Monitor respiratory, thyroid, and neurological function
12. After administering bretylium, keep the client supine and monitor for hypotension
13. Instruct the client to change positions slowly to minimize **orthostatic hypotension**
14. Instruct the client taking amiodarone to use sunscreen and protective clothing to prevent photosensitivity reactions
15. Encourage the client to increase fiber intake to prevent constipation
16. Assess for bradycardia when administering atropine sulfate in low doses or by slow infusion

XVI. ADRENERGIC AGONISTS (Box 58-21)

A. Dobutamine (Dobutrex)
1. Increases myocardial force and **cardiac output** through stimulation of beta receptors
2. Used in CHF and for clients undergoing cardiopulmonary bypass surgery

B. Dopamine hydrochloride (Intropin)
1. Increases **BP** and **cardiac output** through positive inotropic action and increases renal blood flow through its action on alpha and beta receptors
2. Used to treat mild renal failure caused by low **cardiac output**

C. Epinephrine (Adrenalin)
1. Used for cardiac stimulation in cardiac arrest
2. Used for bronchodilation in asthma or allergic reactions
3. Produces mydriasis
4. Produces local vasoconstriction when combined with local anesthetics and prolongs anesthetic action by decreasing blood flow to the site

D. Isoproterenol hydrochloride (Isuprel)
1. Stimulates beta receptors
2. Used for cardiac stimulation and bronchodilation

E. Norepinephrine (levarterenol, Levophed)
1. Stimulates the heart in cardiac arrest
2. Vasoconstricts and increases the **BP** in hypotension and shock

F. Side effects
1. Dysrhythmias
2. Tachycardia
3. Angina

4. Restlessness
5. Urgency or urinary incontinence

G. Implementation
1. Monitor vital signs
2. Monitor lung sounds
3. Monitor urinary output
4. Monitor ECG
5. Administer the medication through a large vein
6. If extravasation occurs, infiltrate the site with normal saline and phentolamine (Regitine)

XVII. ANTILIPEMIC MEDICATIONS

A. Description
1. Reduce serum levels of cholesterol, triglycerides, or low-density lipoprotein (LDL)
2. When cholesterol, triglycerides, and LDL are elevated, the client is at increased risk for coronary artery disease
3. In many cases diet alone will not lower blood lipid levels; therefore, antilipemic medications will be prescribed

B. Bile sequestrants (Box 58-22)
1. Description
   a. Bind with acids in the intestines
   b. Bile acid sequestrants should not be used as the only therapy in clients with elevated triglycerides, because they typically raise triglyceride levels
2. Side effects
   a. Constipation
   b. Peptic ulcer
3. Implementation
   a. Cholestyramine (Questran) comes in a gritty powder that must be mixed thoroughly in juice or water prior to administration
   b. Monitor the client for early signs of peptic ulcer, such as nausea and abdominal discomfort followed by abdominal pain and distention
   c. Instruct the client that the medication must be taken with and followed by sufficient fluids

C. HMG-CoA reductase inhibitors (Box 58-23)
1. Description
   a. Lovastatin (Mevacor) is highly protein bound and should not be administered with anticoagulants
   b. Lovastatin should not be administered with gemfibrozil (Lopid)

BOX 58-21

Adrenergic Agonists

Dobutamine (Dobutrex)
Dopamine (Intropin)
Epinephrine (Adrenalin)
Isoproterenol (Isuprel)
Norepinephrine (levarterenol, Levophed)

BOX 58-22

Bile Acid Sequestrants

Cholestyramine (Questran)
Colestipol (Colestid)

BOX 58-23

HMG-CoA Reductase Inhibitors

Atorvastatin (Lipitor)
Cerivastatin (Baycol)
Fluvastatin (Lescol)
Lovastatin (Mevacor)
Pravastatin (Pravachol)
Simvastatin (Zocor)

BOX 58-24

Other Antilipemic Medications

Clofibrate (Atromid-S)
Fenofibrate (Tricor)
Gemfibrozil (Lopid)
Nicotinic acid (Niacor)

c. Administer lovastatin with caution to the client on immunosuppressive medications
2. Side effects
   a. Nausea
   b. Diarrhea or constipation
   c. Abdominal pain or cramps
   d. Flatulence
   e. Dizziness
   f. Headache
   g. Blurred vision
   h. Rash
   i. Pruritis
   j. Elevated liver enzymes
   k. Causes GI disturbances, headaches, muscle cramps, and fatigue
3. Implementation
   a. Monitor serum liver enzymes
   b. Instruct the client to receive an annual eye exam because the medication causes cataract formation
   c. If lovastatin is not effective in lowering the lipid level after 3 months, it should be discontinued
D. Other antilipemic medications (Box 58-24)
   1. Description
      a. Gemfibrozil should not be taken with anticoagulants because they compete for protein sites, and if the client is on an anticoagulant, the anticoagulant dose should be reduced during antilipemic therapy and the INR monitored closely
      b. Do not administer gemfibrozil with lovastatin
      c. Clofibrate (Atromid-S) should not be used long term because of its side effects such as dysrhythmias, angina, thromboembolism, and gallbladder stones
   2. Implementation
      a. Monitor vital signs
      b. Monitor liver enzyme levels
      c. Monitor serum cholesterol and triglyceride levels
      d. Instruct the client to restrict intake of fats, cholesterol, carbohydrates, and alcohol
      e. Instruct the client to follow an exercise program

f. Instruct the client that it will take several weeks before the lipid level declines
g. Instruct the client to have an annual eye exam and to report any changes in vision
h. Instruct the client with diabetes mellitus who is taking gemfibrozil to monitor blood glucose levels regularly
i. Instruct the client to increase fluid intake
j. Note that nicotinic acid has numerous side effects, which include GI disturbances, flushing of the skin, elevated liver enzymes, hyperglycemia, and hyperuricemia
k. Instruct the client that aspirin may assist in reducing the side effects of nicotinic acid
l. Instruct the client to take nicotinic acid with meals to reduce GI discomfort

PRACTICE QUESTIONS

1. A nurse provides discharge instructions to a postoperative client who is taking warfarin sodium (Coumadin). Which statement, if made by the client, reflects the need for further teaching?
   1. "I will take Ecotrin for my headaches because it is coated."
   2. "I will be certain to limit my alcohol consumption."
   3. "I will take my pills every day at the same time."
   4. "I have already called my family to pick up a Medic-Alert bracelet."

2. A client has a serum potassium (K^+) of 3.0 mEq/L and is complaining of anorexia. A physician orders a digitalis level to rule out digitalis toxicity. A nurse checks the results, knowing that which of the following is the therapeutic serum level for digitalis?
   1. 0.5 to 2.0 ng/mL
   2. 1.2 to 2.8 ng/mL
   3. 3.0 ng/mL
   4. 3.5 ng/mL

3. A client is being treated with procainamide hydrochloride (Pronestyl) for a cardiac dysrhythmia. Following intravenous administration of the medication, the client complains of dizziness. What intervention should the nurse do first?
   1. Administer ordered nitroglycerin tablets
   2. Auscultate the client's apical pulse and obtain a blood pressure

3. Measure heart rate and rhythm on the rhythm strip
4. Obtain a 12-lead ECG immediately

4. A nurse is monitoring a client who is taking propranolol (Inderal). Which of the following assessment data would indicate a potential serious complication associated with propranolol?
   1. A baseline blood pressure of 150/80 mm Hg followed by a blood pressure of 138/72 mm Hg after two doses of the medication
   2. A baseline resting heart rate of 88 beats per minute followed by a resting heart rate of 72 beats per minute after two doses of the medication
   3. The development of audible expiratory wheezes
   4. The development of complaints of insomnia

5. A home health care nurse is visiting an elderly client at home. Furosemide (Lasix) is prescribed for the client. The nurse teaches the client about the medication. Which of the following statements, if made by the client, indicates the need for further teaching?
   1. "I will take my medication every morning with breakfast."
   2. "I will call my doctor if my ankles swell or my rings get tight."
   3. "I need to drink lots of coffee and tea to keep myself healthy."
   4. "I will sit up slowly before standing each morning."

6. A nurse is caring for a client receiving a heparin IV infusion. The nurse anticipates that which laboratory study will be prescribed to monitor the therapeutic effect of heparin?
   1. Prothrombin time (PT)
   2. Activated partial thromboplastin time (APTT)
   3. Hematocrit (Hct)
   4. Hemoglobin (Hgb)

7. A client is diagnosed with an acute myocardial infarction (MI) and is receiving tissue plasminogen activator (t-PA). Which of the following is a priority nursing intervention?
   1. Have heparin sodium available
   2. Monitor for renal failure
   3. Monitor for signs of bleeding
   4. Monitor psychosocial status

8. A home health nurse instructs a client about the use of a nitrate patch. The nurse tells the client which of the following that will prevent client tolerance to nitrates?
   1. Do not remove the patches
   2. Have a 12-hour "no nitrate" time
   3. Have a 24-hour "no nitrate" time
   4. Keep nitrates on 24 hours, then off 24 hours

9. A client is admitted to a medical unit with nausea and bradycardia. The family hands a nurse a small white envelope labeled "heart pill." The envelope is sent to pharmacy and reveals digoxin (Lanoxin). A family member states, "That doctor doesn't know how to take care of my family." The most therapeutic response by the nurse would be:
   1. "You are concerned your loved one receives the best care."
   2. "You're right! I've never seen a doctor put pills in an envelope."
   3. "I think you're wrong. That physician has been in practice over 30 years."
   4. "Don't worry about this. I'll take care of everything."

10. A nurse is caring for a client receiving dopamine (Intropin). Which of the following potential nursing diagnoses is appropriate for this client?
    1. Increased cardiac output
    2. Fluid volume excess
    3. Impaired tissue perfusion
    4. Altered sensory perception

11. A nurse is planning to administer hydrochlorothiazide (HydroDiuril) to a client. The nurse understands that which of the following are concerns related to the administration of this medication?
    1. Hyperkalemia, hypoglycemia, penicillin allergy
    2. Hypouricemia, hyperkalemia
    3. Hypokalemia, hyperglycemia, sulfa allergy
    4. Increased risk of osteoporosis

12. A home health care nurse is visiting a client with elevated triglycerides and a serum cholesterol of 398 mg/dL. The client is taking cholestyramine resin (Questran). Which of the following statements, if made by the client, indicates the need for further education?
    1. "Constipation and bloating might be a problem."
    2. "I'll continue to watch my diet and reduce my fats."
    3. "I'll continue my nicotinic acid from the health food store."
    4. "Walking a mile each day will help the whole process."

13. A client with congestive heart failure is on a 1-g sodium diet. A nurse understands that which medication prescribed for the client promotes sodium excretion while conserving potassium?
    1. Spironolactone (Aldactone)
    2. Furosemide (Lasix)
    3. Ethacrynic acid (Edecrin)
    4. Hydrochlorothiazide (HydroDIURIL)

14. A client has developed paroxysmal nocturnal dyspnea (PND). Which of the following medications does a nurse anticipate will be prescribed by the physician?
    1. Lidocaine (Xylocaine)
    2. Propranolol (Inderal)
    3. Bumetanide (Bumex)
    4. Urokinase (Abbokinase)

15. A client arrives in the emergency department after complaining of unrelieved chest pain for 2 days.

The pain has subsided slightly but never disappeared. When the nurse approaches the client with a 0.4-mg nitroglycerin sublingual tablet, the client states, "I don't need that. My dad takes that for his heart. There's nothing wrong with my heart." The nurse interprets that the client is exhibiting which type of reaction?

1. Obsessive-compulsive
2. Denial
3. Phobic
4. Angry

16. A nurse has admitted a client who has a diagnosis of syncope to a medical unit. The client is taking enalapril (Vasotec), atenolol (Tenormin), and aspirin (ASA) daily. The client admits that the medications were prescribed by different physicians. The admitting physician wrote in the client's order sheet, "Administer medications as taken at home." Which of the following is the most appropriate action for the nurse to take?

1. Administer the medications as ordered by the physician
2. Send the client's medication bottles to the pharmacy for identification and then administer the medications as ordered
3. Call the physician, describe the medications, and request order clarification
4. Refuse to give any medications, and wait until the physician makes rounds to clarify the orders

17. A 66-year-old client complaining of not feeling well is seen in a clinic. The client is taking several medications for the control of heart disease and hypertension. These medications include atenolol (Tenormin), digoxin (Lanoxin) and chlorothiazide (Diuril). A tentative diagnosis of digoxin toxicity is made. Which of the following assessment data would support this diagnosis?

1. Chest pain, hypotension, and paresthesia
2. Constipation, dry mouth, and sleep disorder
3. Double vision, loss of appetite, and nausea
4. Dyspnea, edema, and palpitations

18. A client is being treated for acute congestive heart failure with IV bumetanide (Bumex). The vital signs are as follows: blood pressure, 100/60 mm Hg; pulse, 96 beats per minute; and respirations, 24 breaths per minute. After the initial dose, which of the following is the priority assessment?

1. Monitoring blood pressure
2. Monitoring potassium level
3. Monitoring urine output
4. Monitoring weight loss

19. A client with a diagnosis of congestive heart failure is seen in a clinic. The client is being treated with a variety of medications, including digoxin (Lanoxin) and furosemide (Lasix). Which of the following assessment findings would lead the nurse to suspect that the client is hypokalemic?

1. Diarrhea
2. Intermittent intestinal colic
3. Muscle weakness and leg cramps
4. Tingling of fingers and toes

20. A client is being discharged with a prescription for propranolol hydrochloride (Inderal). In developing a medication teaching plan, a nurse would include which of the following instructions?

1. Exercise will prevent orthostatic hypotension
2. Hot baths and showers are advised to increase vasodilation
3. Medication should be taken on an empty stomach to enhance absorption
4. Medication should be withheld if the pulse rate drops below 60 beats per minute

CRITICAL THINKING: FREE-TEXT ENTRY

A client with coronary artery disease complains of substernal chest pain. After assessing the client's heart rate and blood pressure, a nurse administers nitroglycerin, 0.4 mg, sublingually. After 5 minutes, the client states, "My chest still hurts." The nurse checks the client's vital signs, notes that they have remained stable, and does what priority action next?

Answer: _____

ANSWERS

1. **1**

Rationale: Ecotrin is an aspirin-containing product and should be avoided. Excessive alcohol consumption should be avoided by a client taking warfarin sodium. Taking prescribed medication at the same time increases client compliance. The Medic-Alert bracelet provides health care personnel emergency information.

Test-Taking Strategy: Use the process of elimination. Note the key words "need for further teaching." Recalling that Couma-

din is an anticoagulant and that Ecotrin is an aspirin-containing product will direct you to option 1. Review client teaching points related to Coumadin if you had difficulty with this question.

Level of Cognitive Ability: Application
Client Needs: Health Promotion and Maintenance
Integrated Concept/Process: Teaching/Learning
Content Area: Pharmacology
Reference: Wilson, B., Shannon, M., & Stang, C. (2000). *Nurses drug guide 2000.* Stamford, Conn.: Appleton & Lange, p. 1169.

2. 1
Rationale: Therapeutic levels for digitalis range from 0.5 to 2.0 ng/mL.
Test-Taking Strategy: Knowledge of the therapeutic serum digitalis level will direct you to option 1. If you had difficulty with this question, learn the therapeutic level for digitalis.
Level of Cognitive Ability: Analysis
Client Needs: Physiological Integrity
Integrated Concept/Process: Nursing Process/Analysis
Content Area: Pharmacology
Reference: Cleveland, L., Aschenbrenner, D., Venable, S., & Yensen, J. (1999). *Nursing management in drug therapy.* Philadelphia: Lippincott, p. 1041.

3. 2
Rationale: Signs of toxicity from procainamide include confusion, dizziness, drowsiness, decreased urination, nausea, vomiting, and tachydysrhythmias. If the client complains of dizziness, the nurse should first assess the vital signs.
Test-Taking Strategy: Use the steps of the nursing process to eliminate options 1 and 4. From the remaining options, remember always to assess the client first, not the monitoring devices. Therefore, option 2 is correct. Review the signs of toxicity and the nursing interventions if you had difficulty with this question.
Level of Cognitive Ability: Analysis
Client Needs: Physiological Integrity
Integrated Concept/Process: Nursing Process/Assessment
Content Area: Pharmacology
Reference: Hodgson, B., & Kizior, R. (2001). *Saunders nursing drug handbook 2001.* Philadelphia: W.B. Saunders, p. 862.

4. 3
Rationale: Audible expiratory wheezes may indicate a serious adverse reaction, bronchospasm. Beta blockers may induce this reaction, particularly in clients with COPD or asthma. Normal decreases in blood pressure and heart rate are expected. Insomnia is a frequent mild side effect and should be monitored.
Test-Taking Strategy: Use the process of elimination, eliminating options 1 and 2 because these are expected effects from the medication. Note the key words "potential serious complication." These key words will direct you to option 3. Review the adverse effects of this medication if you had difficulty with this question.
Level of Cognitive Ability: Analysis
Client Needs: Physiological Integrity
Integrated Concept/Process: Nursing Process/Assessment
Content Area: Pharmacology
Reference: Hodgson, B., & Kizior, R. (2001). *Saunders nursing drug handbook 2001.* Philadelphia: W.B. Saunders, pp. 877-880.

5. 3
Rationale: Tea and coffee are stimulants as well as mild diuretics. These are a poor choice for hydration. Taking the medication at the same time each day improves compliance. Since furosemide is a diuretic, the morning is the best time to take the medication so as not to interrupt sleep. Notification of the health care provider is appropriate if edema is noticed in the hands, feet, or face, or if the client is short of breath. Sitting up slowly prevents postural hypotension.
Test-Taking Strategy: Use the process of elimination, noting the key words "need for further teaching." Recalling that tea and coffee are stimulants and that diuretics can potentially worsening dehydration will direct you to option 3. In addition, coffee and tea are not healthy foods. Review client teaching points related to this medication if you had difficulty with this question.
Level of Cognitive Ability: Analysis
Client Needs: Health Promotion and Maintenance
Integrated Concept/Process: Teaching/Learning
Content Area: Pharmacology
Reference: Gutierrez, K. (1999). *Pharmacotherapeutics: Clinical decision-making in nursing.* Philadelphia: W.B. Saunders, pp. 830-831.

6. 2
Rationale: The PT will assess for the therapeutic effect of warfarin sodium (Coumadin), and the APTT will assess the therapeutic effect of heparin. Hct and Hgb assess red blood cell concentrations. Baseline assessment, including an APTT value, should be completed, as well as ongoing daily APTT values while the client is on heparin. Heparin doses are determined on the basis of the result of the APTT.
Test-Taking Strategy: Use the process of elimination. Eliminate options 3 and 4 because they are similar and are unrelated to heparin therapy. From the remaining options, recall the relationship between the PT and Coumadin and the APTT and heparin. Review care of a client on heparin infusion if you had difficulty with this question.
Level of Cognitive Ability: Analysis
Client Needs: Physiological Integrity
Integrated Concept/Process: Nursing Process/Assessment
Content Area: Pharmacology
Reference: Cleveland, L., Aschenbrenner, D., Venable, S., & Yensen, J. (1999). *Nursing management in drug therapy.* Philadelphia: Lippincott, p. 448.

7. 3
Rationale: Tissue plasminogen activator is a thrombolytic. Hemorrhage is a complication of any type of thrombolytic medication. The client is monitored for bleeding. Monitoring for renal failure and monitoring the client's psychosocial status are important but are not the most critical interventions. Heparin is given after thrombolytic therapy, but the question is not asking about follow-up medications.
Test-Taking Strategy: Use the process of elimination. Note the key word "priority." Remember, bleeding is a priority. Review care of the client on t-PA if you had difficulty with this question.
Level of Cognitive Ability: Application
Client Needs: Physiological Integrity
Integrated Concept/Process: Nursing Process/Implementation
Content Area: Pharmacology
Reference: Wilson, B., Shannon, M., & Stang, C. (2000). *Nurses drug guide 2000.* Stamford, Conn.: Appleton & Lange, p. 33.

8. 2
Rationale: To help prevent tolerance, clients need a 12-hour "no nitrate" time, sometimes referred to as a pharmacological vacation away from the medication. Options 1, 3, and 4 are incorrect.
Test-Taking Strategy: Use the process of elimination, focusing on the issue, preventing tolerance to nitrates. This issue and

knowledge regarding administering this medication will direct you to option 2. Review the administration of nitrate patches if you had difficulty with this question.
Level of Cognitive Ability: Application
Client Needs: Physiological Integrity
Integrated Concept/Process: Teaching/Learning
Content Area: Pharmacology
Reference: Wilson, B., Shannon, M., & Stang, C. (2000). *Nurses drug guide 2000.* Stamford, Conn.: Appleton & Lange, p. 999.

9. **1**
Rationale: This is a therapeutic, nonjudgmental response. The statement reflects the family's concern, but remains nonjudgmental. Option 2 creates doubt about the physician's practice without actually knowing the circumstances. Option 3 is argumentative and nontherapeutic. Option 4 dismisses the family's concerns and disempowers the family.
Test-Taking Strategy: Use therapeutic communication techniques. Reflection of the client or family's concerns is the most therapeutic. Review therapeutic communication techniques if you had difficulty with this question.
Level of Cognitive Ability: Application
Client Needs: Psychosocial Integrity
Integrated Concept/Process: Communication and Documentation
Content Area: Pharmacology
Reference: Lindeman, C., & McAthie, M. (1999). *Fundamentals of contemporary nursing practice.* Philadelphia: W.B. Saunders, p. 163.

10. **3**
Rationale: The client receiving dopamine therapy should be assessed for impaired tissue perfusion related to peripheral vasoconstriction. Options 1, 2, and 4 are not directly related to this medication therapy.
Test-Taking Strategy: Use the process of elimination. Recalling that dopamine causes peripheral vasoconstriction will direct you to option 3. Review the action of this medication if you had difficulty with this question.
Level of Cognitive Ability: Analysis
Client Needs: Physiological Integrity
Integrated Concept/Process: Nursing Process/Analysis
Content Area: Pharmacology
Reference: Gutierrez, K. (1999). *Pharmacotherapeutics: Clinical decision-making in nursing.* Philadelphia: W.B. Saunders, p. 176.

11. **3**
Rationale: Thiazide diuretics like hydrochlorothiazide are sulfa-based medications, and a client with a sulfa allergy is at risk for an allergic reaction. Also, clients are at risk for hypokalemia, hyperglycemia, hypercalcemia, hyperlipidemia, and hyperuricemia.
Test-Taking Strategy: Use the process of elimination. Recalling that thiazide diuretics carry a sulfa ring will direct you to option 3. Review the nursing considerations related to administering this medication if you had difficulty with this question.
Level of Cognitive Ability: Analysis
Client Needs: Physiological Integrity
Integrated Concept/Process: Nursing Process/Analysis
Content Area: Pharmacology
Reference: Hodgson, B., & Kizior, R. (2001). *Saunders nursing drug handbook 2001.* Philadelphia: W.B. Saunders, pp. 494-496.

12. **3**
Rationale: Nicotinic acid, even over-the-counter forms, should be avoided because it may lead to liver abnormalities. All lipid-lowering medications can also cause liver abnormalities, so a combination of nicotinic acid and cholestyramine resin is to be avoided. Constipation and bloating are the two most common side effects. Both walking and the reduction of fats in the diet are therapeutic measures to reduce cholesterol and triglyceride levels.
Test-Taking Strategy: Use the process of elimination. Note the key words "need for further education." Remembering that over-the-counter medications should be avoided when a client is taking a prescription medication will direct you to option 3. Review client teaching points related to this medication if you had difficulty with this question.
Level of Cognitive Ability: Analysis
Client Needs: Health Promotion and Maintenance
Integrated Concept/Process: Teaching/Learning
Content Area: Pharmacology
Reference: Hodgson, B., & Kizior, R. (2001). *Saunders nursing drug handbook 2001.* Philadelphia: W.B. Saunders, pp. 215-217.

13. **1**
Rationale: Spironolactone (Aldactone) is a potassium-sparing diuretic that promotes sodium excretion while conserving potassium. Options 2, 3, and 4 identify diuretics that do not conserve potassium.
Test-Taking Strategy: Use the process of elimination. Recalling that spironolactone is a potassium-sparing diuretic will direct you to option 1. Review the potassium-sparing diuretics, if you had difficulty with this question.
Level of Cognitive Ability: Analysis
Client Needs: Physiological Integrity
Integrated Concept/Process: Nursing Process/Analysis
Content Area: Pharmacology
Reference: Gutierrez, K. (1999). *Pharmacotherapeutics: Clinical decision-making in nursing.* Philadelphia: W.B. Saunders, p. 834.

14. **3**
Rationale: Bumex is a diuretic. The PND may be due to increased venous return when the client is lying in bed, and the client needs diuresis. Propranolol is a beta blocker, lidocaine is an antidysrhythmic, and urokinase is a thrombolytic.
Test-Taking Strategy: Use the process of elimination. Knowledge of each medication type and that a diuretic will increase urine output will direct you to option 3. Review the actions of the medications identified in the options, if you had difficulty with this question.
Level of Cognitive Ability: Analysis
Client Needs: Physiological Integrity
Integrated Concept/Process: Nursing Process/Analysis
Content Area: Pharmacology
Reference: Hodgson, B., & Kizior, R. (2001). *Saunders nursing drug handbook 2001.* Philadelphia: W.B. Saunders, p. 127.

15. **2**
Rationale: Denial is the most common reaction when a client has a myocardial infarction or anginal pain. Options 1, 3, and 4 are incorrect.
Test-Taking Strategy: Use the process of elimination. Eliminate options 1 and 3 first because both are psychiatric diagnoses. From the remaining options, recalling that denial is the most

common reaction when a client has chest pain will direct you to option 2. Review behavioral reactions of a client with chest pain if you had difficulty with this question.
Level of Cognitive Ability: Analysis
Client Needs: Psychosocial Integrity
Integrated Concept/Process: Nursing Process/Analysis
Content Area: Pharmacology
Reference: Ignatavicius, D., Workman, M., & Mishler, M. (1999). *Medical-surgical nursing across the health care continuum* (3rd ed.). Philadelphia: W.B. Saunders, p. 906.

16. 3
Rationale: The nurse is responsible for administering the correct medication. When medication orders are vague, the nurse must call the physician to clarify the orders before administering the medication. Waiting for the physician to make rounds delays needed treatment.
Test-Taking Strategy: Use the process of elimination. Options 1 and 2 are similar in that they indicate administering the medication and are eliminated first. Eliminate option 4 next because it is not appropriate to wait to clarify an unclear physician's order. Review the procedures related to clarifying a physician's orders if you had difficulty with this question.
Level of Cognitive Ability: Application
Client Needs: Safe, Effective Care Environment
Integrated Concept/Process: Nursing Process/Implementation
Content Area: Pharmacology
Reference: Lindeman, C., & McAthie, M. (1999). *Fundamentals of contemporary nursing practice.* Philadelphia: W.B. Saunders, pp. 347-348.

17. 3
Rationale: Double vision, loss of appetite, and nausea are early signs of digoxin toxicity. Additional signs of digoxin toxicity include bradycardia, difficulty reading, visual alterations such as green and yellow vision or seeing spots or halos, confusion, vomiting, diarrhea, decreased libido, and impotence.
Test-Taking Strategy: Use the process of elimination. Recalling that gastrointestinal and visual disturbances occur with digoxin toxicity will direct you to option 3. If you had difficulty with this question, review the signs of digoxin toxicity.
Level of Cognitive Ability: Analysis
Client Needs: Physiological Integrity
Integrated Concept/Process: Nursing Process/Assessment
Content Area: Pharmacology
Reference: Gutierrez, K. (1999). *Pharmacotherapeutics: Clinical decision-making in nursing.* Philadelphia: W.B. Saunders, p. 660.

18. 1
Rationale: Hypotension is a common side effect associated with the use of this medication. Options 2, 3, and 4 will also require assessment but are not the priority.
Test-Taking Strategy: Use the process of elimination. Note the key word "priority." Also, note that blood pressure is mentioned in the question and also in option 1. Use of the ABCs—airway, breathing, and circulation—will also direct you to option 1. Review care of the client receiving this medication by the IV route if you had difficulty with this question.
Level of Cognitive Ability: Application
Client Needs: Physiological Integrity
Integrated Concept/Process: Nursing Process/Assessment

Content Area: Pharmacology
Reference: Hodgson, B., & Kizior, R. (2001). *Saunders nursing drug handbook 2001.* Philadelphia: W.B. Saunders, p. 128.

19. 3
Rationale: Clients on potassium-wasting diuretics are at high risk for hypokalemia. Clinical manifestations of hypokalemia include fatigue, anorexia, nausea, vomiting, muscle weakness, leg cramps, decreased bowel motility, paresthesias, and dysrhythmias.
Test-Taking Strategy: Use the process of elimination and knowledge regarding the signs of electrolyte imbalances. Diarrhea and intestinal colic are signs of hyperkalemia. Tingling of the fingers and toes are signs of hypocalcemia. If you had difficulty with this question, review the signs of hypokalemia.
Level of Cognitive Ability: Analysis
Client Needs: Physiological Integrity
Integrated Concept/Process: Nursing Process/Assessment
Content Area: Pharmacology
Reference: Ignatavicius, D., Workman, M., & Mishler, M. (1999). *Medical-surgical nursing across the health care continuum* (3rd ed.). Philadelphia: W.B. Saunders, p. 244.

20. 4
Rationale: Most beta blockers may be administered with food or on an empty stomach, but propranolol is best absorbed if taken with meals or directly after eating. Exercise will not prevent orthostatic hypotension. Hot showers and baths are not advised. The client needs to be instructed in how to take the pulse rate and to notify the physician if the heart rate falls below 60 beats per minute.
Test-Taking Strategy: Use the process of elimination. Recalling that bradycardia can occur with propranolol will direct you to option 4. If you had difficulty with question, review the client teaching points related to this medication.
Level of Cognitive Ability: Application
Client Needs: Health Promotion and Maintenance
Integrated Concept/Process: Teaching/Learning
Content Area: Pharmacology
Reference: Wilson, B., Shannon, M., & Stang, C. (2000). *Nurses drug guide 2000.* Stamford, Conn.: Appleton & Lange, p. 1193.

CRITICAL THINKING: FREE-TEXT ENTRY

Answer: Administers another nitroglycerin tablet
Rationale: The usual protocol for administering nitroglycerin tablets for chest pain is to administer one tablet every 5 minutes PRN for chest pain, for a total dose of three tablets. Since the client is still complaining of chest pain, the nurse would administer a second nitroglycerin tablet.
Test-Taking Strategy: Knowledge regarding the protocol for administering nitroglycerin for chest pain is required to answer this question. Noting that the client's vital signs have remained stable will assist in determining the next priority nursing action. Review care of the client with chest pain and the protocol for the administration of nitroglycerin if you had difficulty with this question.
Level of Cognitive Ability: Application
Client Needs: Physiological Integrity
Integrated Concept/Process: Nursing Process/Implementation
Content Area: Pharmacology
Reference: Hodgson, B., & Kizior, R. (2001). *Saunders nursing drug handbook 2001.* Philadelphia: W.B. Saunders, p. 753.

REFERENCES

Cleveland, L., Aschenbrenner, D., Venable, S., & Yensen, J. (1999). *Nursing management in drug therapy.* Philadelphia: Lippincott.

Gutierrez, K. (1999). *Pharmacotherapeutics: Clinical decision-making in nursing.* Philadelphia: W.B. Saunders.

Hodgson, B., & Kizior, R. (2001). *Saunders nursing drug handbook 2001.* Philadelphia: W.B. Saunders.

Ignatavicius, D., Workman, M., & Mishler, M. (1999). *Medical-surgical nursing across the health care continuum* (3rd ed.). Philadelphia: W.B. Saunders.

Lindeman, C., & McAthie, M. (1999). *Fundamentals of contemporary nursing practice.* Philadelphia: W.B. Saunders.

Wilson, B., Shannon, M., & Stang, C. (2000). *Nurses drug guide 2000.* Stamford, Conn.: Appleton & Lange.

The Adult Client with a Renal System Disorder

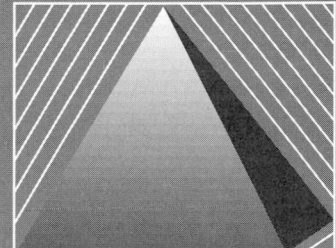

PYRAMID TERMS

acute renal failure (ARF) The sudden loss of kidney function as a result of renal cell damage from ischemia or toxic substances. ARF occurs abruptly and can be reversible. It leads to hypoperfusion, cell death, and decompensation in renal function. The prognosis is dependent on the cause and the condition of the client. Near-normal or normal kidney function may resume gradually.

anuria Urine output of less than 100 mL a day.

arterial steal syndrome Can develop following the insertion of an AV fistula when too much blood is diverted to the vein and arterial perfusion to the hand is compromised.

azotemia The retention of nitrogenous waste products in the blood.

chronic renal failure (CRF) The progressive loss and ongoing deterioration of kidney function that occurs slowly over a period of time. It is irreversible and results in uremia or end-stage renal disease. Chronic renal failure requires dialysis or kidney transplant to maintain life.

disequilibrium syndrome A rapid change in the composition of the extracellular fluid (ECF) occurs during hemodialysis. Solutes are removed from the blood faster than from the cerebrospinal fluid (CSF) and brain. Fluid is pulled into the brain, causing cerebral edema.

hemodialysis The process of cleansing a client's blood. The diffusion of dissolved particles from one fluid compartment into another across a semipermeable membrane. The client's blood flows through one fluid compartment, and the dialysate is in another fluid compartment.

internal arteriovenous fistula (AV fistula) Created surgically when an artery in the arm is anastomosed to a vein. This creates an opening, or fistula, between a large artery and a large vein. The flow of arterial blood into the venous system causes the vein to become engorged (maturity). Maturity is necessary so that the engorged vein can be punctured for the dialysis procedure, using a large-bore needle.

nephrolithiasis The formation of kidney stones. Kidney stones are formed in the renal parenchyma.

oliguria Urine output of less than 400 mL a day.

peritoneal dialysis The peritoneum is the dialyzing membrane (semipermeable membrane) and substitutes for kidney function during kidney failure. Works on the principles of diffusion and osmosis, and the dialysis occurs via the transfer of fluid and solute from the bloodstream through the peritoneum.

renal failure The loss of kidney function. The types of renal failure include ARF and CRF. The signs and symptoms of renal failure are caused by the retention of wastes, the retention of fluids, and the inability of the kidneys to regulate electrolytes.

urolithiasis The formation of urinary stones or calculi. Urinary calculi are formed in the ureter.

PYRAMID TO SUCCESS

Pyramid points focus on ARF and CRF, dialysis procedures such as hemodialysis and continuous ambulatory peritoneal dialysis (CAPD), urinary diversions, and postoperative care following urinary or renal surgery. Focus on the major problems associated with renal failure and the rationale for the prescribed treatment modalities. Be familiar with the complications associated with hemodialysis and peritoneal dialysis, the specific assessment data related to complications, and the expected treatment. Focus on the care of a peritoneal catheter and hemodialysis access devices, the complications associated with these access devices, and the appropriate nursing interventions if a complication is suspected. Review preoperative and postoperative care related to renal transplantation and the assessment data indicating rejection. Be familiar with urinary diversions, care of the client following prostatectomy, and treatment measures for the client with urinary or renal calculi. The Integrated Concepts and Processes addressed in this unit include Nursing Process, Caring, Communication and Documentation, Cultural Awareness, Self-Care, and Teaching/Learning.

▲ CLIENT NEEDS

Safe, Effective Care Environment

Accident prevention related to complications associated with disorder

Asepsis related to wound care and dialysis access devices

Client rights

Confidentiality related to the renal disorder

Consultations with members of the health care team

Establishing priorities

Informed consent related to diagnostic and surgical procedures

Renal organ donation

Standard (universal) precautions related to care of the client

Health Promotion and Maintenance

Expected body image changes

Instructions regarding care to a urinary diversion or a dialysis access device and dialysis procedures

Instructions regarding prescribed treatments related to urinary or renal disorder

Instructions regarding the prevention of the recurrence of a urinary or renal disorder

Instructions regarding postoperative management

Urinary and renal assessment techniques

Psychosocial Integrity

Body image disturbances

Community resources

Coping mechanisms

End of life

Grief and loss

Loss of function of a body part that occurs in clients with a renal disorder

Religious and spiritual influences

Support systems

Physiological Integrity

Adequate rest and sleep

Assessment data indicating rejection of renal transplant

Care related to dialysis access devices

Care related to hemodialysis and peritoneal dialysis

Care of the client following prostatectomy

Comfort interventions

Diagnostic tests and laboratory results

Elimination measures

Fluid and electrolyte and acid-base disorders

Pharmacological therapy

Preoperative and postoperative care related to renal transplantation

Prescribed nutrition and fluid measures

Prevention of complications arising as a result of dialysis

Treatment measures for the client with urinary or renal calculi

Urinary diversions

REFERENCES

Craven, R., & Hirnle, C. (2000). *Fundamentals of nursing: Human health and function* (3rd ed.). Philadelphia: Lippincott.

Harkreader, H. (2000). *Fundamentals of nursing: Caring and clinical judgment.* Philadelphia: W.B. Saunders.

Ignatavicius, D., Workman, M., & Mishler, M. (1999). *Medical-surgical nursing across the health care continuum* (3rd ed.). Philadelphia: W.B. Saunders.

LeMone, P., & Burke, K. (2000). *Medical-surgical nursing: Critical thinking in client care* (2nd ed.). Upper Saddle River, N.J.: Prentice-Hall.

Lewis, S., Heitkemper, M., & Dirksen, S. (2000). *Medical-surgical nursing: Assessment and management of clinical problems* (5th ed.). St. Louis: Mosby.

National Council of State Boards of Nursing (eds.) (2000). *Test Plan for the National Council Licensure Examination for Registered Nurses.* Chicago: Author.

Potter, P., & Perry, A. (2001). *Fundamentals of nursing* (5th ed.). St. Louis: Mosby.

Smeltzer, S., & Bare, B. (2000). *Textbook of medical-surgical nursing* (9th ed.). Philadelphia: Lippincott Williams & Wilkins.

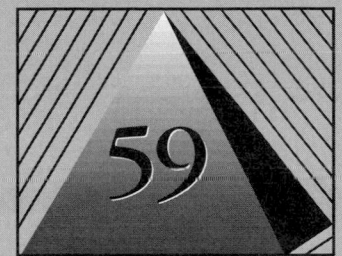

59

Renal System

I. ANATOMY AND PHYSIOLOGY

A. Kidneys
1. There are two; each is attached to the abdominal wall at the level of the last thoracic and first three lumbar vertebrae
2. Enclosed in the renal capsule
3. The cortex is the outer layer of the renal capsule
4. The medulla is surrounded by the cortex
5. The nephron makes up the functional unit of the kidneys
6. Functions of kidneys
   a. Maintain homeostasis of the blood
   b. Excrete end products of body metabolism
   c. Control fluid and electrolyte balance
   d. Excrete bacterial toxins, water-soluble drugs, and drug metabolites
   e. Secrete renin and erythropoietin, which play a role in the function of the parathyroid hormones and vitamin D
7. Nephron
   a. Functional renal unit
   b. Composed of glomerulus and tubules
8. Glomerulus
   a. Is encased in Bowman's capsule
   b. Filters the fluid out of blood
9. Tubules
   a. Include proximal, distal, and Henle's loop
   b. Fluid is converted to urine in the tubules, and then the urine moves to the pelvis of the kidney
   c. The urine flows from the pelvis of the kidney through the ureter, and empties into bladder
B. Bladder
1. The ureterovesical sphincter prevents reflux of urine from the bladder to the ureter
2. The total capacity of the bladder is 1 liter
C. Prostate gland
1. Surrounds the male urethra

2. Contains a duct that opens into the prostatic portion of the urethra and secretes the alkaline portion of seminal fluid
D. Urine production
1. As fluid flows through the proximal tubules, water and solutes are reabsorbed
2. Water and solutes that are not reabsorbed become urine
3. The process of selective reabsorption determines the amount of water and solutes to be secreted
E. Homeostasis of water
1. The antidiuretic hormone (ADH) is primarily responsible for the reabsorption of water by the kidneys
2. ADH is produced by the hypothalamus and secreted from the posterior lobe of the pituitary gland
3. Secretion of ADH is stimulated by dehydration or high sodium intake and by a fall in blood volume
4. ADH increases the permeability to water of the distal convoluted tubules and collecting duct
5. Water is drawn out of the tubules by osmosis into a high salt concentration of fluid in the medulla and its capillaries; water returns to the blood, and concentrated urine remains in the tubule to be excreted
6. When the client lacks ADH, he or she develops diabetes insipidus
7. Clients with diabetes insipidus produce very large amounts of dilute urine and without treatment have difficulty drinking sufficient water to survive
F. Homeostasis of sodium
1. When the amount of sodium increases, extra water is retained to preserve osmotic pressure
2. An increase in sodium and water produces an increase in the blood volume and blood pressure (BP)
3. When the BP increases, glomerular filtration increases, and extra water and sodium are lost;

blood volume is reduced and returns the BP to normal

4. Reabsorption of sodium in the distal convoluted tubules is controlled by the hormones of the renin-angiotensin system
5. Renin is secreted when the BP or concentration of fluid in the distal convoluted tubule is low
6. Renin is an enzyme and splits angiotensin I from angiotensinogen, which converts to angiotensin II as blood flows through the lung
7. Angiotensin II, a potent vasoconstrictor, stimulates the secretion of aldosterone
8. Aldosterone stimulates the distal convoluted tubules to reabsorb sodium and secrete potassium
9. The additional sodium increases water reabsorption and increases blood volume and BP, returning the BP to normal; the stimulus for the secretion of renin is then removed

G. Homeostasis of potassium
1. Increases in potassium stimulate the secretion of aldosterone
2. Aldosterone stimulates the distal convoluted tubules to secrete potassium; this acts to return the potassium concentration to normal

H. Homeostasis of acidity (pH)
1. Blood pH is controlled by maintaining the concentration of buffer systems
2. Carbonic acid and sodium bicarbonate form the most important buffer for neutralizing acids in the plasma
3. The concentration of carbonic acid is controlled by the respiratory system
4. The concentration of sodium bicarbonate is controlled by the kidneys
5. Normal pH is 7.35 to 7.45, maintained by keeping the ratio of concentrations of sodium bicarbonate to carbon dioxide constant at 20:1
6. Strong acids are neutralized by sodium bicarbonate to produce carbonic acid and the sodium salts of the strong acid; this process quickly restores the ratio and thus blood pH
7. The carbonic acid produced dissociates into carbon dioxide and water; because the concentration of carbon dioxide is maintained at a constant level by the respiratory system, the excess carbonic acid is rapidly excreted
8. Sodium combined with the strong acid is actively reabsorbed in the distal convoluted tubules in exchange for hydrogen or potassium ions; the strong acid is neutralized by the secretion of ammonia and is excreted as ammonia or potassium salts

I. Refer to Box 59-1 for risk factors

II. DIAGNOSTIC TESTS (Box 59-2)

A. Refer to Chapter 10 for information regarding normal values for renal function studies

---

BOX 59-1

Risk Factors Associated with Renal Disorders

Associated medical conditions
Contact sports
Family history of renal disease
Frequent urinary tract infections
High-sodium diet
History of hypertension
Medication use
Trauma and injury

BOX 59-2

Normal Renal Function Tests

BUN (blood urea nitrogen), 8 to 25 mg/dL
Serum creatinine, 0.6 to 1.3 mg/dL
Creatinine clearance, 100 to 120 mL/min
Uric acid, serum, 2.5 to 8.0 ng/dL
Uric acid, urine, 250 to 750 mg/24 hr

B. Urinalysis
1. Description: A urine test for evaluation of the renal system and for determining renal disease
2. Implementation
   a. Wash perineal area and use a clean container
   b. Obtain 10 to 15 mL of the first morning sample
   c. Note that refrigerated samples may alter the specific gravity
   d. If the client is menstruating, indicate this on the laboratory requisition form

C. Specific gravity determination
1. Description: A urine test that measures the kidney's ability to concentrate urine
2. Implementation
   a. Can be measured by multiple-test dipstick (most common method), refractometer (an instrument used in the laboratory setting, or urinometer (least accurate method)
   b. Factors that interfere with an accurate reading include radiopaque contrast agents, glucose, and proteins
   c. Cold specimens may produce a false high reading
   d. Normal value is 1.016 to 1.022 (may vary depending on the laboratory)
   e. An increase in specific gravity (more concentrated urine) occurs with insufficient fluid intake, decreased renal perfusion, or the presence of ADH
   f. A decrease in specific gravity (less concentrated urine) occurs with increased fluid intake, diuretic administration, and diabetes insipidus

D. Urine culture and sensitivity
1. Description: A urine test that identifies the presence of microorganisms and determines the specific antibiotics that will appropriately treat the existing microorganism
2. Implementation
   a. Clean perineal area and urinary meatus with bacteriostatic solution
   b. Collect midstream sample in a sterile container
   c. Send the collected specimen to the laboratory immediately
   d. Note that urine from the client who forced fluids may be too dilute to provide a positive culture
   e. Identify any sources of potential contaminants during the collection of the specimen, such as the hands, skin, clothing, hair, or vaginal or rectal secretions
E. Creatinine clearance test
1. Description
   a. A blood and timed urine specimen that evaluates kidney function
   b. Blood is drawn at the start of the test and the morning of the day that the 24-hour urine specimen collection is complete
2. Implementation
   a. Encourage adequate fluids before and during the test
   b. Instruct the client, as prescribed, to avoid tea, coffee, and medications during testing
   c. If the client is taking corticosteroids or thyroid medication, check with the physician regarding the administration of these medications during testing
   d. Maintain the urine specimen on ice or refrigerate, and check with the laboratory regarding the addition of a preservative to the specimen during collection
F. Vanillylmandelic acid (VMA) test
1. Description
   a. A 24-hour urine collection to diagnose pheochromocytoma, a tumor of the adrenal gland
   b. The test identifies an assay of urinary catecholamines in the urine
2. Implementation
   a. Instruct the client to avoid foods such as caffeine, cocoa, vanilla, cheese, gelatin, licorice, and fruits for at least 2 days prior to beginning the urine collection and during the collection, and to avoid taking medications for 2 to 3 days prior to beginning the test, as prescribed
   b. Instruct the client to avoid stress and to maintain adequate food and fluids during the test
   c. Save all urine, label the container, add preservative, and place the specimen on ice or refrigerate

d. Check with the laboratory regarding medication restrictions
G. Uric acid test
1. Description: A 24-hour urine collection to diagnose gout and kidney disease
2. Implementation
   a. Encourage fluids and a regular diet during testing
   b. Place the specimen on ice or refrigerate, and check with the laboratory regarding the addition of a preservative
H. KUB (kidneys, ureters, and bladder) radiograph
1. Description: An x-ray film that views the urinary system and adjacent structures; used to detect urinary calculi
2. Implementation: There is no specific preparation
I. Bladder ultrasonography
1. A noninvasive method of measuring the volume of urine in the bladder
2. May be performed for evaluating urinary frequency or inability to urinate
J. Computed tomography (CT) and magnetic resonance imaging (MRI)
1. Description: Provide cross-sectional views of the kidney and urinary tract
2. Implementation: Refer to Chapter 63
K. Intravenous pyelogram (IVP) ▲
1. Description
   a. The injection of a radiopaque dye that outlines the renal system
   b. Performed to identify abnormalities in the system
2. Preprocedure implementation
   a. Obtain a consent form
   b. Assess the client for allergies to iodine, sea- ▲ food, and radiopaque dyes
   c. Withhold food and fluids after midnight on the night before the test
   d. Administer laxatives as prescribed
   e. Inform the client about possible throat irritation, flushing of the face, warmth, or a salty taste that may be experienced during the test
3. Postprocedure implementation
   a. Monitor vital signs
   b. Instruct the client to drink at least 1 liter of ▲ fluid unless contraindicated
   c. Assess the venipuncture site for bleeding
   d. Monitor urinary output
L. Renal angiography
1. Description: The injection of a radiopaque dye through a catheter for examination of the renal arterial supply
2. Preprocedure implementation
   a. Obtain a consent form
   b. Assess the client for allergies to iodine, sea- ▲ food, and radiopaque dyes
   c. Inform the client about the possible burning ▲

feeling or the feeling of heat along the vessel when the dye is injected

   d. Withhold food and fluids after midnight on the night before the test

   e. Instruct the client to void immediately before the procedure

   f. Administer enemas as prescribed

   g. Shave injection sites as prescribed

   h. Assess and mark the peripheral pulses

  3. Postprocedure implementation

   a. Assess vital signs and peripheral pulses

   b. Provide bed rest and use of a sandbag at the insertion site for 4 to 8 hours

   c. Assess the color and temperature of the involved extremity

   d. Inspect the catheter insertion site for bleeding or swelling

   e. Force fluids unless contraindicated

   f. Monitor urinary output

 M. Renal scan

  1. Description: An IV injection of a radioisotope for visual imaging of renal blood flow

  2. Preprocedure implementation

   a. Obtain a consent form

   b. Assess for allergies

   c. Assist with administering radioisotope as necessary

   d. Instruct the client that he or she will be required to remain motionless

   e. Instruct the client that imaging may be repeated at various intervals before the test is complete

  3. Postprocedure implementation

   a. Encourage fluids unless contraindicated

   b. Assess the client for signs of delayed allergic reaction, such as itching and hives

   c. Note that the radioactivity is eliminated in 24 hours

   d. Follow standard precautions when caring for incontinent clients and double-bag client linens per agency policy

 N. Cystometrogram (CMG)

  1. Description: A graphic recording of the pressures exerted at varying phases of the bladder

  2. Preprocedure implementation: Inform the client of the voiding requirements during the procedure

  3. Postprocedure implementation: Monitor the client's voiding after the procedure

 O. Cystoscopy and biopsy

  1. Description: The bladder mucosa is examined for inflammation, calculi, or tumors by means of a cystoscope; a biopsy may be obtained

  2. Preprocedure implementation

   a. Obtain a consent form

   b. Withhold food and fluids after midnight on the night before the test

   c. Administer enemas and medications as prescribed

  3. Postprocedure implementation

   a. Monitor vital signs

   b. Monitor for postural hypotension

   c. Force fluids as prescribed

   d. Monitor intake and output

   e. Encourage deep-breathing exercises to relieve bladder spasms

   f. Administer analgesics as prescribed

   g. Administer sitz baths for back and abdominal pain

   h. Note that leg cramps are common because of the lithotomy position maintained during the procedure

   i. Assess the urine for color and consistency

   j. Note that pink-tinged or tea-colored urine is common

   k. Monitor for bright red urine or clots, and notify the physician if this occurs

 P. Renal biopsy

  1. Description: Insertion of a needle into the kidney to obtain a sample of tissue for examination

  2. Preprocedure implementation

   a. Assess vital signs

   b. Assess baseline clotting studies

   c. Obtain a consent form

   d. Withhold food and fluids after midnight on the night before the test

  3. Implementation during the procedure: Position the client prone with a pillow under the abdomen and shoulders

  4. Postprocedure implementation

   a. Monitor vital signs

   b. Monitor hemoglobin and hematocrit

   c. Place the client in the supine position and on bed rest for 8 hours as prescribed

   d. Provide pressure to the biopsy site for 30 minutes

   e. Check the biopsy site for bleeding

   f. Force fluids to 1500 to 2000 mL as prescribed

   g. Instruct the client to avoid heavy lifting and strenuous activity for 2 weeks

III. RENAL FAILURE

A. Description

  1. The loss of kidney function

  2. The types of **renal failure** include **acute renal failure** and **chronic renal failure**

  3. The signs and symptoms of **renal failure** are caused by the retention of wastes, the retention of fluids, and the inability of the kidneys to regulate electrolytes

  4. Prerenal causes include intravascular volume depletion, decreased cardiac output, and vascular failure secondary to vasodilation or obstruction

  5. Intrarenal causes include tubular necrosis, nephrotoxicity, and alterations in renal blood flow

  6. Postrenal causes include obstruction of urine

Phases of Acute Renal Failure

Oliguric
Diuretic
Recovery (convalescent)

flow between the kidney and urethral meatus and bladder neck obstruction

B. **Acute renal failure (ARF)** (Box 59-3)
  1. Description
    a. The sudden loss of kidney function; caused by renal cell damage from ischemia or toxic substances
    b. **ARF** occurs abruptly and can be reversible
    c. It leads to hypoperfusion, cell death, and decompensation in renal function
    d. The prognosis is dependent on the cause and the condition of the client
    e. Near-normal or normal kidney function may resume gradually
  2. Causes
    a. Infection
    b. Renal artery occlusion
    c. Obstruction
    d. Acute kidney disease
    e. Dehydration
    f. Diuretic therapy
    g. Ischemia from hypovolemia, heart failure, septic shock, or blood loss
    h. Toxic substances such as medications, particularly antibiotics
  3. Oliguric phase (Table 59-1)
    a. Duration is 8 to 15 days, and the longer the duration, the less chance of recovery
    b. Sudden drop in urine output; urine output less than 400 mL/day
    c. Urine specific gravity of 1.010 to 1.016
    d. Anorexia, nausea, and vomiting
    e. Hypertension
    f. Decreased skin turgor
    g. Pruritus
    h. Tingling of the extremities
    i. Drowsiness progressing to disorientation to coma
    j. Edema
    k. Dysrhythmias
    l. Signs of congestive heart failure (CHF) and pulmonary edema
    m. Signs of pericarditis
    n. Signs of acidosis
  4. Diuretic phase (Table 59-1)
    a. Urine output rises slowly and then diuresis occurs (4 to 5 L/day)
    b. Excessive urine output indicates recovery of damaged nephrons

TABLE 59-1	
Acute Renal Failure	
OLIGURIC PHASE	**DIURETIC PHASE**
Glomerular filtration rate decreases	Glomerular filtration rate begins to increase
Hyperkalemia	Hypokalemia
Sodium level normal or decreased	Hyponatremia
	Hypovolemia
Fluid overload	Gradual decline in BUN and creatinine
Elevated BUN and creatinine	
RECOVERY PHASE (CONVALESCENT)	
BUN is stable and normal	
Complete recovery may take 1 to 2 years	

TABLE 59-2	
Stages of Chronic Renal Failure	
STAGE I: DIMINISHED RENAL RESERVE	
Renal function is reduced	
No accumulation of metabolic wastes	
The healthier kidney compensates	
Nocturia and polyuria occur as a result of decreased ability to concentrate urine	
STAGE II: RENAL INSUFFICIENCY	
Metabolic wastes begin to accumulate	
Oliguria and edema occur as a result of decreased responsiveness to diuretics	
STAGE III: END STAGE	
Excessive accumulation of metabolic wastes	
Kidneys are unable to maintain homeostasis	
Dialysis or other renal replacement therapy is required	

    c. Hypotension
    d. Tachycardia
    e. Improvement in level of consciousness (LOC)
  5. Recovery phase (convalescent) (Table 59-1)
    a. A slow process; complete recovery may take 1 to 2 years
    b. Urine volume is normal
    c. Increase in strength
    d. Increase in LOC
    e. BUN is stable and normal
    f. Client can develop **chronic renal failure**
C. **Chronic renal failure (CRF)**
  1. Description
    a. The progressive loss and ongoing deterioration in kidney function that occurs slowly over a period of time
    b. It occurs in stages, is irreversible, and results in uremia or end-stage renal disease (Table 59-2)
    c. **CRF** affects all of the major body systems

and requires dialysis or kidney transplant to maintain life

   c. Hypervolemia can occur owing to the inability of the kidneys to excrete sodium and water, or hypovolemia can occur owing to the inability of the kidneys to conserve sodium and water

2. Causes
   a. May follow **ARF**
   b. Renal artery occlusion
   c. Chronic urinary obstruction
   d. Recurrent infections
   e. Hypertension
   f. Metabolic disorders
   g. Diabetes mellitus
   h. Autoimmune disorders

3. Assessment
   a. Anorexia and nausea
   b. Headache
   c. Weakness and fatigue
   d. Hypertension
   e. Confusion and lethargy, followed by convulsions and coma
   f. Kussmaul respirations
   g. Diarrhea or constipation
   h. Muscle twitching and numbness of the extremities
   i. Decreased urine output
   j. Decreased urine specific gravity
   k. Proteinuria
   l. Anemia
   m. **Azotemia**
   n. Fluid overload and signs of heart failure
   o. Uremic frost: a layer of urea crystals from evaporated perspiration that appears on the face, eyebrows, axilla, and groin in clients with advanced uremic syndrome

D. Implementation
   1. Monitor vital signs
   2. Monitor urine and I & O (hourly in **ARF**)
   3. Monitor weight, noting that an increase of 0.5 to 1 pound daily indicates fluid retention
   4. Monitor BUN, creatinine, and electrolyte values
   5. Monitor for acidosis and treat with sodium bicarbonate as prescribed
   6. Assess urinalysis for protein, hematuria, casts, and specific gravity
   7. Monitor LOC
   8. Assess for signs of infection, since the client may not demonstrate a temperature or an increased white blood cell (WBC) count
   9. Assess for dysrhythmias, since a potassium level above 6 mEq/L will cause peaked T waves and a widened QRS complex
   10. Monitor for fluid overload; assess lungs for rales and rhonchi
   11. Monitor for edema
   12. Administer prescribed diet; usually a moderate

protein intake (to decrease the workload on the kidneys) and a high-carbohydrate, low-potassium, and low-phosphorus diet is prescribed

13. Restrict sodium intake as prescribed, based on the electrolyte level
14. Daily fluid allowances may be 400 mL to 1000 mL plus measured urinary putput
15. Administer sodium polystyrene sulfonate (Kayexalate) to lower the potassium level as prescribed
16. Be alert to the mechanism for metabolism and excretion of all prescribed medication
17. Be alert to nephrotoxic medications, such as antibiotics, which may be prescribed
18. Prepare the client for dialysis if prescribed

E. Special problems in **renal failure**
   1. Hypertension
      a. Failure of the kidneys to maintain homeostasis of the blood pressure
      b. Monitor vital signs
      c. Maintain fluid and sodium restrictions as prescribed
      d. Administer diuretics and antihypertensives as prescribed
      e. Administer propranolol (Inderal), a beta-adrenergic antagonist, as prescribed, which decreases renin release (renin causes vasoconstriction)
   2. Hypervolemia
      a. Monitor vital signs
      b. Monitor I & O and weight
      c. Monitor for edema
      d. Monitor electrolytes
      e. Monitor for hypertension
      f. Monitor for CHF and pulmonary edema
      g. Enforce fluid restriction
      h. Avoid the administration of IV fluids
      i. Administer diuretics as prescribed
      j. Instruct the client to avoid foods with sodium
      k. Instruct the client to avoid antacids or cold remedies containing sodium bicarbonate
   3. Hypovolemia
      a. Monitor vital signs
      b. Monitor I & O and weight
      c. Monitor electrolytes
      d. Monitor for hypotension
      e. Monitor for dehydration
      f. Provide replacement therapy based on the electrolyte results
      g. Provide sodium supplements as prescribed, depending on the electrolyte value
   4. Potassium retention
      a. Monitor vital signs and apical rate
      b. Monitor potassium level
      c. Monitor for dysrhythmias (peaked T waves

and widened QRS complex) indicating hyperkalemia

d. Provide a low-potassium diet

e. Administer medications as prescribed to lower the potassium level

f. Prepare the client for dialysis

5. Phosphorus retention

a. Phosphorus rises and calcium drops, which leads to stimulation of parathyroid hormone, causing bone demineralization

b. Treatment is aimed at lowering serum phosphorus levels

c. Administer aluminum hydroxide preparations or other phosphate binders, as prescribed, that bind phosphorus in the intestine and allow the phosphorus to be eliminated

d. Administer aluminum hydroxide preparations at meals and not with other medications, because they bind medications in the intestinal tract

e. Administer stools softeners and laxatives as prescribed to prevent constipation, because aluminum hydroxide preparations are constipating

f. Enforce phosphorus restriction in the diet

6. Low calcium

a. Occurs because of the high phosphorus level and because of the inability of the diseased kidney to activate vitamin D

b. The absence of vitamin D causes a poor absorption of calcium from the intestinal tract

c. Monitor calcium level

d. Administer calcium supplements as prescribed

e. Administer activated vitamin D as prescribed

7. Metabolic acidosis

a. The kidneys are unable to excrete hydrogen ions or manufacture bicarbonate, resulting in acidosis

b. Administer alkalyzers such as sodium bicarbonate as prescribed

c. Note that clients with **CRF** adjust to low bicarbonate levels and do not become acutely ill

8. Anemia

a. A decreased rate of production of red blood cells (RBCs) occurs as a result of the diseased kidney and the decreased secretion of erythropoeitin

b. Monitor hemoglobin and hematocrit

c. Administer epoetin alfa (Epogen) as prescribed to stimulate the production of RBCs

d. Administer folic acid (vitamin B$_9$) as prescribed, instead of oral iron, because oral iron is not well absorbed by the GI tract in **CRF** and causes nausea and vomiting

e. Administer blood transfusions if prescribed, but blood transfusions are prescribed only when necessary because they decrease the stimulus to produce RBCs

f. Monitor bleeding

g. Instruct the client to use a soft toothbrush

h. Administer stool softeners as prescribed

i. Avoid the administration of acetylsalicylic acid (aspirin) because the medication is excreted by the kidneys; and if administered, high toxic levels will occur and prolong bleeding time

9. GI bleeding

a. Urea is broken down to ammonia by the intestinal bacteria, and ammonia is a mucosal irritant that causes ulceration and bleeding

b. Monitor hemoglobin and hematocrit levels

c. Monitor stools for occult blood

10. Infection and Injury

a. Infection and injury need to be monitored and avoided because tissue breakdown causes increased potassium levels

b. Monitor for signs of infection

c. Avoid urinary catheters and provide strict asepsis during insertion and catheter care

d. Instruct the client to avoid fatigue, which decreases body resistance

e. Instruct the client to avoid persons with infections

f. Administer antibiotics as prescribed, monitoring for nephrotoxic effects

11. Pruritis

a. Urate crystals are excreted through the skin to rid of excess wastes

b. This deposit of crystals is called uremic frost, and it is seen in advanced stages of **renal failure**

c. Monitor for skin breakdown, rash, and uremic frost

d. Provide good skin care and oral hygiene

e. Avoid the use of soaps

f. Administer antipruritics as prescribed

12. Muscle cramps

a. Occur in the extremities and hands and can be due to electrolyte imbalances

b. Monitor electrolytes

c. Administer electrolyte replacements as prescribed

d. Administer heat and massage as prescribed

13. Ocular irritation

a. Calcium deposits in the conjunctiva cause burning and watering of the eyes

b. Administer medications to control the calcium and phosphate levels as prescribed

c. Administer lubricating eye drops

14. Insomnia and fatigue

a. The diseased kidneys cause a buildup of wastes, causing fatigue in the client

b. Provide adequate rest periods

c. Administer mild CNS depressants as prescribed

15. Neurological changes

a. The buildup of active particles and fluids causes changes in the brain cells and leads to confusion and impairment in decision-making ability

b. Monitor for confusion and monitor LOC

c. Protect the client from injury

d. Provide a safe and hazard-free environment

e. Use side rails as needed

f. Provide a calm and restful environment

g. Provide comfort measures and backrubs

16. Psychosocial problems: Monitor the client for psychological problems such as depression, anxiety, suicidal behavior, denial, dependence/independence conflict, and changes in body image

IV. HEMODIALYSIS

A. Description

1. The diffusion of dissolved particles from one fluid compartment into another across asemipermeable membrane

2. The client's blood flows through one fluid compartment, and the dialysate is in another fluid compartment

B. Functions of **hemodialysis**

1. Cleanses the blood of accumulated waste products

2. Removes the by-products of protein metabolism, such as urea, creatinine, and uric acid

3. Removes excessive fluids

4. Maintains or restores the body's buffer system

5. Maintains or restores electrolyte levels

C. Principles of **hemodialysis**

1. The semipermeable membrane is made of a thin, porous cellophane

2. The pore size of the membrane allows small particles to pass through, such as urea, creatinine, uric acid, and water molecules

3. Proteins, bacteria, and blood cells are too large to pass through the membrane

4. The client's blood flows into the dialyzer; the movement of substances occurs from the blood to the dialysate

5. Diffusion: The movement of particles from an area of greater concentration to one of lesser concentration

6. Osmosis: The movement of fluids across a semipermeable membrane from an area of lesser concentration of particles to an area of greater concentration of particles

7. Ultrafiltration: The movement of fluid across a semipermeable membrane as a result of an artificially created pressure gradient

D. Dialysate bath

1. Composed of water and major electrolytes

2. The dialysate need not be sterile because bacteria are too large to pass through; however, the dialysate must meet specific standards, and water treatment systems are used to ensure a safe water supply

E. Implementation

1. Monitor vital signs

2. Monitor laboratory values before, during, and after dialysis

3. Assess the client for fluid overload prior to the procedure

4. Assess patency of the blood access device

5. Weigh the client before and after the procedure to determine fluid loss

6. Hold antihypertensives and other medications that can affect the BP prior to the procedure, as prescribed

7. Hold medications that could be dialyzed off, such as water-soluble vitamins and certain antibiotics

8. Monitor for shock and hypovolemia during the procedure

9. Provide adequate nutrition (client may eat prior to the procedure)

V. COMPLICATIONS OF HEMODIALYSIS (Box 59-4)

A. **Disequilibrium syndrome**

1. Description

a. A rapid change in the composition of the extracellular fluid (ECF) occurs during **hemodialysis**

b. Solutes are removed from the blood faster than from the cerebrospinal fluid (CSF) and brain; fluid is pulled into the brain, causing cerebral edema

2. Assessment

a. Nausea

b. Vomiting

c. Headache

d. Hypertension

e. Restlessness and agitation

BOX 59-4

Complications of Hemodialysis

Dialysis encephalopathy
Disequilibrium syndrome
Electrolyte changes
Hepatitis
Hypotension and shock
Loss of blood
Muscle cramping
Sepsis

f. Confusion

g. Seizures

3. Implementation

a. Monitor for signs of **disequilibrium syndrome**

b. Notify the physician if signs of **disequilibrium syndrome** occur

c. Reduce environmental stimuli

d. Prepare to dialyze the client for a shorter period at reduced blood flow rates to prevent occurrence

B. **Dialysis encephalopathy**

1. Description: An aluminum toxicity that occurs as a result of aluminum in the H_2O sources used in the dialysate, and the ingestion of aluminum-containing antacids (phosphate binders)

2. Assessment

a. Progressive neurological impairment

b. Mental cloudiness

c. Speech disturbances

d. Dementia

e. Muscle incoordination

f. Bone pain

g. Seizures

3. Implementation

a. Monitor for signs of dialysis encephalopathy

b. Notify the physician if signs of dialysis encephalopathy occur

c. Administer aluminum-chelating agents as prescribed so that the aluminum is freed up and dialyzed from the body

VI. ACCESS FOR HEMODIALYSIS

A. Subclavian and femoral catheter (Fig. 59-1)

1. Description

a. A subclavian (subclavian vein) or femoral (femoral vein) catheter may be inserted for short-term or temporary use in **ARF**

b. May be used until a fistula or graft matures or develops, or when the client has fistula or graft access failure because of infection or clotting

2. Implementation

a. Assess insertion site for hematoma, bleeding, dislodging, and infection

b. Do not use these catheters for any reason other than dialysis

c. Maintain an occlusive dressing

3. Subclavian vein catheter

a. Is usually filled with heparin and capped to maintain patency between dialysis treatments

b. The catheter should not be uncapped

c. The catheter may be left in place for up to 6 weeks if complications do not occur

4. Femoral vein catheter

a. The client should not sit up more than 45 degrees or lean forward, or the catheter may kink and occlude

b. Assess extremity for circulation, temperature, and pulses

c. Prevent pulling or disconnecting of the catheter when giving care

d. Use an IV control pump with microdrip tubing if a heparin infusion is prescribed

B. External arteriovenous shunt (AV shunt) (Fig. 59-1)

1. Description

a. Access is formed by the surgical insertion of two Silastic cannulas into an artery and a vein in the forearm or leg, to form an external blood path

b. The cannulas are connected to form a U shape; blood flows from the client's artery through the shunt into the vein

c. A tube leading to the membrane compartment of the dialyzer is connected to the arterial cannula

d. Blood fills the membrane compartment and flows back to the client by way of a tube connected to the venous cannula

e. When dialysis is complete, the cannulas are clamped and reattached to form their U shape

2. Advantages

a. Can be used immediately following creation

b. No venipuncture is necessary for dialysis

3. Disadvantages

a. External danger of disconnecting or dislodging

b. Risk of hemorrhage, infection, or clotting

c. Skin erosion around the catheter site can occur

4. Implementation

a. Avoid wetting the shunt

b. A dressing is completely wrapped around the shunt and kept dry and intact

c. Cannula clamps need to be available at the client's bedside

d. Do not take a blood pressure, draw blood, place an IV, or administer injections in the shunt extremity

e. Monitor for hemorrhage, infection, and clotting

f. Monitor skin integrity around the insertion site

g. Note that the shunt is patent if it is warm to touch

h. Auscultate and palpate for a bruit, although a bruit may not be heard and is not always felt with the shunt

i. Notify the physician immediately if signs of clotting, hemorrhage, or infection occur

5. Signs of clotting

a. Fold back the dressing to expose the shunt tubing and assess for signs of clotting

b. Fibrin-white flecks noted in the tubing

c. The separation of serum and cells

d. The absence of a previously heard bruit

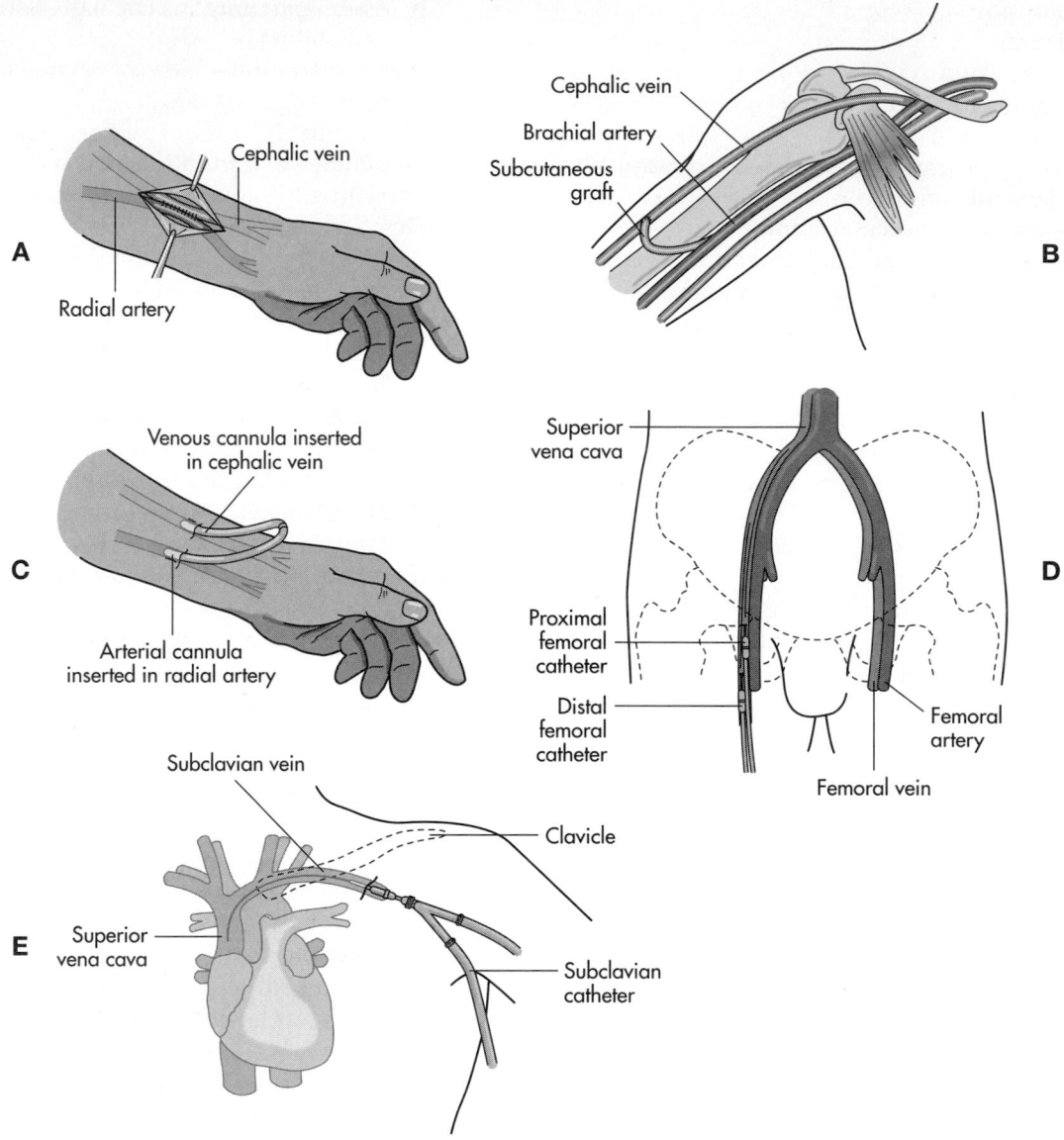

FIG. 59-1   Frequently used means for gaining vascular access for hemodialysis include, **A,** arteriovenous fistula; **B,** arteriovenous graft; **C,** external arteriovenous shunt; **D,** femoral vein catheterization; and, **E,** subclavian vein catheterization. (From Phipps W, Sands J, Marek J: *Medical-surgical nursing: concepts and clinical practice,* ed 6, St Louis, 1999, Mosby.)

e. Coolness of the tubing or extremity

f. Client complaints of a tingling sensation

C. **Internal arteriovenous fistula (AV fistula)** (Fig. 59-1)

1. Description

   a. Access of choice for chronic dialysis clients

   b. Created surgically by anastomosis of an artery in the arm to a vein; this creates an opening or fistula between a large artery and a large vein

   c. The flow of arterial blood into the venous system causes the veins to become engorged (matured or developed)

   d. Maturity takes about 1 to 2 weeks and is required before the fistula can be used, so that the engorged vein can be punctured with a large-bore needle for the dialysis procedure

   e. Subclavian or femoral catheters, **peritoneal dialysis,** or an external AV shunt can be used for dialysis while the fistula is maturing or developing

2. Advantages

   a. Since the fistula is internal, there is less danger of clotting and bleeding

   b. The fistula can be used indefinitely

c. Decreased incidence of infection

d. No external dressing is required

e. Allows freedom of movement

3. Disadvantages

a. Cannot be used immediately after insertion

b. Needle insertions are required for dialysis

c. Infiltration of the needles during dialysis can occur and cause hematomas

d. An aneurysm can form in the fistula

e. **Arterial steal syndrome** can develop (too much blood is diverted to the vein, and arterial perfusion to the hand is compromised)

f. CHF can occur from the increased blood flow in the venous system

D. Internal arteriovenous graft (AV graft) (Fig. 59-1)

1. Description

a. The internal graft is used primarily for chronic dialysis clients who do not have adequate blood vessels for the creation of a fistula

b. An artificial graft made of Gore-Tex or a bovine (cow) carotid artery is used to create an artificial vein for blood flow

c. The procedure involves the anastomosis of the graft to the artery, a tunneling under the skin, and anastomosis to a vein

d. The graft can be used 2 weeks after insertion

e. Complications of the graft include clotting, aneurysms, and infection

2. Advantages

a. Since the graft is internal, there is less danger of clotting and bleeding

b. The graft can be used indefinitely

c. Decreased incidence of infection

d. No external dressing is required

e. Allows freedom of movement

3. Disadvantages

a. Cannot be used immediately after insertion

b. Needle insertions are required for dialysis

c. Infiltration of the needles during dialysis can occur and cause hematomas

d. An aneurysm can form in the graft

e. **Arterial steal syndrome** can develop (too much blood is diverted to the vein, and arterial perfusion to the hand is compromised)

f. CHF can occur from the increased blood flow in the venous system

E. Implementation for **AV fistula** and AV graft

1. Do not measure a blood pressure, draw blood, place an IV, or administer injections in the fistula or graft extremity

2. Monitor for clotting

a. Complaints of tingling or discomfort in the extremity

b. Inability to palpate a thrill or auscultate a bruit over the fistula or graft

3. Monitor for **arterial steal syndrome**

4. Palpate or auscultate for bruit or thrill over the fistula or graft

5. Palpate pulses below the fistula or graft, and monitor for hand swelling as an indication of ischemia

6. Note temperature and capillary refill of the extremity

7. Monitor for infection

8. Monitor lung and heart sounds for signs of CHF

9. Notify the physician immediately if signs of clotting, infection, or **arterial steal syndrome** occur

VII. PERITONEAL DIALYSIS

A. Description

1. The peritoneum is the dialyzing membrane (semipermeable membrane) and substitutes for kidney function during kidney failure

2. Works on the principles of diffusion and osmosis, and the dialysis occurs via the transfer of fluid and solute from the bloodstream through the peritoneum

3. The peritoneal membrane is large and porous, allowing solutes and fluid to move via an osmotic gradient from an area of higher concentration in the body to an area of lower concentration in the dialyzing fluid

4. The peritoneal cavity is rich in capillaries; therefore, it provides a ready access to blood supply

B. Contraindications to **peritoneal dialysis**

1. Peritonitis

2. Recent abdominal surgery

3. Abdominal adhesions

4. Impending renal transplant

C. Dialysate solution

1. Solution is sterile

2. Contains electrolytes and minerals, a specific osmolarity, a specific glucose concentration, and other medication additives as prescribed

3. The higher the glucose concentration, the greater the amount of fluid removed during an exchange

4. Increasing the glucose concentration increases the concentration of active particles that cause osmosis, and increases the rate of ultrafiltration and the amount of fluid removed

5. Potassium: If hyperkalemia is not a problem, potassium may be added to each bag of solution

6. Heparin: Added to the dialysate solution to prevent clotting of the catheter

7. Antibiotics: Prophylactic antibiotics may be added to dialysate to prevent peritonitis

8. Insulin: May be added to the dialysate for the client with diabetes mellitus

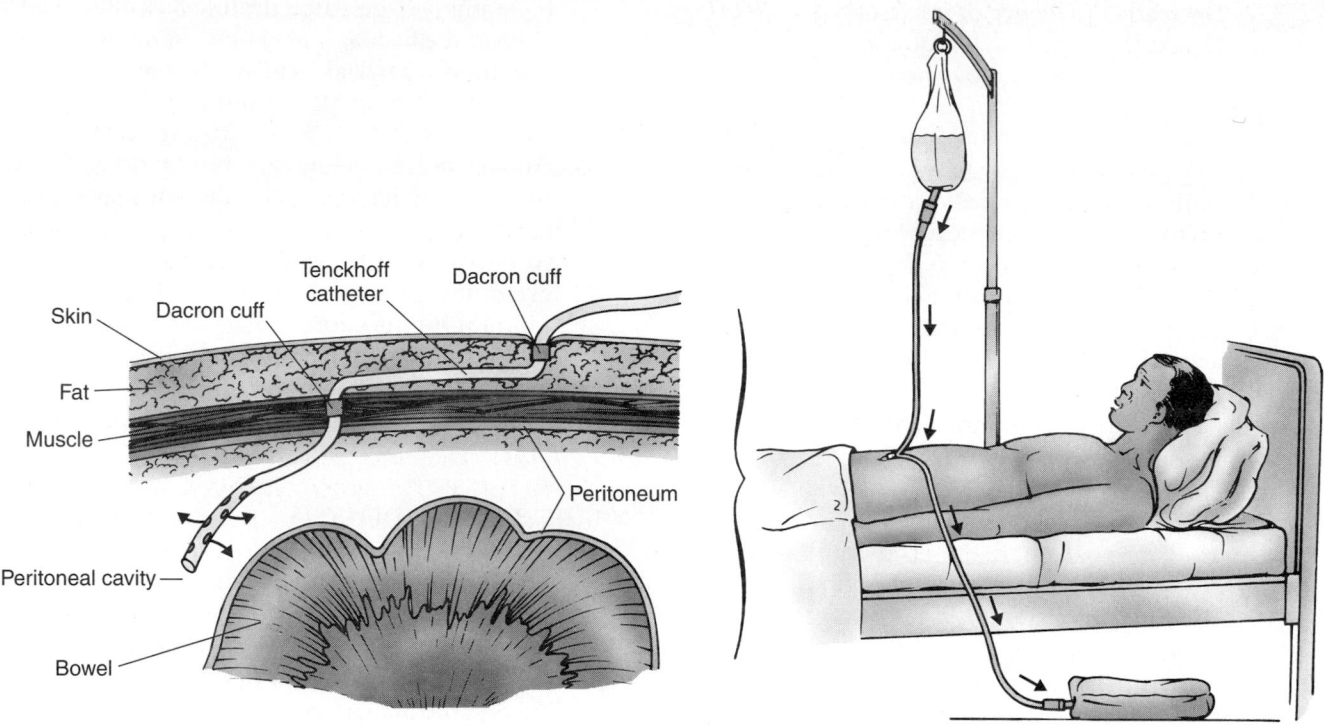

FIG. 59-2 Manual peritoneal dialysis via an implanted abdominal catheter (Tenckhoff catheter). (From Ignatavicius D, Workman M, Mishler M: *Medical surgical nursing across the health care continuum,* ed 3, Philadelphia, 1999, WB Saunders.)

VIII. ACCESS FOR PERITONEAL DIALYSIS
(Fig. 59-2)

A. Description

1. A surgical insertion of a siliconized rubber catheter into the abdominal cavity is required to allow infusion of dialysis fluid

2. The preferred insertion site is 3 to 5 cm below the umbilicus because this area is relatively avascular and has less fascial resistance

3. The catheters are tunneled under the skin to stabilize the catheter and reduce the risk of infection

4. Over a period of 1 to 2 weeks following insertion, there is an ingrowth of fibroblasts and blood vessels into the cuffs of the catheter, which fix the catheter in place and provide an extra barrier against dialysate leakage and bacterial invasion

B. Types of **peritoneal dialysis**

1. Continuous ambulatory **peritoneal dialysis** (CAPD)

a. Closely resembles renal function because it is a continuous process

b. Does not require a machine for the procedure

c. Promotes client independence

d. The client performs self-dialysis 24 hours a day, 7 days a week

e. Usually four dialysis cycles are administered

in 24 hours, including an 8-hour dwell time overnight

f. One and a half to two liters of dialysate is instilled into the abdomen four times daily and allowed to dwell as prescribed

g. The dialysis bag, attached to the catheter, is folded and carried in the client's clothing until time for outflow

h. After dwell, the bag is placed lower than the insertion site so that fluid drains by gravity flow

i. When full, the bag is changed, new dialysate is instilled into the abdomen, and the process continues

2. Automated **peritoneal dialysis** (APD) (Box 59-5)

a. Similar to CAPD in that it is a continuous dialysis process

b. Requires a peritoneal cycling machine

c. Can be done as intermittent **peritoneal dialysis** (IPD), continuous cycling **peritoneal**

d. **dialysis** (CCPD), or nightly **peritoneal dialysis** (NPD)

C. **Peritoneal dialysis** infusion

1. Description

a. One infusion (inflow), dwell, and outflow is considered one exchange

b. Uses an open system that presents a risk of infection

c. Inflow: The infusion of 1 to 2 liters of dialysate as prescribed is infused by gravity into the peritoneal space, which usually takes approximately 10 to 20 minutes

d. Dwell time: The amount of time that the dialysate solution remains in the peritoneal cavity; prescribed by the physician

e. Outflow: Fluid drains out of body by gravity into the drainage bag

2. Implementation before treatment
   a. Monitor vital signs
   b. Obtain weight
   c. Have the client void, if possible
   d. Assess electrolyte and glucose levels

3. Implementation during treatment
   a. Monitor vital signs
   b. Monitor for signs of infection
   c. Monitor for respiratory distress, pain, or discomfort
   d. Monitor for signs of pulmonary edema
   e. Monitor for hypotension and hypertension
   f. Monitor for malaise, nausea, vomiting
   g. Assess the catheter site dressing for wetness or bleeding
   h. Monitor dwell time as prescribed by the physician and initiate outflow
   i. Do not allow dwell time to extend beyond the physician's order because this increases the risk for hyperglycemia
   j. Turn the client from side to side or have the client sit upright if the flow is slow to start
   k. Monitor outflow, which should be a continuous stream after the clamp is opened
   l. Monitor outflow for color and clarity
   m. Monitor I & O accurately
   n. If outflow is less than inflow, the difference is equal to the amount absorbed or retained by the client during dialysis and should be counted as intake

IX. **COMPLICATIONS OF PERITONEAL DIALYSIS**
A. Peritonitis
    1. Maintain meticulous sterile technique when hooking up or clamping off bags, and when caring for the catheter insertion site
    2. Follow institutional procedure for hooking up or clamping off bags, which may include scrubbing the connection sites with an antiseptic solution
    3. Monitor temperature closely
    4. Monitor for fever, cloudy outflow, and rebound abdominal tenderness
    5. If peritonitis is suspected, obtain a culture of the outflow to determine the infective organism
    6. Administer antibiotics as prescribed
B. Abdominal pain
    1. Pain during inflow is common during the first few exchanges, is caused by peritoneal irritation, and usually disappears after a week or two of dialysis treatments
    2. The cold temperature of the dialysate aggravates the discomfort, and the dialysate should be warmed before use, only with a special dialysate warmer pad
    3. Place a heating pad on the abdomen during the inflow to relieve discomfort
C. Insufficient outflow
    1. May be caused by catheter migration out of the peritoneal area; if this occurs, the catheter must be repositioned by the physician
    2. Insufficient outflow can also be caused by a full colon
    3. Maintain the drainage bag below the client's abdomen
    4. Change the client's outflow position by turning or ambulating
    5. Check for kinks in the tubing
    6. Encourage a high-fiber diet
    7. Administer stool softeners as prescribed
D. Leakage around the catheter site
    1. Over a period of 1 to 2 weeks following insertion of the catheter, an ingrowth of fibroblasts and blood vessels into the cuffs of the catheter occurs, which fix the catheter in place and provide an extra barrier against dialysate leakage and bacterial invasion
    2. It may take up to 2 weeks for the client to tolerate a full 2-liter exchange without leaking around the catheter site
E. Characteristics of outflow
    1. During the first or initial exchanges, the outflow may be bloody; outflow should be clear and colorless thereafter

2. A brown outflow indicates bowel perforation
3. If the outflow is same color as urine, this indicates bladder perforation
4. Cloudy outflow indicates peritonitis

X. UREMIC SYNDROME

A. Description
   1. The accumulation of nitrogenous waste products in the blood because of the inability of the kidneys to filter out these waste products
   2. It may occur as a result of **acute** or **chronic renal failure**
B. Assessment
   1. **Oliguria**
   2. The presence of protein, red blood cells, and casts in the urine
   3. A urine specific gravity of 1.010
   4. Elevated levels of urea, uric acid, potassium, and magnesium in the urine
   5. Hypotension or hypertension
   6. Alterations in LOC
   7. Electrolyte imbalances
   8. Stomatitis
   9. Nausea or vomiting
   10. Diarrhea or constipation
C. Implementation
   1. Monitor vital signs
   2. Monitor electrolyte values
   3. Monitor I & O
   4. Provide a diet low in protein unless the client is on **peritoneal dialysis**
   5. Limit sodium, nitrogen, potassium, and phosphate intake as prescribed

XI. CYSTITIS/URINARY TRACT INFECTIONS (UTI)
   (Box 59-6)

A. Description
   1. Inflammation of the bladder from infection or obstruction of the urethra
   2. The most common causative organisms are *Escherichia coli*, *Enterobacter*, *Pseudomonas*, and *Serratia*
   3. More common in women because women have a shorter urethra than men, and the location of the urethra in the woman is close to the rectum
   4. Sexually active and pregnant women are most vulnerable to cystitis
B. Assessment
   1. Frequency and urgency
   2. Burning on urination
   3. Voiding in small amounts
   4. Inability to void
   5. Incomplete emptying of the bladder
   6. Lower abdominal discomfort or back discomfort
   7. Cloudy, dark, foul-smelling urine
   8. Hematuria

BOX 59-6

Causes of Cystitis

Allergens or irritants, such as soaps, sprays, bubble bath, perfumed sanitary napkins
Bladder distention
Calculus
Hormonal changes influencing alterations in vaginal flora
Indwelling urethral catheters
Invasive urinary tract procedures
Loss of bactericidal properties of prostatic secretions in the male
Poor-fitting diaphragms
Sexual intercourse
Synthetic underwear and pantyhose
Urinary stasis
Use of spermicides
Wet bathing suits

---

   9. Bladder spasms
   10. Malaise, chills, fever
   11. Nausea and vomiting
C. Implementation
   1. Obtain a urine specimen for culture and sensitivity, if prescribed, to identify bacterial growth prior to administering prescribed antibiotics
   2. Instruct the client to force fluids up to 3000 mL a day, especially if the client is taking a sulfonamide, because these medications can form crystals in concentrated urine
   3. Administer medications as prescribed, which may include analgesics, antiseptics, antispasmodics, antibiotics, and antimicrobials
   4. Maintain an acid urine pH (5.5) by an acid ash diet; instruct the client in foods to consume on an acid ash diet
   5. Note that if the client is prescribed an aminoglycoside, a sulfonamide, or nitrofurantoin (Macrodantin), the actions of these medications are diminished by acidic urine
   6. Use strict aseptic technique when inserting a urinary catheter into a client
   7. Maintain closed urinary drainage systems for the client with an indwelling catheter
   8. Provide meticulous perineal care for the client with an indwelling catheter
   9. Discourage caffeine products such as coffee, tea, and cola
   10. Instruct the client to avoid alcohol
   11. Provide heat to the abdomen or sitz baths for complaints of discomfort
   12. Instruct the client to take medications as prescribed
   13. Instruct the client to take antibiotics on schedule and to take entire course of medications

---

BOX 59-7

Prevention of Cystitis

Teach the female client good perineal care and to wipe from front to back

Instruct the female client to avoid bubble baths and tub baths and avoid vaginal deodorants or sprays

Instruct the client to void every 2 to 3 hours

Instruct the female client to void and drink a glass of water after intercourse

Instruct the female client to wear cotton pants and to avoid wearing tight clothes or pantyhose with slacks, and to avoid sitting in a wet bathing suit for prolonged periods of time

Teach pregnant women to void every 2 hours

Encourage menopausal women to use estrogen vaginal creams to restore pH

Instruct the female client to use water-soluble lubricants for coitus, especially after menopause

---

as prescribed, which may be a course of 10 to 14 days

14. Instruct the client in the importance of a follow-up urine culture following treatment

15. Preventive measures are listed in Box 59-7

XII. UROSEPSIS

A. Description

1. A gram-negative bacteremia originating in the urinary tract

2. The most common responsible organism is *Escherichia coli*

3. The most common cause is the presence of an indwelling urinary catheter or an untreated UTI in a client who is medically compromised

4. The major problem is the ability of this bacterium to develop resistant strains

5. Urosepsis can lead to septic shock if not treated aggressively

B. Assessment: Fever is the most common and earliest manifestation

C. Implementation

1. Obtain a urine specimen for urine culture and sensitivity

2. Administer IV antibiotics as prescribed, usually until the client has been afebrile for 3 to 5 days

3. Administer oral antibiotics as prescribed after the 3- to 5-day afebrile period

XIII. URETHRITIS

A. Description

1. An inflammation of the urethra commonly associated with sexually transmitted diseases (STD), and may be seen with cystitis

2. In men, it is most often caused by gonorrhea or chlamydial infection

3. In women, it is most often caused by feminine hygiene sprays, perfumed toilet paper or sanitary napkins, spermicidal jellies, UTIs, or changes in the vaginal mucosal lining

B. Assessment

1. Males

a. Burning on urination

b. Frequency

c. Urgency

d. Nocturia

e. Difficulty voiding

f. Discharge from the penis

2. Females

a. Frequency

b. Urgency

c. Nocturia

d. Painful urination

e. Difficulty voiding

f. Lower abdominal discomfort

C. Implementation

1. Encourage fluids

2. Prepare the client for testing to determine if an STD is present

3. Administer antibiotics as prescribed

4. Instruct the client in the administration of sitz baths

5. If stricture occurs, prepare the client for dilation of the urethra and instillation of an antiseptic solution

6. Instruct the client to avoid intercourse until the symptoms subside or treatment of the STD is complete

7. Instruct the female client to avoid the use of perfumed toilet paper or sanitary napkins and feminine hygiene sprays

XIV. URETERITIS AND PYELONEPHRITIS

A. Ureteritis

1. An inflammation of the ureter that is commonly associated with pyelonephritis

2. Chronic pyelonephritis causes the ureter to become fibrotic and narrowed by strictures

B. Pyelonephritis

1. An inflammation of the renal pelvis and the parenchyma, commonly caused by bacterial invasion

2. Acute pyelonephritis often occurs after bacterial contamination of the urethra or following an invasive procedure of the urinary tract

3. Chronic pyelonephritis most commonly occurs following chronic obstruction with reflux or chronic disorders

4. *Escherichia coli* is the most common bacterial causative organism

C. Acute pyelonephritis

1. Usually a short course that recurs as a relapse of a previous infection or as a new infection

2. Can progress to bacteremia or chronic pyelonephritis
3. Assessment
   a. Fever and chills
   b. Nausea
   c. Flank pain on the affected side
   d. Costovertebral angle (CVA) tenderness
   e. Headache
   f. Muscular pain
   g. Dysuria
   h. Frequency and urgency
   i. Cloudy, bloody, or foul-smelling urine
   j. Increased white blood cells in the urine
D. Chronic pyelonephritis
   1. A slow, progressive disease that is usually associated with recurrent acute attacks
   2. Causes contraction of the kidney and dysfunctioning of the nephrons, which are replaced by scar tissue
   3. Can lead to **renal failure**
   4. Assessment
      a. Frequently diagnosed incidentally when a client is being evaluated for hypertension
      b. Poor urine-concentrating ability
      c. Pyuria
      d. **Azotemia**
      e. Proteinuria
      f. Anemia
      g. Acidosis
E. Implementation
   1. Monitor vital signs
   2. Monitor I & O
   3. Monitor weight
   4. Encourage fluids up to 3000 mL a day
   5. Encourage adequate rest
   6. Instruct the client in a high-calorie, low-protein diet
   7. Provide warm moist compresses to the flank area
   8. Encourage the client to take warm baths
   9. Administer analgesics, antipyretics, antibiotics, urinary antiseptics, and antiemetics as prescribed
   10. Monitor for signs of **renal failure**

▲ **XV. GLOMERULONEPHRITIS**
A. Description
   1. A term that includes a variety of disorders, most of which are caused by an immunological reaction
   2. It results in proliferative and inflammatory changes within the glomerular structure
   3. Destruction, inflammation, and sclerosis of the glomeruli of both kidneys occur
   4. The inflammation of the glomeruli results from an antigen-antibody reaction produced from an infection elsewhere in the body
   5. Loss of kidney function develops

B. Causes
   1. Immunological or autoimmune diseases
   2. Streptococcal infection, group A beta-hemolytic ▲
   3. History of pharyngitis or tonsillitis 2 to 3 weeks ▲ prior to symptoms
C. Types
   1. Acute: Occurs 2 to 3 weeks after a streptococcal ▲ infection
   2. Chronic: Can occur after the acute phase or slowly over time
D. Complications
   1. Heart failure
   2. Hypertensive encephalopathy
   3. Pulmonary edema
   4. **Renal failure**
E. Assessment
   1. Gross hematuria ▲
   2. Dark, smoky, cola-colored or red-brown urine ▲
   3. Proteinuria that produces a persistent and ▲ excessive foam in the urine
   4. Urinary debris
   5. Moderately elevated to high specific gravity
   6. Low urinary pH
   7. **Oliguria** or **anuria**
   8. Headache
   9. Chills and fever
   10. Fatigue and weakness
   11. Anorexia, nausea, and vomiting
   12. Pallor
   13. Edema in the face, periorbital area, feet, or generalized
   14. Shortness of breath, ascites, pleural effusion, and CHF
   15. Abdominal or flank pain
   16. Hypertension
   17. Reduced visual acuity
   18. Increased BUN and creatinine levels
   19. Increased antistreptolysin O titer (used to diag- ▲ nose disorders caused by streptococcal infections)
F. Implementation ▲
   1. Monitor vital signs
   2. Monitor I & O and urine closely
   3. Monitor daily weight
   4. Monitor for edema
   5. Monitor for fluid overload, ascites, pulmonary edema, and CHF
   6. Restrict fluid intake as prescribed
   7. Provide a high-calorie and low-protein diet
   8. Restrict sodium intake as prescribed if edema is present
   9. Provide bed rest and limited activity
   10. Instruct the client to obtain treatment for ▲ infections, specifically sore throats and upper respiratory infections
   11. Administer diuretics, antihypertensives, and antibiotics as prescribed

12. Monitor for signs of **renal failure,** cardiac failure, hypertensive encephalopathy
13. Instruct the client to report signs of bloody urine, headache, or edema

XVI. NEPHROTIC SYNDROME

A. Description: A set of clinical manifestations arising from protein wasting secondary to diffuse glomerular damage
B. Assessment
   1. Proteinuria
   2. Hypoalbuminemia
   3. Edema
   4. Hyperlipidemia
   5. Waxy pallor to the skin
   6. Anemia
   7. Anorexia
   8. Malaise
   9. Irritability
   10. Amenorrhea or abnormal menses
   11. Hematuria may be present
   12. Hypertension
C. Implementation
   1. Monitor vital signs
   2. Monitor I & O
   3. Bed rest if severe edema is present
   4. Normal to low-protein diet as prescribed, with adequate carbohydrate and calorie intake
   5. Monitor daily weights
   6. Provide a mild sodium restriction as prescribed
   7. Monitor potassium level; potassium may be restricted from the diet if the potassium rises
   8. Administer diuretics as prescribed
   9. Administer corticosteroids and cytotoxic medications as prescribed
   10. Administer plasma volume expanders, such as albumin, plasma, and dextran, to raise the osmotic pressure
   11. Administer anticoagulants as prescribed for those clients who develop renal vein thrombosis

XVII. HYDRONEPHROSIS

A. Description
   1. Distention of the renal pelvis and calices, caused by an obstruction of normal urine flow
   2. The urine becomes trapped proximal to the obstruction
   3. The causes include calculus, tumors, scar tissue, and kinks in the ureter
B. Assessment
   1. Hypertension
   2. Headache
   3. Flank pain
   4. Electrolyte imbalances
C. Implementation
   1. Monitor vital signs frequently

2. Monitor for fluid and electrolyte imbalances, including dehydration after the obstruction is relieved
3. Monitor for diuresis, which can lead to fluid depletion
4. Monitor daily weights
5. Monitor urine for specific gravity, albumin, and glucose
6. Administer fluid replacement as prescribed

XVIII. GENITOURINARY TUBERCULOSIS

A. Description
   1. Usually a late manifestation of tuberculosis and is caused by the spread of *Mycobacterium tuberculosis* from the lungs through the bloodstream
   2. *Mycobacterium tuberculosis* is the cause of tuberculosis and is most often seen in the poor, the malnourished, those living in close housing, and the immunosuppressed client
B. Assessment
   1. Frequency and pain on urination
   2. Bladder spasms
   3. Fatigue
   4. Weight loss
   5. Tubercle bacilli in the urine culture
   6. Lesions noted on x-ray film
   7. Tuberculosis nodules noted on the prostate
C. Implementation
   1. Administer antitubercular medications as prescribed
   2. Use precautions when handling urine specimens, since the bacillus in the urine is infectious
   3. Instruct the client to use precautions to prevent the spread of the disease
   4. Instruct the client to use condoms during intercourse to prevent the spread of the disease

XIX. POLYCYSTIC KIDNEY DISEASE

A. Description
   1. A cystic formation and hypertrophy of the kidneys, which lead to cystic rupture, infection, the formation of scar tissue, and damaged nephrons
   2. There is no known way to arrest the progress of the destructive cysts
   3. The ultimate result of this disease is renal failure
B. Types
   1. Infantile polycystic disease: An inherited autosomal recessive trait that results in the death of the infant within a few months after birth
   2. Adult polycystic disease: An autosomal dominant trait that results in end-stage renal disease
C. Assessment
   1. Flank, lumbar, or abdominal pain
   2. Fever and chills
   3. UTIs
   4. Hematuria, proteinuria, pyuria

5. Calculi
6. Hypertension
7. Palpable abdominal masses and enlarged kidneys
D. Implementation
1. Monitor for gross hematuria, which indicates cyst rupture
2. Increase sodium and water intake because sodium loss rather than retention occurs
3. Provide bed rest if ruptured cysts and bleeding occur
4. Prepare the client for percutaneous cyst puncture for relief of obstruction, or for draining an abscess
5. Prepare the client for dialysis or renal transplantation
6. Encourage the client to seek genetic counseling

XX. UROLITHIASIS AND NEPHROLITHIASIS
A. Description
1. Calculi or stones can form anywhere in the urinary tract; however, the most frequent site is the kidneys
2. The problems that can occur as a result of calculi are pain, obstruction, and tissue trauma, with secondary hemorrhage and infection
3. Kidneys, ureters, and bladder (KUB) film, intravenous pyelogram (IVP), computed tomography (CT) scan, and renal ultrasonography will determine the stone location
4. A stone analysis will be done after passage to determine the type of stone and assist in determining treatment
5. **Urolithiasis** refers to the formation of urinary stones; urinary calculi are formed in the ureters
6. **Nephrolithiasis** refers to the formation of kidney stones; kidney stones are formed in the renal parenchyma
7. When a calculus occludes the ureter and blocks the flow of urine, the ureter dilates, producing a condition known as hydroureter
8. If the obstruction is not removed, urinary stasis results in infection, impairment of renal function on the side of the blockage, and resultant hydronephrosis and irreversible kidney damage
B. Causes
1. Family history of stone formation
2. Diet high in calcium, vitamin D, milk, protein, oxalate, purines, or alkali
3. A high intake of purine-rich food
4. Obstruction and urinary stasis
5. Dehydration
6. Use of diuretics, which can cause volume depletion
7. UTIs and prolonged urinary catheterization
8. Immobilization
9. Hypercalcemia and hyperparathyroidism
10. Elevated uric acid, such as in gout

C. Assessment
1. Renal colic originates in the lumbar region and radiates around the side and down toward the testicle in men, and to the bladder in the women
2. Ureteral colic radiates toward the genitalia and thigh
3. Sharp, severe pain of sudden onset
4. Dull, aching kidney
5. Nausea and vomiting, pallor, and diaphoresis during acute pain
6. Urinary frequency with alternating retention
7. Signs of a UTI
8. Low-grade fever
9. RBCs, WBCs, and bacteria in the urinalysis
10. Hematuria
D. Implementation
1. Monitor vital signs
2. Monitor I & O
3. Assess for fever, chills, and infection
4. Monitor for nausea, vomiting, and diarrhea
5. Force fluids up to 3000 mL/day, unless contraindicated, to facilitate the passage of the stone and prevent infection
6. Strain all urine for the presence of stones
7. Send stones to the laboratory for analysis
8. Provide warm baths and heat to the flank area
9. Administer analgesics at regularly scheduled intervals as prescribed to relieve pain
10. Assess the client's response to pain medication
11. Administer IV fluids as prescribed to increase the flow of urine and facilitate the passage of the stone
12. Assist the client in performing relaxation techniques to assist in relieving pain
13. Instruct the client in the diet specific to the stone composition
14. Maintain urinary pH depending on the type of stone
15. Turn and reposition immobilized clients
16. Prepare the client for surgical procedures if prescribed
E. Stone composition (Boxes 59-8 and 59-9)
1. Calcium phosphate stones
a. Caused by supersaturation of urine with calcium and phosphate
b. Diet includes acid ash foods because calcium stones have an alkaline chemistry
c. Dietary prescription may include to decrease intake of foods high in calcium and phosphate to reduce urinary calcium content, and to avoid excess vitamin D intake to prevent stones from forming
2. Calcium oxalate stones
a. Caused by supersaturation of urine with calcium and oxalate
b. Diet includes acid ash foods because calcium stones have an alkaline chemistry

BOX 59-8

Alkaline Ash Diet

OUTCOME
Increases the pH
Reduces the acidity of the urine

FOODS TO INCLUDE
Milk
Fruits, except cranberries, plums, and prunes
Rhubarb
Most vegetables
Small amounts of beef, halibut, veal, trout, and salmon allowed

BOX 59-9

Acid Ash Diet

OUTCOME
Decreases the pH
Makes the urine more acidic

FOODS TO INCLUDE
Cheese, eggs
Meat, fish, oysters, poultry
Bread, cereal, whole grains
Pastries
Cranberries, prunes, plums, tomatoes
Corn and legumes

c. Dietary prescription may include decreasing intake of foods high in calcium
d. Dietary prescription may include avoiding oxalate food sources to reduce urinary oxalate content and the formation of stones
e. Oxalate-rich food sources include tea, almonds, cashews, chocolate, cocoa, beans, spinach, and rhubarb
3. Struvite stones
a. Also called triple phosphate stones and are composed of magnesium and ammonium phosphate
b. Caused by urea splitting by bacteria
c. Struvite stones tend to form in alkaline urine
d. Diet includes acid ash foods
e. Dietary prescription includes to limit high-phosphate foods such as dairy products, red and organ meats, and whole grains, to reduce urinary phosphate content
4. Uric acid stones
a. Caused by excess dietary purine or gout
b. Uric acid stones tend to form in acidic urine
c. Dietary prescription may include alkaline ash foods and decreased intake of purine sources, such as organ meats, gravies, red wines, and sardines, to reduce urinary purine content

d. Allopurinol (Zyloprim) may be prescribed to lower uric acid levels
5. Cystine stones
a. Caused by cystine crystal formation
b. Cystine stones tend to form in acidic urine
c. Diet includes alkaline ash foods
d. Dietary prescription may also include a low intake of methionine, an essential amino acid that forms cystine, and the client would be instructed to avoid meat, milk, cheese, and eggs
e. Dietary measures also focus on encouraging fluid intake up to 3 liters a day unless contraindicated, to help dilute the urine and prevent cystine crystals from forming

XXI. SURGICAL MANAGEMENT OF KIDNEY STONES

A. Cystoscopy
1. May be done for stones located in the bladder or lower ureter
2. There is no incision
3. One or two ureteral catheters are inserted past the stone
4. The stone may be manipulated and dislodged by the procedure
5. The catheters may mechanically guide the stones downward as they are removed
6. Catheters are left in place for 24 hours to drain the urine trapped proximal to the stone and to dilate the ureter
7. A continuous chemical irrigation may be prescribed to dissolve the stone

B. Extracorporeal shock wave lithotripsy (ESWL)
1. Noninvasive mechanical procedure for breaking up stones that are located in the kidney or upper ureter so that they can pass spontaneously or be removed by other methods
2. Fluoroscopy is used to visualize the stone
3. There is no incision or drains
4. Ultrasonic waves are delivered through a bath of warm water to the areas of the stone to disintegrate it
5. Stones are passed in the urine within a few days
6. Preprocedure: NPO for 8 hours prior to procedure
7. Postprocedure
a. Monitor vital signs
b. Monitor I & O
c. Monitor for bleeding
d. Monitor for pain and signs of urinary obstruction
e. Instruct the client to increase fluid intake to wash out the stone fragments
f. Inform the client that ambulation is important

C. Percutaneous lithotripsy
1. Performed for stones in the bladder, ureter, or kidney

2. An invasive procedure in which a guide is inserted under fluoroscopy near the area of the stone
3. An ultrasonic wave is aimed at the stone to break it into fragments
4. May be performed via cystoscopy or nephroscopy
5. No incision is required for cystoscopy; however a small flank incision is needed for nephroscopy
6. The client may possibly have an indwelling catheter
7. A nephrostomy tube may be placed to administer chemical irrigations to break up the stone; nephrostomy tube may remain in place for 1 to 5 days
▲ 8. Encourage the client to drink 3000 to 4000 mL of fluid per day following the procedure
▲ 9. Monitor for and instruct the client to monitor for complications of infection, hemorrhage, and extravasation of fluid into the retroperitoneal cavity

D. Ureterolithotomy
1. An open surgical procedure, performed if lithotripsy is not effective
2. Performed if the location of the stone is in the ureter
3. Incision into the ureter is made through a lower abdominal or flank incision to remove the stone
4. The client may have a Penrose drain, a ureteral stent catheter, and an indwelling bladder catheter

E. Pyelolithotomy
1. A flank incision into the kidney is made to remove stones from the renal pelvis
2. A large flank incision is required
3. The client will have a Penrose drain and an indwelling catheter

F. Nephrolithotomy
1. Incision into the kidney is made to remove the stone
2. A large flank incision is required
3. The client may have a nephrostomy tube and an indwelling catheter

G. Partial or total nephrectomy
1. Performed if there is extensive kidney damage, renal infection, or severe obstruction, and to prevent stone recurrence
2. Postoperative implementation
   a. The plan of care will be focused based on the incision location and the type of drainage tubes present
   ▲ b. Monitor incision, particularly if a Penrose drain is in place, because it will drain large amounts of urine
   ▲ c. Protect the skin from urinary drainage
   d. Place an ostomy pouch over the Penrose drain to protect the skin if urinary drainage is excessive
   e. Monitor the nephrostomy tube, which may be attached to a drainage bag for a free flow of urine

f. If urethral catheters are in place, do not ▲ irrigate
g. Monitor indwelling Foley catheter for drainage
h. Encourage fluid intake to ensure a urine ▲ output of 2500 to 3000 mL or more per day
i. Monitor I & O closely
j. Determine the composition of stone from laboratory analysis
k. Instruct the client in dietary restrictions if required
l. Instruct the client about medications that may be needed for long term to reduce the development of calculi
m. Medications prescribed for calcium stones may include phosphates, thiazide diuretics, and allopurinol (Zyloprim)
n. Pyridoxine or magnesium oxide may be prescribed for clients with oxalate stones
o. Allopurinol (Zyloprim) may be prescribed for oxalate and uric acid stones
p. Long-term antibiotics may be prescribed for struvite or cystine stones

XXII. KIDNEY TUMORS

A. Description
1. May be benign or malignant, bilateral or unilateral
2. Common sites of metastasis include bone, lungs, liver, spleen, or other kidney
3. The exact cause of renal carcinoma is unknown

B. Assessment
1. Dull flank pain
2. Palpable renal mass
3. Painless gross hematuria

C. Radical nephrectomy
1. Description
   a. Removal of the entire kidney, adjacent adrenal gland, and renal artery and vein
   b. Radiation therapy and possibly chemotherapy may follow radical nephrectomy
2. Postoperative implementation
   a. Monitor vital signs
   b. Monitor abdomen for distention caused by ▲ bleeding
   c. Observe bed linens under the client for ▲ bleeding
   d. Monitor for hypotension, decreases in urinary ▲ output, and alterations in LOC, as indicating signs of hemorrhage
   e. Monitor for signs of adrenal insufficiency
   f. In clients with adrenal insufficiency, a large ▲ urinary output followed by hypotension and subsequent **oliguria** occurs
   g. Administer IV fluids and packed red blood cells as prescribed
   h. Monitor I & O and daily weight
   i. Monitor for a urinary output of 30 to 50 mL ▲ an hour to ensure adequate renal function

j. Monitor urine for specific gravity

k. Maintain semi-Fowler's position

l. Monitor for signs of respiratory complications related to surgery

m. Encourage coughing and deep-breathing exercises

n. Monitor bowel sounds for paralytic ileus

o. Apply antiembolism stockings as prescribed

p. Do not irrigate or manipulate the nephrostomy tube if in place

q. Administer pain medications as prescribed

XXIII. BLADDER TRAUMA

A. Description

1. Occurs following a blunt or penetrating injury to the lower abdomen

2. Penetrating wounds occur as a result of stabbing, gunshot wound, or other objects piercing the abdominal wall

3. A fractured pelvis that causes bone fragments to puncture the bladder is the most common cause of bladder trauma

4. A blunt trauma causes compression of the abdominal wall and the bladder

B. Assessment

1. **Anuria**

2. Hematuria

3. Pain over the costovertebral area (CVA)

4. Nausea and vomiting

C. Implementation

1. Monitor vital signs

2. Monitor for hematuria, hemorrhage, and signs of shock

3. Promote bed rest

4. Monitor pain level

5. Prepare the client for insertion of a suprapubic catheter to aid in urinary drainage if prescribed

6. Prepare the client for surgical repair of the laceration if prescribed

XXIV. EPIDIDYMITIS

A. Description

1. An acute or chronic inflammation of the epididymis that occurs as a result of a UTI, an STD, prostatitis, or long-term use of a Foley catheter

2. The infective organism passes upward through the urethra and ejaculatory duct, along the vas deferens to the epididymis

B. Assessment

1. Scrotal pain

2. Groin pain

3. Swelling in scrotum and groin

4. Pus and bacteria in the urine

5. Fever and chills

6. Abscess development

C. Implementation

1. Encourage fluid intake

2. Encourage bed rest with the scrotum elevated to prevent traction on the spermatic cord, to facilitate drainage, and to relieve pain

3. Instruct the client in the intermittent application of cold compresses to scrotum

4. Instruct the client in the use of sitz baths

5. Instruct the client in the administration of antibiotics for self and sexual partner if chlamydial or gonorrheal infection is the cause

6. Instruct the client to avoid lifting, straining, and sexual contact until the infection subsides

XXV. PROSTATITIS

A. Description

1. An inflammation of the prostate gland, which can be caused by an infectious agent (bacterial) or by tissue hyperplasia (abacterial)

2. Bacterial type occurs as a result of the organism reaching the prostate via the urethra or the bloodstream

3. Abacterial type usually occurs following a viral illness or a decrease in sexual activity

B. Assessment

1. Bacterial

a. Fever and chills

b. Dysuria

c. Urethral discharge

d. Boggy, tender prostate

e. Urethral discharge on palpation of prostate

f. WBCs found in prostatic secretions

2. Abacterial

a. Backache

b. Dysuria

c. Perineal pain

d. Frequency

e. Hematuria

f. Irregularly enlarged, firm, and tender prostate

C. Implementation

1. Encourage adequate fluid intake

2. Instruct the client in the use of sitz baths to promote comfort

3. Administer antibiotics, analgesics, antispasmodics, and stool softeners as prescribed

4. Inform the client of activities to drain the prostate, such as intercourse, masturbation, and prostatic massage

5. Instruct the client to avoid spicy foods, coffee, alcohol, prolonged automobile rides, and sexual intercourse during an acute inflammation

XXVI. BENIGN PROSTATIC HYPERTROPHY OR HYPERPLASIA (BPH)

A. Description

1. A slow enlargement of the prostate gland, with hypertrophy and hyperplasia of normal tissue

2. The enlargement causes narrowing of the urethra and results in partial or complete obstruction

3. The cause is unknown, and the disorder usually occurs in men older than 50 years

---

BOX 59-10

Surgical Interventions for BPH

Transurethral resection (TUR)
Retropubic prostatectomy
Suprapubic prostatectomy
Perineal prostatectomy

B. Assessment
   1. Urgency, frequency, and hesitancy
   2. Changes in size and force of urinary stream
   3. Retention
   4. Dribbling
   5. Nocturia
   6. Hematuria
   7. Urinary stasis
   8. UTIs
C. Implementation
   1. Encourage fluids of up to 2000 to 3000 mL per day unless contraindicated
   2. Prepare for bladder drainage via urinary catheterization for distention
   3. Avoid administering medications that cause urinary retention, such as anticholinergics, antihistamines, and decongestants
   4. Administer finasteride (Proscar) as prescribed to shrink the prostate gland and improve urine flow
   5. Prepare the client for surgery as prescribed (Box 59-10)
D. Surgical implementation and postoperative care (Refer to Chapter 49)

XXVII. KIDNEY TRANSPLANTATION
A. Description
   1. Implantation of a human kidney from a compatible donor into a recipient
   2. Performed for irreversible kidney failure
   3. Immunosuppressive medications must be taken by the recipient for life
B. Living related donors
   1. Most desirable source of kidneys for transplant is living related donors who match the client closely
   2. Screened for ABO blood group, tissue-specific antigen, human leukocyte antigen (HLA) suitability, and mixed lymphocyte culture index (histocompatibility)
   3. Donor must be in excellent health with two properly functioning kidneys
   4. The emotional well-being of the donor is determined
   5. Complete understanding of the donation process and outcome is necessary
C. Cadaver donors
   1. Must meet criteria of brain death
   2. Must be under 60 years of age

   3. Must have normal renal function
   4. No malignant disease outside of the central nervous system (CNS) can be present
   5. No generalized infection can be present
   6. No abdominal or renal trauma can be present
   7. Potential donor must have a negative hepatitis B antigen and negative HIV antibody
   8. Continuous ventilation and heartbeat are maintained until the kidneys are surgically removed
   9. Normal BP must be present
   10. Once the potential donor has demonstrated cerebral death, it is crucial to restore intravascular volume, wean from vasopressors, and establish diuresis
D. Warm ischemic time
   1. The time elapsed between the cessation of perfusion and cooling of the kidney, and the time required for anastomosis of the kidney
   2. Maximal allowable warm ischemic time is 30 to 60 minutes
   3. Kidney can be cooled, and then the maximum time for transplantation is increased to 24 to 48 hours
E. Preoperative implementation
   1. Verify histocompatibility tests of identical twin or family member
   2. Administer immunosuppressive medications to recipient as prescribed, for 2 days before the transplantation, if this is possible
   3. Maintain protective isolation
   4. Verify that **hemodialysis** of the recipient was completed 24 hours before the transplant
   5. Ensure that the client is free of any infections
   6. Assess renal function studies
   7. Encourage discussion of feelings of both the donor and the recipient
F. Postoperative implementation
   1. Kidney begins to function immediately, or it may be delayed a few days
   2. **Hemodialysis** is performed until adequate kidney function is established
   3. Monitor vital signs
   4. Monitor I & O
   5. Monitor urine output every hour
   6. Monitor daily laboratory studies, urine for blood and specific gravity, daily weight, pulse oximetry, and BUN and creatinine levels
   7. Maintain the client in semi-Fowler's position
   8. Monitor for patency of the Foley catheter
   9. Note that urine is pink and bloody initially but gradually returns to normal within several days to weeks
   10. Monitor for gross hematuria and clots, which are not expected, and notify the physician if they occur
   11. Monitor the three-way bladder irrigation if prescribed, to prevent blood clot formation

12. Note that the Foley catheter should be removed as soon as possible to prevent infection
13. Maintain protective isolation precautions and monitor for infection
14. Monitor IV fluids closely and for fluid overload
15. Begin oral fluids as prescribed
16. Monitor for bowel sounds and initiate diet as prescribed when bowel sounds return
17. Maintain good oral hygiene, monitoring for stomatitis and bacterial and fungal infections
18. Encourage coughing and deep-breathing exercises
19. Maintain strict aseptic technique with wound care
20. Administer medications as prescribed, which may include antifungal medications, antibiotics, immunosuppressive agents, and corticosteroids
21. Assess for organ rejection
22. Promote live donor and recipient relationship
23. Monitor client and recipient for depression

G. Graft rejection: Except for identical twin donor and recipient, the major postoperative complication is graft rejection
   1. Assessment
      a. Fever
      b. Malaise
      c. Elevated WBC count
      d. Graft tenderness
      e. Signs of deteriorating renal function
      f. Acute hypertension
      g. Anemia
   2. Hyperacute rejection
      a. Occurs immediately after surgery to 48 hours postoperatively
      b. Implementation: Removal of rejected kidney
   3. Acute rejection
      a. Occurs within 6 weeks but can occur as late as 2 years
      b. Potentially reversible with increased immunosuppression
      c. Implementation: High doses of corticosteroids; if corticosterois are ineffective, monoclonal antibodies may be administered

4. Chronic rejection
   a. Occurs slowly months to years after transplant
   b. Can be irreversible
   c. Mimics **CRF**
   d. Implementation: Immunosuppressive medications
5. Client instructions following kidney transplant (Box 59-11)

PRACTICE QUESTIONS

1. A nurse is caring for a client who has had a renal biopsy. Which of the following interventions would the nurse avoid in the care of the client after this procedure?
   1. Forcing fluids to at least 3 liters in the first 24 hours
   2. Administering PRN narcotics
   3. Testing serial samples with dipsticks for occult blood
   4. Ambulating the client in the room and hall for short distances

2. A client with urolithiasis has a history of chronic urinary tract infections (UTIs). A nurse concludes that this client most likely has which of the following types of urinary stones?
   1. Calcium oxalate
   2. Uric acid
   3. Struvite
   4. Cystine

3. A client who has a history of gout is also diagnosed with urolithiasis. The stones are determined to be of uric acid type. A nurse gives the client instructions in foods to limit, which include:
   1. Liver
   2. Apples
   3. Carrots
   4. Milk

4. A nurse is receiving in transfer from the postanesthesia care unit a client who has had percutaneous ultrasonic lithotripsy for calculi in the renal pelvis. The nurse anticipates that the client's care will involve monitoring which of the following?
   1. Suprapubic tube
   2. Ureteral stent
   3. Nephrostomy tube
   4. Jackson-Pratt drain

5. A client arrives at an emergency department with complaints of low abdominal pain and hematuria. The client is afebrile. A nurse next assesses the client to determine a history of:
   1. Renal cancer in the client's family
   2. Blow or trauma to the bladder or abdomen
   3. Glomerulonephritis
   4. Pyelonephritis

6. A client is admitted to an emergency department

following a motor vehicle accident. The client was wearing a lap seat belt when the accident occurred. The client has hematuria and lower abdominal pain. To further determine whether the pain is due to bladder trauma, a nurse asks the client if the pain is referred to which of the following areas?
1. Shoulder
2. Umbilicus
3. Costovertebral angle
4. Hip

7. A female client is admitted to an emergency department following a fall from a horse. A physician orders insertion of a Foley catheter. A nurse notes blood at the urinary meatus while preparing for the procedure. The nurse should:
1. Use extra povidone-iodine solution in cleansing the meatus
2. Use a smaller-size catheter
3. Administer pain medication before inserting the catheter
4. Notify the physician

8. A client is admitted with a suspicion of bladder cancer. A nurse assesses the client for which of the following earliest manifestations of the disease?
1. Hematuria with no pain
2. Painful urination and hematuria
3. Pyuria and palpable abdominal mass
4. Proteinuria and dysuria

9. A male client has a tentative diagnosis of urethritis. A nurse assesses the client for which of the following manifestations of the disorder?
1. Hematuria and penile discharge
2. Hematuria and pyuria
3. Dysuria and proteinuria
4. Dysuria and penile discharge

10. A nurse is planning a teaching session with a female client diagnosed with urethritis resulting from infection with chlamydia. The nurse would plan to include which of the following points in the teaching session?
1. The most serious complication of this infection is sterility
2. The infection can be prevented by using spermicide to alter the pH in the perineal area
3. Medication therapy should be continued for 2 weeks without interruption
4. Sexual partners during the last 12 months should be notified and treated

11. A client with chlamydial infection has received instructions on self-care and prevention of further infection. A nurse evaluates that the client needs further reinforcement if the client states to:
1. Reduce the chance of reinfection by limiting the number of sexual partners
2. Use latex condoms to prevent disease transmission

3. Return to the clinic as requested for follow-up culture in 1 week
4. Use doxycycline prophylactically to prevent symptoms of chlamydia

12. A nurse is assessing a client with epididymitis. The nurse anticipates which of the following findings on physical examination?
1. Fever, diarrhea, groin pain, and ecchymosis
2. Fever, nausea and vomiting, and painful scrotal edema
3. Diarrhea, groin pain, and scrotal edema
4. Nausea and vomiting, and scrotal edema with ecchymosis

13. A client has epididymitis as a complication of urinary tract infection. A nurse is giving the client instructions to prevent a recurrence. The nurse would evaluate that the client needs further instruction if the client states to:
1. Drink increased amounts of fluids
2. Continue to take antibiotics until all symptoms are gone
3. Limit the force of the stream during voiding
4. Use condoms to eliminate contracting chlamydia and gonorrhea

14. A client complains of fever, perineal pain, urinary urgency and frequency, and dysuria. To assess whether the client's problem is related to prostatitis, the nurse would look at the results of the prostate examination, which should reveal that the prostate gland is:
1. Tender, indurated, and warm to the touch
2. Boggy, swollen, and warm to the touch
3. Tender and edematous with ecchymosis
4. Reddened, swollen, and boggy

15. A nurse is taking the history of a client who has had benign prostatic hyperplasia (BPH) in the past. To determine if the client is currently experiencing difficulty, the nurse asks the client about the presence of which of the following early symptoms?
1. Urge incontinence
2. Nocturia
3. Decreased force in the stream of urine
4. Urinary retention

16. A client who has a cold is seen in the emergency room with inability to void. Since the client has a history of benign prostatic hyperplasia (BPH), a nurse determines that the client should be questioned about the use of which of the following medications?
1. Diuretics
2. Antibiotics
3. Antitussives
4. Decongestants

17. A client with chronic renal failure (CRF) is at risk for developing dementia related to excessive absorption of aluminum. A nurse teaches the client that

this is the reason that the client is being prescribed which of the following phosphate-binding agents?

1. Alu-Cap
2. Tums
3. Amphojel
4. Basaljel

18. A client newly diagnosed with chronic renal failure has recently begun hemodialysis. Knowing that the client is at risk for disequilibrium syndrome, during dialysis a nurse assesses the client for:
   1. Hypertension, tachycardia, and fever
   2. Hypotension, bradycardia, and hypothermia
   3. Restlessness, irritability, and generalized weakness
   4. Headache, deteriorating level of consciousness, and twitching

19. A client with chronic renal failure has completed a hemodialysis treatment. A nurse would use which of the following standard indicators to evaluate the client's status after dialysis?
   1. Potassium level and weight
   2. Blood urea nitrogen (BUN) and creatinine levels
   3. Vital signs and BUN
   4. Vital signs and weight

20. A hemodialysis client with a left arm fistula is at risk for steal syndrome. A nurse assesses this client for which of the following manifestations?
   1. Warmth, redness, and pain in the left hand
   2. Pallor, diminished pulse, and pain in the left hand
   3. Edema and purplish discoloration of the left arm
   4. Aching pain, pallor, and edema of the left arm

21. A nurse is reviewing a client's record and notes that the physician has documented that the client has a renal disorder. On review of the laboratory results, the nurse would most likely expect to note which of the following?
   1. Elevated blood urea nitrogen (BUN)
   2. Decreased hemoglobin
   3. Decreased red blood cell (RBC) count
   4. Decreased white blood cell (WBC) count

22. A nurse is preparing to care for a client after a renal scan. Which of the following would the nurse include in the plan of care?
   1. Place the client on radiation precautions for 18 hours
   2. Save all urine in a radiation-safe container for 18 hours
   3. Limit contact with the client to 20 minutes per hour
   4. No special precautions except to wear gloves if in contact with the client's urine

23. A client is scheduled for an intravenous pyelogram (IVP). Before the test, the priority nursing action would be to:
   1. Administer an oral preparation of radiopaque dye
   2. Restrict fluids
   3. Determine a history of allergies
   4. Administer a sedative

24. Following a renal biopsy, a client complains of pain at the biopsy site that radiates to the front of the abdomen. A nurse interprets this complaint and further assesses the client for:
   1. Bleeding
   2. Infection
   3. Renal colic
   4. A normal expected pain

25. A client is admitted to the hospital and has a diagnosis of early-stage chronic renal failure (CRF). Which of the following would a nurse expect to note on assessment of the client?
   1. Polyuria
   2. Polydypsia
   3. Oliguria
   4. Anuria

26. A client with chronic renal failure (CRF) returns to the nursing unit following a hemodialysis treatment. On assessment, a nurse notes that the client's temperature is 100.2° F. Which of the following is the most appropriate nursing action?
   1. Encourage fluids
   2. Notify the physician
   3. Monitor the site of the shunt for infection
   4. Continue to monitor vital signs

27. A nurse is performing an assessment on a client who has returned from the dialysis unit following hemodialysis. The client is complaining of a headache and nausea and is extremely restless. Which of the following is the most appropriate nursing action?
   1. Notify the physician
   2. Monitor the client
   3. Elevate the head of the bed
   4. Medicate the client for nausea

28. A nurse is assisting a client on a low-potassium diet to select food items from the menu. Which of the following food items, if selected by the client, would indicate an understanding of this dietary restriction?
   1. Cantaloupe
   2. Spinach
   3. Lima beans
   4. Strawberries

29. A nurse is reviewing the list of components of the peritoneal dialysis solution with a client. The client asks the nurse about the purpose of the glucose contained in the solution. The nurse bases the response on knowledge that the glucose:
   1. Prevents excess glucose from being removed from the client
   2. Decreases the risk of peritonitis
   3. Prevents disequilibrium syndrome

4. Increases osmotic pressure to produce ultra-filtration

30. A nurse is preparing to care for a client receiving peritoneal dialysis. Which of the following would be included in the nursing plan of care to prevent the major complication associated with peritoneal dialysis?
    1. Monitor the client's level of consciousness
    2. Maintain strict aseptic technique
    3. Add heparin to the dialysate solution
    4. Change the catheter site dressing daily

31. A client newly diagnosed with renal failure will be receiving peritoneal dialysis. During the infusion of the dialysate the client complains of abdominal pain. Which action by the nurse is most appropriate?
    1. Slow the infusion
    2. Decrease the amount to be infused
    3. Explain that the pain will subside after the first few exchanges
    4. Stop the dialysis

32. A nurse is instructing a client with diabetes mellitus about peritoneal dialysis. The nurse tells the client that it is important to maintain the dwell time for the dialysis at the prescribed time because of the risk of:
    1. Infection
    2. Hyperglycemia
    3. Fluid overload
    4. Disequilibrium syndrome

33. A nurse is caring for an 88-year-old woman suspected of having a urinary tract infection (UTI). Which of the following, if noted in the client, would alert the nurse to the possibility of the presence of a UTI?
    1. Fever
    2. Frequency
    3. Confusion
    4. Urgency

34. A client passes a urinary stone, and laboratory analysis of the stone indicates that it is composed of calcium oxalate. On the basis of this analysis, which of the following would the nurse include in the dietary instructions?
    1. Increase intake of meat, fish, plums, and cranberries
    2. Avoid citrus fruits and citrus juices
    3. Avoid green leafy vegetables, such as spinach
    4. Increase intake of dairy products

35. A client returns to the nursing unit following a pyelolithotomy for removal of a kidney stone. A Penrose drain is in place. Which of the following would a nurse include in the client's postoperative plan of care?
    1. Sterile irrigation of the Penrose drain
    2. Frequent dressing changes around the Penrose drain

    3. Weighing dressings
    4. Maintaining the client's position on the affected side

36. A nurse is caring for a client following a kidney transplant. The client develops oliguria. Which of the following would the nurse anticipate to be prescribed as the treatment for the oliguria?
    1. Forcing fluids
    2. Administration of diuretics
    3. Irrigation of the Foley catheter
    4. Restricting fluids

37. A week after kidney transplantation, a client develops a fever of 101° F, the blood pressure is elevated, and the kidney is tender. The x-ray results indicate that the transplanted kidney is enlarged. On the basis of these assessment findings, a nurse would suspect which of the following?
    1. Acute rejection
    2. Chronic rejection
    3. Kidney infection
    4. Kidney obstruction

38. A client with benign prostatic hyperplasia (BPH) undergoes a transurethral resection of the prostate (TURP). Postoperatively, the client is receiving continuous bladder irrigations. A nurse assesses the client for signs of transurethral resection (TUR) syndrome. Which of the following assessment data would indicate the onset of this syndrome?
    1. Bradycardia and confusion
    2. Tachycardia and diarrhea
    3. Decreased urinary output and bladder spasms
    4. Increased urinary output and anemia

39. A client is admitted to the hospital with a diagnosis of benign prostatic hyperplasia, and a transurethral resection of the prostate (TURP) is performed. Four hours after surgery, a nurse takes the client's vital signs and empties the urinary drainage bag. Which of the following assessment findings would indicate the need to notify the physician?
    1. Red bloody urine
    2. Urinary output of 200 mL greater than intake
    3. Blood pressure of 100/50 mm Hg, pulse of 130 beats per minute
    4. Pain related to bladder spasms

40. A client is diagnosed with polycystic kidney disease. Which of the following would the nurse not expect to be a component of the treatment plan?
    1. Sodium restriction
    2. Antihypertensive medications
    3. Increased water intake
    4. Genetic counseling

41. A nurse is caring for a client who has undergone renal angiography using the left femoral artery for access. The nurse evaluates that the client is experiencing a complication of the procedure if which of the following observations is made?
    1. Urine output of 50 mL/hr

2. Absence of hematoma in the left groin
3. Blood pressure of 110/74 mm Hg
4. Pallor and coolness of the left leg

42. A nurse has given a client with polycystic kidney disease information about management of the disorder, and prevention and recognition of complications. The nurse determines that the client understands the instructions if the client states that there is no reason to be concerned about:
    1. A lowered blood pressure
    2. Onset of shortness of breath
    3. A fever
    4. Burning on urination

43. A client with prostatitis secondary to kidney infection has received instructions on management of the condition at home and prevention of recurrence. A nurse evaluates that the client understood the instructions if the client verbalized the intention to:
    1. Keep fluid intake to a minimum to decrease the need to void
    2. Exercise as much as possible to stimulate circulation
    3. Stop antibiotic therapy when pain subsides
    4. Use warm sitz baths and analgesics to increase comfort

44. A client with a crush injury to the right lower leg develops acute renal failure (ARF). A nurse interprets that this type of renal failure is due to:
    1. Prerenal causes
    2. Renal causes
    3. Postrenal causes
    4. Extrarenal causes

45. A client with acute renal failure has a serum potassium (K) level of 5.8 mEq/L. A nurse would plan which of the following as a priority action?
    1. Allow an extra 500 mL fluid intake to dilute the electrolyte concentration
    2. Encourage increased vegetables in the diet
    3. Place the client on a cardiac monitor
    4. Check the sodium level

46. A client with chronic renal failure who is scheduled for hemodialysis this morning is due to receive a daily dose of enalapril (Vasotec). A nurse should plan to administer this medication:
    1. Just prior to dialysis
    2. During dialysis
    3. Upon return from dialysis
    4. The day after dialysis

47. A client with chronic renal failure has an indwelling catheter for peritoneal dialysis in the abdomen. The client spills water on the dressing while bathing. A nurse should plan to immediately:
    1. Reinforce the dressing
    2. Change the dressing
    3. Flush the peritoneal dialysis catheter
    4. Scrub the catheter with povidone-iodine

48. A client being hemodialyzed becomes suddenly short of breath and complains of chest pain. The client is tachycardic, pale, and anxious. A nurse suspects air embolism. The nurse should:
    1. Continue dialysis at a slower rate after checking the lines for air
    2. Discontinue dialysis and notify the physician
    3. Monitor vital signs every 15 minutes for the next hour
    4. Bolus the client with 500 mL normal saline to break up the air embolus

49. A nurse has completed client teaching with a hemodialysis client about self-monitoring between hemodialysis treatments. The nurse evaluates that the client best understands the information given if the client states to record on a daily basis:
    1. Pulse, respiratory rate
    2. Intake and output, weight
    3. Blood urea nitrogen and creatinine levels
    4. Activity log

50. A client with an arteriovenous (AV) shunt in place for hemodialysis is at risk for bleeding. A nurse would do which of the following as a priority action to prevent this complication from occurring?
    1. Check the results of the prothrombin time as they are ordered
    2. Observe the site once per shift
    3. Check the shunt for presence of bruit and thrill
    4. Ensure that small clamps are attached to the AV shunt dressing

CRITICAL THINKING: FREE-TEXT ENTRY

A nurse is monitoring a client receiving peritoneal dialysis. The nurse notes that the client's outflow is less than the inflow. Which nursing action is most appropriate initially?

Answer: _____

ANSWERS

1. **4**

Rationale: After renal biopsy, the nurse ensures that the client remains in bed for at least 24 hours. Vital signs and puncture site assessments are done frequently during this time. Forcing fluids is done to reduce possible clot formation at the biopsy site. Serial urine samples are hematested with urine dipsticks to evaluate bleeding. Narcotic analgesics are often needed to manage the renal colic pain that some clients feel after this procedure.

Test-Taking Strategy: Use the process of elimination. Note the key word "avoid." Eliminate options 2 and 3 by recalling that pain and bleeding are potential concerns after this procedure. From the remaining options recall that forcing fluids will reduce clotting at the site, while ambulation could initiate or enhance bleeding at the biopsy site. Review postprocedure care if you had difficulty with this question.

Level of Cognitive Ability: Application
Client Needs: Physiological Integrity
Integrated Concept/Process: Nursing Process/Implementation
Content Area: Adult Health/Renal
Reference: Ignatavicius, D., Workman, M., & Mishler, M. (1999). *Medical-surgical nursing across the health care continuum* (3rd ed.). Philadelphia: W.B. Saunders, pp. 1814-1815.

2. 3
Rationale: Struvite stones are commonly referred to as infection stones, because they form in urine that is alkaline and rich in ammonia, such as with UTI. Calcium oxalate stones result from increased calcium intake or conditions that raise serum calcium concentrations. Uric acid stones occur in clients with gout. Cystine stones are rare, and occur in clients with a genetic defect that results in decreased renal absorption of the amino acid cystine.
Test-Taking Strategy: Use the process of elimination. Focus on the data in the question. Noting that the client has a history of chronic urinary tract infections will direct you to option 3. Review the causes of the various types of stones if you had difficulty with this question.
Level of Cognitive Ability: Analysis
Client Needs: Physiological Integrity
Integrated Concept/Process: Nursing Process/Analysis
Content Area: Adult Health/Renal
Reference: Smeltzer, S., & Bare, B. (2000). *Brunner & Suddarth's textbook of medical-surgical nursing* (9th ed.). Philadelphia: Lippincott Williams & Wilkins, p. 1164.

3. 1
Rationale: Foods containing high amounts of purines should be avoided in the client with uric acid stones. This includes limiting or avoiding organ meats, such as liver, brain, heart, kidney, and sweetbreads. Other foods to avoid include herring, sardines, anchovies, meat extracts, consommés, and gravies. Foods that are low in purines include all fruits, many vegetables, milk, cheese, eggs, refined cereals, sugars and sweets, coffee, tea, chocolate, and carbonated beverages.
Test-Taking Strategy: Use the process of elimination. Begin by examining the options and classifying the types of food sources they represent. Options 2 and 3 represent foods that are grown, while options 1 and 4 represent foods that derive from animal sources. Since purines are end products of protein metabolism, you would eliminate options 2 and 3 first. From the remaining options, recall that organ meats such as liver provide a greater quantity of protein than milk. Review foods high in purines if you had difficulty with this question.
Level of Cognitive Ability: Application
Client Needs: Health Promotion and Maintenance
Integrated Concept/Process: Teaching/Learning
Content Area: Adult Health/Renal
References: Smeltzer, S., & Bare, B. (2000). *Brunner & Suddarth's textbook of medical-surgical nursing* (9th ed.). Philadelphia: Lippincott Williams & Wilkins, p. 1164.

4. 3
Rationale: A nephrostomy tube is put in place after percutaneous ultrasonic lithotripsy to treat calculi in the renal pelvis.

The client may also have a Foley catheter to drain urine produced by the other kidney. The nurse monitors the drainage from each of these tubes, and strains the urine to detect elimination of the calculus fragments.
Test-Taking Strategy: Use the process of elimination. Note that the question states that the calculi are in the renal pelvis. This will direct you to option 3. Review care to the client following this procedure if you had difficulty with this question.
Level of Cognitive Ability: Analysis
Client Needs: Physiological Integrity
Integrated Concept/Process: Nursing Process/Assessment
Content Area: Adult Health/Renal
Reference: Smeltzer, S., & Bare, B. (2000). *Brunner & Suddarth's textbook of medical-surgical nursing* (9th ed.). Philadelphia: Lippincott Williams & Wilkins, p. 1126.

5. 2
Rationale: Bladder trauma or injury should be considered or suspected in the client with low abdominal pain and hematuria. Renal cancer would not cause pain that is felt in the low abdomen; rather it would be in the flank area. Glomerulonephritis and pyelonephritis would be accompanied by fever, and are thus not applicable to the client in this question.
Test-Taking Strategy: Use the process of elimination. Eliminate options 3 and 4, knowing that any inflammatory disease or infection is accompanied by fever. Since this client is afebrile, these are not possible options. Use knowledge of anatomy and pain assessment to select option 2. Pain from renal cancer is a later finding, and is localized in the flank area. Review renal assessment techniques if you had difficulty with this question.
Level of Cognitive Ability: Application
Client Needs: Physiological Integrity
Integrated Concept/Process: Nursing Process/Assessment
Content Area: Adult Health/Renal
Reference: Smeltzer, S., & Bare, B. (2000). *Brunner & Suddarth's textbook of medical-surgical nursing* (9th ed.). Philadelphia: Lippincott Williams & Wilkins, p. 1168.

6. 1
Rationale: Bladder trauma or injury is characterized by lower abdominal pain that may radiate to one of the shoulders. Bladder injury pain does not radiate to the umbilicus, costovertebral angle, or hip.
Test-Taking Strategy: Use the process of elimination. Recall the concepts related to dermatomes of the body, and pain characteristics of bladder trauma. Review the characteristics of bladder trauma if you had difficulty with this question.
Level of Cognitive Ability: Analysis
Client Needs: Physiological Integrity
Integrated Concept/Process: Nursing Process/Assessment
Content Area: Adult Health/Renal
Reference: Smeltzer, S., & Bare, B. (2000). *Brunner & Suddarth's textbook of medical-surgical nursing* (9th ed.). Philadelphia: Lippincott Williams & Wilkins, p. 1168.

7. 4
Rationale: The presence of blood at the urinary meatus may indicate urethral trauma or disruption. The nurse notifies the physician, knowing that the client should not be catheterized until the cause of the bleeding is determined by diagnostic testing.
Test-Taking Strategy: Use the process of elimination. Noting the key words "blood at the urinary meatus" will direct you to option 4. Review the assessment findings in a client with

trauma to the urinary tract if you had difficulty with this question.

Level of Cognitive Ability: Application
Client Needs: Physiological Integrity
Integrated Concept/Process: Nursing Process/Implementation
Content Area: Adult Health/Renal
Reference: Smeltzer, S., & Bare, B. (2000). *Brunner & Suddarth's textbook of medical-surgical nursing* (9th ed.). Philadelphia: Lippincott Williams & Wilkins, p. 1168.

8. **1**
Rationale: The most common earliest manifestation of bladder cancer is hematuria that is not accompanied by pain. The hematuria is intermittent at first. Later symptoms include hematuria with dysuria and frequency resulting from bladder irritation. Pyuria and proteinuria are not part of the clinical picture. A mass is usually not palpable.
Test-Taking Strategy: Use the process of elimination. Note the key word "earliest." Eliminate option 3 first. Since this is not an infectious process, the client should not have pyuria. Knowing that pain and discomfort are later signs helps you to eliminate options 2 and 4 next. Review the early manifestations of bladder cancer if you had difficulty with this question.
Level of Cognitive Ability: Analysis
Client Needs: Physiological Integrity
Integrated Concept/Process: Nursing Process/Assessment
Content Area: Adult Health/Renal
Reference: Smeltzer, S., & Bare, B. (2000). *Brunner & Suddarth's textbook of medical-surgical nursing* (9th ed.). Philadelphia: Lippincott Williams & Wilkins, p. 1171.

9. **4**
Rationale: Urethritis in the male client often results from chlamydial infection, and is characterized by dysuria, which is accompanied by a clear to mucopurulent discharge. Because this disorder often coexists with gonorrhea, diagnostic tests are done for both, and include culture and rapid assays.
Test-Taking Strategy: Use the process of elimination. Recalling that urethritis is generally accompanied by dysuria in the male client will assist in eliminating options 1 and 2. Knowing that the problem originates in the urethra, not the kidney, will assist in eliminating option 3 because proteinuria indicates a problem with kidney function. Review the clinical manifestations of urethritis if you had difficulty with this question.
Level of Cognitive Ability: Application
Client Needs: Physiological Integrity
Integrated Concept/Process: Nursing Process/Assessment
Content Area: Adult Health/Renal
Reference: Ignatavicius, D., Workman, M., & Mishler, M. (1999). *Medical-surgical nursing across the health care continuum* (3rd ed.). Philadelphia: W.B. Saunders, p. 1826.

10. **1**
Rationale: The most serious complication of chlamydial infection is sterility. The infection can be prevented by the use of latex condoms. It is treated with doxycycline for 7 days, or with azithromycin (Zithromax) as a single dose. All sexual partners during the 30 days before diagnosis should be notified, examined, and treated as necessary.
Test-Taking Strategy: Use the process of elimination. Eliminate option 2 first, using principles of infection control. Knowing that most courses of antibiotic therapy extend from 7 to 10 days in general may help to eliminate option 3. From the

remaining options, it is necessary to know either that sterility is a serious and permanent complication or that partners within the last month should be notified and treated as needed. Review the teaching points for the client with chlamydia if you had difficulty with this question.
Level of Cognitive Ability: Application
Client Needs: Physiological Integrity
Integrated Concept/Process: Teaching/Learning
Content Area: Adult Health/Renal
Reference: Smeltzer, S., & Bare, B. (2000). *Brunner & Suddarth's textbook of medical-surgical nursing* (9th ed.). Philadelphia: Lippincott Williams & Wilkins, pp. 1888-1889.

11. **4**
Rationale: Antibiotics are not taken prophylactically to prevent acquisition of urethritis from chlamydia. The risk of reinfection can be reduced by limiting the number of sexual partners and by the use of condoms. In some instances, follow-up culture is requested in 4 to 7 days to confirm a cure.
Test-Taking Strategy: Use the process of elimination. Note the key words "needs further reinforcement." Knowing the basic principles of antibiotic therapy will direct you to option 4, since antibiotics are not used intermittently at will for prophylaxis of this infection. Review client teaching related to chlamydial infection if you had difficulty with this question.
Level of Cognitive Ability: Analysis
Client Needs: Health Promotion and Maintenance
Integrated Concept/Process: Teaching/Learning
Content Area: Adult Health/Renal
Reference: Smeltzer, S., & Bare, B. (2000). *Brunner & Suddarth's textbook of medical-surgical nursing* (9th ed.). Philadelphia: Lippincott Williams & Wilkins, p. 1889.

12. **2**
Rationale: Typical signs and symptoms of epididymitis include scrotal pain and edema, which are often accompanied by fever, nausea and vomiting, and chills. It is most often caused by infection, although sometimes it can be caused by trauma. It needs to be correctly distinguished from testicular torsion.
Test-Taking Strategy: Use the process of elimination. Any disorder that ends in "itis" results from inflammation or infection. Therefore, an expected finding would be elevated temperature. With this in mind, eliminate options 3 and 4, since they do not contain fever as part of the option. Knowing that ecchymosis results from bleeding, which is not part of this clinical picture, directs you to option 2. Review the clinical manifestations of epididymitis if you had difficulty with this question.
Level of Cognitive Ability: Analysis
Client Needs: Physiological Integrity
Integrated Concept/Process: Nursing Process/Assessment
Content Area: Adult Health/Renal
Reference: Ignatavicius, D., Workman, M., & Mishler, M. (1999). *Medical-surgical nursing across the health care continuum* (3rd ed.). Philadelphia: W.B. Saunders, p. 2047.

13. **2**
Rationale: The client who experiences epididymitis from urinary tract infection should increase intake of fluids to flush the urinary system. Since organisms can be forced into the vas deferens and epididymis from strain or pressure during voiding, the client should limit the force of the stream. Condom use can help to prevent urethritis and epididymitis.

Antibiotics are always taken until the full course of therapy is completed.

Test-Taking Strategy: Use the process of elimination. Note the key words "needs further instruction." Careful reading will direct you to option 2. Remember, antibiotics are not stopped when symptoms subside and must be taken until the full course of therapy is completed. Review client instructions regarding epididymitis if you had difficulty with this question.

Level of Cognitive Ability: Analysis

Client Needs: Health Promotion and Maintenance

Integrated Concept/Process: Teaching/Learning

Content Area: Adult Health/Renal

Reference: Ignatavicius, D., Workman, M., & Mishler, M. (1999). *Medical-surgical nursing across the health care continuum* (3rd ed.). Philadelphia: W.B. Saunders, p. 2047.

14. **1**

Rationale: The client with prostatitis has a prostate gland that is swollen and tender, but which is also warm to the touch, firm, and indurated. Systemic symptoms include fever with chills, perineal and low back pain, and signs of urinary tract infection (which often accompany the disorder).

Test-Taking Strategy: Use the process of elimination. Begin to answer this question by reasoning that inflammation of the prostate gland would cause the area to be tender. This would allow you to eliminate options 2 and 4. Recalling that inflammation is accompanied by local warmth will direct you to option 1. Review the signs of prostatitis if you had difficulty with this question.

Level of Cognitive Ability: Analysis

Client Needs: Physiological Integrity

Integrated Concept/Process: Nursing Process/Assessment

Content Area: Adult Health/Renal

Reference: Ignatavicius, D., Workman, M., & Mishler, M. (1999). *Medical-surgical nursing across the health care continuum* (3rd ed.). Philadelphia: W.B. Saunders, p. 2047.

15. **3**

Rationale: Decreased force in the stream of urine is an early sign of BPH. The stream later becomes weak and dribbling. The client may then develop hematuria, frequency, urgency, urge incontinence, and nocturia. If BPH is untreated, complete obstruction and urinary retention can occur.

Test-Taking Strategy: Use the process of elimination. Note the key word "early." If you know that BPH can lead to urinary obstruction, look for the option that identifies the least severe symptom. Review early signs of BPH if you had difficulty with this question.

Level of Cognitive Ability: Application

Client Needs: Physiological Integrity

Integrated Concept/Process: Nursing Process/Assessment

Content Area: Adult Health/Renal

Reference: Ignatavicius, D., Workman, M., & Mishler, M. (1999). *Medical-surgical nursing across the health care continuum* (3rd ed.). Philadelphia: W.B. Saunders, p. 2021.

16. **4**

Rationale: In the client with BPH, episodes of urinary retention can be triggered by certain medications, such as decongestants, anticholinergics, and antidepressants. The client should be questioned about the use of these medications if presenting with urinary retention. Retention can also be precipitated by other factors, such as alcoholic beverages, infection, bed rest, and becoming chilled.

Test-Taking Strategy: Use the process of elimination. The question is asking about medications that could exacerbate or contribute to urinary retention in the client with BPH. Diuretics should help voiding; therefore option 1 is readily eliminated. Antibiotics should have no effect at all, and thus option 2 is eliminated. From the remaining options, recalling that medications that contain anticholinergics may cause urinary retention will direct you to option 4. Review the factors that can precipitate urinary retention in the client with BPH if you had difficulty with this question.

Level of Cognitive Ability: Analysis

Client Needs: Physiological Integrity

Integrated Concept/Process: Nursing Process/Assessment

Content Area: Adult Health/Renal

Reference: Ignatavicius, D., Workman, M., & Mishler, M. (1999). *Medical-surgical nursing across the health care continuum* (3rd ed.). Philadelphia: W.B. Saunders, p. 2024.

17. **2**

Rationale: Phosphate-binding agents that contain aluminum include Alu-Caps, Basaljel, and Amphojel. These products are made from aluminum hydroxide. Tums are made from calcium carbonate, and also bind phosphorus. Tums are prescribed in order to avoid the occurrence of dementia related to high intake of aluminum. Phosphate-binding agents are needed by the client in renal failure because the kidneys cannot eliminate phosphorus.

Test-Taking Strategy: Use the process of elimination. Option 1 may be eliminated, since the name of the medication gives a clue as to its ingredients. Otherwise, specific knowledge of the types of antacids is needed to answer this question accurately. Review the various phosphate-binding agents if you had difficulty with this question.

Level of Cognitive Ability: Application

Client Needs: Physiological Integrity

Integrated Concept/Process: Teaching/Learning

Content Area: Pharmacology

Reference: Smeltzer, S., & Bare, B. (2000). *Brunner & Suddarth's textbook of medical-surgical nursing* (9th ed.). Philadelphia: Lippincott Williams & Wilkins, p. 1150.

18. **4**

Rationale: Disequilibrium syndrome is characterized by headache, mental confusion, decreasing level of consciousness, nausea, vomiting, twitching, and possible seizure activity. It is caused by rapid removal of solutes from the body during hemodialysis. At the same time, the blood-brain barrier interferes with the efficient removal of wastes from brain tissue. As a result, water goes into cerebral cells because of the osmotic gradient, causing brain swelling and onset of symptoms. It most often occurs in clients who are new to dialysis, and is prevented by dialyzing for shorter times or at reduced blood flow rates.

Test-Taking Strategy: Use the process of elimination. Focus on the name of the syndrome, "disequilibrium," to assist in directing you to option 4. Review the manifestations of this syndrome if you had difficulty with this question.

Level of Cognitive Ability: Analysis

Client Needs: Physiological Integrity

Integrated Concept/Process: Nursing Process/Assessment

Content Area: Adult Health/Renal
Reference: Ignatavicius, D., Workman, M., & Mishler, M. (1999). *Medical-surgical nursing across the health care continuum* (3rd ed.). Philadelphia: W.B. Saunders, p. 1903.

19. **4**
Rationale: After dialysis, the client's vital signs are monitored to determine whether the client is remaining hemodynamically stable. Weight is measured and compared with the client's predialysis weight to determine effectiveness of fluid extraction. Laboratory studies are done as per protocol, but are not necessarily done after the hemodialysis treatment has been ended.
Test-Taking Strategy: Use the process of elimination. Note the issue, measures to determine the client's status after dialysis. Recalling the purpose of the dialysis will direct you to option 4. Review postdialysis nursing assessments if you had difficulty with this question.
Level of Cognitive Ability: Analysis
Client Needs: Physiological Integrity
Integrated Concept/Process: Nursing Process/Evaluation
Content Area: Adult Health/Renal
Reference: Ignatavicius, D., Workman, M., & Mishler, M. (1999). *Medical-surgical nursing across the health care continuum* (3rd ed.). Philadelphia: W.B. Saunders, pp. 1901-1902.

20. **2**
Rationale: Steal syndrome results from vascular insufficiency after creation of a fistula. The client exhibits pallor and a diminished pulse distal to the fistula. The client also complains of pain distal to the fistula, which is due to tissue ischemia. Warmth, redness, and pain would more likely characterize a problem with infection. The patterns described in options 3 and 4 are incorrect.
Test-Taking Strategy: It is necessary to understand steal syndrome and know the signs and symptoms to answer this question. Review this syndrome and associated signs and symptoms if you had difficulty with this question.
Level of Cognitive Ability: Application
Client Needs: Physiological Integrity
Integrated Concept/Process: Nursing Process/Assessment
Content Area: Adult Health/Renal
Reference: Ignatavicius, D., Workman, M., & Mishler, M. (1999). *Medical-surgical nursing across the health care continuum* (3rd ed.). Philadelphia: W.B. Saunders, p. 1899.

21. **1**
Rationale: The BUN is the most frequently used laboratory test to determine renal function. The BUN starts to rise when the glomerular filtration rate falls below 40% to 60%. Decreased hemoglobin and RBC count may be noted if bleeding from the urinary tract occurs or if erythropoietic function by the kidney is impaired. An increased WBC is most likely to be noted in renal disease.
Test-Taking Strategy: Use the process of elimination. Recalling the relationship between the BUN and renal function will direct you to option 1. Review significant laboratory tests related to renal function, if you had difficulty with this question.
Level of Cognitive Ability: Analysis
Integrated Concept/Process: Nursing Process/Assessment
Client Needs: Physiological Integrity
Content Area: Adult Health/Renal

Reference: Smeltzer, S., & Bare, B. (2000). *Brunner & Suddarth's textbook of medical-surgical nursing* (9th ed.). Philadelphia: Lippincott Williams & Wilkins, p. 1094.

22. **4**
Rationale: There are no specific precautions following a renal scan. Urination into a commode is acceptable without risk from the small amount of radioactive material to be excreted. The nurse wears gloves to maintain body secretion precautions.
Test-Taking Strategy: Use the process of elimination. Recalling that there is generally no danger from the small amount of radioactive material used in this procedure will direct you to option 4. Review this procedure if you had difficulty with this question.
Level of Cognitive Ability: Application
Client Needs: Safe, Effective Care Environment
Integrated Concept/Process: Nursing Process/Planning
Content Area: Adult Health/Renal
Reference: Smeltzer, S., & Bare, B. (2000). *Brunner & Suddarth's textbook of medical-surgical nursing* (9th ed.). Philadelphia: Lippincott Williams & Wilkins, p. 1095.

23. **3**
Rationale: The iodine-based dye used during the IVP can cause allergic reactions such as itching, hives, rash, a tight feeling in the throat, shortness of breath, and bronchospasm. Assessing for allergies is the priority.
Test-Taking Strategy: Use the process of elimination. Note the key word "priority" in the stem of the question. Use the steps of the nursing process as a guide. Options 1, 2, and 4 address implementation. Option 3 is the only option that addresses assessment. Review preprocedure care for an IVP if you had difficulty with this question.
Level of Cognitive Ability: Application
Client Needs: Physiological Integrity
Integrated Concept/Process: Nursing Process/Assessment
Content Area: Adult Health/Renal
Reference: Fischbach, F. (2000). *A manual of laboratory & diagnostic tests* (6th ed.). Philadelphia: Lippincott Williams & Wilkins, p. 786.

24. **1**
Rationale: If pain originates at the biopsy site and begins to radiate to the flank area and around the front of the abdomen, bleeding should be suspected. Hypotension, a decreasing hematocrit level, and gross or microscopic hematuria would also indicate bleeding. Signs of infection would not appear immediately following a biopsy. Pain of this nature is not normal. There are no data to support the presence of renal colic.
Test-Taking Strategy: Use the process of elimination. Focusing on the data in the question will assist in eliminating options 3 and 4. Recalling that signs of infection may not appear immediately following biopsy will assist in eliminating option 2. Review the complications following renal biopsy if you had difficulty with this question.
Level of Cognitive Ability: Analysis
Client Needs: Physiological Integrity
Integrated Concept/Process: Nursing Process/Analysis
Content Area: Adult Health/Renal
Reference: Ignatavicius, D., Workman, M., & Mishler, M. (1999). *Medical-surgical nursing across the health care continuum* (3rd ed.). Philadelphia: W.B. Saunders, pp. 1814-1815.

25. 1

Rationale: Polyuria occurs early in CRF and if untreated can cause severe dehydration. Polyuria progresses to anuria, and the client loses all normal functions of the kidney. Oliguria and anuria are not early signs, and polydipsia is unrelated to CRF.

Test-Taking Strategy: Use the process of elimination. Note the key word "early" in the question. Eliminate options 3 and 4 because they are similar. From the remaining options select option 1 because this option relates to renal function. Review the early and the late signs of CRF, if you had difficulty with this question.

Level of Cognitive Ability: Analysis
Client Needs: Physiological Integrity
Integrated Concept/Process: Nursing Process/Assessment
Content Area: Adult Health/Renal
Reference: Ignatavicius, D., Workman, M., & Mishler, M. (1999). *Medical-surgical nursing across the health care continuum* (3rd ed.). Philadelphia: W.B. Saunders, p. 1917.

26. 4

Rationale: The client may have an elevated temperature following dialysis because the dialysis machine warms the blood slightly. If the temperature is elevated excessively, and remains elevated, sepsis would be suspected and a blood sample would be obtained as prescribed for culture and sensitivity determinations.

Test-Taking Strategy: Use the process of elimination. Note the key words "most appropriate." Recalling that an elevation in temperature is expected following dialysis will direct you to option 4. Review the normal expected findings following dialysis if you had difficulty with this question.

Level of Cognitive Ability: Application
Client Needs: Physiological Integrity
Integrated Concept/Process: Nursing Process/Implementation
Content Area: Adult Health/Renal
Reference: Ignatavicius, D., Workman, M., & Mishler, M. (1999). *Medical-surgical nursing across the health care continuum* (3rd ed.). Philadelphia: W.B. Saunders, p. 1902.

27. 1

Rationale: Disequilibrium syndrome may be due to the rapid decrease in blood urea nitrogen (BUN) levels during hemodialysis. These changes can cause cerebral edema, which leads to increased intracranial pressure. The client is exhibiting early signs of disequilibrium syndrome, and appropriate treatments with anticonvulsive medications and barbiturates may be necessary to prevent a life-threatening situation. The physician must be notified.

Test-Taking Strategy: Use the process of elimination, and focus on the client's signs and symptoms. Recalling the complications associated with hemodialysis will direct you to option 1. Review the signs and symptoms of disequilibrium syndrome if you had difficulty with this question.

Level of Cognitive Ability: Application
Client Needs: Physiological Integrity
Integrated Concept/Process: Nursing Process/Implementation
Content Area: Adult Health/Renal
Reference: Ignatavicius, D., Workman, M., & Mishler, M. (1999). *Medical-surgical nursing across the health care continuum* (3rd ed.). Philadelphia: W.B. Saunders, p. 1902.

28. 3

Rationale: Cantaloupe (¼ small), spinach (½ cup cooked), and strawberries (1¼ cups) are high potassium foods and average 7 mEq per serving. Lima beans (⅓ cup) average 3 mEq per serving.

Test-Taking Strategy: Use the process of elimination. Remembering that many fruits and green leafy vegetables are high in potassium will assist in directing you to option 3. Review foods that are high in potassium if you had difficulty with this question.

Level of Cognitive Ability: Analysis
Client Needs: Health Promotion and Maintenance
Integrated Concept/Process: Teaching/Learning
Content Area: Adult Health/Renal
Reference: Ignatavicius, D., Workman, M., & Mishler, M. (1999). *Medical-surgical nursing across the health care continuum* (3rd ed.). Philadelphia: W.B. Saunders, p. 1892

29. 4

Rationale: Increasing the glucose concentration makes the solution increasingly more hypertonic. The more hypertonic the solution, the greater the osmotic pressure for ultrafiltration, and thus the greater the amount of fluid removed from the client during an exchange. Options 1, 2, and 3 do not identify the purpose of the glucose.

Test-Taking Strategy: Use the process of elimination. Knowledge regarding the principles related to ultrafiltration will direct you to option 4. If you had difficulty with this question, review dialysate solutions for peritoneal dialysis.

Level of Cognitive Ability: Application
Client Needs: Physiological Integrity
Integrated Concept/Process: Teaching/Learning
Content Area: Adult Health/Renal
Reference: Ignatavicius, D., Workman, M., & Mishler, M. (1999). *Medical-surgical nursing across the health care continuum* (3rd ed.). Philadelphia: W.B. Saunders, p. 1905.

30. 2

Rationale: The major complication of peritoneal dialysis is peritonitis. Strict aseptic technique is required in caring for the client receiving this treatment. Although option 4 may assist in preventing infection, this option relates to an external site. Options 1 and 3 are unrelated to the major complication of peritoneal dialysis.

Test-Taking Strategy: Use the process of elimination. Visualize this procedure and recall the major concern related to peritonitis. This will direct you to option 2. Review the complications associated with peritoneal dialysis if you had difficulty with this question.

Level of Cognitive Ability: Application
Client Needs: Safe, Effective Care Environment
Integrated Concept/Process: Nursing Process/Planning
Content Area: Adult Health/Renal
Reference: Ignatavicius, D., Workman, M., & Mishler, M. (1999). *Medical-surgical nursing across the health care continuum* (3rd ed.). Philadelphia: W.B. Saunders, p. 1906.

31. 3

Rationale: Pain during the inflow of dialysate is common during the first few exchanges because of peritoneal irritation; however, it disappears after a week or two. The infusion amount should not be decreased, and the infusion should not be slowed or stopped.

Test-Taking Strategy: Use the process of elimination. Eliminate options 1, 2, and 4 because they are similar actions. Review the complications associated with peritoneal dialysis and the appropriate nursing actions, if you had difficulty with this question.
Level of Cognitive Ability: Application
Client Needs: Physiological Integrity
Integrated Concept/Process: Nursing Process/Implementation
Content Area: Adult Health/Renal
Reference: Ignatavicius, D., Workman, M., & Mishler, M. (1999). *Medical-surgical nursing across the health care continuum* (3rd ed.). Philadelphia: W.B. Saunders, pp. 1906-1907.

32. **2**
Rationale: An extended dwell time increases the risk of hyperglycemia in the client with diabetes mellitus as a result of absorption of glucose from the dialysate and electrolyte changes. Diabetic clients may require extra insulin when receiving peritoneal dialysis.
Test-Taking Strategy: Use the process of elimination. Noting the client's diagnosis and recalling that the dialysate solution contains glucose will direct you to option 2. Review the complications associated with peritoneal dialysis if you had difficulty with this question.
Level of Cognitive Ability: Application
Client Needs: Health Promotion and Maintenance
Integrated Concept/Process: Self-Care
Content Area: Adult Health/Renal
Reference: Ignatavicius, D., Workman, M., & Mishler, M. (1999). *Medical-surgical nursing across the health care continuum* (3rd ed.). Philadelphia: W.B. Saunders, p. 1907.

33. **3**
Rationale: In an elderly client, the only symptom of a UTI may be something as vague as increasing mental confusion. Frequency and urgency may commonly occur in an elderly client. These symptoms are not specific to UTI in the elderly client. Fever can be associated with a variety of conditions.
Test-Taking Strategy: Use the process of elimination. Note the client's age in the question. Eliminate options 2 and 4 because these symptoms may commonly occur in an elderly client. Eliminate option 1 next because fever can be associated with a variety of conditions. Review the clinical manifestations of UTI that occur in the elderly, if you had difficulty with this question.
Level of Cognitive Ability: Analysis
Client Needs: Physiological Integrity
Integrated Concept/Process: Nursing Process/Assessment
Content Area: Adult Health/Renal
Reference: Phipps, W., Sands, J., & Marek, J. (1999). *Medical-surgical nursing: Concepts & clinical practice* (6th ed.). St. Louis: Mosby, p. 1402.

34. **3**
Rationale: Oxalate is found in dark green foods such as spinach. Other foods that raise urinary oxalate are rhubarb, strawberries, chocolate, wheat bran, nuts, beets, and tea.
Test-Taking Strategy: Use the process of elimination. Remembering that green leafy foods are high in oxalate will assist in directing you to option 3. Review the foods high in oxalate if you had difficulty with this question.
Level of Cognitive Ability: Application
Client Needs: Health Promotion and Maintenance

Integrated Concept/Process: Teaching/Learning
Content Area: Adult Health/Renal
Reference: Ignatavicius, D., Workman, M., & Mishler, M. (1999). *Medical-surgical nursing across the health care continuum* (3rd ed.). Philadelphia: W.B. Saunders, pp 1839, 1843.

35. **2**
Rationale: Frequent dressing changes around the Penrose drain are required to protect the skin against breakdown from the urinary drainage. If urinary drainage is excessive, an ostomy pouch may be placed over the drain to protect the skin. A Penrose drain is not irrigated. Weighing the dressings is not necessary. Placing the client on the affected side will prevent a free flow of urine through the drain.
Test-Taking Strategy: Use the process of elimination. Identify the issue of the question, which relates to the Penrose drain. This should provide you with the clue that drainage is expected. Eliminate option 3 as the least likely answer. Eliminate option 1 because a Penrose drain is not irrigated. Visualize the effect that positioning on the affected side will have on the client. Review postoperative care following a pyelolithotomy, if you had difficulty with this question.
Level of Cognitive Ability: Application
Client Needs: Physiological Integrity
Integrated Concept/Process: Nursing Process/Planning
Content Area: Adult Health/Renal
Reference: Phipps, W., Sands, J., & Marek, J. (1999). *Medical-surgical nursing: Concepts & clinical practice* (6th ed.). St. Louis: Mosby, pp. 520-521.

36. **2**
Rationale: To increase urinary output, diuretics and osmotic agents are administered. The client should be monitored closely because fluid overload can cause hypertension, congestive heart failure, and pulmonary edema. Fluids would not be forced or restricted. Irrigation of the Foley catheter will not assist in alleviating this oliguria.
Test-Taking Strategy: Use the process of elimination. Recalling the definition of oliguria will easily direct you to option 2 as the treatment for this occurrence. If you are unfamiliar with the treatment of oliguria following kidney transplant, review this content.
Level of Cognitive Ability: Analysis
Client Needs: Physiological Integrity
Integrated Concept/Process: Nursing Process/Planning
Content Area: Adult Health/Renal
Reference: LeMone, P., & Burke, K. (2000). *Medical-surgical nursing: Critical thinking in client care* (2nd ed.). Upper Saddle River, N.J.: Prentice-Hall, pp. 1006-1007.

37. **1**
Rationale: Acute rejection most often occurs in the first 2 weeks after transplant. Clinical manifestations include fever, malaise, elevated white blood cell count, acute hypertension, graft tenderness, and manifestations of deteriorating renal function. Chronic rejection occurs gradually during a period of months to years. Although kidney infection or obstruction can occur, the symptoms presented in the question do not specifically relate to these disorders.
Test-Taking Strategy: Use the process of elimination. Note the key words "a week after kidney transplantation." These words should easily direct you to option 1, "acute" rejection. Review

the signs of acute rejection, if you had difficulty with this question.
Level of Cognitive Ability: Analysis
Client Needs: Physiological Integrity
Integrated Concept/Process: Nursing Process/Analysis
Content Area: Adult Health/Renal
Reference: Ignatavicius, D., Workman, M., & Mishler, M. (1999). *Medical-surgical nursing across the health care continuum* (3rd ed.). Philadelphia: W.B. Saunders, p. 1914.

38. 1
Rationale: TUR syndrome is caused by increased absorption of nonelectrolyte irrigating fluid used during surgery. The client may show signs of cerebral edema and increased intracranial pressure, such as increased blood pressure, bradycardia, confusion, disorientation, muscle twitching, visual disturbances, and nausea and vomiting.
Test-Taking Strategy: Use the process of elimination. Recalling that increased intracranial pressure is the concern in this syndrome will direct you to option 1. Review the clinical manifestations of this disorder if you had difficulty with this question.
Level of Cognitive Ability: Analysis
Client Needs: Physiological Integrity
Integrated Concept/Process: Nursing Process/Assessment
Content Area: Adult Health/Renal
Reference: Monahan, F., & Neighbors, M. (1998). *Medical-surgical nursing: Foundations for clinical practice* (2nd ed.). Philadelphia: W.B. Saunders, p. 1712.

39. 3
Rationale: Frank bleeding (arterial or venous) may occur during the first day after surgery. Some hematuria is usual for several days after surgery. A urinary output of 200 mL greater than intake is adequate. Bladder spasms are expected to occur following surgery. A rapid pulse with a low blood pressure is a potential sign of excessive blood loss. The physician should be notified.
Test-Taking Strategy: Use the process of elimination. Focus on the issue, "need to notify the physician." Think about the expected findings following this procedure, and note that the vital signs noted in option 3 are indicative of excessive blood loss. Review the expected findings following TURP if you had difficulty with this question.
Level of Cognitive Ability: Analysis
Client Needs: Physiological Integrity
Integrated Concept/Process: Nursing Process/Analysis
Content Area: Adult Health/Renal
Reference: Ignatavicius, D., Workman, M., & Mishler, M. (1999). *Medical-surgical nursing across the health care continuum* (3rd ed.). Philadelphia: W.B. Saunders, p. 2028.

40. 1
Rationale: Individuals with polycystic kidney disease seem to waste rather than retain sodium. Thus, they need an increased sodium and water intake. Aggressive control of hypertension is essential. Genetic counseling is advisable because of the hereditary nature of the disease.
Test-Taking Strategy: Use the process of elimination. Note the key word "not." Recalling that sodium is wasted in polycystic kidney disease will direct you to option 1. Review the manifestations associated with this disease if you had difficulty with this question.

Level of Cognitive Ability: Analysis
Client Needs: Physiological Integrity
Integrated Concept/Process: Nursing Process/Planning
Content Area: Adult Health/Renal
Reference: LeMone, P., & Burke, K. (2000). *Medical-surgical nursing: Critical thinking in client care* (2nd ed.). Upper Saddle River, N.J.: Prentice-Hall, p. 950.

41. 4
Rationale: Potential complications after renal angiography include allergic reaction to the dye, renal damage from the dye, and a number of vascular complications. These include hemorrhage, thrombosis, or embolism. The nurse detects these complications by noting signs and symptoms of allergic reaction, decreased urine output, hematoma or hemorrhage at the insertion site, or signs of decreased circulation to the affected leg.
Test-Taking Strategy: Use the process of elimination, focusing on the issue, a complication. Eliminate options 1 and 3, since they are normal findings. Since a hematoma is abnormal, then "absence of hematoma" is a normal finding, which eliminates option 2 also. Review the signs of a complication following a renal angioplasty if you had difficulty with this question.
Level of Cognitive Ability: Analysis
Client Needs: Physiological Integrity
Integrated Concept/Process: Nursing Process/Assessment
Content Area: Adult Health/Renal
Reference: Smeltzer, S., & Bare, B. (2000). *Brunner & Suddarth's textbook of medical-surgical nursing* (9th ed.). Philadelphia: Lippincott Williams & Wilkins, p. 1096.

42. 1
Rationale: The client with polycystic kidney disease should report any signs and symptoms of urinary tract infection so that treatment may begin promptly. Lowered blood pressure is not a complication of polycystic kidney disease, and it is an expected effect of antihypertensive therapy. The client would be concerned about rises in blood pressure, because control of hypertension is essential. The client may experience heart failure as a result of hypertension, and thus any symptoms of heart failure, such as shortness of breath, are also a concern.
Test-Taking Strategy: Use the process of elimination. Note the key words "understands" and "no reason to be concerned." Recalling that the client with polycystic kidney disease is likely to be hypertensive will direct you to option 1. Also note that options 2, 3, and 4 identify signs of complications. Review teaching points for the client with polycystic kidney disease if you had difficulty with this question.
Level of Cognitive Ability: Analysis
Client Needs: Health Promotion and Maintenance
Integrated Concept/Process: Teaching/Learning
Content Area: Adult Health/Renal
Reference: Phipps, W., Sands, J., & Marek, J. (1999). *Medical-surgical nursing: Concepts & clinical practice* (6th ed.). St. Louis: Mosby, p. 1413.

43. 4
Rationale: Treatment of prostatitis includes medication with antibiotics, analgesics, and stool softeners. The client is also taught to rest, increase fluid intake, and use sitz baths for comfort. Antimicrobial therapy is always continued until the prescription is completely finished.

Test-Taking Strategy: Use the process of elimination. Eliminate option 3 first, since the stopping medication therapy before the end of the course is contraindicated. Option 1 is also eliminated, since fluid intake should be increased. From the remaining options, recall either that sitz baths provide comfort or that rest is helpful in the healing process. Review home care instructions for the client with prostatitis if you had difficulty with this question.
Level of Cognitive Ability: Analysis
Client Needs: Health Promotion and Maintenance
Integrated Concept/Process: Teaching/Learning
Content Area: Adult Health/Renal
Reference: Smeltzer, S., & Bare, B. (2000). *Brunner & Suddarth's textbook of medical-surgical nursing* (9th ed.). Philadelphia: Lippincott Williams & Wilkins, p. 1305.

44. **2**
Rationale: Crush injuries may cause acute tubular necrosis, from the accumulation of large amounts of myoglobin and hemoglobin that are released from damaged muscle and blood cells. This type of renal failure is said to be due to renal causes—that is, conditions within the kidney itself. Prerenal causes are conditions that interfere with the perfusion of blood to the kidney. Postrenal causes include conditions that cause urinary obstruction distal to the kidney. It is necessary to determine the cause of the type of renal failure, since this knowledge guides the interventions used in treatment to a certain extent.
Test-Taking Strategy: Use the process of elimination and knowledge of the categories of ARF to answer this question. Eliminate option 4 first, since it is not a category of ARF. Next, focus on the nature of the injury and its effect on the kidney to direct you to option 2. Review the causes of ARF if you had difficulty with this question.
Level of Cognitive Ability: Analysis
Client Needs: Physiological Integrity
Integrated Concept/Process: Nursing Process/Analysis
Content Area: Adult Health/Renal
Reference: Ignatavicius, D., Workman, M., & Mishler, M. (1999). *Medical-surgical nursing across the health care continuum* (3rd ed.). Philadelphia: W.B. Saunders, p. 1306.

45. **3**
Rationale: The client with hyperkalemia is at risk for developing cardiac dysrhythmias and cardiac arrest. Because of this, the client should be placed on a cardiac monitor. Fluid intake is not increased, since it contributes to fluid overload and would not significantly affect the serum potassium level. Vegetables are a natural source of potassium in the diet, and their use would not be increased. The nurse may also assess the sodium level, since it is another electrolyte that is commonly measured with the potassium level. However, this is not a priority action of the nurse.
Test-Taking Strategy: First, note that the K level is elevated. Next use the ABCs—airway, breathing, and circulation—to direct you to option 3. Review care to the client with hyperkalemia if you had difficulty with this question.
Level of Cognitive Ability: Application
Client Needs: Physiological Integrity
Integrated Concept/Process: Nursing Process/Planning
Content Area: Adult Health/Renal

Reference: Ignatavicius, D., Workman, M., & Mishler, M. (1999). *Medical-surgical nursing across the health care continuum* (3rd ed.). Philadelphia: W.B. Saunders, p. 248.

46. **3**
Rationale: Antihypertensive medications such as enalapril are given to the client following hemodialysis. This prevents the client from becoming hypotensive during dialysis, and also from having the medication removed from the bloodstream by dialysis. There is no rationale for waiting a full day to resume the medication. This would lead to ineffective control of the blood pressure.
Test-Taking Strategy: Use the process of elimination. Begin to answer this question by thinking about the effects of an antihypertensive medication on the blood pressure when fluid is being removed from the body. Since hypotension is much more likely to occur in this circumstance, eliminate options 1 and 2. Eliminate option 4 because this action would lead to ineffective blood pressure control. Review preprocedure hemodialysis measures if you had difficulty with this question.
Level of Cognitive Ability: Application
Client Needs: Physiological Integrity
Integrated Concept/Process: Nursing Process/Planning
Content Area: Adult Health/Renal
Reference: Smeltzer, S., & Bare, B. (2000). *Brunner & Suddarth's textbook of medical-surgical nursing* (9th ed.). Philadelphia: Lippincott Williams & Wilkins, p. 1114.

47. **2**
Rationale: Clients with peritoneal dialysis catheters are at high risk for infection. A dressing that is wet is a conduit for bacteria to reach the catheter insertion site. The nurse ensures that the dressing is kept dry at all times. Reinforcing the dressing is not a safe practice to prevent infection in this circumstance. Flushing the catheter is not indicated. Scrubbing the catheter with povidone-iodine is done at the time of connection or disconnection of peritoneal dialysis.
Test-Taking Strategy: Use the process of elimination. Note the issue of the question, a wet dressing. Recalling that this client is at risk for infection and knowing that it is better to change a wet dressing than reinforce it will direct you to option 2. Review care of the client receiving peritoneal dialysis if you had difficulty with this question.
Level of Cognitive Ability: Application
Client Needs: Safe, Effective Care Environment
Integrated Concept/Process: Nursing Process/Implementation
Content Area: Adult Health/Renal
Reference: Ignatavicius, D., Workman, M., & Mishler, M. (1999). *Medical-surgical nursing across the health care continuum* (3rd ed.). Philadelphia: W.B. Saunders, p. 1907.

48. **2**
Rationale: If the client experiences air embolus during hemodialysis, the nurse should terminate dialysis immediately, notify the physician, and administer oxygen as needed. All other actions are incorrect. Options 1, 3, and 4 are incorrect.
Test-Taking Strategy: Use the process of elimination. Recalling that air embolus is an emergency situation that affects the cardiopulmonary system suddenly and profoundly will direct you to option 2. Review the emergency care of a client who develops air embolism if you had difficulty with this question.
Level of Cognitive Ability: Application

Client Needs: Physiological Integrity
Integrated Concept/Process: Nursing Process/Implementation
Content Area: Adult Health/Renal
Reference: Smeltzer, S., & Bare, B. (2000). *Brunner & Suddarth's textbook of medical-surgical nursing* (9th ed.). Philadelphia: Lippincott Williams & Wilkins, p. 1114.

49. **2**
Rationale: The client on hemodialysis should monitor fluid status between hemodialysis treatments. This can be accomplished by recording intake and output and measuring weight on a daily basis. Ideally, the hemodialysis client should not gain more than 0.5 kg of weight per day.
Test-Taking Strategy: Use the process of elimination. Recalling the pathophysiology of renal failure and the impact on the client's bodily functions will assist in answering the question. Also, note that option 2 relates to monitoring of fluid retention. Review teaching points for the client receiving hemodialysis if you had difficulty with this question.
Level of Cognitive Ability: Analysis
Client Needs: Health Promotion and Maintenance
Integrated Concept/Process: Self-Care
Content Area: Adult Health/Renal
Reference: Ignatavicius, D., Workman, M., & Mishler, M. (1999). *Medical-surgical nursing across the health care continuum* (3rd ed.). Philadelphia: W.B. Saunders, p. 1902.

50. **4**
Rationale: An AV shunt is a less common form of access site, but carries a risk for bleeding when it is used. This is because two ends of a cannula are tunneled subcutaneously into an artery and a vein, and the ends of the cannula are joined. If accidental disconnection occurs, the client could lose blood rapidly. For this reason, small clamps are attached to the dressing that covers the insertion site for use if needed. The shunt site should also be assessed at least every 4 hours.

Test-Taking Strategy: Use the process of elimination. Focus on the issue, preventing bleeding. Visualize this type of access device. Recalling that the risk of disconnection can occur will direct you to option 4. Review care to the client with an AV shunt if you had difficulty with this question.
Level of Cognitive Ability: Application
Client Needs: Safe, Effective Care Environment
Integrated Concept/Process: Nursing Process/Implementation
Content Area: Adult Health/Renal
Reference: Ignatavicius, D., Workman, M., & Mishler, M. (1999). *Medical-surgical nursing across the health care continuum* (3rd ed.). Philadelphia: W.B. Saunders, p. 1901.

CRITICAL THINKING: FREE-TEXT ENTRY

Answer: Reposition the client
Rationale: If outflow drainage is inadequate, the nurse attempts to stimulate outflow by changing the client's position. Turning the client to the other side or making sure that the client is in good body alignment may assist with outflow drainage.
Test-Taking Strategy: Use the process of elimination. Note the key word "initially." Also note that the issue of the question relates to inadequate outflow and the need for a nursing intervention. Review the nursing interventions related to insufficient flow of dialysate, if you had difficulty with this question.
Level of Cognitive Ability: Application
Client Needs: Physiological Integrity
Integrated Concept/Process: Nursing Process/Implementation
Content Area: Adult Health/Renal
Reference: Ignatavicius, D., Workman, M., & Mishler, M. (1999). *Medical-surgical nursing across the health care continuum* (3rd ed.). Philadelphia: W.B. Saunders, p. 1907.

REFERENCES

Fischbach, F. (2000). *A manual of laboratory & diagnostic tests* (6th ed.). Philadelphia: Lippincott Williams & Wilkins.

Hodgson, B., & Kizior, R. (2001). *Saunders nursing drug handbook 2001*. Philadelphia: W.B. Saunders.

Ignatavicius, D., Workman, M., & Mishler, M. (1999). *Medical-surgical nursing across the health care continuum* (3rd ed.). Philadelphia: W.B. Saunders.

LeMone, P., & Burke, K. (2000). *Medical-surgical nursing: Critical thinking in client care* (2nd ed.). Upper Saddle River, N.J.: Prentice-Hall.

Monahan, F., & Neighbors, M. (1998). *Medical-surgical nursing: Foundations for clinical practice* (2nd ed.). Philadelphia: W.B. Saunders.

Phipps, W., Sands, J., & Marek, J. (1999). *Medical-surgical nursing: Concepts & clinical practice* (6th ed.). St. Louis: Mosby.

Smeltzer, S., & Bare, B. (2000). *Brunner & Suddarth's textbook of medical-surgical nursing* (9th ed.). Philadelphia: Lippincott Williams & Wilkins.

Smith, S., Duell, D., & Martin, B. (2000). *Clinical nursing skills: Basic to advanced skills* (5th ed.). Upper Saddle River, N.J.: Prentice-Hall Health.

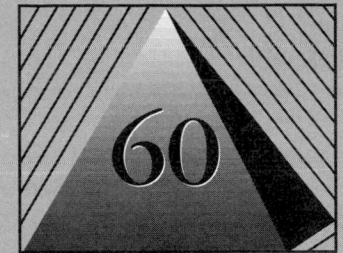

Renal Medications

I. URINARY TRACT ANTISEPTICS (Box 60-1)

A. Description
1. Inhibit the growth of bacteria in the urine
2. Act as disinfectants within the urinary tract
3. Used to treat urinary tract infections
4. These medications do not achieve effective antibacterial concentrations in blood or tissues and therefore cannot be used for infections at sites outside the urinary tract

B. Side effects and nursing considerations
1. Nitrofurantoin
   a. Gastrointestinal effects such as anorexia, nausea, vomiting, and diarrhea; administration with milk or meals will minimize gastrointestinal (GI) distress
   b. Pulmonary reactions such as dyspnea, chest pain, chills, fever, cough, and alveolar infiltrates; these resolve in 2 to 4 days following cessation of treatment
   c. Hematological effects such as agranulocytosis, leukopenia, thrombocytopenia, and megaloblastic anemia
   d. Peripheral neuropathy such as muscle weakness, tingling sensations, and numbness
   e. Neurological effects such as headache, vertigo, drowsiness, nystagmus
   f. Imparts a harmless brown color to the urine
   g. Contraindicated in clients with renal impairment
   h. Instruct the client in the expected side effects and those warranting notifying the physician
2. Methenamine
   a. Relatively safe and well tolerated
   b. May cause gastric distress
   c. Chronic high-dose therapy can cause bladder irritation
   d. Can cause crystalluria and should not be used in clients with renal impairment

e. Decomposition of medication generates ammonia; thus it should not be used for clients with liver dysfunction
   f. Requires acidic urine with pH of 5.5 or less
   g. Ingestion of large amounts of fluid will reduce antibacterial effects by diluting the medication and raising the urinary pH
   h. Should not be combined with sulfonamides because of the risk of crystalluria and urinary tract injury
   i. Clients taking this medication should not be given alkalinizing agents
3. Nalidixic acid
   a. Gastrointestinal disturbances: nausea, vomiting, and abdominal discomfort
   b. Rash
   c. Visual disturbances
   d. Photosensitivity reactions
   e. May produce intracranial hypertension in pediatric clients and should not be administered to children under age 3 months
   f. When used for more than 2 weeks, complete blood cell (CBC) counts and liver function tests should be performed
   g. Can intensify the effects of oral anticoagulants
   h. Contraindicated in clients with a history of convulsive disorders
4. Cinoxacin
   a. Side effects are similar to those of nalidixic acid

BOX 60-1

Urinary Tract Antiseptics

Nitrofurantoin (Furadantin, Furalan, Macrobid)
Nitrofurantoin macrocrystals (Macrodandin)
Methenamine (Mandelamine, Hiprex, Urex)
Nalidixic acid (NegGram)
Cinoxacin (Cinobac)
Norfloxacin (Noroxin)

b. Dosage should be reduced in clients with renal impairment; failure to do so could result in accumulation of the medication to toxic levels

5. Norfloxacin
   a. Can cause fatigue, headache, nausea, constipation, rash, and elevated liver function tests
   b. Encourage the client to consume a high fluid intake
   c. Advise the client to take medication 1 hour before or 2 hours after meals because food may hamper absorption

II. SULFONAMIDES (Box 60-2)
A. Description
1. Suppress bacterial growth by inhibiting the synthesis of folic acid
2. Active against a broad spectrum of microbes
B. Side effect and nursing considerations
1. Hypersensitivity reactions: rash, fever, and photosensitivity
2. Stevens-Johnson syndrome, the most severe hypersensitivity response, producing symptoms that include widespread lesions of the skin and mucous membranes, with fever, malaise, and toxemia
3. Should be discontinued if a rash is observed
4. Can cause hemolytic anemia, agranulocytosis, leukopenia, and thrombocytopenia
5. Instruct the client to take medication on an empty stomach with a full glass of water
6. Instruct the client to avoid prolonged exposure to sunlight, wear protective clothing, and apply a sunscreen to exposed skin
7. Adults should maintain a daily urine output of 1200 mL by consuming 8 to 10 glasses of water each day to minimize the risk of renal damage from the medication
8. Can intensify the effects of warfarin sodium (Coumadin), phenytoin (Dilantin), and oral hypoglycemics
9. Administer with caution in clients with renal impairment

BOX 60-2

Sulfonamides

Sulfadiazine
Sulfadoxine-pyrimethamine (Fansidar)
Sulfamethizole (Thiosulfil Forte)
Sulfamethoxazole (Gantanol, Urobak)
Sulfamethoxazole-phenazopyridine (Azo-Gantanol)
Sulfasalazine (Azulifidine)
Sulfisoxazole (Gantrisin)
Sulfisoxazole-phenazopyridine (Azo-Gantrisin)

---

10. Contraindicated if a hypersensitivity exists to sulfonamides, sulfonylureas, or thiazide or loop diuretics
11. Contraindicated in infants under age 2 months and in pregnant women or mothers who are breast-feeding

III. TRIMETHOPRIM (PROLOPRIM, TRIMPEX)
A. Description
1. Active against a broad spectrum of microbes
2. Suppresses bacterial synthesis of DNA, RNA, and proteins
B. Side effects and nursing considerations
1. Itching and rash are the most frequent side effects
2. GI reactions such as epigastric distress, nausea and vomiting, glossitis, and stomatitis occur occasionally
3. Megaloblastic anemia, thrombocytopenia, and neutropenia may occur in individuals with preexisting folic acid deficiency
4. If early signs of bone marrow suppression occur, such as sore throat, fever or pallor, a CBC should be performed
5. Contraindicated in women who are pregnant or are breast-feeding
6. Contraindicated in clients with a folate deficiency

IV. TRIMETHOPRIM-SULFAMETHOXAZOLE
A. Description
1. A fixed-dose combination product (TMP-SMZ) that is a powerful broad-spectrum antimicrobial preparation
2. Trade names include Bactrim, Cotrim, and Septra
B. Side effects and nursing considerations
1. Nausea, vomiting, and rash are the most common side effects
2. Can cause megaloblastic anemia in clients who are folate deficient
3. Can cause central nervous system (CNS) effects such as headache, depression, and hallucinations
4. Hyperkalemia can occur
5. Toxicity: hypersensitivity reactions, blood dyscrasias, and renal damage
6. Contraindicated during pregnancy and lactation, for infants under age 2 months, in clients with a folate deficiency, and in clients with a history of hypersensitivity to sulfonamides and chemically related medications

V. CHOLINERGIC (Box 60-3)
A. Description
1. Used to treat nonobstructive urinary retention and neurogenic bladder
2. Used to increase bladder tone and function
B. Side effects
1. Headache

2. Hypotension
3. Flushing and sweating
4. Increased salivation
5. Abdominal cramps
6. Nausea and vomiting
7. Diarrhea
8. Urinary urgency
9. Bronchoconstriction
C. Nursing considerations
1. Do not administer if the client has a urinary obstruction
2. Never administer by the intramuscular (IM) or intravenous (IV) route
3. Monitor intake and output (I & O)
4. Monitor for increased bladder tone and function
5. Monitor for cholinergic overdose
6. Have atropine sulfate (antidote) readily available

VI. **ANTISPASMODICS**
A. Description
1. Oxybutynin chloride (Ditropan) relaxes smooth muscles of the urinary tract
2. Propantheline bromide (Pro-Banthine) decreases bladder muscle spasms
B. Oxybutynin chloride (Ditropan)
1. Side effects
a. Leukopenia
b. Anxiety
c. Anorexia, nausea, vomiting
d. Palpitations
e. Sinus bradycardia
2. Nursing considerations
a. Do not administer to clients with known hypersensitivity, GI or genitourinary (GU) obstruction, glaucoma, severe colitis, or myasthenia gravis
b. Instruct the client to avoid hazardous activities
C. Propantheline bromide (Pro-Banthine)
1. Side effects
a. Palpitations
b. Blurred vision
c. Confusion in elderly clients
d. Tachycardia
e. Constipation
f. Dry mouth
g. Urinary hesitancy and urgency
h. Decreased sweating
2. Nursing considerations
a. Monitor I & O

b. Provide gum or hard candy for dry mouth
c. Do not administer to clients with narrow-angle glaucoma, obstructive uropathy, GI disease, or ulcerative colitis

VII. **URINARY ANALGESIC** (Box 60-4)
A. Description
1. Used for pain from urinary tract irritation or infection
2. Administered with an antibiotic because it does not treat infection; it only treats pain
B. Side effects
1. Nausea
2. Headache
3. Vertigo
C. Nursing considerations
1. Instruct the client that the urine will turn red or orange
2. Contraindicated in renal or hepatic disease

VIII. **HEMATOPOIETIC GROWTH FACTOR** (Box 60-5)
A. Description
1. Used to stimulate red blood cell (RBC) production
2. Reverses anemia associated with **chronic renal failure**
3. Initial effects can be seen within 1 to 2 weeks, and the hematocrit reaches normal levels (30% to 33%) in 2 to 3 months
B. Side effect: Major side effect is hypertension
C. Nursing considerations
1. Monitor the CBC
2. Monitor vital signs, especially the blood pressure for hypertension
3. The extent of hypertension is directly related to the rate of rise in the hematocrit
4. Contraindicated in clients with uncontrolled hypertension or hypersensitivity to mammalian cell–derived products or human albumin
5. Use with caution in clients with cancers of myeloid origin

---

BOX 60-4

Urinary Analgesic

Phenazopyridine hydrochloride (Pyridium)

BOX 60-3

Cholinergic

Bethanechol chloride (Duvoid, Urecholine)

BOX 60-5

Hematopoietic Growth Factor

Epoetin alfa (Epogen, Procrit)

▲ IX. PREVENTING ORGAN REJECTION (Box 60-6)

A. Description
1. Cyclosporine acts on T lymphocytes to suppress production of interleukin-2, gamma interferon, and other cytokines
2. Tracrolimus inhibits calcineurin and thereby prevents T cells from producing interleukin-2, gamma interferon, and other cytokines
3. Azathioprine (Imuran) suppresses cell-mediated and humoral immune responses by inhibiting the proliferation of B and T lymphocytes
4. Mycophenolate mofentil causes selective inhibition of B and T lymphocyte proliferation
5. Muromonab-CD3 blocks all T cell functions
6. Therapeutic effect of anti-thymocyte globulin results from a decrease in the number and activity of thymus-derived lymphocytes
7. Daclizumab and basiliximab bind to IL-2 receptors on lymphocytes, resulting in diminished cell-mediated immune reactions

B. Cyclosporine (Sandimmune, Neoral)
1. Used to prevent rejection of allogenic kidney transplant
2. Prednisone is usually administered concurrently
3. Oral administration is preferred; IV administration is reserved for clients who cannot take the medication orally
4. Blood levels should be measured periodically
5. The most common adverse effects are nephrotoxicity, infection, hypertension, tremor, and hirsutism
6. The client should be informed about the possibility of renal damage and liver damage and the need for periodic blood urea nitrogen (BUN), creatinine, and liver function tests
7. The client should be instructed to monitor for early signs of infection and to report these signs immediately
8. Instruct the client to dispense the oral liquid into a glass container by using a specially calibrated pipette, mix well, and drink immediately; rinse the glass container with diluent and drink it to ensure ingestion of the complete dose; dry the outside of the pipette and return to its cover for storage
9. Instruct the client to mix the concentrated medication solution with milk, chocolate milk, or orange juice just before administration
10. Assure the client that hirsutism is reversible
11. Grapefruit juice can raise cyclosporine levels, thereby increasing the risk of toxicity
12. Phenytoin (Dilantin), phenobarbital, rifampin (Rifadin), and TMP-SMZ can decrease cyclosporine levels
13. Ketoconazole (Nizoral), erythromycin, and amphotericin B (Fungizone) can elevate cyclosporine levels
14. Renal damage can be intensified by the concurrent use of other nephrotoxic medications
15. Contraindicated in the presence of hypersensitivity, pregnancy and breast-feeding, recent inoculation with live virus vaccines, and recent contact with an active infection such as chickenpox or herpes zoster
16. Is embryotoxic, and women of childbearing age should use a mechanical form of contraception and avoid oral contraceptives

C. Tacrolimus (Prograf)
1. Nephrotoxicity is the major concern
2. Other common reactions include neurotoxicity, GI effects, hypertension, hyperkalemia, and hyperglycemia
3. Increases the risk of infection and lymphomas
4. Concurrent use of glucocorticoids is recommended

D. Azathioprine (Imuran)
1. Used as an adjunct to cyclosporine and glucocorticoids to help suppress transplant rejection
2. Can cause neutropenia and thrombocytopenia from bone marrow suppression
3. Contraindicated in pregnancy and is associated with an increased incidence of neoplasms

E. Mycophenolate mofetil (CellCept)
1. Used in combination with cyclosporine and glucocorticoids
2. Major adverse effects include diarrhea, severe neutropenia, vomiting, and sepsis
3. Associated with an increased risk of infection and malignancies
4. Absorption is decreased by the use of magnesium and aluminum antacids and by cholestyramine (Questran, Prevalite)
5. Contraindicated in pregnancy

BOX 60-6

Preventing Organ Rejection

IMMUNOSUPPRESSANTS
Cyclosporine (Sandimmune, Neoral)
Tracrolimus (Prograf)

CYTOTOXIC MEDICATIONS
Azathioprine (Imuran)
Mycophenolate Mofetil (CellCept)

GLUCOCORTICOID
Prednisone (Deltasone)

ANTIBODIES
Anti-thymocyte globulin (Atgam)
Basiliximab (Simulect)
Daclizumab (Zenapax)
Muromonab-CD3 (Orthoclone OKT3)

F. Muromonab-CD3 (Orthoclone OKT3)
1. Used to prevent acute allograft rejection of kidney transplants
2. Adverse reactions include fever, chills, dyspnea, chest pain, and nausea and vomiting
G. Anti-thymocyte globulin (Atgam)
1. Used to prevent rejection of renal transplants
2. Usually administered with glucocorticoids and azathioprine
3. Adverse reactions include chills, fever, leukopenia, and skin reactions
H. Daclizumab (Zenapax) and basiliximab (Simulect)
1. Used to prevent acute rejection of transplanted kidneys
2. Used in combination with other immunosuppressants such as cyclosporine and glucocorticoids
3. Administered by the IV route
4. Contraindicated in the client with an allergy to protein
5. Daclizumab (Zenapax)
   a. Initial dose administered within 24 hours prior to transplant
   b. Side effects include chest pain, GI distress, edema, shortness of breath, pain in the joints, and slow wound healing
6. Basiliximab (Simulect)
   a. Initial dose administered within 2 hours prior to transplant
   b. Side effects are similar to those for daclizumab; in addition, headache, insomnia, dizziness, and tremor can occur

PRACTICE QUESTIONS

1. Co-trimoxazole (Bactrim) is prescribed to be administered by IV infusion to a client with a recurrent urinary tract infection. A nurse would plan to administer this medication:
   1. Over 60 to 90 minutes
   2. Over a period of 30 minutes
   3. Piggybacked into the existing infusion of normal saline and potassium chloride
   4. Piggybacked into the peripheral line containing total parenteral nutrition (TPN)

2. Nalidixic acid (NegGram) is prescribed for a client with a urinary tract infection (UTI). On review of the client's record, a nurse notes that the client is taking warfarin sodium (Coumadin) on a daily basis. Which of the following prescriptions would the nurse anticipate because the client is on this oral anticoagulant?
   1. An increase in the anticoagulation dosage
   2. A decrease in the anticoagulation dosage
   3. The need to discontinue the anticoagulant
   4. The need to administer an alternative medication to treat the UTI

3. A nurse is providing discharge instructions to a client receiving sulfisoxazole (Gantrisin). Which of the following would be included in the list of instructions?
   1. Restrict fluid intake
   2. Maintain a high fluid intake
   3. Decrease the dosage when symptoms are improving to prevent an allergic response
   4. If the urine turn dark brown, call the physician immediately

4. Sulfamethoxazole (Gantanol) is prescribed for a client with a urinary tract infection (UTI). The client has diabetes mellitus and is receiving tolbutamide (Orinase). Based on the administration of these two medications in combination, which of the following would the nurse anticipate might be prescribed?
   1. A decreased dosage of the tolbutamide
   2. An increased dosage of the tolbutamide
   3. A decreased dosage of the sulfamethoxazole
   4. An increased dosage of the sulfamethoxazole

5. Trimethoprim-sulfamethoxazole (Bactrim) is prescribed for a client. A nurse would instruct the client to report which of the following symptoms, if developed during the course of this medication therapy?
   1. Headache
   2. Nausea
   3. Diarrhea
   4. Sore throat

6. Phenazopyridine (Pyridium) is prescribed for a client for symptomatic relief of pain resulting from a lower urinary tract infection (UTI). Which of the following would a nurse include in the teaching plan for the client?
   1. Take the medication prior to meals
   2. A reddish orange discoloration of the urine may occur
   3. Discontinue the medication if a headache occurs
   4. Take the medication at bedtime

7. Bethanechol chloride (Urecholine) is prescribed for a client with urinary retention. Which of the following disorders would be a contraindication to the administration of this medication?
   1. Neurogenic atony
   2. Urinary strictures
   3. Gastroesophogeal reflux
   4. Gastric atony

8. A nurse who is administering bethanechol chloride (Urecholine) is monitoring for acute toxicity associated with the medication. Which of the following is not a manifestation associated with toxicity?
   1. Salivation
   2. Sweating
   3. Bradycardia
   4. Severe hypertension

9. Oxybutynin (Ditropan) is prescribed for a client with neurogenic bladder. Which of the following

would indicate a possible toxic effect related to this medication?
1. Bradycardia
2. Pallor
3. Restlessness
4. Drowsiness

10. Propantheline bromide (Pro-Banthine) is prescribed for a client with bladder spasms. Which of the following disorders, if noted in the client's record, would alert a nurse to question the prescription for this medication?
1. Glaucoma
2. Hypothyroidism
3. Myexdema
4. Coronary artery disease

11. Following kidney transplant, cyclosporine (Sandimmune) is prescribed for a client. Which of the following laboratory results would indicate an adverse effect from the use of this medication?
1. Decreased white blood cell count
2. Decreased hemoglobin
3. Elevated blood urea nitrogen (BUN)
4. Decreased creatinine

12. A nurse is providing dietary instructions to a client who has been prescribed cyclosporine (Sandimmune). Which of the following food items would the nurse instruct the client to avoid?
1. Orange juice
2. Grapefruit juice
3. Red meats
4. Green leafy vegetables

13. A nurse is caring for a client who will be receiving amphotericin B (Fungizone). The nurse notes that the client is also taking cyclosporine (Sandimmune) to prevent rejection of a kidney transplant performed 2 years ago. Which of the following prescriptions would the nurse anticipate to be prescribed for this client during the administration of these medications concurrently?
1. An increased amount of amphotericin B
2. A decreased amount of amphotericin B
3. An increased amount of cyclosporine
4. A decreased amount of cyclosporine

14. A nurse provides instructions to a client prescribed to take cyclosporine (Sandimmune) oral solution. Which of the following instructions would the nurse provide to the client?
1. Dilute the concentrate in a Styrofoam cup prior to administration
2. Avoid diluting the concentrate for administration
3. Mix the concentrate with chocolate milk
4. Mix the concentrate with grapefruit juice

15. A nurse is monitoring a client receiving cyclosporine (Sandimmune). Which of the following would indicate to the nurse that the client is experiencing an adverse effect from this medication?
1. Nausea

2. Alopecia
3. Tremors
4. Hypotension

16. Tacrolimus (Prograf) is prescribed for a client. Which of the following disorders, if noted in the client's record, would indicate that the medication needs to be administered with caution?
1. Diabetes insipidus
2. Coronary artery disease
3. Pancreatitis
4. Ulcerative colitis

17. A nurse is reviewing the laboratory results for a client receiving tacrolimus (Prograf). Which of the following would indicate to the nurse that the client is experiencing an adverse effect of the medication?
1. White blood cell (WBC) count of 6000/uL
2. Blood glucose of 200 mg/dL
3. Potassium level of 3.8 mEq/L
4. Platelet count of 300,000 cells/uL

18. Mycophenolate mofetil (CellCept) is prescribed for a client for prophylaxis of organ rejection following allogeneic renal transplant. Which of the following instructions would a nurse provide to the client regarding administration of this medication?
1. Administer following meals
2. Open the capsule and mix with food for administration
3. Contact the physician if a sore throat occurs
4. Take the medication with a magnesium-type antacid

19. A client with chronic renal failure is receiving epoetin alfa (Epogen, Procrit). A nurse is evaluating the laboratory results. Which of the following results would indicate a therapeutic effect of the medication?
1. White blood cell (WBC) count of 6000/uL
2. Hematocrit of 32%
3. Platelet count of 400,000 cells/uL
4. Blood urea nitrogen (BUN) of 15 mg/dL

20. A nurse is instructing a client to administer epoetin alfa (Epogen, Procrit) by the subcutaneous route. Which of the following indicates an accurate description of the instruction?
1. Shake the bottle before use
2. Keep the vial of medication at room temperature
3. Use only 1 dose per vial
4. Use alcohol to clean the top of the vial when reused

CRITICAL THINKING: FREE-TEXT ENTRY

A nurse is administering a dose of bethanechol chloride (Urecholine) subcutaneously to a client with urinary retention. The nurse plans to have what medication (antidote) readily available when administering the bethanechol chloride to the client?

Answer: _____

ANSWERS

1. 1

Rationale: Bactrim may be administered by IV infusion but should not be mixed with any other medications or solutions. It is infused over a period of 60 to 90 minutes, and bolus infusions or rapid infusions must be avoided.

Test-Taking Strategy: Use the process of elimination. Eliminate options 3 and 4 because they both address the issue of mixing the Bactrim with other solutions. From the remaining options, option 1 identifies the longer time frame and is the safe and correct choice. Review administration of this medication by IV if you had difficulty with this question.

Level of Cognitive Ability: Application
Client Needs: Physiological Integrity
Integrated Concept/Process: Nursing Process/Implementation
Content Area: Pharmacology
Reference: Hodgson, B., & Kizior, R. (2001). *Saunders nursing drug handbook 2001.* Philadelphia: W.B. Saunders, p. 263.

2. 2

Rationale: Nalidixic acid can intensify the effects of oral anticoagulants by displacing these agents from binding sites on plasma protein. When an oral anticoagulant is combined with nalidixic acid, a decrease in the anticoagulant dosage may be needed.

Test-Taking Strategy: Knowledge regarding the medication interactions associated with the use of nalidixic acid is needed to answer this question. Review these interactions if you had difficulty with this question.

Level of Cognitive Ability: Analysis
Client Needs: Physiological Integrity
Integrated Concept/Process: Nursing Process/Analysis
Content Area: Pharmacology
Reference: Salerno, E. (1999). *Pharmacology for health professionals.* St. Louis: Mosby, p. 665.

3. 2

Rationale: Each dose of Gantrisin should be administered with a full glass of water, and the client should maintain a high fluid intake. The medication is more soluble in alkaline urine. The client should not be instructed to taper or discontinue the dose. Some forms of Gantrisin, such as Azo-Gantrisin, cause urine to turn dark brown or red. This does not indicate the need to notify the physician.

Test-Taking Strategy: Use the process of elimination. Recalling that this medication is used to treat urinary tract infections will direct you to option 2. Review client instructions regarding this medication if you had difficulty with this question.

Level of Cognitive Ability: Application
Client Needs: Health Promotion and Maintenance
Integrated Concept/Process: Teaching/Learning
Content Area: Pharmacology
Reference: Wilson, B., Shannon, M., & Stang, C. (2000). *Nurses drug guide 2000.* Stamford, Conn.: Appleton & Lange, p. 1316.

4. 1

Rationale: Sulfonamides can intensify the effects of warfarin sodium (Coumadin), phenytoin (Dilantin), and oral hypoglycemics, such as tolbutamide (Orinase). When combined with sulfonamides, these medications may require a reduction in dosage.

Test-Taking Strategy: Use the process of elimination. Recalling that sulfonamides intensify the action of oral hypoglycemics will direct you to option 1. Review the medication interactions

associated with sulfonamides if you had difficulty with this question.

Level of Cognitive Ability: Analysis
Client Needs: Physiological Integrity
Integrated Concept/Process: Nursing Process/Analysis
Content Area: Pharmacology
Reference: Salerno, E. (1999). *Pharmacology for health professionals.* St. Louis: Mosby, p. 664.

5. 4

Rationale: Clients taking trimethoprim-sulfamethoxazole should be informed about early signs of blood disorders that can occur from this medication. These signs include sore throat, fever, and pallor, and the client should be instructed to notify the physician if these symptoms occur. The other options do not require physician notification.

Test-Taking Strategy: Use the process of elimination. Knowledge that this medication can cause blood dyscrasias will direct you to option 4. If you are unfamiliar with this medication, review this content.

Level of Cognitive Ability: Application
Client Needs: Health Promotion and Maintenance
Integrated Concept/Process: Teaching/Learning
Content Area: Pharmacology
Reference: Gutierrez, K. (1999). *Pharmacotherapeutics: Clinical decision-making in nursing.* Philadelphia: W.B. Saunders, pp. 847-848.

6. 2

Rationale: The client should be instructed that a reddish orange discoloration of urine may occur. The client should also be instructed that this discoloration can stain fabric. The medication should be taken after meals to reduce the possibility of gastrointestinal upset. A headache is an occasional side effect of the medication and does not warrant discontinuation of the medication.

Test-Taking Strategy: Use the process of elimination. Eliminate options 1 and 4 first because they are similar in that they both address time schedules for the administration of the medication. From the remaining options, eliminate option 3 because the nurse would not advise the client to discontinue this medication. Review client instructions regarding this medication if you had difficulty with this question.

Level of Cognitive Ability: Application
Client Needs: Health Promotion and Maintenance
Integrated Concept/Process: Teaching/Learning
Content Area: Pharmacology
Reference: Hodgson, B., & Kizior, R. (2001). *Saunders nursing drug handbook 2001.* Philadelphia: W.B. Saunders, p. 813.

7. 2

Rationale: Urecholine can be hazardous to clients with urinary tract obstruction or weakness of the bladder wall. The medication has the ability to contract the bladder and thereby increase pressure within the urinary tract. Elevation of pressure within the urinary tract could rupture the bladder in clients with these conditions

Test-Taking Strategy: Use the process of elimination. Noting that the medication is used for urinary retention may assist in directing you to option 2. Review the contraindications associated with this medication, if you had difficulty with this question.

Level of Cognitive Ability: Analysis
Client Needs: Physiological Integrity

Integrated Concept/Process: Nursing Process/Analysis
Content Area: Pharmacology
Reference: Clark, J., Queener, S., & Karb, V. (2000). *Pharmacologic basis of nursing practice* (6th ed.). St. Louis: Mosby, p. 286.
8. **4**
Rationale: Toxicity (overdose) produces manifestations of excessive muscarinic stimulation, such as salivation, sweating, involuntary urination and defecation, bradycardia, and severe hypotension. Treatment includes supportive measures and the administration of atropine sulfate subcutaneously or by the IV route.
Test-Taking Strategy: Use the process of elimination, noting the key word "not." Recalling the signs of cholinergic overdose will direct you to option 4. Review these signs if you had difficulty with this question.
Level of Cognitive Ability: Analysis
Client Needs: Physiological Integrity
Integrated Concept/Process: Nursing Process/Assessment
Content Area: Pharmacology
Reference: Salerno, E. (1999). *Pharmacology for health professionals.* St. Louis: Mosby, p. 256.
9. **3**
Rationale: Toxicity (overdosage) of this medication produces central nervous system excitation, such as nervousness, restlessness, hallucinations, and irritability. Other signs of toxicity include either hypotension or hypertension, confusion, tachycardia, flushed or red face, and signs of respiratory depression. Drowsiness is a frequent side effect of the medication, but does not indicate overdosage.
Test-Taking Strategy: Knowledge regarding the manifestations related to toxicity is required to answer this question. Review the signs that indicate toxicity if you had difficulty with this question.
Level of Cognitive Ability: Analysis
Client Needs: Physiological Integrity
Integrated Concept/Process: Nursing Process/Assessment
Content Area: Pharmacology
Reference: Hodgson, B., & Kizior, R. (2001). *Saunders nursing drug handbook 2001.* Philadelphia: W.B. Saunders, p. 799.
10. **1**
Rationale: Pro-Banthine is contraindicated in clients with narrow-angle glaucoma, obstructive uropathy, gastrointestinal disease, or ulcerative colitis. The medication decreases bladder muscle spasms.
Test-Taking Strategy: Use the process of elimination. Eliminate options 2 and 3 because they are similar. From the remaining options, it is necessary to know the contraindications associated with the medication. Review these contraindications if you had difficulty with this question.
Level of Cognitive Ability: Analysis
Client Needs: Safe, Effective Care Environment
Integrated Concept/Process: Nursing Process/Analysis
Content Area: Pharmacology
Reference: Deglin, J., & Vallerand, A. (2001). *Davis's drug guide for nurses* (7th ed.). Philadelphia: F.A. Davis, p. 843.
11. **3**
Rationale: Nephrotoxicity can occur from the use of Sandimmune. Nephrotoxicity is evaluated by monitoring for elevated BUN and serum creatinine levels. Sandimmune does not depress the bone marrow.

Test-Taking Strategy: Use the process of elimination. Eliminate options 1 and 2 first because they are unrelated to renal function. Next, eliminate option 4 because the creatinine level would be elevated not decreased. Option 3 is the only option that indicates an increased level of a renal function test. Review the adverse effects related to this medication if you had difficulty with this question.
Level of Cognitive Ability: Analysis
Client Needs: Physiological Integrity
Integrated Concept/Process: Nursing Process/Analysis
Content Area: Pharmacology
Reference: Hodgson, B., & Kizior, R. (2001). *Saunders nursing drug handbook 2001.* Philadelphia: W.B. Saunders, p. 274.
12. **2**
Rationale: A compound present in grapefruit juice inhibits metabolism of cyclosporine. As a result, consuming grapefruit juice can raise cyclosporine levels by 50% to 100%, thereby greatly increasing the risk of toxicity.
Test-Taking Strategy: Use the process of elimination, noting the key word "avoid." Knowledge regarding substances that inhibit the metabolism of cyclosporine will direct you to option 2. If you had difficulty with this question, review this medication and the client instructions regarding its use.
Level of Cognitive Ability: Application
Client Needs: Health Promotion and Maintenance
Integrated Concept/Process: Teaching/Learning
Content Area: Pharmacology
Reference: Hodgson, B., & Kizior, R. (2001). *Saunders nursing drug handbook 2001.* Philadelphia: W.B. Saunders, p. 273.
13. **4**
Rationale: Amphotericin B as well as erythromycin and ketoconazole can elevate cyclosporine levels. When either of these medications is combined with cyclosporine, the dosage of cyclosporine must be reduced to prevent accumulation to toxic levels.
Test-Taking Strategy: Knowledge regarding the medications that elevate cyclosporine levels is required to answer this question. If you are unfamiliar with these medications, review these medication interactions.
Level of Cognitive Ability: Analysis
Client Needs: Physiological Integrity
Integrated Concept/Process: Nursing Process/Analysis
Content Area: Pharmacology
Reference: Hodgson, B., & Kizior, R. (2001). *Saunders nursing drug handbook 2001.* Philadelphia: W.B. Saunders, p. 273.
14. **3**
Rationale: To improve palatability, the client should be taught to mix the concentrated drug solution with chocolate milk or orange juice just before administration. Grapefruit juice is avoided because it can raise cyclosporine levels. The client is instructed to dilute the concentrate in a glass (not styrofoam) to ensure ingestion of the complete dose.
Test-Taking Strategy: Knowledge regarding the administration of the oral concentrate of cyclosporine is required to answer this question. Review the client instructions regarding administering this medication if you had difficulty with this question.
Level of Cognitive Ability: Application
Client Needs: Health Promotion and Maintenance
Integrated Concept/Process: Teaching/Learning

Content Area: Pharmacology
Reference: Hodgson, B., & Kizior, R. (2001). *Saunders nursing drug handbook 2001.* Philadelphia: W.B. Saunders, p. 272.

15. 3

Rationale: The most common adverse effects of cyclosporine are nephrotoxicity, infection, hypertension, tremors, and hirsutism. Of these, nephrotoxicity and infection are the most serious.

Test-Taking Strategy: Knowledge regarding the adverse effects associated with cyclosporine is required to answer this question. If you are unfamiliar with these effects, review this content.

Level of Cognitive Ability: Analysis
Client Needs: Physiological Integrity
Integrated Concept/Process: Nursing Process/Assessment
Content Area: Pharmacology
Reference: Hodgson, B., & Kizior, R. (2001). *Saunders nursing drug handbook 2001.* Philadelphia: W.B. Saunders, pp. 273-274.

16. 3

Rationale: Prograf is used with caution in immunosuppressed clients and in clients with renal, hepatic, or pancreatic function impairment. It is contraindicated in clients with hypersensitivity to this medication or hypersensitivity to cyclosporine.

Test-Taking Strategy: Use the process of elimination. Many medications affect renal, hepatic, and pancreatic function. If you had to select an option and were unsure, select the option that addresses these body systems. Review the cautions and contraindications associated with the administration of this medication, if you had difficulty with this question.

Level of Cognitive Ability: Analysis
Client Needs: Physiological Integrity
Integrated Concept/Process: Nursing Process/Analysis
Content Area: Pharmacology
Reference: Hodgson, B., & Kizior, R. (2001). *Saunders nursing drug handbook 2001.* Philadelphia: W.B. Saunders, p. 960.

17. 2

Rationale: Nephrotoxicity is a major concern with this medication. Other common reactions include neurotoxicity evidenced by headache, tremor, and insomnia, gastrointestinal effects such as diarrhea, nausea, and vomiting, hypertension, hyperkalemia, and hyperglycemia.

Test-Taking Strategy: Use the process of elimination, noting that options 1, 3, and 4 represent normal values. Option 2 is the only abnormal value, reflecting an elevation. Review the adverse effects related to this medication if you had difficulty with this question.

Level of Cognitive Ability: Analysis
Client Needs: Physiological Integrity
Integrated Concept/Process: Nursing Process/Analysis
Content Area: Pharmacology
Reference: Clark, J., Queener, S., & Karb, V. (2000). *Pharmacologic basis of nursing practice* (6th ed.). St. Louis: Mosby, p. 463.

18. 3

Rationale: CellCept should be administered on an empty stomach. The capsules should not be opened or crushed. The client should contact the physician if unusual bleeding or bruising, sore throat, mouth sores, abdominal pain, or fever occurs. Antacids containing magnesium and aluminum may decrease the absorption of the medication and therefore should not be taken with the medication. The medication is given in combination with corticosteroids and cyclosporine.

Test-Taking Strategy: Use the process of elimination. Recalling that neutropenia can occur with the use of this medication will direct you to option 3. Review this medication if you had difficulty with this question.

Level of Cognitive Ability: Application
Client Needs: Health Promotion and Maintenance
Integrated Concept/Process: Teaching/Learning
Content Area: Pharmacology
Reference: Hodgson, B., & Kizior, R. (2001). *Saunders nursing drug handbook 2001.* Philadelphia: W.B. Saunders, p. 709-711.

19. 2

Rationale: Epoetin alfa is used to reverse anemia associated with chronic renal failure. Therapeutic effect is seen when the hematocrit is between 30% and 33%. Options 1, 3, and 4 are not associated with the action of this medication.

Test-Taking Strategy: Use the process of elimination. Relate the name of the medication, "erythropoietin," to the potential action or effect. The only laboratory test that would reflect the effect of this medication is option 2. Review the therapeutic effect of this medication, if you had difficulty with this question.

Level of Cognitive Ability: Analysis
Client Needs: Physiological Integrity
Integrated Concept/Process: Nursing Process/Analysis
Content Area: Pharmacology
Reference: Wilson, B., Shannon, M., & Stang, C. (2000). *Nurses drug guide 2000.* Stamford, Conn.: Appleton & Lange, p. 523.

20. 3

Rationale: The client should be instructed not to shake the bottle. The medication should be refrigerated at all times. All partially used vials should be discarded, and the client should use only 1 dose per vial and not reenter the vial. Unused portions need to be discarded.

Test-Taking Strategy: Use the process of elimination. Note the key words "accurate description." Note that options 3 and 4 are identifying opposite actions. This should provide you with the clue that one of these options may be the correct one. Review the teaching points related to the administration of this medication if you had difficulty with this question.

Level of Cognitive Ability: Application
Client Needs: Health Promotion and Maintenance
Integrated Concept/Process: Teaching/Learning
Content Area: Pharmacology
Reference: Wilson, B., Shannon, M., & Stang, C. (2000). *Nurses drug guide 2000.* Stamford, Conn.: Appleton & Lange, p. 524.

CRITICAL THINKING: FREE-TEXT ENTRY

Answer: Atropine sulfate

Rationale: Cholinergic overdose can occur with bethanechol chloride (Urecholine). The antidote is atropine sulfate, administered subcutaneously or IV, and it should be readily available for use should overdose occur.

Test-Taking Strategy: Knowledge regarding the antidote for bethanechol chloride is required to answer this question. Review this medication and its antidote if you had difficulty with this question.

Level of Cognitive Ability: Application
Client Needs: Physiological Integrity
Integrated Concept/Process: Nursing Process/Planning
Content Area: Pharmacology
Reference: Salerno, E. (1999). *Pharmacology for health professionals.* St. Louis: Mosby, p. 258.

REFERENCES

Clark, J., Queener, S., & Karb, V. (2000). *Pharmacologic basis of nursing practice* (6th ed.). St. Louis: Mosby.

Deglin, J., & Vallerand, A. (2001). *Davis's drug guide for nurses* (7th ed.). Philadelphia: F.A. Davis.

Gutierrez, K. (1999). *Pharmacotherapeutics: Clinical decision-making in nursing.* Philadelphia: W.B. Saunders.

Hodgson, B., & Kizior, R. (2001). *Saunders nursing drug handbook 2001.* Philadelphia: W.B. Saunders.

Kuhn, M. (1998). *Pharmacotherapeutics: A nursing process approach* (4th ed.). Philadelphia: F.A. Davis.

Lehne, R. (1998). *Pharmacology for nursing care* (3rd ed.). Philadelphia: W.B. Saunders.

Salerno, E. (1999). *Pharmacology for health professionals.* St. Louis: Mosby.

Wilson, B., Shannon, M., & Stang, C. (2000). *Nurses drug guide 2000.* Stamford, Conn.: Appleton & Lange.

The Adult Client with an Eye or Ear Disorder

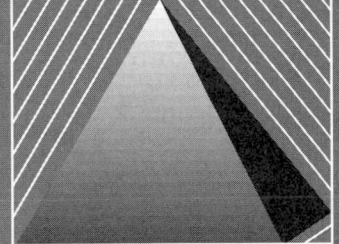

PYRAMID TERMS

accommodation   Process by which a clear visual image is maintained as the gaze is shifted from a distant to a near point.

astigmatism   Corneal curvature; eye may be hyperopic or myopic.

cataracts   An opacity of the lens that distorts the image projected onto the retina and that can progress to blindness.

conductive hearing loss   When sound waves are blocked to the inner ear fibers because of external ear or middle ear disorders. Disorders can often be corrected with no damage to hearing, or minimal permanent hearing loss.

cycloplegia   Refers to the paralysis of the ciliary muscles by medications that block muscarinic receptors. Cycloplegia causes blurred vision because the shape of the lens can no longer be adjusted to near vision.

emmetropia   Term to describe ideal refraction of the eye.

fenestration   Removal of the stapes with a small hole drilled in the footplate, and a prosthesis is connected between the incus and foot plate. Sounds cause the prosthesis to vibrate in the same manner as did the stapes.

glaucoma   Increased intraocular pressure as a result of inadequate drainage of aqueous humor from canal of the Schlemm or overproduction of aqueous humor. The condition damages the optic nerve and can result in blindness.

hyperopia   Farsightedness; objects converge to a point behind the retina. Vision beyond 20 feet is normal, but near vision is poor. Correction is done by a convex lens.

legally blind   If the best visual acuity with corrective lenses in the better eye is 20/200 or less, or if visual acuity is less than 20 degrees of the visual field in the better eye.

Meniere's syndrome   A syndrome also called endolymphatic hydrops, which refers to dilation of the endolymphatic system by either overproduction or decreased reabsorption of endolymphatic fluid. It is characterized by tinnitus, unilateral sensorineural hearing loss, and vertigo.

miosis   Refers to a constricted pupil and is achieved primarily by stimulating the muscarinic receptors of the sphincter muscles.

miotics   Medications that cause contraction of the pupil.

mydriasis   Refers to a dilated pupil and is achieved by blocking the muscarinic receptors of the sphincter muscles or by stimulating the alpha receptors of the dilator muscles.

mydriatics   Medications that dilate the pupil.

myopia   Nearsightedness; rays coming from an object are focused in front of the retina. Near vision is normal, but distant vision is defective. A biconcave lens is used for correction.

otosclerosis   Disease of the labyrinthine capsule of the middle ear that results in a bony overgrowth of tissue surrounding the ossicles. Causes the development of irregular areas of new bone formation and causes fixation of the bones. Stapes fixation leads to a conductive hearing loss.

presbycusis   Common cause of sensorineural hearing loss associated with aging.

refraction   Process of bending light rays so as to focus an image on the retina.

retinal detachment   Occurs when the layers of the retina separate because of the accumulation of fluid between them, or when both retinal layers elevate away from the choroid as a result of a tumor. Partial separation becomes complete if untreated. When detachment becomes complete, blindness occurs.

sensorineural hearing loss   A pathological process of the inner ear or of the sensory fibers that lead to the cerebral cortex. Is often permanent, and measures must be taken to reduce further damage or to attempt to amplify sound as a means of improving hearing to some degree.

PYRAMID TO SUCCESS

Pyramid points focus on nursing interventions for clients with impairment in sight or hearing and on the nursing care related to disorders such as cataracts, glaucoma, and retinal detachment. Pyramid points also focus on emergency interventions for eye and ear disorders and injuries. Review nursing care related to organ donation for the donor and the recipient. Pyramid points also focus on client instructions related to medication administration, sensory perceptual alterations and safety issues, and available support systems. The Integrated Concepts and Processes addressed in this unit include Nursing Process, Caring, Communication and Documentation, Cultural Awareness, Self-Care, and Teaching/Learning.

CLIENT NEEDS

Safe, Effective Care Environment

Accident prevention related to sensory impairments
Asepsis with procedures and treatments
Client rights
Communication techniques for impaired vision or hearing
Consultation with members of the health care team
Establishing priorities
Informed consent for invasive procedures
Organ donation
Standard (universal) precautions

Health Promotion and Maintenance

Aging process
Expected body image changes
Home care instructions following procedures related to the eye or the ear
Instructions regarding the administration of eye and ear medications
Physical assessment of eye and ear disorders
Reinforcement regarding the importance of compliance with the prescribed therapy
The prevention and early detection of health problems and diseases related to the eye or the ear

Psychosocial Integrity

Available community resources
Family support systems
Role changes
Sensory perceptual alterations

The ability to cope with feelings of isolation and loss of independence
The threat of vision or hearing loss

Physiological Integrity

Care of assistive devices such as glasses, contact lens, and hearing aids
Complications related to procedures
Expected responses to therapy
Medical emergencies
Pharmacological therapy
Self-care limitations

REFERENCES

Craven, R., & Hirnle, C. (2000). *Fundamentals of nursing: Human health and function* (3rd ed.). Philadelphia: Lippincott.

Harkreader, H. (2000). *Fundamentals of nursing: Caring and clinical judgment.* Philadelphia: W.B. Saunders.

Ignatavicius, D., Workman, M., & Mishler, M. (1999). *Medical-surgical nursing across the health care continuum* (3rd ed.). Philadelphia: W.B. Saunders.

LeMone, P., & Burke, K. (2000). *Medical-surgical nursing: Critical thinking in client care* (2nd ed.). Upper Saddle River, N.J.: Prentice-Hall.

Lewis, S., Heitkemper, M., & Dirksen, S. (2000). *Medical-surgical nursing: Assessment and management of clinical problems* (5th ed.). St. Louis: Mosby.

National Council of State Boards of Nursing (eds.) (2000). *Test Plan for the National Council Licensure Examination for Registered Nurses.* Chicago: Author.

Potter, P., & Perry, A. (2001). *Fundamentals of nursing* (5th ed.). St. Louis: Mosby.

Smeltzer, S., & Bare, B. (2000). *Textbook of medical-surgical nursing* (9th ed). Philadelphia: Lippincott Williams & Wilkins.

61

The Eye and The Ear

I. ANATOMY AND PHYSIOLOGY OF THE EYE

A. The eye
  1. The eye is 1 inch in diameter
  2. It is located in the anterior portion of the orbit
  3. The orbit is the bony structure of the skull that surrounds the eye and offers protection to the eye

B. Layers of the eye
  1. External layer
     a. The fibrous coat that supports the eye
     b. Contains the sclera, which is an opaque white tissue
     c. Contains the cornea, which is a dense transparent layer
  2. Middle layer
     a. The second layer of the eyeball
     b. Is vascular and heavily pigmented
     c. Consists of the choroid, the ciliary body, and the iris
     d. The choroid is the dark brown membrane located between the sclera and the retina
     e. The choroid lines most of the sclera and is attached to the retina, but can easily detach from the sclera
     f. The choroid contains many blood vessels and supplies nutrients to the retina
     g. The ciliary body connects the choroid with the iris and secretes aqueous humor that helps give the eye its shape
     h. The iris is the colored portion of the eye, is located in front of the lens, and has a central circular opening called the pupil
  3. Internal layer
     a. Consists of the retina
     b. The retina is a thin, delicate structure in which the fibers of the optic nerve are distributed
     c. The retina is bordered externally by the choroid and sclera and internally by the vitreous
     d. The retina contains blood vessels and photoreceptors called rods and cones

C. Vitreous body
  1. Contains a gelatinous substance that occupies the vitreous chamber, which is the space between the lens and the retina
  2. It transmits light and gives shape to the posterior eye

D. Vitreous
  1. A jell-like substance that maintains the shape of the eye
  2. Provides additional physical support to the retina

E. Rods and cones
  1. Rods are responsible for peripheral vision and function at reduced levels of illumination
  2. Cones function at bright levels of illumination and are responsible for color vision and central vision

F. Optic disk
  1. A creamy pink to white depressed area in the retina; the optic nerve enters and exits the eyeball at this area
  2. This area is called the blind spot because it contains only nerve fibers, lacks photoreceptor cells, and is insensitive to light

G. Macula lutea
  1. A small, oval, yellowish pink area located lateral and temporal to the optic disk
  2. The central depressed part of the macula is the fovea centralis, where most acute vision occurs

H. Aqueous humor
  1. A clear watery fluid that fills the anterior and posterior chambers of the eye
  2. Produced by the ciliary processes, and the fluid drains into the canal of Schlemm
  3. The anterior chamber lies between the cornea and the iris
  4. The posterior chamber lies between the iris and the lens

I. Canal of Schlemm
   1. A passageway that extends completely around the eye
   2. Permits fluid to drain out of the eye into the systemic circulation so that a constant intraocular pressure is maintained
J. Lens
   1. A transparent circular structure behind the iris and in front of the vitreous body
   2. Bends rays of light so that the light falls on the retina
K. Pupils
   1. Control the amount of light that enters the eye and reaches the retina
   2. Darkness produces dilation
   3. Light produces constriction
L. Conjunctivae
   1. The thin transparent mucous membranes
   2. Line the posterior surface of each eyelid and located over the sclera
M. Lacrimal gland
   1. Produces tears
   2. Tears are drained through the punctum into the lacrimal duct and sac
N. Eye muscles
   1. Muscles do not work independently but work in conjunction with the muscle that produces the opposite movement
   2. Rectus muscles: exert their pull when the eye turns temporally
   3. Oblique muscles: exert their pull when the eye turns nasally
O. Nerves
   1. Cranial nerve II: optic nerve (nerve of sight)
   2. Cranial nerve III: oculomotor
   3. Cranial nerve IV: trochlear
   4. Cranial nerve VI: abducens
P. Blood vessels
   1. Ophthalmic artery: major artery supplying the structures in the eye
   2. Ophthalmic veins: venous drainage occurs through the veins

II. ASSESSMENT OF VISION

A. Acuity
   1. Visual acuity tests measure the client's distance and near vision
   2. Snellen chart
      a. A simple tool to record visual acuity
      b. The client stands 20 feet from the chart and covers one eye and uses the other eye to read the line that appears most clearly
      c. If the client is able to do this accurately, the client reads the next lower line
      d. This sequence is repeated until the client is unable to correctly identify more than half of the characters on the line
      e. The procedure is repeated for the other eye
      f. The findings are recorded as a comparison between what the client can read at 20 feet and the number of feet normally required by an individual to read the same line
      g. A result of 20/50 means that the client is able to read at 20 feet from the chart what a healthy eye can read at 50 feet
      h. Clients who wear corrective lenses other than for reading should have their vision tested with the lens in place
B. Confrontational test
   1. Performed to examine visual fields or peripheral vision
   2. The examiner and the client sit facing each other
   3. The client is asked to look directly into the eyes of the examiner throughout the test
   4. The examiner covers their right eye while the client covers his or her left eye
   5. The examiner moves a finger from a nonvisible area into the client's line of vision
   6. Both examiner and client should see the object at approximately the same time
   7. When the client sees the object coming into the line of vision, the client informs the examiner
   8. The procedure is repeated on the opposite eye
   9. The test assumes that the examiner has normal peripheral vision
C. Extraocular muscle function
   1. Six cardinal positions of gaze
      a. Client's right (lateral position)
      b. Upward and right (temporal position)
      c. Down and right
      d. Client's left (lateral position)
      e. Upward and left (temporal position)
      f. Down and left
   2. Client holds head still and is asked to move eyes and to follow a small object
   3. The examiner looks for any parallel movements of the eye or for nystagmus, an involuntary rhythmic rapid twitching of the eyeballs
D. Color vision
   1. Tests for color vision involve picking numbers or letters out of a complex and colorful picture
   2. Ishihara chart
      a. Consists of numbers that are composed of colored dots located within a circle of colored dots
      b. Client is asked to read the numbers on the chart
      c. Each eye is tested separately
      d. The test is sensitive for the diagnosis of red/green blindness but not effective for the detection of the discrimination of blue
E. Pupils
   1. Round and of equal size
   2. Increasing light causes pupillary constriction

3. Decreasing light causes pupillary dilation
4. Constriction of both pupils is a normal response to direct light
5. The client is asked to look straight ahead while the examiner quickly brings a beam of light (flashlight) in from the side and directs it onto the eye
6. The constriction of the eye is a direct response to the shining of a light into that eye; constriction of the opposite eye is known as a consensual response

F. Sclera and cornea
1. Normal sclera color is white
2. A yellow color to the sclera may indicate jaundice or systemic problems
3. In a dark-skinned person, the sclera may normally appear yellow; pigmented dots may be present
4. The cornea is transparent, smooth, shiny, and bright
5. Cloudy areas or specks on the cornea may be the result of an accident or eye injury

G. Ophthalmoscopy
1. An instrument is used to examine the external structures and the interior of the eye
2. Darken the room so that the pupil will dilate
3. Hold the instrument with the right hand when examining the right eye and with the left hand when examining the left eye
4. Ask the client to look straight ahead at an object on the wall
5. Approach the client's eye from about 12 to 15 inches away and 15 degrees lateral to the client's line of vision
6. As the instrument is directed at the pupil, a red glare (red reflex) is seen in the pupil
7. The red reflex is the reflection of light on the vascular retina
8. Absence of the red reflex may indicate opacity of the lens
9. The retina, optic disk, optic vessels, fundus, and macula can be examined

III. DIAGNOSTIC TESTS FOR THE EYE

A. Fluorescein angiography
1. Description: detailed imaging and recording of ocular circulation by a series of photographs after the administration of a dye
2. Implementation preprocedure
   a. Assess the client for allergies and previous reactions to dyes
   b. Obtain informed consent
   c. A mydriatic medication, which causes pupil dilation, is instilled in the eye 1 hour before the test
   d. The dye is injected into a vein of the client's arm
   e. Inform the client that the dye may cause the skin to appear yellow for several hours after the test and is gradually eliminated through the urine
   f. The client may experience nausea, vomiting, sneezing, paresthesia of the tongue, or pain at the injection site
   g. If hives appear, oral or intramuscular (IM) antihistamines such as diphenhydramine (Benadryl) are administered as prescribed
3. Implementation postprocedure
   a. Encourage rest
   b. Encourage fluids to assist in eliminating the dye from the client's system
   c. Remind the client that the yellow skin appearance will disappear
   d. Instruct the client that the urine will appear bright green until the dye is excreted
   e. Instruct the client to avoid direct sunlight for a few hours after the test
   f. Instruct the client that the photophobia will continue until pupil size returns to normal

B. Computed tomography
1. Description
   a. A beam of x-ray scans the skull and orbits of the eye
   b. A cross-sectional image is formed by the use of a computer
   c. Contrast material is not usually administered
2. Implementation
   a. No special client preparation or follow-up care is required
   b. Instruct the client that he or she will be positioned in a confined space and need to keep the head still during the procedure

C. Slit lamp
1. Description
   a. Allows examination of the anterior ocular structures under microscopic magnification
   b. The client leans on a chin rest to stabilize the head while a narrowed beam of light is aimed so that it illuminates only a narrow segment of the eye
2. Implementation
   a. Explain the procedure to the client
   b. Advise the client about the brightness of the light and the need to look forward at a point over the examiner's ear

D. Corneal staining
1. Description
   a. Instillation of a topical dye into the conjuctival sac to outline irregularities of the corneal surface that are not easily visible
   b. The eye is viewed through a blue filter, and a bright green color indicates areas of a nonintact corneal epithelium

2. Implementation
   a. If the client wears contact lenses, they must be removed
   b. The client is instructed to blink after the dye has been applied, to distribute the dye evenly across the cornea
E. Tonometry
   1. Description
      a. The test is primarily used to assess for an increase in intraocular pressure and potential **glaucoma**
      b. Normal ocular pressure is 8 to 21 mm Hg
   2. Implementation
      a. Each eye is anesthetized
      b. The client is asked to stare forward at a point above the examiner's ear
      c. A flattened cone is brought into contact with the cornea
      d. The amount of pressure needed to flatten the cornea is measured
      e. The client must be instructed to avoid rubbing the eye following the examination if the eye has been anesthetized, because the potential for scratching the cornea exists

IV. DISORDERS OF THE EYE
A. Risk factors related to eye disorders (Box 61-1)
B. **Legally blind**
   1. Description: If the best visual acuity with corrective lenses in the better eye is 20/200 or less, or a visual field of 20 degrees or less in the better eye
   2. Implementation
      a. When speaking to the client who has limited sight or is blind, the nurse uses a normal tone of voice
      b. Alert the client when approaching
      c. Orient the client to the environment
      d. Use a focal point and provide further orientation to the environment from that focal point
      e. Allow the client to touch objects in the room
      f. Use the clock placement of foods on the meal tray to orient the client
      g. Promote independence as much as is possible
      h. Provide radios, TVs, and clocks that give the time orally, or provide a Braille watch
      i. When ambulating, allow the client to grasp

the nurse's arm at the elbow; the nurse keeps his or her arm close to the body so that the client can detect the direction of movement
   j. Instruct the client to remain one step behind the nurse when ambulating
   k. Instruct the client in the use of the cane used for the blind client, which is differentiated from other canes by its straight shape and white color with red tip
   l. Instruct the client that the cane is held in the dominant hand several inches off the floor
   m. Instruct the client that the cane sweeps the ground where the client's foot will be placed next, to determine the presence of obstacles
C. **Cataracts**
   1. Description
      a. An opacity of the lens that distorts the image projected onto the retina and that can progress to blindness
      b. Causes include the aging process (senile **cataracts**), inherited (congenital **cataracts**), and injury (traumatic **cataracts**); can also occur as a result of another eye disease (secondary **cataracts**)
      c. Intervention is indicated when visual acuity has been reduced to a level that the client finds to be unacceptable or adversely affecting lifestyle
   2. Assessment
      a. Opaque or cloudy white pupil
      b. Gradual loss of vision
      c. Blurred vision
      d. Decreased color perception
      e. Vision that is better in dim light with pupil dilation
      f. Photophobia
      g. Absence of the red reflex
   3. Implementation
      a. Surgical removal of the lens, one eye at a time
      b. Extracapsular extraction: the lens is lifted out without removing the lens capsule; may be performed by phacoemulsification, in which the lens is broken up by ultrasonic vibrations and extracted
      c. Intracapsular extraction: the lens is removed within its capsule through a small incision
      d. A partial iridectomy may be performed with the lens extraction to prevent acute secondary **glaucoma**
      e. A lens implantation may be performed at the time of the surgical procedure
   4. Preoperative implementation
      a. Instruct the client regarding the postoperative measures to prevent or decrease intraocular pressure
      b. Administer preoperative eye medications, including **mydriatics** and **cycloplegics,** as prescribed

---
BOX 61-1

Risk Factors of Eye Disorders

Aging process
Congenital
Diabetes mellitus
Hereditary
Medications
Trauma

5. Postoperative implementation
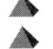
   a. Elevate the head of the bed 30 to 45 degrees
   b. Turn the client to the back or unoperative side
   c. Maintain an eye patch; orient the client to the environment
   d. Position the client's personal belongings on the nonoperative side
   e. Use side rails for safety
   f. Assist with ambulation
6. Client education (Box 61-2)

D. Glaucoma
1. Description
   a. Increased intraocular pressure as a result of inadequate drainage of aqueous humor from the canal of Schlemm or overproduction of aqueous humor
   b. The condition damages the optic nerve and can result in blindness
2. Types
   a. Acute closed-angle or narrow-angle **glaucoma**: results from obstruction to outflow to aqueous humor
   b. Chronic closed-angle **glaucoma**: follows an untreated attack of acute closed-angle **glaucoma**
   c. Chronic open-angle **glaucoma**: results from overproduction or obstruction to the outflow of aqueous humor
   d. Acute: a rapid onset of intraocular pressure greater than 50 to 70 mm Hg
   e. Chronic: a slow, progressive, gradual onset of intraocular pressure greater than 30 to 50 mm Hg

---

BOX 61-2

Client Education Following Cataract Surgery

Avoid eye straining
Avoid rubbing or placing pressure on the eyes
Avoid rapid movements, straining, sneezing, coughing, bending, vomiting, or lifting objects over 5 pounds
Measures to prevent constipation
Dressing changes and prescribed eye drops and medications
Wipe excess drainage or tearing with a sterile wet cotton ball from the inner to the outward canthus
Use an eye shield at bedtime
If a lens implant is not performed, the eye cannot accommodate and glasses must be worn at all times
Cataract glasses act as magnifying glasses and replace central vision only
Cataract glasses magnify, and objects will appear closer; therefore, the client needs to accommodate, judge distance, and climb stairs carefully
Contact lenses provide sharp visual acuity, but dexterity is needed to insert them
Contact the physician for any decrease in vision, severe eye pain, or increase in eye discharge

---

3. Assessment
   a. Progressive loss of peripheral vision followed by loss of central vision
   b. Elevated intraocular pressure (normal pressure is 10 to 21 mm Hg)
   c. Vision worsening in the evening with difficulty adjusting to dark rooms
   d. Blurred vision
   e. Halos around white lights
   f. Frontal headaches
   g. Eye pain
   h. Photophobia
   i. Lacrimation
   j. Progressive loss of central vision
4. Implementation for acute **glaucoma**
   a. Treat as a medical emergency
   b. Administer medications as prescribed to lower intraocular pressure
   c. Prepare the client for peripheral iridectomy, which allows aqueous humor to flow from the posterior to anterior chamber
5. Implementation for chronic **glaucoma**
   a. Instruct the client in the importance of medications: **miotics** to constrict the pupils, carbonic anhydrase inhibitors to decrease the production of aqueous humor, and beta blockers to decrease the production of aqueous humor and intraocular pressure
   b. Instruct the client about the need for lifelong medication use
   c. Instruct the client to wear a Medic-Alert bracelet
   d. Instruct the client to avoid anticholinergic medications
   e. Instruct the client to report eye pain, halos around the eyes, and changes in vision to the physician
   f. Instruct the client that when maximal medical therapy has failed to halt the progression of visual field loss and optic nerve damage, surgery will be recommended
   g. Prepare the client for trabeculoplasty as prescribed to facilitate aqueous humor drainage
   h. Prepare the client for trabeculectomy as prescribed, which allows drainage of aqueous humor into the conjunctival spaces by the creation of an opening

E. Retinal detachment
1. Description
   a. Occurs when the layers of the retina separate because of the accumulation of fluid between them, or when both retinal layers elevate away from the choroid as a result of a tumor
   b. Partial separation becomes complete if untreated
   c. When detachment becomes complete, blindness occurs

2. Assessment
   a. Flashes of light
   b. Floaters
   c. Increase in blurred vision
   d. Sense of a curtain being drawn
   e. Loss of a portion of the visual field
3. Immediate implementation
   a. Provide bed rest
   b. Cover both eyes with patches to prevent further detachment
   c. Speak to the client before approaching
   d. Position the client's head as prescribed
   e. Protect the client from injury
   f. Avoid jerky head movements
   g. Minimize eye stress
   h. Prepare the client for the surgical procedure as prescribed
4. Surgical procedures
   a. Draining fluid from the subretinal space so that the retina can return to the normal position
   b. Sealing retinal breaks by cryosurgery, a cold probe applied to the sclera, to stimulate an inflammatory response leading to adhesions
   c. Diathermy, the use of an electrode needle and heat through the sclera, to stimulate an inflammatory response
   d. Laser therapy, to stimulate an inflammatory response, to seal small retinal tears before the detachment occurs
   e. Scleral buckling, to hold the choroid and retina together with a splint, until scar tissue forms, closing the tear
   f. Insertion of gas or silicone oil to encourage attachment because these agents have a specific gravity less than vitreous or air, and can float against the retina
5. Postoperative implementation
   a. Maintain eye patches bilaterally as prescribed
   b. Monitor for hemorrhage
   c. Prevent nausea and vomiting and monitor for restlessness, which can cause hemorrhage
   d. Monitor for sudden, sharp eye pain (notify the physician)
   e. Encourage deep breathing but avoid coughing
   f. Provide bed rest for 1 to 2 days as prescribed
   g. Position the client as prescribed
   h. If gas has been inserted, position as prescribed on the abdomen and turn the head so unaffected eye is down
   i. Administer eye medications as prescribed
   j. Assist the client with activities of daily living
   k. Avoid sudden head movements or anything that increases intraocular pressure
   l. Instruct the client to limit reading for 3 to 5 weeks
   m. Instruct the client to avoid squinting, straining

and constipation, lifting heavy objects, and bending from the waist
   n. Instruct the client to wear dark glasses during the day and an eye patch at night
   o. Encourage follow-up care because of the danger of recurrence or occurrence in the other eye

F. Hyphema
1. Description
   a. The presence of blood in the anterior chamber
   b. Occurs as a result of an injury
   c. The condition usually resolves in 5 to 7 days
2. Implementation
   a. Encourage rest with the client in semi-Fowler's position
   b. Avoid sudden eye movements for 3 to 5 days to decrease the likelihood of bleeding
   c. Administer cycloplegic eye drops as prescribed to place the eye at rest
   d. Instruct the client in the use of eye shields or eye patches as prescribed
   e. Instruct the client to restrict reading and watching television

G. Contusions
1. Description
   a. Bleeding into the soft tissue as a result of an injury
   b. Causes a black eye and the discoloration disappears in approximately 10 days
   c. Pain, photophobia, edema, and diplopia may occur
2. Implementation
   a. Place ice on the eye immediately
   b. Instruct the client to receive an eye examination

H. Foreign bodies
1. Description: an object such as dust that enters the eye
2. Implementation
   a. Have the client look upward, expose the lower lid, wet a cotton-tipped applicator with sterile normal saline, and gently twist the swab over the particle and remove it
   b. If the particle cannot be seen, have the client look downward, place a cotton applicator horizontally on the outer surface of the upper eye lid, grasp the lashes, and pull the upper lid outward and over the cotton applicator; if the particle is seen, gently twist swab over it to remove

I. Penetrating objects
1. Description: an injury that occurs to the eye in which an object penetrates the eye
2. Implementation
   a. Never remove the object because it may be holding ocular structures in place; the object must be removed by the physician

b. Cover the object with a cup

c. Do not allow the client to bend

d. Do not place pressure on eye

e. Client is to be seen by a physician immediately

J. Chemical burns

1. Description: an eye injury in which a caustic substance enters the eye

2. Implementation

a. Treatment should begin immediately

b. Flush the eyes at the site of injury with water for at least 15 to 20 minutes

c. At the scene of the injury, obtain a sample of the chemical involved

d. At the emergency room, the eye is irrigated with normal saline solution or an ophthalmic irrigation solution

e. The solution is directed across the cornea and toward the lateral canthus

f. Prepare for visual acuity assessment

g. Apply an antibiotic ointment as prescribed

h. Cover the eye with a patch as prescribed

K. Enucleation and exenteration

1. Description

a. Enucleation: removal of the entire eyeball

b. Exenteration: removal of the eyeball and surrounding tissues and bone

c. Performed for the removal of ocular tumors

d. After the eye is removed, a ball implant is inserted to provide a firm base for socket prosthesis and to facilitate the best cosmetic result

e. A prosthesis is fitted approximately 1 month after surgery

2. Preoperative implementation

a. Provide emotional support to the client

b. Encourage the client to verbalize feelings related to loss

3. Postoperative implementation

a. Monitor vital signs

b. Assess pressure patch or dressing

c. Report changes in vital signs or the presence of bright red drainage on the pressure patch or dressing

L. Organ donation

1. Donor eyes

a. Obtained from cadavers

b. Must be enucleated soon after death because of rapid endothelial cell death

c. Must be stored in a preserving solution

d. Storage, handling, and coordination of donor tissue with surgeons is provided by a network of state eye bank associations across the country

2. Care of the deceased client as a potential eye donor

a. Discuss the option of eye donation with the physician and family

b. Raise the head of the bed 30 degrees

c. Instill antibiotic eye drops as prescribed

d. Close the eyes and apply a small ice pack to the closed eyes

3. Preoperative care of the recipient

a. Recipient may be told of the tissue availability only several hours to 1 day before the surgery

b. Assist in alleviating client anxiety

c. Assess eye for signs of infection

d. Report the presence of any redness, watery or purulent drainage, or edema around the eye to the physician

e. Instill antibiotic drops into the eye as prescribed to reduce the number of microorganisms present

f. Administer IV fluids and medications as prescribed

4. Postoperative care to the recipient

a. Eye is covered with a pressure patch and protective shield that are left in place until the next day

b. Do not remove or change the dressing without a physician's order

c. Monitor vital signs

d. Monitor level of consciousness

e. Assess dressing

f. Position the client on the nonoperative side to reduce intraocular pressure

g. Orient the client frequently

h. Monitor for complications of bleeding, wound leakage, infection, and graft rejection

i. Instruct the client in how to apply a patch and eye shield

j. Instruct the client to wear the eye shield at night for 1 month and whenever around small children or pets

k. Advise the client not to rub the eye

5. Graft rejection

a. Can occur at any time

b. Inform the client of the signs of rejection

c. Signs include redness, swelling, decreased vision, and pain (RSVP)

d. Treated with topical corticosteroids

V. ANATOMY AND PHYSIOLOGY OF THE EAR

A. Functions

1. Hearing

2. Maintenance of balance

B. External ear

1. Embedded in the temporal bone bilaterally at the level of the eyes

2. Extends from the auricle through the external canal to the tympanic membrane or eardrum

3. Includes the mastoid process, which is the bony ridge located over the temporal bone

C. Middle ear

1. Consists of the medial side of the tympanic membrane

2. Contains three bony ossicles
   a. Malleus
   b. Incus
   c. Stapes
3. The tympanic membrane is a thick transparent sheet of tissue that provides a barrier between the external and the middle ear
4. The middle ear is protected from the inner ear by the round and the oval window membranes
5. The eustachian tube opens into the middle ear and allows for equalization of pressure on both sides of the tympanic membrane

D. Inner ear
1. Contains the semicircular canals, the cochlea, and the distal end of the eighth cranial nerve
2. The semicircular canals contain fluid and hair cells connected to sensory nerve fibers of the vestibular portion of eighth cranial nerve
3. Maintains sense of balance or equilibrium
4. Cochlea: spiral-shaped organ of hearing
5. Organ of Corti: receptor and organ of hearing
6. Eighth cranial nerve
   a. Cochlear branch: transmits neuroimpulses from the cochlea to the brain, where they are interpreted as sound
   b. Vestibular branch: maintains balance and equilibrium

E. Hearing and equilibrium
1. The external ear conducts sound waves to the middle ear
2. The middle ear, also called the tympanic cavity, conducts sound waves to the inner ear
3. The middle ear is filled with air, which is kept at atmospheric pressure by the opening of the eustachian tube
4. The inner ear contains sensory receptors for sound and for equilibrium
5. The receptors in the inner ear transmit sound waves and changes in body position to the nerve impulses

VI. ASSESSMENT OF THE EAR
A. Otoscopic exam
1. The speculum is never blindly introduced into the external canal because of the risk of perforating the tympanic membrane
2. Tilt the client's head slightly away and hold the otoscope upside down as if it were a large pen, as this permits the examiner's hand to lie against the client's head for support
3. Pull the pinna up and back to straighten the external canal in an adult
4. Visualize the external canal while slowly inserting the speculum
5. The normal external canal is pink and intact without lesions and with various amounts of cerumen and fine little hairs

6. Assess the tympanic membrane for intactness; the normal tympanic membrane is intact, without perforations, and should be free from lesions
7. The tympanic membrane is transparent, opaque, pearly gray, and slightly concave

B. Auditory assessment
1. Sound is transmitted by air conduction and bone conduction
2. Air conduction is two to three times longer than bone conduction
3. Hearing loss is categorized as **conductive, sensorineural**, and mixed **conductive** and **sensorineural**
4. **Conductive hearing loss** is due to any physical obstruction to the transmission of sound waves
5. **Sensorineural hearing loss** is due to a defect in the organ of hearing, in the eighth cranial nerve, or in the brain itself
6. A mixed **conductive, sensorineural hearing loss** results in profound hearing loss

C. Voice test
1. Ask the client to block one external canal
2. The examiner stands 1 to 2 feet away and quietly whispers a statement
3. The client is asked to repeat the whispered statement
4. Each ear is tested separately

D. Watch test
1. A ticking watch is used to test for high-frequency sounds
2. The examiner holds a ticking watch about 5 inches from each ear and asks the client if the ticking is heard

E. Tuning fork tests
1. Weber tuning fork test
   a. Place the vibrating tuning fork stem in the middle of the client's head at the midline of the forehead or above the upper lip over the teeth
   b. Hold the fork by the stem only
   c. The client is asked whether the sound is heard equally in both ears or whether the sound is louder in one ear
   d. Normal test result is hearing the sound equally in both ears
   e. If the client hears the sound louder in one ear, the term lateralization is applied to the side hearing the loudest
   f. Such a finding may indicate that the client has a **conductive hearing loss** in the ear to which the sound is lateralized, or that there is a **sensorineural hearing loss** in the opposite ear
2. Rinne tuning fork test
   a. Compares the client's hearing by air conduction and bone conduction

b. Air conduction is 2 to 3 times longer than bone conduction

c. Place the vibrating tuning fork stem on the client's mastoid process and ask the client to indicate when he or she no longer hears the sound

d. The examiner quickly brings the tuning fork in front of the pinna without touching the client and asks the client to indicate if he or she still hears the sound

e. The client normally continues to hear the sound two times louder in front of the pinna; such results are a positive Rinne test

f. The examiner records the duration of both phases, bone conduction followed by air conduction, and compares the times

g. If the client is unable to hear the sound through the ear in front of the pinna, the client may have a **conductive hearing loss** on the side tested; in this situation, the bone conduction is greater than the air conduction (negative Rinne test)

h. The Rinne test is of no value in determining **sensorineural hearing loss**

F. Vestibular assessment

1. Test for falling

   a. The examiner asks the client to stand with the feet together and arms hanging loosely at the sides and eyes closed

   b. The client normally remains erect with only slight swaying

   c. A significant sway is a positive Romberg sign

2. Test for past pointing

   a. The client sits in front of the examiner

   b. The client closes the eyes and extends the arms in front, pointing both index fingers at the examiner

   c. The examiner holds and touches his or her own extended index fingers under the extended index fingers of the client to give the client a point of reference

   d. The client is instructed to raise both arms and then lower them, attempting to return to the examiner's extended index fingers

   e. The normal test response is that the client can easily return to the point of reference

   f. The client with a vestibular function problem lacks a normal sense of position and is unable to return the extended fingers to the point of reference; instead, the fingers deviate either to the right or the left of the reference point

3. Gaze nystagmus evaluation

   a. Examine the client's eyes as they look straight ahead, 30 degrees to each side, upward and downward

   b. Any spontaneous nystagmus, a constant and involuntary cyclic movement of the eyeball in any direction, represent a problem with the vestibular system

4. Hallpike maneuver

   a. Assesses for positional vertigo or induced dizziness

   b. The client assumes a supine position

   c. The head is rotated to one side for 1 minute

   d. A positive test results in nystagmus after 5 to 10 seconds

VII. DIAGNOSTIC TESTS FOR THE EAR

A. Tomography

1. Description

   a. May be performed with or without contrast medium

   b. Assesses the mastoid, middle ear, and inner ear structures

   c. Multiple x-rays of the head are done

   d. Especially helpful in the diagnosis of acoustic tumors

2. Implementation

   a. All jewelry is removed

   b. Lead eye shields are used to cover the cornea to diminish the radiation dose to the eyes

   c. The client must remain still in a supine position

   d. No follow-up care is required

B. Audiometry

1. Description

   a. Measures hearing acuity

   b. Uses two types, pure tone audiometry and speech audiometry

   c. Pure tone audiometry is used to identify problems with hearing, speech, music, and other sounds in the environment

   d. In speech audiometry, the client's ability to hear spoken words is measured

   e. After testing, audiogram patterns are depicted on a graph to determine the type and level of the hearing loss

2. Implementation

   a. Inform the client regarding the procedure

   b. Instruct the client to identify the sounds as they are heard

C. Electronystagmography

1. Description

   a. A vestibular test that evaluates spontaneous and induced eye movements known as nystagmus

   b. Used to distinguish between normal nystagmus and either medication-induced nystagmus or nystagmus caused by a lesion in the central or peripheral vestibular pathway

   c. Records changing electrical fields with the movement of the eye, as monitored by electrodes placed on the skin around the eye

2. Implementation
   a. The client is instructed to remain NPO for 3 hours before testing
   b. Unnecessary medications are omitted for 24 hours before testing
   c. Instruct the client that this is a long and tiring procedure
   d. The client should bring prescription eyeglasses to the exam
   e. The client sits and is instructed to gaze at lights, focus on a moving pattern, focus on a moving point, and then sit with the eyes closed
   f. While sitting in a chair, the client may be rotated to provide information about vestibular function
   g. In addition, the client's ears are irrigated with both cool and warm water, which may cause nausea and vomiting
   h. Following the procedure, the client begins taking clear fluids slowly and cautiously because nausea and vomiting may occur
   i. Assistance with ambulation may also be necessary following the procedure

D. Caloric test (bithermal test)
   1. Description
      a. Performed to evaluate the client experiencing dizziness
      b. Nystagmus, nausea, vomiting, or ataxia may indicate a pathological condition of the labyrinth system, whereas a decreased response may indicate that the vestibular system is affected
   2. Implementation
      a. Warm water causes a greater response than cold water
      b. Warm water caloric testing (irrigation) precedes cool water caloric testing (irrigation)
      c. The character and duration of the eye movements are measured
      d. The client must assume a supine position with the eyes closed and the head elevated to 30 degrees
      e. Following the procedure, the client begins taking clear fluids slowly and cautiously because nausea and vomiting may occur
      f. Assistance with ambulation may also be necessary following the procedure

VIII. DISORDERS OF THE EAR

A. Risk factors related to ear disorders (Box 61-3)
B. **Conductive hearing loss**
   1. Description
      a. When sound waves are blocked to the inner ear fibers because of external ear or middle ear disorders
      b. Disorders can often be corrected with no

BOX 61 3

Risk Factors of Ear Disorders

Aging process
Infection
Medications
Ototoxicity
Trauma
Tumors

---

damage to hearing, or minimal permanent hearing loss
   2. Causes
      a. Any inflammatory process or obstruction of the external or middle ear
      b. Tumors
      c. **Otosclerosis**
      d. A buildup of scar tissue on the ossicles from previous middle ear surgery

C. **Sensorineural hearing loss**
   1. Description
      a. A pathological process of the inner ear or of the sensory fibers that lead to the cerebral cortex
      b. Is often permanent, and measures must be taken to reduce further damage or to attempt to amplify sound as a means of improving hearing to some degree
   2. Causes
      a. Damage to the inner ear structures
      b. Damage to cranial nerve VIII
      c. Prolonged exposure to loud noise
      d. Medications
      e. Trauma
      f. Inherited disorders
      g. Metabolic and circulatory disorders
      h. Infections
      i. Surgery
      j. **Meniere's syndrome**
      k. Diabetes mellitus
      l. Myxedema

D. Mixed hearing loss
   1. Also known as **conductive-sensorineural hearing loss**
   2. Client has both **sensorineural** and **conductive hearing loss**

E. Signs of hearing loss and facilitating communication (Boxes 61-4 and 61-5)

F. Cochlear implantation
   1. Used for **sensorineural hearing loss**
   2. A small computer converts sound waves into electrical impulses
   3. Electrodes are placed by the internal ear with a computer device attached to the external ear
   4. Electronic impulses directly stimulate nerve fibers

BOX 61-4

Signs of Hearing Loss

Frequently asking people to repeat statements
Straining to hear
Turning head or leaning forward to favor one ear
Shouting in conversation
Ringing in the ears
Failing to respond when not looking in the direction of
the sound
Answering questions incorrectly
Raising the volume of the television or radio
Avoiding large groups
Better understanding of speech when in small groups
Withdrawing from social interactions

BOX 61-5

Facilitating Communication

Use of written words if the client is able to see, read,
and write
Providing plenty of light in the room
Getting the attention of the client before you begin to
speak
Facing the client when speaking
Talking in a room without distracting noises
Moving close to the client and speaking slowly and
clearly
Keeping hands and other objects away from the mouth
when talking to the client
Talking in lower tones, because shouting is not helpful
Rephrasing sentences and repeating information
Validating with the client the understanding of state-
ments made, by asking the client to repeat what was
said
Reading lips
Encouraging the client to wear glasses when talking to
someone to improve vision for lip reading
Using sign language, which combines speech with hand
movements that signify letters, words, or phrases
Using telephone amplifiers
Flashing lights that are activated by ringing of the tele-
phone or doorbell
Specially trained dogs that help the client to be aware of
sound and to alert the client of potential dangers

BOX 61-6

Client Education Regarding a Hearing Aid

Encourage to begin using the hearing aid slowly to
develop an adjustment to the device
Adjust the volume to the minimal hearing level to
prevent feedback squeaking
Teach the client to concentrate on the sounds that are to
be heard and to filter out background noise
Instruct the client to clean the ear mold with mild soap
and water
Avoid excessive wetting of the hearing aid, and try to
keep the hearing aid dry
Clean the ear cannula of the hearing aid with a tooth-
pick or pipe cleaner
Turn off the hearing aid and remove the battery when
not in use
Keep extra batteries on hand
Keep the hearing aid in a safe place
Prevent hair sprays, oils, or other hair and face products
from coming into contact with the receiver of the
hearing aid

G. Hearing aids
  1. Used for the client with **conductive hearing loss**
  2. Can help the client with **sensorineural** loss,
     although it is not as effective
  3. A difficulty that exists in its use is the amplifica-
     tion of background noise as well as voices
  4. Client education (Box 61-6)
▲ H. **Presbycusis**
  1. Description
     a. Associated with aging
     b. Leads to degeneration or atrophy of the
        ganglion cells in the cochlea and a loss of
        elasticity of the basilar membranes
     c. Leads to compromise of the vascular supply to
        the inner ear with changes in several areas of
        the ear structure
  2. Assessment
     a. Hearing loss is gradual and bilateral
     b. Client states that he or she has no problem
        with hearing, but cannot understand what the
        words are
     c. Client thinks that the speaker is mumbling
I. External otitis
  1. Description
     a. Infective inflammatory or allergic responses
        involving the structure of the external auditory
        canal or the auricles
     b. An irritating or infective agent comes into
        contact with the epithelial layer of the exter-
        nal ear
     c. This leads to either an allergic response or
        signs and symptoms of an infection
     d. The skin becomes red, swollen, and tender to
        touch on movement
     e. The extensive swelling of the canal can lead to
        conductive hearing loss because of ob-
        struction
     f. It is more common in children, is termed
        "swimmer's ear," and occurs more often in
        hot, humid environments
     g. Prevention includes the elimination of irritat-
        ing or infecting agents
  2. Assessment
     a. Pain
     b. Itching

c. Plugged feeling in the ear

d. Redness and edema

e. Exudate

f. Hearing loss

3. Implementation

a. Apply heat locally for 20 minutes three times a day

b. Encourage rest to assist in reducing pain

c. Administer antibiotics or steroids as prescribed

d. Administer analgesics such as aspirin or acetaminophen (Tylenol) for the pain as prescribed

e. Instruct the client that the ears should be kept clean and dry

f. Instruct the client to use earplugs for swimming

g. Instruct the client that cotton-tipped applicators should not be used to dry ears because their use can lead to trauma to the canal

h. Instruct the client that irritating agents such as hair products or headphones should be discontinued

J. Otitis media: Refer to Chapter 34

1. Myringotomy

a. Refer to Chapter 34

b. Client education (Box 61-7)

K. Chronic otitis media

1. Description

a. A chronic infective, inflammatory, or allergic response involving the structure of the middle ear

b. Surgical treatment is necessary to restore hearing

c. The type of surgery can vary and include a simple reconstruction of the tympanic membrane, a myringoplasty, or replacement of the ossicles within the middle ear

d. A tympanoplasty, a reconstruction of the middle ear, may be attempted to improve **conductive hearing loss**

2. Preoperative implementation

a. Administer antibiotic drops as prescribed

b. Clean the ear of debris as prescribed; irrigate the ear with a solution of equal parts of vinegar and sterile water as prescribed, to restore the normal pH of the ear

c. Instruct the client to avoid persons with upper respiratory infections

d. Instruct the client to obtain adequate rest, eat a balanced diet, and drink adequate fluids

e. Instruct the client in deep breathing and coughing; forceful coughing, which increases pressure in the middle ear, is avoided postoperatively

3. Postoperative implementation

a. Inform the client that initial hearing after surgery is diminished because of the packing in the ear canal, and that hearing improvement will occur after the ear canal packing is removed

b. Keep dressing clean and dry

c. Keep the client flat with operative ear up for at least 12 hours

d. Administer antibiotics as prescribed

e. Instruct the client that he or she may return to work in approximately 3 weeks postoperatively as prescribed

L. **Mastoiditis**

1. Description

a. May be acute or chronic and results from untreated or inadequately treated chronic or acute otitis media

b. The pain is not relieved by myringotomy

2. Assessment

a. Swelling behind the ear and pain with minimal movement of the head

b. Cellulitus on the skin or external scalp over the mastoid process

c. A reddened, dull, thick, immobile tympanic membrane with or without perforation

d. Tender and enlarged postauricular lymph nodes

e. Low-grade fever

f. Malaise

g. Anorexia

3. Implementation

a. Prepare the client for surgical removal of infected material

b. Monitor for complications

c. Simple or modified radical mastoidectomy

BOX 61-7

Client Education Following Myringotomy

Avoid strenuous activities

Avoid rapid head movements, bouncing, or bending

Avoid straining on bowel movement

Avoid drinking through a straw

Avoid traveling by air

Avoid forceful coughing

Avoid contact with persons with colds

Avoid washing hair, showering, or getting the head wet for 1 week as prescribed

Instruct the client that if he or she needs to blow the nose, to blow one side at a time with mouth open

Instruct the client to keep ears dry by keeping a ball of cotton coated with petroleum jelly in the ear and to change cotton ball daily

Instruct the client to report excessive ear drainage to the physician

with tympanoplasty is the most common treatment
d. Once tissue that is infected is removed, the tympanoplasty is performed to reconstruct the ossicles and the tympanic membranes, in an attempt to restore normal hearing

4. Complications
a. Damage to the abducens and facial cranial nerves
b. Damage exhibited by inability to look laterally (cranial nerve VI) and a drooping of the mouth on the affected side (cranial nerve VII)
c. Meningitis
d. Brain abscess
e. Chronic purulent otitis media
f. Wound infections
g. Vertigo, if the infection spreads into the labyrinth

5. Postoperative implementation
a. Monitor for dizziness
b. Monitor for signs of meningitis as evidenced by a stiff neck and vomiting
c. Prepare for a wound dressing change 24 hours postoperatively
d. Monitor the surgical incision for edema, drainage, and redness
e. Position the client flat with the operative side up
f. Restrict the client to bed with bedside commode privileges for 24 hours as prescribed
g. Assist the client with getting out of bed, to prevent falling or injuries from dizziness
h. With reconstruction of the ossicles via a graft, precautions are taken to prevent dislodging of the graft

M. **Otosclerosis**
1. Description
a. Disease of the labyrinthine capsule of the middle ear that results in a bony overgrowth of the tissue surrounding the ossicles
b. Causes the development of irregular areas of new bone formation and causes the fixation of the bones
c. Stapes fixation leads to a **conductive hearing loss**
d. If the disease involves the inner ear, **sensorineural hearing loss** is present
e. It is not uncommon to have bilateral involvement, although hearing loss may be worse in one ear
f. The cause is unknown, although it is thought to have a familial tendency
g. Nonsurgical intervention promotes the improvement of hearing through amplification
h. Surgical intervention involves removal of the bony growth that is causing the hearing loss

i. A partial stapedectomy or complete stapedectomy with prosthesis (**fenestration**) may be surgically performed

2. Assessment
a. Slowly progressing **conductive hearing loss**
b. Bilateral hearing loss
c. A ringing or roaring type of constant tinnitus
d. Loud sounds heard in the ear when chewing
e. Pinkish discoloration (Schwartze's sign) of the tympanic membrane, which indicates vascular changes within the ear
f. Negative Rinne test
g. Weber test shows lateralization of sound to the ear with the most **conductive hearing loss**

N. **Fenestration**
1. Description
a. Removal of the stapes with a small hole drilled in the footplate, and a prosthesis is connected between the incus and footplate
b. Sounds cause the prosthesis to vibrate in the same manner as did the stapes
c. Complications include complete hearing loss, prolonged vertigo, infection, or facial nerve damage

2. Preoperative implementation
a. Instruct the client in measures to prevent middle ear or external ear infections
b. Instruct the client to avoid excessive nose blowing
c. Instruct the client not to clean the ear canal with cotton-tipped applicators
d. Instruct the client to remove the hearing aid 2 weeks before surgery to ensure the integration of local tissue

3. Postoperative implementation
a. Inform the client that hearing is initially worse after the surgical procedure because of swelling and that no noticeable improvement in hearing may occur for as long as 6 weeks
b. Inform the client that the Gelfoam ear packing interferes with hearing but is used to decrease bleeding
c. Assist with ambulating during the first 1 to 2 days after surgery
d. Provide side rails when the client is in bed
e. Administer antibiotics and antivertiginous and pain medications as prescribed
f. Assess for facial nerve damage, weakness, changes in tactile sensation, changes in taste sensation, vertigo, nausea, and vomiting
g. Instruct the client to move the head slowly when changing positions, to prevent vertigo
h. Instruct the client to avoid persons with upper respiratory tract infections
i. Instruct the client to avoid showering and getting the head and wound wet

j. Instruct the client to refrain from using small objects to clean the external ear canal

k. Instruct the client to avoid rapid, extreme changes in pressure caused by quick head movements, sneezing, nose blowing, straining, and changes in altitude

l. Instruct the client to avoid changes in middle ear pressure because they could dislodge the graft or prosthesis

O. Labyrinthitis

1. Description: Infection of the labyrinth that occurs as a complication of acute or chronic otitis media

2. Assessment

a. Hearing loss that may be permanent on the affected side

b. Tinnitus

c. Spontaneous nystagmus to the affected side

d. Vertigo

e. Nausea and vomiting

3. Implementation

a. Monitor for signs of meningitis, the most common complication, as evidenced by headache, stiff neck, lethargy

b. Administer systemic antibiotics as prescribed

c. Advise the client to rest in bed in a darkened room

d. Administer antiemetics and antivertiginous medications as prescribed

e. Instruct the client that the vertigo subsides as the inflammation resolves

f. Instruct the client that balance problems that persist may require gait training through physical therapy

▲ P. **Meniere's syndrome**

1. Description

a. A syndrome also called endolymphatic hydrops, which refers to dilation of the endolymphatic system by either overproduction or decreased reabsorption of endolymphatic fluid

b. It is characterized by tinnitus, unilateral **sensorineural hearing loss,** and vertigo

c. Symptoms occur in attacks and last for several days, and the client becomes totally incapacitated during the attacks

d. Initial hearing loss is reversible, but as the frequency of attacks continues, hearing loss becomes permanent

e. Repeated damage to the cochlea caused by increased fluid pressure leads to the permanent hearing loss

2. Causes

a. Any factor that increases endolymphatic secretion in the labyrinth

b. Viral and bacterial infections

c. Allergic reactions

d. Biochemical disturbances

e. Vascular disturbance producing changes in the microcirculation in the labyrinth

3. Assessment

a. Feelings of fullness in the ear

b. Tinnitus, as a continuous low-pitched roar or humming sound, is present much of the time, but worsens just before and during severe attacks

c. Hearing loss is worse during an attack

d. Vertigo, as periods of whirling, which might cause the client to fall to the ground

e. Vertigo, which is so intense that even while lying down, the client holds the bed or ground in an attempt to prevent the whirling

f. Nausea and vomiting

g. Nystagmus

h. Severe headaches

4. Nonsurgical implementation

a. Preventing injury during vertigo attacks

b. Providing bed rest in a quiet environment

c. Providing assistance with walking

d. Instruct the client to move the head slowly to prevent worsening of the vertigo

e. Initiate sodium and fluid restrictions as prescribed

f. Instruct the client not to smoke

g. Administer nicotinic acid (niacin) as prescribed for its vasodilatory effect

h. Administer antihistamines as prescribed, which will reduce the production of histamine and the inflammation

i. Administer antiemetics as prescribed

j. Administer tranquilizers and sedatives as prescribed to calm the client and allow the client to rest, and to control vertigo, nausea, and vomiting

5. Surgical implementation

a. Performed when medical therapy is ineffective and the functional level of the client has decreased significantly

b. Endolymphatic drainage and insertion of a shunt may be performed early in the course of the disease to assist with the drainage of excess fluids

c. A resection of the vestibular nerve or total removal of the labyrinth or a labyrinthectomy may be performed

6. Postoperative implementation

a. Assess packing and dressing on the ear

b. Speak to the client on the side of the unaffected ear

c. Perform neurological assessments

d. Maintain side rails

e. Assist with ambulating

f. Encourage the use of a bedside commode

g. Administer antivertiginous and antiemetic medications as prescribed

Q. Acoustic neuroma

1. Description
   a. A benign tumor of the vestibular or acoustic nerve
   b. The tumor may cause damage to hearing and to facial movements and sensations
   c. Treatment includes surgical removal of the tumor via craniotomy
   d. Care is taken to preserve the function of the facial nerve
   e. The tumor rarely recurs after surgical removal
   f. Postoperative nursing care is similar to postoperative craniotomy care

2. Assessment
   a. Symptoms usually begin with tinnitus and progress to gradual **sensorineural hearing loss**
   b. As the tumor enlarges, damage to adjacent cranial nerves occurs

R. Trauma

1. Description
   a. The tympanic membrane has a limited stretching ability and gives way under high pressure
   b. Foreign objects placed in the external canal may exert pressure on the tympanic membrane and cause perforation
   c. If the object continues through the canal, the bony structure of the stapes, incus, and malleus may be damaged
   d. A blunt injury to the basal skull and ear can damage the middle ear structures through fractures extending to the middle ear
   e. Excessive nose blowing and rapid changes of pressure that occur with nonpressurized air flights can increase pressure in the middle ear
   f. Depending on the damage to the ossicles, hearing loss may or may not return

2. Implementation
   a. Tympanic membrane perforations usually heal within 24 hours
   b. Surgical reconstruction of the ossicles and tympanic membrane through tympanoplasty or myringoplasty may be performed to improve hearing

S. Cerumen and foreign bodies

1. Description
   a. Cerumen or wax is the most common cause of impacted canals
   b. Foreign bodies can include vegetables, beads, pencil erasers, and insects

2. Assessment
   a. Sensation of fullness in the ear with or without hearing loss
   b. Pain, itching, or bleeding

3. Cerumen
   a. Removal of wax by irrigation is a slow process
   b. Irrigation is contraindicated in clients with a history of tympanic membrane perforation
   c. To soften cerumen, add 3 drops of glycerin to the ear at bedtime, and 3 drops of hydrogen peroxide twice a day
   d. After several days, the ear is irrigated
   e. 50 to 70 mL of solution is the maximal amount a client can tolerate during an irrigation sitting

4. Foreign bodies
   a. With a foreign object of vegetable matter, irrigation is used with care because this material expands with hydration
   b. Insects are killed before removal, unless they can be coaxed out by flashlight or a humming noise
   c. Mineral oil or alcohol is instilled to suffocate the insect, which is then removed with ear forceps
   d. Use small ear forceps to remove the object, and avoid pushing the object farther into the canal and damaging the tympanic membrane

PRACTICE QUESTIONS

1. A clinic nurse is preparing to test the visual acuity of a client with a Snellen chart. Which of the following identifies the accurate procedure for this visual acuity test?
   1. Both eyes are assessed together, followed by the assessment of the right and then the left eye
   2. The right eye is tested, followed by the left eye; then both eyes are tested
   3. The client is asked to stand at a distance of 40 feet from the chart and to read the largest line on the chart
   4. The client is asked to stand at a distance of 40 feet from the chart and to read the line that can be read 200 feet away by an individual with unimpaired vision

2. A client's vision is tested with a Snellen chart. The results of the tests are documented as 20/60. A nurse interprets this as:
   1. The client can read at a distance of 60 feet what a client with normal vision can read at 20 feet
   2. The client is legally blind
   3. The client's vision is normal
   4. The client can only read at a distance of 20 feet what a client with normal vision can read at 60 feet

3. A clinic nurse notes that after several eye examinations, the physician has documented a diagnosis of legal blindness in a client's chart. The nurse reviews

the results of the Snellen chart test, expecting to note which finding?
1. 20/20 vision
2. 20/40 vision
3. 20/60 vision
4. 20/200 vision

4. Tonometry is performed on a client with a suspected diagnosis of glaucoma. A nurse analyzes the test results as documented in the client's chart and understands that normal intraocular pressure is:
1. 2 to 7 mm Hg
2. 8 to 21 mm Hg
3. 22 to 30 mm Hg
4. 31 to 35 mm Hg

5. A nurse is developing a plan of care for a client scheduled for cataract surgery. The nurse documents which most appropriate nursing diagnosis in the plan of care?
1. Self-care deficit
2. Alteration in nutrition
3. Sensory perceptual alterations
4. Anxiety

6. A nurse is performing an assessment on a client with a suspected diagnosis of cataract. The chief clinical manifestation that the nurse would expect to note in the early stages of cataract formation is:
1. Eye pain
2. Floating spots
3. Blurred vision
4. Diplopia

7. In preparation for cataract surgery, a nurse is to administer prescribed eye drops. The nurse reviews the physician's orders, expecting which type of eye drops to be prescribed?
1. An osmotic diuretic
2. A miotic agent
3. A mydriatic medication
4. A thiazide diuretic

8. During the early postoperative period, a client who had a cataract extraction complains of nausea and severe eye pain over the operative site. The initial nursing action is to:
1. Call the physician
2. Administer the ordered pain medication and antiemetic
3. Reassure the client that this is normal
4. Turn the client on his or her operative side

9. A client is being discharged from the ambulatory care unit after cataract removal. A nurse provides instructions regarding home care. Which of the following, if stated by the client, indicates an understanding of the instructions?
1. "I will take aspirin if I have any discomfort."
2. "I will sleep on the side that I was operated on."
3. "I will wear my eye shield at night and my glasses during the day."

4. "I will not lift anything if it weighs more than 10 pounds."

10. A client with glaucoma asks a nurse if complete vision will return. The most appropriate response is:
1. "Although some vision has been lost and cannot be restored, further loss may be prevented by adhering to the treatment plan."
2. "Your vision will return as soon as the medication begins to work."
3. "Your vision will never return to normal."
4. "Your vision loss is temporary and will return in about 3 to 4 weeks."

11. A nurse is developing a teaching plan for a client with glaucoma. Which of the following instructions would the nurse include in the plan of care?
1. Decrease fluid intake to control the intraocular pressure
2. Avoid overuse of the eyes
3. Decrease the amount of salt in the diet
4. Eye medications will need to be administered lifelong

12. A nurse is performing an admission assessment on a client with a diagnosis of detached retina. Which of the following is associated with this eye disorder?
1. Pain in the affected eye
2. Total loss of vision
3. A sense of a curtain falling across the field of vision
4. A yellow discoloration of the sclera

13. A nurse is caring for a client with a diagnosis of detached retina. Which assessment sign would indicate that bleeding has occurred as a result of the retinal detachment?
1. Complaints of a burst of black spots or floaters
2. A sudden sharp pain in the eye
3. Total loss of vision
4. A reddened conjunctiva

14. A client arrives in the emergency room following an automobile accident. The client's forehead hit the steering wheel, and a hyphema is diagnosed. A nurse places the client in which position?
1. Flat on bed rest
2. Semi-Fowler's on bed rest
3. Lateral on the affected side
4. Lateral on the unaffected side

15. A client sustains a contusion of the eyeball following a traumatic injury with a blunt object. Which intervention is initiated immediately?
1. Notify the physician
2. Irrigate the eye with cool water
3. Apply ice to the affected eye
4. Accompany the client to the emergency room

16. A client arrives in an emergency room with a penetrating eye injury from wood chips produced while the client was cutting wood. The nurse assesses the eye and notes a piece of wood

protruding from the eye. What is the initial nursing action?

1. Remove the piece of wood with a sterile eye clamp
2. Apply an eye patch
3. Perform visual acuity tests
4. Irrigate the eye with sterile saline

17. A client arrives in an emergency room after sustaining a chemical eye injury from a splash of battery acid. The initial nursing action is to:

1. Begin visual acuity testing
2. Irrigate the eye with sterile normal saline
3. Swab the eye with antibiotic ointment
4. Cover the eye with a pressure patch

18. A nurse is caring for a client following enucleation. The nurse notes the presence of bright red drainage on the dressing. Which nursing action is appropriate?

1. Notify the physician
2. Continue to monitor the drainage
3. Document the finding
4. Mark the drainage on the dressing, and monitor for any increase in bleeding

19. A nurse is performing a voice test to assess hearing. Which of the following describes the accurate procedure for performing this test?

1. Stand 4 feet away from the client to ensure that the client can hear at this distance
2. Quietly whisper a statement and ask the client to repeat it
3. Whisper a statement with the examiner's back facing the client
4. Whisper a statement while the client blocks both ears

20. During a hearing assessment, a nurse notes that the sound lateralizes to the client's left ear with the Weber test. The nurse analyses these results as:

1. A normal finding
2. A conductive hearing loss in the right ear
3. A sernorineural or conductive loss
4. The presence of nystagmus

21. A nurse is caring for a client who is hearing impaired. Which of the following approaches will facilitate communication?

1. Speak frequently
2. Speak loudly
3. Speak directly into the impaired ear
4. Speak in a normal tone

22. A client arrives at an emergency room with a foreign body in the left ear, which has been determined to be an insect. Which intervention would the nurse anticipate to be prescribed initially?

1. Irrigation of the ear
2. Instillation of diluted alcohol
3. Instillation of antibiotic ear drops
4. Instillation of corticosteroid ointment

23. A nurse notes that a physician has documented a diagnosis of presbycusis on a client's chart. The nurse plans care, knowing that the condition is:

1. A sensorineural hearing loss that occurs with aging
2. A conductive hearing loss that occurs with aging
3. Tinnitus that occurs with aging
4. Nystagmus that occurs with aging

24. A nurse has conducted discharge teaching for a client who had a fenestration procedure for the treatment of otosclerosis. Which of the following, if stated by the client, would indicate that teaching was effective?

1. "I should drink liquids through a straw for the next 2 to 3 weeks."
2. "It is OK to take a shower and wash my hair."
3. "I will take stool softeners as prescribed by my doctor."
4. "I can resume my tennis lesions starting next week."

25. A client with Meniere's disease is experiencing severe vertigo. Which instruction would the nurse give to the client to assist in controlling the vertigo?

1. Increase fluid intake to 3000 mL a day
2. Avoid sudden head movements
3. Lie still and watch the television
4. Increase sodium in the diet

26. A nurse is reviewing the physician's orders for a client with Meniere's disease. Which diet would most likely be prescribed for the client?

1. Low-cholesterol diet
2. Low-sodium diet
3. Low-carbohydrate diet
4. Low-fat diet

27. A nurse is caring for a client after craniotomy for removal of an acoustic neuroma. Assessment of which of the following cranial nerves would identify a complication specifically associated with this surgery?

1. Cranial nerve I, olfactory
2. Cranial nerve III, oculomotor
3. Cranial nerve IV, trochlear
4. Cranial nerve VII, facial nerve

28. A nurse assesses a client with a blunt head injury sustained from a motor vehicle accident. Which assessment sign would indicate a basal skull fracture as a result of the injury?

1. Purulent drainage from the auditory canal
2. Bloody or clear drainage from the auditory canal
3. Epistaxis
4. Periorbital edema

29. A nurse is performing an otoscopic examination on a client with mastoiditis. On examination of the tympanic membrane, which of the following would the nurse expect to observe?

1. A pink-colored tympanic membrane
2. A pearly colored tympanic membrane
3. A red, dull, thick, and immobile tympanic membrane
4. A transparent and clear tympanic membrane

30. A client is diagnosed with a disorder involving the inner ear. Which of the following is the most common client complaint associated with a disorder involving this part of the ear?
    1. Hearing loss
    2. Pruritus
    3. Tinnitus
    4. Burning in the ear

CRITICAL THINKING: FREE-TEXT ENTRY

A client who underwent cataract extraction returns to the surgical care unit following the procedure. The client is resting on her back in a semi-Fowler's position and asks to be repositioned. The nurse places the client in which position?

Answer: _____

ANSWERS

1. **2**
Rationale: Visual acuity is assessed in one eye at a time, and then in both eyes together, with the client comfortably standing or sitting. The right eye is tested with the left eye covered; then the left eye is tested with the right eye covered. Both eyes are then tested together. Visual acuity is measured with or without corrective lenses, and the client stands at a distance of 20 feet from the chart.
Test-Taking Strategy: Use the process of elimination. Remember that normal visual acuity as measured by a Snellen chart is 20/20 vision. This should assist in eliminating options 3 and 4. From the remaining options, remember that it is best to test each eye separately first, and then test both eyes together. This most accurately assesses visual acuity. Review the procedure for testing visual acuity with a Snellen chart if you had difficulty with this question.
Level of Cognitive Ability: Application
Client Needs: Health Promotion and Maintenance
Integrated Concept/Process: Nursing Process/Implementation
Content Area: Adult Health/Eye
Reference: Jarvis, C. (2000). *Physical examination and health assessment* (3rd ed.). Philadelphia: W.B. Saunders, p. 307.

2. **4**
Rationale: Vision that is 20/20 is normal; that is, the client is able to read from 20 feet what a person with normal vision can read from 20 feet. A client with a visual acuity of 20/60 can only read at a distance of 20 feet what a person with normal vision can read at 60 feet.
Test-Taking Strategy: Use the process of elimination. Focus on the test result, 20/60, to direct you to option 4. If you had difficulty with this question, review interpretation of visual acuity test results.
Level of Cognitive Ability: Analysis
Client Needs: Physiological Integrity
Integrated Concept/Process: Nursing Process/Analysis
Content Area: Adult Health/Eye
Reference: Jarvis, C. (2000). *Physical examination and health assessment* (3rd ed.). Philadelphia: W.B. Saunders, p. 308.

3. **4**
Rationale: Legal blindness is defined as 20/200 or less with corrected vision (glasses or contact lenses), or a visual field of 20 degrees or less in the better eye.
Test-Taking Strategy: Knowledge of the definition of legal blindness is required to answer this question. Review this definition if you had difficulty with this question.
Level of Cognitive Ability: Comprehension
Client Needs: Physiological Integrity
Integrated Concept/Process: Nursing Process/Analysis

Content Area: Adult Health/Eye
Reference: Ignatavicius, D., Workman, M., & Mishler, M. (1999). *Medical-surgical nursing across the health care continuum* (3rd ed.). Philadelphia: W.B. Saunders, p. 1192.

4. **2**
Rationale: Tonometry is the method of measuring intraocular fluid pressure by using a calibrated instrument that indents or flattens the corneal apex. Pressures between 8 and 21 mm Hg are considered within the normal range.
Test-Taking Strategy: Use the process of elimination and knowledge regarding the normal intraocular pressure to answer this question. If you had difficulty with this question, learn this normal value.
Level of Cognitive Ability: Comprehension
Client Needs: Physiological Integrity
Integrated Concept/Process: Nursing Process/Assessment
Content Area: Adult Health/Eye
Reference: Ignatavicius, D., Workman, M., & Mishler, M. (1999). *Medical-surgical nursing across the health care continuum* (3rd ed.). Philadelphia: W.B. Saunders, p. 1181.

5. **3**
Rationale: The most appropriate nursing diagnosis for the client scheduled for cataract surgery is sensory perceptual alteration (visual) related to lens extraction and replacement. Although options 1, 2, and 4 identify nursing diagnoses that may be appropriate, they are not specifically related to cataract surgery.
Test-Taking Strategy: Use the process of elimination. When asked questions regarding nursing diagnosis, use the information presented in the question to select an option. Remember that disorders of the eye or ear relate to sensory perceptual alterations. Review care of the client scheduled for cataract surgery if you had difficulty with this question.
Level of Cognitive Ability: Analysis
Client Needs: Psychosocial Integrity
Integrated Concept/Process: Nursing Process/Planning
Content Area: Adult Health/Eye
Reference: Ignatavicius, D., Workman, M., & Mishler, M. (1999). *Medical-surgical nursing across the health care continuum* (3rd ed.). Philadelphia: W.B. Saunders, p. 1177.

6. **3**
Rationale: A gradual painless blurring of central vision is the chief clinical manifestation of a cataract. Early symptoms include slightly blurred vision and a decrease in color perception. Options 1, 2, and 4 are not signs of a cataract.
Test-Taking Strategy: Use the process of elimination. Remember the pathophysiology related to cataract development. As a cataract develops, the lens of the eye becomes opaque. This description will assist in directing you to the correct option. If

you had difficulty with this question, review the assessment signs associated with cataract development.

Level of Cognitive Ability: Analysis
Client Needs: Physiological Integrity
Integrated Concept/Process: Nursing Process/Assessment
Content Area: Adult Health/Eye
Reference: Ignatavicius, D., Workman, M., & Mishler, M. (1999). *Medical-surgical nursing across the health care continuum* (3rd ed.). Philadelphia: W.B. Saunders, p. 1177.

7. 3

Rationale: A mydriatic medication produces mydriasis or dilation of the pupil. Mydriatic medications are used preoperatively in the cataract client. These medications act by dilating the pupils. They also constrict blood vessels. An osmotic diuretic may be used to decrease intraocular pressure. A miotic medication constricts the pupil. A thiazide diuretic is not likely to be prescribed for a client with a cataract.

Test-Taking Strategy: Use the process of elimination. Read the question carefully, noting that the client is being prepared for eye surgery. Dilation of the eye is necessary prior to cataract extraction. Recalling that a mydriatic dilates will direct you to option 3. Review preoperative care for cataract surgery if you had difficulty with this question.

Level of Cognitive Ability: Analysis
Client Needs: Physiological Integrity
Integrated Concept/Process: Nursing Process/Analysis
Content Area: Adult Health/Eye
Reference: Ignatavicius, D., Workman, M., & Mishler, M. (1999). *Medical-surgical nursing across the health care continuum* (3rd ed.). Philadelphia: W.B. Saunders, p. 1178.

8. 1

Rationale: Severe pain or pain accompanied by nausea is an indicator of increased intraocular pressure and should be reported to the physician immediately. Options 2, 3, and 4 are inappropriate actions.

Test-Taking Strategy: Use the process of elimination. Note the key word "severe." Eliminate option 3 because this is not a normal condition. The client should not be turned to his or her operative side; therefore eliminate option 4. From the remaining options, focusing on the key word will direct you to option 1. If you had difficulty with this question, review the postoperative complications of cataract surgery requiring physician notification.

Level of Cognitive Ability: Analysis
Client Needs: Physiological Integrity
Integrated Concept/Process: Nursing Process/Implementation
Content Area: Adult Health/Eye
Reference: Ignatavicius, D., Workman, M., & Mishler, M. (1999). *Medical-surgical nursing across the health care continuum* (3rd ed.). Philadelphia: W.B. Saunders, p. 1178.

9. 3

Rationale: The client is instructed to wear a metal or plastic shield to protect the eye from accidental injury and is instructed not to rub the eye. Glasses may be worn during the day. Aspirin or medications containing aspirin are not to be administered or taken by the client, and the client is instructed to take acetaminophen (Tylenol) as needed for pain. The client is instructed not to sleep on the side of the body that was operated on. The client is not to lift more than 5 pounds.

Test-Taking Strategy: Use the process of elimination, noting the key words "understanding of the instructions." Recalling that the operative site needs to be protected will direct you to option 3. If you had difficulty with this question, review the discharge instructions for the client following cataract extraction.

Level of Cognitive Ability: Application
Client Needs: Health Promotion and Maintenance
Integrated Concept/Process: Teaching/Learning
Content Area: Adult Health/Eye
Reference: Ignatavicius, D., Workman, M., & Mishler, M. (1999). *Medical-surgical nursing across the health care continuum* (3rd ed.). Philadelphia: W.B. Saunders, p. 1179.

10. 1

Rationale: Vision loss to glaucoma is irreparable. The client should be reassured that although some vision has been lost and cannot be restored, further loss may be prevented by adhering to the treatment plan. Option 3 does not provide reassurance to the client.

Test-Taking Strategy: Use the process of elimination and therapeutic communication techniques. Also note that option 1 is global, addressing the importance of compliance with the treatment plan. Review the effects of glaucoma and therapeutic communication techniques if you had difficulty with this question.

Level of Cognitive Ability: Application
Client Needs: Psychosocial Integrity
Integrated Concept/Process: Communication and Documentation
Content Area: Adult Health/Eye
Reference: Ignatavicius, D., Workman, M., & Mishler, M. (1999). *Medical-surgical nursing across the health care continuum* (3rd ed.). Philadelphia: W.B. Saunders, p. 1181.

11. 4

Rationale: The administration of eye drops is a critical component of the treatment plan for the client with glaucoma. The client needs to be instructed that medications will need to be taken for the rest of his or her life. Options 1, 2, and 3 are not accurate instructions.

Test-Taking Strategy: Use the process of elimination. Recalling that medications are an integral component of the treatment plan will assist in directing you to the correct option. Review the treatment associated with the care of the client with glaucoma, if you had difficulty with this question.

Level of Cognitive Ability: Application
Client Needs: Health Promotion and Maintenance
Integrated Concept/Process: Teaching/Learning
Content Area: Adult Health/Eye
Reference: Ignatavicius, D., Workman, M., & Mishler, M. (1999). *Medical-surgical nursing across the health care continuum* (3rd ed.). Philadelphia: W.B. Saunders, p. 1181.

12. 3

Rationale: A characteristic manifestation of retinal detachment described by the client is the feeling that a shadow or curtain is falling across the field of vision. There is no pain associated with detachment of the retina. Options 2 and 4 are not characteristics of this disorder. A retinal detachment is an ophthalmic emergency and even more so if visual acuity is still normal.

Test-Taking Strategy: Use the process of elimination, focusing on the diagnosis. It is necessary to recall the characteristic manifestations associated with this disorder to answer correctly. Review the manifestations associated with this condition, if you had difficulty with this question.
Level of Cognitive Ability: Analysis
Client Needs: Physiological Integrity
Integrated Concept/Process: Nursing Process/Assessment
Content Area: Adult Health/Eye
Reference: Ignatavicius, D., Workman, M., & Mishler, M. (1999). *Medical-surgical nursing across the health care continuum* (3rd ed.). Philadelphia: W.B. Saunders, p. 1185.

13. **1**
Rationale: Complaints of a sudden burst of black spots or floaters indicates that bleeding has occurred as a result of the detachment. Options 2, 3, and 4 are not signs of bleeding.
Test-Taking Strategy: Recalling the complications associated with retinal detachment is necessary to answer this question. Review the manifestations associated with the complications of a detached retina, if you had difficulty with this question.
Level of Cognitive Ability: Analysis
Client Needs: Physiological Integrity
Integrated Concept/Process: Nursing Process/Assessment
Content Area: Adult Health/Eye
Reference: Ignatavicius, D., Workman, M., & Mishler, M. (1999). *Medical-surgical nursing across the health care continuum* (3rd ed.). Philadelphia: W.B. Saunders, p. 1185.

14. **2**
Rationale: A hyphema is the presence of blood in the anterior chamber. It is produced when a force is sufficient to break the integrity of the blood vessels in the eye. It can be caused by direct injury, such as a penetrating injury from a BB pellet, or indirectly, such as from striking the forehead on a steering wheel during an accident. The client is treated by bed rest in a semi-Fowler's position to assist gravity in keeping the hyphema away from the optical center of the cornea.
Test-Taking Strategy: Use the process of elimination to answer this question. Remember, placing the client flat will produce an increase in pressure at the injured site. Also, note that option 2 is the option that identifies a position different from the other options. Review care of the client with hyphema, if you had difficulty with this question.
Level of Cognitive Ability: Application
Client Needs: Physiological Integrity
Integrated Concept/Process: Nursing Process/Implementation
Content Area: Adult Health/Eye
Reference: Ignatavicius, D., Workman, M., & Mishler, M. (1999). *Medical-surgical nursing across the health care continuum* (3rd ed.). Philadelphia: W.B. Saunders, p. 1188.

15. **3**
Rationale: Treatment for a contusion begins at the time of injury. Ice is applied immediately. The client should then be seen by a physician and receive a thorough eye examination to rule out the presence of other eye injuries.
Test-Taking Strategy: Use the process of elimination. Focus on the key word "immediately." Recalling the principles related to initial treatment of injuries will direct you to option 3. Review emergency treatment of eye injuries if you had difficulty with this question.

Level of Cognitive Ability: Application
Client Needs: Physiological Integrity
Integrated Concept/Process: Nursing Process/Implementation
Content Area: Adult Health/Eye
Reference: Ignatavicius, D., Workman, M., & Mishler, M. (1999). *Medical-surgical nursing across the health care continuum* (3rd ed.). Philadelphia: W.B. Saunders, p. 1188.

16. **3**
Rationale: If the laceration is the result of a penetrating injury, an object may be noted protruding from the eye. This object must never be removed except by the ophthalmologist, because it may be holding ocular structures in place. Application of an eye patch or irrigation of the eye may disrupt the foreign body and cause further tearing of the cornea.
Test-Taking Strategy: Use the process of elimination to answer this question. Note the key word "penetrating." This should indicate that a laceration has occurred and that interventions are directed at preventing further disruption of the integrity of the eye. The only option that will prevent further disruption is to assess visual acuity. Review emergency eye care, if you had difficulty with this question.
Level of Cognitive Ability: Application
Client Needs: Physiological Integrity
Integrated Concept/Process: Nursing Process/Implementation
Content Area: Adult Health/Eye
Reference: Ignatavicius, D., Workman, M., & Mishler, M. (1999). *Medical-surgical nursing across the health care continuum* (3rd ed.). Philadelphia: W.B. Saunders, pp. 1188-1189.

17. **2**
Rationale: Emergency care after a chemical burn to the eye includes irrigating the eye immediately with sterile normal saline or ocular irrigating solution. The irrigation should be maintained for at least 10 minutes. Following this emergency treatment, visual acuity is assessed. Options 3 and 4 are not components of initial care.
Test-Taking Strategy: Read the question carefully, noting the type of injury to the eye. Noting the key word "splash" will direct you to option 2. Review emergency eye care if you had difficulty with this question.
Level of Cognitive Ability: Application
Client Needs: Physiological Integrity
Integrated Concept/Process: Nursing Process/Implementation
Content Area: Adult Health/Eye
Reference: Phipps, W., Sands, J., & Marek, J. (1999). *Medical-surgical nursing: Concepts & clinical practice* (6th ed.). St. Louis: Mosby, pp. 1831-1832.

18. **1**
Rationale: If the nurse notes the presence of bright red drainage on the dressing, it must be reported to the physician because this can indicate hemorrhage. Options 2, 3, and 4 are inappropriate.
Test-Taking Strategy: Use the process of elimination. Note the key words "bright red." Remember, bright red drainage indicates active bleeding. Review postoperative complications associated with an enucleation, if you had difficulty with this question.
Level of Cognitive Ability: Application
Client Needs: Physiological Integrity
Integrated Concept/Process: Nursing Process/Implementation
Content Area: Adult Health/Eye

Reference: Phipps, W., Sands, J., & Marek, J. (1999). *Medical-surgical nursing: Concepts & clinical practice* (6th ed.). St. Louis: Mosby, p. 1848.

19. 2

Rationale: The examiner stands 1 to 2 feet away from the client and asks the client to block one external ear canal. The nurse quietly whispers a statement and asks the client to repeat it. Each ear is tested separately.

Test-Taking Strategy: Use the process of elimination. Eliminate options 3 and 4 because they are not measures that would effectively assess hearing. Eliminate option 1 because distance hearing is not the issue of the question. Review the procedure for performing a voice test if you had difficulty with this question.

Level of Cognitive Ability: Application
Client Needs: Health Promotion and Maintenance
Integrated Concept/Process: Nursing Process/Implementation
Content Area: Adult Health/Ear
Reference: Jarvis, C. (2000). *Physical examination and health assessment* (3rd ed.). Philadelphia: W.B. Saunders, p. 357.

20. 3

Rationale: In the Weber tuning fork test, the nurse places the vibrating tuning fork in the middle of the client's head at the midline of the forehead, or above the upper lip over the teeth. Normally, the sound is heard equally in both ears by bone conduction. If the client has a sensorineural hearing loss in one ear, the sound is heard in the other ear. If the client has a conductive hearing loss in one ear, the sound is heard in that ear.

Test-Taking Strategy: Use the process of elimination. This is a difficult question. Knowledge regarding analyzing the results of the Weber tuning fork test is required to answer this question. If you had difficulty with this question, review this hearing test. Also, review the Rinne tuning fork test.

Level of Cognitive Ability: Analysis
Client Needs: Physiological Integrity
Integrated Concept/Process: Nursing Process/Analysis
Content Area: Adult Health/Ear
Reference: Jarvis, C. (2000). *Physical examination and health assessment* (3rd ed.). Philadelphia: W.B. Saunders, p. 357.

21. 4

Rationale: It is important to speak in a normal tone to the client with impaired hearing. It is also important not to shout. The nurse should talk directly to the client while facing the client and speak clearly. If the client does not seem to understand what is said, the nurse should express it differently. Moving closer to the client and toward the better ear may facilitate communication, but the nurse should avoid talking directly into the impaired ear.

Test-Taking Strategy: Use the process of elimination and knowledge regarding effective communication techniques for the hearing impaired to answer this question. If you had difficulty with this question, review these techniques.

Level of Cognitive Ability: Application
Client Needs: Psychosocial Integrity
Integrated Concept/Process: Nursing Process/Implementation
Content Area: Adult Health/Ear
Reference: Smeltzer, S., & Bare, B. (2000). *Brunner & Suddarth's textbook of medical-surgical nursing* (9th ed.). Philadelphia: Lippincott Williams & Wilkins, p. 1588.

22. 2

Rationale: Insects are killed before removal unless they can be coaxed out by a flashlight or a humming noise. Mineral oil or diluted alcohol is instilled into the ear to suffocate the insect, which is then removed by using ear forceps. When the foreign object is vegetable matter, irrigation is not used because this material expands with hydration and the impaction becomes worse.

Test-Taking Strategy: Use the process of elimination. Focusing on the key words "foreign body" and "insect" will direct you to option 2. If you had difficulty with this question, review care of the client with a foreign body in the ear.

Level of Cognitive Ability: Analysis
Client Needs: Physiological Integrity
Integrated Concept/Process: Nursing Process/Planning
Content Area: Adult Health/Ear
Reference: Ignatavicius, D., Workman, M., & Mishler, M. (1999). *Medical-surgical nursing across the health care continuum* (3rd ed.). Philadelphia: W.B. Saunders, p. 1212.

23. 1

Rationale: Presbycusis is a type of hearing loss that occurs with aging. It is a gradual sensorineural loss caused by nerve degeneration in the inner ear or auditory nerve. Options 2, 3, and 4 are incorrect.

Test-Taking Strategy: Knowledge regarding the description of presbycusis is required to answer this question. If you are unfamiliar with this condition, review this age-related disorder.

Level of Cognitive Ability: Comprehension
Client Needs: Physiological Integrity
Integrated Concept/Process: Nursing Process/Planning
Content Area: Adult Health/Ear
Reference: Ignatavicius, D., Workman, M., & Mishler, M. (1999). *Medical-surgical nursing across the health care continuum* (3rd ed.). Philadelphia: W.B. Saunders, p. 1196.

24. 3

Rationale: After ear surgery, the client needs to avoid straining when having a bowel movement. The client needs to be instructed to avoid drinking with a straw for 2 to 3 weeks, air travel, and coughing excessively. The client needs to avoid getting his or her head wet, washing hair, showering for 1 week, and rapidly moving the head, bouncing, and bending over for 3 weeks.

Test-Taking Strategy: Use the process of elimination. Note the key words "teaching was effective." Consider the anatomical area of the client's condition and the surgical procedure in eliminating the incorrect options. If you had difficulty with this question, review client instructions following ear surgery.

Level of Cognitive Ability: Analysis
Client Needs: Health Promotion and Maintenance
Integrated Concept/Process: Teaching/Learning
Content Area: Adult Health/Ear
Reference: Smeltzer, S., & Bare, B. (2000). *Brunner & Suddarth's textbook of medical-surgical nursing* (9th ed.). Philadelphia: Lippincott Williams & Wilkins, p. 1593.

25. 2

Rationale: The nurse instructs the client to make slow head movements to prevent worsening of the vertigo. Dietary changes such as salt and fluid restrictions that reduce the amount of endolymphatic fluid are sometimes prescribed. Lying still and watching television will not control vertigo.

Test-Taking Strategy: Use the process of elimination. Identify the issue, vertigo. Note the relationship between vertigo and avoiding sudden head movements in the correct option. If you had difficulty with this question, review the measures that will reduce vertigo in the client with Meniere's disease.

Level of Cognitive Ability: Application
Client Needs: Physiological Integrity
Integrated Concept/Process: Nursing Process/Implementation
Content Area: Adult Health/Ear
Reference: Ignatavicius, D., Workman, M., & Mishler, M. (1999). *Medical-surgical nursing across the health care continuum* (3rd ed.). Philadelphia: W.B. Saunders, 1217.

26. 2

Rationale: Dietary changes such as salt and fluid restrictions that reduce the amount of endolymphatic fluid are sometimes prescribed. Options 1, 3, and 4 are not specific to the client with Meniere's disease.

Test-Taking Strategy: Use the process of elimination. Recalling the pathophysiology related to Meniere's disease will direct you to option 2. Review the pathophysiology related to this condition and the treatment measures if you had difficulty with this question

Level of Cognitive Ability: Analysis
Client Needs: Physiological Integrity
Integrated Concept/Process: Nursing Process/Planning
Content Area: Adult Health/Ear
Reference: Ignatavicius, D., Workman, M., & Mishler, M. (1999). *Medical-surgical nursing across the health care continuum* (3rd ed.). Philadelphia: W.B. Saunders, p. 1217.

27. 4

Rationale: Treatment for acoustic neuroma is surgical removal via a craniotomy. Extreme care is taken to preserve remaining hearing and preserve the function of the facial nerve. Acoustic neuromas rarely occur following surgical removal.

Test-Taking Strategy: Use the process of elimination and knowledge regarding the anatomical location of an acoustic neuroma to direct you to option 4. If you had difficulty with this question, review the complications associated with this surgical procedure.

Level of Cognitive Ability: Analysis
Client Needs: Physiological Integrity
Integrated Concept/Process: Nursing Process/Assessment
Content Area: Adult Health/Ear
Reference: Ignatavicius, D., Workman, M., & Mishler, M. (1999). *Medical-surgical nursing across the health care continuum* (3rd ed.). Philadelphia: W.B. Saunders, p. 1218.

28. 2

Rationale: Bloody or clear watery drainage from the auditory canal indicates a cerebrospinal fluid leak following trauma and suggests a basal skull fracture. This warrants immediate attention. Options 1, 3, and 4 are not specific to a basal skull fracture.

Test-Taking Strategy: Use the process of elimination. Recalling the concern related to leakage of cerebrospinal fluid will direct you to option 2. If you had difficulty with this question, review these assessment signs.

Level of Cognitive Ability: Analysis
Client Needs: Physiological Integrity
Integrated Concept/Process: Nursing Process/Assessment

Content Area: Adult Health/Ear
Reference: Smeltzer, S., & Bare, B. (2000). *Brunner & Suddarth's textbook of medical-surgical nursing* (9th ed.). Philadelphia: Lippincott Williams & Wilkins, p. 1675.

29. 3

Rationale: Otoscopic examination in a client with mastoiditis reveals a red, dull, thick, and immobile tympanic membrane with or without perforation. Postauricular lymph nodes are tender and enlarged. Clients also have a low-grade fever, malaise, anorexia, swelling behind the ear, and pain with minimal movement of the head.

Test-Taking Strategy: Knowledge regarding the pathophysiology associated with mastoiditis is required to answer this question. If you had difficulty with this question, review the assessment findings associated with this disorder.

Level of Cognitive Ability: Analysis
Client Needs: Physiological Integrity
Integrated Concept/Process: Nursing Process/Assessment
Content Area: Adult Health/Ear
Reference: Ignatavicius, D., Workman, M., & Mishler, M. (1999). *Medical-surgical nursing across the health care continuum* (3rd ed.). Philadelphia: W.B. Saunders, pp. 1214-1215.

30. 3

Rationale: Tinnitus is the most common complaint of clients with otological disorders, especially disorders involving the inner ear. Symptoms of tinnitus range from mild ringing in the ear, which can go unnoticed during the day, to a loud roaring in the ear, which can interfere with the client's thinking process and attention span. Options 1, 2, and 4 are not specifically associated with disorders of the inner ear.

Test-Taking Strategy: Use the process of elimination. Recalling the function of the inner ear will direct you to option 3. Review the manifestations associated with an inner ear disorder if you had difficulty with this question.

Level of Cognitive Ability: Analysis
Client Needs: Physiological Integrity
Integrated Concept/Process: Nursing Process/Assessment
Content Area: Adult Health/Ear
Reference: Ignatavicius, D., Workman, M., & Mishler, M. (1999). *Medical-surgical nursing across the health care continuum* (3rd ed.). Philadelphia: W.B. Saunders, p. 1216.

CRITICAL THINKING: FREE-TEXT ENTRY

Answer: On the nonoperative side

Rationale: Postoperatively, cataract extraction clients should be positioned on their backs in semi-Fowler's position or on the nonoperative side to prevent edema in the surgical site.

Test-Taking Strategy: Remember that edema to the surgical site can occur following the trauma of surgery. Think about the principles of gravity and the prevention of the accumulation of fluid around the surgical site in answering the question. If you had difficulty with this question, review postoperative care of a client following cataract surgery.

Level of Cognitive Ability: Application
Client Needs: Physiological Integrity
Integrated Concept/Process: Nursing Process/Implementation
Content Area: Adult Health/Eye
Reference: Ignatavicius, D., Workman, M., & Mishler, M. (1999). *Medical-surgical nursing across the health care continuum* (3rd ed.). Philadelphia: W.B. Saunders, p. 1179.

REFERENCES

Ignatavicius, D., Workman, M., & Mishler, M. (1999). *Medical-surgical nursing across the health care continuum* (3rd ed.). Philadelphia: W.B. Saunders.

Jarvis, C. (2000). *Physical examination and health assessment* (3rd ed.). Philadelphia: W.B. Saunders.

LeMone, P., & Burke, K. (2000). *Medical-surgical nursing: Critical thinking in client care* (2nd ed.). Upper Saddle River, N.J.: Prentice-Hall.

Phipps, W., Sands, J., & Marek, J. (1999). *Medical-surgical nursing: Concepts & clinical practice* (6th ed.). St. Louis: Mosby.

Potter, P., & Perry, A. (2001). *Fundamentals of nursing* (5th ed.). St. Louis: Mosby.

Smeltzer, S., & Bare, B. (2000). *Brunner & Suddarth's textbook of medical-surgical nursing* (9th ed.). Philadelphia: Lippincott Williams & Wilkins.

Ophthalmic and Otic Medications

62

I. OPHTHALMIC MEDICATION ADMINISTRATION
(Box 62-1)

A. Guidelines for the use of eye medications

1. Eye medications are usually in the form of drops or ointments
2. To prevent overflow of medication into the nasal and pharyngeal passages, thus reducing systemic absorption, instruct the client to occlude the nasolacrimal duct with one finger for 1 to 2 minutes after instilling the medication
3. When two or more eye medications are to be administered, wait at least 3 minutes between medications
4. Wash hands before administering eye medications to avoid contaminating the eye or medication dropper or applicator, and after administering eye medications to rinse off any residue
5. Use a separate bottle or tube of medication for each client to avoid accidental cross contamination
6. Place prescribed dose of eye medication in the lower conjunctival sac, never directly onto the cornea
7. Avoid touching any part of the eye with the dropper or applicator
8. Administer drops or liquid preparations before ointments
9. Administer glucocorticoid preparations before other medications
10. Monitor the pulse of the client receiving an ophthalmic beta blocker, and instruct the client to do the same; if the pulse is below 50 to 60 beats per minute (adult), withhold the next dose of eye medication and notify the physician
11. Instruct the client in how to instill medication correctly, and supervise instillation until the client can do it safely
12. Instruct the client to read the medication labels carefully to ensure administration of the correct medication and correct strength
13. Remind the client to keep these medications out of the reach of children
14. Instruct the client to avoid driving or operating hazardous equipment if vision is blurred
15. Inform the client that he or she may be unable to drive home after eye examinations when medications to dilate the pupil (**mydriatics**) or medications to paralyze the ciliary muscle (**cycloplegics**) are used
16. If photophobia occurs, instruct the client to wear sunglasses and avoid bright lights
17. Instruct the client to administer a missed dose of the eye medication as soon as remembered, unless the next dose is scheduled to be administered in 1 to 2 hours
18. Inform the client with **glaucoma** that the disorder cannot be cured, only controlled
19. Reinforce the importance of using medications to treat **glaucoma** as prescribed and not to discontinue these medications without consulting the physician
20. Inform the client that medications used to treat **glaucoma** may cause pain and blurred vision, especially when therapy is begun
21. Instruct the client to report the development of any eye irritation
22. Inform the client using eye gel to store the gel at room temperature or in the refrigerator but not to freeze it
23. Instruct the client to discard unused eye gel kept at room temperature after 8 weeks
24. Inform the client that soft contact lenses may absorb certain eye medications and that preservatives in eye medications may discolor the contact lenses

---

BOX 62-1

Abbreviations

Left eye (OS)
Right eye (OD)
Both eyes (OU)

BOX 62-2

Mydriatic/Cycloplegic Eye Medications

Atropine sulfate (Isopto-Atropine, Ocu-Tropine, Atropair, Atropisol)
Scopolamine hydrobromide (Isopto-Hyoscine)
Cyclopentolate hydrochloride (Cyclogyl, AK-Pentolate, Pentolair)
Homatropine hydrobromide (Isopto Homatrine, AK-Homatropine, Spectro-Homatrine)
Tropicamide (Mydriacyl, I-Picamide, Tropicacyl)
Phenylephrine hydrochloride (AK-Dilate, Dilatair, Mydfrin, Ocu-Phrin)

---

25. Advise the client wearing contact lenses to question the physician carefully about special precautions to observe
26. In infants, inform the parents that atropine sulfate eye drops may contribute to abdominal distention
27. Instruct the parents to keep a record of the bowel movements of the infant being administered atropine sulfate eye drops
28. Auscultate bowel sounds of the infant or child receiving atropine sulfate eye drops

▲ B. Instillation of eye medications
1. Drops
   a. Wash hands
   b. Put gloves on
   c. Check the name, strength, and expiration date of the medication
   d. Instruct the client to tilt the head backward, open the eyes, and look up
   e. Pull the lower lid down against the cheekbone
   f. Hold the bottle like a pencil with the tip downward
   g. Holding the bottle, gently rest the wrist of the hand on the client's cheek
   h. Squeeze the bottle gently to allow the drop to fall into the conjunctival sac
   i. Instruct the client to close the eyes gently and not to squeeze the eyes shut
   j. Wait 3 to 5 minutes before instilling another drop, if more than one drop is prescribed, to promote maximal absorption of the medication
   k. Do not allow the medication bottle, dropper, or applicator to come into contact with the eyeball
2. Ointments
   a. Hold the ointment tube near, but not touching, the eye or eyelashes
   b. Squeeze a thin ribbon of ointment along the lining of the lower conjunctival sac from the inner to the outer canthus
   c. Instruct the client to close the eyes gently
   d. Instruct the client that vision may be blurred by the ointment

▲ II. MYDRIATIC/CYCLOPLEGIC AND ANTICHOLINERGIC MEDICATIONS (Box 62-2)
A. Description
   1. **Mydriatics** and **cycloplegics** dilate the pupils

(**mydriasis**) and relax the ciliary muscles (**cycloplegia**)
2. Anticholinergics block responses of the sphincter muscle in the ciliary body, producing **mydriasis** and **cycloplegia**
3. Used preoperatively or for eye examinations to produce **mydriasis**
4. Contraindicated in clients with **glaucoma** because of the risk of increased intraocular pressure
5. **Mydriatics** are contraindicated in cardiac dysrhythmias and cerebral atherosclerosis and should be used with caution in the elderly and in clients with prostatic hypertrophy, diabetes mellitus, or parkinsonism
B. Side effects
   1. Tachycardia
   2. Photophobia
   3. Conjunctivitis
   4. Dermatitis
C. Atropine toxicity
   1. Dry mouth
   2. Blurred vision
   3. Photophobia
   4. Tachycardia
   5. Fever
   6. Urinary retention
   7. Constipation
   8. Headache, brow pain
   9. Confusion
   10. Hallucinations, delirium
   11. Coma
   12. Worsening of narrow-angle **glaucoma**
D. Systemic reactions of anticholinergics
   1. Dry mouth and skin
   2. Fever
   3. Thirst
   4. Confusion
   5. Hyperactivity
E. Implementation
   1. Monitor for allergic response
   2. Assess for risk of injury
   3. Assess for constipation and urinary retention

BOX 62-3

Antiinfective Eye Medications

ANTIBACTERIAL
Chloramphenicol (Chloromycetin, Chloroptic)
Ciprofloxacin hydrochloride (Cipro)
Erythromycin (Ilotycin)
Gentamicin sulfate (Garamycin, Genoptic)
Norfloxacin (Chibroxin)
Tobramycin (Nebcin, Tobrex)
Silver nitrate 1%

ANTIFUNGAL
Natamycin (Natacyn Ophthalmic)

ANTIVIRAL
Idoxuridine (Herplex Liquifilm)
Trifluridine (Viroptic)
Vidarabine (Vira-A Ophthalmic)

BOX 62-4

Antiinflammatory Eye Medications

Dexamethasone (Maxidex)
Diclofenac (Voltaren)
Flurbiprofen sodium (Ocufen)
Suprofen (Profenal)
Ketorolac tromethamine (Acular)
Prednisolone acetate (Predforte, Econopred)
Prednisolone sodium phosphate (AK-Pred, Inflamase)
Rimaxolone (Vexol)

BOX 62-5

Topical Anesthetics for the Eye

Proparacaine hydrochloride (Ophthaine, Ophthetic)
Tetracaine hydrochloride (Pontocaine)

---

4. Instruct the client that a burning sensation may occur on instillation
5. Instruct the client not to drive or operate machinery for 24 hours after instillation of the medication unless otherwise directed by the physician
6. Instruct the client to wear sunglasses until the effects of the medication wear off
7. Instruct the client to notify the physician if blurring of vision, loss of sight, difficulty in breathing, sweating, or flushing occurs
8. Instruct the client to report eye pain to the physician
F. Alpha-adrenergic blocker
  1. Medication: dapiprazole hydrochloride (Rev-Eyes)
  2. Use: to counteract **mydriasis**

III. ANTIINFECTIVE EYE MEDICATIONS (Box 62-3)
A. Description: Kill or inhibit the growth of bacteria, fungi, and viruses
B. Side effects
  1. Superinfection
  2. Global irritation
C. Implementation
  1. Assess for risk of injury
  2. Instruct the client in how to apply the eye medication
  3. Instruct the client to continue treatment as prescribed
  4. Instruct the client to wash hands thoroughly and frequently
  5. Advise the client that if improvement does not occur, to notify the physician

IV. ANTIINFLAMMATORY EYE MEDICATIONS (Box 62-4)
A. Description
  1. Control inflammation, thereby reducing vision loss and scarring

2. Used for uveitis, allergic conditions, and inflammation of the conjunctiva, cornea, and lids
B. Side effects
  1. **Cataracts**
  2. Increased intraocular pressure
  3. Impaired healing
  4. Masking signs and symptoms of infection
C. Implementation
  1. Refer to Implementation, Antiinfective Eye Medications
  2. Note that dexamethasone (Maxidex) should not be used for eye abrasions and wounds

V. TOPICAL ANESTHETICS FOR THE EYE (Box 62-5)
A. Description
  1. Produce corneal anesthesia
  2. Used for anesthesia for eye examinations, for surgery, or to remove foreign bodies from the eye
B. Side effects
  1. Temporary stinging or burning of the eye
  2. Temporary loss of corneal reflex
C. Implementation
  1. Assess for risk of injury
  2. Note that the medications should not be given to the client for home use and are not to be self-administered by the client
  3. Note that the blink reflex is temporarily lost and that the corneal epithelium needs to be protected
  4. Provide an eye patch to protect the eye from injury until the corneal reflex returns

VI. EYE LUBRICANTS (Box 62-6)
A. Description
  1. Replace tears or add moisture to the eyes
  2. Moisten contact lenses or an artificial eye
  3. Protect the eyes during surgery or diagnostic procedures
  4. Used for keratitis, during anesthesia, or in a

BOX 62-6

Eye Lubricants

Hydroxypropyl methylcellulose (Lacril, Isopto Plain)
Petroleum-based ointment (Artificial Tears, Liquifilm Tears)

BOX 62-7

Miotics

Acetylcholine chloride (Miochol)
Carbachol (Miostat)
Pilocarpine hydrochloride (Isopto Carpine, Pilocar)
Pilocarpine nitrate (Pilofrin, Liquifilm, Pilagan)
Echothiophate iodide (Phospholine Iodide)
Demecarium bromide (Humorsol)
Isoflurophate (Floropryl)

---

disorder that results in unconsciousness or decreased blinking

B. Side effects
1. Burning on instillation
2. Discomfort or pain on instillation

C. Implementation
1. Inform the client that burning may occur on instillation
2. Be alert to allergic responses to the preservatives in the lubricants

▲ **VII. MIOTICS** (Box 62-7)

A. Description
1. Reduce intraocular pressure by constricting the pupil and contracting the ciliary muscle, thereby increasing the blood flow to the retina and decreasing retinal damage and loss of vision
2. Open the anterior chamber angle and increase the outflow of aqueous humor
3. **Miotic** cholinergic medications reduce intraocular pressure by mimicking the action of acetylcholine
4. **Miotic** acetylcholine inhibitors reduce intraocular pressure by inhibiting the action of cholinesterase
5. Used for chronic open-angle **glaucoma** or acute and chronic closed-angle **glaucoma**
6. Used to achieve **miosis** during eye surgery
7. Contraindicated in clients with **retinal detachment,** adhesions between the iris and lens, or inflammatory diseases
8. Use with caution in clients with asthma, hypertension, corneal abrasion, hyperthyroidism, coronary vascular disease, urinary tract obstruction, gastrointestinal (GI) obstruction, ulcer disease, parkinsonism, or bradycardia

B. Side effects
1. **Myopia**
2. Headache
3. Eye pain
4. Decreased vision in poor light
5. Local irritation
6. Systemic effects
   a. Flushing
   b. Diaphoresis
   c. GI upset and diarrhea
   d. Frequent urination
   e. Increased salivation
   f. Muscle weakness
   g. Respiratory difficulty
7. Toxicity
   a. Vertigo and syncope
   b. Bradycardia
   c. Hypotension
   d. Cardiac dysrhythmias
   e. Tremors
   f. Seizures

C. Implementation
1. Assess vital signs
2. Assess for risk of injury
3. Assess the client for the degree of diminished vision
4. Monitor for side effects and toxic effects
5. Monitor for postural hypotension and instruct the client to change positions slowly
6. Assess breath sounds for rales and rhonchi because cholinergic medications can cause bronchospasms and increased bronchial secretions
7. Maintain oral hygiene because of the increase in salivation
8. Have atropine sulfate available as an antidote for pilocarpine
9. Instruct the client or family regarding the correct administration of eye medications
10. Instruct the client not to stop the medication suddenly
11. Instruct the client to avoid activities such as driving while vision is impaired
12. Instruct clients with **glaucoma** to read labels on over-the-counter medications and to avoid atropine-like medications because atropine will increase intraocular pressure

VIII. OCUSERT SYSTEM

A. Description
1. Ocusert is a thin eye wafer (disk) impregnated with time-release pilocarpine
2. It is devised to overcome the frequent application of pilocarpine
3. It is placed in the upper or lower cul-de-sac of the eye
4. The pilocarpine is released over 1 week

5. The disk is replaced every 7 days
6. Drawbacks of its use include sudden leakage of pilocarpine, migration of the system over the cornea, and unnoticed loss of the system

B. Implementation
   1. Assess the client's ability to insert the medication disk
   2. Store the medication in the refrigerator
   3. Instruct the client to discard damaged or contaminated disks
   4. Inform the client that temporary stinging is expected but to notify the physician if blurred vision or brow pain occurs
   5. Instruct the client to check for the presence of the disk in the conjunctival sac daily at bedtime and upon arising
   6. Since vision may change in the first few hours after the eye system is inserted, instruct the client to replace the disk at bedtime

IX. BETA-ADRENERGIC BLOCKING EYE MEDICATIONS (Box 62-8)

A. Description
   1. Reduce intraocular pressure by decreasing sympathetic impulses and decreasing aqueous humor production without affecting **accommodation** or pupil size
   2. Used to treat chronic open-angle **glaucoma**
   3. Contraindicated in the client with asthma because systemic absorption can cause increased airway resistance
   4. Use with caution in the client receiving oral beta-blockers

B. Side effects
   1. Ocular irritation
   2. Visual disturbances
   3. Bradycardia
   4. Hypotension
   5. Bronchospasm

C. Implementation
   1. Monitor vital signs, especially blood pressure and pulse, before administering medication
   2. If the pulse is 60 or below or if the systolic blood pressure is below 90 mm Hg, withhold the medication and contact the physician
   3. Monitor for shortness of breath
   4. Assess for risk of injury
   5. Monitor I & O
   6. Instruct the client to notify the physician if shortness of breath occurs
   7. Instruct the client not to discontinue the medication abruptly
   8. Instruct the client to change positions slowly to avoid orthostatic hypotension
   9. Instruct the client to avoid hazardous activities
   10. Instruct the client to avoid over-the-counter medications without the physician's approval

---

BOX 62-8

Beta-Adrenergic Blocking Eye Medications

Betaxolol hydrochloride (Betoptic)
Carteolol hydrochloride (Ocupress)
Levobunolol hydrochloride (Betagan)
Metipranolol (Optipranolol)
Timolol maleate (Timoptic)

BOX 62-9

Adrenergic Medications

Apraclonidine hydrochloride (Iopidine)
Brimonidine tartrate (Alphagan)
Dipivefrin hydrochloride (Propine)
Epinephrine borate (Epinal, Eppy)
Epinephrine hydrochloride (Epifrin, Glaucon)

D. Adrenergic medications (Box 62-9)
   1. Decrease the production of aqueous humor and lead to a decrease in intraocular pressure
   2. Used to treat **glaucoma**

X. CARBONIC ANHYDRASE INHIBITORS (Box 62-10)

A. Description
   1. Interfere with the production of carbonic acid, which leads to decreased aqueous humor formation and decreased intraocular pressure
   2. Used for long-term treatment of open-angle **glaucoma**
   3. Contraindicated in the client allergic to sulfonamides

B. Side effects
   1. Appetite loss
   2. GI upset
   3. Paresthesias in the fingers, toes, and face
   4. Polyuria
   5. Hypokalemia
   6. Renal calculi
   7. Photosensitivity
   8. Lethargy and drowsiness
   9. Depression

C. Implementation
   1. Monitor vital signs
   2. Assess visual acuity
   3. Assess for risk of injury
   4. Monitor I & O
   5. Monitor weight
   6. Maintain oral hygiene
   7. Monitor for side effects such as lethargy, anorexia, drowsiness, polyuria, nausea, and vomiting
   8. Monitor electrolytes for hypokalemia

BOX 62-10

Carbonic Anhydrase Inhibitors: Eye Medications

Acetazolamide (Diamox, AK-Zol)
Dichlorphenamide (Daranide)
Dorzolamide hydrochloride (Trusopt)
Methazolamide (Neptazane)
Brinzolamide (Azopt)

BOX 62-10

Carbonic Anhydrase Inhibitors: Eye Medications

Acetazolamide (Diamox, AK-Zol)
Dichlorphenamide (Daranide)
Dorzolamide hydrochloride (Trusopt)
Methazolamide (Neptazane)
Brinzolamide (Azopt)

BOX 62-11

Osmotic Medications for the Eye

Glycerin (Glyrol, Osmoglyn)
Mannitol (Osmitrol)
Urea (Ureaphil)

BOX 62-12

Medications That Affect Hearing

ANTIBIOTICS
Amikacin (Amikin)
Chloramphenicol (Chloromycetin, Chloroptic, Ophthoclor)
Erythromycin (E-Mycin, ERYC, Ery-Tab, PCE Dispertabs, Ilotycin)
Gentamicin (Garamycin)
Streptomycin sulfate (Streptomycin)
Tobramycin sulfate (Nebcin)
Vancomycin (Vancocin)

DIURETICS
Acetazolamide (Diamox)
Furosemide (Lasix)
Ethacrynic acid (Edecrin)

OTHERS
Cisplatin (Platinol, Platinol-AQ)
Nitrogen mustard
Quinine (Quinamm)
Quinidine (Cardioquin, Quinaglute, Quinidex)

9. Increase fluid intake unless contraindicated
10. Advise the client to avoid prolonged exposure to sunlight
11. Encourage the use of artificial tears for dry eyes
12. Instruct the client not to discontinue the medication abruptly
13. Instruct the client to avoid hazardous activities while vision is impaired

XI. OSMOTIC MEDICATIONS (Box 62-11)
A. Description
  1. Lower intraocular pressure
  2. Used in emergency treatment of acute closed-angle **glaucoma**
  3. Used preoperatively and postoperatively to decrease vitreous humor volume
B. Side effects
  1. Headache
  2. Nausea, vomiting, diarrhea
  3. Disorientation
  4. Electrolyte imbalances
C. Implementation
  1. Assess vital signs
  2. Assess visual acuity
  3. Assess for risk of injury
  4. Monitor I & O
  5. Monitor weight
  6. Monitor electrolyte imbalances
  7. Increase fluid intake unless contraindicated
  8. Monitor for changes in level of orientation

XII. OTIC MEDICATION ADMINISTRATION
  (Box 62-12)
A. Administering drops
  1. In an adult, pull the pinna up and back to straighten the external canal to instill ear drops
  2. Pull the pinna down and back for infants and children younger than 3 years of age; up and back for older children

B. Irrigation of the ear
  1. Irrigation of the ear needs to be prescribed by the physician
  2. Ensure that there is direct visualization of the tympanic membrane
  3. Warm irrigating solution to 100° F because solutions that are not close to the client's body temperature will cause ear injury, nausea, and vertigo
  4. Irrigation must be done gently to avoid damage to the eardrum
  5. When irrigating, do not direct irrigation solution directly toward the eardrum
  6. If a perforation of the eardrum is suspected, irrigation is not done

XIII. ANTIINFECTIVE EAR MEDICATIONS
  (Box 62-13)
A. Description
  1. Kill or inhibit the growth of bacteria
  2. Used for otitis media or otitis externa
  3. Contraindicated if a prior hypersensitivity exists
B. Side effects: Overgrowth of nonsusceptible organisms
C. Implementation
  1. Monitor vital signs
  2. Assess for allergies
  3. Assess for pain
  4. Monitor for nephrotoxicity
  5. Instruct the client to report dizziness, fatigue, fever, or sore throat, which may be indicative of a superimposed infection

BOX 62-13

Antiinfective Ear Medications

Amoxicillin (Amoxil)
Ampicillin trihydrate (Polycillin)
Cefaclor (Ceclor)
Clindamycin hydrochloride (Cleocin)
Trimethoprim (TMP) and Sulfamethoxazole (SMZ)
  (Bactrim, Cotrim, and Septra)
Erythromycin (Ilotycin, E-Mycin)
Penicillin V potassium (Pen-V)
Loracarbef (Lorabid)
Clarithromycin (Biaxin)
Chloramphenicol (Chloromycetin Otic)
Polymyxin B sulfate (Aerosporin)
Tetracycline hydrochloride (Achromycin)
Acetic acid and aluminum acetate (Otic Domeboro)

BOX 62-14

Antihistamines and Decongestants

Triprolidine and pseudoephedrine (Actifed)
Naphazoline hydrochloride (Allerest, Albalon)
Chlorpheniramine (Chlor-Trimeton, Teldrin)
Brompheniramine (Bromphen, Dimetane)
Terfenadine (Seldane)
Clemastine (Tavist)
Cetirizine (Zyrtec)
Astemizole (Hismanal)

BOX 62-15

Ceruminolytic Medications

Carbamide peroxide (Debrox)
Boric acid (Ear-Dry)
Trolamine polypeptide oleate-condensate (Cerumenex)

6. Instruct the client to complete the entire course of the medication
7. Instruct the client to keep ear canals dry

XIV. ANTIHISTAMINES AND DECONGESTANTS (Box 62-14)
A. Description
 1. Produce vasoconstriction
 2. Stimulate the receptors of the respiratory mucosa
 3. Reduce respiratory tissue hyperemia and edema to open obstructed eustachian tubes
 4. Used for acute otitis media
B. Side effects
 1. Drowsiness
 2. Blurred vision
 3. Dry mucous membranes
C. Implementation
 1. Inform the client that drowsiness, blurred vision, and a dry mouth may occur
 2. Instruct the client to increase fluid intake unless contraindicated and to suck on hard candy to alleviate the dry mouth
 3. Instruct the client to avoid hazardous activities if drowsiness occurs

XV. LOCAL ANESTHETICS
A. Description
 1. Block nerve conduction at or near the application site to control pain
 2. Used for pain associated with ear infections
B. Medication: Benzocaine (Americaine Otic; Tympagesic)
C. Side effects
 1. Allergic reaction
 2. Irritation
D. Implementation
 1. Monitor for effectiveness if used for pain relief
 2. Assess for irritation or allergic reaction

XVI. CERUMINOLYTIC MEDICATIONS (Box 62-15)
A. Description
 1. Emulsify and loosen cerumen deposits
 2. Used to loosen and remove impacted wax from the ear canal
B. Side effects
 1. Irritation
 2. Redness or swelling of the ear canal
C. Implementation
 1. Instruct the client not to use drops more often than prescribed
 2. Moisten a cotton plug with medication before insertion
 3. Keep the container tightly closed and away from moisture
 4. Avoid touching the ear with the dropper
 5. Thirty minutes after instillation, gently irrigate the ear as prescribed with warm water, using a soft rubber bulb ear syringe
 6. Irrigation may be done with hydrogen peroxide solution as prescribed, to flush cerumen deposits out of the ear canal
 7. For a chronic cerumen impaction, 1 to 2 drops of mineral oil will soften the wax
 8. Instruct the client to notify physician if redness, pain or swelling persists

PRACTICE QUESTIONS

1. In preparation for cataract surgery, a nurse is to administer cyclopentolate (Cyclogel) eye drops. The nurse prepares to administer the eye drops, knowing that the purpose of this medication is to:
 1. Provide lubrication to the operative eye
 2. Produce miosis of the operative eye

3. Dilate the pupil of the operative eye
4. Constrict the pupil of the operative eye

2. A home health nurse visits a client at home and instructs the client in the administration of the prescribed eye drops. Which of the following statements by the client indicates a need for further education?
1. "I can tilt my head back, pull down on the lower lid, and place the drop in the lower lid."
2. "I can lie down, pull down on the lower lid, and place the drop in the lower lid."
3. "I can lie down, pull up on the upper lid, and place the drop in the lower lid."
4. "I can lie on my side opposite to the eye I am going to place the drop. Put the drop in the corner of the lid nearest my nose, and then slowly turn to my other side while blinking."

3. Ear drops are prescribed for an infant with otitis media. The most appropriate method to administer the ear drops to the infant is to:
1. Pull up and back on the pinna and direct the solution onto the eardrum
2. Pull down and back on the pinna and direct the solution onto the eardrum
3. Pull down and back on the ear and direct the solution toward the wall of the canal
4. Pull up and back on the earlobe and direct the solution toward the wall of the canal

4. A nurse is providing instructions to a client who will be self-administering eye drops. To minimize the systemic effects that eye drops can produce, the nurse instructs the client to:
1. Eat prior to instilling the drops
2. Swallow several times after instilling the drops
3. Blink vigorously to encourage tearing after instilling the drops
4. Occlude the nasolacrimal duct with a finger for several minutes after instilling the drops

5. A client is receiving both epinephrine hydrochloride (Epifrin, Glaucon) and timolol maleate (Timoptic) eye drops. When instructing the client in the administration of the eye drops, the nurse tells the client to:
1. Administer the epinephrine hydrochloride first, followed by the timolol maleate
2. Administer the timolol maleate first, followed by the epinephrine hydrochloride
3. Administer epinephrine hydrochloride in the morning and the timolol maleate in the evening
4. Wait 3 minutes between the instillation of each medication

6. A nurse is caring for a client with glaucoma. Which of the following medications, if prescribed for the client, would the nurse question?
1. Carbachol (Miostat)

2. Pilocarpine HCl (Isopto Carpine)
3. Pilocarpine nitrate (Ocusert Pilo-20, Pilo-40)
4. Atropine sulfate (Buf Opto-Atropine, Isopto-Atropine)

7. A miotic medication has been prescribed for a client with glaucoma. The client asks the nurse about the purpose of the medication. The nurse tells the client:
1. "The medication will lower the pressure in the eye and increase the blood flow to the retina."
2. "The medication will help to dilate the eye to prevent pressure from occurring."
3. "The medication will relax the muscles of the eyes and prevent blurred vision."
4. "The medication will help to block the responses that are sent to the muscles in the eye."

8. Pilocarpine hydrochloride (Isopto Carpine) is prescribed for a client with glaucoma. Which of the following medications does the nurse plan to have available in the event of systemic toxicity?
1. Naloxone hydrochloride (Narcan)
2. Pindolol (Visken)
3. Atropine sulfate
4. Mesoridazine besylate (Serentil)

9. Betaxolol (Betoptic) eye drops have been prescribed for a client with glaucoma. Which of the following nursing actions is most appropriate related to monitoring for the side effects of this medication?
1. Monitor temperature
2. Monitor blood pressure
3. Assess blood glucose level
4. Assess peripheral pulses

10. A nurse prepares a client for an ear irrigation as prescribed by a physician. In performing the procedure, the nurse:
1. Positions the client to turn her head so that the ear to be irrigated in facing upward
2. Warms the irrigating solution to 100° F
3. Directs a slow steady stream of irrigation solution toward the eardrum
4. Positions the client with the affected side up following the irrigation

CRITICAL THINKING: FREE-TEXT ENTRY

A nurse is providing instructions to a client with glaucoma regarding the procedure for administering eye drops. The nurse tells the client to perform what specific action following administration of the eye drops to prevent systemic absorption?

Answer: _____

ANSWERS

1. 3

Rationale: Cyclopentolate is a rapidly acting mydriatic and cycloplegic medication. It is effective in 25 to 75 minutes, and accommodation returns in 6 to 24 hours. Cyclopentolate is used for preoperative mydriasis.

Test-Taking Strategy: Use the process of elimination. Options 2 and 4 are similar and are eliminated first. Miosis refers to constricted pupil. Note that the question identifies a client being prepared for eye surgery. The pupil would need to be dilated for the surgical procedure. Review the action and purpose of this medication, if you had difficulty with this question.

Level of Cognitive Ability: Application
Client Needs: Physiological Integrity
Integrated Concept/Process: Nursing Process/Implementation
Content Area: Adult Health/Eye
Reference: Clark, J., Queener, S., & Karb, V. (2000). *Pharmacologic basis of nursing practice* (6th ed.). St. Louis: Mosby, p. 859.

2. 3

Rationale: The client can either lie down or sit with the head tilted back. The lower lid should be pulled downward with the thumb or fingers. The client holds the bottle like a pencil, with the tip downward, and squeezes the bottle gently, allowing 1 drop to fall into the sac. The client gently closes the eye. Options 1, 2, and 4 identify correct methods for administering eye drops.

Test-Taking Strategy: Use the process of elimination. Note the key words "need for further education." Knowing that the client places drops into the eye by pulling down on the lower lid will direct you to the correct option. Review the procedure for the administration of eye medications, if you had difficulty with this question.

Level of Cognitive Ability: Analysis
Client Needs: Health Promotion and Maintenance
Integrated Concept/Process: Teaching/Learning
Content Area: Adult Health/Eye
Reference: Clark, J., Queener, S., & Karb, V. (2000). *Pharmacologic basis of nursing practice* (6th ed.). St. Louis: Mosby, p. 65.

3. 3

Rationale: In a child younger than 3 years, pull the ear down and straight back. The infant should be turned on the side, with the affected ear uppermost. With the nondominant hand pull down and back on the earlobe. Rest the wrist of the dominant hand on infant's head. Administer the medication by aiming it at the wall of the canal rather than directly onto the eardrum. The infant should remain with the affected ear uppermost for 10 to 15 minutes to retain the solution. In the adult or a child older than 3 years, pull up and back on the pinna to straighten the auditory canal.

Test-Taking Strategy: Use the process of elimination. Eliminate options 1 and 2 because you would not direct ear solution directly onto the eardrum. Remember that in a child younger than 3 years, pulling the ear down and straight back is the correct procedure for administering ear medications. Review the procedure for the administration of ear medications, if you had difficulty with this question.

Level of Cognitive Ability: Application
Client Needs: Physiological Integrity
Integrated Concept/Process: Nursing Process/Implementation

Content Area: Child Health
Reference: Clark, J., Queener, S., & Karb, V. (2000). *Pharmacologic basis of nursing practice* (6th ed.). St. Louis: Mosby, p. 67.

4. 4

Rationale: Applying pressure on the nasolacrimal duct prevents systemic absorption of the medication. Options 1, 2, and 3 will not prevent systemic absorption.

Test-Taking Strategy: Use the process of elimination. Eating and swallowing are similar options and are not related to the systemic absorption of an eye medication. Blinking vigorously to produce tearing may result in the loss of the administered medication. Review the procedure for administering eye drops to prevent systemic absorption if you had difficulty with this question.

Level of Cognitive Ability: Application
Client Needs: Health Promotion and Maintenance
Integrated Concept/Process: Teaching/Learning
Content Area: Adult Health/Eye
Reference: Wilson, B., Shannon, M., & Stang, C. (2000). *Nurses drug guide 2000.* Stamford, Conn.: Appleton & Lange, p. 1124.

5. 4

Rationale: When two or more eye drop medications are to be administered, the client should wait 3 minutes between instillations. Options 1, 2, and 3 are incorrect.

Test-Taking Strategy: Use the process of elimination. Note that option 4 is different and provides specific information related to medication administration. Review the procedures for administering eye medications if you had difficulty with this question.

Level of Cognitive Ability: Application
Client Needs: Health Promotion and Maintenance
Integrated Concept/Process: Teaching/Learning
Content Area: Adult Health/Eye
Reference: Clark, J., Queener, S., & Karb, V. (2000). *Pharmacologic basis of nursing practice* (6th ed.). St. Louis: Mosby, p. 961.

6. 4

Rationale: Options 1, 2, and 3 are miotic agents used in the treatment of glaucoma. Option 4 is a mydriatic and cycloplegic medication, and its use is contraindicated in clients with glaucoma. Mydriatic medications dilate the pupil and can cause an increase in intraocular pressure.

Test-Taking Strategy: Use the process of elimination. Knowledge regarding the classifications of the medications identified in the options will assist in answering the question. Remember that mydriatics dilate and that these medications are contraindicated in glaucoma. Review the contraindications related to medications in the client with glaucoma if you had difficulty with this question.

Level of Cognitive Ability: Analysis
Client Needs: Physiological Integrity
Integrated Concept/Process: Nursing Process/Analysis
Content Area: Adult Health/Eye
Reference: Salerno, E. (1999). *Pharmacology for health professionals.* St. Louis: Mosby, p. 257.

7. 1

Rationale: Miotics are used to lower the intraocular pressure, thereby increasing blood flow to the retina and decreasing retinal damage and loss of vision. Miotics cause a contraction of the ciliary muscle and a widening of trabecular meshwork. Options 2, 3, and 4 are incorrect.

Test-Taking Strategy: Use the process of elimination. Note that the client has glaucoma. Recall that prevention of increased intraocular pressure is the goal in the client with glaucoma. Options 2, 3, and 4 all describe actions related to mydriatic medications, which primarily dilate the pupils and relax the ciliary muscles. Review the action of a miotic medication if you had difficulty with this question.
Level of Cognitive Ability: Application
Client Needs: Health Promotion and Maintenance
Integrated Concept/Process: Teaching/Learning
Content Area: Adult Health/Eye
Reference: Salerno, E. (1999). *Pharmacology for health professionals.* St. Louis: Mosby, p. 514.

8. **3**
Rationale: Systemic absorption of pilocarpine hydrochloride can produce toxicity, which includes manifestations of vertigo, bradycardia, tremors, hypotension, syncope, cardiac dysrhythmias, and seizures. Atropine sulfate must be available in the event of systemic toxicity. Mesoridazine besylate is an antipsychotic medication. Pindolol is a beta-adrenergic blocker. Naloxone hydrochloride is an opioid antagonist used to reverse narcotic-induced respiratory depression.
Test-Taking Strategy: Use the process of elimination and knowledge regarding antidotes related to various medications to answer this question. Remember that atropine sulfate is the antidote for systemic reactions that occur with pilocarpine. Review antidotes if you had difficulty with this question.
Level of Cognitive Ability: Analysis
Client Needs: Physiological Integrity
Integrated Concept/Process: Nursing Process/Planning
Content Area: Adult Health/Eye
Reference: Wilson, B., Shannon, M., & Stang, C. (2000). *Nurses drug guide 2000.* Stamford, Conn.: Appleton & Lange, p. 111.

9. **2**
Rationale: Hypotension, dizziness, nausea, diaphoresis, headache, fatigue, constipation, and diarrhea are systemic effects of the medication. Nursing interventions include monitoring the blood pressure for hypotension and assessing the pulse for strength, weakness, irregular rate, and bradycardia. Options 1, 3, and 4 are not side effects of this medication.
Test-Taking Strategy: Use the ABCs—airway, breathing, and circulation—to direct you to option 2. Although option 4, peripheral pulses, is also related to circulation monitoring, the blood pressure is the more global option. Review the side effect of this medication if you had difficulty with this question.
Level of Cognitive Ability: Analysis
Client Needs: Physiological Integrity
Integrated Concept/Process: Nursing Process/Assessment

Content Area: Adult Health/Eye
Reference: Hodgson, B., & Kizior, R. (2001). *Saunders nursing drug handbook 2001.* Philadelphia: W.B. Saunders, pp. 109-111.

10. **2**
Rationale: Irrigation solutions that are not close to the client's body temperature can be uncomfortable and may cause injury, nausea, and vertigo. Position the client so that the ear to be irrigated is facing downward, because this allows gravity to assist in the removal of the ear wax and solution. After the irrigation, the client is to lie on the affected side to finish the drainage of the irrigating solution. A slow, steady stream of solution should be directed toward the upper wall of the ear canal and not toward the eardrum. Too much force could cause the tympanic membrane to rupture.
Test-Taking Strategy: Use the process of elimination. Read each option carefully, and remember that the nurse's concern is to prevent damage to the tympanic membrane. In addition, remember that the client should be positioned with the affected side downward to allow drainage of the irrigation solution. Review the procedure for performing an ear irrigation if you had difficulty with this question.
Level of Cognitive Ability: Application
Client Needs: Physiological Integrity
Integrated Concept/Process: Nursing Process/Implementation
Content Area: Adult Health/Ear
Reference: Smith, S., Duell, D., & Martin, B. (2000). *Clinical nursing skills: Basic to advanced skills* (5th ed.). Upper Saddle River, N.J.: Prentice-Hall Health, pp. 417-418.

CRITICAL THINKING: FREE-TEXT ENTRY

Answer: Occlude the nasolacrimal duct
Rationale: To prevent overflow of the medication into nasal and pharyngeal passages, thus reducing systemic absorption, the client is taught to occlude the nasolacrimal duct with one finger for 1 to 2 minutes following administration of the medication.
Test-Taking Strategy: Focus on the issue, to prevent systemic absorption following administration of the eye drops. Visualize the procedure to determine what specific action will prevent this occurrence. If you are unfamiliar with the procedure for administering eye medications, review these guidelines.
Level of Cognitive Ability: Application
Client Needs: Health Promotion and Maintenance
Integrated Concept/Process: Teaching/Learning
Content Area: Adult Health/Eye
Reference: Clark, J., Queener, S., & Karb, V. (2000). *Pharmacologic basis of nursing practice* (6th ed.). St. Louis: Mosby, p. 855.

REFERENCES

Clark, J., Queener, S., & Karb, V. (2000). *Pharmacologic basis of nursing practice* (6th ed.). St. Louis: Mosby.

Hodgson, B., & Kizior, R. (2001). *Saunders nursing drug handbook 2001.* Philadelphia: W.B. Saunders.

LeMone, P., & Burke, K. (2000). *Medical-surgical nursing: Critical thinking in client care* (2nd ed.). Upper Saddle River, N.J.: Prentice-Hall.

Salerno, E. (1999). *Pharmacology for health professionals.* St. Louis: Mosby.

Smith, S., Duell, D., & Martin, B. (2000). *Clinical nursing skills: Basic to advanced skills* (5th ed.). Upper Saddle River, N.J.: Prentice-Hall Health.

Wilson, B., Shannon, M., & Stang, C. (2000). *Nurses drug guide 2000.* Stamford, Conn.: Appleton & Lange.

The Adult Client with a Neurological Disorder

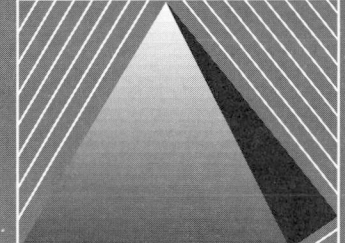

PYRAMID TERMS

agnosia   The inability to use an object correctly.

apraxia   The inability to carry out a purposeful activity.

autonomic dysreflexia   Also known as hyperreflexia. Caused by visceral distention from a distended bladder or impacted rectum. A neurological emergency, and must be treated immediately to prevent a hypertensive stroke. It occurs after the period of spinal shock is complete. Occurs with lesions or injuries above T6.

Babinski reflex   Indicates a disruption of the pyramidal tract. Dorsiflexion of the ankle and great toe with fanning of the other toes.

Brudzinski's sign   Flexion of the head causes flexion of both thighs at the hips and knee flexion. Indicates meningeal irritation.

decerebrate posturing   Client stiffly extends one or both arms and possibly the legs. Indicates a brainstem lesion.

decorticate posturing   Client flexes one or both arms on the chest and may stiffly extend the legs. Indicates a nonfunctioning cortex.

flaccid posturing   Client displays no motor response in any extremity.

Glasgow Coma Scale   A method of assessing a client's neurological condition. A scoring system based on a scale of 1 to 15 points. A score below 8 indicates that coma is present. Eye opening is the most important indicator.

halo traction   Pins or screws are inserted into the client's skull, and a circular fixation device and halo jacket or cast are applied.

hemianopia   Blindness in half the visual field.

homonymous hemianopia   Blindness in the same visual field of both eyes.

increased intracranial pressure   An increase in intracranial pressure caused by trauma, hemorrhage, growths or tumors, hydrocephalus, edema, or inflammation. Can impede circulation to the brain and absorption of cerebrospinal fluid (CSF), and affect the functioning of nerve cells and lead to brainstem compression and death.

Kernig's sign   Flex thigh and knee to right angle, and when they are extended, spasm of hamstring and pain occur. Indicates meningeal irritation.

skull tongs   Skull tongs are inserted into the outer aspect of the client's skull, just above the ears, and traction is applied.

spinal shock   Also known as neurogenic shock. A sudden depression of reflex activity in the spinal cord below the level of injury (areflexia). Occurs within the first hour of injury and lasts days to months. The muscles become completely paralyzed and flaccid, and reflexes are absent.

Tensilon test   Test done to diagnose myasthenia gravis and to differentiate between myasthenic crisis and cholinergic crisis.

unconscious client   A state of depressed cerebral functioning, with unresponsiveness to sensory and motor function. Some of the causes include head trauma, cerebral toxins, shock, hemorrhage, tumor, and infections.

PYRAMID TO SUCCESS

Pyramid points related to neurological disorders focus on monitoring for increased intracranial pressure, assessing level of consciousness, positioning clients, head injuries, spinal cord injuries, spinal shock, autonomic dysreflexia, implementation during a seizure, the client with a cerebrovascular accident (CVA), Parkinson's disease, myasthenia gravis, and the Tensilon test. Altered body image and psychosocial issues that occur as a result of a neurological disorder are also a focus of the Pyramid to Success. The Integrated Concepts and Processes addressed in this unit include Nursing Process, Caring, Communication and Documentation, Cultural Awareness, Self-Care, and Teaching/Learning.

CLIENT NEEDS
Safe, Effective Care Environment

Accident prevention related to neurological deficits
Advance directives
Advocacy
Asepsis with procedures and treatments
Client rights
Confidentiality
Consultation with members of the health care team

Establishing priorities
Informed consent for invasive procedures
Referrals
Standard (universal) precautions

Health Promotion and Maintenance

Expected body image changes resulting from neurological deficits
Home care instructions regarding care related to neurological disorder
Neurological assessment
Prevention and early detection of health problems associated with neurological deficits
Reinforcement regarding the importance of prescribed therapy

Psychosocial Integrity

Ability to cope with feelings of isolation and loss of independence
Cultural, religious, and spiritual influences
End-of-life issues
Grief and loss
Mobilizing coping mechanisms
Sensory and perceptual alterations
Support systems and utilization of community resources
Unexpected body image changes

Physiological Integrity

Alterations in body systems
Complications related to procedures

Emergency care
Fluid and electrolyte imbalances
Measures to promote comfort
Pharmacological therapy
Promoting normal elimination patterns
Promoting self-care measures
Use of assistive devices for mobility

REFERENCES

Craven, R., & Hirnle, C. (2000). *Fundamentals of nursing: Human health and function* (3rd ed.). Philadelphia: Lippincott.

Harkreader, H. (2000). *Fundamentals of nursing: Caring and clinical judgment.* Philadelphia: W.B. Saunders.

Ignatavicius, D., Workman, M., & Mishler, M. (1999). *Medical-surgical nursing across the health care continuum* (3rd ed.). Philadelphia: W.B. Saunders.

LeMone, P., & Burke, K. (2000). *Medical-surgical nursing: Critical thinking in client care* (2nd ed.). Upper Saddle River, N.J.: Prentice-Hall.

Lewis, S., Heitkemper, M., & Dirksen, S. (2000). *Medical-surgical nursing: Assessment and management of clinical problems* (5th ed.). St. Louis: Mosby.

National Council of State Boards of Nursing (eds.) (2000). *Test Plan for the National Council Licensure Examination for Registered Nurses.* Chicago: Author.

Potter, P., & Perry, A. (2001). *Fundamentals of nursing* (5th ed.). St. Louis: Mosby.

Smeltzer, S., & Bare, B. (2000). *Textbook of medical-surgical nursing* (9th ed.) Philadelphia: Lippincott Williams & Wilkins.

Neurological System

I. ANATOMY AND PHYSIOLOGY OF THE BRAIN AND SPINAL CORD

A. Cerebrum
1. Consists of the right and left hemispheres
2. Each hemisphere receives sensory information from the opposite side of the body and controls the skeletal muscles of the opposite side
3. Governs sensory and motor activity
4. Governs thought and learning
B. Cerebral cortex (Box 63-1)
1. Outer gray layer
2. Divided into four lobes
3. Responsible for the conscious activities of the cerebrum
C. Basal ganglia
1. Cell bodies in white matter
2. Assists cerebral cortex in producing smooth voluntary movements
D. Diencephalon
1. Thalamus
a. Relays sensory impulses to the cortex
b. Provides a thalamic pain gate
c. Part of the reticular activating system
2. Hypothalamus
a. Regulates autonomic responses of the sympathetic and parasympathetic nervous systems
b. Regulates stress response, sleep, appetite, body temperature, fluid balance, and emotions
c. Responsible for the production of hormones secreted by the pituitary gland and hypothalamus
E. Brainstem
1. Midbrain
a. Responsible for motor coordination
b. Visual reflex and auditory relay centers

BOX 63-1

Cerebral Cortex

FRONTAL LOBE
Broca's area for speech
Prefontal lobe controls morals, emotions, and judgments

PARIETAL LOBE
Interprets pain, touch, temperature, and pressure

TEMPORAL LOBE
Auditory center
Wenicke's area for sensory and speech

OCCIPITAL LOBE
Visual area

---

2. Pons
a. Contains respiratory centers
b. Regulates breathing
3. Medulla oblongata
a. Contains all afferent and efferent tracts
b. Contains cardiac, respiratory, vomiting, and vasomotor centers
c. Controls heart rate, respiration, blood vessel diameter, sneezing, swallowing, vomiting, and coughing
F. Cerebellum
1. Coordinates smooth muscle movement
2. Coordinates posture, equilibrium, and muscle tone
G. Spinal cord
1. Provides neuron and synapse networks to produce involuntary responses to sensory stimulation
2. Allows for control of the number of pain impulses that pass through the spinal cord on their way to the brain

3. Carries sensory information to, and motor information from, the brain
4. Extends from the first cervical to the second lumbar vertebra
5. Protected by the meninges, cerebrospinal fluid, and adipose tissue
6. Horns
    a. Inner column of gray matter contains two anterior and two posterior horns
    b. Posterior horns connect with afferent (sensory) nerve fibers
    c. Anterior horns contain efferent (motor) nerve fibers
7. Nerve tracts
    a. White matter contains the nerve tract
    b. Ascending tracts (sensory pathway)
    c. Descending tract (motor pathway)
H. Meninges
   1. Dura mater is the tough and fibrous membrane
   2. Arachnoid membrane is the delicate membrane and contains subarachnoid fluid
   3. Pia mater is the vascular membrane
   4. Subarachnoid space is formed by the arachnoid membrane and the pia mater
I. Cerebrospinal fluid
   1. Secreted in the ventricles and circulates through the ventricles to the subarachnoid layer of the meninges, where it is reabsorbed
   2. Circulates in the subarachnoid space
   3. Normal pressure is 50 to 175 mm H_2O
   4. Normal volume is 125 to 150 mL
   5. Acts as a protective cushion
   6. Aids in the exchange of nutrients and wastes
J. Ventricles
   1. Four ventricles
   2. Communicate between the subarachnoid spaces
   3. Produce and circulate cerebrospinal fluid
K. Blood supply
   1. Right and left internal carotids
   2. Right and left vertebral arteries
   3. These arteries supply the brain via an anastamosis at the base of the brain called the circle of Willis
L. Neurotransmitters
   1. Acetylcholine
   2. Norepinephrine
   3. Dopamine
   4. Serotonin
   5. Amino acids
   6. Polypeptides
M. Neurons
   1. The cell body
   2. Contains the axons and dendrites
   3. Neurons carrying impulses to the central nervous system (CNS) are called sensory neurons
   4. Neurons carrying impulses away from the central nervous system (CNS) are called motor neurons

5. Synapse is the chemical transmission of impulses from one neuron to another
N. Axons and dendrites
   1. The axon conducts impulses from the cell body
   2. The dendrites receive stimuli from the body and transmit them to the axon
   3. Protected and insulated by Schwann's cells
   4. The Schwann's cell sheath is called the neurolemma
   5. Neurons do not reproduce after the neonatal period
   6. If an axon or dendrite is damaged, it will die and be slowly replaced only if the neurolemma is intact and the cell body has not died
O. Spinal nerves
   1. Thirty-one pairs of spinal nerves
   2. Mixed nerve fibers are formed by the joining of the anterior motor and posterior sensory roots
   3. Posterior roots contain afferent (sensory) nerve fibers
   4. Anterior roots contain efferent (motor) nerve fibers
P. Autonomic nervous system
   1. Sympathetic (adrenergic) fibers dilate pupils, increase heart rate and rhythm, contract blood vessels, and relax smooth muscles of the bronchi
   2. Parasympathetic (cholinergic) fibers produce the opposite effect

II. DIAGNOSTIC TESTS
A. Skull and spinal x-ray
   1. Description
       a. X-rays of the skull reveal the size and shape of the skull bones, suture separation in infants, fractures or bony defects, erosion, or calcification
       b. Spinal x-rays identify fractures, dislocation, compression, curvature, erosion, narrowed spinal cord, and degenerative processes
   2. Implementation preprocedure
       a. Provide nursing support for the confused, combative, or ventilator-dependent client
       b. Maintain immobilization of the neck if a ▲ spinal fracture is suspected
       c. Remove metal items from body parts
       d. If the client has thick and heavy hair, this should be documented, because it may affect interpretation of the x-ray film
   3. Implementation postprocedure: Maintain immo- ▲ bilization until results are known
B. Computed tomography (CT) scan
   1. Description
       a. A type of brain scanning that may or may not require an injection of a dye
       b. Used to detect intracranial bleeding, space-occupying lesions, cerebral edema, infarc-

tions, hydrocephalus, cerebral atrophy, and shifts of brain structures

2. Implementation preprocedure
   a. Obtain a consent if a dye is used
   b. Assess for allergies to iodine, contrast dyes, or shellfish if a dye is used
   c. Instruct the client in the need to lie still and flat during the test
   d. Instruct the client to hold his or her breath when requested
   e. Initiate an IV if prescribed
   f. Remove objects from the head, such as wigs, barrettes, earrings, and hairpins
   g. Assess for claustrophobia
   h. Inform the client of possible mechanical noises as the scanning occurs
   i. Inform the client that there may be a hot, flushed sensation and a metallic taste in the mouth when the dye is injected
   j. Note that some clients may be given the dye even if they report an allergy, and are treated with an antihistamine and corticosteroids prior to the injection, to reduce the severity of a reaction

3. Implementation postprocedure
   a. Provide replacement fluids because diuresis from the dye is expected
   b. Monitor for an allergic reaction to dye
   c. Assess dye injection site for bleeding or hematoma, and monitor extremity for color, warmth, and the presence of distal pulses

C. Magnetic resonance imaging (MRI)
   1. Description
      a. A noninvasive procedure that identifies types of tissues, tumors, and vascular abnormalities
      b. Similar to the CT scan but provides more detailed pictures and does not expose the client to ionizing radiation
   2. Implementation preprocedure
      a. Remove all metal objects from the client
      b. Determine if the client has a pacemaker, implanted defibrillator, or metal implants such as a hip prosthesis or vascular clips because these clients cannot have this test performed
      c. Remove IV fluid pumps during the test
      d. Provide precautions for the client who is attached to pulse oximetry because it can cause a burn during testing if coiled around the body or a body part
      e. Provide an assessment of the client with claustrophobia
      f. Administer medication as prescribed for the client with claustrophobia
      g. Determine if a contrast agent is to be used, and follow the prescription related to the administration of food, fluids, and medications

   h. Instruct the client that he or she will need to remain still during the procedure
   3. Implementation postprocedure
      a. Client may resume normal activities
      b. Expect diuresis if a contrast agent was used

D. Lumbar puncture
   1. Description
      a. Insertion of a spinal needle through L3-L4 interspace into the lumbar subarachnoid space to obtain cerebrospinal fluid (CSF), measure CSF fluid or pressure, or instill air, dye, or medications
      b. Contraindicated in clients with **increased intracranial pressure**, because the procedure will cause a rapid decrease in pressure within the CSF around the spinal cord, leading to brain herniation
   2. Implementation preprocedure
      a. Obtain a consent
      b. Have the client empty the bladder
   3. Implementation during the procedure
      a. Position the client in a lateral recumbent position and have the client draw knees up to the abdomen and chin onto the chest
      b. Assist with the collection of specimens (label the specimens in sequence)
      c. Maintain strict asepsis
   4. Implementation postprocedure
      a. Monitor vital signs and neurological signs
      b. Position the client flat as prescribed
      c. Force fluids
      d. Monitor I & O

E. Myelogram
   1. Description: Injection of dye or air into the subarachnoid space to detect abnormalities of the spinal cord and vertebrae
   2. Implementation preprocedure
      a. Obtain a consent
      b. Provide hydration for at least 12 hours before the test
      c. Assess for allergies to iodine
      d. If the client is taking a phenothiazine, hold the medication because this medication lowers the seizure threshold
      e. Premedicate for sedation as prescribed
   3. Implementation postprocedure
      a. Vital signs and neurological assessment frequently as prescribed
      b. If a water-based dye is used, elevate the head 15 to 30 degrees for 8 hours as prescribed
      c. If an oil-based dye is used, keep the client flat 6 to 8 hours as prescribed
      d. If air is used, keep the head lower than the trunk as prescribed
      e. Administer analgesics for headache or backache as prescribed

f. Force fluids

g. Monitor I & O

h. Assess for bladder distention and voiding

F. Cerebral angiography

1. Description: Injection of contrast through the femoral artery into the carotid arteries to visualize the cerebral arteries and assess for lesions

2. Implementation preprocedure

a. Obtain a consent

b. Assess the client for allergies to iodine and shellfish

c. Encourage hydration for 2 days before the test

d. NPO 4 to 6 hours prior to the test as prescribed

e. Obtain a baseline neurological assessment

f. Mark the peripheral pulses

g. Remove metal items from the hair

h. Administer premedication as prescribed

3. Implementation postprocedure

a. Monitor neurological status and vital signs frequently until stable

b. Monitor for swelling in the neck and for difficulty swallowing and notify the physician if these symptoms occur

c. Maintain bed rest for 12 hours as prescribed

d. Elevate the head of the bed 15 to 30 degrees only if prescribed

e. Keep the bed flat if the femoral artery is used, as prescribed

f. Assess peripheral pulses

g. Immobilize the puncture site for 12 hours as prescribed

h. Apply sandbags and a pressure dressing to the injection site as prescribed

i. Place ice on the puncture site as prescribed

j. Force fluids

G. Electroencephalography (EEG)

1. Description: A graphic recording of the electrical activity of the superficial layers of the cerebral cortex

2. Implementation preprocedure

a. Wash the client's hair

b. Inform the client that electrodes are attached to the head and that electricity does not enter the head

c. Withhold stimulants, antidepressants, tranquilizers, and anticonvulsants for 24 to 48 hours prior to the test as prescribed

d. Allow the client to have breakfast if prescribed

e. Premedicate for sedation as prescribed

3. Implementation postprocedure

a. Wash the client's hair

b. Maintain side rails and safety precautions if the client was sedated

H. Caloric testing (oculovestibular testing)

1. Description: Provides information about the function of the vestibular portion of the eighth cranial nerve and aids in the diagnosis of cerebellum and brainstem lesions

2. Procedure

a. Patency of the external canal is confirmed

b. Cold or warm water is introduced into the external auditory canal

c. Stimulation of the auditory canal with warm water produces a horizontal nystagmus toward the side of the irrigated ear when the vestibular eighth cranial nerve is normal

d. Stimulation of the auditory canal with cold water produces a horizontal nystagmus away from the side of the irrigated ear if the brainstem is intact

III. NEUROLOGICAL ASSESSMENT

A. Assessment of risk factors

1. Trauma

2. Hemorrhage

3. Tumors

4. Infection

5. Toxicity

6. Metabolic disorders

7. Hypoxic conditions

8. Deficiency conditions

9. Hypertension

10. Cigarette smoking

11. Stress

B. Assessment of the cranial nerves

1. Cranial nerve I (olfactory): Sensory, smell

a. Have the client close eyes and occlude one nostril with finger

b. Ask the client to identify nonirritating odors such as coffee, tea, cloves, soap, chewing gum, and peppermint

c. Repeat the test on the other nostril

2. Cranial nerve II (optic): Sensory, vision

a. Assess visual acuity with a Snellen chart or newspaper, or ask the client to count how many fingers the examiner is holding up

b. Check visual fields by confrontation

c. Have the client sit directly in front of examiner and stare at examiner's nose

d. Examiner slowly moves his or her finger from the periphery toward the center until the client says it can be seen

e. Check color vision by asking the client to name the colors of several nearby objects

3. Cranial nerve III (oculomotor); cranial nerve IV (trochlear); cranial nerve VI (abducens)

a. The motor functions of these nerves overlap; therefore, they need to be tested together

b. First, inspect the eyelids for ptosis (drooping); then assess ocular movements and note any eye deviation

c. Test accommodation and direct and consensual light reflexes

d. Cranial nerve III (oculomotor): Motor; assesses pupillary constriction, upper eyelid elevation, and most eye movement

e. Cranial nerve IV (trochlear): Motor; assesses downward and inward eye movement

f. Cranial nerve VI (abducens): Assesses lateral eye movement

4. Cranial nerve V (trigeminal): Sensory and motor

a. Assesses sensation to the cornea, nasal and oral mucosa, facial skin, and mastication

b. To test motor function, ask the client to close jaws tightly, and then try to separate the clenched jaw

c. Test the corneal reflex by lightly touching the client's cornea with a cotton wisp

d. Check sensory function by asking the client to close the eyes; then lightly touch the forehead, cheeks, and chin, noting if the touch can be felt equally on both sides

5. Cranial nerve VII (facial): Sensory and motor

a. Test taste perception on the anterior two thirds of the tongue

b. Have the client show the teeth

c. Attempt to close the client's eyes against resistance, and ask the client to puff out the cheeks

d. Place sugar, salt, or vinegar on the front of the tongue, and have the client identify these substances by their tastes

6. Cranial nerve VIII (acoustic): Sensory

a. The ability to hear tests the cochlear portion

b. The sense of equilibrium tests the vestibular portion

c. Check the client's ability to hear a watch ticking or a whisper

d. Observe the client's balance, and observe for swaying when walking or standing

7. Cranial nerve IX (glossopharyngeal): Sensory and motor

a. Assesses swallowing ability

b. Assesses sensation to the pharyngeal soft palate and tonsillar mucosa, and taste perception on the posterior third of the tongue and salivation

8. Cranial nerve X (vagus): Sensory and motor

a. Assesses swallowing and phonation, sensation to the exterior ear's posterior wall, and sensation behind the ear

b. Assesses sensation to the thoracic and abdominal viscera

9. Cranial nerve IX (glossopharyngeal); cranial nerve X (vagus)

a. Have the client identify a taste at the back of the tongue

b. Inspect the soft palate and observe for symmetrical elevation when the client says "aah"

c. Touch the posterior pharyngeal wall with a tongue depressor to elicit a gag reflex

10. Cranial nerve XI (spinal accessory): Motor

a. Assesses uvula and soft palate movement, sternocleidomastoid and trapezius muscles

b. Assesses upper portion of the trapezius muscle, which governs shoulder movement and neck rotation

c. Palpate and inspect the sternocleidomastoid muscle as the client pushes the chin against the examiner's hand

d. Palpate and inspect the trapezius muscle as the client shrugs the shoulders against the examiner's resistance

11. Cranial nerve XII (hypoglossal): Motor

a. Assesses tongue movements involved in swallowing and speech

b. Observe the tongue for asymmetry, atrophy, deviation to one side, and fasciculations

c. Ask the client to push the tongue against a tongue depressor, then have the client move the tongue rapidly in and out and from side to side

C. Assessment of level of consciousness ▲

a. Assesses cerebral function

b. Assess client behavior to determine level of consciousness, such as confusion, delirium, unconsciousness, stupor, and coma

D. Assessment of vital signs: Monitor for blood pressure or pulse changes, which may indicate **increased intracranial pressure** (ICP)

E. Assessment of respirations (Box 63-2) ▲

F. Assessment of temperature ▲

1. An elevated temperature increases the brain's metabolic rate

2. An elevation in temperature may indicate a dysfunction of the hypothalamus or brainstem

3. A slow rise in temperature may indicate infection

G. Assessment of pupils ▲

1. Size

2. Equality

3. Reactions to light: described as brisk, slow, or fixed

4. Unusual eye movements

5. Unilateral pupil dilation indicates compression of the third cranial nerve

6. Midposition fixed pupil indicates midbrain injury

7. Pinpoint fixed pupil indicates pontine damage

H. Assessment of motor function ▲

1. Muscle tone, including strength and equality

2. Voluntary and involuntary movements

3. Purposeful and nonpurposeful movements

I. Assessment for posturing (Fig. 63-1) ▲

1. Posturing indicates a deterioration of the condition

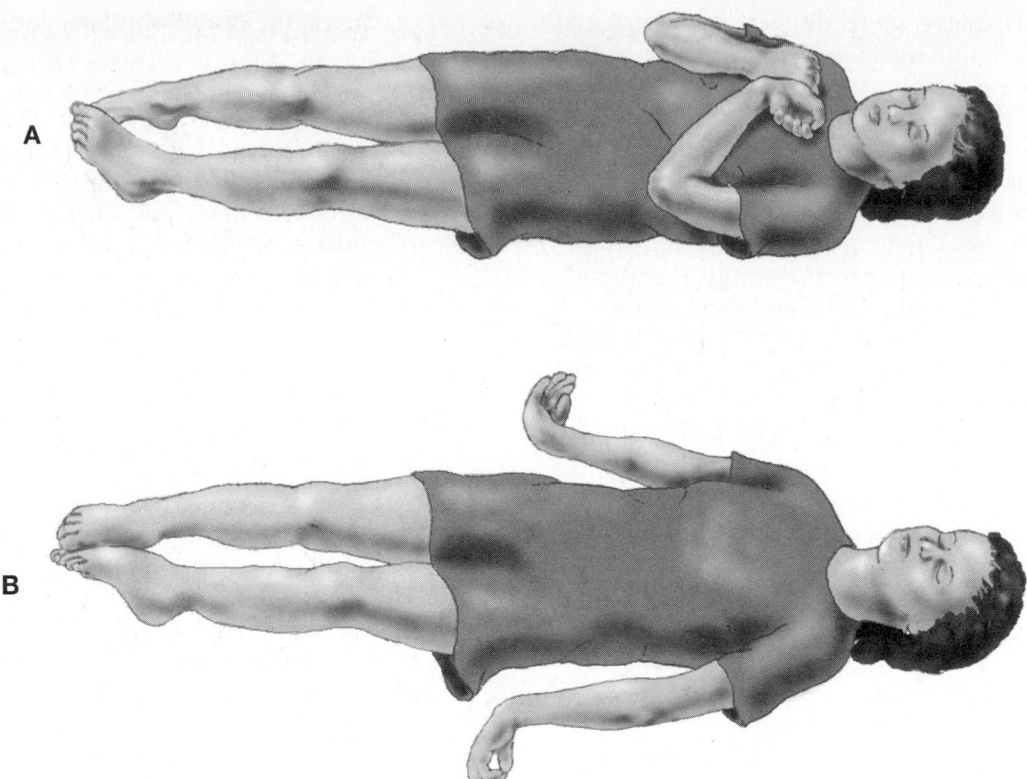

FIG. 63-1   Posturing. **A,** Decorticate posturing. **B,** Decerebrate posturing. (From Ignatavicius D, Workman M, Mishler M: *Medical-surgical nursing across the health care continuum,* ed 3, Philadelphia, 1999, WB Saunders.)

BOX 63-2

Assessment of Respirations

CHEYNE-STOKES
Rhythmical with periods of apnea
Can indicate a metabolic dysfunction or dysfunction in the cerebral hemisphere or basal ganglia

NEUROGENIC HYPERVENTILATION
Regular rapid and deep sustained respirations
Indicates a dysfunction in the low midbrain and middle pons

APNEUSTIC
Irregular respirations with pauses at the end of inspiration and expiration
Indicates a dysfunction in the middle or caudal pons

ATAXIC
Totally irregular in rhythm and depth
Indicates a dysfunction in the medulla

CLUSTER
Clusters of breaths with irregularly spaced pauses
Indicates a dysfunction in the medulla and pons

---

2. Flexor **(decorticate posturing)**
   a. Client flexes one or both arms on the chest and may stiffly extend the legs
   b. Indicates a nonfunctioning cortex
3. Extensor **(decerebrate posturing)**
   a. Client stiffly extends one or both arms and possibly the legs
   b. Indicates a brainstem lesion
4. **Flaccid posturing:** Client displays no motor response in any extremity
J. Assessment of reflexes (Box 63-3)
K. Assessment of meningeal irritation (Box 63-4)
   1. Nuchal rigidity
   2. Irritability
   3. Fever
L. Assessment of the autonomic system
   1. Sympathetic functions/adrenergic responses
      a. Increased pulse and blood pressure
      b. Dilated pupils
      c. Decreased peristalsis
      d. Increased perspiration
   2. Parasympathetic function/cholinergic responses
      a. Decreased pulse and blood pressure
      b. Constricted pupils

BOX 63-3

Assessment of Reflexes

BABINSKI REFLEX
Dorsiflexion of the ankle and great toe with fanning of the other toes
Indicates a disruption of the pyramidal tract

CORNEAL REFLEX
Loss of the blink reflex
Indicates a dysfunction of cranial nerve V

GAG REFLEX
Loss of the gag reflex
Indicates a dysfunction of cranial nerves IX and X

BOX 63-4

Assessment of Meningeal Irritation

BRUDZINSKI'S SIGN
Flexion of the head causes flexion of both thighs at the hips, and knee flexion

KERNIG'S SIGN
Flexion of the thigh and knee to right angles, and when extended, causes spasm of hamstring and pain

---

BOX 63-5

Glasgow Coma Scale

MOTOR RESPONSE POINTS
Obeys a simple response = 6
Localizes painful stimuli = 5
Normal flexion (withdrawal) = 4
Abnormal flexion (decorticate posturing) = 3
Extensor response (decerebrate posturing) = 2
No motor response to pain = 1

VERBAL RESPONSE POINTS
Oriented = 5
Confused conversation = 4
Inappropriate words = 3
Responds with incomprehensible sounds = 2
No verbal response = 1

EYE-OPENING POINTS
Spontaneous = 4
In response to sound = 3
In response to pain = 2
No response even to painful stimuli = 1

---

c. Increased salivation
d. Increased peristalsis
e. Dilated blood vessels
f. Bladder contraction

M. Assessment of sensory function
1. Touch
2. Pressure
3. Pain
4. Bladder control
5. Bowel control

N. **Glasgow coma scale** (Box 63-5)
1. A method of assessing a client's neurological condition
2. A scoring system based on a scale of 1 to 15 points
3. A score below 8 indicates coma is present
4. Eye opening is the most important indicator

IV. THE UNCONSCIOUS CLIENT
A. Description
1. A state of depressed cerebral functioning with unresponsiveness to sensory and motor function
2. Some of the causes include head trauma, cerebral toxins, shock, hemorrhage, tumor, and infection
B. Assessment
1. Unarousable
2. Primitive or no response to painful stimuli

3. Altered respirations
4. Decreased cranial nerve and reflex activity
C. Implementation (Box 63-6)

V. INCREASED INTRACRANIAL PRESSURE (ICP)
A. Description
1. An increase in **ICP** caused by trauma, hemorrhage, growths or tumors, hydrocephalus, edema, or inflammation
2. Can impede circulation to the brain, impede the absorption of CSF, affect the functioning of nerve cells, and lead to brainstem compression and death
B. Assessment
1. Assess level of consciousness (LOC), which is the most sensitive and earliest indication of **increasing intracranial pressure**
2. Declining LOC from restlessness to confusion and coma
3. Headache
4. Abnormal respirations
5. Rise in blood pressure with widening pulse pressure
6. Slowing of pulse
7. Elevated temperature
8. Vomiting
9. Pupil changes
10. Changes in motor function from weakness to hemiplegia, a positive **Babinski reflex, decorticate** or **decerebrate posturing,** and seizures
11. Late signs of **increased ICP** include increased

BOX 63-6

Care of the Unconscious Client

Assess patency of airway and keep an airway and emergency equipment at the bedside
Monitor blood pressure, pulse, and heart sounds
Assess respiratory and circulatory status
Maintain a patent airway and ventilation because a high CO_2 level increases intracranial pressure
Assess lung sounds for the accumulation of secretions
Suction PRN
Assess neurological status, including LOC, pupillary reactions, motor and sensory function
Place the client in semi-Fowler's position
Change position of the client every 2 hours, avoiding injury when turning
Avoid Trendelenburg position
Use side rails at all times
Assess for edema
Monitor for dehydration
Monitor I & O and daily weight
Maintain NPO status until consciousness returns
Maintain nutrition as prescribed, and monitor fluid and electrolyte balance
Check the gag and swallowing reflex before resuming diet, and begin with ice chips and fluids
Provide intravenous or enteral feedings as prescribed
Assess bowel sounds
Monitor elimination patterns
Monitor for constipation, impaction, and paralytic ileus
Maintain urinary output to prevent stasis, infection, and calculus formation
Monitor the status of skin integrity
Initiate measures to prevent skin breakdown
Provide frequent mouth care
Remove dentures and contact lenses
Assess the eyes for corneal reflex and irritation, and instill artificial tears or cover the eyes with eye patches
Monitor drainage from the ears or nose for the presence of cerebrospinal fluid
Assume that the unconscious client can hear
Avoid restraints
Do not leave the client unattended if unstable
Initiate seizure precautions if necessary
Provide range-of-motion exercises to prevent contractures
Use a footboard or high-top sneakers to prevent foot drop
Use splints to prevent wrist deformities
Initiate physical therapy as appropriate

BOX 63-7

Medications for ICP

MANNITOL (OSMITROL)
Hyperosmotic agent
Increases intravascular pressure by drawing fluid from the interstitial spaces and from the brain cells
Monitor renal function
Diuresis is expected

CORTICOSTEROIDS
Stabilize the cell membrane and reduce the leakiness in the blood-brain barrier
Decrease cerebral edema
A histamine blocker may be administered to counteract the excess gastric secretion that occurs with the corticosteroid
Clients must be withdrawn slowly from corticosteroid therapy to reduce the risk of adrenal crisis

BLOOD PRESSURE MEDICATION
May be required to maintain cerebral perfusion at a normal level
Notify the physician if the blood pressure range is below 100 or above 150 mm Hg systolic

ANTIPYRETICS AND MUSCLE RELAXANTS
Temperature reduction decreases metabolism, cerebral blood flow, and thus ICP
Muscle relaxants prevent shivering

ANTICONVULSANTS
May be given prophylactically to prevent seizures
Seizures increase metabolic requirements and cerebral blood flow and volume, thus increasing ICP

IV FLUIDS
Administered via infusion pump to control the amount of IV fluid administered
Hypertonic IV solutions are avoided because of the risk of promoting additional cerebral edema

systolic blood pressure, widened pulse pressure, and slowed heart rate

C. Implementation
  1. Elevate the head of the bed 30 to 40 degrees as prescribed
  2. Avoid Trendelenburg position
  3. Prevent flexion of the neck and hips
  4. Monitor respiratory status and prevent hypoxia
  5. Avoid the administration of morphine sulfate to prevent the occurrence of hypoxia
  6. Maintain mechanical ventilation as prescribed, maintaining the $Paco_2$ at 30 to 35 mm Hg, which will result in vasoconstriction of the cerebral blood vessels, decreased blood flow, and therefore decreased **ICP**
  7. Maintain body temperature
  8. Prevent shivering, which can raise **ICP**
  9. Decrease environmental stimuli
  10. Monitor electrolyte levels and acid-base balance
  11. Monitor I & O
  12. Limit fluid intake to 1200 mL/day

BOX 63-8

Surgical Intervention for ICP

VENTRICULOPERITONEAL SHUNT
Description
Shunts CSF from the ventricles into the peritoneum
Implementation Postprocedure
Position the client supine and turn from back to non-operative side
Monitor for signs of increasing ICP resulting from shunt failure
Monitor for signs of infection

BOX 63-9

Medications to Prevent Shivering

CHLORPROMAZINE HYDROCHLORIDE (THORAZINE)
Depresses thermoregulation in the hypothalamus and reduces peripheral vasoconstriction, muscle tone, and shivering

MEPERIDINE HYDROCHLORIDE (DEMEROL)
Relaxes the smooth muscle and reduces shivering

---

13. Instruct the client to avoid straining activities such as coughing and sneezing
14. Instruct the client to avoid Valsalva maneuver
D. Medications (Box 63-7)
E. Surgical intervention (Box 63-8)

VI. HYPERTHERMIA
A. Description
  1. A temperature of 106° F, which increases the cerebral metabolism and increases the risk of hypoxia
  2. The causes include infection, heat stroke, exposure to high environmental temperatures, and dysfunction of the thermoregulatory center
B. Assessment
  1. Temperature of 106° F
  2. Shivering
  3. Nausea and vomiting
C. Implementation
  1. Maintain a patent airway
  2. Initiate seizure precautions
  3. Monitor I & O and assess skin and mucous membranes for signs of dehydration
  4. Monitor lung sounds
  5. Monitor for dysrhythmias
  6. Assess peripheral pulses for systemic blood flow
  7. Induce normothermia with fluids, cool baths, fans, or hypothermia blanket
D. Inducing normothermia
  1. Prevent shivering, which will increase CSF pressure and oxygen consumption
  2. Administer medications as prescribed to prevent shivering
  3. Monitor neurological status
  4. Monitor for infection and respiratory complications because hypothermia may mask signs of infection
  5. Monitor for cardiac dysrhythmias
  6. Monitor I & O
  7. Prevent trauma to the skin and tissues
  8. Apply lotion to the skin frequently
  9. Inspect for frostbite
E. Medications to prevent shivering (Box 63-9)

VII. HEAD INJURY
A. Description
  1. A trauma to the skull resulting in mild to extensive damage to the brain
  2. Immediate complications include cerebral bleeding, hematomas, uncontrolled **increased ICP**, infections, and seizures
  3. Changes in personality or behavior, cranial nerve deficits, and any other residual deficits depend on the area of the brain damage and the extent of the damage
B. Types of head injuries (Box 63-10)
  1. Open
    a. Scalp lacerations
    b. Fractures in the skull
    c. Interruption of the dura mater
  2. Closed
    a. Concussions
    b. Contusions
    c. Fractures
C. Hematoma
  1. Description: Can occur as a result of a subarachnoid hemorrhage or an intracerebral hemorrhage
  2. Assessment
    a. Assessment findings will be dependent on the injury
    b. Clinical manifestations usually result from **increased ICP**
    c. Changing neurological signs in the client
    d. Changes in level of consciousness
    e. Airway and breathing pattern
    f. Vital signs for signs of **increasing ICP**
    g. Headache, nausea, and vomiting
    h. Visual disturbances, pupillary changes, papilledema, and extraocular eye movements
    i. Nuchal rigidity
    j. CSF drainage from the ears or nose
    k. Weakness and paralysis
    l. Posturing
    m. Decreased sensation or absence of feeling
    n. Reflex activity
    o. Seizure activity

BOX 63-10

Types of Head Injuries

CONCUSSION
A jarring of the brain within the skull with temporary loss of consciousness

CONTUSION
A bruising type of injury to the brain
It may occur with subdural or extradural collections of blood

SKULL FRACTURES
Linear
Depressed
Compound
Comminuted

EPIDURAL HEMATOMA
The most serious type of hematoma; forms rapidly and results from an arterial bleed
Forms between the dura and the skull from a tear in the meningeal artery
A surgical emergency

SUBDURAL HEMATOMA
Forms slowly and results from a venous bleed
It occurs under the dura, as a result of tears in the veins crossing the subdural space

SUBARACHNOID HEMORRHAGE
Bleeding directly into the brain, the ventricles, or the subarachnoid space

INTRACEREBRAL HEMORRHAGE
Multiple hemorrhages around a contused area

3. Implementation
  a. Monitor respiratory status and maintain a patent airway because increased CO_2 levels increase cerebral edema
  b. Monitor neurological status and vital signs, including temperature
  c. Monitor for **increased ICP**
  d. Maintain head elevation to reduce venous pressure
  e. Prevent neck flexion
  f. Initiate normothermia measures for increased temperature
  g. Assess cranial nerve function, reflexes, and motor and sensory function
  h. Initiate seizure precautions
  i. Monitor for pain and restlessness
  j. Avoid the administration of morphine sulfate because it is a respiratory depressant and may **increase ICP**
  k. Monitor for drainage from the nose or ears because this fluid may be CSF

  l. Do not attempt to clean the nose, suction, or allow the client to blow the nose if drainage occurs
  m. Do not clean the ear if drainage is noted, but apply a loose, dry sterile dressing
  n. Check drainage for the presence of CSF
  o. Notify the physician if drainage from ears or nose is noted
  p. Instruct the client to avoid coughing because this increases **ICP**
  q. Monitor for signs of infection
  r. Prevent complications of immobility

D. Craniotomy
  1. Description
    a. A surgical procedure that involves an incision through the cranium to remove accumulated blood or a tumor
    b. Complications of the procedure include **increased ICP** from cerebral edema, hemorrhage, or obstruction of the normal flow of CSF
    c. Additional complications include hematomas, hypovolemic shock, hydrocephalus, respiratory and neurogenic complications, pulmonary edema, and wound infections
    d. Complications related to fluid and electrolyte imbalances include diabetes insipidus and inappropriate secretion of antidiuretic hormone
  2. Implementation preoperatively
    a. Explain the procedure to the client and family
    b. Ensure that a consent has been obtained
    c. Prepare to shave the client's head as prescribed and cover the head with appropriate covering
    d. Stabilize the client prior to surgery
  3. Implementation postoperatively (Box 63-11)
  4. Postoperative positioning (Box 63-12)

VIII. SPINAL CORD INJURY

A. Description
  1. Trauma to the spinal cord causing partial or complete disruption of the nerve tracts and neurons
  2. The injury can involve contusion, laceration, or compression of the cord
  3. Spinal cord edema develops, and necrosis of the spinal cord can develop as a result of compromised capillary circulation and venous return
  4. Loss of motor function, sensation, reflex activity, and bowel and bladder control may result
  5. The most common causes include motor vehicle accidents, falls, sporting and industrial accidents, and gunshot or stab wounds
  6. Complications related to the injury include respiratory failure, **autonomic dysreflexia, spinal shock,** further cord damage, and death

BOX 63-11

Nursing Care Following Craniotomy

Monitor vital signs and neurological status every 30 minutes to 1 hour

Monitor for increased ICP

Monitor for decreased LOC, motor weakness or paralysis, aphasia, visual changes, and personality changes

Maintain mechanical ventilation and slight hyperventilation for the first 24 to 48 hours as prescribed to prevent increased ICP

Assess the physician's orders regarding client positioning

Avoid extreme hip or neck flexion, and maintain the head in a midline neutral position

Provide a quiet environment

Monitor the head dressing frequently for signs of drainage

Mark the area of drainage once each nursing shift for baseline comparison

Monitor the Hemovac or Jackson-Pratt drain, which may be in place for 24 hours

Maintain suction on the Hemovac or Jackson-Pratt drain

Measure drainage from the Hemovac or Jackson-Pratt drain every 8 hours, and record the amount and color

Notify the physician if drainage is greater than the normal of 30 to 50 mL per shift

Notify the physician immediately of excessive amounts of drainage or a saturated head dressing

Record strict measurement of hourly I & O

Maintain fluid restriction at 1500 mL/day as prescribed

Monitor electrolyte values

Monitor for dysrhythmias, which may occur as a result of fluid and electrolyte imbalance

Apply ice packs or cool compresses as prescribed for periorbital edema and ecchymosis of one or both eyes, which is not an unusual occurrence

Provide range-of-motion exercises every 8 hours

Place antiembolism stockings on the client as prescribed

Administer anticonvulsants, antacids, corticosteroids, and antibiotics as prescribed

Administer analgesics such as codeine sulfate and acetaminophen (Tylenol) as prescribed for pain

BOX 63-12

Client Positioning Following Craniotomy

Positions prescribed following craniotomy vary with the type of surgery and the specific postoperative physician's orders

Always check the physician's orders regarding client positioning

Incorrect positioning may cause serious and possibly fatal complications

REMOVAL OF A BONE FLAP FOR DECOMPRESSION

To facilitate brain expansion, the client should be turned from the back to the nonoperative side, but not to the side operated on

POSTERIOR FOSSA SURGERY

To protect the operative site from pressure and minimize tension on the suture line, position the client on the side, with a pillow under the head for support, and not on the back

INFRATENTORIAL SURGERY

Involves surgery below the brain's tentorium

The physician may order a flat position without head elevation or may order the head of the bed to be elevated at 30 to 45 degrees

Do not elevate the head of the bed in the acute phase of care following surgery without a physician's order

SUPRATENTORIAL SURGERY

Involves surgery above the brain's tentorium

The physician may order the head of the bed to be elevated at 30 degrees to promote venous outflow through the jugular veins

Do not lower the head of the bed in the acute phase of care following surgery without a physician's order

---

B. Most frequently involved vertebrae
   1. Cervical 5, 6, and 7
   2. Thoracic 12
   3. Lumbar 1
C. Transection of the cord
   1. Complete transection of the cord
      a. The spinal cord is completely severed, with total loss of sensation, movement, and reflex activity below the level of injury
      b. If the cord has not suffered irreparable damage, early treatment is needed to prevent partial damage from developing into total and permanent damage
   2. Partial transection of the cord
      a. The spinal cord is partially damaged or severed

   b. The symptoms depend on the extent and location of the damage
D. Types of injuries
   1. Anterior cord syndrome
      a. Damage to the anterior portion of the gray and white matter of the spinal cord
      b. Motor function, pain, and temperature sensation are lost below the level of injury; however, the sensations of touch, position, and vibration remain intact
   2. Posterior cord injury
      a. Damage to the posterior portion of the gray and white matter of the spinal cord
      b. Motor function remains intact, but the client experiences a loss of vibratory sense, crude touch, and position sensation
   3. Central cord syndrome
      a. Occurs from a lesion in the central portion of the spinal cord
      b. Loss of motor function is more pronounced in

BOX 63-13
Effects of the Spinal Cord Injury

QUADRIPLEGIA
Injury occurring from C1 through C8
Paralysis involving all four extremities

PARAPLEGIA
Injury occurring from T1 through L4
Paralysis involving only the lower extremities

the upper extremities, and varying degrees and patterns of sensation remain intact
4. Brown-Séquard syndrome
   a. Results from penetrating injuries that cause hemisection of the spinal cord or injuries that affect half of the cord
   b. Motor function, proprioception, vibration, and deep touch sensations are lost on the same side of the body (ipsilateral) as the lesion
   c. On the opposite side of the body (contralateral) from the injury, the sensations of pain, temperature, and light touch are affected

E. Assessment of spinal cord injuries (Box 63-13)
   1. Depends on the level of the cord injury
   2. The level of spinal cord injury is the lowest spinal cord segment with intact motor and sensory function
   3. Respiratory status changes
   4. Motor and sensory changes below the level of injury
   5. Total sensory loss and motor paralysis below the level of injury
   6. Loss of reflexes below the level of injury
   7. Loss of bladder and bowel control
   8. Urinary retention and bladder distention
   9. Presence of sweat, which does not occur on paralyzed areas

F. Cervical injuries
   1. C2 to C3 injury is usually fatal
   2. C4 is the major innervation to the diaphragm by the phrenic nerve
   3. Involvement above C4 causes respiratory difficulty and paralysis of all four extremities
   4. Client may have movement in the shoulder if the injury is at C5 or below

G. Thoracic level injuries
   1. Loss of movement of the chest, trunk, bowel, bladder, and legs, depending on the level of injury
   2. Leg paralysis (paraplegia)
   3. **Autonomic dysreflexia** with lesions or injuries above T6 and in cervical lesions
   4. Visceral distention from a distended bladder or impacted rectum may cause reactions such as

sweating, bradycardia, hypertension, nasal stuffiness, and gooseflesh

H. Lumbar and sacral level injuries
   1. Loss of movement and sensation of the lower extremities
   2. S2 and S3 center on micturation; therefore, below this level, the bladder will contract but not empty (neurogenic bladder)
   3. Injury above S2 in males allows them to have an erection, but they are unable to ejaculate because of sympathetic nerve damage
   4. Injury between S2 and S4 damages the sympathetic and parasympathetic response, preventing erection or ejaculation

I. Emergency implementation
   1. Emergency management is critical because improper handling can cause further damage and loss of neurological function
   2. Maintain a patent airway
   3. Always suspect spinal cord injury until this injury is ruled out
   4. Immobilize the client on a spinal backboard with the head in a neutral position to prevent an incomplete injury from becoming complete
   5. Prevent head flexion, rotation, or extension
   6. During immobilization, maintain traction and alignment on the head by placing hands on either side of the head by the ears
   7. Maintain an extended position
   8. Logroll the client
   9. No part of the body should be twisted or turned, and the client is not allowed to assume a sitting position
   10. In the emergency room, a client who has sustained a severe cervical injury should be placed immediately in skeletal traction via **skull tongs** or **halo traction** to immobilize the cervical spine and reduce the fracture and dislocation

J. Implementation during hospitalization
   1. Respiratory system
      a. Assess respiratory status because paralysis of the intercostal and abdominal muscles occurs with C4 injuries
      b. Monitor arterial blood gases and maintain mechanical ventilation if prescribed to prevent respiratory arrest, especially with cervical injuries
      c. Encourage deep breathing and the use of an incentive spirometer
      d. Monitor for signs of infection, particularly pneumonia
   2. Cardiovascular system
      a. Monitor for cardiac dysrhythmias
      b. Assess for signs of hemorrhage or bleeding around the fracture site
      c. Assess for signs of shock, such as hypotension, tachycardia, and a weak and thready pulse

d. Assess the lower extremities for deep vein thrombosis

e. Measure circumferences of calf and thigh

f. Apply thigh-high antiembolism stockings as prescribed

g. Remove antiembolism stockings daily to assess the skin

h. Monitor for orthostatic hypotension when repositioning the client

3. Neuromuscular system

a. Assess neurological status

b. Assess motor and sensory status to determine the level of injury

c. Assess motor ability by testing the client's ability to squeeze hands, spread the fingers, move the toes, and turn the feet

d. Assess sensation by pinching skin or pricking with a pin, starting at shoulders and working down the extremities

e. Monitor for signs of **autonomic dysreflexia** and **spinal shock**

f. Immobilize the client to promote healing and prevent further injury

g. Assess pain

h. Initiate measures to reduce pain

i. Administer analgesics as prescribed

j. Monitor for complications of immobility

k. Prepare the client for decompression laminectomy, spinal fusion, or insertion of steel rods if prescribed

l. Collaborate with the physical therapist and occupational therapist to determine appropriate exercise techniques, to assess the need for hand and wrist splints, and to develop an appropriate plan to prevent footdrop

4. Gastrointestinal system

a. Assess abdomen for distention and hemorrhage

b. Monitor bowel sounds and assess for paralytic ileus

c. Prevent bowel retention

d. Initiate a bowel control program as appropriate

e. Maintain adequate nutrition and a high-fiber diet

5. Renal system

a. Prevent bladder retention

b. Initiate a bladder control program as appropriate

c. Maintain fluid and electrolyte balance

d. Maintain adequate fluid intake of 2000 mL daily

e. Monitor for urinary tract infection and calculi

6. Integumentary system

a. Assess skin integrity

b. Turn the client every 2 hours

7. Psychosocial integrity

a. Assess psychosocial status

b. Encourage the client to express feelings of anger and depression

c. Discuss the sexual concerns of the client

d. Promote self-care, setting realistic goals based on the client's potential functional level

e. Encourage contact with appropriate community resources

K. **Spinal shock** ▲

1. Description

a. Also known as neurogenic shock

b. A sudden depression of reflex activity in the spinal cord below the level of injury (areflexia)

c. Occurs within the first hour of injury and can last days to months

d. The muscles become completely paralyzed and flaccid and reflexes are absent

e. **Spinal shock** ends when the reflexes are regained

2. Assessment

a. Flaccid paralysis

b. Hypotension

c. Bradycardia

d. Loss of reflex activity below the level of injury

e. Paralytic ileus

3. Implementation

a. Monitor for signs of **spinal shock** following a spinal cord injury

b. Monitor for hypotension and bradycardia

c. Monitor for reflex activity

d. Assess bowel sounds

e. Monitor for bowel and bladder retention

f. Provide supportive measures as prescribed, based on the presence of symptoms

g. Monitor for the return of reflexes

L. **Autonomic dysreflexia** ▲

1. Description

a. Also known as hyperreflexia

b. Commonly caused by visceral distention from a distended bladder or impacted rectum

c. A neurological emergency and must be treated immediately to prevent a hypertensive stroke

d. It generally occurs after the period of **spinal shock** is resolved

e. Occurs with lesions or injuries above T6 and in cervical lesions

2. Assessment

a. Hypertension

b. Bradycardia

c. Flushing of the face and neck

d. Severe, throbbing headache

e. Nasal stuffiness

f. Piloerection (gooseflesh)

g. Sweating

h. Nausea

i. Restlessness

j. Dilated pupils and blurred vision

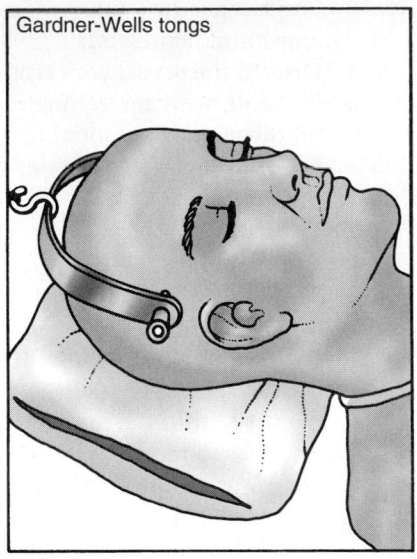
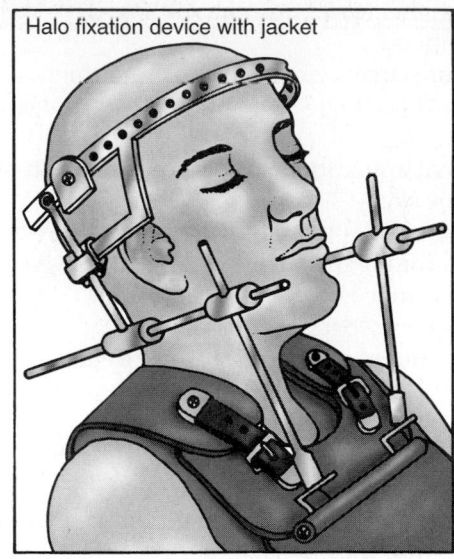

FIG. 63-2 Types of cervical spine traction. (From Ignatavicius D, Workman M, Mishler M: *Medical-surgical nursing across the health care continuum,* ed 3, Philadelphia, 1999, WB Saunders.)

3. Implementation
   a. Notify the physician if signs of **autonomic dysreflexia** occur
   b. Assess for the potential cause and remove the stimulus
   c. Monitor vital signs, particularly blood pressure, every 15 minutes
   d. Raise the head of the bed to high-Fowler's
   e. Loosen tight clothing
   f. Assess for bladder distention, and prepare for urinary catheterization
   g. If a urinary catheter is present, check for kinks in the tubing and for drainage
   h. Assess for a fecal impaction and disimpact immediately
   i. Administer antihypertensives as prescribed
M. Cervical traction for cervical injuries (Fig. 63-2)
   1. Description
      a. Skeletal traction is used to stabilize fractures or dislocations of the cervical or upper thoracic spine
      b. Two types of equipment used for cervical traction are **skull (cervical) tongs** and **halo traction (halo fixation device)**
   2. Skull tongs
      a. **Skull tongs** are inserted into the outer aspect of the client's skull, and traction is applied
      b. Weights are attached to the **tongs** and the client is used as countertraction
      c. Monitor neurological status of the client
      d. Determine the amount of weight prescribed to be added to the traction
      e. Ensure that weights hang securely and freely at all times
      f. Ensure that the ropes for the traction remain within the pulley

   g. Maintain body alignment and maintain care of the client on a special bed (Roto-Rest bed, Stryker, or Foster frame) as prescribed
   h. Turn the client every 2 hours
   i. Assess insertion site of the **tongs** for infection
   j. Provide sterile pin site care as prescribed
3. **Halo traction**
   a. A static traction device that consists of a headpiece with four pins, two anterior and two posterior, inserted into the client's skull
   b. The metal halo ring may be attached to a vest (jacket) or cast when the spine is stable, allowing increased client mobility
   c. Monitor the client's neurological status for changes in movement or decreased strength
   d. Never move or turn the client by holding or pulling on the **halo** device
   e. Assess for tightness of the jacket by ensuring that one finger can be placed under the jacket
   f. Assess skin integrity to ensure that the jacket or cast is not causing pressure
   g. Provide sterile pin site care as prescribed
4. Client education for **halo** fixation device (Box 63-14)
N. Implementation for thoracic and lumbar/sacral injuries
   1. Bed rest
   2. Immobilization with a body cast
   3. Use of a brace or corset when the client is out of bed
O. Surgical implementation for thoracic and lumbar/sacral injuries
   1. Decompressive laminectomy
      a. Removal of one or more laminae
      b. Allows for cord expansion from edema

BOX 63-14

Client Education for a Halo Fixation Device

Notify the physician if the halo vest (jacket) or ring bolts loosen

Use fleece or foam inserts to relieve pressure points

Keep the vest lining dry

Clean the pin site daily

Notify the physician if redness, swelling, drainage, open areas, pain, tenderness, or a clicking sound occurs from the pin site

A sponge bath or tub bath is allowed; showers are prohibited

Assess the skin under the vest daily for breakdown, using a flashlight

Do not use any products other than shampoo on the hair

When shampooing the hair, cover the vest with plastic

When getting out of bed, roll onto the side and push on the mattress with the arms

Never use the metal frame for turning or lifting

Use a rolled towel or pillowcase between the back of the neck and the bed, or next to the cheek when lying on the side, and raise the head of the bed to increase sleep comfort

Adapt clothing to fit over the halo device

Eat foods high in protein and calcium to promote bone healing

Have the correct-size wrench available at all times for an emergency

If cardiopulmonary resuscitation is required, the anterior portion of the vest will be loosened and the posterior portion will remain in place to provide stability

---

    c. Performed if conventional methods fail to prevent neurological deterioration

  2. Spinal fusion and rod insertion

    a. Used for thoracic spinal injuries

    b. Insertion of a metal or steel rod, such as Harrington rods, to stabilize the thoracic spine

  3. Implementation postoperatively

    a. Monitor for respiratory impairment

    b. Monitor vital signs, motor function, sensation, and circulatory status in the lower extremities

    c. Encourage breathing exercises

    d. Assess for signs of fluid and electrolyte imbalance

    e. Observe for complications of immobility

    f. Keep the client flat

    g. Provide cast care if the client is in a full body cast

    h. Turn and reposition frequently by logrolling side to back to side, using turning sheets and pillows between the legs to maintain alignment

    i. Administer pain medication as prescribed

    j. Maintain NPO status until the client is actively passing flatus

    k. Monitor bowel sounds

    l. Provide the use of a fracture bedpan

    m. Monitor I & O

    n. Maintain nutritional status

P. Medications

  1. Dexamethasone (Decadron)

    a. Used for its antiinflammatory and edema-reducing effects

    b. May interfere with healing

  2. Dextran

    a. A plasma expander

    b. Used to increase capillary blood flow within the spinal cord and to prevent or treat hypotension

  3. Dantrolene (Dantrium)/Baclofen (Lioresal)

    a. Used for clients with upper motor neuron injuries

    b. Controls muscle spasticity

IX. CEREBRAL ANEURYSM

A. Description

  1. Dilation of the walls of a weakened cerebral artery

  2. Can lead to rupture

B. Assessment

  1. Headache

  2. Pain

  3. Diplopia

  4. Blurred vision

  5. Tinnitus

  6. Nausea

  7. Hemiparesis

  8. Nuchal rigidity

  9. Irritability

  10. Seizures

C. Implementation

  1. Maintain a patent airway (suction only with a physician's order)

  2. Administer oxygen as prescribed

  3. Monitor vital signs and for hypertension or dysrhythmias

  4. Avoid rectal temperatures

  5. Maintain bed rest in semi-Fowler's position or side-lying position

  6. Maintain a darkened room without stimulation

  7. Limit visitors

  8. Maintain fluid restrictions

  9. Monitor I & O

  10. Avoid stimulants in the diet

X. SEIZURES

A. Description

  1. An abnormal sudden excessive discharge of electrical activity within the brain

  2. Epilepsy is a disorder characterized by chronic seizure activity and indicates brain or central nervous system (CNS) irritation

  3. Causes include genetic factors, trauma, tumors,

TABLE 63-1

Types of Seizures

Generalized Seizures	Partial Seizures
TONIC-CLONIC May begin with an aura The tonic phase involves the stiffening or rigidity of the muscles of the arms and legs and usually lasts 10 to 20 seconds, followed by loss of consciousness The clonic phase consists of hyperventilation and jerking of the extremities and usually lasts about 30 seconds Full recovery from the seizure may take several hours	**SIMPLE PARTIAL** Produces sensory symptoms accompanied by motor symptoms that are localized or confined to a specific area The client remains conscious and may report an aura
ABSENCE Brief seizure lasting seconds, and the individual may or may not lose consciousness No loss or change in muscle tone occurs Seizures may occur several times during a day The victim appears to be daydreaming This type of seizure is more common in children	**COMPLEX PARTIAL** A psychomotor seizure The area of the brain most involved is the temporal lobe Characterized by periods of altered behavior that the client is not aware of The client loses consciousness for a few seconds
MYOCLONIC A seizure that presents as a brief generalized jerking or stiffening of extremities The victim may fall to ground from the seizure	
ATONIC OR AKINETIC (DROP ATTACKS) A sudden momentary loss of muscle tone The victim may fall to ground as a result of the seizure	

circulatory or metabolic disorders, toxicity, and infections

4. Status epilepticus involves a rapid succession of epileptic spasms without intervals of consciousness; it is a potential complication that can occur with any type of seizure, and brain damage may result

B. Types of seizures (Table 63-1)
  1. Generalized seizures
    a. Tonic-clonic (grand mal)
    b. Absence (petit mal)
    c. Myoclonic
    d. Atonic or akinetic (drop attacks)
  2. Partial seizures
    a. Simple partial
    b. Complex partial

C. Assessment
  1. Seizure history
  2. Type of seizure
  3. Occurrences before, during, and after the seizure
  4. Prodromal signs, such as mood changes, irritability, and insomnia
  5. Aura, a sensation that warns the client of the impending seizure
  6. Loss of motor activity or bowel and bladder function, or loss of consciousness during the seizure

7. Occurrences during the postictal state, such as headache, loss of consciousness, sleepiness, and impaired speech or thinking

D. Implementation
  1. Note the time and duration of the seizure
  2. Assess behavior at the onset of the seizure: if the client experienced an aura, if a change in facial expression occurred, or if a sound or cry occurred from the client
  3. If the client is standing, place the client on the floor and protect the head and body
  4. Maintain a patent airway (do not force the jaws open)
  5. Administer oxygen
  6. Prepare to suction
  7. Turn the client's head to the side
  8. Prevent injury during the seizure
  9. Remain with the client
  10. Do not restrain the client
  11. Loosen restrictive clothing
  12. Note the type, character, and progression of the movements during the seizure
  13. Monitor for incontinence
  14. Administer medications such as IV diazepam (Valium), phenytoin (Dilantin), and phenobarbital sodium (Luminal) as prescribed to stop the seizure

15. Document the characteristics of the seizure
16. Monitor behavior following the seizure, such as the state of consciousness, motor ability, and speech ability
17. Instruct the client about the importance of lifelong medication and the need for follow-up medication blood levels
18. Instruct the client to avoid alcohol, excessive stress, and fatigue
19. Encourage the client to contact available community resources, such as the Epilepsy Foundation of America

XI. CEREBROVASCULAR ACCIDENT (CVA)

A. Description
   1. A sudden focal neurological deficit caused by cerebrovascular disease
   2. A syndrome in which the cerebral circulation is interrupted, causing neurological deficits
   3. Cerebral anoxia lasting longer than 10 minutes causes cerebral infarction with irreversible change
   4. Surrounding cerebral edema and congestion cause further dysfunction
   5. Diagnosis is determined by CT scan, EEG, and cerebral arteriography
   6. The permanent disability cannot be determined until the cerebral edema subsides
   7. The order in which function may return is facial, swallowing, lower limb, speech, and arms
B. Causes
   1. Thrombosis
   2. Embolism
   3. Hemorrhage from rupture of a vessel
   4. Transient ischemic attack (TIA)
C. Risk factors
   1. Atherosclerosis
   2. Hypertension
   3. Anticoagulation therapy
   4. Diabetes mellitus
   5. Stress
   6. Obesity
   7. Oral contraceptives
D. Assessment (Table 63-2; Boxes 63-15 and 63-16)
   1. Airway patency
   2. Pulse (may be slow and bounding)
   3. Respirations (Cheyne-Stokes)
   4. Blood pressure (hypertension)
   5. Headache, nausea, and vomiting
   6. Facial drooping
   7. Nuchal rigidity
   8. Visual changes
   9. Ataxia
   10. Dysarthria
   11. Dysphagia
   12. Speech changes
   13. Decreased sensation to pressure, heat, and cold

TABLE 63-2

Left and Right Hemisphere Lesions

Assessment findings depend on the area of the brain affected
Lesions in the cerebral hemisphere result in manifestations on the contralateral side, which is the side of the body opposite the cerebral accident

Left Hemisphere Lesion	Right Hemisphere Lesion
Aphasia both expressive and receptive	Disoriented to time, place, and person
Agraphia: difficulty writing	Cannot recognize faces
Alexia: reading problems	Spatial: perceptual deficits
No memory deficit	Neglect of left side
Deficits in the right visual field as reading problems and inability to discriminate words and letters	Client unaware of paralyzed side
	Loss of depth perception
No hearing deficit	Impulsive
Behavior slow, cautious, and disorganized	Unaware of neurological deficits
	Confabulates
Anxious when attempting a new task	Euphoric, impaired sense of humor
Depression	Constantly smiles
Sense of guilt	Denies illness
Quick anger and frustration	Poor judgment
Feelings of worthlessness	Overestimates ability
Worries over the future	Loss of ability to hear tonal variations

---

BOX 63-15

Neurological Assessment in CVA

Changes in level of consciousness (LOC)
Signs of increasing intracranial pressure (ICP)
Assessment of cranial nerves V, VII, IX, X, XII
Cranial nerve V: difficulty with chewing
Cranial nerve VII: facial paralysis or paresis
Cranial nerves IX and X: dysphagia
Cranial nerve IX: absent gag reflex
Cranial nerve XII: impaired tongue movement

BOX 63-16

Assessment Findings in a CVA

AGNOSIA
Inability to use an object correctly

APRAXIA
Inability to carry out a purposeful activity

HEMIANOPSIA
Blindness in half of the visual field

HOMONYMOUS HEMIANOPSIA
Blindness in the same side of both eyes
NOTE: With visual problems, client must turn the head to scan the complete range of vision

14. Bowel and bladder dysfunctions
15. Paralysis
E. Aphasia
   1. Expressive
      a. Damage in Broca's area of the frontal brain
      b. Client understands what is said but is unable to communicate verbally
   2. Receptive
      a. Injury involving Wernicke's area in the temporoparietal area
      b. Client is unable to understand the spoken and often the written word
   3. Global or mixed: Language dysfunction in both areas of expression and reception
   4. Implementation for aphasia
      a. Provide repetitive directions
      b. Break tasks down to one step at a time
      c. Repeat names of objects frequently used
      d. Use a picture board or communication board
F. Implementation during the acute phase of CVA
   1. Maintain a patent airway and administer oxygen as prescribed
   2. Monitor vital signs
   3. Maintain a blood pressure of 150/100 mm Hg to maintain cerebral perfusion
   4. Suction as prescribed, but never suction nasally and for no longer than 10 seconds, to prevent **increasing ICP**
   5. Monitor for **increasing ICP** because the client is at most risk during the first 72 hours following the CVA
   6. Position the client on the side, with head of bed elevated 15 to 30 degrees as prescribed
   7. Monitor LOC, pupillary response, motor and sensory response, cranial nerve function, and reflexes
   8. Maintain a quiet environment and provide minimal handling of the client to prevent further bleeding
   9. Insert a Foley catheter as prescribed
   10. Administer IVs as prescribed
   11. Maintain fluid and electrolyte balance
   12. Prepare to administer anticoagulants, antiplatelets, diuretics, antihypertensives, and anticonvulsants as prescribed
   13. Establish a form of communication
G. Implementation in the postacute phase of a CVA
   1. Continue with implementation from the acute phase
   2. Position the client 2 hours on the unaffected side, 20 minutes on the affected side
   3. Position the client in the prone position if prescribed, for 30 minutes three times daily
   4. Provide skin, mouth, and eye care
   5. Perform passive range-of-motion exercises to prevent contractures
   6. Place antiembolism stockings on client

7. Measure thighs and calves for an increase in size, and assess for positive Homans' sign
8. Monitor gag reflex and ability to swallow
9. Provide sips of fluids and slowly advance diet to foods that are easy to chew and swallow
10. Provide soft and semisoft foods and fluids rather than liquids, because the CVA client is better able to tolerate these types of food
11. When the client is eating, position the client sitting in a chair, or sitting up in bed with the head and neck positioned slightly forward and flexed
12. Place food in the back of the mouth on the unaffected side to prevent trapping of food in the affected cheek
H. Implementation in the chronic phase of CVA
   1. Approach the client from the unaffected side
   2. Place the client's personal objects within the visual field
   3. Instruct the client with visual problems to turn the head from side to side (scan the environment)
   4. Provide eye care for visual deficits
   5. Place a patch over the affected eye if the client has diplopia
   6. Increase mobility as tolerated
   7. Encourage fluids and a high-fiber diet
   8. Administer stool softeners as prescribed
   9. Encourage the client to express feelings
   10. Encourage independence in activities of daily living
   11. Assess the need for assistive devices such as a cane, walker, splints, or braces
   12. Teach transfer technique from bed to chair, and chair to bed
   13. Provide gait training
   14. Initiate physical and occupational therapy
   15. Refer to speech and language pathologist

XII. MULTIPLE SCLEROSIS (MS)

A. Description
   1. A chronic, progressive, noncontagious, degenerative disease of the CNS, characterized by demyelinization of the neurons
   2. It usually occurs between the ages of 20 and 40 and consists of periods of remissions and exacerbations
   3. The causes are unknown, but the disease is thought to be a result of autoimmune response or viral infection
   4. Precipitating factors include pregnancy, fatigue, stress, infection, and trauma
   5. EEG findings are abnormal
   6. A lumbar puncture indicates increased gamma globulin, but the serum globulin level is normal
B. Assessment
   1. Fatigue and weakness

2. Ataxia and vertigo
3. Tremors and spasticity of the lower extremities
4. Parasthesias
5. Blurred vision and diplopia
6. Nystagmus
7. Dysphasia
8. Decreased perception to pain, touch, and temperature
9. Bladder and bowel disturbances, including urgency, frequency, retention, and incontinence
10. Abnormal reflexes, including hyperreflexia, absent reflexes, and a positive **Babinski reflex**
11. Emotional changes such as apathy, euphoria, irritability, and depression
12. Memory changes and confusion

C. Implementation
1. Provide bed rest during exacerbation
2. Protect the client from injury by providing safety measures
3. Place an eye patch on the eye for diplopia
4. Monitor for potential complications such as urinary tract infections, calculi, decubitus ulcers, respiratory tract infections, and contractures
5. Promote regular elimination by bladder and bowel training
6. Encourage independence
7. Assist the client to establish a regular exercise and rest program
8. Instruct the client to balance moderate activity with rest periods
9. Assess the need for and provide assistive devices
10. Initiate physical and speech therapy
11. Instruct the client to avoid fatigue, stress, infection, overheating, and chilling
12. Instruct the client to increase fluids and eat a balanced diet, including low-fat, high-fiber foods and foods high in potassium
13. Instruct the client in safety measures related to sensory loss, such as regulating the temperature of bath water and avoiding heating pads
14. Instruct the client in safety measures related to motor loss, such as avoiding the use of scatter rugs and using assistive devices
15. Instruct the client in the self-administration of prescribed medications (Box 63-17)
16. Provide information about the National Multiple Sclerosis Society

XIII. MYASTHENIA GRAVIS

A. Description
1. A neuromuscular disease characterized by marked weakness and abnormal fatigue of the voluntary muscles
2. A defect in the transmission of nerve impulses at the myoneural junction occurs
3. Causes include insufficient secretion of acetylcholine, excessive secretion of cholinesterase, and

---

BOX 63-17

Medications Used with Multiple Sclerosis

CORTICOSTEROIDS
Corticotropin (ACTH) (Acthar)
Methylprednisolone Sodium Succinate (Solu-Medrol)
Used to reduce edema and the inflammatory response
Used to decrease the length of time the client's symptoms are exacerbated and improve the degree of recovery

IMMUNOSUPPRESSIVES
Used for the treatment of chronic progressive MS to stabilize the disease process

BACLOFEN (LIORESAL), DANTROLENE (DANTRIUM), OR DIAZEPAM (VALIUM)
Used to lessen muscle spasticity

CARBAMAZEPINE (TEGRETOL)
Used to treat paresthesia

PROPRANOLOL (INDERAL) AND CLONAZEPAM (CLONOPIN)
Used to treat cerebellar ataxia

BETHANECHOL (URECHOLINE)
Used to prevent urinary retention

OXYBUTYNIN CHLORIDE (DITROPAN)
Used to increase bladder capacity

---

unresponsiveness of the muscle fibers to acetylcholine

B. Assessment
1. Weakness and fatigue
2. Difficulty chewing
3. Dysphagia
4. Ptosis
5. Diplopia
6. Weak, hoarse voice
7. Difficulty breathing
8. Diminished breath sounds
9. Respiratory paralysis and failure

C. Implementation
1. Monitor respiratory status and ability to cough and deep breathe adequately
2. Monitor for respiratory failure
3. Maintain suctioning and emergency equipment at the bedside
4. Monitor vital signs
5. Monitor speech and swallowing abilities to prevent aspiration
6. Encourage the client to sit up when eating
7. Assess muscle status
8. Instruct the client to conserve strength
9. Plan short activities that coincide with times of maximal muscle strength
10. Monitor for myasthenic and cholinergic crises

11. Administer anticholinesterase medications as prescribed
12. Instruct the client to avoid stress, infection, fatigue, and over-the counter medications
13. Instruct the client to wear a Medic-Alert bracelet
14. Inform the client about services from the Myasthenia Gravis Foundation

D. Anticholinesterase medications
   1. Action: Increase levels of acetycholine at the myoneural junction
   2. Medications
      a. Neostigmine bromide (Prostigmin)
      b. Pyridostigmine bromide (Mestinon, Regonol)
      c. Edrophonium chloride (Tensilon)
   3. Side effects
      a. Sweating
      b. Salivation
      c. Nausea
      d. Diarrhea and abdominal cramps
      e. Bradycardia
      f. Hypotension
   4. Implementation
      a. Administer medications on time
      b. Administer medication 30 minutes before meals with milk and crackers to reduce gastrointestinal upset
      c. Monitor and record muscle strength
      d. Note that excessive doses lead to cholinergic crisis
      e. Have the antidote (atropine sulfate) available

E. Myasthenic crisis
   1. Description
      a. Acute exacerbation of disease
      b. Caused by a rapid, unrecognized progression of the disease, an inadequate amount of medication, infection, fatigue, or stress
   2. Assessment
      a. Restlessness
      b. Weakness
      c. Dyspnea
      d. Dysphagia
      e. Difficulty speaking
   3. Implementation
      a. Assess for signs of myasthenic crisis
      b. Increase anticholinesterase medication

F. Cholinergic crisis
   1. Description
      a. Depolarization of the motor end plates
      b. Caused by overmedication with anticholinesterase
   2. Assessment
      a. Restlessness
      b. Weakness
      c. Dysphagia
      d. Dyspnea
      e. Nausea, vomiting, and diarrhea
      f. Fasciculations

      g. Sweating
      h. Salivation
      i. Increased bronchial secretions
   3. Implementation
      a. Hold anticholinesterase medication
      b. Prepare to administer the antidote, atropine sulfate, if prescribed

G. **Tensilon test**   ▲
   1. Description: Performed to diagnose myasthenia gravis and to differentiate between myasthenic crisis and cholinergic crisis
   2. To diagnose myasthenia gravis
      a. Tensilon injection is administered to the client
      b. Positive for myasthenia gravis: Client shows improvement in muscle strength after the administration of Tensilon
      c. Negative for myasthenia gravis: Client shows no improvement in muscle strength, and strength may even deteriorate after injection of Tensilon
   3. To differentiate crisis
      a. Myasthenic crisis: Tensilon is administered, and if strength improves, the client needs more medication
      b. Cholinergic crisis: Tensilon is administered, and if weakness is more severe, the client is overmedicated; administer atropine sulfate, the antidote, as prescribed

XIV. **PARKINSON'S DISEASE**   ▲
A. Description
   1. A degenerative disease caused by the depletion of dopamine, which interferes with the inhibition of excitatory impulses
   2. It results in a dysfunction of the extrapyramidal system
   3. It is a slow, progressive disease that results in a crippling disability
   4. The debilitation can result in falls, self-care deficits, failure of body systems, and depression
   5. Mental deterioration occurs late in the disease
B. Assessment
   1. Bradykinesia, abnormal slowness of movement, and sluggishness of physical and mental responses
   2. Aching shoulders and arms
   3. Monotonous speech
   4. Handwriting that becomes progressively smaller
   5. Tremors in hands and fingers at rest (pill rolling)
   6. Tremors increasing when fatigued and decreasing with purposeful activity or sleep
   7. Rigidity with jerky interrupted movements
   8. Restlessness and pacing
   9. Blank facial expression
   10. Drooling
   11. Difficulty swallowing and speaking

12. Loss of coordination and balance
13. Shuffling steps, stooped position, and propulsive gait
C. Implementation
    1. Assess neurological status
    2. Assess ability to swallow and chew
    3. Provide high-calorie, high-protein, high-fiber soft diet with small frequent feedings
    4. Increase fluids to 2000 mL/day
    5. Monitor for constipation
    6. Promote independence along with safety measures
    7. Avoid rushing the client with activities
    8. Assist with ambulation
    9. Provide assistive devices
    10. Instruct the client to wear low-heeled shoes
    11. Encourage the client to lift feet when walking and to avoid prolonged sitting
    12. Provide a firm mattress, and position the client prone, without a pillow, to facilitate proper posture
    13. Instruct in proper posture by teaching the client to hold the hands behind the back to keep the spine and neck erect
    14. Promote physical therapy and rehabilitation
    15. Administer anticholinergic medications as prescribed to treat tremors and rigidity and to inhibit the action of acetylcholine
    16. Administer antiparkinsonian medications to increase the level of dopamine in the CNS
    17. Instruct the client to avoid foods high in vitamin B_6 because they block the effects of antiparkinsonian medications
    18. Instruct the client to avoid monoamine oxidase (MAO) inhibitors because they will precipitate hypertensive crisis
    19. Refer to Chapter 64 regarding medication to treat Parkinson's disease

XV. TRIGEMINAL NEURALGIA
A. Description
    1. A sensory disorder of the fifth cranial nerve
    2. Results in severe, recurrent, sharp, facial pain along the trigeminal nerve
B. Assessment
    1. Pain on the lips, gums, or nose, or across the cheeks
    2. Situations that stimulate symptoms, such as cold, washing the face, chewing, or food or fluids of extreme temperatures
C. Implementation
    1. Instruct the client to avoid hot or cold foods and fluids
    2. Provide small feedings of liquid and soft foods
    3. Instruct the client to chew food on the unaffected side
    4. Administer medications as prescribed (Box 63-18)

BOX 63-18

Medications to Treat Trigeminal Neuralgia

Carbamazepine (Tegretol)
Phenytoin (Dilantin)
Baclofen (Lioresal)
Amitriptyline (Elavil)
Diazepam (Valium)

D. Surgical implementation
    1. An alcohol injection along the affected portion of the nerve to produce anesthesia of the nerve may provide relief of pain for up to 16 months
    2. Retrogasserian rhizotomy or total severance of the sensory root of the trigeminal nerve
    3. Jannetta procedure, which surgically relocates the artery that is compressing the trigeminal nerve
    4. Electrocoagulation or percutaneous radiofrequency rhizotomy to create a heat lesion

XVI. BELL'S PALSY (FACIAL PARALYSIS)
A. Description
    1. A lower motor neuron lesion of the seventh cranial nerve that may occur as a result of trauma, hemorrhage, meningitis, or a tumor
    2. It results in paralysis of one side of the face
    3. Recovery usually occurs in a few weeks without residual effects
B. Assessment
    1. Flaccid facial muscles
    2. Inability to raise the eyebrows, frown, smile, close the eyelids, or puff out the cheeks
    3. Upward movement of the eye occurs when attempting to close the eyelid
    4. Loss of taste
C. Implementation
    1. Encourage active facial exercises to prevent the loss of muscle tone
    2. Provide a face sling to prevent stretching of weak muscles
    3. Protect the eyes from dryness and prevent injury
    4. Promote frequent oral care
    5. Instruct the client to chew on the unaffected side
    6. Administer analgesics and corticosteroids as prescribed

XVII. GUILLAIN-BARRÉ SYNDROME
A. Description
    1. An acute infectious neuronitis of the cranial and peripheral nerves
    2. The immune system overreacts to the infection and destroys the myelin sheath
    3. It is usually preceded by a mild upper respiratory infection or gastroenteritis

4. The recovery is a slow process and can take years
5. The major concern is difficulty breathing

B. Assessment
1. Paresthesias
2. Weakness of lower extremities
3. Gradual progressive weakness of upper extremities and facial muscles
4. Can progress to respiratory failure
5. Cardiac dysrhythmias
6. Cerebrospinal fluid reveals an elevated protein level
7. EEG is abnormal

C. Implementation
1. Care is directed toward the treatment of symptoms
2. Monitor respiratory status
3. Provide respiratory treatments
4. Prepare to initiate respiratory support
5. Monitor cardiac status
6. Assess for complications of immobility
7. Provide the client and family with support

XVIII. AMYOTROPHIC LATERAL SCLEROSIS

A. Description
1. Also known as Lou Gehrig's disease
2. A progressive degenerative disease involving the motor system
3. The sensory and autonomic systems are not involved, and mental status changes do not result from the disease
4. The cause of the disease may be related to an excess of glutamate, a chemical responsible for relaying messages between the motor neurons
5. As the disease progresses, muscle weakness and atrophy develop until a flaccid quadriplegia develops
6. Eventually the respiratory muscles become affected, leading to respiratory compromise, pneumonia, and death
7. There is no known cure, and the treatment is symptomatic

B. Assessment
1. Fatigue
2. Fatigue while talking
3. Muscle weakness and atrophy
4. Tongue atrophy
5. Dysphagia
6. Weakness of the hands and arms
7. Fasciculations of the face
8. Nasal quality of speech
9. Dysarthria

C. Implementation
1. Care is directed toward the treatment of symptoms
2. Monitor respiratory status
3. Provide respiratory treatments

4. Prepare to initiate respiratory support
5. Assess for complications of immobility
6. Provide the client and family with support

XIX. ENCEPHALITIS

A. Description
1. An inflammation of the brain parenchyma and often the meninges
2. Affects the cerebrum, the brainstem, and/or the cerebellum
3. Most often caused by a viral agent, although bacteria, fungi, or parasites may also be involved
4. Viral encephalitis is almost always preceded by a viral infection

B. Transmission
1. Arboviruses can be transmitted to humans through the bite of an infected mosquito or tick
2. Echovirus, coxsackievirus, poliovirus, herpes zoster, and viruses that cause mumps and chickenpox are common enteroviruses associated with encephalitis
3. Herpes simplex type 1 virus can cause viral encephalitis
4. Amebic meningoencephalitis can enter the nasal mucosa of people swimming in warm fresh water, ponds, and lakes

C. Assessment
1. Presence of cold sores, lesions, or ulcerations of the oral cavity
2. History of insect bites and swimming in fresh water
3. Exposure to infectious diseases
4. Travel to areas where the disease in prevalent
5. Fever
6. Nausea and vomiting
7. Stiff neck
8. Changes in LOC and mental status
9. Signs of **increased ICP**
10. Motor dysfunction and focal neurological deficits

D. Implementation
1. Monitor vital and neurological signs
2. Assess LOC using the **Glasgow Coma Scale**
3. Assess for mental status changes and personality and behavior changes
4. Assess for signs of **increased ICP**
5. Assess for the presence of nuchal rigidity and a positive **Kernig's** or **Brudzinski's sign,** indicating meningeal irritation
6. Assist the client to turn, cough, and deep breathe frequently
7. Elevate the head of the bed 30 to 45 degrees
8. Assess for muscle and neurological deficits
9. Administer acyclovir (Zovirax) as prescribed
10. Initiate rehabilitation as needed for motor dysfunction or neurological deficits

XX. MENINGITIS

A. Description
1. Inflammation of the arachnoid and pia mater of the brain and spinal cord
2. Caused by bacterial and viral organisms, although fungal and protozoal meningitis also occurs
3. Predisposing factors include skull fractures, brain or spinal surgery, sinus or upper respiratory infections, the use of nasal sprays, and individuals with a compromised immune system
4. CSF fluid is analyzed to determine the diagnosis and the type of meningitis

B. Transmission
1. Direct contact, including droplet spread
2. Occurs in areas of high population density, crowded living areas, and prisons

C. Assessment
1. Mild lethargy
2. Memory changes
3. Short attention span
4. Personality and behavior changes
5. Severe headache
6. Generalized muscle aches and pains
7. Nausea and vomiting
8. Fever and chills
9. Tachycardia
10. Deterioration in the LOC
11. Photophobia
12. Signs of meningeal irritation such as nuchal rigidity and positive **Kernig's sign** and **Brudzinski's sign**
13. Red, macular rash with meningococcal meningitis
14. Abdominal and chest pain with viral meningitis

D. Implementation
1. Monitor vital signs and neurological signs
2. Assess for signs of **increasing ICP**
3. Initiate seizure precautions
4. Monitor for seizure activity
5. Monitor for signs of meningeal irritation
6. Perform cranial nerve assessment
7. Assess vascular status
8. Maintain isolation precautions as necessary with bacterial meningitis
9. Maintain urine and stool precautions with viral meningitis
10. Maintain respiratory isolation for the client with pneumococcal meningitis
11. Elevate the head of the bed 30 degrees, and avoid neck flexion and extreme hip flexion
12. Prevent stimulation and restrict visitors
13. Administer analgesics as prescribed
14. Administer antibiotics as prescribed

PRACTICE QUESTIONS

1. A client has an impairment of cranial nerve II. Specific to this impairment, the nurse would plan to do which of the following to ensure client safety?
   1. Provide a clear path for ambulation without obstacles
   2. Test the temperature of the shower water
   3. Speak loudly to the client
   4. Check the temperature of the food on the dietary tray

2. A client has a neurological deficit involving the limbic system. Specific to this type of deficit, the nurse would document which of the following information related to the client's behavior?
   1. Demonstrates inability to add and subtract; does not know who is president
   2. Cannot recall what was eaten for breakfast today
   3. Disoriented to person, place, and time
   4. Affect flat, with periods of emotional lability

3. A nurse is planning to test the function of the trigeminal nerve (cranial nerve V). The nurse would gather which of the following items to perform the test?
   1. Flashlight, pupil size chart or millimeter ruler
   2. Tuning fork and audiometer
   3. Safety pin, hot and cold water in test tubes, cotton wisp
   4. Snellen's chart, ophthalmoscope

4. A nurse is testing the coordinated functioning of cranial nerves III, IV, and VI. To do this correctly, the nurse would test the:
   1. Corneal reflex
   2. Six cardinal fields of gaze
   3. Pupil response to light
   4. Pupil response to light and accommodation

5. A nurse is assessing the motor function of an unconscious client. The nurse would plan to use which of the following to test the client's peripheral response to pain?
   1. Sternal rub
   2. Pressure on the orbital rim
   3. Squeezing of the sternocleidomastoid muscle
   4. Nail bed pressure

6. A client admitted with a neurological problem indicates to the nurse that magnetic resonance imaging (MRI) may be done. The nurse interprets that the client may be ineligible for this diagnostic procedure based on the client's history of:
   1. Hypertension
   2. Chronic obstructive pulmonary disorder
   3. Heart failure
   4. Prosthetic valve replacement

7. A client is having a lumbar puncture (LP) performed. The nurse would plan to place the client in which position for the procedure?
   1. Side-lying, with legs pulled up and head bent down onto chest

2. Side-lying, with a pillow under the hip
3. Prone, in slight Trendelenburg
4. Prone, with a pillow under the abdomen

8. A client has just undergone computerized tomography (CT) scanning with a contrast medium. The nurse would evaluate that the client understands postprocedure care if the client stated that he or she needed to:
   1. Eat lightly for the remainder of the day
   2. Rest quietly for the remainder of the day
   3. Hold medications for at least 4 hours
   4. Force fluids for the day

9. A nurse is assisting with caloric testing of the oculovestibular reflex of an unconscious client. Cold water is injected into the left auditory canal. The client exhibits horizontal nystagmus toward the right. The nurse understands that this indicates the client has:
   1. A cerebral lesion
   2. A temporal lesion
   3. An intact brainstem
   4. Brain death

10. A nurse is admitting the client to the short stay unit after a myelogram. A water-based contrast agent was used. The nurse would plan which of the following activity restrictions for the client?
    1. Bed rest for 6 to 8 hours, with the head of bed elevated 15 to 30 degrees
    2. Bed rest for 2 to 4 hours, with the head of bed elevated 15 to 30 degrees
    3. Bed rest for 6 to 8 hours, with the head of bed flat
    4. Bed rest for 2 to 4 hours, with the head of bed flat

11. A nurse is caring for the client with increased intracranial pressure (ICP). The nurse would assess which of the following trends in vital signs if the intracranial pressure were rising?
    1. Increasing temperature, increasing pulse, increasing respirations, decreasing blood pressure (BP)
    2. Increasing temperature, decreasing pulse, decreasing respirations, increasing BP
    3. Decreasing temperature, decreasing pulse, increasing respirations, decreasing BP
    4. Decreasing temperature, increasing pulse, decreasing respirations, increasing BP

12. A nurse is positioning a client with increased intracranial pressure (ICP). Which of the following positions would the nurse avoid?
    1. Head turned to the side
    2. Head midline
    3. Neck in neutral position
    4. Head of bed elevated 30 to 45 degrees

13. A client recovering from a head injury is arousable and participating in care. The nurse would evaluate that the client understands measures to prevent elevations in intracranial pressure (ICP) if the nurse

observed the client doing which of the following activities?
   1. Exhaling during repositioning
   2. Isometric exercises
   3. Blowing the nose
   4. Coughing vigorously

14. A client has clear fluid leaking from the nose after a basilar skull fracture. The nurse assesses that this is cerebrospinal fluid (CSF) if the fluid:
    1. Clumps together on the dressing and has a pH of 7
    2. Separates into concentric rings and tests positive for glucose
    3. Is grossly bloody in appearance and has a pH of 6
    4. Is clear in appearance and tests negative for glucose

15. A client with a head injury has begun putting out copious amounts of urine through the Foley catheter. The client's urine output for the previous shift was 3000 mL. The nurse implements a new physician order to administer:
    1. Desmopressin (DDAVP, Stimate)
    2. Dexamethasone (Decadron)
    3. Ethacrynic acid (Edecrin)
    4. Mannitol (Osmitrol)

16. A nurse is caring for a client in the emergency department following a head injury. The client momentarily lost consciousness at the time of the injury, then regained it. The client has now lost consciousness again. The nurse takes quick action, knowing this is compatible with:
    1. Skull fracture
    2. Concussion
    3. Subdural hematoma
    4. Epidural hematoma

17. A nurse is evaluating the status of a client who had a craniotomy 3 days ago. The nurse would suspect that the client is developing meningitis as a complication of surgery if the client exhibits:
    1. A positive Brudzinski's sign
    2. A negative Kernig's sign
    3. Absence of nuchal rigidity
    4. A Glasgow Coma Scale score of 15

18. A client with a cervical spine injury has Crutchfield tongs applied in the emergency department. The nurse would avoid which of the following when planning care for this client?
    1. Use of a Roto-Rest bed
    2. Assessment of the integrity of the weights and pulleys
    3. Comparing the amount of ordered traction with the amount in use
    4. Removing the weights to reposition the client

19. A nurse has completed discharge instructions for a client with application of a Halo vest. The nurse

would evaluate that the client needs further clarification of the instructions if the client stated that he or she should:

1. Use caution since the vest alters balance
2. Wash the skin daily under the lamb's wool liner of the vest
3. Use a straw for drinking
4. Drive only during the daytime

20. A nurse is caring for a client who suffered a spinal cord injury 48 hours ago. The nurse monitors for gastrointestinal complications by assessing for:
    1. A flattened abdomen
    2. Hematest-positive nasogastric tube (NGT) drainage
    3. Hyperactive bowel sounds
    4. A history of diarrhea

21. A client with paraplegia has a nursing diagnosis of Risk for Injury related to spasticity of the leg muscles. Which of the following items would the nurse not include in a plan to minimize the risk of injury to the client?
    1. Removing potentially harmful objects near the spastic limbs
    2. Performing range-of-motion exercises to the affected limbs
    3. Use of padded restraints to immobilize the limb
    4. Use of PRN orders for muscle relaxants such as baclofen (Lioresal)

22. A nurse is caring for a client who has suffered a spinal cord injury. The nurse further assesses the client for other signs of autonomic dysreflexia if the client experiences:
    1. Severe, throbbing headache
    2. Pallor of the face and neck
    3. Sudden tachycardia
    4. Severe and sudden hypotension

23. The family of a client with a spinal cord injury rushes to the nursing station saying that the client needs immediate help. Upon entering the room, the nurse notes that the client is diaphoretic with a flushed face and neck, and complains of a severe headache. The pulse rate is 40 beats per minute and the blood pressure (BP) is 230/100 mm Hg. The nurse acts quickly, knowing that the client is experiencing:
    1. Spinal shock
    2. Malignant hypertension
    3. Pulmonary embolism
    4. Autonomic dysreflexia

24. A client with a spinal cord injury is prone to experiencing autonomic dysreflexia. The nurse would avoid which of the following measures to minimize the risk of recurrence?
    1. Strict adherence to a bowel retraining program
    2. Limiting bladder catheterization to once every 12 hours

3. Keeping the linen wrinkle-free under the client
4. Avoiding unnecessary pressure on the lower limbs

25. A nurse is planning care for a client in spinal shock. Which of the following actions would be least helpful in minimizing the effects of vasodilatation below the level of the injury?
    1. Monitoring vital signs before and during position changes
    2. Using vasopressor medications as prescribed
    3. Moving the client quickly as one unit
    4. Applying TEDs or compression stockings

26. A nurse is caring for a client admitted with spinal cord injury. The nurse minimizes the risk of compounding the injury most effectively by:
    1. Keeping the client on a stretcher
    2. Logrolling the client on a firm mattress
    3. Logrolling the client on a soft mattress
    4. Placing the client on a Stryker frame

27. A nurse is evaluating the neurological signs of a male client in spinal shock after spinal cord injury. Which of the following observations by the nurse indicates that spinal shock persists?
    1. Presence of bulbospongiosis reflex
    2. Hyperreflexia
    3. Inability to elicit a Babinski reflex
    4. Reflex emptying of the bladder

28. A nurse is assessing a client who is experiencing seizure activity. The nurse would not need to determine information about which of the following items as part of routine assessment of seizures?
    1. Duration of the seizure
    2. What the client ate in the 2 hours preceding seizure activity
    3. Seizure progression and type of movements
    4. Changes in pupil size or eye deviation

29. A nurse is planning to institute seizure precautions for a client who is being admitted from the emergency department. Which of the following measures would the nurse avoid in planning for the client's safety?
    1. Placing an airway, oxygen, and suction equipment at the bedside
    2. Padding the side rails of the bed
    3. Putting a padded tongue blade at the head of the bed
    4. Having IV equipment ready for insertion of an IV access

30. A nurse is caring for a client who begins to experience seizure activity while in bed. Which of the following actions by the nurse would be contraindicated?
    1. Loosening restrictive clothing
    2. Removing the pillow and raising padded side rails
    3. Restraining the client's limbs

4. Positioning the client to the side if possible, with head flexed forward

31. A nurse has given medication instructions to a client who is receiving phenytoin (Dilantin). The nurse evaluates that the client has an adequate understanding if the client states that:
    1. The medication dose may be self-adjusted depending on side effects
    2. Alcohol is not contraindicated while taking this medication
    3. Good oral hygiene is needed, including brushing and flossing
    4. The morning dose of the medication should be taken before a serum drug level is drawn

32. A nurse is planning care for a client with hemiparesis of the right arm and leg. The nurse incorporates in the care plan the statement that objects should be placed:
    1. Within the client's reach, on the right side
    2. Within the client's reach, on the left side
    3. Just out of the client's reach, on the right side
    4. Just out of the client's reach, on the left side

33. A client with a cerebrovascular accident (CVA) has residual dysphagia. When a diet order is initiated, the nurse avoids doing which of the following?
    1. Giving the client thin liquids
    2. Thickening liquids to the consistency of oatmeal
    3. Placing food on the unaffected side of the mouth
    4. Allowing plenty of time for chewing and swallowing

34. A nurse has instructed the family of a client with a cerebrovascular accident who has homonymous hemianopsia about measures to help the client overcome the deficit. The nurse would evaluate that the family understands the measures to use if they stated that they should:
    1. Place objects in the client's impaired field of vision
    2. Approach the client from the impaired field of vision
    3. Remind the client to turn the head to scan the lost visual field
    4. Discourage the client from wearing own eyeglasses

35. A nurse is assessing the adaptation of a client to changes in functional status after a cerebrovascular accident (CVA). The nurse assesses that the client is adapting most successfully if the client:
    1. Experiences bouts of depression and irritability
    2. Consistently uses adaptive equipment in dressing self
    3. Has difficulty in using modified feeding utensils
    4. Gets angry with family if they interrupt a task

36. A nurse has formulated a nursing diagnosis of unilateral neglect for a client with a cerebrovascular accident (CVA). Which of the following strate-gies would not be used by the nurse in planning to help the client adapt to this deficit?
    1. Move the commode and chair to the affected side
    2. Place the bedside articles on the affected side
    3. Approach the client from the unaffected side
    4. Teach the client to scan the environment

37. A nurse is trying to communicate with a cerebrovascular accident (CVA) client with aphasia. Which of the following actions by the nurse would be least helpful to the client?
    1. Speaking to the client at a slower rate
    2. Completing the sentences that the client cannot finish
    3. Looking directly at the client during attempts at speech
    4. Allowing plenty of time for the client to respond

38. A client with diplopia has been taught to use an eye patch to promote better vision and prevent injury. The nurse would evaluate that the client has correct understanding of the use of the patch if the client states that he or she should:
    1. Use the patch only when vision is especially troublesome
    2. Wear the patch for 1 hour at a time
    3. Wear the patch continuously, alternating eyes each day
    4. Wear the patch continuously, alternating eyes each week

39. A client receives a dose of edrophonium (Tensilon) intravenously. The client shows improvement in muscle strength for a period of time following the injection. The nurse interprets that this finding is compatible with:
    1. Multiple sclerosis
    2. Amyotrophic lateral sclerosis
    3. Myasthenia gravis
    4. Muscular dystrophy

40. A client with myasthenia gravis is having difficulty in speaking. The speech is dysarthric and has a nasal tone. The nurse would plan to avoid using which of the following communication strategies when working with this client?
    1. Repeating what the client said to verify the message
    2. Encouraging the client to speak quickly
    3. Using a communication board when necessary
    4. Asking yes and no questions when able

41. A client with myasthenia gravis has nursing diagnoses of Risk for Ineffective Airway Clearance and Risk for Ineffective Breathing Pattern. The nurse would keep which of the following available at the client's bedside?
    1. Incentive spirometer and cough pillow
    2. Oxygen and metered dose inhaler
    3. Pulse oximeter and a cardiac monitor
    4. Ambu bag and suction equipment

42. A client has experienced an episode of myasthenic crisis. The nurse would assess whether the client has precipitating factors such as:
    1. Too little exercise
    2. Increased intake of fatty foods
    3. Omitted doses of medication
    4. Excess medication

43. A nurse is teaching a client with myasthenia gravis about prevention of myasthenic and cholinergic crises. The nurse tells the client that this is most effectively done by:
    1. Doing all chores early in the day while less fatigued
    2. Taking medications on time to maintain therapeutic blood levels
    3. Doing muscle strengthening exercises
    4. Eating large, well balanced meals

44. A home health nurse is visiting a client with myasthenia gravis and is discussing methods to minimize the risk of aspiration during meals because of decreased muscle strength. Which of the following suggestions would the nurse avoid giving to the client?
    1. Sit straight up in the chair while eating
    2. Cut food into very small pieces, chewing thoroughly
    3. Swallow when the chin is tipped slightly downward to the chest
    4. Lift the head while swallowing liquids

45. A nurse has instructed a client with myasthenia gravis about ways to manage health at home. The nurse would evaluate that the client needs more information if the client made which of the following statements?
    1. "I should take my medications an hour before mealtime."
    2. "I've made arrangements to get a portable resuscitation bag and home suction equipment."
    3. "Going to the beach will be a nice, relaxing form of activity."
    4. "Here's the Medic-Alert bracelet I obtained."

46. A client with Parkinson's disease has a nursing diagnosis of Risk for Falls related to an abnormal gait documented in the nursing care plan. The nurse assesses the client, expecting to observe which type of gait?
    1. Broad based and waddling
    2. Accelerating with walking on toes
    3. Unsteady and staggering
    4. Shuffling and propulsive

47. A client with Parkinson's disease is embarrassed about the symptoms of the disorder, and is bored and lonely. The nurse would plan which of the following approaches as most therapeutic in assisting the client to cope with the disease?
    1. Plan only a few activities for the client during the day

2. Assist the client with activities of daily living (ADLs) as much as possible
3. Encourage and praise perseverance in exercising and performing ADLs
4. Cluster activities at the end of the day when the client is most bored

48. A nurse has given instructions to a client with Parkinson's disease about maintaining mobility. The nurse would evaluate that the client understood the directions if the client stated he or she should:
    1. Exercise in the evening to combat fatigue
    2. Rock back and forth to start movement with bradykinesia
    3. Sit in soft, deep chairs
    4. Buy clothes with many buttons to maintain finger dexterity

49. A nurse has given suggestions to a client with trigeminal neuralgia about strategies to minimize episodes of pain. The nurse would evaluate that the client needs reinforcement of information if the client made which of the following statements?
    1. "I will wash my face with cotton pads."
    2. "I'll have to start chewing on the unaffected side."
    3. "I should rinse my mouth sometimes if tooth brushing is painful."
    4. "I'll try to eat my food either very warm or very cold."

50. A client with Bell's palsy asks a nurse what caused this problem to occur. The nurse's response is based on an understanding that the etiology is:
    1. Unknown, but possibly includes ischemia, viral infection, or an autoimmune problem
    2. Unknown, but possibly includes long-term tissue malnutrition and cellular hypoxia
    3. Primarily genetic in origin, but triggered by exposure to neurotoxins
    4. Primarily genetic in origin, but triggered by exposure to meningitis

51. A client with an onset of Bell's palsy is very upset and crying about the change in facial appearance. The nurse plans to emotionally support the client by telling the client that:
    1. This is similar to a cerebrovascular accident (CVA), but all symptoms will reverse without treatment
    2. This is not a CVA, and many clients recover in 3 to 5 weeks
    3. This is caused by a small tumor, which can be easily removed
    4. This is a temporary problem, with treatment similar to that for migraine headaches

52. A nurse is reinforcing information given to a client with Bell's palsy about medications used to decrease edema of nerve tissue. The nurse gives the client specific information about which of the following medications?
    1. Acetylsalicylic acid (aspirin)

2. Ibuprofen (Motrin)
3. Dexamethasone (Decadron)
4. Prednisone (Deltasone)

53. A nurse has given a client with Bell's palsy instructions on preserving muscle tone in the face and preventing denervation. The nurse evaluates that the client needs additional information if the client states that he or she should:
   1. Expose the face to cold and drafts
   2. Massage the face with a gentle upward motion
   3. Wrinkle the forehead, blow out the cheeks, and whistle
   4. Use a device for electrical stimulation of the face

54. A client is admitted to the hospital with a diagnosis of Guillain-Barré syndrome. The nurse inquires during the nursing admission interview whether the client has a history of:
   1. Back injury or trauma to the spinal cord
   2. Seizures or trauma to the brain
   3. Respiratory or gastrointestinal (GI) infection during the previous month
   4. Meningitis during the last 5 years

55. A client with Guillain-Barré syndrome has ascending paralysis and is intubated and receiving mechanical ventilation. Which of the following strategies would the nurse incorporate in the plan of care to help the client cope with this illness?
   1. Giving client full control over care decisions and restricting visitors
   2. Providing information, giving positive feedback, and using distraction
   3. Providing IV sedatives, reducing distractions, and limiting visitors
   4. Providing positive feedback and encouraging active range of motion (ROM)

56. A nurse is admitting a client with Guillain-Barré syndrome to the nursing unit. The client has an ascending paralysis to the level of the waist. Knowing the complications of the disorder, the nurse brings which of the following items into the client's room?
   1. Nebulizer and pulse oximeter
   2. Flashlight and incentive spirometer
   3. ECG monitoring electrodes and intubation tray
   4. Blood pressure cuff and flashlight

57. A nurse is evaluating the respiratory outcomes for a client with Guillain-Barré syndrome. The nurse

would evaluate that which of the following is the least optimal outcome for the client?
   1. Adventitious breath sounds
   2. Spontaneous breathing
   3. Oxygen saturation 98%
   4. Vital capacity within normal range

58. A client is admitted with an exacerbation of multiple sclerosis (MS). The nurse is assessing the client for possible precipitating risk factors. Which of the following factors, if stated by the client, would the nurse assess as being unrelated to the exacerbation?
   1. A stressful week at work
   2. Ingestion of more fruits and vegetables
   3. A recent bout of the flu
   4. Inability to sleep well

59. A client with multiple sclerosis (MS) is experiencing muscle weakness, spasticity, and an ataxic gait. Based on this information, the nurse would formulate which of the following nursing diagnoses for the client?
   1. Impaired Physical Mobility
   2. Activity Intolerance
   3. Impaired Tissue Integrity
   4. Self-Care Deficit

60. A nurse is planning care for a client with a neurogenic bladder due to multiple sclerosis (MS). Which of the following plans for fluid administration of at least 2000 mL/day would be most helpful to this client?
   1. 400 to 500 mL with each meal, additional fluids in the morning, but not after mid-day
   2. 400 to 500 mL with each meal, 500 to 600 mL in the evening prior to bedtime
   3. 400 to 500 mL with each meal, 200 to 250 mL at midmorning, midafternoon, and late afternoon
   4. 400 to 500 mL with each meal, with all extra fluid concentrated in the afternoon and evening

CRITICAL THINKING: FREE-TEXT ENTRY

A client with a spinal cord injury suddenly experiences an episode of autonomic dysreflexia. After checking the vital signs, what is a nurse's next immediate action?

Answer: _____

ANSWERS

1. **1**

Rationale: Cranial nerve II is the optic nerve, which governs vision. The nurse can provide safety for the visually impaired client by clearing the path of obstacles when ambulating. Testing the shower water temperature would be useful if there were impairment of peripheral nerves. Speaking loudly may help overcome a deficit of cranial nerve VIII (vestibuloco-

chlear). Cranial nerve VII (facial) and IX (glossopharyngeal) control taste from the anterior 2/3 and posterior 1/3 of the tongue, respectively.

Test-Taking Strategy: Use the process of elimination. Recalling that cranial nerve II is the optic nerve will easily direct you to option 1. Review the function of this nerve if you had difficulty with this question.

Level of Cognitive Ability: Application

Client Needs: Safe, Effective Care Environment
Integrated Concept/Process: Nursing Process/Planning
Content Area: Adult Health/Neurological
Reference: Smeltzer, S., & Bare, B. (2000) *Brunner & Suddarth's textbook of medical-surgical nursing* (9th ed.). Philadelphia: Lippincott Williams & Wilkins, p. 1614.

2. 4

Rationale: The limbic system is responsible for feelings (affect) and emotions. Calculation ability and knowledge of current events relates to function of the frontal lobe. The cerebral hemispheres, with specific regional functions, control orientation. Recall of recent events is controlled by the hippocampus.

Test-Taking Strategy: Use the process of elimination. Recall that the limbic system is responsible for feelings and emotions to direct you to option 4. Review the function of the limbic system if you had difficulty with this question.

Level of Cognitive Ability: Application
Client Needs: Psychosocial Integrity
Integrated Concept/Process: Communication and Documentation
Content Area: Adult Health/Neurological
Reference: Smeltzer, S., & Bare, B. (2000). *Brunner & Suddarth's textbook of medical-surgical nursing* (9th ed.). Philadelphia: Lippincott Williams & Wilkins, p. 75.

3. 3

Rationale: The trigeminal nerve has a motor and sensory division. The motor division innervates the muscles for chewing (mastication). The sensory division innervates the entire face, scalp, cornea, and nasal and oral cavities. The sensations of pain, temperature, and touch can be assessed by use of each of the respective items noted in option 3. The corneal reflex (motor division) can also be tested using the cotton wisp. The supplies noted in options 1, 2, and 4 are used for testing cranial nerves III, VIII, and II respectively.

Test-Taking Strategy: Use the process of elimination. Recalling the function of cranial nerve V will direct you to option 3. Review the function of this nerve if you had difficulty with this question.

Level of Cognitive Ability: Application
Client Needs: Health Promotion and Maintenance
Integrated Concept/Process: Nursing Process/Assessment
Content Area: Adult Health/Neurological
Reference: Smeltzer, S., & Bare, B. (2000). *Brunner & Suddarth's textbook of medical-surgical nursing* (9th ed.). Philadelphia: Lippincott Williams & Wilkins, p. 1615.

4. 2

Rationale: Cranial nerves III (oculomotor), IV (trochlear), and VI (abducens) have only motor components, and control, in a coordinated manner, the six cardinal fields of gaze. This is tested by moving an object in six directions (involving horizontal and diagonal movements). Corneal reflex is the function of the trigeminal nerve (cranial nerve V). Pupillary response and accommodation is the function of cranial nerve III alone.

Test-Taking Strategy: If you look at this question carefully, you will see that each of the incorrect options has to do with pupillary reactions of some type. The correct option is the one that is different from the others. Being able to move the eyes through the six cardinal fields of gaze is a coordinated effort of three cranial nerves. Review cranial nerve testing if you had difficulty with this question.

Level of Cognitive Ability: Application
Client Needs: Health Promotion and Maintenance
Integrated Concept/Process: Nursing Process/Assessment
Content Area: Adult Health/Neurological
Reference: Smeltzer, S., & Bare, B. (2000). *Brunner & Suddarth's textbook of medical-surgical nursing* (9th ed.). Philadelphia: Lippincott Williams & Wilkins, p. 1615.

5. 4

Rationale: Motor testing of the unconscious client can be done only by testing response to painful stimuli. Nailbed pressure tests a basic peripheral response. Cerebral responses to pain are tested by sternal rub, placing upward pressure on the orbital rim, or squeezing the clavicle or sternocleidomastoid muscle.

Test-Taking Strategy: If you evaluate this question from the viewpoint of the location of each of the body parts described, you can easily determine the correct option. The nailbeds are the most distal of all the choices, and is therefore the most peripheral. Each of the other options may elicit a generalized response, but not a localized one. Review the process of peripheral testing if you had difficulty with this question.

Level of Cognitive Ability: Application
Client Needs: Safe, Effective Care Environment
Integrated Concept/Process: Nursing Process/Assessment
Content Area: Adult Health/Neurological
Reference: Phipps, W., Sands, J., & Marek, J. (1999). *Medical-surgical nursing: Concepts & clinical practice* (6th ed.). St. Louis: Mosby, p. 1768.

6. 4

Rationale: The client having a MRI has all metallic objects removed, because of the magnetic field generated by the device. A careful history is done to determine if any metal objects are inside the client, such as orthopedic hardware, pacemakers, artificial heart valves, aneurysm clips, or intrauterine devices. These may heat up, become dislodged, or malfunction during this procedure. The client may be ineligible if there is significant risk.

Test-Taking Strategy: Use the process of elimination, noting the key word "ineligible." You will note that each of the incorrect options is a medical disorder. The correct option is the name of a surgical procedure where an artificial valve (sometimes metal) is implanted. An important concept with regard to MRI is the avoidance of any metal objects in the vicinity of the machine. Review the contraindications related to this procedure if you had difficulty with this question.

Level of Cognitive Ability: Analysis
Client Needs: Physiological Integrity
Integrated Concept/Process: Nursing Process/Assessment
Content Area: Adult Health/Neurological
Reference: Smeltzer, S., & Bare, B. (2000). *Brunner & Suddarth's textbook of medical-surgical nursing* (9th ed.). Philadelphia: Lippincott Williams & Wilkins, p. 1627.

7. 1

Rationale: The client undergoing LP is positioned lying on the side, with the legs pulled up to the abdomen, and with the head bent down onto the chest. This position helps to open the spaces between the vertebrae.

Test-Taking Strategy: Use the process of elimination. Recall that an LP is the introduction of a needle into the subarachnoid space. The correct option is the only position that flexes

the vertebrae for easier needle insertion. Review positioning procedures for an LP if you had difficulty with this question.
Level of Cognitive Ability: Application
Client Needs: Physiological Integrity
Integrated Concept/Process: Nursing Process/Implementation
Content Area: Adult Health/Neurological
Reference: Smeltzer, S., & Bare, B. (2000). *Brunner & Suddarth's textbook of medical-surgical nursing* (9th ed.). Philadelphia: Lippincott Williams & Wilkins, p. 1631.

8. **4**
Rationale: After CT scanning, the client may resume all usual activities. The client should be encouraged to consume extra fluids to replace those lost with diuresis from the contrast dye.
Test-Taking Strategy: Use the process of elimination. Noting the key words "scanning with a contrast medium" will direct you to option 4. Review the procedure related to CT scanning if you had difficulty with this question.
Level of Cognitive Ability: Analysis
Client Needs: Health Promotion and Maintenance
Integrated Concept/Process: Self-Care
Content Area: Adult Health/Neurological
Reference: Smeltzer, S., & Bare, B. (2000). *Brunner & Suddarth's textbook of medical-surgical nursing* (9th ed.). Philadelphia: Lippincott Williams & Wilkins, pp. 1626-1627.

9. **3**
Rationale: Caloric testing provides information about the vestibular portion of cranial nerve VIII, which aids in differentiating between cerebellar and brainstem lesions. After patency of the ear canal has been determined, either warm or cold water is injected into the auditory canal. Normally, nystagmus occurs in the same direction as the irrigated ear if warm water is used and away from the irrigated ear if cold water is used. Nystagmus indicates that the brain- stem is intact. If death of the brainstem has occurred, nystagmus will not occur.
Test-Taking Strategy: In order to answer this question correctly, you must understand the purpose and nature of the test. It will be helpful to remember that this test is used as an adjunct to determine brain death. This would limit the choices to options 3 or 4. Knowledge of the test results and their meaning is needed to differentiate between the remaining options. Review this test if you had difficulty with this question.
Level of Cognitive Ability: Analysis
Client Needs: Physiological Integrity
Integrated Concept/Process: Nursing Process/Analysis
Content Area: Adult Health/Neurological
Reference: Phipps, W., Sands, J., & Marek, J. (1999). *Medical-surgical nursing: Concepts & clinical practice* (6th ed.). St. Louis: Mosby, p. 1695.

10. **1**
Rationale: After a myelogram, the client is placed on bed rest for 6 to 8 hours after the procedure. When a water-based contrast medium is used, the client is positioned with the head of bed elevated 15 to 30 degrees. With use of an oil-based medium, the head of the bed is positioned flat (even though the contrast is aspirated out after the procedure).
Test-Taking Strategy: Use the process of elimination. With a myelogram procedure, remember that the longer the bedrest, the less likelihood of complications. This will assist in

eliminating options 2 and 4. If you can remember "oil rises, so keep the head low," you will be able to choose correctly. Review postprocedure care following a myelogram if you had difficulty with this question.
Level of Cognitive Ability: Application
Client Needs: Physiological Integrity
Integrated Concept/Process: Nursing Process/Planning
Content Area: Adult Health/Neurological
Reference: LeMone, P., & Burke, K. (2000). *Medical-surgical nursing: Critical thinking in client care* (2nd ed.). Upper Saddle River, N.J.: Prentice-Hall, p. 1803.

11. **2**
Rationale: A change in vital signs may be a late sign of increased ICP. Trends include increasing temperature and blood pressure, and decreasing pulse and respirations. Respiratory irregularities may also arise.
Test-Taking Strategy: This question looks complex but can be logically answered. If you remember that the temperature rises, then you are able to eliminate options 3 and 4. If you know that the client becomes bradycardic, or know that the BP rises, you are able to select the correct option. Review the signs of increased intracranial pressure, if you had difficulty with this question.
Level of Cognitive Ability: Analysis
Client Needs: Physiological Integrity
Integrated Concept/Process: Nursing Process/Assessment
Content Area: Adult Health/Neurological
Reference: Smeltzer, S., & Bare, B. (2000). *Brunner & Suddarth's textbook of medical-surgical nursing* (9th ed.). Philadelphia: Lippincott Williams & Wilkins, p. 1643.

12. **1**
Rationale: The head of the client with increased ICP should be positioned so the head is in a neutral, midline position. The nurse should avoid flexing or extending the neck, or turning the neck side to side. The head of bed should be raised to 30 to 45 degrees. Use of proper positions promotes venous drainage from the cranium to keep intracranial pressure down.
Test-Taking Strategy: Use the process of elimination, noting the key word "avoid." Select the position that interferes either with arterial circulation to the brain or with venous drainage from the brain. The only position that meets one of those criteria is option 1. Review client positioning with ICP if you had difficulty with this question.
Level of Cognitive Ability: Application
Client Needs: Physiological Integrity
Integrated Concept/Process: Nursing Process/Implementation
Content Area: Adult Health/Neurological
Reference: Ignatavicius, D., Workman, M., & Mishler, M. (1999). *Medical-surgical nursing across the health care continuum* (3rd ed.). Philadelphia: W. B. Saunders, p. 1133.

13. **1**
Rationale: Activities that increase intrathoracic and intraabdominal pressures cause an indirect elevation of the ICP. Some of these activities include isometric exercises, Valsalva maneuver, coughing, sneezing, and blowing the nose. Exhaling during activities such as repositioning or pulling up in bed opens the glottis, which prevents intrathoracic pressure from rising.
Test-Taking Strategy: Use the process of elimination. Evaluate each of the options in terms of the tension it puts on the body.

Doing so will help you eliminate each of the incorrect options systematically. Review the measures that will reduce or prevent increased intracranial pressure if you had difficulty with this question.

Level of Cognitive Ability: Analysis
Client Needs: Health Promotion and Maintenance
Integrated Concept/Process: Nursing Process/Evaluation
Content Area: Adult Health/Neurological
Reference: Phipps, W., Sands, J., & Marek, J. (1999). *Medical-surgical nursing: Concepts & clinical practice* (6th ed.). St. Louis: Mosby, p. 1708.

14. 2

Rationale: Leakage of CSF from the ears or nose may accompany basilar skull fracture. It can be distinguished from other body fluids because the drainage will separate into bloody and yellow concentric rings on dressing material, called halo sign. It also tests positive for glucose.

Test-Taking Strategy: Use the process of elimination and knowledge about the characteristics of CSF. Recalling that CSF contains glucose, while other secretions, such as mucus, do not, and knowing that CSF separates into rings will also help you with this particular question. Review testing for CSF fluid if you had difficulty with this question.

Level of Cognitive Ability: Analysis
Client Needs: Physiological Integrity
Integrated Concept/Process: Nursing Process/Assessment
Content Area: Adult Health/Neurological
Reference: Ignatavicius, D., Workman, M., & Mishler, M. (1999). *Medical-surgical nursing across the health care continuum* (3rd ed.). Philadelphia: W. B. Saunders, p. 1131.

15. 1

Rationale: A complication of head injury is diabetes insipidus (DI). This can occur with insult to the hypothalamus, the antidiuretic hormone storage vesicles, or the posterior pituitary gland. Urine output that exceeds 9 L per day generally requires treatment with desmopressin. Dexamethasone, a glucocorticoid, is administered to treat cerebral edema. This medication may already be ordered for a client with a head injury. Ethacrynic acid and mannitol are both diuretics, which would be contraindicated.

Test-Taking Strategy: Use the process of elimination, recalling that a complication of head injury is DI. Knowing that DI results in excretion of very large amounts of dilute urine, you can eliminate options 3 and 4 immediately. From the remaining options, select option 1 because of its action. Review the action and purpose of desmopressin if you had difficulty with this question.

Level of Cognitive Ability: Analysis
Client Needs: Physiological Integrity
Integrated Concept/Process: Nursing Process/Implementation
Content Area: Pharmacology
Reference: Phipps, W., Sands, J., & Marek, J. (1999). *Medical-surgical nursing: Concepts & clinical practice* (6th ed.). St. Louis: Mosby, pp. 1068-1069.

16. 4

Rationale: The changes in neurological signs from an epidural hematoma begin with loss of consciousness as arterial blood collects in the epidural space and exerts pressure. The client regains consciousness as the cerebrospinal fluid is rapidly reabsorbed to compensate for the rising intracranial pressure

(ICP). As the compensatory mechanisms fail, even small amounts of additional blood cause the ICP to rise rapidly, and the client's neurological status deteriorates quickly.

Test-Taking Strategy: Use the process of elimination. Begin to answer this question by ruling out skull fracture and concussion as responsible for fluctuating neurological signs. Recall that a subdural hematoma is a collection of venous blood, which may accumulate more slowly and cause a steadier deterioration of neurological signs. This will help you discriminate between epidural and subdural hematomas. Review the clinical manifestations associated with the various types of head injury, if you had difficulty with this question.

Level of Cognitive Ability: Analysis
Client Needs: Physiological Integrity
Integrated Concept/Process: Nursing Process/Assessment
Content Area: Adult Health/Neurological
Reference: Phipps, W., Sands, J., & Marek, J. (1999). *Medical-surgical nursing: Concepts & clinical practice* (6th ed.). St. Louis: Mosby, pp. 1728-1729.

17. 1

Rationale: Signs of meningeal irritation compatible with meningitis include nuchal rigidity, positive Brudzinski's sign, and positive Kernig's sign. Nuchal rigidity is characterized by a stiff neck and soreness, which are especially noticeable when the neck is flexed. Kernig's sign is positive when the client feels pain and spasm of the hamstring muscles when the knee is straightened while the hip is flexed at a 90-degree angle. Brudzinski's sign is positive when the client flexes the hips and knees in response to the nurse gently flexing the head and neck onto the chest. A Glasgow coma scale score of 15 is a perfect score, and indicates the client is awake and alert with no neurological deficits.

Test-Taking Strategy: Use the process of elimination, focusing on the client's diagnosis, meningitis. Options 2, 3, and 4 can be eliminated because they are normal findings. Review the signs of meningitis if you had difficulty with this question.

Level of Cognitive Ability: Analysis
Client Needs: Physiological Integrity
Integrated Concept/Process: Nursing Process/Assessment
Content Area: Adult Health/Neurological
Reference: Phipps, W., Sands, J., & Marek, J. (1999). *Medical-surgical nursing: Concepts & clinical practice* (6th ed.). St. Louis: Mosby, pp. 1733-1734.

18. 4

Rationale: After holes have been drilled in the client's skull under local anesthesia, Crutchfield tongs are applied. Weights are attached to the tongs, which exert pulling pressure on the longitudinal axis of the cervical spine. Serial radiographs of the cervical spine are taken, with weights being gradually added until the radiograph reveals that the vertebral column is realigned. After that, weights may be gradually reduced to a point that maintains alignment. The client with Crutchfield tongs is placed on a Stryker frame or Roto-Rest bed. The nurse ensures that weights hang freely and that the amount of weight matches the current order. The nurse also inspects the integrity and position of the ropes and pulleys. The nurse does not remove the weights to administer care.

Test-Taking Strategy: Use the process of elimination, noting the key word "avoid." Recalling the basics related to the care of a client in traction will direct you to option 4. Review nursing

care related to the client with cervical tongs if you had difficulty with this question.
Level of Cognitive Ability: Application
Client Needs: Safe, Effective Care Environment
Integrated Concept/Process: Nursing Process/Planning
Content Area: Adult Health/Neurological
Reference: LeMone, P., & Burke, K. (2000). *Medical-surgical nursing: Critical thinking in client care* (2nd ed.). Upper Saddle River, N.J.: Prentice-Hall, p. 1794.

19. **4**
Rationale: The halo device alters balance and can cause fatigue due to its weight. The client should cleanse the skin daily under the vest to protect the skin from ulceration, and should use powder or lotions sparingly or not at all. The wool liner should be changed if odor becomes a problem. The client should have food cut into small pieces to facilitate chewing and use straws for drinking. Pin care is done as instructed. The client may not drive, because the device impairs the range of vision.
Test-Taking Strategy: Use the process of elimination and note the key words "needs further clarification." Visualize this device to answer correctly. The inability to turn the head without turning the torso would make driving contraindicated. Review client education points related to a halo device if you had difficulty with this question
Level of Cognitive Ability: Analysis
Client Needs: Health Promotion and Maintenance
Integrated Concept/Process: Self-Care
Content Area: Adult Health/Neurological
Reference: LeMone, P., & Burke, K. (2000). *Medical-surgical nursing: Critical thinking in client care* (2nd ed.). Upper Saddle River, N.J.: Prentice-Hall, pp. 1794-1795.

20. **2**
Rationale: After spinal cord injury, the client can develop paralytic ileus, which is characterized by the absence of bowel sounds and abdominal distention. Development of a stress ulcer can be detected by Hematest-positive NGT aspirate or stool. A history of diarrhea is irrelevant.
Test-Taking Strategy: Use the process of elimination, focusing on the client's diagnosis and the signs of a GI complication. Review this information if you had difficulty with this question.
Level of Cognitive Ability: Application
Client Needs: Physiological Integrity
Integrated Concept/Process: Nursing Process/Assessment
Content Area: Adult Health/Neurological
Reference: LeMone, P., & Burke, K. (2000). *Medical-surgical nursing: Critical thinking in client care* (2nd ed.). Upper Saddle River, N.J.: Prentice-Hall, p. 1793.

21. **3**
Rationale: Range-of-motion exercises are beneficial in stretching muscles, which may diminish spasticity. Removing potentially harmful objects is a good safety measure. Use of muscle relaxants is also indicated if the spasms cause discomfort to the client or pose a risk to the client's safety. Use of limb restraints will not alleviate spasticity and could harm the client.
Test-Taking Strategy: Use the process of elimination. Noting the key word "not" should easily direct you to option 3. Review care of the paraplegic client if you had difficulty with this question.

Level of Cognitive Ability: Application
Client Needs: Safe, Effective Care Environment
Integrated Concept/Process: Nursing Process/Planning
Content Area: Adult Health/Neurological
Reference: LeMone, P., & Burke, K. (2000). *Medical-surgical nursing: Critical thinking in client care* (2nd ed.). Upper Saddle River, N.J.: Prentice-Hall, p. 1796.

22. **1**
Rationale: A client with spinal cord injury is at risk for autonomic dysreflexia with an injury above the level of T6. It is characterized by severe, throbbing headache, flushing of the face and neck, bradycardia, and sudden severe hypertension. Other signs include nasal stuffiness, blurred vision, nausea, and sweating. It is a life-threatening syndrome triggered by a noxious stimulus below the level of the injury.
Test-Taking Strategy: Use the process of elimination. Recalling that a massive sympathetic nervous system response occurs, causing the severe hypertension, the throbbing headache, and flushing of the face and neck will direct you to the correct option. Review the signs of autonomic dysreflexia if you had difficulty with this question.
Level of Cognitive Ability: Application
Client Needs: Physiological Integrity
Integrated Concept/Process: Nursing Process/Assessment
Content Area: Adult Health/Neurological
Reference: Smeltzer, S., & Bare, B. (2000). *Brunner & Suddarth's textbook of medical-surgical nursing* (9th ed.). Philadelphia: Lippincott Williams & Wilkins, p. 1693.

23. **4**
Rationale: A client with a spinal cord injury is at risk for autonomic dysreflexia. Autonomic dysreflexia is characterized by severe, throbbing headache, flushing of the face and neck, bradycardia, and sudden severe hypertension. Other signs include nasal stuffiness, blurred vision, nausea, and sweating. It is a life-threatening syndrome triggered by a noxious stimulus below the level of the injury.
Test-Taking Strategy: Use the process of elimination. Begin by eliminating options 1 and 3. The client in spinal shock would be hypotensive (not hypertensive), and the client's clinical picture does not correlate with pulmonary embolism. (It may be useful to know also that autonomic dysreflexia does not occur until spinal shock resolves). Recalling that malignant hypertension occurs with anesthesia will assist in eliminating option 2. Review the signs of autonomic dysreflexia if you had difficulty with this question.
Level of Cognitive Ability: Analysis
Client Needs: Physiological Integrity
Integrated Concept/Process: Nursing Process/Analysis
Content Area: Adult Health/Neurological
Reference: Smeltzer, S., & Bare, B. (2000). *Brunner & Suddarth's textbook of medical-surgical nursing* (9th ed.). Philadelphia: Lippincott Williams & Wilkins, p. 1693.

24. **2**
Rationale: The most frequent cause of autonomic dysreflexia is a distended bladder. Straight catheterization should be done every 4 to 6 hours, and Foley catheters should be checked frequently to prevent kinks in the tubing. Constipation and fecal impaction are other causes, so maintaining bowel regularity is important. Other causes include stimulation of the skin from tactile, thermal, or painful stimuli. The nurse administers care to minimize risk in these areas.

Test-Taking Strategy: Use the process of elimination. Remember that autonomic dysreflexia is caused by noxious stimuli to the bowel, bladder, or skin. With this in mind, you can easily eliminate each of the incorrect options. Review the measures to minimize the risk of autonomic dysreflexia if you had difficulty with this question.
Level of Cognitive Ability: Application
Client Needs: Physiological Integrity
Integrated Concept/Process: Nursing Process/Implementation
Content Area: Adult Health/Neurological
Reference: Smeltzer, S., & Bare, B. (2000). *Brunner & Suddarth's textbook of medical-surgical nursing* (9th ed.). Philadelphia: Lippincott Williams & Wilkins, pp. 1693-1694.
25. **3**
Rationale: Reflex vasodilatation below the level of the spinal cord injury places the client at risk of orthostatic hypotension, which can be profound. Measures to minimize this include measuring vital signs before and during position changes, use of a tilt-table with early mobilization, and changing the client's position slowly. Venous pooling can be reduced by using TEDs (compression stockings) or pneumatic boots. Vasopressor medications are administered as per protocol.
Test-Taking Strategy: Use the process of elimination. Note the key words "least helpful." Note the word "quickly" in option 3. Knowing that quick position changes and movement would aggravate hypotension will direct you to this option. Review care of the client with spinal shock if you had difficulty with this question.
Level of Cognitive Ability: Application
Client Needs: Physiological Integrity
Integrated Concept/Process: Nursing Process/Planning
Content Area: Adult Health/Neurological
Reference: Smeltzer, S., & Bare, B. (2000). *Brunner & Suddarth's textbook of medical-surgical nursing* (9th ed.). Philadelphia: Lippincott Williams & Wilkins, p. 1693.
26. **4**
Rationale: Spinal immobilization is necessary after spinal cord injury to prevent further damage and insult to the spinal cord. Whenever possible, the client is placed on a Stryker frame, which allows the nurse to turn the client to prevent complications of immobility, while maintaining alignment of the spine. If a Stryker frame is not available, a firm mattress with a bedboard under it should be used.
Test-Taking Strategy: Use the process of elimination, focusing on the issue, which is preventing further injury. This will easily direct you to option 4. If you are unfamiliar with a Stryker frame, review this content.
Level of Cognitive Ability: Application
Client Needs: Safe, Effective Care Environment
Integrated Concept/Process: Nursing Process/Implementation
Content Area: Adult Health/Neurological
Reference: LeMone, P., & Burke, K. (2000). *Medical-surgical nursing: Critical thinking in client care* (2nd ed.). Upper Saddle River, N.J.: Prentice-Hall, p. 1792.
27. **3**
Rationale: Resolution of spinal shock is occurring when there is return of reflexes (especially flexors to noxious cutaneous stimuli), a state of hyperreflexia rather than flaccidity, return of bulbospongiosis reflex in the male, and a positive Babinski reflex.

Test-Taking Strategy: Use the process of elimination. Recall that spinal shock is characterized by the loss of movement of skeletal muscles, bowel or bladder wall, or by reflex action. Return of any of these indicates that spinal shock is beginning to resolve. The inability to elicit a Babinski reflex indicates that spinal shock is ongoing. Thus, this is the correct option. Review signs of spinal shock if you had difficulty with this question.
Level of Cognitive Ability: Analysis
Client Needs: Physiological Integrity
Integrated Concept/Process: Nursing Process/Assessment
Content Area: Adult Health/Neurological
Reference: LeMone, P., & Burke, K. (2000). *Medical-surgical nursing: Critical thinking in client care* (2nd ed.). Upper Saddle River, N.J.: Prentice-Hall, p. 1792.
28. **2**
Rationale: Typically, seizure assessment includes the time the seizure began, part(s) of the body affected, the type of movements and progression of the seizure, changes in pupil size, eye deviation or nystagmus, client condition during the seizure, and postictal status.
Test-Taking Strategy: Use the process of elimination, noting the key word "not." The option about the client's intake prior to the seizure suggests concern about vomiting and subsequent aspiration. The nurse is concerned about aspiration, not from vomiting, but from inhalation of the client's own saliva. Since all of the other options are standard assessments, this is the answer to the question. Review nursing assessment during a seizure if you had difficulty answering this question.
Level of Cognitive Ability: Application
Client Needs: Physiological Integrity
Integrated Concept/Process: Nursing Process/Assessment
Content Area: Adult Health/Neurological
Reference: Smeltzer, S., & Bare, B. (2000). *Brunner & Suddarth's textbook of medical-surgical nursing* (9th ed.). Philadelphia: Lippincott Williams & Wilkins, pp. 1738-1739.
29. **3**
Rationale: Seizure precautions may vary somewhat from agency to agency, but they generally have some commonalities. Usually an airway, oxygen, and suctioning equipment are kept available at the bedside. The side rails of the bed are padded, and the bed is kept in the lowest position. The client has an IV access in place to have a readily accessible route if IV anticonvulsant medications must be administered. The use of padded tongue blades is highly controversial, and they should not be kept at the bedside. Forcing a tongue blade into the mouth during a seizure will more likely harm the client who bites down during seizure activity. Risks include blocking the airway from improper placement, chipping the client's teeth, and subsequent risk of aspirating tooth fragments. If the client has an aura before the seizure, it may give the nurse enough time to place an oral airway before seizure activity begins.
Test-Taking Strategy: Use the process of elimination, noting the key word "avoid." Evaluate this question from the perspective of causing possible harm. No harm can come to the client from any of the options except for the tongue blade. Review seizure precautions if you had difficulty with this question
Level of Cognitive Ability: Application
Client Needs: Safe, Effective Care Environment
Integrated Concept/Process: Nursing Process/Planning

Content Area: Adult Health/Neurological
Reference: Smeltzer, S., & Bare, B. (2000). *Brunner & Suddarth's textbook of medical-surgical nursing* (9th ed.). Philadelphia: Lippincott Williams & Wilkins, p. 1739.

30. 3

Rationale: Nursing actions during a seizure include providing for privacy, loosening restrictive clothing, removing the pillow and raising side rails in bed, and placing the client on one side with the head flexed forward, if possible, to allow the tongue to fall forward and facilitate drainage. The limbs are never restrained, because the strong muscle contractions could cause the client harm. If the client is not in bed when seizure activity begins, the nurse lowers the client to the floor if possible, protects the head from injury, and moves furniture that may injure the client. Other aspects of care are as described for the client who is in bed.

Test-Taking Strategy: Use the process of elimination and note the key word "contraindicated." Evaluate this question from the perspective of causing possible harm. No harm can come to the client from any of the options except for restraining the limbs. Remember, avoid restraints. Review care of a client during a seizure if you had difficulty with this question.

Level of Cognitive Ability: Application
Client Needs: Safe, Effective Care Environment
Integrated Concept/Process: Nursing Process/Implementation
Content Area: Adult Health/Neurological
Reference: Smeltzer, S., & Bare, B. (2000). *Brunner & Suddarth's textbook of medical-surgical nursing* (9th ed.). Philadelphia: Lippincott Williams & Wilkins, p. 1740.

31. 3

Rationale: Typical anticonvulsant medication instructions include taking the dose daily to keep the blood level of the drug constant and having a serum drug level drawn before taking the morning dose. The client is taught not to abruptly stop the medication; avoid alcohol; check with the physician before taking over-the-counter medications; avoid activities where alertness and coordination are required until medication effects are known; provide good oral hygiene and obtain regular dental care. The client should also wear a Medic-Alert bracelet.

Test-Taking Strategy: Use the process of elimination. Using knowledge of general principles related to the medication administration will assist in eliminating options 1 and 2. From the remaining options, recall that medications are not generally taken just before therapeutic serum level tests are drawn, because the results would be artificially high. This leaves oral hygiene as the correct option, because of the risk of gingival hyperplasia. Review client education related to phenytoin (Dilantin) if you had difficulty with this question.

Level of Cognitive Ability: Analysis
Client Needs: Health Promotion and Maintenance
Integrated Concept/Process: Self-Care
Content Area: Adult Health/Neurological
Reference: Smeltzer, S., & Bare, B. (2000). *Brunner & Suddarth's textbook of medical-surgical nursing* (9th ed.). Philadelphia: Lippincott Williams & Wilkins, p. 1742.

32. 2

Rationale: Hemiparesis is a weakness of the face, arm, and leg on one side. The client with one-sided hemiparesis benefits from having objects placed on the unaffected side and within reach. Other helpful activities with hemiparesis include range

of motion exercises to the affected side, and muscle strengthening exercises to the unaffected side.

Test-Taking Strategy: Use the process of elimination Begin to answer by eliminating options 3 and 4 as potentially hazardous to the client. Also, distinguish between hemiparesis and unilateral neglect to answer this question. The client with hemiparesis has weakness on one side, and therefore objects should be placed on the stronger side. With unilateral neglect, objects are placed on the affected side to train the client to attend to that part of the environment. Knowing this, select option 2. Review care of the client with hemiparesis if you had difficulty with this question.

Level of Cognitive Ability: Application
Client Needs: Safe, Effective Care Environment
Integrated Concept/Process: Nursing Process/Planning
Content Area: Adult Health/Neurological
Reference: Smeltzer, S., & Bare, B. (2000). *Brunner & Suddarth's textbook of medical-surgical nursing* (9th ed.). Philadelphia: Lippincott Williams & Wilkins, p. 1653.

33. 1

Rationale: Before the client with dysphagia is started on a diet, the gag and swallow reflexes must have returned. The client is assisted with meals as needed, and is given ample time to chew and swallow. Food is placed on the unaffected side of the mouth. Liquids are thickened to avoid aspiration.

Test-Taking Strategy: Use the process of elimination, noting the key word "avoids." Option 4 is generally a good action for all clients. Option 3 is correct because the client has better sensation and motion on the unaffected side of the mouth. Remember that thickened liquids are easier for the client with impaired facial motion and swallowing ability to manage. Knowing this enables you to choose option 1 as the action to avoid. Review care of the client with residual dysphagia if you had difficulty with this question.

Level of Cognitive Ability: Application
Client Needs: Physiological Integrity
Integrated Concept/Process: Nursing Process/Implementation
Content Area: Adult Health/Neurological
Reference: Smeltzer, S., & Bare, B. (2000). *Brunner & Suddarth's textbook of medical-surgical nursing* (9th ed.). Philadelphia: Lippincott Williams & Wilkins, p. 1659.

34. 3

Rationale: Homonymous hemianopsia is loss of one half of the visual field. The client with homonymous hemianopsia should have objects placed in the intact field of vision, and the nurse should also approach the client from the intact side. The nurse instructs the client to scan the environment to overcome the visual deficit, and does client teaching from within the intact field of vision. The nurse encourages the use of personal eyeglasses, if they are available.

Test-Taking Strategy: Use the process of elimination. Recalling the definition of homonymous hemianopsia will easily direct you to option 3. Review the concept of homonymous hemianopsia if you are unfamiliar with it.

Level of Cognitive Ability: Analysis
Client Needs: Health Promotion and Maintenance
Integrated Concept/Process: Teaching/Learning
Content Area: Adult Health/Neurological
Reference: Smeltzer, S., & Bare, B. (2000). *Brunner & Suddarth's textbook of medical-surgical nursing* (9th ed.). Philadelphia: Lippincott Williams & Wilkins, p. 1658.

35. 2

Rationale: Clients are evaluated as coping successfully with lifestyle changes after a CVA if they make appropriate lifestyle alterations, use the assistance of others, and have appropriate social interactions. Options 1, 3, and 4 are not adaptive behaviors.

Test-Taking Strategy: Use the process of elimination, focusing on the key words "adapting most successfully." Options 1 and 4 are behaviors that may be expected in the client with a CVA, but they are not adaptive responses. Rather, they are a result of the insult to the brain. Options 2 and 3 indicate that the client is trying to adapt, but option 2 has the best outcome. Review care of the client with a CVA if you had difficulty with this question.

Level of Cognitive Ability: Analysis
Client Needs: Psychosocial Integrity
Integrated Concept/Process: Nursing Process/Evaluation
Content Area: Adult Health/Neurological
Reference: Smeltzer, S., & Bare, B. (2000). *Brunner & Suddarth's textbook of medical-surgical nursing* (9th ed.). Philadelphia: Lippincott Williams & Wilkins, p. 1660.

36. 3

Rationale: Unilateral neglect is an unawareness of the paralyzed side of the body, which increases the client's risk for injury. The nurse's role is to refocus the client's attention to the affected side. The nurse moves personal care items and belongings to the affected side, as well as the bedside chair and commode. The nurse teaches the client to scan the environment to become aware of that half of the body, and approaches the client from that side to further increase awareness.

Test-Taking Strategy: Use the process of elimination, noting the key word "not." Recall that with unilateral neglect the client loses awareness of the affected side. If you know that the client needs to be trained to attend to that side, you can eliminate each of the incorrect options. Review care of the client with unilateral neglect if you had difficulty with this question.

Level of Cognitive Ability: Application
Client Needs: Safe, Effective Care Environment
Integrated Concept/Process: Nursing Process/Planning
Content Area: Adult Health/Neurological
Reference: Smeltzer, S., & Bare, B. (2000). *Brunner & Suddarth's textbook of medical-surgical nursing* (9th ed.). Philadelphia: Lippincott Williams & Wilkins, p. 1658.

37. 2

Rationale: Clients with aphasia after CVA often fatigue easily and have a short attention span. General guidelines when trying to communicate with the aphasic client include speaking more slowly and allowing adequate response time, listening to and watching attempts to communicate, and trying to put the client at ease with a caring and understanding manner. Avoid shouting (since the client is not deaf), appearing rushed for a response, and letting family members provide all the responses for the client.

Test-Taking Strategy: Use the process of elimination, noting the key words "least helpful." This question tests a fundamental concept in communicating with the aphasic client. If this question was difficult, review these communication strategies.

Level of Cognitive Ability: Application
Client Needs: Psychosocial Integrity
Integrated Concept/Process: Communication and Documentation
Content Area: Adult Health/Neurological
Reference: Smeltzer, S., & Bare, B. (2000). *Brunner & Suddarth's textbook of medical-surgical nursing* (9th ed.). Philadelphia: Lippincott Williams & Wilkins, p. 1660.

38. 3

Rationale: Placing an eye patch over one eye in the client with diplopia removes the second image and restores more normal vision. The patch is alternated daily to maintain the strength of the extraocular muscles of the eyes.

Test-Taking Strategy: Use the process of elimination. Knowing that an eye patch will help diplopia only while it is worn will assist in eliminating options 1 and 2. Recalling that the extraocular muscles weaken with eye patch use will direct you to option 3. Review instructions for the client with diplopia if you had difficulty with this question.

Level of Cognitive Ability: Analysis
Client Needs: Physiological Integrity
Integrated Concept/Process: Self-Care
Content Area: Adult Health/Neurological
Reference: Ignatavicius, D., Workman, M., & Mishler, M. (1999). *Medical-surgical nursing across the health care continuum* (3rd ed.). Philadelphia: W. B. Saunders, p. 1096.

39. 3

Rationale: Myasthenia gravis can often be diagnosed on the basis of clinical signs and symptoms. The diagnosis can be confirmed by injecting the client with a dose of Tensilon. This medication inhibits the breakdown of an enzyme in the neuromuscular junction, so more acetylcholine binds onto receptors. If the muscle is strengthened for 3 to 5 minutes after this injection, it confirms a diagnosis of myasthenia gravis. Another medication, neostigmine (Prostigmin) may also be used because its effect lasts for 1 to 2 hours, giving a better analysis. For either medication, atropine sulfate should be available as the antidote.

Test-Taking Strategy: Use the process of elimination. Knowledge of the purpose and expected findings of the Tensilon test is required to answer this question. Review the Tensilon test if you are unfamiliar with it.

Level of Cognitive Ability: Analysis
Client Needs: Physiological Integrity
Integrated Concept/Process: Nursing Process/Analysis
Content Area: Pharmacology
Reference: Ignatavicius, D., Workman, M., & Mishler, M. (1999). *Medical-surgical nursing across the health care continuum* (3rd ed.). Philadelphia: W. B. Saunders, p. 1093.

40. 2

Rationale: The client has speech that is nasal in tone and dysarthric because of cranial nerve involvement of the muscles governing speech. The nurse listens attentively and verbally, verifies what the client has said, asks questions requiring a yes or no response, and develops alternative communication methods (letter board, picture board, pen and paper, flash cards). Encouraging the client to speak quickly is unsuccessful and counterproductive.

Test-Taking Strategy: Use the process of elimination, noting the key word "avoid." Options 3 and 4 are classic examples of alternative communication methods that are useful, and are eliminated first. Since option 1 is also helpful, this leaves option 2 as the correct option. Speaking quickly is difficult for a client with a speech impairment. Review communication strategies for the client with speaking difficulty if this question was difficult.

Level of Cognitive Ability: Application
Client Needs: Psychosocial Integrity
Integrated Concept/Process: Nursing Process/Planning
Content Area: Adult Health/Neurological
Reference: Ignatavicius, D., Workman, M., & Mishler, M. (1999). *Medical-surgical nursing across the health care continuum* (3rd ed.). Philadelphia: W. B. Saunders, p. 1096.

41. 4

Rationale: The client with myasthenia gravis may experience episodes of respiratory distress if excessively fatigued, or if the client develops myasthenic crisis or cholinergic crisis. For this reason, an Ambu bag, intubation tray, and suction equipment should be available at the bedside.

Test-Taking Strategy: Use the process of elimination. Note that there are two items in each option. In order for the option to be correct, both parts of the option must be correct. Knowing that the client with myasthenia gravis is at risk for aspiration and respiratory failure helps you select option 4 over each of the others. Additionally, option 4 addresses the maintenance of a patent airway. Review care of the client with myasthenia gravis if you had difficulty with this question.

Level of Cognitive Ability: Application
Client Needs: Safe, Effective Care Environment
Integrated Concept/Process: Nursing Process/Implementation
Content Area: Adult Health/Neurological
Reference: Ignatavicius, D., Workman, M., & Mishler, M. (1999). *Medical-surgical nursing across the health care continuum* (3rd ed.). Philadelphia: W. B. Saunders, p. 1093.

42. 3

Rationale: Myasthenic crisis is often caused by undermedication, and responds to the administration of cholinergic medications such as neostigmine (Prostigmin) and pyridostigmine (Mestinon). Cholinergic crisis (the opposite problem) is caused by excess medication and responds to withholding of medications. Too little exercise and fatty food intake are incorrect. Overexertion and overeating could possibly trigger myasthenic crisis.

Test-Taking Strategy: Use the process of elimination. Recalling that undermedication is a common cause of myasthenic crisis will easily direct you to option 3. Review the causes of myasthenic crisis if you had difficulty with this question.

Level of Cognitive Ability: Application
Client Needs: Physiological Integrity
Integrated Concept/Process: Nursing Process/Assessment
Content Area: Adult Health/Neurological
Reference: Ignatavicius, D., Workman, M., & Mishler, M. (1999). *Medical-surgical nursing across the health care continuum* (3rd ed.). Philadelphia: W. B. Saunders, p. 1094.

43. 2

Rationale: Clients with myasthenia gravis are taught to space out activities over the day to conserve energy and restore muscle strength. It is very important to take medications correctly to maintain blood levels that are not too low or too high. Muscle strengthening exercises are not helpful and can fatigue the client. Overeating is a cause of exacerbation of symptoms, as well as exposure to heat, crowds, erratic sleep habits, and emotional stress.

Test-Taking Strategy: Use the process of elimination. Recalling that the common causes of myasthenic and cholinergic crises are undermedication and overmedication, respectively, will assist in eliminating each of the incorrect options. No other option would prevent both of those complications. Review measures to prevent myasthenic and cholinergic crises if you are unfamiliar with them.

Level of Cognitive Ability: Application
Client Needs: Health Promotion and Maintenance
Integrated Concept/Process: Teaching/Learning
Content Area: Adult Health/Neurological
Reference: Ignatavicius, D., Workman, M., & Mishler, M. (1999). *Medical-surgical nursing across the health care continuum* (3rd ed.). Philadelphia: W. B. Saunders, p. 1096.

44. 4

Rationale: The client avoids swallowing any type of food or drink with the head lifted upward, which could actually cause aspiration by opening the glottis. The client should be advised to sit bolt upright while eating, not to talk with food in the mouth (glottis is open), cut food into very small pieces, chew thoroughly, and tip the chin downward to swallow.

Test-Taking Strategy: Use the process of elimination, noting the key word "avoid." If you look at the construct of this question, you will note that options 3 and 4 oppose each other. This makes it likely that one of the two is correct. In examining each of them, option 4 is the better choice. Lifting the head opens the airway, which will increase the risk of aspiration during drinking or eating. Review care of the client with myasthenia gravis if you had difficulty with this question.

Level of Cognitive Ability: Application
Client Needs: Health Promotion and Maintenance
Integrated Concept/Process: Teaching/Learning
Content Area: Adult Health/Neurological
Reference: Ignatavicius, D., Workman, M., & Mishler, M. (1999). *Medical-surgical nursing across the health care continuum* (3rd ed.). Philadelphia: W. B. Saunders, p. 1096.

45. 3

Rationale: Most ongoing treatment for myasthenia gravis is done in outpatient settings, and the client needs to be aware of the lifestyle changes needed to maintain independence. Taking medications an hour before mealtime gives greater muscle strength for chewing, and is indicated. The client should have portable suction equipment and a portable resuscitation bag available in case of respiratory distress. The client should carry medical identification about the presence of the condition. The client should avoid activities that could worsen the symptoms, including stress, infection, heat, surgery or alcohol.

Test-Taking Strategy: Use the process of elimination, noting the key words "needs more information." Options 2 and 4 are very reasonable courses of action, and so they are eliminated first. To discriminate between the remaining options, recall that premedication an hour before meals gives strength to the muscles (for chewing and swallowing), and that heat and infection (crowds at the beach) trigger myasthenic crisis. Review client education points with myasthenia gravis if you had difficulty with this question.

Level of Cognitive Ability: Analysis
Client Needs: Health Promotion and Maintenance
Integrated Concept/Process: Teaching/Learning

Content Area: Adult Health/Neurological
Reference: Ignatavicius, D., Workman, M., & Mishler, M. (1999). *Medical-surgical nursing across the health care continuum* (3rd ed.). Philadelphia: W. B. Saunders, p. 1097.

46. 4

Rationale: The Parkinsonian gait is characterized by short, accelerating, shuffling steps. The client leans forward with the head, hips, and knees flexed, and has difficulty starting and stopping. A dystrophic gait is broad-based and waddling. A festinating gait is accelerating with walking on toes. An ataxic gait is staggering and unsteady.

Test-Taking Strategy: Use the process of elimination. Recall that the client has difficulty in initiating movement and bradykinesia. The gait is difficult to start, but it accelerates once it has begun. This will assist in eliminating options 1 and 3. From the remaining options, recall that the client with Parkinson's disease shuffles but does not walk on the toes. Review the characteristics associated with Parkinson's disease if you had difficulty with this question.

Level of Cognitive Ability: Analysis
Client Needs: Physiological Integrity
Integrated Concept/Process: Nursing Process/Assessment
Content Area: Adult Health/Neurological
Reference: Phipps, W., Sands, J., & Marek, J. (1999). *Medical-surgical nursing: Concepts & clinical practice* (6th ed.). St. Louis: Mosby, p. 1765.

47. 3

Rationale: The client with Parkinson's disease tends to become withdrawn and depressed, and should become an active participant in his or her own care to prevent this. There should be planned activities throughout the day to inhibit daytime sleeping and boredom. The nurse gives the client encouragement and praises the client for perseverance. Exercise helps prevent progression of the disease and self-care improves self-esteem.

Test-Taking Strategy: Use the process of elimination, focusing on the issue. Options 1 and 4 are the least plausible of all available options, and are eliminated first. Option 2 is well-intentioned, but it is not therapeutic in helping the client to cope with the disease. Option 3 is the best choice. Review care of the client with Parkinson's disease if you had difficulty with this question.

Level of Cognitive Ability: Application
Client Needs: Psychosocial Integrity
Integrated Concept/Process: Nursing Process/Planning
Content Area: Adult Health/Neurological
Reference: Phipps, W., Sands, J., & Marek, J. (1999). *Medical-surgical nursing: Concepts & clinical practice* (6th ed.). St. Louis: Mosby, p. 1766.

48. 2

Rationale: The client with Parkinson's disease should exercise in the morning when energy levels are highest. The client should avoid sitting in soft, deep chairs, because they are difficult to get up from. The client can rock back and forth to initiate movement. The client should buy clothes with Velcro fasteners and slide-locking buckles to support the ability to dress.

Test-Taking Strategy: Use the process of elimination. Option 1 is not useful to clients with fatigue from any disorder, so this option is eliminated first. Knowing that the client with

Parkinson's has difficulty with movement and dexterity helps to eliminate options 3 and 4 next. Review client-teaching points with Parkinson's disease if you had difficulty with this question.

Level of Cognitive Ability: Analysis
Client Needs: Health Promotion and Maintenance
Integrated Concept/Process: Teaching/Learning
Content Area: Adult Health/Neurological
Reference: Phipps, W., Sands, J., & Marek, J. (1999). *Medical-surgical nursing: Concepts & clinical practice* (6th ed.). St. Louis: Mosby, p. 1767.

49. 4

Rationale: Using cotton pads to wash the face, and using room temperature water can minimize facial pain. The client should chew on the unaffected side of the mouth, eat a soft diet, and take in foods and beverages at room temperature. If tooth brushing triggers pain, sometimes an oral rinse after meals is helpful instead.

Test-Taking Strategy: Use the process of elimination. Recall that the pain of trigeminal neuralgia is triggered by mechanical or thermal stimuli. This will help you eliminate each of the incorrect options systematically. Very hot or cold foods are likely to trigger the pain, not relieve it. Review client education points if you had difficulty with this question.

Level of Cognitive Ability: Analysis
Client Needs: Health Promotion and Maintenance
Integrated Concept/Process: Teaching/Learning
Content Area: Adult Health/Neurological
Reference: Ignatavicius, D., Workman, M., & Mishler, M. (1999). *Medical-surgical nursing across the health care continuum* (3rd ed.). Philadelphia: W. B. Saunders, p. 1105.

50. 1

Rationale: Bell's palsy is a one-sided facial paralysis from compression of the facial nerve. The exact cause is unknown. Possible causes include vascular ischemia, exposure to viruses such as herpes zoster or simplex, autoimmune disease, or a combination of these items.

Test-Taking Strategy: Use the process of elimination. If you know that the etiology of Bell's palsy is uncertain, you are able to eliminate options 3 and 4. Recalling that viruses and the immune system may have an effect in causing this disorder will direct you to option 1. Review the etiology of Bell's palsy if you had difficulty with this question.

Level of Cognitive Ability: Comprehension
Client Needs: Physiological Integrity
Integrated Concept/Process: Nursing Process/Analysis
Content Area: Adult Health/Neurological
Reference: Smeltzer, S., & Bare, B. (2000). *Brunner & Suddarth's textbook of medical-surgical nursing* (9th ed.). Philadelphia: Lippincott Williams & Wilkins, p. 1752.

51. 2

Rationale: Clients with Bell's palsy should be reassured that they have not experienced a CVA and that symptoms often disappear spontaneously in 3 to 5 weeks. The client is given supportive treatment for symptoms. It is not usually caused by a tumor, and the treatment is not similar to that for migraine headaches.

Test-Taking Strategy: Use the process of elimination. Bell's palsy is not similar to CVA, which eliminates option 1 first. It is not caused by an easily removed tumor, nor is it treated like

a migraine headache, which eliminates each of the other incorrect options. Review the characteristics of Bell's palsy if you had difficulty with this question.
Level of Cognitive Ability: Application
Client Needs: Psychosocial Integrity
Integrated Concept/Process: Caring
Content Area: Adult Health/Neurological
Reference: Smeltzer, S., & Bare, B. (2000). *Brunner & Suddarth's textbook of medical-surgical nursing* (9th ed.). Philadelphia: Lippincott Williams & Wilkins, p. 1754.

52. 4
Rationale: Bell's palsy is typically treated with prednisone. The medication reduces inflammation and edema, allowing return of normal circulation to the nerve. If given early, the medication reduces the severity of the palsy, reduces pain, and preserves substantial, if not all, nerve function. Options 1, 2, and 3 are incorrect.
Test-Taking Strategy: Use the process of elimination. It is useful to know that the corticosteroid medications are helpful in the treatment of nervous system disorders. This eliminates option 1 and 2. Recalling how Bell's palsy is treated will direct you to option 4. Review Bell's palsy and the action and purposes of these medications, if you had difficulty with this question.
Level of Cognitive Ability: Application
Client Needs: Physiological Integrity
Integrated Concept/Process: Teaching/Learning
Content Area: Pharmacology
Reference: Smeltzer, S., & Bare, B. (2000). *Brunner & Suddarth's textbook of medical-surgical nursing* (9th ed.). Philadelphia: Lippincott Williams & Wilkins, p. 1754.

53. 1
Rationale: Prevention of muscle atrophy with Bell's palsy is accomplished with the use of facial massage, facial exercises, and electrical stimulation of the nerves. Exposure to cold or drafts is avoided. Local application of heat to the face may improve blood flow and provide comfort.
Test-Taking Strategy: Use the process of elimination, noting the key words "needs additional information." Evaluate each of the options with regard to its effect on preserving muscle tone in the face. Option 1 is unrelated to muscle tone and is also contraindicated in clients with this condition. Review teaching points for the client with Bell's palsy if you had difficulty with this question.
Level of Cognitive Ability: Analysis
Client Needs: Health Promotion and Maintenance
Integrated Concept/Process: Teaching/Learning
Content Area: Adult Health/Neurological
Reference: Smeltzer, S., & Bare, B. (2000). *Brunner & Suddarth's textbook of medical-surgical nursing* (9th ed.). Philadelphia: Lippincott Williams & Wilkins, p. 1754.

54. 3
Rationale: Guillain-Barré syndrome is a clinical syndrome of unknown origin that involves cranial and peripheral nerves. Many clients report a history of respiratory or GI infection in the 1 to 4 weeks before the onset of neurological deficits. Occasionally, it has been triggered by vaccination or surgery.
Test-Taking Strategy: Use the process of elimination and knowledge about the etiology related to this disorder. If you are unfamiliar with Guillain-Barré syndrome, review this disorder.

Level of Cognitive Ability: Analysis
Client Needs: Physiological Integrity
Integrated Concept/Process: Nursing Process/Assessment
Content Area: Adult Health/Neurological
Reference: Smeltzer, S., & Bare, B. (2000). *Brunner & Suddarth's textbook of medical-surgical nursing* (9th ed.). Philadelphia: Lippincott Williams & Wilkins, p. 1755.

55. 2
Rationale: The client with Guillain-Barré syndrome experiences fear and anxiety from the ascending paralysis and sudden onset of the disorder. The nurse can alleviate these fears by providing accurate information about the client's condition, giving expert care, giving positive feedback to the client, and encouraging relaxation and distraction. The family can become involved with selected care activities and provide diversion for the client, as well.
Test-Taking Strategy: Use the process of elimination. Option 1 should be eliminated first, because it is not practical to think that the client would be given full control over all care decisions. The client who is paralyzed cannot participate in active ROM, which eliminates option 4. Of the remaining options, option 2 is more beneficial in assisting the client to cope than option 3. Review care of the client with Guillain-Barré syndrome if you had difficulty with this question.
Level of Cognitive Ability: Application
Client Needs: Psychosocial Integrity
Integrated Concept/Process: Caring
Content Area: Adult Health/Neurological
Reference: Smeltzer, S., & Bare, B. (2000). *Brunner & Suddarth's textbook of medical-surgical nursing* (9th ed.). Philadelphia: Lippincott Williams & Wilkins, p. 1756.

56. 3
Rationale: The client with Guillain-Barré syndrome is at risk for respiratory failure because of ascending paralysis. An intubation tray should be available for use. Another complication of this syndrome is cardiac dysrhythmia, which necessitates the use of ECG monitoring. Because the client is immobilized, the nurse should routinely assess for deep vein thrombosis and pulmonary embolism.
Test-Taking Strategy: Use the process of elimination. With an ascending paralysis, the client is at risk for involvement of respiratory muscles and subsequent respiratory failure. Option 3 is the only option that includes an intubation tray, which would be needed if the client status deteriorated to needing intubation and mechanical ventilation. This option most directly addresses airway. Review care of the client with Guillain-Barré syndrome if you had difficulty with this question.
Level of Cognitive Ability: Application
Client Needs: Physiological Integrity
Integrated Concept/Process: Nursing Process/Implementation
Content Area: Adult Health/Neurological
Reference: Smeltzer, S., & Bare, B. (2000). *Brunner & Suddarth's textbook of medical-surgical nursing* (9th ed.). Philadelphia: Lippincott Williams & Wilkins, p. 1756.

57. 1
Rationale: Satisfactory respiratory outcomes include clear breath sounds on auscultation, spontaneous breathing, normal vital capacity, and normal arterial blood gases and pulse oximetry.

Test-Taking Strategy: Use the process of elimination, noting the key words "least optimal." There is only one option that does not represent full respiratory function. This should help you eliminate each of the incorrect options. Review care of the client with Guillain-Barré syndrome if you had difficulty with this question.
Level of Cognitive Ability: Analysis
Client Needs: Physiological Integrity
Integrated Concept/Process: Nursing Process/Evaluation
Content Area: Adult Health/Neurological
Reference: Smeltzer, S., & Bare, B. (2000). *Brunner & Suddarth's textbook of medical-surgical nursing* (9th ed.). Philadelphia: Lippincott Williams & Wilkins, p. 1757.

58. **2**
Rationale: The onset or exacerbation of MS is preceded by a number of different factors. These include emotional stress, fatigue, infection, physical injury, and pregnancy. There are no known methods of primary prevention. Intake of fruit and vegetables is an unrelated item.
Test-Taking Strategy: Use the process of elimination. If you examine each of the options, all but option 2 involve physiological or psychological stress. Since this is the option that is different than the others, it is a likely choice for being the correct option. Review the precipitating risk factors associated with MS, if you had difficulty with this question.
Level of Cognitive Ability: Analysis
Client Needs: Physiological Integrity
Integrated Concept/Process: Nursing Process/Assessment
Content Area: Adult Health/Neurological
Reference: Smeltzer, S., & Bare, B. (2000). *Brunner & Suddarth's textbook of medical-surgical nursing* (9th ed.). Philadelphia: Lippincott Williams & Wilkins, p. 1718.

59. **1**
Rationale: Impaired Physical Mobility has been defined by the North American Nursing Diagnosis Association (NANDA) as "a state in which the individual experiences a limitation of ability for independent physical movement." The client's muscle weakness, muscle spasticity, and ataxic gait meet the defining characteristics for this nursing diagnosis. In addition, neuromuscular impairment is listed as a related factor.
Test-Taking Strategy: Use the process of elimination. Focusing on the data provided in the question will easily direct you to option 1. Review care of the client with MS if you had difficulty with this question.
Level of Cognitive Ability: Analysis
Client Needs: Physiological Integrity

Integrated Concept/Process: Nursing Process/Analysis
Content Area: Adult Health/Neurological
Reference: Smeltzer, S., & Bare, B. (2000). *Brunner & Suddarth's textbook of medical-surgical nursing* (9th ed.). Philadelphia: Lippincott Williams & Wilkins, p. 1720.

60. **3**
Rationale: Spacing fluid intake over the day helps the client with a neurogenic bladder to establish regular times for successful voiding. Omitting intake after the evening meal minimizes incontinence or the need to empty the bladder during the night.
Test-Taking Strategy: Use the process of elimination. Options 2 and 4 should be eliminated first, because they could cause or aggravate nocturia. From the remaining options, option 3 provides fluids at times that coincide with toileting schedules for bladder training. Review care of the client with MS if you had difficulty with this question.
Level of Cognitive Ability: Application
Client Needs: Physiological Integrity
Integrated Concept/Process: Nursing Process/Implementation
Content Area: Adult Health/Neurological
Reference: LeMone, P., & Burke, K. (2000). *Medical-surgical nursing: Critical thinking in client care* (2nd ed.). Upper Saddle River, N.J.: Prentice-Hall, p. 1836.

CRITICAL THINKING: FREE-TEXT ENTRY

Answer: Raise the head of the bed and remove the noxious stimulus
Rationale: Immediate nursing actions are to sit the client up in bed and remove the noxious stimulus. Antihypertensive medication will be prescribed to minimize cerebral hypertension.
Test-Taking Strategy: Note the word "immediate" in the stem of the question. Thinking about the causes and the effects of autonomic dysreflexia will assist in determining the immediate nursing actions. If you know to raise the head of the client's bed first (to try to minimize cerebral hypertension), then this eliminates each of the incorrect options. Review immediate nursing interventions for the client experiencing autonomic dysreflexia, if you had difficulty with this question.
Level of Cognitive Ability: Application
Client Needs: Physiological Integrity
Integrated Concept/Process: Nursing Process/Implementation
Content Area: Adult Health/Neurological
Reference: Smeltzer, S., & Bare, B. (2000). *Brunner & Suddarth's textbook of medical-surgical nursing* (9th ed.). Philadelphia: Lippincott Williams & Wilkins, p. 1694.

REFERENCES

Deglin, J., & Vallerand, A. (2001). *Davis's drug guide for nurses* (7th ed.). Philadelphia: F.A. Davis.

Fischbach, F. (2000). *A manual of laboratory & diagnostic tests* (6th ed.). Philadelphia: Lippincott Williams & Wilkins.

Hodgson, B., & Kizior, R. (2001). *Saunders nursing drug handbook 2001.* Philadelphia: W.B. Saunders.

Ignatavicius, D., Workman, M., & Mishler, M. (1999). *Medical-surgical nursing across the health care continuum* (3rd ed.). Philadelphia: W.B. Saunders.

LeMone, P., & Burke, K. (2000). *Medical-surgical nursing: Critical thinking in client care* (2nd ed.). Upper Saddle River, N.J.: Prentice-Hall.

Phipps, W., Sands, J., & Marek, J. (1999). *Medical-surgical nursing: Concepts & clinical practice* (6th ed.). St. Louis: Mosby.

Smeltzer, S., & Bare, B. (2000). *Brunner & Suddarth's textbook of medical-surgical nursing* (9th ed.). Philadelphia: Lippincott Williams & Wilkins.

Neurological Medications

I. ANTIMYASTHENIC MEDICATIONS

A. Description

1. Relieve muscle weakness associated with myasthenia gravis by blocking acetycholine breakdown at the neuromuscular junction
2. Used to treat or diagnose myasthenia gravis or to distinguish cholinergic crisis from myasthenic crisis
3. Neostigmine bromide (Prostigmin), pyridostigmine bromide (Mestinon), ambenonium (Mytelase) are used to control myasthenic symptoms
4. Edrophonium chloride (Tensilon) is used to diagnose myasthenia gravis and to distinguish cholinergic crisis from myasthenic crisis

B. Medications (Box 64-1)

C. Side effects: Cholinergic crisis (Box 64-2)

D. Implementation

1. Assess neuromuscular status, including reflexes, muscle strength, and gait
2. Monitor the client for signs and symptoms of medication overdose (cholinergic crisis) and underdose (myasthenic crisis)
3. Instruct the client to take medications on time to prevent weakness, because weakness can impair the client's ability to breath and swallow
4. Instruct the client to take the medication before meals for best absorption
5. Instruct the client to wear a Medic-Alert bracelet
6. Note that antimyasthenic therapy is lifelong therapy
7. Evaluate for medication effectiveness, which is based on the improvement of neuromuscular symptoms or strength without cholinergic signs and symptoms
8. When administering edrophonium (Tensilon), have emergency resuscitation equipment on hand and atropine sulfate available for cholinergic crisis

---

BOX 64-1

Antimyasthenic Medications

Edrophonium chloride (Tensilon, Enlon)
Neostigmine bromide (Prostigmin Bromide)
Pyridostigmine bromide (Mestinon)
Ambenonium chloride (Mytelase)

BOX 64-2

Signs of Cholinergic Crisis

GI disturbances
Abdominal cramps
Nausea, vomiting, diarrhea
Increased salivation and tearing
Increased bronchial secretions
Sweating
Miosis
Hypertension

E. **Tensilon test**

1. Tensilon is injected by IV
2. The **Tensilon test** can cause ventricular fibrillation and cardiac arrest
3. Atropine sulfate is the antidote for overdose
4. Diagnosis of myasthenia gravis: Most myasthenic clients will show a marked improvement in muscle tone within 30 to 60 seconds after injection, and the muscle improvement lasts 4 to 5 minutes
5. Diagnosis of cholinergic crisis (overdose with anticholinesterase) or myasthenic crisis (undermedication)
   a. In cholinergic crisis, muscle tone does not improve after the administration of Tensilon, and muscle twitching may be noted around the eyes and face
   b. A tensilon injection makes the client in

cholinergic crisis temporarily worse (negative **Tensilon test**)

   c. A tensilon injection temporarily improves the condition when the client is in myasthenic crisis (positive **Tensilon test**)

II. ANTIPARKINSONIAN MEDICATIONS

A. Description

   1. Restore the balance of the neurotransmitters acetylcholine and dopamine in the central nervous system (CNS), decreasing the signs and symptoms of Parkinson's disease

   2. These medications include the dopaminergics, which stimulate the dopamine receptors, and the anticholinergics, which block the cholinergic receptors

   3. Used for drug-induced parkinsonism, in which neuroleptic agents block dopamine receptors in the CNS, leading to functional loss of dopamine activity

   4. Used for Parkinson's disease, in which dopamine-containing neurons in the basal ganglia are destroyed or deficient, which causes loss of fine motor control

B. Dopaminergic medications

   1. Description

     a. Stimulate the dopamine receptors

     b. Increase the amount of dopamine available in the CNS or enhance neurotransmission of dopamine

     c. Contraindicated in cardiac, renal, or psychiatric disorders

     d. Levodopa taken with a monoamine oxidase inhibitor (MAOI) antidepressant can cause a hypertensive crisis

   2. Medications (Box 64-3)

   3. Side effects

     a. Dyskinesia

     b. Involuntary body movements

     c. Tachycardia

     d. Nausea and vomiting

     e. Urinary retention

     f. Constipation

     g. Dizziness

     h. Orthostatic hypotension

     i. Confusion

     j. Mood changes

     k. Hallucinations

   4. Implementation

     a. Assess vital signs

     b. Assess for risk of injury

     c. Instruct the client to take the medication with food if nausea and vomiting occur

     d. Assess for signs and symptoms of parkinsonism, such as rigidity, tremors, akinesia, and bradykinesia; a stooped forward posture; shuffling gait; and masked facies

---

BOX 64-3

Medications to Treat Parkinson's Disease

MEDICATIONS AFFECTING THE AMOUNT OF DOPAMINE
Amantadine (Symmetrel)
Bromocriptine (Parlodel)
Carbidopa-levodopa (Sinemet)
Levodopa (Larodopa, Dopar)
Pergolide mesylate (Permax)
Pramipexole (Mirapex)
Ropinirole (Requip)
Selegiline hydrochloride (Carbex, Eldepryl)
Tolcapone (Tasmar)

ANTICHOLINERGICS
Benztropine mesylate (Cogentin)
Biperiden hydrochloride (Akineton)
Ethopropazine hydrochloride (Parsidol)
Procyclidine hydrochloride (Kemadrin)
Trihexyphenidyl hydrochloride (Artane)

ANTIHISTAMINE
Diphenhydramine hydrochloride (Benadryl)

---

     e. Monitor for signs of dyskinesia

     f. Instruct the client who is taking carbidopa-levodopa (Sinemet) to eat low-protein foods, because high-protein diets interfere with medication transport to the CNS

     g. Instruct the client to change positions slowly to minimize orthostatic hypotension

     h. Instruct the client not to discontinue the medication abruptly

     i. Instruct the client to report side effects and symptoms of dyskinesia

     j. Instruct the client to avoid alcohol

     k. Monitor the client for improvement in signs and symptoms of parkinsonism without the development of severe side effects from the medications

     l. Inform the client that urine or perspiration may be discolored and that this is harmless, but it may stain the clothing

     m. Advise the client with diabetes mellitus that glucose testing should not be done through urine testing because the results will not be reliable

     n. When administering levodopa, instruct the client to avoid excessive vitamin B$_6$ intake to prevent medication reactions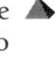

C. Anticholinergic medications

   1. Description

     a. Block the cholinergic receptors in the CNS, thereby suppressing acetylcholine activity

     b. Reduce the rigidity and some of the tremors but have a minimal effect on the bradykinesia

     c. Contraindicated in clients with glaucoma

d. The client with chronic obstructive lung disease can develop dry, thick mucus secretions
2. Medications (Box 64-3)
3. Side effects
   a. Blurred vision
   b. Dry mouth and dry secretions
   c. Increased pulse rate
   d. Constipation
   e. Urinary retention
   f. Restlessness and confusion
   g. Photophobia
4. Implementation
   a. Monitor vital signs
   b. Assess for risk of injury
   c. Assess for signs and symptoms of parkinsonism, such as rigidity, tremors, akinesia, and bradykinesia; a stooped forward posture; shuffling gait; and masked facies
   d. Monitor the client for improvement in signs and symptoms
   e. Assess the client's bowel and urinary function, and monitor for urinary retention and constipation
   f. Monitor for involuntary movements
   g. Encourage the client to avoid alcohol, smoking, caffeine, and aspirin to decrease gastric acidity
   h. Instruct the client to consult with the physician before taking any nonprescription medications
   i. Instruct the client to minimize dry mouth by increasing fluid intake and by using ice chips, hard candy, or gum
   j. Instruct the client to prevent constipation by increasing fluid and fiber in the diet
   k. Instruct the client to use sunglasses in direct sun because of possible photophobia
   l. Instruct the client to have routine eye examinations to assess for intraocular pressure

III. ANTICONVULSANT MEDICATIONS (Table 64-1)

A. Description
1. Used to depress abnormal neuronal discharges and prevent the spread of seizures
2. Used with caution in clients on anticoagulants, aspirin, sulfonamides, cimetidine (Tagamet), or antipsychotics
3. Absorption is decreased with the use of antacids, calcium preparations, and antineoplastic medications
B. Implementation for clients on anticonvulsants
1. Initiate seizure precautions
2. Monitor urinary output
3. Monitor liver and renal function tests
4. Monitor for signs of medication toxicity, which would include CNS depression, ataxia, nausea, vomiting, drowsiness, dizziness, restlessness, and visual disturbances

---

TABLE 64-1

Anticonvulsant Medications

Medication	Therapeutic Serum Range
Phenytoin (Dilantin)	10-20 µg/mL
Carbamazepine (Tegretol)	3-14 µg/mL
Mephenytoin (Mesantoin)	25-40 µg/mL
Ethotoin (Peganone)	10-50 µg/mL
Phenobarbital (Luminal)	15-40 µg/mL
Primidone (Mysoline)	5-10 µg/mL
Amobarbital (Amytal)	1-5 µg/mL
Mephobarbital (Mebaral)	15-40 µg/mL
Clonazepam (Klonopin)	20-80 ng/mL
Lorazepam (Ativan)	50-240 ng/mL
Ethosuximide (Zarontin)	40-100 µg/mL
Valproic acid (Depakene)	40-100 µg/mL

BOX 64-4

Client Education: Anticonvulsants

Take anticonvulsant with food to decrease GI irritation, but avoid milk and antacids, which impair absorption
If taking liquid medication, shake well before ingesting
Do not discontinue medication
Avoid alcohol
Avoid over-the-counter medications
Wear a Medic-Alert bracelet
Use caution when driving or performing activities that require alertness
Maintain good oral hygiene and use a soft toothbrush
Importance of preventive dental checkups
Importance of follow-up with periodic blood studies related to determining toxicity
Monitor serum glucose levels (diabetes mellitus)
Urine may be a harmless pink-red or red-brown color
Report symptoms of sore throat, bruising, and nosebleeds, which may indicate a blood dyscrasia
Inform the physician if adverse reactions occur, such as gingivitis, nystagmus, slurred speech, rash, or dizziness

---

5. If a seizure occurs, assess seizure activity, including location and duration
6. Protect client from hazards in the environment during a seizure
C. Client education (Box 64-4)
D. Hydantoins (Box 64-5)
1. Used to treat seizures
2. Phenytoin (Dilantin) is also used to treat dysrhythmias
3. Side effects
   a. Gingival hyperplasia
   b. Reddened gums that bleed easily
   c. Slurred speech
   d. Confusion
   e. Depression
   f. Nausea and vomiting

BOX 64-5

Hydantoins

Phenytoin (Dilantin)
Mephenytoin (Mesantoin)
Ethotoin (Peganone)
Fosphenytoin (Cerebyx)

BOX 64-6

Barbiturates

Phenobarbital
Primidone (Mysoline)
Amobarbital (Amytal)
Mephobarbital (Mebaral)

BOX 64-7

Benzodiazepines

Clonazepam (Klonopin)
Clorazepate (Tranxene)
Diazepam (Valium)
Lorazepam (Ativan)

BOX 64-8

Succinimides

Ethosuximide (Zarontin)
Methsuximide (Celontin)
Phensuximide (Milontin)

BOX 64-9

Oxazolidinediones

Paramethadione (Paradione)
Trimethadione (Tridione)

BOX 64-10

Valproates

Valproic acid (Depakene)
Divalproex sodium (Depakote)

g. Constipation
h. Headaches
i. Blood dyscrasias: Decreased platelet count and decreased white blood cell (WBC) count
j. Elevated blood glucose
k. Alopecia
l. Hirsutism
4. Implementation
a. Oral tube feedings may interfere with the absorption of oral phenytoin and diminish the medication's effectiveness; therefore, feedings should be scheduled as far as possible from the phenytoin administration
b. Monitor therapeutic serum levels to assess for toxicity
c. Monitor for signs of toxicity
d. When administering IV phenytoin, dilute in normal saline, because dextrose causes the medication to precipitate
e. When administering IV phenytoin, infuse no faster than 50 mg per minute; otherwise hypotension and cardiac dysrhythmias can occur
f. Instruct the client about the importance of good oral hygiene and regular dental examinations
g. Instruct the client to consult with the physician before taking other medications, to ensure compatibility with anticonvulsants
E. Barbiturates (Box 64-6)
1. Used for tonic-clonic seizures and acute episodes of seizures resulting from status epilepticus
2. May also be used as adjuncts to anesthesia
3. Side effects
a. Drowsiness
b. Dizziness
c. Hypotension
d. Respiratory depression
e. Tolerance to the medication
F. Benzodiazepines (Box 64-7)
1. To treat absence seizures
2. Diazepam (Valium) is used to treat status epilepticus, anxiety, and skeletal muscle spasms
3. Clorazepate (Tranxene) is used as adjunctive therapy for partial seizures
4. Side effects
a. Ataxia
b. Respiratory and cardiac depression
c. Medication tolerance and drug dependency

G. Succinimides (Box 64-8)
1. Used to treat absence seizures
2. Side effects
a. Anorexia, nausea, vomiting
b. Blood dyscrasias
H. Oxazolidinediones (Box 64-9)
1. Used for absence seizures
2. Side effects
a. Sedation
b. Photophobia
I. Valproates (Box 64-10)
1. Used to treat tonic-clonic, partial, myoclonic, and psychomotor seizures
2. Side effects
a. Nausea
b. Vomiting

BOX 64-11

Other Anticonvulsants

Carbamazepine (Tegretol)
Felbamate (Felbatol)
Gabapentin (Neurontin)
Lamotrigine (Lamictal)
Tiagabine (Gabitril)
Topiramate (Topamax)

BOX 64-12

Amphetamines

Amphetamine sulfate
Dextroamphetamine sulfate (Dexedrine)
Methamphetamine hydrochloride (Desoxyn)
Methylphenidate hydrochloride (Ritalin)
Pemoline (Cylert)

BOX 64-13

Anorexiants

Diethylpropion hydrochloride (Tenuate, Tepanil,)
Mazindol (Sanorex, Mazanor)
Phendimetrazine (Anorex, Bontril, Melfiat, Obalan)
Phentermine hydrochloride (Fastin, Adipex, Zantril)
Benzphetamine hydrochloride (Didrex)
Phenylpropanolamine (Acutrim, Dexatrim, Phenyldrine)
Sibutramine (Meridia)

BOX 64-14

Treating Respiratory Depression

Aminophylline
Caffeine
Doxapram (Dopram)
Theophylline

c. Abdominal cramps
d. Diarrhea
e. Constipation
f. Hepatotoxicity
J. Iminostilbenes (Box 64-11)
   1. Used to treat seizure disorders that have not responded to other anticonvulsants
   2. Used to treat trigeminal neuralgia
   3. Side effects
      a. Drowsiness
      b. Dizziness
      c. Nausea
      d. Vomiting
      e. Constipation or diarrhea
      f. Visual abnormalities
      g. Dry mouth
      h. Headache

IV. CENTRAL NERVOUS SYSTEM STIMULANTS
A. Description
   1. Amphetamines and caffeine stimulate the cerebral cortex of the brain (Box 64-12)
   2. Analeptics and caffeine act on the brainstem and medulla to stimulate respiration
   3. Anorexiants act on the cerebral cortex and hypothalamus to suppress appetite (Box 64-13)
   4. Used to treat narcolepsy and attention deficit hyperactivity disorders
   5. Used to treat respiratory depression (Box 64-14)
   6. Used as adjunctive therapy for exogenous obesity
B. Side effects
   1. Irritability
   2. Restlessness
   3. Tremors
   4. Insomnia
   5. Heart palpitations
   6. Tachycardia
   7. Hypertension
   8. Dry mouth
   9. Anorexia
   10. Weight loss
   11. Diarrhea or constipation
   12. Impotence
   13. Dependence and tolerance
C. Implementation
   1. Monitor vital signs
   2. Assess mental status
   3. Assess height, weight, and growth of the child
   4. Monitor complete blood count (CBC) and white blood cell (WBC) and platelet counts before and during therapy
   5. Monitor for side effects
   6. Monitor sleep patterns
   7. Monitor for withdrawal symptoms such as nausea, vomiting, weakness, and headache
   8. Instruct the client to take the medication before meals
   9. Instruct the client to avoid foods and beverages containing caffeine to prevent additional stimulation
   10. Instruct the client to read labels on over-the-counter products because many contain caffeine
   11. Instruct the client to avoid alcohol
   12. Instruct the client not to discontinue the medication abruptly
   13. Instruct the client to take the last daily dose of the CNS stimulant at least 6 hours before bedtime to prevent insomnia
   14. Monitor for drug dependence and abuse with amphetamines
   15. If a child is taking a CNS stimulant, instruct the parents to notify the school nurse

16. Monitor for calming effects of CNS stimulants within 3 to 4 weeks on children with attention deficit hyperactivity disorder
17. Monitor growth in the child on long-term therapy with methylphenidate hydrochloride (Ritalin)

V. NONNARCOTIC ANALGESICS

A. Nonsteroidal antiinflammatory drugs (NSAIDs) (Box 64-15)
   1. Description
      a. NSAIDs are aspirin and aspirin-like medications that inhibit the synthesis of prostaglandins
      b. They act as an analgesic to relieve pain, as an antipyretic to reduce body temperature, and as an anticoagulant to inhibit platelet aggregation
      c. Used to relieve inflammation and pain and in the treatment of rheumatoid arthritis, bursitis, tendinitis, osteoarthritis, and acute gout
      d. Contraindicated in hypersensitivity or liver or renal disease
      e. Aspirin should not be taken by children with flu symptoms because of the risk of Reye's syndrome
      f. Aspirin should not be taken if the client is on an anticoagulant
      g. Aspirin and an NSAID should not be taken together because aspirin decreases the blood level and the effectiveness of the NSAID
      h. NSAIDs can increase the effects of warfarin (Coumadin), sulfonamides, cephalosporins, and phenytoin (Dilantin)
      i. Hypoglycemia can result if ibuprofen (Motrin) is taken with insulin or an oral hypoglycemic medication
      j. A high risk of toxicity exists if ibuprofen is taken concurrently with calcium blockers
   2. Side effects (Table 64-2)
   3. Implementation
      a. Assess client for allergies
      b. Obtain a medication history and medical history on the client
      c. Assess for history of gastric upset or bleeding or liver disease
      d. Assess the client for GI upset during medication administration
      e. Monitor for edema
      f. Monitor serum salicylate (aspirin) level when the client is taking high doses
      g. Monitor for signs of bleeding, such as tarry stools, bleeding gums, petechiae, ecchymosis, and purpura
      h. Instruct the client to take the medication with water, milk, or food
      i. Enteric-coated form or buffered form of aspirin can be taken to decrease gastric distress

---

BOX 64-15

Nonsteroidal Antiinflammatory Drugs (NSAIDs)

ACETAMINOPHEN
Acetaminophen (Tylenol)

ASPIRIN AND OTHER SALICYLATES
Aspirin (acetylsalicylic acid) (ASA, Aspergum, Bayer, Ecotrin)
Aspirin (acetylsalicylic acid), buffered (Alka-Seltzer, Bufferin)
Choline salicylate (Arthropan)
Diflunisal (Dolobid)
Magnesium salicylate (Doan's, Magan)
Olsalazine (Dipentum)
Salsalate (Amigesic, Disalcid)
Sulfasalazine (Azulfidine)

PROPIONIC ACID DERIVATIVES
Fenoprofen (Nalfon)
Flurbipofen (Ansaid)
Ibuprofen (Motrin, Advil, Nuprin, Medipren)
Ketoprofen (Orudis)
Naproxen (Anaprox, Naprosyn)
Oxaprozin (Daypro)

OTHER NSAIDS
Diclofenac (Voltaren)
Etodolac (Lodine)
Indomethacin (Indocin)
Ketorolac tromethamine (Toradol)
Meclofenamate (Meclomen)
Mefenamic acid (Ponstel)
Nabumetone (Relafen)
Phenylbutazone (Butazolidin, Butazone)
Piroxicam (Feldene)
Sulindac (Clinoril)
Tolmetin (Tolectin)

TABLE 64-2

Side Effects of Aspirin and NSAIDs

Aspirin	NSAIDs
Drowsiness	Hypotension
Tinnitus	Sodium and water retention
Headaches	Gastric irritation
Flushing	Blood dyscrasias
Dizziness	Dizziness
GI symptoms	Tinnitus
Visual changes	Pruritus

j. Instruct the client that enteric-coated tablets cannot be crushed or broken
k. Advise the client to inform other health care professionals if he or she is taking high doses of aspirin
l. Note that aspirin should be discontinued 3 to

7 days prior to surgery to reduce the risk of bleeding

   m. Instruct the client to avoid alcoholic beverages

B. Acetaminophen (Tylenol)

  1. Description

    a. Inhibits prostaglandin synthesis

    b. Used to decrease pain and fever

    c. Contraindicated in hepatic or renal disease, alcoholism, and hypersensitivity

  2. Side effects

    a. Anorexia, nausea, vomiting

    b. Rash

    c. Hypoglycemia

    d. Oliguria

    e. Hepatotoxicity

  3. Implementation

    a. Monitor vital signs

    b. Assess client for history of liver dysfunction

    c. Monitor for hepatic damage, which includes nausea, vomiting, diarrhea, and abdominal pain

    d. Monitor liver enzyme tests

    e. Instruct the client that self-medication should not be used longer than 10 days for an adult and 5 days for a child

    f. Note that the antidote for Tylenol is acetylcysteine (Mucomyst)

    g. Evaluate for the effectiveness of the medication

VI. NARCOTIC ANALGESICS

A. Description

  1. Suppress pain impulses but can suppress respiration and coughing by acting on the respiratory and cough center in the medulla of the brainstem

  2. Can produce euphoria and sedation

  3. Can cause physical dependence

  4. Used for relief of mild, moderate, or severe pain

B. Medications (Box 64-16)

  1. Codeine sulfate

    a. Effective cough suppressant at low doses

    b. Can cause constipation

  2. Hydromorphone hydrochloride (Dilaudid)

    a. Can decrease respiration

    b. Can cause constipation

  3. Meperidine hydrochloride (Demerol)

    a. Can cause hypotension and dizziness

    b. Used for acute pain and as a preoperative medication

    c. Can **increase intracranial pressure** in head injuries

    d. Contraindicated in head injuries and **increased intracranial pressure**, respiratory disorders, hypotension, shock, severe hepatic and renal disease, and in clients taking monoamine oxidase inhibitors

---

BOX 64-16

Narcotic Analgesics

Codeine sulfate; codeine phosphate
Hydromorphone hydrochloride (Dilaudid, Hydrostat IR, PMS-Hydromorphone)
Meperidine hydrochloride (Demerol)
Morphine sulfate
Oxycodone hydrochloride with acetaminophen (Percocet)
Oxycodone with aspirin (Percodan)
Propoxyphene napsylate (Darvon-N)
Buprenorphine hydrochloride (Buprenex)
Butorphanol tartrate (Stadol, Stadol NS)
Dezocine (Dalgan)
Nalbuphine hydrochloride (Nubain)
Methadone hydrochloride (Dolophine, Methadose)
Pentazocine hydrochloride (Talwin)
Hydrocodone (Hycodan)
Levorphanol tartrate (Levo-Dromoran)
Fentanyl (Duragesic, Sulimaze)
Sufentanil citrate (Sufenta)
Oxycodone (Roxicodone)
Oxymorphone hydrochloride (Numorphan)
Tramadol hydrochloride (Ultram)

---

    e. Should not be taken with alcohol or sedative hypnotics because it may increase the CNS depression

  4. Morphine sulfate

    a. Can cause respiratory depression, orthostatic hypotension, and constipation

    b. May cause nausea and vomiting because of increased vestibular sensitivity

    c. Used for acute pain resulting from myocardial infarction (MI) or cancer, for dyspnea resulting from pulmonary edema, and as a preoperative medication

    d. Contraindicated in severe respiratory disorders, head injuries, **increased intracranial pressure**, severe renal disease, or seizure activity

    e. Used with caution in clients with shock or blood loss

  5. Oxycodone with aspirin (Percodan)

    a. Should not be taken by a client allergic to aspirin

    b. Can cause gastric irritation and should be taken with food or plenty of liquids

  6. Propoxyphene hydrochloride (Darvon) and propoxyphene napsylate (Darvon-N)

    a. Darvon compound contains aspirin and should not be taken by a client allergic to aspirin

    b. Darvocet-N contains acetaminophen

  7. Nalbuphine hydrochloride (Nubain): Preferable for treating the pain of an MI because it reduces

the oxygen needs of the heart without reducing blood pressure

8. Methadone hydrochloride (Dolophine)
   a. Dilute doses of oral concentrate with at least 90 mL of water
   b. Dilute dispersible tablets in at least 120 mL of water, orange juice, or acidic fruit beverage
   c. Used as a replacement medication for opiate dependence or to facilitate withdrawal
9. Hydrocodone (Hycodan): Frequently used for cough suppression

C. Implementation for narcotic analgesics
   1. Monitor vital signs
   2. Assess the client thoroughly before administering pain medication
   3. Initiate nursing measures such as massage, distraction, deep breathing and relaxation exercises, the application of heat or cold as prescribed, and providing care and comfort prior to administering the narcotic analgesic
   4. Administer medications 30 to 60 minutes before painful activities
   5. Monitor respiratory rate, and if the rate is less than 12 breaths per minute in an adult, withhold the medication unless ventilatory support is being provided
   6. Monitor pulse, and if bradycardia develops, hold the dose and notify the physician
   7. Monitor blood pressure for hypotension
   8. Auscultate breath sounds because narcotic analgesics suppress the cough reflex
   9. Encourage activities such as turning, deep breathing, and incentive spirometry to prevent atelectasis and pneumonia
   10. Monitor level of consciousness (LOC)
   11. Initiate safety precautions such as side rails, a night-light, and supervised ambulation
   12. Monitor I & O
   13. Assess for urinary retention
   14. Instruct the client to take oral doses with milk or a snack to reduce gastric irritation
   15. Instruct the client to avoid alcohol
   16. Instruct the client to avoid activities that require alertness
   17. Note effectiveness of medication
   18. Have the narcotic antagonist, oxygen, and resuscitation equipment available

D. Morphine sulfate
   1. Side effects
      a. Respiratory depression
      b. Orthostatic hypotension
      c. Urinary retention
      d. Nausea
      e. Vomiting
      f. Constipation
      g. Cough suppression
      h. Reduction in pupillary size
      i. Miosis
   2. Implementation
      a. Have naxolone (Narcan) available for overdose
      b. Assess vital signs
      c. Note rate and depth of respirations
      d. Withhold the medication if the respiratory rate is less than 12 breaths per minute; respirations of less than 10 breaths per minute can indicate respiratory distress
      e. Monitor urinary output, which should be at least 600 mL/day
      f. Monitor bowel sounds for decreased peristalsis because constipation can occur
      g. Monitor for pupil changes because pinpoint pupils can indicate morphine overdose
      h. Avoid alcohol or CNS depressants because they can cause respiratory depression
      i. Instruct the client to report dizziness or difficulty breathing
      j. To administer IV, dilute in at least 5 mL of sterile water or normal saline for injection and administer at a rate of 15 mg or less over 4 to 5 minutes

E. Meperidine hydrochloride (Demerol)
   1. Side effects
      a. Respiratory depression
      b. Hypotension
      c. Tachycardia
      d. Drowsiness
      e. Constipation
      f. Urinary retention
      g. Nausea
      h. Vomiting
      i. Tremors
   2. Implementation
      a. Monitor vital signs
      b. Monitor for respiratory dysfunction and hypotension
      c. Have naloxone (Narcan) available for overdose
      d. Monitor for urinary retention
      e. Monitor bowel sounds and for constipation
      f. To administer IV, dilute in at least 5 mL of sterile water or normal saline for injection and administer the dose over 4 to 5 minutes

VII. NARCOTIC ANTAGONISTS (Box 64-17)
A. Used to treat respiratory depression from narcotic overdose
B. Implementation
   1. Monitor blood pressure, pulse, and respiratory rate every 5 minutes initially, tapering to every 15 minutes, and then every 30 minutes until stable
   2. Place the client on a cardiac monitor and monitor cardiac rhythm

BOX 64-17

Narcotic Antagonists

Nalmefene (Revex)
Naloxone hydrochloride (Narcan)
Naltrexone (ReVia)

BOX 64-18

Osmotic Diuretics

Mannitol (Osmitrol)
Urea (Ureaphil)

3. Auscultate breath sounds
4. Have resuscitation equipment available
5. Do not leave the client unattended
6. Monitor the client closely for several hours because when the effects of the antagonist wears off, the client may again display signs of narcotic overdose

VIII. OSMOTIC DIURETICS (Box 64-18)

A. Description
   1. Increase osmotic pressure of the glomerular filtrate, inhibiting reabsorption of water and electrolytes
   2. Used for oliguria and to prevent renal failure
   3. Used to decrease intracranial pressure
   4. Used to decrease intraocular pressure in narrow-angle glaucoma
   5. Mannitol is used with chemotherapy to induce diuresis
B. Side effects
   1. Fluid and electrolyte imbalances
   2. Pulmonary edema from the rapid shifts of fluid
   3. Nausea and vomiting
   4. Tachycardia from the rapid fluid loss
   5. Hyponatremia and dehydration
C. Implementation
   1. Monitor vital signs
   2. Monitor weight
   3. Monitor urine output
   4. Monitor electrolyte levels
   5. Monitor lungs and heart sounds for signs of pulmonary edema
   6. Monitor for signs of dehydration
   7. Monitor neurological status
   8. Assess for signs of decreasing intracranial pressure if appropriate
   9. Change the client's position slowly to prevent orthostatic hypotension
   10. Monitor for crystallization in the vial of mannitol prior to administering the medication; if crystallization is noted, do not administer the medication

PRACTICE QUESTIONS

1. In the emergency room, a nurse is caring for a client diagnosed with Bell's palsy. The client has been taking acetaminophen (Tylenol), and a Tylenol overdose is suspected. The nurse anticipates that the antidote to be prescribed is:
   1. Auranofin (Ridaura)
   2. Fludarabine (Fludara)
   3. Acetylcysteine (Mucomyst)
   4. Pentostatin (Nipent)
2. A client with trigeminal neuralgia tells the nurse that he or she takes acetaminophen (Tylenol) on a frequent daily basis for the relief of generalized discomfort. Which of the following laboratory values would indicate toxicity associated with the medication?
   1. Platelet count of 400,000 cells/μL
   2. Direct bilirubin level of 2 mg/dL
   3. Prothrombin time of 12 seconds
   4. Sodium of 140 mEq/L
3. A client is suspected of having myasthenia gravis. Edrophonium (Tensilon) 2 mg IV is administered to determine the diagnosis. Which of the following indicates that the client has myasthenia gravis?
   1. An increase in muscle strength within 1 to 3 minutes following administration of the medication
   2. A decrease in muscle strength within 1 to 3 minutes following administration of the medication
   3. Joint pain following administration of the medication
   4. Feelings of faintness, dizziness, hypotension, and signs of flushing in the client
4. A client with myasthenia gravis becomes increasingly weaker. The physician prepares to identify whether the client is reacting to an overdose of the medication (cholinergic crisis) or an increasing severity of the disease (myasthenic crisis). An injection of edrophonium (Tensilon) is administered. Which of the following would indicate that the client is in cholinergic crisis?
   1. An improvement of the weakness
   2. A temporary worsening of the condition
   3. No change is the condition
   4. Complaints of muscle spasms
5. A client with myasthenia gravis verbalizes complaints of feeling much weaker than normal. The physician plans to implement a diagnostic test to determine if the client is experiencing a myasthenic crisis. The physician administers edrophonium (Tensilon). Which of the following would indicate that the client is experiencing a myasthenic crisis?
   1. Increasing weakness
   2. No change in the condition
   3. A temporary improvement in the condition
   4. An increase in muscle spasms

6. Levodopa (Carbidopa) is prescribed for a client with Parkinson's disease. The nurse monitors the client for adverse reactions to the medication. Which of the following would indicate that the client is experiencing an adverse reaction?
   1. Pruritus
   2. Hypertension
   3. Tachycardia
   4. Impaired voluntary movements

7. Phenytoin (Dilantin), 100 mg PO three times daily, has been prescribed for a client for seizure control. The home health nurse visits the client and provides teaching about the medication. Which of the following statements, if made by the client, would indicate effective teaching?
   1. "It's OK to break the capsules to make it easier for me to swallow them."
   2. "I will use a soft toothbrush to brush my teeth."
   3. "If I forget to take my medication, I can wait until the next dose and eliminate that dose."
   4. "If my throat becomes sore, it's a normal effect of the medication and it's nothing to be concerned about."

8. A client is taking phenytoin (Dilantin) for seizure control. A blood specimen for serum drug level is drawn and the nurse reviews the results. Which of the following would indicate a therapeutic serum drug range?
   1. 5 to 10 µg/mL
   2. 10 to 20 µg/mL
   3. 20 to 30 µg/mL
   4. 30 to 40 µg/mL

9. A nurse is preparing an IV infusion of phenytoin (Dilantin) as prescribed by the physician for a client with seizures. Which of the following solutions will the nurse plan to use to dilute this medication?
   1. Lactated Ringer's
   2. 5% dextrose
   3. 5% dextrose and ½ normal saline
   4. Normal saline solution

10. A home health nurse visits a client who is taking phenytoin (Dilantin) for control of seizures. During the assessment, the nurse notes that the client is taking birth control pills. Which of the following information should the nurse include in the teaching plan?
    1. The increased risk of thrombophlebitis while taking phenytoin and birth control pills together
    2. The potential decreased effectiveness of the birth control pills while taking phenytoin
    3. A client may stop the medication if it is causing severe gastrointestinal effects
    4. That pregnancy should be avoided while taking phenytoin

11. A client with trigeminal neuralgia is being treated with carbamazepine (Tegretol), 400 mg PO daily. Which of the following indicates that the client is experiencing an adverse reaction to the medication?
    1. White blood cell (WBC) count, 3000/µL
    2. Blood urea nitrogen (BUN), 15 mg/dL
    3. Sodium, 140 mEq/L
    4. Uric acid, 5.0 ng/dL

12. A nurse is caring for a client receiving morphine sulfate, 10 mg subcutaneously (SC) every 4 hours, for pain. Because this medication has been prescribed for this client, which nursing action would be included in the plan of care?
    1. Monitor the client's temperature
    2. Force fluids
    3. Maintain the client in a supine position
    4. Encourage the client to cough and deep-breathe

13. Meperidine hydrochloride (Demerol) is prescribed for a client with pain. Which of the following would the nurse monitor for as a side effect of this medication?
    1. Hypertension
    2. Bradycardia
    3. Diarrhea
    4. Urinary retention

14. A nurse is caring for a client with severe back pain. Codeine sulfate has been prescribed for the client. Which of the following does the nurse specifically include in the plan of care while the client is taking this medication?
    1. Monitor for hypertension
    2. Monitor fluid balance
    3. Monitor the bowel activity
    4. Monitor peripheral pulses

15. Dantrolene (Dantrium) is prescribed for a client with spinal cord injury for discomfort caused by spasticity. Which of the following laboratory values would the nurse monitor while the client is taking this medication?
    1. Sedimentation rate
    2. White blood cell count
    3. Liver function studies
    4. Creatinine

16. A client with epilepsy is taking the prescribed dose of phenytoin (Dilantin) to control seizures. Results of a phenytoin blood level study reveal a level of 35 µg/mL. Which of the following symptoms would be expected as a result of this laboratory result?
    1. No symptoms because this is a normal therapeutic level
    2. Slurred speech
    3. Tachycardia
    4. Tachypnea

17. Mannitol (Osmitrol) is prescribed for a client with increased intracranial pressure after a head injury. The nurse prepares to administer this medication, knowing that the therapeutic action is to:
    1. Induce diuresis by raising the osmotic pressure

of glomerular filtrate, thereby inhibiting tubular reabsorption of water and solutes

2. Induce diuresis by promoting the reabsorption of sodium and water in the loop of Henle

3. Prevent the filtration of sodium and water through the kidneys

4. Prevent the filtration of sodium and potassium through the kidneys

18. Dexamethasone (Decadron) IV is prescribed for a client with cerebral edema. The nurse prepares the medication for administration and plans to:
   1. Mix the medication in 100 mL of lactated Ringers solution
   2. Mix the medication in 1000 mL of 5% dextrose
   3. Prepare an undiluted direct injection of the medication
   4. Dilute the medication in lactated Ringer's solution and administer as a direct injection

19. A client arrives at the emergency department complaining of back spasms. The client states "I have been taking two to three aspirin every 4 hours for the last week and it hasn't helped my back." Aspirin intoxication is suspected and the nurse assesses the client for which of the following?
   1. Diarrhea

2. Constipation
3. Tinnitus
4. Photosensitivity

20. A client with multiple sclerosis is receiving diazepam (Valium), a centrally acting skeletal muscle relaxant. Which of the following, if noted during assessment of the client, would indicate that the client is experiencing a side effect related to this medication?
   1. Headache
   2. Increased salivation
   3. Urinary retention
   4. Drowsiness

CRITICAL THINKING: FREE-TEXT ENTRY

A client with myasthenia gravis is receiving pyridostigmine (Mestinon), and a nurse is monitoring the client for signs and symptoms of cholinergic crisis that can occur as a result of overdose of the medication. The nurse plans to have the antidote for cholinergic crisis available and obtains which medication from the pharmacy?

Answer: _____

ANSWERS

1. **3**
Rationale: The antidote for acetaminophen is acetylcysteine (Mucomyst). The normal therapeutic acetaminophen serum level is 5 to 20 mg/µL. A toxic level is greater than 50 µg/mL, and levels of greater than 200 µg/mL could indicate hepatotoxicity. Auranofin (Ridaura) is a gold preparation used to treat rheumatoid arthritis (RA). Fludarabine (Fludara) and Pentostatin (Nipent) are antineoplastic agents.
Test-Taking Strategy: Use the process of elimination. Eliminate options 2 and 4 first because they are similar (antineoplastic agents). Recalling that auranofin is used to treat RA will direct you to option 3. Review the antidote for Tylenol if you had difficulty with this question.
Level of Cognitive Ability: Analysis
Client Needs: Physiological Integrity
Integrated Concept/Process: Nursing Process/Analysis
Content Area: Pharmacology
Reference: Cleveland, L., Aschenbrenner, D., Venable, S., & Yensen, J. (1999). *Nursing management in drug therapy.* Philadelphia: Lippincott, pp. 490-492.

2. **2**
Rationale: In adults, overdose of acetaminophen causes liver damage. Option 2 is an indicator of liver function and is the only option that indicates an abnormal laboratory value. The normal direct bilirubin is 0 to 0.3 mg/dL. The normal platelet count is 150,000 to 400,000 cells/µL. The normal prothrombin time is 10 to 13 seconds. The normal sodium is 135 to 145 mEq/L.

Test-Taking Strategy: Use the process of elimination. Knowledge that acetaminophen causes liver damage and knowledge of normal laboratory results will assist in answering this question. Option 2 is the only abnormal value. Also, of all of the options, the bilirubin is the laboratory value most directly related to liver function. Review the effects of toxicity from Tylenol and normal laboratory values if you had difficulty with this question.
Level of Cognitive Ability: Analysis
Client Needs: Physiological Integrity
Integrated Concept/Process: Nursing Process/Analysis
Content Area: Pharmacology
Reference: Clark, J., Queener, S., & Karb, V. (2000). *Pharmacologic basis of nursing practice* (6th ed.). St. Louis: Mosby, p. 366.

3. **1**
Rationale: Edrophonium is a short-acting acetylcholinesterase inhibitor used as a diagnostic agent. When a client with suspected myasthenia gravis is given 2 mg of the medication intravenously, an increase in muscle strength should be seen in 1 to 3 minutes. If no response occurs, another 4 to 10 mg of edrophonium is given over the next 2 minutes, and muscle strength is again tested. If no increase in muscle strength occurs with this higher dose, the muscle weakness is not caused by myasthenia gravis. Clients receiving injections of this medication commonly demonstrate a drop in blood pressure, feel faint and dizzy, and are flushed.
Test-Taking Strategy: Use the process of elimination. Recalling that the client with myasthenia gravis is treated with medication to improve muscle strength will assist in directing you to

option 1. Review this medication as a diagnostic tool for suspected myasthenia gravis if you had difficulty with this question.

Level of Cognitive Ability: Analysis
Client Needs: Physiological Integrity
Integrated Concept/Process: Nursing Process/Analysis
Content Area: Pharmacology
Reference: Karch, A. (2000). *Focus on nursing pharmacology.* Philadelphia: Lippincott, p. 368.

4. 2
Rationale: An edrophonium injection makes the client in cholinergic crisis temporarily worse. This in known as a negative Tensilon test.

Test-Taking Strategy: Use the process of elimination. Recalling that a cholinergic crisis indicates an overdose to medication, it seems reasonable that a worsening of the condition will occur when medication is administered. Review cholinergic crisis if you had difficulty with this question.

Level of Cognitive Ability: Analysis
Client Needs: Physiological Integrity
Integrated Concept/Process: Nursing Process/Analysis
Content Area: Pharmacology
Reference: Gutierrez, K. (1999). *Pharmacotherapeutics: Clinical decision-making in nursing.* Philadelphia: W. B. Saunders, p. 449.

5. 3
Rationale: Edrophonium is administered to determine whether the client is reacting to an overdose of a medication (cholinergic crisis) or an increasing severity of the disease (myasthenic crisis). When the edrophonium injection is given and the condition improves temporarily, the client is in myasthenic crisis. This in known as a positive Tensilon test.

Test-Taking Strategy: Use the process of elimination. Recall that myasthenic crisis is treated with medication. It seems reasonable then that the client's condition will improve when medication is administered. Review this diagnostic test and the differences between cholinergic and myasthenic crisis if you had difficulty with this question.

Level of Cognitive Ability: Analysis
Client Needs: Physiological Integrity
Integrated Concept/Process: Nursing Process/Analysis
Content Area: Pharmacology
Reference: Gutierrez, K. (1999). *Pharmacotherapeutics: Clinical decision-making in nursing.* Philadelphia: W. B. Saunders, p. 449.

6. 4
Rationale: Dyskinesia and impaired voluntary movement can occur with high levodopa dosages. Nausea, anorexia, dizziness, orthostatic hypotension, bradycardia, and akinesia (the temporary muscle weakness that lasts 1 minute to 1 hour, also know as "on-off phenomenon") are frequent side effects of the medication.

Test-Taking Strategy: Use the process of elimination. Options 2 and 3 are similar and are cardiac-related options, so these options can be eliminated first. Note that the question asks for an adverse reaction; therefore, select option 4 over option 1 because it is neurologically related. Review the adverse effects of levodopa if you had difficulty with this question.

Level of Cognitive Ability: Analysis
Client Needs: Physiological Integrity

Integrated Concept/Process: Nursing Process/Analysis
Content Area: Pharmacology
Reference: Salerno, E. (1999). *Pharmacology for health professionals.* St. Louis: Mosby, p. 292.

7. 2
Rationale: Phenytoin is an anticonvulsant. Gingival hyperplasia, bleeding, swelling, and tenderness of the gums can occur with the use of this medication. The client needs to be taught good oral hygiene, gum massage, and the need for regular dentist visits. The client should not skip medication doses because this could precipitate a seizure. Capsules should not be chewed or broken, and they must be swallowed. The client needs to be instructed to report a sore throat, fever, glandular swelling, or any skin reaction, because this indicates hematological toxicity.

Test-Taking Strategy: Use the process of elimination. Note the key words "indicate effective teaching." Eliminate option 3 because the client needs to be encouraged to take medications on time. Also, eliminate option 4 because the client needs to report these symptoms to the physician. Remember, Dilantin capsules should not be broken. Review the client teaching points related to phenytoin if you had difficulty with this question.

Level of Cognitive Ability: Analysis
Client Needs: Health Promotion and Maintenance
Integrated Concept/Process: Teaching/Learning
Content Area: Pharmacology
Reference: Karch, A. (2000). *Focus on nursing pharmacology.* Philadelphia: Lippincott, p. 258.

8. 2
Rationale: The therapeutic serum drug level range for phenytoin is 10 to 20 µg/mL.

Test-Taking Strategy: Use the process of elimination. A helpful pyramid point may be to remember that the theophylline therapeutic range and the acetaminophen therapeutic range are the same as the phenytoin therapeutic range. Remembering this may assist you when answering questions related to these three medications. Review this medication if you had difficulty with this question.

Level of Cognitive Ability: Analysis
Client Needs: Physiological Integrity
Integrated Concept/Process: Nursing Process/Analysis
Content Area: Pharmacology
Reference: Wilson, B., Shannon, M., & Stang, C. (2000). *Nurses' drug guide 2000.* Stamford, Conn: Appleton & Lange, p. 1117.

9. 4
Rationale: Intravenous infusion of phenytoin should be administered by injection into a large vein. The medication may be diluted in normal saline solution; however, dextrose solution should be avoided because of medication precipitation. The medication is administered as intermittent doses. Continuous IV infusions should not be used. Infusion rates of more than 50 mg/min may cause hypotension or cardiac dysrhythmias, especially in elderly and debilitated clients.

Test-Taking Strategy: Use the process of elimination. In most, but not all, situations, medications can be diluted in normal saline, so this would be the best option to select if you were unfamiliar with the IV administration of this medication. Review this procedure if you had difficulty with this question.

Level of Cognitive Ability: Application

Client Needs: Physiological Integrity
Integrated Concept/Process: Nursing Process/Planning
Content Area: Pharmacology
Reference: Wilson, B., Shannon, M., & Stang, C. (2000). *Nurses' drug guide 2000.* Stamford, Conn.: Appleton & Lange, p. 1117.

10. 2

Rationale: Phenytoin enhances the rate of estrogen metabolism, which can decrease the effectiveness of some birth control pills. Options 1, 3, and 4 are inappropriate instructions.

Test-Taking Strategy: Use the process of elimination. Option 1 would cause anxiety in the client. A client should not be instructed to stop anticonvulsant medication, as indicated in option 3. Pregnancy does not need to be "avoided." Review medication interactions related to phenytoin if you had difficulty with this question.

Level of Cognitive Ability: Application
Client Needs: Health Promotion and Maintenance
Integrated Concept/Process: Teaching/Learning
Content Area: Pharmacology
Reference: Wilson, B., Shannon, M., & Stang, C. (2000). *Nurses' drug guide 2000.* Stamford, Conn.: Appleton & Lange, p. 1116.

11. 1

Rationale: Adverse effects of carbamazepine appear as blood dyscrasias, including aplastic anemia, agranulocytosis, thrombocytopenia, leukopenia, cardiovascular disturbances, thrombophlebitis, dysrhythmias, and dermatological effects.

Test-Taking Strategy: Use the process of elimination. If you are familiar with normal laboratory values, you will note that the only option that indicates an abnormal value is option 1. Review the signs of adverse reactions related to this medication if you had difficulty with this question.

Level of Cognitive Ability: Analysis
Client Needs: Physiological Integrity
Integrated Concept/Process: Nursing Process/Analysis
Content Area: Pharmacology
Reference: Hodgson, B., & Kizior, R. (2001). *Saunders nursing drug handbook 2001.* Philadelphia: W. B. Saunders, p. 145.

12. 4

Rationale: Morphine sulfate suppresses the cough reflex. Clients need to be encouraged to cough and deep breath to prevent pneumonia. Options 1, 2, and 3 are not specifically associated with the use of this medication.

Test-Taking Strategy: Use the process of elimination. The question specifically asks about a nursing action related to this medication. Recalling that morphine sulfate suppresses the cough reflex and the respiratory reflex will direct you to the correct option. Additionally, use the ABCs, airway, breathing, and circulation, when selecting the correct option. Review the nursing considerations when administering this medication if you had difficulty with this question.

Level of Cognitive Ability: Application
Client Needs: Physiological Integrity
Integrated Concept/Process: Nursing Process/Planning
Content Area: Pharmacology
Reference: Hodgson, B., & Kizior, R. (2001). *Saunders nursing drug handbook 2001.* Philadelphia: W. B. Saunders, p. 706.

13. 4

Rationale: Side effects of this medication include respiratory depression, orthostatic hypotension, tachycardia, drowsiness and mental clouding, constipation, and urinary retention.

Test-Taking Strategy: Use the process of elimination. It is necessary to know the side effects associated with specific narcotic analgesics to answer the question. Review the side effects of this medication if you had difficulty with this question.

Level of Cognitive Ability: Analysis
Client Needs: Physiological Integrity
Integrated Concept/Process: Nursing Process/Assessment
Content Area: Pharmacology
Reference: Clark, J., Queener, S., & Karb, V. (2000). *Pharmacologic basis of nursing practice* (6th ed.). St. Louis: Mosby, p. 385.

14. 3

Rationale: While the client is taking codeine sulfate, the nurse would monitor vital signs and assess for hypotension. The nurse should also increase fluid intake, palpate the bladder for urinary retention, auscultate bowel sounds, and monitor the pattern of daily bowel activity and stool consistency. The nurse should monitor respiratory status and initiate breathing and coughing exercises. Additionally, the nurse monitors the effectiveness of the pain medication.

Test-Taking Strategy: Use the process of elimination. Note the key word "specifically" and recall that codeine sulfate can cause constipation. If you had difficulty with this question, review nursing measures related to the administration of codeine sulfate.

Level of Cognitive Ability: Application
Client Needs: Physiological Integrity
Integrated Concept/Process: Nursing Process/Planning
Content Area: Pharmacology
Reference: Hodgson, B., & Kizior, R. (2001). *Saunders nursing drug handbook 2001.* Philadelphia: W. B. Saunders, p. 251.

15. 3

Rationale: Dantrolene can cause liver damage, and the nurse should monitor the liver function studies. Baseline liver function studies are done before therapy starts, and regular liver function studies are performed throughout therapy. Dantrolene is discontinued if no relief of spasticity is achieved in 6 weeks.

Test-Taking Strategy: Use the process of elimination. Knowledge that this medication is hepatotoxic will direct you to the correct option. If you had difficulty with this question, review the adverse effects of this medication.

Level of Cognitive Ability: Analysis
Client Needs: Physiological Integrity
Integrated Concept/Process: Nursing Process/Assessment
Content Area: Pharmacology
Reference: Clark, J., Queener, S., & Karb, V. (2000). *Pharmacologic basis of nursing practice* (6th ed.). St. Louis: Mosby, p. 751.

16. 2

Rationale: The therapeutic phenytoin level is 10 to 20 µg/mL. At greater than 20 µg/mL, involuntary movements of the eyeballs (nystagmus) appear. At greater than 30 µg/mL, ataxia and slurred speech arise.

Test-Taking Strategy: Use the process of elimination and knowledge about the therapeutic phenytoin level. From this point it is necessary to know the symptoms that would be noted in the client when the phenytoin level is 35 µg/mL. Review therapeutic levels and associated symptoms if you had difficulty with this question.

Level of Cognitive Ability: Analysis

Client Needs: Physiological Integrity

Integrated Concept/Process: Nursing Process/Assessment

Content Area: Pharmacology

Reference: Clark, J., Queener, S., & Karb, V. (2000). *Pharmacologic basis of nursing practice* (6th ed.). St. Louis: Mosby, p. 729.

17. 1

Rationale: Mannitol is an osmotic diuretic that induces diuresis by raising the osmotic pressure of glomerular filtrate, thereby inhibiting tubular reabsorption of water and solutes. It is used to reduce intracranial pressure in the client with head trauma.

Test-Taking Strategy: Use the process of elimination. Read the question carefully, noting that it identifies a client with increased intracranial pressure. The only option that suggests an action that will produce diuresis and thus reduce intracranial pressure is option 1. If you had difficulty with this question, review the action of mannitol.

Level of Cognitive Ability: Analysis

Client Needs: Physiological Integrity

Integrated Concept/Process: Nursing Process/Analysis

Content Area: Pharmacology

Reference: Wilson, B., Shannon, M., & Stang, C. (2000). *Nurses' drug guide 2000*. Stamford, Conn.: Appleton & Lange, p. 833.

18. 3

Rationale: Dexamethasone may be given by direct IV injection or IV infusion. It may be mixed with normal saline or 5% dextrose. If administered as an infusion, a minimum amount of diluting solution is needed.

Test-Taking Strategy: Use the process of elimination. Eliminate option 2 because 1000 mL of solution is a very large amount to use to dilute this medication, particularly in a client with cerebral edema. Eliminate options 1 and 4 because they are similar, addressing the use of lactated Ringer's solution. If you had difficulty with this question, review the administration of dexamethasone.

Level of Cognitive Ability: Application

Client Needs: Physiological Integrity

Integrated Concept/Process: Nursing Process/Planning

Content Area: Pharmacology

Reference: Hodgson, B., & Kizior, R. (2001). *Saunders nursing drug handbook 2001*. Philadelphia: W. B. Saunders, p. 296-297.

19. 3

Rationale: Mild intoxication with acetylsalicylic acid (aspirin) is called salicylism and is commonly experienced when the daily dosage is more than 4 grams. Tinnitus (ringing in the ears) is the most frequent effect noted with intoxication. Hyperventilation may occur because salicylate stimulates the respiratory center. Fever may result because salicylate inter-

feres with the metabolic pathways coupling oxygen consumption and heat production. Options 1, 2, and 4 are not specifically associated with toxicity.

Test-Taking Strategy: Use the process of elimination. Note that the question refers to aspirin intoxication. Options 1 and 2 relate to gastrointestinal symptoms, are similar, and are eliminated first. From the remaining options, it is necessary to know that tinnitus occurs. If you had difficulty with this question, review aspirin intoxication.

Level of Cognitive Ability: Analysis

Client Needs: Physiological Integrity

Integrated Concept/Process: Nursing Process/Assessment

Content Area: Pharmacology

Reference: Hodgson, B., & Kizior, R. (2001). *Saunders nursing drug handbook 2001*. Philadelphia: W. B. Saunders, p. 76.

20. 4

Rationale: Lack of coordination and drowsiness are common side effects resulting from this medication. Options 1, 2, and 3 are unrelated to the use of this medication.

Test-Taking Strategy: Use the process of elimination. Note that the question addresses a centrally acting skeletal muscle relaxant. This will assist in directing you to option 4. If you had difficulty with this question, review the side effects associated with Valium.

Level of Cognitive Ability: Analysis

Client Needs: Physiological Integrity

Integrated Concept/Process: Nursing Process/Assessment

Content Area: Pharmacology

Reference: Hodgson, B., & Kizior, R. (2001). *Saunders nursing drug handbook 2001*. Philadelphia: W. B. Saunders, p. 308.

CRITICAL THINKING: FREE: TEXT ENTRY

Answer: Atropine sulfate

Rationale: The antidote for cholinergic crisis is atropine sulfate.

Test-Taking Strategy: Recall that atropine sulfate is an anticholinergic agent. Since the client is at risk for cholinergic crisis, it would seem reasonable that the antidote would have to contain anticholinergic properties. If you are unfamiliar with cholinergic crisis and its antidote, review this information.

Level of Cognitive Ability: Application

Client Needs: Physiological Integrity

Integrated Concept/Process: Nursing Process/Planning

Content Area: Pharmacology

Reference: Deglin, J., & Vallerand, A. (2001). *Davis's drug guide for nurses* (7th ed.). Philadelphia: F.A. Davis, p. 82.

REFERENCES

Clark, J., Queener, S., & Karb, V. (2000). *Pharmacologic basis of nursing practice* (6th ed.). St. Louis: Mosby.

Cleveland, L., Aschenbrenner, D., Venable, S., & Yensen, J. (1999). *Nursing management in drug therapy*. Philadelphia: Lippincott.

Gutierrez, K. (1999). *Pharmacotherapeutics: Clinical decision-making in nursing*. Philadelphia: W.B. Saunders.

Hodgson, B., & Kizior, R. (2001). *Saunders nursing drug handbook 2001*. Philadelphia: W.B. Saunders.

Karch, A. (2000). *Focus on nursing pharmacology*. Philadelphia: Lippincott.

Salerno, E. (1999). *Pharmacology for health professionals*. St. Louis: Mosby.

Wilson, B., Shannon, M., & Stang, C. (2000). *Nurses' drug guide 2000*. Stamford, Conn.: Appleton & Lange.

The Adult Client with a Musculoskeletal Disorder

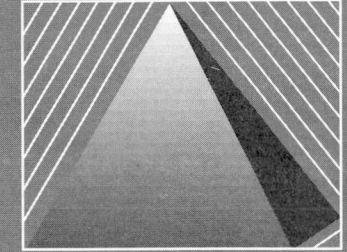

PYRAMID TERMS

casts   Made of plaster or fiberglass to provide immobilization of bone and joints after a fracture or injury.

compartment syndrome   Increased pressure within one or more compartments causing massive compromise of circulation to an area and causing irreversible neuromuscular damage within 4 to 6 hours of its onset if not treated.

external fixation   Stabilization of a fracture by the use of an external frame, with multiple pins applied through the bone.

fat embolism   An embolism that can occur 24 to 48 hours or within the first 72 hours following a fracture.

internal fixation   Stabilization of a fracture that involves the application of screws, plates, pins, or nails to hold the fragments in alignment.

reduction   The procedure that restores the bone to proper alignment.

traction   Force applied in two directions to reduce and immobilize a fracture.

‣ PYRAMID TO SUCCESS

The Pyramid to Success focuses on the emergency care for a client who sustains a fracture or other musculoskeletal injury, monitoring for complications related to fractures, and interventions if complications occur. Nursing care related to casts and traction is emphasized. Skill related to instructing the client in the use of an assistive device such as a cane, a walker, or crutches is a pyramid point. Pyramid points also include postoperative care following hip surgery or amputation, and care of the client with rheumatoid arthritis or osteoporosis. Focus on the points related to the psychosocial effects as a result of the musculoskeletal disorder, such as unexpected body image changes, and the appropriate and available support services needed for the client. The Integrated Concepts and Processes addressed in this unit include Nursing Process, Caring, Communication and Documentation, Cultural Awareness, Self-Care, and Teaching/Learning.

CLIENT NEEDS
Safe, Effective Care Environment

Asepsis related to wounds
Client rights
Confidentiality regarding disorder and plan of care
Dietary consultation
Handling hazardous and infectious materials
Informed consent for diagnostic treatments and surgical procedures
Physical therapy and occupational therapy referrals
Preventing injury from accidents
Standard (universal) precautions

Health Promotion and Maintenance

Aging process and disease prevention
Expected body image changes
Health promotion related to diet and activity
Home care instructions regarding care related to musculoskeletal disorder
Physical assessment related to the musculoskeletal system
Reinforcement regarding the importance of prescribed therapy

Psychosocial Integrity

Ability to cope with feelings of isolation and loss of independence
Available support systems and utilization of community resources
Cultural, religious, and spiritual influences
Grief and loss related to mobility limitations and restrictions
Mobilizing coping mechanisms
Sensory and perceptual alterations
Situational role changes as a result of musculoskeletal disorder
Unexpected body image changes as a result of injury or disease

Physiological Integrity

Care related to casts and traction
Complications of a fracture
Complications related to procedures or injuries
Emergency care for a fracture or other injury
Measures to promote comfort
Pharmacological therapy
Postoperative interventions
Promoting normal elimination patterns
Promoting self-care measures
Use of assistive devices for mobility such as canes, walkers, and crutches

REFERENCES

Craven, R., & Hirnle, C. (2000). *Fundamentals of nursing: Human health and function* (3rd ed.). Philadelphia: Lippincott.

Harkreader, H. (2000). *Fundamentals of nursing: Caring and clinical judgment.* Philadelphia: W.B. Saunders.

Ignatavicius, D., Workman, M., & Mishler, M. (1999). *Medical-surgical nursing across the health care continuum* (3rd ed.). Philadelphia: W.B. Saunders.

LeMone, P., & Burke, K. (2000). *Medical-surgical nursing: Critical thinking in client care* (2nd ed.). Upper Saddle River, N.J.: Prentice-Hall.

Lewis, S., Heitkemper, M., & Dirksen, S. (2000). *Medical-surgical nursing: Assessment and management of clinical problems* (5th ed.). St. Louis: Mosby.

National Council of State Boards of Nursing (eds.) (2000). *Test Plan for the National Council Licensure Examination for Registered Nurses.* Chicago: Author.

Potter, P., & Perry, A. (2001). *Fundamentals of nursing* (5th ed.). St. Louis: Mosby.

Smeltzer, S., & Bare, B. (2000). *Textbook of medical-surgica nursing* (9th ed). Philadelphia: Lippincott Williams & Wilkins.

Musculoskeletal System

I. ANATOMY AND PHYSIOLOGY

A. Skeleton
  1. Axial portion
     a. Cranium
     b. Vertebrae
     c. Ribs
  2. Appendicular portion
     a. Limbs
     b. Shoulders
     c. Hips
B. Types of bones (Box 65-1)
  1. Spongy bone
     a. Located in the ends of long bones and the center of flat and irregular bones
     b. Can withstand forces applied in many directions
  2. Dense (compact) bone
     a. Covers spongy bone
     b. Cylinder around a central marrow cavity
     c. Can withstand force predominantly in one direction
  3. Characteristics of the bones
     a. Support and protect structures of the body
     b. Provide attachments for muscles, tendons, and ligaments
     c. Contain tissue in the central cavities, which aids in the formation of blood cells
     d. Assists in regulating calcium and phosphate concentrations
  4. Bone growth
     a. The length of bone growth is a result of the ossification of the epiphyseal cartilage at the ends of bones, and bone growth stops between the ages of 18 and 25 years
     b. The width of bone growth is a result of the activity of osteoblasts and occurs throughout life but does slow down with the aging process

BOX 65-1
Types of Bones
Long
Short
Flat
Irregular

     c. Bone absorption around the bone marrow continues throughout life; therefore, bones become weaker with aging
C. Types of joints (Table 65-1)
  1. Characteristics of the joints
     a. Allow the movement between bones
     b. Formed where two bones join
     c. Surfaces are covered with cartilage
     d. Enclosed in a capsule
     e. Contain a cavity filled with synovial fluid
     f. Ligaments hold the bone and joint in the correct position
     g. Articulation is the meeting point of two or more joints
  2. Synovial fluid
     a. Found in the joint capsule
     b. Formed by synovial membrane, which lines the joint capsule
     c. Lubricates the cartilage
     d. Cushion for shocks
D. Muscles
  1. Characteristics of muscles
     a. Made up of bundles of muscle fibers
     b. Provide the force to move bones
     c. Assist in maintaining posture
     d. Assist with heat production
  2. The process of contraction and relaxation
     a. Muscle contraction and relaxation require large amounts of adenosine triphosphate (ATP)

TABLE 65-1

Types of Joints

Type	Description
Synarthrosis	Fibrous or fixed joints
	No movement associated with these joints
Amphiarthrosis	Cartilaginous joints
	Slightly movable joints
Diarthrosis	Synovial joints
	Ball-and-socket joints
Condyloid	Freely movable joints
	Allow frictionless, painless movement

BOX 65-2

Risk Factors Associated with Musculoskeletal Disorders

Autoimmune disorders
Calcium deficiency
Degenerative conditions
Falls
Hyperuricemia
Infection
Medications
Metabolic disorders
Neoplastic disorders
Obesity
Postmenopausal states
Trauma and injury

b. Contraction also requires calcium, which functions as a catalyst
c. Acetylcholine released by the motor end plate of the motor neuron initiates an action potential
d. Acetylcholine is then destroyed by acetylcholinesterase
e. Calcium is required to contract muscle fibers and acts as a catalyst for the enzyme needed for the sliding together action of actin and myosin
f. Following contraction, ATP transports calcium out, in order to allow actin and myosin to slide apart and allow the muscle to relax

3. Skeletal muscles
a. Are attached to two bones and cross at least one joint
b. The point of origin is the point of attachment on the bone closest to the trunk
c. The point of insertion is the point of attachment on the bone farthest from the trunk
d. Skeletal muscles act in groups
e. Prime movers contract to produce movement
f. Antagonists relax
g. Synergists contract to stabilize
h. Nerves activate and control the muscles

II. RISK FACTORS ASSOCIATED WITH MUSCULOSKELETAL DISORDERS (Box 65-2)

III. DIAGNOSTIC TESTS
A. X-rays
1. Description: a commonly used procedure to diagnose disorders of the musculoskeletal system
2. Implementation
a. Handle injured area carefully
b. Administer analgesics as prescribed prior to the procedure, particularly if the client is in pain
c. Remove any radiopaque objects, such as jewelry

d. Shield client's testes, ovaries, or pregnant abdomen
e. The client must lie still during an x-ray
f. Inform the client that exposure to radiation is minimal and not dangerous
g. Health care provider is to wear a lead apron if staying in the room with the client

B. Arthrocentesis
1. Description
a. Involves aspirating synovial fluid, blood, or pus via a needle inserted into a joint cavity
b. Medication may be instilled into the joint if necessary to alleviate inflammation
2. Implementation
a. Obtain a consent form
b. Apply a compress bandage postprocedure as prescribed
c. Instruct the client to rest the joint for 8 to 24 hours postprocedure
d. Instruct the client to notify the physician if a fever or swelling of the joint occurs

C. Arthrogram
1. Description
a. A radiographic examination of the soft tissues of the joint structures: used to diagnose trauma to the joint capsule or ligaments
b. A local anesthetic is used for the procedure
c. A contrast medium or air is injected into the joint cavity, and the joint is moved through range of motion as a series of x-rays are taken
2. Implementation
a. Instruct the client to fast from food and fluids for 8 hours prior to the procedure
b. Assess the client for allergies to iodine or seafood prior to the procedure
c. Obtain a consent form
d. Inform the client of the need to remain as still as possible, except when asked to reposition

c. Minimize the use of the joint for 12 hours after the procedure

f. Instruct the client that the joint may be edematous and tender for 1 to 2 days after the procedure and may be treated with ice packs and analgesics as prescribed

g. Instruct the client that if edema and tenderness last longer than 2 days, to notify the physician

h. If knee arthrography was performed, an Ace wrap over the knee may be prescribed for 3 to 4 days

i. If air was used for injection, crepitus may be felt in the joint for up to 2 days

D. Arthroscopy

1. Description

a. Provides an endoscopic examination of various joints

b. Articular cartilage abnormalities can be assessed, loose bodies can be removed, and the cartilage can be trimmed

c. A biopsy may be performed during the procedure

2. Implementation

a. Instruct the client to fast for 8 to 12 hours prior to the procedure

b. Obtain a consent form

c. Administer pain medication as prescribed postprocedure

d. An elastic wrap should be worn for 2 to 4 days as prescribed postprocedure

e. Instruct the client that walking without weight bearing is usually permitted after sensation returns but to limit activity for 1 to 4 days as prescribed following the procedure

f. Instruct the client to elevate the extremity as often as possible for 2 days following the procedure, and to place ice on the site to minimize swelling

g. Reinforce instructions regarding the use of crutches, which may be used for 5 to 7 days postprocedure when walking

h. Advise the client to notify the physician if fever or increased knee pain occurs or if edema continues for more than 3 days postprocedure

E. Bone scan

1. Description

a. Radioisotope is injected IV and will collect in areas that indicate abnormal bone metabolism and some fractures, if they exist

b. The isotope is excreted in the urine and feces within 48 hours and is not harmful to others

2. Implementation

a. Hold fluids for 4 hours prior to the procedure

b. Obtain a consent form

c. Remove all jewelry and metal objects

d. Following the injection of the radioisotope, the client must drink 32 ounces of water (if not contraindicated) to promote renal filtering of the excess isotope

e. From 1 to 3 hours after the injection, have the client void, and then the scanning procedure is performed

f. Inform the client of the need to lie supine during the procedure and that the procedure is not painful

g. No special precautions are required after the procedure because a minimal amount of radioactivity exists in the radioisotope

h. Monitor the injection site for redness and swelling

i. Encourage oral fluid intake following the procedure

F. Bone or muscle biopsy

1. Description: may be done during surgery or through aspiration, or punch or needle biopsy

2. Implementation

a. Obtain a consent form

b. Monitor for bleeding, swelling, hematoma, or severe pain

c. Elevate the site for 24 hours following the procedure to reduce edema

d. Apply ice packs as prescribed following the procedure to prevent the development of a hematoma

e. Monitor for signs of infection following the procedure

f. Inform the client that mild to moderate discomfort is normal following the procedure

G. Electromyography (EMG)

1. Description

a. Measures electrical potential associated with skeletal muscle contractions

b. Needles are inserted into the muscle, and recordings of muscular electrical activity are traced on recording paper through an oscilloscope

2. Implementation

a. Obtain a consent form

b. Instruct the client that the needle insertion is uncomfortable

c. Instruct the client not to take any stimulants or sedatives for 24 hours prior to the procedure

d. Inform the client that slight bruising may occur at the needle insertion sites

H. Myelogram

1. Description: injection of dye or air into the subarachnoid space to detect abnormalities of the spinal cord and vertebrae

2. Implementation preprocedure

a. Obtain a consent form

b. Provide hydration for at least 12 hours before the test

c. Assess for allergies to iodine
d. Premedicate for sedation as prescribed
3. Implementation postprocedure
a. Perform vital signs and neurological assessment frequently as prescribed
b. If a water-base dye is used, elevate the head 15 to 30 degrees for 8 hours as prescribed
c. If an oil-base dye is used, keep the client flat 6 to 8 hours as prescribed
d. If air is used, keep the head lower than the trunk
e. Force fluids and monitor I & O

IV. INJURIES
A. Strains
1. An excessive stretching of a muscle or tendon
2. Management involves cold and heat applications, exercise with activity limitations, antiinflammatory medications, and muscle relaxants
3. Surgical repair may be required for a severe strain (ruptured muscle or tendon)
B. Sprains
1. An excessive stretching of a ligament; usually caused by a twisting motion
2. Characterized by pain and swelling
3. Management involves rest, ice, and a compression bandage to reduce swelling and provide joint support
4. Casting may be required for moderate sprains to allow the tear to heal
5. Surgery may be necessary for severe ligament damage
C. Rotator cuff injuries
1. Musculotendinous or rotator cuff of the shoulder sustains a tear, usually as a result of trauma
2. Characterized by shoulder pain and the inability to maintain abduction of the arm at the shoulder (drop arm test)
3. Management involves nonsteroidal antiinflammatory drugs (NSAIDs), physical therapy, sling support, and ice/heat applications
4. Surgery may be required if medical management is unsuccessful or for those who have a complete tear

V. FRACTURES
A. Description: A break in the continuity of the bone caused by trauma, twisting as a result of muscle spasm or indirect loss of leverage, or bone decalcification and disease that result in osteopenia
B. Types of fractures (Box 65-3)
C. Assessment of a fracture of an extremity
1. Pain or tenderness over the involved area
2. Loss of function
3. Obvious deformity
4. Crepitation

BOX 65-3

Types of Fractures

Closed or simple: skin over the fractured area remains intact
Greenstick: one side of the bone is broken and the other is bent; most commonly seen in children
Transverse: the bone is fractured straight across
Oblique: the break extends in an oblique direction
Spiral: the break partially encircles bone
Comminuted: the bone is splintered or crushed, with three or more fragments
Complete: the bone is completely separated by a break into two parts
Incomplete: a partial break in the bone
Open or compound: the bone is exposed to air through a break in the skin, and soft tissue injury and infection are common
Impacted: a part of the fractured bone is driven into another bone
Depressed: bone fragments are driven inward
Compression: a fractured bone compressed by other bone
Pathological: a fracture that results from weakening of the bone structure by pathological processes, such as neoplasia or osteomalacia; also called spontaneous fracture

---

BOX 65-4

Interventions for a Fracture

Reduction
Fixation
Traction
Casts

---

5. Erythema, edema, ecchymosis
6. Muscle spasm and impaired sensation
D. Initial care of a fracture of an extremity
1. Immobilize affected extremity
2. If a compound fracture exists, splint the extremity and cover the wound with a sterile dressing
E. Interventions for a fracture (Box 65-4)
F. **Reduction:** Restoring the bone to proper alignment
1. Closed **reduction**
a. Performed by manual manipulation
b. May be performed under local or general anesthesia
c. A **cast** may be applied following **reduction**
2. Open **reduction**
a. Involves a surgical intervention
b. May be treated with **internal fixation** devices
c. The client may be placed in **traction** or a **cast** following the procedure

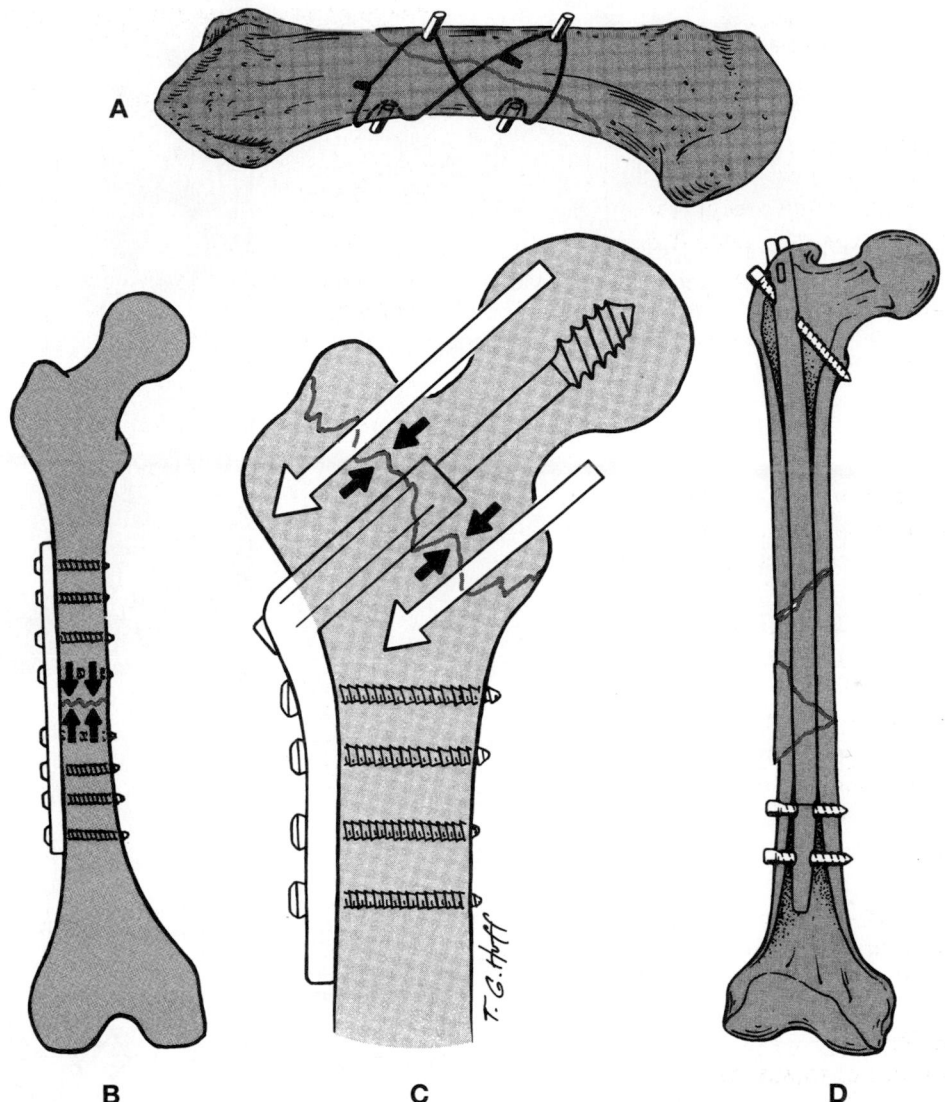

FIG. 65-1 Examples of internal fixation. **A,** Tension band wiring technique using Kirschner wires for fracture of a phalanx. **B,** Compression plate to the lateral aspect of the femur. **C,** Sliding hip screw. **D,** Static locked intramedullary and fixed to both proximal and distal fragments of the femur. (From Browner BD et al: *Skeletal trauma,* Philadelphia, 1992, WB Saunders.)

G. **Fixation**
1. **Internal fixation** (Fig. 65-1)
   a. Follows open **reduction**
   b. Involves the application of screws, plates, pins, or nails to hold the fragments in alignment
   c. May involve the removal of damaged bone and replacement with a prosthesis
   d. Provides immediate bone strength
   e. Risk of infection is associated with the procedure
2. **External fixation** (Fig. 65-2)
   a. An external frame is utilized with multiple pins applied through the bone
   b. Provides more freedom of movement than with **traction**

H. **Traction** (Fig. 65-3)
1. Description
   a. The exertion of a pulling force applied in two directions to reduce and immobilize a fracture
   b. Provides proper bone alignment and reduces muscle spasms
2. Implementation
   a. Maintain proper body alignment
   b. Ensure that the weights hang freely and do not touch the floor
   c. Do not remove or lift the weights without a physician's order

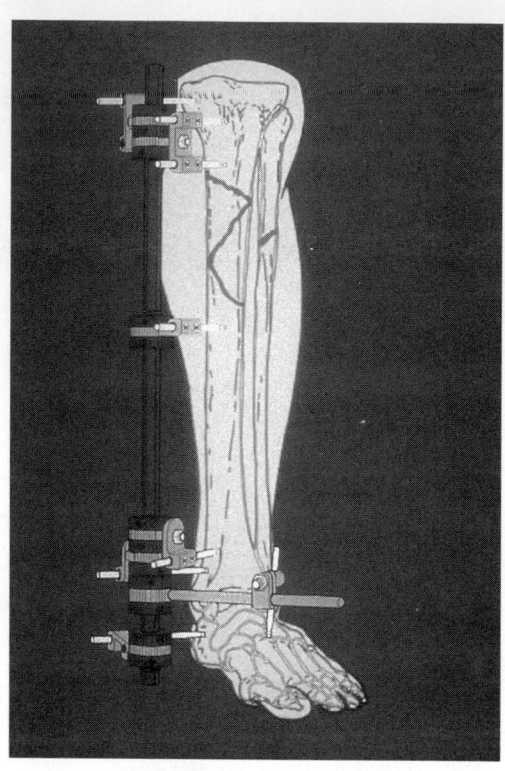

FIG. 65-2 The Hex-Fix external fixation system for tibial fractures. (Courtesy Smith & Nephew, Inc, Orthopaedic Division, Memphis, Tenn. From Ignatavicius D, Workman M, Mishler M: *Medical-surgical nursing across the health care continuum,* ed 3, Philadelphia, 1999, WB Saunders.)

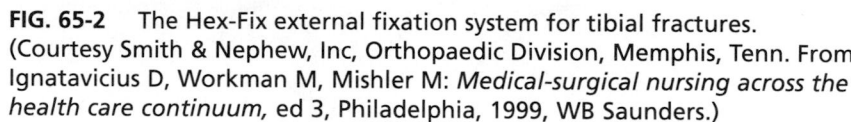

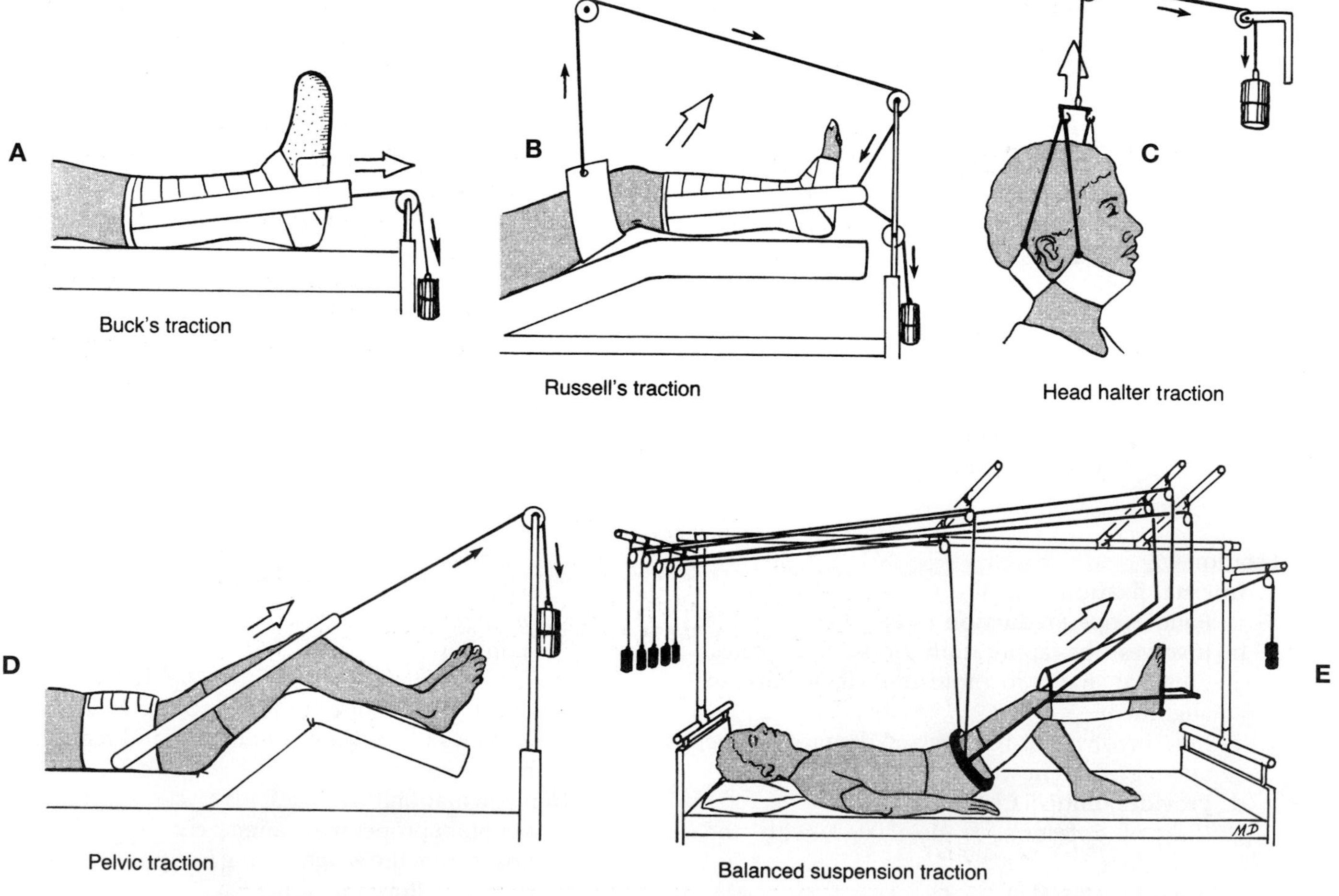

A Buck's traction

B Russell's traction

C Head halter traction

D Pelvic traction

E Balanced suspension traction

FIG. 65-3 Examples of common types of traction. **A,** Buck's traction. **B,** Russell's traction. **C,** Head halter traction. **D,** Pelvic traction. **E,** Balanced suspension traction. (From deWit S: *Essentials of medical-surgical nursing,* ed 4, Philadelphia, 1998, WB Saunders.)

d. Ensure that pulleys are not obstructed and that ropes in the pulleys move freely

e. Place knots in the ropes to prevent slipping

f. Check the ropes for fraying

I. Skeletal **traction** (Fig. 65-4)

　1. Description: mechanically applied to the bone with pins, wires, or tongs

　2. Implementation

　　a. Monitor color, motion, and sensation (CMS) of the affected extremity

　　b. Monitor the insertion sites for redness, swelling, or drainage

　　c. Provide insertion site care as prescribed

　3. Cervical tongs and a halo fixation device (refer to Chapter 63 regarding care of the client with these types of devices)

J. Skin **traction** (Box 65-5)

　1. Description: **traction** applied by the use of elastic bandages or adhesive

　2. Cervical skin **traction** (Fig. 65-3)

　　a. Relieves muscle spasms and compression in the upper extremities and neck

　　b. Uses a head halter and a chin pad to attach the **traction**

　　c. Use powder to protect the ears from friction rub

d. Position the client with the head of the bed elevated 30 to 40 degrees, and attach the weights to a pulley system over the head of the bed

3. Buck's skin **traction** (Fig. 65-3)

　a. Used to alleviate muscle spasms; immobilizes a lower limb by maintaining a straight pull on the limb with the use of weights

　b. A boot appliance is applied to attach to the **traction**

　c. Weight is attached to a pulley; allow the weights to hang freely over the edge of bed

　d. Not more than 8 to 10 pounds of weight should be applied

　e. Elevate the foot of the bed to provide the **traction**

4. Bryant's and Russell's skin **traction** (refer to Chapter 41 regarding information related to these types of **traction**)

5. Pelvic skin **traction** (Fig. 65-3)

　a. Used to relieve low back, hip, or leg pain and to reduce muscle spasm

　b. Apply the **traction** snugly over the pelvis and iliac crest and attach to the weights

　c. Use measures as prescribed to prevent the client from slipping down in bed

K. Balanced suspension (Fig. 65-3)

　1. Description

　　a. Used with skin or skeletal **traction**

　　b. Used to approximate fractures of the femur, tibia, or fibula

　　c. Produced by a counterforce other than client

　2. Implementation

　　a. Position the client in low Fowler's, on either the side or the back

　　b. Maintain a 20-degree angle from the thigh to the bed

BOX 65-5

Types: Skin Traction

Cervical traction
Buck's traction
Bryant's traction
Pelvic traction
Russell's traction

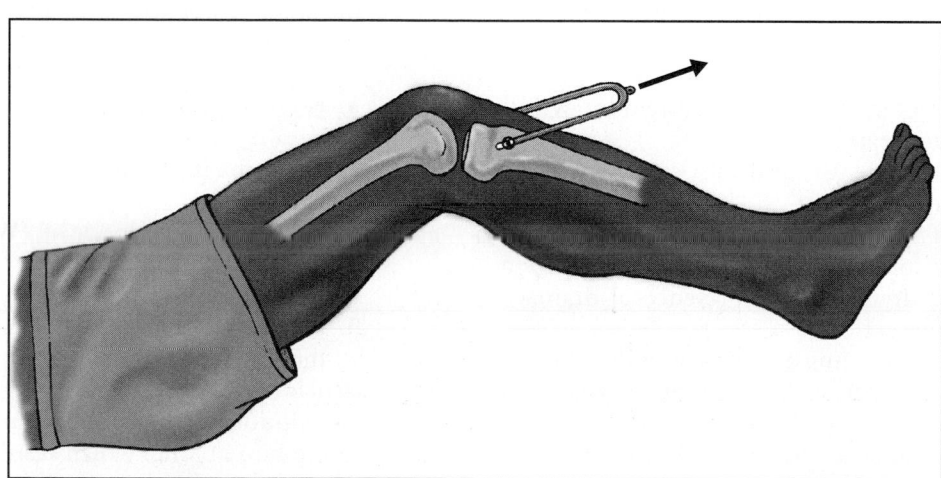

FIG. 65-4　Skeletal traction (Steinmann pin). (From Monahan FD, Neighbors M: *Medical-surgical nursing: foundations for clinical practice*, ed 2, Philadelphia, 1998, WB Saunders.)

c. Protect the skin from breakdown

d. Provide pin care if pins are used with the skeletal **traction**

e. Clean the pin sites with sterile normal saline and hydrogen peroxide or Betadine as prescribed or per agency procedure

L. Dunlop's **traction**

1. Description: horizontal **traction** to align fractures of the humerus; vertical **traction** maintains the forearm in proper alignment

2. Implementation: nursing care is similar to that for Buck's **traction**

M. **Casts**

1. Description: made of plaster or fiberglass to provide immobilization of bone and joints after a fracture or injury

2. Implementation

a. Keep the **cast** and extremity elevated

b. Allow a wet **cast** 24 to 48 hours to dry (synthetic **casts** dry in 20 minutes)

c. Handle a wet **cast** with the palms of the hand until dry

d. Turn the extremity unless contraindicated, so that all sides of the wet **cast** will dry

e. Heat can be used to dry the **cast**

f. The **cast** will change from a dull to a shiny substance when dry

g. Examine the skin and **cast** for pressure areas

h. Monitor the extremity for circulatory impairment such as pain, swelling, discoloration, tingling, numbness, coolness, or diminished pulse

i. Notify the physician immediately if circulatory compromise occurs

j. Prepare for bivalving or cutting the **cast** if circulatory impairment occurs

k. Petal the **cast;** maintain smooth edges around the **cast** to prevent crumbling of the **cast** material

l. Monitor the client's temperature

m. Monitor for the presence of a foul odor, which may indicate infection

n. Monitor drainage and circle the area of drainage on the **cast**

o. Monitor for warmth on the **cast**

p. Monitor for wet spots, which may indicate a need for drying, or the presence of drainage under the **cast**

q. If an open draining area exists on the affected extremity, a cut-out portion of the **cast** or a window will be made by the physician

r. Instruct the client not to stick objects inside the **cast**

s. Teach the client to keep the **cast** clean and dry

t. Instruct the client in isometric exercises to prevent muscle atrophy

VI. **COMPLICATIONS OF FRACTURES** (Box 65-6)

A. **Fat embolism**

1. Description

a. An embolism originating in the bone marrow that occurs after a fracture

b. Clients with long bone fractures are at the greatest risk for the development of **fat embolism**

c. Usually occurs within 48 hours following the injury

2. Assessment

a. Restlessness

b. Mental status changes

c. Tachycardia, tachypnea, and hypotension

d. Dyspnea

e. Petechial rash over the upper chest and neck

3. Implementation

a. Notify the physician immediately

b. Treat symptoms as prescribed to prevent respiratory failure and death

B. **Compartment syndrome**

1. Description

a. Increased pressure within one or more compartments causing massive compromise of circulation to an area

b. Leads to decreased perfusion and tissue anoxia

c. Within 4 to 6 hours after the onset of **compartment syndrome,** neuromuscular damage is irreversible

2. Assessment

a. Increased pain and swelling

b. Pain with passive motion

c. Inability to move joints

d. Loss of sensation (paresthesia)

e. Pulselessness

3. Implementation: Notify the physician immediately

C. Infection and osteomyelitis

1. Description: Can be caused by the interruption of the integrity of the skin; the infection invades bone tissue

2. Assessment

a. Fever

b. Pain

c. Erythema in the area surrounding the fracture

d. Tachycardia

e. Elevated white blood cell (WBC) count

3. Implementation

a. Notify the physician

b. Prepare to initiate aggressive IV antibiotic therapy

D. Avascular necrosis

1. Description: An interruption in the blood supply to the bony tissue, which results in the death of the bone

2. Assessment

a. Pain

b. Decreased sensation

3. Implementation
   a. Notify the physician if pain or decreased sensation occurs
   b. Prepare the client for removal of necrotic tissue because it serves as a focus for infection

E. Pulmonary embolism
   1. Description: Caused by immobility precipitated by a fracture
   2. Assessment
      a. Restlessness and apprehension
      b. Dyspnea
      c. Diaphoresis
      d. Arterial blood gas changes
   3. Implementation
      a. Notify the physician if signs of emboli are present
      b. Prepare to administer anticoagulant therapy

BOX 65-6

Complications of Fractures

Compartment syndrome
Fat emboli
Infection and osteomyelitis
Avascular necrosis
Pulmonary emboli

VII. CRUTCH WALKING
A. Description
   1. An accurate measurement of the client for crutches is important because an incorrect measurement could damage the brachial plexus
   2. The distance between the axillae and the arm pieces on the crutches should be two fingerwidths in the axilla space
   3. The elbows should be slightly flexed, 20 to 30 degrees, when the client is walking
   4. When ambulating with the client, stand on the affected side
   5. Instruct the client never to rest the axilla on the axillary bars
   6. Instruct the client to look up and outward when ambulating
   7. Instruct the client to stop ambulation if numbness or tingling in the hands or arms occurs

B. Crutch gaits (Fig. 65-5)
C. Assisting the client with crutches to sit and stand
   1. Place the unaffected leg against the front of the chair
   2. Move the crutches to the affected side, and grasp the chair's arm with the hand on the unaffected side
   3. Flex the knee of the unaffected leg to lower self

Gait	Description	Pattern
Four-point gait	Sequence 1. Advance left crutch. 2. Advance right foot. 3. Advance right crutch. 4. Advance left foot. Advantages: most stable crutch gait. Requirements: partial weight bearing on both legs.	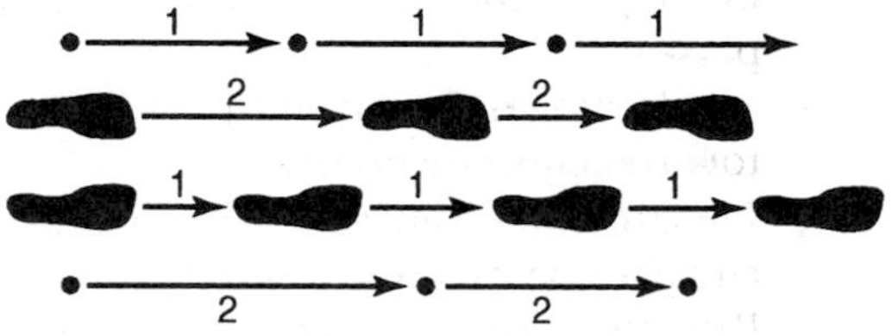
Three-point gait	Sequence 1. Advance both crutches forward with the affected leg and shift weight to crutches. 2. Advance unaffected leg and shift weight onto it. Advantages: allows the affected leg to be partially or completely free of weight bearing. Requirements: full weight bearing on one leg, balance, and upper-body strength.	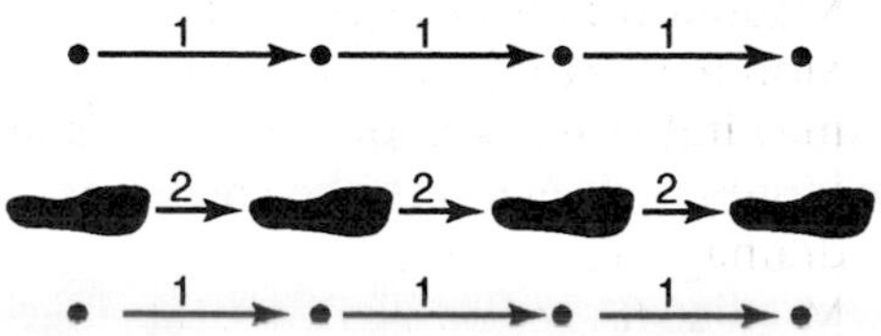
Two-point gait	Sequence 1. Advance left crutch and right foot. 2. Advance right crutch and left foot. Advantages: Faster version of the four-point gait, more normal walking pattern (arms and legs moving in opposition). Requirements: Partial weight bearing on both legs, balance.	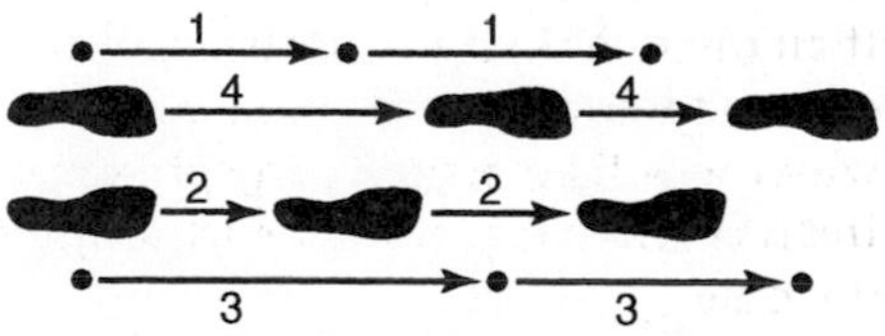

FIG. 65-5 Crutch gaits. (From deWit S: *Essentials of medical-surgical nursing*, ed 4, Philadelphia, 1998, WB Saunders.)

into the chair while placing the affected leg straight out in front

4. Reverse the steps to move from a sitting to a standing position

D. Going up and down stairs
   1. Up the stairs
      a. The client moves the unaffected leg up first
      b. The client moves the affected leg and the crutches up
   2. Down the stairs
      a. The client moves the crutches and the affected leg down
      b. The client moves the unaffected leg down

VIII. CANES AND WALKERS

A. Description: Made of a lightweight material with a rubber tip at the bottom

B. Implementation
   1. Stand at the affected side of the client when ambulating
   2. The handle should be at the level of the client's greater trochanter
   3. The client's elbow should be flexed at a 25- to 30-degree angle
   4. Instruct the client to hold the cane close to the body
   5. Instruct the client to hold the cane in the hand on the unaffected side so that the cane and weaker leg can work together with each step
   6. Instruct the client to move the cane at the same time as the affected leg
   7. Instruct the client to inspect the rubber tips regularly for worn places

C. Hemicanes or quadripod canes
   1. Used for clients who have the use of only one upper extremity
   2. Hemicanes provide more security than a quadripod cane; however, both types provide more security than a single-tipped cane
   3. Position the cane at the client's unaffected side, with the straight nonangled side adjacent to the body
   4. Position the cane 6 inches from client's side, with the hand grips level with the greater trochanter

D. Walker
   1. Stand adjacent to the client on the affected side
   2. Instruct the client to put all four points of the walker flat on the floor before putting weight on the hand pieces
   3. Instruct the client to move the walker forward and to walk into it

IX. FRACTURED HIP

A. Types
   1. Intracapsular
      a. Bone is broken inside the joint

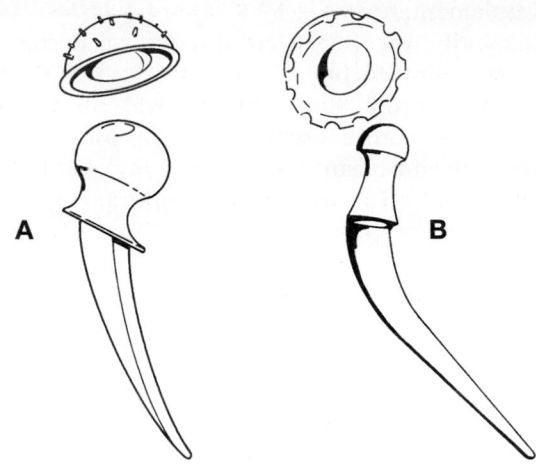

FIG. 65-6   Hip prostheses. **A,** The McKee-Farrar procedure involves replacement of the femoral head and acetabulum with a metal prosthesis. **B,** The Charnley prosthesis involves total prosthetic replacement of the hip joint. (From deWit S: *Essentials of medical-surgical nursing,* ed 4, Philadelphia, 1998, WB Saunders.)

   b. Skin **traction** is applied preoperatively to immobilize and prevent pain
   c. Treatment includes a total hip replacement or **internal fixation** with replacement of the femoral head with a prosthesis (Fig. 65-6)
   d. Avoid hip flexion to prevent displacement ▲
   2. Extracapsular
      a. Fracture can occur at the greater trochanter or can be an intertrochanteric fracture
      b. Trochanteric fracture is outside the joint
      c. Preoperative treatment includes balanced suspension **traction**
      d. Avoid hip flexion to prevent displacement ▲
      e. Surgical treatment includes **internal fixation** with nail plate, screws, or wires

B. Implementation postoperatively ▲
   1. Maintain leg and hip in proper alignment
   2. Prevent flexion or external or internal rotation
   3. Turn the client from back to unaffected side
   4. Do not position to the affected side unless prescribed by the physician
   5. Maintain leg abduction to prevent internal or external rotation
   6. Use a trochanter roll to prevent external rotation
   7. Ensure that the hip flexion angle does not exceed 60 to 80 degrees
   8. Elevate the head of the bed 30 to 45 degrees for meals only
   9. Ambulate as prescribed by the physician
   10. Avoid weight bearing on the affected leg as prescribed; instruct the client in the use of a walker to avoid weight bearing
   11. Keep the operative leg extended, supported, and elevated when getting client out of bed

12. Avoid hip flexion greater than 90 degrees and avoid low chairs when out of bed
13. Monitor the wound for infection or hemorrhage
14. Monitor circulation and sensation of the affected side
15. Maintain the Hemovac or Jackson-Pratt drain if in place; maintain compression to facilitate drainage and monitor and record output of drainage
16. Drainage should continuously decrease in amount, and by 48 hours postoperatively, drainage should be approximately 30 mL in an 8-hour period
17. Maintain the use of antiembolism stockings, and encourage the client to flex and extend the feet and ankles
18. Instruct the client to avoid crossing the legs and bending-over activities
19. Physical therapy will begin postoperatively as prescribed by the physician

X. TOTAL KNEE REPLACEMENT
A. Description: Implantation of a device to substitute for the femoral condyles and the tibial joint surfaces
B. Implementation postoperatively
1. Monitor the incision for drainage and infection
2. Maintain the Hemovac or Jackson-Pratt drain if in place
3. Begin continuous passive motion (CPM) 24 to 48 hours postoperatively as prescribed to exercise the knee and provide moderate flexion and extension
4. Administer analgesics before CPM to decrease pain
5. The leg should not be dangled, to prevent dislocation
6. Prepare the client for out-of-bed activities as prescribed
7. Avoid weight bearing and instruct the client in crutch walking

XI. HERNIATION: INTERVERTEBRAL DISK
A. Description: Nucleus of the disk protrudes into the annulus, causing nerve compression
B. Cervical disk
1. Occurs at C5 to C6 and C6 to C7 interspaces
2. Causes pain and stiffness in the neck, top of the shoulders, scapula, upper extremities, and head
3. Produces paresthesia and numbness of the upper extremities
4. Implementation
   a. Provide bed rest to relieve pressure and reduce inflammation and edema
   b. Provide immobilization as prescribed via cervical collar, **traction,** or brace

   c. Apply hot, moist compresses as prescribed to increase the blood flow and relax spasms
   d. Instruct the client to avoid flexing, extending, or rotating the neck
   e. Instruct the client that while sleeping, to avoid the prone position and keep the head, spine, and hip in alignment
   f. Instruct the client to avoid long periods of sitting
   g. Instruct the client in the use of analgesics, sedatives, antiinflammatory agents, and corticosteroids as prescribed
   h. Prepare the client for a corticosteroid injection into the epidural space if prescribed
   i. Assist the client with the application of a cervical collar or cervical **traction** as prescribed
5. Cervical collar
   a. Used for cervical disk herniation
   b. Holds the head in a neutral or slightly flexed position
   c. The client may have to wear a cervical collar 24 hours a day
   d. Inspect the skin under the collar for irritation
   e. When the pain subsides, the client is taught cervical isometric exercises to strengthen the muscles
C. Lumbar disk
1. Most often occurs at L4 to L5 or L5 to S1 interspaces
2. Postural deformity occurs
3. Produces muscle weakness, sensory loss, and alteration of the tendon reflexes
4. The client experiences low back pain and muscle spasms with radiation of the pain into one hip and down the leg (sciatica)
5. Pain is aggravated by bending, lifting, straining, sneezing, and coughing, and is relieved by bed rest
6. Implementation
   a. Provide bed rest as prescribed
   b. Apply moist heat and massage as prescribed
   c. Instruct the client to sleep on the side, with the knees and hips in a position of flexion and with a pillow between the legs
   d. Apply pelvic **traction** as prescribed to relieve muscle spasms
   e. Begin ambulation gradually as the inflammation and edema subside
   f. Instruct the client in the use of muscle relaxants, antiinflammatory medications, and corticosteroids as prescribed
   g. Instruct the client in the use of a corset or brace as prescribed
   h. Instruct the client regarding correct posture while sitting, standing, walking, and working

i. Instruct the client to lift objects by bending the knees and keeping the back straight, avoiding lifting anything above the elbows

j. Instruct the client regarding a weight-control program as prescribed

k. Instruct the client in an exercise program as prescribed to strengthen abdominal and back muscles

D. Disk surgery (Box 65-7)

1. Implementation preoperatively
   a. Reassure the client that surgery will not weaken the back
   b. Instruct the client regarding coughing and deep-breathing exercises
   c. Instruct the client about logrolling and range-of-motion exercises

2. Implementation postoperatively: cervical disk
   a. Monitor for respiratory difficulty
   b. Encourage coughing and deep breathing
   c. Monitor for hoarseness and inability to cough effectively because this may indicate laryngeal nerve damage
   d. Use throat sprays or lozenges for sore throat, and do not use those that may numb the throat, to avoid choking
   e. Monitor the wound for drainage
   f. Provide a soft diet if the client complains of dysphagia
   g. Monitor for sudden return of radicular pain, which may indicate that the cervical spine has become unstable

3. Implementation postoperatively: lumbar disk
   a. Monitor for wound hemorrhage
   b. Monitor sensation and motor ability of the lower extremities as well as color, temperature, and sensation of toes
   c. Monitor for urinary retention, paralytic ileus, and constipation
   d. Initiate measures to prevent constipation, such as a high-fiber diet, increased fluids, and stool softeners, as prescribed
   e. When turning and repositioning the client, place the bed in a flat position and a pillow between the legs; turn the client as a unit (logroll) without twisting the client's back

f. When positioning the client, a pillow is placed under the head with the knees slightly flexed

g. Avoid extreme knee flexion when the client is lying on the side

h. To assist the client out of bed, raise the head of the bed while the client lies on the side; the client's head and shoulders are supported by the first nurse, the client pushes self to a sitting position, and the second nurse eases the legs over the side of the bed

i. Instruct the client to avoid sitting because it places a strain on the surgical site

j. Administer narcotics and sedatives as prescribed to relieve pain and anxiety

k. Encourage early ambulation

l. Assist the client with the use of a back brace or corset if prescribed

XII. AMPUTATION OF A LOWER EXTREMITY (Fig. 65-7)

A. Description: The surgical removal of a lower limb or part of the limb

B. Implementation postoperatively
1. Monitor vital signs
2. Monitor for infection and hemorrhage
3. Mark bleeding and drainage on the dressing if it occurs
4. Keep a tourniquet at the bedside

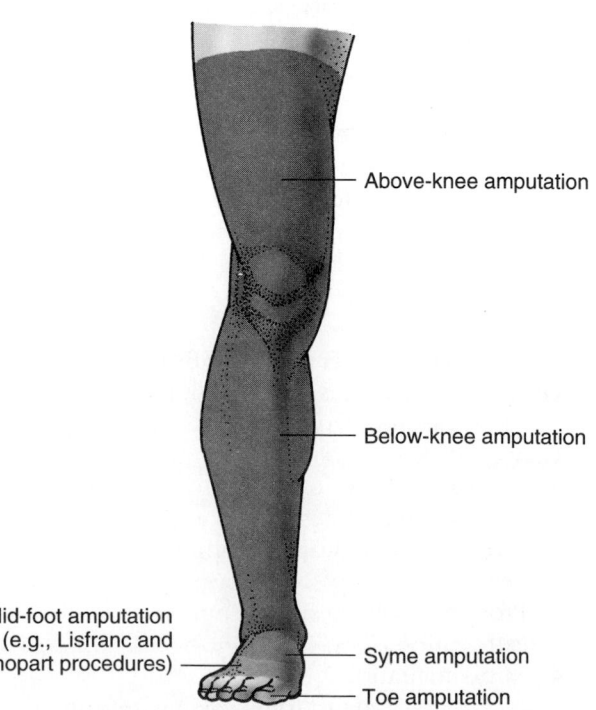

FIG. 65-7 Common levels of lower-extremity amputation. (From Ignatavicius D, Workman M, Mishler M: *Medical-surgical nursing across the health care continuum,* ed 3, Philadelphia, 1999, WB Saunders.)

BOX 65-7

Types of Disk Surgery

Chemolysis: injections to dissolve affected disk
Diskectomy: removal of herniated disk tissue and related matter
Diskectomy with fusion: fusion of vertebrae with bone graft
Laminotomy: division of the lamina of a vertebra
Laminectomy: removal of the lamina

5. Monitor for pulmonary emboli
6. Observe for and prevent contractures
7. Monitor for signs of necrosis and neuroma
8. Evaluate for phantom limb sensation and pain; explain sensation and pain to the client, and medicate the client as prescribed
9. Check the physician's orders regarding positioning
10. If prescribed, during the first 24 hours, elevate the foot of the bed to reduce edema; then keep the bed flat to prevent hip flexion contractures
11. Do not elevate the stump itself because elevation can cause flexion contracture of the hip joint
12. After 24 and 48 hours postoperatively, position the client prone if prescribed, to stretch the muscles and prevent flexion contractures of hip
13. In the prone position, place a pillow under the abdomen and stump and keep the legs close together to prevent abduction
14. Maintain application of an Ace wrap or elastic stump shrinker as prescribed, to provide stump shrinkage
15. Remove and rewrap the Ace bandage or elastic stump shrinker three or four times daily as prescribed
16. Wash the stump with mild soap and water and apply lanolin to the skin if prescribed
17. Massage the skin toward the suture line to increase circulation
18. Prepare for a **cast** application if prescribed, to prepare the stump for prosthesis
19. Encourage the client to look at the stump
20. Encourage verbalization regarding loss of the body part, and assist the client to identify coping mechanisms to deal with the loss

C. Implementation for below-the-knee amputation
1. Prevent edema
2. Do not allow the stump to hang over the edge of the bed
3. Do not allow the client to sit for long periods of time, to prevent contractures

D. Implementation for above-the-knee amputation
1. Prevent internal or external rotation of the limb
2. Place a sandbag or rolled towel along the outside of the thigh to prevent rotation

E. Rehabilitation
1. Instruct the client in crutch walking
2. Prepare the stump for prosthesis
3. Prepare the client for the fitting of the stump for prosthesis
4. Instruct the client in exercises to maintain range of motion
5. Provide psychosocial support to the client

XIII. RHEUMATOID ARTHRITIS (RA)
A. Description
1. Chronic systemic inflammatory disease; the etiol-

ogy may be related to a combination of environmental and genetic factors
2. Leads to destruction of connective tissue and synovial membrane within the joints
3. Weakens and leads to dislocation of the joint and permanent deformity
4. Formation of pannus occurs at the junction of synovial tissue and articular cartilage, projecting into the joint cavity and causing necrosis
5. Exacerbations are increased by physical or emotional stress
6. Risk factors include exposure to infectious agents; fatigue and stress can exacerbate the condition
7. Vasculitis can cause malfunction and eventual failure of an organ or system

B. Assessment
1. Inflammation, tenderness, and stiffness of the joints
2. Moderate to severe pain and morning stiffness lasting longer than 30 minutes
3. Joint deformities, muscle atrophy, and decreased range of motion
4. Spongy, soft feeling in the joints
5. Low-grade temperature, fatigue, and weakness
6. Anorexia, weight loss, and anemia
7. Elevated sedimentation rate and positive rheumatoid factor
8. X-ray showing joint deterioration
9. Synovial tissue biopsy presents inflammation

C. Rheumatoid (RA) factor
1. A blood test used to diagnose rheumatoid arthritis
2. Values
a. Nonreactive: 0 to 39 IU/mL
b. Weakly reactive: 40 to 79 IU/mL
c. Reactive: greater than 80 IU/mL

D. Pain
1. Salicylates (acetylsalicyic acid [aspirin])
a. Monitor for side effects, including tinnitus, gastrointestinal (GI) upset, and prolonged bleeding time
b. Administer with meals or a snack
c. Monitor for abnormal bleeding or bruising
2. Nonsteroidal antiinflammatory drugs (NSAIDs)
a. May be prescribed in combination with salicylates if pain and inflammation have not decreased within 6 to 12 weeks following salicylate therapy
b. Monitor for side effects such as GI upset, CNS manifestations, skin rash, hypertension, fluid retention, and changes in renal function
3. Corticosteroids: Administer as prescribed during exacerbations or when commonly used agents are ineffective
4. Antineoplastic medications: Administer as prescribed in clients with life-threatening RA
5. Gold salts: Administer as prescribed in combina-

tion with salicylates and NSAIDS to induce remission and decrease pain and inflammation

E. Physical mobility
   1. Preserve joint function
   2. Provide ROM exercises to maintain joint motion and muscle strengthening
   3. Balance rest and activity
   4. Splints during acute inflammation to prevent deformity
   5. Prevent flexion contractures
   6. Apply heat or cold therapy as prescribed to joints
   7. Apply paraffin baths and massage as prescribed
   8. Encourage consistency with exercise program
   9. Instruct the client to stop exercise if pain increases
   10. Exercise only to the point of pain
   11. Avoid weight bearing on inflamed joints

F. Self-care (Box 65-8)
   1. Assess the need for assistive devices such as higher toilet seats, chairs, and wheelchairs to facilitate mobility
   2. Collaborate with occupational therapy to obtain assistive or adaptive devices
   3. Instruct the client in alternative strategies for providing activities of daily living

G. Fatigue
   1. Identify factors that may contribute to fatigue
   2. Monitor for signs of anemia
   3. Administer iron, folic acid, and vitamin supplements as prescribed
   4. Monitor for drug-related blood loss by testing the stool for occult blood
   5. Instruct the client in measures to conserve energy, such as pacing activities and obtaining assistance when possible

H. Body image disturbance
   1. Assess the client's reaction to the body change
   2. Encourage the client to verbalize feelings

BOX 65-8

Client Education for RA and DJD

Assist the client to identify and correct hazards in the home
Instruct the client in the correct use of assistive or adaptive devices
Instruct in energy conservation measures
Review prescribed exercise program
Instruct the client to sit in a chair with a high, straight back
Instruct the client to use a small pillow, only when lying down
Instruct the client in measures to protect the joints
Instruct the client regarding the prescribed medications
Stress the importance of follow-up visits with the health care provider

---

   3. Assist the client with self-care activities and grooming
   4. Encourage the client to wear street clothes

I. Surgical implementation
   1. Synovectomy: Surgical removal of the synovia to help maintain joint function
   2. Arthrodesis: Bony fusion of a joint to regain some mobility
   3. Joint replacement (arthroplasty): Surgical replacement of diseased joints with artificial joints; performed to restore motion to a joint and function to the muscles, ligaments, and other soft tissue structures that control a joint

XIV. OSTEOARTHRITIS (DEGENERATIVE JOINT DISEASE, DJD)

A. Description
   1. Progressive degeneration of the joints as a result of wear and tear
   2. Causes the formation of bony buildup and the loss of articular cartilage in peripheral and axial joints
   3. Affects the weight-bearing joints and joints that receive the greatest stress, such as the knees, toes, and lower spine
   4. The cause is unknown but may be trauma, fractures, infections, or obesity

B. Assessment
   1. Joint pain that early in the disease process diminishes after rest and intensifies after activity
   2. As the disease progresses, pain occurs with slight motion or even at rest
   3. Symptoms are aggravated by temperature change and humidity
   4. Crepitus
   5. Joint enlargement
   6. Presence of Heberden's nodes or Bouchard's nodes
   7. Limited ROM
   8. Difficulty getting up after prolonged sitting
   9. Skeletal muscle atrophy
   10. Inability to perform activities of daily living
   11. Compression of the spine as manifested by radiating pain, stiffness, and muscle spasms in one or both extremities

C. Pain
   1. Administer NSAIDs, salicylates, and muscle relaxants as prescribed
   2. Prepare the client for corticosteroid injections into joints as prescribed
   3. Place affected joint in a functional position
   4. Immobilize the affected joint with a splint or brace
   5. Avoid large pillows under the head or knees
   6. Provide a bed or foot cradle
   7. Position the client prone twice a day
   8. Instruct the client in the importance of moist

heat, hot packs or compresses, and paraffin dips as prescribed

9. Apply cold applications as prescribed when the joint is acutely inflamed

10. Encourage adequate rest, recommending 10 hours of sleep at night and a 1- to- 2 hour nap in the afternoon

D. Nutrition
1. Encourage a well-balanced diet
2. Encourage weight loss if necessary

E. Physical mobility
1. Reinforce the exercise program and the importance of participating in the program
2. Instruct the client that exercises should be active rather than passive and to exercise only to the point of pain
3. Instruct the client to stop exercise if pain is increased with exercising
4. Instruct the client to decrease the number of repetitions in an exercise when the inflammation is severe

F. Surgical management
1. Osteotomy: The bone is cut to correct joint deformity and promote realignment
2. Total joint replacement (TJR)
   a. Performed when all measures of pain relief have failed
   b. Hips and knees are most commonly replaced
   c. Contraindicated in the presence of infection, advanced osteoporosis, or severe inflammation

XV. OSTEOPOROSIS

A. Description
1. An age-related metabolic disease
2. Bone demineralization results in the loss of bone mass, leading to fragile and porous bones and subsequent fractures
3. Greater bone resorption than bone formation occurs
4. Occurs most commonly in the wrist, hip, and vertebral column
5. Can occur postmenopausally or as a result of a metabolic disorder or calcium deficiency

B. Assessment
1. Back pain after lifting, bending, or stooping
2. Back pain that increases with palpation
3. Pelvic or hip pain, especially with weight bearing
4. Problems with balance
5. Decline in height from vertebral compression
6. Kyphosis of the dorsal spine
7. Constipation, abdominal distention, and respiratory impairment as a result of movement restriction and spinal deformity
8. Pathological fractures
9. Appearance of thin porous bone on x-ray

C. Implementation
1. Assess risk for injury

2. Provide a safe and hazard-free environment, and assist the client to identify hazards in the home environment

3. Use side rails to prevent falls

4. Move the client gently when turning and repositioning

5. Encourage ambulation; assist with ambulation if the client is unsteady

6. Instruct in the use of assistive devices such as a cane or walker

7. Provide ROM exercises

8. Instruct in the use of good body mechanics

9. Instruct the client in exercises to strengthen abdominal and back muscles in order to improve posture and provide support for the spine

10. Instruct the client to avoid activities that can cause vertebral compression

11. Apply a back brace as prescribed during an acute phase to immobilize the spine and provide spinal column support

12. Encourage the use of a firm mattress

13. Provide a diet high in protein, calcium, vitamins C and D, and iron

14. Encourage adequate fluid intake to prevent renal calculi

15. Instruct the client to avoid alcohol and coffee

16. Administer estrogen or androgens to decrease the rate of bone resorption as prescribed

17. Administer calcium, vitamin D, and phosphorus as prescribed for bone metabolism

18. Administer calcitonin as prescribed to inhibit bone loss

19. Administer analgesics, muscle relaxants, and antiinflammatory medications as prescribed

XVI. GOUT

A. Description
1. A systemic disease in which urate crystals deposit in joints and other body tissues
2. Leads to abnormal amounts of uric acid in the body
3. Primary gout results from a disorder of purine metabolism
4. Secondary gout involves excessive uric acid in the blood that is caused by another disease

B. Phases
1. Asymptomatic
   a. No symptoms
   b. Serum uric acid is elevated
2. Acute: Excruciating pain and inflammation of one or more small joints, especially the great toe
3. Intermittent: Asymptomatic period between acute attacks
4. Chronic
   a. Results from repeated episodes of acute gout
   b. Results in deposits of urate crystals under the

skin and within the major organs, especially the renal system

C. Assessment
1. Excruciating pain in the involved joints
2. Swelling and inflammation of the joints
3. Tophi (hard, fairly large, and irregularly shaped deposits in the skin) that may break open and discharge a yellow gritty substance
4. Low-grade fever
5. Malaise and headache
6. Pruritis
7. Presence of renal stones
8. Elevated uric acid levels

D. Implementation
1. Provide a low-purine diet as prescribed
2. Instruct the client to avoid foods such as organ meats, wines, aged cheese
3. Encourage a high fluid intake of 2000 mL to prevent stone formation
4. Encourage weight-reduction diet if required
5. Instruct the client to avoid alcohol and starvation diets because they may precipitate a gout attack
6. Increase urinary pH (above 6) by eating alkaline ash foods such as citrus fruits and juices, milk, and other dairy products
7. Provide bed rest during the acute attacks
8. Monitor joint ROM ability and appearance of joints
9. Position the joint in mild flexion during acute attack
10. Elevate the affected extremity
11. Protect the affected joint from excessive movement or direct contact with sheets or blankets
12. Provide heat or cold for local treatments to affected joint as prescribed
13. Administer NSAIDs and antigout medications as prescribed

PRACTICE QUESTIONS

1. A client is treated in a physician's office after a fall that sprained an ankle. X-ray examination has ruled out a fracture. Before sending the client home, the nurse plans to teach the client to avoid which of the following in the next 24 hours?
   1. Application of a heating pad
   2. Application of an Ace wrap
   3. Resting the foot
   4. Elevating the ankle on a pillow while sitting or lying down

2. A nurse has given dietary instructions to a client to minimize the risk of osteoporosis. The nurse would evaluate that the client understands the recommended dietary changes if the client stated he or she should increase intake of which food?
   1. Rice
   2. Yogurt

3. Sardines
4. Chicken

3. A nurse is conducting health screening for osteoporosis. The nurse would interpret that which of the following clients is at greatest risk of developing this disorder?
   1. A 36-year-old male who has asthma
   2. A 25-year-old female who jogs
   3. A sedentary 65-year-old female who smokes cigarettes
   4. A 70-year-old male who consumes excess alcohol

4. A home health nurse is planning to teach a client with osteoporosis about home modifications to reduce the risk of falls. Which of the following recommendations would be unnecessary to include in the teaching plan?
   1. Use of staircase railings
   2. Use of night-lights
   3. Removing wall-to-wall carpeting
   4. Placing handrails in the bathroom

5. A nurse is providing care to a client after bone biopsy. Which action by the nurse is not needed in the care of this client?
   1. Monitoring site for swelling, bleeding, or hematoma
   2. Administering intramuscular narcotic analgesics
   3. Elevating the limb for 24 hours
   4. Monitoring vitals signs every 4 hours

6. A nurse has given instructions to a client returning home after arthroscopy of a knee. The nurse would evaluate that the client understands the instructions if the client states to:
   1. Stay off the leg entirely for the rest of the day
   2. Resume regular exercise the following day
   3. Refrain from eating food for the remainder of the day
   4. Report fever or site inflammation to the physician

7. A nurse is caring for a client who is going to have an arthrogram with a contrast medium. Which assessment by the nurse would be of highest priority?
   1. Allergy to iodine or shellfish
   2. Ability of the client to remain still during the procedure
   3. Whether the client has any remaining questions about the procedure
   4. Whether the client wishes to void before the procedure

8. A client with possible rib fracture has never had a chest radiograph. The nurse would plan to tell the client which of the following items about the procedure?
   1. The x-rays stimulate a small amount of pain
   2. It is necessary to remove jewelry and any other metal objects
   3. A client will be asked to breathe in and out as the radiograph is taken

4. The x-ray technologist will stand next to the client during the procedure

9. A client has had a bone scan done. The nurse would evaluate that the client understands the elements of follow-up care if the client states that he or she should:
   1. Report any feelings of nausea or flushing
   2. Ambulate at least three times before the end of the day
   3. Eat only small meals for the remainder of the day
   4. Drink plenty of water for a day or two following the procedure

10. A client seeks treatment in the emergency room for a lower leg injury. There is visible deformity of the lower aspect of the leg, and the injured leg appears shorter than the other. The area is painful, swollen, and beginning to become ecchymotic. The nurse interprets that this client has experienced a:
    1. Contusion
    2. Fracture
    3. Sprain
    4. Strain

11. A nurse is one of several people who witness a vehicle hit a pedestrian at fairly low speed on a small street. The person is dazed and tries to get up. The leg appears fractured. The nurse would plan to:
    1. Stay with the person and encourage the person to remain still
    2. Assist the person to get up and walk to the sidewalk
    3. Leave the person for a few moments to call an ambulance
    4. Try to manually reduce the fracture

12. A nurse is planning to teach a client with a left arm cast about measures to keep the left shoulder from becoming stiff and frozen. Which suggestion would the nurse include in the teaching plan?
    1. Lift the left arm up over the head
    2. Lift the right arm up over the head
    3. Make a fist with the hand of the casted arm
    4. Use a sling on the left arm

13. A client has a fiberglass (nonplaster) cast applied to the lower leg. The client asks the nurse when the client will be able to walk on the cast. The nurse replies that the client will be able to bear weight on the cast:
    1. Within 20 to 30 minutes of application
    2. In approximately 8 hours
    3. In 24 hours
    4. In 48 hours

14. A nurse has given a client with a nonplaster (fiberglass) leg cast instructions on cast care at home. The nurse would evaluate that the client needs further instruction if the client makes which of the following statements?
    1. "I should avoid walking on wet, slippery floors."
    2. "It's OK to wipe dirt off the top of the cast with a damp cloth."
    3. "I'm not supposed to scratch the skin underneath the cast."
    4. "If the cast gets wet, I can dry it with a hair dryer turned to the warmest setting."

15. A client with a hip fracture asks the nurse why Buck's extension traction is being applied before surgery. The nurse's response is based on the understanding that Buck's extension traction primarily:
    1. Provides rigid immobilization of the fracture site
    2. Provides comfort by reducing muscle spasms, and provides fracture immobilization
    3. Lengthens the fractured leg to prevent severing of blood vessels
    4. Allows bony healing to begin before surgery

16. A client in skeletal leg traction with an overbed frame is not allowed to turn from side to side. Which action by the nurse would be most useful in trying to provide good skin care to the client?
    1. Ask the client to lift up by digging into the mattress with the unaffected leg
    2. Push down on the mattress of the bed while administering care
    3. Have another nurse tilt the client anyway
    4. Ask the client to pull up on a trapeze to lift the hips off the bed

17. A nurse is evaluating the pin sites of a client in skeletal traction. The nurse would be least concerned with which of the following findings?
    1. Purulent drainage
    2. Serous drainage
    3. Pain at a pin site
    4. Inflammation

18. A client immobilized in skeletal leg traction complains of being bored and restless. Based on these complaints, the nurse formulates which of the following nursing diagnoses for this client?
    1. Diversional Activity Deficit
    2. Powerlessness
    3. Self-Care Deficit
    4. Impaired Physical Mobility

19. A client has Buck's extension traction applied to the right leg. The nurse would plan which of the following interventions to prevent complications of the device?
    1. Massage the skin of the right leg with lotion every 8 hours
    2. Give pin care once a shift
    3. Inspect the skin on the right leg at least once every 8 hours
    4. Release the weights on the right leg for range of motion exercises daily

20. A nurse is caring for a client who had skeletal traction applied to the left leg. The client is complaining of severe left leg pain. Which of the following actions should the nurse take first?
    1. Medicate the client with an analgesic
    2. Provide pin care

3. Call the physician
4. Check the client's alignment in bed

21. A nurse is assessing the casted extremity of a client. The nurse would assess for which of the following signs and symptoms indicative of infection?
    1. Coolness and pallor of the extremity
    2. Presence of a "hot spot" on the cast
    3. Diminished distal pulse
    4. Dependent edema

22. A client has sustained a closed fracture and has just had a cast applied to the affected arm. The client is complaining of intense pain. The nurse has elevated the limb, applied an ice bag, and administered an analgesic with very little relief. The nurse interprets that this pain may be due to:
    1. Impaired tissue perfusion
    2. The newness of the fracture
    3. The anxiety of the client
    4. Infection under the cast

23. A nurse is admitting a client with multiple trauma to the nursing unit. The client has a leg fracture and had a plaster cast applied. In positioning the casted leg, the nurse should:
    1. Keep the leg in a level position
    2. Keep the leg level for 3 hours, and elevate it for 1 hour
    3. Elevate the leg on pillows continuously for 24 to 48 hours
    4. Elevate the leg for 3 hours, and put it flat for 1 hour

24. A client is complaining of skin irritation from the edges of a cast applied the previous day. The nurse should take which of the following actions?
    1. Massage the skin at the rim of the cast
    2. Apply lotion to the skin at the rim of the cast
    3. Use a rough file to smooth the cast edges
    4. Petal the cast edges with adhesive tape

25. A client is being discharged to home after application of a plaster leg cast. The nurse would evaluate that the client understands proper care of the cast if the client states that he or she should:
    1. Avoid getting the cast wet
    2. Use the fingertips to lift and move the leg
    3. Cover the casted leg with warm blankets
    4. Use a padded coat hanger end to scratch under the cast

26. A client being measured for crutches asks the nurse why the crutches cannot rest up underneath the arm for extra support. The nurse's response is based on the understanding that this could result in:
    1. Impaired range of motion while the client ambulates
    2. Skin breakdown in the area of the axilla
    3. Injury to the brachial plexus nerves
    4. A fall and further injury

27. A nurse is planning to teach a client how to stand on crutches. The nurse plans to incorporate into written instructions that the client should be told to place the crutches:
    1. 8 inches to the front and side of the client's toes
    2. 3 inches to the front and side of the client's toes
    3. 20 inches to the front and side of the client's toes
    4. 15 inches to the front and side of the client's toes

28. A nurse has given a client instructions about crutch safety. The nurse evaluates that the client needs reinforcement of information if the client states:
    1. The need to have spare crutches and tips available
    2. That crutch tips will not slip even when wet
    3. Not to use someone else's crutches
    4. That crutch tips should be inspected periodically for wear

29. A client with right-sided weakness needs to learn how to use a cane. The nurse plans to teach the client to position the cane by holding it with the:
    1. Left hand and placing the cane in front of the left foot
    2. Right hand and placing the cane in front of the right foot
    3. Left hand and 6 inches lateral to the left foot
    4. Right hand and 6 inches lateral to the right foot

30. A nurse is evaluating a client's use of a cane for left-sided weakness. The nurse would intervene and correct the client if the nurse observed that the client:
    1. Holds the cane on the right side
    2. Keeps the cane 6 inches out to the side of the right foot
    3. Moves the cane when the right leg is moved
    4. Leans on the cane when the right leg swings through

31. A client with a fractured femur experiences sudden dyspnea. A set of arterial blood gas tests reveal the following: pH, 7.35; $Paco_2$, 43; Pao_2, 58; HCO_3^-, 23. A nurse interprets that the client probably has experienced fat embolus because of the result of the:
    1. $Paco_2$
    2. Pao_2
    3. HCO_3^-
    4. pH

32. A client with a fat embolus is experiencing respiratory distress. The nurse plans to assist with which of the following therapies?
    1. Administration of bronchodilators, intubation, mechanical ventilation
    2. Administration of plasma expanders, oxygen mask, and suctioning
    3. Administration of corticosteroids, intubation, mechanical ventilation with positive-end expiratory pressure (PEEP)
    4. Administration of antihypertensives, high flow

oxygen, continuous positive airway pressure (CPAP) mask

33. A nurse is caring for a client being treated for fat embolus after multiple fractures. Which of the following data would the nurse evaluate as the most favorable indication of resolution of the fat embolus?
   1. Arterial oxygen level of 78 mm Hg
   2. Minimal dyspnea
   3. Clear chest radiograph
   4. Oxygen saturation of 85%

34. A nurse is caring for a client who develops compartment syndrome from a severely fractured arm. The client asks the nurse how this can happen. The nurse's response is based on the understanding that:
   1. An injured artery causes impaired arterial perfusion through the compartment
   2. The fascia expands with injury, causing pressure on underlying nerves and muscles
   3. A bone fragment has injured the nerve supply in the area
   4. Bleeding and swelling cause increased pressure in an area that cannot expand

35. A nurse has conducted teaching with a client in an arm cast about signs and symptoms of compartment syndrome. The nurse would evaluate that the client understands the information if the client stated that he or she should report which of the following early symptoms of compartment syndrome?
   1. Pain that is relieved only by oxycodone and aspirin (Percodan)
   2. Pain that increases when the arm is dependent
   3. Cold, bluish colored fingers
   4. Numbness and tingling in the fingers

36. A nurse is repositioning a client who has returned to the nursing unit after internal fixation of a fractured right hip. The nurse should use a:
   1. Pillow to keep the right leg abducted during turning
   2. Pillow to keep the right leg adducted during turning
   3. Trochanter roll to prevent external rotation while turning
   4. Trochanter roll to prevent abduction while turning

37. A nurse has an order to get a client out of bed to a chair on the first postoperative day after total knee replacement (TKR). The nurse would plan to do which of the following to protect the knee joint?
   1. Apply a knee immobilizer before getting the client up and elevate the client's surgical leg while sitting
   2. Apply an Ace wrap around the dressing and put ice on the knee while sitting
   3. Lift the client to the bedside chair, leaving the

continuous passive motion (CPM) machine in place
   4. Obtain a walker to minimize weight bearing by the client on the affected leg

38. A nurse has completed giving discharge instructions to a client after total knee replacement (TKR) with a metal prosthesis. The nurse would evaluate that the instructions are not fully understood if the client says he or she should:
   1. Report fever, redness, or increased pain
   2. Ignore changes in the shape of the knee
   3. Report bleeding gums or tarry stools
   4. Tell future caregivers about the metal implant

39. A client with diabetes mellitus has had a right below-the-knee amputation. The nurse would specifically assess for which of the following signs and symptoms due to the history of diabetes?
   1. Edema of the stump
   2. Hemorrhage
   3. Separation of wound edges
   4. Slight redness of incision

40. A client is admitted to the nursing unit after a left below-the-knee amputation following a crush injury to the foot and lower leg. The client tells the nurse "I think I'm going crazy. I can feel my left foot itching." The nurse interprets the client's statement to be:
   1. A normal response, and indicates the presence of phantom limb sensation
   2. A normal response, and indicates the presence of phantom limb pain
   3. An abnormal response, and indicates that the client needs more psychological support
   4. An abnormal response, and indicates that the client is in denial about the limb loss

41. A nurse is planning to teach the client with below-the-knee amputation about care to prevent skin breakdown. Which of the following points would the nurse include while developing the teaching plan?
   1. A stump sock must be worn at all times and changed twice a week
   2. The residual limb is washed gently and dried every other day
   3. The socket of the prosthesis is washed with a harsh bactericidal agent daily
   4. The socket of the prosthesis must be dried carefully before using it

42. A nurse is caring for a client who had an above-the-knee amputation 2 days ago. The residual limb was wrapped with an elastic compression bandage, which has come off. The nurse immediately:
   1. Calls the physician
   2. Rewraps the stump with an elastic compression bandage
   3. Applies ice to the site

   4. Applies a dry sterile dressing and elevates it on one pillow
43. A client is complaining of low back pain that radiates down the left posterior thigh. The nurse further assesses the client to see if the pain is worsened or aggravated by:
   1. Bed rest
   2. Application of heat
   3. Bending or lifting
   4. Ibuprofen (Motrin)
44. A client has just undergone spinal fusion after experiencing herniated lumbar disk. The nurse would avoid which of the following to maintain client safety after this procedure?
   1. Logrolling technique for repositioning
   2. Pillows under the length of the legs
   3. Head of bed flat
   4. Overhead trapeze
45. A nurse has taught a client with a herniated lumbar disk about proper body mechanics and other items pertinent to low back care. The nurse evaluates that the client needs further instruction if the client says he or she should:
   1. Get out of bed by sitting straight up and swinging the legs over the side of the bed
   2. Increase fiber and fluids in the diet
   3. Strengthen the back muscles by swimming or walking
   4. Bend at the knees to pick up objects
46. A nurse is caring for a client who has had spinal fusion with insertion of hardware. The nurse would be especially concerned with which of the following assessment findings?
   1. Complaints of discomfort during repositioning
   2. Temperature of 101.6° F orally
   3. Old bloody drainage outlined on the surgical dressing
   4. Discomfort during coughing and deep breathing exercises
47. A client has several fractures of the lower leg and has been placed in an external fixation device. The client is upset about the appearance of the leg, which is very edematous. The nurse formulates which of the following nursing diagnoses for the client?
   1. Body Image Disturbance
   2. Activity Intolerance
   3. Risk for Impaired Physical Mobility
   4. Social Isolation
48. A client has been placed in Buck's extension traction. The nurse can provide for countertraction to reduce shear and friction by:
   1. Slightly elevating the head of the bed
   2. Slightly elevating the foot of the bed
   3. Providing an overhead trapeze
   4. Using a footboard
49. A nurse is caring for a client with a diagnosis of gout. Which of the following laboratory values would the nurse expect to note in the client?
   1. Uric acid level of 8.0 mg/dL
   2. Calcium level of 9.0 mg/dL
   3. Phosphorus level of 3.0 mg/dL
   4. Potassium level of 4.0 mEq/L
50. A nurse is caring for a client with osteoarthritis. The nurse performs an assessment knowing that which of the following is a clinical manifestation associated with the disorder?
   1. Pain that is most severe later in the day
   2. An elevated platelet count
   3. Dull aching pain in the affected joints
   4. Elevated antinuclear antibody levels

CRITICAL THINKING: FREE-TEXT ENTRY

A client with a left arm fracture exhibits loss of sensation in the left fingers, pallor, poor capillary refill, and a diminished left radial pulse. On the basis of these assessment findings, a nurse would take which take which priority action?

Answer: _____

ANSWERS

1. **1**

Rationale: Soft tissue injuries such as sprains are treated by RICE (*r*est, *i*ce, *c*ompression, and *e*levation) for the first 24 hours after the injury. Ice is applied intermittently for 20 to 30 minutes at a time. Heat is not used in the first 24 hours because it could increase venous congestion, which would increase edema and pain.

Test-Taking Strategy: Use the process of elimination. Note the key word "avoid." It is likely that sprains should be rested and elevated, so options 3 and 4 are eliminated. Use of an Ace wrap is also helpful in reducing the pain and swelling, so option 2 is eliminated. Review treatment measures for a sprain if you had difficulty with this question.

Level of Cognitive Ability: Application
Client Needs: Physiological Integrity
Integrated Concept/Process: Self-Care
Content Area: Adult Health/Musculoskeletal
Reference: Ignatavicius, D., Workman, M., & Mishler, M. (1999). *Medical-surgical nursing across the health care continuum* (3rd ed.). Philadelphia: W. B. Saunders, p. 1308.

2. **2**

Rationale: A client at risk for osteoporosis needs to increase intake of calcium. The major dietary source of calcium is dairy food, including milk, yogurt, and a variety of cheeses. Calcium may also be added to certain products, such as orange juice, which is then advertised as being "fortified" with calcium. Calcium supplements are available and recommended for those with typically low calcium intake. Options 1, 3, and 4 are not food sources high in calcium.

Test-Taking Strategy: Use the process of elimination. Recall that the client at risk for osteoporosis needs to increase intake of calcium. Knowing that dairy products are high in calcium will direct you to option 2. Review osteoporosis and food sources of calcium if you had difficulty with this question.
Level of Cognitive Ability: Analysis
Client Needs: Health Promotion and Maintenance
Integrated Concept/Process: Teaching/Learning
Content Area: Adult Health/Musculoskeletal
Reference: Ignatavicius, D., Workman, M., & Mishler, M. (1999). *Medical-surgical nursing across the health care continuum* (3rd ed.). Philadelphia: W. B. Saunders, p. 223.

3. 3
Rationale: Risk factors for osteoporosis include being female, postmenopausal, of advanced age, low calcium diet, excessive alcohol intake, being sedentary, and smoking cigarettes. Long-term use of corticosteroids, anticonvulsants, and furosemide also increases risk.

Test-Taking Strategy: Use the process of elimination. Option 2 is eliminated first. The 25-year-old female who jogs (exercise using the long bones) has negligible risk. The 36-year-old male with asthma is eliminated next because his only risk factor might be long-term corticosteroid use. Of the two remaining options, the 65-year-old female has more risk (age, gender, postmenopausal, sedentary, smoking) than the 70-year-old male (age, alcohol consumption). Review the risk factors associated with osteoporosis if you had difficulty with this question.
Level of Cognitive Ability: Analysis
Client Needs: Health Promotion and Maintenance
Integrated Concept/Process: Nursing Process/Assessment
Content Area: Adult Health/Musculoskeletal
Reference: Ignatavicius, D., Workman, M., & Mishler, M. (1999). *Medical-surgical nursing across the health care continuum* (3rd ed.). Philadelphia: W. B. Saunders, p. 1244.

4. 3
Rationale: Home modifications to reduce the risk for falls include use of railings on all staircases, ample lighting, removing scatter rugs, and placing hand rails in the bathroom. Removal of wall-to-wall carpeting is not necessary.

Test-Taking Strategy: Use the process of elimination. Begin to answer this question by eliminating options 1 and 4. Both of these items provide physical support to the client and are needed. Use of night-lights will enhance vision for the client getting up at night to use the bathroom, and is also warranted. Wall-to-wall carpeting does not pose a risk to the client and does not need to be removed. Review home care measures to ensure safety if you had difficulty with this question.
Level of Cognitive Ability: Application
Client Needs: Health Promotion and Maintenance
Integrated Concept/Process: Teaching/Learning
Content Area: Adult Health/Musculoskeletal

Reference: Ignatavicius, D., Workman, M., & Mishler, M. (1999). *Medical-surgical nursing across the health care continuum* (3rd ed.). Philadelphia: W. B. Saunders, pp. 1248-1249.

5. 2
Rationale: Nursing care after bone biopsy includes monitoring the site for swelling, bleeding, and hematoma formation. The biopsy site is elevated for 24 hours to reduce edema. The vital signs are monitored every 4 hours for 24 hours. The client usually requires mild analgesics; more severe pain usually indicates that complications are arising.

Test-Taking Strategy: Use the process of elimination. Note the key words "not needed." Recalling that this procedure is done under local anesthesia will direct you to option 2. Review nursing care following a bone biopsy if you had difficulty with this question.
Level of Cognitive Ability: Application
Client Needs: Physiological Integrity
Integrated Concept/Process: Nursing Process/Implementation
Content Area: Adult Health/Musculoskeletal
Reference: Ignatavicius, D., Workman, M., & Mishler, M. (1999). *Medical-surgical nursing across the health care continuum* (3rd ed.). Philadelphia: W. B. Saunders, p. 1239.

6. 4
Rationale: After arthroscopy, the client can usually walk carefully on the leg once sensation has returned. The client is instructed to avoid strenuous exercise for at least a few days. The client may resume the usual diet. Signs and symptoms of infection should be reported to the physician.

Test-Taking Strategy: Use the process of elimination. Recalling the client teaching points related to surgical procedures will direct you to option 4. Review client teaching points following arthroscopy if you had difficulty with this question.
Level of Cognitive Ability: Analysis
Client Needs: Health Promotion and Maintenance
Integrated Concept/Process: Teaching/Learning
Content Area: Adult Health/Musculoskeletal
Reference: Ignatavicius, D., Workman, M., & Mishler, M. (1999). *Medical-surgical nursing across the health care continuum* (3rd ed.). Philadelphia: W. B. Saunders, p. 1240.

7. 1
Rationale: Because of the risk of allergy to contrast dye, the nurse places highest priority on assessing whether the client has an allergy to iodine or shellfish. The nurse also reinforces information about the test, tells the client about the need to remain still during the procedure, and encourages the client to void before the procedure for comfort.

Test-Taking Strategy: Use the process of elimination. Note the key words "highest priority." This tells you that more than one or all of the options are correct (in fact, they all are). Use Maslow's hierarchy of needs theory. While options 2, 3, and 4 all compete for priority, option 1 (allergy to iodine or shellfish) takes first preference. The consequence of possible anaphylactic shock (physiological risk) makes this the correct option. Review client preparation for an arthrogram if you had difficulty with this question.
Level of Cognitive Ability: Analysis
Client Needs: Physiological Integrity
Integrated Concept/Process: Nursing Process/Assessment
Content Area: Adult Health/Musculoskeletal

Reference: Ignatavicius, D., Workman, M., & Mishler, M. (1999). *Medical-surgical nursing across the health care continuum* (3rd ed.). Philadelphia: W. B. Saunders, p. 1238.

8. **2**

Rationale: A radiograph is a photographic image of a part of the body on a special film, which is used to diagnose a wide variety of conditions. The x-ray itself is painless; any discomfort would arise from repositioning a painful part for filming. The nurse may want to premedicate a client who is at risk for pain. Any radiopaque objects such as jewelry or other metal must be removed. The client is asked to breathe in deeply, and then hold the breath while the chest radiograph is taken. To minimize risk of radiation exposure, the x-ray technologist stands in a separate area protected by a lead wall. The client also wears a lead shield over the gonads.

Test-Taking Strategy: Use the process of elimination. Recalling that radiopaque objects need to be removed will direct you to option 2. Review client preparation for a chest radiograph if you had difficulty with this question.

Level of Cognitive Ability: Application
Client Needs: Physiological Integrity
Integrated Concept/Process: Teaching/Learning
Content Area: Adult Health/Musculoskeletal
Reference: Ignatavicius, D., Workman, M., & Mishler, M. (1999). *Medical-surgical nursing across the health care continuum* (3rd ed.). Philadelphia: W. B. Saunders, p. 1327.

9. **4**

Rationale: There are no special restrictions after a bone scan. The client is encouraged to drink large amounts of water for 24 to 48 hours to flush the radioisotope from the system. There are no hazards to the client or staff from the minimal amount of radioactivity of the isotope.

Test-Taking Strategy: Use the process of elimination. There is no purpose for options 2 or 3, so eliminate these options first. Nausea and flushing could accompany dye injection during a procedure, but this procedure uses radioisotopes. Additionally, the question relates to care after the procedure. Remember, fluids hasten elimination of the isotope from the client's system. Review care following a bone scan if you had difficulty with this question.

Level of Cognitive Ability: Analysis
Client Needs: Health Promotion and Maintenance
Integrated Concept/Process: Teaching/Learning
Content Area: Adult Health/Musculoskeletal
Reference: Ignatavicius, D., Workman, M., & Mishler, M. (1999). *Medical-surgical nursing across the health care continuum* (3rd ed.). Philadelphia: W. B. Saunders, p. 1241.

10. **2**

Rationale: Typical signs and symptoms of fracture include pain, loss of function in the area, deformity, shortening of the extremity, crepitus, swelling, and ecchymosis. Not all fractures lead to the development of every sign. A contusion results from a blow to soft tissue and causes pain, swelling, and ecchymosis. A sprain is an injury to a ligament caused by a wrenching or twisting motion. Symptoms include pain, swelling, and inability to use the joint or bear weight normally. A strain results from a pulling force on the muscle. Symptoms include soreness and pain with muscle use.

Test-Taking Strategy: Use the process of elimination. Within the list of signs and symptoms in the question, note the one

stating that one leg is shorter than another. Only a fractured bone (which shortens with displacement) could cause this sign. This makes it easy to eliminate each of the incorrect options. Review signs of a fracture if you had difficulty with this question.

Level of Cognitive Ability: Analysis
Client Needs: Physiological Integrity
Integrated Concept/Process: Nursing Process/Assessment
Content Area: Adult Health/Musculoskeletal
Reference: Ignatavicius, D., Workman, M., & Mishler, M. (1999). *Medical-surgical nursing across the health care continuum* (3rd ed.). Philadelphia: W. B. Saunders, p. 1285.

11. **1**

Rationale: With a suspected fracture, the client is not moved unless it is dangerous to remain in that spot. The nurse should remain with the client and have someone else call for emergency help. A fracture is not reduced at the scene. Before the client is moved, the site of fracture is immobilized to prevent further injury.

Test-Taking Strategy: Use the process of elimination. Options 2 and 4 are eliminated first because either of these options could result in further injury to the client. Of remaining options, the more prudent action would be for the nurse to remain with the client and have someone else call for emergency assistance. Review care to the client with a fracture if you had difficulty with this question.

Level of Cognitive Ability: Application
Client Needs: Physiological Integrity
Integrated Concept/Process: Nursing Process/Implementation
Content Area: Adult Health/Musculoskeletal
Reference: Ignatavicius, D., Workman, M., & Mishler, M. (1999). *Medical-surgical nursing across the health care continuum* (3rd ed.). Philadelphia: W. B. Saunders, p. 1289.

12. **1**

Rationale: Immobility and the weight of a casted arm may cause the shoulder above an arm fracture to become stiff. The shoulder of a casted arm should be lifted over the head periodically as a preventive measure. The use of slings further immobilizes the shoulder and may be contraindicated. Making fists with the left hand provides good isometric exercise to maintain muscle strength. Range of motion of the affected fingers is also a useful general measure. Lifting the right arm is of no particular value.

Test-Taking Strategy: Use the process of elimination. Imagine each of the movements and think about the muscle groups that are moved with each. Options 2 and 4 provide for no movement of the left arm and are eliminated first. Making a fist with the hand on the casted arm provides good isometric exercise to the muscles surrounding the fracture, but again does nothing for the shoulder. The only viable option is raising the arm over the head, which provides some range of motion for the shoulder joint. Review teaching points for a client with a casted arm if you had difficulty with this question.

Level of Cognitive Ability: Application
Client Needs: Health Promotion and Maintenance
Integrated Concept/Process: Teaching/Learning
Content Area: Adult Health/Musculoskeletal
Reference: Jarvis, C. (2000). *Physical examination and health assessment* (3rd ed.). Philadelphia: W. B. Saunders, p. 644.

13. 1

Rationale: A fiberglass cast is made of water-activated polyure-thane materials that are dry to the touch within minutes and reach full rigid strength in about 20 minutes. Because of this, the client can bear weight on the cast within 20 to 30 minutes.

Test-Taking Strategy: Use the process of elimination. Note the key word "nonplaster." Options 3 and 4 should be eliminated first, because these timeframes are similar to the drying times for plaster casts. Recalling that the nonplaster type of cast is lighter and dries quickly may help you to choose the 20 to 30 minute time frame as correct. Review client teaching points related to a nonplaster cast if you had difficulty with this question.

Level of Cognitive Ability: Application
Client Needs: Health Promotion and Maintenance
Integrated Concept/Process: Teaching/Learning
Content Area: Adult Health/Musculoskeletal
Reference: Ignatavicius, D., Workman, M., & Mishler, M. (1999). *Medical-surgical nursing across the health care continuum* (3rd ed.). Philadelphia: W. B. Saunders, pp. 1286-1287.

14. 4

Rationale: Client instructions should include avoiding walking on wet, slippery floors to prevent falls. Surface soil on a cast can be removed with a damp cloth. If the cast gets wet, it can be dried with a hair dryer set to a cool setting to prevent skin breakdown. If the skin under the cast itches, cool air from a hair dryer may be used to relieve it. The client should never scratch under a cast because of the risk of skin breakdown and ulcer formation.

Test-Taking Strategy: Use the process of elimination. Note the key words "needs further instruction." Remember never to use a hair dryer on a cast or on the skin under any cast, with the dryer set at the warmest setting; only cool settings are used to prevent burns. Review client teaching points about a cast if you had difficulty with this question.

Level of Cognitive Ability: Analysis
Client Needs: Health Promotion and Maintenance
Integrated Concept/Process: Self-Care
Content Area: Adult Health/Musculoskeletal
Reference: Ignatavicius, D., Workman, M., & Mishler, M. (1999). *Medical-surgical nursing across the health care continuum* (3rd ed.). Philadelphia: W. B. Saunders, pp. 1286-1287.

15. 2

Rationale: Buck's extension traction is a type of skin traction often applied after hip fracture before the fracture is reduced in surgery. It reduces muscle spasms and helps to immobilize the fracture. It does not lengthen the leg for the purpose of preventing blood vessel severance. It also does not allow for bony healing to begin.

Test-Taking Strategy: Use the process of elimination. Focus on the client's diagnosis, hip fracture. Read each option carefully. Noting the words "provides fracture immobilization" will direct you to option 2. Review the purpose of Buck's traction if you had difficulty with this question.

Level of Cognitive Ability: Application
Client Needs: Physiological Integrity
Integrated Concept/Process: Nursing Process/Implementation
Content Area: Adult Health/Musculoskeletal
Reference: Ignatavicius, D., Workman, M., & Mishler, M. (1999). *Medical-surgical nursing across the health care continuum* (3rd ed.). Philadelphia: W. B. Saunders, p. 1289.

16. 4

Rationale: If the client in skeletal traction may not turn from side to side, the nurse should have the client pull up on a trapeze and try to lift the hips off the bed for skin care, bed pan use, and linen changes. If the client is unable to pull up on a trapeze, the nurse can push down on the mattress with one hand while administering care with the other.

Test-Taking Strategy: Use the process of elimination. Option 3 is contraindicated because it ignores a medical order. Option 1 is not feasible as stated. The client cannot lift up from the bed using only one foot. Options 2 and 4 are both acceptable alternatives. Since the question asks which would be "most useful," the answer is option 4. Providing care to the client who can lift the hips off the bed by use of a trapeze is easier and more efficient than providing care to one who cannot. Review care to the client in skeletal leg traction if you had difficulty with this question.

Level of Cognitive Ability: Application
Client Needs: Physiological Integrity
Integrated Concept/Process: Nursing Process/Implementation
Content Area: Adult Health/Musculoskeletal
Reference: Smeltzer, S., & Bare, B. (2000). *Brunner & Suddarth's textbook of medical-surgical nursing* (9th ed.). Philadelphia: Lippincott Williams & Wilkins, p. 1790.

17. 2

Rationale: A small amount of serous oozing is expected at pin insertion sites. Signs of infection such as inflammation, purulent drainage, and pain at the pin site are not expected findings, and should be reported to the physician.

Test-Taking Strategy: Use the process of elimination. Note the key words "least concerned." Options 1 and 4 seem to indicate an infectious problem, and are eliminated first. From the remaining options, note that the complaint of pain is at "a pin site" only. It gives no indication that the pain is related to the fracture or to muscle spasm. Since serous drainage is an expected finding, select option 2. Review expected findings in the client with skeletal traction if you had difficulty with this question.

Level of Cognitive Ability: Analysis
Client Needs: Physiological Integrity
Integrated Concept/Process: Nursing Process/Evaluation
Content Area: Adult Health/Musculoskeletal
Reference: Ignatavicius, D., Workman, M., & Mishler, M. (1999). *Medical-surgical nursing across the health care continuum* (3rd ed.). Philadelphia: W. B. Saunders, p. 1290.

18. 1

Rationale: A major defining characteristic of Diversional Activity Deficit is expression of boredom by the client. The question does not identify difficulties with coordination, range of motion, or muscle strength, which would indicate Impaired Physical Mobility. The question also does not relate client feelings of inability to perform activities of daily living (Self-Care Deficit) or lack of control (Powerlessness).

Test-Taking Strategy: Use the process of elimination. When asked about a nursing diagnosis, focus on the information in the question to direct you to the correct option. Review the defining characteristics of Diversional Activity Deficit if you had difficulty with this question.

Level of Cognitive Ability: Analysis
Client Needs: Psychosocial Integrity

Integrated Concept/Process: Nursing Process/Analysis
Content Area: Adult Health/Musculoskeletal
Reference: Johnson, M., Bulechek, G., Dochterman, J., Maas, M., & Moorhead, S. (2001). *Nursing diagnoses, outcomes, and interventions.* St. Louis: Mosby, p. 102.

19. **3**
Rationale: Buck's extension traction is a type of skin traction. The nurse inspects the skin of the limb in traction at least once every 8 hours for irritation or inflammation. Massaging the skin with lotion is not indicated. The nurse never releases the weights of traction unless specifically ordered by the physician. There are no pins to care for with skin traction.
Test-Taking Strategy: Use the process of elimination and the steps of the nursing process to answer this question. Option 3 is the only option that relates to assessment. Review care to the client in Buck's traction if you had difficulty with this question.
Level of Cognitive Ability: Application
Client Needs: Physiological Integrity
Integrated Concept/Process: Nursing Process/Implementation
Content Area: Adult Health/Musculoskeletal
Reference: Ignatavicius, D., Workman, M., & Mishler, M. (1999). *Medical-surgical nursing across the health care continuum* (3rd ed.). Philadelphia: W. B. Saunders, p. 1289.

20. **4**
Rationale: A client who complains of severe pain may need realignment, or may have traction weights ordered that are too heavy. The nurse realigns the client, and if that is ineffective, then calls the physician. Severe leg pain, once traction has been established, indicates a problem. Medicating the client should be done after one has tried to determine and treat the cause. Providing pin care is unrelated to the problem as described.
Test-Taking Strategy: Use the process of elimination. Note the key word "first." Use the steps of the nursing process to direct you to option 4. This is the only option that addresses assessment. Review care of the client in traction if you had difficulty with this question.
Level of Cognitive Ability: Application
Client Needs: Physiological Integrity
Integrated Concept/Process: Nursing Process/Implementation
Content Area: Adult Health/Musculoskeletal
Reference: Ignatavicius, D., Workman, M., & Mishler, M. (1999). *Medical-surgical nursing across the health care continuum* (3rd ed.). Philadelphia: W. B. Saunders, p. 1290.

21. **2**
Rationale: Signs and symptoms of infection under a casted area include odor or purulent drainage from the cast, or the presence of "hot spots," which are areas of the cast that are warmer than others. The physician should be notified if any of these occur. Signs of impaired circulation in the distal limb include coolness and pallor of the skin, diminished arterial pulse, and edema.
Test-Taking Strategy: Use the process of elimination. Answer this question thinking about what you would expect to note with infection: redness, swelling, heat, and purulent drainage. With this in mind, options 1 and 3 can be eliminated easily. From the remaining options, remember "dependent edema" is not necessarily indicative of infection. Swelling would be continuous. The "hot spot" on the cast could signify infection underneath that area, and is the correct answer to the question.

Review signs of infection in an extremity with a cast if you had difficulty with this question.
Level of Cognitive Ability: Analysis
Client Needs: Physiological Integrity
Integrated Concept/Process: Nursing Process/Assessment
Content Area: Adult Health/Musculoskeletal
Reference: Ignatavicius, D., Workman, M., & Mishler, M. (1999). *Medical-surgical nursing across the health care continuum* (3rd ed.). Philadelphia: W. B. Saunders, p. 1288.

22. **1**
Rationale: Most pain associated with fractures can be minimized with rest, elevation, application of cold, and administration of analgesics. Pain that is not relieved by these measures should be reported to the physician, because it may result from impaired tissue perfusion, tissue breakdown, or necrosis. Since this is a new closed fracture and cast, infection would not have had time to set in.
Test-Taking Strategy: Use the process of elimination. Focus on the issue, intense pain. Use of the ABCs, airway, breathing, and circulation will direct you to option 1. Review care to the client with a fracture and new cast if you had difficulty with this question.
Level of Cognitive Ability: Analysis
Client Needs: Physiological Integrity
Integrated Concept/Process: Nursing Process/Evaluation
Content Area: Adult Health/Musculoskeletal
Reference: Smeltzer, S., & Bare, B. (2000). *Brunner & Suddarth's textbook of medical-surgical nursing* (9th ed.). Philadelphia: Lippincott Williams & Wilkins, p. 1780.

23. **3**
Rationale: A casted extremity is elevated continuously for the first 24 to 48 hours to minimize swelling and to promote venous drainage. Options 1, 2, and 4 are incorrect.
Test-Taking Strategy: Use the process of elimination. Recalling that edema is a concern and knowledge of the effects of gravity on edema will direct you to option 3. Review care to the client with a new cast if you had difficulty with this question.
Level of Cognitive Ability: Application
Client Needs: Physiological Integrity
Integrated Concept/Process: Nursing Process/Implementation
Content Area: Adult Health/Musculoskeletal
Reference: Smeltzer, S., & Bare, B. (2000). *Brunner & Suddarth's textbook of medical-surgical nursing* (9th ed.). Philadelphia: Lippincott Williams & Wilkins, p. 1782.

24. **4**
Rationale: The nurse petals the edges of the cast with tape to minimize skin irritation. If a client has a cast applied and returns home, the client can be taught to do the same.
Test-Taking Strategy: Use the process of elimination. Options 1 and 2 are similar, and neither helps to get rid of the cause of the irritation, so they are eliminated first. Imagine the use of a "rough file"; it would create plaster chips and dust that could go underneath the cast. By the process of elimination, the nurse would petal the cast to cushion the skin from the irritating cast material. Review care to the client with a cast if you had difficulty with this question.
Level of Cognitive Ability: Application
Client Needs: Physiological Integrity
Integrated Concept/Process: Nursing Process/Implementation
Content Area: Adult Health/Musculoskeletal

Reference: Smeltzer, S., & Bare, B. (2000). *Brunner & Suddarth's textbook of medical-surgical nursing* (9th ed.). Philadelphia: Lippincott Williams & Wilkins, p. 1782.

25. **1**

Rationale: A plaster cast must remain dry to keep its strength. The cast should be handled with the palms of the hands, not the fingertips, until fully dry. Air should circulate freely around the cast to help it dry; the cast also gives off heat as it dries. The client should never scratch under the cast; a cool hair dryer may be used to eliminate an itch.

Test-Taking Strategy: Use the process of elimination. Knowing that a wet cast can be dented with the fingertips, causing pressure underneath, helps you to eliminate option 2 first. Knowing that the cast needs to dry helps to eliminate option 3 next. Option 4 is dangerous to skin integrity and is immediately eliminated. Remember plaster casts, once they have dried after application, should not become wet. Review care to the client with a cast if you had difficulty with this question.

Level of Cognitive Ability: Analysis
Client Needs: Health Promotion and Maintenance
Integrated Concept/Process: Teaching/Learning
Content Area: Adult Health/Musculoskeletal
Reference: Smeltzer, S., & Bare, B. (2000). *Brunner & Suddarth's textbook of medical-surgical nursing* (9th ed.). Philadelphia: Lippincott Williams & Wilkins, p. 1782.

26. **3**

Rationale: Crutches are measured so that the tops are 3 to 4 fingerbreadths or 1 to 2 inches from the axillae. This assures that the client's axillae are not resting on the crutch or bearing the weight of the crutch. This could result in injury to the nerves of the brachial plexus.

Test-Taking Strategy: Use the process of elimination. Recalling the risk associated with brachial nerve plexus injury will direct you to option 3. Review the complications associated with the use of crutches if you had difficulty with this question.

Level of Cognitive Ability: Analysis
Client Needs: Physiological Integrity
Integrated Concept/Process: Teaching/Learning
Content Area: Adult Health/Musculoskeletal
Reference: Smeltzer, S., & Bare, B. (2000). *Brunner & Suddarth's textbook of medical-surgical nursing* (9th ed.). Philadelphia: Lippincott Williams & Wilkins, p. 132.

27. **1**

Rationale: The classic tripod position is taught to the client before one gives instructions on gait. The crutches are placed anywhere from 6 to 10 inches in front and to the side of the client, depending on the client's body size. This provides a wide enough base of support to the client and improves balance.

Test-Taking Strategy: Use the process of elimination. Three inches (option 2) and 20 inches (option 3) seem excessively short and long, respectively, and are eliminated first. Visualize the descriptions in the options. Eight inches seems more in keeping with the normal length of a stride than 15 inches for someone with crutches. Review the points related to client instructions for the use of crutches if you had difficulty with this question.

Level of Cognitive Ability: Application
Client Needs: Health Promotion and Maintenance
Integrated Concept/Process: Teaching/Learning

Content Area: Adult Health/Musculoskeletal
Reference: Potter, P., & Perry, A. (2001). *Fundamentals of nursing* (5th ed.). St. Louis: Mosby, p. 1009.

28. **2**

Rationale: Crutch tips should remain dry. Water could cause slipping by decreasing the surface friction of the rubber tip on the floor. If crutch tips get wet, the client should dry them with a cloth or paper towel. The client should use only crutches measured for the client. The tips should be inspected for wear, and spare crutches and tips should be available if needed.

Test-Taking Strategy: Use the process of elimination. Note the key words "needs reinforcement of information." Remember, crutch tips can slip when they get wet, posing a possible threat to the unsuspecting client. Review client teaching points related to safety and the use of crutches if you had difficulty with this question.

Level of Cognitive Ability: Analysis
Client Needs: Health Promotion and Maintenance
Integrated Concept/Process: Nursing Process/Evaluation
Content Area: Adult Health/Musculoskeletal
Reference: Potter, P., & Perry, A. (2001). *Fundamentals of nursing* (5th ed.). St. Louis: Mosby, p. 1009.

29. **3**

Rationale: The client is taught to hold the cane on the side opposite from the weakness. The reason is that, with normal walking, the opposite arm and leg move together (called reciprocal motion). The cane is placed 6 inches lateral to the fifth toe.

Test-Taking Strategy: Use the process of elimination. Knowing that the cane is held at the client's side, not in front, helps you to eliminate options 1 and 2 first. Knowing that the preferred method is to have the cane positioned on the stronger side helps you to choose option 3 over option 4. Review client teaching points related to the use of a cane if you had difficulty with this question.

Level of Cognitive Ability: Application
Client Needs: Health Promotion and Maintenance
Integrated Concept/Process: Self Care
Content Area: Adult Health/Musculoskeletal
Reference: Potter, P., & Perry, A. (2001). *Fundamentals of nursing* (5th ed.). St. Louis: Mosby, p. 1008.

30. **3**

Rationale: The cane is held on the stronger side to minimize stress on the affected extremity and provide a wide base of support. The cane is held 6 inches lateral to the fifth toe. The cane is moved forward with the affected leg. The client leans on the cane for added support while the stronger side swings through.

Test-Taking Strategy: Use the process of elimination. Note the key word "intervene." Knowing that the cane is held on the stronger side helps you eliminate options 1 and 2 first. Recalling that the client moves the cane with the weaker leg and leans on it for support when the stronger leg swings through will direct you to option 3. Review client instructions about the use of a cane if you had difficulty with this question.

Level of Cognitive Ability: Analysis
Client Needs: Health Promotion and Maintenance
Integrated Concept/Process: Self-Care
Content Area: Adult Health/Musculoskeletal

Reference: Potter, P., & Perry, A. (2001). *Fundamentals of nursing* (5th ed.). St. Louis: Mosby, p. 1008.

31. 2

Rationale: A key feature of fat embolism is a significant degree of hypoxemia, with a Pao_2 often less than 60 mm Hg. Options 1, 3, and 4 are normal blood gas results.

Test-Taking Strategy: Use the process of elimination. Recall that fat embolus causes significant hypoxemia. Also note that the values of the $Paco_2$, HCO_3^-, and pH are normal. Review the clinical manifestations of fat embolism if you had difficulty with this question.

Level of Cognitive Ability: Analysis
Client Needs: Physiological Integrity
Integrated Concept/Process: Nursing Process/Evaluation
Content Area: Adult Health/Musculoskeletal
Reference: Phipps, W., Sands, J., & Marek, J. (1999). *Medical-surgical nursing: Concepts & clinical practice* (6th ed.). St. Louis: Mosby, p. 1934.

32. 3

Rationale: Respiratory failure is the most common cause of death after fat embolus. The client may be intubated and mechanically ventilated with PEEP to treat the significant hypoxemia and pulmonary edema. Corticosteroids are given to treat inflammatory lung reactions and control cerebral edema.

Test-Taking Strategy: Use the process of elimination. Fat embolus does not cause bronchoconstriction or bronchospasm, which may help to eliminate option 1. The question makes no mention of hypovolemia, so the plasma expanders in option 2 have no use. From the remaining options it is helpful to know that corticosteroids are used for the inflammatory lung reaction, and that hypertension may not be part of the clinical picture. Review the complications associated with fat embolism and manifestations of respiratory failure if you had difficulty with this question.

Level of Cognitive Ability: Application
Client Needs: Physiological Integrity
Integrated Concept/Process: Nursing Process/Planning
Content Area: Adult Health/Musculoskeletal
Reference: Phipps, W., Sands, J., & Marek, J. (1999). *Medical-surgical nursing: Concepts & clinical practice* (6th ed.). St. Louis: Mosby, p. 1934.

33. 3

Rationale: A clear chest radiograph is a good indicator that fat embolus is resolving. When fat embolism occurs, there is a "snowstorm" appearance to the chest radiograph. Eupnea, not minimal dyspnea, is a normal sign. Arterial oxygen levels should be 80 to 100 mm Hg. Oxygen saturation should be greater than 95%.

Test-Taking Strategy: Use the process of elimination. Note the key words "most favorable indication." Knowing that the arterial oxygen and oxygen saturation levels are below normal helps you to eliminate options 1 and 4. Dyspnea, even at a minimal level, is not normal, so option 2 is eliminated. Review the expected outcomes in a client being treated for fat embolism if you had difficulty with this question.

Level of Cognitive Ability: Analysis
Client Needs: Physiological Integrity
Integrated Concept/Process: Nursing Process/Evaluation
Content Area: Adult Health/Musculoskeletal

Reference: Phipps, W., Sands, J., & Marek, J. (1999). *Medical-surgical nursing: Concepts & clinical practice* (6th ed.). St. Louis: Mosby, p. 1934.

34. 4

Rationale: Compartment syndrome is caused by bleeding and swelling within a compartment, which is lined by fascia and does not expand. The bleeding and swelling put pressure on the nerves, muscles, and blood vessels in the compartment, triggering the symptoms. Options 1, 2, and 3 are inaccurate descriptions of compartment syndrome.

Test-Taking Strategy: Use the process of elimination. Note the name of the syndrome and the relationship of the name to the description in option 4. Review the pathophysiology related to compartment syndrome if you had difficulty with this question.

Level of Cognitive Ability: Analysis
Client Needs: Physiological Integrity
Integrated Concept/Process: Nursing Process/Implementation
Content Area: Adult Health/Musculoskeletal
Reference: Phipps, W., Sands, J., & Marek, J. (1999). *Medical-surgical nursing: Concepts & clinical practice* (6th ed.). St. Louis: Mosby, p. 1935.

35. 4

Rationale: The earliest symptom of compartment syndrome is paresthesia (numbness and tingling in the fingers). Other symptoms include pain unrelieved by narcotics, pain that increases with limb elevation, and pallor and coolness to the distal limb. Cyanosis is a late sign.

Test-Taking Strategy: Use the process of elimination. Note the key word "early." Knowing that compartment syndrome is characterized by insufficient circulation and ischemia secondary to pressure will direct you to option 4. Review the early signs of compartment syndrome if you had difficulty with this question.

Level of Cognitive Ability: Analysis
Client Needs: Health Promotion and Maintenance
Integrated Concept/Process: Nursing Process/Evaluation
Content Area: Adult Health/Musculoskeletal
Reference: Phipps, W., Sands, J., & Marek, J. (1999). *Medical-surgical nursing: Concepts & clinical practice* (6th ed.). St. Louis: Mosby, p. 1935.

36. 1

Rationale: Following internal fixation of a hip fracture, the client is turned to the affected side or the unaffected side as prescribed by the surgeon. Before moving the client, the nurse places a pillow between the client's legs to keep the affected leg in abduction. The client is then repositioned while proper alignment and abduction are maintained. A trochanter roll is useful in preventing external rotation, but it is used once the client has been repositioned. It is not used while the client is being turned.

Test-Taking Strategy: Use the process of elimination. Visualizing each description in the options and recalling that the affected leg remains abducted will direct you to option 1. Review care to the client following a hip pinning if you had difficulty with this question.

Level of Cognitive Ability: Application
Client Needs: Physiological Integrity
Integrated Concept/Process: Nursing Process/Implementation
Content Area: Adult Health/Musculoskeletal

Reference: Ignatavicius, D., Workman, M., & Mishler, M. (1999). *Medical-surgical nursing across the health care continuum* (3rd ed.). Philadelphia: W. B. Saunders, p. 1298.

37. 1

Rationale: The nurse assists the client to get out of bed after putting a knee immobilizer on the affected joint for stability. The surgeon orders the weight-bearing limits on the affected leg. To minimize edema, the leg is elevated while the client is sitting in the chair. The CPM machine is used while the client is in bed.

Test-Taking Strategy: Use the process of elimination. A compression dressing should already be in place on the wound, so option 2 can be eliminated. Since the CPM machine is used while the client is in bed, option 3 is eliminated. From the remaining options, recalling that ambulation is not started until the second postoperative day will direct you to option 1. Also, a knee immobilizer is most appropriate to protect a knee joint. Review care to the client following TKR if you had difficulty with this question.

Level of Cognitive Ability: Application
Client Needs: Physiological Integrity
Integrated Concept/Process: Nursing Process/Planning
Content Area: Adult Health/Musculoskeletal
Reference: Ignatavicius, D., Workman, M., & Mishler, M. (1999). *Medical-surgical nursing across the health care continuum* (3rd ed.). Philadelphia: W. B. Saunders, p. 413.

38. 2

Rationale: After TKR, the client should report signs and symptoms of infection and any changes in the shape of the knee. Any of these could indicate developing complications. With a metal implant, the client must be on anticoagulant therapy and should report adverse effects of this therapy, including bleeding from a variety of sources. With a metal implant, the client must notify caregivers, because certain diagnostic tests (magnetic resonance imaging) will need to be avoided, and the client will need antibiotic prophylaxis for invasive procedures.

Test-Taking Strategy: Use the process of elimination. The question states that there is a metal prosthesis, which indicates that the client is receiving anticoagulant therapy. This would make options 3 and 4 correct. It is important to report signs and symptoms of infection, so option 1 is eliminated. Recalling that changes in the shape of the knee could indicate developing complications with the prosthesis will direct you to option 2. Review client teaching points after this surgical procedure if you had difficulty with this question.

Level of Cognitive Ability: Analysis
Client Needs: Health Promotion and Maintenance
Integrated Concept/Process: Teaching/Learning
Content Area: Adult Health/Musculoskeletal
Reference: Smeltzer, S., & Bare, B. (2000). *Brunner & Suddarth's textbook of medical-surgical nursing* (9th ed.). Philadelphia: Lippincott Williams & Wilkins.

39. 3

Rationale: Clients with diabetes mellitus are more prone to wound infection and delayed wound healing due to the disease. Postoperative stump edema and hemorrhage are complications in the immediate postoperative period that apply to any client with an amputation. Slight redness of the incision is considered normal, as long it is dry and intact.

Test-Taking Strategy: Use the process of elimination. Recalling that diabetes mellitus increases the client's chances of developing infection and delayed wound healing will direct you to option 3. Review the complications associated with an amputation in the client with diabetes mellitus if you had difficulty with this question.

Level of Cognitive Ability: Application
Client Needs: Physiological Integrity
Integrated Concept/Process: Nursing Process/Assessment
Content Area: Adult Health/Musculoskeletal
Reference: Smeltzer, S., & Bare, B. (2000). *Brunner & Suddarth's textbook of medical-surgical nursing* (9th ed.). Philadelphia: Lippincott Williams & Wilkins.

40. 1

Rationale: Phantom limb sensations are felt in the area of the amputated limb. These can include itching, warmth, and cold. The sensations are due to intact peripheral nerves in the area amputated. Whenever possible, the client should be prepared for these sensations. The client may also feel painful sensations in the amputated limb, called phantom limb pain. The origin of the pain is less well understood, but the client should be prepared for this, too, whenever possible.

Test-Taking Strategy: Use the process of elimination. Knowing that sensation and pain may be felt in the residual limb helps you to eliminate options 3 and 4 first, because the sensations are not abnormal responses. Select option 1 because the client has described an itching sensation, but has not complained of pain in the residual limb. Review expected findings following amputation if you had difficulty with this question.

Level of Cognitive Ability: Analysis
Client Needs: Psychosocial Integrity
Integrated Concept/Process: Nursing Process/Assessment
Content Area: Adult Health/Musculoskeletal
Reference: Ignatavicius, D., Workman, M., & Mishler, M. (1999). *Medical-surgical nursing across the health care continuum* (3rd ed.). Philadelphia: W. B. Saunders, p. 1301.

41. 4

Rationale: A stump sock must be worn at all times to absorb perspiration and is changed daily. The residual limb is washed, dried, and inspected for breakdown twice each day. The socket of the prosthesis is cleansed with a mild detergent and rinsed and dried carefully each day. A harsh bactericidal agent would not be used.

Test-Taking Strategy: Use the process of elimination. Eliminate options 1 and 2 because of the lengthy time frames. Eliminate option 3 because of the word "harsh." Review client teaching related to skin care following an amputation if you had difficulty with this question.

Level of Cognitive Ability: Application
Client Needs: Health Promotion and Maintenance
Integrated Concept/Process: Teaching/Learning
Content Area: Adult Health/Musculoskeletal
Reference: Ignatavicius, D., Workman, M., & Mishler, M. (1999). *Medical-surgical nursing across the health care continuum* (3rd ed.). Philadelphia: W. B. Saunders, p. 1305.

42. 2

Rationale: If the client with an amputation has a cast or elastic compression bandage that slips off, the nurse must immediately wrap the stump with another elastic compression bandage. Otherwise, excessive edema will rapidly form, which could cause a significant delay in rehabilitation. If the client had a cast that slipped off, the nurse would have to call the physician so a new one could be applied. Elevation on one pillow is not going to greatly impede the development of edema once compression is released. Ice would be of limited value in controlling edema from this cause. If the physician were called, the order would likely be to reapply the compression dressing anyway.

Test-Taking Strategy: Use the process of elimination. Recalling that excessive edema can form rapidly will direct you to option 2. Review care to the client after amputation if you had difficulty with this question.

Level of Cognitive Ability: Application
Client Needs: Physiological Integrity
Integrated Concept/Process: Nursing Process/Implementation
Content Area: Adult Health/Musculoskeletal
Reference: Ignatavicius, D., Workman, M., & Mishler, M. (1999). *Medical-surgical nursing across the health care continuum* (3rd ed.). Philadelphia: W. B. Saunders, p. 1304.

43. **3**

Rationale: Low back pain that radiates into one leg (sciatica) is consistent with herniated lumbar disc. The nurse assesses the client to see if the pain is aggravated either by events that increase intraspinal pressure, such as bending, lifting, sneezing, coughing, or by lifting the leg straight up while supine (straight leg raising test).

Test-Taking Strategy: Use the process of elimination. Recall that bed rest, heat (or sometimes ice), and nonsteroidal antiinflammatory agents usually relieve back pain, while bending, lifting, and straining aggravate it. Review the causes of back pain and the factors that alleviate or aggravate pain if you had difficulty with this question.

Level of Cognitive Ability: Application
Client Needs: Physiological Integrity
Integrated Concept/Process: Nursing Process/Assessment
Content Area: Adult Health/Musculoskeletal
Reference: Ignatavicius, D., Workman, M., & Mishler, M. (1999). *Medical-surgical nursing across the health care continuum* (3rd ed.). Philadelphia: W. B. Saunders, p. 1058.

44. **4**

Rationale: After spinal fusion, the head of bed is generally kept flat. The client is logrolled from side to side as ordered. Pillows may be placed under the entire length of the legs by surgeon preference to relieve tension on the lower back. The use of an overhead trapeze is contraindicated because its use could promote twisting of the spine after surgery.

Test-Taking Strategy: Use the process of elimination. Note the key word "avoid." After spinal surgery, the nurse utilizes positioning techniques and aids that will keep the spine in good alignment. Thus, options 1 and 3 are indicated. From the remaining options, recall that using pillows under the length of the legs promotes slight flexion of the spine, while avoiding pressure on the popliteal space (which predisposes to thrombophlebitis). Using an overbed trapeze could allow the client to twist the spine, which is directly contraindicated. Review care to the client after spinal fusion if you had difficulty with this question.

Level of Cognitive Ability: Application
Client Needs: Safe, Effective Care Environment
Integrated Concept/Process: Nursing Process/Implementation

Content Area: Adult Health/Musculoskeletal
Reference: Ignatavicius, D., Workman, M., & Mishler, M. (1999). *Medical-surgical nursing across the health care continuum* (3rd ed.). Philadelphia: W. B. Saunders, p. 1061.

45. **1**

Rationale: Clients are taught to get out of bed by sliding near the edge of the mattress. The client then rolls onto one side and pushes up from the bed using one or both arms. The back is kept straight and the legs are swung over the side. Increasing fluids and dietary fiber helps prevent straining at stool, thereby preventing increases in intraspinal pressure. Walking and swimming are excellent exercises for strengthening lower back muscles. Proper body mechanics includes bending at the knees, not the waist, to lift objects.

Test-Taking Strategy: Use the process of elimination. Note the key words "needs further instruction." Recall that the client with low back pain should avoid events that increase intraspinal pressure. This will direct you to option 1. Review client teaching about body mechanics if you had difficulty with this question.

Level of Cognitive Ability: Analysis
Client Needs: Health Promotion and Maintenance
Integrated Concept/Process: Teaching/Learning
Content Area: Adult Health/Musculoskeletal
Reference: Smeltzer, S., & Bare, B. (2000). *Brunner & Suddarth's textbook of medical-surgical nursing* (9th ed.). Philadelphia: Lippincott Williams & Wilkins, p. 1751.

46. **2**

Rationale: The nursing assessment conducted after spinal surgery is similar to that done after other surgical procedures. For this specific type of surgery, the nurse assesses the neurovascular status of the lower extremities, watches for signs and symptoms of infection, and inspects the surgical site for evidence of cerebrospinal fluid leakage (drainage is clear, tests positive for glucose). A mild temperature is expected after insertion of hardware, but a temperature of 101.6° F should be reported.

Test-Taking Strategy: Use the process of elimination. Note the key words "especially concerned." Thus, you are looking for the option that has the greatest deviation from normal. Options 1 and 4 are expected after surgery, and although the nurse tries to minimize discomfort, the client is likely to have some discomfort even with proper analgesic use. The words "old" and "outlined" in option 3 indicate that this is not a new occurrence. This leaves the temperature of 101.6°, which is excessive, and should be reported. Review the signs of complications following this surgical procedure if you had difficulty with this question.

Level of Cognitive Ability: Analysis
Client Needs: Physiological Integrity
Integrated Concept/Process: Nursing Process/Assessment
Content Area: Adult Health/Musculoskeletal
Reference: Ignatavicius, D., Workman, M., & Mishler, M. (1999). *Medical-surgical nursing across the health care continuum* (3rd ed.). Philadelphia: W. B. Saunders, p. 1067.

47. **1**

Rationale: The client experiences a Body Image Disturbance related to a change in the structure and function of the affected leg. There are no data in the question to support a diagnosis of (actual) Activity Intolerance or Social Isolation. The client does have an actual Impaired Physical Mobility because of the fixation device.

Test-Taking Strategy: Use the process of elimination. Note the key words "upset about the appearance." This should direct you to option 1. Review the defining characteristics for Body Image Disturbance if you had difficulty with this question.

Level of Cognitive Ability: Analysis
Client Needs: Psychosocial Integrity
Integrated Concept/Process: Nursing Process/Analysis
Content Area: Adult Health/Musculoskeletal
Reference: Johnson, M., Bulechek, G., Dochterman, J., Maas, M., & Moorhead, S. (2001). *Nursing diagnoses, outcomes, and interventions.* St. Louis: Mosby, p. 54.

48. **2**
Rationale: The part of the bed under an area in traction is usually elevated to aid in countertraction. For the client in Buck's extension traction (which is applied to a leg), the foot of the bed is elevated.

Test-Taking Strategy: Use the process of elimination. Recalling the principles of traction and countertraction will assist in eliminating option 3. Knowing that Buck's extension traction is applied to the leg helps to eliminate option 1. From the remaining options, option 4 places undue pressure on the client's unaffected foot. Furthermore, a footboard is not used for the purpose of providing countertraction. Review the principles of traction and countertraction if you had difficulty with this question.

Level of Cognitive Ability: Application
Client Needs: Physiological Integrity
Integrated Concept/Process: Nursing Process/Implementation
Content Area: Adult Health/Musculoskeletal
Reference: Ignatavicius, D., Workman, M., & Mishler, M. (1999). *Medical-surgical nursing across the health care continuum* (3rd ed.). Philadelphia: W. B. Saunders, p. 1289.

49. **1**
Rationale: In addition to the presence of clinical manifestations, gout is diagnosed by the presence of persistent hyperuricemia of greater than 7 mg/dL. Options 2, 3, and 4 all indicate normal laboratory values. Additionally, the presence of uric acid in an aspirated sample of synovial fluid confirms the diagnosis.

Test-Taking Strategy: Use the process of elimination and knowledge of normal laboratory values. Recalling that increased uric acid levels occur in gout and noting that option 1 is the only abnormal value will assist in answering the question. Review the manifestations of gout and the normal uric acid level if you had difficulty with this question.

Level of Cognitive Ability: Analysis
Client Needs: Physiological Integrity
Integrated Concept/Process: Nursing Process/Assessment
Content Area: Adult Health/Musculoskeletal

Reference: Smeltzer, S., & Bare, B. (2000). *Brunner & Suddarth's textbook of medical-surgical nursing* (9th ed.). Philadelphia: Lippincott Williams & Wilkins, p. 1430.

50. **3**
Rationale: The stiffness and joint pain that occur in osteoarthritis increase with lack of activity, are usually more severe in the morning, and may be aggravated by cold, damp weather. No specific laboratory findings are useful in diagnosing osteoarthritis. The client may have a normal or slightly elevated sedimentation rate. Dull aching pain occurs in the affected joints and, unlike rheumatoid arthritis, systemic manifestations are absent and joint involvement is not symmetric. Elevated white blood cell counts, platelet counts, and antinuclear antibodies occur in rheumatoid arthritis.

Test-Taking Strategy: Use the process of elimination and knowledge about the differences between osteoarthritis and rheumatoid arthritis to answer this question. Review the characteristics of osteoarthritis if you had difficulty with the question.

Level of Cognitive Ability: Analysis
Client Needs: Physiological Integrity
Integrated Concept/Process: Nursing Process/Assessment
Content Area: Adult Health/Musculoskeletal
Reference: Smeltzer, S., & Bare, B. (2000). *Brunner & Suddarth's textbook of medical-surgical nursing* (9th ed.). Philadelphia: Lippincott Williams & Wilkins, p. 1429.

CRITICAL THINKING: FREE-TEXT ENTRY

Answer: Contact the physician and report the findings
Rationale: The client with pallor, slow capillary refill, weakened or lost pulse, and absence of sensation or motion in the distal limb may have arterial damage from a lacerated, contused, thrombosed, or severed artery. These signs can occur with constriction from a tight cast as well. Regardless of the cause, the nurse notifies the physician immediately. Emergency intervention is needed, which could include removal of the constricting bandage, fracture reduction, or surgery to repair the area.

Test-Taking Strategy: Focus on the assessment data presented in the question. Recall that these signs indicate insufficient arterial circulation that can lead to irreversible ischemia and damage. The physician needs to be notified. Review the complications associated with a fracture of an extremity and the associated nursing interventions if you had difficulty with this question.

Level of Cognitive Ability: Application
Client Needs: Physiological Integrity
Integrated Concept/Process: Nursing Process/Implementation
Content Area: Adult Health/Musculoskeletal
Reference: Ignatavicius, D., Workman, M., & Mishler, M. (1999). *Medical-surgical nursing across the health care continuum* (3rd ed.). Philadelphia: W.B. Saunders, p. 1288.

REFERENCES

Fortinash, K., & Holoday-Worret, P. (2000). *Psychiatric mental health nursing* (2nd ed.). St. Louis: Mosby.

Hodgson, B., & Kizior, R. (2001). *Saunders nursing drug handbook 2001.* Philadelphia: W.B. Saunders.

Ignatavicius, D., Workman, M., & Mishler, M. (1999). *Medical-surgical nursing across the health care continuum* (3rd ed.). Philadelphia: W.B. Saunders.

Jarvis, C. (2000). *Physical examination and health assessment* (3rd ed.). Philadelphia: W.B. Saunders.

Johnson, M., Bulechek, G., Dochterman, J. Maas, M., Moorhead, S. (2001). *Nursing diagnoses, outcomes, and interventions.* St. Louis: Mosby.

Phipps, W., Sands, J., & Marek, J. (1999). *Medical-surgical nursing: Concepts & clinical practice* (6th ed.). St. Louis: Mosby.

Potter, P., & Perry, A. (2001). *Fundamentals of nursing* (5th ed.). St. Louis: Mosby.

Smeltzer, S., & Bare, B. (2000). *Brunner & Suddarth's textbook of medical-surgical nursing* (9th ed.). Philadelphia: Lippincott Williams & Wilkins.

Musculoskeletal Medications

I. SKELETAL MUSCLE RELAXANTS (Box 66-1)

A. Description
1. Act directly on the neuromuscular junction or indirectly on the central nervous system (CNS)
2. Centrally acting muscle relaxants depress neuron activity in the spinal cord or brain
3. Peripherally acting muscle relaxants act directly on the skeletal muscles
4. Used to prevent or relieve muscle spasms, to treat spasticity associated with spinal cord disease or lesions, for painful musculoskeletal conditions, and for chronic debilitating disorders, such as multiple sclerosis, cerebrovascular accident (CVA), or cerebral palsy
5. Contraindicated in severe liver, renal, or heart disease
6. Should not be taken with CNS depressants, such as barbiturates, narcotics, and alcohol; sedatives; hypnotics; or tricyclic antidepressants

B. Side effects
1. Dizziness and hypotension
2. Drowsiness
3. Dry mouth
4. Gastrointestinal (GI) upset
5. Photosensitivity
6. Liver toxicity

C. Implementation
1. Obtain a medical history
2. Monitor vital signs
3. Monitor for CNS side effects
4. Assess for risk of injury
5. Assess involved joints and muscles for pain and mobility
6. Monitor liver function tests because hepatotoxicity can occur
7. Monitor renal function studies
8. Instruct the client to take the medication with food to decrease GI upset

9. Instruct the client to report side effects
10. Instruct the client to avoid alcohol and CNS depressants
11. Instruct the client to avoid activities requiring alertness

D. Nursing considerations
1. Baclofen (Lioresal)
   a. Causes CNS effects such as drowsiness, dizziness, weakness, and fatigue
   b. Frequently causes nausea, constipation, and urinary retention
   c. Can be administered by the physician by intrathecal infusion using an implantable pump
2. Dantrolene (Dantrium)
   a. Acts directly on skeletal muscles to relieve spasticity
   b. Liver damage is the most serious adverse effect
   c. Liver function tests should be monitored prior to the initiation of treatment and during treatment
   d. Can cause GI bleeding, urinary frequency, impotence, photosensitivity, and rash

---

BOX 66-1

Skeletal Muscle Relaxants

Baclofen (Lioresal)
Carisoprodol (Soma, Vanadom)
Cyclobenzaprine (Flexeril, Cycoflex)
Dantrolene (Dantrium)
Diazepam (Valium)
Metaxalone (Skelaxin)
Methocarbamol (Robaxin, Carbacot, Skelex)
Orphenadrine (Norflex, Flexoject)
Chlorzoxazone (Paraflex, Parafon Forte, Relaxone)
Chlorphenesin (Maolate)
Tizanidine (Zanaflex)

c. Instruct the client to wear protective clothing when in the sun

f. Instruct the client to notify physician if rash, bloody or tarry stool, or yellow discoloration of the skin or eyes occurs

3. Cyclobenzaprine (Flexeril, Cycoflex)
   a. Contraindicated in clients who have received monoamine oxidase (MAO) inhibitors within 14 days of initiation of cyclobenzaprine therapy, and in clients with cardiac disorders
   b. Used with caution in clients with a history of urinary retention, angle-closure glaucoma, or increased intraocular pressure
   c. Should be used only for short term (2 to 3 weeks of therapy)
4. Methocarbamol (Robaxin, Carbocot, Skelex)
   a. Parenteral form is contraindicated in clients with renal impairment
   b. Parenteral form can cause hypotension, bradycardia, anaphylaxis, and seizures
   c. May cause urine to turn brown, black, or green
   d. Inform the client to notify the physician if blurred vision, nasal congestion, urticaria, or rash occurs
5. Chlorzoxazone (Paraflex, Parafon Forte, Relaxone)
   a. Monitor for hypersensitivity reactions such as urticaria, redness or itching, and possibly angioedema
   b. May cause malaise and urine discoloration
6. Carisoprodol (Soma, Vanadom)
   a. Advise the client to take the medication with food to prevent GI upset
   b. Instruct the client to report any rash or hypersensitivity to the physician

II. ANTIGOUT MEDICATIONS (Box 66-2)
A. Description
   1. Decrease inflammation
   2. Reduce uric acid production and increase uric acid excretion to prevent or relieve gout or to manage hyperuricemia
   3. Used cautiously in clients with GI, renal, cardiac, or hepatic disease
   4. Allopurinol (Lopurin, Zyloprim) can increase the effect of warfarin and oral hypoglycemic agents
B. Side effects
   1. Headaches
   2. Nausea, vomiting, and diarrhea
   3. Blood dyscrasias such as bone marrow depression
   4. Flushed skin and skin rash
   5. Uric acid kidney stones
   6. Sore gums
   7. Metallic taste
C. Implementation
   1. Assess serum uric acid levels

BOX 66-2
Antigout Medications

Allopurinol (Lopurin, Zyloprim)
Colchicine
Probenecid (Benemid)
Sulfinpyrazone (Anturane)

---

2. Monitor intake and output (I & O)
3. Maintain a fluid intake of at least 2000 to 3000 mL a day to avoid kidney stones
4. Monitor complete blood cell count (CBC) and renal and liver function studies
5. Instruct the client to avoid alcohol and caffeine because these products can increase uric acid levels
6. Instruct the client not to take large doses of vitamin C while taking allopurinol (Zyloprim) because kidney stones may occur
7. Encourage the client to comply with therapy to prevent elevated uric acid levels, which can trigger a gout attack
8. Instruct the client to avoid foods high in purine, such as wine, alcohol, organ meats, sardines, salmon, and gravy
9. Instruct the client to take the medication with food
10. Instruct the client to report side effects to the physician
11. Advise the client to have a yearly eye examination because visual changes can occur from prolonged use of allopurinol
12. Caution the client not to take aspirin with these medications because this could trigger a gout attack
13. Concurrent use of aspirin causes elevated uric acid levels; the client should be instructed to take acetaminophen (Tylenol)

III. ANTIARTHRITIC MEDICATIONS (Box 66-3)
A. Nonsteroidal antiinflammatory medications (NSAIDs) (refer to Chapter 64)
B. Gold therapy
   1. Description
      a. Referred to as chrysotherapy or heavy-metal therapy
      b. Depresses migration of leukocytes and suppresses prostaglandin activity
      c. Reduces inflammation by decreasing enzyme release and altering the immune response
      d. Primarily used for palliative relief of symptoms in rheumatoid arthritis
      e. Contraindications are listed in Box 66-4
   2. Side effects
      a. Dizziness
      b. Urticaria and rash

BOX 66-3

Antiarthritic Medications

Auranofin (Ridura)
Aurothioglucose (Solganal)
Azathioprine (Imuran)
Gold sodium thiomalate (Myochrysine)
Hydroxychloroquine sulfate (Plaquenil)
Methotrexate (Rheumatrex)
Penicillamine (Cuprimine)
Sulfasalazine (Azulfidine)

BOX 66-4

Contraindications to Gold Therapy

Eczema
Urticaria
Colitis
Hemorrhagic conditions
Systemic lupus erythematosus
Renal or hepatic dysfunction
Uncontrolled diabetes mellitus
Congestive heart failure
Recent radiation therapy

    c. Erythema and dermatitis
    d. Alopecia
    e. Stomatitis
    f. Diarrhea
    g. Hepatitis
    h. Metallic taste in the mouth
    i. Blood dyscrasias such as bone marrow suppression
    j. Photosensitivity reactions
    k. Gold toxicity
  3. Implementation
    a. Obtain the client's medical history
    b. Monitor for blood dyscrasias before and during therapy
    c. Monitor for proteinuria and hematuria before and during therapy
    d. When administering the gold injection, monitor the client for 30 minutes after injection for possible allergic reaction
    e. Instruct the client to maintain good oral hygiene
    f. Instruct the client to use sunscreen and protective clothing to prevent photosensitivity reactions
    g. Teach the client about the signs and symptoms of gold toxicity, which include pruritis, skin rash, metallic taste, stomatitis, and diarrhea
    h. If toxicity occurs, dimercaprol (BAL in oil) may be prescribed to enhance gold excretion

PRACTICE QUESTIONS

1. Allopurinol (Zyloprim) has been prescribed for a client. The nurse prepares to administer this medication knowing that which of the following information is accurate about this medication?
   1. It is used for the lysis of thrombi obstructing coronary arteries
   2. It prevents calcium ion entry across cell membranes of the cardiac smooth muscle
   3. It decreases sympathetic outflow from the central nervous system
   4. It decreases uric acid production and reduces uric acid concentrations in both the serum and urine

2. A community health nurse visits a client at home. The client is taking allopurinol (Zyloprim) 400 mg PO daily. The nurse instructs the client:
   1. That the effect of the medication will occur immediately
   2. To drink 3000 mL of fluid per day
   3. To take medication on an empty stomach
   4. That if swelling of the lips occurs, this is a normal expected response

3. Colchicine is prescribed for a client with a diagnosis of gout. The nurse reviews the client's record knowing that this medication would be contraindicated in which of the following disorders?
   1. Renal failure
   2. Hypothyroidism
   3. Diabetes mellitus
   4. Myxedema

4. A home health nurse is caring for a client who is taking probenecid (Benemid). The client has been instructed to restrict the diet to low-purine foods. Which of the following foods would the nurse instruct the client to avoid?
   1. Potatoes
   2. Ice cream
   3. Spinach
   4. Scallops

5. A physician prescribes auranofin (Ridaura) for a client with rheumatoid arthritis. Which of the following would indicate to the nurse that the client is experiencing toxicity related to the medication?
   1. Constipation
   2. A metallic taste in the mouth
   3. Ringing in the ears
   4. Joint pain

6. Diclofenac (Voltaren) is prescribed for a client with osteoarthritis. Which of the following medications, if noted on the client's record, would alert the nurse to consult with the physician?
   1. Warfarin sodium (Coumadin)
   2. Mesoridazine besylate (Serentil)
   3. Primidone (Mysoline)
   4. Trifluoperazine hydrochloride (Stelazine)

7. A film-coated form of diflunisal (Dolobid) has been prescribed for a client for the treatment of chronic

rheumatoid arthritis. The client calls the clinic nurse because of difficulty swallowing the tablets. Which of the following instructions would the nurse provide to the client?
1. Crush the tablets and mix with food
2. Open the tablet and mix the contents with food
3. Swallow the tablets with large amounts of water or milk
4. Notify the physician for a medication change

8. Baclofen (Lioresal) is prescribed for a client with multiple sclerosis. The nurse monitors the client, knowing that the primary therapeutic effect of this medication is which of the following?
1. Increased muscle tone
2. Decreased muscle spasms
3. Decreased local pain and tenderness
4. Increased range of motion

9. A nurse is monitoring a client receiving baclofen (Lioresal) for side effects related to the medication. Which of the following would indicate that the client is experiencing a side effect?
1. Drowsiness
2. Diarrhea
3. Polyuria
4. Muscular excitability

10. A nurse is providing discharge instructions to a client receiving baclofen (Lioresal). Which of the following would be included in the teaching plan?
1. Restrict fluid intake
2. Avoid the use of alcohol
3. Stop the medication if diarrhea occurs
4. Notify the physician if fatigue occurs

11. An adult client with muscle spasms is taking an oral maintenance dose of baclofen (Lioresal). Which of the following represents a safe maintenance dose for this medication?
1. 15 mg qid
2. 25 mg qid
3. 30 mg qid
4. 40 mg qid

12. A client with acute muscle spasms has been taking baclofen (Lioresal). The client calls the clinic nurse because of continuous feelings of weakness and fatigue and asks the nurse about discontinuing the medication. Which of the following responses to the client would be most appropriate?
1. "It is best that you taper the dose if you intend to stop the medication."
2. "Weakness and fatigue commonly occur and will diminish with continued medication use."
3. "It is all right to stop the medication if you think that you can tolerate the muscle spasms."
4. "You should never stop the medication."

13. Dantrolene sodium (Dantrium) is prescribed for the client experiencing flexor spasms. The nurse monitors the client, knowing that which of the following is the therapeutic action of this medication?
1. Acts within the spinal cord to suppress hyperactive reflexes
2. Acts on the central nervous system (CNS) to suppress spasms
3. Acts directly on the skeletal muscle to relieve spasticity
4. Depresses spinal reflexes

14. A nurse is analyzing the laboratory studies on a client receiving dantrolene sodium (Dantrium). Which of the following laboratory tests would identify an adverse effect associated with the administration of this medication?
1. Blood urea nitrogen
2. Creatinine
3. Liver function tests
4. Platelet count

15. A physician is planning to administer a skeletal muscle relaxant to a client with a spinal cord injury. The medication is going to be administered intrathecally (within the spinal column). Which of the following medications would the nurse expect to be prescribed and administered by this route?
1. Cyclobenzaprine hydrochloride (Flexeril)
2. Chlorzoxazone (Paraflex)
3. Dantrolene sodium (Dantrium)
4. Baclofen (Lioresal)

16. A nurse is reviewing the record of a client who has been prescribed baclofen (Lioresal). Which of the following disorders, if noted in the client's history, would alert the nurse to contact the physician?
1. Coronary artery disease
2. Diabetes mellitus
3. Seizure disorders
4. Hyperthyroidism

17. Cyclobenzaprine hydrochloride (Flexeril) is prescribed for a client for muscle spasms. The nurse is reviewing the client's record. Which of the following disorders, if noted in the record, would indicate a need to contact the physician about the administration of this medication?
1. Glaucoma
2. Hypothyroidism
3. Emphysema
4. Diabetes mellitus

18. A client is to receive a prescription for methocarbamol (Robaxin). The nurse provides instructions to the client about the medication. Which of the following client statements would indicate a need for further education?
1. "My urine may turn brown or green."
2. "If my vision becomes blurred I don't need to be concerned about it."
3. "I might get some nasal congestion from this medication."

4. "This medication is prescribed to help relieve my muscle spasms."

19. A nurse is administering an IV dose of methocarbamol (Robaxin) to a client with multiple sclerosis. Which of the following adverse effects would the nurse monitor for?
   1. Hypertension
   2. Tachycardia
   3. Rapid pulse
   4. Bradycardia

20. A nurse is reviewing a physician's orders for an adult client who has been admitted to the hospital following a back injury. Carisoprodol (Soma) is prescribed for the client to relieve the muscle spasms. The physician has prescribed 350 mg to be administered qid. The nurse determines that this dosage is:
   1. The normal adult dosage

2. A lower than normal dosage
3. A higher than normal dosage
4. A dosage requiring further clarification

CRITICAL THINKING: FREE-TEXT ENTRY

A nurse is caring for a hospitalized client who is taking allopurinol (Zyloprim) for a history of gout. The nurse reviews the physician's orders and notes that the physician has prescribed the following medications: pentazocine (Talwin), warfarin sodium (Coumadin), and ergonovine maleate (Ergotrate). Which of these prescribed medications would the nurse question?

Answer: _____

ANSWERS

1. 4
Rationale: Allopurinol (Zyloprim) is an antigout medication. It decreases uric acid production by inhibiting xanthine oxidase, an enzyme, and reduces uric acid concentrations in both serum and urine.
Test-Taking Strategy: Use the process of elimination. Note that options 1 and 2 are similar in that they both address a cardiac situation. Knowledge that this medication is in the antigout classification will assist in directing you to the correct option. If you had difficulty with this question, review the action of allopurinol (Zyloprim).
Level of Cognitive Ability: Analysis
Client Needs: Physiological Integrity
Integrated Concept/Process: Nursing Process/Planning
Content Area: Pharmacology
Reference: Hodgson, B., & Kizior, R. (2001). *Saunders nursing drug handbook 2001.* Philadelphia: W. B. Saunders, p. 24.

2. 2
Rationale: Clients taking allopurinol are encouraged to drink 3000 mL of fluid a day. A full therapeutic effect may take 1 or more weeks. Allopurinol is to be given with, or immediately after, meals or milk. A client who develops a rash, irritation of the eyes, or swelling of the lips or mouth should contact the physician, because this may indicate hypersensitivity.
Test-Taking Strategy: Use the process of elimination. Option 4 can be easily eliminated because it indicates hypersensitivity, which is not a normal expected response. From the remaining options, recalling that this medication is used to treat gout will direct you to option 2. If you had difficulty with this question, review the client instructions related to allopurinol.
Level of Cognitive Ability: Analysis
Client Needs: Health Promotion and Maintenance
Integrated Concept/Process: Teaching/Learning
Content Area: Pharmacology
Reference: Hodgson, B., & Kizior, R. (2001). *Saunders nursing drug handbook 2001.* Philadelphia: W. B. Saunders, p. 25.

3. 1
Rationale: Colchicine is contraindicated in severe gastrointestinal, renal, hepatic, or cardiac disorders, and in clients with blood dyscrasias. Clients with impaired renal function may exhibit myopathy and neuropathy manifested as generalized weakness. This medication should be used with caution in clients with impaired hepatic function, the elderly, and the debilitated.
Test-Taking Strategy: Use the process of elimination. Note that options 2, 3, and 4 are all endocrine-related disorders. Option 1, the correct option, is different from the others. Review the contraindications associated with this medication if you had difficulty with this question.
Level of Cognitive Ability: Analysis
Client Needs: Physiological Integrity
Integrated Concept/Process: Nursing Process/Analysis
Content Area: Pharmacology
Reference: Salerno, E. (1999). *Pharmacology for health professionals.* St. Louis: Mosby, p. 434.

4. 4
Rationale: Uric acid is produced when purine is catabolized. Probenecid is a medication used for clients with gout to inhibit the reabsorption of uric acid by the kidney and promote excretion of uric acid in the urine. Clients are instructed to modify their diets and limit excessive purine intake. High-purine foods to avoid or limit include organ meats, roe, sardines, scallops, anchovies, broth, mincemeat, herring, shrimp, mackerel, gravy, and yeast.
Test-Taking Strategy: Use the process of elimination. Options 1 and 3 are high-nutrient foods, so eliminate these options first. From this point, use your knowledge about the purpose of the medication, the treatment for gout, and food sources high in purine to select the correct option. If you had difficulty with this question, review foods that are high in purine.
Level of Cognitive Ability: Application
Client Needs: Health Promotion and Maintenance
Integrated Concept/Process: Teaching/Learning

Content Area: Pharmacology
Reference: Clark, J., Queener, S., & Karb, V. (2000). *Pharmacologic basis of nursing practice* (6th ed.). St. Louis: Mosby, p. 375.

5. 2
Rationale: Auranofin is the one gold preparation that is given orally rather than by injection. Gastrointestinal reactions including diarrhea, abdominal pain, nausea, and loss of appetite are common early in therapy, but usually subside in the first 3 months. Early symptoms of toxic reactions include a rash, purple blotches, pruritus, mouth lesions and a metallic taste in the mouth.
Test-Taking Strategy: Recalling that auranofin is a gold preparation will assist you in answering the question. Noting that the question is asking for a toxic effect will direct you to option 2. Remember, gold is a metal. If you had difficulty with this question, review toxicity related to gold compounds.
Level of Cognitive Ability: Analysis
Client Needs: Physiological Integrity
Integrated Concept/Process: Nursing Process/Assessment
Content Area: Pharmacology
Reference: Salerno, E. (1999). *Pharmacology for health professionals.* St. Louis: Mosby, p. 150.

6. 1
Rationale: Voltaren is a nonsteroidal antiinflammatory drug (NSAID). Interactions may occur with anticoagulants. The nurse should consult with the physician about a potential medication interaction. Serentil is an antipsychotic medication. Mysoline is an anticonvulsant, and Stelazine is an antipsychotic. These medications are not contraindicated when administering diclofenac.
Test-Taking Strategy: Use the process of elimination. Recall that diclofenac is an NSAID and knowledge of the adverse reactions related to these medications will direct you to option 1. Review the contraindications associated with this medication if you had difficulty with this question.
Level of Cognitive Ability: Analysis
Client Needs: Physiological Integrity
Integrated Concept/Process: Nursing Process/Analysis
Content Area: Pharmacology
Reference: Monahan, F., & Neighbors, M. (1998). *Medical-surgical nursing: Foundations for clinical practice* (2nd ed.). Philadelphia: W. B. Saunders, p. 893.

7. 3
Rationale: Dolobid may be given with water, milk, or meals. The tablets should not be crushed or broken open.
Test-Taking Strategy: Use the process of elimination. Eliminate option 4 first as the least likely option. Note the words "film coated" to eliminate options 1 and 2. Additionally, these options are similar in that they both suggest breaking the tablets. If you had difficulty with this question, review the procedure for administration.
Level of Cognitive Ability: Application
Client Needs: Health Promotion and Maintenance
Integrated Concept/Process: Teaching/Learning
Content Area: Pharmacology
Reference: Hodgson, B., & Kizior, R. (2001). *Saunders nursing drug handbook 2001.* Philadelphia: W. B. Saunders, p. 322.

8. 2
Rationale: Baclofen is a skeletal muscle relaxant and acts at the spinal cord level to decrease the frequency and amplitude of muscle spasms in clients with spinal cord injuries or diseases, and multiple sclerosis.
Test-Taking Strategy: Use the process of elimination. Knowledge that this medication is a skeletal muscle relaxant will easily direct you to option 2. Review this medication if you had difficulty with this question.
Level of Cognitive Ability: Analysis
Client Needs: Physiological Integrity
Integrated Concept/Process: Nursing Process/Assessment
Content Area: Pharmacology
Reference: Cleveland, L., Aschenbrenner, D., Venable, S., & Yensen, J. (1999). *Nursing management in drug therapy.* Philadelphia: Lippincott, p. 372.

9. 1
Rationale: Baclofen is a central nervous system (CNS) depressant and frequently causes drowsiness, dizziness, weakness, and fatigue. It can also cause nausea, constipation, and urinary retention. Clients should be warned about the possible reactions.
Test-Taking Strategy: Use the process of elimination. Knowledge that baclofen is a CNS depressant used to treat muscle spasticity will easily direct you to option 1. If you had difficulty with this question, review the side effects of this medication.
Level of Cognitive Ability: Analysis
Client Needs: Physiological Integrity
Integrated Concept/Process: Nursing Process/Assessment
Content Area: Pharmacology
Reference: Cleveland, L., Aschenbrenner, D., Venable, S., & Yensen, J. (1999). *Nursing management in drug therapy.* Philadelphia: Lippincott, p. 373.

10. 2
Rationale: Baclofen is a central nervous system (CNS) depressant. The client should be cautioned against the use of alcohol and other CNS depressants, because baclofen potentiates the depressant activity of these agents. Constipation rather than diarrhea is an adverse effect. It is not necessary to restrict fluids, but the client should be warned that urinary retention can occur. Fatigue is related to a CNS effect that is most intense during the early phase of therapy and diminishes with continued medication use. It is not necessary that the client notify the physician.
Test-Taking Strategy: Use the process of elimination. Knowledge that baclofen is a CNS depressant will easily direct you to option 2. If you were unsure of the correct option, use general principles related to medication administration. Alcohol should be avoided with the use of many medications. Review client teaching points related to this medication if you had difficulty with this question.
Level of Cognitive Ability: Application
Client Needs: Health Promotion and Maintenance
Integrated Concept/Process: Teaching/Learning
Content Area: Pharmacology
Reference: Cleveland, L., Aschenbrenner, D., Venable, S., & Yensen, J. (1999). *Nursing management in drug therapy.* Philadelphia: Lippincott, p. 374.

11. 1
Rationale: Baclofen is dispensed in tablets of 10 and 20 mg for oral use. Dosages are low initially and then gradually increased. Maintenance doses range from 15 to 20 mg administered 3 to 4 times a day.

Test-Taking Strategy: Knowledge about the normal adult maintenance dosage is required to answer this question. This may be a difficult question and if you are unfamiliar with this maintenance dosage, review this content.
Level of Cognitive Ability: Analysis
Client Needs: Physiological Integrity
Integrated Concept/Process: Nursing Process/Analysis
Content Area: Pharmacology
Reference: Lehne, R. (1998). *Pharmacology for nursing care* (3rd ed.). Philadelphia: W. B. Saunders. pp. 222-223.

12. **2**
Rationale: The client should be instructed that symptoms such as drowsiness, weakness, and fatigue are more intense in the early phase of therapy and diminish with continued medication use. The client should be instructed never to abruptly withdraw or stop the medication because abrupt withdrawal can cause visual hallucinations, paranoid ideation, and seizures. It is best for the nurse to inform the client that these symptoms will subside and encourage the client to continue the use of the medication.
Test-Taking Strategy: Use the process of elimination. Note the key words "most appropriate." Eliminate option 4 first because, it is a rather extreme nursing response. Next, eliminate options 1 and 3 because these responses do not represent the scope of nursing practice. Review the effects of this medication if you had difficulty with this question.
Level of Cognitive Ability: Application
Client Needs: Health Promotion and Maintenance
Integrated Concept/Process: Teaching/Learning
Content Area: Pharmacology
Reference: Hodgson, B., & Kizior, R. (2001). *Saunders nursing drug handbook 2001*. Philadelphia: W. B. Saunders, p. 96.

13. **3**
Rationale: Dantrium acts directly on skeletal muscle to relieve muscle spasticity. The primary action is the suppression of calcium release from the sarcoplasmic reticulum. This in turn decreases the ability of the skeletal muscle to contract.
Test-Taking Strategy: Use the process of elimination. Options 1, 2, and 4 are all similar in that they address the CNS and the depression of reflexes. Therefore, eliminate these options. Review the action of medication if you had difficulty with this question.
Level of Cognitive Ability: Analysis
Client Needs: Physiological Integrity
Integrated Concept/Process: Nursing Process/Assessment
Content Area: Pharmacology
Reference: Salerno, E. (1999). *Pharmacology for health professionals*. St. Louis: Mosby, p. 304.

14. **3**
Rationale: Dose-related liver damage is the most serious adverse effect of dantrolene. To reduce the risk of liver damage, tests of liver function should be performed prior to treatment and throughout the treatment interval. It is administered in the lowest effective dosage for the shortest time necessary.
Test-Taking Strategy: Use the process of elimination. Eliminate options 1 and 2 because these tests both assess kidney function. From the remaining options, it is necessary to recall that this medication affects liver function. Review this medication if you had difficulty with this question.
Level of Cognitive Ability: Analysis

Client Needs: Physiological Integrity
Integrated Concept/Process: Nursing Process/Analysis
Content Area: Pharmacology
Reference: Wilson, B., Shannon, M., & Stang, C. (2000). *Nurses drug guide 2000*. Stamford, Conn.: Appleton & Lange, p. 402.

15. **4**
Rationale: Baclofen is the only skeletal muscle relaxant that can be administered intrathecally within the spinal column.
Test-Taking Strategy: Knowledge about intrathecal administration of muscle relaxants is required to answer this question. If you are unfamiliar with this form of therapy, review this content.
Level of Cognitive Ability: Analysis
Client Needs: Physiological Integrity
Integrated Concept/Process: Nursing Process/Analysis
Content Area: Pharmacology
Reference: Clark, J., Queener, S., & Karb, V. (2000). *Pharmacologic basis of nursing practice* (6th ed.). St. Louis: Mosby, p. 750.

16. **3**
Rationale: Clients with seizure disorders may have a lowered seizure threshold when baclofen is administered. Concurrent therapy may require an increase in the anticonvulsive medication.
Test-Taking Strategy: Use the process of elimination and knowledge about the contraindications and the cautions associated with the administration of baclofen. If you are unfamiliar with these contraindications and cautions, review this content.
Level of Cognitive Ability: Analysis
Client Needs: Physiological Integrity
Integrated Concept/Process: Nursing Process/Analysis
Content Area: Pharmacology
Reference: Wilson, B., Shannon, M., & Stang, C. (2000). *Nurses drug guide 2000*. Stamford, Conn.: Appleton & Lange, p. 131.

17. **1**
Rationale: Because this medication has anticholinergic effects, it should be used with caution in clients with a history of urinary retention, glaucoma, and increased intraocular pressure. Flexeril should be used only for a short term 2 to 3 week period.
Test-Taking Strategy: Use the process of elimination. Knowledge that this medication has anticholinergic effects will direct you to option 1. If you are unfamiliar with this medication and the contraindications associated with its administration, review this content.
Level of Cognitive Ability: Analysis
Client Needs: Physiological Integrity
Integrated Concept/Process: Nursing Process/Analysis
Content Area: Pharmacology
Reference: Clark, J., Queener, S., & Karb, V. (2000). *Pharmacologic basis of nursing practice* (6th ed.). St. Louis: Mosby, p. 753.

18. **2**
Rationale: The client needs to be told that the urine may turn brown, black, or green. Other adverse effects include blurred vision, nasal congestion, urticaria, and rash. The client needs to be instructed that if these adverse effects occur the physician needs to be notified.
Test-Taking Strategy: Use the process of elimination. Note the key words "need for further education." This will assist in directing you to option 2. If you had difficulty with this question, review this medication.

Level of Cognitive Ability: Analysis
Client Needs: Health Promotion and Maintenance
Integrated Concept/Process: Teaching/Learning
Content Area: Pharmacology
Reference: Wilson, B., Shannon, M., & Stang, C. (2000). *Nurses drug guide 2000*. Stamford, Conn.: Appleton & Lange, p. 884.

19. **4**
Rationale: Intravenous administration of methocarbamol can cause hypotension and bradycardia. The nurse needs to monitor for these side effects.
Test-Taking Strategy: Use the process of elimination. Eliminate options 2 and 3 first because they are similar. Knowledge about the specific side effects related to the IV use of this medication will direct you to option 4. Review this medication if you had difficulty with this question!
Level of Cognitive Ability: Analysis
Client Needs: Physiological Integrity
Integrated Concept/Process: Nursing Process/Assessment
Content Area: Pharmacology
Reference: Wilson, B., Shannon, M., & Stang, C. (2000). *Nurses drug guide 2000*. Stamford, Conn.: Appleton & Lange, p. 883.

20. **1**
Rationale: The normal adult dosage for Soma is 350 mg po 3 to 4 times daily.
Test-Taking Strategy: Use the process of elimination. This question may be difficult if you are not familiar with the normal medication dosage. Review this medication if you had difficulty with this question.
Level of Cognitive Ability: Analysis
Client Needs: Physiological Integrity
Integrated Concept/Process: Nursing Process/Analysis
Content Area: Pharmacology
Reference: Hodgson, B., & Kizior, R. (2001). *Saunders nursing drug handbook 2001*. Philadelphia: W. B. Saunders, p. 1187.

CRITICAL THINKING: FREE-TEXT ENTRY

Answer: Warfarin sodium (Coumadin)
Rationale: Allopurinol is an antigout medication that may increase the effects of oral anticoagulants. Warfarin sodium is an anticoagulant, and if this medication was prescribed for the client, the nurse would verify the order. Ergonovine maleate is an antimigraine medication. Pentazocine is an opioid analgesic.
Test-Taking Strategy: Recalling the interactive effect between allopurinol and warfarin sodium will assist in answering the question. If you had difficulty with this question, review the medication interactions associated with this medication.
Level of Cognitive Ability: Analysis
Client Needs: Safe, Effective Care Environment
Integrated Concept/Process: Nursing Process/Implementation
Content Area: Pharmacology
Reference: Hodgson, B., & Kizior, R. (2001). *Saunders nursing drug handbook 2001*. Philadelphia: W.B. Saunders, p. 25.

REFERENCES

Clark, J., Queener, S., & Karb, V. (2000). *Pharmacologic basis of nursing practice* (6th ed.). St. Louis: Mosby.

Cleveland, L., Aschenbrenner, D., Venable, S., & Yensen, J. (1999). *Nursing management in drug therapy*. Philadelphia: Lippincott.

Hodgson, B., & Kizior, R. (2001). *Saunders nursing drug handbook 2001*. Philadelphia: W.B. Saunders.

Ignatavicius, D., Workman, M., & Mishler, M. (1999). *Medical-surgical nursing across the health care continuum* (3rd ed.). Philadelphia: W.B. Saunders.

Karch, A. (2000). *Focus on nursing pharmacology*. Philadelphia: Lippincott.

Lehne, R. (1998). *Pharmacology for nursing care* (3rd ed.). Philadelphia: W.B. Saunders.

Monahan, F., & Neighbors, M. (1998). *Medical-surgical nursing: Foundations for clinical practice* (2nd ed.). Philadelphia: W.B. Saunders.

Salerno, E. (1999). *Pharmacology for health professionals*. St. Louis: Mosby.

Wilson, B., Shannon, M., & Stang, C. (2000). *Nurses drug guide 2000*. Stamford, Conn.: Appleton & Lange.

The Adult Client with an Immune Disorder

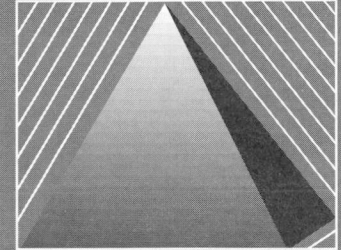

PYRAMID TERMS

acquired immunity   Received passively from the mother's antibodies, animal serum, or the production of antibodies in response to a disease. Immunization produces active acquired immunity.

allergy   An abnormal, individual response to certain substances that normally do not trigger such an exaggerated reaction.

cellular response   A delayed response; also called delayed hypersensitivity. Active against slowly developing bacterial infections.

humoral response   An immediate response that provides protection against acute, rapidly developing bacterial and viral infections.

immune deficiency   The absence or inadequate production of immune bodies.

natural immunity   Also called innate immunity. Is present at birth.

▶ PYRAMID TO SUCCESS

Pyramid points focus on the effects of and complications associated with an immune deficiency. Specific focus relates to the nursing care related to the disorder, the impact of the treatment or disorder, and client adaptation. Acquired immunodeficiency syndrome is a pyramid focus, along with protecting the client from infection, and preventing the transmission of infection to other individuals. Psychosocial issues relate to social isolation and the body image disturbances that can occur as a result of an immune disorder. The Integrated Concepts and Processes addressed in this unit include Nursing Process, Caring, Communication and Documentation, Cultural Awareness, Self-Care, and Teaching/Learning.

CLIENT NEEDS

Safe, Effective Care Environment

Advance directives
Advocacy related to client's decisions
Asepsis
Client rights
Confidentiality regarding diagnosis
Consultation with members of the health care team
Establishing priorities
Handling hazardous and infectious materials
Informed consent for treatments and procedures
Standard (universal) and protective precautions

Health Promotion and Maintenance

Client lifestyle choices
Expected body image changes
Health promotion programs
Health screening measures
Immunizations
Prevention of disease related to infection

Psychosocial Integrity

Ability to cope, adapt, and/or problem solve during illness or stressful events
Assisting in mobilizing appropriate support and resource systems
Assisting the client and family to cope
Grief and loss related to death and the dying process
Promoting a positive environment to maintain optimal quality of life
Religious, spiritual, and cultural preferences

Physiological Integrity

Diagnostic tests and laboratory values

Managing pain

Medical emergencies

Monitoring for the expected and unexpected responses
  to treatments

Promoting nutrition

Protecting the client from the infection

Providing basic care and comfort

REFERENCES

Craven, R., & Hirnle, C. (2000). *Fundamentals of nursing: Human health and function* (3rd ed.). Philadelphia: Lippincott.

Harkreader, H. (2000). *Fundamentals of nursing: Caring and clinical judgment*. Philadelphia: W.B. Saunders.

Ignatavicius, D., Workman, M., & Mishler, M. (1999). *Medical-surgical nursing: Across the health care continuum* (3rd ed.). Philadelphia: W.B. Saunders.

LeMone, P., & Burke, K. (2000). *Medical-surgical nursing: Critical thinking in client care* (2nd ed.). Upper Saddle River, N.J.: Prentice-Hall.

Lewis, S., Heitkemper, M., & Dirksen, S. (2000). *Medical-surgical nursing: Assessment and management of clinical problems* (5th ed.). St. Louis: Mosby.

National Council of State Boards of Nursing (eds.) (2000). *Test Plan for the National Council Licensure Examination for Registered Nurses.* Chicago: Author.

Potter, P., & Perry, A. (2001). *Fundamentals of nursing* (5th ed.). St. Louis: Mosby.

Smeltzer, S., & Bare, B. (2000). *Textbook of medical-surgical nursing* (9th ed.). Philadelphia: Lippincott Williams & Wilkins.

Immune Disorders

I. FUNCTIONS OF THE IMMUNE SYSTEM
A. Provides protection against invasion from outside the body, such as from microorganisms
B. Protects the body from internal threats
C. Maintains the internal environment by removing dead or damaged cells

II. IMMUNE RESPONSE
A. T lymphocytes and B lymphocytes
  1. Migrate to lymphoid tissue, where they wait to form either sensitized lymphocytes for **cellular** immunity or antibodies for **humoral** immunity
  2. Some B lymphocytes lie dormant until a specific antigen enters the body, at which time they greatly increase in number and are available for defense
  3. T lymphocytes are responsible for rejection of transplanted tissue
  4. Both T and B lymphocytes are necessary for a normal immune response
B. **Humoral response**
  1. An immediate response
  2. Provides protection against acute, rapidly developing bacterial and viral infections
C. **Cellular response**
  1. A delayed response; also called delayed hypersensitivity
  2. Active against slowly developing bacterial infections
  3. Also involved in autoimmune response, some allergic reactions, and rejection of foreign cells

▲ III. IMMUNITY
A. **Natural immunity**
  1. Also called innate immunity
  2. Present at birth
B. **Acquired immunity**
  1. Received passively from the mother's antibodies, animal serum, or the production of antibodies in response to a disease
  2. Immunization produces active **acquired immunity**

IV. IMMUNIZATIONS (Refer to Chapter 45)

V. LABORATORY STUDIES
A. Antinuclear antibody (ANA)
  1. A blood test used in the differential diagnosis of rheumatic diseases, and to detect antinucleoprotein factors and patterns associated with certain autoimmune diseases
  2. Positive at a titer of 1:20 or 1:40, depending on the laboratory
  3. A positive result does not necessarily confirm a disease
B. Anti-dsDNA antibody test
  1. A blood test done specifically to identify or differentiate DNA antibodies found in systemic lupus erythematosus (SLE) or other rheumatic diseases
  2. Supports a diagnosis, monitors disease activity and response to therapy, and establishes a prognosis for systemic lupus erythematosus (SLE)
  3. Values
    a. Negative: Less than 70 units by ELISA
    b. Borderline: 70 to 200 units
    c. Positive: More than 200 units
C. Refer to Chapter 10 for testing related to acquired immunodeficiency syndrome (AIDS)

VI. IMMUNE DEFICIENCY
A. Description
  1. Absence or inadequate production of immune bodies
  2. Can be congenital (primary) or acquired (secondary)
  3. Treatment depends on the inadequacy of immune bodies and its primary cause

B. Assessment
1. Factors that decrease immune function
2. Frequent infections
3. Nutritional status
4. Medication history such as corticosteroids
5. History of alcohol or drug abuse
C. Implementation
1. Protect from infection
2. Promote balanced, adequate nutrition
3. Use strict aseptic technique for all procedures
4. Provide psychosocial care regarding lifestyle changes and role changes
5. Instruct the client in measures to prevent infection

▲ VII. HYPERSENSITIVITY AND ALLERGY
A. Description
1. An **allergy** is an abnormal, individual response to certain substances that normally do not trigger such an exaggerated reaction
2. In most types of allergies, a reaction occurs only on second and subsequent contacts with the allergen
3. Skin testing may be done to determine the allergen
B. Assessment
1. History of exposure to allergens
2. Itching, tearing, and burning of eyes
3. Itching and burning of the skin
4. Rashes
5. Nose twitching, nasal stuffiness
C. Implementation
1. Identification of the specific allergen
2. Managing the symptoms with the use of antihistamines, antiinflammatory agents, or corticosteroids
3. Salves, wet compresses, and soothing baths for local reactions
4. Desensitization programs

▲ VIII. ANAPHYLAXIS
A. Description
1. A serious and dramatic allergic reaction, with the release of histamine from the damaged cells
2. Can cause shock and death if not treated immediately
B. Assessment
1. Identification of allergies
2. Difficulty breathing
3. Difficulty swallowing
4. Complaints of a swollen tongue
5. Facial edema and swelling of the lips
6. Skin redness
7. Presence of a rash
C. Implementation
1. Establish a patent airway
2. Prepare for the administration of epinephrine

(Adrenalin), diphenhydramine hydrochloride (Benadryl), or corticosteroids
3. Provide measures to control shock
4. Provide emotional support
5. Instruct the client to wear a Medic-Alert bracelet
6. Instruct the client in the use of prescribed medication for immediate treatment of a reaction

IX. LATEX ALLERGY
A. Description
1. A hypersensitivity to latex
2. The source of the allergic reaction is thought to be the proteins in the natural rubber latex or the various chemicals used in the manufacturing process of the latex, from a liquid substance into the finished product
3. Symptoms of the **allergy** can range from mild contact dermatitis to moderately severe symptoms of rhinitis, conjunctivitis, urticaria, and bronchospasm, to severe, life-threatening anaphylaxis
B. Common routes of exposure (Box 67-1)
1. Cutaneous: Wearing natural latex gloves
2. Percutaneous and parenteral: IV lines and catheters; hemodialysis equipment
3. Mucosal: Use of latex condoms, catheters, airways, and nipples
4. Aerosol: Aerosolization of powder from latex gloves can occur when gloves are dispensed from the box or when gloves are removed from the hands

---

BOX 67-1

Common Products that Contain Natural Rubber Latex

Ace bandages (brown)
Adhesive bandages
Ambu bag
Balloons
Band-Aid dressings
Blood pressure cuff (tubing and bladder)
Catheters
Catheter leg bag straps
Condoms
Diaphragms
Elastic pressure stockings
ECG pads
Feminine hygiene pads
Gloves
IV catheters, tubing, and rubber injection ports
Levine tubes
Pads for crutches
Prepackaged enema kits
Rubber stoppers on medication vials
Stethoscopes
Syringes

C. At-risk individuals
  1. Health care workers
  2. Individuals who work with manufacturing of latex products
  3. Females
  4. Individuals with spina bifida
  5. Individuals who wear gloves frequently, such as food handlers, hairdressers, and auto mechanics
  6. Individuals who are allergic to kiwis, bananas, pineapples, tropical fruits, avocados, potatoes, or chestnuts
D. Assessment
  1. Anaphylactic hypersensitivity
    a. Rapid onset
    b. Urticaria, wheezing, dyspnea, laryngeal edema, bronchospasm, tachycardia, angioedema, hypotension, and cardiac arrest
  2. Delayed-type hypersensitivity: Includes symptoms of contact dermatitis, such as pruritus, edema, erythema, vesicles, papules, and crusting and thickening of the skin
E. Implementation
  1. Ask the client about a known **allergy** to latex when performing the initial assessment
  2. Identify risk factors to a latex **allergy** in the client
  3. Individuals with an **allergy**
    a. Avoid latex products
    b. Obtain an emergency medical kit that contains antihistamines and epinephrine
    c. Wear a Medic-Alert bracelet
    d. Inform health care providers and local and paramedic ambulance companies about the **allergy**
    e. Advise the individual to place a warning label in the car window to alert police and paramedics of the **allergy,** in case of a car accident
    f. Provide information about local support groups and resources for alternative products

X. AUTOIMMUNE DISEASE
A. Description
  1. Body is unable to recognize its own cells as a part of itself
  2. Can affect collagenous tissue
B. Systemic lupus erythematosus (SLE)
  1. Description
    a. A chronic progressive systemic inflammatory disease that can cause major organs and systems to fail
    b. Connective tissue and fibrin deposits in blood vessels, collagen fibers, and organs
    c. Leads to necrosis and/or inflammation of blood vessels, lymph nodes, gastrointestinal (GI) tract, pleura
    d. There is no cure for the disease
  2. Causes
    a. The cause is unknown, although the disease is thought to be due to a defect in the immunological mechanisms or to have a genetic origin
    b. Precipitating factors include medications, stress, genetic factors, sunlight or ultraviolet light, and pregnancy
  3. Assessment
    a. Precipitating factors such as sunlight, stress, and medications
    b. Dry scaly raised rash on the face or upper body
    c. Fever
    d. Weakness, malaise, and fatigue
    e. Anorexia
    f. Weight loss
    g. Photosensitivity
    h. Joint pain
    i. Erythema of the palms
    j. Butterfly erythema of the face
    k. Anemia
    l. Positive antinuclear antibodies (ANA) and LE prep
    m. Elevated sedimentation rate
  4. Implementation
    a. Monitor skin integrity and provide frequent oral care
    b. Instruct the client to clean skin with a mild soap, avoiding harsh and perfumed substances
    c. Assist with the use of ointments and creams for rash as prescribed
    d. Identify factors contributing to fatigue
    e. Administer iron, folic acid, or vitamin supplements as prescribed if anemia occurs
    f. Provide a high-vitamin and high-iron diet
    g. Provide a high-protein diet if there is no evidence of kidney disease
    h. Instruct in measures to conserve energy, such as pacing activities and balancing rest with exercise
    i. Administer topical or systemic corticosteroids, salicylates, and nonsteroidal antiinflammatory drugs (NSAIDs) as prescribed for pain and inflammation
    j. Administer hydroxychloroquine (Plaquenil) as prescribed to decrease the inflammatory response
    k. Instruct the client to avoid exposure to sunlight and ultraviolet light
    l. Monitor for proteinuria and red cell casts in the urine
    m. Monitor for bruising, bleeding, and injury
    n. Assist with plasmapheresis as prescribed to remove autoantibodies and immune complexes from the blood before organ damage occurs
    o. Monitor for signs of organ involvement, such as pleuritis, nephritis, pericarditis, neuritis, anemia, and peritonitis

p. Note that lupus nephritis occurs early in the disease process

q. Provide supportive therapy as major organs become affected

r. Provide emotional support and encourage the client to verbalize feelings

s. Provide information regarding support groups, and encourage utilization of community resources

C. Scleroderma (progressive systemic sclerosis)

1. Description
   a. A chronic connective tissue disease, similar to SLE, characterized by inflammation, fibrosis, and sclerosis
   b. Affects the connective tissue throughout the body
   c. Causes fibrotic changes involving the skin, synovial membranes, esophagus, heart, lungs, kidneys, and GI tract
   d. Treatment is directed toward forcing the disease into remission and slowing its progress

2. Assessment
   a. Pain
   b. Stiffness and muscle weakness
   c. Pitting edema of the hands and fingers, which progresses to the rest of the body
   d. Taut and shiny skin that is free from wrinkles
   e. Skin tissue is tight, hard, and thick, and loses its elasticity
   f. Masklike hard skin that adheres to underlying structures
   g. Dysphagia
   h. Decreased range of motion
   i. Joint contractures
   j. Inability to perform activities of daily living

3. Implementation
   a. Encourage activity as tolerated
   b. Maintain a constant room temperature
   c. Provide small frequent meals, eliminating foods that stimulate gastric secretions, such as spicy foods, caffeine, and alcohol
   d. Advise the client to sit up for 1 to 2 hours after meals if esophageal involvement exists
   e. Provide supportive therapy as the major organs become affected
   f. Administer corticosteroids as prescribed for inflammation
   g. Provide emotional support and encourage the use of resources as necessary

D. Polyarteritis nodosa

1. Description
   a. A collagen disease that causes inflammation of the arteries and thickening and impairment of the circulation
   b. Treatment is similar to treatment for SLE
   c. Affects middle-aged men and involves every body system

d. The cause is unknown and the prognosis is poor

e. Renal disorders and cardiac involvement are the most frequent causes of death

2. Assessment
   a. Malaise and weakness
   b. Low-grade fever
   c. Severe abdominal pain
   d. Bloody diarrhea
   e. Weight loss
   f. Elevated sedimentation rate

3. Implementation
   a. Provide supportive care as required
   b. Provide a well-balanced diet
   c. Administer corticosteroids and analgesics to control pain and inflammation
   d. Provide emotional support and encourage the client to verbalize feelings
   e. Initiate support services for the client

E. Pemphigus

1. Description
   a. A rare disease that occurs predominately between middle and old age
   b. The cause is unknown and the disorder is potentially fatal
   c. Initial lesions occur on the oral mucosa and then progress to a generalized distribution
   d. Treatment is aimed at suppressing the immune response that causes blister formation

2. Assessment
   a. Lesions appear as fragile flaccid bullae
   b. Partial-thickness wounds that bleed, weep, and form crusts when bullae are disrupted
   c. Debilitation, malaise, and pain
   d. Chewing and swallowing difficulties
   e. Nikolsky's sign: Separation of the epidermis caused by rubbing the skin
   f. Leukocytosis, eosinophilia, foul-smelling discharge from skin

3. Implementation
   a. Provide supportive care
   b. Provide oral hygiene and increase fluid intake
   c. Soothe oral lesions
   d. Assist with oatmeal or potassium permanganate baths as prescribed for relief of symptoms
   e. Administer topical or systemic antibiotics as prescribed for secondary infections
   f. Administer corticosteroids and cytotoxic agents as prescribed to bring about remission

XI. ACQUIRED IMMUNODEFICIENCY SYNDROME (AIDS)

A. Description

1. An infectious disease characterized by severe deficits in cellular function
2. Manifested clinically by opportunistic infection and/or unusual neoplasms
3. Etiology: human immunodeficiency virus (HIV)

4. The disease has a long incubation period, sometimes up to 10 years or more
5. Manifestations may not appear until late in the infection

B. AIDS-related complex (ARC)
1. Similar to AIDS
2. Two or more symptoms or two or more laboratory findings characteristic of immunodeficiency
3. Client is not as ill as the AIDS client
4. May lead to AIDS

C. High-risk groups
1. Male homosexuals or bisexuals
2. Intravenous drug abusers
3. Persons receiving blood transfusions (hemophiliacs, surgical clients)
4. Those individuals with frequent exposure to blood and body fluids
5. Heterosexual contact with high-risk individuals
6. Babies born to infected mothers

D. Assessment
1. Malaise, weight loss
2. Lymphadenopathy of at least 3 months
3. Leukopenia
4. Diarrhea
5. Fatigue
6. Night sweats
7. Presence of opportunistic infections
8. *Pneumocystis carinii* pneumonia (major source of mortality)
9. Kaposi's sarcoma: Purplish red lesions on internal organs and skin
10. Candidiasis
11. Fungal infections
12. Cytomegalovirus (CMV)

E. Implementation
1. Provide respiratory support
2. Administer respiratory treatments as prescribed
3. Administer oxygen as prescribed
4. Maintain fluid and electrolyte balance
5. Monitor for signs of infection
6. Prevent the spread of infection
7. Initiate standard (universal) precautions
8. Provide comfort as necessary
9. Provide meticulous skin care
10. Provide adequate nutritional support as prescribed
11. Refer to Chapters 25 and 42 for additional information on AIDS

PRACTICE QUESTIONS

1. A client is suspected of having systemic lupus erythematosus (SLE). The nurse monitors the client, knowing that which of the following is a characteristic sign of SLE?
   1. Rash on the face across the bridge of the nose and on the cheeks
   2. Fatigue
   3. Fever
   4. Elevated red blood cell count

2. A nurse is providing home care instructions to a client with systemic lupus erythematous (SLE). Which of the following would not be on the list of instructions for the client about methods to manage fatigue?
   1. To avoid long periods of rest
   2. To sit whenever possible
   3. To take a hot bath in the evening
   4. To engage in moderate low-impact exercise when not fatigued

3. A client has requested and undergone testing for human immunodeficiency virus (HIV). The client now asks what will be done next, since the results of two enzyme-linked immunosorbent assay (ELISA) tests have been positive. The nurse's response is based on the understanding that:
   1. The client will probably have a bone marrow biopsy done
   2. A Western blot will be done to confirm these findings
   3. A CD4 cell count will be done to measure T-helper lymphocytes
   4. The client will be definitively diagnosed as HIV positive at this point

4. A nurse is caring for a client with acquired immunodeficiency syndrome (AIDS). The nurse detects early infection with *Pneumocystis carinii* by monitoring the client for which of the following clinical manifestations?
   1. Dyspnea on exertion
   2. Dyspnea at rest
   3. Fever
   4. Cough

5. A client with acquired immunodeficiency syndrome (AIDS) has a concurrent diagnosis of histoplasmosis. The nurse notes, during the assessment, that the client has enlarged lymph nodes. The nurse interprets that:
   1. The client has disseminated histoplasmosis infection
   2. This is a side effect of the medications given to treat AIDS
   3. This indicates that the histoplasmosis is resolving
   4. The client probably has yet another infection that is developing

6. A nurse is caring for the client with acquired immunodeficiency syndrome (AIDS) who is experiencing night fever and night sweats. Which of the following nursing interventions would be the least helpful in managing this symptom?
   1. Keep a change of bed linens nearby in case they are needed
   2. Administer an antipyretic after the client spikes the fever
   3. Make sure the pillow has a plastic cover
   4. Keep liquids at the bedside

7. A client exposed to human immunodeficiency virus (HIV) approximately 3 months ago has seroconverted to an HIV positive status. The nurse anticipates that the client will experience which of the following at this time?
   1. Oral lesions
   2. Purplish skin lesions
   3. Chronic cough
   4. No signs and symptoms

8. A client with acquired immunodeficiency syndrome (AIDS) has raised, dark purplish lesions on the trunk of the body. The nurse anticipates that which of the following procedures will be done to confirm whether these lesions are result from Kaposi's sarcoma?
   1. Enzyme-linked immunosorbent assay (ELISA)
   2. Western blot
   3. Skin biopsy
   4. Lung biopsy

9. A nurse participating in a health fair is setting up a booth on prevention of human immunodeficiency virus (HIV) transmission. A poster is planned that will list sexual behaviors in one of two columns, rated "safe" and "not safe." Which of the following behaviors would the nurse place in the "not safe" column?
   1. Use of latex condoms
   2. Use of "natural skin" condoms
   3. Abstinence
   4. Mutual monogamy

10. A client with acquired immunodeficiency syndrome (AIDS) is experiencing nausea and vomiting. The nurse would make which of the following dietary alterations for this client to enhance nutritional intake?
   1. Avoid dairy products and red meat
   2. Plan large, nutritious meals
   3. Add spices to food for added flavor
   4. Serve foods while they are very warm

11. A client with acquired immunodeficiency syndrome (AIDS) has a respiratory infection from *Pneumocystis carinii*. In evaluating the documented plan of care for the nursing diagnosis Impaired Gas Exchange, which of the following would not be considered by the nurse to be a positive outcome criterion for this client?
   1. Is free of complaints of shortness of breath
   2. Expectorates secretions easily
   3. Has clear breath sounds
   4. Limits fluid intake

12. A client with pemphigus vulgaris is being seen in the clinic on a regular basis. The nurse plans care based on which of the following descriptions of this condition?
   1. The presence of skin vesicles found along the nerve caused by a virus
   2. An autoimmune disease that causes blistering in the epidermis

3. The presence of red raised papules and large plaques covered by silvery scales
   4. The presence of tiny red vesicles

13. A nurse is providing dietary instructions to a client with systemic lupus erythematosus (SLE). Which of the following dietary items would the nurse instruct the client to avoid?
   1. Cantaloupe
   2. Broccoli
   3. Turkey
   4. Steak

14. A client is brought to the emergency room and is experiencing an anaphylaxis reaction from eating shellfish. The nurse prepares for which of the following initial actions?
   1. Administering epinephrine (Adrenalin)
   2. Administering a corticosteroid
   3. Maintaining a patent airway
   4. Instructing the client on the importance of obtaining a Medic-Alert bracelet

15. A nurse is assisting in planning care for a client with a diagnosis of immune deficiency. The nurse would incorporate which of the following as a priority in the plan of care?
   1. Providing emotional support to decrease fear
   2. Protecting the client from infection
   3. Encouraging discussion about lifestyle changes
   4. Identifying factors that decreased the immune function

16. A client calls the emergency room and tells the nurse that he was just stung by a bumblebee while gardening. The client is afraid of a severe reaction because the client's neighbor experienced such a reaction just a week ago. The most appropriate nursing action is to:
   1. Ask the client if he ever received a bee sting in the past
   2. Tell the client to call an ambulance for transport to the emergency room
   3. Advise the client to soak the site in hydrogen peroxide
   4. Tell the client not to worry about the sting unless difficulty breathing occurs

17. A nurse is assisting in administering immunizations at a health care clinic. The nurse understands that an immunization will provide:
   1. Natural immunity from disease
   2. Acquired immunity from disease
   3. Innate immunity from disease
   4. Protection from all diseases

18. A nurse is assigned to care for a client with systemic lupus erythematosus (SLE). The nurse plans care knowing that this disorder is:
   1. A local rash that occurs as a result of allergy
   2. An inflammatory disease of collagen contained in connective tissue
   3. A disease caused by overexposure to sunlight

4. A disease caused by the continuous release of histamine in the body

19. A nurse is assigned to care for a client admitted to the hospital with a diagnosis of systemic lupus erythematosus (SLE). The nurse reviews the physician's orders, expecting to note that which of the following medications is prescribed?
   1. Antibiotic
   2. Narcotic analgesic
   3. Antidiarrheal
   4. Corticosteroid

20. A nurse administers an injection to a client with a diagnosis of acquired immunodeficiency syndrome (AIDS). After administering the medication, the nurse disposes the used needle by:
   1. Placing it in a puncture-resistant container
   2. Laying the needle and syringe on the bedside table and carefully recapping the needle.
   3. Asking the client to recap the needle
   4. Recapping the needle before placing it in a puncture-resistant container

21. A community health nurse, conducting a research study, is identifying clients in the community at risk for latex allergy. Which client population is at most risk for developing this type of allergy?
   1. The homeless
   2. Persons living in a group home
   3. Children in day-care centers
   4. Hairdressers

22. A clinic nurse is providing home care instructions to a client who has been diagnosed with a latex allergy. The nurse most appropriately instructs the client to avoid:
   1. Outdoor activities as much as possible
   2. Going to parties
   3. The use of condoms
   4. Sunlight

23. A home care nurse is performing an assessment on a client who has been diagnosed with an allergy to latex. In determining the client's risk factors associated with the allergy, the nurse questions the client about an allergy to which food item?
   1. Milk
   2. Bananas
   3. Yogurt
   4. Eggs

24. A home care nurse is assigned to visit a client who returned to home from the emergency room after treatment for a sprained ankle. The nurse notes that the client was sent home with crutches and needs instructions about crutch walking. On admission assessment, the nurse discovers that the client has an allergy to latex. Before providing instructions about crutch walking, the nurse most appropriately:
   1. Contacts the physician
   2. Covers the crutch pads with cloth
   3. Tells the client that the crutches must be removed from the house immediately
   4. Calls the local medical supply store and asks for a cane to be delivered

25. A home care nurse is ordering dressing supplies for a client who has an allergy to latex. The nurse asks the medical supply personnel to deliver which of the following?
   1. Adhesive bandages
   2. Band-Aid dressings
   3. Cotton pads and silk tape
   4. Brown Ace bandages

CRITICAL THINKING: FREE-TEXT ENTRY

A home care nurse is assigned to visit a client who has a diagnosis of hypertension. The client was just discharged from the hospital to home. On assessment of the client, the nurse discovers that the client has an allergy to latex. The nurse realizes that the blood pressure equipment contains latex. What action will the nurse take in regard to obtaining the client's blood pressure?

Answer: _____

ANSWERS

1. **1**
Rationale: Skin lesions or rash on the face across the bridge of the nose and on the cheeks is a characteristic sign of SLE. Fever and fatigue may potentially occur before and during exacerbation. Anemia is most likely to occur in SLE.
Test-Taking Strategy: Use the process of elimination. Note the key words "characteristic sign." Recalling the characteristic butterfly rash associated with SLE will easily direct you to option 1. If you are unfamiliar with this disorder, review this content.
Level of Cognitive Ability: Analysis
Client Needs: Physiological Integrity
Integrated Concept/Process: Nursing Process/Assessment

Content Area: Adult Health/Immune
Reference: Monahan, F., & Neighbors, M. (1998). *Medical-surgical nursing: Foundations for clinical practice* (2nd ed.). Philadelphia: W. B. Saunders, p.1491.

2. **3**
Rationale: To help reduce fatigue in the client with SLE, the nurse should instruct the client to sit whenever possible, to avoid hot baths, to schedule moderate low-impact exercises when not fatigued, and to maintain a balanced diet. The client is instructed to avoid long periods of rest because they promote joint stiffness.
Test-Taking Strategy: Note the key words "not" and "manage fatigue." By the process of elimination, you should easily be directed to option 3 as the action that would exacerbate

fatigue. If you had difficulty with this question, review measures to prevent fatigue in a client with SLE.

Level of Cognitive Ability: Application
Client Needs: Health Promotion and Maintenance
Integrated Concept/Process: Teaching/Learning
Content Area: Adult Health/Immune
Reference: Monahan, F., & Neighbors, M. (1998). *Medical-surgical nursing: Foundations for clinical practice* (2nd ed.). Philadelphia: W. B. Saunders, p. 1493.

3. 2
Rationale: If the results of two ELISA tests are positive, the Western blot is done to confirm the findings. If the result of the Western blot is positive, then the client is considered to be positive for HIV and infected with the HIV virus. Options 1, 3, and 4 are incorrect.
Test-Taking Strategy: Knowledge of the procedural steps in diagnosing HIV is needed to answer this question. If you are unfamiliar with these diagnostic tests, review this content.
Level of Cognitive Ability: Analysis
Client Needs: Physiological Integrity
Integrated Concept/Process: Nursing Process/Implementation
Content Area: Adult Health/Immune
Reference: Smeltzer, S., & Bare, B. (2000). *Brunner & Suddarth's textbook of medical-surgical nursing* (9th ed.). Philadelphia: Lippincott Williams & Wilkins, p. 1359.

4. 4
Rationale: The client with *Pneumocystis carinii* infection usually has cough as the first symptom, which begins as nonproductive, then progresses to productive. Later signs include fever, dyspnea on exertion, and finally dyspnea at rest.
Test-Taking Strategy: Use the process of elimination, noting the key word "early." While all of these symptoms may appear at some point in the client with *Pneumocystis carinii*, knowing that the cough appears first helps you to eliminate each of the other options. Review the early signs of *Pneumocystis carinii* infection if you had difficulty with this question.
Level of Cognitive Ability: Analysis
Client Needs: Physiological Integrity
Integrated Concept/Process: Nursing Process/Assessment
Content Area: Adult Health/Immune
Reference: Smeltzer, S., & Bare, B. (2000). *Brunner & Suddarth's textbook of medical-surgical nursing* (9th ed.). Philadelphia: Lippincott Williams & Wilkins, p. 1367.

5. 1
Rationale: Histoplasmosis usually starts as a respiratory infection in the client with AIDS. It then becomes a disseminated infection, with enlargement of lymph nodes, spleen, and liver. Options 2, 3, and 4 are incorrect.
Test-Taking Strategy: Knowing that lymph nodes may enlarge with generalized infection helps you eliminate options 2 and 3. Since the question contains no information that indicates that option 4 is true, option 1 is the correct option by elimination. Review disseminated infections in the client with AIDS if you had difficulty with this question.
Level of Cognitive Ability: Analysis
Client Needs: Physiological Integrity
Integrated Concept/Process: Nursing Process/Analysis
Content Area: Adult Health/Immune
Reference: Ignatavicius, D., Workman, M., & Mishler, M. (1999). *Medical-surgical nursing: Across the health care continuum* (3rd ed.). Philadelphia: W. B. Saunders, p. 446.

6. 2
Rationale: For clients with AIDS who experience night fever and night sweats, it is useful to offer the client an antipyretic of choice prior to going to sleep. It is also helpful to keep a change of bed linens and nightclothes nearby for use. The pillow should have a plastic cover, and a towel may be placed over the pillowcase if there is profuse diaphoresis. The client should have liquids at the bedside to drink.
Test-Taking Strategy: Use the process of elimination, noting the key words "least helpful." Options 1 and 3 are helpful from an environmental viewpoint, so they are eliminated first as answers to this question. Knowing that liquids will help prevent dehydration will assist in eliminating this option next. Since night fever and sweats occur serially, it is most helpful to give the antipyretic before sleep as a prophylactic measure.
Level of Cognitive Ability: Application
Client Needs: Physiological Integrity
Integrated Concept/Process: Nursing Process/Implementation
Content Area: Adult Health/Immune
Reference: Ignatavicius, D., Workman, M., & Mishler, M. (1999). *Medical-surgical nursing: Across the health care continuum* (3rd ed.). Philadelphia: W. B. Saunders, p. 445.

7. 4
Rationale: The client in stage 1 (seroconversion) acute HIV infection has laboratory documentation of HIV positive status, but is asymptomatic. Following introduction of the infection and seroconversion in stage 1, the client may remain asymptomatic for a period of 6 months to in excess of 10 years (stage 2: chronic asymptomatic status). The client's T4 cell count is normal during these two stages. The client will begin to show symptoms in stage 3: symptomatic stage, when the T4 cell count drops below 500/cu mm. At this time, the client experiences opportunistic infections, including oral lesions (thrush) and skin lesions (Kaposi's sarcoma). The client may also experience signs of respiratory infection in stage 3.
Test-Taking Strategy: Use the process of elimination. Read the question carefully noting the 3-month time period between exposure and seroconversion. This will direct you to option 4. Review the clinical manifestations associated with HIV if you had difficulty with this question.
Level of Cognitive Ability: Analysis
Client Needs: Physiological Integrity
Integrated Concept/Process: Nursing Process/Assessment
Content Area: Adult Health/Immune
Reference: Phipps, W., Sands, J., & Marek, J. (1999). *Medical-surgical nursing: Concepts & clinical practice* (6th ed.). St. Louis: Mosby, p. 2192.

8. 3
Rationale: The skin biopsy is the procedure of choice to diagnose Kaposi's sarcoma, which frequently complicates the clinical picture of the client with AIDS. Lung biopsy would confirm *Pneumocystis carinii* infection. The ELISA and Western blot are tests to diagnose HIV status.
Test-Taking Strategy: Use the process of elimination. Eliminate options 1 and 2, which are used to diagnose whether or not the client is HIV positive. Knowledge of the meaning of Kaposi's sarcoma, or attention to the words "lesions" and "trunk" will help you to choose correctly between the remaining options. Review the diagnostic testing to confirm Kaposi's sarcoma if you had difficulty with this question.
Level of Cognitive Ability: Analysis

Client Needs: Physiological Integrity
Integrated Concept/Process: Nursing Process/Analysis
Content Area: Adult Health/Immune
Reference: Phipps, W., Sands, J., & Marek, J. (1999). *Medical-surgical nursing: Concepts & clinical practice* (6th ed.). St. Louis: Mosby, p. 2217.

9. **2**
Rationale: Abstinence is the safest way to avoid HIV infection. The next most reliable method is participation in a mutually monogamous relationship. The use of latex condoms is considered safe, because the latex prevents the transmission of the HIV virus as long as the condom is used properly and remains in place. The use of "natural skin" condoms is not considered safe because the pores in the condom are large enough for the virus to pass through.
Test-Taking Strategy: Use the process of elimination, noting the issue of the question, sexual behaviors that are not safe. Recalling that condoms not made of latex will not protect the individual from sexually transmitted diseases will direct you to option 2. Review these preventive measures if you had difficulty with this question.
Level of Cognitive Ability: Application
Client Needs: Health Promotion and Maintenance
Integrated Concept/Process: Teaching/Learning
Content Area: Adult Health/Immune
Reference: Phipps, W., Sands, J., & Marek, J. (1999). *Medical-surgical nursing: Concepts & clinical practice* (6th ed.). St. Louis: Mosby, p. 1644.

10. **1**
Rationale: The AIDS client with nausea and vomiting should avoid fatty products such as diary products and red meat. Meals should be small and frequent to lessen the chance of vomiting. Spices and odorous foods should be avoided, since they aggravate nausea. Foods are best tolerated either cold or at room temperature.
Test-Taking Strategy: Use the process of elimination and basic principles for treating nausea and vomiting to answer this question. Doing so will guide you to option 1. Review nutritional support for the client with AIDS if you had difficulty with this question.
Level of Cognitive Ability: Application
Client Needs: Physiological Integrity
Integrated Concept/Process: Nursing Process/Implementation
Content Area: Adult Health/Immune
Reference: Phipps, W., Sands, J., & Marek, J. (1999). *Medical-surgical nursing: Concepts & clinical practice* (6th ed.). St. Louis: Mosby, p. 2200.

11. **4**
Rationale: The status of the client with a diagnosis of Impaired Gas Exchange would be evaluated against the standard outcome criteria for this nursing diagnosis. These would include the fact that the client states that breathing is easier, coughs up secretions effectively, and has clear breath sounds. The client should not limit fluid intake, because fluids are needed to decrease the viscosity of secretions for expectoration.
Test-Taking Strategy: Use the process of elimination and note the key words "not" and "positive outcome." This will easily direct you to option 4. Review care of the client with AIDS if you had difficulty with this question.

Level of Cognitive Ability: Analysis
Client Needs: Physiological Integrity
Integrated Concept/Process: Nursing Process/Analysis
Content Area: Adult Health/Immune
Reference: Phipps, W., Sands, J., & Marek, J. (1999). *Medical-surgical nursing: Concepts & clinical practice* (6th ed.). St. Louis: Mosby, pp. 2211-2212.

12. **2**
Rationale: Pemphigus vulgaris is an autoimmune disease that causes blistering in the epidermis. The clients have large flaccid blisters (bullae). Because the blisters are in the epidermis, they have a very tiny covering of skin and break easily, leaving large denuded areas of skin. On initial examination, clients may have crusting areas instead of intact blisters. Option 1 describes herpes zoster. Option 3 describes psoriasis, and option 4 describes eczema.
Test-Taking Strategy: Use the process of elimination. Recalling that pemphigus vulgaris is an autoimmune disorder will easily direct you to option 2. If you had difficulty with this question, review the characteristics of this disorder.
Level of Cognitive Ability: Analysis
Client Needs: Physiological Integrity
Integrated Concept/Process: Nursing Process/Planning
Content Area: Adult Health/Immune
Reference: Beare, P., & Myers, J. (1998). *Adult health nursing* (3rd ed.). St. Louis: Mosby, p. 1767.

13. **4**
Rationale: The client with SLE is at risk for cardiovascular disorders, such as coronary artery disease and hypertension. The client is advised of lifestyle changes to reduce these risks, which include smoking cessation and prevention of obesity and hyperlipidemia. The client is advised to reduce salt, fat, and cholesterol intake.
Test-Taking Strategy: Use the process of elimination. Note the key word "avoid" in the question. Knowledge about the risks associated with SLE will assist in answering this question. Use knowledge about basic nutritional components of food items to help direct you to option 4. If you had difficulty with this question, review therapeutic management of SLE.
Level of Cognitive Ability: Application
Client Needs: Health Promotion and Maintenance
Integrated Concept/Process: Teaching/Learning
Content Area: Adult Health/Immune
Reference: Smeltzer, S., & Bare, B. (2000). *Brunner & Suddarth's textbook of medical-surgical nursing* (9th ed.). Philadelphia: Lippincott Williams & Wilkins, p. 1424-1425.

14. **3**
Rationale: The initial action would be to maintain a patent airway. The client would then receive epinephrine. Corticosteroids may also be prescribed. The client will need to be instructed about wearing a Medic-Alert bracelet, but this is not the initial action.
Test-Taking Strategy: Focus on the key word "initial." This key word tells you that you need to prioritize your nursing actions. Use the ABCs, airway, breathing, and circulation, to answer the question. Airway is always the priority. Review care to the client experiencing an anaphylaxis reaction if you had difficulty with this question.
Level of Cognitive Ability: Application
Client Needs: Physiological Integrity

Integrated Concept/Process: Nursing Process/Implementation
Content Area: Adult Health/Immune
Reference: Smeltzer, S., & Bare, B. (2000). *Brunner & Suddarth's textbook of medical-surgical nursing* (9th ed.). Philadelphia: Lippincott Williams & Wilkins, p. 1916.

15. **2**
Rationale: The client with immune deficiency has inadequate immune bodies or their absence, and is at risk for infection. The priority nursing intervention is to protect the client from infection. Options 1, 3, and 4 may be components of care but are not the priority.
Test-Taking Strategy: Use Maslow's hierarchy of needs theory to answer the question. Remember that physiological needs are the priority. This will easily direct you to option 2. Review the care of a client with immune deficiency if you had difficulty with this question.
Level of Cognitive Ability: Application
Client Needs: Physiological Integrity
Integrated Concept/Process: Nursing Process/Planning
Content Area: Adult Health/Immune
Reference: Smeltzer, S., & Bare, B. (2000). *Brunner & Suddarth's textbook of medical-surgical nursing* (9th ed.). Philadelphia: Lippincott Williams & Wilkins, p. 1347.

16. **1**
Rationale: In most types of allergies, a reaction occurs only on second and subsequent contacts with the allergen. The most appropriate action therefore, would be to ask the client if he ever received a bee sting in the past. Option 2 is unnecessary. Option 3 is not appropriate advice. The client should not be told not to worry.
Test-Taking Strategy: Use the steps of the nursing process to answer the question. Option 1 is the only option that addresses assessment. Review information related to allergic reactions if you had difficulty with this question.
Level of Cognitive Ability: Application
Client Needs: Physiological Integrity
Integrated Concept/Process: Nursing Process/Implementation
Content Area: Adult Health/Immune
Reference: Smeltzer, S., & Bare, B. (2000). *Brunner & Suddarth's textbook of medical-surgical nursing* (9th ed.). Philadelphia: Lippincott Williams & Wilkins, p. 1387.

17. **2**
Rationale: Acquired immunity can occur by receiving an immunization that causes antibodies to a specific pathogen to form. Natural (innate) immunity is present at birth. There is no immunization that protects the client from all diseases.
Test-Taking Strategy: Use the process of elimination and knowledge about immunity to disease to answer the question. Eliminate option 4 first because of the absolute word "all." Next eliminate options 1 and 3 because they are similar. Review natural and acquired immunity if you had difficulty with this question.
Level of Cognitive Ability: Comprehension
Client Needs: Physiological Integrity
Integrated Concept/Process: Nursing Process/Implementation
Content Area: Adult Health/Immune
Reference: Smeltzer, S., & Bare, B. (2000). *Brunner & Suddarth's textbook of medical-surgical nursing* (9th ed.). Philadelphia: Lippincott Williams & Wilkins, p. 1331.

18. **2**
Rationale: SLE is an inflammatory disease of collagen contained in connective tissue. Options 1, 3, and 4 are not associated with this disease.
Test-Taking Strategy: Use the process of elimination. Eliminate option 1 because SLE is a systemic disorder, not a local one. Next eliminate option 4 because of its similarity to option 1. From the remaining options, select option 2 because of its systemic characteristic. If you are unfamiliar with this disorder, review its characteristics.
Level of Cognitive Ability: Application
Client Needs: Physiological Integrity
Integrated Concept/Process: Nursing Process/Planning
Content Area: Adult Health/Immune
Reference: Smeltzer, S., & Bare, B. (2000). *Brunner & Suddarth's textbook of medical-surgical nursing* (9th ed.). Philadelphia: Lippincott Williams & Wilkins, p. 1424.

19. **4**
Rationale: Treatment of SLE is based on the systems involved and symptoms. Treatment normally consists of antiinflammatory agents, corticosteroids, and immunosuppressants. Options 1, 2, and 3 are not standard components of medication therapy.
Test-Taking Strategy: Use the process of elimination. Recalling that SLE is an inflammatory disorder will direct you to option 4. If you are unfamiliar with the treatments normally prescribed in this disease, review this content.
Level of Cognitive Ability: Analysis
Client Needs: Physiological Integrity
Integrated Concept/Process: Nursing Process/Analysis
Content Area: Adult Health/Immune
Reference: Smeltzer, S., & Bare, B. (2000). *Brunner & Suddarth's textbook of medical-surgical nursing* (9th ed.). Philadelphia: Lippincott Williams & Wilkins, p. 1425.

20. **1**
Rationale: The correct procedure for needle disposal is to dispose of uncapped needles and sharps in a hard-wall, puncture-resistant container, immediately after use. Needles are not recapped.
Test-Taking Strategy: Use the process of elimination and principles related to the safe disposal of needles and syringes to answer the question. Note that options 2, 3, and 4 are similar in that they all address recapping the needle. Review these principles if you had difficulty with this question.
Level of Cognitive Ability: Application
Client Needs: Safe, Effective Care Environment
Integrated Concept/Process: Nursing Process/Implementation
Content Area: Adult Health/Immune
Reference: Potter, P., & Perry, A. (2001). *Fundamentals of nursing* (5th ed.). St. Louis: Mosby, p. 948.

21. **4**
Rationale: Individuals at risk for developing a latex allergy include health care workers; individuals who work with manufacturing latex products; females; individuals with spina bifida; persons who wear gloves frequently, such as food handlers, hairdressers, and auto mechanics; and persons allergic to kiwis, bananas, pineapples, passion fruits, avocados, and chestnuts.
Test-Taking Strategy: Focus on the issue, a latex allergy. Recalling the cause and the source of the allergic reaction will

easily direct you to option 4. Review the cause of this type of allergy and the individuals at risk if you had difficulty with this question.

Level of Cognitive Ability: Analysis
Client Needs: Health Promotion and Maintenance
Integrated Concept/Process: Nursing Process/Assessment
Content Area: Adult Health/Immune
Reference: Smeltzer, S., & Bare, B. (2000). *Brunner & Suddarth's textbook of medical-surgical nursing* (9th ed.). Philadelphia: Lippincott Williams & Wilkins, p. 1401.

22. **3**
Rationale: Mucosal exposure to latex can occur on contact with latex condoms. The nurse would most appropriately provide instructions to the client about the need to avoid the use of condoms unless they are latex-free. There is no reason to avoid outdoor activities or sunlight. There is also no reason to avoid parties; however, the client should be informed that certain kinds of balloons are made of latex.
Test-Taking Strategy: Use the process of elimination. Note the key word "avoid." Eliminate options 1 and 4 first because they are similar. From the remaining options, focusing on the issue will direct you to option 3. Review home-care instructions for the client with a latex allergy if you had difficulty with this question.
Level of Cognitive Ability: Application
Client Needs: Health Promotion and Maintenance
Integrated Concept/Process: Teaching/Learning
Content Area: Adult Health/Immune
Reference: Smeltzer, S., & Bare, B. (2000). *Brunner & Suddarth's textbook of medical-surgical nursing* (9th ed.). Philadelphia: Lippincott Williams & Wilkins, pp. 1402-1403.

23. **2**
Rationale: People who are allergic to bananas, avocados, tropical fruits, kiwis, potatoes, and chestnuts are at risk for developing a latex allergy. This is thought to be due to a possible cross-reaction between the food and the latex allergen. Options 1, 3, and 4 are unrelated to latex allergy.
Test-Taking Strategy: Use the process of elimination and knowledge about the food items related to a latex allergy. Eliminate options 1, 3, and 4 because they are similar and all relate to dairy products. Review the food items that are associated with a risk for latex allergy if you had difficulty with this question.
Level of Cognitive Ability: Analysis
Client Needs: Health Promotion and Maintenance
Integrated Concept/Process: Nursing Process/Assessment
Content Area: Adult Health/Immune
Reference: Phipps, W., Sands, J., & Marek, J. (1999). *Medical-surgical nursing: Concepts & clinical practice* (6th ed.). St. Louis: Mosby, p. 511.

24. **2**
Rationale: Pads used on crutches contain latex. If the client requires the use of crutches, the nurse can cover the pads with a cloth to prevent cutaneous contact. Option 3 is inappropriate and may alarm the client. The nurse cannot order a cane for

a client. Additionally, this type of assistive device may not be appropriate, considering this client's injury. There is no reason to contact the physician at this time.
Test-Taking Strategy: Use the process of elimination and knowledge about the alternative resources that can be used for a client with an allergy to latex. There are no data in the question that support the need to contact the physician. The nurse should not prescribe assistive devices for the client. Option 3 is not a therapeutic action. Review care of the client with a latex allergy if you had difficulty with this question.
Level of Cognitive Ability: Application
Client Needs: Safe, Effective Care Environment
Integrated Concept/Process: Nursing Process/Implementation
Content Area: Adult Health/Immune
Reference: Smeltzer, S., & Bare, B. (2000). *Brunner & Suddarth's textbook of medical-surgical nursing* (9th ed.). Philadelphia: Lippincott Williams & Wilkins, p. 1402.

25. **3**
Rationale: Cotton pads and plastic or silk tape are latex-free products. The items identified in options 1, 2, and 4 are all products that contain latex.
Test-Taking Strategy: Use the process of elimination and knowledge about the products that contain latex to answer this question. Noting the key words "cotton" and "silk" in option 3 may assist in answering correctly. Review the list of products that contain latex if you had difficulty with this question.
Level of Cognitive Ability: Application
Client Needs: Safe, Effective Care Environment
Integrated Concept/Process: Nursing Process/Implementation
Content Area: Adult Health/Immune
Reference: Smeltzer, S., & Bare, B. (2000). *Brunner & Suddarth's textbook of medical-surgical nursing* (9th ed.). Philadelphia: Lippincott Williams & Wilkins, p. 1402.

CRITICAL THINKING: FREE-TEXT ENTRY

Answer: Obtain the blood pressure by placing the equipment over the client's clothing
Rationale: Both a blood pressure cuff and a stethoscope contain latex. If available, a nylon or vinyl cuff that is latex free can be used to obtain the blood pressure. An alternative to this method is to wrap stockinette over the equipment or obtain the blood pressure by placing the equipment over the client's clothing.
Test-Taking Strategy: Recall that a source of exposure to latex is cutaneous. Avoiding skin contact with the blood pressure equipment will prevent a reaction. Covering the skin will prevent cutaneous contact.
Level of Cognitive Ability: Application
Client Needs: Safe, Effective Care Environment
Integrated Concept/Process: Nursing Process/Implementation
Content Area: Adult Health/Immune
Reference: Smeltzer, S., & Bare, B. (2000). *Brunner & Suddarth's textbook of medical-surgical nursing* (9th ed.). Philadelphia: Lippincott Williams & Wilkins, p. 1402.

REFERENCES

Beare, P., & Myers, J. (1998). *Adult health nursing* (3rd ed.). St. Louis: Mosby.

Ignatavicius, D., Workman, M., & Mishler, M. (1999). *Medical-surgical nursing: Across the health care continuum* (3rd ed.). Philadelphia: W.B. Saunders.

Monahan, F., & Neighbors, M. (1998). *Medical-surgical nursing: Foundations for clinical practice* (2nd ed.). Philadelphia: W.B. Saunders.

Phipps, W., Sands, J., & Marek, J. (1999). *Medical-surgical nursing: Concepts & clinical practice* (6th ed.). St. Louis: Mosby.

Potter, P., & Perry, A. (2001). *Fundamentals of nursing* (5th ed.). St. Louis: Mosby.

Smeltzer, S., & Bare, B. (2000). *Brunner & Suddarth's textbook of medical-surgical nursing* (9th ed.). Philadelphia: Lippincott Williams & Wilkins.

Immunologic Medications

I. **HUMAN IMMUNODEFICIENCY VIRUS (HIV) AND ACQUIRED IMMUNODEFICIENCY SYNDROME (AIDS)** (Box 68-1)

A. Antiinflammatory medications
1. Sulfasalazine (Azulfidine)
a. Used to treat toxoplasmosis or nocardiasis
b. Administered orally
c. Can cause renal toxicity
d. Suppresses bone marrow function
e. Increases photosensitivity
f. Monitor urine output and complete blood count (CBC)
g. Monitor the client for sore throat, pallor, purpura, jaundice, and weakness
h. Encourage fluid intake
i. Advise the client to avoid exposure to the sun

B. Antiinfective medications
1. Pentamidine isethionate (Pentam 300)
a. Used to treat *Pneumocystis carinii* pneumonia
b. Administered by intramuscular (IM) or intravenous (IV) route
c. Can cause nephrotoxicity
d. Monitor blood pressure and heart rate (may cause hypotension)
e. Monitor for hypoglycemia
f. Is hepatotoxic and immunosuppressive
g. Monitor liver function tests and CBC
2. Metronidazole (Flagyl)
a. Used to treat cryptosporidiosis and giardiasis
b. Administered orally or by the IV route
c. Administer with food or milk
d. Monitor for dry mouth, dizziness, or fungal infection
e. Instruct the client to avoid alcohol during treatment

BOX 68-1

Medications for HIV and AIDS

ANTIINFLAMMATORY MEDICATIONS
Sulfasalazine (Azulfidine)

ANTIINFECTIVE MEDICATIONS
Pentamidine isethionate (Pentam 300)
Metronidazole (Flagyl)

ANTIFUNGAL MEDICATIONS
Ketonazole (Nizoral)
Fluconazole (Dilfulcan)
Amphotericin B (Fungizone)

ANTIVIRALS
Ganciclovir (Cytovene)
Acyclovir (Zovirax)
Foscarnet (Foscavir)

ANTIRETROVIRALS (NUCLEOSIDE REVERSE TRANSCRIPTASE INHIBITORS)
Zidovudine (Retrovir, AZT)
Didanosine (Videx)
Lamivudine (Epivir)
Zalcitabine (ddC)

ANTIRETROVIRALS (PROTEASE INHIBITORS)
Saquinavir (Invirase)
Ritonavir (Norvir)
Stavudine (d4T, Zerit)

ANTIFUNGAL, ANTI-INFECTIVE, ANTIPROTOZOAL
Dapsone (Avlosulfon, DDS)

ANTIMALARIAL, ANTIPROTOZOAL
Pyrimethamine (Daraprim)

C. Antifungal medications
 1. Ketonazole (Nizoral)
   a. Used in the treatment of candidiasis, coccidioidomycosis, or histoplasmosis
   b. Administered orally
   c. Administer with food or milk
   d. Instruct the client to avoid antacids for 2 hours after taking the medication because gastric acid is needed to activate the medication
   e. Is hepatotoxic
   f. Monitor hepatic function
   g. Instruct the client to avoid exposure to the sun because the medication increases photosensitivity
   h. Instruct the client to avoid alcohol during treatment
 2. Fluconazole (Dilfulcan)
   a. Used to treat candidiasis
   b. Administered orally
   c. Is hepatotoxic
   d. Monitor for abdominal pain, fever, and diarrhea
   e. Monitor hepatic function
 3. Amphotericin B (Fungizone)
   a. Used to treat candidiasis and other fungal infections
   b. Administered by the IV route
   c. Is nephrotoxic
   d. Can cause thrombophlebitis
   e. Suppresses bone marrow function
   f. Monitor renal function
   g. Monitor infusion site
   h. Monitor CBC
D. Antivirals
 1. Ganciclovir (Cytovene)
   a. Used to treat cytomegalovirus retinitis
   b. Administered orally or by the IV route
   c. Suppresses bone marrow function
   d. Monitor neutrophil and platelet count
   e. Administer with food
 2. Acyclovir (Zovirax)
   a. Used to treat herpes simplex, herpes zoster, or varicella zoster
   b. May be administered orally or by the IV route
   c. Is nephrotoxic
   d. Monitor renal function
   e. Encourage fluid intake
   f. Is irritating to a blood vessel when administered by the IV route
 3. Foscarnet (Foscavir)
   a. Used in the treatment of cytomegalovirus retinitis in human immunodeficiency virus (HIV)–infected clients
   b. Administered by the IV route
   c. Is nephrotoxic
   d. Monitor renal function

4. Zidovudine (Retrovir, AZT)
   a. Antiretroviral (nucleoside reverse transcriptase inhibitor)
   b. Indicated for clients with HIV seropositivity
   c. Administered orally
   d. Suppresses bone marrow function
   e. Is hepatotoxic and nephrotoxic
   f. Monitor CBC and hepatic and renal function studies
   g. Monitor for dizziness because the medication crosses the blood-brain barrier
   h. Instruct the client that medication must be administered around the clock
5. Didanosine (Videx)
   a. Antiretroviral (nucleoside reverse transcriptase inhibitor)
   b. Indicated for clients with HIV seropositivity
   c. Administered orally
   d. Administer on an empty stomach to enhance absorption
   e. Instruct the client to chew or crush tablet
   f. Monitor for dizziness, neuropathy, and pancreatitis
6. Lamivudine (Epivir)
   a. Antiretroviral (nucleoside reverse transcriptase inhibitor)
   b. Indicated for clients with HIV seropositivity
   c. Used as prophylaxis for occupational exposure
   d. Administered orally
   e. Can cause severe pancreatitis
   f. Instruct the client to avoid fatty foods
7. Zalcitabine (ddC)
   a. Antiretroviral (nucleoside reverse transcriptase inhibitor)
   b. Used in the management of HIV infection with other antiretrovirals, such as AZT, because of the synergistic effect
   c. It has also been used as a single agent in clients who are intolerant of other regimens
   d. Administered orally (with AZT)
   e. Can cause serious liver damage
   f. Monitor liver function studies
8. Saquinavir (Invirase)
   a. Antiretroviral (protease inhibitor)
   b. Used in combination with other antiretroviral medications in the management of HIV infection
   c. Administered orally
   d. Administered with meals
   e. Is best absorbed if the client consumes high-calorie, high-fat meals
   f. It can cause photosensitivity, and the client is instructed to avoid sun exposure
9. Ritonavir (Norvir)
   a. Antiretroviral (protease inhibitor)
   b. Used in combination with other antiretrovi-

ral medications in the management of HIV infection

   c. Administered orally

   d. Administered 1 hour before or 2 hours after meals because it is best absorbed in a fasting state

   e. Can increase triglyceride levels

   f. Monitor triglyceride levels

10. Stavudine (d4T, Zerit)

   a. Antiretroviral (protease inhibitor)

   b. Used in the management of HIV infection in clients who do not respond to or cannot tolerate conventional therapy

   c. Administered orally

   d. Can cause peripheral neuropathy

   e. Monitor the client's gait

   f. Ask the client about paresthesias

E. Dapsone (Avlosulfon, DDS)

   1. Antifungal, antiinfective, antiprotozoal

   2. Used for the treatment of toxoplasmosis

   3. Administered orally

   4. Suppresses bone marrow activity

   5. Can cause anemia, peripheral motor weakness, liver damage

   6. Monitor the CBC

   7. Monitor for fever, sore throat, purpura, or jaundice

F. Pyrimethamine (Daraprim)

   1. Antimalarial, antiprotozoal

   2. Used in the treatment of toxoplasmosis or *Pneumocystis carinii* pneumonia

   3. Administered orally

   4. Suppresses bone marrow function

   5. Monitor complete blood count (CBC) and platelet count

   6. Administer with food or milk

II. SYSTEMIC LUPUS ERYTHEMATOSUS (Box 68-2)

A. Medications are used to control symptoms and to prevent or control serious complications that occur as a result of organ damage by the inflammatory process

B. Azathioprine (Imuran)

   1. Glucocorticoid-sparing effect

   2. Potentiates the immunosuppressive action of glucocorticoids and thereby allows a lower dosage of glucocorticoid to have a greater immunosuppressive action

   3. Monitor CBC and liver function tests

C. Cyclophosphamide (Cytoxan)

   1. Immunosuppressive treatment of diffuse proliferative nephritis and other organ inflammation unresponsive to glucocorticoids

   2. Reserved for use in severe cases because of the adverse side effects

D. Hydroxychloroquine sulfate (Plaquenil)

   1. An antimalarial used to prevent the recurrence of an exacerbation

---

> **BOX 68-2**
>
> **Medications for Systemic Lupus Erythematosus**
>
> Azathioprine (Imuran)
> Cyclophosphamide (Cytoxan)
> Hydroxychloroquine sulfate (Plaquenil)
> Prednisone (Deltasone)
> Nonsteroidal antiinflammatory drugs

   2. An eye examination should be performed initially and 6 months after treatment

   3. Administer with meals or a glass of milk

E. Prednisone (Deltasone)

   1. Used at high doses to treat exacerbations and at low doses to control symptoms when other medications do not work

   2. Refer to Chapter 52 for information on glucocorticoids

F. Nonsteroidal antiinflammatory drugs (NSAIDs)

   1. Used to control fever and arthralgia

   2. Refer to Chapter 64 for information on NSAIDs

III. IMMUNIZATIONS (Refer to Chapter 45)

PRACTICE QUESTIONS

1. Dapsone (DDS) is prescribed for a client with acquired immunodeficiency syndrome (AIDS) for the treatment of toxoplasmosis. The nurse reinforces medication instructions and tells the client to:

   1. Discontinue the medication if nausea and vomiting develop

   2. Plan to take the medication every 6 hours around the clock

   3. Contact the physician if fever or a sore throat occurs

   4. Report to the clinic weekly for the injections

2. Pyrimethamine (Daraprim) has been added to the medication regimen for a client with acquired immunodeficiency syndrome (AIDS). On review of the client's record, the nurse notes this new prescription and plans care, knowing that this has been prescribed for the treatment of:

   1. Toxoplasmosis

   2. Cardiac irregularities

   3. Kaposi's sarcoma

   4. Nausea and vomiting

3. Saquinavir (Invirase) is prescribed for the client who is seropositive for human immunodeficiency virus (HIV). The nurse reinforces medication instructions and tells the client to:

   1. Take the medication on an empty stomach

   2. Eat low-calorie foods

   3. Eat foods that are low in fat

   4. Avoid sun exposure

4. A clinic nurse is providing medication instructions to a client who will be receiving hydroxychloroquine sulfate (Plaquenil) for the treatment of systemic lupus erythematosus. The nurse instructs the client about the importance of returning to the clinic in 6 months for which of the following?
   1. Dental examination
   2. Eye examination
   3. Chest radiograph
   4. Sigmoidoscopy

5. A client who is seropositive for human immunodeficiency virus (HIV) has been taking Stavudine (d4T, Zerit). The nurse monitors which of the following most closely while the client is taking this medication?
   1. Appetite
   2. Gait
   3. Gastrointestinal function
   4. Level of consciousness (LOC)

6. A client who is seropositive for human immunodeficiency virus (HIV) has been taking zalcitabine (ddC) as a component of treatment. The nurse plans to monitor which of the following most closely while the client is taking this medication?
   1. Liver function studies
   2. Platelet count
   3. Red blood cell count
   4. Glucose level

7. A nurse is assigned to care for a client with cytomegalovirus retinitis and acquired immunodeficiency syndrome (AIDS) who is receiving foscavir (Foscarnet). The nurse checks the latest results of which of the following laboratory studies while the client is taking this medication?
   1. Serum albumin
   2. Serum creatinine
   3. CD4 cell count
   4. Lymphocyte count

8. A client with acquired immunodeficiency syndrome (AIDS) and *Pneumocystis carinii* infection has been receiving pentamidine (Pentam 300). The

client develops a fever of 101° F. The nurse does further monitoring of the client, knowing that this sign would most likely indicate:
   1. The dose of the medication is too low
   2. The client is experiencing toxic effects of the medication
   3. The client has developed inadequacy of thermoregulation
   4. This is a result of another infection, caused by leukopenic effects of the medication

9. A client with acquired immunodeficiency syndrome (AIDS) has been started on therapy with zidovudine (AZT, Retrovir). The nurse carefully monitors which of the following laboratory results during treatment with this medication?
   1. Complete blood count (CBC)
   2. Blood urea nitrogen (BUN)
   3. Blood culture
   4. Blood glucose level

10. A nurse is reviewing the results of serum laboratory studies drawn on a client with acquired immunodeficiency syndrome (AIDS) who is receiving didanosine (Videx). The nurse interprets that the client may have the medication discontinued by the physician if which of the following significantly elevated results is noted?
    1. Serum cholesterol
    2. Serum amylase
    3. Blood glucose
    4. Serum protein

CRITICAL THINKING: FREE-TEXT ENTRY

A client who is human immunodeficiency virus (HIV) seropositive has been taking ritonavir (Norvir). The client returns to a clinic for follow-up laboratory blood tests. A nurse reviews the client's record and expects to note a physician's order for which specific laboratory blood test?

Answer: _____

ANSWERS

1. **3**
Rationale: Dapsone may be prescribed for the treatment of toxoplasmosis. The medication is taken orally on a daily basis. The medication suppresses bone marrow activity and the complete blood count (CBC) is monitored closely. If the client develops fever, sore throat, purpura, or jaundice, the physician is notified. Medications are available to treat nausea and vomiting, and the client should not discontinue the medication if these symptoms occur, but should contact the physician.
Test-Taking Strategy: Use the process of elimination. Eliminate option 1 first because the nurse would not tell the client to

discontinue the medication. Next, eliminate options 2 and 4, knowing that the medication is administered orally on a daily basis. Review this medication if you had difficulty with this question.
Level of Cognitive Ability: Application
Client Needs: Health Promotion and Maintenance
Integrated Concept/Process: Teaching/Learning
Content Area: Adult Health/Immune
Reference: Deglin, J., & Vallerand, A. (1999). *Davis's drug guide for nurses* (6th ed.). Philadelphia: F. A. Davis, p. 1132.
2. **1**
Rationale: Daraprim is an antimalarial and antiprotozoal medication. It is used in the treatment of toxoplasmosis or

Pneumocystis carinii pneumonia. It is not used to treat nausea, vomiting, cardiac irregularities, or Kaposi's sarcoma.

Test-Taking Strategy: Use the process of elimination. If you knew that this medication is an antimalarial and antiprotozoal medication, then you would easily be directed to option 1. Review this medication if you had difficulty with this question.

Level of Cognitive Ability: Analysis
Client Needs: Physiological Integrity
Integrated Concept/Process: Nursing Process/Planning
Content Area: Adult Health/Immune
Reference: Deglin, J., & Vallerand, A. (1999). *Davis's drug guide for nurses* (6th ed.). Philadelphia: F. A. Davis, p. 877.

3. 4

Rationale: Invirase is an antiretroviral (protease inhibitor) used in combination with other antiretroviral medications in the management of HIV infection. It is administered with meals and is best absorbed if the client consumes high-calorie, high-fat meals. It can cause photosensitivity, and the client is instructed to avoid sun exposure.

Test-Taking Strategy: Use the process of elimination. Options 2 and 3 can be eliminated first because these dietary measures would not likely be prescribed. From the remaining options, it is necessary to know that this medication can cause photosensitivity. Review this medication if you had difficulty with this question.

Level of Cognitive Ability: Application
Client Needs: Health Promotion and Maintenance
Integrated Concept/Process: Teaching/Learning
Content Area: Adult Health/Immune
Reference: Ignatavicius, D., Workman, M., & Mishler, M. (1999). *Medical-surgical nursing: Across the health care continuum* (3rd ed.). Philadelphia: W. B. Saunders, p. 453.

4. 2

Rationale: Ocular toxicity is an adverse reaction to the use of hydroxychloroquine sulfate. An eye examination should be performed when medication therapy is started and after 6 months of therapy. Options 1, 3, and 4 are unrelated to the use of this medication.

Test-Taking Strategy: To answer this question, it is necessary to recall that this medication causes retinopathy. If you are unfamiliar with this medication, review its toxic effects.

Level of Cognitive Ability: Application
Client Needs: Health Promotion and Maintenance
Integrated Concept/Process: Teaching/Learning
Content Area: Adult Health/Immune
Reference: Clark, J., Queener, S., & Karb, V. (2000). *Pharmacologic basis of nursing practice* (6th ed.). St. Louis: Mosby, p. 488.

5. 2

Rationale: Stavudine is an antiretroviral (protease inhibitor) used in the management of HIV infection in clients who do not respond to or who cannot tolerate conventional therapy. The medication can cause peripheral neuropathy, and the nurse should closely monitor the client's gait and ask the client about paresthesia.

Test-Taking Strategy: Knowledge that this medication causes peripheral neuropathy is needed to answer this question. If you are not familiar with this medication and the important assessment measures, review this content.

Level of Cognitive Ability: Application
Client Needs: Physiological Integrity

Integrated Concept/Process: Nursing Process/Assessment
Content Area: Adult Health/Immune
Reference: Ignatavicius, D., Workman, M., & Mishler, M. (1999). *Medical-surgical nursing: Across the health care continuum* (3rd ed.). Philadelphia: W. B. Saunders, p. 453.

6. 1

Rationale: Zalcitabine is an antiretroviral (nucleoside reverse transcriptase inhibitor) used to manage HIV infection with other antiretrovirals. It has also been used as a single agent in clients who are intolerant of other regimens. It can cause serious liver damage, and liver function studies should be monitored closely. Options 2, 3, and 4 are not specifically associated with the use of this medication.

Test-Taking Strategy: Recalling that this medication is hepatotoxic will direct you to option 1. If you are unfamiliar with this medication, review this content.

Level of Cognitive Ability: Application
Client Needs: Physiological Integrity
Integrated Concept/Process: Nursing Process/Assessment
Content Area: Adult Health/Immune
Reference: Ignatavicius, D., Workman, M., & Mishler, M. (1999). *Medical-surgical nursing: Across the health care continuum* (3rd ed.). Philadelphia: W. B. Saunders, p. 453.

7. 2

Rationale: Foscavir is very toxic to the kidneys. Serum creatinine is monitored prior to therapy, 2 to 3 times per week during induction therapy, and at least weekly during maintenance therapy. It can also cause decreased levels of calcium, magnesium, phosphorus, and potassium. Thus, these levels are also measured with the same frequency.

Test-Taking Strategy: Use the process of elimination. Recalling that this medication is nephrotoxic will easily direct you to option 2. Review this medication if you are unfamiliar with it.

Level of Cognitive Ability: Application
Client Needs: Physiological Integrity
Integrated Concept/Process: Nursing Process/Assessment
Content Area: Adult Health/Immune
Reference: Deglin, J., & Vallerand, A. (1999). *Davis's drug guide for nurses* (6th ed.). Philadelphia: F. A. Davis, p. 411.

8. 4

Rationale: Frequent side effects of this medication include leukopenia, thrombocytopenia, and anemia. The client should be routinely monitored for signs and symptoms of infection. Options 1, 2, and 3 are inaccurate interpretations.

Test-Taking Strategy: Use the process of elimination, focusing on the key words "develops a fever." Note the relationship between these key words and option 4. Review the side effects of this medication if you had difficulty with this question.

Level of Cognitive Ability: Analysis
Client Needs: Physiological Integrity
Integrated Concept/Process: Nursing Process/Analysis
Content Area: Adult Health/Immune
Reference: Deglin, J., & Vallerand, A. (1999). *Davis's drug guide for nurses* (6th ed.). Philadelphia: F. A. Davis, p. 300.

9. 1

Rationale: A common side effect of this medication therapy is agranulocytopenia and anemia. The nurse monitors the CBC results for these changes. Options 2, 3, and 4 are unrelated to the use of this medication.

Test-Taking Strategy: Recalling that AZT causes anemia will direct you to option 1. Review this medication if you had difficulty with this question.
Level of Cognitive Ability: Application
Client Needs: Physiological Integrity
Integrated Concept/Process: Nursing Process/Assessment
Content Area: Adult Health/Immune
Reference: Deglin, J., & Vallerand, A. (1999). *Davis's drug guide for nurses* (6th ed.). Philadelphia: F. A. Davis, p. 1051.
10. **2**
Rationale: A serum amylase level that is increased 1.5 to 2 times normal may signify pancreatitis in the AIDS client, which is potentially fatal. The medication may have to be discontinued. The medication is also hepatotoxic, and can result in liver failure.
Test-Taking Strategy: Recalling that this medication can cause damage to the pancreas and is hepatotoxic will direct you to the correct option. Review this medication if you had difficulty with this question.
Level of Cognitive Ability: Analysis
Client Needs: Physiological Integrity
Integrated Concept/Process: Nursing Process/Assessment

Content Area: Adult Health/Immune
Reference: Deglin, J., & Vallerand, A. (1999). *Davis's drug guide for nurses* (6th ed.). Philadelphia: F. A. Davis, p. 270.

CRITICAL THINKING: FREE-TEXT ENTRY

Answer: Triglyceride level
Rationale: Norvir is an antiretroviral (protease inhibitor) used in combination with other antiretroviral medications in the management of HIV infection. It can increase the triglyceride level, and therefore this level should be monitored. Liver function studies are also monitored.
Test-Taking Strategy: It is necessary to be familiar with the adverse effects related to this medication to answer this question. Remember that Norvir increases the triglyceride level. If you are unfamiliar with this medication, review this information.
Level of Cognitive Ability: Analysis
Client Needs: Physiological Integrity
Integrated Concept/Process: Nursing Process/Analysis
Content Area: Adult Health/Immune
Reference: Hodgson, B., & Kizior, R. (2001). *Saunders nursing drug handbook 2001*. Philadelphia: W.B. Saunders, p. 913.

REFERENCES

Clark, J., Queener, S., & Karb, V. (2000). *Pharmacologic basis of nursing practice* (6th ed.). St. Louis: Mosby.

Deglin, J., & Vallerand, A. (1999). *Davis's drug guide for nurses* (6th ed.). Philadelphia: F.A. Davis.

Hodgson, B., & Kizior, R. (2001). *Saunders nursing drug handbook 2001*. Philadelphia: W.B. Saunders.

Ignatavicius, D., Workman, M., & Mishler, M. (1999). *Medical-surgical nursing: Across the health care continuum* (3rd ed.). Philadelphia: W.B. Saunders.

Salerno, E. (1999). *Pharmacology for health professionals*. St. Louis: Mosby.

Smeltzer, S., & Bare, B. (2000). *Brunner & Suddarth's textbook of medical-surgical nursing* (9th ed.). Philadelphia: Lippincott Williams & Wilkins.

The Adult Client with a Mental Health Disorder

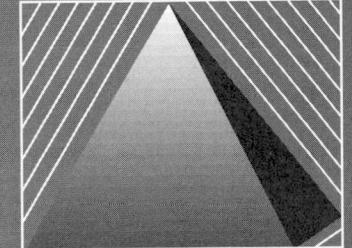

PYRAMID TERMS

abuse An act of misuse, deceit, or exploitation. The wrong or improper use of or action toward another individual that results in injury, damage, maltreatment, or corruption.

addiction Also known as drug dependence. Incorporates the concepts of loss of control with respect to the use of a drug, taking the drug despite related problems and complications, and a tendency to relapse.

coping mechanisms Methods of adjusting to environmental stress without altering one's own goals or purposes. Can include both conscious and unconscious mechanisms.

crisis A temporary state of disequilibrium in which an individual's usual coping mechanisms or problem-solving methods fail. It can result in personality growth or personality disorganization.

defense mechanisms Coping mechanisms (protective defenses) of the ego that attempt to protect the individual from feelings of inadequacy and worthlessness and prevent awareness of anxiety. When anxiety is too painful, the individual copes by using defense mechanisms to protect the ego and decrease anxiety.

milieu The physical and social environment in which an individual lives. Milieu therapy focuses on positive physical and social environmental manipulation in order to produce positive change.

restraints Physical restraints include any manual method or mechanical device, material, or equipment that inhibits free movement. Chemical restraints include the administration of medications for the specific purpose of inhibiting a specific behavior or movement.

seclusion Placing a client alone in a specially designed room for protection and close supervision. It is the last measure in a process to maximize safety of the client and others.

suicide The ultimate act of self-destruction, in which an individual purposefully ends his or her own life.

suicide attempt Any willfull, self-inflicted, life-threatening action by an individual that has not led to death.

PYRAMID TO SUCCESS

The Pyramid to Success focuses on the therapeutic nurse-client relationship, client rights, hospital admission procedures, and the ethical and legal issues related to the care of the client with a mental health disorder. Pyramid points focus on the use of restraints, seclusion, and electroconvulsive therapy (ECT). Focus on care of the client with an addiction, such as an eating disorder or a drug or alcohol disorder. Additional focus areas include anxiety, depression, suicide, abuse and violence, rape crisis interventions, posttraumatic stress disorders, obsessive-compulsive disorders, schizophrenia, and bipolar disorders. Pyramid points address the use of medications prescribed for a client with a mental health disorder, particularly lithium and the benzodiazepines. The Integrated Concepts and Processes addressed in this unit include Nursing Process, Caring, Communication and Documentation, Cultural Awareness, Self-Care, and Teaching/Learning.

CLIENT NEEDS
Safe, Effective Care Environment

Client advocacy
Client rights
Confidentiality
Informed consent related to treatments, such as restraints, seclusion, and electroconvulsive therapy (ECT)
Legal responsibilities related to reporting incidences of violence and abuse
Psychiatric consultations and referrals
Providing safety to client and others
Use of restraints and seclusion

Health Promotion and Maintenance

Health promotion programs related to addictions
Individual lifestyle choices
Psychosocial assessment techniques

Psychosocial Integrity

Abuse/neglect
Behavioral interventions

Chemical dependency
Coping mechanisms
Counseling techniques
Crisis intervention
Domestic violence
End-of-life issues
Grief and loss
Religious and spiritual influences on health
Sexual abuse/rape
Stress management
Support systems
Therapeutic nurse-client relationship
Therapeutic milieu

Physiological Integrity

Abusive and self-destructive behavior
Alterations in body systems related to addictions
Elimination
Expected and untoward effects of medications
Laboratory values related to medication therapy

Medication administration
Nutrition
Pathophysiology related to mental health disorders
Personal hygiene measures
Potential complications related to medications and electroconvulsive therapy
Rest and sleep

REFERENCES

Fortinash, K., & Holoday-Worret, P. (2000). *Psychiatric mental health nursing* (2nd ed.). St. Louis: Mosby.

Glod, C.A. (1998). *Contemporary psychiatric-mental health nursing.* Philadelphia: F.A. Davis.

Keltner, N., Schwecke, L., & Bostrom, C. (1999). *Psychiatric nursing* (3rd ed.). St. Louis: Mosby.

National Council of State Boards of Nursing (eds.) (2000). *Test Plan for the National Council Licensure Examination for Registered Nurses.* Chicago: Author.

Stuart, G.W., & Laraia, M.T. (1998). *Principles and practice of psychiatric nursing.* (6th ed.). St. Louis: Mosby.

Varcarolis, E. (1998). *Foundations of psychiatric mental health nursing* (3rd ed.). Philadelphia: W.B. Saunders.

Foundations of Psychiatric Mental Health Nursing

I. MENTAL HEALTH

A. A lifelong process of successful adaptation to a changing internal and external environment
B. The individual is in contact with reality and the environment and possesses the ability to love, work, and resolve conflicts within a framework of reasonability
C. The individual has psychobiological resilience

II. PSYCHIATRIC/MENTAL HEALTH ILLNESS

A. Description
  1. Loss of the ability to respond to the environment in ways that are in accord with oneself or society's expectations
  2. Characterized by thought or behavior patterns that impair functioning and cause the individual distress
B. Personality characteristics
  1. Is unaccepting of self and dislikes self
  2. Has an unrealistic perception of strengths and weaknesses
  3. Thoughts and perceptions may not be reality based
  4. Is unable to find meaning and purpose in life
  5. Lacks direction and productivity in life
  6. Has difficulty in meeting own needs
  7. Depends on others for thought and actions
C. Adaptations to stress
  1. Feels out of control with self and with the environment
  2. Has a negative perception of the environment
  3. Has ineffective **coping mechanisms**
D. Interpersonal relationships
  1. Is unable to love and care for others
  2. Is unable to feel loved by others or accept feelings from others

III. COPING AND DEFENSE MECHANISMS

A. **Coping mechanisms**
  1. Coping involves any effort to decrease the stress response
  2. **Coping mechanisms** can be either constructive or destructive in nature; they can be task oriented and related to direct problem solving, or they can be defense-oriented regulating responses to protect oneself
  3. Destructive **coping mechanisms** often cause a mental health disorder because the problem that causes the disorder is avoided
  4. Neurotic or psychotic behaviors can typically result when **coping mechanisms** become destructive
B. **Defense mechanisms** (Box 69-1)
  1. **Coping mechanisms** (protective defenses) of the ego that attempt to protect the individual from feelings of inadequacy and worthlessness and prevent awareness of anxiety
  2. When anxiety is too painful, the individual copes by using **defense mechanisms** to protect the ego and decrease anxiety
C. Implementation
  1. Assess the client's use of the **defense mechanism**
  2. Determine if the use of the **defense mechanism** characterizes unhealthy adjustment
  3. Facilitate appropriate use of **defense mechanisms**
  4. Avoid criticizing the behavior and the use of **defense mechanisms**
  5. Assist the client to identify the source of the anxiety
  6. Assist the client to explore methods to reduce the anxiety

999

BOX 69-1

Types of Defense Mechanisms

COMPENSATION
Putting forth extra effort to achieve in areas in which one has a real or imagined deficiency

CONVERSION
The expression of emotional conflicts through physical symptoms

DENIAL
Disowning consciously intolerable thoughts and impulses

DISPLACEMENT
Feelings toward one person are directed to another who is less threatening, thereby satisfying an impulse with a substitute object

DISSOCIATION
The blocking off of an anxiety-provoking event or period of time from the conscious mind

FANTASY
Gratification by imaginary achievements and wishful thinking

FIXATION
Never advancing to the next level of emotional development and organization; the persistence in later life of interests and behavior patterns appropriate to an earlier age

IDENTIFICATION
The unconscious attempt to change oneself to resemble an admired person

INSULATION
Withdrawing into passivity and becoming inaccessible in order to avoid further threatening situations

INTELLECTUALIZATION
Excessive reasoning to avoid feeling; the thinking is disconnected from feelings, and situations are dealt with at a cognitive level

INTROJECTION
A type of identification in which the individual incorporates the traits or values of another into self

ISOLATION
Response in which a person blocks feelings associated with an unpleasant experience

PROJECTION
Transferring one's internal feelings, thoughts, and unacceptable ideas and traits to someone else

RATIONALIZATION
An attempt to make unacceptable feelings and behavior acceptable by justifying the behavior

REACTION FORMATION
Developing conscious attitudes and behaviors and acting out behaviors opposite to what one really feels

REGRESSION
Returning to an earlier developmental stage to express an impulse in order to deal with reality

REPRESSION
An unconscious process in which the client blocks undesirable and unacceptable thoughts from conscious expression

SUBLIMATION
Replacement of an unacceptable need, attitude, or emotion with one more socially acceptable

SUBSTITUTION
The replacement of a valued unacceptable object with an object that is more acceptable to the ego

SUPPRESSION
The conscious, deliberate forgetting of unacceptable or painful thoughts, ideas, and feelings

SYMBOLIZATION
The conscious use of an idea or object to represent another actual event or object; many times the meaning is not clear because the symbol may be representative of something unconscious

UNDOING
Engaging in behavior that is considered to be the opposite of a previous unacceptable behavior, thought, or feeling

IV. THE NURSE-CLIENT RELATIONSHIP
A. Principles
  1. Respect the client and value the client as an individual
  2. Care for the client in a holistic manner
  3. Maintain appropriate limits
  4. Remember that empathy is therapeutic and sympathy is nontherapeutic
  5. Maintain honest and open communication
  6. Encourage expression of the client's feelings
  7. Assist the client to develop resources
B. Phases of the therapeutic relationship
  1. Orientation/initiation phase
    a. Establish boundaries and trust with the client
    b. Identify the expectations of the relationship

c. Assess the anxiety in the client
d. Define goals with the client
2. Working/continuation phase
   a. Promote an attitude of acceptance
   b. Assist the client to express feelings
   c. Identify problems
   d. Continue to assess and evaluate problems
   e. Promote insight and the use of constructive **coping mechanisms**
   f. Increase the client's independence
3. Termination/separation phase
   a. Prepare the client for termination and separation on initial contact
   b. Evaluate progress and achievement of goals
   c. Identify and deal with termination and separation issues
   d. Encourage the client to discuss feelings about termination
   e. Transfer the client to other support systems
   f. Do not promise the client that the relationship will be continued

▲ **V. THERAPEUTIC COMMUNICATION PROCESS**
A. Principles
   1. Communication includes both verbal and nonverbal expression
   2. Successful communication includes appropriateness, efficiency, flexibility, and feedback
   3. Anxiety in either the nurse or the client impedes communication
   4. Communication needs to be goal directed within a professional framework
B. Therapeutic communication techniques and blocks to communication (Table 69-1)

VI. DIAGNOSTIC AND STATISTICAL MANUAL OF MENTAL DISORDERS
A. A nomenclature of psychiatric diagnoses developed by the American Psychiatric Association
B. A system used in clinical, research, and educational settings, in which diagnostic criteria are inclusive for each diagnosis but allow for individualized differences within a pattern of behavior
C. Knowledge of the criteria for a particular psychiatric diagnosis will assist the nurse in making a clinical decision about a nursing diagnosis

▲ **VII. TYPES OF MENTAL HEALTH ADMISSIONS AND DISCHARGES** (Box 69-2)
A. Voluntary admission
   1. Any citizen of lawful age may apply in writing (usually on a standard admission form) for admission to the hospital
   2. Sought by the client or the client's guardian if the client is too ill but voluntarily seeks assistance
   3. Client agrees to accept treatment
   4. Civil rights are fully retained by the client

TABLE 69-1

Therapeutic Communication Techniques and Blocks to Communication

Therapeutic Techniques	Blocks
Listening	Giving advice
Being silent	Changing the subject
Respecting the client	Giving approval or disapproval
Providing recognition and acknowledgment	Challenging the client
Providing feedback	Making stereotypical comments
Offering to assist	Making value judgments
Focusing and refocusing	Providing false reassurance
Clarifying and validating	Placing the client's feelings on hold
Reflecting	Asking the client "Why?"
Making observations	Being defensive
Giving information	
Presenting reality	
Summarizing	
Using open-ended questions	
Providing nonverbal encouragement	
Maintaining neutral responses	
Encouraging formulation of plan of action	

BOX 69-2

Client Rights

Right to accessible health care
Right to a coordination and continuity of health care
Right to courteous and individualized health care
Right to information about the qualifications, names, and titles of personnel delivering care
Right to refuse observation by those not directly involved in care
Right to privacy and confidentiality
Right to informed consent
Right to treatment
Right to refuse treatment
Right to treatment in the least restrictive setting
Right not to be subjected to unnecessary restraints
Right to habeas corpus; may request a hearing at any time to be released from the hospital
Right to information about diagnosis, prognosis, and treatment
Right to information on the charges for service
Right to communicate with people outside the hospital through written correspondence, telephone, and personal visits
Right to keep clothing and personal effects
Right to be employed
Right to religious freedom
Right to execute wills
Right to retain licenses, privileges, or permits established by the law, such as a driver's or professional license

5. Client is free to sign him or herself out of the hospital

B. Involuntary admission

1. Involuntary admission may be necessary when a person is mentally ill, is a danger to self or others, or is in need of psychiatric treatment or physical care

2. An admission status in which a person who has the legal capacity to consent to mental health treatment refuses to do so and is involuntarily detained for treatment by the state

3. The client who is involuntarily admitted does not lose his or her right of informed consent

4. The length of time for hospitalization is specified by the state and varies from state to state

5. The client is considered legally competent until he or she has been declared incompetent through a legal proceeding

6. If the nurse believes that a client lacks competency, action should be initiated to have a legal guardian appointed from the court

7. Categories
   a. Evaluation and emergency care
   b. Certification for observation and treatment
   c. Extended or indeterminate commitment

C. Release from the hospital

1. Description
   a. Depends on the client's admission status
   b. The client who sought voluntary admission has the right to demand and receive release
   c. Some states provide for conditional release of voluntary clients, which enables the treating physician or administrator to order continued treatment on an outpatient basis if the clinical needs of the client would warrant further care

2. Conditional release
   a. Usually requires outpatient treatment for a specified period to determine the client's compliance with medication protocol, ability to meet basic needs, and ability to reintegrate into the community
   b. A voluntary client who is conditionally released cannot be reinstitutionalized without the client's consent, unless the institution complies with the procedures for involuntary admission
   c. An involuntary client who is conditionally released may be reinstitutionalized while the commitment is still in effect without recommencement of formal admission procedures

3. Discharge
   a. Discharge (unconditional release) is the termination of the client-institution relationship
   b. This release may be ordered by the psychiatrist, court ordered, or administratively ordered

c. The administration officer of an institution has the discretion to discharge clients

d. In most states, clients can institute a court proceeding to seek a judicial discharge (writ of habeas corpus)

e. Discharge planning and follow-up care are important for the continued well-being of the client with a mental health disorder

f. After-care case managers are needed to facilitate the client's adaptation back into the community and to provide early referral if the treatment plan is not followed

PRACTICE QUESTIONS

1. Unresolved feelings related to loss may be most likely recognized during which phase of the therapeutic nurse-client relationship?
   1. Orientation
   2. Working
   3. Termination
   4. Trusting

2. A client with a diagnosis of major depression who attempted suicide says to the nurse, "I should have died. I've always been a failure. Nothing ever goes right for me." The most therapeutic response to the client is:
   1. "I don't see you as a failure."
   2. "Feeling like this is all part of being ill."
   3. "You've been feeling like a failure for a while?"
   4. "You have everything to live for."

3. A community health nurse visits a client at home. The client states, "I haven't slept at all the last couple of nights." Which response by the nurse illustrates the most therapeutic communication technique for this client?
   1. "Go on..."
   2. "Sleeping?"
   3. "The last couple of nights?"
   4. "You're having difficulty sleeping?"

4. A nurse is performing an admission assessment on a client and is attempting to obtain subjective data about the client's sexual and reproductive status. The client states, "I don't want to discuss this; it's private and personal." Which statement, if made by the nurse, indicates that the nurse is therapeutic?
   1. "I hate being asked these sorts of questions too."
   2. "I am a professional nurse and as such I'll have you know that all information is kept confidential."
   3. "I know that some of these questions are difficult for you but, as a professional nurse, I must legally respect your confidentiality."
   4. "This is difficult for you to speak about, but I am trying to perform a complete assessment and I need this information."

5. A nurse is caring for a Native American client who says, "I don't want you to touch me. I'll take care of myself!" Which nursing response is most therapeutic?
   1. "OK. If that's what you want. I'll just leave this cup for you to collect your urine in. After breakfast, I will take more blood from you."
   2. "If you didn't want our care, why did you come here?"
   3. " Why are you being so difficult? I only want to help you."
   4. "It sounds as though you want to take care of yourself. Let's work together so you can do things for yourself."
6. A client admitted to the mental health unit is experiencing Altered Thought Processes. The client believes that the food is being poisoned. Which communication technique does the nurse plan to use to encourage the client to express feelings?
   1. Using open-ended questions and silence
   2. Offering opinions about the necessity of adequate nutrition
   3. Identifying the reasons that the client may not want to eat
   4. Focusing on self-disclosure about food preferences
7. A nurse is working with a client who has sought counseling after trying to rescue a neighbor involved in a house fire. In spite of the client's efforts, the neighbor died. Which action does the nurse engage in with the client during the working phase of the nurse-client relationship?
   1. Exploring the client's potential for self-harm
   2. Exploring the client's ability to function
   3. Inquiring about the client's perception or appraisal of the neighbor's death
   4. Inquiring about and examining the client's feelings that may block adaptive coping
8. A client who has just been sexually assaulted is very quiet and calm. The nurse analyzes this behavior as indicative of which defense mechanism?
   1. Denial
   2. Projection
   3. Rationalization
   4. Intellectualization
9. A nurse completes the initial assessment of a client admitted to the mental health unit. The nurse analyzes the data obtained on assessment and determines that which of the following presents a priority concern?
   1. The presence of bruises on the client's body
   2. The client's report of not eating or sleeping
   3. The client's report of suicidal thoughts
   4. The significant other's disapproving of the treatment
10. Laboratory work is prescribed for a client who has been experiencing delusions. When the nurse approaches the client to obtain a specimen of the client's blood, the client begins to shout, "You're all vampires. Let me out of here!" The most appropriate nursing response is which of the following?
    1. "I am not going to hurt you, I am going to help you!"
    2. "What makes you think that I am a vampire?"
    3. "I'll leave and come back later for your blood."
    4. "It must be fearful to think others want to hurt you."
11. An inebriated client is brought to the emergency department by the local police. The client is told that the physician will be in to see the client in about 30 minutes. The client becomes very loud and offensive and wants to be seen by the physician immediately. The most appropriate nursing intervention is which of the following?
    1. Attempt to talk with the client to deescalate behavior
    2. Watch the behavior escalate before intervening
    3. Inform the client that he or she will be asked to leave if the behavior continues
    4. Offer to take the client to an examination room until he or she can be treated
12. A client is admitted to a mental health unit for treatment of psychotic behavior. The client is at the locked exit door and is shouting, "Let me out. There's nothing wrong with me. I don't belong here." The nurse analyzes this behavior as:
    1. Projection
    2. Denial
    3. Regression
    4. Rationalization
13. A home health nurse is talking to the spouse of a client taking an antidepressant. The spouse says, "Now that my husband is responding to the antidepressant, the suicidal risk is over and you can stop making these home visits." After analyzing this statement, which of the following is the most appropriate nursing response?
    1. "I agree with you. Clients who want to kill themselves are only suicidal for a limited time. No one can feel self-destructive forever."
    2. "I need to continue with my visits. Your comment reflects a lack of knowledge that this disease runs in families."
    3. "I agree with you. The suicidal threats were really attention seeking. Continuing to visit would reinforce your husband's use of manipulation".
    4. "I need to continue with my visits. Most suicides occur within 3 months after improvement begins because the client now has the energy to carry out the suicidal intentions."
14. A supervisor reprimands the nurse in charge of a nursing unit because the charge nurse has not

adhered to the unit budget. Later that afternoon, the charge nurse accuses the nursing staff of wasting supplies. This behavior is an example of:
1. Denial
2. Repression
3. Suppression
4. Displacement

15. A client says to the nurse, "I'm going to die, and I wish my family would stop hoping for a cure! I get so angry when they carry on like this! After all, I'm the one who's dying." The most therapeutic response by the nurse is:
1. "You're feeling angry that your family continues to hope for you to be cured?"
2. "I think we should talk more about your anger with your family."
3. "Well, it sounds like you're being pretty pessimistic. After all, years ago people died of pneumonia."
4. "Have you shared your feelings with your family?"

16. A nurse employed in a mental health unit is assigned to care for a client admitted to the unit 2 days ago. On review of the client's record, the nurse notes that the admission was a voluntary admission. Based on this type of admission, the nurse anticipates which of the following?
1. The client will be very resistant to treatment measures
2. The client's family will be very resistant to treatment measures
3. The client will be angry and will refuse care
4. The client will participate in the planning of the care and treatment plan

17. A nurse enters a client's room and the client is demanding release from the hospital. The nurse reviews the client's record and notes that the client was admitted 2 days ago for treatment of an anxiety disorder and that the admission was voluntary. Which of the following actions will the nurse take?
1. Tell the client that discharge is not possible at this time
2. Call the client's family
3. Contact the physician
4. Persuade the client to stay a few more days

18. A client is admitted to the mental health unit. On admission assessment, the nurse notes that the client is admitted by involuntary status. Based on this type of admission, the nurse would most likely expect that the client:
1. Presents a harm to self
2. Requested the admission
3. Consented to the admission
4. Provided written application to the facility for admission

19. A nurse is caring for a client who is scheduled for electroconvulsive therapy (ECT). The nurse notes that an informed consent has not been obtained for the procedure. On review of the record, the nurse notes that the admission was an involuntary hospitalization. Based on this information, the nurse determines:
1. That an informed consent does not need to be obtained
2. That an informed consent should be obtained from the family
3. That an informed consent needs to be obtained from the client
4. That the physician will obtain the informed consent

20. After a group therapy session, a client approaches a nurse and verbalizes a need for seclusion because of uncontrollable feelings. The most appropriate nursing action would be to:
1. Inform the client that seclusion has not been prescribed
2. Obtain an informed consent
3. Call the client's family
4. Place the client in seclusion immediately

21. A nurse is providing care to a client admitted to the hospital with a diagnosis of acute anxiety disorder. The nurse is conversing with the client. The client says to the nurse "I have a secret that I want to tell you. You won't tell anyone about it, will you?" The most appropriate nursing response is which of the following?
1. "No, I won't tell anyone."
2. "I cannot promise to keep a secret."
3. "If you tell me the secret, I will tell it to your doctor."
4. "If you tell me the secret, I will need to document it in your record."

22. A nurse employed in a mental health clinic is greeted by a neighbor in a local grocery store. The neighbor says to the nurse, "How is Carol doing? She is my best friend and is seen at your clinic every week." The most appropriate nursing response is which of the following?
1. "I'm not supposed to discuss this, but since you are my neighbor, I can tell you that she is doing great!"
2. "I'm not supposed to discuss this, but since you are my neighbor, I can tell you that she really has some problems!"
3. "If you want to know about Carol, you need to ask her yourself."
4. "I cannot discuss any client situation with you."

23. A client was involuntarily admitted to the mental health unit because of episodes of extremely violent behavior. The client is demanding to be discharged from the hospital. The nurse does not allow the client to leave. Which of the following represent the

legal ramifications associated with the nurse's behavior?

1. The nurse will be charged with imprisonment
2. The nurse will be charged with assault
3. The nurse will be charged with slander
4. No charge will be made against the nurse because the nurse's actions are reasonable

24. A nurse is preparing a client for the termination phase of the nurse-client relationship. The nurse prepares to implement which nursing task that is most appropriate for this phase?
    1. Identifying expected outcomes
    2. Planning short-term goals
    3. Making appropriate referrals
    4. Developing realistic solutions

25. During the termination phase of the nurse-client relationship, the clinic nurse observes that the client continuously demonstrates bursts of anger. The most appropriate interpretation of the behavior is that the client:
    1. Requires further treatment and is not ready to be discharged

2. Is displaying typical behaviors that can occur during termination
3. Needs to be admitted to the hospital
4. Needs to be referred to the psychiatrist as soon as possible

CRITICAL THINKING: FREE-TEXT ENTRY

A nurse employed in an inpatient mental health unit has been meeting with a client with depression for therapy sessions on a regular basis. The client says to the nurse, "When I get out of the hospital, I want to be a nurse just like you." At the end of the session, the nurse documents that the client used which defense mechanism when making this statement?

Answer: _____

ANSWERS

1. **3**

Rationale: In the termination phase, the relationship comes to a close. Ending treatment can sometimes be traumatic for clients who have come to value the relationship and the help. Since loss is an issue, any unresolved feelings related to loss may resurface during this phase. Options 1, 2, and 4 are incorrect.

Test-Taking Strategy: Note the key words "unresolved," "loss," and "recognized" in the question. Considering the phases of the therapeutic nurse-client relationship directs you to option 3. Review these phases and the nursing implications if you had difficulty with this question.

Level of Cognitive Ability: Analysis
Client Needs: Psychosocial Integrity
Integrated Concept/Process: Caring
Content Area: Mental Health
Reference: Fortinash, K., & Holoday-Worret, P. (2000). *Psychiatric mental health nursing* (2nd ed.). St. Louis: Mosby, p. 19.

2. **3**

Rationale: Responding to the feelings expressed by a client is an effective therapeutic communication technique. The correct option is an example of the use of restating. Options 1, 2, and 4 block communication because they minimize the client's experience and do not facilitate exploration of the client's expressed feelings.

Test-Taking Strategy: Use the process of elimination and therapeutic communication techniques to direct you to the option that directly addresses client feelings and concerns. Also, option 3 is the only option that is stated in the form of a question and is open-ended, thus will encourage the verbaliza-

tion of feelings. Review therapeutic communication techniques if you had difficulty with this question.

Level of Cognitive Ability: Application
Client Needs: Psychosocial Integrity
Integrated Concept/Process: Communication and Documentation
Content Area: Mental Health
Reference: Fortinash, K., & Holoday-Worret, P. (2000). *Psychiatric mental health nursing* (2nd ed.). St. Louis: Mosby, p. 159.

3. **4**

Rationale: The most therapeutic nursing communication technique is restatement. Although it is a technique that has a prompting component to it, it repeats the client's major theme, which assists the nurse to obtain a more specific perception of the problem from the client. Options 1, 2, and 3 are not therapeutic responses.

Test-Taking Strategy: Use the process of elimination. Option 1 is a general lead and allows the client to direct the discussion. Option 2 uses reflection that simply repeats the client's last words to prompt further discussion. Option 3 focuses on the number of nights rather than the specific problem of sleep. Option 4 will provide the perception of the problem from the client's perspective. Review therapeutic communication techniques if you had difficulty with this question.

Level of Cognitive Ability: Application
Client Needs: Psychosocial Integrity
Integrated Concept/Process: Communication and Documentation
Content Area: Mental Health
Reference: Fortinash, K., & Holoday-Worret, P. (2000). *Psychiatric mental health nursing* (2nd ed.). St. Louis: Mosby, p. 159.

4. 3

Rationale: Option 3 is the only option that identifies a therapeutic response. In option 1, the nurse's feelings are the focus. This response clearly ignores the fact that the issue is about the client and the client's discomfort, not about the nurse. In option 2, the nurse becomes pompous and a bit angry and supercilious, which is not therapeutic. In option 4, the nurse begins correctly with an empathic stance but then becomes demanding.

Test-Taking Strategy: Use of the process of elimination and therapeutic communication techniques will easily direct you to option 3. Review therapeutic communication techniques if you had difficulty with this question.

Level of Cognitive Ability: Analysis

Client Needs: Psychosocial Integrity

Integrated Concept/Process: Communication and Documentation

Content Area: Mental Health

References: Fortinash, K., & Holoday-Worret, P. (2000). *Psychiatric mental health nursing* (2nd ed.). St. Louis: Mosby, p. 159.

Glod, C. A. (1998). *Contemporary psychiatric-mental health nursing.* Philadelphia: F. A. Davis, pp. 58-60.

5. 4

Rationale: Native Americans view touch very differently from other Americans. The most therapeutic response is the one that reflects the client's feelings and empowers the client by offering self control over one's own care. In option 1, the nurse uses avoidance and information giving. Option 2 is an aggressive and nontherapeutic communication technique. Option 3 labels the client's behavior and is likely to provoke anger.

Test-Taking Strategy: Use the process of elimination and knowledge about the use of therapeutic communication techniques. Focus on the client's cultural heritage and the client's feelings to direct you to option 4. Review therapeutic communication techniques and cultural considerations if you had difficulty with this question.

Level of Cognitive Ability: Analysis

Client Needs: Psychosocial Integrity

Integrated Concept/Process: Cultural Awareness

Content Area: Mental Health

Reference: Keltner, N., Schwecke, L., & Bostrom, C. (1999). *Psychiatric nursing* (3rd ed.). St. Louis: Mosby, pp. 202-203.

6. 1

Rationale: Open-ended questions and silence are strategies used to encourage clients to discuss their problem. Options 2 and 3 are not helpful to the client because they do not encourage the client to express feelings. The nurse should not offer opinions and should encourage the client to identify the reasons for the behavior. Option 4 is not a client-centered intervention.

Test-Taking Strategy: Use the process of elimination. Eliminate options 2 and 3 first, because they do not support client expression of feelings. Eliminate option 4 next, because it is not a client-centered response. Focusing on the client's feelings will easily direct you to option 1. Review therapeutic communication techniques if you had difficulty with this question.

Level of Cognitive Ability: Application

Client Needs: Psychosocial Integrity

Integrated Concept/Process: Communication and Documentation

Content Area: Mental Health

Reference: Fortinash, K., & Holoday-Worret, P. (2000). *Psychiatric mental health nursing* (2nd ed.). St. Louis: Mosby, p. 159.

7. 4

Rationale: The client must first deal with feelings and negative responses before being able to work through the meaning of the crisis. Option 4 pertains directly to the client's feelings. Options 1, 2, and 3 do not directly address the client's feelings.

Test-Taking Strategy: Focus on the issue of the question, the working phase of the nurse-client relationship. Use the process of elimination, focusing on this issue and on the option that focuses on the feelings of the client. Review the phases of the nurse-client relationship if you had difficulty with this question.

Level of Cognitive Ability: Application

Client Needs: Psychosocial Integrity

Integrated Concept/Process: Caring

Content Area: Mental Health

Reference: Fortinash, K., & Holoday-Worret, P. (2000). *Psychiatric mental health nursing* (2nd ed.). St. Louis: Mosby, p. 160.

8. 1

Rationale: Denial is an adaptive and protective reaction and may be a response by a victim of sexual abuse. Projection is transferring one's internal feelings, thoughts, and unacceptable ideas and traits to someone else. Rationalization is justifying the unacceptable attributes about oneself. Intellectualization is the excessive use of abstract thinking or generalizations to decrease painful thinking.

Test-Taking Strategy: Use the process of elimination. Note the key words "calm" and "quiet." These behaviors are indicative of denial in a sexually abused victim. If you had difficulty with this question, review content related to the sexually abused victim and defense mechanisms.

Level of Cognitive Ability: Analysis

Client Needs: Psychosocial Integrity

Integrated Concept/Process: Nursing Process/Analysis

Content Area: Mental Health

Reference: Fortinash, K., & Holoday-Worret, P. (2000). *Psychiatric mental health nursing* (2nd ed.). St. Louis: Mosby, p. 10.

9. 3

Rationale: The client's thoughts are extremely important when verbalized. A client's report of suicidal thoughts is of highest priority. Options 1, 2, and 4 will all affect the treatment of the client but are not of greatest importance at this time.

Test-Taking Strategy: The client is the focus of the question; therefore eliminate option 4. Use the process of elimination and principles related to prioritizing to select the correct option. The life-threatening concern is identified in option 3. Review the techniques of assessment and analysis of assessment data from a client with a mental health disorder if you had difficulty with this question.

Level of Cognitive Ability: Analysis

Client Needs: Psychosocial Integrity

Integrated Concept/Process: Nursing Process/Analysis

Content Area: Mental Health

Reference: Fortinash, K., & Holoday-Worret, P. (2000). *Psychiatric mental health nursing* (2nd ed.). St. Louis: Mosby, pp. 662-663.

10. **4**

Rationale: Option 4 helps the client to focus on the emotion underlying the delusion but does not argue with it. Option 3 avoids the client. Option 2 places the client in a position that requires a response. Option 1 is an attempt to convince the client to believe another thought. This response may cause the client to hold the delusion more strongly.

Test-Taking Strategy: Use the process of elimination and therapeutic communication techniques to answer the question. Option 4 is the only option that recognizes the client's need and focuses on the client's feelings. Review therapeutic communication techniques if you had difficulty with this question.

Level of Cognitive Ability: Analysis
Client Needs: Psychosocial Integrity
Integrated Concept/Process: Caring
Content Area: Mental Health
Reference: Keltner, N., Schwecke, L., & Bostrom, C. (1999). *Psychiatric nursing* (3rd ed.). St. Louis: Mosby, p. 132.

11. **4**

Rationale: Safety of the client, other clients, and staff is of prime concern. Option 1 is not appropriate, given the fact that the client is inebriated and may not be able to be reasoned with. Option 2 is inaccurate because waiting to intervene could cause the client to become even more agitated and a threat to others. Option 3 would further aggravate an already agitated individual. Option 4 is in effect an isolation technique that allows for separation from others and provides a less stimulating environment where the client can maintain dignity.

Test-Taking Strategy: Focus on the issue, an inebriated client. Use this information and the process of elimination in selecting the correct option. Option 4 most directly addresses the situation and the behavior and feelings of the client. Review therapeutic communication techniques if you had difficulty with this question.

Level of Cognitive Ability: Analysis
Client Needs: Psychosocial Integrity
Integrated Concept/Process: Communication and Documentation
Content Area: Mental Health
Reference: Fortinash, K., & Holoday-Worret, P. (2000). *Psychiatric mental health nursing* (2nd ed.). St. Louis: Mosby, p. 364.

12. **2**

Rationale: Denial is refusal to admit to a painful reality, which is treated as if it does not exist. In projection, a person unconsciously rejects emotionally unacceptable features and attributes them to other people, objects, or situations. In regression, the client returns to an earlier, more comforting, although less mature way of behaving. Rationalization is justifying illogical or unreasonable ideas, actions, or feelings by developing acceptable explanations that satisfy the teller as well as the listener.

Test-Taking Strategy: Use the process of elimination. The key words in the question that should direct you to the correct option are "There's nothing wrong with me." Select the option that recognizes the client's attempt to avoid looking at the reality of the situation. If you had difficulty with this question, review defense mechanisms.

Level of Cognitive Ability: Analysis

Client Needs: Psychosocial Integrity
Integrated Concept/Process: Nursing Process/Analysis
Content Area: Mental Health
Reference: Keltner, N., Schwecke, L., & Bostrom, C. (1999). *Psychiatric nursing* (3rd ed.). St. Louis: Mosby, pp. 31-32.

13. **4**

Rationale: Most suicides occur within 3 months after the beginning of the improvement, when the client has the energy to carry out the suicidal intentions. Options 1, 2, and 3 are incorrect.

Test-Taking Strategy: Use the process of elimination and knowledge of the facts about suicide to answer the question. Recalling that a critical time for a suicidal client is when the client has energy will direct you to option 4. Review the concepts related to suicide and therapeutic communication techniques if you had difficulty with this question.

Level of Cognitive Ability: Application
Client Needs: Physiological Integrity
Integrated Concept/Process: Nursing Process/Implementation
Content Area: Mental Health
Reference: Fortinash, K., & Holoday-Worret, P. (2000). *Psychiatric mental health nursing* (2nd ed.). St. Louis: Mosby, p. 662.

14. **4**

Rationale: Ego defense mechanisms are operations outside a person's awareness that the ego calls into play to protect against anxiety. Displacement is the discharging of pent-up feelings on persons less dangerous than those who initially aroused the emotion. Denial is the blocking out of painful or anxiety-inducing events or feelings. Repression is unconsciously keeping unacceptable feelings out of awareness. Suppression is consciously keeping unacceptable feelings and thoughts out of awareness.

Test-Taking Strategy: Use the process of elimination. Read the behavior identified in the question to assist you in determining the type of ego defense mechanism or behavior used. If you had difficulty with this question, review defense mechanisms.

Level of Cognitive Ability: Analysis
Client Needs: Psychosocial Integrity
Integrated Concept/Process: Nursing Process/Analysis
Content Area: Mental Health
Reference: Fortinash, K., & Holoday-Worret, P. (2000). *Psychiatric mental health nursing* (2nd ed.). St. Louis: Mosby, p. 10.

15. **1**

Rationale: Restating is the therapeutic communication technique in which the nurse repeats what the client says to show understanding and to review what was said. Option 1 uses the therapeutic technique of restating. In option 2, the nurse attempts to use focusing, but the attempt to discuss central issues is premature. In option 3, the nurse makes a judgment and is nontherapeutic in the one-to-one relationship. In option 4, the nurse is attempting to assess the client's ability to openly discuss feelings with family members.

Test-Taking Strategy: Use therapeutic communication techniques to answer the question. Option 1 is the only option that identifies the use of a therapeutic technique and focuses on the client's feelings. Review these techniques if you had difficulty with this question.

Level of Cognitive Ability: Application
Client Needs: Psychosocial Integrity

Integrated Concept/Process: Communication and Documentation

Content Area: Mental Health

Reference: Fortinash, K., & Holoday-Worret, P. (2000). *Psychiatric mental health nursing* (2nd ed.). St. Louis: Mosby, p. 159.

16. 4

Rationale: Generally, voluntary admission is sought by the client. A voluntary admission permits a client to make a written application for admission. If the client seeks voluntary admission, the most likely expectation is that the client will participate in the treatment program. Options 1, 2, and 3 are not characteristics of this type of admission.

Test-Taking Strategy: Use the process of elimination. Note the key words "voluntary admission." This should direct you to option 4. Additionally, note that options 1, 2, and 3 are similar. Review the various types of hospital admission processes if you had difficulty with this question.

Level of Cognitive Ability: Analysis

Client Needs: Psychosocial Integrity

Integrated Concept/Process: Nursing Process/Analysis

Content Area: Mental Health

Reference: Varcarolis, E. (1998). *Foundations of psychiatric mental health nursing* (3rd ed.). Philadelphia: W. B. Saunders, p. 99.

17. 3

Rationale: Generally, voluntary admission is sought by the client. Voluntary clients have the right to demand and obtain release. If the client is a minor, the release may be contingent on the consent of the parents or guardian. The nurse needs to be familiar with the state and facility policies and procedures. Many states require that the client submit a written release notice to the facility staff, who reevaluate the client's condition for possible conversion to involuntary status, according to criteria established by laws. The best nursing action is to contact the physician.

Test-Taking Strategy: Use the process of elimination. Noting the type of hospital admission will assist in eliminating option 1. It is inappropriate to "persuade" a client to stay in the hospital. Option 2 should be eliminated simply on the issue of client rights and the issue of confidentiality. Review the various types of hospital admission and discharge processes if you had difficulty with this question.

Level of Cognitive Ability: Application

Client Needs: Safe, Effective Care Environment

Integrated Concept/Process: Nursing Process/Implementation

Content Area: Mental Health

Reference: Varcarolis, E. (1998). *Foundations of psychiatric mental health nursing* (3rd ed.). Philadelphia: W. B. Saunders, p. 99.

18. 1

Rationale: Involuntary admission is made without the client's consent. Involuntary admission is necessary when a person is a danger to self or others or is in need of psychiatric treatment or physical care. Options 2, 3, and 4 describe the process of voluntary admission.

Test-Taking Strategy: Use the process of elimination. Note the key words "involuntary status." This should easily direct you to option 1. Also, note that options 2, 3, and 4 are all similar. Review the process of involuntary admission if you had difficulty with this question.

Level of Cognitive Ability: Analysis

Client Needs: Psychosocial Integrity

Integrated Concept/Process: Nursing Process/Analysis

Content Area: Mental Health

Reference: Keltner, N., Schwecke, L., & Bostrom, C. (1999). *Psychiatric nursing* (3rd ed.). St. Louis: Mosby, p. 48.

19. 3

Rationale: Clients who are involuntarily admitted do not lose their right to informed consent. Clients must be considered legally competent until they have been declared incompetent through a legal proceeding. The informed consent needs to be obtained from the client.

Test-Taking Strategy: Knowledge about the hospital admission processes and client's rights is necessary to answer this question. If you had difficulty with this question, focus on the issue of client rights to direct you to option 3. Review client rights if you had difficulty with this question.

Level of Cognitive Ability: Analysis

Client Needs: Safe, Effective Care Environment

Integrated Concept/Process: Nursing Process/Analysis

Content Area: Mental Health

Reference: Keltner, N., Schwecke, L., & Bostrom, C. (1999). *Psychiatric nursing* (3rd ed.). St. Louis: Mosby, p. 52.

20. 2

Rationale: A client may request to be secluded or restrained. Federal laws require the consent of the client, unless an emergency situation exists in which an immediate risk to the client or others can be documented. The use of seclusion and restraint is permitted only on the written order of a physician, which must be reviewed and renewed every 24 hours, and which also must specify the type of restraint to be used.

Test-Taking Strategy: Use the process of elimination and knowledge about the issue of client's rights to direct you to option 2. There is no reason to call the family at this time; therefore, eliminate option 3. Knowing that a physician's written order is necessary will assist in eliminating option 4. Option 1 is not the best option, because this information, if given to a client experiencing uncontrollable feelings, may cause escalation of the feelings. Review the nursing implications about seclusion and restraint if you had difficulty with this question.

Level of Cognitive Ability: Application

Client Needs: Safe, Effective Care Environment

Integrated Concept/Process: Nursing Process/Implementation

Content Area: Mental Health

Reference: Keltner, N., Schwecke, L., & Bostrom, C. (1999). *Psychiatric nursing* (3rd ed.). St. Louis: Mosby, p. 61.

21. 2

Rationale: The nurse should never promise to keep a secret. Secrets are appropriate in a social relationship but not in a therapeutic one. The nurse needs to be honest with the client and tell the client that a promise cannot be made to keep the secret. Options 1, 3, and 4 are inappropriate responses.

Test-Taking Strategy: Use the process of elimination. Option 1 can be easily eliminated because it is inappropriate. Options 3 and 4 are not only inappropriate but are to an extent threatening and may even block further communication. Review therapeutic communication techniques and nurse client relationships if you had difficulty with this question.

Level of Cognitive Ability: Application

Client Needs: Safe, Effective Care Environment

Integrated Concept/Process: Communication and Documentation

Content Area: Mental Health
Reference: Fortinash, K., & Holoday-Worret, P. (2000). *Psychiatric mental health nursing* (2nd ed.). St. Louis: Mosby, p. 86.

22. 4
Rationale: A nurse is required to maintain confidentiality about the client and his or her care. Confidentiality is basic to the therapeutic relationship and is a client's right. The most appropriate response to the neighbor is option 4. Option 3 is correct in a sense; however, it is a rather blunt statement. Both options 1 and 2 identify statements that do not maintain client confidentiality. Option 4 is most direct and correct.
Test-Taking Strategy: Focus on the issue of the question, maintaining confidentiality. This should easily assist in eliminating options 1 and 2. From the remaining options, select option 4 over option 3 because it is most direct and correct. Option 3 is a rather blunt and somewhat rude statement. Review confidentiality issues if you had difficulty with this question.
Level of Cognitive Ability: Application
Client Needs: Safe, Effective Care Environment
Integrated Concept/Process: Nursing Process/Implementation
Content Area: Mental Health
Reference: Keltner, N., Schwecke, L., & Bostrom, C. (1999). *Psychiatric nursing* (3rd ed.). St. Louis: Mosby, p. 58.

23. 4
Rationale: False imprisonment is an act with the intent to confine a person to a specific area. A nurse can be charged with false imprisonment if the nurse prohibits a client from leaving the hospital if the client was voluntarily admitted and if there are no agency or legal policies for detaining the client. On the other hand, if the client was involuntarily admitted or had agreed to an evaluation before discharge, the nurse's actions are reasonable.
Test-Taking Strategy: Noting the key words "involuntarily admitted" will assist in eliminating option 1 and direct you to option 4. Options 2 and 3 are unrelated to the issue of the question and can be easily eliminated. Review the issues related to false imprisonment and hospital admissions if you had difficulty with this question.
Level of Cognitive Ability: Analysis
Client Needs: Safe, Effective Care Environment
Integrated Concept/Process: Nursing Process/Analysis
Content Area: Mental Health
Reference: Keltner, N., Schwecke, L., & Bostrom, C. (1999). *Psychiatric nursing* (3rd ed.). St. Louis: Mosby, p. 60.

24. 3
Rationale: Tasks of the termination phase include evaluating client performance, evaluating achievement of expected outcomes, evaluating future needs, making appropriate referrals, and dealing with the common behaviors associated with termination. Options 1, 2, and 4 identify the tasks of the working phase of the relationship.

Test-Taking Strategy: Use the process of elimination. Noting the key words "termination phase" should easily direct you to option 3. If you are unfamiliar with the appropriate tasks of the phases of the nurse-client relationship, review this content.
Level of Cognitive Ability: Analysis
Client Needs: Psychosocial Integrity
Integrated Concept/Process: Nursing Process/Planning
Content Area: Mental Health
Reference: Keltner, N., Schwecke, L., & Bostrom, C. (1999). *Psychiatric nursing* (3rd ed.). St. Louis: Mosby, p. 131.

25. 2
Rationale: In the termination phase of a relationship, it is normal for a client to demonstrate a number of regressive behaviors that can be disturbing to the nurse. Typical behaviors include return of symptoms, anger, withdrawal, and minimizing the relationship. The anger that the client is experiencing is a normal behavior during the termination phase and does not necessarily indicate the need for hospitalization or treatment.
Test-Taking Strategy: Note the key words "termination phase." This alone may assist in directing you to option 2. Additionally, note the similarity between options 1, 3, and 4. These options address the need for further supervised treatment. If you are unfamiliar with the client behaviors associated with the termination phase, review this content.
Level of Cognitive Ability: Analysis
Client Needs: Psychosocial Integrity
Integrated Concept/Process: Nursing Process/Analysis
Content Area: Mental Health
Reference: Keltner, N., Schwecke, L., & Bostrom, C. (1999). *Psychiatric nursing* (3rd ed.). St. Louis: Mosby, p. 131.

CRITICAL THINKING: FREE-TEXT ENTRY

Answer: Identification
Rationale: Identification is the unconscious attempt to change oneself to resemble an admired person. This client's statement reflects the use of the defense mechanism known as identification.
Test-Taking Strategy: Focus on the client's statement. Noting the client's words "I want to be a nurse just like you" will assist in identifying the defense mechanism used by the client. Review defense mechanisms if you had difficulty with this question.
Level of Cognitive Ability: Analysis
Client Needs: Psychosocial Integrity
Integrated Concept/Process: Communication and Documentation
Content Area: Mental Health
Reference: Keltner, N., Schwecke, L., & Bostrom, C. (1999). *Psychiatric nursing* (3rd ed.). St. Louis: Mosby, p. 31.

REFERENCES

Fortinash, K., & Holoday-Worret, P. (2000). *Psychiatric mental health nursing* (2nd ed.). St. Louis: Mosby.
Glod, Carol. A. (1998). *Contemporary psychiatric-mental health nursing.* Philadelphia: F.A. Davis.
Keltner, N., Schwecke, L., & Bostrom, C. (1999). *Psychiatric nursing* (3rd ed.). St. Louis: Mosby.
Stuart, G.W., & Laraia, M.T. (1998). *Principles and practice of psychiatric nursing.* (6th ed.). St. Louis: Mosby.
Varcarolis, E. (1998). *Foundations of psychiatric mental health nursing* (3rd ed.). Philadelphia: W.B. Saunders.

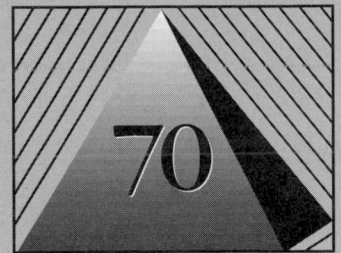

Models of Care

I. MILIEU THERAPY

A. Description
 1. **Milieu** is the physical and social environment in which an individual lives
 2. Provides a safe environment that is adapted to the individual client's needs and also provides greater comfort and freedom of expression than has been experienced in the past by the client
 3. Staffed by persons trained to provide support and understanding and individual attention
 4. All members contribute to the planning and functioning of the setting
 5. The power hierarchy is diminished because all members are viewed as significant and valuable members of the community

B. Focus
 1. Positive environmental manipulation, both physical and social, in order to effect a positive change
 2. Client's rights through involvement in setting goals, freedom of movement, and informal relationships with staff
 3. Group and social interaction
 4. Use of community meetings, activity groups, social skills groups, and physical exercise programs

II. PSYCHOTHERAPY

A. Description
 1. Use of a group of techniques to modify feelings, attitudes, and behaviors in clients
 2. Therapist uses both verbal and nonverbal means of communication to build a relationship with the client

B. Focus
 1. The basic concept involves understanding
 2. The focus in on issues of importance to the client, the purpose of the interaction, identification of the roles of the therapist and the client, and the use of primarily verbal means of communication

 3. Nonverbal techniques include silence, body language, facial expressions, and respect for personal space

C. Levels of psychotherapy
 1. Supportive therapy
  a. Allows the client to express feelings, explore alternatives, and make decisions in a safe, caring environment
  b. It may be needed briefly or over a period of years
  c. There is no plan to introduce new methods of coping; instead the therapist reinforces the client's existing **coping mechanisms**
 2. Reeducative therapy
  a. Involves learning new ways of perceiving and behaving
  b. The client explores alternatives in a planned, systematic way, which requires a longer period than supportive therapy requires
  c. The client enters into a contract that specifies desired changes of behavior
  d. Reeducative therapy includes short-term psychotherapy, reality therapy, cognitive restructuring, and behavior modification
 3. Reconstructive therapy
  a. Involves deep psychotherapy or psychoanalysis
  b. It may require 2 to 5 years of therapy or more and focuses on all aspects of the client's life
  c. Emotional and cognitive restructuring of self takes place
  d. Positive outcomes include a greater understanding of self and others, more emotional freedom, and the development of potential abilities

III. BEHAVIOR AND BEHAVIOR MODIFICATION

A. Behavior therapy
 1. An approach to bring about behavioral change

2. It includes a group of diversified approaches for dealing with maladaptive behavior
3. The belief is that most behaviors are learned
4. Maladaptive behavior is a way of dealing with stress, and the therapy is an approach to bringing about a change in the behavior

B. Self-control therapy
   1. Combination of cognitive and behavioral approaches
   2. A basic theme is that talking to oneself can direct and control actions more effectively
   3. Useful to deal with stress

C. Desensitization
   1. The reduction of intense reactions to a stimulus by repeated exposure to the stimulus in a weaker and milder form
   2. Gradually over a period of time, exposure is increased until the fear of the object or situation has ceased

D. Aversion therapy
   1. Negative reinforcement is a technique to change behavior
   2. A stimulus attractive to the client is paired with an unpleasant event in hopes of endowing the stimulus with negative properties

E. Modeling: The therapist provides a role model for specified identified behaviors, and the client learns through imitation

F. Operant conditioning: Entails rewarding a client for desired behaviors and is the basis for behavior modification

IV. COGNITIVE THERAPY

1. An active, directive, time-limited, structured approach used to treat a variety of psychiatric disorders
2. Therapeutic techniques are designed to identify reality testing and correct distorted conceptualization and the dysfunctional belief underlying these cognitions
3. The client learns to master problems in situations that he or she previously considered insuperable, by evaluating and correcting his or her thinking
4. The cognitive therapist helps the client to think and act more realistically and adaptively about his or her psychological problems so as to reduce symptoms
5. Various cognitive and behavioral strategies are used in cognitive therapy

V. GROUP AND GROUP THERAPY

A. Stages of group development
   1. Initial stage
      a. Involves superficial rather than open and trusting communication
      b. Members are becoming acquainted with each other and are searching for similarity between themselves and other group members
      c. Members may be unclear about the purpose or goals of the group
      d. A certain amount of structuring of group norms, roles, and responsibilities takes place
   2. Working stage
      a. During this stage, the real work of the group is accomplished
      b. Members are familiar with each other, the group leader, and the group roles, and they feel free to approach their problems and to attempt to solve their problems
      c. Conflict and cooperation surface during the group's work
   3. Termination stage
      a. The group evaluates the experience and explores members' feelings about it and the impending separation
      b. Provides an opportunity for members who have difficulty with termination to learn to deal more realistically and comfortably with this normal part of human experience

B. Psychoanalytical group psychotherapy
   1. Therapist holds a main position
   2. Each client in the group has a relationship with the therapist
   3. Communication is focused on three levels: unconscious, semiconscious, and conscious information

C. Transactional analysis (TA)
   1. The three ego states of the individual, the parent, the child, and the adult, are examined in TA groups
   2. The goal is that individuals in the group will communicate from the proper ego states for the situation and the responses of others, thereby lessening conflict and promoting mature relationships

D. Rational emotive therapy: The therapist designs activities to eliminate the irrational ideas of the members of the group

E. Rogerian therapy
   1. The therapist's goal is to help the members express their feelings toward one another during group sessions
   2. The therapist's role is one of encouraging the expression of feelings, clarifying these feelings with clients, and accepting clients and their feelings nonjudgmentally

F. Gestalt therapy
   1. Emphasis is on the "here and now"
   2. Emphasizes self-expression, self-exploration, and self-awareness in the present
   3. The client and the therapist focus on everyday problems and try to solve them
   4. The individual becomes aware of the total self and the surrounding environment

5. Awareness of the problem renders the client capable of change
6. The therapist's role is to help the members express their feelings and grow from their experiences

G. Interpersonal group therapy: To promote the individual's comfort with others in the group, which then transfers to other relationships

▲ H. Psychodrama groups
1. Explore truth through dramatic methods
2. The individual produces a topic to be explored
3. The therapist directs the individual through role playing
4. The audience experiences the feelings and identifies with the action on the stage
5. A catharsis occurs for the individual and the object

▲ I. Community support groups
1. Promote identification, clarification, understanding, role modeling, feelings of togetherness, and group cohesion
2. Prevent the individual member from feeling lonely and isolated
3. Help members decrease levels of stress and increase levels of self-acceptance
4. Members are better able to deal with the problems that they brought to the group
5. The outcome is rewarding, and the members develop new or more effective patterns of behavior
6. Some groups evolve into educational models that enhance communication, self-image, body image, problem solving, decision making, and growth processes

J. Family therapy
1. Specific intervention mode based on the premise that the members, with the presenting symptoms, signal the presence of pain in the entire family
2. The therapist works to assist the family members to identify and express their thoughts and feelings, define family roles and rules, try new, more productive styles of relating, and restore strength to the family

PRACTICE QUESTIONS

1. An 18-year-old woman is admitted to an inpatient unit with the diagnosis of anorexia nervosa. A cognitive behavioral approach is used as part of her treatment plan. The nurse understands that the purpose of this approach is to:
   1. Help the client identify and examine dysfunctional thoughts and beliefs
   2. Emphasize social interaction with clients who withdraw
   3. Provide a supportive environment
   4. Examine intrapsychic conflicts and past issues

2. A nurse is preparing to provide reminiscence therapy for a group of clients. Which of the following clients would the nurse select for this group?
   1. A client who exhibits profound depression with moderate cognitive impairment
   2. A catatonic, immobile client with moderate cognitive impairment
   3. An undifferentiated schizophrenic client with moderate cognitive impairment
   4. A client with mild depression who demonstrates normal cognition

3. A client with major depression is considering cognitive therapy. The client says to the nurse, "How does this treatment work?" The nurse responds and tells the client that:
   1. " This type of treatment helps you examine how your thoughts and feelings contribute to your difficulties."
   2. "This type of treatment helps you examine how your past life has contributed to your problems."
   3. "This type of treatment helps you confront your fears by gradually exposing you to them."
   4. "This type of treatment will help you relax and develop new coping skills."

4. A client asks a nurse about milieu therapy. The nurse responds, knowing that the primary locus of milieu therapy can best be described as which of the following?
   1. A form of behavior modification therapy
   2. A cognitive approach to changing behavior
   3. A living, learning, or working environment
   4. A behavioral approach to changing behavior

5. A nurse is caring for a client with a phobia who is being treated for the condition. The client is introduced to short periods of exposure to the phobic object while in a relaxed state. The nurse understands that this form of behavior modification can best be described as:
   1. Systematic desensitization
   2. Self-control therapy
   3. Milieu therapy
   4. Aversion therapy

6. A client with an eating disorder is planning to attend group meetings with Overeaters Anonymous. The nurse describes this group to the client, knowing that which of the following is not a characteristic of this form of self-help group?
   1. People who have a similar problem are able to help others
   2. It is designed to serve people who have a common problem
   3. The members provide support to each other
   4. The leader is a nurse or psychiatrist

7. A client is preparing to attend a Gamblers Anonymous meeting for the first time. The prototype used by this group is the 12-step program developed by Alcoholics Anonymous. The nurse tells the client

that the first step in the 12-step program is which of the following?

1. Stating that the gambling will be stopped
2. Discontinuing relationships with friends who are gamblers
3. Substituting gambling for other activities
4. Admitting to having a problem

8. A nurse is conducting a group therapy session and a client with a manic disorder is monopolizing the group. The most appropriate nursing action is which of the following?

1. Suggest that the client stop talking and try listening to others
2. Ask the client to leave
3. Tell the client to stop monopolizing the group
4. Refer the client to another group

9. A nurse is planning to formulate a psychotherapy group. Several clients are interested in attending the session. The nurse plans the group, knowing that the maximum number of group members to include in this group is:

1. 10
2. 12
3. 14
4. 16

10. A nurse is monitoring a group therapy session. During this session, the members are identifying tasks and boundaries. The nurse determines that these activities are characteristic of which stage of group development?

1. Forming
2. Storming
3. Norming
4. Performing

CRITICAL THINKING: FREE-TEXT ENTRY

A nurse is providing information to a client about the use of disulfiram (Antabuse) for the treatment of alcohol abuse. The nurse understands that this form of treatment works on the principle of which therapy?

Answer: _____

ANSWERS

1. 1

Rationale: Cognitive behavioral therapy is used to help clients to identify and examine dysfunctional thoughts as well as to identify and examine values and beliefs that maintain these thoughts. Options 2, 3, and 4 are incorrect.

Test-Taking Strategy: Use the process of elimination. Note the key words "cognitive behavioral." Focusing on these key words should direct you to option 1. If you are unfamiliar with this type of therapy and its purpose, review this content.

Level of Cognitive Ability: Analysis

Client Needs: Psychosocial Integrity

Integrated Concept/Process: Nursing Process/Analysis

Content Area: Mental Health

Reference: Keltner, N., Schwecke, L., & Bostrom, C. (1999). *Psychiatric nursing* (3rd ed.). St. Louis: Mosby, p. 36.

2. 4

Rationale: Reminiscence therapy is best for clients who meet the following criteria: normal to mild cognitive impairment; mild to moderate depression; withdrawn, socially isolated, understimulated behavior.

Test-Taking Strategy: Use the process of elimination, focusing on the type of therapy addressed in the question. Options 1, 2, and 3 describe clients whose cognitive impairment would not be improved with this form of therapy. If you had difficulty with this question, review the characteristics of reminiscence therapy.

Level of Cognitive Ability: Analysis

Client Needs: Health Promotion and Maintenance

Integrated Concept/Process: Nursing Process/Analysis

Content Area: Mental Health

Reference: Glod, C. A. (1998). *Contemporary psychiatric-mental health nursing.* Philadelphia: F. A. Davis, pp. 203-211.

3. 1

Rationale: Cognitive therapy is frequently used with clients who have depression. This type of therapy is based on exploring the client's subjective experience. It includes examining the client's thoughts and feelings about situations as well as how these thoughts and feelings contribute to and perpetuate the client's difficulties and mood.

Test-Taking Strategy: Focusing on the word "cognitive" will assist in selecting the correct option. Look for a similar word used in the question and repeated in one of the options. Option 1 uses the word "thought" in describing the treatment. Review this form of therapy if you had difficulty with this question.

Level of Cognitive Ability: Application

Client Needs: Health Promotion and Maintenance

Integrated Concept/Process: Teaching/Learning

Content Area: Mental Health

Reference: Fortinash, K., & Holoday-Worret, P. (2000). *Psychiatric mental health nursing* (2nd ed.). St. Louis: Mosby, p. 55.

4. 3

Rationale: Milieu therapy, or "therapeutic community," has as its locus a living, learning, or working environment. Such therapy may be based on any number of therapeutic modalities, from structured behavioral therapy to spontaneous, humanistically oriented approaches. Although milieu may include behavioral approaches, its primary focus is described in option 3.

Test-Taking Strategy: Use the process of elimination. Note that options 1, 2, and 4 are similar and that option 3 identifies a global description. Review milieu therapy if you had difficulty with this question.

Level of Cognitive Ability: Comprehension

Client Needs: Health Promotion and Maintenance

Integrated Concept/Process: Self-Care
Content Area: Mental Health
Reference: Fortinash, K., & Holoday-Worret, P. (2000). *Psychiatric mental health nursing* (2nd ed.). St. Louis: Mosby, p. 808.
5. **1**
Rationale: Systematic desensitization is a form of therapy used when the client is introduced to short periods of exposure to the phobic object while in a relaxed state. Gradually, exposure is increased until the anxiety about or fear of the object or situation has ceased. Options 2, 3, and 4 are incorrect.
Test-Taking Strategy: Use the process of elimination. Focus on the key words "introduced to short periods of exposure." This should assist in directing you to the correct option. If you had difficulty with this question, review systematic desensitization.
Level of Cognitive Ability: Comprehension
Client Needs: Psychosocial Integrity
Integrated Concept/Process: Nursing Process/Implementation
Content Area: Mental Health
Reference: Fortinash, K., & Holoday-Worret, P. (2000). *Psychiatric mental health nursing* (2nd ed.). St. Louis: Mosby, pp. 52-53.
6. **4**
Rationale: The sponsor of a self-help group is an experienced member of the group. A nurse or psychiatrist may be asked by the group to serve as a resource but would not be the leader of the group. Options 1, 2, and 3 are characteristics of a self-help group.
Test-Taking Strategy: Use the process of elimination and focus on the issue, self-help group. Note the key word "not" in the stem of the question. Note that options 1, 2, and 3 are all similar. This should easily direct you to option 4, the correct option. Review the characteristics of a self-help group, if you had difficulty with this question.
Level of Cognitive Ability: Application
Client Needs: Psychosocial Integrity
Integrated Concept/Process: Nursing Process/Implementation
Content Area: Mental Health
Reference: Varcarolis, E. (1998). *Foundations of psychiatric mental health nursing* (3rd ed.). Philadelphia: W. B. Saunders, p. 258.
7. **4**
Rationale: The first step in the 12-step program is to admit that a problem exists. Options 1 and 2 are unrealistic as a first step in the process to recovery. Although option 3 may be a strategy, it is not the first step.
Test-Taking Strategy: Use the process of elimination. Note the key words "first step" in the question. This will assist in directing you to option 4. If you are unfamiliar with the 12-step program, review this content.
Level of Cognitive Ability: Application
Client Needs: Psychosocial Integrity
Integrated Concept/Process: Teaching/Learning
Content Area: Mental Health
Reference: Keltner, N., Schwecke, L., & Bostrom, C. (1999). *Psychiatric nursing* (3rd ed.). St. Louis: Mosby, p. 536.
8. **1**
Rationale: If a client is monopolizing the group, it is important that the nurse be direct and decisive. The best action is to suggest that the client stop talking and try listening to others.

Although option 3 may be a direct response, option 1 is the most therapeutic direct statement. Options 2 and 4 are inappropriate.
Test-Taking Strategy: Use the process of elimination. Eliminate options 2 and 4 first because they are similar. Use therapeutic communication techniques to assist in directing you to option 1. If you had difficulty with this question, review therapeutic communication techniques for the client with a manic disorder.
Level of Cognitive Ability: Application
Client Needs: Psychosocial Integrity
Integrated Concept/Process: Nursing Process/Implementation
Content Area: Mental Health
Reference: Keltner, N., Schwecke, L., & Bostrom, C. (1999). *Psychiatric nursing* (3rd ed.). St. Louis: Mosby, p. 179.
9. **1**
Rationale: The ideal number of clients in a psychotherapy group ranges from 7 to 10. Having more than 10 members is not recommended because the group will subdivide, which is counterproductive. Too large a group can also create more opportunities for acting out, as opposed to working through issues.
Test-Taking Strategy: Knowledge about the general guidelines related to establishing a psychotherapy group is required to answer this question. If you are unfamiliar with these guidelines, review this content.
Level of Cognitive Ability: Comprehension
Client Needs: Psychosocial Integrity
Integrated Concept/Process: Nursing Process/Planning
Content Area: Mental Health
Reference: Varcarolis, E. (1998). *Foundations of psychiatric mental health nursing* (3rd ed.). Philadelphia: W. B. Saunders, p. 261.
10. **1**
Rationale: In the forming or initial stage, the members are identifying tasks and boundaries. Storming involves responding emotionally to tasks. In the norming stage, members express intimate personal opinions and feelings around personal tasks. In the performing stage, members direct group energy toward the completion of tasks.
Test-Taking Strategy: Use the process of elimination and focus on the issue. Note the key word "identifying" in the question. This key word should assist in directing you to option 1. If you had difficulty with this question, review the stages of group development.
Level of Cognitive Ability: Analysis
Client Needs: Psychosocial Integrity
Integrated Concept/Process: Nursing Process/Analysis
Content Area: Mental Health
Reference: Varcarolis, E. (1998). *Foundations of psychiatric mental health nursing* (3rd ed.). Philadelphia: W. B. Saunders, p. 264.

CRITICAL THINKING: FREE-TEXT ENTRY

Answer: Aversion therapy
Rationale: Aversion therapy, also known as aversion conditioning or negative reinforcement, is a technique used to change behavior. In this therapy, a stimulus attractive to the client is paired with an unpleasant event in hopes of endowing the stimulus with negative properties.

Test-Taking Strategy: Focus on the issue, the use of disulfiram (Antabuse) for the treatment of alcohol abuse. Recalling the purpose and use of disulfiram will assist in identifying the use of aversion therapy. If you had difficulty with this question, review this form of therapy.
Level of Cognitive Ability: Comprehension

Client Needs: Psychosocial Integrity
Integrated Concept/Process: Teaching/Learning
Content Area: Mental Health
Reference: Keltner, N., Schwecke, L., & Bostrom, C. (1999). *Psychiatric nursing* (3rd ed.). St. Louis: Mosby, p. 572.

REFERENCES

Fortinash, K., & Holoday-Worret, P. (2000). *Psychiatric mental health nursing* (2nd ed.). St. Louis: Mosby.

Glod, C.A. (1998). *Contemporary psychiatric-mental health nursing.* Philadelphia: F.A. Davis.

Keltner, N., Schwecke, L., & Bostrom, C. (1999). *Psychiatric nursing* (3rd ed.). St. Louis: Mosby.

Varcarolis, E. (1998). *Foundations of psychiatric menta health nursing* (3rd ed.). Philadelphia: W.B. Saunders.

Psychiatric Disorders

I. ANXIETY
A. Description
 1. A subjective, individual experience
 2. A normal response to stress
 3. A feeling of apprehension, uneasiness, uncertainty, or dread
 4. Occurs as a result of threats that may be misperceived or misinterpreted
 5. Occurs as a result of a threat to identity or self-esteem
 6. May result when values are threatened
 7. May precede new experiences
B. Types of anxiety
 1. Normal: A healthy type of anxiety
 2. Acute: Precipitated by imminent loss or change that threatens the sense of security
 3. Chronic: Anxiety that the individual has lived with for a long time
C. Levels of anxiety
 1. Mild
  a. Associated with the tension of every day life
  b. The individual is alert
  c. The perceptual field is increased
  d. Can be motivating, produce growth and creativity, and increase learning
 2. Moderate
  a. The focus is on immediate concerns
  b. Narrows the perceptual field
  c. Selective inattentiveness occurs
  d. Learning and problem-solving still take place
 3. Severe
  a. A feeling that something bad is about to happen
  b. A significant reduction in perceptual field occurs
  c. Focus is on specific details or scattered details

 d. All behavior is directed at relieving the anxiety
 e. Learning and problem solving are not possible
 f. The individual needs direction to focus
 4. Panic
  a. Associated with dread and terror and a sense of impending doom
  b. The personality is disorganized
  c. The individual is unable to communicate or function effectively
  d. Increased motor activity occurs
  e. Loss of rational thoughts, with distorted perception
  f. Inability to concentrate
  g. If prolonged, panic can lead to exhaustion and death
D. Implementation: General nursing measures
 1. Recognize the anxiety
 2. Establish trust
 3. Protect the client
 4. Do not attack **coping mechanisms**
 5. Do not force the client into situations that provoke anxiety
 6. Decrease stimulation in the environment
 7. Modify the environment by setting limits or limiting the interaction with others
 8. Provide creative outlets
 9. Provide activities that limit the amount of time for destructive behavior
 10. Promote relaxation techniques
 11. Administer antianxiety medications as prescribed
E. Implementation: Mild to moderate levels
 1. Help the client identify the anxiety
 2. Encourage the client to talk about feelings and concerns
 3. Help the client identify thoughts and feelings that occurred prior to the onset of anxiety

4. Encourage problem solving
5. Encourage gross motor exercise

▲ F. Implementation: Severe to panic levels
▲ 1. Reduce the anxiety quickly
2. Use a calm manner
3. Always remain with the client
4. Minimize environmental stimuli
5. Provide clear, simple statements
6. Use a low-pitched voice
7. Attend to the physical needs of the client
▲ 8. Provide gross motor activity
9. Administer antianxiety medications as prescribed

II. GENERALIZED ANXIETY DISORDER

A. Description
1. An unrealistic anxiety in which the cause can usually be identified
2. Physical symptoms occur
B. Assessment
1. Restlessness and inability to relax
2. Episodes of trembling and shakiness
3. Chronic muscular tension
4. Dizziness
5. Inability to concentrate
6. Chronic fatigue and sleep problems
7. Inability to recognize the connection between the anxiety and physical symptoms
8. The client is focused on the physical discomfort
▲ C. Panic disorder
1. Description
a. The cause usually cannot be identified
b. It produces a sudden onset, with feelings of intense apprehension and dread
c. Severe, recurrent, intermittent anxiety attacks, lasting 5 to 30 minutes, occur
2. Assessment
a. Choking sensation
b. Labored breathing
c. Pounding heart
d. Chest pain
e. Dizziness
f. Nausea
g. Blurred vision
h. Numbness or tingling of the extremities
i. A sense of unreality and helplessness
j. A fear of being trapped
k. A fear of dying
3. Implementation
▲ a. Attend to physical symptoms
b. Assist the client to identify the thoughts that aroused the anxiety and to identify the basis for these thoughts
c. Assist the client to change the unrealistic thoughts to more realistic thoughts
d. Use cognitive restructuring
e. Administer antianxiety medications as prescribed

III. POST-TRAUMATIC STRESS DISORDER (PTSD)

A. Description: After experiencing a psychologically traumatic event, outside the range of usual experience, the individual reexperiences the event via recurrent and intrusive dreams or flashbacks
B. Stressors
1. A natural disaster
2. Combat experiences
3. Victim of rape
4. Accidents
5. Victim of crime or violence
6. Victim of sexual, physical, or emotional **abuse**
7. Reexperiencing the event as flashbacks
C. Assessment
1. Emotional numbness
2. Detachment
3. Depression
4. Anxiety
5. Sleep disturbances and nightmares
6. Hypervigilance
7. Guilt about surviving the event
8. Poor concentration and avoidance of activities that trigger the memory of the event
D. Implementation
1. Desensitization through gradual exposure to the ▲ event or situations similar to the event
2. Instruct the client in relaxation techniques
3. Provide individual therapy that addresses loss-of-control issues or anger
4. Use of support groups
5. Use of hypnotherapy

IV. PHOBIAS

A. Description
1. An irrational fear of an object or situation that persists even though the person may recognize it as unreasonable
2. Is associated with panic-level anxiety if the object, situation, or activity cannot be avoided
3. **Defense mechanisms** commonly used include repression and displacement
B. Types
1. Agoraphobia
a. Fear of being alone in open or public places where escape might be difficult
b. The individual may not leave home
c. The individual experiences fear or a sense of helplessness or embarrassment if the phobic attack occurs
d. The individual avoids situations that may trigger the phobic attack
2. Social phobia
a. Fear of situations in which one might be embarrassed or criticized and the fear of making a fool of oneself
b. Can include the fear of eating in public, public speaking, or performing

3. Specific phobia: A fear of a single object, activity, or situation, such as snakes, closed spaces, and flying

▲ C. Implementation
   1. Stay with the client when the anxiety is high to promote safety and security
   2. Identify the basis of the anxiety
   3. Allow the client to verbalize feelings about the anxiety-producing object or situation; frequently talking about the feared object is the first step in the desensitization process
   4. Desensitization by gradually introducing the individual to the feared object or situation in small doses
   5. Teach relaxation techniques such as breathing exercises, muscle relaxation exercises, and visualization of pleasant situations
   6. Do not force contact with the phobic object or situation

V. OBSESSIVE-COMPULSIVE DISORDER

▲ A. Obsessions: Preoccupation with persistent intrusive thoughts and ideas

▲ B. Compulsions
   1. Repeated performance of rituals or purposeless behaviors designed to prevent some event, divert unacceptable thoughts, and decrease anxiety
   2. Obsessions and compulsions often occur together and can disrupt normal activities
   3. Anxiety occurs if obsessions or compulsions are resisted, and from being powerless to resist the thoughts or rituals
   4. Obsessive thoughts can involve issues of violence, aggression, sexual behavior, orderliness, or religion and can uncontrollably interrupt conscious thoughts and the ability to function

▲ C. Compulsive behavior patterns
   1. Decrease the anxiety
   2. Are associated with the obsessive thoughts
   3. Neutralize the thought
   4. During stressful times, the ritualistic behavior increases
   5. **Defense mechanisms** include repression, displacement, and undoing

▲ D. Implementation
   1. Identify the situations that precipitate the behavior
   2. Do not interrupt the compulsive behaviors
   3. Allow time for the client to perform the compulsive rituals
   4. Provide for client safety related to the behaviors
   5. Implement a schedule for the client that distracts from the behaviors
   6. Set limits on the rituals that may interfere with the client's physical well-being, to protect the client from physical harm

   7. Encourage the client to verbalize concerns
   8. Establish a written contract that will assist the client to gradually decrease the frequency of compulsive behaviors

VI. SOMATOFORM DISORDERS

A. Description (Box 71-1)
   1. Characterized by persistent worry or complaints regarding physical illness when there are no supporting physical findings
   2. The client focuses on the physical signs and symptoms and is unable to control the signs and symptoms
   3. The physical signs and symptoms increase with psychosocial stressors
   4. The anxiety is redirected into a somatic concern

B. Somatization disorder
   1. Description
      a. The client has multiple physical complaints involving multiple body systems
      b. The emotional stress can result from anxiety, fear, depression, worry, or repressed anger
      c. The client may unconsciously use somatization for secondary gains such as increased attention and decreased responsibilities
   2. Assessment
      a. Physical complaints of abdominal pain, denial of emotional problems, signs of anxiety, fear, and low self-esteem
      b. Psychosexual symptoms
      c. Secondary gain

C. Hypochondriasis
   1. Description
      a. The preoccupation with fears of having a serious disease
      b. No evidence of physical illness exists
      c. Causes significantly impaired social and occupational functioning
   2. Assessment
      a. Preoccupation with physical functioning
      b. Frequent somatic complaints
      c. Complaints of fatigue and insomnia
      d. Anxiety
      e. Difficulty expressing feelings
      f. Extensive use of home remedies or nonprescription medications
      g. Repeatedly visiting the doctor
      h. Secondary gain

BOX 71-1

Types of Somatoform Disorders

Somatization disorder
Hypochondriasis
Conversion disorder

▲ D. Conversion disorder
  1. Description
     a. A physical symptom or a deficit suggesting loss or altered body function related to psychological conflict or a neurological disorder
     b. An expression of a psychological conflict or need
     c. The most common conversion symptoms are blindness, deafness, paralysis, and the inability to talk
     d. There is no organic cause
     e. Symptoms are not intentionally produced by the client
     f. Symptoms are directly related to conflict and decrease anxiety
  2. Assessment
     a. "La belle indifference": Unconcerned with symptoms
     b. Physical limitation or disability
     c. Feelings of guilt, anxiety, or frustration
     d. Low self-esteem and feelings of inadequacy
     e. Unexpressed anger or conflict
     f. Secondary gain
  E. Implementation
     1. Obtain a nursing history and assess for physical problems
  ▲ 2. Do not reinforce the sick role
     3. Discourage verbalization about physical symptoms by not responding with positive reinforcement
     4. Explore with the client the needs being met by the physical symptoms
     5. Assist the client to identify alternative ways of meeting needs
     6. Assist the client to relate feelings and conflicts to the physical symptoms
  ▲ 7. Allow a specific time period to discuss physical complaints because the client will feel less threatened if this behavior is limited rather than stopped completely
  ▲ 8. Convey understanding that the physical symptoms are real to the client
     9. Assure the client that physical illness has been ruled out
     10. Explore the source of anxiety and stimulate verbalization of anxiety
     11. Encourage the use of relaxation techniques as the anxiety increases
     12. Implement pain-reduction measures as required
     13. Report and assess any new physical complaint
  ▲ 14. Encourage diversional activities to decrease the client's focus on self
     15. Provide positive feedback for accomplishments to increase self-esteem
     16. Assist the client in recognizing his or her own feelings and emotions

     17. Establish a written contract with the client that will redirect the client's thoughts and feelings
     18. Administer antianxiety medications as prescribed

VII. DISSOCIATIVE DISORDER

A. Description
  1. A disruption in integrative functions of memory, consciousness, or identity
  2. Associated with exposure to a traumatic event
B. Dissociative identity disorder (multiple personality)
  1. Description
     a. Two or more fully developed distinct and unique personalities within the person
     b. The personalities may take full control of the client, one at a time
     c. The personalities may or may not be aware of each other
  2. Assessment
     a. The inability to recall important information (unrelated to ordinary forgetfulness)
     b. Transition from one personality to the other is related to stress and is sudden
     c. Dissociation is used as a method of distancing and defending self from anxiety and traumatizing experiences
C. Dissociative amnesia
  1. Description
     a. Inability to recall important personal information because it is anxiety provoking
     b. Memory impairment may be partial or almost complete
  2. Assessment
     a. Localized: The client blocks out all memories about a specified period
     b. Selective: The client recalls some but not all memories about a specified period
     c. Generalized: Loss of all memory about past life
D. Dissociative fugue
  1. Description
     a. The assumption of a new identity in a new environment
     b. The disorder may occur suddenly
  2. Assessment
     a. May drift from place to place
     b. Develops few social relationships
     c. When the fugue lifts, the client returns home and is unable to recall the fugue state
E. Depersonalization disorder
  1. Description: An altered self-perception in which one's own reality is temporarily lost or changed
  2. Assessment
     a. Feelings of detachment
     b. Intact reality testing

F. Implementation
1. Develop a trusting relationship with the client
2. Encourage verbal expression of painful experiences, anxieties, and concerns
3. Explore methods of coping
4. Identify sources of conflict
5. Focus on the client's strengths and skills
6. Orient the client
7. Provide nondemanding, simple routines
8. Allow the client to progress at his or her own pace
9. Use stress-reduction techniques
10. Plan for individual, group, and/or family psychotherapy to integrate dissociated aspects of personality or memory and to expand self-awareness

▲ VIII. BIPOLAR DISORDER
A. Description (Box 71-2)
1. Characterized by episodes of mania and depression with periods of normal mood and activity in between
2. The medication of choice is lithium carbonate, which can be toxic and therefore necessitates the regular monitoring of serum lithium levels

▲ B. Implementation for mania
1. Remove hazardous objects from the environment
2. Assess the client closely for fatigue
3. Use comfort measures to promote sleep
4. Provide frequent rest periods
5. Monitor the client's sleep patterns
6. Provide a private room if possible
7. Administer a hypnotic or sedative medication as prescribed
8. Encourage the client to ventilate feelings
9. Use calm, slow interactions
10. Help the client focus on one topic during the conversation
11. Ignore or distract the client from grandiose thinking
12. Present reality to the client
13. Don't argue with the client
14. Limit group activities and assess the client's tolerance level
▲ 15. Provide high-calorie finger foods and fluids
16. Supervise the client's choice of clothing
17. Reduce environmental stimuli
18. Set limits on inappropriate behaviors
▲ 19. Provide physical activities and outlets for tension
▲ 20. Avoid competitive games
▲ 21. Provide gross motor activities, such as walking
22. Provide structured activities or one-to-one activities with the nurse
23. Provide simple and direct explanations for routine procedures
▲ 24. Supervise the administration of medication

BOX 71-2

Assessment of Bipolar Disorder

MANIA
Inappropriate affect
Restlessness
Flight of ideas
Inability to eat or sleep because of involvement in more important things
Extroverted personality
Delusional self-confidence
Initiation of activity
High and unstable affect
Becomes angry quickly
Pressure of speech
Grandiose and persecutory delusions
Inappropriate dress
Urgent motor activity
Significant decrease in appetite
Inability to sleep yet still active
Sexually promiscuous
Distracted by environmental stimuli
Unlimited energy

DEPRESSION
Decreased emotion and physical activity
Inability to make quick decisions
Introverted personality
Lack of initiative
Lack of self-confidence
Internalizing hostility
Loss of interest in appearance
Lack of energy
Easily fatigued
Withdrawn from groups
Lack of sexual interest

IX. SCHIZOPHRENIA
A. Descrption
1. A group of mental disorders characterized by psychotic features, inability to trust others, disordered thought processes, and disrupted interpersonal relationships
2. Disturbances in affect, mood, behavior, and thought processes
B. Assessment
1. Physical characteristics
a. Disheveled appearance
b. Body image distortions
c. Preoccupied with somatic complaints
d. Neglects eating, sleeping, and elimination
2. Motor activity (Box 71-3)
a. Catatonic posturing: holding bizarre postures for long periods of time
b. Catatonic excitement: Moving excitedly with no environmental stimuli present
c. May be totally immobilized

BOX 71-3
Abnormal Motor Behaviors

DESCRIPTION
Abnormal motor behavior or activity, displayed by the mentally ill client, occurring as a result of a psychiatric disorder

TYPES OF ABNORMAL MOTOR BEHAVIORS
Akathisia
Displaying motor restlessness and muscular quivering; the client is unable to sit or lie quietly
Echolalia
Repeating the speech of another person
Echopraxia
Repeating the movements of another person
Parkinson-Like Symptoms
Making mask-like faces, drooling, and having shuffling gait, tremors, and muscular rigidity
Waxy Flexibility
Having one's arms or legs placed in a certain position and holding that same position for hours
Dyskinesia
Impairment of the power of voluntary movements

BOX 71-4
Abnormal Thought Processes

DESCRIPTION
Abnormal thought processes, displayed by the mentally ill client, occurring as a result of a psychiatric disorder

NEOLOGISMS
Words that an individual makes up that have meaning only for the individual; often part of a delusional system

LOOSENESS OF ASSOCIATION
The individual's thinking is haphazard, illogical, and confused, and connections in thought are interrupted; seen mostly in schizophrenic disorders

FLIGHT OF IDEAS
A constant flow of speech in which the individual jumps from one topic to another in rapid succession; there is a connection between topics, although it is sometimes difficult to identify; seen in manic states

BLOCKING
A sudden cessation of a thought in the middle of a sentence; the client is unable to continue the train of thought; often sudden new thoughts, unrelated to the topic, come up

CIRCUMSTANTIALITY
Before getting to the point or answering a question, the individual gets caught up in countless details and explanations

CONFABULATION
Filling a memory gap with detailed fantasy believed by the teller; the purpose of confabulation is to maintain self-esteem; seen in organic conditions such as Korsakoff's psychosis

WORD SALAD
A mixture of words and phrases that have no meaning

---

d. Unable to respond to commands, or responds only to commands
e. Waxy flexibility
f. Movements may be repetitive or stereotyped
g. Motor activity may be increased, as evidenced by agitation, pacing, inability to sleep, loss of appetite and weight, and impulsiveness
h. May be unable to initiate activity, known as lack of volition or anergia
3. Emotional characteristics
   a. Mistrust
   b. Views the world as threatening and unsafe
   c. Feelings not easily interpreted
   d. Ambivalence manifested as compulsive rituals, negativism, and overcompliance
   e. May display feelings of helplessness, anxiety, anger, guilt and depression, and decreased self-esteem
4. Compulsive rituals: Attempts to solve conflicting feelings by constant, repetitive activity, which may be stereotyped or seem meaningless
5. Overcompliance: Attempts to deny responsibility for any action by doing only what another exactly instructs
6. Affective disturbances
   a. Flat affect or inappropriate affect
   b. Altered thought processes
7. Thought processes (Box 71-4)
   a. Impaired reality testing
   b. Fragmentation of thoughts
   c. Blocking

d. Loose associations
e. Autistic thinking
f. Perceives environment in a totally self-centered way
g. Neologisms
h. Magical thinking
i. Unable to conceptualize meaning in words or thoughts
j. Unable to organize facts logically
k. Delusions
8. Types of delusions (Box 71-5)
   a. Loss of reference, in which the client believes that certain events, situations, or interactions are directly related to self
   b. Delusions of persecution, in which the client

BOX 71-5

Delusions

DESCRIPTION
A false belief held to be true even when there is evidence to the contrary

TYPES
Persecution
The thought that one is being singled out for harm by others
Grandeur
The false belief that one is a very powerful and important person
Jealousy
The false belief that one's partner or mate is going out with other people

BOX 71-6

Preoccupation in Thought Content

HALLUCINATION
A sense perception for which no external stimuli exist; can have an organic or a functional etiology

TYPES
Visual
Seeing things that are not there
Auditory
Hearing voices when none are present
Olfactory
Smelling smells that do not exist
Tactile
Feeling touch sensations in the absence of stimuli
Gustatory
Experiencing taste in the absence of stimuli

believes that he or she is being harassed, threatened, or persecuted by some powerful force
   c. Delusions of grandeur, in which the client attaches special significance to self in relation to others or the universe and has an exaggerated sense of self that has no basis in reality
   d. Somatic delusions, in which the client believes that his or her body is changing or responding in an unusual way, which has no basis in reality
9. Perceptual distortions
   a. Illusions that may be brief experiences with a misinterpretation or exaggeration of reality
   b. Hallucinations such as perceiving objects, sensations, or images with no basis in reality (Box 71-6)
10. Language and communication disturbances (Box 71-7)
   a. Related to disorders in thought process
   b. Unable to organize language
   c. Difficulty communicating clearly
   d. Inappropriate responses to a situation
   e. A single word or phrase may represent the whole meaning of the conversation, and the client may feel that he or she has communicated adequately
   f. May develop private language
C. Types of schizophrenia (Box 71-8)
   1. Paranoid schizophrenia
      a. Suspiciousness
      b. Hostility
      c. Delusions
      d. Auditory hallucinations
      e. Anxiety and anger
      f. Aloofness
      g. Persecutory themes
      h. Violence

BOX 71-7

Language and Communication Disturbance

Neologism: a new word devised that has special meaning only to the client
Echolalia: repetition of words or phrases heard from another person
Verbigeration: purposeless repetition of words or phrases
Metonymic speech: mental confusion exhibited by the use of a word that is not the precise term intended but is of similar meaning
Clang association: repetition of words or phrases that are similar in sound but in no other way
Word salad: form of speech in which words or phrases are connected meaninglessly
Stilted language: an inappropriate and overly formal communication pattern, usually written, that seems artificial and intellectual
Pressured speech: person speaks as if the words were being forced out quickly
Mutism: absence of verbal speech

BOX 71-8

Types of Schizophrenia

Paranoid
Disorganized
Catatonic
Undifferentiated
Residual

   2. Disorganized schizophrenia
      a. Extreme social withdrawal
      b. Disorganized speech or behavior
      c. Flat or inappropriate affect
      d. Silliness unrelated to speech
      e. Stereotyped behaviors

f. Grimacing mannerisms

g. Inability to perform activities of daily living (ADLs)

3. Catatonic schizophrenia
   a. Marked psychomotor disturbances
   b. Immobility
   c. Stupor
   d. Waxy flexibility
   e. Excessive purposeless motor activity
   f. Echolalia
   g. Automatic obedience
   h. Stereotyped or repetitive behavior

4. Undifferentiated schizophrenia
   a. Does not meet the criteria for paranoid, disorganized, or catatonic schizophrenia
   b. Delusions and hallucinations
   c. Disorganized speech
   d. Disorganized or catatonic behavior
   e. Flat affect
   f. Social withdrawal

5. Residual schizophrenia
   a. Diagnosed as schizophrenic in the past
   b. Time limited between attacks but may last for many years
   c. The client exhibits marked social isolation and withdrawal and impaired role functioning

D. Implementation: Refer to Box 71-9

E. Implementation: Active hallucinations
   1. Monitor for hallucination cues
   2. Intervene with a one-on-one contact
   3. Decrease stimuli or move the client to another area
   4. Avoid conveying to the client that others are also experiencing the hallucination
   5. Respond verbally to anything real that the client talks about
   6. Avoid touching the client
   7. Encourage the client to express feelings
   8. During a hallucination, attempt to engage the client's attention through a concrete activity
   9. Accept and do not joke about or judge the client's behavior
   10. Provide easy activities and a structured environment with routine ADLs
   11. Monitor for signs of increasing fear, anxiety, or agitation
   12. Provide **seclusion** as necessary
   13. Administer medications as prescribed

F. Implementation: Delusions
   1. Interact on the basis of reality
   2. Encourage the client to express feelings
   3. Do not dispute with the client or try to convince the client that delusions are false
   4. Initially initiate activities on a one-on-one basis
   5. Alter hospital routines as necessary, such as using canned or packaged food or food from home

BOX 71-9

Implementation for Schizophrenia

Assess the client's physical needs
Set limits on the client's behavior when it interferes with others and becomes disruptive
Maintain a safe environment
Initiate one-on-one interaction and progress to small groups as tolerated
Spend time with the client even if client is unable to respond
Monitor for altered thought processes
Maintain ego boundaries and avoid touching the client
Limit the time of interaction with the client
Avoid an overly warm approach; a neutral approach is less threatening
Do not make promises to the client that cannot be kept
Establish daily routines
Assist the client to improve grooming and accept responsibility for personal care
Sit with the client in silence if necessary
Provide brief and frequent contact with the client
Tell the client when you are leaving
Tell the client when you don't understand
Do not "go along" with the client's delusions or hallucinations
Provide simple, concrete activities such as puzzles or word games
Reorient the client as necessary
Help the client establish what is real and unreal
Stay with the client if the client is frightened
Speak to the client in a simple, direct, and concise manner
Reassure the client that the environment is safe
Remove the client from group situations if client behavior is too bizarre, disturbing, or dangerous to others
Set realistic goals
Initially do not offer choices to the client, and gradually assist the client in making own decisions
Use containers for food, especially with the paranoid schizophrenic client
Provide a radio or tape player at night for insomnia
Explain to the client everything that is being done
Set limits on the client's behavior if the client is unable to do so
Decrease excessive stimuli in the environment
Monitor for suicide risk
Assist the client to use alternative means to express feelings, through music or art therapy or writing

6. Recognize accomplishments and provide positive feedback for successes

X. PARANOID DISORDERS

A. Description
   1. The client demonstrates suspiciousness and mistrust of others
   2. The client is often viewed by others as hostile, stubborn, and defensive

3. Concrete, pervasive delusional system characterized by persecutory and grandiose beliefs

▲ B. Behaviors
1. Suspicious and mistrustful
2. Emotionally distant
3. Distorts reality
4. Poor insight
5. Hypervigilance
6. Low self-esteem
7. Highly sensitive, difficulty in admitting own error, and takes pride in being correct
8. Hypercritical and intolerant of others
9. Hostile, aggressive, and quarrelsome
10. Evasive
11. Concrete thinking

▲ C. Delusions
1. Serves a purpose in establishing identity and self-esteem
2. Grandiose and persecutory delusions
3. Process of delusion includes denial, projection, and rationalization
4. As trust in others increases, the need for delusions decreases

D. Types (Box 71-10)
1. Paranoid personality
   a. Suspicious
   b. Nonpsychotic
   c. No hallucinations or delusions
   d. No symptoms of schizophrenia
2. Paranoid state
   a. Onset abrupt in response to stress and subsides when stress decreases
   b. No hallucinations but experiences paranoid delusions
   c. May be sensitive and suspicious before the development of delusions
   d. Psychotic state
   e. No symptoms of schizophrenia
3. Paranoia
   a. Client appears normal except for delusional system
   b. Single, highly organized delusional system
   c. Not bizarre
   d. No hallucinations
   e. Reserved and sensitive before onset
   f. Psychotic state
   g. No symptoms of schizophrenia
4. Paranoid schizophrenia
   a. Prior to the onset client becomes cold, withdrawn, distrustful, resentful, argumentative, sarcastic, and defiant
   b. Bizarre, numerous, and changeable delusions
   c. Delusions become less logical as the client becomes more disorganized
   d. Persecutory hallucinations
   e. Psychotic state
   f. All symptoms of schizophrenia are present

E. Implementation (Box 71-11)

BOX 71-10

Types of Paranoid Disorders

Paranoid personality
Paranoid state
Paranoia
Paranoid schizophrenia

BOX 71-11

Implementation: Paranoid Disorders

Assess for suicide risk
Diminish suspicious behavior
Establish a trusting relationship
Promote increased self-esteem
Remain calm, nonthreatening, and nonjudgmental
Provide continuity of care
Respond honestly to the client
Follow through on commitments made to the client
Acknowledge the client's feelings, but tell the client that you do not share his or her interpretation of an event
Provide a daily schedule of activities
Assist the client to identify diversionary activities
Gradually introduce the client to groups
Refocus conversation to reality-based topics
Use role playing to help the client identify thoughts and feelings
Provide positive reinforcement for successes
Do not argue with delusions
Use concrete, specific words
Do not be secretive with the client
Do not whisper in the client's presence
Assure the client that he or she will be safe
Involve the client in noncompetitive tasks
Provide the client opportunity to complete small tasks
Monitor eating, drinking, sleeping, and elimination patterns
Limit physical contact
Monitor for agitation and decrease stimuli as needed

XI. PERSONALITY DISORDERS

A. Description
1. Include various inflexible maladaptive behavior patterns or traits that may impair functioning and relationships
2. The individual usually remains in touch with reality and typically has a lack of insight into his or her behavior
3. Stress exacerbates manifestations of the personality disorder
4. In severe cases, the personality disorder may deteriorate to a psychotic state

B. Characteristics
1. Poor impulse control
   a. Acting out to manage internal pain
   b. Forms of acting out include physical and

verbal attacks, manipulation, substance **abuse,** promiscuous sexual behaviors, and **suicide attempts**
2. Mood characteristics
   a. Experiences abandonment and depression
   b. Moods include rage, guilt, fear, and emptiness
3. Impaired judgment
   a. Has difficulty with problem solving
   b. Unable to perceive the consequences of behavior
4. Impaired reality testing: Distorts reality and often projects own feelings onto others
5. Impaired object relations: Rigid and inflexible and has difficulty in intimate relationships
6. Impaired self-perception: Distorted self-perception and experiences self-hate or self-idealization
7. Impaired thought processes
   a. Concrete or diffuse thinking
   b. Difficulty concentrating
   c. Impaired memory
8. Impaired stimulus barrier
   a. Unable to regulate incoming sensory stimuli
   b. Increased excitability
   c. Excessive response to noise and light
   d. Poor attention span
   e. Agitated
   f. Insomnia
C. Schizoid personality disorder
1. Description: Characterized by an inability to form warm, close social relationships
2. Assessment
   a. Social detachment and lack of close relationships
   b. Interest in solitary activities
   c. Aloof and indifferent
   d. Restricted expression of emotions
   e. Lack of interest in others
D. Schizotypal personality disorder
1. Description: Exhibits abnormal or highly unusual thoughts, perceptions, speech, and behavior patterns
2. Assessment
   a. Suspicious
   b. Paranoia
   c. Magical thinking
   d. Odd thinking and speech
   e. Relationship deficits
E. Paranoid personality disorder
1. Description: Characterized by suspiciousness and mistrust of others
2. Assessment
   a. Suspicious and distrusting
   b. Argumentative
   c. Hostile aloofness
   d. Rigid, critical, and controlling of others
   e. Grandiosity

F. Histrionic personality disorder
1. Description
   a. Characterized by overly dramatic and intensely expressive behavior
   b. The client is lively and dramatic and enjoys being the center of attention
   c. Interpersonal relations may be poor
2. Assessment
   a. Attention seeking
   b. Needs to be the center of attention
   c. Sexually seductive or provocative
   d. Self-dramatizing and theatrical
   e. Overly concerned with appearance
   f. Has romantic fantasies and controls partners
   g. Bores easily
   h. Displays dependency
G. Narcissistic personality disorder
1. Description
   a. Characterized by an increased sense of self-importance
   b. The client is preoccupied with fantasies and unlimited success and has a constant need for attention and admiration
2. Assessment
   a. Grandiosity
   b. Requires admiration and inflated accomplishments
   c. Overestimates abilities and underestimates contributions of others
   d. Lacks empathy and sensitivity to needs of others
H. Avoidant personality disorder
1. Description: Characterized by social withdrawal and extreme sensitivity to potential rejection
2. Assessment
   a. Feelings of inadequacy
   b. Hypersensitive to reactions of others and reacts poorly to criticism
   c. Social inhibition
   d. Lack of support system
I. Dependent personality disorder
1. Description
   a. The individual lacks self-confidence and the ability to function independently
   b. Passively allows others to make decisions and assume responsibility for major areas in his or her life
2. Assessment
   a. Difficulty making decisions
   b. Lacks autonomy
   c. Cannot tolerate being alone and must always have a close relationship
   d. Needs others to assume responsibility and make decisions
J. Obsessive-compulsive personality disorder
1. Description: The client has difficulty expressing warm and tender emotions and reflects perfectionism, stubbornness, the need to control others, and a devotion to work

2. Assessment
   a. Orderliness and perfectionism
   b. Overly conscientious
   c. Inflexible and preoccupied with details and rules
   d. Devoted to work and lacks leisure activities and friendships
   e. Miserly and stubborn
   f. Hoards worthless objects
K. Antisocial personality disorder
   1. Description
      a. A pattern of irresponsible and antisocial behavior
      b. Characterized by selfishness, inability to maintain lasting relationships, poor sexual adjustment, failure to accept social norms, irritability, and aggressiveness
   2. Assessment
      a. Perceives the world as hostile
      b. Superficial charm and hostility
      c. No shame or guilt
      d. Self-centered
      e. Unreliable
      f. Easily bored
      g. Poor work history
      h. Unable to tolerate frustration
      i. Views others as objects to be manipulated
      j. Poor judgment
      k. Impulsive
L. Borderline personality disorder
   1. Description
      a. Characterized by instability in interpersonal relationships, mood, and self-image
      b. Behavior may be impulsive and unpredictable
   2. Assessment
      a. Unclear identity
      b. Unstable and intense
      c. Extreme shifts in mood
      d. Easily angered
      e. Easily bored
      f. Argumentative
      g. Depression
      h. Self-destructive behavior
      i. Manipulation
      j. Unable to tolerate anxiety
      k. Chronic feelings of emptiness and fear of being alone
      l. Splitting
M. Passive-aggressive personality disorder
   1. Description
      a. Characterized by passively expressing covert aggression rather than dealing with it directly
      b. The behavior can interfere with both social and work activities
   2. Assessment
      a. Procrastination
      b. Stubbornness

   c. Intentional inefficiency
   d. Forgetfulness
   e. Dependency
N. Implementation
   1. Maintain safety against self-destructive behaviors
   2. Allow the client to make choices and be as independent as possible
   3. Encourage the client to discuss feelings rather than act them out
   4. Provide consistency in response to the client's acting-out behaviors
   5. Discuss expectations and responsibilities with the client
   6. Discuss the consequences that will follow certain behaviors
   7. Inform the client that harm to self, others, and property is unacceptable
   8. Identify splitting behavior
   9. Assist the client to deal directly with anger
   10. Develop a written contract with the client
   11. Encourage the client to keep a journal recording daily feelings
   12. Encourage the client to participate in group activities, and praise nonmanipulative behavior
   13. Set and maintain limits to decrease manipulative behavior
   14. Remove the client from group situations in which attention-seeking behaviors occur
   15. Provide realistic praise for positive behaviors in social situations

XII. ELECTROCONVULSIVE THERAPY (ECT)
A. Description
   1. An effective treatment for depression that consists of inducing a grand mal (tonic-clonic) seizure by passing an electrical current through electrodes that are attached to the temples
   2. The administration of a muscle relaxant minimizes seizure activity, preventing damage to long bones and cervical vertebrae
   3. The usual course is 6 to 12 treatments given two to three times per week
   4. Maintenance ECT once a month may help to decrease the relapse rate for the client with recurrent depression
   5. ECT is not a permanent cure
   6. Not necessarily effective in clients with dysrhythmic depression or those with depression and personality disorders, those with drug dependence, or those with depression secondary to situational or social difficulties
   7. At-risk clients include those with recent myocardial infarction, cerebral vascular accident, or cerebral vascular malformation, or clients with intracranial mass lesions

B. Uses
1. Clients with major depressive and bipolar depressive disorders, especially when psychotic symptoms are present such as delusions of guilt, somatic delusions, and delusions of infidelity
2. Clients who have depression with marked psychomotor retardation and stupor
3. Manic clients whose conditions are resistant to lithium and antipsychotic medications and clients who are rapid cyclers (a client with a bipolar disorder who has many episodes of mood swings close together)
4. Clients with schizophrenia (especially catatonia), those with schizoaffective syndromes, and psychotic clients

C. Indications for use
1. When antidepressant medications have no effect
2. When there is a need for a rapid definitive response, such as when a client is suicidal or homicidal
3. The client is in extreme agitation or stupor
4. The risks of other treatments outweigh the risk of ECT
5. The client has a history of poor medication response, a history of good ECT response, or both
6. The client prefers it

D. Preprocedure
1. Explain the procedure to the client
2. Encourage the client to discuss feelings, including myths regarding ECT
3. Teach the client and family what to expect
4. Informed consent must be obtained when voluntary clients are being treated
5. For involuntary clients, when informed consent cannot be obtained, permission may be obtained from the next of kin, although in some states the permission for ECT must be obtained from the court
6. NPO after midnight or at least 4 hours prior to treatment
7. Baseline vital signs are taken
8. The client is requested to void
9. Hairpins, contact lenses, and dentures are removed
10. Administer preoperative medication if prescribed; glycopyrrolate (Robinul) or atropine sulfate may be prescribed to prevent the potential for aspiration and to minimize bradydysrhythmias in response to electrical stimulants

E. During the procedure
1. Place a blood pressure cuff on one of the client's arms
2. An IV line is inserted, and EEG and ECG electrodes are attached
3. A pulse oximeter is placed onto the client's finger
4. Blood pressure is monitored throughout the treatment

5. Medications administered may include a short-acting anesthetic such as methohexital sodium (Brevital Sodium) or thiopental sodium (Pentothal) and a muscle relaxant such as succinylcholine (Anectine)
6. 100% oxygen by mask via positive pressure is administered throughout the procedure
7. An airway or bite block is placed to prevent biting of the tongue
8. Electrical stimulus is administered, and the seizure should last 30 to 60 seconds

F. Postprocedure
1. The client will be transported to a recovery room with the blood pressure cuff and oximeter in place, where oxygen, suction, and other emergency equipment are available
2. Once the client is awake, talk to the client and take vital signs
3. The client may be confused; provide frequent orientation (brief, distinct, and simple) and reassurance
4. The client returns to the nursing unit when a 90% oxygen saturation level is maintained, vital signs are stable, and mental status is satisfactory
5. Assess the gag reflex prior to giving the client fluids, food, or medication

G. Potential side effects
1. Major side effects with bilateral treatment are confusion, disorientation, and short-term memory loss
2. The client may be confused and disorientated upon awakening
3. Memory deficits may occur, but memory usually recovers completely, although some clients have memory loss lasting up to 6 months

XIII. COGNITIVE IMPAIRMENT DISORDERS
A. Autism: Refer to Chapter 33
B. Attention deficit hyperactivity disorder (ADHD): Refer to Chapter 33
C. Tourette's disorder: Refer to Chapter 33
D. Dementia and Alzheimer's disease
1. Dementia
a. Organic syndrome with progressive deterioration in intellectual functioning
b. Long- and short-term memory loss occurs, with impairment in judgment, abstract thinking, problem-solving ability, and behavior
c. Results in a self-care deficit
d. The most common type of dementia is Alzheimer's disease
2. Alzheimer's disease (Box 71-12)
a. An irreversible form of senile dementia resulting from nerve cell deterioration
b. Individuals with Alzheimer's disease experience cognitive deterioration and progressive loss of ability to carry out ADLs

---

BOX 71-12

Alzheimer's Disease

Amnesia: inability to learn new information or to recall previously learned information

Agnosia: failure to recognize or identify objects despite intact sensory function

Aphasia: language disturbance in understanding and expressing the spoken word

Apraxia: inability to perform motor activities despite intact motor function

---

c. The client experiences a steady decline in physical and mental functioning and usually requires nursing home placement in the final stages of the illness

3. Implementation
   a. Identify and reinforce retained skills
   b. Provide continuity of care
   c. Orient to the environment
   d. Furnish environment with familiar possessions
   e. Acknowledge the client's feelings
   f. Assist the client and family members to manage memory deficits and behavior changes
   g. Encourage the family members to express feelings about caregiving
   h. Provide the caregiver support, and identify the resources and support groups available
   i. Monitor ADLs
   j. Remind the client how to perform self-care activities
   k. Maintain independence
   l. Provide consistent routines
   m. Provide exercise, such as walking with an escort
   n. Avoid activities that tax the memory
   o. Allow plenty of time to complete a task
   p. Use constant encouragement in a step-by-step approach
   q. Provide activities that distract and occupy time, such as listening to music, coloring, and watching TV
   r. Provide mental stimulation with simple games or activities

4. Wandering
   a. Provide a safe environment
   b. Prevent unsafe wandering
   c. Provide close supervision
   d. Close and secure doors
   e. Use identification bracelets and electronic surveillance

5. Communication
   a. Adapt to the communication level of the client
   b. Use a firm volume and a low-pitched voice to communicate

c. Stand directly in front of the client and maintain eye contact
d. Call the client by name and identify self; wait for a response
e. Use a calm and reassuring voice
f. Use pantomime gestures if the client is unable to understand spoken words
g. Use slow, clear, verbal communication techniques
h. Use short words and simple sentences
i. Ask only one question at a time, and give one direction at a time
j. Repeat questions if necessary, but do not rephrase

6. Impaired judgment
   a. Remove throw rugs, toxic substances, and dangerous electrical appliances from the environment
   b. Reduce hot water heater temperature

7. Altered thought processes
   a. Call the client by name
   b. Orient the client frequently
   c. Use familiar objects in the room
   d. Place a calendar and a clock in a visible place
   e. Maintain familiar routines
   f. Allow the client to reminisce
   g. Make tasks simple
   h. Allow time for the client to complete a task
   i. Provide positive reinforcement for positive behaviors

8. Altered sleep patterns
   a. Allow the client to wander in a safe place until he or she becomes tired
   b. Prevent shadows in the room
   c. Avoid the use of hypnotics, as they cause confusion and aggravate the sundown effect

9. Agitation
   a. Assess the precipitant of the agitation
   b. Reassure the client
   c. Remove items that can be hazardous during the time of agitation
   d. Approach the client slowly and calmly from the front; then speak, gesture, and move slowly
   e. Remove the client to a less stressful environment
   f. Use touch gently
   g. Do not argue with the client or restrain the client
   h. Distract the client with questions about the problem, and gradually turn the attention to something else

XIV. PSYCHOSEXUAL ALTERATIONS
A. Sexuality
   1. One's sense of being a sexual individual
   2. Includes how one looks, behaves, and relates to others

B. Sexual expression
1. Heterosexuality: Male-female sexual relationships
2. Homosexuality: Sexual attraction to a member of the same sex
3. Bisexuality: Sexual attraction to and activity with both sexes
4. Transvestism: Obsession with wearing clothing of the opposite sex

C. Alterations in sexual behavior
1. Transsexualism: Feeling that one's sex is inappropriate and desiring to acquire sexual characteristics of the opposite sex
2. Exhibitionism: Sexual urges and fantasies and exposing genitals to strangers
3. Fetishism: Using nonliving objects for sexual gratification
4. Pedophelia: Desiring sexual activity with a child under age 13
5. Sexual masochism: Sexual gratification that involves receiving pain
6. Sexual sadism: Sexual gratification that involves inflicting pain
7. Voyeurism: Sexual gratification through observing others disrobing or engaging in sexual activity
8. Zoophilla: Intense sexual arousal or desire for sexual contact with animals
9. Frotteurism: Intense sexual arousal or desire when rubbing against a nonconsenting person

D. Implementation
1. Assessment of sexual history and precipitating event for sexual disorder
2. Encourage the client to explore personal beliefs
3. Provide a nonjudgmental attitude
4. Provide supportive psychotherapy
5. Initiate psychoanalysis as prescribed

PRACTICE QUESTIONS

1. A nurse is planning activities for a client who has bipolar disorder with aggressive social behavior. Which of the following activities would be most appropriate for this client?
   1. Ping-Pong
   2. Writing
   3. Chess
   4. Basketball

2. A client is admitted to the hospital with a diagnosis of "major depression: severe, single episode." The nurse assesses the client and identifies the client's altered nutrition related to poor nutritional intake as a major concern. What is the most appropriate nursing intervention related to this diagnosis?
   1. Explaining to the client the importance of a good nutritional intake
   2. Weighing the client three times per week before breakfast
   3. Reporting the nutritional concern to the psychiatrist and obtaining a nutritional consultation as soon as possible
   4. Consulting with the nutritionist, offering the client several small, frequent meals per day, and scheduling brief nursing interactions with the client during these times

3. When planning activities for the depressed client, especially during the early stages of hospitalization, which of the following plans is best?
   1. Providing an activity that is quiet and solitary in nature to avoid increased fatigue, such as working on a puzzle or reading a book
   2. Planning nothing until the client asks to participate in the milieu
   3. Offering the client a menu of daily activities and insisting that the client participate in all of them
   4. Providing a structured daily program of activities and encouraging the client to participate

4. A depressed client verbalizes feelings of low self-esteem and self-worth with statements such as, "I'm such a failure . . . I can't do anything right!" What would the best nursing response be?
   1. Telling the client that this is not true and that we all have a purpose in life
   2. Remaining with the client and sitting in silence; this will encourage the client to verbalize feelings
   3. Reassuring the client that you know how the client is feeling and that things will get better
   4. Identifying recent behaviors or accomplishments that demonstrate skill ability

5. A client with a diagnosis of "major depression: recurrent with psychotic features" is admitted to the mental health unit. To create a safe environment for the client, the nurse most importantly devises a plan of care that deals specifically with the client's:
   1. Altered thought processes
   2. Altered nutrition
   3. Self-care deficit
   4. Knowledge deficit

6. A depressed client is ready for discharge. The nurse feels comfortable that the client has a good understanding of the disease process when the client states which of the following?
   1. "I'll never let this happen to me again. I won't let my boss or my job or my family get to me!"
   2. "It's important for me to eat well, exercise, and to take my medication. If I begin to lose my appetite or not sleep well, I've got to get in to see my doctor."
   3. "I've learned that I am a good person and that I am worthy of giving and receiving love. I don't need anyone, I have myself to rely on!"
   4. "I don't know what happened to me. I've always been able to make decisions for myself and for my business. I don't ever want to feel so weak or vulnerable again!"

7. A nurse assesses a client with the admitting diagnosis of "bipolar affective disorder: mania."

Which of the following symptoms presented by the client requires the nurse's immediate intervention?

1. Outlandish behaviors and inappropriate dress
2. Grandiose delusions of being a royal descendent of King Arthur
3. Nonstop physical activity and poor nutritional intake
4. Incessant talking that includes sexual innuendoes and teasing of the staff

8. A nurse reviews the activity schedule for the day and plans which activity for the manic client?
   1. Brown-bag luncheon and a book review
   2. Tetherball
   3. Paint-by-number activity
   4. Deep-breathing and progressive relaxation group

9. A client who is delusional says to the nurse, "The federal guards were sent to kill me." What is the nurse's best response?
   1. "The guards are not out to kill you."
   2. "I don't believe this is true."
   3. "I don't know anything about the guards. Do you feel afraid that people are trying to hurt you?"
   4. "What makes you think the guards were sent to hurt you?"

10. A woman comes into the emergency room in a severe state of anxiety after a car accident. What is the most appropriate nursing intervention?
    1. Remaining with the client
    2. Putting the client in a quiet room
    3. Teaching the client deep-breathing
    4. Encouraging the client to talk about her feelings and concerns

11. A male client with delirium becomes disoriented and confused in his room at night. What is the most appropriate initial nursing intervention?
    1. Using a night-light and turning off the television
    2. Keeping the television and a soft light on during the night
    3. Moving the client next to the nurse's station
    4. Playing soft music during the night and maintaining a well-lit room

12. A hospitalized client is being considered for electroconvulsive therapy (ECT). The client appears calm, but the family is anxious. The client's mother begins to cry and states, "My son's brain will be destroyed. How can the doctor do this to him?" What is the nurse's best response?
    1. "It sounds as though you need to speak to the psychiatrist."
    2. "Your son has decided to have this treatment. You should be supportive of him."
    3. "Perhaps you'd like to see the ECT room and speak to the staff."
    4. "It sounds as though you have some concerns about the ECT procedure. Why don't we all sit down together and discuss any concerns you may have."

13. A nurse is performing an assessment on a client with dementia. Which data gathered during the assessment would indicate a potential complication associated with dementia?
    1. Presence of personal hygienic care
    2. Improvement in sleeping
    3. Absence of sundowner's syndrome
    4. Confabulation

14. The community health nurse visits a client who recently retired. The client states, "Lately I'm getting forgetful about things. Do you think I'm getting Alzheimer's disease?" Which response by the nurse would be the most therapeutic?
    1. "Tell me more about your forgetfulness. It isn't unusual for forgetfulness to occur if memory is not exercised. Are you staying socially active?"
    2. "Oh, I'm certain it's not Alzheimer's disease, because there's no family history of it."
    3. "Now, I'm not going to discuss this with you because I think you're just normal."
    4. "I am so forgetful, too. I have to make out lists now to go shopping."

15. A nurse is discharging a client with a history of command hallucinations to harm self or others. The nurse provides instructions to the client about interventions for hallucinations and anxiety and determines that the client understands these instructions if the client states which of the following?
    1. "My medications won't make me anxious."
    2. "I can call my therapist when I'm hallucinating so that I can talk about my feelings and plans and not hurt anyone."
    3. "I'll go to support group and talk so that I don't hurt anyone."
    4. "I won't get anxious or hear things if I get enough sleep and eat well."

16. A nurse develops a nursing diagnosis of self-care deficit for an elderly client with dementia. Which of the following is the most appropriate goal for this client?
    1. The client will be admitted to a long-term care facility to have activities of daily living (ADLs) needs met
    2. The client will function at the highest level of independence possible
    3. The client will complete all ADLs independently within a 1-hour time frame
    4. The nursing staff will attend to all of the client's ADL needs during the hospital stay

17. A nurse observes that a client is pacing, agitated, and presenting aggressive gestures. The client's speech pattern is rapid and affect is belligerent. Based on these observations, what is the nurse's immediate priority of care?
    1. Providing safety for the client and other clients on the unit
    2. Offering the client a less stimulating area in which to calm down and gain control

3. Providing the clients on the unit with a sense of comfort and safety
4. Assisting the staff in caring for the client in a controlled environment

18. A nurse is caring for a male client diagnosed with catatonic stupor. The client is lying on the bed, with his body pulled into a fetal position. Which of the following is the most appropriate nursing intervention?
    1. Leaving the client alone and intermittently checking on him
    2. Taking the client into the day room with other clients so that they can help watch him
    3. Sitting quietly beside the client and asking occasional open-ended questions
    4. Asking direct questions to encourage the client to talk

19. A client is admitted to the mental health unit with a diagnosis of schizophrenia. A nursing diagnosis formulated for the client is "altered thought process secondary to paranoia." In formulating nursing interventions with the members of the health care team, the nurse provides instructions to do which of the following?
    1. Avoid laughing or whispering in front of the client
    2. Increase socialization of the client with peers
    3. Have the client sign a release of information to appropriate parties so that adequate data can be obtained for assessment purposes
    4. Begin to educate the client about social supports in the community

20. A client is admitted with a diagnosis of depression. A nurse develops a plan of care for the client. Which of the following is the most appropriate activity to be included in the plan of care?
    1. An activity that is quiet and solitary in nature to avoid increased fatigue, such as working on a puzzle or reading a book
    2. Nothing until the client asks to participate in the milieu
    3. A menu of daily activities, with the nurse insisting that the client participate in all of them
    4. A structured daily program of activities, with the nurse encouraging the client to participate

21. When planning the discharge of a client with chronic anxiety, a nurse directs the goals at promoting a safe environment at home. The most appropriate maintenance goal should focus on which of the following?
    1. Continued contact with a crisis counselor
    2. Identifying anxiety-producing situations
    3. Ignoring feelings of anxiety
    4. Eliminating all anxiety from daily situations

22. A client is unwilling to go out of the house for fear of "doing something crazy in public." Because of this fear, the client remains homebound except when accompanied outside by the spouse. Based on this data, the nurse determines that the client is experiencing which of the following?
    1. Social phobia
    2. Agoraphobia
    3. Claustrophobia
    4. Hypochondriasis

23. A nurse is developing a plan of care for a client who is scheduled to have electroconvulsive therapy (ECT). Which nursing diagnosis is a priority for this client?
    1. Fear
    2. Anxiety
    3. Risk for aspiration
    4. Body image disturbance

24. A client is admitted to a medical nursing unit with a diagnosis of acute blindness. Many tests are performed, and there seems to be no organic reason why this client cannot see. A nurse later learns that the client became blind after witnessing a hit-and-run car accident, when a family of three was killed. The nurse suspects that the client may be experiencing which of the following?
    1. Psychosis
    2. A conversion disorder
    3. A dissociative disorder
    4. Repression

25. A manic client announces to everyone in the day room that a stripper is coming to perform this evening. When the nurse firmly states that this will not happen, the manic client becomes verbally abusive and threatens physical violence to the nurse. Based on the analysis of this situation, the nurse determines that the most appropriate action would be to do which of the following?
    1. With assistance, escort the manic client to a room and administer PRN haloperidol (Haldol)
    2. Tell the client that smoking privileges are revoked for 24 hours
    3. Orient the client to time, person, and place
    4. Tell the client that the behavior is not appropriate

CRITICAL THINKING: FREE-TEXT ENTRY

A female client in a manic state emerges from her room. She is topless and is making sexual remarks and gestures toward the staff and peers. What is the best initial nursing action?

Answer: _____

ANSWERS

1. 2

Rationale: Solitary activities that require a short attention span with mild physical exertion are the most appropriate activities for a client who is exhibiting aggressive behavior. Writing (journaling), walks with staff, and finger painting are activities that minimize stimuli and provide a constructive release for tension. Competitive games should be avoided, because they can stimulate aggression and increase psychomotor activity.

Test-Taking Strategy: Use the process of elimination. Options 1, 3, and 4 are similar in that they are activities that the client cannot do alone. Option 2 identifies a solitary activity. Review care to the client with aggressive behavior if you had difficulty with this question.

Level of Cognitive Ability: Application
Client Needs: Psychosocial Integrity
Integrated Concept/Process: Nursing Process/Planning
Content Area: Mental Health
Reference: Keltner, N., Schwecke, L., & Bostrom, C. (1999). *Psychiatric nursing* (3rd ed.). St. Louis: Mosby, p. 413.

2. 4

Rationale: Change in appetite is one of the major symptoms of depression. Other symptoms include a depressed mood; increased fatigue; feelings of worthlessness; diminished ability to think or indecisiveness; and psychomotor agitation or retardation. Option 1 is incorrect, because the client is experiencing poor concentration; hence, even if the client does understand the rationale, he or she still may not be able to complete tasks. Weighing the client does not address a way to increase nutritional intake. Reporting to the psychiatrist and the nutritionist is to some degree correct, but that option lacks the method as to how one might increase the client's food intake.

Test-Taking Strategy: Use the process of elimination, and focus on the issue of poor nutritional status. Option 4 is the only option that directly addresses altered nutrition and provides a method in which the client will feasibly increase the nutritional intake. Review care of the client with depression if you had difficulty with this question.

Level of Cognitive Ability: Application
Client Needs: Physiological Integrity
Integrated Concept/Process: Nursing Process/Implementation
Content Area: Mental Health
Reference: Fortinash, K., & Holoday-Worret, P. (2000). *Psychiatric mental health nursing* (2nd ed.). St. Louis: Mosby, p. 268.

3. 4

Rationale: A depressed person experiences a depressed mood and is often withdrawn. Also, the person experiences difficulty concentrating, loss of interest or pleasure, low energy, fatigue, and feelings of worthlessness and poor self-esteem. The plan of care needs to provide successful experiences in a stimulating yet structured environment. Options 1 and 2 provide little or no structure, and option 3 is a forceful and absolute approach.

Test-Taking Strategy: Use the process of elimination. Recall that the depressed client requires a structured and stimulating program. Eliminate options 1 and 2, because these provide little or no structure and stimulation. Option 3 is eliminated because of the word "all." Review care to the client with depression if you had difficulty with this question.

Level of Cognitive Ability: Application

Client Needs: Safe, Effective Care Environment
Integrated Concept/Process: Nursing Process/Planning
Content Area: Mental Health
Reference: Fortinash, K., & Holoday-Worret, P. (2000). *Psychiatric mental health nursing* (2nd ed.). St. Louis: Mosby, p. 268.

4. 4

Rationale: Feelings of low self-esteem and worthlessness are common symptoms of the depressed client. An effective plan of care to enhance the client's personal self-esteem is to provide experiences for the client that are challenging but that will not be met with failure. Reminders of the client's past accomplishments or personal successes are ways to interrupt the client's negative self-talk and distorted cognitive view of self. Silence may be interpreted as agreement. Options 1 and 3 give advice and devalue the client's feelings.

Test-Taking Strategy: Use the process of elimination and therapeutic communication techniques. Focus on the client's diagnosis. Options 1 and 3 can be easily eliminated. From the remaining options, focusing on the client's diagnosis will direct you to option 4. Review care of the client with depression if you had difficulty with this question.

Level of Cognitive Level: Application
Client Needs: Psychosocial Integrity
Integrated Concept/Process: Nursing Process/Implementation
Content Area: Mental Health
Reference: Fortinash, K., & Holoday-Worret, P. (2000). *Psychiatric mental health nursing* (2nd ed.). St. Louis: Mosby, p. 268.

5. 1

Rationale: The diagnosis of "major depression: recurrent with psychotic features" alerts the nurse that, in addition to the criteria that designates the diagnosis of major depression, he or she also must deal with the client's psychosis. Psychosis is defined as a state in which a person's mental capacity to recognize reality and to communicate and relate to others is impaired; this obviously interferes with the person's capacity to deal with life's demands. Altered thought processes generally indicate a state of increased anxiety, where hallucinations and delusions prevail. Although all of the nursing diagnoses may be appropriate because the client is experiencing psychosis, option 1 is the correct option.

Test-Taking Strategy: Use the process of elimination. All of the nursing diagnoses listed may be appropriate for a client diagnosed with major depression. The key to the correct option lies with the specifier "psychotic features," which suggests that the client often experiences altered thought processes such as hallucinations and delusions. Review appropriate nursing diagnoses for the client with major depression and psychotic features if you had difficulty with this question.

Level of Cognitive Ability: Analysis
Client Needs: Safe, Effective Care Environment
Integrated Concept/Process: Nursing Process/Planning
Content Area: Mental Health
Reference: Fortinash, K., & Holoday-Worret, P. (2000). *Psychiatric mental health nursing* (2nd ed.). St. Louis: Mosby, pp. 267-268.

6. 2

Rationale: The exact cause of depression is not known, but it is believed to be related to a biochemical disruption of neurotransmitters in the brain. Diet, exercise, and medication are recognized treatments of the disease process. Options 1, 3, and 4 offer no insight into the disease process. In addition, option 1 reflects possible blaming or personal failure, and option 3 reflects an unwillingness to reach out to others.

Test-Taking Strategy: Use the process of elimination, and look for the global option. Option 2 is the only option that incorporates a holistic treatment approach, which includes good nutrition, exercise, medication, and the client's knowledge of the signs of possible relapse. Review concepts related to depression if you had difficulty with this question.

Level of Cognitive Ability: Analysis
Client Needs: Health Promotion and Maintenance
Integrated Concept/Process: Nursing Process/Evaluation
Content Area: Mental Health
Reference: Fortinash, K., & Holoday-Worret, P. (2000). *Psychiatric mental health nursing* (2nd ed.). St. Louis: Mosby, p. 260.

7. 3

Rationale: Mania is a mood characterized by excitement, euphoria, hyperactivity, excessive energy, decreased need for sleep, and impaired ability to concentrate or stay with a single train of thought. It is a period when the mood is predominantly elevated, expansive, or irritable. All of the options reflect a client's possible symptomatology. Option 3, however, clearly presents a problem that compromises one's physiological integrity and needs to be addressed immediately.

Test-Taking Strategy: Use the process of elimination and Maslow's hierarchy of needs theory to assist in answering the question. Option 3 is the only option that reflects a physiological need. Review care of the client with mania if you had difficulty with this question.

Level of Cognitive Ability: Analysis
Client Needs: Physiological Integrity
Integrated Concept/Process: Nursing Process/Assessment
Content Area: Mental Health
Reference: Fortinash, K., & Holoday-Worret, P. (2000). *Psychiatric mental health nursing* (2nd ed.). St. Louis: Mosby, p. 271.

8. 2

Rationale: A person who is experiencing mania is overactive, full of energy, lacks concentration, and has poor impulse control. The client needs an activity that will allow him or her to use excess energy but to not endanger others during the process. Options 1, 3, and 4 are relatively sedate activities that require concentration, which is a quality that is lacking during the manic state. Such activities may lead to increased frustration and anxiety for the client. Tetherball is an exercise that uses the large muscle groups of the body, and it is a great way to expend the increased energy that this client is experiencing.

Test-Taking Strategy: Use the process of elimination. Eliminate options 1, 3, and 4, because they are similar and relatively sedate activities. Review the appropriate interventions for a manic client if you had difficulty with this question.

Level of Cognitive Ability: Analysis
Client Needs: Physiological Integrity
Integrated Concept/Process: Nursing Process/Planning
Content Area: Mental Health
Reference: Fortinash, K., & Holoday-Worret, P. (2000). *Psychiatric mental health nursing* (2nd ed.). St. Louis: Mosby, p. 274.

9. 3

Rationale: It is most therapeutic for the nurse to empathize with the client's experience. Disagreeing with delusions may make the client more defensive, and the client may cling to the delusions even more. Encouraging discussion about the delusion is inappropriate.

Test-Taking Strategy: Use therapeutic communication techniques. Eliminate options 1 and 2, because they are similar and disagree with the client. Option 4 encourages discussion about the delusion. Review communication techniques with the client experiencing delusions if you had difficulty with this question.

Level of Cognitive Ability: Application
Client Needs: Psychosocial Integrity
Integrated Concept/Process: Communication and Documentation
Content Area: Mental Health
Reference: Keltner, N., Schwecke, L., & Bostrom, C. (1999). *Psychiatric nursing* (3rd ed.). St. Louis: Mosby, p. 132.

10. 1

Rationale: If a client with severe anxiety is left alone, he or she may feel abandoned and become overwhelmed. Placing the client in a quiet room is also important, but the nurse must stay with the client. It is not possible to teach the client deep-breathing or relaxation exercises until the anxiety decreases. Encouraging the client to discuss concerns and feelings would not take place until the anxiety has decreased.

Test-Taking Strategy: Use the process of elimination. Note the key words "most appropriate" and "severe state." Eliminate options 3 and 4 first, knowing that these actions are not possible when the client is in a severe state of anxiety. From the remaining options, the most appropriate action is to remain with the client. Review care of the client with severe anxiety if you had difficulty with this question.

Level of Cognitive Ability: Application
Client Needs: Psychosocial Integrity
Integrated Concept/Process: Nursing Process/Implementation
Content Area: Mental Health
Reference: Fortinash, K., & Holoday-Worret, P. (2000). *Psychiatric mental health nursing* (2nd ed.). St. Louis: Mosby, pp. 250-251.

11. 1

Rationale: It is important to provide a consistent daily routine and a low-stimulation environment when the client is disorientated. Noise, including radio and television, may add to the confusion and disorientation. Moving the client next to the nurses' station is not the initial action.

Test-Taking Strategy: Use the process of elimination. Note the key word "initial" in the stem of the question. Eliminate options 2 and 4 first because they are similar. Focusing on the key word will easily direct you to option 1. Review measures related to the client that is disoriented and confused if you had difficulty with this question.

Level of Cognitive Ability: Application
Client Needs: Psychosocial Integrity
Integrated Concept/Process: Nursing Process/Implementation
Content Area: Mental Health
Reference: Fortinash, K., & Holoday-Worret, P. (2000). *Psychiatric mental health nursing* (2nd ed.). St. Louis: Mosby, pp. 410-411.

12. 4

Rationale: In option 4, the nurse encourages the client and the family to verbalize fears and concerns. Options 1, 2, and 3 avoid dealing with concerns and are blocks to communication.

Test-Taking Strategy: Use the process of elimination and therapeutic communication techniques. Option 4 is the only therapeutic option. Options 1, 2, and 3 are blocks to communication. Review these therapeutic techniques if you had difficulty with this question.

Level of Cognitive Ability: Analysis
Client Needs: Psychosocial Integrity
Integrated Concept/Process: Communication and Documentation
Content Area: Mental Health
Reference: Varcarolis, E. (1998). *Foundations of psychiatric mental health nursing* (3rd ed.). Philadelphia: W. B. Saunders, p. 579.

13. **4**

Rationale: The clinical picture of dementia varies from the development of mild cognitive defects to severe, life-threatening alterations in neurological functioning. It is not unusual for the client to employ confabulation or the fabrication of events or experiences to fill in memory gaps. Often a lack of inhibition on the part of the client may constitute the first indication of anything being "wrong" to the client's significant others (the client may undress in front of people or demonstrate slovenly table manners, whereas in the past the client was very well-mannered). As the dementia progresses, the client will have episodes of wandering or sundowning.

Test-Taking Strategy: Use the process of elimination. Knowledge about the manifestations associated with dementia is required to answer this question. Focusing on the issue of a potential complication will direct you to option 4. If you had difficulty with this question, review the complications associated with dementia.

Level of Cognitive Ability: Analysis
Client Needs: Physiological Integrity
Integrated Concept/Process: Nursing Process/Assessment
Content Area: Mental Health
Reference: Glod, C. A. (1998). *Contemporary psychiatric-mental health nursing.* Philadelphia: F. A. Davis, pp. 233-258.

14. **1**

Rationale: The most effective communication technique is the one in which the nurse is giving information. With regard to memory functioning, the normal older adult who ages will find that the time required for memory scanning is longer for both recent and remote memory recall. Dementia of the Alzheimer's type involves a disorder that is characterized by a syndrome of symptomatology with a slow and insidious onset and a generally progressive and deteriorating course. In option 2, the nurse gives false reassurance, which devalues the client's feelings and discourages the client from expressing feelings due to the client's anticipation of ridicule. In option 3, the nurse is rejecting the client by refusing to consider the client's ideas or demonstrating ridicule or contempt for the client's ideas or behavior. In option 4, the nurse makes a social (not a professional) comment and belittles the client's concerns, which will discourage the expression of feelings.

Test-Taking Strategy: Use the process of elimination and knowledge about therapeutic communication techniques. Option 1 is the only option that identifies the use of a

therapeutic communication technique. Review these techniques if you had difficulty with this question.

Level of Cognitive Ability: Application
Client Needs: Psychosocial Integrity
Integrated Concept/Process: Communication and Documentation
Content Area: Mental Health
Reference: Fortinash, K., & Holoday-Worret, P. (2000). *Psychiatric mental health nursing* (2nd ed.). St. Louis: Mosby, p. 387.

15. **2**

Rationale: There may be an increased risk for impulsive and/or aggressive behavior if a client is receiving command hallucinations to harm self or others. The client should be asked about his or her intentions to hurt. Talking about auditory hallucinations can interfere with the subvocal muscular activity associated with a hallucination. Options 1, 3, and 4 will aid in wellness, but they are not specific interventions for hallucinations.

Test-Taking Strategy: Use the process of elimination. Options 1, 3, and 4 are all interventions that a client can do to aid wellness. Option 2 is a specific agreement to seek help and evidences self-responsible commitment and control over one's own behavior. Review teaching points for a client with a history of hallucinations if you had difficulty with this question.

Level of Cognitive Ability: Analysis
Client Needs: Health Promotion and Maintenance
Integrated Concept/Process: Nursing Process/Evaluation
Content Area: Mental Health
Reference: Keltner, N., Schwecke, L., & Bostrom, C. (1999). *Psychiatric nursing* (3rd ed.). St. Louis: Mosby, p. 132.

16. **2**

Rationale: All clients, regardless of age, need to be encouraged to perform at the highest level of independence possible. This contributes to the client's sense of control and well-being. Option 1 is incorrect, because one does not know what the "self-care deficit" entails. To assume that the client requires long-term care on such little data would be erroneous. Options 3 and 4 are absolute statements.

Test-Taking Strategy: Use the process of elimination. Eliminate options 3 and 4 first because of the absolute word "all." From the remaining options, select option 2, because it is the global option. Review care of the client with dementia if you had difficulty with this question.

Level of Cognitive Ability: Application
Client Needs: Health Promotion and Maintenance
Integrated Concept/Process: Nursing Process/Planning
Content Area: Mental Health
Reference: Fortinash, K., & Holoday-Worret, P. (2000). *Psychiatric mental health nursing* (2nd ed.). St. Louis: Mosby, p. 400.

17. **1**

Rationale: Safety of the client and other clients is the priority. Option 1 is the only option that addresses the client and other clients' safety needs. Option 2 addresses only the client's needs. Option 3 addresses only other clients' needs. Option 4 is not client-centered.

Test-Taking Strategy: Use the process of elimination and Maslow's hierarchy of needs theory to prioritize. Note the words "agitated, aggressive, and belligerent." Safety is the key issue. Option 1 is the global option and addresses the safety of

all. Review nursing interventions to provide safety to clients if you had difficulty with this question.
Level of Cognitive Ability: Application
Client Needs: Safe, Effective Care Environment
Integrated Concept/Process: Nursing Process/Implementation
Content Area: Mental Health
Reference: Keltner, N., Schwecke, L., & Bostrom, C. (1999). *Psychiatric nursing* (3rd ed.). St. Louis: Mosby, pp. 313, 321.

18. **3**
Rationale: Clients who are withdrawn may be immobile and mute and require consistent, repeated approaches. Communication with withdrawn clients requires much patience from the nurse. Interventions include the establishment of interpersonal contact. The nurse facilitates communication with the client by sitting in silence, asking open-ended questions, and pausing to provide opportunities for the client to respond.
Test-Taking Strategy: Use the process of elimination. Eliminate option 1, because the client would not be left alone. Option 2 relies on other clients to care for this client, and this is an inappropriate expectation. Asking direct questions to this client is not therapeutic. Option 3 is the best action, because it provides for client supervision and communication as appropriate.
Level of Cognitive Ability: Application
Client Needs: Safe, Effective Care Environment
Integrated Concept/Process: Nursing Process/Implementation
Content Area: Mental Health
Reference: Keltner, N., Schwecke, L., & Bostrom, C. (1999). *Psychiatric nursing* (3rd ed.). St. Louis: Mosby, p. 399.

19. **1**
Rationale: "Altered thought process secondary to paranoia" is the client's problem, and the plan of care must address this problem. The client is experiencing paranoia and is distrustful and suspicious of others. The members of the health care team need to establish rapport and trust with the client, so laughing or whispering in front of the client would be counterproductive. Options 2, 3, and 4 ask the client to trust on a multitude of levels; these options are actions that are too intrusive for a client who is paranoid.
Test-Taking Strategy: Use the process of elimination and knowledge about this disorder to answer the question. Noting that the client has paranoia will direct you to option 1. Review this disorder if you had difficulty with this question.
Level of Cognitive Ability: Application
Client Needs: Psychosocial Integrity
Integrated Concept/Process: Nursing Process/Implementation
Content Area: Mental Health
Reference: Fortinash, K., & Holoday-Worret, P. (2000). *Psychiatric mental health nursing* (2nd ed.). St. Louis: Mosby, p. 280.

20. **4**
Rationale: A client with depression often has a depressed mood and is often withdrawn. Also, the person experiences difficulty concentrating, loss of interest or pleasure, low energy, fatigue, and feelings of worthlessness and poor self-esteem. The plan of care needs to provide successful experiences in a stimulating yet structured environment. Options 1, 2, and 3 are too restrictive and offer little or no structure or stimulation.
Test-Taking Strategy: Use the process of elimination. Recall that the depressed client requires a structured and stimulating

program in a safe environment. Option 4 is the only option that will provide a safe and effective environment. Review care of the client with depression if you had difficulty with this question.
Level of Cognitive Ability: Application
Client Needs: Safe, Effective Care Environment
Integrated Concept/Process: Nursing Process/Planning
Content Area: Mental Health
Reference: Fortinash, K., & Holoday-Worret, P. (2000). *Psychiatric mental health nursing* (2nd ed.). St. Louis: Mosby, p. 279.

21. **2**
Rationale: Recognizing situations that produce anxiety allows the client to prepare to cope with anxiety or avoid specific stimuli. Counselors will not be available for all anxiety-producing situations, and this option does not encourage the development of internal strengths. Ignoring feelings will not resolve anxiety. It is impossible to eliminate all anxiety from life.
Test-Taking Strategy: Use the process of elimination. Eliminate option 4 first because of the word "all." Eliminate option 3 next, because feelings should not be ignored. From the remaining options, select option 2, because this option is more client-centered and provides the preparation for the client to deal with anxiety should it occur. Review home care planning for the client with chronic anxiety if you had difficulty with this question.
Level of Cognitive Ability: Application
Client Needs: Health Promotion and Maintenance
Integrated Concept/Process: Nursing Process/Planning
Content Area: Mental Health
Reference: Fortinash, K., & Holoday-Worret, P. (2000). *Psychiatric mental health nursing* (2nd ed.). St. Louis: Mosby, pp. 250-251.

22. **2**
Rationale: Agoraphobia is a fear of open spaces and the fear of being trapped in a situation from which there may not be an escape. Agoraphobia includes the possibility of experiencing a sense of helplessness or embarrassment if an attack occurs. Avoidance of such situations usually results in reduction of social and professional interactions. Social phobia focuses more on specific situations such as the fear of speaking, performing, or eating in public. Claustrophobia is a fear of closed places. Clients with hypochondriacal symptoms focus their anxiety on physical complaints and are preoccupied with their health.
Test-Taking Strategy: Use the process of elimination. Focusing on the key words "remains homebound" will direct you to option 2. If you had difficulty with this question, review phobia types and associated client behaviors.
Level of Cognitive Ability: Analysis
Client Needs: Psychosocial Integrity
Integrated Concept/Process: Nursing Process/Assessment
Content Area: Mental Health
Reference: Fortinash, K., & Holoday-Worret, P. (2000). *Psychiatric mental health nursing* (2nd ed.). St. Louis: Mosby, p. 241.

23. **3**
Rationale: Aspiration is safeguarded against by keeping the client NPO for 6 to 8 hours before ECT, removing dentures, and administering preprocedure medications as prescribed. Although options 1 and 2 could also be appropriate nursing

diagnoses, they are not the priority. There is no reason to assume that option 4 is even a consideration.

Test-Taking Strategy: Use the process of elimination and Maslow's hierarchy of needs theory to answer this question. Physiological needs must come first. Additionally, use the ABCs (airway, breathing, and circulation). Airway is the concern when there is a risk of aspiration. If you had difficulty with this question, review the procedures related to ECT.

Level of Cognitive Ability: Analysis
Client Needs: Physiological Integrity
Integrated Concept/Process: Nursing Process/Analysis
Content Area: Mental Health
Reference: Keltner, N., Schwecke, L., & Bostrom, C. (1999). *Psychiatric nursing* (3rd ed.). St. Louis: Mosby, p. 581.

24. 2

Rationale: A conversion disorder is the alteration or loss of a physical function that cannot be explained by any known pathophysiological mechanism. It is thought to be an expression of a psychological need or conflict. In this situation, the client witnessed an accident that was so psychologically painful that the client became blind. A dissociative disorder is a disturbance or alteration in the normally integrative functions of identity, memory, or consciousness. Psychosis is a state in which a person's mental capacity to recognize reality, communicate, and relate to others is impaired, thereby interfering with the person's capacity to deal with life demands. Repression is a coping mechanism in which unacceptable feelings are kept out of awareness.

Test-Taking Strategy: Use the process of elimination. The key to the correct option lies in the fact that the client presents no organic reason to account for the blindness, which suggests a conversion disorder. If you had difficulty with this question, review defense mechanisms and the concepts associated with a conversion disorder.

Level of Cognitive Ability: Analysis
Client Needs: Psychosocial Integrity
Integrated Concept/Process: Nursing Process/Analysis
Content Area: Mental Health
Reference: Fortinash, K., & Holoday-Worret, P. (2000). *Psychiatric mental health nursing* (2nd ed.). St. Louis: Mosby, p. 245.

25. 1

Rationale: The client is at risk for injury to self and others and therefore should be escorted out of the day room. Antipsy-

chotic medications are useful to manage the manic client. Hyperactive and agitated behavior usually responds to haloperidol (Haldol). Option 2 may increase the agitation that already exists in this client. Orientation will not halt the behavior. Telling the client that the behavior is not appropriate has already been attempted by the nurse.

Test-Taking Strategy: Use the process of elimination and Maslow's hierarchy of needs theory to answer the question. Look for the option that promotes safety of the client, other clients, and staff. If you had difficulty with this question, review the appropriate interventions for dealing with a manic client.

Level of Cognitive Ability: Analysis
Client Needs: Psychosocial Integrity
Integrated Concept/Process: Nursing Process/Implementation
Content Area: Mental Health
Reference: Fortinash, K., & Holoday-Worret, P. (2000). *Psychiatric mental health nursing* (2nd ed.). St. Louis: Mosby, pp. 281-282.

CRITICAL THINKING: FREE-TEXT ENTRY

Answer: Quietly approach the client, escort her to her room, and assist her in getting dressed

Rationale: A person who is experiencing mania lacks insight and judgment, has poor impulse control, and is highly excitable. The nurse must take control without creating increased stress or anxiety in the client. A quiet, firm approach while distracting the client (walking her to her room and assisting her to get dressed) achieves the goal of having her dressed appropriately and preserving her psychosocial integrity.

Test-Taking Strategy: Focus on the data provided in the question. Note the key word "initial." Recalling that a primary nursing responsibility is to protect the client will assist in determining the best nursing action. Review care of the client with mania if you had difficulty with this question.

Level of Cognitive Ability: Application
Client Needs: Psychosocial Integrity
Integrated Concept/Process: Nursing Process/Implementation
Content Area: Mental Health
Reference: Fortinash, K., & Holoday-Worret, P. (2000). *Psychiatric mental health nursing* (2nd ed.). St. Louis: Mosby, p. 274.

REFERENCES

Clark, J., Queener, S., & Karb, V. (2000). *Pharmacologic basis of nursing practice* (6th ed.). St. Louis: Mosby.

Fortinash, K., & Holoday-Worret, P. (2000). *Psychiatric mental health nursing* (2nd ed.). St. Louis: Mosby.

Glod, C.A. (1998). *Contemporary psychiatric-mental health nursing.* Philadelphia: F.A. Davis.

Keltner, N., Schwecke, L., & Bostrom, C. (1999). *Psychiatric nursing* (3rd ed.). St. Louis: Mosby.

Varcarolis, E. (1998). *Foundations of psychiatric mental health nursing* (3rd ed.). Philadelphia: W.B. Saunders.

Addictions

I. EATING DISORDERS

A. Description: Characterized by uncertain self-identification and grossly disturbed eating habits

B. Compulsive overeating
1. Binge-like overeating without purging
2. Food consumption is out of the individual's control and occurs in a stereotyped fashion
3. Client may be repulsed by eating, and the eating relieves tension but does not produce pleasure
4. Is aware that eating patterns are abnormal and feels depressed after eating
5. Eats secretly during a binge and consumes high-calorie and easily digestible food
6. Repeatedly tries to diet but without success
7. Lacks interest in exercise programs and feels helpless and hopeless about weight
8. When experiencing guilt, anger, depression, boredom, loneliness, inadequacy, or ambivalence, responds by eating

C. Anorexia nervosa
1. Description
   a. The onset is often associated with a stressful life event
   b. The client intensely fears obesity
   c. Body image is distorted, and the client has a disturbed self-concept
   d. Preoccupied with foods that prevent weight gain and has a phobia against foods that produce weight gain
   e. The eating disorder can be life threatening
   f. Death can occur from starvation, **suicide,** or electrolyte imbalance
2. Assessment
   a. Refusal to eat and appetite loss
   b. Appetite denial
   c. Feelings of lack of control
   d. Self-induced vomiting and self-administered enemas
   e. Exercises compulsively
   f. Overachiever and perfectionist
   g. Decreased temperature, pulse, and blood pressure
   h. Weight loss
   i. Gastrointestinal (GI) disturbances
   j. Constipation
   k. Electrolyte imbalances
   l. Scaly, dry skin
   m. Sleep disturbances
   n. Hormone deficiencies
   o. Amenorrhea for at least three consecutive menstrual periods
   p. Teeth and gum deterioration
   q. Cyanosis and numbness of extremities
   r. Esophageal varices from vomiting
   s. Bone degeneration

D. Bulimia nervosa
1. Description
   a. The client indulges in eating binges followed by purging behaviors
   b. Most clients remain within a normal weight range but feel that their lives are dominated by the eating-related conflict
2. Assessment
   a. Preoccupied with body shape and weight
   b. Consumes high-calorie food in secret; guilt about secretive eating
   c. Binge-purge syndrome
   d. Attempts to lose weight through diets, vomiting, enemas, cathartics, and amphetamines or diuretics
   e. Needs to control yet experiences feelings of powerlessness or loss of control
   f. Low self-esteem
   g. Poor interpersonal relationships
   h. Mood swings
   i. Self-mutilating behavior; **suicide** thoughts and attempts at **suicide**

j. Electrolyte imbalances

k. Loss of tooth enamel and dental decay

l. Stomach ulcers and rectal bleeding

m. Esophageal varices from vomiting

n. Cardiac disease and hypertension

▲ E. Implementation: Clients with an eating disorder

1. Assess the client's nutritional status

2. Establish a contract with the client concerning the diet plan for the day

3. Assist the client in identifying precipitators of the eating disorder

4. Encourage the client to state feelings about the eating behavior

5. Be accepting and nonjudgmental, expressing neither approval nor disapproval of the behavior

6. Encourage behavior modification techniques

7. Provide praise and positive reinforcement for accomplishments

8. Supervise the client during mealtimes and for a specified period after meals

9. Set a time limit for each meal

10. Provide a pleasant, relaxed environment for eating

11. Monitor for signs of physical complications related to the eating disorder

12. Record intake and output (I & O)

13. Weigh the client daily at the same time, using the same scale, after the client voids

14. When weighing the client, ensure that the client is wearing the same clothing as when the previous weight was taken

15. Monitor and restore fluid and electrolyte balance

16. Monitor elimination patterns

17. Assess and limit the client's activity level

18. Encourage the client to participate in diversional activities

19. Assess the client's suicidal potential

20. Administer antidepressant medication as prescribed

21. Encourage psychotherapy as prescribed

22. Refer the client to support groups

II. SUBSTANCE ABUSE DISORDERS

A. Description: Behavioral changes associated with regular substance **abuse** that affects the central nervous system (CNS)

B. Substance dependence (Box 72-1)

1. Pattern of repeated use of a substance, which usually results in tolerance, withdrawal, and compulsive drug-taking behavior

2. Client takes substances in larger amounts and over longer periods of time than were intended

3. Client has the desire to cut down but has unsuccessful efforts to decrease or discontinue use

4. Daily activities revolve around the use of a substance

BOX 72-1

CAGE Screening Test

C: Have you ever felt the need to cut down on your drinking or drug use?

A: Have you ever been annoyed at criticism of your drinking or drug use?

G: Have you ever felt guilty about something you have done when you have been drinking or taking drugs?

E: Have you ever had an eye opener, drinking or taking drugs first thing in the morning to get going or to avoid withdrawal symptoms?

C. Substance tolerance: The need for increased amounts of the substance to achieve the desired effect

D. Substance **abuse**   ▲

1. Client recurrently uses substances

2. Client experiences recurrent, significant harmful consequences related to the use of substances

3. Client has legal problems related to substance **abuse**

E. Substance withdrawal   ▲

1. Physiological and/or substance-specific cognitive symptoms

2. Occurs when blood levels decrease in an individual with prolonged heavy use of a substance

F. Precipitating factors of substance **abuse**

1. Rebellion and peer group pressure in adolescence

2. Pleasure-seeking experience, as the substance decreases physical and emotional pain

3. Group influence and peer pressure

4. Depression

5. Loss and grieving

G. Dysfunctional behaviors of substance **abuse**

1. Insensitive to self and others

2. Manipulative

3. Impulsiveness

4. Anger, including physical and verbal **abuse**

5. Avoidance of relationships, with physical and emotional distancing

6. Sense of self-importance and requiring special treatment

7. Denial, blaming everything but the substance

8. Codependent and expects others to accept behavior

9. Low self-esteem

10. Depression

III. ALCOHOL ABUSE   ▲

A. Description

1. Alcohol is a central nervous system (CNS) depressant affecting all body tissues

2. Physical dependence is a biological need for alcohol to avoid physical withdrawal symptoms

3. Psychological dependence is a craving for the subjective effect of alcohol

B. Risk factors
1. Biological predisposition
2. Depressed and highly anxious characteristics
3. Low self-esteem
4. Poor self-control
5. History of rebelliousness, poor school performance, delinquency
6. Poor parental relationships
C. Assessment
1. Slurred speech
2. Uncoordinated movements
3. Unsteady gait
4. Restlessness
5. Belligerence
6. Confusion
7. Sneaking drinks, drinking in the morning, and experiencing blackouts
8. Binge drinking
9. Arguments about drinking
10. Missing work
11. Increased tolerance to alcohol
12. Intoxication, with blood alcohol levels of 0.08% to 0.1% (80 to 100 mg alcohol/dL blood) or higher
D. Psychological symptoms
1. Depression
2. Hostility
3. Suspiciousness
4. Rationalization
5. Irritability
6. Isolation
7. Decrease in inhibitions
8. Decrease in self-esteem
9. Denial that a problem exists
▲ E. Complications associated with chronic alcohol use
1. Vitamin deficiencies
a. Vitamin B deficiency causing peripheral neuropathies
b. Thiamine deficiency causing Korsakoff's syndrome
2. Alcohol-induced persistent amnesiac disorder causing severe memory problems
3. Wernicke's encephalopathy, causing confusion, ataxia, and abnormal eye movements
4. Hepatitis; cirrhosis of the liver
5. Esophagitis and gastritis
6. Pancreatitis
7. Anemias
8. Immune system dysfunctions
9. Brain damage
10. Peripheral neuropathy
11. Cardiac disorders

▲ IV. ALCOHOL WITHDRAWAL
A. Description
1. Occurs when an addicted person stops ingesting alcohol
2. Can occur 6 to 8 hours after drinking has ended

or decreased, and symptoms can last 5 days or longer
3. Alcohol withdrawal is highly individual, and some clients experience mild withdrawal symptoms requiring minimal medical supervision; others experience severe systems that can be life threatening
B. Stages of withdrawal
1. Stage 1
a. May begin 6 to 8 hours after last ingestion or a significant decrease in usual consumption of alcohol
b. Anxiety
c. Anorexia
d. Insomnia
e. Tremors
f. Hyperalertness
g. Internal shaking
h. Nausea and vomiting
i. Headache
j. Increased pulse and blood pressure
k. Depression
2. Stage 2
a. May begin 8 to 12 hours after the last ingestion or a significant decrease in usual consumption of alcohol
b. Profound confusion
c. Gross tremors
d. Nervousness
e. Disorientation
f. Illusions
g. Auditory and visual hallucinations
h. Nightmares
3. Stage 3
a. May begin 12 to 48 hours after the last ingestion or a significant decrease in usual consumption of alcohol
b. Severe hallucinations
c. Seizures
4. Stage 4
a. May begin 3 to 5 days after the last ingestion or a significant decrease in usual alcohol consumption
b. Confusion, disorientation, clouding of consciousness, and delirium
c. Hypertension, diaphoresis, tachycardia
d. Visual and tactile hallucinations
e. Fluctuating levels of consciousness
f. Fever (103° to 104° F)
g. Tremors
h. Uncontrolled tachycardia
i. Severe psychomotor activity
j. Agitation
k. Hallucinations
l. Sleeplessness
m. A medical emergency
C. Implementation
1. Initiate seizure precautions

2. Administer chlordiazepoxide (Librium) as prescribed for withdrawal and anticonvulsive effects
3. Administer diazepam (Valium) or pentobarbital (phenobarbital) as prescribed to produce sedation and control withdrawal
4. Administer phenytoin (Dilantin) to prevent seizures
5. Administer vitamin B_1 (thiamine) as prescribed for malnutrition
6. Administer magnesium sulfate as prescribed to increase the effectiveness of vitamin B_1 and help reduce postwithdrawal seizures
7. Hydrate the client
8. Monitor vital signs frequently
9. Monitor I & O
10. Orient client frequently
11. Maintain minimal stimuli
12. Approach client in an accepting and nonjudgmental manner
13. Assist client to use assertive techniques rather than manipulation to meet needs
14. Set limits on manipulative behavior
15. Direct client to focus on the substance **abuse** problem
16. Limit the client's blame-placing or rationalizing to explain the substance **abuse** problem
17. Encourage the client to participate in group therapy and support groups
18. Encourage the client to attend weekly Alcoholics Anonymous (AA) meetings

▲ D. Disulfiram (Antabuse) therapy
  1. Description
    a. An alcohol deterrent used for alcoholic dependence
    b. The medication sensitizes the client to alcohol, so a disulfiram-alcohol reaction occurs if alcohol is ingested
    c. The client must abstain from alcohol for at least 12 hours before the initial dose is administered
    d. The client must avoid drinking for 14 days after disulfiram therapy has been discontinued; otherwise the client is at risk for disulfiram-alcohol reaction
  2. Negative physiological responses
    a. Throbbing headache
    b. Flushing
    c. Nausea
    d. Copious vomiting
    e. Diaphoresis
    f. Dizziness
    g. Blurred vision and confusion
    h. Hypotension
    i. Dyspnea
    j. Palpitations and tachycardia
    k. Chest pain

BOX 72-2

Hallucinogens

Lysergic acid diethylamide (LSD)
Mescaline
Peyote
Phencyclidine (PCP)
Psilocybin (derived from mushrooms)

---

3. Client education
  a. Educate as to the effects of the medication
  b. Instruct the client that the effects of the medication may occur for several days after discontinuance
  c. Ensure that the client agrees to abstain from alcohol and any alcohol-containing substances
  d. Instruct the client to avoid the use of substances that contain alcohol, such as cough medicines, rubbing compounds, vinegar, mouthwashes, and aftershave lotions

V. HALLUCINOGENS (Box 72-2)
A. Cause psychosis, with distorted perception, heightened sense of awareness, grandiosity, hallucinations, mystical experiences, and distortions of time and space
B. May harm self when under the influence
C. No withdrawal syndrome when discontinued, but flashbacks may occur for several months after use stops
D. Bad trips may result in panic and unpredictable psychotic behaviors

VI. CANNABIS
A. Can include marijuana, "pot," hashish
B. Causes altered state of awareness, relaxation, and mild euphoria
C. Decreases inhibitions
D. Decreased motivation from prolonged use
E. Can cause possible psychosis
F. Physiological effects include slowed reflexes
G. Causes drying of mucous membranes and reddening of eyes

VII. OPIOIDS (Box 72-3)
A. Description
  1. Cause mental and physical deterioration
  2. High risk for infection with human immunodeficiency virus (HIV) or hepatitis virus if taken intravenously
  3. Cause decreased response to pain, respiratory depression, constriction of pupils, euphoria, apathy, impaired judgment
B. Withdrawal
  1. Methadone blocks the action of opioids and may be used to assist with withdrawal

---

BOX 72-3

Opioids

Codeine
Heroin ("China white," synthetic heroin)
Meperidine hydrochloride (Demerol)
Methadone
Morphine sulfate
Opium

BOX 72-5

Central Nervous System Stimulants

Amphetamines
Benzedrine inhalers
Caffeine
Cocaine, "crack"
Diet pills
Methylenedioxylmethamphetamine (Ecstasy)

BOX 72-4

Central Nervous System Depressants

Barbiturates
Benzodiazapines
Methaqualone (quaaludes, "sopers")

BOX 72-6

Therapies for Substance Abuse Clients

Community treatment programs
Family counseling
Psychotherapy
Self-help groups
Transitional living programs

---

2. Signs of withdrawal include anxiety; yawning; diaphoresis; cramping; rhinorrhea; achiness and muscle twitching; anorexia; insomnia; increased temperature, respiration, and blood pressure; nausea, vomiting, and diarrhea; and restlessness
3. Overdose of opioids can lead to coma, respiratory depression, and death

VIII. CENTRAL NERVOUS SYSTEM DEPRESSANTS
(Box 72-4)
A. Description
1. Act as a depressant, sedative, and hypnotic
2. Cause physical and psychological dependence
3. Cause euphoria
4. Can cause depression and hostility
5. Impaired judgment and lack of coordination can occur
6. Slurring of speech and decreased inhibitions can occur
7. Tolerance can develop
B. Withdrawal: Causes increased temperature, tachycardia, postural hypotension, insomnia, tremors, agitation, apprehension, weakness, seizures, and psychosis

IX. CENTRAL NERVOUS SYSTEM STIMULANTS
(Box 72-5)
A. Description
1. Stimulants lead to alertness and extra energy
2. Effects include euphoria, hyperactivity, insomnia, anorexia and weight loss, tachycardia and hypertension, psychotic behavior
3. Psychological dependence and tolerance can occur
4. Sudden death has been associated with cocaine **abuse**

B. Withdrawal
1. Crash
2. Depression
3. Lack of energy

X. IMPLEMENTATION: WITHDRAWAL
1. Initiate seizure precautions
2. Hydrate the client
3. Monitor vital signs every hour
4. Monitor I & O
5. Orient client frequently
6. Maintain minimal stimuli
7. Approach client in an accepting and nonjudgmental manner
8. Direct client's focus to the substance **abuse** problem
9. Identify with client situations that precipitate angry feelings
10. Limit client's blame-placing or rationalizing to explain the substance **abuse** problem
11. Assist client to use assertive techniques rather than manipulation to meet needs
12. Set limits on manipulative behavior and verbal and physical **abuse**
13. Hold client firmly to reasonable limits, consistently reinforcing rules, with reasonable consequences for breaking rules
14. Hold client accountable for all behaviors
15. Assist client to explore strengths and weaknesses
16. Encourage time-out if client is losing control
17. Encourage client to participate in unit activities
18. Encourage client to participate in group therapy and support groups
19. See Box 72-6 for a list of therapies
20. Box 72-7 delineates nursing care for clients

BOX 72-7

Withdrawal: Nursing Care

Obtain information regarding the drug type and amount consumed
Assess vital signs
Remove unnecessary objects from the environment
Provide one-to-one supervision if necessary
Provide a quiet, calm environment with minimal stimuli
Maintain client orientation
Ensure client's safety by implementing seizure precautions
Use restraints, if necessary and prescribed, to prevent client from harming self and others
Provide for physical needs
Provide food and fluids as tolerated
Administer medications as prescribed to decrease withdrawal symptoms
Collect blood and urine samples for drug screening

PRACTICE QUESTIONS

1. A nurse is caring for a female client who was recently admitted for anorexia nervosa. The nurse enters the client's room and notes that the client is engaged in rigorous push-ups. Which nursing action is most appropriate?
   1. Allowing the client to complete her exercise program
   2. Telling the client that she is not allowed to exercise rigorously
   3. Interrupting the client and offering to take her for a walk
   4. Interrupting the client and weighing her immediately

2. A nurse is caring for a client with anorexia nervosa. The nurse is monitoring the behavior of the client and understands that the client with anorexia nervosa manages anxiety by doing which of the following?
   1. Always reinforcing self-approval
   2. Having the need to always make the right decision
   3. Engaging in immoral acts
   4. Observing rigid rules and regulations

3. A nurse is developing a plan of care for a hospitalized client with bulimia nervosa. Which of the following would not be included in the plan of care?
   1. Monitoring intake and output
   2. Monitoring electrolyte levels
   3. Observing for excessive exercise
   4. Checking for the presence of laxatives and diuretics in the client's belongings

4. A nurse is monitoring a client who abuses alcohol for signs of alcohol withdrawal. Which of the following would alert the nurse to the potential for delirium tremors (DTs)?
   1. Hypertension, changes in level of consciousness, and hallucinations
   2. Hypotension, ataxia, and vomiting
   3. Stupor, agitation, and muscular rigidity
   4. Hypotension, coarse hand tremor, and agitation

5. The spouse of a client admitted for alcohol withdrawal says to a nurse, "I should get out of this bad situation." What would be the most helpful response for the nurse to give?
   1. "I agree with you. You should get out of this situation."
   2. "What do you find difficult about this situation?"
   3. "Why don't you tell your husband about this?"
   4. "This is not the best time to make that decision."

6. A home health nurse visits a client at home and determines that the client is dependent on drugs. Which of the following assessment questions would assist the nurse to provide appropriate nursing care?
   1. "Why did you get started on these drugs?"
   2. "How long did you think you could take these drugs without someone finding out?"
   3. "How much do you use and what effect does it have on you?"
   4. The nurse does not ask any questions in fear that the client is in denial and will throw the nurse out of the home

7. A client with a diagnosis of anorexia nervosa, who is in a state of starvation, is in a two-bed room. A newly admitted client will be assigned to this client's room. Which of the following clients would be an appropriate choice as this client's roommate?
   1. A client with pneumonia
   2. A client receiving diagnostic tests
   3. A client who could benefit from the anorexic client's assistance at mealtime
   4. A client who thrives on managing others

8. A female client with anorexia nervosa is a member of a predischarge group/support group. The client verbalizes that she would like to buy some new clothes, but her finances are limited. Group members brought some used clothes to the client to replace the client's old clothes. The client believed that the new clothes were much too tight, and she reduced her calorie intake to 800 calories daily. The nurse analyzes this behavior as:
   1. Normal behavior
   2. Indicative of the client's ambivalence about hospital discharge
   3. Evidence of the client's altered/distorted body image
   4. Regression as the client is moving toward the community

9. A nurse determines that the wife of an alcoholic client is benefiting from attending an Al-Anon

group when the nurse hears the wife say which of the following?

1. "My attendance at the meetings has helped me to see that I provoke my husband's violence."
2. "I no longer feel that I deserve the beatings my husband inflicts on me."
3. "I can tolerate my husband's destructive behaviors now that I know they are common with alcoholics."
4. "I enjoy attending the meetings because they get me out of the house and away from my husband."

10. A client has been hospitalized and has participated in substance abuse therapy group sessions. Upon discharge, the client has consented to participate in Alcoholics Anonymous (AA) community groups. The nurse is monitoring the client's response to the substance abuse sessions. Which statement by the client best indicates that the client has well assimilated session topics and coping response styles and has processed information effectively for self-use?

1. "I know I'm ready to be discharged; I feel like I can say "no" and leave a group of friends if they are drinking. No problem."
2. "This group has really helped a lot. I know it will be different when I go home. I'm sure that my family and friends will all help me like the people in this group have . . . they'll all help me . . . I know they will . . . they won't let me go back to old ways."
3. "I'm looking forward to leaving here. I know that I will miss all of you, so I'm happy and I'm sad, I'm excited and I'm scared. I know that I have to work hard to be strong and that everyone isn't going to be as helpful as you all have been."
4. "I'll keep all my of appointments, go to all of my

AA groups, and do everything I'm supposed to do. Nothing will go wrong that way."

11. A hospitalized client with a history of alcohol abuse tells a nurse, "I'm leaving now. I have to go. I don't want any more treatment. I have things that I have to do right away." The client has not been discharged. In fact, the client is scheduled for an important diagnostic test to be performed an hour later. After discussing the client's concerns with the client, the client dresses and begins to walk out of the hospital room. What is the most important nursing action?

1. Restraining the client until the physician can be reached
2. Calling security to block all exit areas
3. Telling the client that they cannot return to this hospital again if they leave now
4. Calling the nursing supervisor

12. A nurse is performing an admission assessment on a client with a diagnosis of bulimia nervosa. The nurse gathers assessment data knowing that which of the following is not a characteristic finding of a client with this disorder?

1. Loss of tooth enamel
2. Dental decay
3. Electrolyte imbalances
4. Body weight well below ideal range

CRITICAL THINKING: FREE-TEXT ENTRY

A client who has been drinking alcohol on a regular basis admits to having "a problem." The client is asking for assistance with the problem. A nurse would support the client to attend which self-help community group?

Answer: _____

ANSWERS

1. 3

Rationale: Clients with anorexia nervosa are frequently preoccupied with rigorous exercise and push themselves beyond normal limits to work off caloric intake. The nurse must provide for appropriate exercise and place limits on rigorous activities. Options 1, 2, and 4 are inappropriate nursing actions.

Test-Taking Strategy: Use the process of elimination. Focus on the key words "most appropriate." Also, focus on the need for the nurse to set firm limits with clients who have this disorder. If you had difficulty with this question, review interventions for the client with anorexia nervosa.

Level of Cognitive Ability: Application
Client Needs: Physiological Integrity
Integrated Concept/Process: Nursing Process/Implementation

Content Area: Mental Health
Reference: Fortinash, K., & Holoday-Worret, P. (2000). *Psychiatric mental health nursing* (2nd ed.). St. Louis: Mosby, p. 453.

2. 4

Rationale: Clients with anorexia nervosa have the desire to please others. Their need to be correct or perfect interferes with rational decision-making processes. These clients are moralistic. Rules and rituals help the clients manage their anxiety.

Test-Taking Strategy: Use the process of elimination and focus on the issue of managing anxiety. Eliminate options 1 and 2 because of the absolute word "always." Option 3 is not characteristic of the client with anorexia. Review the characteristics associated with this disorder if you had difficulty with this question.

Level of Cognitive Ability: Analysis
Client Needs: Psychosocial Integrity

Integrated Concept/Process: Nursing Process/Assessment
Content Area: Mental Health
Reference: Fortinash, K., & Holoday-Worret, P. (2000). *Psychiatric mental health nursing* (2nd ed.). St. Louis: Mosby, p. 453.

3. 3

Rationale: Excessive exercise is a characteristic of clients with anorexia nervosa; it is not a characteristic of clients with bulimia. Frequent vomiting, in addition to laxative and diuretic abuse, may lead to dehydration and electrolyte imbalance. Assessing for dehydration and electrolyte imbalance are important nursing actions. Option 3 is the only option that is not a characteristic of bulimia.

Test-Taking Strategy: Use the process of elimination. Note the key word "not" in the stem of the question. Options 1, 2, and 4 are similar and directly or indirectly infer concern about fluid and electrolyte balance. Option 3 is different from the other options. Review the characteristics associated with bulimia nervosa if you had difficulty with this question.
Level of Cognitive Ability: Analysis
Client Needs: Physiological Integrity
Integrated Concept/Process: Nursing Process/Planning
Content Area: Mental Health
Reference: Fortinash, K., & Holoday-Worret, P. (2000). *Psychiatric mental health nursing* (2nd ed.). St. Louis: Mosby, p. 456.

4. 1

Rationale: The symptoms associated with DTs typically are anxiety, insomnia, anorexia, hypertension, disorientation, visual or tactile hallucinations, changes in level of consciousness, agitation, fever, and delusions.

Test-Taking Strategy: Use the process of elimination. Review each option carefully to ensure that all of the symptoms are contained in the correct option. Eliminate options 2 and 4 first knowing that hypertension rather than hypotension occurs. From the remaining options, recalling that the client who is stuporous is not likely to exhibit agitation will direct you to option 1. Review these symptoms if you had difficulty with this question.
Level of Cognitive Ability: Analysis
Client Needs: Physiological Integrity
Integrated Concept/Process: Nursing Process/Assessment
Content Area: Mental Health
Reference: Keltner, N., Schwecke, L., & Bostrom, C. (1999). *Psychiatric nursing* (3rd ed.). St. Louis: Mosby, p. 516.

5. 2

Rationale: The most helpful response is one that encourages the client to problem-solve. Giving advice implies that the nurse knows what is best and can also foster dependency. The nurse should not agree with the client, nor should the nurse request that the client provide explanations.

Test-Taking Strategy: Use therapeutic communication techniques. Eliminate option 3 because of the word "why," which should be avoided in communication. Eliminate option 1, because the nurse is agreeing with the client. Eliminate option 4, because this option places the client's feelings on hold. Option 2 is the only option that addresses the client's feelings. Review therapeutic communication techniques if you had difficulty with this question.
Level of Cognitive Ability: Application
Client Needs: Psychosocial Integrity
Integrated Concept/Process: Communication and Documentation

Content Area: Mental Health
Reference: Varcarolis, E. (1998). *Foundations of psychiatric mental health nursing* (3rd ed.). Philadelphia: W. B. Saunders, p. 191.

6. 3

Rationale: Whenever the nurse employs an assessment for a client who is dependent on drugs, it is best for the nurse to attempt to elicit information by being nonjudgmental and direct. Option 1 is incorrect, because it is judgmental, off-focus, and reflects the nurse's bias. Option 2 is incorrect, because it is judgmental, insensitive, and aggressive, all of which are nontherapeutic. Option 4 is incorrect, because it indicates passivity on the nurse's part and uses rationalization to avoid the therapeutic nursing intervention.

Test-Taking Strategy: Use the process of elimination and therapeutic communication techniques to answer the question. Also, focus on the issue of providing "appropriate care." Review the assessment of a client who is a substance abuser if you had difficulty with this question.
Level of Cognitive Ability: Analysis
Client Needs: Health Promotion and Maintenance
Integrated Concept/Process: Nursing Process/Assessment
Content Area: Mental Health
Reference: Glod, C. A. (1998). *Contemporary psychiatric-mental health nursing.* Philadelphia: F. A. Davis, pp. 289-293.

7. 2

Rationale: A client receiving diagnostic tests is an acceptable roommate. The client with anorexia is most likely experiencing hematological complications such as leukopenia. Having a roommate with pneumonia would place the client with anorexia nervosa at risk for infection. The client with anorexia nervosa should not be put into a situation in which he or she is able to focus on the nutritional needs of others or being managed by others, because this may contribute to sublimation and suppression of the client's own hunger.

Test-Taking Strategy: Use the process of elimination and note the key words "in a state of starvation." Recalling the characteristics associated with anorexia nervosa will direct you to option 2. Review care of the client with anorexia nervosa if you had difficulty with this question.
Level of Cognitive Ability: Analysis
Client Needs: Safe, Effective Care Environment
Integrated Concept/Process: Nursing Process/Analysis
Content Area: Mental Health
Reference: Stuart, G. W., & Laraia, M. T. (1998). *Principles and practice of psychiatric nursing.* (6th ed.). St. Louis: Mosby, p. 527.

8. 3

Rationale: Altered/distorted body image is a concern with clients with anorexia nervosa. Although the client may struggle with ambivalence and present with regressed behavior, the client's coping pattern relates to the basic issue of distorted body image. The nurse should address this need in the support group.

Test-Taking Strategy: Use the process of elimination, and focus on the information provided in the question, which is directly related to an altered body image. This should direct you to the correct option. Review the needs of the client with anorexia nervosa if you had difficulty with this question.
Level of Cognitive Ability: Analysis
Client Needs: Physiological Integrity

Integrated Concept/Process: Nursing Process/Analysis
Content Area: Mental Health
Reference: Fortinash, K., & Holoday-Worret, P. (2000). *Psychiatric mental health nursing* (2nd ed.). St. Louis: Mosby, pp. 459-460.

9. **2**
Rationale: Al-Anon support groups are a protected, supportive opportunity for spouses and significant others to learn what to expect and to obtain excellent pointers about successful behavioral changes. Option 2 is the most healthy response, because it exemplifies an understanding that the alcoholic partner is responsible for his behavior and cannot be allowed to blame family members for loss of control. With regard to option 1, the nonalcoholic partner should not feel responsible when the spouse loses control. Option 3 indicates that the wife remains codependent. Option 4 indicates that the group is being seen as an escape, not a place to work on issues.
Test-Taking Strategy: Use the process of elimination. Identify the client of the question, and identify the option that most directly addresses the issue of the question, which is the benefit gained from attending an Al-Anon group; this will direct you to option 2. Review the purpose of this group if you had difficulty with this question.
Level of Cognitive Ability: Analysis
Client Needs: Physiological Integrity
Integrated Concept/Process: Nursing Process/Evaluation
Content Area: Mental Health
Reference: Fortinash, K., & Holoday-Worret, P. (2000). *Psychiatric mental health nursing* (2nd ed.). St. Louis: Mosby, p. 381.

10. **3**
Rationale: In the defense mechanism of denial, the person denies reality. Option 1 identifies denial. In option 2, the client is relying heavily on others, and the client's focus of control is external. In option 4, the client is concrete and procedure-oriented; again, the client maintains that "nothing will go wrong" if the client follows all directions. In option 3, the client is expressing real concern and ambivalence about discharge from the hospital. The client also demonstrates reality in the statement.
Test-Taking Strategy: Use the process of elimination. Focus on the issue, and select the option that identifies the most realistic client verbalization. Review the expected client outcomes from group therapy if you had difficulty with this question.
Level of Cognitive Ability: Analysis
Client Needs: Psychosocial Integrity
Integrated Concept/Process: Nursing Process/Analysis
Content Area: Mental Health
Reference: Keltner, N., Schwecke, L., & Bostrom, C. (1999). *Psychiatric nursing* (3rd ed.). St. Louis: Mosby, p. 504.

11. **4**
Rationale: A nurse can be charged with false imprisonment if a client is made to wrongfully believe that he or she cannot leave the hospital. Most health care facilities have documents that the client is asked to sign that relate to the client's responsibilities when they leave against medical advice (AMA). The client should be asked to sign this document before leaving. The nurse should request that the client wait to speak to the physician before leaving, but if the client refuses to do so, the nurse cannot hold the client against his or her will. Restraining the client and calling security to block exits constitutes false imprisonment. Any client has a right to health care and cannot be told otherwise.
Test-Taking Strategy: Use the process of elimination. Keeping the concept of false imprisonment in mind, eliminate options 1 and 2 because they are similar. Eliminate option 3, knowing that any client has a right to health care. From the options presented, the best action is option 4. Review the points related to false imprisonment if you had difficulty with this question.
Level of Cognitive Ability: Application
Client Needs: Safe, Effective Care Environment
Integrated Concept/Process: Nursing Process/Implementation
Content Area: Mental Health
Reference: Keltner, N., Schwecke, L., & Bostrom, C. (1999). *Psychiatric nursing* (3rd ed.). St. Louis: Mosby, p. 60.

12. **4**
Rationale: Clients with bulimia nervosa may not initially appear to be physically or emotionally ill. They are often at or slightly below ideal body weight. On further inspection, the client demonstrates dental decay and loss of tooth enamel, which is a result of the client inducing vomiting. Electrolyte imbalances are present.
Test-Taking Strategy: Use the process of elimination. Eliminate options 1 and 2 because they are similar. From the remaining options, recall that in anorexia nervosa the body weight is normally below 85% of ideal body weight. Option 4 is a characteristic sign of anorexia nervosa, not bulimia nervosa. Review the characteristics of these disorders if you had difficulty with this question.
Level of Cognitive Ability: Analysis
Client Needs: Physiological Integrity
Integrated Concept/Process: Nursing Process/Assessment
Content Area: Mental Health
Reference: Keltner, N., Schwecke, L., & Bostrom, C. (1999). *Psychiatric nursing* (3rd ed.). St. Louis: Mosby, p. 560.

CRITICAL THINKING: FREE-TEXT ENTRY

Answer: Alcoholics Anonymous
Rationale: Alcoholics Anonymous is a major self-help organization for the treatment of alcoholism.
Test-Taking Strategy: Focus on the issue and the client's problem identified in the question. Familiarize yourself with the purpose of specific support groups if you had difficulty with this question.
Level of Cognitive Ability: Application
Client Needs: Health Promotion and Maintenance
Integrated Concept/Process: Self-Care
Content Area: Mental Health
Reference: Keltner, N., Schwecke, L., & Bostrom, C. (1999). *Psychiatric nursing* (3rd ed.). St. Louis: Mosby, p. 535.

REFERENCES

Fortinash, K., & Holoday-Worret, P. (2000). *Psychiatric mental health nursing* (2nd ed.). St. Louis: Mosby.

Glod, C.A. (1998). *Contemporary psychiatric-mental health nursing.* Philadelphia: F.A. Davis.

Keltner, N., Schwecke, L., & Bostrom, C. (1999). *Psychiatric nursing* (3rd ed.). St. Louis: Mosby.

Stuart, G.W., & Laraia, M.T. (1998). *Principles and practice of psychiatric nursing.* (6th ed.). St. Louis: Mosby.

Varcarolis, E. (1998). *Foundations of psychiatric mental health nursing* (3rd ed.). Philadelphia: W.B. Saunders.

Crisis Theory and Intervention

I. CRISIS INTERVENTION

A. Description
1. **Crisis** is a temporary state of severe emotional disorganization resulting from failure of **coping mechanisms** and/or lack of support
2. Decision making and problem solving are inadequate
3. Treatment is immediate, supportive, and directly responsive to the immediate **crisis** to assist the client and/or the family through the stressful situation

B. Phases of a **crisis**
1. Phase 1: External precipitating event
2. Phase 2
   a. Perception of threat
   b. Increase in anxiety
   c. Client may cope or resolve **crisis**
3. Phase 3
   a. Failure of coping
   b. Increasing disorganization
   c. Physical symptoms emerge
   d. Relationship problems
4. Phase 4
   a. Mobilization of internal and external resources
   b. Resolutions related to precrisis functioning include functioning at a higher level, at the same level, or at a lower level

C. **Crisis** intervention
1. Treatment is immediate, supportive, and directly responsive to the immediate **crisis**
2. Goal-directed intervention
3. Feelings of the client are acknowledged
4. Provides opportunities for expression and validation of feelings
5. Connections are made between the meaning of the event and the **crisis**

6. Explores alternative **coping mechanisms** and tries out new behaviors

II. GRIEVING

A. Description
1. A normal human process that occurs in response to a loss
2. Progresses through various stages, and the entire process may take up to 3 years

B. Assessment
1. Crying
2. Guilt and anger
3. Fatigue and lethargy
4. Insomnia
5. Depression
6. Agitation
7. Anorexia
8. Ambivalence
9. Somatic complaints
10. Sense of detachment and unreality
11. Denial

C. Implementation
1. Assess the client's progress through the grieving process
2. Encourage the client to express feelings about the loss and its significance to the client's life
3. Encourage expression of angry feelings
4. Explain the normal stages of the grieving process to the client
5. Assist the client to make appropriate future plans related to changes caused by the loss
6. Encourage the client to work through the feelings associated with the loss

III. DEPRESSION

A. Description
1. Affects feelings, thoughts, and behaviors
2. Can occur after a loss, including loss of self-

esteem, the end of a significant relationship, the death of a loved one, or a traumatic event
3. The loss is followed by grief and mourning, and if this process does not resolve, depression results
4. Depression may be mild, moderate, or severe
5. Treatment includes counseling, antidepressant medication, and electroconvulsive therapy (ECT)

B. Mild depression
1. Triggered by an external event, and the experience follows the normal grief reaction
2. Lasts less than 2 weeks
3. Feeling sad
4. Feeling let down or disappointed
5. Mild alterations in sleep patterns
6. Feeling less alert
7. Irritability
8. Not interested in spending time with others
9. Increased use of alcohol or drugs

C. Moderate depression
1. Persists over time
2. The person experiences a sense of change and often seeks help
3. Despondent and gloomy
4. Feels dejected
5. Low self-esteem
6. Helplessness and powerlessness
7. May experience intense anxiety and anger
8. Diurnal variation: May feel better at a certain time of the day, such as in the morning
9. Slow thought processes and difficulty in concentrating
10. Rumination: Persistent thinking about and discussion of a particular subject
11. Negative thinking and suicidal thoughts
12. Sleep disturbances
13. Social withdrawal
14. Anorexia, weight loss, and fatigue
15. Somatic complaints
16. Menstrual changes
17. Increased use of alcohol or drugs

D. Severe depression
1. Intense and pervasive
2. Despair and hopelessness
3. Guilt and worthlessness
4. Flat affect
5. May show agitation and pace about
6. Poor posture and unkempt appearance
7. Decreased speech
8. Self-destructive thoughts; however, client may lack energy to act on thought
9. Social withdrawal
10. Poor concentration and overwhelmed by simple tasks
11. Severe psychomotor retardation
12. Anorexia and marked weight loss
13. Constipation and urinary retention
14. Lack of sexual interest

15. Terminal insomnia
16. Diurnal variation: The person feels worse in the morning and better as the day goes on
17. Delusions and hallucinations

E. Implementation
1. Altered thought processes
   a. Encourage the client to discuss losses or changes in life situation
   b. Encourage the client to express sadness or anger, and allow adequate time for verbal responses
   c. Assist in developing short-term goals
   d. Encourage the use of problem solving and positive thinking
   e. Limit decision making
   f. Spend short periods of time throughout the day with the client
   g. Be on time when a schedule is planned with the client
   h. Sit in silence with clients who are not verbalizing
   i. Use simple, concrete words when communicating
   j. Avoid a cheerful attitude
2. Risk for self-harm
   a. Assess for **suicide** clues, and intervene to provide safety precautions as necessary
   b. Ask client directly, "Have you thought of hurting yourself?"
   c. Assess lethality of plans
   d. Do not leave alone for extended periods
   e. If the client has a suicidal plan, place on one-to-one supervision
   f. Develop a contract with the client
3. Activity intolerance
   a. Encourage daily exercise
   b. Assist with activities of daily living (ADLs) if the client is unable to perform them
   c. Begin with one-to-one activities
   d. Provide activities for easy mastery to increase self-esteem and assist in alleviating guilt feelings
   e. Provide activities that require little orientation (card games, drawing)
   f. Engage in gross motor activities (walking)
   g. Eventually bring the client into small group activities, and then large groups
4. Altered nutrition
   a. Ensure adequate nutrition
   b. Offer small, high-calorie, high-protein snacks and fluids throughout the day
   c. Stay with the client during meals
   d. Weigh the client weekly
   e. Assess bowel patterns for constipation
5. Sleep pattern disturbance
   a. Ensure adequate sleep
   b. Provide rest periods after activities

c. Encourage the client to dress and stay out of bed during the day
d. Provide relaxation measures at bedtime
e. Decrease environmental stimuli at bedtime
f. Spend time with the client before bedtime

IV. SUICIDAL BEHAVIOR

A. Description
1. Suicidal clients characteristically have feelings of worthlessness, guilt, and hopelessness that are so overwhelming that they feel unable to go on with life and unfit to live
2. The nurse caring for a depressed client always considers the possibility of **suicide**

B. High-risk groups
1. Those with a history of previous **suicide attempts**
2. Family history of **suicide attempts**
3. Adolescents
4. Elderly clients
5. Disabled or terminally ill adults
6. Clients with personality disorders
7. Clients with organic brain syndrome or dementia
8. Depressed or psychotic clients
9. Substance **abusers**

C. Clues
1. Giving away personal, special, and prized possessions
2. Canceling social engagements
3. Making out or changing a will
4. Taking out or changing insurance policies
5. Positive or negative changes in behavior
6. Poor appetite
7. Sleeping difficulties
8. Feelings of hopelessness
9. Difficulty in concentrating
10. Loss of interest in activities
11. Client statements that indicate an intent to attempt **suicide**
12. Sudden calmness or improvement in a depressed client
13. Client questions about poisons, guns, or other lethal objects

D. Assessment
1. The plan
a. Does the client have a plan?
b. What is the plan, how lethal is the plan, and how likely is death to occur?
c. Does the client have the means to carry out the plan?
2. Client history of attempts
a. **Suicide attempts** in the past and the outcomes
b. Was the client accidentally rescued?
c. Have the past attempts and methods been the same, or have methods increased in lethality?
3. Psychosocial
a. Is the client alone or alienated from others?

b. Is hostility or depression present?
c. Do hallucinations exist?
d. Is substance **abuse** present?
e. Any recent losses or physical illness?
f. Any environmental or lifestyle changes?

E. Implementation
1. Initiate **suicide** precautions
2. Remove harmful objects
3. Do not leave the client alone
4. Provide one-to-one supervision at all times
5. Provide a nonjudgmental, caring attitude
6. Develop a contract that is written, dated, and signed and indicates alternative behavior at times of suicidal thoughts
7. Encourage the client to talk about feelings and to identify positive aspects about self
8. Encourage active participation in own care
9. Keep the client active by assigning simple tasks
10. Check that visitors do not leave harmful objects in the client's room
11. Identify support systems
12. Do not allow the client to leave the unit unless accompanied by a staff member
13. Continue to assess the client's **suicide** potential

V. ABUSIVE BEHAVIORS

A. Anger
1. A feeling of annoyance that may be displaced onto an object or person
2. Is used to avoid anxiety and gives a feeling of power in situations in which the person feels out of control
B. Violence: The physical force that is threatening to the safety of self and others
C. Aggression: Can be harmful and destructive when not controlled
D. Assessment
1. History of violence or self-harm
2. Poor impulse control and low tolerance of frustration
3. Defiant and argumentative
4. Verbal threats
5. Increased pacing and agitation
6. Muscle rigidity
7. Flushed face
8. Glaring
9. Loud voice
E. Implementation
1. Acknowledge anger
2. Set limits on behavior
3. Listen actively and assist client to deal with consequences of anger
4. Provide safety for expressing anger and safety to others
F. **Restraints** and **seclusion**
1. Description
a. Physical **restraint**: Any manual method or

mechanical device, material, or equipment that inhibits free movement

b. **Seclusion:** The last step in a process to maximize safety of a client and others, in which a client is placed alone in a specially designed room for protection and close supervision

c. Chemical **restraint:** Medication given for a very specific purpose of inhibiting a specific behavior or movement; has an impact on the client's ability to relate to the environment

2. Use of **restraints** and **seclusion**

a. Should never be used as punishment or for the convenience of the health care staff

b. The least restrictive means of **restraint** for the shortest duration should be used

c. Used when behavior is physically harmful to the client or others

d. Used when the disruptive behavior presents a danger to the facility

e. Used when alternative or less restrictive measures are insufficient in protecting the client or others from harm

f. Used when the client anticipates that a controlled environment would be helpful and requests **seclusion**

g. Requires a written order of a physician, which must be reviewed and renewed every 24 hours and which also must specify the type of **restraint** to be used

h. In an emergency, the charge nurse may place a client in **restraint** or **seclusion** and obtain a written or verbal order as soon as possible thereafter

i. Laws require the consent of the client unless an emergency situation exists and can be documented

j. The client must be removed from **restraint** or **seclusion** when safer and quieter behavior is observed

k. While in **restraint** or **seclusion**, the client must be protected from all sources of harm

l. The nurse must document the behavior leading to **restraint** or **seclusion** and the time the client is placed in and released from **restraint** or **seclusion**

m. The client in **restraint** or **seclusion** must be assessed every 15 to 30 minutes for physical needs, safety, and comfort, and these observations are also documented

VI. FAMILY VIOLENCE

A. Description

1. The violence begins with threats or verbal or physical minor assaults, and the victim attempts to comply with the requests of the **abuser**

2. The **abuser** loses control and becomes destructive and harmful while the victim attempts to protect himself or herself; the **abuser** then becomes loving and attempts to make peace

3. The behavior of the **abuser** may be an attempt for closeness and companionship

4. The **abuser** believes that violence is normal and that the victim is responsible for the **abuse**

5. Outsiders are not aware of what is happening in the family, and when outsiders try to enter the family, the family feels assaulted

6. Family members are socially isolated and lack autonomy and trust among each other

7. Caring and intimacy in the family are absent

8. Family members expect other members of the family to meet their needs, but none are able to do so

9. The **abuser** threatens to abandon the family

B. Characteristics of **abusers**

1. Impaired self-esteem

2. Strong dependency needs

3. Narcissistic and suspicious

4. History of sexual **abuse** during childhood

5. Perceive victims as their property and believe that they are entitled to **abuse** them

C. Characteristics of victims

1. Feel trapped, dependent, helpless, and powerless

2. Depressed

3. Low self-esteem and blame themselves for the problems

D. Implementation

1. Report cases of suspected **abuse**

2. Assess situations associated with family violence

3. Assess for evidence of physical injuries

4. Ensure privacy and confidentiality during assessment, and provide a nonjudgmental and empathetic approach to foster trust

5. Assist in resolving family dysfunction with prescribed therapies

6. Encourage psychotherapy, counseling, group therapy, and support groups to assist family members to develop coping strategies

7. Encourage individual therapy for victims that promotes coping with the trauma and prevents further psychological conflict

8. Provide individual therapy for **abusers** that focuses on preventing violent behavior and repairing relationships

9. Ensure that the victim is not left alone with **abuser**

10. Assist the victim to understand his or her participation in the **abuse**

11. Assist the victim to develop self-protective abilities and other problem-solving abilities

12. Provide support and assistance in coping with contacting the legal system

13. Assist the family to identify an access to community and personal resources

▲ **VII. CHILD ABUSE** (Refer to Chapter 33)
  A. Description: Involves emotional or physical **abuse** or neglect, as well as sexual exploitation or molestation by caretakers or other individuals
  B. Assessment
    1. Physical **abuse**
       a. Unexplained bruises, burns, or fractures
       b. Bald spots on scalp
       c. Apprehensive child
       d. Extreme aggressiveness or withdrawal
       e. Fear of parents
       f. Lack of crying when approached by a stranger
    2. Physical neglect
       a. Inadequate weight gain
       b. Poor hygiene
       c. Consistent hunger
       d. Inconsistent school attendance
       e. Constant fatigue
       f. Reports of lack of child supervision
       g. Delinquency
    3. Emotional **abuse**
       a. Speech disorders
       b. Habit disorders, such as sucking, biting, rocking
       c. Psychoneurotic reactions
       d. Learning disorders
       e. **Suicide attempts**
    4. Sexual **Abuse**
       a. Difficulty walking or sitting
       b. Torn, stained, or bloody underclothing
       c. Pain, swelling, or itching of the genitals
       d. Bruises, bleeding, or lacerations in the genital or anal area
       e. Unwillingness to change clothes or unwillingness to participate in gym activities
       f. Poor peer relations
       g. Delinquency
       h. Changes in sleep performance
       i. Self-disruptive behavior
▲ C. Implementation
▲   1. Report cases of suspected **abuse**
    2. Support the child during a thorough physical assessment
    3. Assess injuries
    4. Place the child in an environment that is safe, thereby preventing further injury
    5. Move slowly around the child
    6. Avoid loud noises around the child
    7. Communicate with the child at the child's eye level
    8. Reassure the child that he or she is not a bad person, that the child is loved and not responsible for the **abuser's** behavior
    9. Do not rescue the child from the parents
    10. Document in an objective manner information related to the suspected **abuse**
    11. Assess parents' strengths and weaknesses, nor-

mal **coping mechanisms,** and presence or absence of support systems
    12. Assist the family in identifying stressors and alternative ways to express feelings
    13. Provide education to the parents, and refer parents to **crisis** hotlines and community support systems

VIII. ELDER ABUSE
  A. Description
    1. **Abuse** can be physical, sexual, psychological, or financial
    2. Neglect can include unintentional failure to care for the elder person's needs or an intentional neglect, such as abandonment
    3. Victims may attempt to dismiss injuries as accidental, and **abusers** may prevent victims from receiving proper medical care to avoid discovery
    4. Victims are often socially isolated
    5. Victims may be care providers for the **abusers**
  B. Assessment
    1. Physical **abuse**
       a. Fractures
       b. Lacerations
       c. Punctures
       d. Bruises
       e. Burns
    2. Sexual **abuse**
       a. Torn or stained underclothing
       b. Discomfort or bleeding in the genital area
       c. Difficulty in walking or sitting
       d. Unexplained genital infections or disease
    3. Psychological **abuse**
       a. Confusion
       b. Fearful and agitated
       c. Changes in appetite and weight
       d. Withdrawn and loss of interest in self and social activities
    4. Financial **abuse**
       a. Fearful when discussing finances
       b. Confused, inaccurate, or no knowledge of finances
       c. Inability to pay bills
    5. Neglect
       a. Disheveled appearance
       b. Dehydration and malnutrition
       c. Dressed inadequately or inappropriately
       d. Lacking physical needs, such as glasses, hearing aids, and dentures
       e. Skin breaks
       f. Signs of medication overdose
  C. Implementation
    1. Report cases of suspected **abuse**
    2. Assess for physical injuries
    3. Assist with providing care to treat physical injuries

4. Assist with legal procedures, such as police reports, order of protection, and court-ordered counseling
5. Explore alternative living arrangements that are least restrictive and disruptive to the victim
6. Assist with financial management protection
7. Encourage counseling and provide referrals to emergency community resources
8. Refer to protective services for adults
9. Arrange counseling and treatment for the **abuser**

▲ IX. RAPE AND SEXUAL ASSAULT

A. Description
   1. Engaging another person in a sexual act and/or sexual intercourse through the use of force and without the consent of the sexual partner
   2. The victim is not required by law to report the rape or assault
   3. The victim is often blamed by others and often receives no support from significant others
   4. Acquaintance rapes involve someone known to the victim
   5. Statutory rape is the act of sexual intercourse with someone under the age of legal consent even if there is consent from the minor
B. Assessment
   1. Female client
      a. Obtain the date of the last menstrual period
      b. Determine form of birth control used and last act of intercourse before rape
      c. Duration of intercourse, orifices violated, and penile penetration
      d. Use of condom by perpetrator
   2. Shame, embarrassment, and humiliation
   3. Anger and revenge
   4. Fear of telling others for fear of not being believed
C. Rape trauma syndrome
   1. Sleep disturbances, nightmares
   2. Loss of appetite
   3. Fears, anxiety, phobias, suspicion
   4. Decrease in activities and motivation
   5. Disruptions in relationships with partner, family, friends
   6. Self-blame, guilt, shame
   7. Lowered self-esteem, feelings of worthlessness
   8. Somatic complaints
▲ D. Implementation
   1. Encourage the client not to shower, bathe, douche (female), or change clothing
   2. Assist with the female pelvic examination and obtaining specimens to detect semen
   3. Preserve any evidence
   4. Treat physical injuries
   5. Provide client safety
   6. Assist client to refrain from self-blame

7. Reinforce to the client that surviving the assault is most important; if the victim survived the rape, then he or she did exactly what was necessary to stay alive
8. Refer to **crisis** intervention and support groups

PRACTICE QUESTIONS

1. A nurse is reviewing the assessment data of a client admitted to the mental health unit. The nurse notes that the admission nurse has documented that the client is experiencing anxiety as a result of a situational crisis. The nurse determines that this type of crisis could be caused by which of the following?
   1. A fire that destroyed the client's home
   2. A recent rape episode experienced by the client
   3. The death of a loved one
   4. Witnessing a murder

2. A nurse is conducting an initial assessment of a client in crisis. When assessing the client's perception of the precipitating event that led to the crisis, what is the most appropriate question for the nurse to ask?
   1. "What leads you to seek help now?"
   2. "Who is available to help you?"
   3. "What do you usually do to feel better?"
   4. "With whom do you live?"

3. A nurse is developing a plan of care for a client in a crisis state. When developing the plan, the nurse considers which of the following?
   1. Presenting symptoms in a crisis situation are similar for all individuals experiencing a crisis.
   2. A crisis state indicates that the individual is suffering from an emotional illness
   3. A crisis state indicates that the individual is suffering from a mental illness
   4. A client's response to a crisis is individualized, and what constitutes a crisis for one person may not constitute a crisis for another person

4. A nurse observes that a client with a potential for violence is agitated, pacing up and down the hallway, and making aggressive and belligerent gestures at other clients. Which statement would be most appropriate to make to this client?
   1. "What is causing you to become agitated?"
   2. "You need to stop that behavior now!"
   3. "You will need to be restrained if you do not change your behavior."
   4. "You will need to be placed in seclusion."

5. During a conversation with a depressed client on an inpatient unit, the client says to the nurse, "My family would be better off without me." Which of the following is the nurse's best response?
   1. "Everyone feels this way when they are depressed."

2. "Have you talked to your family about this?"

3. "You sound very upset. Are you thinking of hurting yourself?"

4. "You will feel better once your medication begins to work."

6. A nurse has been closely observing a client that has been displaying aggressive behaviors. The nurse observes that the behavior displayed by the client is escalating. Which nursing intervention is least helpful to this client at this time?

   1. Acknowledging the client's behavior

   2. Maintaining a safe distance from the client

   3. Assisting the client to an area that is quiet

   4. Initiating confinement measures

7. Which behavior observed by the nurse indicates reason for suspicion that a depressed female adolescent client may be suicidal?

   1. The client becomes angry while speaking on the telephone and slams the receiver down on the hook

   2. The client runs out of the therapy group, swearing at the group leader, and runs to her room

   3. The client gets angry with her roommate when the roommate borrows the client's clothes without asking

   4. The client gives away a prized compact disc and a cherished autograph picture of the performer.

8. A client is admitted to the mental health unit after a serious suicide attempt by hanging. The nurse's most important aspect of care is to maintain client safety, which is best accomplished by which of the following?

   1. Assigning a staff member to the client who will remain with the client at all times

   2. Admitting the client to a seclusion room where all potentially dangerous articles are removed

   3. Removing the client's clothing and placing the client in a hospital gown

   4. Requesting that a peer remain with the client at all times

9. The police arrive at the emergency room with a client who has seriously lacerated both wrists. What is the initial nursing action?

   1. Examining and treating the wound sites

   2. Securing and recording a detailed history

   3. Encouraging and assisting the client to ventilate feelings

   4. Administering an antianxiety agent

10. The nursing care plan indicates a nursing diagnosis of "high risk for violence, self-directed, suicidal ideations with a plan." An expected outcome of this plan of care would be that the client does which of the following?

    1. Develops adequate coping and problem-solving skills

2. Displays less anxiety and agitation

3. Establishes a relationship with staff and peers

4. Denies suicidal ideation and identifies options to deal with stressors

11. A nurse receives a telephone call from a male client who states that he wants to kill himself and that he has a bottle of sleeping pills in front of him. What is the most appropriate nursing action?

    1. Insisting that the client give you his name and address so that you can get the police there immediately

    2. Keeping the client talking and allowing him to ventilate his feelings

    3. Using therapeutic communication techniques, especially the reflection of feelings

    4. Keeping the client talking and signaling to another staff member to trace the call so that appropriate help can be sent

12. A client is admitted to the hospital with a nursing diagnosis of "dysfunctional grieving related to the loss of a spouse." The client progresses well and is approaching discharge. Which of the following is an appropriate outcome for this nursing diagnosis?

    1. The client verbalizes the stages of grief and plans to attend a community grief group

    2. The client verbalizes the connections between significant losses and low self-esteem

    3. The client verbalizes a decreased desire for self-harm and discusses two alternatives to suicide

    4. The client reports three additional coping strategies

13. A client in a severe major depressive episode is unable to address activities of daily living (ADLs). What is the most appropriate nursing intervention?

    1. Feeding, bathing, and dressing the client as needed until the client can perform these activities independently

    2. Structuring the client's day so that adequate time can be devoted to the client's assuming responsibility for the ADLs

    3. Offering the client choices and consequences to the failure to comply with the expectation of maintaining ADLs

    4. Having the client's peers confront the client about how the noncompliance in addressing ADLs affects the milieu

14. A nurse is preparing a hospitalized client with a diagnosis of depression for discharge. In evaluating the coping strategies learned during hospitalization, the nurse would recognize which of the following statements, if made by the client, as an indication that further teaching needs to occur?

    1. "I have learned ways to deal with the stresses in my life."

    2. "I know that I won't become depressed again."

3. "I know that I can't be all things to all people."
4. "I need to take my medications just as prescribed."

15. A nurse is monitoring a client that is in seclusion. The nurse determines that the client is safe to come out of seclusion when the client states which of the following?
 1. "I am no longer a threat to myself or others."
 2. "I need to go to the bathroom."
 3. "I want to be alone for a while in my own room."
 4. "I can't breathe in here. The walls are closing in on me."

16. A nurse is preparing a discharge plan for the client who attempted suicide. The plan of care should focus on which of the following?
 1. Follow-up appointments
 2. Contracts and immediately available crisis resources
 3. Encouraging the family to always be with the client
 4. Providing the hospital phone number

17. An elderly male client who is a victim of elder abuse and his family have been attending weekly counseling sessions. Which of the following statements, if made by the abusive family member, would indicate that he or she has learned positive coping skills?
 1. "I will be more careful to make sure that my father's needs are met."
 2. "I am so sorry and embarrassed that the abusive event occurred. It won't happen again."
 3. "I feel better able to care for my father now that I know where to obtain assistance."
 4. "Now that my father is moving into my home, I will need to change my ways."

18. A moderately depressed client who was admitted 2 days ago suddenly begins smiling and reporting that the crisis is over. The client says to the nurse, "I'm finally cured." The nurse interprets this behavior as a cue to modify the treatment plan by doing which of the following?
 1. Allowing the client off unit privileges as needed
 2. Suggesting a reduction of medication
 3. Allowing increased "in room" activities
 4. Increasing the level of suicide precautions

19. A nurse is planning care for a client who attempted suicide and who is being admitted to the nursing unit. Which of the following priority nursing interventions will the nurse include in the plan of care?
 1. Check the whereabouts of the client every 15 minutes
 2. Suicide precautions with 30-minute checks
 3. One-to-one suicide precautions
 4. Ask the client to report suicidal thoughts immediately

20. An emergency room nurse is caring for a client who has been identified as a victim of physical abuse. In planning care for the client, which of the following is the priority nursing action?
 1. Adhering to the mandatory abuse reporting laws
 2. Obtaining treatment for the abusing family member
 3. Notifying the case worker of the family situation
 4. Removing the client from any immediate danger

21. An emergency room nurse is caring for an adult client who is a victim of family violence. Which of the following priority instructions would be included in the discharge instructions?
 1. Explaining the importance of leaving the violent situation
 2. Information about shelters
 3. Instructions about self-defense classes
 4. Instructions about calling the police

22. A female victim of a sexual assault is being seen in the crisis center. The client states that she still feels "as though the rape just happened yesterday," even though it has been a few months since the incident. Which of the following is the most appropriate nursing response?
 1. "What do you think that you can do to alleviate some of your fears about being raped again?"
 2. "Tell me what it is about the incident that causes you to feel like the rape just occurred."
 3. "It will take some time to get over these feelings about your rape."
 4. "You need to try to be realistic. The rape did not just occur."

23. A nurse in the emergency department is caring for a young female victim of sexual assault. The client's physical assessment is complete, and physical evidence has been collected. The nurse notes that the client is withdrawn, confused, and at times physically immobile. These behaviors are interpreted by the nurse as which of the following?
 1. Evidence that the client is a high suicide risk
 2. Indicative of the need for hospital admission
 3. Signs of depression
 4. Normal reactions to a devastating event

24. A nurse has been working with a victim of rape in a clinic setting for the past 4 weeks. Which of the following short-term initial goals will not be a component of the plan of care?
 1. The client will resolve feelings of fear and anxiety related to the rape trauma.
 2. Physical wounds will heal.
 3. The client will verbalize feelings about the event.
 4. The client will participate in the treatment plan.

25. A client comes to a clinic after losing all of his personal belongings in a hurricane. The nurse develops a nursing diagnosis of "ineffective individual coping." Which of the following is the least realistic goal for this client?
 1. The client will identify a realistic perception of stressors

2. The client will develop adaptive coping patterns
3. The client will express and share feelings about the present crisis
4. The client will stop blaming himself for the lack of insurance

CRITICAL THINKING: FREE-TEXT ENTRY

A nurse who is caring for a client with severe depression is planning activities for the client. The nurse goes to the activity room and finds a puzzle, a checkers board game, a paint-by-number picture, and drawing supplies. Which activity would be most appropriate for this client?

Answer: _____

ANSWERS

1. **3**
Rationale: A situational crisis arises from external rather than internal sources. External situations that could precipitate crisis include the loss of or change of a job; the death of a loved one; an abortion; a change in financial status; divorce; the addition of new family members; pregnancy; and severe illness. Options 1, 2, and 4 identify adventitious crisis, which is not a part of every day life and is unplanned and accidental.
Test-Taking Strategy: Use the process of elimination. Eliminate options 1, 2, and 4, because they are similar types of occurrences. If you had difficulty with this question, review the types of crises.
Level of Cognitive Ability: Analysis
Client Needs: Psychosocial Integrity
Integrated Concept/Process: Nursing Process/Analysis
Content Area: Mental Health
Reference: Fortinash, K., & Holoday-Worret, P. (2000). *Psychiatric mental health nursing* (2nd ed.). St. Louis: Mosby, p. 596.

2. **1**
Rationale: A nurse's initial task when assessing a client in crisis is to assess the individual or family and the problem. The more clearly the problem can be defined, the better the chance that a solution can be found. Option 1 will assist in determining data related to the precipitating event that led to the crisis. Options 2 and 4 assess situational supports. Option 3 assesses personal coping skills.
Test-Taking Strategy: Use the process of elimination. Note the key words "precipitating event." Focus on these key words when selecting the correct option. Eliminate options 2 and 4, because this data will determine support systems. Eliminate option 3, because this question would be asked when determining coping skills. Review assessment techniques for the client in crisis if you had difficulty with this question.
Level of Cognitive Ability: Application
Client Needs: Psychosocial Integrity
Integrated Concept/Process: Nursing Process/Assessment
Content Area: Mental Health
Reference: Fortinash, K., & Holoday-Worret, P. (2000). *Psychiatric mental health nursing* (2nd ed.). St. Louis: Mosby, p. 598.

3. **4**
Rationale: Although each crisis response can be described in similar terms as far as presenting symptoms are concerned, what constitutes a crisis for one person may not constitute a crisis for another person, because each person is a unique individual. Being in the crisis state does not mean that the client is suffering from an emotional or mental illness.
Test-Taking Strategy: Use the process of elimination. Eliminate option 1 because of the word "all." Next, eliminate options 2 and 3, because a crisis does not indicate "illness." Review the characteristics of a crisis state if you had difficulty with this question.
Level of Cognitive Ability: Analysis
Client Needs: Psychosocial Integrity
Integrated Concept/Process: Nursing Process/Planning
Content Area: Mental Health
Reference: Fortinash, K., & Holoday-Worret, P. (2000). *Psychiatric mental health nursing* (2nd ed.). St. Louis: Mosby, p. 598.

4. **1**
Rationale: The best option is to ask the client what is causing the agitation; this will help the client to become aware of the behavior, and it may assist the nurse in planning appropriate interventions for the client. Option 2 is demanding behavior that could cause increased agitation in the client. Options 3 and 4 are threats to the client and are inappropriate.
Test-Taking Strategy: Use the process of elimination. Eliminate option 2 because of the demand that it places on the client. Eliminate options 3 and 4 because they indicate threats to the client. Review appropriate nursing actions for the agitated client if you had difficulty with this question.
Level of Cognitive Ability: Application
Client Needs: Psychosocial Integrity
Integrated Concept/Process: Communication and Documentation
Content Area: Mental Health
Reference: Keltner, N., Schwecke, L., & Bostrom, C. (1999). *Psychiatric nursing* (3rd ed.). St. Louis: Mosby, p. 163.

5. **3**
Rationale: Clients who are depressed may be at risk for suicide. It is critical for the nurse to assess suicidal ideation and plan. Ask the client directly if a plan for self-harm exists. Options 1, 2, and 4 do not directly deal with the client's feelings.
Test-Taking Strategy: Using therapeutic communication techniques will assist in directing you to the correct option. Option 3 is the only option that deals directly with the client's feelings. Additionally, clients at risk for suicide need to be directly assessed about the potential for self-harm. Review care to the client at risk for suicide if you had difficulty with this question.
Level of Cognitive Ability: Application
Client Needs: Psychosocial Integrity

Integrated Concept/Process: Communication and Documentation
Content Area: Mental Health
Reference: Keltner, N., Schwecke, L., & Bostrom, C. (1999). *Psychiatric nursing* (3rd ed.). St. Louis: Mosby, p. 416.

6. 4

Rationale: During the escalation period, the client's behavior is moving toward loss of control. Nursing actions include taking control; maintaining a safe distance; acknowledging behavior; moving the client to a quiet area; and medicating the client, if appropriate. It is not appropriate during this period to initiate confinement measures; confinement measures are most appropriate during the crisis period.

Test-Taking Strategy: Note the key words "behavior," "escalating," and "least helpful." Recalling that the least restrictive measures should be used will direct you to option 4. Review care to the client with aggressive behavior if you had difficulty with this question.

Level of Cognitive Ability: Application
Client Needs: Psychosocial Integrity
Integrated Concept/Process: Nursing Process/Implementation
Content Area: Mental Health
Reference: Fortinash, K., & Holoday-Worret, P. (2000). *Psychiatric mental health nursing* (2nd ed.). St. Louis: Mosby, p. 172.

7. 4

Rationale: A depressed, suicidal client often gives away that which is of value as a way of saying good-bye and wanting to be remembered. Options 1, 2, and 3 deal with anger and acting out behaviors, which are often typical of any adolescent.

Test-Taking Strategy: Use the process of elimination. Eliminate options 1, 2, and 3 because they are similar. Option 4 is different and describes an action that could indicate that the client may be "saying good-bye." Review behaviors that indicate suicidal intent if you had difficulty with this question.

Level of Cognitive Ability: Analysis
Client Needs: Psychosocial Integrity
Integrated Concept/Process: Nursing Process/Assessment
Content Area: Mental Health
Reference: Fortinash, K., & Holoday-Worret, P. (2000). *Psychiatric mental health nursing* (2nd ed.). St. Louis: Mosby, p. 662.

8. 1

Rationale: Hanging is a serious suicide attempt. The plan of care must reflect action that will promote the client's safety. Constant observation status (one-to-one) with a staff member who is never less than an arm's length away is the best selection. Seclusion should not be the initial intervention, and the least restrictive measure should be used. Placing the client in a hospital gown and requesting that a peer remain with the client will not ensure a safe environment.

Test-Taking Strategy: Use the process of elimination. Eliminate option 2, because seclusion should not be the initial intervention. Eliminate option 4 next, because the responsibility to safeguard a client is not the peer's responsibility. Eliminate option 3, because removing the client's clothing will not maximize all possible safety strategies. Review nursing interventions for the client at risk for suicide if you had difficulty with this question.

Level of Cognitive Ability: Application
Client Needs: Safe, Effective Care Environment
Integrated Concept/Process: Nursing Process/Implementation

Content Area: Mental Health
Reference: Keltner, N., Schwecke, L., & Bostrom, C. (1999). *Psychiatric nursing* (3rd ed.). St. Louis: Mosby, p. 416.

9. 1

Rationale: The initial nursing action is to assess and treat the self-inflicted injuries. Injuries from lacerated wrists can lead to a life-threatening situation. Other interventions may follow after the client has been treated medically.

Test-Taking Strategy: Use Maslow's hierarchy of needs theory to prioritize; physiological needs come first. Option 1 addresses the physiological need. Review care of the client who attempted suicide if you had difficulty with this question.

Level of Cognitive Ability: Application
Client Needs: Physiological Integrity
Integrated Concept/Process: Nursing Process/Implementation
Content Area: Mental Health
Reference: Fortinash, K., & Holoday-Worret, P. (2000). *Psychiatric mental health nursing* (2nd ed.). St. Louis: Mosby, pp. 664-665.

10. 4

Rationale: A suicidal client may have numerous diagnoses that encompass inadequate coping skills, anxiety, and strained interpersonal relationships. The question, however, directly and clearly designates that the problem that needs to be dealt with is the "high risk for violence, self-directed" and that the client has both the ideation and a plan. The expected outcome is that the client no longer has suicidal ideations and has identified options to deal with stress. Options 1, 2, and 3 are not directly related to the nursing diagnosis as stated in the question.

Test-Taking Strategy: When presented with a question that identifies a nursing diagnosis, use the information in the question to assist in directing you to the correct option. Option 4 is the only option that offers a resolution to the nursing diagnosis of "suicidal ideation with a plan" in that the client "denies suicidal ideation and identifies options." Review the appropriate plan of care for a suicidal client if you had difficulty with this question.

Level of Cognitive Ability: Analysis
Client Needs: Health Promotion and Maintenance
Integrated Concept/Process: Nursing Process/Evaluation
Content Area: Mental Health
Reference: Keltner, N., Schwecke, L., & Bostrom, C. (1999). *Psychiatric nursing* (3rd ed.). St. Louis: Mosby, p. 416.

11. 4

Rationale: In a crisis, the nurse must take an authoritative, active role to promote the client's safety. A bottle of sleeping pills in front of a client who verbalizes that he wants to kill himself is a crisis. The client's safety is of prime concern. Keeping the client on the phone and getting help to the client is the best intervention. Insisting that the client provide his name may anger the client, and he might hang up. Option 2 lacks the authoritative action stance of securing the client's safety. Using therapeutic communication techniques is important, but overuse of reflection may sound uncaring or superficial and is lacking direction and solutions to the immediate problem of the client's safety.

Test-Taking Strategy: Use the process of elimination, and focus on the issue of the client's safety. Option 4 is the global option that most directly addresses the safety of the client.

Review care of the suicidal client if you had difficulty with this question.

Level of Cognitive Ability: Application
Client Needs: Safe, Effective Care Environment
Integrated Concept/Process: Nursing Process/Implementation
Content Area: Mental Health
Reference: Keltner, N., Schwecke, L., & Bostrom, C. (1999). *Psychiatric nursing* (3rd ed.). St. Louis: Mosby, p. 417.

12. **1**

Rationale: The question is focused on the nursing diagnosis of dysfunctional grieving. The only option that deals with grief is option 1. Options 2, 3, and 4 are unrelated to this nursing diagnosis.

Test-Taking Strategy: When presented with a question that identifies a nursing diagnosis, use the information in the question to assist with directing you to the correct option. Option 1 is the only option that is focused on the nursing diagnosis of dysfunctional grieving. Additionally, note the word "grieving" in the question and the word "grief" in the correct option. Review expected outcomes for the client experiencing dysfunctional grieving if you had difficulty with this question.

Level of Cognitive Ability: Analysis
Client Needs: Health Promotion and Maintenance
Integrated Concept/Process: Nursing Process/Evaluation
Content Area: Mental Health
Reference: Fortinash, K., & Holoday-Worret, P. (2000). *Psychiatric mental health nursing* (2nd ed.). St. Louis: Mosby, p. 683.

13. **1**

Rationale: The symptoms of major depression includes depressed mood, loss of interest or pleasure, changes in appetite and sleep patterns, psychomotor agitation or retardation, fatigue, feelings of worthlessness/guilt, diminished ability to think or concentrate, and recurrent thoughts of death. Often the clients do not have the energy or interest to complete activities of daily living. Option 3 may lead to increased feelings of worthlessness as the client fails to meet expectations. Option 4 will increase the client's feelings of poor self-esteem and unworthiness.

Test-Taking Strategy: Use the process of elimination. Note the key words "severe major depressive episode." Remember that severely depressed clients are unable to perform even the simplest of activities of daily living. Review care to the client with severe depression if you had difficulty with this question.

Level of Cognitive Ability: Application
Client Needs: Physiological Integrity
Integrated Concept/Process: Nursing Process/Implementation
Content Area: Mental Health
Reference: Keltner, N., Schwecke, L., & Bostrom, C. (1999). *Psychiatric nursing* (3rd ed.). St. Louis: Mosby, p. 398.

14. **2**

Rationale: Depression may be a recurring illness for some people. The client needs to understand the symptoms and recognize when or if treatment needs to begin again. Options 1, 3, and 4 indicate that the client has learned some coping skills such as setting limits and taking medications. Option 2 is an unrealistic statement and indicates that further teaching is needed.

Test-Taking Strategy: Use the process of elimination, and note the key words "further teaching needs to occur." Review

expected outcomes for the client with depression if you had difficulty with this question.

Level of Cognitive Ability: Analysis
Client Needs: Health Promotion and Maintenance
Integrated Concept/Process: Nursing Process/Evaluation
Content Area: Mental Health
Reference: Fortinash, K., & Holoday-Worret, P. (2000). *Psychiatric mental health nursing* (2nd ed.). St. Louis: Mosby, p. 276.

15. **1**

Rationale: The client in seclusion must be assessed at regular intervals (usually every 15 to 30 minutes) for physical needs, safety, and comfort. Option 2 indicates a physical need that could be met with a urinal or a bedpan, if necessary; it does not indicate that the client has calmed down enough to leave the seclusion room. Option 3 could be an attempt to manipulate the nurse; there is no indication that the client will control him- or herself when alone in their room. Option 4 indicates the need for supportive communication or possibly a PRN medication; it does not necessitate discontinuing seclusion.

Test-Taking Strategy: The issue of the question specifically relates to safety. Use the process of elimination and focus on the issue to direct you to option 1. Review seclusion procedures if you had difficulty with this question.

Level of Cognitive Ability: Analysis
Client Needs: Safe, Effective Care Environment
Integrated Concept/Process: Nursing Process/Evaluation
Content Area: Mental Health
Reference: Fortinash, K., & Holoday-Worret, P. (2000). *Psychiatric mental health nursing* (2nd ed.). St. Louis: Mosby, p. 89.

16. **2**

Rationale: Crisis times may occur between appointments. Contracts facilitate the client feeling a responsibility for keeping a promise; this gives the client control. Option 3 is unrealistic. Providing phone numbers will not ensure available and immediate crisis intervention.

Test-Taking Strategy: Use the process of elimination. The issue of the question relates to the availability of immediate resources for the client, if needed. Eliminate option 3 first, because this is unrealistic. Options 1 and 4 will not necessarily provide immediate resources. Also, note the word "immediate" in the correct option. Review care of the client who has attempted suicide if you had difficulty with this question.

Level of Cognitive Ability: Application
Client Needs: Health Promotion and Maintenance
Integrated Concept/Process: Self-Care
Content Area: Mental Health
Reference: Fortinash, K., & Holoday-Worret, P. (2000). *Psychiatric mental health nursing* (2nd ed.). St. Louis: Mosby, p. 598.

17. **3**

Rationale: Elder abuse is sometimes the result of family members who are being expected to care for their aging parents. This care can cause the family to become overextended, frustrated, or financially depleted. Knowing where to turn in the community for assistance with caring for aging family members can bring much-needed relief. These alternatives are positive coping strategies that many families use.

Test-Taking Strategy: Use the process of elimination. Note the key words "positive coping skills." Option 3 identifies a means of coping with the issues. The other options identify statements of good faith or promises, which may or may not be kept in the future. Only option 3 outlines a definitive plan for how to handle the pressure associated with the father's care. Review coping mechanisms if you had difficulty with this question.

Level of Cognitive Ability: Analysis
Client Needs: Health Promotion and Maintenance
Integrated Concept/Process: Nursing Process/Evaluation
Content Area: Mental Health
Reference: Fortinash, K., & Holoday-Worret, P. (2000). *Psychiatric mental health nursing* (2nd ed.). St. Louis: Mosby, p. 643.

18. **4**
Rationale: A client who is moderately depressed and has only been in the hospital for 2 days is very unlikely to have such a dramatic cure. When a mood suddenly lifts, it is very likely that the client may have made the decision to harm him- or herself. Suicide precautions are necessary to keep the client safe.
Test-Taking Strategy: Use the process of elimination. Options 1 and 2 support the client's notion that a cure has occurred. Option 3 allows the client to increase isolation, and that would present a threat to the treatment plan. Safety is of the utmost importance; therefore, option 4 is the correct option. Review care to the client with depression if you had difficulty with this question.
Level of Cognitive Ability: Analysis
Client Needs: Safe, Effective Care Environment
Integrated Concept/Process: Nursing Process/Planning
Content Area: Mental Health
Reference: Fortinash, K., & Holoday-Worret, P. (2000). *Psychiatric mental health nursing* (2nd ed.). St. Louis: Mosby, p. 664.

19. **3**
Rationale: One-to-one suicide precautions are required for the client who has attempted suicide. Options 1 and 2 may be appropriate, but they are not appropriate at the present time, considering the situation. Option 4 may also be an appropriate nursing intervention, but the priority is identified in option 3. The best intervention is constant supervision so that the nurse may intervene as needed if the client attempts to cause harm to self.
Test-Taking Strategy: Use the process of elimination, and note the key words "attempted suicide." Option 3 is the only option that provides a safe environment. Review interventions for the suicidal client if you had difficulty with this question.
Level of Cognitive Ability: Application
Client Needs: Safe, Effective Care Environment
Integrated Concept/Process: Nursing Process/Implementation
Content Area: Mental Health
Reference: Fortinash, K., & Holoday-Worret, P. (2000). *Psychiatric mental health nursing* (2nd ed.). St. Louis: Mosby, p. 672.

20. **4**
Rationale: Whenever the abused client remains in the abusive environment, priority must be placed on ascertaining whether the person is in any immediate danger. If so, emergency action must be taken to remove the client from the abusing situation. Options 1, 2, and 3 may be appropriate interventions, but they are not the priority.
Test-Taking Strategy: Use Maslow's hierarchy of needs theory, and remember that if a physiological need is not present, then safety is the priority. This guide should direct you to option 4,

which is the only option that directly addresses client safety. Review care to the client who is a victim of physical abuse if you had difficulty with this question.
Level of Cognitive Ability: Application
Client Needs: Safe, Effective Care Environment
Integrated Concept/Process: Nursing Process/Planning
Content Area: Mental Health
Reference: Fortinash, K., & Holoday-Worret, P. (2000). *Psychiatric mental health nursing* (2nd ed.). St. Louis: Mosby, p. 628.

21. **2**
Rationale: Tertiary prevention of family violence includes assisting the victim after the abuse has already occurred. The nurse should provide the client with information about where to obtain help; this includes a specific plan for removing the client from the abuser, information about escaping, hot line numbers, and the location of shelters. An abused person is usually reluctant to call the police. Teaching the victim to fight back is not the appropriate action for the victim who is dealing with a violent person.
Test-Taking Strategy: Use the process of elimination. Focus on the issue of the question, which relates to providing the client with a safe environment. Use Maslow's hierarchy of needs theory to assist in directing you to option 2. If you had difficulty with this question, review the nursing measures for caring for a victim of family violence.
Level of Cognitive Ability: Application
Client Needs: Safe, Effective Care Environment
Integrated Concept/Process: Self-Care
Content Area: Mental Health
Reference: Fortinash, K., & Holoday-Worret, P. (2000). *Psychiatric mental health nursing* (2nd ed.). St. Louis: Mosby, p. 629.

22. **2**
Rationale: Option 2 allows the client to express her ideas and feelings more fully and portrays a nonhurried, nonjudgmental, supportive attitude. Clients need to be reassured that their feelings are normal and that they may freely express their concerns in a safe, caring environment. Option 1 places the problem solving totally on the client. Option 3 places the client's feelings on hold. Option 4 immediately blocks communication.
Test-Taking Strategy: Use the process of elimination. Option 2 is the only option that addresses the client's feelings. Always address the client's feelings first. Review therapeutic communication techniques if you had difficulty with this question.
Level of Cognitive Ability: Application
Client Needs: Psychosocial Integrity
Integrated Concept/Process: Caring
Content Area: Mental Health
Reference: Keltner, N., Schwecke, L., & Bostrom, C. (1999). *Psychiatric nursing* (3rd ed.). St. Louis: Mosby, p. 595.

23. **4**
Rationale: During the acute phase of the rape crisis, the client can display a wide range of emotional and somatic responses. The symptoms noted indicate a normal reaction to an intensely difficult crisis event.
Test-Taking Strategy: Use the process of elimination and knowledge about client responses to devastating events to answer the question. Focus on the symptoms noted in the question to direct you to option 4. If you had difficulty with this question, review normal and abnormal client responses to dealing with devastating crisis events.

Level of Cognitive Ability: Analysis
Client Needs: Psychosocial Integrity
Integrated Concept/Process: Nursing Process/Analysis
Content Area: Mental Health
Reference: Fortinash, K., & Holoday-Worret, P. (2000). *Psychiatric mental health nursing* (2nd ed.). St. Louis: Mosby, p. 649.

24. **1**
Rationale: Short-term goals will include the beginning stages of dealing with the rape trauma. Clients will be expected initially to keep appointments, participate in care, begin to explore feelings, and begin to heal any physical wounds that were inflicted at the time of the rape.
Test-Taking Strategy: Use the process of elimination. Note the key words "not" and "short-term initial goals." Use the process of elimination, and consider each option and the reality of the option statement being achieved over the short term. Note the word "resolve" in option 1; this word should provide you with the clue that this option is a long-term goal. Review expected outcomes in the plan of care for the client who has been raped if you had difficulty with this question.
Level of Cognitive Ability: Application
Client Needs: Psychosocial Integrity
Integrated Concept/Process: Nursing Process/Planning
Content Area: Mental Health
Reference: Keltner, N., Schwecke, L., & Bostrom, C. (1999). *Psychiatric nursing* (3rd ed.). St. Louis: Mosby, p. 595.

25. **4**
Rationale: Options 1, 2, and 3 identify a positive movement toward increased self-esteem and problem solving. Option 4 places undue pressure on the client by implying that the client was negligent and contributed to the loss.
Test-Taking Strategy: Use the process of elimination. Note the key words "least realistic." The words "realistic," "adaptive," and "express and share feelings" in options 1, 2, and 3, respectively, identify positive goals; this should assist in directing you to option 4. Additionally, there is nothing in the question that indicates that the client lacked insurance as is reflected in option 4. Review expected outcomes for the client who experienced a crisis if you had difficulty with this question.
Level of Cognitive Ability: Application
Client Needs: Psychosocial Integrity
Integrated Concept/Process: Nursing Process/Planning
Content Area: Mental Health
Reference: Keltner, N., Schwecke, L., & Bostrom, C. (1999). *Psychiatric nursing* (3rd ed.). St. Louis: Mosby, p. 153.

CRITICAL THINKING: FREE-TEXT ENTRY

Answer: Drawing
Rationale: Concentration and memory are poor in severe depression. When a client has a diagnosis of severe depression, the nurse needs to provide activities that require little concentration. Activities that have no right or wrong choices or that do not require decisions minimize opportunities for the client to put himself or herself down.
Test-Taking Strategy: Note that the client's diagnosis is severe depression. Remember that clients with depression have difficulty concentrating and need activities that require little concentration. Review care of the client with severe depression if you had difficulty with this question.
Level of Cognitive Ability: Application
Client Needs: Psychosocial Integrity
Integrated Concept/Process: Nursing Process/Implementation
Content Area: Mental Health
Reference: Keltner, N., Schwecke, L., & Bostrom, C. (1999). *Psychiatric nursing* (3rd ed.). St. Louis: Mosby, p. 399.

REFERENCES

Fortinash, K., & Holoday-Worret, P. (2000). *Psychiatric mental health nursing* (2nd ed.). St. Louis: Mosby.

Glod, C.A. (1998). *Contemporary psychiatric-mental health nursing.* Philadelphia: F.A. Davis.

Keltner, N., Schwecke, L., & Bostrom, C. (1999). *Psychiatric nursing* (3rd ed.). St. Louis: Mosby.

National Council of State Boards of Nursing (eds.) (2000). *Test Plan for the National Council Licensure Examination for Registered Nurses.* Chicago: Author.

Stuart, G.W., & Laraia, M.T. (1998). *Principles and practice of psychiatric nursing.* (6th ed.). St. Louis: Mosby.

Varcarolis, E. (1998). *Foundations of psychiatric mental health nursing* (3rd ed.). Philadelphia: W.B. Saunders.

Psychiatric Medications

I. SELECTIVE SEROTONIN REUPTAKE INHIBITORS (SSRIs) (Box 74-1)

A. Description
1. Inhibit serotonin uptake
2. Produce an antidepressant response

B. Side effects
1. Nausea and diarrhea
2. Dry mouth
3. Central nervous system (CNS) stimulation
4. Photosensitivity
5. Insomnia
6. Nervousness
7. Headache
8. Dizziness
9. Weight loss

C. Implementation
1. Monitor vital signs
2. Monitor weight
3. Initiate safety precautions, particularly if dizziness occurs
4. Instruct the client to take a single dose in the morning to prevent insomnia
5. Administer with a snack or with meals to reduce the risk of dizziness and lightheadedness
6. Monitor the suicidal client, especially during improved mood and increased energy levels
7. Instruct the client on fluoxetine (Prozac) to take the medication early in the day to avoid interference with sleep
8. For the client on long-term therapy, monitor liver and renal function tests
9. Monitor white blood cell (WBC) and neutrophil counts and discontinue the medication, as prescribed, if levels fall below normal
10. If priapism (painful, prolonged penile erection) occurs, discontinue the medication immediately and notify the physician

11. Instruct the client to change positions slowly to avoid hypotensive effect
12. Instruct the client to avoid alcohol
13. Instruct the client to report any visual changes to the physician

II. TRICYCLIC ANTIDEPRESSANTS (Box 74-2)

A. Description
1. Block the reuptake of norepinephrine and serotonin at the presynaptic neuron
2. Used to treat depression
3. May reduce seizure threshold
4. May reduce effectiveness of antihypertensive agents
5. Concurrent use with alcohol or antihistamines can cause CNS depression
6. Concurrent use with monoamine oxidase inhibitors (MAOIs) can cause hypertensive crisis

B. Side effects
1. Anticholinergic effects
2. Dry mouth
3. Decreased gastrointestinal (GI) motility and constipation
4. Difficulty voiding
5. Dilated pupils and blurred vision
6. Photosensitivity
7. Cardiovascular disturbances

BOX 74-2

Tricyclic Antidepressants

Amitriptyline hydrochloride (Elavil)
Amoxapine (Asendin)
Bupropion (Wellbutrin, Zyban)
Clomipramine (Anafranil)
Desipramine hydrochloride (Norpramin)
Doxepin hydrochloride (Sinequan)
Fluoxetine hydrochloride (Prozac)
Imipramine hydrochloride (Tofranil)
Maprotiline (Ludiomil)
Mirtazapine (Remeron)
Nefazodone (Serzone)
Nortriptyline hydrochloride (Aventyl)
Protriptyline hydrochloride (Vivactil)
Trazodone (Desyrel)
Trimipramine maleate (Surmontil)

BOX 74-3

Monoamine Oxidase Inhibitors (MAOIs)

Isocarboxazid (Marplan)
Phenelzine sulfate (Nardil)
Tranylcypromine sulfate (Parnate)

---

8. Tachycardia, dysrhythmias
9. Orthostatic hypotension
10. Sedation
11. Weight gain
12. Anxiety, restlessness, and irritability
13. Decreased or increased libido, with ejaculatory and erection disturbances

C. Implementation
1. Instruct the client that the medication may take several weeks to produce the desired effect (client response may not occur until 2 to 4 weeks after the first dose)
2. Monitor the suicidal client, especially during improved mood and increased energy levels
3. Instruct the client to change positions slowly to avoid hypotensive effect
4. Monitor pattern of daily bowel activity
5. Assess for urinary retention
6. For the client on long-term therapy, monitor liver and renal function tests
7. Administer with food or milk if GI distress occurs
8. Administer the entire daily oral dose at one time, preferably at bedtime
9. Instruct the client to avoid alcohol and nonprescription medications, to prevent adverse medication interactions
10. Instruct the client to avoid driving and other activities requiring alertness
11. When the medication is discontinued, it should be tapered gradually

III. MONOAMINE OXIDASE INHIBITORS (MAOIs) (Box 74-3)
A. Description
1. Inhibit MAO enzyme, which is present in the brain, blood platelets, liver, spleen, and kidneys
2. Inhibition of the MAO enzyme metabolizes

amines, norepinephrine, and serotonin, and the concentrations of these amines increase
3. Used for depression in the client who has not responded to other antidepressant therapies, including electroconvulsive therapy
4. Concurrent use with amphetamines, antidepressants, dopamine, epinephrine, guanethidine, levodopa, methyldopa, nasal decongestants, norepinephrine, reserpine, tyramine-containing foods, or vasoconstrictors may cause hypertensive crisis
5. Concurrent use with narcotic analgesics may cause hypertension, hypotension, coma, or seizures

B. Side effects
1. Orthostatic hypotension
2. Restlessness
3. Insomnia
4. Dizziness
5. Weakness, lethargy
6. GI upset
7. Dry mouth
8. Weight gain
9. Peripheral edema
10. Anticholinergic effects
11. CNS stimulation, including anxiety, agitation, and mania
12. Delay in ejaculation

C. Hypertensive crisis
1. Hypertension
2. Occipital headache radiating frontally
3. Neck stiffness and soreness
4. Nausea and vomiting
5. Sweating
6. Fever and chills
7. Clammy skin
8. Dilated pupils
9. Palpitations, tachycardia, or bradycardia
10. Constricting chest pain
11. Antidote for hypertensive crisis: 5 to 10 mg phentolamine (Regitine) by IV injection

D. Implementation
1. Monitor blood pressure frequently for hypertension
2. Monitor for signs of hypertensive crisis
3. If palpitations or frequent headaches occur, discontinue the medication and notify the physician

BOX 74-4

Tyramine Foods to Avoid

Cheese, especially aged, except cottage cheese
Sour cream
Pickled herring
Avocados
Bananas
Papaya
Broad beans
Figs
Overripe fruit
Brewer's yeast
Meat extracts and tenderizers
Yogurt
Sausage, bologna, pepperoni, salami
Soy sauce
Raisins
Red wine, beer, sherry
Beef or chicken liver
Caffeine as coffee, tea, or chocolate

---

4. Administer with food if GI distress occurs
5. Instruct the client that the medication effect may be noted during the first week of therapy, but maximum benefit may take up to 3 weeks
6. Instruct the client to report headache, neck stiffness, or neck soreness immediately
7. Instruct the client to change positions slowly to prevent orthostatic hypotension
8. Instruct the client to avoid caffeine or over-the-counter preparations such as weight-reducing pills or medications for hay fever and colds
9. Monitor for client compliance with medication administration
10. Instruct the client to carry a Medic-Alert card indicating that an MAOI medication has been prescribed
11. Avoid administering the medication in the evening because insomnia may result
12. MAO inhibitors should be tapered and discontinued 7 to 14 days before surgery
13. When the medication is discontinued, it should be discontinued gradually
14. Instruct the client to avoid foods that require bacteria or molds for their preparation or preservation or those that contain tyramine (Box 74-4)

▲ **IV. ANTIMANIC MEDICATIONS** (Box 74-5)
A. Description
   1. Affect cellular transport mechanism and alter both the presynaptic and postsynaptic events affecting serotonin, thus enhancing serotonin function
   2. Concurrent use with diuretics, fluoxetine, methyldopa, or nonsteroidal antiinflammatory medi-

BOX 74-5

Antimanic Medications

Lithium carbonate (Eskalith, Lithane, Lithobid)
Lithium citrate (Cibalith-Si)

---

cations increases lithium reabsorption by the kidney, or inhibits lithium excretion, either of which increases the risk of lithium toxicity
   3. Acetazolamide, aminophylline, phenothiazines, or sodium bicarbonate may increase renal excretion of lithium, reducing its effectiveness
   4. The therapeutic dose is only slightly less than the amount producing toxicity
   5. The therapeutic drug serum level of lithium is 0.6 to 1.2 mEq/L
   6. The causes of an increase in lithium level include decreased sodium intake, fluid and electrolyte loss associated with severe sweating, dehydration, diarrhea, or diuretic therapy, illness, and overdose
   7. Serum lithium levels should be checked every 1 to 2 months or whenever any behavioral change suggests an altered serum level
   8. Blood samples to check serum lithium levels should be drawn in the morning, 12 hours after the last dose was taken
B. Side effects
   1. Polyuria
   2. Polydipsia
   3. Anorexia, nausea
   4. Dry mouth
   5. Mild thirst
   6. Weight gain
   7. Abdominal bloating
   8. Soft stools or diarrhea
   9. Fine hand tremors
   10. Inability to concentrate
   11. Muscle weakness
   12. Lethargy
   13. Fatigue
   14. Headache
   15. Hair loss
C. Implementation
   1. Monitor the suicidal client, especially during improved mood and increased energy levels
   2. Administer the medication with food to minimize GI irritation
   3. Instruct the client to maintain a fluid intake of 6 to 8 glasses of water a day
   4. Instruct the client to avoid excessive amounts of coffee, tea, or cola, which have a diuretic effect
   5. Instruct the client to maintain an adequate salt intake
   6. Do not administer diuretics while the client is taking lithium

7. Instruct the client to avoid alcohol
8. Instruct the client to avoid over-the-counter medications
9. Instruct the client that he or she may take a missed dose within 2 hours of the scheduled time; otherwise the client should skip the missed dose and take the next dose at the scheduled time
10. Instruct the client not to adjust the dosage without consulting the physician, because lithium should be tapered off and not discontinued abruptly
11. Instruct the client in the signs and symptoms of lithium toxicity
12. Instruct the client to notify the physician if polyuria, prolonged vomiting, diarrhea, or fever occurs
13. Instruct the client that the therapeutic response to the medication will be noted in 1 to 3 weeks
14. Monitor electrocardiogram (ECG), renal function tests, and thyroid tests

D. Lithium toxicity
 1. Description
    a. Occurs when ingested lithium cannot be detoxified and excreted by the kidneys
    b. Symptoms of toxicity begin to appear when the serum lithium level is 1.5 to 2.0 mEq/L
 2. Mild toxicity
    a. Serum lithium level at 1.5 mEq/L
    b. Apathy
    c. Lethargy
    d. Diminished concentration
    e. Mild ataxia
    f. Coarse hand tremors
    g. Slight muscle weakness
 3. Moderate toxicity
    a. Serum lithium level of 1.5 to 2.5 mEq/L
    b. Nausea, vomiting
    c. Severe diarrhea
    d. Mild to moderate ataxia and incoordination
    e. Slurred speech
    f. Tinnitus
    g. Blurred vision
    h. Muscle twitching
    i. Irregular tremor
 4. Severe toxicity
    a. Serum lithium level above 2.5 mEq/L
    b. Nystagmus
    c. Muscle fasciculations
    d. Deep tendon hyperreflexia
    e. Visual or tactile hallucinations
    f. Oliguria or anuria
    g. Impaired level of consciousness (LOC)
    h. Grand mal seizure or coma leading to death
 5. Implementation for lithium toxicity
    a. Hold lithium and notify the physician
    b. Monitor vital signs and LOC

BOX 74-6
Benzodiazepines

Alprazolam (Xanax)
Chlordiazepoxide (Librium)
Clonazepam (Klonopin)
Clorazepate (Tranxene)
Diazepam (Valium)
Estazolam (ProSom)
Flurazepam (Dalmane)
Halazepam (Paxipam)
Lorazepam (Ativan)
Oxazepam (Serax)
Prazepam (Centrax)
Quazepam (Doral)
Temazepam (Restoril)
Triazolam (Halcion)

    c. Monitor cardiac status
    d. Prepare to obtain lithium level; electrolyte, blood urea nitrogen (BUN), and creatinine counts; and complete blood cell (CBC) count
    e. Monitor for suicidal tendencies and institute **suicide** precautions

V. ANTIANXIETY OR ANXIOLYTIC MEDICATIONS
A. Description
 1. Depress the CNS, thereby increasing the effects of gamma-aminobutyric acid (GABA), which produces relaxation and may depress the limbic system
 2. Benzodiazepines have anxiety-reducing (anxiolytic), sedative-hypnotic, muscle-relaxing, and anticonvulsant actions (Box 74-6)
B. Side effects
 1. Daytime sedation
 2. Ataxia
 3. Dizziness
 4. Headaches
 5. Blurred or double vision
 6. Hypotension
 7. Tremor
 8. Amnesia
 9. Slurred speech
 10. Urinary incontinence
 11. Constipation
 12. Paradoxical CNS excitement
C. Acute toxicity
 1. Somnolence
 2. Confusion
 3. Diminished reflexes and coma
 4. Flumazenil (Romazicon), a benzodiazepine antagonist, administered IV, will reverse benzodiazepine intoxication in 5 minutes
 5. The client being treated for an overdose of a benzodiazepine may experience agitation, restlessness, discomfort, and anxiety

▶ D. Implementation
1. Monitor for motor responses such as agitation, trembling, and tension
2. Monitor for autonomic responses such as cold, clammy hands and sweating
3. Monitor for paradoxical CNS excitement during early therapy, particularly in elderly or debilitated individuals
4. Monitor for visual disturbances, since the medications can worsen glaucoma
5. Monitor liver and renal function tests and blood counts
6. Reduce the medication dose, as prescribed, for the older adult client and for the client with impaired liver function
7. Initiate safety precautions because the older adult client is at risk for falling when taking the medication for sleep or anxiety
8. Assist with ambulation if drowsiness or light-headedness occurs
9. Instruct the client that drowsiness usually disappears during continued therapy
10. Instruct the client to avoid tasks that require alertness until the response to the medication is established
11. Instruct the client to avoid alcohol
12. Instruct the client not to take other medications without consulting the physician
13. Instruct the client not to withdraw the medication abruptly

▶ E. Withdrawal
1. To lessen withdrawal symptoms, the dosage of a benzodiazepine should be tapered gradually over 2 to 6 weeks
2. Abrupt or too rapid withdrawal results in:
   a. Restlessness
   b. Irritability
   c. Insomnia
   d. Hand tremors
   e. Abdominal or muscle cramps
   f. Sweating
   g. Vomiting
   h. Seizures

VI. MEDICATIONS FOR INSOMNIA AND ANXIETY
(Box 74-7)
A. Description
1. Depress the reticular activating system by promoting the inhibitory synaptic action of the neurotransmitter GABA
2. Used for short-term treatment of insomnia or for sedation to relieve anxiety, tension, and apprehension
B. Side effects
1. Confusion
2. Irritability
3. Allergic reactions

BOX 74-7

Barbiturates and Sedative-Hypnotic Anxiolytics

BARBITURATES
Amobarbital (Amytal)
Aprobarbital (Alurate)
Butabarbital (Butisol)
Pentobarbital (Nembutal)
Phenobarbital (Luminal)
Secobarbital (Seconal)

SEDATIVE-HYPNOTIC ANXIOLYTICS
Busparone (BuSpar)
Chloral hydrate (Noctec)
Ethchlorvynol (Placidyl)
Hydroxyzine hydrochloride (Atarax)
Meprobamate (Equanil)
Zolpidem tartrate (Ambien)

---

4. Agranulocytosis
5. Thrombocytopenic purpura
6. Megaloblastic anemia
C. Overdose
1. Tachycardia
2. Hypotension
3. Cold and clammy skin
4. Dilated pupils
5. Weak and rapid pulse
6. Signs of shock
7. Depressed respirations
8. Absent reflexes
9. Coma and death may result from respiratory and cardiovascular collapse
D. Withdrawal
1. Severe withdrawal symptoms begin within 24 hours after the medication is discontinued in an individual with severe drug dependence
2. Gradual withdrawal is used to detoxify a dependent person
3. Anxiety
4. Insomnia
5. Nightmares
6. Daytime agitation
7. Tremors
8. Delirium
9. Seizures
E. Implementation
1. Administer lower doses as prescribed for the elderly client
2. Medications should be used with caution in the client who has suicidal tendencies or has a history of drug **addiction**
3. Maintain safety by supervising ambulation and using side rails at night
4. Instruct the client to take medication as directed
5. Instruct the client to avoid driving or operating

hazardous equipment if drowsiness, dizziness, or unsteadiness occurs

6. Instruct the client to avoid alcohol
7. For insomnia, instruct the client to take the medication 30 minutes before bedtime
8. Instruct the client that a hangover effect may occur in the morning
9. Instruct the client not to discontinue the medication abruptly
10. Instruct the client taking chloral hydrate to take the medication with food or a full glass of water, fruit juice, or ginger ale to improve the taste and to prevent gastric irritation

VII. ANTIPSYCHOTIC MEDICATIONS (Box 74-8)

A. Description
  1. Improve the thought processes and the behavior of the client with psychotic symptoms, especially the client with schizophrenia
  2. Block dopamine receptors in the brain, thereby reducing the psychotic symptoms
  3. Block the chemoreceptor trigger zone and vomiting center in the brain, producing an antiemetic effect
  4. Phenothiazines lower the seizure threshold
  5. Antipsychotics should not be given with other antipsychotic or antidepressant medications

B. Side effects
  1. Anticholinergic effects
  2. Dry mouth
  3. Increased heart rate
  4. Urinary retention
  5. Constipation
  6. Hypotension
  7. Drowsiness
  8. Blood dyscrasias
  9. Pruritis
  10. Photosensitivity

C. Extrapyramidal syndrome
  1. Parkinsonism
    a. Tremors
    b. Mask-like facies
    c. Rigidity
    d. Shuffling gait
  2. Dystonia
    a. Facial grimacing
    b. Abnormal or involuntary eye movements
  3. Akathisia
    a. Restlessness
    b. Constant moving about
  4. Tardive dyskinesia
    a. Protrusion of the tongue
    b. Chewing motion
    c. Involuntary movement of the body and extremities

D. Implementation
  1. Monitor vital signs

BOX 74-8

Antipsychotic Medications

PHENOTHIAZINES
Acetophenazine maleate (Tindal)
Chlorpromazine hydrochloride (Thorazine)
Fluphenazine hydrochloride (Prolixin)
Perphenazine (Trilafon)
Prochlorperazine (Compazine)
Promazine hydrochloride (Sparine)
Thioridazine hydrochloride (Mellaril)
Trifluoperazine (Stelazine)
Triflupromazine hydrochloride (Vesprin)

OTHER ANTIPSYCHOTICS
Clozapine (Clozaril)
Haloperidol (Haldol)
Loxapine (Loxitane)
Molindone hydrochloride (Moban)
Olanzapine (Zyprexa)
Risperidone (Risperdal)
Thiothixene hydrochloride (Navane)

---

2. Monitor for extrapyramidal syndrome
3. Monitor for symptoms of neuroleptic malignant syndrome
4. Monitor urine output
5. Monitor serum glucose
6. Note that the client taking an antipsychotic medication may require long-term medication for parkinsonian symptoms
7. Administer the medication with food or milk to decrease gastric irritation
8. For oral use, the liquid form might be preferred because some clients hide tablets in the mouth to avoid taking them
9. Note that the absorption rate is faster with the liquid form
10. Avoid skin contact with the liquid concentrate to prevent contact dermatitis
11. Protect the liquid concentrate from light
12. Dilute the liquid concentrate with fruit juice
13. Inform the client that a full therapeutic effect of the medication may not be evident for 3 to 6 weeks following initiation of therapy; however, an observable therapeutic response may be apparent after 7 to 10 days
14. Inform the client that phenothiazines may cause a harmless pinkish to red-brown urine color
15. Instruct the client to use sunscreen, hats, and protective clothing when outdoors
16. Instruct the client to avoid alcohol or other CNS depressants
17. Instruct the client to change positions slowly to avoid orthostatic hypotension

18. Instruct the client to report signs of agranulocytosis, including sore throat, fever, and malaise
19. Instruct the client to report signs of liver dysfunction, including jaundice, malaise, fever, and right upper abdominal pain
20. When antipsychotics are discontinued, the medication dosage should be reduced gradually to avoid sudden recurrence of psychotic symptoms

▲ **VIII. NEUROLEPTIC MALIGNANT SYNDROME**

A. Description
   1. A potentially fatal syndrome that may occur at any time during therapy with neuroleptic medications (antipsychotic or antischizophrenic medications)
   2. Although it is rare, it is more commonly seen at the initiation of therapy, after the client is changed from one medication to another, after a dosage increase, or when a combination of medications is used

B. Assessment
   1. Dyspnea or tachypnea
   2. Tachycardia or irregular pulse rate
   3. Fever
   4. High or low blood pressure
   5. Increased sweating
   6. Loss of bladder control
   7. Skeletal muscle rigidity
   8. Pale skin
   9. Excessive weakness or fatigue
   10. Altered level of consciousness
   11. Seizures
   12. Severe extrapyramidal side effects
   13. Difficulty swallowing
   14. Excessive salivation
   15. Oculogyric crisis
   16. Dyskinesia
   17. Elevated WBC count
   18. Elevated liver function tests
   19. Elevated creatinine phosphokinase (CPK) level

C. Implementation
   1. Notify the physician
   2. Monitor vital signs
   3. Initiate safety and seizure precautions
   4. Discontinue the neuroleptic medication
   5. Monitor LOC
   6. Administer antipyretics as prescribed
   7. Use a cooling blanket to lower the body temperature
   8. Monitor electrolytes and administer IV fluids as prescribed

IX. MEDICATIONS TO TREAT ATTENTION DEFICIT HYPERACTIVITY DISORDER (ADHD) (Box 74-9)

A. Children with ADHD may require medication to reduce hyperactive behavior and lengthen attention span

---

BOX 74-9

Medications to Treat Attention Deficit Hyperactivity Disorder (ADHD)

Amphetamine
Dextroamphetamine (Dexedrine)
Methamphetamine (Desoxyn)
Methylphenidate (Ritalin)
Pemoline (Cylert)

B. Medications that are most effective in controlling this disorder are CNS stimulants
C. CNS stimulants, which increase agitation and activity in adults, have a calming effect on children with ADHD and increase alertness and sensitivity to stimuli
D. Implementation
   1. Monitor for CNS side effects
   2. Instruct the client and the parents that over-the-counter medications need to be avoided
   3. Instruct the client and the parents that the last dose of the day should be taken at least 6 hours before bedtime (14 hours for extended-released forms) to prevent insomnia
   4. Monitor height and weight (particularly in children)
   5. Reinforce that several weeks of therapy may be necessary before the therapeutic effect can be evaluated
   6. Instruct the client and the parents that a drug-free period may be prescribed to allow growth of the child if the medication has caused growth retardation
   7. Methylphenidate (Ritalin) should be taken on an empty stomach, 30 to 45 minutes before a meal or snack

X. MEDICATIONS TO TREAT ALZHEIMER'S DISEASE

A. Acetylcholinesterase inhibitors may be used to treat Alzheimer's disease to improve cognitive functions in the early stages
B. Donepezil (Aricept)
   1. A reversible inhibitor of acetylcholinesterase
   2. Used to treat mild to moderate dementia of Alzheimer's disease
   3. Common side effects include nausea and diarrhea
   4. Can slow the heart rate through its vagotonic effect
C. Tacrine (Cognex)
   1. A centrally acting acetylcholinesterase inhibitor
   2. Used to treat mild to moderate dementia of Alzheimer's disease
   3. Side effects include ataxia, loss of appetite, nausea, vomiting, and diarrhea

4. An adverse effect is hepatotoxicity; liver function studies need to be monitored

PRACTICE QUESTIONS

1. A client who is receiving lithium carbonate (Lithobid) complains of loose, watery stools and difficulty walking. The nurse would expect the serum lithium level to be which of the following?
   1. 0.7 mEq/L
   2. 1.0 mEq/L
   3. 1.3 mEq/L
   4. 1.8 mEq/L

2. A nurse is teaching a client who is being started on imipramine hydrochloride (Tofranil) about the medication. The nurse informs the client that the maximum desired effects may:
   1. Start during the first week of administration
   2. Start during the second week of administration
   3. Not occur for 2 to 3 weeks after the start of administration
   4. Not occur until after a month after the start of administration

3. A client who is receiving thioridazine hydrochloride (Mellaril) complains that he feels very faint when trying to get out of bed in the morning. The nurse recognizes this complaint as a symptom of which of the following?
   1. Psychosomatic symptoms
   2. Cardiac dysrhythmias
   3. Respiratory insufficiency
   4. Postural hypotension

4. A client receiving tricyclic antidepressants arrives at the mental health clinic. Which observation would indicate that the client is correctly following the medication plan?
   1. The client reports sleeping 12 hours per night and 3 to 4 hours during the day
   2. The client arrives at the clinic neat and appropriate in appearance
   3. The client reports not having gone to work for this past week
   4. The client complains of not being able to "do anything" anymore

5. A nurse is performing a follow-up teaching session with a client discharged 1 month ago. The client is taking fluoxetine (Prozac). What information would be important for the nurse to obtain during this client visit about the side effects related to the medication?
   1. Problems with excessive sweating
   2. Gastrointestinal (GI) dysfunctions
   3. Cardiovascular symptoms
   4. Problems with mouth dryness

6. A client who has been taking buspirone hydrochloride (BuSpar) for 1 month returns to the clinic for a follow-up assessment. A nurse determines that the medication is effective if the absence of which manifestation(s) has occurred?
   1. Alcohol withdrawal symptoms
   2. Paranoid thought process
   3. Rapid heartbeat or anxiety
   4. Thought broadcasting or delusions

7. A client taking lithium carbonate (Eskalith) reports vomiting, abdominal pain, diarrhea, blurred vision, tinnitus, and tremors. The client's lithium level is 2.5 mEq/L. The nurse interprets this level as which of the following?
   1. Normal
   2. Slightly above normal
   3. Excessively below normal
   4. Toxic

8. A hospitalized client is placed on chloral hydrate (Noctec). A nurse includes which action in the plan of care?
   1. Monitor apical heart rate every 2 hours
   2. Monitor blood pressure every 4 hours
   3. Instruct the client to call for ambulation assistance
   4. Clear a path to the bathroom at bedtime

9. A home health nurse visits a client. The client gives the nurse a bottle of clomipramine hydrochloride (Anafranil), and the nurse notes that the medication has not been taken by the client for the last 2 months. What behaviors observed in the client would validate noncompliance with this medication?
   1. Frequent handwashing with hot, soapy water
   2. Complaints of hunger and fatigue
   3. A pulse rate below 60 beats per minute
   4. Complaints of insomnia

10. A mental health clinic nurse is discussing the past week's activities with a client receiving amitriptyline hydrochloride (Elavil). The nurse evaluates that the medication is most effective for this client if the client reports which of the following?
    1. Ability to get to work on time each day
    2. Having difficulty concentrating on an activity
    3. Sleeping 14 to 16 hours a day
    4. Decrease in appetite

11. A client with schizophrenia has been started on medication therapy with haloperidol (Haldol). A nurse determines that the client is experiencing the intended effects of the medication if which of the following client behaviors is observed?
    1. Decreased appetite and food intake
    2. Taking sips of water for dry mouth
    3. Presence of a fixed stare
    4. Absence of delusional statements

12. A hospitalized client has begun taking bupropion (Wellbutrin) as an antidepressant agent. The nurse monitors this client for which adverse effect that indicates that the client is taking an excessive amount of medication?
    1. Dizziness when getting upright

2. Seizure activity
3. Increased weight
4. Constipation

13. A client has been started on medication therapy with alprazolam (Xanax). When a nurse teaches the client that the medication should not be discontinued abruptly, the client asks why. The nurse incorporates which of the following when formulating a reply?
    1. Rebound central nervous system (CNS) excitation could occur and cause feelings of restlessness and irritability
    2. It will make the medication much less effective if it must be restarted
    3. The client is likely to become resistant to medication effects
    4. The client is likely to suffer irreversible damage to the kidneys

14. A client's medication sheet contains an order for sertraline hydrochloride (Zoloft). To ensure safe administration of the medication, the nurse would administer the dose:
    1. Evenly spaced around the clock
    2. At the same time each evening
    3. When the client has an empty stomach
    4. On an as-needed basis when the client complains of depression

15. A client with schizophrenia has been started on medication therapy with clozapine (Clozaril). A nurse assesses the results of which laboratory study to monitor for adverse effects from this medication?
    1. White blood cell (WBC) count
    2. Platelet count
    3. Blood glucose
    4. Liver function studies

16. A client is scheduled for discharge and will be taking phenobarbital sodium (Luminal) for an extended period of time. A nurse would place highest priority on teaching the client which of the following points that directly relates to client safety?
    1. Avoid drinking alcohol while taking this medication
    2. Take the medication only with meals
    3. Take medication at the same time each day
    4. Use a dose container to help prevent missed doses

17. A 26-year-old female client with schizophrenia has been prescribed chlorpromazine (Thorazine). The client calls the mental health clinic and tells a nurse that her urine has become dark in color but that she has no other urinary symptoms. What does the nurse tell the client?
    1. To increase the intake of acid ash foods and liquids
    2. To seek treatment for a urinary tract infection
    3. That this is an expected side effect of the medication
    4. That this indicates medication toxicity

18. A client is receiving fluphenazine hydrochloride (Prolixin) on a daily basis. A nurse would teach the client to do which of the following to minimize common side effects of this medication?
    1. Have the blood pressure checked once a week
    2. Monitor the temperature on a daily basis
    3. Eat snacks at mid-morning and at bedtime
    4. Use hard sour candy or sugarless gum

19. A nurse is describing the medication side effects to a client who is taking oxazepam (Serax). The nurse incorporates in discussions with the client the need to do which of the following?
    1. Take antidiarrheal agents if diarrhea occurs
    2. Rest if the heart begins to beat rapidly
    3. Consume a low-fiber diet
    4. Increase fluids and bulk in the diet

20. A nurse is administering thioridazine hydrochloride (Mellaril) in oral concentrate form. The nurse prepares this medication by mixing it in which of the following just before giving it to the client?
    1. Milk
    2. Fruit juice
    3. Pudding
    4. Applesauce

CRITICAL THINKING: FREE-TEXT ENTRY

A hospitalized client is started on phenelzine sulfate (Nardil) for the treatment of depression. At lunchtime, a tray is delivered to the client that contains yogurt, tossed salad, crackers, and oatmeal cookies. Which of these food items will a nurse remove from the client's tray?

Answer: _____

ANSWERS

1. **4**

Rationale: The therapeutic serum level of lithium is 1.0 to 1.5 mEq/L for clients with acute mania and 0.6 to 1.2 mEq/L for maintenance levels. Serum lithium concentrations of 1.5 to 2.0 mEq/L may produce vomiting, diarrhea, drowsiness, incoordination, muscle weakness, and slurred speech.

Test-Taking Strategy: Focusing on the client's symptoms will assist in answering this question. Review the normal lithium level and signs of toxicity if you had difficulty with this question.
Level of Cognitive Ability: Analysis
Client Needs: Physiological Integrity
Integrated Concept/Process: Nursing Process/Analysis

Content Area: Pharmacology
Reference: Wilson, B., Shannon, M., & Stang, C. (2000). *Nurses' drug guide 2000*. Stamford, Conn.: Appleton & Lange, p. 806.

2. **3**

Rationale: The maximum therapeutic effects of imipramine hydrochloride may not occur for 2 to 3 weeks after the antidepressant therapy has been initiated.

Test-Taking Strategy: Focus on the key word "maximum." Recalling that it takes 2 to 3 weeks for a maximum therapeutic effect to occur with most antidepressants will direct you to option 3. Review this medication if you had difficulty with this question.

Level of Cognitive Ability: Application
Client Needs: Health Promotion and Maintenance
Integrated Concept/Process: Teaching/Learning
Content Area: Pharmacology
Reference: Hodgson, B., & Kizior, R. (2001). *Saunders nursing drug handbook 2001*. Philadelphia: W. B. Saunders, p. 522.

3. **4**

Rationale: Mellaril, an antipsychotic, can cause postural hypotension. The client needs to be taught to get out of bed slowly and to rise from a sitting position slowly because of this untoward effect related to the medication. Options 1, 2, and 3 are not related to this medication.

Test-Taking Strategy: Use the process of elimination. Note the key words "feels very faint"; this should direct you to option 4. Review the side effects of this medication if you had difficulty with this question.

Level of Cognitive Ability: Analysis
Client Needs: Psychosocial Integrity
Integrated Concept/Process: Nursing Process/Assessment
Content Area: Pharmacology
Reference: Hodgson, B., & Kizior, R. (2001). *Saunders nursing drug handbook 2001*. Philadelphia: W. B. Saunders, p. 987.

4. **2**

Rationale: Depressed individuals will sleep for long periods, are not able to go to work, and feel as if they cannot "do anything." After they have had some therapeutic effect from their medication, they will report the resolution of many of these complaints and demonstrate an improvement in their appearance.

Test-Taking Strategy: Use the process of elimination. The client's behaviors or reports identified in options 1, 3, and 4 are all symptoms of depression. The improvement in appearance indicates a therapeutic response to the medication and, so, compliance with the medication regime. Review the expected effect of a tricyclic antidepressant if you had difficulty with this question.

Level of Cognitive Ability: Analysis
Client Needs: Physiological Integrity
Integrated Concept/Process: Nursing Process/Evaluation
Content Area: Pharmacology
Reference: Cleveland, L., Aschenbrenner, D., Venable, S., & Yensen, J. (1999). *Nursing management in drug therapy*. Philadelphia: Lippincott, p. 306.

5. **2**

Rationale: The most common side effects related to this medication include central nervous system and GI system dysfunction. Fluoxetine affects the GI system by causing nausea and vomiting, cramping, and diarrhea. Excessive sweating, dry mouth, and cardiovascular symptoms are not associated side effects of this medication.

Test-Taking Strategy: Use the process of elimination. Recalling that this medication causes GI problems will direct you to option 2. Review the side effects related to this medication if you had difficulty with this question.

Level of Cognitive Ability: Application
Client Needs: Physiological Integrity
Integrated Concept/Process: Nursing Process/Assessment
Content Area: Pharmacology
Reference: Clark, J., Queener, S., & Karb, V. (2000). *Pharmacologic basis of nursing practice* (6th ed.). St. Louis: Mosby, p. 702.

6. **3**

Rationale: Buspirone hydrochloride is not recommended for the treatment of drug or alcohol withdrawal, thought disorders, or schizophrenia. Buspirone hydrochloride is most often indicated for the treatment of anxiety and aggression.

Test-Taking Strategy: Use the process of elimination. Recalling that buspirone hydrochloride is an antianxiety agent will direct you to the correct option. Review the action and use of this medication if you had difficulty with this question.

Level of Cognitive Ability: Analysis
Client Needs: Physiological Integrity
Integrated Concept/Process: Nursing Process/Evaluation
Content Area: Pharmacology
Reference: Clark, J., Queener, S., & Karb, V. (2000). *Pharmacologic basis of nursing practice* (6th ed.). St. Louis: Mosby, p. 672.

7. **4**

Rationale: Maintenance serum levels are 0.6 to 1.2 mEq/L. Symptoms of toxicity begin to appear at levels of 1.5 mEq/L to 2.0 mEq/L. Lithium toxicity requires immediate medical attention with lavage and possible peritoneal dialysis or hemodialysis.

Test-Taking Strategy: Use the process of elimination. Recalling that the high end of the maintenance level is 1.2 mEq/L will direct you to option 4. Review the maintenance level and signs of toxicity if you had difficulty with this question.

Level of Cognitive Ability: Analysis
Client Needs: Physiological Integrity
Integrated Concept/Process: Nursing Process/Analysis
Content Area: Pharmacology
Reference: Clark, J., Queener, S., & Karb, V. (2000). *Pharmacologic basis of nursing practice* (6th ed.). St. Louis: Mosby, p. 707.

8. **3**

Rationale: Chloral hydrate is a sedative. This medication does not affect cardiac function. Blood pressure changes are not significant with the use of this medication. The client should call for assistance to the bathroom at night. Additionally, there may be residual daytime sedation; therefore, the client is also instructed to call for ambulation assistance during the daytime hours.

Test-Taking Strategy: Use the process of elimination. Recalling that this medication is a sedative will easily direct you to option 3. Review nursing considerations related to this medication if you had difficulty with this question.

Level of Cognitive Ability: Application
Client Needs: Safe, Effective Care Environment
Integrated Concept/Process: Nursing Process/Planning
Content Area: Pharmacology

Reference: Deglin, J. & Vallerand, A. (2001). *Davis's drug guide for nurses* (7th ed.). Philadelphia: F. A. Davis, p. 185.

9. 1

Rationale: Clomipramine hydrochloride is a tricyclic antidepressant used in the treatment of obsessive-compulsive disorder. Weight gain and tachycardia are side effects of this medication. Sedation sometimes occurs, and insomnia is a rare side effect.

Test-Taking Strategy: Recalling that this medication is a tricyclic antidepressant used in the treatment of obsessive-compulsive disorder will direct you to option 1. Review the purpose and use of this medication if you had difficulty with this question.

Level of Cognitive Ability: Analysis
Client Needs: Physiological Integrity
Integrated Concept/Process: Nursing Process/Evaluation
Content Area: Pharmacology
Reference: Deglin, J., & Vallerand, A. (2001). *Davis's drug guide for nurses* (7th ed.). Philadelphia: F. A. Davis, p. 209.

10. 1

Rationale: Depressed individuals will sleep for extended periods, have a change in appetite, are unable to go to work, and have difficulty concentrating. They may also experience increased fatigue, feelings of guilt or worthlessness, loss of interest in activities, and possible suicidal tendencies. After they have had some therapeutic effect from their medication, they will report the resolution of many of these complaints and demonstrate an improvement in their appearance.

Test-Taking Strategy: Use the process of elimination. Note the key words "most effective." The symptoms stated in options 2, 3, and 4 are all symptoms of depression. The ability to report to work indicates a therapeutic response to the medication. Review the action and expected effects of amitriptyline if you had difficulty with this question.

Level of Cognitive Ability: Analysis
Client Needs: Physiological Integrity
Integrated Concept/Process: Nursing Process/Evaluation
Content Area: Pharmacology
Reference: Hodgson, B. & Kizior, R. (2001). *Saunders nursing drug handbook 2001.* Philadelphia: W. B. Saunders, p. 49.

11. 4

Rationale: Haloperidol (Haldol) is an antipsychotic used in the management of psychotic disorder. Hallucinations, delusions, and altered thought processes are characteristics of a psychotic disorder and should decrease with effective treatment. Fixed stare (option 3) and dry mouth (option 2) are side effects of therapy. Option 1 is unrelated to this medication.

Test-Taking Strategy: Use the process of elimination. Recalling that this medication is an antipsychotic will direct you to option 4. Review the purpose of this medication if you had difficulty with this question.

Level of Cognitive Ability: Analysis
Client Needs: Physiological Integrity
Integrated Concept/Process: Nursing Process/Evaluation
Content Area: Pharmacology
Reference: Hodgson, B., & Kizior, R. (2001). *Saunders nursing drug handbook 2001.* Philadelphia: W. B. Saunders, p. 486.

12. 2

Rationale: The nurse monitors for signs of toxicity. Seizure activity is common in bupropion dosages of more than 450

mg daily. This medication does not cause significant orthostatic blood pressure changes. Weight gain is an occasional side effect, and constipation is a common side effect of this medication.

Test-Taking Strategy: Use the process of elimination. Note the key words "adverse effect" and "excessive amount"; these key words will direct you to option 2. Review this medication if you had difficulty with this question.

Level of Cognitive Ability: Analysis
Client Needs: Physiological Integrity
Integrated Concept/Process: Nursing Process/Evaluation
Content Area: Pharmacology
Reference: Hodgson, B., & Kizior, R. (2001). *Saunders nursing drug handbook 2001.* Philadelphia: W. B. Saunders, p. 130.

13. 1

Rationale: The abrupt withdrawal of alprazolam could result in seizure activity from rebound CNS excitation. All clients receiving this medication should be warned of this danger. The other options are incorrect.

Test-Taking Strategy: Use the process of elimination. Remember that options that are similar are not likely to be correct. With this in mind, eliminate options 2 and 3 first. From the remaining options, recalling the adverse effects will direct you to option 1. If this question was difficult, review the adverse effects associated with this medication.

Level of Cognitive Ability: Application
Client Needs: Health Promotion and Maintenance
Integrated Concept/Process: Teaching/Learning
Content Area: Pharmacology
Reference: Hodgson, B., & Kizior, R. (2001). *Saunders nursing drug handbook 2001.* Philadelphia: W. B. Saunders, p. 28.

14. 2

Rationale: Zoloft is classified as an antidepressant. It is generally administered once every 24 hours. It may be administered in the morning or evening, but evening administration may be preferable, because drowsiness is a side effect. The medication may be administered without food or with food if gastrointestinal distress occurs. It is not ordered for PRN use.

Test-Taking Strategy: Use the process of elimination. Recalling that this medication is administered on a daily basis will direct you to option 2. Review this medication if you had difficulty with this question.

Level of Cognitive Ability: Application
Client Needs: Physiological Integrity
Integrated Concept/Process: Nursing Process/Implementation
Content Area: Pharmacology
Reference: Deglin, J., & Vallerand, A. (2001). *Davis's drug guide for nurses* (7th ed.). Philadelphia: F. A. Davis, p. 917.

15. 1

Rationale: The client taking clozapine may experience agranulocytosis, which is monitored for by reviewing the results of the WBC count. Treatment is interrupted if the WBC count drops below 3000/mm^3. Agranulocytosis could be fatal if undetected and untreated. The other options are not specifically related to the use of this medication.

Test-Taking Strategy: Use the process of elimination. Recalling that this medication causes agranulocytosis will direct you to option 1. Review the adverse effects of this medication if you had difficulty with this question.

Level of Cognitive Ability: Analysis
Client Needs: Physiological Integrity
Integrated Concept/Process: Nursing Process/Assessment
Content Area: Pharmacology
Reference: Kuhn, M. (1998). *Pharmacotherapeutics a nursing process approach* (4th ed.). Philadelphia: F. A. Davis, p. 395.

16. **1**
Rationale: Phenobarbital sodium is an anticonvulsant and a hypnotic agent. The client should avoid taking any other central nervous system depressants (such as alcohol) while taking this medication. The medication may be given without regard to meals. Taking the medication at the same time each day enhances compliance and maintains more stable blood levels of the medication. Using a dose container or "pill box" may be helpful for some clients.
Test-Taking Strategy: Use the process of elimination. Focus on the issue of client safety. Note the key words "highest priority"; this tells you that more than one or all of the options may be partially or totally correct and that you must prioritize your answer. Remember, alcohol should not be consumed when taking hypnotics. Review client teaching points related to this medication if you had difficulty with this question.
Level of Cognitive Ability: Analysis
Client Needs: Health Promotion and Maintenance
Integrated Concept/Process: Teaching/Learning
Content Area: Pharmacology
Reference: Hodgson, B., & Kizior, R. (2001). *Nursing drug handbook 2001*. Philadelphia: W. B. Saunders, pp. 815-816.

17. **3**
Rationale: Chlorpromazine is an antipsychotic medication. A side effect of this medication is that the urine may darken in color. The client should be aware that this effect is harmless. The other options are incorrect.
Test-Taking Strategy: Use the process of elimination. Eliminate options 1 and 2 first, because the question states that the client exhibits no other urinary symptoms. From the remaining options, it is necessary to know the side effects of this medication. Review the side effects of this medication if you had difficulty with this question.
Level of Cognitive Ability: Application
Client Needs: Physiological Integrity
Integrated Concept/Process: Nursing Process/Implementation
Content Area: Pharmacology
Reference: Hodgson, B., & Kizior, R. (2001). *Nursing drug handbook 2001*. Philadelphia: W. B. Saunders, p. 213.

18. **4**
Rationale: Dry mouth is a common side effect. Frequent mouth rinsing with water, sucking on hard candy, and chewing sugarless gum will alleviate this common side effect. Hypotension and hypertension are rare side effects of fluphenazine. Mild leukopenia may occur, but the temperature does not need to be taken daily. Weight gain is a common side effect, and frequent snacks will worsen the problem.
Test-Taking Strategy: Use the process of elimination, and note the key words "common side effect." Eliminate options 1 and 2, because they are assessments rather than interventions; as such, they cannot minimize a side effect. From the remaining options, it is necessary to recall that dry mouth is a side effect. Review the common side effects

related to this medication if you had difficulty with this question.
Level of Cognitive Ability: Application
Client Needs: Health Promotion and Maintenance
Integrated Concept/Process: Teaching/Learning
Content Area: Pharmacology
Reference: Hodgson, B., & Kizior, R. (2001). *Nursing drug handbook 2001*. Philadelphia: W. B. Saunders, p. 435.

19. **4**
Rationale: Oxazepam causes constipation, and the client is instructed to increase fluids and bulk (high fiber) in the diet. If the heart begins to beat fast, the physician is notified, because this could indicate overdose. Additionally, diarrhea could indicate an incomplete intestinal obstruction, and if this occurs, the physician is notified.
Test-Taking Strategy: Use the process of elimination. Recalling that constipation is a side effect of this medication will direct you to option 4. Review the side effects and adverse effects of oxazepam if you had difficulty with this question.
Level of Cognitive Ability: Application
Client Needs: Health Promotion and Maintenance
Integrated Concept/Process: Teaching/Learning
Content Area: Pharmacology
Reference: Hodgson, B., & Kizior, R. (2001). *Nursing drug handbook 2001*. Philadelphia: W. B. Saunders, p. 779.

20. **2**
Rationale: The oral concentrate form of Mellaril should be diluted in water or fruit juice just before administration to the client. The other options are incorrect.
Test-Taking Strategy: Knowledge about the nursing considerations related to the administration of Mellaril is required to answer this question. If you are unfamiliar with this medication, review the concepts related to the administration of this medication.
Level of Cognitive Ability: Application
Client Needs: Physiological Integrity
Integrated Concept/Process: Nursing Process/Implementation
Content Area: Pharmacology
Reference: Wilson, B., Shannon, M., & Stang, C. (2000). *Nurses drug guide 2000*. Stamford, CT: Appleton & Lange, p. 1359.

CRITICAL THINKING: FREE-TEXT ENTRY

Answer: Yogurt
Rationale: Phenelzine sulfate is a monoamine oxidase inhibitor (MAOI). The client should avoid taking in foods that are high in tyramine. Use of these foods could trigger a potentially fatal hypertensive crisis. Foods to avoid include yogurt, aged cheeses, smoked or processed meats, red wines, and fruits such as avocados, raisins, or figs.
Test-Taking Strategy: Recall that phenelzine sulfate is an MAOI and that foods high in tyramine need to be avoided. Next, from the food items listed in the question, identify the food that contains tyramine. Review the food items to avoid with MAOIs if you had difficulty with this question.
Level of Cognitive Ability: Application
Client Needs: Physiological Integrity
Integrated Concept/Process: Nursing Process/Implementation
Content Area: Pharmacology
Reference: Fortinash, K., & Holoday-Worret, P. (2000). *Psychiatric mental health nursing* (2nd ed.). St. Louis: Mosby, p. 285.

REFERENCES

Cleveland, L., Aschenbrenner, D., Venable, S., & Yensen, J. (1999). *Nursing management in drug therapy.* Philadelphia: Lippincott.

Corbett, J. (2000). *Laboratory tests and diagnostic procedures* (5th ed.). Upper Saddle River, N.J.: Prentice-Hall.

Fortinash, K., & Holoday-Worret, P. (2000). *Psychiatric mental health nursing* (2nd ed.). St. Louis: Mosby.

Deglin, J., & Vallerand, A. (2001). *Davis's drug guide for nurses* (7th ed.). Philadelphia: F.A. Davis.

Hodgson, B., & Kizior, R. (2001). *Saunders nursing drug handbook 2001.* Philadelphia: W.B. Saunders.

Kuhn, M. (1998). *Pharmacotherapeutics: A nursing process approach* (4th ed.). Philadelphia: F.A. Davis.

Wilson, B., Shannon, M., & Stang, C. (2000). *Nurses drug guide 2000.* Stamford, Conn.: Appleton & Lange.

The Gerontological Client

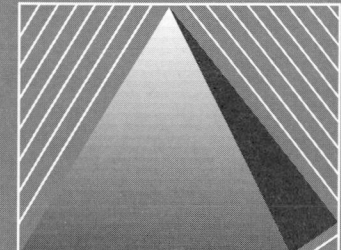

PYRAMID TERMS

abuse   The willful infliction of pain, injury, or mental anguish. Unreasonable confinement or willful deprivation of services, including medical care. Abuse can include failure to prevent injury, verbal assaults, the demand to perform demeaning tasks, theft, or mismanagement of personal belongings.

aging   The biopsychosocial process of change occurring between birth and death.

Alzheimer's disease   An irreversible form of senile dementia. Individuals with Alzheimer's disease experience cognitive deterioration and progressive loss of ability to carry out the activities of daily living. The client experiences a steady decline in physical and mental functioning that frequently requires caregivers to seek outside resources for assistance.

dementia   Organic syndrome identified by gradual and progressive deterioration in intellectual functioning. Long- and short-term memory loss occurs, with impairment in judgment, abstract thinking, problem-solving ability, and behavior. Results in a self-care deficit. The most common type of dementia is Alzheimer's disease.

depression   A functional disorder of mood that is not linked with aging. It may be precipitated by losses related to aging. Depression can be manifested by cognitive impairment or may be the cause of a decline in mental status. Depression can be identified by feelings of sadness, hopelessness, and worthlessness, and decreased interest in activities.

exploitation   Illegal or improper use of an individual's resources.

gerontology   The study of the process of aging.

neglect   The lack of provision of services necessary for physical or mental health.

self-neglect   A person's choosing to avoid medical care or other services that could promote his or her optimal functioning. Unless declared legally incompetent, an individual has the right to refuse care.

◤ PYRAMID TO SUCCESS

The Pyramid to Success focuses on safety issues, the prevention of injury, restraints, abuse and neglect, depression, dementia, and Alzheimer's disease. Pyramid points also focus on methods of communication, particularly when deficits exist. When a question is presented on the NCLEX-RN, if an age is identified in the case of the question, note the age. If the age represents an elderly client, consider gerontological nursing concepts when answering the question. The Integrated Concepts and Processes addressed in this unit include Nursing Process, Caring, Communication and Documentation, Cultural Awareness, Self-Care, and Teaching/Learning.

CLIENT NEEDS
Safe, Effective Care Environment

Accident prevention
Advance directives
Client rights and advocacy
Confidentiality
Consultation with members of the health care team
Continuity of care
Establishing priorities
Ethical practice
Informed consent
Safety
The use of restraints

Health Promotion and Maintenance

Aging process
Client and family education
Expected body image changes
Family systems
Lifestyle choices
Prevention and early detection of disorders associated with aging
The safe use of medications
The importance of follow-up visits to the physician

Psychosocial Integrity

Abuse and neglect
Adjustment to potential deterioration in physical and mental health and well-being

Changes and adjustment in role function
Coping mechanisms
End of life
Grief and loss
Loss of the quantity and quality of relationships
Religious and spiritual resources
Sensory/perceptual alterations
Situational role changes
Threat to independent functioning
Use of resources for the client and family

Physiological Integrity

Alterations in body systems and the related risks
  resulting from the aging process
Assistive devices
Elimination
Mobility and immobility
Nutrition and oral hydration
Personal hygiene

Rest and sleep
Safe medication administration

REFERENCES

Harkreader, H. (2000). *Fundamentals of nursing: Caring and clinical judgment.* Philadelphia: W.B. Saunders.

Ignatavicius, D., Workman, M., & Mishler, M. (1999). *Medical-surgical nursing across the health care continuum* (3rd ed.). Philadelphia: W.B. Saunders.

Leuckenotte, A. (2000). Gerontologic Nursing (2nd ed.). St. Louis: Mosby.

Lewis, S., Heitkemper, M., & Dirksen, S. (2000). *Medical-surgical nursing: Assessment and management of clinical problems* (5th ed.). St. Louis: Mosby.

National Council of State Boards of Nursing (eds.) (2000). *Test Plan for the National Council Licensure Examination for Registered Nurses.* Chicago: Author.

Potter, P., & Perry, A. (2001). *Fundamentals of nursing* (5th ed.). St. Louis: Mosby.

Tyson R. (1999). *Gerontological nursing care.* Philadelphia: W.B. Saunders.

Care of the Gerontological Client

I. PHYSIOLOGICAL CHANGES OF AGING

A. Integumentary system
1. Loss of pigment in hair and skin
2. Increased nail thickness and decreased nail growth
3. Thinning of the epidermis
4. Easy bruising and tearing of the skin
5. Reduction in blood flow to the skin
6. Decreased skin turgor
7. Loss of elasticity and subcutaneous fat
8. Wrinkling of the skin
9. Dry, itchy, cracked skin
10. Inadequate sweating
11. Seborrheic dermatitis and keratosis formation

B. Neurological system
1. Changes in mental status
2. Slowed reflexes
3. Loss of balance
4. Dizziness and syncope
5. Slight tremors
6. Difficulty with fine motor movement
7. Changes in sleep patterns, such as decreased total sleep with earlier risings
8. Increased susceptibility to hypothermia and hyperthermia

C. Musculoskeletal system
1. Posture and stature changes causing a decrease in height
2. Kyphosis of the dorsal spine
3. Muscle mass decreases and muscles atrophy
4. Joint capsule components deteriorate
5. Decreased mobility, range of motion, flexibility, and stability
6. Increased stiffness
7. Decrease in physical strength
8. Decrease in muscular coordination
9. Change of gait, with shortened step and wider base
10. Increased brittleness of the bones
11. Decrease in deep tendon reflexes

D. Cardiopulmonary system
1. Energy and endurance diminish
2. Lowered tolerance to exercise
3. Decreased stretch and compliance of the chest wall
4. Decreased rib mobility and lung tone
5. Decreased strength and function of respiratory muscles
6. Decreased depth of respirations and oxygen intake
7. Decreased ability to cough and expectorate sputum
8. Decreased size and number of alveoli
9. Decreased compliance of the heart muscle
10. Heart valves become thicker and more rigid
11. Decreased efficiency of blood return to the heart and decreased cardiac output
12. Decreased resting heart rate
13. Increased blood pressure
14. Susceptible to postural hypotension

E. Hematological and immune systems
1. Hemoglobin and hematocrit levels remain within normal range but average toward the low end of normal
2. Lymphocyte counts tend to be low
3. Decreased resistance to infection and disease
4. Prone to increased blood clotting

F. Gastrointestinal system
1. Decreased appetite, thirst, and oral intake
2. Decreased need for calories
3. Digestive disturbances
4. Decreased stomach-emptying time
5. Increased tendency toward constipation

6. Tooth loss
7. Difficulty in chewing and swallowing food
8. Decreased absorption of carbohydrates, proteins, fats, and vitamins
9. Decreased lean body weight

G. Endocrine system
1. Decreased secretion of hormones, with specific changes related to each hormone function
2. Decreased metabolic rate
3. Decreased glucose tolerance
4. Resistance to insulin in peripheral tissues

H. Renal system
1. Decreased kidney size, function, and ability to concentrate urine
2. Decreased glomerular filtration rate
3. Decreased capacity of the bladder
4. Increased residual urine and increased incidence of infection and incontinence
5. Impaired medication excretion

I. Reproductive system
1. Decreased testosterone production and decreased size of testes
2. Changes in the prostate leading to urinary problems
3. Decreased secretion of hormones with the cessation of menses
4. Vaginal changes, including decreased muscle tone and lubrication

J. Special senses
1. Decreased visual acuity
2. Decreased accommodation in eyes
3. Decreased peripheral vision and increased sensitivity to glare
4. Increased adjustment time to changes in light
5. Presbyopia and cataract formation
6. Possible loss of hearing ability
7. Inability to discern taste of food
8. Decreased smell acuity
9. Changes in touch
10. Decreased pain awareness

II. PSYCHOSOCIAL ASPECTS OF AGING (Box 75-1)

A. Adjustment to retirement and loss of income
B. Changes in role function
C. Coping with change and new life situations
D. Changes in social life
E. Diminished quantity and quality of relationships
F. Coping with loss
G. Adjustment to potential deterioration in physical and mental health and well-being
H. Threat to independent functioning
I. Loss of skills and competencies developed early in life

III. ELDER ABUSE AND NEGLECT

A. Description
1. Involves physical, psychological, financial, and social **abuse**

BOX 75-1
Concerns of the Older Population
Adequate income
Functional limitations from chronic illness or disability
Ability to maintain independence
Becoming a burden to loved ones
Isolation
Dependence on governmental and social systems
Access to social support systems

2. Can involve a violation of the client's rights
3. Individuals at most risk include those who are dependent because of immobility or altered mental status
4. Factors that contribute to **abuse** and **neglect** include long-standing family violence, caregiver stress, and the individual's increasing dependence

B. Types
1. **Abuse**
   a. The willful infliction of pain, injury, or mental anguish
   b. Unreasonable confinement or willful deprivation of services, including medical care
   c. Can include failure to prevent injury, verbal assaults, the demand to perform demeaning tasks, theft, or mismanagement of personal belongings
2. **Neglect:** The lack of provision of services necessary for physical or mental health
3. **Self-neglect**
   a. The person chooses to avoid medical care or other services that would promote optimal functioning
   b. Unless declared legally incompetent, an individual has the right to refuse care
4. **Exploitation:** Illegal or improper use of an individual's resources
5. Assessment of **abuse** and **neglect**
   a. Abrasions, lacerations, and bruises
   b. Burns
   c. Sprains, fractures, or dislocations
   d. Pressure sores
   e. Injuries inconsistent with history
   f. Frequent falls
   g. Untreated medical problems
   h. Inappropriate dress and poor hygiene
   i. Excessive drowsiness
   j. Overmedication or undermedication
   k. Malnutrition
   l. Dehydration
   m. Expression of fear in response to touch
6. Implementation
   a. Assess for signs of **abuse** and **neglect**
   b. Report cases of **abuse** and **neglect,** as mandated by all states

c. Initiate protective services

d. Assess for dysfunctional family systems

e. Promote family functioning and initiate appropriate contact with resources

IV. USE OF RESTRAINTS

A. Physical restraints used to prevent injury are to be avoided, and alternative methods to provide safety must be assessed prior to the use of physical restraints

B. A physician's order must be obtained for the use of restraints

C. Discuss the use of restraints with the client and family

D. Obtain client and family consent for the use of restraints

E. Use the least restrictive device for restraint

F. Use only restraints that have been manufactured as a safety restraint

G. Observe the client frequently, and monitor for alterations in skin integrity and circulation as a result of the restraints

H. Restraints need to be removed at frequent intervals (per agency policy) to assess for complications and to allow for mobility and range of motion

I. Always follow the institutional policy regarding the use of restraints

V. MEDICATIONS

A. Major problems with prescription medications include adverse affects, medication interactions, medication errors, noncompliance, and the cost

B. Determine the client's use of over-the-counter medications

C. Keep the use of medications to a minimum

D. Medication dosages are normally prescribed at one third to one half of the normal adult dosages

E. Closely monitor for adverse effects and response to therapy because of the increased risk for medication toxicity

F. Note that a common sign of an adverse reaction in the elderly is an acute change in mental status

G. Assess for medication interactions in client taking multiple medications

H. Advise the client to use one pharmacy and to notify the consulting physicians of the medications taken

I. Administration of medications
1. Place the client in a sitting position when administering medication
2. Check for mouth dryness because medication may stick and dissolve in the mouth
3. Administer liquid preparations if the client has difficulty swallowing tablets
4. Crush tablets if necessary and give with textured food (nectar, applesauce) if not contraindicated
5. Do not crush enteric-coated tablets and do not open capsules
6. If administering a suppository, do not insert suppository immediately after removing from the refrigerator
7. A suppository may take longer to dissolve because of decreased body core temperature
8. When administering parenteral medication, monitor the site because it may ooze medication or bleed because of decreased tissue elasticity
9. Do not use an immobile limb for administering parenteral medication
10. Monitor client compliance with taking prescribed medications
11. Monitor for safety in correctly taking medications
12. Use a medication cassette to facilitate proper administration of medication

VI. DEMENTIA

A. Description
1. Organic syndrome with progressive deterioration in intellectual functioning
2. Long- and short-term memory loss occurs, with impairment in judgment, abstract thinking, problem-solving ability, and behavior
3. Results in a self-care deficit
4. The most common type of **dementia** is **Alzheimer's disease**

B. **Alzheimer's disease**
1. An irreversible form of senile **dementia**
2. Individuals with **Alzheimer's disease** experience cognitive deterioration and progressive loss of ability to carry out the activities of daily living
3. The client experiences a steady decline in physical and mental functioning that frequently requires caregivers to seek outside resources for assistance

C. Assessment
1. Begins with mild memory impairment
2. The client has difficulty remembering names, appointments, and where things are
3. The client is indifferent and occasionally irritable
4. As the disease progresses, moderate memory impairment, particularly of recent events, occurs
5. The client develops a decrease in orientation, is restless, and paces about
6. As the progression of the disease continues, the client develops severely impaired cognitive function, disorientation, delusions, and agitation
7. Limb rigidity and flexion posture
8. Urinary and fecal incontinence

D. Implementation
1. Identify and reinforce retained skills
2. Assist the client and family members to manage memory deficits and behavior changes
3. Encourage the family members to express feelings about caregiving
4. Provide caregiver support and identify the resources and support groups available
5. Provide continuity of care

6. Orient the client to the environment
7. Furnish the environment with familiar possessions
8. Acknowledge the client's feelings
9. Monitor activities of daily living
10. Remind the client how to perform self-care activities
11. Maintain independence as much as possible
12. Provide consistent routines
13. Provide exercise with supervision, such as walking with an escort
14. Avoid activities that tax the memory
15. Allow plenty of time to complete a task
16. Use constant encouragement in a step-by-step approach
17. Provide mental stimulation with simple games or activities
18. Provide activities that distract and occupy time, such as listening to music, coloring, and watching TV

E. Implementation for specific behaviors
▲ 1. Wandering
   a. Provide a safe environment
   b. Prevent unsafe wandering
   c. Provide close supervision
   d. Close and secure doors
   e. Use identification bracelets and electronic surveillance devices
▲ 2. Communication
   a. Adapt to the communication level of the client
   b. Use a calm and reassuring voice
   c. Use pantomime gestures if the client is unable to understand spoken words
   d. Use slow, clear, verbal communication techniques
   e. Use short words and simple sentences
   f. Call the client by name, identify self, and wait for a response
   g. Ask only one question at a time and give one direction at a time
   h. Repeat questions if necessary, but do not rephrase because this may cause confusion in the client
   i. Stand directly in front of the client and maintain eye contact
   j. Listen and observe the emotion expressed by the client
▲ 3. Impaired judgment
   a. Eliminate throw rugs, toxic substances, dangerous electrical appliances, or any other objects that can present a risk of injury
   b. Reduce hot water heater temperature
▲ 4. Altered thought processes
   a. Orient the client frequently
   b. Place a calendar and a clock in a visible place
   c. Call the client by name
   d. Place familiar objects in the room

e. Maintain familiar routines
f. Make tasks simple and allow time for the client to complete a task
g. Allow the client to reminisce
5. Altered sleep patterns ▲
   a. Allow the client to wander in a safe place until he or she becomes tired
   b. Prevent shadows in the room
   c. Avoid the use of hypnotics and sedatives because they cause confusion and aggravate the sundown effect
6. Agitation ▲
   a. Assess the precipitant of the agitation
   b. Reassure the client
   c. Remove items that can be hazardous during the time of agitation
   d. Approach the client slowly and calmly from the front; then speak, gesture, and move slowly
   e. Use touch gently
   f. Take the client to a less stressful environment
   g. Distract the client with questions about the problem, and gradually turn the attention to something else
   h. Do not argue with the client or restrain the client

VII. DEPRESSION ▲

A. Description
   1. A functional disorder of mood that is not linked with **aging**
   2. The **depression** may be manifested by cognitive impairment or may be the cause of a decline in mental status
   3. **Depression** can be identified by feelings of sadness, hopelessness, and worthlessness, and decreased interest in activities
B. Assessment
   1. Difficulty concentrating
   2. Feelings of inadequacy and sadness
   3. Difficulty sleeping or excessive sleeping
   4. Weight gain or loss
   5. Vegetative symptoms
   6. Constipation
   7. Loss of interest in activities
   8. Decreased endurance and energy
   9. Preoccupation with physical health
   10. Thoughts of death or suicide
C. Implementation
   1. Assess for signs associated with **depression**
   2. Monitor for the risk of suicide and notify the physician
   3. Implement safety precautions for suicide risk
   4. Provide and reinforce positive experiences
   5. Provide variation in the daily schedule, but limit changes, because change is anxiety producing for the older client

6. Allow the client to talk and reminisce
7. Maintain reality
8. Initiate counseling as appropriate
9. Refer to Chapter 74 for information about the prescribed medications for **depression**

▲ VIII. PAIN
A. Description
   1. Pain can occur from numerous causes and most often occurs as a result of degenerative changes in the musculoskeletal system
   2. The failure to alleviate pain in the older client can lead to functional limitations affecting the ability to function independently
B. Assessment
   1. Agitation
   2. Moaning
   3. Crying
   4. Restlessness
   5. Verbal reporting of pain
C. Implementation
   1. Monitor the client for signs of pain
   2. Identify the pattern of pain
   3. Identify the precipitating factor(s) for the pain
   4. Monitor the impact of the pain on activities of daily living
   5. Provide pain relief through measures such as distraction, relaxation, massage, and biofeedback
   6. Administer pain medication as prescribed and instruct the client in their use
   7. Evaluate the effects of pain-reducing measures

IX. IMPAIRED VISION AND HEARING
A. Description
   1. Because of the physiological changes that occur with the **aging** process, clients develop decreased visual and hearing acuity
   2. Such conditions as loss of sight and hearing, cataracts, glaucoma, and presbyopia can develop
B. Assessment and implementation: Refer to Chapter 61

X. ALTERED SKIN INTEGRITY
A. Description
   1. Physiological changes include thinning of the epidermis, easy bruising and tearing of the skin, and the reduction in blood flow to the skin
   2. Altered skin integrity often occurs in the bedridden or immobile client
B. Assessment and implementation: Refer to Chapter 47 regarding information on decubitus

XI. IMPAIRED MOBILITY
A. Description
   1. Usually occurs as a result of multiple types of problems and diseases
   2. Impaired mobility can occur as a result of decreased physical function related to cardiovascular, pulmonary, musculoskeletal, or neurological disease, or accidents
B. Assessment
   1. Existing disease processes
   2. Ambulation ability
   3. Ability to care for self
C. Implementation
   1. Assess risk of injury
   2. Determine cause of mobility restriction
   3. Assess mobility restrictions related to disease processes
   4. Monitor limitations related to all self-care activities
   5. Maintain activity through exercise and guided activities
   6. Provide rest periods between activities and in the afternoon
   7. Break activities up to last no longer than 20 minutes
   8. Perform activities that require a high level of energy in the morning
   9. Determine the best assistive aid or adaptive device for the client
   10. Demonstrate and monitor the safe use of the assistive device
   11. Monitor skin for integrity
   12. Provide range-of-motion exercises to prevent deformities and contractures
   13. Monitor respiratory status and encourage deep breathing to promote lung expansion
D. Assistive devices: Refer to Chapter 65 for information on canes and walkers ▲

XII. FRACTURED HIP
A. Description
   1. The most disabling type of fracture for the older adult
   2. Usually caused by falls with direct trauma to the hip
B. Assessment and implementation: Refer to Chapter 65

XIII. PNEUMONIA
A. Description: The causes of pneumonia in the older client include the effects of the **aging** process on the respiratory system, weakness and the inability to cough, malnutrition, and the use of medications
B. Assessment
   1. Acute change in mental status
   2. Confusion
   3. Cough
   4. Fever
   5. Increased respiratory rate
   6. Chest pain
   7. Dyspnea
   8. Chest radiograph confirmation

C. Implementation
1. Monitor vital signs
2. Assess lung sounds
3. Administer oxygen as prescribed
4. Administer respiratory therapy as prescribed
5. Administer antibiotics as prescribed
6. Provide adequate rest with some progressive activity
7. Mobilize the bed rest client as soon as possible
8. Provide adequate nutrition and hydration
9. Encourage the client to receive immunization against influenza and pneumococcal pneumonia to prevent infection

XIV. NUTRITIONAL INTAKE

A. Description
1. Physiological requirements decrease with age
2. The older client is at risk for inadequate nutritional and fluid intake because of inability to prepare food, loss of dentition, loss of appetite, lack of exercise, loss of taste and smell sensation, loss of interest in eating, **depression,** or lack of financial resources

B. Assessment
1. Appetite
2. Hydration status
3. Body weight
4. Ability to feed self
5. Ability to chew and swallow
6. Fluid and calorie intake
7. Ability to prepare food and mobilize the resources to shop

C. Implementation
1. Assess appetite
2. Monitor for signs of dehydration and malnutrition
3. Monitor body weight
4. Assess ability to chew and swallow
5. Monitor intake of food and fluids
6. Assess food likes and dislikes
7. Provide small, frequent, nutritious meals
8. Offer nutritious between-meal drinks and snacks
9. Assess ability to prepare food and to shop for food
10. Provide resources necessary to supply the client with adequate food

XV. CONSTIPATION

A. Description
1. Normal elimination does not occur because of a structural problem or disease state
2. Constipation is a frequent complaint regarding bowel function of older people

B. Assessment
1. Frequency of defecation
2. Usual time for defecation
3. Dietary habits
4. Use of laxatives or enemas

C. Implementation
1. Determine the cause of constipation
2. Reestablish typical bowel habits
3. Maintain regular defecation
4. Promote comfort and privacy during defecation
5. Increase fluid intake
6. Add fiber to the diet
7. Provide anal lubricant
8. Administer stool softeners as prescribed
9. Use suppositories sparingly, limiting the type to glycerin or Dulcolax as prescribed
10. Use enemas sparingly, limiting their use to small cleansing enemas such as Fleet, as prescribed
11. Avoid the use of mineral oil as a laxative because of problems associated with the absorption of fat-soluble vitamins and the risk of aspiration

XVI. DIARRHEA

A. Description
1. Frequent defecation of loose or liquid stools
2. Infections may cause diarrhea
3. Fecal impaction may cause overflow diarrhea, with stool oozing around the impaction
4. Antibiotic-associated diarrhea, such as that caused by *Clostridium difficile*, is a problem for older individuals, particularly if they are hospitalized

B. Assessment
1. Frequency of defecation
2. Usual time for defecation
3. Dietary habits
4. Use of laxatives or enemas
5. Stool oozing
6. Signs of dehydration
7. Electrolyte values

C. Implementation
1. Assess causative factor
2. Initiate interventions, as prescribed, based on causative factor
3. Assess for fluid deficit and dehydration
4. Monitor intake and output (I & O) and electrolyte levels
5. Increase dietary bulk and fiber
6. Monitor skin around anal area

XVII. URINARY INCONTINENCE

A. Description
1. The involuntary release or leakage of urine
2. The physiological changes that occur in the kidney and bladder as a result of the **aging** process may lead to the urinary incontinence problems experienced by some older clients

B. Assessment
1. Contributing factors

BOX 75-2

Kegel exercises

Contract pubococcygeus muscle
Hold contraction for 10 seconds
Relax for 10 seconds
Work up to 25 repetitions three times a day

---

2. I & O
3. Urinary incontinence patterns
4. Urinary retention
5. Signs of urinary infection, such as burning, frequency, foul odor, or confusion
6. Urinalysis results

C. Implementation
   1. Monitor I & O
   2. Monitor urinary patterns
   3. Assess contributing factors such as a bladder infection, the distance to the bathroom, difficulty ambulating or removing clothing, or coughing, sneezing, or laughing
   4. Establish a toileting schedule, such as every 2 hours or before and after activities, meals, sleep, and rest periods
   5. Provide easy access to bathroom
   6. Ensure adequate fluid intake
   7. Provide a protection plan for accidents to avoid embarrassment
   8. Instruct the client about the use of incontinence aids such as pads or briefs
   9. Provide skin care and monitor for skin breakdown
   10. Teach Kegel exercises to control stress and urge incontinence (Box 75-2)

PRACTICE QUESTIONS

1. A nurse is providing instructions to a nursing assistant about care to an elderly client with hearing loss. The nurse tells the assistant that the clients with a hearing loss:
   1. Are often distracted
   2. Respond to low-pitched tones
   3. Have middle-ear changes
   4. Develop moist cerumen production

2. An elderly male client is admitted to the hospital with a diagnosis of malnutrition. Which of the following laboratory data indicates that the client is experiencing a protein deficiency?
   1. Creatinine 0.6 mg/dL
   2. Transferrin 90 mg/dL
   3. Calcium 10 mg/dL
   4. Sodium 138 mEq/L

3. A nurse is providing an educational session to new employees, and the topic is elder abuse. The nurse tells the employees that which client is most characteristic of a victim of elder abuse?
   1. A 90-year-old woman with advanced Parkinson's disease
   2. A 68-year-old man with newly diagnosed cataracts
   3. A 70-year-old woman with early diagnosed Lyme's disease
   4. A 75-year-old man with moderate hypertension

4. An elderly female client confides to the visiting nurse that she is afraid she will fall while going to the bathroom at night. Which suggestion, if made by the nurse, indicates that the nurse understands the visual changes affecting the elderly?
   1. "Use a bell to call your daughter if you need to get up."
   2. "Keep a red light on in the bathroom at night."
   3. "Use a commode in your bedroom at night."
   4. "Limit your fluid intake during the day."

5. A nurse is caring for an agitated elderly client with Alzheimer's disease. Which nursing intervention would most likely calm the client?
   1. Playing a radio
   2. Turning the lights out
   3. Putting an arm around the client's waist
   4. Encouraging group participation

6. A nurse who volunteers at a senior citizens' center is planning activities for the members who attend the center. Which activity would best promote health and maintenance for these senior citizens?
   1. Gardening every day for an hour
   2. Cycling three times a week for twenty minutes
   3. Sculpting once a week for forty minutes
   4. Walking three to five times a week for thirty minutes

7. A nurse is working with elderly clients in a long-term care facility. Which of the following activities performed by the nurse fosters reminiscence among these clients?
   1. Displaying calendars and clocks
   2. Encouraging client participation in pottery class
   3. Setting up pet therapy sessions
   4. Having story telling hours

8. A home care nurse is performing an environmental assessment in the home of an elderly client. Which of the following, if observed by the nurse, requires immediate attention?
   1. An operable smoke detector
   2. A prefilled medication cassette
   3. Unsecured scatter rugs
   4. Clear exit passageways

9. A nurse is teaching an elderly client about measures to prevent constipation. Which statement, if made by the client, indicates that further teaching about bowel elimination is necessary?
   1. "I drink 6 to 8 glasses of water per day."
   2. "I walk 1 to 2 miles per day."

3. "I need to decrease fiber in my diet."

4. "I have a bowel movement every other day."

10. A nurse educator is providing an information session to nursing assistants about caring for the older adult. The nurse educator tells the nursing assistants that which of the following situations portrays ageism?
    1. Accepting differences among older adults
    2. Allowing older adults to make decisions
    3. Informing the older adults of their rights
    4. Advising older adults to forego aggressive treatment

11. A nurse is providing medication instructions to an elderly client who is taking digoxin (Lanoxin) daily. The nurse bears in mind that which age-related body changes could place the client at risk for digitalis toxicity?
    1. Decreased cough efficiency and decreased vital capacity
    2. Decreased lean body mass and decreased glomerular filtration rate
    3. Decreased salivation and decreased gastrointestinal motility
    4. Decreased muscle strength and loss of bone density

12. A nurse employed in a long-term care facility is caring for an elderly male client. Which of the following nursing actions would contribute to encouraging autonomy in the client?
    1. Scheduling his barber appointments
    2. Allowing him to choose social activities
    3. Decorating his room
    4. Planning his meals

13. A nurse assigned to care for an elderly client places an extra blanket in the client's room. The nurse understands that the elderly client is less able to regulate hot and cold bodily changes due to alterations in the activity of the:
    1. Parotid glands
    2. Thymus gland
    3. Pineal gland
    4. Sweat glands

14. A home care nurse is visiting an elderly female client whose husband died 6 months ago. Which behavior by the client indicates ineffective coping?
    1. Visiting her husband's grave once a month
    2. Participating in a senior citizens program
    3. Looking at old snapshots of her family
    4. Neglecting her personal grooming

15. A nurse is preparing to communicate with an elderly client who is hearing impaired. The most appropriate initial nursing action is to:
    1. Stand in front of the client
    2. Exaggerate lip movements
    3. Obtain a sign language interpreter
    4. Pantomime and write the client notes

16. A nurse is performing an assessment of an elderly client who is having difficulty sleeping at night. Which statement, if made by the client, indicates that teaching about improving sleep is necessary?
    1. "I drink hot chocolate before bedtime."
    2. "I have stopped smoking cigars."
    3. "I swim three times a week."
    4. "I read for 40 minutes before bedtime."

17. A visiting nurse observes that an elderly male client is confined by his daughter-in-law to his room. When the nurse suggests he walk to the den and join the family, he says, "I'm in everyone's way, my son needs for me to stay here." The most important action for the nurse to take is to:
    1. Suggest to the client and daughter-in-law that they consider a nursing home for the client
    2. Suggest appropriate resources to the client and daughter-in-law such as respite care and senior citizens' centers
    3. Say nothing, as it is best for the nurse to remain neutral and wait to be asked for help
    4. Say to the son, "Confining your father to his room is inhuman."

18. A nurse is performing an assessment of an older adult client. Which assessment data would indicate a potential complication associated with the skin of this client?
    1. Wrinkling
    2. Thinning and loss of elasticity in the skin
    3. Deepening of expression lines
    4. Crusting

19. A home care nurse provides medication instructions to an elderly hypertensive client who is taking lisinopril (Prinivil, Zestril) 20 mg po daily. Which statement, if made by the client, indicates that further teaching is necessary?
    1. "I take the pill after breakfast each day."
    2. "I need to change my position slowly."
    3. "If I get a bad headache, I should call my doctor immediately."
    4. "I can skip a dose once a week."

20. A nurse is caring for an elderly client who is on bed rest. The nurse plans which intervention to prevent respiratory complications?
    1. Monitoring vital signs every shift
    2. Decreasing oral fluid intake
    3. Changing the client's position every 2 hours
    4. Instructing the client to bear down every hour and hold the breath

CRITICAL THINKING: FREE-TEXT ENTRY

A nurse is caring for an elderly client with dysphagia who is at risk for aspiration. When preparing the client for eating, a nurse places the client in which best position?

Answer: _____

ANSWER

1. 2

Rationale: Presbycusis refers to age-related irreversible degenerative changes of the inner ear leading to decreased hearing acuity. As a result of these changes, the elderly have a decreased response to high-frequency sounds. Low-pitched tones of voice are more easily heard and interpreted by the elderly. Options 1, 3, and 4 are not accurate.

Test-Taking Strategy: Use the process of elimination. Recalling that a client with a hearing loss responds to low-pitched tones will direct you to option 2. If you had difficulty with this question, review the characteristics associated with presbycusis and hearing loss.

Level of Cognitive Ability: Application
Client Needs: Physiological Integrity
Integrated Concept/Process: Teaching/Learning
Content Area: Adult Health/Ear
Reference: Phipps, W., Sands, J., & Marek, J. (1999). *Medical-surgical nursing: Concepts & clinical practice* (6th ed.). St. Louis: Mosby, p. 1855.

2. 2

Rationale: Serum transferrin is an iron-transport protein that can be measured directly or calculated as an indirect measurement of total iron-binding capacity. It is a more sensitive indicator of protein status than albumin. When serum transferrin is less than 100 mg/dL, the level of visceral protein depletion is severe. Options 1, 3, and 4 identify normal laboratory values.

Test-Taking Strategy: Use the process of elimination. Note the key word "protein." The only option that refers to the analysis of protein is option 2. Additionally, eliminate options 1, 3, and 4 because these are normal laboratory values. Review these laboratory values if you had difficulty with this question.

Level of Cognitive Ability: Analysis
Client Needs: Physiological Integrity
Integrated Concept/Process: Nursing Process/Analysis
Content Area: Fundamental Skills
Reference: Lueckenotte, A. (2000). *Gerontologic nursing* (2nd ed.). St. Louis: Mosby, p. 409.

3. 1

Rationale: Elder abuse is widespread and occurs among all subgroups of the population. It includes physical and psychological abuse, misuse of property, and violation of rights. The typical abuse victim is a woman of advanced age with few social contacts and at least one physical or mental impairment that limits the ability to perform activities of daily living. In addition, the client usually lives alone or with the abuser, and depends on the abuser for care.

Test-Taking Strategy: Use the process of elimination. Read each option carefully and identify the client that is most defenseless as the result of the disease process. If you had difficulty with this question, review content related to elder abuse.

Level of Cognitive Ability: Application
Clients Needs: Psychosocial Integrity
Integrated Concept/Process: Teaching/Learning
Content Area: Mental Health
Reference: Ignatavicius, D., Workman, M., & Mishler, M. (1999). *Medical-surgical nursing across the health care continuum* (3rd ed.). Philadelphia: W. B. Saunders, pp. 69-70.

4. 2

Rationale: Because it takes longer to adapt to changes from dark to light and vice versa, older people are at a greater risk of falls and injuries. Any place where there is a sudden change from dark to light or from light to dark can be dangerous. Getting up during the night is a hazardous situation for an elderly client. Eyes adapt to the dark by using the rod receptors, which are sensitive to short blue-green wavelengths. Red wavelengths are longer and are perceived by the cones. Thus, a red light in the bathroom at night will allow for adequate vision to function in the dark without the need for adaptation.

Test-Taking Strategy: Use the process of elimination, focusing on the issue. Eliminate options 1 and 3 because they do not meet the client's need for independence. Additionally, there is no information in the question that the client lives with the daughter. Option 4 is incorrect because the elderly need to be encouraged to drink at least 2 liters of fluid a day to prevent dehydration. Review the physiological changes in the eye that occur with aging if you had difficulty with this question.

Level of Cognitive Ability: Analysis
Clients Needs: Physiological Integrity
Integrated Concept/Process: Nursing Process/Implementation
Content Area: Adult Health/Eye
Reference: Ignatavicius, D., Workman, M., & Mishler, M. (1999). *Medical-surgical nursing across the health care continuum* (3rd ed.). Philadelphia: W. B. Saunders, p. 1157.

5. 3

Rationale: Nursing interventions for the Alzheimer client who is angry, frustrated, or hostile include decreasing environmental stimuli, approaching the client calmly and with assurance, not demanding anything from the client, and distracting the client. It is important that the nurse reach out, touch, hold a hand, put an arm around the waist, or in some way maintain physical contact. Playing a radio may increase stimuli and turning the lights out may produce more agitation. The client with Alzheimer's disease would not be a candidate for group work if he or she is agitated.

Test-Taking Strategy: Use the process of elimination, recalling the need to decrease environmental stimuli and avoid further agitation. These concepts will direct you to option 3. Review care of the client with Alzheimer's disease if you had difficulty with this question.

Level of Cognitive Ability: Application
Clients Needs: Safe, Effective Care Environment
Integrated Concept/Process: Caring
Content Area: Mental Health
Reference: Ignatavicius, D., Workman, M., & Mishler, M. (1999). *Medical-surgical nursing across the health care continuum* (3rd ed.). Philadelphia: W. B. Saunders, p. 1048.

6. 4

Rationale: Exercise and activity are essential for health promotion and maintenance in the older adult and to achieve an optimal level of functioning. Approximately half of the physical deterioration of the elderly is caused by disuse rather than by the aging process or disease. One of the best exercises for an older adult is walking, progressing to 30-minute sessions three to five times each week. Swimming and dancing are also beneficial.

Test-Taking Strategy: Use the process of elimination, noting the key word "best." Options 1, 2, and 3, although possible, are not the best activities. Remember, walking is one of the best forms of exercise. Review this content if you had difficulty with this question.

Level of Cognitive Ability: Application
Clients Needs: Health Promotion and Maintenance
Integrated Concept/Process: Nursing Process/Planning
Content Area: Fundamental Skills
Reference: Ignatavicius, D., Workman, M., & Mishler, M. (1999). *Medical-surgical nursing across the health care continuum* (3rd ed.). Philadelphia: W. B. Saunders, pp. 63-64.

7. 4

Rationale: Clients who like to retell stories or past events need to be provided the opportunity to do so. This phenomenon is called life review or reminiscence. In a sense, it is a way for the elder client to relive and restructure life experiences, and is a part of achieving ego identity. Option 1 indicates reality orientation techniques. Options 2 and 3 indicate socialization and physical activity.

Test-Taking Strategy: Use the process of elimination. Focusing on the key word reminiscence, and recalling the definition of this word will direct you to option 4. Review this form of activity if you had difficulty with this question.

Level of Cognitive Ability: Application
Clients Needs: Physiological Integrity
Integrated Concept/Process: Caring
Content Area: Mental Health
Reference: Potter, P., & Perry, A. (2001). *Fundamentals of nursing* (5th ed.). St. Louis: Mosby, p. 549.

8. 3

Rationale: Trauma to the elderly in the home may be caused by a variety of factors. Some of these factors include an unsteady gait, the presence of unsecured scatter rugs, cluttered passageways, inoperable smoke detectors, or a history of previous falls.

Test-Taking Strategy: Use the process of elimination. Note the key words "requires immediate attention." Focusing on the issue and looking for the item that identifies an unsafe condition will direct you to option 3. Review the components of an environmental assessment if you had difficulty with this question.

Level of Cognitive Ability: Analysis
Clients Needs: Safe, Effective Care Environment
Integrated Concept/Process: Nursing Process/Assessment
Content Area: Fundamental Skills
Reference: Potter, P., & Perry, A. (2001). *Fundamentals of nursing* (5th ed.). St. Louis: Mosby, p. 1021.

9. 3

Rationale: Adequate dietary fiber is an important factor in aiding bowel function. Dietary fiber increases fecal weight and water content and accelerates the transit of fecal mass through the gastrointestinal tract. The retention of water by the fiber has the ability to soften stools and promote regularity. Fluid intake and exercise also facilitate bowel elimination.

Test-Taking Strategy: Note the key words "further teaching about bowel elimination is necessary." Use the process of elimination and basic principles related to preventing constipation. If you had difficulty with this question, review these basic principles.

Level of Cognitive Ability: Analysis
Clients Needs: Health Promotion and Maintenance

Integrated Concept/Process: Teaching/Learning
Content Area: Fundamental Skills
Reference: Leahy, J., & Kizilay, P. (1998). *Foundations of nursing practice: A nursing process approach.* Philadelphia: W. B. Saunders, p. 928.

10. 4

Rationale: Ageism is a form of prejudice in which older adults are stereotyped by characteristics found in only a few members of their group. Fundamental to ageism is the view that older people are different from "me" and will remain different from "me." Therefore, they are portrayed as not experiencing the same desires, needs, and concerns. Options 1, 2, and 3 identify supportive roles that the nurse engages in when dealing with the older adult. Option 4 suggests that the older adult is not worthy of aggressive treatment and demonstrates ageism.

Test-Taking Strategy: Use the process of elimination and focus on the issue, ageism. Recalling the definition of ageism will direct you to option 4. Review this concept if you had difficulty with this question.

Level of Cognitive Ability: Comprehension
Clients Needs: Health Promotion and Maintenance
Integrated Concept/Process: Caring
Content Area: Fundamental Skills
Reference: Smeltzer, S., & Bare, B. (2000). *Brunner & Suddarth's textbook of medical-surgical nursing* (9th ed.). Philadelphia: Lippincott Williams & Wilkins, p. 150.

11. 2

Rationale: The elderly client is at risk for medication toxicity because of decreased lean body mass and age-associated decreased glomerular filtration rate. Although options 1, 3, and 4 identify age-related changes that occur in the elderly client, they are not specifically associated with this risk.

Test-Taking Strategy: Use the process of elimination and focus on the issue, an age-related body change that could place the client at risk for medication toxicity. Note that option 2 is the only option that addresses renal excretion. If you had difficulty with this question, review the physiological changes associated with aging.

Level of Cognitive Ability: Analysis
Clients Needs: Physiological Integrity
Integrated Concept/Process: Teaching/Learning
Content Area: Fundamental Skills
Reference: Ignatavicius, D., Workman, M., & Mishler, M. (1999). *Medical-surgical nursing across the health care continuum* (3rd ed.). Philadelphia: W. B. Saunders, pp. 54-55.

12. 2

Rationale: Autonomy is the personal freedom to direct one's own life as long as it does not impinge on the rights of others. An autonomous person is capable of rational thought. This individual can identify problems, search for alternatives, and select solutions that allow continued personal freedom as long as the rights and property of others are not harmed. Loss of autonomy, and therefore of independence, is a very real fear among the elderly. Option 2 is the only option that allows the client to be a decision-maker.

Test-Taking Strategy: Use the process of elimination, focusing on the issue, encouraging autonomy. Recalling the definition of autonomy will direct you to the correct option. Remember, to promote independence in clients, it is essential to give the

client choices. Review the concept of autonomy if you had difficulty with this question.
Level of Cognitive Ability: Application
Clients Needs: Safe, Effective Care Environment
Integrated Concept/Process: Caring
Content Area: Fundamental Skills
Reference: Ignatavicius, D., Workman, M., & Mishler, M. (1999). *Medical-surgical nursing across the health care continuum* (3rd ed.). Philadelphia: W. B. Saunders, p. 181.

13. **4**
Rationale: Functions of the skin include protection, sensory reception, homeostasis, and temperature regulation. The skin helps regulate the body temperature in two ways, by dilation and constriction of blood vessels and by the activity of the sweat glands. As aging progresses, alterations in sweat gland activity make the glands less effective in temperature regulation, so the aging person is less able to regulate hot and cold bodily changes. The parotid glands are responsible for the drainage of saliva, which plays an important role in digestion. The pineal gland is a major site of melatonin biosynthesis. The thymus gland plays an immunological role throughout life.
Test-Taking Strategy: Use the process of elimination and focus on the issue, temperature regulation. Recalling the function of the skin and that the sweat glands control temperature regulation will direct you to the correct option. Review the age-related changes that occur in the elderly if you had difficulty with this question.
Level of Cognitive Ability: Comprehension
Clients Needs: Physiological Integrity
Integrated Concept/Process: Nursing Process/Implementation
Content Area: Fundamental Skills
Reference: Jarvis, C. (2000). *Physical examination and health assessment* (3rd ed.). Philadelphia: W. B. Saunders, p. 216.

14. **4**
Rationale: Coping mechanisms are behaviors used to decrease stress and anxiety. In response to a death, ineffective coping is manifested by an extreme behavior that in some instances may be harmful to the individual either physically or psychologically. Option 4 is indicative of an ineffective coping behavior in the grieving process.
Test-Taking Strategy: Use the process of elimination and note the issue, an ineffective coping behavior. Eliminate options 1, 2, and 3 because they are similar and are positive activities that the individual is engaging in to get on with her life. Review coping mechanisms in response to grief and loss if you had difficulty with this question.
Level of Cognitive Ability: Analysis
Clients Needs: Psychosocial Integrity
Integrated Concept/Process: Nursing Process/Assessment
Content Area: Mental Health
Reference: Potter, P., & Perry, A. (2001). *Fundamentals of nursing* (5th ed.). St. Louis: Mosby, pp. 618-619.

15. **1**
Rationale: The nurse would ensure that the hearing-impaired client can see the nurse when he or she is speaking by providing adequate lighting and by standing in front of the client. The nurse should enunciate words clearly but not exaggerate lip movements. If the client is profoundly hearing impaired and uses signing, a sign language interpreter should be obtained. If a client cannot understand by reading lips, the

nurse would try using gestures, pantomiming, or writing notes.
Test-Taking Strategy: Note the key words "initial nursing action." To communicate effectively with a hearing impaired client, the nurse first makes sure that the client can see her or him. If you had difficulty with this question, review the nursing interventions for the hearing impaired.
Level of Cognitive Ability: Application
Clients Needs: Health Promotion and Maintenance
Integrated Concept/Process: Nursing Process/Implementation
Content Area: Fundamental Skills
Reference: Potter, P., & Perry, A. (2001). *Fundamentals of nursing* (5th ed.). St. Louis: Mosby, p. 1651.

16. **1**
Rationale: Many nonpharmacological sleep aids can be used to influence sleep. The client should avoid caffeinated beverages and stimulants such as tea, cola, and chocolate, and foods with tyrosine such as cheddar cheese. The client should exercise regularly, because exercise enhances sleep by burning off tension that accumulates during the day. A 20- to 30-minute walk, swim, or bicycle ride three times a week is helpful. The client should sleep on a bed with a firm mattress. Smoking and alcohol should be avoided. The client should avoid large meals, peanuts, beans, fruit and raw vegetables that produce gas, and snacks high in fat that are difficult to digest.
Test-Taking Strategy: Focus on the issue, that teaching is necessary. Options 2, 3, and 4 are positive statements indicating that the client understands the methods of improving sleep. Review the factors that can interfere with sleep if you had difficulty with this question.
Level of Cognitive Ability: Analysis
Clients Needs: Physiological Integrity
Integrated Concept/Process: Teaching/Learning
Content Area: Fundamental Skills
Reference: Smeltzer, S., & Bare, B. (2000). *Brunner & Suddarth's textbook of medical-surgical nursing* (9th ed.). Philadelphia: Lippincott Williams & Wilkins, p. 1462.

17. **2**
Rationale: Assisting clients and families to become knowledgeable of community supports systems that are available is a role and responsibility of the nurse. Option 1 suggests that the client be admitted to a nursing home and is a premature action on the nurse's part. While the data provided tell the nurse that this client requires nursing care, the nurse does not know the extent of nursing care. Observing that the client has begun to be confined to his room makes it necessary for the nurse to intervene legally and ethically so option 3 is not appropriate and is passive in terms of advocacy. Option 4 is incorrect and judgmental.
Test-Taking Strategy: Use the process of elimination. Note the key words "most important action." Using principles related to the ethical and legal responsibility of the nurse and knowledge of the nurse's role will direct you to option 2. Review these principles if you had difficulty with this question.
Level of Cognitive Ability: Application
Client Needs: Safe, Effective Care Environment
Integrated Concept/Process: Nursing Process/Implementation
Content Area: Fundamental Skills

Reference: Ignatavicius, D., Workman, M., & Mishler, M. (1999). *Medical-surgical nursing across the health care continuum* (3rd ed.). Philadelphia: W. B. Saunders, pp. 69-70.

18. 4

Rationale: The normal physiological changes that occur in the skin of older adults include thinning, loss of elasticity, deepening of expression lines, becoming smooth, and wrinkling. Crusting noted on the skin would indicate a potential complication.

Test-Taking Strategy: Use the process of elimination and note the key words "potential complication." Think about the normal physiological changes that occur in the aging process to direct you to option 4. Review these age-related skin changes if you had difficulty with this question.

Level of Cognitive Ability: Analysis

Client Needs: Physiological Integrity

Integrated Concept/Process: Nursing Process/Assessment

Content Area: Fundamental Skills

Reference: Ignatavicius, D., Workman, M., & Mishler, M. (1999). *Medical-surgical nursing across the health care continuum* (3rd ed.). Philadelphia: W. B. Saunders, p. 54.

19. 4

Rationale: Lisinopril is an antihypertensive, angiotensin-converting enzyme inhibitor (ACE inhibitor). The usual dosage range is 20 to 40 mg daily. Adverse effects include headache, dizziness, fatigue, orthostatic hypotension, tachycardia, and angioedema. Specific client teaching points include taking one pill a day, not stopping the medication without consulting the physician, and monitoring for side effects and adverse reactions. The client should notify the physician if side effects occur.

Test-Taking Strategy: Use the process of elimination. Note the key words "further teaching is necessary." Basic principles related to the administration of prescribed medications will direct you to option 4. If you had difficulty with this question, review teaching points related to medication administration.

Level of Cognitive Ability: Analysis

Clients Needs: Health Promotion and Maintenance

Integrated Concept/Process: Teaching/Learning

Content Area: Pharmacology

Reference: Hodgson, B. & Kizior, R. (2001). *Saunders nursing drug handbook 2001.* Philadelphia: W. B. Saunders, pp. 596-598.

20. 3

Rationale: Frequent position change helps to mobilize lung secretions and prevent pooling. This is the only intervention identified in the options that will prevent respiratory complications. The nurse should assess the client's vital signs every 4 hours to identify an elevated temperature that may suggest infection. The nurse would encourage fluid intake to thin secretions and thus enable the client to expectorate more easily. It is important to encourage coughing and deep breathing to mobilize lung secretions. The client should be instructed to avoid the Valsalva maneuver or any activity involving holding the breath.

Test-Taking Strategy: Use the process of elimination. Note the key words "prevent respiratory complications." Changing the position of the immobilized client every 2 hours will help prevent pooling of lung secretions. The other options do not assist the client to improve ventilatory efforts or prevent respiratory complications. Review nursing interventions to prevent respiratory complications in the client who is immobilized if you had difficulty with this question.

Level of Cognitive Ability: Application

Clients Needs: Physiological Integrity

Integrated Concept/Process: Nursing Process/Implementation

Content Area: Fundamental Skills

Reference: Ignatavicius, D., Workman, M., & Mishler, M. (1999). *Medical-surgical nursing across the health care continuum* (3rd ed.). Philadelphia: W. B. Saunders, pp. 1076-1077.

CRITICAL THINKING: FREE-TEXT ENTRY

Answer: Upright in a chair

Rationale: It is best to assist the client out of bed and to have the client sitting in a chair for meals. This position facilitates chewing and swallowing and prevents reflux of stomach contents.

Test-Taking Strategy: Focusing on the issue, aspiration, will assist in answering the question. Also note that the client has dysphagia. It is best to place the client in an upright position. Review the nursing interventions to prevent aspiration if you had difficulty with this question.

Level of Cognitive Ability: Application

Clients Needs: Safe, Effective Care Environment

Integrated Concept/Process: Nursing Process/Implementation

Content Area: Fundamental Skills

Reference: Ignatavicius, D., Workman, M., & Mishler, M. (1999). *Medical-surgical nursing across the health care continuum* (3rd ed.). Philadelphia: W.B. Saunders, p. 604.

REFERENCES

Hodgson, B., & Kizior, R. (2001). *Saunders nursing drug handbook 2001.* Philadelphia: W.B. Saunders.

Ignatavicius, D., Workman, M., & Mishler, M. (1999). *Medical-surgical nursing across the health care continuum* (3rd ed.). Philadelphia: W.B. Saunders.

Jarvis, C. (2000). *Physical examination and health assessment* (3rd ed.). Philadelphia: W.B. Saunders.

Lueckenotte, A. (2000). *Gerontologic nursing* (2nd ed.). St. Louis: Mosby.

Phipps, W., Sands, J., & Marek, J. (1999). *Medical-surgical nursing: Concepts & clinical practice* (6th ed.). St. Louis: Mosby.

Potter, P., & Perry, A. (2001). *Fundamentals of nursing* (5th ed.). St. Louis: Mosby.

Smeltzer, S., & Bare, B. (2000). *Brunner & Suddarth's textbook of medical-surgical nursing* (9th ed.). Philadelphia: Lippincott Williams & Wilkins.

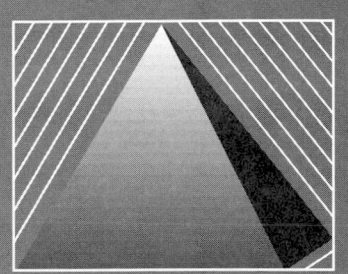

1. A nurse is assessing a child with a diagnosis of suspected appendicitis. In assessing the intensity and progression of the pain, the nurse palpates the child at McBurney's point. In performing this assessment, the nurse knows that McBurney's point is located midway between the:
   1. Right anterior inferior iliac crest and the umbilicus
   2. Left anterior superior iliac crest and the umbilicus
   3. Right anterior superior iliac crest and the umbilicus
   4. Left anterior superior iliac crest and the umbilicuo

2. A nurse is caring for a client with a burn injury to the lower legs. Nitrofurazone (Furacin) is prescribed to be applied to the sites of injury. The nurse documents which of the following in the plan of care as the appropriate method to apply this medication?
   1. Apply dressings soaked with saline solution over the medication
   2. Apply 1-inch film directly to the burn sites
   3. Apply $^1/_{16}$-inch film directly to the burn sites
   4. Apply $^1/_2$-inch film directly to the burn sites

3. A client suspected of having an abdominal tumor is scheduled for a computerized tomography (CT) scan with dye injection. A nurse tells the client that:
   1. The test may be painful
   2. The dye injected may cause a warm, flushing sensation
   3. Fluids will be restricted following the test
   4. The test takes approximately 2 hours

4. A nurse is caring for a client whose magnesium level is 3.5 mg/dL. On the basis of this magnesium level, which assessment sign or symptom would the nurse most likely expect to note?
   1. Tetany
   2. Twitches
   3. Positive Trousseau's sign
   4. Loss of deep tendon reflexes

5. A nurse is caring for a client with a diagnosis of hyperthyroidism. Laboratory studies are performed, and the serum calcium level is 12.0 mg/dL. Which medication would the nurse anticipate to be prescribed for the client?
   1. Calcium gluconate
   2. Calcium chloride
   3. Calcitonin (Calcimar)
   4. Large doses of vitamin D

6. A nurse prepares to administer sodium polystyrene sulfonate (Kayexalate) to the client. Before administering the medication, the nurse reviews the action of the medication and understands that it releases:
   1. Bicarbonate in exchange for primarily sodium ions
   2. Sodium ions in exchange for primarily bicarbonate ions
   3. Sodium ions in exchange for primarily potassium ions
   4. Potassium ions in exchange for primarily sodium ions

7. Which of the following clients is least likely to be at risk for the development of third spacing?
   1. A client with cirrhosis
   2. A client with diabetes mellitus
   3. A client with liver failure
   4. A client with renal failure

8. A nurse is preparing to care for a client after a gastroscopy procedure. The nurse includes which most appropriate component in the nursing care plan?
   1. Place the client in a supine position to provide comfort
   2. Monitor the client's vital signs every hour for 4 hours
   3. Provide saline gargles immediately on return to the unit to aid in comfort
   4. Check the gag reflex by using a tongue depressor to stroke the back of the client's throat

9. Ringer's lactate solution IV is prescribed for a postoperative client. A nursing instructor asks a nursing student who is caring for the client about the tonicity of the prescribed IV solution. The nursing student responds correctly by stating that this solution is:
   1. Isotonic
   2. Normotonic
   3. Hypotonic
   4. Hypertonic

10. A nurse reviews the arterial blood gas results of a client with Guillain-Barré syndrome. The pH is 7.35 and the P_{CO_2} is 50 mm Hg. The nurse interprets that this client is experiencing which acid-base imbalance?
    1. Respiratory acidosis
    2. Respiratory alkalosis
    3. Metabolic acidosis
    4. Metabolic alkalosis

11. A client is admitted 24 hours after an aspirin overdose. A nurse assesses this client for which signs and symptoms indicating the acid-base disturbance that can occur in the client?
    1. Bradycardia and hyperactivity
    2. Restlessness, confusion, and a positive Trousseau's sign
    3. Headache, nausea, vomiting, and diarrhea
    4. Bradypnea, dizziness, and paresthesias

12. An adult client with hepatic encephalopathy has a serum ammonia level of 95 μg/dL, and receives treatment with lactulose syrup. A nurse would evaluate that the client had the best and most realistic response if the serum ammonia level changed to which of the following after medication administration?
    1. 80 μg/dL
    2. 40 μg/dL
    3. 10 μg/dL
    4. 5 μg/dL

13. A client who suffered a crush injury to the leg has a highly positive urine myoglobin level. A nurse assesses this particular client carefully for signs of:
    1. Cerebrovascular accident
    2. Acute tubular necrosis
    3. Respiratory failure
    4. Myocardial infarction

14. An adult male client admitted with shock has received fluid volume replacement. A nurse evaluates that the client has had adequate fluid resuscitation if the client's repeat hematocrit level has decreased to which of the following values in the normal range?
    1. 56%
    2. 48%
    3. 39%
    4. 34%

15. A nurse is formulating a plan of care for a client receiving enteral feedings. Which nursing diagnosis is of highest priority for this client?
    1. Altered nutrition, less than body requirements
    2. High risk for aspiration
    3. High risk for fluid volume deficit
    4. Diarrhea

16. A client who has a gastrostomy tube for feeding refuses to participate in the plan of care, will not make eye contact, and does not speak to family or visitors. A nurse assesses that this client is using which type of coping mechanism?
    1. Self-control
    2. Problem solving
    3. Accepting responsibility
    4. Distancing

17. A nurse conducting a weight-loss program prepares to monitor a client's weight loss. What method would most accurately assess the effectiveness of weight loss?
    1. Daily weights
    2. Serum protein levels
    3. Calorie counts
    4. Daily intake and output

18. A clinic nurse is monitoring a client with anorexia nervosa. Which statement, if made by the client, would indicate to the nurse that treatment has been effective?
    1. "I no longer have a weight problem."
    2. "I don't want to starve myself anymore."
    3. "I'll eat until I don't feel hungry."
    4. "My friends and I went out to lunch today."

19. A nurse is preparing a diet plan for a postgastrectomy client with dumping syndrome. Which of the following would not be a component of this teaching plan?
    1. Lie down after eating
    2. Drink liquids with meals
    3. Eat small meals six times daily
    4. Avoid concentrated sweets

20. A client has been diagnosed with pernicious anemia. In planning care for the client, a nurse anticipates that the client will be treated with:
    1. Thiamine
    2. Iron
    3. Vitamin B_{12}
    4. Folic acid

21. An elderly postoperative client has been tolerating a full-liquid diet, and a nurse plans to advance the diet to solid food as prescribed. Which assessment is most important for the nurse to make before advancing the diet to solids?
    1. Food preferences
    2. Cultural preferences
    3. Presence of bowel sounds
    4. Ability to chew

22. A diabetic client has been instructed in the dietary exchange system. The client asks a nurse if bacon is allowed in the diet. Which nursing response is most appropriate?
    1. "Bacon is much too high in fat."
    2. "Bacon is not allowed."
    3. "One strip of bacon may be eaten if you eliminate 1 teaspoon of butter."
    4. "Bacon may be eaten if you eliminate one meat item from your diet."

23. A client with heart disease is provided instructions regarding a low-fat diet. A nurse evaluates that the client understands the diet if the client states that a food item to avoid is:
    1. Apples
    2. Oranges
    3. Avocado
    4. Cherries

24. A client with liver cancer who is receiving chemotherapy tells a nurse that some foods on the meal tray taste bitter. The nurse would try to limit which of the following foods that are most likely to cause this taste for the client?
    1. Beef
    2. Potatoes
    3. Custard
    4. Cantaloupe

25. A nursing student is caring for a client who has been admitted to the hospital with malnutrition. The student is reviewing with a nursing instructor

the results of the various laboratory tests performed on the client. Which statement, if made by the nursing student, indicates an understanding of the interpretation of the results?

1. "An elevated creatinine level indicates respiratory problems."
2. "A normal hemoglobin level indicates that iron and protein intake is sufficient."
3. "An elevated albumin level indicates a definite dehydration."
4. "A normal red blood cell level indicates adequate vitamin B_6 intake."

26. A nurse notes that an infant with a diagnosis of hydrocephalus has a head that is heavier than that of the average infant. The nurse determines that special safety precautions are needed for moving an infant with hydrocephalus. Which statement would the nurse plan to include in the discharge teaching with the parents to reflect this safety need?

1. "When picking up your infant, support the infant's neck and head with the open palm of your hand."
2. "Feed your infant in a side-lying position."
3. "Place a helmet on your infant when in bed."
4. "Hyperextend your infant's head with a rolled blanket under the neck area."

27. A nurse is performing an admission assessment on a child with a seizure disorder. The nurse is interviewing the child's parents to determine their adjustment to caring for a child who has a chronic illness. Which statement, if made by the parents, would indicate a need for further teaching?

1. "Our child is involved in a swim program with neighbors and friends."
2. "Our child sleeps in our bedroom at night."
3. "Our baby-sitter just completed cardiopulmonary resuscitation (CPR) training."
4. "We worry about injuries when our child has a seizure."

28. A nurse is reviewing the results of a serum carbamazepine (Tegretol) level, drawn from a child who is receiving Tegretol for the control of seizures. The results indicate a level of 10 µg/mL. The nurse analyzes the results and anticipates that the child's physician will prescribe:

1. An increase in the dose of the medication
2. A decrease in the dose of the medication
3. Discontinuation of the medication
4. Continuation of the presently prescribed dosage

29. A nursing student is asked to describe the corpus of the uterus. Which of the following responses, if made by the student, indicates an understanding of the anatomy of the uterus?

1. "It is the lower portion of the uterus."
2. "It is the uppermost part of the uterus."
3. "It is the area where the cervix meets the external os."
4. "It is the area where the vagina meets the uterus."

30. A nurse instructs a client with diabetes mellitus about blood glucose monitoring and monitoring for signs of hypoglycemia. The nurse informs the client that hypoglycemia is a blood glucose level of less than:

1. 120 mg/dL
2. 110 mg/dL
3. 90 mg/dL
4. 60 mg/dL

31. A client newly diagnosed with diabetes mellitus is instructed by the physician to obtain glucagon for emergency home use. The client asks a home care nurse about the purpose of the medication. The nurse instructs the client that the purpose of the medication is to treat:

1. Hypoglycemia from insulin overdose
2. Hyperglycemia from insufficient insulin
3. Lipoatrophy from insulin injections
4. Lipohypertrophy from inadequate insulin absorption

32. A nurse is providing care to a Cuban-American client who is terminally ill. Numerous family members are present most of the time, and many of the family members are very emotional. The most appropriate action is to:

1. Restrict the number of family members visiting at one time
2. Inform the family that emotional outbursts are to be avoided
3. Request permission to move the client to a private room and allow the family members to visit
4. Contact the physician to speak to the family regarding their behaviors

33. A nurse is instructing a postpartum client with endometritis about preventing the spread of infection to her newborn infant. The nurse would tell the client that:

1. Hands should be washed thoroughly before holding the infant
2. The newborn infant will not be allowed in the mother's room at all
3. There is no danger of the newborn contracting the disease
4. Visitors are not allowed to hold the baby

34. A client presents to an emergency department with upper gastrointestinal (GI) bleeding and is in moderate distress. In planning priorities for care, which nursing action would be the first priority for this client?

1. Thorough investigation of precipitating events
2. Insertion of a nasogastric tube and performance of a hematest of emesis

3. Complete abdominal examination
4. Assessment of vital signs

35. A nurse is caring for a client with possible cholelithiasis who is being prepared for an intravenous cholangiogram. The nurse teaches the client about the procedure. Which client statement indicates that the client understands the purpose of this test?
    1. "They are going to 'look at' my gallbladder and ducts."
    2. "This procedure will drain my gallbladder."
    3. "My gallbladder will be irrigated."
    4. "They will put medication in my gallbladder."

36. A nurse provides instructions to a malnourished client regarding iron supplementation during pregnancy. Which statement, if made by the client, would indicate an understanding of the instructions?
    1. "The iron is best absorbed if taken on an empty stomach."
    2. "Meat does not provide iron and should be avoided."
    3. "Iron supplements will give me diarrhea."
    4. "My body has all the iron it needs, and I don't need to take supplements."

37. A nurse has given discharge instructions to a client who underwent vein ligation and stripping early in the day. The nurse evaluates that the client understands activity and positioning limitations if the client states that it is most appropriate to:
    1. Lie down with the legs elevated and avoid sitting
    2. Cross the legs at the ankle only, and not at the knee
    3. Sit in a chair three times a day for 3 hours at a time
    4. Walk upright as much as possible each day

38. Octreotide acetate (Sandostatin) is prescribed for a client with acromegaly. A nurse monitors the client, knowing that which side effect is associated with the administration of this medication?
    1. Constipation
    2. Polyuria
    3. Abdominal pain
    4. Hypotension

39. Levothyroxine (Synthroid) is prescribed for a client diagnosed with hypothyroidism. A nurse reviews the client's record and notes that the client is presently taking warfarin (Coumadin). The nurse contacts the physician, anticipating that the physician will prescribe which of the following?
    1. An increased dosage of Coumadin
    2. A decreased dosage of Coumadin
    3. An increased dosage of Synthroid
    4. A decreased dosage of Synthroid

40. A nurse is teaching a client with emphysema about positions that help breathing during dyspneic episodes. The nurse instructs the client to avoid which of the following positions, which will aggravate breathing?
    1. Sitting up with the elbows resting on knees
    2. Standing and leaning against a wall
    3. Lying on the back in low Fowler's position
    4. Sitting up and leaning on a table

41. A client is about to undergo a lumbar puncture (LP). A nurse explains to the client that which of the following positions will be used during the procedure?
    1. Side-lying, with the legs pulled up and the head bent down onto the chest
    2. Side-lying, with a pillow under the hip
    3. Prone, with a pillow under the abdomen
    4. Prone, in slight Trendelenburg position

42. A nurse recognizes that which of the following interventions is unlikely to facilitate effective communication between a dying client and his or her family?
    1. The nurse encourages the client and family to identify and discuss feelings openly
    2. The nurse makes decisions for the client and family to relieve them of unnecessary demands
    3. The nurse assists the client and family in carrying out spiritually meaningful practices
    4. The nurse maintains a calm attitude and one of acceptance when the family or client expresses anger

43. A client with acute pancreatitis is experiencing severe pain from the disorder. The nurse determines that the client understood suggestions for positioning to reduce pain if the client avoided:
    1. Leaning forward
    2. Drawing the legs up to the chest
    3. Sitting up
    4. Lying flat

44. A client has had surgery to repair a fractured left hip. A nurse obtains which of the following most important items from the unit storage area to use when repositioning the client from side to side in bed?
    1. Abductor splint
    2. Adductor splint
    3. Bed pillow
    4. Overhead trapeze

45. A nurse is preparing to care for a client who has undergone myelography for which an oil-based contrast agent was used. The nurse plans to position the client on bed rest for:
    1. 6 to 8 hours, with the head of the bed flat
    2. 6 to 8 hours, with the head of the bed elevated 15 to 30 degrees
    3. 2 to 4 hours, with the head of the bed flat
    4. 2 to 4 hours, with head of bed elevated 15 to 30 degrees

46. A nurse has given activity guidelines to a client

with chronic low back pain. The nurse evaluates that the client understood the instructions if the client states to avoid which of the following positions?

1. Lying on the side with knees and hips bent
2. Lying prone
3. Standing with one foot on a step or stool
4. Sitting using a lumbar roll or pillow

47. A nurse has just admitted to the nursing unit a client with a basilar skull fracture who is at risk for increased intracranial pressure (ICP). Pending specific physician orders, a nurse would avoid placing the client in which of the following positions?

1. Neck in neutral position
2. Head of the bed elevated 30 to 45 degrees
3. Flat, with the head turned to the side
4. Head midline

48. A nurse reviews the arterial blood gas (ABG) results of an assigned client and notes that the laboratory report indicates a pH of 7.30, a P_{CO_2} of 58 mm Hg, a P_{O_2} of 80 mm Hg, and an HCO_3 of 27 mEq/L. The nurse interprets that the client has which acid-base disturbance?

1. Metabolic acidosis
2. Metabolic alkalosis
3. Respiratory acidosis
4. Respiratory alkalosis

49. Cortisone acetate (Cortone Acetate) is prescribed for a client with adrenal insufficiency. A nurse provides instructions to the client regarding the medication. Which statement, if made by the client, indicates a need for further instruction?

1. "I will eat a good breakfast every day."
2. "I will avoid people with colds."
3. "I will limit my sodium intake."
4. "I will stop the medication when I feel better."

50. A hospitalized client with diabetes mellitus received NPH insulin in the morning. A nurse monitors the client for hypoglycemia, knowing that the peak action occurs:

1. 2 to 4 hours after administration
2. 4 to 12 hours after administration
3. 12 to 16 hours after administration
4. 18 to 24 hours after administration

51. A nurse has admitted a client to a clinical nursing unit following modified right radical mastectomy for the treatment of breast cancer. The nurse plans to place the right arm in which of the following positions?

1. Elevated above shoulder level
2. Elevated on a pillow
3. Level with the right atrium
4. Dependent to the right atrium

52. On the second postpartum day, a woman complains of burning on urination, urgency, and frequency of urination. A urinalysis is performed, and the results indicate the presence of a urinary tract infection. A nurse instructs the new mother regarding measures to take for the treatment of the infection. Which of the following statements, if made by the mother, would indicate a need for further instructions?

1. "The prescribed medication must be taken until it is completed."
2. "My fluid intake should be increased to at least 3000 mL daily."
3. "I need to urinate frequently throughout the day."
4. "Foods and fluids that will increase urine alkalinity should be consumed."

53. A registered nurse is beginning a new job in a clinic and is attending an orientation session. After the orientation session, another new employee asks the registered nurse to describe case management, a component of the discussions in the orientation session, because the employee did not clearly understand the concept. The registered nurse responds that:

1. "Case management requires an experienced nurse, since it represents a primary health prevention focus and is managed by a single nurse."
2. "Case management saves money for the institution, because clients with similar problems are all treated in the same manner."
3. "Case management is an important concept, but it doesn't promote appropriate use of personnel."
4. "Case management will maximize hospital revenues and at the same time provide optimal outcome of client care."

54. A nurse provides dietary instructions to a client with diabetes mellitus regarding the prescribed diabetic diet. Which statement, if made by the client, indicates a need for further teaching?

1. "I need to drink diet soft drinks."
2. "I'll eat a balanced meal plan."
3. "I need to purchase special dietetic foods."
4. "I'll snack on fruit instead of cake."

55. A client received 20 units of NPH insulin subcutaneously at 8:00 A.M. The nurse should assess the client for a hypoglycemic reaction at:

1. 10:00 A.M.
2. 11:00 A.M.
3. 5:00 P.M.
4. 11:00 P.M.

56. A community health nurse is working with disaster relief in a local community after a hurricane that ruined many homes in the community. The nurse is working to find housing for the survivors and is organizing counseling services. These actions of the nurse represent which level of prevention?

1. The primary level of prevention

2. The secondary level of prevention

3. The tertiary level of prevention

4. The fourth level of prevention

57. A pregnant woman in her second trimester calls a prenatal clinic nurse to report a recent exposure to a child with rubella. Which of the following responses by the nurse would be most appropriate and supportive to the woman?

1. "There is no need to be concerned if you don't have a fever or rash within the next 2 days."

2. "Be sure to tell the doctor on your next prenatal visit, but there is little risk in the second trimester."

3. "You should avoid all school-aged children during pregnancy."

4. "You were wise to call. I will check your rubella titer screening results, and we can immediately determine whether future interventions are needed."

58. The breastfeeding mother of an infant with lactose intolerance asks a nurse about dietary measures. The nurse tells the mother to avoid:

1. Hard cheeses

2. Green leafy vegetables

3. Dried beans

4. Egg yolk

59. A diabetic client is told that amputation of a leg is necessary to sustain life. The client is very upset and states to the nurse, "This is all the doctor's fault! I have done everything that the doctor has asked me to do!" The nurse interprets the client's statement as:

1. An expected coping mechanism

2. A need to notify the hospital lawyer

3. An expression of guilt on the part of the client

4. An ineffective coping mechanism

60. A client brought to the emergency department is dead on arrival (DOA). A family member of the client tells the physician that the client had a terminal cancer. The emergency department physician examines the client and asks a nurse to contact the medical examiner regarding an autopsy. The family of the client tells the nurse that they do not want an autopsy performed. Which of the following responses to the family is most appropriate?

1. "It is required by federal law. Why don't we talk about it, and why don't you tell me why you don't want the autopsy done?"

2. "The decision is made by the medical examiner."

3. "I will contact the medical examiner regarding your request."

4. "An autopsy is mandatory for any client who is DOA."

61. A pregnant woman who is positive for human immunodeficiency virus (HIV) delivers a newborn infant. A nurse provides instructions to help the mother regarding newborn infant care. Which statement would not be included in the instructions to this client?

1. "Be sure to wash your hands before and after bathroom use."

2. "Support groups are available to assist with the impact of the diagnosis of HIV."

3. "Breastfeeding is encouraged, especially for the first 6 weeks postpartum."

4. "The newborn infant should receive antiviral medications for the first 6 weeks after delivery."

62. A pregnant woman has a positive history of genital herpes but has not had lesions during this pregnancy. A nurse should plan to provide which of the following information to the client?

1. "You will be isolated from your newborn infant following delivery."

2. "You will be evaluated at the time of delivery for herpetic genital tract lesions, and if they are present, a cesarean delivery will be needed."

3. "There is little risk to your newborn infant during this pregnancy and birth and following delivery."

4. "Vaginal deliveries can reduce neonatal infection risks, even if you have an active lesion at the time of the birth."

63. A 7-year-old child is diagnosed with viral conjunctivitis. Antibiotic eye drops are prescribed for the child. The mother asks a nurse when the child can return to school. The most appropriate response is:

1. "The child can return to school immediately."

2. "The child should be kept home until the antibiotic eye drops have been administered for 24 hours."

3. "The child should be kept home until the antibiotic eye drops have been administered for 72 hours."

4. "The child cannot return to school until seen by the physician in 1 week."

64. An adolescent is diagnosed with conjunctivitis. The adolescent asks a nurse if it is all right to wear contact lenses. Which of the following is not an appropriate instruction to the adolescent?

1. Contacts can be worn if they are cleaned as directed

2. Contact lenses should not be worn

3. New contact lenses should be obtained

4. Old contact lenses should be discarded

65. A pregnant client is seen in a health care clinic and asks a nurse what causes the breasts to change in size and appearance during pregnancy. The nurse plans to base the response on which of the following?

1. The breast changes result from the secretion of estrogen and progesterone

2. The breasts become stretched because of the weight gain

3. The increased metabolic rate causes the breasts to become larger

4. Cortisol secreted by the adrenal glands plays a role in increasing the size and changing the appearance of the breasts

66. A nurse is caring for a client receiving bolus feedings via a Levin type of nasogastric tube. As the nurse is finishing the feeding, the client asks for the bed to be positioned flat to sleep. The nurse understands that the most appropriate position for this client at this time is which of the following?

1. Head of the bed flat with the client in the supine position for at least 30 minutes

2. Head of the bed elevated 30 to 45 degrees with the client in the right lateral position for 60 minutes

3. Head of the bed elevated 45 to 60 degrees with the client in the supine position for 30 minutes

4. Head of the bed in semi-Fowler's with the client in the left lateral position for 60 minutes

67. Before administering an intermittent tube feeding through a nasogastric tube, a nurse assesses for gastric residuum. The nurse understands that this procedure is important to:

1. Confirm proper nasogastric tube placement

2. Observe the digestion of formula

3. Assess fluid and electrolyte status

4. Evaluate absorption of the last feeding

68. A 4-year-old child is diagnosed with otitis media. The mother asks the nurse about the causes of this illness. The nurse responds, knowing that which of the following is not a risk factor associated with otitis media?

1. Household smoking

2. Bottle feeding

3. Exposure to illness in other children

4. A history of urinary tract infections (UTIs)

69. A pediatric nurse assists a physician in performing a lumbar puncture on a 3-year-old child with leukemia suspected of central nervous system (CNS) metastasis. The nurse places the child in which position for this procedure?

1. Prone with the knees flexed to the abdomen and the head bent, with the chin resting on the chest

2. Modified Sims' position

3. Lateral recumbent with the knees flexed to the abdomen and the head bent, with the chin resting on the chest

4. Lithotomy position

70. A client with diabetes mellitus is self-administering NPH insulin from a vial that is kept at room temperature. The client asks a nurse about the length of time an unrefrigerated vial of insulin will maintain its potency. The most appropriate response to the client is which of the following?

1. Two weeks

2. One month

3. Two months

4. Six months

71. A nurse is caring for a client scheduled for a transsphenoidal hypophysectomy. Which of the following would be the most important statement to include in the preoperative teaching plan?

1. "Your hair will need to be shaved."

2. "Deep breathing and coughing will be needed after surgery."

3. "Toothbrushing will not be permitted for at least 2 weeks following surgery."

4. "You will receive spinal anesthesia."

72. A nurse caring for a client with Addison's disease would expect to note which of the following on assessment of the client?

1. Obesity

2. Edema

3. Hypotension

4. Hirsutism

73. A nurse is conducting a prepared childbirth class and is instructing pregnant women about the method of effleurage. The nurse instructs the women to perform the procedure by:

1. Contracting and then consciously relaxing different muscle groups

2. Contracting an area of the body such as an arm or leg and then concentrating on letting tension go from the rest of the body

3. Massaging the abdomen during contractions, using both hands in a circular motion

4. Instructing the significant other to stroke or massage a tightened muscle by the use of touch

74. During a routine prenatal visit, a client complains of gums that bleed easily with brushing. A nurse performs an assessment and then teaches the client about proper nutrition to minimize this problem. Which statement, if made by the client, indicates an understanding of the proper nutrition to minimize this problem?

1. "I will eat three servings of cracked wheat bread each day."

2. "I will eat fresh fruits and vegetables for snacks and for dessert each day."

3. "I will drink 8 ounces of water with each meal."

4. "I will eat two saltine crackers before I get up each morning."

75. A 6-year-old child has just been diagnosed with localized Hodgkin's disease, and chemotherapy is planned to begin immediately. The mother of the child asks the nurse about radiation therapy because it was not prescribed as a part of

treatment. The most appropriate and supportive response to the mother is:

1. "I'm not sure. I'll discuss it with the physician."
2. "The child is too young to have radiation therapy."
3. "It's very costly, and chemotherapy works just as well."
4. "The physician would prefer that you discuss treatment options with the oncologist."

76. A diagnostic workup is being performed on a 1-year-old child, and a diagnosis of neuroblastoma is suspected. A nurse reviews the results of the diagnostic tests and understands that which finding is most specifically related to this type of tumor?

1. Elevated vanillylmandelic acid (VMA) urinary levels
2. The presence of blast cells in the bone marrow
3. Projectile vomiting occurring most often in the morning
4. Positive Babinski's sign

77. A nurse is developing a postoperative plan of care for a 40-year-old male Filipino client scheduled for an appendectomy. The nurse most appropriately includes in the plan of care to:

1. Inform the client that he will need to ask for pain medication when needed
2. Offer pain medication when nonverbal signs of discomfort are identified
3. Offer pain medication on a regular basis as prescribed
4. Allow the client to maintain control and request pain medication on his own

78. A nurse provides instructions regarding home care to the parents of a 3-year-old child hospitalized with hemophilia. Which statement, if made by the parents, indicates a need for further instructions?

1. "We will supervise the child closely."
2. "We will pad corners of the furniture."
3. "We will remove household items that can easily fall over."
4. "We will avoid having the child receive immunizations and cancel the scheduled dental appointments."

79. A nurse is planning to instruct a Mexican American client about nutrition and dietary restrictions. When developing the plan, the nurse is aware that this ethnic group:

1. Enjoys foods that lack color, flavor, and texture
2. Primarily eats raw fish
3. Enjoys eating red meat
4. Views food as a primary form of socialization

80. A registered nurse is planning the client assignments for the day. Which of the following is the most appropriate assignment for the nursing assistant?

1. A client with bladder cancer who will be receiving chemotherapy

2. A client scheduled for a barium enema who requires tap water enemas until clear
3. A new diabetic mellitus client scheduled for discharge
4. A client scheduled to receive a blood transfusion

81. Propythiouracil (PTU) is prescribed for a client with hyperthyroidism. A nurse provides instructions to the client regarding the medication. The nurse instructs the client to notify the physician if which of the following signs occurs?

1. Drowsiness
2. Sore throat
3. Increased urination
4. Dry mouth

82. A client who has been taking iodine solution (Lugol solution, potassium iodide solution) is admitted to an emergency department, and an iodine overdose is suspected. Gastric lavage is initiated to remove the iodine from the stomach. In addition to treatment with gastric lavage, a nurse anticipates that which of the following will be administered?

1. Calcium gluconate
2. Vitamin K
3. Acetylcysteine (Mucomyst)
4. Sodium thiosulfate

83. A nurse is interviewing a 16-year-old client during her initial prenatal clinic visit. The client is beginning week 18 of her first pregnancy. Which statement, if made by the client, indicates an immediate need for further investigation?

1. "I don't like my face anymore. I always look like I have been crying."
2. "I don't like my breasts anymore. These silver lines are ugly."
3. "I don't like my stomach anymore. That brown line is disgusting."
4. "I don't like my figure anymore. My clothes are all too tight."

84. A client seen in a health care clinic has tested positive for gonorrhea. A nurse anticipates that which medication will be prescribed for the client on the basis of this finding?

1. Ceftriaxone (Rocephin)
2. Benzathine penicillin G (Bicillin)
3. Acyclovir (Zovirax)
4. Azithromycin (Zithromax)

85. A client is brought into an emergency department in ventricular fibrillation (VF). The advanced cardiac life support (ACLS) nurse prepares to defibrillate by placing conductive gel pads on which parts of the chest?

1. The upper and lower halves of the sternum
2. The right of the sternum just below the clavicle and to the left of the precordium
3. The right shoulder and in the back of the left shoulder

4. Parallel between the umbilicus and the right nipple

86. A rubella vaccine is prescribed to be administered to a client who is 2 days postpartum. The nurse preparing to administer the vaccine develops a list of the potential risks associated with this vaccine. The nurse reviews the list with the client and cautions the client to avoid:
   1. Sunlight for 3 days
   2. Scratching the injection site
   3. Pregnancy for 2 to 3 months after the vaccination
   4. Sexual intercourse for 2 to 3 months after the vaccination

87. A client has undergone mastectomy. A nurse interprets that the client is making the best adjustment to the loss of the breast if which of the following behaviors is observed?
   1. Participating in the care of the surgical drain
   2. Reading a postoperative care booklet
   3. Refusing to look at the wound
   4. Asking for pain medication when needed

88. A client is preparing for discharge 10 days after radical vulvectomy. A nurse plans to teach this client that which of the following activities is acceptable after discharge because it will not precipitate complications?
   1. Sexual activity
   2. Walking
   3. Sitting for lengthy periods
   4. Driving a car

89. A child with croup is being discharged from the hospital. A nurse provides instructions to the mother and advises the mother to bring the child to the emergency department if the child:
   1. Appears tired
   2. Takes fluids poorly
   3. Is irritable
   4. Develops stridor

90. An emergency department nurse is caring for a child suspected of having epiglottitis. The nurse has ensured that the child has a patent airway. The next priority in the care of this child would be to:
   1. Prepare the child for a chest x-ray evaluation
   2. Assist the physician with intubation
   3. Prepare the child for tracheotomy
   4. Prepare to administer epinephrine

91. A nurse reviews the plan of care for a client at 37 weeks of gestation who has sickle cell anemia. The nurse determines that which nursing diagnosis listed in the nursing care plan will receive the highest priority?
   1. Activity intolerance
   2. Body image disturbance
   3. Potential alteration in comfort
   4. Fluid volume deficit

92. A mother arrives at a clinic with her 3-year-old child. The mother tells a nurse that the child has had a fever and a cough for the past 2 days, and that this morning the child began to wheeze. Viral pneumonia is diagnosed. On the basis of the diagnosis, the nurse anticipates that which of the following will be a component of the treatment plan?
   1. Oral antibiotics
   2. Hospitalization and IV antibiotics
   3. Supportive treatment
   4. IV fluid administration

93. The mother of a child with cystic fibrosis (CF) asks a clinic nurse about the disease. The nurse tells the mother that CF is:
   1. A disease that causes the formation of multiple cysts in the lungs
   2. A chronic multisystem disorder affecting the exocrine glands
   3. Transmitted as an autosomal dominant trait
   4. A disease that causes dilation of the passageways of many organs

94. Minoxidil solution (Rogaine) is prescribed for a client to treat hair loss. A nurse tell the client that the usual dosage for this medication is:
   1. 1 mL applied six times daily
   2. 1 mL applied at bedtime
   3. 1 mL applied two times a day
   4. 1 mL applied four times a day

95. Collagenase (Santyl) is prescribed for a client with a severe burn to the hand. A home care nurse provides instructions to the client regarding the use of the medication. Which client statement indicates an accurate understanding of the use of this medication?
   1. "I will apply the ointment once a day and leave it open to the air."
   2. "I will apply the ointment once a day and cover it with a sterile dressing."
   3. "I will apply the ointment twice a day and leave it open to the air."
   4. "I will apply the ointment at bedtime and in the morning and cover it with a sterile dressing."

96. The mother of an infant diagnosed with Hirschsprung's disease asks a nurse about the disorder. The nurse tells the mother that this disease is a:
   1. Congenital aganglionosis or megacolon
   2. Complete small intestinal obstruction
   3. Condition that causes the pyloric valve to remain open
   4. Severe inflammation of the gastrointestinal tract

97. A nurse is preparing to care for a newborn infant who will be returning from surgery with a colostomy that was created for imperforate anus. When the newborn infant returns from surgery, the nurse assesses the stoma and notes that it is red and edematous. Which of the following is the most appropriate nursing intervention?
   1. Call the physician

2. Document the findings

3. Apply ice immediately

4. Elevate the buttocks

98. A nurse is developing a plan of care for a preterm newborn infant and is addressing measures to provide skin care. The nurse develops measures, knowing that the preterm newborn infant's skin appears:

    1. Reddened, translucent, and gelatinous with decreased amounts of subcutaneous fat

    2. Thin and gelatinous with increased subcutaneous fat

    3. Thin and gelatinous with increased amounts of brown fat

    4. With fine downy hair on thin epidermal and dermal layers with increased amounts of brown fat

99. A nurse in the labor room is performing an initial assessment on a newborn infant. On assessment of the newborn infant's head, the nurse notes that the ears are low set. Which of the following nursing actions would be most appropriate?

    1. Cover the ears with gauze pads

    2. Document the findings

    3. Arrange for hearing testing

    4. Notify the physician

100. A clinic nurse is assessing the status of jaundice in a child with hepatitis. Which anatomical area will provide the best data regarding the presence of jaundice?

    1. The nailbeds

    2. The skin in the abdominal area

    3. The skin in the sacral area

    4. The membranes in the ear canal

101. A perinatal client with a history of heart disease has been instructed in care at home. Which statement, if made by the client, would indicate that the client understands her needs?

    1. "There is no restriction on people who visit me."

    2. "I should avoid stressful situations."

    3. "My weight gain is not important."

    4. "I should rest on my right side."

102. A prenatal client has acquired the sexually transmitted infection human papillomavirus. When planning care, a nurse would anticipate that which of the following interventions would be prescribed because of its safety during pregnancy?

    1. Cryotherapy

    2. Use of cytotoxic agents

    3. Treatment with imiquimod

    4. Treatment with podophyllin

103. A home care nurse is assigned to visit a Mexican American client to perform an admission assessment. On initial meeting of the client, the nurse should plan to:

    1. Greet the client with a handshake

    2. Avoid touching the client

    3. Avoid any affirmative nods during the conversations with the client

    4. Smile and use humor throughout the entire admission assessment

104. Russell's traction is prescribed for a child with a lower leg fracture. The mother of the child asks the nurse about the purpose of the traction. The nurse explains to the mother that this type of traction primarily:

    1. Reduces or realigns a fracture site

    2. Keeps the child from moving around in bed

    3. Provides a form of restraint for the child

    4. Will relieve the child's pain

105. A home care nurse's assignment is to visit a new mother at home 24 to 48 hours after discharge. What finding would the nurse expect in a healthy mother who is breastfeeding her newborn infant?

    1. A mother breastfeeding with the infant in a tummy-to-tummy position, without signs of cracked nipples; the baby demonstrates bursts of sucking followed by a pause and swallow

    2. A mother breastfeeding the infant with the infant's head turned toward her breast, with the body flat in her arms; mother with sore nipples and infant with a suck blister

    3. A mother complaining of breast engorgement, with the infant demonstrating difficulty in latching onto the breast

    4. A mother with cracked nipples feeding the infant with a supplemental bottle

106. A nurse is assigned to care for a client who is in traction. The nurse prepares a plan of care for the client and includes which nursing action in the plan?

    1. Monitoring the weights to be sure that they are resting on a firm surface

    2. Checking the weights to be sure that they are off of the floor

    3. Making sure that the knots are at the pulleys

    4. Making sure the head of the bed is kept at a 45- to 90-degree angle

107. A nurse is conducting a diet history with an elderly client living alone. The nurse finds that the client's typical 24-hour food intake consists of eggs and sausage for breakfast, a fast food lunch of hamburger and French fries, takeout fried chicken for dinner, and ice cream in the evening. To decrease the risk of cancer, what statement would the nurse make to the client?

    1. "You should not eat eggs."

    2. "You should not eat sausage."

    3. "Excessive tobacco use increases the risk of liver cancer."

    4. "A high-fat diet increases your risk of colon cancer."

108. A private duty nurse has been caring for a terminally ill client whose death is imminent. The nurse has developed a close relationship with the

family of the client. Which of the following nursing interventions will the nurse avoid in dealing with the family during this difficult time?

1. Making the decisions for the family
2. Encouraging family discussion of feelings
3. Facilitating the use of spiritual practices identified by the family
4. Accepting the family's expressions of anger

109. A nurse is reviewing the record of a pregnant client and notes that the physician has documented the presence of Chadwick's sign. The nurse understands that the hormone responsible for the development of this sign is which of the following?

1. Human chorionic gonadotropin (hCG)
2. Estrogen
3. Progesterone
4. Prolactin

110. A nurse is caring for an elderly client who has been placed in Buck's extension traction following a hip fracture. On assessment of the client, the nurse notes that the client is disoriented. The most appropriate nursing intervention is to:

1. Ask the family to stay with the client
2. Apply restraints to the client
3. Ask the laboratory to perform electrolyte studies
4. Reorient the client frequently and place a clock and a calendar in the client's room

111. A nurse is preparing a plan of care for a client who is in skin traction. The nurse includes in the plan that a priority intervention is to assess the client frequently for:

1. The presence of bowel sounds
2. Signs of infection around the pin sites
3. Signs of skin breakdown
4. Urinary incontinence

112. A contraction stress test is scheduled for a pregnant client. The client asks a nurse about the test. The nurse tells the client that:

1. Small amounts of oxytocin (Pitocin) are administered during internal fetal monitoring to stimulate uterine contractions
2. An external fetal monitor is attached and the woman ambulates on a treadmill until contractions begin
3. The uterus is stimulated to contract either by small amounts of oxytocin (Pitocin) or by nipple stimulation
4. Uterine contractions are stimulated by Leopold's maneuvers

113. A mother arrives at a well-baby clinic with her 1-month-old infant. She expresses concern because one of the infant's eyes appears to be crossed. The most appropriate and supportive response by the nurse is which of the following?

1. "The infant will probably need surgery."

2. "This condition is probably permanent."
3. "It bears watching because the other eye may do the same thing."
4. "This is normal in the young infant but should not be present after about age 4 months."

114. A physician prescribes "patching" for a child with strabismus of the right eye. A nurse instructs the mother regarding this procedure. Which of the following will the nurse include in the instructions?

1. Place the patch on the right eye
2. Place the patch on both eyes
3. Place the patch on the left eye
4. Alternate the patch from the right to the left eye hourly

115. A nonstress test is performed on a client who is pregnant, and the results of the test indicate nonreactive findings. The physician prescribes a contraction stress test. The test is performed, and the nurse notes that the physician has documented the results as negative. The nurse interprets this finding as indicating:

1. A high risk for fetal demise
2. A normal test result
3. The need for a cesarean delivery
4. An abnormal test result

116. A nurse has developed a plan of care for a client who is in traction and documents a nursing diagnosis of Self-Care Deficit. The nurse evaluates the plan of care and determines that which of the following observations indicates a successful outcome?

1. The client allows the nurse to complete the care on a daily basis
2. The client allows the family to assist in the care
3. The client refuses care
4. The client assists in self-care as much as possible

117. A home care nurse is visiting a client who is in a body cast. The nurse is performing an assessment that includes the psychosocial adjustment of the client to the cast. During the assessment, the nurse would most appropriately include:

1. The type of transportation available for follow-up care
2. The ability to perform activities of daily living
3. The need for sensory stimulation
4. The amount of home care support available

118. A maternity nurse is providing an inservice educational session to nursing students regarding the process of conception. The nurse instructs the nursing students that fertilization of a mature ovum occurs in which of the following areas?

1. Uterus
2. Ovary
3. Distal third of the fallopian tube
4. Wall of the myometrium

119. A nurse is preparing to teach a client how to safely use crutches. Before initiating the teaching, the nurse performs an assessment on the client. The priority nursing assessment should include which of the following?
    1. The client's fear related to the use of the crutches
    2. The client's understanding of the need for increased mobility
    3. The client's vital signs, muscle strength, and previous activity level
    4. The client's feelings about the restricted mobility

120. A nurse is assessing for a Kernig sign in a child with a suspected diagnosis of meningitis. The nurse performs this test by:
    1. Bending the head toward the knees and hips and assessing for pain
    2. Tapping the facial nerve and assessing for spasm
    3. Compressing the upper arm and assessing for tetany
    4. Raising the leg with the knee flexed and then extending the leg at the knee and assessing for pain

121. A physician has written an order to start progressive ambulation as tolerated for a hospitalized client who experiences periods of confusion resulting from bed rest and prolonged confinement to the hospital room. Which nursing intervention would be most appropriate to implement the physician's order and in addressing the needs of the client?
    1. Ambulate the client in the room for short distances frequently
    2. Ambulate the client to the bathroom in the client's room three times a day
    3. Progressively ambulate the client in the hall three times a day
    4. Assist with range-of-motion exercises three times a day to increase strength

122. A client is seen in a health care clinic, and a vitamin K deficiency is suspected. On assessment of the client, a nurse would expect to note which of the following if this vitamin deficiency were present?
    1. Client complaints of night blindness
    2. Signs of clotting problems
    3. Scaly skin
    4. Client complaints of skeletal pain

123. A nurse is caring for a postterm, small-for-gestational age (SGA) newborn infant immediately after admission to the nursery. The priority nursing action would be to monitor:
    1. Urinary output
    2. Total bilirubin levels
    3. Blood glucose levels
    4. Hemoglobin and hematocrit levels

124. A nurse is performing an initial assessment on a large-for-gestational age (LGA) newborn infant. Which physical assessment technique would the nurse perform to assess for the evidence of birth trauma?
    1. Palpate the clavicles for a fracture
    2. Auscultate the heart for a cardiac defect
    3. Blanch the skin for evidence of jaundice
    4. Perform Ortolani's maneuver for hip dislocation

125. Somatropin (Humatrope), a growth hormone, is prescribed for a client. The nurse reviews the assessment data in the client's health record, knowing that the medication is contraindicated in which of the following conditions?
    1. A child with growth hormone deficiency
    2. A child with pituitary dwarfism
    3. A 20-year-old with growth failure
    4. A child with growth failure

126. A nurse is caring for a client who is receiving growth hormone replacement therapy. The nurse monitors the client for which side effect of this therapy?
    1. Hyperglycemia
    2. Hyperthyroidism
    3. Hypoglycemia
    4. Hypocalciuria

127. A nurse is assessing a client with a diagnosis of goiter. Which of the following would the nurse expect to note during the assessment of the client?
    1. Client complaints of slow wound healing
    2. Client complaints of chronic fatigue
    3. An enlarged thyroid gland
    4. The presence of heart damage

128. A fasting blood glucose screening is performed on a pregnant client. The results indicate that the blood glucose is 140 mg/dL. Which of the following would a nurse anticipate to be prescribed for the mother?
    1. Administration of an oral hypoglycemic agent
    2. Administration of NPH insulin on a daily basis
    3. A 3-hour glucose tolerance test (GTT)
    4. A sliding-scale Regular insulin dose

129. A pregnant client seen in a health care clinic has tested positive for human immunodeficiency virus (HIV). On the basis of this information, a nurse determines that:
    1. The client has the herpes simplex virus
    2. HIV antibodies are detected on the ELISA test
    3. The neonate will definitely develop this disease after birth
    4. This client has contracted an airborne disease

130. During a wellness fair, an adult client admits to a nurse of not eating a well-balanced diet. According

to the Food Guide Pyramid, which of the following instructions would the nurse provide to the client?

1. "Your diet should consist of 6 to 11 servings of bread, cereal, pasta, and rice a day."
2. "Your diet should consist of 2 to 4 servings of vegetables a day."
3. "Your diet should consist of 4 to 5 servings of milk, yogurt, and cheese a day."
4. "Your diet should consist of 4 to 6 servings of meat, poultry, fish, dry beans, and nuts a day."

131. An 85-year-old client is hospitalized for a right fractured hip. During the postoperative period, the client's appetite is poor and the client refuses to get out of bed. Which nursing statement would be most appropriate to make to the client?

1. "It is important for you to get out of bed so that calcium will go back into the bone."
2. "We need to increase your calcium intake because you are spending too much time in bed."
3. "We need to give you iodine so that it will help in hemoglobin synthesis."
4. "You need to remember to turn yourself in bed every 2 hours to keep from getting so stiff."

132. Lindane (Kwell) is prescribed for the treatment of scabies. A nurse reviews the client's record, knowing that the medication therapy is contraindicated if the client is:

1. A 42-year-old female
2. An elderly client
3. A 6-year-old child
4. A 52-year-old male with hypertension

133. DuoDerm is prescribed for a client with a leg ulcer. A home health nurse is preparing a plan of care for the client and most appropriately documents to:

1. Change the DuoDerm daily
2. Apply the DuoDerm over a dry sterile dressing
3. Change the DuoDerm weekly
4. Apply the DuoDerm over a normal saline–soaked dressing

134. A nurse is performing an initial assessment on a large-for-gestational age (LGA) newborn infant. The nurse understands that the LGA infant is at most risk for which type of birth trauma?

1. Shoulder dystocia
2. Transposition of the great vessels
3. Jaundice
4. Hip dislocation

135. A pregnant woman in her second trimester has been exposed to a child with rubella. The nurse anticipates that a rubella titer screen will be performed, knowing that:

1. The incubation period begins immediately following exposure
2. There is little risk in the second trimester as a result of exposure
3. The woman should avoid all school-aged children during pregnancy
4. Congenital anomalies can occur as a result of infection

136. A nursing instructor is providing a session on cultural beliefs related to health. After the session, the instructor asks a nursing student to describe the beliefs of an Appalachian client in regard to health care providers. Which of the following would be the most appropriate response by the nursing student?

1. "The Appalachian client will evaluate the nurse's effectiveness on the basis of professional competency."
2. "The Appalachian client expects an impersonal relationship with the nurse."
3. "The Appalachian client is most comfortable with impersonal relationships with health care providers."
4. "The Appalachian client will evaluate the nurse's effectiveness on the basis of interpersonal skills."

137. A pregnant woman has a positive history of genital herpes. The nurse provides information to the woman about delivery and determines that the woman understands if she states:

1. "I will be isolated from my newborn infant following delivery."
2. "I may need a cesarean delivery."
3. "There is little risk to my newborn infant."
4. "I can deliver vaginally even if I have an active lesion at birth."

138. A registered nurse (RN) is planning assignments for the clients on a nursing unit. The RN needs to assign four clients and has a registered nurse, a licensed practical (vocational) nurse, and two nursing assistants on a nursing team. Which of the following clients would the nurse most appropriately assign to the licensed practical (vocational) nurse?

1. A client who requires a 24-hour urine collection
2. An elderly client requiring assistance with a bed bath and frequent ambulation
3. A client on a mechanical ventilator who requires frequent assessment and suctioning
4. A client with an abdominal wound requiring wound irrigations and dressing changes every 3 hours

139. A nursing instructor asks a nursing student to define a critical path. Which of the following

statements if made by the student indicates a need for further understanding regarding critical paths?
1. "They are developed through the collaborative efforts of all members of the health care team."
2. "They provide an effective way to monitor care and for reducing or controlling the length of hospital stay for the client."
3. "They are developed based on appropriate standards of care."
4. "They are nursing care plans and use the steps of the nursing process."

140. A nurse is caring for an 18-month-old child who has been vomiting. The most appropriate position for the child during naps and sleep time is:
1. Side-lying position
2. Prone with the face turned to the side
3. Supine
4. Prone with the head elevated

141. The parents of a child with a cleft lip are concerned and ask a nurse when the lip will be repaired. The nurse supportively tells the parents that:
1. Cleft lip repair is usually performed between 6 months and 2 years
2. Cleft lip repair is usually performed by 6 months of age
3. Cleft lip repair is usually performed during the first weeks of life
4. Cleft lip cannot be repaired

142. A nurse is assessing a client for signs of postpartum depression. Which of the following if noted in the new mother would indicate the need for further assessment related to this form of depression?
1. The mother is caring for the infant in a loving manner
2. The mother constantly complains of tiredness and fatigue
3. The mother demonstrates an interest in the surroundings
4. The mother looks forward to visits from the father of the newborn

143. A postpartum client is attempting to breastfeed for the first time. A nurse notes that the client has inverted nipples. What nursing action can the nurse take to assist the client in breastfeeding the newborn infant?
1. Provide breast shells and assist the mother with using a breast pump before each feeding to make the nipples easier for the newborn infant to grasp
2. Have the mother grasp the nipples between the thumb and forefinger and tug firmly to get them to protrude
3. Massage the breast, applying gentle pressure on the areola
4. Take a cool shower, allowing the water to run over the breasts because this will encourage the nipples to protrude

144. A nurse instructs a client in breast self-examination (BSE). The nurse tells the client to lie down and to examine the left breast. The nurse instructs the client that while examining the left breast, to place a pillow:
1. Under the right shoulder
2. Under the left shoulder
3. Under the small of the back
4. Under the right scapula

145. A nurse is teaching breast self-examination (BSE) to a client who had a hysterectomy. The most appropriate instruction regarding when the BSE should be performed is:
1. 7 to 10 days after menses
2. Just before menses begin
3. At ovulation time
4. On a specific day of the month and on that same day every month thereafter

146. A nursing instructor asks a nursing student to describe Montgomery's tubercles of the breast. The student indicates an understanding of this anatomical structure if the student states that Montgomery's tubercles are:
1. Sebaceous glands that are located in the areola
2. Lobes of glandular tissue that secrete milk
3. Small sacs that contain acinar cells to secrete milk
4. Ducts containing milk from all areas of the breast

147. A 32-year-old female client has a history of fibrocystic disorder of the breasts. A nurse interviewing the client asks whether the breast lumps are more noticeable:
1. In the spring months
2. In the autumn
3. After menses
4. Before menses

148. A 1-year-old child is diagnosed with intussusception. The mother of the child asks a nurse to describe the disorder. The nurse tells the mother that this disorder is:
1. An acute bowel obstruction
2. A condition that occurs when a proximal segment of the bowel prolapses into a distal segment of the bowel
3. A condition that occurs when a distal segment of the bowel prolapses into a proximal segment of the bowel
4. A condition that causes an acute inflammatory process in the bowel

149. A 3-year-old child is seen in a health care clinic, and a diagnosis of encopresis is made. A nurse reviews the assessment findings, expecting to note documentation of which sign of this disorder?
1. Nausea and vomiting
2. Diarrhea
3. Evidence of soiled clothing
4. Malaise and anorexia

150. A nurse is teaching a client who had a laryngectomy for laryngeal cancer how to use an artificial larynx. The nurse tells the client to:
    1. Insert the device into the tracheostomy
    2. Hold the device alongside the neck
    3. Hold the device over the upper portion of the sternum
    4. Swallow air into the esophagus to make speech

151. A client is scheduled for a Papanicolaou (Pap) smear at the next scheduled clinic visit. A nurse provides instructions to the client regarding preparation for this test. The nurse tells the client that:
    1. The test can be performed during menstruation
    2. Fluids are restricted on the day of the test
    3. The test is painless
    4. Vaginal douching is required 2 hours before the test

152. A nurse witnesses an accident on a highway and stops to provide assistance to the victim. The nurse notes that the client sustained a head injury and a compound fracture to the left leg. The nurse provides the appropriate care before transport of the victim to the hospital by ambulance. The client develops a severe bone infection at the site of the fracture, which requires amputation of the leg, and files suit against the nurse who provided care at the scene of the accident. Which of the following is accurate regarding the nurse's immunity from this suit?
    1. The Good Samaritan Law will protect the nurse
    2. The Good Samaritan Law will not protect the nurse
    3. The Good Samaritan Law will provide immunity from suit even if the nurse accepted compensation for the care provided
    4. The Good Samaritan Law protects lay persons and not professional health care providers

153. A client is seen in a clinic for complaints of thirst, frequent urination, and headaches. Following diagnostic studies, diabetes insipidus in diagnosed. Lypressin (Diapid) is prescribed. A nurse instructs the client that the medication is prescribed to:
    1. Relieve the headaches
    2. Increase water reabsorption
    3. Decrease the production of the antidiuretic hormone
    4. Stimulate the production of aldosterone

154. Somatrem (Protropin) is prescribed for a client with pituitary dwarfism. A nurse explains to the client that the expected outcome of the medication is:
    1. Growth that begins in 4 to 5 years
    2. An increase in height that will begin in late adulthood
    3. An immediate increase in growth
    4. Growth spurts that occur every 2 years

155. A nurse manager attends a conference, and the topic of discussion is leadership styles. The nurse is seeking a leadership style that will best empower staff toward excellence. Which leadership style would the nurse select to achieve this goal?
    1. Autocratic
    2. Situational
    3. Democratic
    4. Laissez-faire

156. A community health nurse is working with disaster relief following a tornado. The nurse's goal with the overall community is to prevent as much injury and death as possible from the uncontrollable event. Finding safe housing for survivors, providing support to families, organizing counseling, and securing physical care when needed are all examples of which type of prevention?
    1. The primary level of prevention.
    2. The secondary level of prevention.
    3. The tertiary level of prevention.
    4. Aggregate care prevention

157. A nursing instructor asks a nursing student about the physiology related to the cessation of ovulation that occurs during pregnancy. Which of the following responses if made by the student indicates an understanding of this physiological process?
    1. "Ovulation ceases during pregnancy because the circulating levels of estrogen and progesterone are high."
    2. "Ovulation ceases during pregnancy because the circulating levels of estrogen and progesterone are low."
    3. "The low levels of estrogen and progesterone increase the release of the follicle-stimulating hormone and the luteinizing hormone."
    4. "The high levels of estrogen and progesterone promote the release of the follicle-stimulating hormone and the luteinizing hormone."

158. Calcifediol (Calderol) is prescribed for a client with hypoparathyroidism in the management of hypocalcemia. The client arrives at a clinic for a follow-up visit and complains of chronic constipation. Which of the following would not be a component of the teaching plan to alleviate the constipation?
    1. Increase daily fluid intake
    2. Add one-half ounce of mineral oil to the daily diet
    3. Increase high-fiber foods
    4. Increase activity level as tolerated

159. Etidronate (Didronel), an antihypercalcemic medication, is prescribed for a client. A nurse instructs the client to take the medication:
    1. Two hours before meals
    2. With meals
    3. With milk
    4. With an antacid

160. A client was hospitalized for a cervical radiation implant. The implant is removed, and a nurse provides home care instructions to the client. Which statement made by the client indicates a need for further instructions?
    1. "Cream may be used to relieve dryness or itching."
    2. "Foul-smelling vaginal discharge is a sign of an infection."
    3. "Sexual intercourse may be resumed after 7 to 10 days."
    4. "Some vaginal bleeding is expected for 1 to 3 months."

161. A nurse teaches skin care to a client receiving external radiation therapy. Which of the following statements, if made by the client, would indicate the need for further instruction?
    1. "I will handle the area gently."
    2. "I will avoid the use of deodorants."
    3. "I will limit sun exposure to 1 hour daily."
    4. "I will wear loose-fitting clothing."

162. A nurse manager is planning to implement a change in the nursing unit from team nursing to primary nursing. The nurse anticipates that there will be resistance to the change during the change process. The primary technique that the nurse would use in implementing this change is which of the following?
    1. Introduce the change gradually
    2. Confront the individuals involved in the change process
    3. Use coercion to implement the change
    4. Manipulate the participants in the change process

163. Lispro insulin (Humalog), a rapid-acting form of insulin, is prescribed for a client. The client is instructed to administer the insulin before meals. A nurse instructs the client to administer the insulin:
    1. Immediately before eating
    2. 30 minutes before eating
    3. 45 minutes before eating
    4. 60 minutes before eating

164. An emergency department nurse is caring for a client admitted with diabetic ketoacidosis. The physician prescribes IV insulin. The nurse plans to prepare which type of insulin for the client?
    1. NPH
    2. Regular
    3. Lente
    4. Ultralente

165. A client has an order for a set of arterial blood gases (ABGs) to be drawn on "room air." The client is currently receiving oxygen by nasal cannula at a delivery rate of 3 liters per minute. After reading the order, the nurse takes which of the following actions?
    1. Removes the oxygen for 15 minutes; then has the ABGs drawn
    2. Leaves the nasal cannula in place for 15 minutes; then has the ABGs drawn
    3. Changes the nasal cannula to a Venturi face mask; then has the ABGs drawn
    4. Changes the nasal cannula to a shovel face mask; then has the ABGs drawn

166. Metformin (Glucophage) is prescribed for a client with type 2 diabetes mellitus. The nurse tells the client that the most common side effect of the medication is:
    1. Hypoglycemia
    2. Gastrointestinal (GI) disturbances
    3. Weight gain
    4. Flushing and palpitations

167. A nurse encourages a pregnant human immuno-deficiency virus (HIV)–positive client to report any early signs of vaginal discharge or perineal tenderness to the health care providers immediately. The client asks the nurse about the importance of this action, and the nurse responds by telling the client that this is necessary to:
    1. Relieve anxiety for the pregnant client
    2. Eliminate the need for further, unnecessary screenings
    3. Assist in identifying potential infections that may need to be treated
    4. Minimize the financial cost of caring for an HIV-positive client

168. A pregnant client who is anemic tells a nurse that she is concerned about her baby's condition following delivery. Which nursing response would best support the client?
    1. "You will not have any problems if you follow all the advice the doctor has given you."
    2. "Your baby will need to spend a few days in the neonatal intensive care unit following delivery."
    3. "Don't worry about your baby; complications are rare."
    4. "The effects of anemia on your baby are difficult to predict, but let's review your plan of care to ensure that you are providing the best nutrition and growth potential."

169. A diabetic nurse specialist conducts a teaching session for a group of nursing students regarding sulfonylureas, oral hypoglycemic medications used for type 2 diabetes mellitus. The nurse specialist tells the students that the primary action of these medications is to:
    1. Decrease glucose production by the liver
    2. Inhibit carbohydrate digestion
    3. Promote insulin secretion by the pancreas
    4. Decrease insulin resistance

170. A male client with diabetes mellitus calls a clinic and tells a nurse that he has been nauseated during the night. The client asks the nurse if the morning insulin should be administered. Which

of the following is the most appropriate nursing response?

1. Omit the insulin
2. Administer half of the prescribed dose
3. Administer the full dose as prescribed
4. Wait until noontime before making a decision

171. A client with Cushing's syndrome verbalizes concern to a nurse regarding the appearance of the buffalo hump that has developed. Which statement by the nurse is most appropriate?

1. "This is permanent, but looks are deceiving and not that important."
2. "Don't be concerned; this problem can be covered with clothing."
3. "Try not to worry about it; there are other things to be concerned about."
4. "Usually these physical changes slowly improve following treatment."

172. A nurse is caring for a client following thyroidectomy. The nurse notes that calcium gluconate is prescribed for the client. The nurse determines that this medication has been prescribed to:

1. Treat thyroid storm
2. Prevent cardiac irritability
3. Stimulate release of parathyroid hormone
4. Treat hypocalcemic tetany

173. A pregnant human immunodeficiency virus (HIV)–positive woman delivers a newborn infant. A nurse provides instructions to the mother regarding the newborn infant care. Which statement by the mother indicates a need for further instructions?

1. "I will wash my hands frequently."
2. "Support groups are available to me."
3. "I will breastfeed."
4. "My infant should be on antiviral medications for the first 6 weeks after delivery."

174. A client with type 1 diabetes mellitus is to begin an exercise program, and a nurse is providing instructions to the client regarding the program. Which of the following does the nurse include in the teaching plan?

1. Exercise is best performed during peak times of insulin
2. Administer insulin after exercising
3. Take a blood glucose test before exercising
4. Try to exercise before mealtime

175. A nursery room nurse is assessing a newborn infant who was born to a mother who abuses alcohol. Which of the following assessment findings would the nurse expect to note?

1. Lethargy
2. Higher than normal birth weight
3. Irritability
4. A greater than normal appetite when feeding

176. A postpartum nurse is teaching a mother how to provide a bath to the newborn infant. Which of the following instructions would not be a component of the plan of care?

1. To bathe the newborn infant after a feeding
2. To fill a clean basin or sink with 2 to 3 inches of water and then check the temperature by using the wrist
3. To never leave the newborn infant in the tub of water alone
4. To gather all supplies before the bath is started

177. A 13-year-old child is diagnosed with a Ewing sarcoma of the femur. After a course of radiation and chemotherapy, it has been decided that leg amputation is necessary. After the amputation, the child becomes very frightened because of aching and cramping felt in the missing limb. Which nursing statement would be most appropriate to assist in alleviating the child's fear?

1. "This aching and cramping is normal and temporary and will subside."
2. "This normally occurs after the surgery, and we will teach you ways to deal with it."
3. "The pain medication that I give you will take these feelings away."
4. "This pain is not real pain, and relaxation exercises will help it go away."

178. Oral iron supplements are prescribed for a 6-year-old child with iron deficiency anemia (IDA). A nurse instructs the mother to administer the iron with which of the following food items?

1. Water
2. Milk
3. Apple juice
4. Orange juice

179. A client with diabetes mellitus is being discharged following treatment for hyperglycemic hyperosmolar nonketotic syndrome (HHNS) precipitated by acute illness. The client tells the nurse, "I will call the doctor next time I can't eat for more than a day or so." Which of the following statements reflects the most appropriate analysis of this client's level of knowledge?

1. The client needs immediate education before discharge
2. The client's statement is accurate, but knowledge should be evaluated further
3. The client's statement is inaccurate, and the client should be scheduled for outpatient diabetic counseling
4. The client requires follow-up teaching regarding the administration of insulin

180. A client with type 1 diabetes mellitus is having trouble remembering the types, duration, and onset of action of insulin. The client tells a nurse that family members have not been supportive. The nurse's best response to the client is:

1. "You can't always depend on your family to help."

2. "Let me go over the types of insulin with you again."

3. "It's not really necessary for you to remember this."

4. "What is it that you don't understand?"

181. A nursing student is asked to specify the size of the uterus in a nonpregnant client. The student responds correctly by stating that the uterus in a nonpregnant client:
1. Weighs about 2 ounces
2. Weighs about 2.2 pounds
3. Has a capacity of about 50 mL
4. Is round in shape and weighs approximately 1000 g

182. Fludrocortisone (Florinef) is prescribed for a client with Addison's disease. A nurse prepares to administer the medication, knowing that the primary action of this medication is to:
1. Enhance the reabsorption of sodium and chloride ions in the distal tubules of the kidney
2. Promote the retention of potassium in the distal tubules of the kidney
3. Promote the retention of hydrogen ions in the distal tubules of the kidney
4. Promote the excretion of water in the distal tubules of the kidney

183. A nurse is performing an assessment on a pregnant client at 16 weeks of gestation. The nurse would expect that the fundus of the uterus would be located at which of the following areas?
1. Midway between the symphysis pubis and the umbilicus
2. At the umbilicus
3. Just above the symphysis pubis
4. At the level of the xiphoid process

184. A nursing instructor asks a nursing student to identify the priorities of care for an assigned client. The student correctly identifies the client needs that are the priority by telling the nursing instructor that:
1. Actual or life-threatening concerns are the priority
2. Time constraints related to the client's needs are the priority
3. Obtaining needed supplies to care for the client is the priority
4. Completing care in a reasonable time frame is the priority

185. A nurse employed in a prenatal clinic is performing prenatal assessments on clients who are in the first trimester of pregnancy. The nurse is concerned with identifying clients who may be at risk for the development of postpartum complications. Which of the following clients would be least likely at risk for the development of thromboembolitic disorders in the postpartum period?
1. A 39-year-old woman who reports that she smokes

2. A 37-year-old woman in her fourth pregnancy who is overweight

3. A 26-year-old woman with a family history of thrombophlebitis

4. A woman who is 22 years old with a first pregnancy and who states that oral contraceptives taken in the past have caused thrombophlebitis

186. A client arrives at a clinic complaining of fatigue, a lack of energy, constipation, and depression. After diagnostic studies, hypothyroidism is diagnosed. Levothyroxine (Synthroid) is prescribed. A nurse instructs the client that the expected outcome of the medication is to:
1. Increase energy levels
2. Achieve normal thyroid hormone levels
3. Increase blood glucose levels
4. Alleviate depression

187. A client diagnosed with hypothyroidism is taking levothyroxine (Synthroid). The client returns to the clinic 1 week after beginning the medication and tells the nurse that the medication has not helped. The most appropriate nursing response to the client is based on which of the following?
1. A higher dosage is required
2. The medication may need to be changed
3. Full therapeutic effect may take 1 to 3 weeks
4. Full therapeutic effect may take up to 4 months

188. A nurse has provided instructions for a mother who is at risk for thrombosis regarding measures to prevent its occurrence. Which of the following statements if made by the mother indicates a need for further education?
1. "I should perform regularly scheduled exercise such as walking."
2. "I should avoid prolonged standing or sitting in one position."
3. "I should avoid using pillows under my knees, to prevent pressure in the back of my knee area."
4. "I should apply my antiembolism stockings after my shower in the morning."

189. A nurse is preparing to administer an IV insulin injection. The vial of Regular insulin has been refrigerated. On inspection of the vial, the nurse finds the medication frozen. The nurse should:
1. Wait for the insulin to thaw at room temperature
2. Check the temperature settings of the refrigerator
3. Discard the insulin and obtain another vial
4. Rotate the vial between the hands until the medication becomes liquid

190. In a prenatal clinic, a nurse is interviewing a new client for the health history information. The nurse plans to do which of the following to most

appropriately elicit accurate responses to questions that refer to sexually transmitted diseases?
1. Establish a therapeutic relationship
2. Use specific closed-ended questions
3. Omit this area of questions because it is highly personal
4. Apologize for the embarrassment that these questions will cause the client

191. A clinic nurse is teaching a pregnant client about the warning signs in pregnancy. Which of the following, if identified as a warning sign by the client, would indicate a need for further education?
1. Visual disturbances
2. Rapid weight gain
3. Generalized or facial edema
4. The presence of irregular painless contractions

192. A nurse is preparing to discharge a client who has had a parathyroidectomy. The discharge instructions include administration of oral calcium supplements that the client will need daily. Which statement by the nurse would be appropriate regarding the oral calcium supplement therapy?
1. Store the tablets in the refrigerator to maintain potency
2. Check the pulse daily; if it is below 60 beats per minute, do not take the tablets
3. Take the tablets after a meal
4. Avoid sunlight because the medication can cause skin color change

193. A nurse is providing instructions to a client with hypophosphatemia. The nurse instructs the client to avoid:
1. Fish
2. Chicken
3. Organ meats
4. Cheese

194. A nurse is assessing the learning readiness of a client newly diagnosed with diabetes mellitus. Which client behavior indicates to the nurse that the client is not ready to learn?
1. The client complains of fatigue whenever the nurse plans a teaching session
2. The client asks if the spouse can attend the teaching session
3. The client asks for written materials about diabetes mellitus before class
4. The client asks appropriate questions about what will be taught

195. A young male client with type 1 diabetes mellitus tells a nurse that he might lose his job because he has been having frequent hypoglycemic reactions. His boss thinks that he is drunk during these episodes, and that he has been drinking on the job. Which action by the nurse would best assist this client to meet his needs?
1. Contact the local employment office to help him find another job

2. Ask the client if he indeed has been drinking at work
3. Examine factors with the client that may be causing frequent hypoglycemic episodes
4. Ask the client what he does to treat his hypoglycemia

196. A nurse in a newborn nursery is assessing a neonate who was born of a mother addicted to cocaine. Which of the following would the nurse not expect to note in the neonate?
1. Tremors
2. Bradycardia
3. Irritability
4. Hypertension

197. Thyroid replacement therapy is prescribed for a client diagnosed with hypothyroidism. The client asks a nurse when the medication will no longer be needed. The most appropriate nursing response is which of the following?
1. "You will need to ask your physician."
2. "Most clients require medication therapy for about 1 year."
3. "It depends on the results of the laboratory tests."
4. "The medication will need to be continued for life."

198. An adult client with hypothyroidism is admitted to the hospital. On admission assessment, a nurse notes that the client is taking a maintenance dose of levothyroxine (Synthroid). The nurse transcribes the medication order, knowing that the normal adult maintenance dose of this medication is:
1. 0.025 to 0.05 mg daily
2. 0.075 to 0.1 mg daily
3. 0.05 to 0.075 mg daily
4. 0.1 to 0.2 mg daily

199. A nurse is performing a physical assessment on a client during her first prenatal visit to the clinic. The nurse takes the client's temperature and notes that it is 99.2° F. On the basis of this finding, which nursing action is most appropriate?
1. Document the temperature
2. Retake the temperature by the rectal route
3. Notify the physician
4. Inform the client that the temperature is elevated and that antibiotics may be required

200. A physician orders a 24-hour urine collection for vanillylmandelic acid (VMA). A community health nurse visits the client at home and instructs the client in the procedure for the collection of the urine. Which statement, if made by the client, would indicate a need for further instruction?
1. "I will start the collection in 2 days. Starting now, I cannot eat or drink any tea, chocolate, vanilla, or fruit until the test is completed."
2. "When I start the collection, I will urinate and discard that specimen."

3. "I will pour the urine in the collection bottle each time I urinate and refrigerate the urine."

4. "I can take medication if I need to during the collection."

201. A client with pheochromocytoma is scheduled for surgery and says to the nurse, "I'm not sure that surgery is the best thing to do." The most appropriate response by the nurse is which of the following?
1. "You have concerns about the surgical treatment for your condition?"
2. "There is no reason to worry. Your doctor is a wonderful surgeon."
3. "You are very ill. Your physician has made the correct decision."
4. "I think you are making the right decision to have the surgery."

202. A nurse has inserted a nasogastric (NG) tube to the level of the oropharynx and has repositioned the client's head in a flexed-forward position. The client has been asked to begin swallowing. The nurse starts to slowly advance the nasogastric tube with each swallow. The client begins to cough, gag, and choke. Which nursing action would least likely result in proper tube insertion and promote client relaxation?
1. Continuing to advance the tube to the desired distance
2. Pulling the tube back slightly
3. Checking the back of the pharynx by using a tongue blade and flashlight
4. Instructing the client to breathe slowly

203. A maternity nurse is describing the ovarian cycle to a group of nursing students. The instructor asks a nursing student to identify the phases of the cycle. Which of the following, if identified as a phase of the cycle by the nursing student, indicates a need to further research this area?
1. Follicular phase
2. Ovulatory phase
3. Luteal phase
4. Proliferative phase

204. A client seen in a health care clinic is diagnosed with mild anemia. The anemia is believed to be a result of the menstrual period. The woman asks a nurse how much blood is lost during a menstrual period. The nurse plans to base the response on which of the following amounts of blood lost during this time?
1. 40 mL
2. 60 mL
3. 80 mL
4. 100 mL

205. A nurse is caring for a client with acute pancreatitis and is monitoring the client for paralytic ileus.

Which assessment data would alert the nurse to this occurrence?
1. Firm, nontender mass palpable at the lower right costal margin
2. Severe, constant pain with rapid onset
3. Inability to pass flatus
4. Loss of anal sphincter control

206. A nurse inspects the color of the drainage from a nasogastric tube on a postoperative client approximately 24 hours after a laparotomy. Which of the following findings would indicate the need to notify the physician?
1. Light yellowish brown drainage
2. Dark red drainage
3. Dark brown drainage
4. Greenish tinged drainage

207. A nurse is preparing to discontinue a client's nasogastric (NG) tube. The client is positioned properly, and the tube has been flushed with 15 mL of air to clear secretions. Before removing the tube, the nurse makes which statement to the client?
1. "Take a deep breath when I tell you and breathe normally while I remove the tube."
2. "Take a deep breath when I tell you and bear down while I remove the tube."
3. "Take a deep breath when I tell you and slowly exhale while I remove the tube."
4. "Take a deep breath when I tell you and hold it while I remove the tube."

208. A nurse is caring for a client with a nasogastric (NG) tube connected to continuous suction. During the assessment, the nurse observes that the client is mouth breathing, has dry mucous membranes, and has a foul breath odor. In planning care, which of the following would be the most appropriate to maintain the integrity of this client's oral mucosa?
1. Offer small sips of water frequently
2. Encourage the client to suck on sour, hard candy
3. Brush teeth frequently; use mouthwash and water
4. Use lemon-glycerin swabs to provide oral hygiene

209. A client with a small bowel obstruction asks a nurse to explain the purpose of the nasogastric tube and continuous gastric suction. After the teaching is completed, the nurse determines that the client understands if the client states that the purpose of the continuous gastric suction is to:
1. Provide nourishment
2. Relieve the bronchi of mucus
3. Withdraw gastric contents for laboratory analysis
4. Remove gas and fluids from the stomach and intestine

210. A client with a history of lung disease is at risk for developing respiratory acidosis. A nurse assesses this client for which signs and symptoms characteristic of this disorder?
    1. Bradycardia and hyperactivity
    2. Decreased respiratory rate and depth
    3. Headache, restlessness, and confusion
    4. Bradypnea, dizziness, and paresthesias

211. A nurse is caring for a client with a resolved intestinal obstruction who has a nasogastric (NG) tube in place. The client has tolerated the tube being clamped every 2 hours for 1 hour. The physician has now ordered the NG tube to be removed. Before removing the tube, the nurse assesses for:
    1. Proper NG tube placement
    2. Normal serum electrolyte levels
    3. The presence of bowel sounds in all four quadrants
    4. Normal pH of the gastric aspirate

212. A nurse has administered approximately half of an enema solution when the client complains of pain and cramping. Which nursing action is the most appropriate?
    1. Raise the enema bag so that the solution can be completed quickly
    2. Clamp the tubing for 30 seconds and restart the flow at a slower rate
    3. Reassure the client and continue the flow
    4. Discontinue the enema and notify the physician

213. A nurse is preparing to administer an enema. The nurse positions the client in the:
    1. Left lateral position with the right leg acutely flexed
    2. Right Sims' position
    3. Dorsal recumbent position
    4. Right lateral position with the left leg acutely flexed

214. A nurse aspirates 40 mL of undigested formula from a client's nasogastric tube. Before administering an intermittent tube feeding, the nurse understands that the 40 mL of gastric aspirate should be:
    1. Discarded properly and recorded as output on the client's I & O record
    2. Poured into the nasogastric tube through a syringe with the plunger removed
    3. Mixed with the formula and poured into the nasogastric tube through a syringe with the plunger removed
    4. Diluted with water and injected into the nasogastric tube by putting pressure on the plunger

215. A client experiencing a great deal of stress and anxiety is being taught to use self-control therapy. The nurse teaching the client understands that which of the following is not a characteristic of this form of therapy?
    1. An advantage of this technique is that change is likely to last
    2. This form of therapy can be applied to new situations
    3. Talking to oneself is a basic component of this form of therapy
    4. It provides a negative reinforcement when the stimulus is produced

216. A nurse caring for a client with a chronic mental illness is using a behavior modification approach (operant conditioning). The nurse understands that which of the following is not a characteristic of this form of therapy?
    1. It uses negative reinforcement
    2. It increases the level of self-care in the client
    3. It increases social behaviors in the client
    4. It uses positive reinforcement

217. A nurse is speaking with a group of family members at a local support group regarding the importance of medication compliance. The nurse tells the group that which of the following is not known to increase medication compliance?
    1. Working with the psychiatrist to find the right medication at the right dose that produces the fewest side effects
    2. Giving all medications just once per day
    3. Providing clients with the injectable, long-acting form of the medication
    4. Including the family in the medication planning process so that compliance can be reinforced at home

218. An infant returns to the nursing unit after surgery for a diagnosis of esophageal atresia with tracheo-oesophageal fistula (TEF). The infant is receiving IV fluids, and a gastrostomy tube is in place. Following assessment, the nurse positions the infant and:
    1. Connects the gastrostomy to the feeding pump
    2. Attaches the gastrostomy tube to low suction
    3. Tapes the gastrostomy tube to the bed linens
    4. Elevates the gastrostomy tube

219. A depressed client is found unconscious on the floor in the day room. A nurse finds several empty bottles of a prescribed tricyclic antidepressant lying near the client. The immediate action of the nurse is to:
    1. Call a "Code," as this incident presents a medical emergency
    2. Induce vomiting and contact the physician for further orders
    3. Call the Poison Control Center
    4. Try to figure out the number of pills taken

220. A client is scheduled for an upper gastrointestinal (GI) endoscopy. Which of the following assess-

ments is essential to include in the plan of care following the procedure?

1. Monitoring for rectal bleeding
2. Assessing pulses
3. Monitoring urine output
4. Assessing for the presence of the gag reflex

221. A nurse is preparing to insert a nasogastric tube (NG) into a client. What nursing measure will best facilitate easy insertion of the tube?
    1. Placing the NG tube in warm water
    2. Removing the tube if any resistance to insertion is met
    3. Asking the client to swallow as the tube is being advanced
    4. Hyperextending the head to insert the tube

222. Epoetin alfa (Epogen, Procrit) has been prescribed for a client with chronic renal failure (CRF). A nurse will prepare to administer this medication by which of the following routes?
    1. Orally
    2. Intramuscularly (IM)
    3. Intradermally
    4. Subcutaneously (SC)

223. A client is returned to the nursing unit with chest tubes in place after thoracic surgery. During the first few hours postoperatively, the nurse assesses for drainage and expects to note that it is:
    1. Serous
    2. Serosanguineous
    3. Bloody
    4. Bloody with frequent small clots

224. A client has had radical neck dissection, and begins to hemorrhage at the incision site. Which action by the nurse would be contraindicated?
    1. Lowering the head of the bed to a flat position
    2. Applying manual pressure over the site
    3. Monitoring the client's airway
    4. Calling the physician immediately

225. A nurse has an order to begin administering foscavir (Foscarnet) to a client with cytomegalovirus retinitis and acquired immunodeficiency syndrome (AIDS). Before administering the dose, the nurse assesses the latest results of which of the following laboratory studies?
    1. Serum albumin
    2. Serum creatinine
    3. CD4 cell count
    4. Lymphocyte count

226. A client with tuberculosis (TB) asks a nurse about precautions to take after discharge to prevent infection of others. The nurse develops a response to the client's question based on the understanding that:
    1. The client should maintain enteric precautions only
    2. The disease is transmitted by droplet nuclei

3. Clothing and sheets should be bleached after each use
4. Deep pile carpet should be removed from the home

227. A nurse is caring for a client after pulmonary angiography with catheter insertion via the left groin. The nurse assesses for allergic reaction to the contrast medium by noting the presence of:
    1. Hematoma in the left groin
    2. Discomfort in the left groin
    3. Stridor
    4. Hypothermia

228. A sexually active 20-year-old client has developed viral hepatitis. Which of the following statements, if made by the client, would indicate a need for further teaching?
    1. "A condom should be used for sexual intercourse."
    2. "I can never drink alcohol again."
    3. "I won't go back to work right away."
    4. "My close friends should get the vaccine."

229. A nurse is planning care for a client who is being hospitalized because the client has been displaying violent behavior and represents a risk for potential harm to others. Which of the following would not be a component of the plan of care?
    1. Keep the door to the client's room open when providing care to the client
    2. Assign the client to a room at the end of the hall to avoid disturbing the other clients
    3. Face the client when providing care
    4. Ensure that a security officer is within the immediate area

230. A nurse is administering a dose of isoproterenol hydrochloride (Isuprel) to a client. The nurse monitors for which of the following side effects of this medication?
    1. Increased pulse and blood pressure
    2. Drowsiness
    3. Hyperglycemia
    4. Hypokalemia

231. A nurse is preparing to care for a client who will be weaned from a tracheostomy tube. The nurse is planning to use a tracheostomy plug and plans to insert it into the opening in the outer cannula. Which of the following nursing interventions is required before plugging the tube?
    1. Suction the client
    2. Deflate the cuff
    3. Ensure that the client is able to swallow
    4. Ensure that the client is able to speak

232. Cinoxacin (Cinobac), a urinary antiseptic, is prescribed for a client. A nurse checks the client's record, knowing that this medication is used with caution in which of the following disorders?
    1. Hepatic disease

2. Renal disease

3. Diabetes insipidus

4. Congestive heart failure

233. Bethanechol chloride (Urecholine) is prescribed for a client. A nurse instructs the client to take the medication:

1. With meals

2. Two hours after meals

3. With a snack in the afternoon

4. At bedtime with crackers and cheese

234. A client is diagnosed with glaucoma. Which of the following assessment data gathered by a nurse identify a risk factor associated with this eye disorder?

1. A history of migraine headaches

2. Frequent urinary tract infections

3. Cardiovascular disease

4. Frequent upper respiratory infections

235. A client with retinal detachment is admitted to a nursing unit in preparation for a scleral buckling procedure. Which of the following would a nurse anticipate to be prescribed?

1. Bathroom privileges only

2. Elevating the head of the bed to 45 degrees

3. Placing an eye patch over the client's affected eye

4. Wearing dark glasses to read or watch television

236. A nurse is caring for a client who is on strict bed rest. The nurse develops a plan of care and develops goals related to the prevention of deep vein thrombosis (DVT) and pulmonary emboli. Which of the following nursing actions would be most helpful to prevent these disorders from developing?

1. Applying a heating pad to the lower extremities

2. Encouraging active range-of-motion (ROM) exercises

3. Placing a pillow under the knees

4. Restricting fluids

237. A nurse is caring for a suicidal client. The most appropriate nursing intervention in dealing with this client is to:

1. Demonstrate confidence in the client's ability to deal with stressors

2. Provide hope and reassurance that the problems will resolve themselves

3. Display an attitude of detachment, confrontation, and efficiency

4. Provide authority, action, and participation

238. A client with tuberculosis (TB), whose status is being monitored in an ambulatory care clinic, asks a nurse when it will be permissible to return to work. The nurse replies that the client may resume employment when:

1. Two sputum cultures are negative

2. Five sputum cultures are negative

3. A sputum culture and a chest x-ray evaluation are negative

4. A sputum culture and a Mantoux test are negative

239. A nurse is admitting to a nursing unit a client who is suspected of having tuberculosis (TB). The nurse plans to admit the client to a room that has:

1. Ultraviolet light and three air exchanges per hour

2. Ten air exchanges per hour and venting to the outside

3. Venting to the outside and ultraviolet light

4. Venting to the outside, six air exchanges per hour, and ultraviolet light

240. Methenamine mandelate (Mandelamine) is prescribed for a client with a gram-positive urinary tract infection. Which of the following conditions, if noted in the client's record, would alert the nurse to question the order for this prescribed medication?

1. Cirrhosis of the liver

2. Diabetes mellitus

3. Peripheral vascular disease

4. Hypothyroidism

241. Laboratory analysis of a urine specimen for culture and sensitivity reveals a gram-negative bacterial infection. The client is treated with nalidixic acid (NegGram). Which of the following existing disorders in the client would alert a nurse to question the prescription for this medication?

1. Diabetes mellitus

2. Seizure disorder

3. Coronary artery disease

4. Peptic ulcer disease

242. A client comes to an emergency department after an assault. The client is extremely agitated and is trembling and hyperventilating. The most appropriate initial nursing action would be to:

1. Encourage the client to discuss the assault

2. Place the client in a quiet room alone to decrease stimulation

3. Remain with the client until the anxiety decreases

4. Begin to teach relaxation techniques

243. A nasogastric (NG) tube has been inserted into a client, and the physician prescribes that the tube be attached to intermittent suction. A nurse attaches the suction, noting that the pressure should not exceed:

1. 10 mm Hg

2. 20 mm Hg

3. 25 mm Hg

4. 30 mm Hg

244. The client is diagnosed with a gastrointestinal (GI) bleed, and the bleeding has been controlled. Antacids are prescribed to be administered every

hour. A nurse administers the antacids and plans to maintain a gastric pH of approximately:

1. 3
2. 6
3. 9
4. 15

245. A nurse provides instructions regarding the administration of cyclosporine (Sandimmune) to a client. Which of the following statements, if made by the client, would indicate the need for further instruction?

1. "I need to mix the concentrate well and drink it immediately."
2. "After taking the medication, I need to rinse the container with diluent and drink it to ensure that I have taken the complete dose."
3. "I will purchase a dropper from the pharmacist to calibrate the amount of medication that I need."
4. "I will mix the concentrate with orange juice to improve the taste."

246. A nurse is caring for a client admitted to the hospital with a suspected diagnosis of acute appendicitis. Which of the following laboratory results would the nurse expect to note if the client does indeed have appendicitis?

1. Leukopenia with a shift to the right
2. Leukocytosis with a shift to the right
3. Leukocytosis with a shift to the left
4. Leukopenia with a shift to the left

247. A client with acute pancreatitis is experiencing severe pain from the disorder. A nurse would teach the client to avoid which of the following positions that could aggravate the pain?

1. Sitting up
2. Lying flat
3. Leaning forward
4. Flexing the left leg

248. A client is admitted to the hospital with acute viral hepatitis. On the basis of this diagnosis, which of the following signs or symptoms would the nurse expect to note?

1. Spider angiomas
2. Fatigue
3. Pale urine
4. Weight gain

249. A woman comes into the emergency department following an assault. She presents with hyperventilation, pacing, rapid speech, and headache. A nurse correctly assesses the level of anxiety to be:

1. Panic
2. Severe
3. Moderate
4. Psychotic

250. A nurse is caring for a client who has been taking hydrocodone (Hycodan) for the last 3 months.

The nurse assesses the client for which of the following side effects of this medication?

1. Psychological and physical dependence
2. Tachycardia and hypertension
3. Diarrhea and abdominal cramping
4. Increased respiratory rate and bronchospasm

251. Cromolyn sodium (Intal) is prescribed for a client with allergic asthma. A nurse understands that this medication acts to:

1. Inhibit the release of mediators from mast cells after exposure to an antigen
2. Promote the migration of eosinophils into the inflammatory site
3. Increase the number of eosinophils
4. Dilate the bronchi

252. A clinic nurse is preparing to evaluate the peripheral vision of a client by the confrontational method. Which of the following describes the accurate procedure to perform this test?

1. The examiner and the client cover the same eyes and stare at each other's uncovered eye, and a small object is brought into the visual field
2. The examiner and the client cover the eyes directly opposite to one another and stare at each other's uncovered eye, and a small object is brought into the visual field
3. The client is asked to discriminate numbers from a chart composed of colored dots
4. The room is darkened, and the client is asked to identify colored blocks and shapes when they appear in the visual field

253. A nurse prepares to administer acetylcysteine (Mucomyst) to a client with an overdose of acetaminophen (Tylenol). Which of the following are appropriate actions in administering this antidote?

1. Mixing the medication in a flavored ice drink and allowing the client to drink the medication
2. Administering the medication intravenously (IV), mixed in 50 mL of normal saline and piggybacked through the main IV line
3. Administering the medication intramuscularly (IM) in the gluteal muscle
4. Administering the medication subcutaneously (SC) in the deltoid muscle

254. A client is receiving baclofen (Lioresal) for muscle spasms resulting from a spinal cord injury. The nurse monitors the client for which side effect related to this medication?

1. Photosensitivity
2. Slurred speech
3. Hypertension
4. Muscle pain

255. A home care nurse visits a client with unstable angina. The client is taking acetylsalicylic acid (aspirin) on a daily basis to reduce the risk of

myocardial infarction (MI). Which of the following medication doses would the nurse expect the client to be taking?
1. 3 g daily
2. 300 to 325 mg daily
3. 1.3 g daily
4. 650 to 700 mg daily

256. Transcutaneous electrical nerve stimulation (TENS) is prescribed for a client with pain. The client asks a nurse about the purpose of the TENS unit. Which of the following would not be a component of the nurse's response to the client?
1. "Electrodes are attached to the skin."
2. "The unit relieves pain."
3. "The unit will reduce the need for analgesics."
4. "Hospitalization is required because the unit is not portable."

257. A nurse is developing a plan of care for a client experiencing anxiety following the loss of a job. The client is verbalizing concerns regarding the ability to meet role expectations and financial obligations. The most appropriate nursing diagnosis for this client is:
1. Altered family process
2. Altered thought process
3. Potential for anxiety
4. Ineffective individual coping

258. A nurse is monitoring the chest tube drainage system in a client with a chest tube. The nurse notes intermittent bubbling in the water seal compartment. Which of the following is the most appropriate action?
1. Change the chest tube drainage system
2. Document the findings
3. Check for an air leak
4. Notify the physician

259. A nurse is preparing to perform an otoscopic examination on an adult client. The nurse does which of the following to perform this examination?
1. Pulls the pinna up and back before inserting the speculum
2. Pulls the earlobe down and back before inserting the speculum
3. Uses the smallest speculum available to decrease the discomfort of the examination
4. Tilts the client's head forward and down before inserting the speculum

260. Cinoxacin (Cinobac) is prescribed for a client with a urinary tract infection. A clinic nurse is instructing the client regarding the administration of the medication. The nurse tells the client to administer the medication:
1. One hour before meals
2. With meals

3. At bedtime
4. In the morning before breakfast

261. A client who has just suffered a large flail chest is experiencing severe pain and dyspnea. The client's central venous pressure (CVP) is rising, and the arterial blood pressure is falling. A nurse interprets that the client is experiencing:
1. Mediastinal flutter
2. Mediastinal shift
3. Hypovolemic shock
4. Fat embolism

262. A nurse is caring for a client who is suspected of having lung cancer. The nurse assesses the client for which most frequent early symptom of lung cancer?
1. Hemoptysis
2. Cough
3. Hoarseness
4. Pleuritic pain

263. A client arrives in the emergency department in a crisis state. The client demonstrates signs of profound anxiety and is unable to focus on anything but the object of the crisis and the impact on self. The initial nursing assessment would focus on:
1. The object of the crisis
2. The presence of support systems
3. The physical condition of the client
4. The client's coping mechanisms

264. After performing an initial abdominal assessment on a client with a diagnosis of cholelithiasis, a nurse documents that the bowel sounds are normal. Which of the following best describes "normal bowel sounds?"
1. Waves of loud gurgles auscultated in all four quadrants
2. Very high-pitched loud rushes auscultated especially in one or two quadrants
3. Relatively high-pitched clicks or gurgles auscultated in all four quadrants
4. Low-pitched swishing auscultated in one or two quadrants

265. A nurse is evaluating a client in crisis and is determining the potential for self-harm. Which of the following assessment data would indicate that the client is a very high risk for suicide?
1. The client is disorganized
2. The client is impulsive
3. The client has a history of suicide attempts
4. The client has an immediate plan for a suicide attempt

266. Lomotil (diphenoxylate hydrochloride and atropine sulfate) is prescribed for the client with ulcerative colitis. The nurse monitors the client, knowing that which of the following is a therapeutic effect of this medication?
1. Elimination of peristalsis

2. Decreased diarrhea
3. Decreased cramping
4. Improved intestinal tone

267. Sulfasalazine (Azulfidine) is prescribed for a client with a diagnosis of ulcerative colitis. A nurse instructs the client about the medication. Which statement made by the client indicates a need for further education?
    1. "Sensitivity to sunlight may occur."
    2. "I need to take the medication with meals."
    3. "This medication should be taken as prescribed."
    4. "The medication will cause constipation."

268. A client with cirrhosis has ascites and a fluid volume excess. Which measure will the nurse prepare to include in the plan of care for this client?
    1. Increase the amount of sodium in the diet
    2. Restrict the amount of fluids consumed
    3. Encourage frequent ambulation
    4. Administer magnesium antacids

269. Lactulose (Chronulac) is prescribed for a client with a diagnosis of hepatic encephalopathy. Which assessment finding indicates that the client is responding to this medication therapy as anticipated?
    1. The fecal pH is acidic
    2. The client experiences diarrhea
    3. The client is able to tolerate a full diet
    4. Vomiting occurs

270. Cholestyramine resin (Questran Lite) is prescribed for a client with an elevated serum cholesterol level. A nurse would instruct the client to administer the medication:
    1. After meals
    2. Mixed with fruit juice
    3. Via a rectal suppository
    4. At least 3 hours before meals

271. Pancreatin (Viokase) is prescribed for a client with postgastrectomy syndrome. Which of the following assessment findings would indicate a therapeutic effect of this medication?
    1. The client's appetite improves
    2. The client experiences a weight loss
    3. Vitamin B_{12} deficiency is controlled
    4. Stool is less fatty and decreases in frequency

272. A nurse is evaluating the plan of care for a client with peptic ulcer disease (PUD) and a nursing diagnosis of Pain. The nurse would determine that the client has not met the expected outcomes if the client reports:
    1. Pain is relieved with histamine H_2-receptor antagonists
    2. Irritating foods have been eliminated from the diet
    3. Being awakened at 2 A.M. with heartburn
    4. Absence of pain before meals

273. A home health nurse visits an older adult client who has recently lost her husband. The client says, "No one cares about me anymore. All the people I loved are dead." Which of the following is the most appropriate response?
    1. "That seems rather unlikely to me."
    2. "You must be feeling all alone at this point."
    3. "I don't believe that and neither do you."
    4. "Right! Why not just 'pack it in'?"

274. A nurse is caring for a client who has just returned from the postanesthesia care unit after radical neck dissection. The nurse assesses the type of drainage from the wound for which of the following, which is expected in the immediate postoperative period?
    1. Serosanguineous
    2. Grossly bloody
    3. Serous
    4. Serous with sputum

275. A depressed client who appeared sullen, distraught, and hopeless a few days ago now suddenly appears calm, relaxed, and more energetic. A nurse's best action in regard to the client's changes in behavior is to:
    1. Feel comfortable that the client is adapting to the unit and is feeling safe
    2. Continue to assess the client's behaviors and document clearly in the chart
    3. Notify the health care team of these observations, and alert them to the suspicion that the client is contemplating suicide
    4. Engage the client in one-to-one supervision, share with the client the observations that have been made, and ask whether the client is thinking about suicide

276. A nurse is teaching a client about an upcoming colonoscopy procedure. The nurse would include in the instructions that the client will be placed in which of the following positions for the procedure?
    1. Left Sims'
    2. Right Sims'
    3. Knee-chest
    4. Lithotomy

277. A nurse has given a client with tuberculosis (TB) instructions for proper handling and disposal of respiratory secretions. The nurse concludes that the client understands the instructions if the client verbalizes an intention to:
    1. Wash hands at least four times a day
    2. Turn the head to the side if coughing or sneezing
    3. Discard used tissues in a plastic bag
    4. Brush the teeth and rinse the mouth once a day

278. Ultrasonography of the gallbladder is scheduled for a client with a suspected diagnosis of chole-

cystitis. A nurse explains to the client that this test:

1. Requires that the client lie still for short intervals
2. Requires that the client be NPO for 24 hours
3. Is proceeded by the administration of oral tablets
4. Is uncomfortable

279. A nurse is caring for a client who had a Mantoux skin test implanted 48 hours ago on admission to the nursing unit. The nurse reads the result as positive. Which action by the nurse has the highest priority?

1. Call the physician
2. Call the radiology department for a chest x-ray evaluation
3. Document the finding in the client's record
4. Call the employee health service department

280. Cyclosporine (Sandimmune) is prescribed for a client after a kidney transplant. A nurse would be most concerned if it was noted that the client is presently taking which of the following prescribed medications?

1. Digoxin (Lanoxin)
2. Propranolol (Inderal)
3. Phenytoin (Dilantin)
4. Prednisone (Deltasone)

281. A nurse is performing an assessment on a 16-year-old female client who has been diagnosed with anorexia nervosa. Which statement, if made by the client, would the nurse identify as a priority requiring further assessment?

1. "I exercise 3 to 4 hours every day to keep my slim figure."
2. "My best friend was in the hospital with this disease a year ago."
3. "I've been told that I am 10% below ideal body weight."
4. "I check my weight every day without fail."

282. A nurse is consulting with a dietitian and is planning a menu for a client who is on a regular diet and is a strict vegetarian. Which of the following food items would the nurse and the dietitian plan for the client's meal?

1. Chocolate milkshake
2. Buttered wheat toast
3. Stir-fried vegetables
4. Scrambled eggs

283. A nurse is preparing to administer a prescribed dose of cyclosporine (Sandimmune) by IV. Which of the following priority items would the nurse have available during administration of this medication?

1. Oral airway
2. Epinephrine
3. A code cart
4. A suction catheter

284. Cyclosporine (Sandimmune) is prescribed to be administered by the IV route. Which of the following indicates an inappropriate action in regard to preparing and administering this medication?

1. Mixing 1 mL of concentrate in 10 mL of 0.9% sodium chloride and administering by bolus injection
2. Mixing the solution and covering it with a paper bag
3. Mixing 1 mL of concentrate in 50 mL of 0.9% sodium chloride
4. Administering the medication over a period of 2 to 6 hours

285. Muromonab-CD3 (Orthoclone OKT3) is prescribed for a client to manage allograft rejection following a renal transplant. The nurse understands that the primary mechanism of action of this medication is that it:

1. Binds to the CD3 site and blocks all T cell functions
2. Inhibits the proliferation of B lymphocytes
3. Cross links DNA, causing cell injury and death
4. Suppresses B lymphocytes

286. A client taking brompheniramine maleate (Dimetane) is scheduled for allergy skin testing and tells a nurse in the physician's office that a dose was taken this morning. The nurse interprets that:

1. A smaller dose of allergen should be injected
2. A larger dose of allergen should be injected
3. The client should have the skin test read a day later than usual
4. The client should reschedule the appointment

287. A nurse has an order to administer acetylcysteine (Mucomyst) to a client admitted with acetaminophen (Tylenol) overdose. Before giving this medication, the nurse would ensure that the:

1. Client knows how to use a nebulizer
2. Antidote to acetylcysteine is readily available
3. Stomach is empty as a result of emesis or lavage
4. Solution is given full strength

288. A postoperative client has received a dose of naloxone hydrochloride (Narcan) for respiratory depression shortly after transfer to the nursing unit from the postanesthesia care unit. After administration of the medication, the nurse assesses the client for:

1. Pupillary changes
2. Sudden episodes of vomiting
3. Sudden increase in pain
4. Scattered lung wheezes

289. A client with a history of gastric ulcer suddenly complains of a sharp, severe pain in the mid-epigastric area, which then spreads over the entire abdomen. The client's abdomen is rigid and boardlike to palpation, and the client obtains most comfort from lying in the knee-chest posi-

tion. A nurse calls the physician immediately, suspecting that the client is experiencing which of the following complications of peptic ulcer disease?

1. Perforation
2. Obstruction
3. Hemorrhage
4. Intractability

290. A client is admitted with dehydration following creation of an ileostomy. A nurse assesses that the client has lost 3 pounds of weight, has poor skin turgor, and has concentrated urine. The nurse interprets that the client's clinical picture correlates most closely with recent intake of which of the following medications, which is contraindicated for the ileostomy client?

1. Ferrous sulfate (Feosol)
2. Folate (folic acid)
3. Phenolphthalein (Ex-Lax)
4. Cyanocobalamin (vitamin B_{12})

291. A Penrose drain is in place on the first day following a cholecystectomy. Serosanguineous drainage is noted on the dressing covering the drain. Which nursing intervention is most appropriate?

1. Notify the physician
2. Change the dressing
3. Circle the amount on the dressing with a pen
4. Continue to monitor the drainage

292. A client has a chest tube attached to a Pleurevac drainage system. As part of routine nursing care, a nurse would ensure that:

1. The connection between the chest tube and the drainage system is taped and that an occlusive dressing is maintained at the insertion site
2. The amount of drainage into the chest tube is noted and recorded every 24 hours in the client's record
3. The suction control chamber has sterile water added every shift and that the system is kept below waist level
4. The water seal chamber has continuous bubbling and that assessment for crepitus is done once a shift

293. An infant is born to a mother with hepatitis B. Which of the following would be indicated as prophylaxis for the infant?

1. Immune globulin (IG) given as soon as possible after delivery
2. Hepatitis B immune globulin (HBIG) within 14 days after birth
3. Hepatitis B immune globulin (HBIG) and hepatitis B vaccine within 12 hours of birth
4. Hepatitis B vaccine within 24 hours of birth

294. A nurse is planning care for a client scheduled for insertion of a tracheostomy. What equipment should the nurse plan to have at the bedside when the client returns from surgery?

1. Oral airway
2. Epinephrine
3. Obturator
4. Tracheostomy set with the next larger size

295. A nurse is caring for a client with an endotracheal tube attached to a ventilator. The high-pressure alarm sounds on the ventilator. Which of the following is the most appropriate nursing intervention?

1. Assess for a disconnection
2. Evaluate the cuff for a leak
3. Notify the respiratory therapist
4. Suction the client

296. A nurse is caring for a client with a chest tube drainage system. The nurse notes a fluctuating water level on inspiration and expiration in the submerged tube in the water seal chamber of the chest tube system. Which nursing action is most appropriate?

1. No action is necessary
2. Encourage coughing and deep breathing
3. Suction the client
4. Increase the suction

297. A nurse is caring for a client with a chest tube drainage system. The nurse notes constant bubbling in the water seal chamber. Which of the following nursing actions is most appropriate?

1. Reposition the client
2. Change the chest tube drainage system
3. Notify the physician
4. This is a normal, expected finding and no action is necessary

298. A client with acquired immunodeficiency syndrome (AIDS) has been started on therapy with zidovudine (AZT, Retrovir). A nurse carefully assesses which of the following laboratory results during treatment with this medication?

1. Complete blood count (CBC)
2. Blood urea nitrogen (BUN)
3. Blood culture
4. Blood glucose level

299. A nurse in an ambulatory clinic is preparing to administer a Mantoux test to a client who may have been exposed to an individual with tuberculosis (TB). The client reports having had the bacille Calmette-Guérin (BCG) vaccine before moving to the United States from a foreign country. The nurse interprets that:

1. The client's test will be negative, and will require a sputum culture to diagnose
2. The client's test will be positive, and will require a chest x-ray evaluation

3. The client has no risk of acquiring TB, and needs no further workup

4. The client is at increased risk of acquiring TB, and needs immediate medication therapy

300. A client with an order to take theophylline (Slo-Bid) daily has been given medication instructions by a nurse. The nurse concludes that the client needs further information on the medication if the client states an intention to:

1. Avoid changing brands of the medication without physician approval

2. Avoid over-the-counter (OTC) cough and cold medications unless approved by the physician

3. Drink at least 2 liters of fluid per day

4. Take the daily dose at bedtime

ANSWERS

1. 3

Rationale: McBurney's point is midway between the right anterior superior iliac crest and the umbilicus. It is usually the location of greatest pain in a child with appendicitis.

Test-Taking Strategy: Use the process of elimination. Knowledge that the appendix is located in the right side of the abdomen will assist in eliminating options 2 and 4. From this point, attempt to visualize this assessment procedure. This will assist in directing you to option 3. Review the location of McBurney's point if you had difficulty with this question.

Level of Cognitive Ability: Comprehension
Client Needs: Health Promotion and Maintenance
Integrated Concept/Process: Nursing Process/Assessment
Content Area: Child Health
Reference: Ball, J., & Bindler, R. (1999). *Pediatric nursing: Caring for children* (2nd ed.). Stamford, Conn.: Appleton & Lange, p. 618.

2. 3

Rationale: Furacin is applied topically to the burn and has a broad spectrum of antibiotic activity. It is used in burns in which bacterial resistance to other agents is a real or potential problem. A $1/16$-inch film of furacin is applied directly to the burn. Dressings soaked with saline solution are not used.

Test-Taking Strategy: Use the process of elimination. Option 1 can be eliminated because infection is a major concern with a burn client, and a wet dressing can more easily harbor bacteria. Recalling that a very thin film is required will easily direct you to option 3. Review the use of this medication for burn therapy if you had difficulty with this question.

Level of Cognitive Ability: Application
Client Needs: Physiological Integrity
Integrated Concept/Process: Communication and Documentation
Content Area: Pharmacology
Reference: Kuhn, M. (1998). *Pharmacotherapeutics: A nursing process approach* (4th ed.). Philadelphia: F.A. Davis, p. 998.

3. 2

Rationale: The CT scan causes no pain and can take 15 to 60 minutes to perform. The dye may cause a warm, flushing sensation when injected. Fluids are encouraged after the procedure. If an iodine dye is used, the client should be asked about allergies to seafood or iodine.

Test-Taking Strategy: Use the process of elimination. Note the key words *dye injection* in the question. This should provide you with the clue that the issue relates to the dye. If you are unfamiliar with this diagnostic test, review the important teaching points related to it.

Level of Cognitive Ability: Application
Client Needs: Physiological Integrity
Integrated Concept/Process: Nursing Process/Implementation
Content Area: Adult Health/Oncology
Reference: Leahy, J., & Kizilay, P. (1998). *Foundations of nursing practice: A nursing process approach.* Philadelphia: W.B. Saunders, pp. 755-756.

4. 4

Rationale: The normal magnesium level is 1.6 to 2.6 mg/dL. A client with a magnesium level of 3.5 mg/dL is experiencing hypermagnesemia. Assessment signs and symptoms include neurological depression, drowsiness and lethargy, loss of deep tendon reflexes, respiratory insufficiency, bradycardia, and hypotension. Tetany, twitches, and a positive Trousseau's sign are seen in a client with hypomagnesemia.

Test-Taking Strategy: First, it is necessary to determine that the client is experiencing hypermagnesemia. Next, use the process of elimination, noting that options 1, 2, and 3 are similar in that they reflect neurological excitability. If you had difficulty with this question, review the assessment signs and symptoms found in magnesium imbalances.

Level of Cognitive Ability: Analysis
Client Needs: Physiological Integrity
Integrated Concept/Process: Nursing Process/Assessment
Content Area: Fundamental Skills
Reference: Ignatavicius, D., Workman, M., & Mishler, M. (1999). *Medical-surgical nursing across the health care continuum* (3rd ed.). Philadelphia: W.B. Saunders, p. 263.

5. 3

Rationale: The normal serum calcium level is 8.6 to 10.0 mg/dL. This client is experiencing hypercalcemia. Calcium gluconate and calcium chloride are medications used in the treatment of tetany that occurs from acute hypocalcemia. In hypercalcemia, large doses of vitamin D need to be avoided. Calcitonin (Calcimar), a thyroid hormone, decreases the plasma calcium level by increasing the incorporation of calcium into the bones, thus keeping it out of the serum.

Test-Taking Strategy: First, you need to determine that the client is experiencing hypercalcemia. With this knowledge you can easily eliminate options 1 and 2, because you would not administer medication that would add calcium to the body. Remembering that excessive vitamin D is a causative factor of hypercalcemia will assist in eliminating option 4. If you had difficulty with this question, review the treatment for hypercalcemia.

Level of Cognitive Ability: Analysis
Client Needs: Physiological Integrity
Integrated Concept/Process: Nursing Process/Planning

Content Area: Pharmacology

Reference: Ignatavicius, D., Workman, M., & Mishler, M. (1999). *Medical-surgical nursing across the health care continuum* (3rd ed.). Philadelphia: W.B. Saunders, p. 258.

6. 3

Rationale: Sodium polystyrene sulfonate is a cation exchange resin used in the treatment of hyperkalemia. The resin either passes through the intestine or is retained in the colon. It releases sodium ions in exchange for primarily potassium ions. The therapeutic effect occurs 2 to 12 hours after oral administration and longer after rectal administration.

Test-Taking Strategy: Use the process of elimination. Looking closely at the name of the medication (Kayexalate) may provide you with assistance regarding the action of the medication. If you had difficulty with this question, review the action of this very important medication.

Level of Cognitive Ability: Comprehension

Client Needs: Physiological Integrity

Integrated Concept/Process: Nursing Process/Planning

Content Area: Pharmacology

Reference: Hodgson, B., & Kizior, R. (2001). *Saunders nursing drug handbook 2001.* Philadelphia: W.B. Saunders, p. 935.

7. 2

Rationale: Fluid that shifts into the interstitial spaces and remains there is called *third space fluid.* Common sites for third spacing include the abdomen, the pleural cavity, the peritoneal cavity, and the pericardial sac. Third space fluid is physiologically useless because it does not circulate to provide nutrients for the cells. Risk factors include liver or kidney disease, major trauma, burns, sepsis, wound healing or major surgery, malignancy, gastrointestinal malabsorption, malnutrition, and alcoholic or elderly clients.

Test-Taking Strategy: Use the process of elimination and note the key words *least likely.* Eliminate options 1 and 3 first because they are similar. From the remaining options, focusing on the key words will direct you to option 2. Review the risk factors associated with third spacing if you had difficulty with this question.

Level of Cognitive Ability: Analysis

Client Needs: Physiological Integrity

Integrated Concept/Process: Nursing Process/Assessment

Content Area: Fundamental Skills

Reference: LeMone, P., & Burke, K. (2000). *Medical-surgical nursing: Critical thinking in client care* (2nd ed.). Upper Saddle River, N.J.: Prentice-Hall, p. 101.

8. 4

Rationale: Before the gastroscopy procedure, medication is given to prevent a gag reflex. On return from the procedure, the nurse must test the client's gag reflex to ensure that it is present to prevent aspiration of contents. The client must be placed in a side-lying or semi-Fowler's position to avoid aspiration. Vital signs should be taken every 30 minutes for 2 hours to detect abnormalities. Saline gargles must only be administered when the presence of the gag reflex has been confirmed.

Test-Taking Strategy: Use the process of elimination. Use of the ABCs—airway, breathing, and circulation—will assist in answering the question. Option 4 is the only option that addresses airway. If you had difficulty with this question, review the care of a client following a gastroscopy procedure.

Level of Cognitive Ability: Application

Client Needs: Physiological Integrity

Integrated Concept/Process: Nursing Process/Planning

Content Area: Adult Health/Gastrointestinal

Reference: Leahy, J., & Kizilay, P. (1998). *Foundations of nursing practice: A nursing process approach.* Philadelphia: W.B. Saunders, p. 756.

9. 1

Rationale: Ringer's lactate solution is an isotonic solution. Other isotonic solutions include 5% dextrose in water (5% D/W), 0.9% saline (NS), and 5% dextrose in 0.225% saline (5% D/¼ NS); 0.45% saline (½ NS) is hypotonic; 10% dextrose in water (10% D/W), 5% dextrose in 0.9% saline (5% D/NS), and 5% dextrose in 0.45% saline (5% D/½ NS) are hypertonic solutions.

Test-Taking Strategy: Use the process of elimination and knowledge regarding the tonicity of the various IV solutions. If you had difficulty with this question, review this content.

Level of Cognitive Ability: Comprehension

Client Needs: Physiological Integrity

Integrated Concept/Process: Nursing Process/Evaluation

Content Area: Fundamental Skills

Reference: LeMone, P., & Burke, K. (2000). *Medical-surgical nursing: Critical thinking in client care* (2nd ed.). Upper Saddle River, N.J.: Prentice-Hall, p. 110.

10. 1

Rationale: The normal pH is 7.35 to 7.45. The normal P_{CO_2} is 35 to 45 mm Hg. In respiratory acidosis the pH is low and the P_{CO_2} is elevated. This is an expected finding in a client with a neuromuscular disorder such as Guillain-Barré syndrome, because the client may retain carbon dioxide as a result of ventilatory failure as paralysis ensues.

Test-Taking Strategy: Remember that in a respiratory imbalance you will find an opposite response between the pH and the P_{CO_2}. Also remember that the pH is down in an acidotic condition. Recalling this information will allow you to eliminate each of the incorrect options. Review interpretation of blood gas results if you had difficulty with this question.

Level of Cognitive Ability: Analysis

Client Needs: Physiological Integrity

Integrated Concept/Process: Nursing Process/Analysis

Content Area: Fundamental Skills

Reference: Smeltzer, S., & Bare, B. (2000). *Brunner & Suddarth's textbook of medical-surgical nursing* (9th ed.). Philadelphia: Lippincott Williams & Wilkins, pp. 232-234.

11. 3

Rationale: The client who ingests a large amount of aspirin (acetylsalicylic acid) is at risk for developing metabolic acidosis 24 hours after the poisoning. If metabolic acidosis occurs, the client may exhibit hyperpnea with Kussmaul's respirations, headache, nausea, vomiting, diarrhea, fruity-smelling breath because of improper fat metabolism, central nervous system depression, twitching, convulsions, and hyperkalemia. In the very early hours following aspirin overdose, the client may exhibit respiratory alkalosis as a compensatory mechanism. By 24 hours after overdose, however, the compensatory mechanism fails and the client reverts to metabolic acidosis.

Test-Taking Strategy: Knowledge about the clinical manifestations of metabolic acidosis will easily direct you to option 3.

Use the process of elimination, recalling the significant gastrointestinal symptoms that can occur in this disorder. Review the clinical manifestations of metabolic acidosis if this question was difficult.

Level of Cognitive Ability: Analysis
Client Needs: Physiological Integrity
Integrated Concept/Process: Nursing Process/Assessment
Content Area: Fundamental Skills
Reference: Ignatavicius, D., Workman, M., & Mishler, M. (1999). *Medical-surgical nursing across the health care continuum* (3rd ed.). Philadelphia: W.B. Saunders, p. 299.

12. 2
Rationale: The normal serum ammonia level is 35 to 65 µg/dL. In the client with hepatic encephalopathy, the serum level is not likely to drop below normal, nor is it likely to drop into the low-normal range. The most optimal yet realistic change would be to 40 µg/dL, which falls into the normal range. A level of 80 µg/dL represents insufficient effect of the medication.

Test-Taking Strategy: Use the process of elimination and knowledge of the normal serum ammonia level. Option 2 is the only option that identifies a normal ammonia level. Review this test briefly, and the desirable effects of this medication if you had difficulty with this question.

Level of Cognitive Ability: Analysis
Client Needs: Physiological Integrity
Integrated Concept/Process: Nursing Process/Evaluation
Content Area: Adult Health/Gastrointestinal
Reference: Corbett, J. (2000). *Laboratory tests and diagnostic procedures* (5th ed.). Upper Saddle River, N.J.: Prentice-Hall, p. 248.

13. 2
Rationale: The normal urine myoglobin level is negative. After extensive muscle destruction or damage, myoglobin is released into the bloodstream, where it is cleared from the body by the kidneys. When there is a large amount of myoglobin being cleared from the body, there is a risk of the renal tubules being clogged with myoglobin, causing acute tubular necrosis. This is one form of acute renal failure.

Test-Taking Strategy: Use the process of elimination. Note the relationship between the word *urine* in the question and *acute tubular necrosis* in the correct option. Review the significance of myoglobin in the urine if you had difficulty with this question.

Level of Cognitive Ability: Analysis
Client Needs: Physiological Integrity
Integrated Concept/Process: Nursing Process/Assessment
Content Area: Adult Health/Renal
Reference: Phipps, W., Sands, J., & Marek, J. (1999). *Medical-surgical nursing: Concepts & clinical practice* (6th ed.). St. Louis: Mosby, p. 1402.

14. 2
Rationale: The normal hematocrit level for an adult male is 42% to 52%. The client who is in shock has an elevated hematocrit level because of hemoconcentration. The client's hematocrit may be expected to drift back down to within the normal range once fluid volume has been adequately restored. Thus option 2 is the only correct choice. Option 1 is too high, whereas options 3 and 4 are low.

Test-Taking Strategy: Use the process of elimination. Recalling that the normal hematocrit level is 42% to 52% will direct you to option 2. Since this is a very common laboratory study, it would be useful to have this one committed to memory.

Level of Cognitive Ability: Analysis
Client Needs: Physiological Integrity
Integrated Concept/Process: Nursing Process/Evaluation
Content Area: Fundamental Skills
Reference: Fischbach, F. (2000). *A manual of laboratory & diagnostic tests* (6th ed.). Philadelphia: Lippincott Williams & Wilkins, p. 73.

15. 2
Rationale: Any condition in which gastrointestinal motility is slowed or esophageal reflux is possible places a client at risk for aspiration. Options 1 and 4 may be appropriate nursing diagnoses but are not of highest priority. Option 3 is not likely to occur in this client.

Test-Taking Strategy: Note the key words *highest priority.* Use the ABCs—airway, breathing, and circulation. Option 2 addresses airway management. Options 1, 3, and 4 are potential problems, but none is as high a priority as airway maintenance.

Level of Cognitive Ability: Analysis
Client Needs: Physiological Integrity
Integrated Concept/Process: Nursing Process/Analysis
Content Area: Fundamental Skills
Reference: Lewis, S., Heitkemper, M., & Dirksen, S. (2000). *Medical-surgical nursing: Assessment and management of clinical problems* (5th ed.). St. Louis: Mosby, p. 1058.

16. 4
Rationale: Self-control is demonstrated by stoicism and hiding feelings. Problem solving involves making plans and verbalizing what will be done. Accepting responsibility places the responsibility for a situation on oneself. Distancing is an unwillingness or inability to discuss events.

Test-Taking Strategy: Note the key words *refuses, will not,* and *does not.* These words indicate ineffective coping. Option 4, distancing, is the one option that is indicative of ineffective coping. Review coping mechanisms if you had difficulty with this question.

Level of Cognitive Ability: Analysis
Client Needs: Psychosocial Integrity
Integrated Concept/Process: Nursing Process/Assessment
Content Area: Adult Health/Gastrointestinal
Reference: Ignatavicius, D., Workman, M., & Mishler, M. (1999). *Medical-surgical nursing across the health care continuum* (3rd ed.). Philadelphia: W.B. Saunders, p. 102.

17. 1
Rationale: The most accurate way to measure weight loss is to weigh the client daily, at the same time, in the same clothes, and with the same scale. Options 2, 3, and 4 assist in monitoring nutrition and hydration status rather than actual loss of pounds.

Test-Taking Strategy: Note the key words *most accurately.* Also note the issue of the question and the similar words in the question and the correct option. If you had difficulty with this question, review the methods of monitoring weight loss.

Level of Cognitive Ability: Comprehension
Client Needs: Physiological Integrity
Integrated Concept/Process: Nursing Process/Assessment
Content Area: Fundamental Skills

Reference: Craven, R., & Hirnle, C. (2000). *Fundamentals of nursing: Human health and function* (3rd ed.). Philadelphia: Lippincott Williams & Wilkins, p. 370.

18. 4

Rationale: In anorexia nervosa, the client tries to establish identity and control by self-imposed starvation. Options 1, 2, and 3 are verbalizations of the client's intentions. Option 4 is a measurable action that can be verified.

Test-Taking Strategy: Note the key words *that treatment has been effective*. With this in mind, use the process of elimination and select the option that is measurable. Option 4 is the only measurable action.

Level of Cognitive Ability: Analysis
Client Needs: Psychosocial Integrity
Integrated Concept/Process: Nursing Process/Evaluation
Content Area: Fundamental Skills
Reference: Ignatavicius, D., Workman, M., & Mishler, M. (1999). *Medical-surgical nursing across the health care continuum* (3rd ed.). Philadelphia: W.B. Saunders, p. 1352.

19. 2

Rationale: The client with dumping syndrome should be placed on a high-protein, moderate-fat, and high-calorie diet. The client should lie down after eating and should avoid drinking liquids with meals. Frequent, small meals are encouraged, and the client should avoid concentrated sweets.

Test-Taking Strategy: Note the key word *not* in the stem of the question. Think about this disorder and use the process of elimination, selecting option 2 as the item that will contribute to the problems associated with dumping syndrome. If you had difficulty with this question, review the diet associated with this syndrome.

Level of Cognitive Ability: Application
Client Needs: Physiological Integrity
Integrated Concept/Process: Teaching/Learning
Content Area: Adult Health/Gastrointestinal
Reference: Grodner, M., Anderson, S., & DeYoung, S. (2000). *Foundations and clinical applications of nutrition: A nursing approach.* St. Louis: Mosby, p. 501.

20. 3

Rationale: Pernicious anemia is caused by a deficiency of vitamin B_{12}. Treatment consists of monthly injections of vitamin B_{12}. Thiamine is most often prescribed for the client with alcoholism. Iron is administered for iron-deficiency anemia and folic acid for folic-acid deficiency.

Test-Taking Strategy: Knowledge regarding the relationship between pernicious anemia and vitamin B_{12} is required to answer this question. Review the treatment for this disorder if you had difficulty with this question.

Level of Cognitive Ability: Analysis
Client Needs: Physiological Integrity
Integrated Concept/Process: Nursing Process/Planning
Content Area: Adult Health/Gastrointestinal
Reference: Grodner, M., Anderson, S., & DeYoung, S. (2000). *Foundations and clinical applications of nutrition: A nursing approach.* St. Louis: Mosby, p. 169.

21. 4

Rationale: It may be necessary to modify a client's diet of solid food to a soft or mechanically chopped diet if the client has difficulty chewing. Food and cultural preferences should be ascertained on admission. Bowel sounds should have previously been assessed and present before introducing any diet.

Test-Taking Strategy: Note the key words *elderly* and *tolerating a full liquid diet*. Eliminate options 1 and 2 first because they are similar. Eliminate option 3 next because the client has been tolerating a full-liquid diet; therefore bowel sounds have been present. The issue relates to consistency of food. Option 4 is the only option that addresses a factor affecting food consistency.

Level of Cognitive Ability: Comprehension
Client Needs: Physiological Integrity
Integrated Concept/Process: Nursing Process/Assessment
Content Area: Fundamental Skills
Reference: Craven, R., & Hirnle, C. (2000). *Fundamentals of nursing: Human health and function* (3rd ed.). Philadelphia: Lippincott Williams & Wilkins, p. 620.

22. 3

Rationale: Bacon is a component of the fat group in the exchange system: 1 teaspoon of butter is equal to 1 teaspoon of margarine, 1 teaspoon of any oil, 1 tablespoon of salad dressing, 1 strip of bacon, 5 large olives, or 10 whole peanuts.

Test-Taking Strategy: Note the key words *most appropriate* in the stem of the question. Eliminate options 1 and 2 because they are similar. Select option 3 over option 4 knowing that bacon is an item of the fat group. Review foods in the exchange system if you had difficulty with this question.

Level of Cognitive Ability: Application
Client Needs: Health Promotion and Maintenance
Integrated Concept/Process: Teaching/Learning
Content Area: Adult Health/Endocrine
Reference: LeMone, P., & Burke, K. (2000). *Medical-surgical nursing: Critical thinking in client care* (2nd ed.). Upper Saddle River, N.J.: Prentice-Hall, p. 746.

23. 3

Rationale: Fruits and vegetables—except avocado, olives, and coconut—contain minimal amounts of fat.

Test-Taking Strategy: Use the process of elimination. Options 1 and 2 can be easily eliminated based on general knowledge regarding nutrition. From the remaining two options, remember that avocado is high in fat content. Review the food items high in fat content if you had difficulty with this question.

Level of Cognitive Ability: Analysis
Client Needs: Health Promotion and Maintenance
Integrated Concept/Process: Nursing Process/Evaluation
Content Area: Adult Health/Cardiovascular
Reference: Grodner, M., Anderson, S., & DeYoung, S. (2000). *Foundations and clinical applications of nutrition: A nursing approach.* St. Louis: Mosby, p. 850.

24. 1

Rationale: Chemotherapy may cause distortion of taste. Frequently beef and pork are reported to taste bitter or metallic. The nurse can promote client nutrition by assisting the client to choose alternative sources of protein in the diet. Options 2, 3, and 4 are not likely to cause distortion of taste.

Test-Taking Strategy: The issue of the question relates to management of a change in taste sensation. To answer this question accurately, you must be familiar with the most troublesome foods. If you had difficulty with this question review interventions related to nutrition in a client receiving chemotherapy.

Level of Cognitive Ability: Application

Client Needs: Health Promotion and Maintenance
Integrated Concept/Process: Nursing Process/Implementation
Content Area: Adult Health/Oncology
Reference: Grodner, M., Anderson, S., & DeYoung, S. (2000). *Foundations and clinical applications of nutrition: A nursing approach.* St. Louis: Mosby, pp. 620-621.

25. 2
Rationale: Normal hemoglobin levels indicate that iron and protein intake is sufficient. Elevated creatinine levels indicate kidney problems, which is not considered a nutritional disorder. Elevated albumin levels may falsely indicate dehydration. Normal red blood cell levels indicates adequate vitamin B_{12} intake.
Test-Taking Strategy: Knowledge regarding the interpretation of the common laboratory test findings is required to answer this question. Review these common laboratory tests if you had difficulty with this question.
Level of Cognitive Ability: Analysis
Client Needs: Physiological Integrity
Integrated Concept/Process: Nursing Process/Evaluation
Content Area: Fundamental Skills
Reference: Leahy, J., & Kizilay, P. (1998). *Foundations of nursing practice: A nursing process approach.* Philadelphia: W.B. Saunders, pp. 757-758.

26. 1
Rationale: Hydrocephalus is a condition characterized by enlargement of the cranium as a result of an abnormal accumulation of cerebrospinal fluid within the cerebral ventricular system. This characteristic causes an increase in the weight of the infant's head, and significant head enlargement may occur. Care must be exercised to see that the head is well supported when the infant is fed or moved to prevent extra strain on the infant's neck, and measures must be taken to prevent the development of pressure areas. Supporting the infant's head and neck when picking it up will prevent hyperextension of the neck area and prevent the infant from falling backward. The infant should be fed with the head elevated for proper motility of food processing. A helmet could suffocate an unattended infant during rest and sleep times, and hyperextension of the infant's head can put pressure on the neck vertebrae, causing injury.
Test-Taking Strategy: Use the process of elimination and focus on the issue of the question: moving an infant with an enlarged head size. Visualizing each of the options will assist in directing you to option 1, the safe measure. If you had difficulty with this question review care of an infant with hydrocephalus.
Level of Cognitive Ability: Application
Client Needs: Safe, Effective Care Environment
Integrated Concept/Process: Teaching/Learning
Content Area: Child Health
Reference: Wong, D. (1999). *Whaley & Wong's Nursing care of infants and children* (6th ed.). St. Louis: Mosby, p. 499.

27. 2
Rationale: Parents are especially concerned about seizures that might go undetected at night. The nurse needs to decrease parental overprotection and should suggest the use of a baby monitor for nighttime. Options 1 and 3 identify parental understanding of the disorder. Option 4 is a common

concern. The parents need to be reminded that as the child grows, they cannot always observe their child, but that their knowledge of seizure activity and care is appropriate to minimize complications.
Test-Taking Strategy: Note the key words *need for further teaching.* Use the process of elimination, recalling that parental overprotection needs to be discouraged. Option 2 identifies a need to provide the parents with an alternate manner to monitor for night seizures. Review parental home care instructions for a child with a seizure disorder if you had difficulty with this question.
Level of Cognitive Ability: Analysis
Client Needs: Health Promotion and Maintenance
Integrated Concept/Process: Nursing Process/Evaluation
Content Area: Child Health
Reference: Wong, D. (1999). *Whaley & Wong's Nursing care of infants and children* (6th ed.). St. Louis: Mosby, p. 1822.

28. 4
Rationale: When carbamazepine is administered, blood levels need to be drawn periodically to check for the child's absorption of the medication. The amount of the medication prescribed is based on the blood level achieved. Tegretol's therapeutic serum range is 3 to 14 µg/mL. The nurse would anticipate that the physician would continue the presently prescribed dosage.
Test-Taking Strategy: It is necessary to know the therapeutic serum drug level of carbamazepine to answer the question. Recalling that the therapeutic level is 3 to 14 µg/mL will direct you to option 4, because a result of 10 µg/mL is within the therapeutic range. If you had difficulty with this question, learn the therapeutic serum drug level of carbamazepine.
Level of Cognitive Ability: Analysis
Client Needs: Physiological Integrity
Integrated Concept/Process: Nursing Process/Analysis
Content Area: Pharmacology
Reference: Hodgson, B., & Kizior, R. (2001). *Saunders nursing drug handbook 2001.* Philadelphia: W.B. Saunders, pp. 144-146.

29. 2
Rationale: The uterus has three divisions, the corpus, isthmus, and the cervix. The upper division is the corpus or the body of the uterus. The uppermost part of the uterine corpus, above the area where the fallopian tubes enter the uterus, is the fundus of the uterus. Options 1, 3, and 4 are incorrect.
Test-Taking Strategy: Use the process of elimination. Knowledge regarding the divisions of the uterus is required to answer this question. If you had difficulty with this question, review the anatomical structure of the uterus.
Level of Cognitive Ability: Comprehension
Client Needs: Physiological Integrity
Integrated Concept/Process: Nursing Process/Evaluation
Content Area: Maternity
Reference: Gorrie, T., McKinney, E. & Murray, S. (1998). *Foundations of maternal-newborn nursing* (2nd ed.). Philadelphia: W.B. Saunders, p. 61.

30. 4
Rationale: Hypoglycemia is a blood glucose level of less than 50 to 60 mg/dL.
Test-Taking Strategy: Recalling the normal blood glucose level will assist in eliminating options 1, 2, and 3. If you are

unfamiliar with the normal blood glucose level or the concept of hypoglycemia, review this content.
Level of Cognitive Ability: Application
Client Needs: Health Promotion and Maintenance
Integrated Concept/Process: Teaching/Learning
Content Area: Pharmacology
Reference: Lehne, R. (1998). *Pharmacology for nursing care* (3rd ed.). Philadelphia: W.B. Saunders, p. 593.

31. 1
Rationale: Glucagon is used to treat hypoglycemia resulting from insulin overdose. The family of the client is instructed in how to administer the medication. In an unconscious client, arousal usually occurs within 20 minutes of glucagon injection. Once consciousness has been regained, oral carbohydrates should be given. Lipoatrophy and lipohypertrophy result from insulin injections.
Test-Taking Strategy: Use the process of elimination. Noting the word *glucagon* will assist in determining that the medication contains some form of glucose. This relationship should easily direct you to option 1. Review the purpose of this medication if you are unfamiliar with it.
Level of Cognitive Ability: Application
Client Needs: Health Promotion and Maintenance
Integrated Concept/Process: Teaching/Learning
Content Area: Pharmacology
Reference: Wilson, B., Shannon, M., & Stang, C. (2000). *Nurses drug guide 2000.* Stamford, Conn.: Appleton & Lange, p. 641.

32. 3
Rationale: In the Cuban American culture, loud crying and other physical manifestations of grief are considered socially acceptable. Of the options provided, option 3 is the only option that identifies a culturally sensitive approach on the part of the nurse. Options 1, 2, and 4 are inappropriate nursing interventions.
Test-Taking Strategy: Focus on the clients of the question: the family members. Use the process of elimination and therapeutic nursing interventions, recalling the characteristics of the culture and the importance of cultural sensitivity. This will easily direct you to option 3. If you had difficulty with this question, review the characteristics of this culture.
Level of Cognitive Ability: Application
Client Needs: Psychosocial Integrity
Integrated Concept/Process: Cultural Awareness
Content Area: Fundamental Skills
Reference: Purnell, L., & Paulanka, B. (1998). *Transcultural health care: A culturally competent approach.* Philadelphia: F.A. Davis, p. 203.

33. 1
Rationale: Transmission of infectious diseases can occur through contaminated items such as hands and bed linens in clients with endometritis. An important method of preventing infection is to break the chain of infection. Hand washing is one of the most effective methods of preventing the transmission of infectious diseases. The newborn infant is allowed in the mother's room and visitors are allowed to hold the newborn infant, as long as hand washing and other protective measures are instituted.
Test-Taking Strategy: Use the process of elimination. Eliminate options 2, 3, and 4 because of the absolute terms *at all, no,* and *not.* Review content related to the transmission of infection if you had difficulty with this question.

Level of Cognitive Ability: Application
Client Needs: Safe, Effective Care Environment
Integrated Concept/Process: Teaching/Learning
Content Area: Maternity
Reference: Gorrie, T., McKinney, E., & Murray, S. (1998). *Foundations of maternal newborn nursing* (2nd ed.) Philadelphia: W. B. Saunders, p. 800.

34. 4
Rationale: The priority nursing action is to assess vital signs. These data would indicate the amount of blood loss that has occurred and also provide a baseline by which to monitor the progress of treatment. The client may not be able to provide subjective data until the immediate physical needs are met. Although an abdominal examination and assessment of the precipitating events may be necessary, these actions are not the priority.
Test-Taking Strategy: Note the key words *first priority.* Use the process of elimination and the ABCs of airway, breathing, and circulation. This will direct you to option 4. Review care of a client with a GI bleed if you had difficulty with this question.
Level of Cognitive Ability: Application
Client Needs: Physiological Integrity
Integrated Concept/Process: Nursing Process/Implementation
Content Area: Adult Health/Gastrointestinal
Reference: Lewis, S., Heitkemper, M., & Dirksen, S. (2000). *Medical-surgical nursing: Assessment and management of clinical problems* (5th ed.). St. Louis: Mosby, p. 1106.

35. 1
Rationale: An IV cholangiogram is for diagnostic purposes. It outlines both the gallbladder and the ducts, so gallstones that have moved into the ductal system can be detected. X-ray films are used to visualize the biliary duct system after IV injection of radiopaque dye. This test is diagnostic and does not involve irrigation, instillation of medications, or draining of the gallbladder.
Test-Taking Strategy: Use the process of elimination. Eliminate option 2, 3, and 4 because they are similar. If you are unfamiliar with this procedure, review its purpose.
Level of Cognitive Ability: Analysis
Client Needs: Physiological Integrity
Integrated Concept/Process: Nursing Process/Evaluation
Content Area: Adult Health/Gastrointestinal
Reference: Monahan, F., & Neighbors, M. (1998). *Medical-surgical nursing: Foundations for clinical practice* (2nd ed.). Philadelphia: W.B. Saunders, p. 972.

36. 1
Rationale: Iron is needed both to allow for transfer of adequate iron to the fetus and to permit expansion of the maternal red blood cell mass. During pregnancy, the relative excess of plasma causes a decrease in the hemoglobin concentration and hematocrit level, known as *physiologic anemia of pregnancy.* This is a normal adaptation during pregnancy. Meats are an excellent source of iron. Iron supplements usually cause constipation. Iron is best absorbed if taken on an empty stomach.
Test-Taking Strategy: Use the process of elimination, focusing on the key words *understanding of the instructions.* Knowledge of basic principles related to nutrition during pregnancy will assist in eliminating options 2 and 4. From the remaining options, remember that iron causes constipation. Review client teaching points related to iron supplementation if you had difficulty with this question.

Level of Cognitive Ability: Analysis
Client Needs: Physiological Integrity
Integrated Concept/Process: Nursing Process/Evaluation
Content Area: Maternity
Reference: Lowdermilk, D., Perry, S., & Bobak, I. (2000). *Maternity & women's health care* (7th ed.). St. Louis: Mosby, p. 355; 362-363; 372.

37. 1
Rationale: The client who has had vein ligation and stripping should avoid standing or sitting for prolonged periods. The client should remain lying down unless performing a specific activity for the first few days following the procedure. Prolonged standing and sitting increases the risk of edema in the legs by decreasing blood return to the heart. The client should avoid crossing the legs at any level for the same reason.
Test-Taking Strategy: Use the process of elimination and principles associated with gravity and blood flow to answer this question. Eliminate option 2 first because of the absolute term *only*. Knowing that prolonged standing or sitting is harmful helps you to eliminate options 3 and 4. Review client instructions following a vein ligation and stripping if you had difficulty with this question.
Level of Cognitive Ability: Analysis
Client Needs: Health Promotion and Maintenance
Integrated Concept/Process: Nursing Process/Evaluation
Content Area: Adult Health/Cardiovascular
Reference: Lewis, S., Heitkemper, M., & Dirksen, S. (2000). *Medical-surgical nursing: Assessment and management of clinical problems* (5th ed.). St. Louis: Mosby, p. 1005.

38. 3
Rationale: Sandostatin is used to reduce growth hormone levels in clients with acromegaly. The most common side effects of Sandostatin include diarrhea, nausea, gallstone formation, and abdominal discomfort. Hypertension, although rare, may occur. Polyuria is not associated with this medication.
Test-Taking Strategy: Knowledge regarding the side effects associated with Sandostatin is required to answer the question. Review these side effects if you had difficulty with this question.
Level of Cognitive Ability: Analysis
Client Needs: Physiological Integrity
Integrated Concept/Process: Nursing Process/Assessment
Content Area: Pharmacology
Reference: Hodgson, B., & Kizior, R. (2001). *Saunders nursing drug handbook 2001*. Philadelphia: W.B. Saunders, p. 764.

39. 2
Rationale: Synthroid accelerates the degradation of vitamin K–dependent clotting factors. As a result, the effects of Coumadin are enhanced. Therefore, if thyroid hormone replacement therapy is instituted in a client who has been taking warfarin (Coumadin), the dosage of Coumadin should be reduced.
Test-Taking Strategy: Use the process of elimination recalling that Synthroid enhances the effects of Coumadin. Review these medication interactions if you had difficulty with this question.
Level of Cognitive Ability: Analysis
Client Needs: Safe, Effective Care Environment
Integrated Concept/Process: Nursing Process/Analysis
Content Area: Pharmacology

Reference: Salerno, E. (1999). *Pharmacology for health professionals*. St. Louis: Mosby, p. 550.

40. 3
Rationale: The client should use the positions outlined in options 1, 2, and 4. These allow for maximal chest expansion. The client should not lie on the back, because it reduces movement of a large area of the chest wall. Sitting is better than standing whenever possible. If no chair is available, then leaning against a wall while standing allows accessory muscles to be used for breathing, and not posture control.
Test-Taking Strategy: Use the process of elimination, noting the key words *dyspneic episodes* and *avoid*. Also note that options 1, 2, and 4 are similar in that they all address upright positions. If you had difficulty with this question, review client teaching points related to emphysema.
Level of Cognitive Ability: Application
Client Needs: Health Promotion and Maintenance
Integrated Concept/Process: Self-Care
Content Area: Adult Health/Respiratory
Reference: Ignatavicius, D., Workman, M., & Mishler, M. (1999). *Medical-surgical nursing across the health care continuum* (3rd ed.). Philadelphia: W.B. Saunders, p. 616.

41. 1
Rationale: The client undergoing LP is positioned lying on the side, with the legs pulled up to the abdomen, and with the head bent down onto the chest. This position helps to open the spaces between the vertebrae and allows for easier needle insertion by the physician. Each of the other options identifies incorrect positions for this procedure.
Test-Taking Strategy: Use the process of elimination. Recalling that an LP is the introduction of a needle into the subarachnoid space will direct you to option 1. It is reasonable that the position of the client must facilitate this and the correct option is the only position, which flexes the vertebrae and widens the spaces between them. Review care of a client undergoing an LP if you had difficulty with this question.
Level of Cognitive Ability: Application
Client Needs: Physiological Integrity
Integrated Concept/Process: Nursing Process/Implementation
Content Area: Adult Health/Neurological
Reference: Altman, G., Buchsel, P., & Coxon, V. (2000). *Delmar's Fundamental & advanced nursing skills*. Albany, NY: Delmar, p. 1345.

42. 2
Rationale: Maintaining effective and open communication among family members affected by death and grief is of the greatest importance. Option 1 describes encouraging discussion of feelings and is likely to enhance communications. Option 3 is also an effective intervention, because spiritual practices give meaning to life and have an impact on how people react to crisis. Option 4 is also an effective technique, as the client and family need to know that someone will be there who is supportive and nonjudgmental. Option 2 describes the nurse removing autonomy and decision-making from the client and family, who are already experiencing feelings of loss of control in that they cannot change the process of dying. This is an ineffective intervention, which can further impair communication.
Test-Taking Strategy: Use the process of elimination, noting the key words *unlikely to facilitate*. Understanding that people in crisis usually feel helpless and unable to control their

circumstances can assist in identifying option 2 as a response that further removes control. Review these therapeutic interventions if you had difficulty with this question.
Level of Cognitive Ability: Comprehension
Client Needs: Psychosocial Integrity
Integrated Concept/Process: Caring
Content Area: Fundamental Skills
Reference: Kozier, B., Erb, G., Berman, A., & Burke, K. (2000). *Fundamentals of nursing: Concepts, process, and practice* (6th ed.). Upper Saddle River, N.J.: Prentice-Hall, pp. 979-980.

43. 4
Rationale: The pain of pancreatitis is aggravated by lying supine or by walking. This is because the pancreas is located retroperitoneally, and the edema and inflammation intensify the irritation of the posterior peritoneal wall with these positions or movements. The fetal position (with the legs drawn up to the chest) may decrease the abdominal pain of pancreatitis. Positions such as sitting up, leaning forward, and flexing the legs (especially the left leg) will also alleviate some of the pain associated with pancreatitis.
Test-Taking Strategy: Use the process of elimination and note the key word *avoided*. Use your critical thinking skills to visualize the anatomy of the pancreas and the potential effects from stretching associated with the various positions identified in the options. Also, remember that options that are similar are not likely to be correct. This will help you to eliminate options 1, 2, and 3. Review care of a client with pancreatitis if you had difficulty with this question.
Level of Cognitive Ability: Analysis
Client Needs: Health Promotion and Maintenance
Integrated Concept/Process: Nursing Process/Evaluation
Content Area: Adult Health/Gastrointestinal
Reference: Ignatavicius, D., Workman, M., & Mishler, M. (1999). *Medical-surgical nursing across the health care continuum* (3rd ed.). Philadelphia: W.B. Saunders, p. 1509.

44. 1
Rationale: After surgery to repair a fractured hip, an abductor splint is used to maintain the affected extremity in good alignment when the client is turned side to side. An overhead trapeze and bed pillow may also be used in the postoperative period, but they are not the priority items to be used in repositioning.
Test-Taking Strategy: Use the process of elimination noting the key words *most important*. Also, focus on the issue: repositioning the client from side to side in the postoperative period. Use principles of client safety and knowledge of this surgical procedure to direct you to option 1. Review care of a client with a fractured hip if you had difficulty with this question.
Level of Cognitive Ability: Application
Client Needs: Safe, Effective Care Environment
Integrated Concept/Process: Nursing Process/Implementation
Content Area: Adult Health/Musculoskeletal
Reference: Lewis, S., Heitkemper, M., & Dirksen, S. (2000). *Medical-surgical nursing: Assessment and management of clinical problems* (5th ed.). St. Louis: Mosby, p. 1790.

45. 1
Rationale: If an oil-based dye is used during a myelogram, the dye is removed at the end of the procedure. The client is positioned flat in bed for 6 to 8 hours after the dye is removed. When a water-based dye is used, the client is positioned with the head of bed elevated for at least 8 hours to keep the dye from irritating the cerebral meninges.
Test-Taking Strategy: Use the process of elimination. Note the key words *oil-based contrast agent*. Use knowledge regarding care of a client following this procedure to direct you to option 1. Review this procedure if you had difficulty with this question.
Level of Cognitive Ability: Application
Client Needs: Physiological Integrity
Integrated Concept/Process: Nursing Process/Planning
Content Area: Adult Health/Neurological
Reference: Corbett, J. (2000). *Laboratory tests and diagnostic procedures* (5th ed.). Upper Saddle River: N.J.: Prentice-Hall, p. 554.

46. 2
Rationale: The client should avoid positions or activities that place strain on the lower back. The client should not sleep on the abdomen (prone), or on the side if the hips and knees are straight. The client should not lean forward without bending the knees, stand in one position for lengthy amounts of time, or lift anything above elbow level. It may be helpful for the client to stand with a foot elevated on a stool, or sit using a form of lumbar support.
Test-Taking Strategy: Use the process of elimination noting the key word *avoid*. Use knowledge of body mechanics and low back injury to answer the question. If you had difficulty with this question, review client teaching points related to low back pain.
Level of Cognitive Ability: Analysis
Client Needs: Health Promotion and Maintenance
Integrated Concept/Process: Nursing Process/Evaluation
Content Area: Adult Health/Musculoskeletal
Reference: Lewis, S., Heitkemper, M., & Dirksen, S. (2000). *Medical-surgical nursing: Assessment and management of clinical problems* (5th ed.). St. Louis: Mosby, p. 1806.

47. 3
Rationale: The head of the client at risk for or with increased ICP should be positioned so the head is in a neutral, midline position. The nurse should avoid flexing or extending the neck or turning the head side to side. The head of the bed should be raised to 30 to 45 degrees. Use of proper positions promotes venous drainage from the cranium to keep ICP down.
Test-Taking Strategy: Use the process of elimination noting the key words *at risk for increased intracranial pressure* and *avoid*. Visualize each of the positions identified in the options and identify the position that is detrimental to the client with increased ICP. This would be the position that interferes either with arterial circulation to the brain, or with venous drainage from the brain. The only position that meets one of those criteria is option 3. Review care of a client at risk for or with increased ICP if you had difficulty with this question.
Level of Cognitive Ability: Application
Client Needs: Physiological Integrity
Integrated Concept/Process: Nursing Process/Implementation
Content Area: Adult Health/Neurological
Reference: Ignatavicius, D., Workman, M., & Mishler, M. (1999). *Medical-surgical nursing across the health care continuum* (3rd ed.). Philadelphia: W.B. Saunders, p. 1133.

48. 3
Rationale: The normal pH is 7.35 to 7.45. The normal Pco_2 is 35 to 45 mm Hg. In respiratory acidosis the pH is low and the

Pco_2 is elevated. Options 1, 2, and 4 are incorrect interpretation of the values identified in the question.

Test-Taking Strategy: Remember that in a respiratory imbalance you will find an opposite response between the pH and the Pco_2. Also remember that the pH is down in an acidotic condition. Recalling this information will allow you to eliminate each of the incorrect options. Review interpretation of blood gas results if you had difficulty with this question.

Level of Cognitive Ability: Analysis
Client Needs: Physiological Integrity
Integrated Concept/Process: Nursing Process/Analysis
Content Area: Fundamental Skills
Reference: LeMone, P., & Burke, K. (2000). *Medical-surgical nursing: Critical thinking in client care* (2nd ed.). Upper Saddle River, N.J.: Prentice-Hall, p. 153.

49. 4
Rationale: To prevent acute adrenal insufficiency, glucocorticoids should not be abruptly discontinued. These medications can cause sodium and water retention and the loss of potassium, and clients should be instructed to limit sodium intake and consume potassium-rich foods. Adequate dietary intake is also important. These medications can increase the risk of infection, and the client should avoid contact with persons who are ill.

Test-Taking Strategy: Use the process of elimination. Note the key words *indicates a need for further instruction*. You should easily be able to eliminate options 1, 2, and 3 remembering that the client should not stop these medications, or in fact, any medication, without physician approval. Review the administration of glucocorticoids if you had difficulty with this question.

Level of Cognitive Ability: Analysis
Client Needs: Health Promotion and Maintenance
Integrated Concept/Process: Nursing Process/Evaluation
Content Area: Pharmacology
Reference: Clark, J., Queener, S., & Karb, V. (2000). *Pharmacologic basis of nursing practice* (6th ed.). St. Louis: Mosby, p. 471.

50. 2
Rationale: NPH insulin is an intermediate-acting insulin. Its onset of action is 3 to 4 hours, it peaks in 4 to 12 hours, and its duration of action is 16 to 20 hours.

Test-Taking Strategy: Read the question carefully, noting that the question is about NPH insulin. Knowledge regarding the onset of action, peak, and duration of action is required to answer the question. Review these points regarding both NPH and regular insulin if you had difficulty with this question.

Level of Cognitive Ability: Analysis
Client Needs: Physiological Integrity
Integrated Concept/Process: Nursing Process/Analysis
Content Area: Pharmacology
Reference: Salerno, E. (1999). *Pharmacology for health professionals.* St. Louis: Mosby, p. 567.

51. 2
Rationale: The client's operative arm should be positioned so that it is elevated on a pillow, not exceeding shoulder elevation. This promotes optimal drainage from the limb without impairing the circulation to the arm. If the arm is positioned flat (option 3) or dependent (option 4), this could increase the edema in the arm, which is contraindicated because of lymphatic disruption caused by surgery.

Test-Taking Strategy: Use the process of elimination. Read each option carefully and attempt to visualize the position identified in the option. Using the principles of circulation and gravity will easily direct you to option 2. Option 2 is the option that avoids the two extremes of height in positioning the limb affected by surgery. Review care of a client following mastectomy if you had difficulty with this question.

Level of Cognitive Ability: Application
Client Needs: Physiological Integrity
Integrated Concept/Process: Nursing Process/Planning
Content Area: Adult Health/Oncology
Reference: Ignatavicius, D., Workman, M., & Mishler, M. (1999). *Medical-surgical nursing across the health care continuum* (3rd ed.). Philadelphia: W.B. Saunders, p. 1969.

52. 4
Rationale: A woman with a urinary tract infection must be encouraged to take the medication for the entire time it is prescribed; she should also be instructed to drink at least 3000 mL of fluid each day to flush the infection from the bladder and to urinate frequently throughout the day. Foods and fluids that acidify the urine should be encouraged.

Test-Taking Strategy: Use the process of elimination. Note the key words *indicate a need for further instructions*. Recall that foods and fluids that acidify the urine should be consumed rather that foods and fluids that cause urine alkalinity. If you had difficulty with this question, review nursing considerations for the client with a urinary tract infection.

Level of Cognitive Ability: Analysis
Client Needs: Health Promotion and Maintenance
Integrated Concept/Process: Nursing Process/Evaluation
Content Area: Maternity
Reference: Gorrie, T., McKinney, E., & Murray, S. (1998). *Foundations of maternal-newborn nursing* (2nd ed.). Philadelphia: W.B. Saunders, p. 800.

53. 4
Rationale: Case management represents an interdisciplinary health care delivery system to promote appropriate use of hospital personnel and material resources to maximize hospital revenues while providing for optimal outcome of client care. Options 1, 2, and 3 are inaccurate statements regarding case management.

Test-Taking Strategy: Use the process of elimination and knowledge regarding the characteristics of case management. Review the characteristics of case management if you had difficulty with this question.

Level of Cognitive Ability: Application
Client Needs: Safe, Effective Care Environment
Integrated Concept/Process: Communication and Documentation
Content Area: Fundamental Skills
Reference: Rocchiccioli, J., & Tilbury, M. (1998). *Clinical leadership in nursing.* Philadelphia: W.B. Saunders, pp. 38-39.

54. 3
Rationale: It is important to emphasize to the client and family that they are not eating a diabetic diet but rather a balanced meal plan. Adherence to nutrition principles is an important component of diabetic management and an individualized meal plan should be developed for the client. It is not necessary for the client to purchase special dietetic foods.

Test-Taking Strategy: Use the process of elimination. Note the key words *indicates a need for further teaching.* Careful reading of this question and the options will easily direct you to the correct option. Review dietary instructions for the client with diabetes mellitus if you had difficulty with this question.
Level of Cognitive Ability: Analysis
Client Needs: Health Promotion and Maintenance
Integrated Concept/Process: Nursing Process/Evaluation
Content Area: Adult Health/Endocrine
Reference: Smeltzer, S., & Bare, B. (2000). *Brunner & Suddarth's Textbook of medical-surgical nursing* (9th ed.). Philadelphia: Lippincott Williams & Wilkins, p. 984.

55. 3
Rationale: NPH is an intermediate-acting insulin. The onset of action is 3 to 4 hours, it peaks in 4 to 12 hours, and its duration of action is 16 to 20 hours. Hypoglycemic reactions most likely occur during peak time.
Test-Taking Strategy: Use the process of elimination and knowledge regarding the onset, peak, and duration of action for NPH insulin. Recalling that peak action is between 4 and 12 hours will easily direct you to option 3. Review the characteristics of NPH insulin if you had difficulty with this question.
Level of Cognitive Ability: Analysis
Client Needs: Physiological Integrity
Integrated Concept/Process: Nursing Process/Analysis
Content Area: Adult Health/Endocrine
Reference: Smeltzer, S., & Bare, B. (2000). *Brunner & Suddarth's Textbook of medical-surgical nursing* (9th ed.). Philadelphia: Lippincott Williams & Wilkins, p. 987.

56. 3
Rationale: Tertiary prevention involves the reduction of the amount and degree of disability, injury, and damage following a crisis. Primary prevention means keeping the crisis from ever occurring and secondary prevention focuses on reducing the intensity and duration of the crisis during the crisis itself. There is no known fourth care prevention level.
Test-Taking Strategy: Identify the scenario in the question and the role of the nurse in the question. Focus on these nursing roles and use knowledge regarding the various levels of prevention to answer the question. If you had difficulty with this question review the levels of prevention.
Level of Cognitive Ability: Comprehension
Client Needs: Safe, Effective Care Environment
Integrated Concept/Process: Caring
Content Area: Fundamental Skills
Reference: Craven, R., & Hirnle, C. (2000). *Fundamentals of nursing: Human health and function* (3rd ed.). Philadelphia: Lippincott, p. 665.

57. 4
Rationale: Rubella virus is spread by aerosol droplet transmission through the upper respiratory tract and has an incubation period of 14 to 21 days. The risk of maternal and subsequent fetal infection during the second trimester include hearing loss and congenital anomalies. Rubella titer determination is a standard antenatal test for childbearing women during their initial screening and entry into the health care delivery system. Option 4 helps to clarify maternal concerns with accurate information based on the acquisition of rubella infection and potential fetal side effects

Test-Taking Strategy: Use the process of elimination and knowledge regarding the transmission of rubella virus to the fetus. Use of therapeutic communication techniques will direct you to option 4. Option 4 addresses the client's concerns. Review concepts related to exposure to rubella during pregnancy if you had difficulty with this question.
Level of Cognitive Ability: Application
Clients Needs: Psychosocial Integrity
Integrated Concept/Process: Caring
Content Area: Maternity
Reference: Sherwen, L., Scoloveno, M.A., & Weingarten, C. (1999). *Maternity nursing: Care of the childbearing family* (3rd ed.). Stamford, Conn.: Appleton & Lange, p. 619.

58. 1
Rationale: Breastfeeding mothers need to be encouraged to limit dairy products. Cheese is a dairy product. Alternative calcium sources that can be consumed by the mother include egg yolk, green leafy vegetables, dried beans, cauliflower, and molasses.
Test-Taking Strategy: Use the process of elimination. Note the key word *avoid* in the stem of the question. Knowledge that lactose is the sugar found in dairy products will easily direct you to option 1. Review the dietary management for the infant with lactose intolerance if you had difficulty with this question.
Level of Cognitive Ability: Application
Client Needs: Health Promotion and Maintenance
Integrated Concept/Process: Teaching/Learning
Content Area: Child Health
Reference: Wong, D. (1999). *Whaley & Wong's Nursing care of infants and children* (6th ed.). St. Louis: Mosby, p. 638.

59. 1
Rationale: The nurse needs to be aware of the effective and ineffective coping mechanisms that can occur in a client when loss is anticipated. The expression of anger is known to be a normal response to impending loss, and the anger may be directed toward the self, God or other spiritual being, or the caregivers. Notifying the hospital lawyer is inappropriate. Guilt may or may not be a component of the client's feelings, and the data in the question do not provide an indication that guilt is present.
Test-Taking Strategy: Focus on the data provided in the question. Note that options 1 and 4 address coping mechanisms. This provides you with the clue that one of these options may be the correct response. Additionally, knowledge of the stages of grief associated with loss will easily direct you to option 1. Review these stages and expected client responses if you had difficulty with this question.
Level of Cognitive Ability: Analysis
Client Needs: Psychosocial Integrity
Integrated Concept/Process: Nursing Process/Analysis
Content Area: Fundamental Skills
Reference: Harkreader, H. (2000). *Fundamentals of nursing: Caring and clinical judgment.* Philadelphia: W.B. Saunders, p. 1366.

60. 3
Rationale: An autopsy is required by state law in certain circumstances, including the sudden death of a client and a death that occurs under suspicious circumstances. A client may have provided oral or written instructions regarding an

autopsy following death. If an autopsy is not required by law, these oral or written requests will be granted. If no oral or written instructions were provided, state law determines who has the authority to consent for an autopsy. Most often, the decision rests with the surviving relative or next of kin.

Test-Taking Strategy: Note the key words *most appropriate*. Use knowledge regarding the laws and issues surrounding autopsy and therapeutic communication techniques to answer the question. Eliminate options 1 and 4 because these statements are not completely accurate. From the remaining options, option 3 is the most therapeutic and appropriate response to the family. Review the issues and laws surrounding autopsy if you had difficulty with this question.

Level of Cognitive Ability: Application
Client Needs: Safe, Effective Care Environment
Integrated Concept/Process: Caring
Content Area: Fundamental Skills
Reference: Kozier, B., Erb, G., Berman, A., & Burke, K. (2000). *Fundamentals of nursing: Concepts, process, and practice* (6th ed.). Upper Saddle River, N.J.: Prentice-Hall, p. 985.

61. **3**
Rationale: The mode of perinatal transmission of HIV to the fetus or neonate of an HIV-positive woman can occur during the antenatal, intrapartal, or postpartum periods. HIV transmission can occur during breastfeeding; therefore HIV-positive clients should be encouraged to bottle-feed their neonates. Frequent handwashing is encouraged. Support groups and community agencies can be identified to assist the parents with the newborn infant's home care, the impact of the diagnosis of HIV infection, and available financial resources. Newborn infants of HIV-positive clients are recommended to receive antiviral medications for the first 6 weeks of life.

Test-Taking Strategy: Use the process of elimination. Note the key word *not* in the stem of the question. Recalling that breastfeeding is discouraged in the HIV-positive woman will easily direct you to the correct option. Review home care measures for the HIV-client if you had difficulty with this question.

Level of Cognitive Ability: Application
Clients Needs: Safe, Effective Care Environment
Integrated Concept/Process: Teaching/Learning
Content Area: Maternity
Reference: Sherwen, L., Scoloveno, M.A., & Weingarten, C. (1999). *Maternity nursing: Care of the childbearing family* (3rd ed.). Stamford, Conn.: Appleton & Lange, pp. 998; 1033.

62. **2**
Rationale: When active herpetic genital lesions are present, cesarean delivery can reduce neonatal infection risks. In the absence of active genital lesions, vaginal delivery is indicated unless there are other indications for cesarean delivery. Maternal isolation is not necessary, but a culture should be performed on potentially exposed newborn infants on the day of delivery.

Test-Taking Strategy: Use the process of elimination. Knowledge regarding the transmission of genital herpes to the newborn infant is required to answer this question. If you had difficulty with this question, review this content area.

Level of Cognitive Ability: Application
Clients Needs: Safe, Effective Care Environment
Integrated Concept/Process: Teaching/Learning

Content Area: Maternity
Reference: Olds, S., London. M., & Ladewig, P. (2000). *Maternal-newborn nursing: A family and community-based approach* (6th ed.). Upper Saddle River, N.J.: Prentice-Hall Health, p. 432.

63. **2**
Rationale: Viral conjunctivitis is extremely contagious. The child should be kept home from school or day care until the child has received antibiotic eye drops for 24 hours.

Test-Taking Strategy: Use the process of elimination. Recalling that viral conjunctivitis is highly contagious will assist in eliminating option 1. Eliminate option 4 next, because this time frame is rather lengthy. From the remaining options, knowledge regarding the action of antibiotics will assist in directing you to option 2. Review infection control measures related to viral conjunctivitis if you had difficulty with this question.

Level of Cognitive Ability: Application
Client Needs: Health Promotion and Maintenance
Integrated Concept/Process: Teaching/Learning
Content Area: Child Health
Reference: Ball, J. & Bindler, R. (1999). *Pediatric nursing: Caring for children* (2nd ed.). Stamford, Conn.: Appleton & Lange, p. 715.

64. **1**
Rationale: If the child wears contact lenses, the child should be instructed to discontinue wearing them until the infection has completely cleared. Securing new contact lenses will eliminate the chance of reinfection from contaminated contact lenses and will also lessen the risk of a corneal ulceration.

Test-Taking Strategy: Use the process of elimination. Note the key word *not* in the stem of the question. Options 2, 3, and 4 are similar in that they relate to avoiding the use of contact lenses during infection. If you had difficulty with this question, review treatment measures for conjunctivitis.

Level of Cognitive Ability: Application
Client Needs: Health Promotion and Maintenance
Integrated Concept/Process: Teaching/Learning
Content Area: Child Health
Reference: Ashwill, J. & Droske, S. (1997). *Nursing care of children: Principles and practice.* Philadelphia: W.B. Saunders, p. 1337.

65. **1**
Rationale: During pregnancy, the breasts change in both size and appearance. The increase in size is caused by the effects of estrogen and progesterone. Estrogen stimulates the growth of mammary ductal tissue and progesterone promotes the growth of lobes, lobules, and alveoli. A delicate network of veins is often visible just beneath the surface of the skin. Options 2, 3, and 4 are incorrect.

Test-Taking Strategy: Use the process of elimination. Knowledge regarding the physiological changes that occur during pregnancy is required to answer this question. If you are unfamiliar with the effects of hormones and the changes that occur, review this content.

Level of Cognitive Ability: Comprehension
Client Needs: Physiological Integrity
Integrated Concept/Process: Nursing Process/Planning
Content Area: Maternity

Reference: Lowdermilk, D., Perry, S., & Bobak, I. (2000). *Maternity & women's health care* (7th ed.). St. Louis: Mosby, p. 341.

66. **2**

Rationale: Aspiration is a possible complication associated with NG tube feeding. The head of the bed is elevated 30 to 45 degrees for at least 30 minutes after a bolus tube feeding to prevent vomiting and aspiration. The right lateral position uses gravity to facilitate gastric retention to prevent vomiting. The flat supine position is to be avoided for the first 30 minutes after a tube feeding.

Test-Taking Strategy: Use the process of elimination. Note that there are three components to each answer: the level of elevation of the head, the client's position, and duration. Option 1 can be eliminated immediately, because this position could result in aspiration. Options 2 and 4 are the same elevation, but the right lateral position is the correct position and 60 minutes is the correct duration. Option 3 is eliminated because of the supine position and the duration. Review care of a client receiving a bolus tube feeding if you had difficulty with this question.

Level of Cognitive Ability: Application
Client Needs: Physiological Integrity
Integrated Concept/Process: Nursing Process/Implementation
Content Area: Adult Health/Gastrointestinal
Reference: Smith, S., Duell, D., & Martin, B. (2000). *Clinical nursing skills: Basic to advanced skills* (5th ed.). Upper Saddle River, N.J.: Prentice-Hall Health, p. 477.

67. **4**

Rationale: All the stomach contents are aspirated and measured before administering a tube feeding. This procedure measures the gastric residuum. The gastric residuum is assessed to confirm whether undigested formula from a previous feeding remains, thereby evaluating absorption of the last feeding. It is important to assess gastric residuum, because administration of a tube feeding to a full stomach could result in overdistention, thus predisposing the client to regurgitation and possible aspiration. Options 1, 2, and 3 do not relate to the purpose of assessing residuum.

Test-Taking Strategy: Use the process of elimination. Focusing on the issue, the purpose of assessing residuum, will direct you to option 4. Review the purpose of this procedure if you had difficulty with this question

Level of Cognitive Ability: Comprehension
Client Needs: Physiological Integrity
Integrated Concept/Process: Nursing Process/Assessment
Content Area: Adult Health/Gastrointestinal
Reference: Altman, G., Buchsel, P., & Coxon, V. (2000). *Delmar's Fundamental & advanced nursing skills.* Albany, NY: Delmar, pp. 655-657.

68. **4**

Rationale: Factors that increase the risk of otitis media include exposure to illness in other children in day care centers, household smoking, bottle-feeding and congenital conditions such as Down's syndrome and cleft palate. The use of a pacifier beyond age 6 months has also been identified as a risk factor. Allergies are also thought to precipitate otitis media.

Test-Taking Strategy: Use the process of elimination. Note the key word *not* in the stem of the question. Careful reading of each of the options will quickly direct you to option 4. If you had difficulty with this question, review the risk factors associated with otitis media.

Level of Cognitive Ability: Comprehension
Client Needs: Physiological Integrity
Integrated Concept/Process: Nursing Process/Assessment
Content Area: Child Health
Reference: Wong, D. (1999). *Whaley & Wong's Nursing care of infants and children* (6th ed.). St. Louis: Mosby, p. 1469.

69. **3**

Rationale: A lateral recumbent position with the knees flexed to the abdomen and the head bent with the chin resting on the chest is assumed for a lumbar puncture. This position separates the spinal processes and facilitates needle insertion into the subarachnoid space. Options 1, 2, and 4 are incorrect positions.

Test-Taking Strategy: Use the process of elimination. Note the key word *lumbar* in the question. Visualize each of the descriptions of positions described in the options and focus on the key word to direct you to option 3. Review this procedure if you are unfamiliar with it.

Level of Cognitive Ability: Application
Client Needs: Physiological Integrity
Integrated Concept/Process: Nursing Process/Implementation
Content Area: Child Health
Reference: Altman, G., Buchsel, P., & Coxon, V. (2000). *Delmar's Fundamental & advanced nursing skills.* Albany, NY: Delmar, p. 1345.

70. **2**

Rationale: An insulin vial in current use can be kept at room temperature for up to 1 month without significant loss of activity. Direct sunlight and heat must be avoided.

Test-Taking Strategy: Use the process of elimination. Note the key word *unrefrigerated* in the question. This word will assist in directing you to the correct option. If you are unfamiliar with the concepts related to insulin stability, review this information.

Level of Cognitive Ability: Application
Client Needs: Health Promotion and Maintenance
Integrated Concept/Process: Self-Care
Content Area: Pharmacology
Reference: Lehne, R. (1998). *Pharmacology for nursing care* (3rd ed.). Philadelphia: W.B. Saunders, p. 583.

71. **3**

Rationale: Based on the location of the surgical procedure, spinal anesthesia would not be used. Additionally, the hair would not be shaved. Although coughing and deep breathing is important, specific to this procedure is avoiding toothbrushing to prevent disruption of the surgical site.

Test-Taking Strategy: Consider the anatomical location and the surgical procedure itself to eliminate options 1 and 4. Although you may be tempted to select option 2, note the key words *most important*. Because of the anatomical location of the surgery, option 3 is most important. Review this surgical procedure if you had difficulty with this question.

Level of Cognitive Ability: Application
Client Needs: Physiological Integrity
Integrated Concept/Process: Teaching/Learning
Content Area: Adult Health/Endocrine
Reference: Smeltzer, S., & Bare, B. (2000). *Brunner & Suddarth's Textbook of medical-surgical nursing* (9th ed.). Philadelphia: Lippincott Williams & Wilkins, p. 1669.

72. 3

Rationale: Common manifestations of Addison's disease include postural hypotension from fluid loss, syncope, muscle weakness, anorexia, nausea and vomiting, abdominal cramps, weight loss, depression and irritability. Options 1, 2, and 4 are not specific to this disorder.

Test-Taking Strategy: Use the process of elimination and knowledge regarding the clinical manifestations associated with Addison's disease to answer this question. If you had difficulty with this question, review the clinical manifestations of this disorder.

Level of Cognitive Ability: Analysis
Client Needs: Physiological Integrity
Integrated Concept/Process: Nursing Process/Assessment
Content Area: Adult Health/Endocrine
Reference: Monahan, F., & Neighbors, M. (1998). *Medical-surgical nursing: Foundations for clinical practice* (2nd ed.). Philadelphia: W.B. Saunders, p. 1278.

73. 3

Rationale: Effleurage is massage of the abdomen during contractions. Women learn to do effleurage using both hands in a circular motion. Progressive relaxation involves contracting and then consciously releasing different muscle groups. Neuromuscular disassociation helps the woman relax her body even when one group of muscles is strongly contracted. In this procedure, the woman contracts an area such as an arm or leg then concentrates on letting tension go from the rest of the body. Touch relaxation helps the woman to learn to loosen taut muscles when she is touched by her partner.

Test-Taking Strategy: Use the process of elimination focusing on the issue, effleurage. It is necessary to know the procedure for this technique to answer the question correctly. If you had difficulty with this question or are unfamiliar with this cutaneous stimulation technique, review these techniques.

Level of Cognitive Ability: Application
Client Needs: Physiological Integrity
Integrated Concept/Process: Self-Care
Content Area: Maternity
Reference: Sherwen, L., Scoloveno, M.A., & Weingarten, C. (1999). *Maternity nursing: Care of the childbearing family* (3rd ed.). Stamford, Conn.: Appleton & Lange, p. 709.

74. 2

Rationale: Fresh fruits and vegetables will provide vitamins and minerals needed for healthy gums. Cracked wheat bread may abrade the tender gums; drinking water with meals has no direct effect on gums; saltine crackers before arising helps decrease nausea.

Test-Taking Strategy: Use the process of elimination and focus on the issue of the question. Eliminate options 1 and 4 first because these measures could produce irritation to any fragile gums. From the remaining options, eliminate option 3 remembering that drinking water with meals has no direct effect on gums. Review measures that promote dental health during pregnancy if you had difficulty with this question.

Level of Cognitive Ability: Analysis
Client Needs: Physiological Integrity
Integrated Concept/Process: Nursing Process/Evaluation
Content Area: Maternity
Reference: Lowdermilk, D., Perry, S., & Bobak, I. (2000). *Maternity & women's health care* (7th ed.). St. Louis: Mosby, p. 417.

75. 2

Rationale: Whenever possible, radiation therapy is usually delayed until a child is 8 years of age to prevent retardation of bone growth and soft tissue development. Options 1, 3, and 4 are inappropriate responses to the mother.

Test-Taking Strategy: Note the age of the child in the question. Additionally, use therapeutic communication techniques and knowledge regarding the effects of radiation to answer this question. Options 1 and 4 are nontherapeutic and place the mother's inquiry on hold. From the remaining options, use the child's age as a guide in directing you to option 2. Review the effects of radiation therapy if you had difficulty with this question.

Level of Cognitive Ability: Application
Client Needs: Physiological Integrity
Integrated Concept/Process: Caring
Content Area: Child Health
Reference: Bowden, V., Dickey, S., & Greenberg, C. (1998). *Children and their families: the continuum of care.* Philadelphia: W.B. Saunders, p. 1494.

76. 1

Rationale: Neuroblastoma is a solid tumor found only in children. It arises from neural crest cells that develop in the sympathetic nervous system and the adrenal medulla. Typically, the tumor compresses adjacent normal tissue and organs. Neuroblastoma cells may excrete catecholamines and their metabolites. Urine samples will indicate elevated VMA levels. The presence of blast cells in the bone marrow occurs in leukemia. Projectile vomiting occurring most often in the morning and a positive Babinski's sign are clinical manifestations of a brain tumor.

Test-Taking Strategy: Use the process of elimination. If you are unfamiliar with this type of tumor, recall that blast cells are noted in leukemia and eliminate option 2. Next, eliminate options 3 and 4, noting that these manifestations are found in the child with a brain tumor. Review the manifestations associated with neuroblastoma if you had difficulty with this question.

Level of Cognitive Ability: Analysis
Client Needs: Physiological Integrity
Integrated Concept/Process: Nursing Process/Assessment
Content Area: Child Health
Reference: Wong, D. (1999). *Whaley & Wong's Nursing care of infants and children* (6th ed.). St. Louis: Mosby, p. 1746.

77. 3

Rationale: Filipinos view pain as part of living an honorable life. The client may appear stoic and be tolerant of a high degree of pain. Health care providers need to offer, and in fact encourage pain relief interventions for the Filipino client who does not complain of pain despite physiological indicators. Option 3 is the most appropriate intervention to include in the plan of care.

Test-Taking Strategy: Note the key words *most appropriately*. Use the process of elimination and knowledge of cultural responses to pain in the Filipino client to answer this question. If you had difficulty with this question, review the characteristics of this culture.

Level of Cognitive Ability: Application
Client Needs: Physiological Integrity
Integrated Concept/Process: Cultural Awareness
Content Area: Fundamental Skills

Reference: Purnell, L. & Paulanka, B. (1998). *Transcultural health care: A culturally competent approach.* Philadelphia: F.A. Davis, p. 256.

78. **4**

Rationale: The nurse needs to stress the importance of immunizations, dental hygiene, and routine well-child care. Options 1, 2, and 3 are appropriate. The parents are also instructed in measures to implement in the event of blunt trauma, especially trauma involving the joints, and to apply prolonged pressure to superficial wounds until the bleeding has stopped.

Test-Taking Strategy: Use the process of elimination. Note the key words *indicates a need for further instructions.* Knowledge that bleeding is a concern in this disorder will assist in eliminating options 1, 2, and 3, which include measures of protection and safety for the child. If you had difficulty with this question, review home care instructions for the child with hemophilia.

Level of Cognitive Ability: Analysis
Client Needs: Health Promotion and Maintenance
Integrated Concept/Process: Nursing Process/Evaluation
Content Area: Child Health
Reference: Wong, D. (1999). *Whaley & Wong's Nursing care of infants and children* (6th ed.). St. Louis: Mosby, p. 1684.

79. **4**

Rationale: Mexican foods are rich in color, flavor, texture, and spiciness. In the Mexican American culture, any occasion is seen as a time to celebrate with food and enjoy the companionship of family and friends. Because food is a primary form of socialization in the Mexican culture, Mexican Americans may have difficulty adhering to a prescribed diet. Asian Americans eat raw fish, rice, and soy sauce. European Americans prefer carbohydrates and red meat.

Test-Taking Strategy: Use the process of elimination and knowledge regarding the food practices and preferences and the meaning of food in the Mexican American culture. If you had difficulty with this question, review the food preferences associated with this culture.

Level of Cognitive Ability: Comprehension
Client Needs: Physiological Integrity
Integrated Concept/Process: Cultural Awareness
Content Area: Fundamental Skills
Reference: Purnell, L., & Paulanka, B. (1998). *Transcultural health care: A culturally competent approach.* Philadelphia: F.A. Davis, p. 407.

80. **2**

Rationale: The nurse must determine the most appropriate assignment based on the skills of the staff member and the needs of the client. In this case, the most appropriate assignment for a nursing assistant would be to care for a client scheduled for a barium enema who requires tap water enemas until clear. The nursing assistant is skilled in administering tap water enemas. The client receiving chemotherapy and the client receiving a blood transfusion requires the assessment skills that a licensed nurse can perform. The client with diabetes mellitus who is being discharged will require predischarge review of diabetic management instructions and potentially coordination of necessary home care services.

Test-Taking Strategy: Note the key words *most appropriate* in the stem of the question. Use the process of elimination and recall

the principles of delegation and supervision of the work of others in answering the question. Work that is delegated to others must be consistent with the individual's level of expertise and licensure or lack of licensure. Review the principles of delegation if you had difficulty with this question.

Level of Cognitive Ability: Application
Client Needs: Safe, Effective Care Environment
Integrated Concept/Process: Nursing Process/Planning
Content Area: Fundamental Skills
Reference: Yoder-Wise, P. (1999). *Leading and managing in nursing* (2nd ed.). St. Louis: Mosby, pp. 310-311.

81. **2**

Rationale: An adverse effect of PTU is agranulocytosis. The client needs to be informed of the early signs of this adverse effect, which includes fever or sore throat. Drowsiness is an occasional side effect of the medication. Increased urination and dry mouth are unrelated to this medication.

Test-Taking Strategy: Use the process of elimination. Recalling that agranulocytosis is an adverse effect of PTU will direct you to option 2. Review the adverse effects of this medication if you had difficulty with this question.

Level of Cognitive Ability: Application
Client Needs: Health Promotion and Maintenance
Integrated Concept/Process: Self-Care
Content Area: Pharmacology
Reference: Wilson, B., Shannon, M., & Stang, C. (2000). *Nurses drug guide 2000.* Stamford, Conn.: Appleton & Lange, p. 1198.

82. **4**

Rationale: Iodine solution can cause iodine toxicity. Iodine is corrosive and overdose will injure the gastrointestinal tract. Symptoms include abdominal pain, vomiting, and diarrhea. Swelling of the glottis may result in asphyxiation. Treatment consists of gastric lavage to remove iodine from the stomach and administration of sodium thiosulfate to reduce iodine to iodide. Calcium gluconate is used for acute hypocalcemia. Mucomyst is the antidote for acetaminophen (Tylenol) overdose. Vitamin K is the antidote for warfarin (Coumadin).

Test-Taking Strategy: Use the process of elimination. Knowledge of the specific antidotes for medication overdose is required to answer this question. You should be able to easily eliminate options 1, 2, and 3 because these medications should be familiar to you. If they are not familiar and you are unsure of these antidotes, review this content.

Level of Cognitive Ability: Analysis
Client Needs: Physiological Integrity
Integrated Concept/Process: Nursing Process/Analysis
Content Area: Pharmacology
Reference: Lehne, R. (1998). *Pharmacology for nursing care* (3rd ed.). Philadelphia: W.B. Saunders, p. 604.

83. **1**

Rationale: In option 1, there is an implication of periorbital and facial edema which could be indicative of pregnancy-induced hypertension (PIH). Since the question identifies an adolescent who has not sought early prenatal care, she is at higher risk for the development of PIH. Options 2, 3, and 4 also deal with body image and although these comments should not be ignored, the need for follow-up is not urgent.

Test-Taking Strategy: Use the process of elimination. Note the week of the first prenatal visit (week 18). Also note the key words *immediate need.* Although all of the options identify a potential alteration in body image, option 1 is the only option that identifies data that could indicate a complication of the pregnancy. Review assessment signs related to PIH if you had difficulty with this question.

Level of Cognitive Ability: Analysis
Client Needs: Physiological Integrity
Integrated Concept/Process: Nursing Process/Analysis
Content Area: Maternity
Reference: Gorrie, T., McKinney, E.S., & Murray, S.S. (1998). *Foundations of maternal-newborn nursing* (2nd ed.) Philadelphia: W.B. Saunders, p. 682.

84. 1

Rationale: Treatment for gonorrhea consists of antibiotic therapy with ceftriaxone 125 mg IM once plus oral doxycycline (Vibramycin) 100 mg bid for 7 days; therefore, option 1 is correct. Option 2 is the treatment for syphilis, option 3 is the treatment for genital herpes simplex virus, and option 4 is the treatment for chlamydia.

Test-Taking Strategy: The issue of the question is the specific subject content: in this case, the specific medication required to treat the disease. Review content regarding gonorrhea and the medication used to treat this sexually transmitted disease if you had difficulty with this question.

Level of Cognitive Ability: Analysis
Client Needs: Physiological Integrity
Integrated Concept/Process: Nursing Process/Analysis
Content Area: Maternity
Reference: Lowdermilk, D., Perry, S., & Bobak, I. (2000). *Maternity & women's health care* (7th ed.). St. Louis: Mosby, p. 150.

85. 2

Rationale: The ACLS nurse would place one gel pad to the right of the sternum just below the clavicle and the other gel pad to the left of the precordium. The nurse would then place the electrode paddles over the pads. Options 1, 3, and 4 identify incorrect positions.

Test-Taking Strategy: Use the process of elimination, considering the anatomical location of the heart. This will easily assist in eliminating options 1, 3, and 4. If you had difficulty with this question, review the correct placement of pads for defibrillation.

Level of Cognitive Ability: Application
Client Needs: Physiological Integrity
Integrated Concept/Process: Nursing Process/Implementation
Content Area: Adult Health/Cardiovascular
Reference: Lewis, S., Heitkemper, M., & Dirksen, S. (2000). *Medical-surgical nursing: Assessment and management of clinical problems* (5th ed.). St. Louis: Mosby, p. 935.

86. 3

Rationale: Rubella vaccine is a live, attenuated virus that evokes an antibody response that provides immunity for 15 years. Because rubella is a live vaccine, it will act as the virus and is potentially teratogenic in the organogenesis phase of fetal development. The client needs to be informed about the potential effects that this vaccine may have and the need to avoid becoming pregnant for a period of 2 to 3 months after receiving the vaccine. Abstinence from sexual intercourse is not necessary, unless another form of effective contraception is not being used. The vaccine may cause local or systemic reactions, but all are mild and short lived. Sunlight has no effect on the person who is vaccinated.

Test-Taking Strategy: Use the process of elimination. Recalling that rubella is a live vaccine will easily direct you to option 3. Review the risks associated with the administration of this vaccine if you had difficulty with this question.

Level of Cognitive Ability: Application
Client Needs: Safe, Effective Care Environment
Integrated Concept/Process: Teaching/Learning
Content Area: Maternity
Reference: Clark, J., Queener, S., & Karb, V. (2000). *Pharmacologic basis of nursing practice* (6th ed.). St. Louis: Mosby, p. 450.

87. 1

Rationale: The client demonstrates the best adaptation by participating in own care. This would include care of surgical drains that would be in place for a short time after discharge. Asking for pain medication is also an action-oriented option, but it does not relate to acceptance of the loss of the breast. Reading the postoperative care booklet is useful, but is not the best of the options presented here. Refusing to look at the wound indicates no adaptation to the loss.

Test-Taking Strategy: Use the process of elimination. Note the key word *best*. This tells you that more than one or all of the options may be partially or totally correct. Use prioritizing ability to determine the best option of those presented, keeping in mind the issue: best adjustment. Review psychosocial adaptation to the loss of a breast if you had difficulty with this question.

Level of Cognitive Ability: Analysis
Client Needs: Psychosocial Integrity
Integrated Concept/Process: Caring
Content Area: Adult Health/Oncology
Reference: Beare, P., & Myers, J. (1998). *Adult health nursing* (3rd ed.). St. Louis: Mosby, p. 1692.

88. 2

Rationale: The client should resume activity slowly, but walking is a beneficial activity. The client should know to rest when fatigue occurs. Activities to be avoided include driving, heavy housework, wearing tight clothing, crossing the legs, and prolonged standing or sitting. Sexual activity is prohibited for 4 to 6 weeks after surgery.

Test-Taking Strategy: Use the process of elimination. Note the key words *not precipitate complications*. With this in mind, evaluate each of the options in terms of the stress or harm it could cause to the perineal area. Review home care measures following vulvectomy if you had difficulty with this question.

Level of Cognitive Ability: Application
Client Needs: Physiological Integrity
Integrated Concept/Process: Teaching/Learning
Content Area: Adult Health/Oncology
Reference: Beare, P., & Myers, J. (1998). *Adult health nursing* (3rd ed.). St. Louis: Mosby, p. 1684.

89. 4

Rationale: The mother should be instructed to bring the child to the emergency department if the child develops stridor at rest, cyanosis, severe agitation or fatigue, moderate to severe retractions, or is unable to take oral fluids.

Test-Taking Strategy: Use the ABCs, airway, breathing, and circulation, to answer the question. If you had difficulty with this question, review home care instructions for the child with croup.

Level of Cognitive Ability: Application

Client Needs: Health Promotion and Maintenance
Integrated Concept/Process: Teaching/Learning
Content Area: Child Health
Reference: Ball, J., & Bindler, R. (1999). *Pediatric nursing: Caring for children* (2nd ed.). Stamford, Conn.: Appleton & Lange, p. 419.

90. 1

Rationale: When epiglottitis is suspected, the priorities are to maintain a patent airway and to obtain a chest x-ray film to confirm the diagnosis. If epiglottitis is present, the child is taken promptly to the operating room for tracheal intubation or immediate surgical airway. Epinephrine is not used in the treatment of epiglottitis.

Test-Taking Strategy: Use the process of elimination. Note the key word *suspected* in the question. This should assist in directing you to option 1. Confirmation of the diagnosis is necessary to determine the appropriate management. If you had difficulty with this question, review the treatment of this life threatening condition.

Level of Cognitive Ability: Application
Client Needs: Physiological Integrity
Integrated Concept/Process: Nursing Process/Implementation
Content Area: Child Health
Reference: Ball, J., & Bindler, R. (1999). *Pediatric nursing: Caring for children* (2nd ed.). Stamford, Conn.: Appleton & Lange, p. 425.

91. 4

Rationale: For a client with sickle cell anemia, dehydration will precipitate sickling of the red blood cells. Sickling can lead to life-threatening consequences for the pregnant woman and for the fetus, such as an interruption of blood flow to the placenta. Options 1, 2, and 3 may also be appropriate nursing diagnoses for a client with sickle cell anemia but are not the priority.

Test-Taking Strategy: Use Maslow's Hierarchy of Needs theory, remembering that physiological needs come first. Using this principle, eliminate options 1 and 2. From the remaining options, select option 4 because it identifies an actual rather than a potential nursing diagnosis. Review sickle cell anemia if you had difficulty with this question.

Level of Cognitive Ability: Analysis
Client Needs: Physiological Integrity
Integrated Concept/Process: Nursing Process/Analysis
Content Area: Maternity
Reference: Olds, S., London. M., & Ladewig, P. (2000). *Maternal-newborn nursing: A family and community-based approach* (6th ed.). Upper Saddle River, N.J.: Prentice-Hall Health, pp. 368-369.

92. 3

Rationale: With viral pneumonia, treatment is supportive. More severely ill children may be hospitalized and given oxygen, chest physiotherapy, and IV fluids. Antibiotics are not given. Bacterial pneumonia however, is treated with antibiotic therapy.

Test-Taking Strategy: Use the process of elimination. Note the key word *viral* in the question. Recalling that antibiotics are not effective in treating viruses will assist in eliminating options 1 and 2. There are no data in the question to support the need for IV fluid administration. Option 3 is also the most global response. Review the care of a child with viral pneumonia if you had difficulty with this question.

Level of Cognitive Ability: Analysis
Client Needs: Physiological Integrity
Integrated Concept/Process: Nursing Process/Analysis
Content Area: Child Health
Reference: Wong, D. (1999). *Whaley & Wong's Nursing care of infants and children* (6th ed.). St. Louis: Mosby, p. 1482.

93. 2

Rationale: CF is a chronic multisystem disorder affecting the exocrine glands. The mucus produced by these glands (particularly those of the bronchioles, small intestine, and the pancreatic and bile ducts) is abnormally thick, causing obstruction of the small passageways of these organs. It is transmitted as an autosomal recessive trait.

Test-Taking Strategy: Use the process of elimination. Recalling that this is a multisystem disorder will direct you to option 2. In addition, option 2 is the most global response. Review this disorder if you are unfamiliar with it.

Level of Cognitive Ability: Application
Client Needs: Physiological Integrity
Integrated Concept/Process: Teaching/Learning
Content Area: Child Health
Reference: Wong, D. (1999). *Whaley & Wong's Nursing care of infants and children* (6th ed.). St. Louis: Mosby, p. 1518.

94. 3

Rationale: A 2% minoxidil solution is used for topical treatment of baldness. The usual dosage is 1 mL applied two times a day.

Test-Taking Strategy: Use the process of elimination. Eliminate options 1 and 4 because of the excessiveness of application. From the remaining options, it is necessary to know the usual dosage for this medication. Review this medication if you had difficulty with this question.

Level of Cognitive Ability: Application
Client Needs: Physiological Integrity
Integrated Concept/Process: Teaching/Learning
Content Area: Pharmacology
Reference: Lehne, R. (1998). *Pharmacology for nursing care* (3rd ed.). Philadelphia: W.B. Saunders, p. 1061.

95. 2

Rationale: Santyl is used to promote debridement of dermal lesions and severe burns. It is applied once daily and covered with a sterile dressing.

Test-Taking Strategy: Use the process of elimination. Note the key words *indicates an accurate understanding* in the stem of the question. Eliminate options 3 and 4 first, because they are similar. Recalling that the client with a burn is at risk for infection will direct you to option 2, the option that indicates covering the wound. Review this medication if you are unfamiliar with it.

Level of Cognitive Ability: Analysis
Client Needs: Health Promotion and Maintenance
Integrated Concept/Process: Nursing Process/Evaluation
Content Area: Pharmacology
Reference: Lehne, R. (1998). *Pharmacology for nursing care* (3rd ed.). Philadelphia: W.B. Saunders, p. 1061.

96. 1

Rationale: Hirschsprung's disease, also known as congenital aganglionosis or megacolon, is the result of an absence of ganglion cells in the rectum and to varying degrees upward in the colon. Options 2, 3, and 4 are incorrect.

Test-Taking Strategy: Use the process of elimination and knowledge regarding the pathophysiology associated with Hirschsprung's disease to answer this question. If you are unfamiliar with this disorder, review the pathophysiology associated with it.
Level of Cognitive Ability: Application
Client Needs: Physiological Integrity
Integrated Concept/Process: Teaching/Learning
Content Area: Child Health
Reference: Ball, J., & Bindler, R. (1999). *Pediatric nursing: Caring for children* (2nd ed.). Stamford, Conn.: Appleton & Lange, p. 613.

97. **2**
Rationale: A fresh colostomy stoma will be red and edematous, but these characteristics will decrease with time. The colostomy site will then be pink without evidence of abnormal drainage, swelling, or skin breakdown. The nurse would document these findings since this is a normal expectation. Options 1, 3, and 4 are inappropriate interventions.
Test-Taking Strategy: Use the process of elimination. Note the key words *returning from surgery.* You would expect redness and edema at this time. Review postoperative colostomy assessment if you had difficulty with this question.
Level of Cognitive Ability: Application
Client Needs: Physiological Integrity
Integrated Concept/Process: Nursing Process/Implementation
Content Area: Child Health
Reference: Ashwill, J., & Droske, S. (1997). *Nursing care of children: Principles and practice.* Philadelphia: W.B. Saunders, p. 748.

98. **1**
Rationale: The skin of a newborn infant plays a significant role in thermoregulation and as a barrier against infection. The skin of a preterm newborn infant is immature in contrast to a term newborn infant. The skin of a preterm newborn is thin and gelatinous. There are decreased amounts of subcutaneous fat, brown fat, and glycogen stores. In addition, preterm newborn infants lose heat because of the high body surface area in relation to their weight and because their posture is more relaxed with less flexion. For these reasons preterm newborn infants are less able to generate heat. This places the preterm newborn at risk for increased heat loss and increased fluid requirements.
Test-Taking Strategy: Use the process of elimination. Focus on the issue, preterm newborn infant. Options 2, 3, and 4 are similar and address an "increased" amount of fat. Review the characteristics of a preterm newborn infant if you had difficulty with this question.
Level of Cognitive Ability: Application
Client Needs: Physiological Integrity
Integrated Concept/Process: Nursing Process/Planning
Content Area: Maternity
Reference: Ladewig, P., London. M., & Olds, S. (1998). *Maternal-newborn nursing care: The nurse, the family, and the community* (4th ed.). Menlo Park, Calif.: Addison Wesley Longman, p. 636.

99. **4**
Rationale: Low or oddly placed ears are associated with a variety of congenital defects and should be reported immedi-

ately. Although the findings would be documented, the most appropriate action would be to notify the physician. Options 1, 2, and 3 are inaccurate and inappropriate nursing actions.
Test-Taking Strategy: Use the process of elimination. Recalling that low set ears is an abnormal finding will easily direct you to option 4. Review normal assessment findings in a newborn if you had difficulty with this question.
Level of Cognitive Ability: Application
Client Needs: Physiological Integrity
Integrated Concept/Process: Nursing Process/Implementation
Content Area: Maternity
Reference: Lowdermilk, D., Perry, S., & Bobak, I. (2000). *Maternity & women's health care* (7th ed.). St. Louis: Mosby, p. 1092.

100. **1**
Rationale: Jaundice, if present, is best assessed in the sclera, nailbeds, and mucous membranes. Generalized jaundice will appear in the skin throughout the body. Option 4 is not an appropriate area to assess for the presence of jaundice.
Test-Taking Strategy: Use the process of elimination. Note the key word *best* in the stem of the question. Option 2 and 3 can be eliminated first because jaundice present in the skin is generalized. From the remaining options, recalling that skin discoloration can best be assessed in the nailbeds will direct you to option 1. Review assessment findings related to jaundice if you had difficulty with this question.
Level of Cognitive Ability: Comprehension
Client Needs: Health Promotion and Maintenance
Integrated Concept/Process: Nursing Process/Assessment
Content Area: Child Health
Reference: Ball, J., & Bindler, R. (1999). *Pediatric nursing: Caring for children* (2nd ed.). Stamford, Conn.: Appleton & Lange, p. 386.

101. **2**
Rationale: Stress causes increased heart workload and the client should be instructed to avoid stress. To avoid infections, individuals with active infections should not be allowed to visit the client. Otherwise restrictions are not required. Too much weight gain can place further demands on the heart. Resting should be on the left side to promote blood return.
Test-Taking Strategy: Use the process of elimination. Note the key words *heart disease* and *the client understands her needs* in the question. Using principles related to the therapeutic management of cardiac disease in general will assist in directing you to option 2. If you had difficulty with this question, review the measures for the pregnant client with cardiac disease.
Level of Cognitive Ability: Analysis
Client Needs: Health Promotion and Maintenance
Integrated Concept/Process: Nursing Process/Evaluation
Content Area: Maternity
Reference: Gorrie, T., McKinney, E., & Murray, S. (1998). *Foundations of maternal newborn nursing* (2nd ed.) Philadelphia: W. B. Saunders, p. 724.

102. **1**
Rationale: Cryotherapy is a procedure that is safe to perform on the pregnant client. Cytotoxic agents are contraindicated during pregnancy because of their toxic effects. Imiquimod

and podophyllin are agents used to treat human papillomavirus however their use in pregnancy is contraindicated.

Test-Taking Strategy: Use the process of elimination. Eliminate options 2, 3, and 4 because they are similar in that they are identify pharmacological measures. Review the treatment modalities for human papillomavirus in the pregnant client if you had difficulty with this question.

Level of Cognitive Ability: Analysis
Client Needs: Physiological Integrity
Integrated Concept/Process: Nursing Process/Planning
Content Area: Maternity
Reference: Lowdermilk, D., Perry, S., & Bobak, I. (2000). *Maternity & women's health care* (7th ed.). St. Louis: Mosby, p. 151.

103. 1

Rationale: To demonstrate respect, compassion, and understanding, health care providers should greet Mexican American clients with a handshake. On establishing rapport, providers may further demonstrate approval and respect through touch, smiling, and affirmative nods of the head. Given the diversity of dialects and the nuances of language, culturally congruent use of humor is difficult to accomplish and therefore should be avoided.

Test-Taking Strategy: Use the process of elimination and knowledge regarding the cultural communication patterns of the Mexican American. Review the characteristics of this cultural group if you had difficulty with this question.

Level of Cognitive Ability: Application
Client Needs: Psychosocial Integrity
Integrated Concept/Process: Cultural Awareness
Content Area: Fundamental Skills
Reference: Purnell, L., & Paulanka, B. (1998). *Transcultural health care: A culturally competent approach.* Philadelphia: F.A. Davis, p. 401.

104. 1

Rationale: Russell's traction uses skin traction to realign a fracture in the lower extremity and immobilize the hip and knee in a flexed position. It is important to keep the hip flexion at the prescribed angle to prevent fracture malalignment. The traction may also relieve pain by reducing muscle spasms, but this is not the primary reason for this traction. The child can still move in bed with some restriction as a result of the traction. Traction is never used to restrain a child.

Test-Taking Strategy: Use the process of elimination and eliminate options 2 and 3 first because they are similar. Recalling the purpose of this type of traction and noting the key word *primarily* will assist in directing you to option 1. If you had difficulty with this question, review Russell's traction.

Level of Cognitive Ability: Application
Client Needs: Physiological Integrity
Integrated Concept/Process: Nursing Process/Implementation
Content Area: Child Health
Reference: Wong, D. (1999). *Whaley & Wong's Nursing care of infants and children* (6th ed.). St. Louis: Mosby, p. 1921.

105. 1

Rationale: The infant should be positioned completely facing the mother with head, neck, and spine aligned. Poor positioning increases the number of attempts for latching on. Option 2 is incorrect because it demonstrates improper positioning. Options 3 and 4 are the result of improper

positioning. Additionally, options 2, 3, and 4 all identify complications (sore nipples, breast engorgement, cracked nipples).

Test-Taking Strategy: Use the process of elimination. Options 2, 3, and 4 are similar and all identify complications (sore nipples, breast engorgement, cracked nipples). Option 1 is the only option that identifies a normal expectation. Review normal expectations of a mother who is breastfeeding if you had difficulty with this question.

Level of Cognitive Ability: Analysis
Client Needs: Health Promotion and Maintenance
Integrated Concept/Process: Nursing Process/Evaluation
Content Area: Maternity
Reference: Sherwen, L., Scoloveno, M.A., & Weingarten, C. (1999). *Maternity nursing: Care of the childbearing family* (3rd ed.). Stamford, Conn.: Appleton & Lange, pp. 1002-1003.

106. 2

Rationale: To achieve proper traction, weights need to be free-hanging with knots kept away from the pulleys. Weights are not to be kept resting on a firm surface. The head of the bed is usually kept low to provide countertraction.

Test-Taking Strategy: Use the process of elimination. Attempt to visualize the traction recalling that there must be weight to exert the pull from the traction setup. This concept will assist in eliminating options 1 and 3. Recalling that countertraction is needed will assist in eliminating option 4. Review care of a client in traction if you had difficulty with this question.

Level of Cognitive Ability: Application
Client Needs: Physiological Integrity
Integrated Concept/Process: Nursing Process/Planning
Content Area: Adult Health/Musculoskeletal
Reference: Smeltzer, S., & Bare, B. (2000). *Brunner & Suddarth's Textbook of medical-surgical nursing* (9th ed). Philadelphia: Lippincott Williams & Wilkins, p. 1789.

107. 4

Rationale: A diet high in fat may be a factor in the development of breast, colon, and prostate cancer. High fiber diets may reduce the risk of colon cancer. Excessive tobacco use may increase the risk of cancer of the lung, larynx, throat, esophagus, and bladder.

Test-Taking Strategy: Use the process of elimination. Eliminate option 3 first because the question does not address tobacco. Although the food items identified in options 1 and 2 are addressed in the question, option 4 is the global response and addresses both options 1 and 2. Review dietary measures and the risks of cancer if you had difficulty with this question.

Level of Cognitive Ability: Application
Client Needs: Health Promotion and Maintenance
Integrated Concept/Process: Teaching/Learning
Content Area: Adult Health/Oncology
Reference: Phipps, W., Sands, J., & Marek, J. (1999). *Medical-surgical nursing: Concepts & clinical practice* (6th ed.). St. Louis: Mosby, pp. 259-260.

108. 1

Rationale: Maintaining effective and open communication among family members affected by death and grief is of utmost importance. The nurse needs to maintain and enhance communication as well as preserve the family's sense of self-direction and control. Option 1 removes autonomy and decision-making from the family at a time when they are already experiencing feelings of loss of control. This is an ineffective intervention that can impair communication. Option 2 is likely to enhance communications. Option 3 is an effective intervention because spiritual practices give meaning to life and have an impact on how people react to crisis. Option 4 is also an effective technique and the family needs to know that someone will be there who is supportive and nonjudgmental.

Test-Taking Strategy: Note the key word "avoid" in the stem of the question. Use the process of elimination, focusing on therapeutic communication techniques to direct you to option 1. Review therapeutic techniques for individuals in crisis if you had difficulty with this question.

Level of Cognitive Ability: Application
Client Needs: Psychosocial Integrity
Integrated Concept/Process: Caring
Content Area: Fundamental Skills
Reference: Kozier, B., Erb, G., Berman, A., & Burke, K. (2000). *Fundamentals of nursing: Concepts, process, and practice* (6th ed.). Upper Saddle River, N.J.: Prentice-Hall, pp. 979-980.

109. 2
Rationale: The cervix undergoes significant changes following conception. The most obvious changes occur in color and consistency. In response to the increasing levels of estrogen, the cervix becomes congested with blood resulting in the characteristic bluish color that extends to include the vagina and labia. This discoloration, referred to as Chadwick's sign, is one of the earliest signs of pregnancy.

Test-Taking Strategy: Use the process of elimination. Knowledge regarding physiological changes and the hormones responsible for these changes is required to answer this question. If you are unfamiliar with the physiological changes, review this content.

Level of Cognitive Ability: Comprehension
Client Needs: Physiological Integrity
Integrated Concept/Process: Nursing Process/Assessment
Content Area: Maternity
Reference: Sherwen, L., Scoloveno, M.A., & Weingarten, C. (1999). *Maternity nursing: Care of the childbearing family* (3rd ed.). Stamford, Conn.: Appleton & Lange, pp. 430-431.

110. 4
Rationale: An inactive elderly person may become disoriented due to lack of sensory stimulation. The most appropriate nursing intervention would be to frequently reorient the client and to place objects such as a clock and a calendar in the client's room to maintain orientation. The family can assist with orientation of the client but it is not appropriate to ask the family to stay with the client. It is not within the scope of nursing practice to prescribe laboratory studies. Restraints may cause further disorientation and should not be applied unless specifically prescribed and agency policies and procedures should be followed before the application of restraints.

Test-Taking Strategy: Use the process of elimination. Note the key words *most appropriate*. Eliminate option 3 first, because it is not within the realm of nursing practice to prescribe laboratory studies. Next, eliminate option 2, because restraints may add to the disorientation the client is experiencing. It is not appropriate to place the responsibility of the client on the family; therefore eliminate option 1. Note the relationship between the words *disoriented* in the question and *reorient* in the correct option. Review the measures related to caring for a client who is disoriented if you had difficulty with this question.

Level of Cognitive Ability: Application
Client Needs: Psychosocial Integrity
Integrated Concept/Process: Nursing Process/Implementation
Content Area: Adult Health/Musculoskeletal
Reference: Leahy, J., & Kizilay, P. (1998). *Foundations of nursing practice: A nursing process approach.* Philadelphia: W.B. Saunders, p. 1045.

111. 3
Rationale: Skin traction is achieved by ace wraps, boots, and slings that apply a direct force on the client's skin. Skin traction is usually removed and reapplied once a day. Traction is maintained with 5 to 8 pounds of weight and this type of traction can cause skin breakdown. There are no pin sites with skin traction. Urinary incontinence is not related to the use of skin traction. Although constipation can occur as a result of immobility and that assessment of bowel sounds may be a component of the assessment, this intervention is not the priority assessment.

Test-Taking Strategy: Use the process of elimination. Note the key word *priority* in the stem of the question. Eliminate option 2 first because there are no pin sites with skin traction. Visualizing the traction setup and knowledge of the complications associated with this type of traction will easily direct you to option 3. Review the complications associated with skin traction and the priority nursing interventions if you had difficulty with this question.

Level of Cognitive Ability: Application
Client Needs: Physiological Integrity
Integrated Concept/Process: Nursing Process/Planning
Content Area: Adult Health/Musculoskeletal
Reference: Smeltzer, S., & Bare, B. (2000). *Brunner & Suddarth's Textbook of medical-surgical nursing* (9th ed.). Philadelphia: Lippincott Williams & Wilkins, p. 1789.

112. 3
Rationale: A contraction stress test assesses placental oxygenation and function, determines fetal ability to tolerate labor, determines fetal well-being, and is performed if the nonstress test is abnormal. The fetus is exposed to the stressor of contractions to assess the adequacy of placental perfusion under simulated labor conditions. An external fetal monitor is applied to the mother and a 20 to 30 minute baseline strip is recorded. The uterus is stimulated to contract either by the administration of a dilute dose of oxytocin (Pitocin) or by having the mother use nipple stimulation until 3 palpable contractions with a duration of 40 seconds or more in a 10 minute period have been achieved. Frequent maternal blood pressure readings are done and the client is monitored closely while increasing doses of oxytocin are given. Options 1, 2, and 4 are inaccurate.

Test-Taking Strategy: Use the process of elimination. Eliminate option 1 because of the words *internal fetal monitoring*. Eliminate option 2 because a treadmill is not used to stimulate contractions. From the remaining options, recalling that the uterus is stimulated to contract by either small amounts of oxytocin (Pitocin) or by nipple stimulation will direct you to option 3. If you had difficulty answering this question, review the contraction stress test.

Level of Cognitive Ability: Application
Client Needs: Physiological Integrity
Integrated Concept/Process: Nursing Process/Implementation
Content Area: Maternity
Reference: Lowdermilk, D., Perry, S., & Bobak, I. (2000). *Maternity & women's health care* (7th ed.). St. Louis: Mosby, p. 811.

113. **4**

Rationale: Strabismus, also called lazy eye, is a condition in which the eyes are not aligned due to lack of coordination of the extraocular muscles. It is normal in the young infant but should not be present after about age 4 months. Options 1, 2, and 3 are not appropriate responses to the mother of a 1-month-old infant.

Test-Taking Strategy: Use the process of elimination and note the key words *1-month-old infant* and *most appropriate*. Also, use therapeutic communication techniques. Options 1, 2, and 3 may cause fear and concern in the mother. If you had difficulty with this question, review this disorder.

Level of Cognitive Ability: Application
Client Needs: Psychosocial Integrity
Integrated Concept/Process: Caring
Content Area: Child Health
Reference: Wong, D. (1999). *Whaley & Wong's Nursing care of infants and children* (6th ed.). St. Louis: Mosby, p. 1098.

114. **3**

Rationale: Patching may be used in the treatment of strabismus to strengthen the weak eye. In this treatment, the "good" eye is patched. This encourages the child to use the weaker eye. It is most successful when done during the preschool years. The schedule for patching is individualized and is prescribed by the ophthalmologist.

Test-Taking Strategy: Use the process of elimination. Remembering that this condition is a "lazy eye" will direct you to the correct option. It makes sense to patch the unaffected eye in order strengthen the muscles in the affected eye. Review the procedure for patching if you had difficulty with this question.

Level of Cognitive Ability: Application
Client Needs: Physiological Integrity
Integrated Concept/Process: Teaching/Learning
Content Area: Child Health
Reference: Ball, J., & Bindler, R. (1999). *Pediatric nursing: Caring for children* (2nd ed.). Stamford, Conn.: Appleton & Lange, p. 718.

115. **2**

Rationale: Contraction stress test results may be interpreted as negative (normal), positive (abnormal), or equivocal. A negative test result indicates that no late decelerations occurred in the fetal heart rate, although the fetus was stressed by three contractions of at least 40 seconds duration in a 10-minute period. Repetitive late decelerations render the test results positive.

Test-Taking Strategy: Use the process of elimination noting that options 1, 3, and 4 are similar in that they indicate an abnormal test result finding. If you had difficulty with this question and are unfamiliar with the interpretation of the results of a contraction stress test, review this content.

Level of Cognitive Ability: Analysis
Client Needs: Physiological Integrity

Integrated Concept/Process: Nursing Process/Analysis
Content Area: Maternity
Reference: Gorrie, T., McKinney, E., & Murray, S. (1998). *Foundations of maternal-newborn nursing* (2nd ed.). Philadelphia: W.B. Saunders, p. 237.

116. **4**

Rationale: A successful outcome for the nursing diagnosis of Self-Care Deficit is for the client to do as much of the self-care as possible. The nurse should promote independence in the client and allow the client to perform as much self-care as is optimal considering the client's condition. The nurse would determine that the outcome is unsuccessful if the client refused care or allows others to do the care.

Test-Taking Strategy: Use the process of elimination. Focusing on the key words *successful outcome* will assist in eliminating the incorrect options. Additionally, note that options 1 and 2 are similar and should be eliminated. Review successful outcomes related to the nursing diagnosis of Self-Care Deficit if you had difficulty with this question.

Level of Cognitive Ability: Analysis
Client Needs: Health Promotion and Maintenance
Integrated Concept/Process: Nursing Process/Evaluation
Content Area: Adult Health/Musculoskeletal
Reference: Smeltzer, S., & Bare, B. (2000). *Brunner & Suddarth's Textbook of medical-surgical nursing* (9th ed.). Philadelphia: Lippincott Williams & Wilkins, pp. 1791-1792.

117. **3**

Rationale: A psychosocial assessment of the client who is immobilized would most appropriately include the need for sensory stimulation. This assessment should also include such factors as body image, past and present coping skills, and the coping methods used during the period of immobilization. Although transportation, home care support, and the ability to perform activities of daily living are components of an assessment, they are not as specifically related to psychosocial adjustment, as is the need for sensory stimulation.

Test-Taking Strategy: Use the process of elimination and focus on the key words *psychosocial* and *most appropriately*. Option 2 can be eliminated first because it relates to physiological integrity rather than psychosocial integrity. Next eliminate options 1 and 4 because they are most closely related to physical supports rather than psychosocial needs of the client. Review the components of a psychosocial assessment if you had difficulty with this question.

Level of Cognitive Ability: Analysis
Client Needs: Psychosocial Integrity
Integrated Concept/Process: Nursing Process/Assessment
Content Area: Adult Health/Musculoskeletal
Reference: Smeltzer, S., & Bare, B. (2000). *Brunner & Suddarth's Textbook of medical-surgical nursing* (9th ed.). Philadelphia: Lippincott Williams & Wilkins, pp. 1791.

118. **3**

Rationale: The mature ovum is transported through the fallopian tube by the muscular action of the tube and the movement of the cilia within the tube. Fertilization normally occurs in the distal third of the fallopian tube near the ovaries. The ovum, fertilized or not, enters the uterus about three days after its release from the ovum. Options 1, 2, and 4 are incorrect.

Test-Taking Strategy: Use the process of elimination. Knowledge regarding the process of fertilization is required to answer this question. Remember that fertilization occurs in the fallopian tube. Review the process of fertilization if you are unfamiliar with it.
Level of Cognitive Ability: Application
Client Needs: Physiological Integrity
Integrated Concept/Process: Teaching/Learning
Content Area: Maternity
Reference: Gorrie, T., McKinney, E., & Murray, S. (1998). *Foundations of maternal-newborn nursing* (2nd ed.). Philadelphia: W.B. Saunders, p. 100.

119. **3**
Rationale: Vitals signs provide a baseline to determine how well the client will tolerate activity. Assessing muscle strength will help determine if the client has enough strength for crutch walking and if muscle-strengthening exercises are necessary. Previous activity level will provide information related to the tolerance of activity. Options 1, 2, and 4 are also a component of the assessment but physiological needs take precedence over psychosocial needs.
Test-Taking Strategy: Note the key word *priority* in the stem of the question. Use Maslow's Hierarchy of Needs theory to prioritize. Remember that physiological needs take precedence over psychosocial needs. This should easily direct you to option 3. Review assessment of the client's readiness to use crutches if you had difficulty with this question.
Level of Cognitive Ability: Analysis
Client Needs: Physiological Integrity
Integrated Concept/Process: Nursing Process/Assessment
Content Area: Adult Health/Musculoskeletal
Reference: Potter, P., & Perry, A. (2001). *Fundamentals of nursing* (5th ed.). St. Louis: Mosby, pp. 1006-1008.

120. **4**
Rationale: To test for Kernig sign, the leg is raised with the knee flexed. Then, the leg is extended at the knee. If any resistance is noted or pain is felt, the result is a positive Kernig sign. This is a common finding in meningitis. Brudzinski's sign occurs when flexion of the head causes flexion of the hips and knees. Chvostek's sign, seen in tetany, is a spasm of the facial muscles elicited by tapping the facial nerve in the region of the parotid gland. Trousseau's sign is a sign for tetany in which carpal spasm can be elicited by compressing the upper arm and causing ischemia to the nerves distally.
Test-Taking Strategy: Knowledge regarding the appropriate procedure to elicit Kernig sign is required to answer the question. Use the process of elimination and assessment techniques to direct you to option 4. If you had difficulty with this question, review these signs, their significance, and the procedure to elicit these signs.
Level of Cognitive Ability: Application
Client Needs: Health Promotion and Maintenance
Integrated Concept/Process: Nursing Process/Assessment
Content Area: Child Health
Reference: Ball, J., & Bindler, R. (1999). *Pediatric nursing: Caring for children* (2nd ed.). Stamford, Conn.: Appleton & Lange, p. 768.

121. **3**
Rationale: The cause of the client's confusion in this situation is due to bedrest and decreased sensory stimulation from prolonged confinement. Therefore, it is best to ambulate the client in the hall. This will increase sensory stimulation and may decrease confusion. Options 1 and 2 will not address the client's need for sensory stimulation. Option 4 is an action that should have been performed in preparation for ambulation while the client was on bedrest.
Test-Taking Strategy: Use the process of elimination. Focus on the issue, "confusion resulting from bed rest and prolonged confinement." Eliminate option 4 first because this action should have been performed in preparation for ambulation while the client was on bed rest. Next eliminate options 1 and 2 because they are similar in that they both address ambulating the client in the hospital room. Review interventions related to promoting sensory stimulation if you had difficulty with this question.
Level of Cognitive Ability: Application
Client Needs: Psychosocial Integrity
Integrated Concept/Process: Nursing Process/Implementation
Content Area: Fundamental Skills
Reference: Maher, A., Salmond, S., & Pellino, T. (1998). *Orthopaedic nursing* (2nd ed.). Philadelphia: W.B. Saunders, p. 109.

122. **2**
Rationale: Vitamin K is associated with the production of prothrombin, which helps the blood properly clot. Vitamin A deficiency is associated with night blindness. Vitamin B_2 (Riboflavin) deficiency is associated with scaly skin. Vitamin D deficiency can cause skeletal pain.
Test-Taking Strategy: Knowledge regarding the clinical manifestations associated with a vitamin K deficiency is required to answer this question. Recalling that vitamin K is the antidote for warfarin (Coumadin), an anticoagulant medication, will assist in directing you to option 2. Review the clinical manifestations associated with vitamin K deficiency if you had difficulty with this question.
Level of Cognitive Ability: Analysis
Client Needs: Physiological Integrity
Integrated Concept/Process: Nursing Process/Assessment
Content Area: Fundamental Skills
Reference: Leahy, J., & Kizilay, P. (1998). *Foundations of nursing practice: A nursing process approach.* Philadelphia: W.B. Saunders, pp. 741.

123. **3**
Rationale: The most common metabolic complication in the SGA newborn infant is hypoglycemia, which can produce central nervous system abnormalities and mental retardation if not corrected immediately. Urinary output, although important, is not the highest priority action because the post-term SGA infant is typically dehydrated due to placental dysfunction. Hemoglobin and hematocrit levels are monitored because the post-term SGA infant exhibits polycythemia, although this also does not require immediate attention. The polycythemia contributes to increased bilirubin levels, usually beginning on the second day after delivery.
Test-Taking Strategy: Use the process of elimination and knowledge regarding the SGA newborn infant. Recalling that the most common metabolic complication in the SGA newborn infant is hypoglycemia will direct you to option 3. Review the SGA newborn content if you had difficulty with this question.

Level of Cognitive Ability: Application
Client Needs: Physiological Integrity
Integrated Concept/Process: Nursing Process/Implementation
Content Area: Maternity
Reference: Lowdermilk, D., Perry, S., & Bobak, I. (2000). *Maternity & women's health care* (7th ed.). St. Louis: Mosby, p. 1127.

124. 1
Rationale: Because of the newborn infant's large size, there is an increased risk for shoulder dystocia. This may result in fractured clavicles and/or brachial plexus palsy. Other complications related to birth trauma include facial paralysis, phrenic nerve palsy, depressed skull fractures, hematomas, and bleeding. Option 2 would not be related to birth trauma even though there is an increase in cardiac defects in the LGA newborn infant, such as transposition of the great vessels. Jaundice would not be present initially. Hip dislocation is congenital disorder and is not caused by birth trauma.
Test-Taking Strategy: Use the process of elimination, focusing on the key words *birth trauma*. Think of trauma is an injury. Option 1 is the only option that identifies an injury. Review the risks associated with delivery of an LGA newborn infant if you had difficulty with this question.
Level of Cognitive Ability: Analysis
Client Needs: Health Promotion and Maintenance
Integrated Concept/Process: Nursing Process/Assessment
Content Area: Maternity
Reference: Ladewig, P., London. M., & Olds, S. (1998). *Maternal-newborn nursing care: The nurse, the family, and the community* (4th ed.). Menlo Park, Calif.: Addison Wesley Longman, p. 624

125. 3
Rationale: Humatrope should not be administered during or after epiphyseal closure. Efficacy of therapy declines as the client grows older and is usually lost entirely by age 20 to 24 years.
Test-Taking Strategy: Use the process of elimination and note the key word *contraindicated*. Note the similarity between options 1, 2, and 4. These options all relate to growth failure. Note the difference in option 3, as it identifies a particular age of a client. Review the contraindications associated with the administration of Humatrope if you had difficulty with this question.
Level of Cognitive Ability: Analysis
Client Needs: Physiological Integrity
Integrated Concept/Process: Nursing Process/Assessment
Content Area: Pharmacology
Reference: Clark, J., Queener, S., & Karb, V. (2000). *Pharmacologic basis of nursing practice* (6th ed.). St. Louis: Mosby, p. 764.

126. 1
Rationale: Hyperglycemia can occur from the administration of growth hormone particularly in a client with diabetes mellitus. Growth hormone therapy is associated with a decline in thyroid function. Hypercalciuria can occur particularly during the first 2 to 3 months of therapy. Glucose and thyroid hormone levels should be monitored.
Test-Taking Strategy: Knowledge regarding the side effects associated with growth hormone replacement therapy is required to answer the question. Review these side effects if you are unfamiliar with them.

Level of Cognitive Ability: Analysis
Client Needs: Physiological Integrity
Integrated Concept/Process: Nursing Process/Assessment
Content Area: Pharmacology
Reference: Hodgson, B., & Kizior, R. (2001). *Saunders nursing drug handbook 2001*. Philadelphia: W.B. Saunders, p. 939.

127. 3
Rationale: An enlarged thyroid gland occurs in the client with goiter because an excessive amount of thyroxine occurs in the thyroid gland causing it to enlarge. Slow wound healing occurs with zinc deficiency. Chronic fatigue occurs with iron deficiency. Heart damage occurs with selenium deficiency. Additionally, heart damage would not likely be noted during the nursing assessment. Further diagnostic tests, in addition to the assessment would be necessary to determine heart damage.
Test-Taking Strategy: Use the process of elimination. Thinking about the anatomical location of a goiter will easily direct you to option 3. Review the manifestations associated with this disorder if you had difficulty with this question.
Level of Cognitive Ability: Analysis
Client Needs: Physiological Integrity
Integrated Concept/Process: Nursing Process/Assessment
Content Area: Adult Health/Endocrine
Reference: Leahy, J., & Kizilay, P. (1998). *Foundations of nursing practice: A nursing process approach*. Philadelphia: W.B. Saunders, pp. 744.

128. 3
Rationale: A maternal glucose level is performed to screen for gestational diabetes. A 50-g oral glucose load may be prescribed and is followed by a serum glucose determination 1 hour later. If the test is given without regard for fasting, 140 mg/dL is the upper limit of normal. If the test is given when the woman is fasting, the upper acceptable limit is 135 mg/dL. Clients exceeding these limits should be further evaluated with a 3-hour GTT. Options 1, 2, and 4 would not be prescribed based solely on the maternal glucose levels. Further follow-up would be implemented.
Test-Taking Strategy: Use the process of elimination. Eliminate options 1, 2, and 4 because they are similar in that they all identify the administration of medication to treat the elevated blood glucose. Option 2 is the only option that identifies further evaluation of the client. Review measures to evaluate and treat elevated blood glucose levels in a pregnant client if you had difficulty with this question.
Level of Cognitive Ability: Analysis
Client Needs: Physiological Integrity
Integrated Concept/Process: Nursing Process/Analysis
Content Area: Maternity
Reference: Sherwen, L., Scoloveno, M.A., & Weingarten, C. (1999). *Maternity nursing: Care of the childbearing family* (3rd ed.). Stamford, Conn.: Appleton & Lange, p. 600.

129. 2
Rationale: Diagnosis of HIV depends on serological studies to detect HIV antibodies. The most commonly used test is performed by enzyme-linked immunosorbent assay (ELISA) test. Options 1 and 4 are incorrect because HIV primarily occurs through the exchange of body fluids. Option 3 is incorrect. A neonate born to an HIV-positive mother is at risk for developing the virus.

Test-Taking Strategy: Use the process of elimination. Eliminate option 3 first because of the absolute word *definitely*. Next eliminate options 1 and 4 because HIV primarily occurs through the exchange of body fluids. Review the significance of an HIV test in a pregnant client if you had difficulty with this question.
Level of Cognitive Ability: Analysis
Client Needs: Physiological Integrity
Integrated Concept/Process: Nursing Process/Analysis
Content Area: Maternity
Reference: Sherwen, L., Scoloveno, M.A., & Weingarten, C. (1999). *Maternity nursing: Care of the childbearing family* (3rd ed.). Stamford, Conn.: Appleton & Lange, p. 98.

130. **1**
Rationale: The Food Guide Pyramid is a guide for healthy clients to get the proper amounts of nutrition. A nutritious diet for a healthy client should consist of 55% to 58% of foods containing carbohydrates. Six to eleven servings of the bread, cereal, pasta, and rice is the correct amount. The correct servings of vegetables is 3 to 5. The correct servings of milk, yogurt, and cheese is 2 to 3. The correct servings of meat, poultry, fish, dry beans, and nuts is 2 to 3. Additionally, 2 to 4 servings from the fruit group is recommended.
Test-Taking Strategy: Knowledge regarding the components of the Food Guide Pyramid is required to answer this question. If you had difficulty with this question and are unfamiliar with the components of the Food Guide Pyramid, review this dietary food guide.
Level of Cognitive Ability: Application
Client Needs: Physiological Integrity
Integrated Concept/Process: Teaching/Learning
Content Area: Fundamental Skills
Reference: Potter, P., & Perry, A. (2001). *Fundamentals of nursing* (5th ed.). St. Louis: Mosby, p. 1336.

131. **1**
Rationale: Early ambulation in the postoperative period is important because if a client does not increase activity, the bones will suffer from loss of calcium. Increasing calcium intake would cause elevated amounts of calcium in the blood that could lead to kidney stones. Iron, not iodine, is recommended for hemoglobin synthesis because oxygen is necessary for wound healing. Clients who are not turned in bed will develop pressure ulcers. A client who is immobile and is 85-years-old needs to be turned every two hours by the nursing staff. The client should not be expected to turn self.
Test-Taking Strategy: Use the process of elimination. Option 4 should be eliminated first because in this statement, the nurse is not accepting responsibility for the client's care. Next eliminate option 3 because iodine is not useful in hemoglobin synthesis. From the remaining options, select option 1 over option 2 because of the importance of the client to get out of bed. Review the complications associated with immobility if you had difficulty with this question.
Level of Cognitive Ability: Application
Client Needs: Physiological Integrity
Integrated Concept/Process: Teaching/Learning
Content Area: Fundamental Skills
Reference: Leahy, J., & Kizilay, P. (1998). *Foundations of nursing practice: A nursing process approach.* Philadelphia: W.B. Saunders, pp. 749-750.

132. **3**
Rationale: Lindane can penetrate the intact skin and can cause convulsions if absorbed in sufficient quantities. Clients at highest risk for convulsions are premature infants, children, and clients with pre-existing seizure disorders. Lindane should not be used on pediatric clients unless safer medications have failed to control infection.
Test-Taking Strategy: Use the process of elimination. Remembering that the medication can cause seizures will direct you to option 3. Review the contraindications associated with the use of this medication if you had difficulty with this question.
Level of Cognitive Ability: Analysis
Client Needs: Physiological Integrity
Integrated Concept/Process: Nursing Process/Analysis
Content Area: Pharmacology
Reference: Gutierrez, K. (1999). *Pharmacotherapeutics; Clinical decision-making in nursing.* Philadelphia: W.B. Saunders, p. 579.

133. **3**
Rationale: Duo-Derm contains hydroactive particles embedded in a polymer base, which are softened by wound moisture and act as a protective gel over healing tissue. It is applied directly to the wound and can be left in place up to 7 days.
Test-Taking Strategy: Use the process of elimination. Recall the purpose of this type of dressing to assist in directing you to option 3. Review the nursing interventions associated with the use of a protective dressing if you had difficulty with this question.
Level of Cognitive Ability: Application
Client Needs: Physiological Integrity
Integrated Concept/Process: Communication and Documentation
Content Area: Pharmacology
Reference: Gutierrez, K. (1999). *Pharmacotherapeutics; Clinical decision-making in nursing.* Philadelphia: W.B. Saunders, p. 1340.

134. **1**
Rationale: Because of the newborn infant's large size, there is an increased risk for shoulder dystocia. This may result in fractured clavicles and/or brachial plexus palsy. Other complications related to birth trauma include facial paralysis, phrenic nerve palsy, depressed skull fractures, hematomas, and bleeding. Option 2 is not related to birth trauma even though there is an increase in cardiac defects in the LGA newborn infant. Jaundice would not be present initially. Hip dislocation is congenital disorder and is not caused by birth trauma.
Test-Taking Strategy: Use the process of elimination focusing on the key words "birth trauma." Think of trauma is an injury. Option 1 is the only option that identifies an injury. Review the risks associated with delivery of an LGA newborn infant if you had difficulty with this question.
Level of Cognitive Ability: Analysis
Client Needs: Physiological Integrity
Integrated Concept/Process: Nursing Process/Assessment
Content Area: Maternity
Reference: Ladewig, P., London. M., & Olds, S. (1998). *Maternal-newborn nursing care: The nurse, the family, and the community* (4th ed.). Menlo Park, Calif.: Addison Wesley Longman, p. 624.

135. 4

Rationale: Rubella virus has an incubation period of 14 to 21 days. The risk of maternal and subsequent fetal infection during the second trimester include hearing loss and congenital anomalies. Rubella titer determination is a standard antenatal test for childbearing women during their initial screening and entry into the health care delivery system. All school-aged children cannot be avoided.

Test-Taking Strategy: Use the process of elimination. Eliminate options 1, 2, and 3 because of the words "immediately," "little risk," and "all," respectively, in these options. Review concepts related to exposure to rubella during pregnancy if you had difficulty with this question.

Level of Cognitive Ability: Analysis
Clients Needs: Psychosocial Integrity
Integrated Concept/Process: Nursing Process/Planning
Content Area: Maternity
Reference: Sherwen, L., Scoloveno, M.A., & Weingarten, C. (1999). *Maternity nursing: Care of the childbearing family* (3rd ed.). Stamford, Conn.: Appleton & Lange, p. 619.

136. 4

Rationale: Appalachian clients traditionally have close family interaction patterns that often lead them to expect close personal relationships with health care providers. The Appalachian client may evaluate the nurse's effectiveness on the basis of interpersonal skills rather than on professional competency. Appalachian clients are likely to be uncomfortable with the impersonal, bureaucratic orientation of health care institutions.

Test-Taking Strategy: Use the process of elimination. Eliminate options 2 and 3 first because they are similar. From this point, knowledge that interpersonal relationships are important will assist in directing you to the correct option. If you had difficulty with the question, review the characteristics of the Appalachian culture.

Level of Cognitive Ability: Analysis
Client Needs: Psychosocial Integrity
Integrated Concept/Process: Cultural Awareness
Content Area: Fundamental Skills
Reference: Giger, J., & Davidhizar, R. (1999). *Transcultural nursing: Assessment & Intervention* (3rd ed.) St. Louis: Mosby, p. 262.

137. 2

Rationale: With active herpetic genital lesions, cesarean delivery can reduce neonatal infection risks. In the absence of active genital lesions, vaginal delivery is indicated unless there are other indications for cesarean delivery. Maternal isolation is not necessary, but potentially exposed newborn infants should be cultured on the day of delivery.

Test-Taking Strategy: Use the process of elimination. Knowledge regarding the transmission of genital herpes to the newborn infant is required to answer this question. If you had difficulty with this question, review this content area.

Level of Cognitive Ability: Analysis
Clients Needs: Safe, Effective Care Environment
Integrated Concept/Process: Nursing Process/Evaluation
Content Area: Maternity

Reference: Olds, S., London. M., & Ladewig, P. (2000). *Maternal-newborn nursing: A family and community-based approach* (6th ed.). Upper Saddle River, N.J.: Prentice-Hall Health, p. 432.

138. 4

Rationale: When delegating nursing assignments, the nurse needs to consider the skills and educational level of the nursing staff. Collecting a 24-hour urine and frequent ambulation can most appropriately be provided by the nursing assistant considering the clients identified in each of the options. The client on the mechanical ventilator requiring frequent assessment and suctioning should most appropriately be cared for by the registered nurse. The licensed practical (vocational nurse) is skilled in wound irrigations and dressing changes and this client would be assigned to this staff member.

Test-Taking Strategy: Use the principles related to delegation and assignments and consider the education and job position as described by the nurse practice act and employee guidelines. Note the key word *assessment* in option 3. This should alert you that this client should be assigned to the registered nurse. Options 1 and 2 can be eliminated because a nursing assistant can easily perform these tasks. This should assist in directing you to option 4. If you had difficulty with this question, review the principles related to delegation and assignment making.

Level of Cognitive Ability: Application
Client Needs: Safe, Effective Care Environment
Integrated Concept/Process: Nursing Process/Planning
Content Area: Fundamental Skills
Reference: Rocchiccioli, J., & Tilbury, M. (1998). *Clinical leadership in nursing.* Philadelphia: W.B. Saunders, p. 140.

139. 4

Rationale: Critical paths are not specifically nursing care plans however they can take the place of a nursing care plan and actually map out the desired clinical progress of a client during acute care admission. Options 1, 2, and 3 appropriately describe the use of a critical path.

Test-Taking Strategy: Use the process of elimination and knowledge regarding the definition and purpose of critical paths to direct you to option 4. Note the key words in the question, *a need for further understanding.* If you had difficulty with this question, review critical paths.

Level of Cognitive Ability: Analysis
Client Needs: Safe, Effective Care Environment
Integrated Concept/Process: Nursing Process/Evaluation
Content Area: Fundamental Skills
Reference: Rocchiccioli, J., & Tilbury, M. (1998). *Clinical leadership in nursing.* Philadelphia: W.B. Saunders, p. 39.

140. 1

Rationale: The vomiting child should be placed in an upright or side-lying position to prevent aspiration. Options 2, 3, and 4 will place the child at risk for aspiration if vomiting occurs.

Test-Taking Strategy: Use the process of elimination. Eliminate options 2 and 4 first because they are similar. Additionally, these positions would place the child at risk for aspiration if vomiting occurred. Visualize the remaining two positions. Option 3 is also inappropriate and would cause aspiration.

Review appropriate positioning techniques if you had difficulty with this question.
Level of Cognitive Ability: Application
Client Needs: Safe, Effective Care Environment
Integrated Concept/Process: Nursing Process/Implementation
Content Area: Child Health
Reference: Wong, D. (1999). *Whaley & Wong's Nursing care of infants and children* (6th ed.). St. Louis: Mosby, p. 1328.

141. 3
Rationale: Cleft lip repair is usually performed during the first few weeks of life. Early repair may improve bonding and makes feeding much easier. Revisions may be required at a later age. Options 1, 2, and 4 are incorrect
Test-Taking Strategy: Use the process of elimination. Option 4 can be easily eliminated first. Eliminate options 1 and 2 next, because they are similar. Review the management of cleft lip repair if you had difficulty with this question.
Level of Cognitive Ability: Application
Client Needs: Psychosocial Integrity
Integrated Concept/Process: Caring
Content Area: Child Health
Reference: Wong, D. (1999). *Whaley & Wong's Nursing care of infants and children* (6th ed.). St. Louis: Mosby, p. 516.

142. 2
Rationale: Postpartum depression is not the normal depression that many new mothers experience from time to time. The woman experiencing depression shows less interest in her surroundings and a loss of her usual emotional response toward the family. The woman is also unable to show pleasure or love, and may have intense feelings of unworthiness, guilt, and shame. The woman often expresses a sense of loss of self. Generalized fatigue, complaints of ill health, and difficulty in concentrating are also present. The mother would have little interest in food and experience sleep disturbances.
Test-Taking Strategy: Focus on the issue of the question to assist in answering. Note the key words *need for further assessment.* Use the process of elimination noting that options 1, 3, and 4 identify positive maternal behaviors. If you had difficulty with this question, review the clinical manifestations of postpartum depression.
Level of Cognitive Ability: Analysis
Client Needs: Psychosocial Integrity
Integrated Concept/Process: Nursing Process/Analysis
Content Area: Maternity
Reference: Gorrie, T., McKinney, E., & Murray, S. (1998). *Foundations of maternal-newborn nursing* (2nd ed.). Philadelphia: W.B. Saunders, p. 805.

143. 1
Rationale: Wearing breast shells and using a breast pump before each feeding will make it easier for the newborn infant to grasp the nipple. True inverted nipples will retract if the areola is pressed between the thumb and forefinger making option 2 incorrect. Option 3 is an appropriate instruction for the mother suffering from engorgement. Option 4 will only make the mother cold, and it has no effect on inverted nipples.
Test-Taking Strategy: Use the process of elimination. Focus on the key words *inverted nipples* to assist in directing you to option 1. Review the concepts related to breastfeeding if you had difficulty with this question.
Level of Cognitive Ability: Application

Client Needs: Health Promotion and Maintenance
Integrated Concept/Process: Self-Care
Content Area: Maternity
Reference: Sherwen, L., Scoloveno, M.A., & Weingarten, C. (1999). *Maternity nursing: Care of the childbearing family* (3rd ed.). Stamford, Conn.: Appleton & Lange, p. 998.

144. 2
Rationale: The nurse would instruct the client to lie down and place a towel or pillow under the shoulder on the side of the breast to be examined. If the left breast it to be examined, the pillow would be placed under the left shoulder.
Test-Taking Strategy: Use the process of elimination. Attempt to visualize this procedure to select the correct option. Remember to examine the left, the pillow is placed under the left; to examine the right, the pillow is placed under the right If you are unfamiliar with the procedure for performing BSE, review this important self-examination.
Level of Cognitive Ability: Application
Client Needs: Health Promotion and Maintenance
Integrated Concept/Process: Self-Care
Content Area: Adult Health/Oncology
Reference: Leahy, J., & Kizilay, P. (1998). *Foundations of nursing practice: A nursing process approach.* Philadelphia: W.B. Saunders, pp. 332-333.

145. 4
Rationale: If the client has had a hysterectomy or is no longer menstruating, the BSE should be performed on the same day every month. Options 1 and 2 are inappropriate because the client who had a hysterectomy would not be menstruating. It is best not to perform the BSE at ovulation time because of the hormonal changes that occur.
Test-Taking Strategy: Use the process of elimination. Note the key word *hysterectomy* in the question to eliminate options 1 and 2. Eliminate option 3 because of the hormonal changes that occur at this time. If you are unfamiliar with the procedure for performing BSE review this important self-examination.
Level of Cognitive Ability: Application
Client Needs: Health Promotion and Maintenance
Integrated Concept/Process: Self-Care
Content Area: Adult Health/Oncology
Reference: Leahy, J., & Kizilay, P. (1998). *Foundations of nursing practice: A nursing process approach.* Philadelphia: W.B. Saunders, pp. 332-333.

146. 1
Rationale: Montgomery's tubercles are sebaceous glands located in the areola. They are inactive and not obvious except during pregnancy and lactation, when they enlarge and secrete a substance that keeps the nipple soft. Within each breast are lobes of glandular tissue that secrete milk. Alveoli are small sacs that contain acinar cells to secrete milk. The alveoli drain into lactiferous ducts, which connect to drain milk from all areas of the breast.
Test-Taking Strategy: Use the process of elimination and knowledge regarding the anatomy and physiology of the breast to answer this question. If you are unfamiliar with the structures of the female breast, review these structures.
Level of Cognitive Ability: Comprehension
Client Needs: Physiological Integrity
Integrated Concept/Process: Nursing Process/Evaluation
Content Area: Maternity

Reference: Gorrie, T., McKinney, E., & Murray, S. (1998). *Foundations of maternal-newborn nursing* (2nd ed.). Philadelphia: W.B. Saunders, p. 68.

147. 4

Rationale: The nurse assesses the client with fibrocystic breast disorder for worsening of symptoms (breast lumps, painful breasts, and possible nipple discharge) before the onset of menses. This is associated with cyclical hormone changes.

Test-Taking Strategy: Use the process of elimination. Note the key words *more noticeable*. This implies that there is a predictable variation in symptoms. Use knowledge of the effects of various hormones in the body to select the correct option. Review the characteristics of fibrocystic breast disease if you had difficulty with this question.

Level of Cognitive Ability: Application
Client Needs: Physiological Integrity
Integrated Concept/Process: Nursing Process/Assessment
Content Area: Adult Health/Oncology
Reference: Beare, P., & Myers, J. (1998). *Adult health nursing* (3rd ed.). St. Louis: Mosby, p. 1685.

148. 2

Rationale: Intussusception occurs when a proximal segment of the bowel prolapses into a distal segment of the bowel. It is a common cause of acute bowel obstruction in infants and young children. It is not an inflammatory process.

Test-Taking Strategy: Use the process of elimination. Recalling that this condition it a telescoping of the bowel will assist in eliminating options 1 and 4. Use the principles of gravity to assist in directing you to the correct option. Review this disorder if you had difficulty with this question.

Level of Cognitive Ability: Application
Client Needs: Physiological Integrity
Integrated Concept/Process: Teaching/Learning
Content Area: Child Health
Reference: Bowden, V., Dickey, S., & Greenberg, C. (1998). *Children and their families: The continuum of care.* Philadelphia: W.B. Saunders, p. 1072.

149. 3

Rationale: Encopresis is defined as fecal incontinence and is a major concern if the child is constipated. Signs include evidence of soiling clothing, scratching or rubbing the anal area due to irritation, fecal odor without apparent awareness by the child, and social withdrawal.

Test-Taking Strategy: Use the process of elimination and knowledge regarding the definition of encopresis to direct you to option 3. Review the assessment findings in this disorder if you had difficulty with this question.

Level of Cognitive Ability: Analysis
Client Needs: Physiological Integrity
Integrated Concept/Process: Nursing Process/Assessment
Content Area: Child Health
Reference: Ball, J., & Bindler, R. (1999). *Pediatric nursing: Caring for children* (2nd ed.). Stamford, Conn.: Appleton & Lange, p. 974.

150. 2

Rationale: The artificial larynx is an electronic device that assists the client after laryngectomy to produce speech. There are two types; one is held at the side of the neck and the other is inserted into the mouth. The vibration produces a mechanical-sounding speech that is monotone in quality but is intelligible.

Test-Taking Strategy: Use the process of elimination. Focus on the key words *artificial larynx*. To answer this question accurately, it is necessary to be generally familiar with these devices. Review the available devices that assist with speech if you had difficulty with this question.

Level of Cognitive Ability: Application
Client Needs: Physiological Integrity
Integrated Concept/Process: Teaching/Learning
Content Area: Adult Health/Oncology
Reference: Ignatavicius, D., Workman, M., & Mishler, M. (1999). *Medical-surgical nursing across the health care continuum* (3rd ed.). Philadelphia: W.B. Saunders, p. 602.

151. 3

Rationale: A Pap smear is usually painless. The test cannot be performed during menstruation. The client needs to be instructed to avoid douching for at least 24 hours before the test. There is no reason to restrict fluids on the day of the test.

Test-Taking Strategy: Use the process of elimination. Eliminate option 2 first as an unlikely preparation measure. Eliminate options 1 and 4 next because both menstruation and douching will affect the results of the test. Review client preparation for a Pap test if you had difficulty with this question.

Level of Cognitive Ability: Application
Client Needs: Physiological Integrity
Integrated Concept/Process: Teaching/Learning
Content Area: Adult Health/Oncology
Reference: LeMone, P., & Burke, K. (2000). *Medical-surgical nursing: Critical thinking in client care* (2nd ed.). Upper Saddle River, N.J.: Prentice-Hall, p. 2030.

152. 1

Rationale: A Good Samaritan Law is passed by a state legislator to encourage nurses and other health care providers to provide care to a person when an accident, emergency, or injury occurs, without fear of being sued for the care provided. Its protection lies in the inability to sue the nurse or other health care provider for negligence in the care provided at the scene of the accident or during the emergency, even if further injury occurred due to the health care providers' care. Called immunity from suit, this protection usually applies only if all of the conditions of the law are met, such as the heath care provider receives no compensation for the care provided, and the care given is not willfully and wantonly negligent.

Test-Taking Strategy: Use the process of elimination. Eliminate options 2 and 4 because they are similar. There are no data in the question regarding the issue of compensation; therefore the best option is option 1. Review the Good Samaritan law if you had difficulty with this question.

Level of Cognitive Ability: Comprehension
Client Needs: Safe, Effective Care Environment
Integrated Concept/Process: Nursing Process/Evaluation
Content Area: Fundamental Skills
Reference: Leahy, J., & Kizilay, P. (1998). *Foundations of nursing practice: A nursing process approach.* Philadelphia: W.B. Saunders. p. 73.

153. 2

Rationale: Lypressin is an antidiuretic hormone used in the treatment of diabetes insipidus. It promotes renal conservation of water by acting on the collecting ducts of the kidney to increase the permeability to water, which results in increased water reabsorption. Options 1, 3, and 4 are not actions of the medication.

Test-Taking Strategy: Note the diagnosis identified in the question. Recalling the pathophysiology associated with the disorder will assist in the process of elimination and in directing you to the correct option. Review the action of lypressin if you had difficulty with this question.

Level of Cognitive Ability: Application
Client Needs: Physiological Integrity
Integrated Concept/Process: Teaching/Learning
Content Area: Pharmacology
Reference: Clark, J., Queener, S., & Karb, V. (2000). *Pharmacologic basis of nursing practice* (6th ed.). St. Louis: Mosby, p. 762.

154. 3
Rationale: Protropin is a growth hormone used in the treatment of dwarfism. When treatment is started, height may be increased by as much as 6 inches. To monitor treatment, height and weight should be measured monthly. Options 1, 2, and 4 are incorrect.

Test-Taking Strategy: Use the process of elimination. Options 1, 2, and 4 are similar in that each identifies lengthy and specific time frames related to the expected outcome of the medication. Review the expected outcome of Protropin if you had difficulty with this question.

Level of Cognitive Ability: Application
Client Needs: Physiological Integrity
Integrated Concept/Process: Teaching/Learning
Content Area: Pharmacology
Reference: Lehne, R. (1998). *Pharmacology for nursing care* (3rd ed.). Philadelphia: W.B. Saunders. p. 611.

155. 3
Rationale: Democratic styles best empower staff toward excellence because this style of leadership allows nurses an opportunity to grow professionally. The autocratic style is task orientated and directive. Situational leadership style utilizes a style depending on the situation and events. Laissez-faire allows staff to work without assistance, direction, or supervision.

Test-Taking Strategy: Note the key words *empower staff toward excellence*. Use the process of elimination and knowledge of the characteristics of the various leadership styles to direct you to option 3. If you had difficulty with this question review the various leadership styles.

Level of Cognitive Ability: Application
Client Needs: Safe, Effective Care Environment
Integrated Concept/Process: Nursing Process/Planning
Content Area: Fundamental Skills
Reference: Rocchiccioli, J., & Tilbury, M. (1998). *Clinical leadership in nursing.* Philadelphia: W.B. Saunders, pp. 103-104.

156. 3
Rationale: Tertiary prevention involves the reduction of the amount and degree of disability, injury, and damage following a crisis. Primary prevention means keeping the crisis from ever occurring, and secondary prevention focuses on reducing the intensity and duration of a crisis during the crisis itself. There is no known aggregate care prevention level.

Test-Taking Strategy: Identify the scenario in the question. Focus on this scenario and use knowledge regarding the various levels of prevention to answer the question. If you had difficulty with this question, review the levels of prevention.

Level of Cognitive Ability: Comprehension
Client Needs: Safe, Effective Care Environment
Integrated Concept/Process: Caring
Content Area: Fundamental Skills
Reference: Craven, R., & Hirnle, C. (2000). *Fundamentals of nursing: Human health and function* (3rd ed.). Philadelphia: Lippincott, p. 665.

157. 1
Rationale: Ovulation ceased during pregnancy because the circulating levels of estrogen and progesterone are high, inhibiting the release of follicle-stimulating hormones and luteinizing hormones which are necessary for ovulation. Options 2, 3, and 4 are incorrect.

Test-Taking Strategy: Use the process of elimination. Knowledge regarding the hormonal changes that occur during the menstrual cycle and during pregnancy is required to answer this question. If you are unfamiliar with these physiological changes, review this content.

Level of Cognitive Ability: Comprehension
Client Needs: Physiological Integrity
Integrated Concept/Process: Nursing Process/Evaluation
Content Area: Maternity
Reference: Gorrie, T., McKinney, E. & Murray, S. (1998). *Foundations of maternal-newborn nursing* (2nd ed.). Philadelphia: W.B. Saunders, pp. 123-124.

158. 2
Rationale: Clients taking antihypocalcemic medications should be instructed to avoid the use of mineral oil as a laxative because it decreases vitamin D absorption and vitamin D is needed to assist in the absorption of calcium. Options 1, 3, and 4 are basic measures to alleviate constipation.

Test-Taking Strategy: Note the key word *not* in the stem of the question. Use the process of elimination and eliminate options 1, 3, and 4 because they are general and basic teaching measures that will assist in alleviating constipation. If you had difficulty with this question, review these basic measures and review the contraindications associated with the administration of calcifediol.

Level of Cognitive Ability: Application
Client Needs: Health Promotion and Maintenance
Integrated Concept/Process: Self-Care
Content Area: Pharmacology
Reference: Kuhn, M. (1998). *Pharmacotherapeutics: A nursing process approach* (4th ed.). Philadelphia: F.A. Davis, p. 684.

159. 1
Rationale: Didronel should be taken on an empty stomach 2 hours before meals. It should not be taken within 2 hours of vitamins, mineral supplements, antacids, or medications high in calcium, magnesium, iron, or albumin.

Test-Taking Strategy: Use the process of elimination. Eliminate options 2, 3, and 4 because they are similar. Note that each of these options suggest administering the medication with another substance. Option 1 is the only option that reflects administering the medication on an empty stomach. Review concepts related to the administration of this medication if you had difficulty with this question.

Level of Cognitive Ability: Application
Client Needs: Health Promotion and Maintenance
Integrated Concept/Process: Self-Care

Content Area: Pharmacology
Reference: Hodgson, B., & Kizior, R. (2001). *Saunders nursing drug handbook 2001*. Philadelphia: W.B. Saunders, p. 393.

160. 2

Rationale: Foul-smelling vaginal discharge is expected and will occur for some time following removal of a cervical radiation implant. Options 1, 3, and 4 are accurate discharge instructions.

Test-Taking Strategy: Use the process of elimination. Note the key words *need for further instructions*. Knowledge regarding the client teaching points related to radiation implants is required to answer the question. Review these points if you had difficulty with this question.

Level of Cognitive Ability: Analysis
Client Needs: Health Promotion and Maintenance
Integrated Concept/Process: Teaching/Learning
Content Area: Adult Health/Oncology
Reference: Monahan, F., & Neighbors, M. (1998). *Medical-surgical nursing: Foundations for clinical practice* (2nd ed.). Philadelphia: W. B. Saunders, p. 1835.

161. 3

Rationale: The client needs to be instructed to avoid exposure to the sun. Options 1, 2, and 4 are accurate measures in the care of a client receiving external radiation therapy.

Test-Taking Strategy: Use the process of elimination. Note the key words *need for further instruction*. Eliminate option 1 because of the word *gently* and option 4 because of the word *loose*. From the remaining options, recalling that sun exposure is to be avoided will assist in answering the question. Review skin care measures for the client receiving external radiation if you had difficulty with this question.

Level of Cognitive Ability: Analysis
Client Needs: Health Promotion and Maintenance
Integrated Concept/Process: Self-Care
Content Area: Adult Health/Oncology
Reference: Monahan, F., & Neighbors, M. (1998). *Medical-surgical nursing: Foundations for clinical practice* (2nd ed.). Philadelphia: W. B. Saunders, p. 1523.

162. 1

Rationale: The primary technique that can used to handle resistance to change during the change process is to introduce the change gradually. Confrontation is an important strategy used to meet resistance when it occurs. Coercion is another strategy that can be used to decrease resistance to change but is not always a successful technique for managing resistance. Manipulation usually involves a covert action such as leaving out pieces of vital information that the participants might negatively receive. It is not the best method of implementing a change.

Test-Taking Strategy: Use the process of elimination and knowledge regarding techniques used to handle resistance during the change process to direct you to option 1. Note the key words *primary technique* in the question. If you had difficulty with this question, review the techniques that can be used to deal with resistance during the change process.

Level of Cognitive Ability: Application
Client Needs: Safe, Effective Care Environment
Integrated Concept/Process: Nursing Process/Planning
Content Area: Fundamental Skills

Reference: Harkreader, H. (2000). *Fundamentals of nursing: Caring and clinical judgment*. Philadelphia: W.B. Saunders, p. 357.

163. 1

Rationale: The effect of Lispro insulin begins within 10 minutes of SC injection, peaks in 1 hour, and its duration of action is 3 hours. Lispro insulin acts more rapidly that Regular insulin and has a shorter duration of action. Because of its rapid onset, it can be administered immediately before eating. In contrast, Regular insulin is generally administered 30 to 60 minutes before meals.

Test-Taking Strategy: Use the process of elimination. Note the key words *rapid-acting*. This will assist in eliminating options 3 and 4. From the remaining options, remember that the question is asking about Lispro, not Regular insulin. This should direct you to option 1. Review the characteristics of Lispro insulin if you had difficulty with this question.

Level of Cognitive Ability: Application
Client Needs: Health Promotion and Maintenance
Integrated Concept/Process: Self-Care
Content Area: Pharmacology
Reference: Lehne, R. (1998). *Pharmacology for nursing care* (3rd ed.). Philadelphia: W.B. Saunders, p. 583.

164. 2

Rationale: Since Regular insulin forms a true solution, it is safe for IV use. It is the only type of insulin that can be administered by the IV route.

Test-Taking Strategy: Remember that Regular insulin is the only type of insulin that can be administered by the IV route. If you had difficulty with this question, review the different types of insulin and their methods of administration.

Level of Cognitive Ability: Application
Client Needs: Physiological Integrity
Integrated Concept/Process: Nursing Process/Planning
Content Area: Pharmacology
Reference: Hodgson, B., & Kizior, R. (2001). *Saunders nursing drug handbook 2001*. Philadelphia: W.B. Saunders, p. 531.

165. 1

Rationale: The client should have the oxygen removed for at least 15 minutes before the ABGs are drawn. This allows enough time for the client's system to equilibrate, and the ABG results will accurately reflect client status without the supplemental oxygen. This order may be given when the physician is trying to decide whether to discontinue oxygen therapy, and allows staff to see how the client tolerates oxygen removal.

Test-Taking Strategy: Use the process of elimination noting the key words *room air*. Also note the similarity between options 2, 3, and 4. All of these options indicate leaving oxygen on the client. Review the procedures for drawing ABGs if you had difficulty with this question.

Level of Cognitive Ability: Application
Client Needs: Physiological Integrity
Integrated Concept/Process: Nursing Process/Implementation
Content Area: Fundamental Skills
Reference: Phipps, W., Sands, J., & Marek, J. (1999). *Medical-surgical nursing: Concepts & clinical practice* (6th ed.). St. Louis: Mosby, p. 852.

166. 2

Rationale: The most common side effect of Glucophage is GI disturbances including decreased appetite, nausea, and diarrhea. These generally subside over time. This medication does not cause weight gain; in fact, clients lose an average of 7 to 8 pounds because the medication causes nausea and decreased appetite. Although hypoglycemia can occur, it is not the most common side effect.

Test-Taking Strategy: Use the process of elimination noting the key words *most common side effect.* Review these side effects if you had difficulty with this question.

Level of Cognitive Ability: Application
Client Needs: Physiological Integrity
Integrated Concept/Process: Teaching/Learning
Content Area: Pharmacology
Reference: Wilson, B., Shannon, M., & Stang, C. (2000). *Nurses drug guide 2000.* Stamford, Conn.: Appleton & Lange, p. 874.

167. 3

Rationale: The HIV compromised client may be at high-risk for superimposed infections during pregnancy. Among these include *Candida* infections, genital herpes, and anogenital condyloma. Early reporting of symptoms may alert the members of the health care team that further assessment and testing is needed to diagnose and manage additional maternal and fetal physiological risks. Options 1, 2, and 4 do represent possible outcomes of this nursing intervention, but are not the priority of care when promoting maternal-fetal well-being.

Test-Taking Strategy: Focus on the issue of the question and use Maslow's Hierarchy of Needs theory. Option 3 is the only option that addresses physiological integrity. Review teaching points related to the pregnant HIV client if you had difficulty with this question.

Level of Cognitive Ability: Application
Client Needs: Health Promotion and Maintenance
Integrated Concept/Process: Teaching/Learning
Content Area: Maternity
Reference: Sherwen, L., Scoloveno, M.A., & Weingarten, C. (1999). *Maternity nursing: Care of the childbearing family* (3rd ed.). Stamford, Conn.: Appleton & Lange, pp. 621-622.

168. 4

Rationale: The effects of maternal iron-deficiency anemia on the developing fetus and neonate are unclear. In general, it is believed that the fetus will receive adequate maternal stores of iron, even if a deficiency is present. Neonates of severely anemic mothers have been reported to experience reduced red cell volume, hemoglobin, and iron stores. Options 1 and 3 provide a false reassurance to the client. Option 2 will cause further concern in the client. Option 4 provides the most realistic support for the client and allows the nurse an opportunity to review the client's plan of care to clarify information and reassure the mother.

Test-Taking Strategy: Use the process of elimination and therapeutic communication techniques to answer the question. Eliminate options 1 and 3 because these options provide a false reassurance to the client. Eliminate option 2 next because this response will cause further concern in the client. If you had difficulty with this question, review therapeutic communication technique and the effects of maternal anemia on the fetus.

Level of Cognitive Ability: Application
Client Needs: Psychosocial Integrity

Integrated Concept/Process: Caring
Content Area: Maternity
Reference: Gorrie, T., McKinney, E., & Murray, S. (1998). *Foundations of maternal newborn nursing* (2nd ed.). Philadelphia: W. B. Saunders, pp. 727-729.

169. 3

Rationale: Sulfonylureas promote insulin secretion by the pancreas and may also increase tissue response to insulin. Biguanides decrease glucose production by the liver. Alpha-glucosidase inhibitors inhibit carbohydrate digestion. Thiazolidinediones decrease insulin resistance.

Test-Taking Strategy: Knowledge regarding the specific action of the sulfonylureas is required to answer this question. Review this classification of medications if you had difficulty with this question.

Level of Cognitive Ability: Application
Client Needs: Physiological Integrity
Integrated Concept/Process: Teaching/Learning
Content Area: Pharmacology
Reference: Lehne, R. (1998). *Pharmacology for nursing care* (3rd ed.). Philadelphia: W.B. Saunders, p. 587.

170. 3

Rationale: When the client with diabetes mellitus becomes ill, control is more difficult. Insulin is not omitted and the client is encouraged to consume liquid carbohydrates if unable to eat regular meals. The client is instructed to notify the physician if vomiting or diarrhea occurs, or if the illness progresses past 2 days.

Test-Taking Strategy: Use the process of elimination. You can easily eliminate options 1, 2, and 4 because it is not within the legal parameters of nursing responsibilities to adjust or alter medication dosages. If you had difficulty with this question, review the client teaching points related to the administration of insulin on "sick days."

Level of Cognitive Ability: Application
Client Needs: Health Promotion and Maintenance
Integrated Concept/Process: Self-Care
Content Area: Pharmacology
Reference: Kuhn, M. (1998). *Pharmacotherapeutics: A nursing process approach* (4th ed.). Philadelphia: F.A. Davis, p. 670.

171. 4

Rationale: The client with Cushing's syndrome should be reassured that most physical changes resolve with treatment. Options 1, 2, and 3 are not therapeutic responses.

Test-Taking Strategy: Use the process of elimination. If you are unfamiliar with this disorder, you can easily eliminate options 1, 2, and 3 because these statements are not therapeutic responses to a client. Review the effects of treatment in a client with Cushing's syndrome if you had difficulty with this question.

Level of Cognitive Ability: Application
Client Needs: Psychosocial Integrity
Integrated Concept/Process: Caring
Content Area: Adult Health/Endocrine
Reference: Lewis, S., Heitkemper, M., & Dirksen, S. (2000). *Medical-surgical nursing: Assessment and management of clinical problems* (5th ed.). St. Louis: Mosby, p. 1439.

172. 4

Rationale: Hypocalcemia can develop after thyroidectomy if the parathyroid glands are accidentally removed during surgery. Manifestations develop 1 to 7 days after surgery. If the client develops numbness and tingling around the mouth, fingertips or toes, muscle spasms, or twitching, the physician is notified immediately. Calcium gluconate should be kept at the bedside.

Test-Taking Strategy: Use the process of elimination. Noting the name of the medication (calcium gluconate) should easily direct you to option 4. Calcium would be given if hypocalcemic tetany occurs. Review care of a client following thyroidectomy if you had difficulty with this question.

Level of Cognitive Ability: Analysis
Client Needs: Physiological Integrity
Integrated Concept/Process: Nursing Process/Analysis
Content Area: Adult Health/Endocrine
Reference: Lewis, S., Heitkemper, M., & Dirksen, S. (2000). *Medical-surgical nursing: Assessment and management of clinical problems* (5th ed.). St. Louis: Mosby, p. 1422.

173. 3
Rationale: HIV transmission can occur during breastfeeding. Therefore, HIV-positive clients should be encouraged to bottle-feed their neonates. Frequent hand washing is encouraged. Support groups and community agencies can be identified to assist the parent's with the newborn infant's home care, the impact of the diagnosis of HIV infection, and available financial resources. Newborn infants of HIV-positive clients are recommended to receive antiviral medications for the first 6 weeks of life.

Test-Taking Strategy: Use the process of elimination. Note the key words *need for further instructions* in the stem of the question. Recalling that breastfeeding is discouraged in the HIV-positive woman will easily direct you to the correct option. Review home care measures for the HIV-client if you had difficulty with this question.

Level of Cognitive Ability: Analysis
Clients Needs: Safe, Effective Care Environment
Integrated Concept/Process: Teaching/Learning
Content Area: Maternity
Reference: Sherwen, L., Scoloveno, M.A., & Weingarten, C. (1999). *Maternity nursing: Care of the childbearing family* (3rd ed.). Stamford, Conn.: Appleton & Lange, pp. 998, 1033.

174. 3
Rationale: A blood glucose test performed before exercising provides the client with information regarding the need to consume a snack before exercising. Exercising during the peak times of insulin or before meal time places the client at risk for hypoglycemia. Insulin should be administered as prescribed.

Test-Taking Strategy: Focus on the issue, the occurrence of a hypoglycemic reaction. Use the process of elimination keeping this issue in mind and the action of insulin to eliminate options 1, 2, and 4. Review client instructions for implementing an exercise program if you had difficulty with this question.

Level of Cognitive Ability: Application
Client Needs: Health Promotion and Maintenance
Integrated Concept/Process: Teaching/Learning
Content Area: Adult Health/Endocrine
Reference: Monahan, F., & Neighbors, M. (1998). *Medical-surgical nursing: Foundations for clinical practice* (2nd ed.). Philadelphia: W.B. Saunders, p. 1234.

175. 3
Rationale: Characteristic behaviors of the fetal alcohol syndrome (FAS) newborn infant are not unlike behaviors common to the drug exposed newborn infant. These behaviors include irritability, tremors, poor feeding, and hypersensitivity to stimuli. Newborn infants with FAS are smaller at birth and present with failure to thrive. Head circumference and weight are most affected.

Test-Taking Strategy: Use the process of elimination. Recalling that the behaviors of the FAS newborn infant are not unlike behaviors common to the drug exposed newborn infant will assist in directing you to option 3. If you had difficulty with this question, review characteristics in the newborn infant with FAS.

Level of Cognitive Ability: Analysis
Client Needs: Physiological Integrity
Integrated Concept/Process: Nursing Process/Assessment
Content Area: Maternity
Reference: Lowdermilk, D., Perry, S., & Bobak, I. (2000). *Maternity & women's health care* (7th ed.). St. Louis: Mosby, p. 1060.

176. 1
Rationale: It is not advisable to bathe a newborn infant after a feeding because handling may cause regurgitation. Since bathing is thought to be relaxing to the infant, before feeding may be the best time. Options 2, 3, and 4 are appropriate interventions in teaching the mother how to bathe a newborn.

Test-Taking Strategy: Use the process of elimination. Note the key word *not* in the stem of the question. Recalling that handling the baby may cause regurgitation will assist in directing you to option 1. Review teaching points regarding bathing of a newborn if you had difficulty with this question.

Level of Cognitive Ability: Application
Client Needs: Health Promotion and Maintenance
Integrated Concept/Process: Teaching/Learning
Content Area: Maternity
Reference: Olds, S., London. M., & Ladewig, P. (2000). *Maternal-newborn nursing: A family and community-based approach* (6th ed.). Upper Saddle River, N.J.: Prentice-Hall Health, pp. 996-997.

177. 1
Rationale: Following amputation, phantom limb pain is a temporary condition that some children may experience. This sensation of burning, aching, or cramping in the missing limb is most distressing to the child. The child needs to be reassured that the condition is normal and only temporary. Options 2, 3 and 4 are not appropriate responses to the child.

Test-Taking Strategy: Use therapeutic communication techniques. Note that the issue of the question relates to alleviating the child's fear. Option 1 is the only option that will alleviate fear. Options 2, 3, and 4 infer that this pain may be permanent.

Level of Cognitive Ability: Application
Client Needs: Psychosocial Integrity
Integrated Concept/Process: Caring
Content Area: Child Health
Reference: Wong, D. (1999). *Whaley & Wong's Nursing care of infants and children* (6th ed.). St. Louis: Mosby, p. 1749.

178. 4
Rationale: Vitamin C (ascorbic acid) increases the absorption of iron by the body. The mother should be instructed to

administer the medication with a citrus fruit or juice high in vitamin C. From the options presented, option 4 is the option that identifies the item highest in vitamin C.

Test-Taking Strategy: Use the process of elimination. Recalling that vitamin C increases the absorption of iron will assist in eliminating options 1 and 2. From the remaining options, select option 4 because this food item contains the highest amount of vitamin C. Review foods high in vitamin C if you had difficulty with this question.

Level of Cognitive Ability: Application
Client Needs: Health Promotion and Maintenance
Integrated Concept/Process: Teaching/Learning
Content Area: Child Health
Reference: Wong, D. (1999). *Whaley & Wong's Nursing care of infants and children* (6th ed.). St. Louis: Mosby, p. 1665.

179. 1

Rationale: If the client becomes ill and cannot retain fluids or food for a period of 4 hours, the physician should be notified. The client's statement in this question indicates a need for immediate education to prevent HHNS, a life threatening emergency situation.

Test-Taking Strategy: Use the process of elimination and focus on the issue. Eliminate option 2 first because the client's statement is inaccurate. Eliminate option 3 next because the client requires immediate education. Eliminate option 4 because HHNS most commonly occurs with type 2 diabetes mellitus and insulin is not the issue of the question. Review diabetic management during times of illness if you had difficulty with this question.

Level of Cognitive Ability: Analysis
Client Needs: Health Promotion and Maintenance
Integrated Concept/Process: Nursing Process/Analysis
Content Area: Adult Health/Endocrine
Reference: Monahan, F., & Neighbors, M. (1998). *Medical-surgical nursing: Foundations for clinical practice* (2nd ed.). Philadelphia: W.B. Saunders, pp. 1240-1241.

180. 2

Rationale: Reinforcement of knowledge and behaviors is vital to the success of the client's self-care. Options 1, 3, and 4 do not address the need for client instructions and are not therapeutic responses.

Test-Taking Strategy: Use the process of elimination and therapeutic communication techniques. Option 1 devalues a client's family, option 3 places the client's issue on "hold," and option 4 requests an explanation from the client. Option 2 validates and clarifies previous information. Review therapeutic communication techniques if you had difficulty with this question.

Level of Cognitive Ability: Application
Client Needs: Psychosocial Integrity
Integrated Concept/Process: Teaching/Learning
Content Area: Adult Health/Endocrine
Reference: Leahy, J., & Kizilay, P. (1998). *Foundations of nursing practice: A nursing process approach.* Philadelphia: W.B. Saunders, pp. 222-225.

181. 1

Rationale: Before conception, the uterus is a small pear-shaped cavity contained entirely in the pelvic cavity. Before pregnancy, the uterus weighs approximately 60 grams (2 oz) and has a capacity of about 10 mL (one third of an ounce). At the end of pregnancy, the uterus weighs approximately 1000 g (2.2 pounds) and has a sufficient capacity for the fetus, placenta, and amniotic fluid, a total of about 5000 mL.

Test-Taking Strategy: Use the process of elimination and knowledge regarding the structure of the uterus to answer this question. Note the key word *nonpregnant* to assist in directing you to the correct option. Attempt to visualize each of the items identified in the options. Review the anatomical structure of the uterus if you had difficulty with this question.

Level of Cognitive Ability: Comprehension
Client Needs: Physiological Integrity
Integrated Concept/Process: Teaching/Learning
Content Area: Maternity
Reference: Gorrie, T., McKinney, E. & Murray, S. (1998). *Foundations of maternal-newborn nursing* (2nd ed.). Philadelphia: W.B. Saunders, p. 122.

182. 1

Rationale: Florinef has mineralocorticoid activity and also has a modest glucocorticoid effect. It acts primarily on the kidneys distal tubules, enhancing the reabsorption of sodium and chloride ions and the excretion of potassium and hydrogen ions. It promotes water retention.

Test-Taking Strategy: Use the process of elimination and knowledge regarding the action of Florinef. If you are unfamiliar with this medication, try to recall the pathophysiology associated with Addison's disease to assist in answering the question. Review this medication action if you are unfamiliar with it.

Level of Cognitive Ability: Analysis
Client Needs: Physiological Integrity
Integrated Concept/Process: Nursing Process/Planning
Content Area: Pharmacology
Reference: Salerno, E. (1999). *Pharmacology for health professionals.* St. Louis: Mosby, p. 561.

183. 1

Rationale: At 12 weeks of gestation, the uterus extends out of the maternal pelvis and can be palpated above the symphysis pubis. At 16 weeks, the fundus reaches midway between the symphysis pubis and the umbilicus. At 20 weeks, the fundus is located at the umbilicus. By 36 weeks, the fundus reaches its highest level at the xiphoid process.

Test-Taking Strategy: Use the process of elimination and knowledge regarding the patterns of uterine growth to answer this question. Focus on the weeks of gestations identified in the question to assist in directing you to the correct option. If you are unfamiliar with the patterns of uterine growth during pregnancy, review this content.

Level of Cognitive Ability: Comprehension
Client Needs: Physiological Integrity
Integrated Concept/Process: Nursing Process/Assessment
Content Area: Maternity
Reference: Gorrie, T., McKinney, E., & Murray, S. (1998). *Foundations of maternal-newborn nursing* (2nd ed.). Philadelphia: W.B. Saunders, p. 122.

184. 1

Rationale: Setting priorities means deciding which client needs or problems require immediate action and which ones could be delayed until a later time because they are not urgent. Client problems that involve actual or life-threatening concerns are always considered first. Although time constraints, obtaining needed supplies, and completing care in a reasonable time frame are components of time management, these items are not the priority in planning care for the client, based on the options provided.

Test-Taking Strategy: Use the process of elimination and principles related to prioritizing to answer the question. Noting the key words *life-threatening* in option 1 will assist in directing you to this option. Review the principles related to prioritizing if you had difficulty with this question.

Level of Cognitive Ability: Comprehension
Client Needs: Safe, Effective Care Environment
Integrated Concept/Process: Nursing Process/Planning
Content Area: Fundamental Skills
Reference: Harkreader, H. (2000). *Fundamentals of nursing: Caring and clinical judgment.* Philadelphia: W.B. Saunders, p. 242.

185. 3
Rationale: Certain factors create a risk for the development of thromboembolitic disorders. These factors include smoking, varicose veins, obesity, a history of thrombophlebitis, women older than 35 years, or who have had more than 3 pregnancies, and women who have had a cesarean birth. From the options presented, a 26-year-old woman with a family history of thrombophlebitis is least likely to develop thromboembolitic disorders in the postpartum period.

Test-Taking Strategy: Use the process of elimination. Note the key words *least likely* in the stem of the question. Knowing that a woman older than 35 years of age is at risk will assist in eliminating options 1 and 2. From the remaining options, select option 3 because the woman described in option 4 actually has a history of thrombophlebitis. If you had difficulty with this question, review the predisposing factors and risks associated with thromboembolitic disorders.

Level of Cognitive Ability: Analysis
Client Needs: Physiological Integrity
Integrated Concept/Process: Nursing Process/Assessment
Content Area: Maternity
Reference: Gorrie, T., McKinney, E., & Murray, S. (1998). *Foundations of maternal-newborn nursing* (2nd ed.). Philadelphia: W.B. Saunders, p. 793.

186. 2
Rationale: Laboratory determinations of serum thyroid stimulating hormone (TSH) are an important means of evaluation. Successful therapy will cause elevated TSH levels to fall. These levels will begin their decline within hours of the onset of therapy and will continue to drop as plasma levels of thyroid hormone build up. If an adequate dosage is administered, TSH levels will remain suppressed for the duration of the therapy.

Test-Taking Strategy: Use the process of elimination. Note the key words *expected outcome*. Relate the diagnosis hypo*thyroid*ism with *thyroid* hormone levels in the correct option. If you had difficulty with this question, review the therapeutic effect of Synthroid.

Level of Cognitive Ability: Application
Client Needs: Physiological Integrity
Integrated Concept/Process: Teaching/Learning
Content Area: Pharmacology
Reference: Lehne, R. (1998). *Pharmacology for nursing care* (3rd ed.). Philadelphia: W.B. Saunders, p. 601.

187. 3
Rationale: Synthroid is used in the treatment of hypothyroidism. Although therapy with Synthroid may begin with small doses that are gradually increased, the most appropriate response is to inform the client that full therapeutic effect may take 1 to 3 weeks.

Test-Taking Strategy: Use the process of elimination. Eliminate options 1 and 2 first because they are similar. Next, eliminate option 4 because the time frame is lengthy. If you had difficulty with this question, review the therapeutic effects of this medication.

Level of Cognitive Ability: Application
Client Needs: Physiological Integrity
Integrated Concept/Process: Teaching/Learning
Content Area: Pharmacology
Reference: Hodgson, B., & Kizior, R. (2001). *Saunders nursing drug handbook 2001.* Philadelphia: W.B. Saunders. p. 590.

188. 4
Rationale: The nurse should instruct the client to apply antiembolism stockings before the client rises in the morning to prevent the venous congestion that will begin as soon as the mother gets up. Circulation can be improved with a regular schedule of activity preferably walking, and the mother should be instructed to avoid prolonged standing or sitting in one position. The mother should also be encouraged to maintain a fluid intake of at least 2500 mL a day to prevent dehydration and consequent sluggish circulation.

Test-Taking Strategy: Use the process of elimination. Note the key words *need for further education*. Knowledge regarding the application of antiembolism stockings will assist in directing you to option 4. If you had difficulty with this question, review measures to prevent thrombosis in the postpartum woman.

Level of Cognitive Ability: Analysis
Client Needs: Health Promotion and Maintenance
Integrated Concept/Process: Nursing Process/Evaluation
Content Area: Maternity
Reference: Gorrie, T., McKinney, E., & Murray, S. (1998). *Foundations of maternal-newborn nursing* (2nd ed.). Philadelphia: W.B. Saunders, p. 794.

189. 3
Rationale: Insulin should not be frozen. If the nurse notes that the vial of insulin is frozen, the insulin is discarded and a new vial is obtained. Options 1, 2, and 4 are incorrect actions.

Test-Taking Strategy: Use the process of elimination. Eliminate options 1 and 4 because they are similar. From the remaining options, option 3 is most directly related to the issue of the question. Review insulin storage principles if you had difficulty with this question.

Level of Cognitive Ability: Application
Client Needs: Physiological Integrity
Integrated Concept/Process: Nursing Process/Implementation
Content Area: Adult Health/Endocrine
Reference: Lehne, R. (1998). *Pharmacology for nursing care* (3rd ed.). Philadelphia: W.B. Saunders, p. 583.

190. 1
Rationale: The initial assessment interview establishes the therapeutic relationship between the nurse and the pregnant woman. It is planned, purposeful communication that focuses on specific content. Options 2, 3, and 4 are incorrect and would not lend themselves to eliciting accurate information from the client.

Test-Taking Strategy: Use the process of elimination focusing on the issue of the question.

Remember establishing a therapeutic relationship is most meaningful. Review therapeutic communication techniques and care of the client with a sexually transmitted disease if you had difficulty with this question.
Level of Cognitive Ability: Application
Client Needs: Psychosocial Integrity
Integrated Concept/Process: Communication and Documentation
Content Area: Maternity
Reference: Sherwen, L., Scoloveno, M.A., & Weingarten, C. (1999). *Maternity nursing: Care of the childbearing family* (3rd ed.). Stamford, Conn.: Appleton & Lange, pp. 83-84.
191. 4
Rationale: Visual disturbances, rapid weight gain, and generalized or facial edema are warning signs in pregnancy. Braxton Hicks contractions are the normal, irregular, painless contractions of the uterus that may occur throughout the pregnancy. Additional warning signs in pregnancy include vaginal bleeding, premature rupture of the membranes, preterm uterine contractions that are normal and regular, change in or absence of fetal activity, severe headache, epigastric pain, persistent vomiting, abdominal pain, and signs of infection.
Test-Taking Strategy: Use the process of elimination noting the key words *need for further education.* Recalling that Braxton Hicks contractions are irregular, painless contractions will assist in directing you to option 4. If you had difficulty with this question, review the warning signs in pregnancy.
Level of Cognitive Ability: Analysis
Client Needs: Health Promotion and Maintenance
Integrated Concept/Process: Nursing Process/Evaluation
Content Area: Maternity
Reference: Sherwen, L., Scoloveno, M.A., & Weingarten, C. (1999). *Maternity nursing: Care of the childbearing family* (3rd ed.). Stamford, Conn.: Appleton & Lange, p. 454.
192. 3
Rationale: Oral calcium supplements need to be administered with food to enhance its absorption as well as decrease gastrointestinal irritation. Options 1, 2, and 4 are unrelated to oral calcium therapy.
Test-Taking Strategy: Use the process of elimination focusing on the medication being addressed in the question. Recalling that oral calcium supplements need to be administered with food will direct you to option 3. Review the administration of oral calcium supplements if you had difficulty with this question.
Level of Cognitive Ability: Application
Client Needs: Health Promotion and Maintenance
Integrated Concept/Process: Teaching/Learning
Content Area: Adult Health/Endocrine
Reference: Hodgson, B., & Kizior, R. (2001). *Saunders nursing drug handbook 2001.* Philadelphia: W.B. Saunders, p. 139.
193. 4
Rationale: Diet therapy for hypophosphatemia consists primarily of an increased intake of phosphorus-rich foods while decreasing the intake of calcium-rich foods. Options 1, 2, and 3 identify food items allowed, while option 4 should be avoided because it is a calcium-rich food.
Test-Taking Strategy: Note the key word *avoid.* Recalling that the client with hypophosphatemia needs to decrease the intake of calcium-rich foods will direct you to option 4. If you

had difficulty with the question, review the dietary measures for the client with hypophosphatemia.
Level of Cognitive Ability: Application
Client Needs: Health Promotion and Maintenance
Integrated Concept/Process: Teaching/Learning
Content Area: Fundamental Skills
Reference: Ignatavicius, D., Workman, M., & Mishler, M. (1999). *Medical-surgical nursing across the health care continuum* (3rd ed.). Philadelphia: W.B. Saunders, p. 261.
194. 1
Rationale: Physical symptoms can interfere with an individual's ability to learn and can also indicate to the teacher that the learner lacks motivation to learn, if the symptoms repeatedly recur when teaching is initiated. Options 2, 3, and 4 identify active client participation in learning.
Test-Taking Strategy: Use the process of elimination and note the key words *not ready to learn.* Options 2, 3, and 4 identify the client as actively seeking information. Option 1 suggest avoidance on the part of the client. Review teaching/learning concepts if you had difficulty with this question.
Level of Cognitive Ability: Analysis
Client Needs: Psychosocial Integrity
Integrated Concept/Process: Teaching/Learning
Content Area: Adult Health/Endocrine
Reference: Potter, P., & Perry, A. (2001). *Fundamentals of nursing* (5th ed.). St. Louis: Mosby, p. 473.
195. 3
Rationale: Hypoglycemic reactions present adrenergic symptoms of tremor, shakiness and nervousness which are similar to the signs of alcohol intoxication. The best strategy to assist the client to meet his needs is to decrease the episodes of hypoglycemia by first identifying and then eliminating those factors that precipitate this event. Options 1 and 2 are inappropriate. Option 4 is not directly related to the issue of the question.
Test-Taking Strategy: Use the process of elimination and therapeutic communication techniques. Option 1 presumes that the problem is unavoidable and thus the client is at fault. Option 2 presumes that the client may be drinking, and option 4 avoids the issue of the question. Review therapeutic communication techniques if you had difficulty with this question.
Level of Cognitive Ability: Analysis
Client Needs: Psychosocial Integrity
Integrated Concept/Process: Nursing Process/Implementation
Content Area: Adult Health/Endocrine
Reference: Smeltzer, S., & Bare, B. (2000). *Brunner & Suddarth's Textbook of medical-surgical nursing* (9th ed.). Philadelphia: Lippincott Williams & Wilkins, p. 1003.
196. 2
Rationale: Clinical symptoms at birth in neonates exposed to cocaine in utero include tremors, tachycardia, marked irritability, muscular rigidity, hypertension, and exaggerated startle reflex. These infants are difficult to console and exhibit an inability to respond to voices or environmental stimuli. They are often poor feeders and have episodes of diarrhea.
Test-Taking Strategy: Use the process of elimination. Think about the effects of the drug to assist in directing you to the correct option. Also note the similarity between options 1, 3,

and 4. If you had difficulty with this question, review the effects of cocaine on the fetus and the neonate.

Level of Cognitive Ability: Analysis
Client Needs: Physiological Integrity
Integrated Concept/Process: Nursing Process/Assessment
Content Area: Maternity
Reference: Gorrie, T., McKinney, E., & Murray, S. (1998). *Foundations of maternal-newborn nursing* (2nd ed.). Philadelphia: W.B. Saunders, p. 651.

197. 4

Rationale: For most hypothyroid clients, replacement therapy must be continued for life. Treatment provides symptomatic relief but does not produce a cure. The client should be told that although therapy will cause symptoms to improve, these improvements do not constitute a reason to interrupt or discontinue the medication. Options 2 and 3 are incorrect. Option 1 places the client's question on hold.

Test-Taking Strategy: Use the process of elimination. Eliminate option 1 first because it places the client's question on hold. Next eliminate options 2 and 3 because they are similar. Review this disorder and the medication therapy associated with it if you had difficulty with this question.

Level of Cognitive Ability: Application
Client Needs: Health Promotion and Maintenance
Integrated Concept/Process: Teaching/Learning
Content Area: Pharmacology
Reference: Cleveland, L., Aschenbrenner, D., Venable, S., & Yensen, J. (1999). *Nursing management in drug therapy.* Philadelphia: Lippincott, pp. 634-635.

198. 4

Rationale: The normal maintenance dose of Synthroid in an adult is 0.1 to 0.2 mg daily. Maintenance dose for infants 0 to 6 months of age is 0.025 to 0.05 mg daily; children 1 to 5 years of age is 0.075 to 0.1 mg daily; and children 6 to 12 months of age is 0.05 to 0.075 mg daily.

Test-Taking Strategy: Knowledge regarding the normal adult dosage of Synthroid is required to answer the question. Learn this dosage range if you had difficulty with this question.

Level of Cognitive Ability: Analysis
Client Needs: Safe, Effective Care Environment
Integrated Concept/Process: Communication and Documentation
Content Area: Pharmacology
Reference: Hodgson, B., & Kizior, R. (2001). *Saunders nursing drug handbook 2001.* Philadelphia: W.B. Saunders, pp. 589-590.

199. 1

Rationale: The normal temperature during pregnancy is 36.2° to 37.6° C (98 to 99.6 degrees F). A temperature above this level may suggest infection that might require medical management. Options 2, 3, and 4 are unnecessary.

Test-Taking Strategy: Use the process of elimination. Recalling that the normal body temperature in the prenatal period is 98° to 99.6° F will direct you to option 1. Review the normal vital signs during pregnancy if you had difficulty with this question.

Level of Cognitive Ability: Application
Client Needs: Physiological Integrity
Integrated Concept/Process: Nursing Process/Implementation
Content Area: Maternity

Reference: Olds, S., London. M., & Ladewig, P. (2000). *Maternal-newborn nursing: A family and community-based approach* (6th ed.). Upper Saddle River, N.J.: Prentice-Hall Health, p. 259.

200. 4

Rationale: Since a 24-hour urine collection is a timed quantitative determination, it is essential that the client start the test with an empty bladder. Therefore the client is instructed to void, discard the first urine, note the time, and start the test. The 24-hour urine specimen collection bottle must be kept on ice or refrigerated. In a VMA collection, the client is instructed to avoid tea, chocolate, vanilla, and all fruits for 2 days before urine collection begins. Also, clients are reminded not to take medications for 2 to 3 days before the test.

Test-Taking Strategy: Use the process of elimination. Note the key words *a need for further instruction.* Use knowledge regarding the basic procedure for collecting a 24-hour urine to answer the question. Review this procedure if you had difficulty with this question.

Level of Cognitive Ability: Analysis
Client Needs: Safe, Effective Care Environment
Integrated Concept/Process: Teaching/Learning
Content Area: Adult Health/Endocrine
Reference: Ignatavicius, D., Workman, M., & Mishler, M. (1999). *Medical-surgical nursing across the health care continuum* (3rd ed.). Philadelphia: W.B. Saunders, p. 1611.

201. 1

Rationale: Paraphrasing is restating the client's messages in the nurse's own words. Option 1 addresses the therapeutic communication technique of paraphrasing. In option 2, the nurse is offering a false reassurance and this type of response will block communication. Option 3 also represents a communication block in that it reflects a lack of the client's right to an opinion. In option 4, the nurse is expressing approval, which can be harmful to a nurse-client relationship.

Test-Taking Strategy: Use the process of elimination and therapeutic communication techniques. Select the option that will enhance communication. Always address the client's concerns and feelings. Review therapeutic communication techniques if you had difficulty with this question.

Level of Cognitive Ability: Application
Client Needs: Psychosocial Integrity
Integrated Concept/Process: Caring
Content Area: Adult Health/Endocrine
Reference: Leahy, J., & Kizilay, P. (1998). *Foundations of nursing practice: A nursing process approach.* Philadelphia: W.B. Saunders. pp. 229-231.

202. 1

Rationale: As the nasogastric tube is passed through the oropharynx, the gag reflex is stimulated, which may cause coughing, gagging, and/or choking. Instead of passing through to the esophagus, the nasogastric tube may coil around itself in the oropharynx, or it may enter the larynx and obstruct the airway. Since the tube may enter the larynx and obstruct the airway, pulling the tube back slightly will remove it from the larynx; advancing the tube might position it in the trachea. Swallowing closes the epiglottis over the trachea and helps move the tube into the esophagus. Slow breathing helps the client relax to reduce the gag response. The nurse should check the back of the client's throat to note If the tube has coiled. The tube may be advanced after the client relaxes.

Test-Taking Strategy: Use the process of elimination. Note the key words *least likely*. Options 2, 3, and 4 all aim at assessing and promoting relaxation whereas option 1 could result in an unsafe malposition of the nasogastric tube into the trachea. Review the procedure for inserting an NG tube if you had difficulty with this question.

Level of Cognitive Ability: Application
Client Needs: Physiological Integrity
Integrated Concept/Process: Nursing Process/Implementation
Content Area: Adult Health/Gastrointestinal
Reference: Potter, P., & Perry, A. (2001). *Fundamentals of nursing* (5th ed.). St. Louis: Mosby, p. 1474.

203. 4

Rationale: The ovarian cycle consists of three phases, the follicular phase, ovulatory phase, and luteal phase. The proliferative phase is a phase of the endometrial cycle.

Test-Taking Strategy: Use the process of elimination. Note the key words *indicates a need to further research*. Also focus on the issue of the question, the ovarian cycle. Review the phases of the ovarian cycle if you had difficulty with this question.

Level of Cognitive Ability: Comprehension
Client Needs: Physiological Integrity
Integrated Concept/Process: Teaching/Learning
Content Area: Maternity
Reference: Gorrie, T., McKinney, E., & Murray, S. (1998). *Foundations of maternal- nursing* (2nd ed.). Philadelphia: W.B. Saunders, p. 67.

204. 1

Rationale: During a menstrual period, a woman loses about 40 mL of blood. Because of the recurrent loss of blood, many women become mildly anemic during their reproductive years, especially if their diets are low in iron.

Test-Taking Strategy: Use the process of elimination. Knowledge regarding the menstrual phase of the menstrual cycle and the amount of blood lost during a menstrual period is required to answer this question. If you are unfamiliar with the menstrual phase, review this content area.

Level of Cognitive Ability: Comprehension
Client Needs: Physiological Integrity
Integrated Concept/Process: Nursing Process/Planning
Content Area: Maternity
Reference: Gorrie, T., McKinney, E., & Murray, S. (1998). *Foundations of maternal-newborn nursing* (2nd ed.). Philadelphia: W.B. Saunders, p. 68.

205. 3

Rationale: An inflammatory reaction such as acute pancreatitis can cause paralytic ileus; the most common form of nonmechanical obstruction. Inability to pass flatus is a clinical manifestation of paralytic ileus. Option 1 is the description of the physical finding of liver enlargement. The liver is usually enlarged in cases of cirrhosis or hepatitis. Although this client may have an enlarged liver, an enlarged liver is not a sign of paralytic ileus or intestinal obstruction. Pain is associated with paralytic ileus, but the pain usually presents as a more constant generalized discomfort. Pain that is severe, constant, and rapid in onset is more likely caused by strangulation of the bowel. Loss of sphincter control is not a sign of paralytic ileus.

Test-Taking Strategy: Use the process of elimination. Noting

the word *paralytic* will assist in directing you to option 3. Review the clinical manifestations of paralytic ileus if you had difficulty with this question.

Level of Cognitive Ability: Analysis
Client Needs: Physiological Integrity
Integrated Concept/Process: Nursing Process/Assessment
Content Area: Adult Health/Gastrointestinal
Reference: Monahan, F., & Neighbors, M. (1998). *Medical-surgical nursing: Foundations for clinical practice* (2nd ed.). Philadelphia: W.B. Saunders, p. 1076.

206. 2

Rationale: For the first 12 hours after a laparotomy, the NG tube drainage may be dark brown to dark red. Later, the drainage should change to a light yellowish brown color. The presence of bile may cause a greenish tinge. The physician should be notified if dark red drainage is noted.

Test-Taking Strategy: Focus on the issue *need to notify the physician*. Use the process of elimination and recall that bleeding is a concern in the postoperative client. This concept will easily direct you to option 2. Review the signs of postoperative complications following a laparotomy if you had difficulty with this question.

Level of Cognitive Ability: Analysis
Client Needs: Physiological Integrity
Integrated Concept/Process: Communication and Documentation
Content Area: Adult Health/Gastrointestinal
Reference: Ignatavicius, D., Workman, M., & Mishler, M. (1999). *Medical-surgical nursing across the health care continuum* (3rd ed.). Philadelphia: W.B. Saunders, p. 367.

207. 3

Rationale: The client should take a deep breath because the client's airway will be temporarily obstructed during tube removal. The client is then told to exhale slowly and the tube is withdrawn during exhalation. Bearing down could inhibit the removal of the tube. Breathing normally could result in aspiration of gastric secretions during inhalation. Holding the breath does not facilitate tube removal.

Test-Taking Strategy: Use the process of elimination. Attempt to visualize the process of tube removal to direct you to option 3. Remember, exhaling slowly will facilitate the process of removal. Review the procedure for removal of an NG tube if you had difficulty with this question.

Level of Cognitive Ability: Application
Client Needs: Physiological Integrity
Integrated Concept/Process: Nursing Process/Implementation
Content Area: Adult Health/Gastrointestinal
Reference: Monahan, F., & Neighbors, M. (1998). *Medical-surgical nursing: Foundations for clinical practice* (2nd ed.). Philadelphia: W. B. Saunders, p. 980.

208. 3

Rationale: After an NG tube is in place, mouth care is extremely important. With one nares occluded, the client tends to mouth breathe, drying the mucous membranes. Small sips of water are contraindicated when the client is on gastric suction. Hard candy would increase the salivation, but would not be useful in cleaning the oral cavity. Lemon-glycerin swabs have a drying and irritating effect on the mucous membranes.

Test-Taking Strategy: Focus on the issue, maintaining the integrity of the oral mucosa. Options 1, 2, and 4 are unrelated to this issue and can be easily eliminated. Review the basic measures related to maintaining the integrity of oral mucosa if you had difficulty with this question.

Level of Cognitive Ability: Application
Client Needs: Health Promotion and Maintenance
Integrated Concept/Process: Nursing Process/Planning
Content Area: Fundamental Skills
Reference: Lewis, S., Heitkemper, M., & Dirksen, S. (2000). *Medical-surgical nursing: Assessment and management of clinical problems* (5th ed.). St. Louis: Mosby, p. 1167.

209. **4**
Rationale: Treatment of intestinal obstruction is directed toward decompression of the intestine by removal of gas and fluid. Nasogastric tubes may be used to decompress the bowel. Continuous gastric suction does not provide nourishment. Option 2 is the purpose for tracheal suctioning. Although gastric contents may be sent for laboratory analysis, it is not the main purpose for continuous gastric suction.
Test-Taking Strategy: Use the process of elimination. Option 2 can be eliminated first, because it is unrelated to a GI disorder. Eliminate option 1 next recalling that a client with a bowel obstruction is NPO. From the remaining options, focusing on the client's diagnosis will direct you to option 4. Review the treatment for a client with a bowel obstruction if you had difficulty with this question.
Level of Cognitive Ability: Analysis
Client Needs: Physiological Integrity
Integrated Concept/Process: Teaching/Learning
Content Area: Adult Health/Gastrointestinal
Reference: Lewis, S., Heitkemper, M., & Dirksen, S. (2000). *Medical-surgical nursing: Assessment and management of clinical problems* (5th ed.). St. Louis: Mosby, p. 1167.

210. **3**
Rationale: When the client is experiencing respiratory acidosis, in an attempt to compensate, the respiratory rate and depth increase. The client also experiences headache, restlessness, mental status changes, such as drowsiness and confusion, visual disturbances, diaphoresis, cyanosis as the hypoxia becomes more acute, hyperkalemia, a rapid, irregular pulse and dysrhythmias.
Test-Taking Strategy: Use the process of elimination and knowledge of the signs and symptoms of respiratory acidosis to answer the question. Remember that restlessness and confusion occurs in respiratory acidosis. If this question was difficult, review the clinical manifestations associated with respiratory acidosis.
Level of Cognitive Ability: Analysis
Client Needs: Physiological Integrity
Integrated Concept/Process: Nursing Process/Assessment
Content Area: Fundamental Skills
Reference: Lewis, S., Heitkemper, M., & Dirksen, S. (2000). *Medical-surgical nursing: Assessment and management of clinical problems* (5th ed.). St. Louis: Mosby, pp. 344.

211. **3**
Rationale: Distention, vomiting, and abdominal pain are a few of the symptoms associated with intestinal obstruction. Nasogastric tubes may be used to remove gas and fluid from the stomach, thus relieving distention and vomiting. Bowel sounds return to normal as the obstruction is resolved and normal bowel function is restored. Discontinuing the nasogas-

tric tube before normal bowel function may result in a return of the symptoms necessitating reinsertion of the nasogastric tube. Serum electrolyte levels, tube placement, and pH of gastric aspirate are important assessments for the client with a nasogastric tube in place, but would not assist in determining the readiness for removing the nasogastric tube.
Test-Taking Strategy: Use the process of elimination. Eliminate options 1 and 4 first because they are similar. Assessing the pH of gastric aspirate is one method of assessing tube placement. From the remaining options, focus on the issue and the client's diagnosis to direct you to option 3. Review abdominal assessment in the client with an intestinal obstruction if you had difficulty with this question.
Level of Cognitive Ability: Analysis
Client Needs: Physiological Integrity
Integrated Concept/Process: Nursing Process/Assessment
Content Area: Adult Health/Gastrointestinal
Reference: Lewis, S., Heitkemper, M., & Dirksen, S. (2000). *Medical-surgical nursing: Assessment and management of clinical problems* (5th ed.). St. Louis: Mosby, p. 1167.

212. **2**
Rationale: The enema fluid should be administered slowly. If the client complains of fullness or pain, the flow is stopped for 30 seconds and restarted at a slower rate. Slow enema administration and stopping the flow temporarily, if necessary, will decrease the likelihood of intestinal spasm and premature ejection of the solution. The higher the solution container is held above the rectum, the faster the flow and the greater the force in the rectum. There is no need to discontinue the enema and notify the physician at this time. Although client reassurance is important, continuing the flow is inappropriate.
Test-Taking Strategy: Use the process of elimination. Eliminate options 1 and 3 first because they are similar. From the remaining options, focusing on the issue will direct you to option 2. Review the procedure for administering an enema if you had difficulty with this question.
Level of Cognitive Ability: Application
Client Needs: Physiological Integrity
Integrated Concept/Process: Nursing Process/Implementation
Content Area: Fundamental Skills
Reference: Kozier, B., Erb, G., & Blais, K. (1998). *Fundamentals of nursing: Concepts, process, and practice* (5th ed.). Reading, Mass.: Addison-Wesley, pp. 1203, 1205.

213. **1**
Rationale: The sigmoid and descending colon are located on the left side. Therefore the left lateral position uses gravity to facilitate the flow of solution into the sigmoid and descending colon. Acute flexion of the right leg allows for adequate exposure of the anus. Options 2, 3, and 4 are incorrect positions.
Test-Taking Strategy: Knowledge of the anatomy of the rectum will assist in eliminating options 2 and 4. Attempt to visualize the remaining positions to eliminate option 3. Review the procedure for administering an enema if you had difficulty with this question.
Level of Cognitive Ability: Application
Client Needs: Physiological Integrity
Integrated Concept/Process: Nursing Process/Implementation
Content Area: Fundamental Skills

Reference: Kozier, B., Erb, G., & Blais, K. (1998). *Fundamentals of nursing: Concepts, process, and practice* (5th ed.). Reading, Mass.: Addison-Wesley, p. 1204.

214. 2

Rationale: After checking residual feeding contents, the gastric contents are reinstilled into the stomach by removing the syringe bulb or plunger, and pouring the gastric contents into the syringe and through the nasogastric tube. Gastric contents should be reinstilled in order to maintain the client's electrolyte balance. The gastric contents should be poured into the nasogastric tube through a syringe without a plunger and not injected by pushing on the plunger. Gastric contents do not need to be mixed with water, nor should it be discarded.

Test-Taking Strategy: Use the process of elimination. Eliminate option 4 because of the words *putting pressure*. Recalling that gastric contents need to be reinstilled to maintain electrolyte balance will assist in eliminating options 1 and 3. Review care of a client with an NG tube and NG tube feedings if you had difficulty with this question.

Level of Cognitive Ability: Application
Client Needs: Physiological Integrity
Integrated Concept/Process: Nursing Process/Implementation
Content Area: Adult Health/Gastrointestinal
Reference: Kozier, B., Erb, G., & Blais, K. (1998). *Fundamentals of nursing: Concepts, process, and practice* (5th ed.). Reading, Mass.: Addison-Wesley, p. 1050.

215. 4

Rationale: Option 4 describes aversion therapy. Options 1, 2, and 3 are characteristics of self control therapy.

Test-Taking Strategy: Use the process of elimination. Note the key word *not* in the stem of the question. Think about the issue *self-control*. This issue should easily direct you to option 4. If you are unfamiliar with self-control therapy, review this content.

Level of Cognitive Ability: Comprehension
Client Needs: Psychosocial Integrity
Integrated Concept/Process: Self-Care
Content Area: Mental Health
Reference: Varcarolis, E. (1998). *Foundations of psychiatric mental health nursing* (3rd ed.). Philadelphia: W.B. Saunders, p. 58.

216. 1

Rationale: Operant conditioning entails rewarding a client for desired behaviors and is the basis for behavior modification. It uses a positive reinforcement approach. Options 2, 3, and 4 are accurate characteristics of this form of therapy.

Test-Taking Strategy: Use the process of elimination. Note the key word *not* in the stem of the question. Note the similarity between options 2, 3, and 4. This should easily direct you to the correct option. If you had difficulty with this question, review the characteristics of operant conditioning.

Level of Cognitive Ability: Comprehension
Client Needs: Psychosocial Integrity
Integrated Concept/Process: Nursing Process/Implementation
Content Area: Mental Health
Reference: Fortinash, K., & Holoday-Worret, P. (2000). *Psychiatric mental health nursing* (2nd ed.). St. Louis: Mosby, p. 188.

217. 2

Rationale: Finding the right medication at the right dose that provides the fewest side effects for the client, providing clients with the injectable, long-acting form of the medication, and including the family in the medication planning process are measures that will promote compliance. Not all medications can be given on a once per day dosing regimen because of their short half-life.

Test-Taking Strategy: Use the process of elimination. Focus on the issue, medication compliance and note the key words *not known to increase*. Avoid selecting options that contain absolute words, such as *all* in option 2. Review the issues related to medication compliance if you had difficulty with this question.

Level of Cognitive Ability: Application
Client Needs: Health Promotion and Maintenance
Integrated Concept/Process: Self-Care
Content Area: Mental Health
Reference: Keltner, N., Schwecke, L., & Bostrom, C. (1999). *Psychiatric nursing* (3rd ed.). St. Louis: Mosby, p. 536.

218. 4

Rationale: In the immediate postoperative period, the gastrostomy tube is elevated, allowing gastric contents to pass to the small intestine and air to escape. This promotes comfort and decreases the risk of leakage at the anastomosis. Options 1, 2, and 3 are incorrect.

Test-Taking Strategy: Option 3 can be easily eliminated because this action could cause accidental removal of the tube. Option 2 can be eliminated next with the concept that suction on a surgical site could disrupt the repair. Recalling that feedings are not initiated in the immediate postoperative period will assist in directing you to the correct option. Review postoperative nursing care if you had difficulty with this question.

Level of Cognitive Ability: Application
Client Needs: Safe, Effective Care Environment
Integrated Concept/Process: Nursing Process/Implementation
Content Area: Child Health
Reference: Wong, D. (1999). *Whaley & Wong's Nursing care of infants and children* (6th ed.). St. Louis: Mosby, p. 525.

219. 1

Rationale: Tricyclic antidepressants can be fatal when taken as an overdose regardless of the amount ingested. Serious, life-threatening symptoms can develop after an overdose. Immediate emergency medical attention and cardiac monitoring is necessary with an overdose of tricyclics.

Test-Taking Strategy: Use the process of elimination. Note the key word *immediate* in the stem of the question. Options 2, 3, and 4 would delay measures in providing immediate treatment. Additionally, vomiting is not induced in a client who is unconscious. Review care of a client with an overdose if you had difficulty with this question.

Level of Cognitive Ability: Application
Client Needs: Physiological Integrity
Integrated Concept/Process: Nursing Process/Implementation
Content Area: Mental Health
Reference: Fortinash, K., & Holoday-Worret, P. (2000). *Psychiatric mental health nursing* (2nd ed.). St. Louis: Mosby, pp. 279-280.

220. 4

Rationale: Following the procedure, the client remains NPO until the gag reflex returns which is usually in 1 to 2 hours. Options 1, 2, and 3 are not specific assessments related to this procedure.

Test-Taking Strategy: Use the process of elimination. Note the key words *upper GI endoscopy*. The only option that relates to the anatomical location of this procedure is option 4. Review postprocedure care following endoscopy if you had difficulty with this question.

Level of Cognitive Ability: Application
Client Needs: Physiological Integrity
Integrated Concept/Process: Nursing Process/Assessment
Content Area: Adult Health/Gastrointestinal
Reference: Monahan, F., & Neighbors, M. (1998). *Medical-surgical nursing: Foundations for clinical practice* (2nd ed.). Philadelphia: W. B. Saunders, p. 973.

221. 3
Rationale: To best facilitate insertion, when the tube reaches the pharynx, the client is encouraged to lower the head slightly, swallow, and if allowed take sips of water. The NG tube would be iced so that it is stiff to ease insertion. If resistance is met, the tube is withdrawn and repassed. Option 3 is the only option that would facilitate insertion.
Test-Taking Strategy: Use the process of elimination. Focus on the issue, facilitating easy insertion of the NG tube. Next, visualize the procedure to direct you to option 3. Review this procedure if you had difficulty with this question.
Level of Cognitive Ability: Application
Client Needs: Physiological Integrity
Integrated Concept/Process: Nursing Process/Implementation
Content Area: Adult Health/Gastrointestinal
Reference: Monahan, F., & Neighbors, M. (1998). *Medical-surgical nursing: Foundations for clinical practice* (2nd ed.). Philadelphia: W. B. Saunders, p. 978.

222. 4
Rationale: Epoetin alfa is administered parenterally by either the IV or the SC route. Administration is by IV bolus for dialysis clients and by IV bolus or SC injection for nondialysis clients. It cannot be given orally because it is a glycoprotein and would be degraded in the gastrointestinal tract.
Test-Taking Strategy: Knowledge regarding the administration of this medication is required to answer this question. Review the routes of administration of this medication if you had difficulty with this question.
Level of Cognitive Ability: Application
Client Needs: Physiological Integrity
Integrated Concept/Process: Nursing Process/Planning
Content Area: Pharmacology
Reference: Gutierrez, K. (1999). *Pharmacotherapeutics; Clinical decision-making in nursing.* Philadelphia: W.B. Saunders, p. 874.

223. 3
Rationale: In the first few hours after surgery, the drainage from the chest tube is bloody. After several hours, it becomes serosanguineous. The client should not experience frequent clotting. Proper chest tube function should allow for drainage of blood before it has the chance to clot in the chest or the tubing.
Test-Taking Strategy: Recall that after thoracic surgery, there may be considerable capillary oozing for some hours in the postoperative period. This would lead you to choose the bloody drainage over serous or serosanguineous. Knowing that patent chest tubes do not allow blood to collect in the pleural space eliminates the option of blood with clots.

Review the assessment measures required in the care of a client with a chest tube if you had difficulty with this question.
Level of Cognitive Ability: Analysis
Client Needs: Physiological Integrity
Integrated Concept/Process: Nursing Process/Assessment
Content Area: Adult Health/Respiratory
Reference: Ignatavicius, D., Workman, M., & Mishler, M. (1999). *Medical-surgical nursing across the health care continuum* (3rd ed.). Philadelphia: W.B. Saunders, p. 649.

224. 1
Rationale: If the client begins to hemorrhage from the surgical site following radical neck dissection, the nurse elevates the head of the bed to maintain airway patency and prevent aspiration. The nurse applies pressure over the bleeding site, and calls the physician immediately.
Test-Taking Strategy: Use the process of elimination, noting the key word *contraindicated*. Options 2 and 3 are indicated if the client is hemorrhaging. Calling the physician is also indicated immediately, while lowering the head of bed does not help with airway maintenance. Review nursing actions if a client begins to hemorrhage if you had difficulty with this question.
Level of Cognitive Ability: Application
Client Needs: Physiological Integrity
Integrated Concept/Process: Nursing Process/Implementation
Content Area: Adult Health/Respiratory
Reference: Smeltzer, S., & Bare, B. (2000). *Brunner & Suddarth's Textbook of medical-surgical nursing* (9th ed.). Philadelphia: Lippincott Williams & Wilkins, p. 819.

225. 2
Rationale: Foscavir is very toxic to the kidneys. Serum creatinine is monitored before therapy, 2 to 3 times per week during induction therapy, and at least weekly during maintenance therapy. It also may cause decreased levels of calcium, magnesium, phosphorus, and potassium. Thus these levels are also measured with the same frequency.
Test-Taking Strategy: Use the process of elimination. Recalling that Foscavir is nephrotoxic will direct you to option 2. Review the adverse effects of this medication if you had difficulty with this question.
Level of Cognitive Ability: Analysis
Client Needs: Physiological Integrity
Integrated Concept/Process: Nursing Process/Assessment
Content Area: Adult Health/Immune
Reference: Hodgson, B., & Kizior, R. (2001). *Saunders nursing drug handbook 2001.* Philadelphia: W.B. Saunders, pp. 447-448.

226. 2
Rationale: TB is spread by droplet nuclei, or the airborne route. The disease is not carried on objects such as clothing, eating utensils, linens, or furniture. Bleaching of clothing and linens is unnecessary, although the client and family members should use good hand washing technique. It is unnecessary to remove carpeting from the home.
Test-Taking Strategy: Knowing that TB is not carried on inanimate objects helps you to eliminate options 3 and 4 first. To discriminate between options 1 and 2, recall that the disease is transmitted by the airborne route. If you had difficulty with this question, review the transmission mode of TB.

Level of Cognitive Ability: Application
Client Needs: Safe, Effective Care Environment
Integrated Concept/Process: Teaching/Learning
Content Area: Adult Health/Respiratory
Reference: Ignatavicius, D., Workman, M., & Mishler, M. (1999). *Medical-surgical nursing across the health care continuum* (3rd ed.). Philadelphia: W.B. Saunders, p. 675.

227. **3**

Rationale: Signs of allergic reaction to the contrast dye include early signs such as localized itching and edema, which are then followed by more severe symptoms such as respiratory distress, stridor, and decreased blood pressure.

Test-Taking Strategy: Focus on the issue, an allergic reaction. Hypothermia is an unrelated event and is eliminated first. Discomfort is expected, and is eliminated next. Hematoma formation is a complication of the procedure, but does not indicate allergic reaction, and is therefore eliminated. The remaining option is stridor, which is a sign of a severe allergic reaction, and possible anaphylaxis. Review the signs of an allergic reaction to the contrast medium if you had difficulty with this question.

Level of Cognitive Ability: Analysis
Client Needs: Physiological Integrity
Integrated Concept/Process: Nursing Process/Assessment
Content Area: Adult Health/Respiratory
Reference: Black, J., & Matassarin-Jacobs, E. (1997). *Medical-surgical nursing: Clinical management for continuity of care* (5th ed.). Philadelphia: W. B. Saunders. pp. 638, 1062.

228. **2**

Rationale: To prevent transmission of hepatitis, a condom is advised during sexual intercourse as well as vaccination of the partner. Alcohol should be avoided for 1 year since it is detoxified in the liver and may interfere with recovery. Rest is especially important until laboratory studies show that the liver function has returned to normal. The client's activity is increased gradually.

Test-Taking Strategy: Use the process of elimination, focusing on the key words *need for further teaching*. Noting the key word *never* in option 2 will direct you to this option. Review client instructions regarding hepatitis if you had difficulty with this question.

Level of Cognitive Ability: Analysis
Client Needs: Physiological Integrity
Integrated Concept/Process: Teaching/Learning
Content Area: Adult Health/Gastrointestinal
Reference: Lewis, S., Heitkemper, M., & Dirksen, S. (2000). *Medical-surgical nursing: Assessment and management of clinical problems* (5th ed.). St. Louis: Mosby, p. 1202.

229. **2**

Rationale: The client should be placed in a room near the nurses' station and not at the end of a long, relatively unprotected corridor. The nurse should not isolate self with a potentially violent client. The door to the client's room should be kept open and the nurse should never turn away from the client. A security officer should be within immediate call should a suspicion of violence is imminent.

Test-Taking Strategy: Use the process of elimination. Note the key word *not* in the stem of the question. Keeping in mind that safety is the issue, you should easily be able to select the correct option. If you had difficulty with this question, review guidelines in caring for the violent client.

Level of Cognitive Ability: Application
Client Needs: Safe, Effective Care Environment
Integrated Concept/Process: Nursing Process/Planning
Content Area: Mental Health
Reference: Keltner, N., Schwecke, L., & Bostrom, C. (1999). *Psychiatric nursing* (3rd ed.). St. Louis: Mosby, p. 132.

230. **1**

Rationale: Isoproterenol is an adrenergic bronchodilator. Side effects can include tachycardia, hypertension, chest pain, dysrhythmias, nervousness, restlessness, and headache, among others. The nurse monitors for these effects during therapy.

Test-Taking Strategy: Use the process of elimination. Recall that this medication is an adrenergic agent. Thus it causes bronchodilation but also increases pulse and blood pressure due to its cardiovascular effects. With this in mind, you can eliminate each of the incorrect options. Remembering that tachycardia is a side effect should assist in selecting the option that identifies an increased pulse, option 1. Review the side effects of this medication if you had difficulty with this question.

Level of Cognitive Ability: Application
Client Needs: Physiological Integrity
Integrated Concept/Process: Nursing Process/Assessment
Content Area: Pharmacology
Reference: Hodgson, B., & Kizior, R. (2001). *Saunders nursing drug handbook 2001.* Philadelphia: W.B. Saunders, p. 554.

231. **2**

Rationale: Plugging a tracheostomy tube is usually done by inserting the tracheostomy plug (decanullation stopper) into the opening of the outer cannula. This closes off the tracheostomy and air flow and respiration occurs normally through the nose and mouth. When plugging a cuffed tracheostomy tube, the cuff must be deflated. If it remains inflated, ventilation cannot occur and respiratory arrest could result. Suctioning may or may not be needed but this is not the required action from the options presented.

Test-Taking Strategy: Note the key word *required* in the question. This should assist in directing you to the option that addresses a priority physiological need. Use the process of elimination to direct you to option 2, because an inflated cuff would cause airway obstruction. Review this procedure if you had difficulty with this question.

Level of Cognitive Ability: Application
Client Needs: Physiological Integrity
Integrated Concept/Process: Nursing Process/Implementation
Content Area: Adult Health/Respiratory
Reference: Lewis, S., Heitkemper, M., & Dirksen, S. (2000). *Medical-surgical nursing: Assessment and management of clinical problems* (5th ed.). St. Louis: Mosby, p. 593.

232. **2**

Rationale: Cinoxacin should be administered with caution in clients with renal impairment. The dosage should be reduced, and failure to do so could result in accumulation of Cinoxacin to toxic levels.

Test-Taking Strategy: Use the process of elimination. Knowledge that this medication is used with caution in clients with renal impairment will direct you to option 2. If you are unfamiliar with this medication, review its cautions and contraindications.

Level of Cognitive Ability: Analysis
Client Needs: Physiological Integrity
Integrated Concept/Process: Nursing Process/Analysis
Content Area: Pharmacology
Reference: Wilson, B., Shannon, M., & Stang, C. (2000). *Nurses drug guide 2000.* Stamford, Conn.: Appleton & Lange, p. 323.

233. 2
Rationale: Administration of urecholine with food can cause nausea and vomiting in the client. To avoid this problem, oral doses should be administered 1 hour before meals or 2 hours after meals.

Test-Taking Strategy: Use the process of elimination. Note that options 1, 3, and 4 are similar in that they all suggest administering the medication with a food item. Review client teaching points related to this medication if you had difficulty with this question.

Level of Cognitive Ability: Application
Client Needs: Health Promotion and Maintenance
Integrated Concept/Process: Teaching/Learning
Content Area: Pharmacology
Reference: Hodgson, B., & Kizior, R. (2001). *Saunders nursing drug handbook 2001.* Philadelphia: W.B. Saunders, p. 112.

234. 3
Rationale: Hypertension, cardiovascular disease, diabetes mellitus, and obesity are associated with the development of glaucoma. Options 1, 2, and 4 do not identify risk factors associated with this eye disorder.

Test-Taking Strategy: Use the process of elimination. Focusing on the issue, a risk factor associated with glaucoma, will direct you to option 3. If you had difficulty with this question, review the risk factors associated with this disorder.

Level of Cognitive Ability: Analysis
Client Needs: Health Promotion and Maintenance
Integrated Concept/Process: Nursing Process/Assessment
Content Area: Adult Health/Eye
Reference: Ignatavicius, D., Workman, M., & Mishler, M. (1999). *Medical-surgical nursing across the health care continuum* (3rd ed.). Philadelphia: W.B. Saunders, p. 1180.

235. 3
Rationale: The nurse places an eye patch over the client's affected eye to reduce eye movement. Some clients may need bilateral patching. Depending on the location and size of the retinal break, activity restrictions may be needed immediately. These restrictions are necessary to prevent further tearing or detachment and to promote drainage of any subretinal fluid. The nurse positions the client as prescribed by the physician.

Test-Taking Strategy: Use the process of elimination. Remember that the eye needs to be protected and rested. This should direct you option 3. If you had difficulty with this question, review care of a client with retinal detachment.

Level of Cognitive Ability: Analysis
Client Needs: Physiological Integrity
Integrated Concept/Process: Nursing Process/Analysis
Content Area: Adult Health/Eye
Reference: Ignatavicius, D., Workman, M., & Mishler, M. (1999). *Medical-surgical nursing across the health care continuum* (3rd ed.). Philadelphia: W.B. Saunders, p. 1186.

236. 2
Rationale: Persons at greatest risk for pulmonary emboli are immobilized clients. Basic preventive measures include early ambulation, leg elevation, active leg exercises, elastic stockings, and intermittent pneumatic calf compression. Keeping the client well hydrated is essential because dehydration predisposes to clotting. A pillow under the knees may cause venous stasis. Heat should not be applied without a physician's prescription.

Test-Taking Strategy: Use the process of elimination and basic principles related to the care of the immobile client to answer this question. If you are unfamiliar with these basic measures, review this content.

Level of Cognitive Ability: Application
Client Needs: Physiological Integrity
Integrated Concept/Process: Nursing Process/Planning
Content Area: Adult Health/Respiratory
Reference: Monahan, F., & Neighbors, M. (1998). *Medical-surgical nursing: Foundations for clinical practice* (2nd ed.). Philadelphia: W.B. Saunders, 682.

237. 4
Rationale: A crisis is an acute time-limited state of disequilibrium resulting from situational, developmental, or societal sources of stress. A person in this state is temporarily unable to cope with or adapt to the stressor by using previous coping mechanisms. One who intervenes in this situation (the nurse) "takes over" for the client who is not in control and devises a plan (action) to secure and maintain the client's safety. Once this has occurred, the nurse works collaboratively with the client (participates) in developing new coping and problem-solving strategies.

Test-Taking Strategy: Use the process of elimination. The client who experiences a "suicidal crisis" is in a state of acute disequilibrium. Remember, in a "crisis," an authority figure must emerge to take action. Review care of a client in crisis if you had difficulty with this question.

Level of Cognitive Ability: Application
Client Needs: Psychosocial Integrity
Integrated Concept/Process: Nursing Process/Implementation
Content Area: Mental Health
Reference: Keltner, N., Schwecke, L., & Bostrom, C. (1999). *Psychiatric nursing* (3rd ed.). St. Louis: Mosby, pp. 109-110.

238. 1
Rationale: The client must have sputum cultures performed every 2 to 4 weeks after initiation of anti-tuberculosis drug therapy. The client may return to work when the results of two sputum cultures are negative, because the client is considered noninfectious at that point.

Test-Taking Strategy: Use the process of elimination. Knowing that a positive Mantoux test never reverts to negative helps you eliminate option 4. From the remaining options, it is necessary to know that two negative sputum cultures are required. If this question was difficult, review these concepts related to TB.

Level of Cognitive Ability: Application
Client Needs: Health Promotion and Maintenance
Integrated Concept/Process: Teaching/Learning
Content Area: Adult Health/Respiratory
Reference: Ignatavicius, D., Workman, M., & Mishler, M. (1999). *Medical-surgical nursing across the health care continuum* (3rd ed.). Philadelphia: W.B. Saunders, p. 677.

239. **4**

Rationale: The client is admitted to a private room that has at least six air exchanges per hour, and which has negative pressure in relation to surrounding areas. The room should be vented to the outside, and should have ultraviolet lights installed.

Test-Taking Strategy: Use the process of elimination. Knowing that the air must vent to the outside helps to eliminate option 1. Knowing that ultraviolet light is useful in killing these organisms helps you to eliminate option 2. From the remaining options, recall that there must be an air flow system that allows for at least 6 air exchanges per hour. Review care of the hospitalized client with TB if you had difficulty with this question.

Level of Cognitive Ability: Application
Client Needs: Safe, Effective Care Environment
Integrated Concept/Process: Nursing Process/Planning
Content Area: Adult Health/Respiratory
Reference: Potter, P., & Perry, A. (2001). *Fundamentals of nursing* (5th ed.). St. Louis: Mosby, pp. 858-859.

240. **1**

Rationale: Mandelamine is contraindicated in clients with renal or hepatic disease or clients with severe dehydration. The nurse would question the physician's prescription for this medication in the client with cirrhosis of the liver.

Test-Taking Strategy: Use the process of elimination. Knowledge that this medication is contraindicated in hepatic disease will easily direct you to option 1. If you are unfamiliar with this medication and its contraindications, review this content.

Level of Cognitive Ability: Analysis
Client Needs: Safe, Effective Care Environment
Integrated Concept/Process: Nursing Process/Analysis
Content Area: Pharmacology
Reference: Salerno, E. (1999). *Pharmacology for health professionals.* St. Louis: Mosby, p. 665.

241. **2**

Rationale: NegGram is used for acute and chronic urinary tract infections, especially gram-negative bacterial infections. The medication is contraindicated in clients with a history of seizures. It is used with caution in clients with liver or renal disorders.

Test-Taking Strategy: Use the process of elimination and knowledge regarding the contraindications associated with this medication to answer the question. Review this medication if you had difficulty with this question.

Level of Cognitive Ability: Analysis
Client Needs: Physiological Integrity
Integrated Concept/Process: Nursing Process/Analysis
Content Area: Pharmacology
Reference: Salerno, E. (1999). *Pharmacology for health professionals.* St. Louis: Mosby, p. 665.

242. **3**

Rationale: This client is in a severe state of anxiety. When a client is in a severe or panic state of anxiety, it is critical for the nurse to remain with the client. Processing the anxiety at this point will further increase the client's level of anxiety. The client in a severe state of anxiety would not be able to learn relaxation techniques.

Test Taking Strategy: Use the process of elimination and note the key words *most appropriate initial.* The best action in this situation is to remain with the client. If you are unfamiliar with the symptoms of the different levels of anxiety and the interventions that are indicated, review this information.

Level of Cognitive Ability: Application
Client Needs: Psychosocial Integrity
Integrated Concept/Process: Nursing Process/Implementation
Content Area: Mental Health
Reference: Keltner, N., Schwecke, L., & Bostrom, C. (1999). *Psychiatric nursing* (3rd ed.). St. Louis: Mosby, p. 427.

243. **3**

Rationale: When an NG tube is attached to suction, it may be continuous or intermittent, with a pressure not exceeding 25 mm Hg. The specific pressure and the intervals are prescribed by the physician. Options 1, 2, and 4 are incorrect.

Test-Taking Strategy: Knowledge regarding the restrictions related to the amount of pressure with suction on a GI tube is required to answer this question. If you are unfamiliar with the care of a client with an NG tube attached to suction, review this content.

Level of Cognitive Ability: Application
Client Needs: Physiological Integrity
Integrated Concept/Process: Nursing Process/Implementation
Content Area: Adult Health/Gastrointestinal
Reference: Monahan, F., & Neighbors, M. (1998). *Medical-surgical nursing: Foundations for clinical practice* (2nd ed.). Philadelphia: W. B. Saunders, p. 978.

244. **2**

Rationale: During the first few days after hemorrhage, gastric pH should be increased to between 5.5 and 7.0 and maintained at this level to control secretory activity. Ranitidine (Zantac) or cimetidine (Tagamet) may be prescribed in addition to antacids to accomplish this. The use of antacids complements the effectiveness of histamine H_2-receptor antagonists for maintaining the pH level of gastric secretions.

Test-Taking Strategy: Use the process of elimination and knowledge regarding the treatment goals following a GI bleed to answer this question. Remembering that gastric secretions are acidic will assist in eliminating option 1. Options 3 and 4 identify an alkaline pH. Therefore option 2 is the best choice. Review care of a client with a GI bleed if you had difficulty with this question.

Level of Cognitive Ability: Analysis
Client Needs: Physiological Integrity
Integrated Concept/Process: Nursing Process/Planning
Content Area: Adult Health/Gastrointestinal
Reference: Ignatavicius, D., Workman, M., & Mishler, M. (1999). *Medical-surgical nursing across the health care continuum* (3rd ed.). Philadelphia: W.B. Saunders, p. 1390.

245. **3**

Rationale: The client needs to be instructed to dispense the oral liquid into a glass container using a specially calibrated pipette. The client should not use any other type of dropper to calibrate the amount of prescribed medication. Options 1, 2, and 4 are correct.

Test-Taking Strategy: Use the process of elimination. Note the key words *indicate the need for further instruction.* Knowledge regarding the administration of the oral concentrate will direct you to option 3. Review the client instructions regarding administering this medication if you had difficulty with this question.

Level of Cognitive Ability: Analysis
Client Needs: Health Promotion and Maintenance
Integrated Concept/Process: Nursing Process/Evaluation
Content Area: Pharmacology
Reference: Lehne, R. (1998). *Pharmacology for nursing care* (3rd ed.). Philadelphia: W.B. Saunders, p. 734.

246. 3
Rationale: Laboratory findings do not establish the diagnosis of appendicitis, but there is often a moderate elevation of the white blood cell count (leukocytosis) to 10,000 to 18,000/mm^3 with a "shift to the left" (an increased number of immature WBCs.).
Test-Taking Strategy: Use the process of elimination. Knowledge that an inflammatory process causes a rise in the WBC count will assist in eliminating options 1 and 4. From the remaining options, it is necessary to understand the significance of a "shift to the left." If you are unfamiliar with the meaning of "shift to the left," review this content.
Level of Cognitive Ability: Analysis
Client Needs: Physiological Integrity
Integrated Concept/Process: Nursing Process/Assessment
Content Area: Adult Health/Gastrointestinal
Reference: Ignatavicius, D., Workman, M., & Mishler, M. (1999). *Medical-surgical nursing across the health care continuum* (3rd ed.). Philadelphia: W.B. Saunders, p. 1434.

247. 2
Rationale: Positions such as sitting up, leaning forward, and flexing the legs (especially the left leg) may alleviate some of the pain associated with pancreatitis. The pain is aggravated by lying supine or walking. This is because the pancreas is located retroperitoneally, and the edema and inflammation intensify the irritation of the posterior peritoneal wall with these positions.
Test-Taking Strategy: Note the key word *avoid*. Use the process of elimination and your critical thinking skills to visualize the pancreas, and the potential effects from stretching associated with the various positions listed. Remember also that options that are similar are not likely to be correct. This will help you to eliminate at least options 1 and 3. Review pain reduction measures for the client with pancreatitis if you had difficulty with this question.
Level of Cognitive Ability: Application
Client Needs: Physiological Integrity
Integrated Concept/Process: Teaching/Learning
Content Area: Adult Health/Gastrointestinal
Reference: Phipps, W., Sands, J., & Marek, J. (1999). *Medical-surgical nursing: Concepts & clinical practice* (6th ed.). St. Louis: Mosby, pp. 1384-1385.

248. 2
Rationale: Common signs of acute viral hepatitis include weight loss, dark urine, and fatigue. The client is anorexic, possibly from a toxin produced by the diseased liver, and finds food distasteful. The urine darkens because of excess bilirubin being excreted by the kidneys. Fatigue occurs during all phases of hepatitis. Spider angiomas (small, dilated blood vessels) are commonly seen in cirrhosis of the liver.
Test-Taking Strategy: Use the process of elimination. Recalling the function of the liver will direct you to the correct option. If you had difficulty with this question, review content associated with hepatitis.

Level of Cognitive Ability: Analysis
Client Needs: Physiological Integrity
Integrated Concept/Process: Nursing Process/Assessment
Content Area: Adult Health/Gastrointestinal
Reference: Ignatavicius, D., Workman, M., & Mishler, M. (1999). *Medical-surgical nursing across the health care continuum* (3rd ed.). Philadelphia: W.B. Saunders, p. 1480-1481.

249. 2
Rationale: The client who has severe anxiety has significant somatic complaints, ineffective functioning, loud or rapid speech, and purposeless activity. The client symptoms in the question do not relate to options 1, 3, and 4.
Test-Taking Strategy: Use the process of elimination. Note the client's symptoms in the question to answer the question correctly. Review the signs and symptoms associated with each level of anxiety if you had difficulty with this question.
Level of Cognitive Ability: Analysis
Client Needs: Psychosocial Integrity
Integrated Concept/Process: Nursing Process/Assessment
Content Area: Mental Health
Reference: Fortinash, K., & Holoday-Worret, P. (2000). *Psychiatric mental health nursing* (2nd ed.). St. Louis: Mosby, p. 238.

250. 1
Rationale: Hydrocodone is an opioid analgesic that also has antitussive properties. Side effects of this medication include physical and psychological dependence, bradycardia and hypotension, respiratory depression, nausea, vomiting, constipation, sedation, and confusion.
Test-Taking Strategy: Use the process of elimination. Recalling that this medication is an opioid analgesic will direct you to option 1. If this question was difficult, review information on the implications of opioid use and the side effects of this medication.
Level of Cognitive Ability: Application
Client Needs: Psychosocial Integrity
Integrated Concept/Process: Nursing Process/Assessment
Content Area: Pharmacology
Reference: Deglin, J., & Vallerand, A. (2001). *Davis's drug guide for nurses* (7th ed.). Philadelphia: F.A. Davis, p. 483.

251. 1
Rationale: Cromolyn sodium (Intal) is an antiasthmatic, antiallergic, and a mast cell stabilizer that inhibits the release of mediators from mast cells after exposure to an antigen. It can also interrupt the migration of eosinophils into the inflammatory site and decrease the number of eosinophils. These actions decrease airway hyperresponsiveness in some clients with asthma. It has no bronchodilating action.
Test-Taking Strategy: Use the process of elimination. Eliminate options 2 and 3 first because they are similar. From the remaining options, it is helpful to know that cromolyn sodium (Intal) has no bronchodilating action. Also, note the relationship between the words *antigen* in the correct option and *allergic* in the question. Review the action of this medication if you had difficulty with this question.
Level of Cognitive Ability: Analysis
Client Needs: Physiological Integrity
Integrated Concept/Process: Nursing Process/Analysis
Content Area: Pharmacology
Reference: Salerno, E. (1999). *Pharmacology for health professionals.* St. Louis: Mosby, p. 464.

252. 2

Rationale: The confrontational method assumes that the examiner has normal peripheral vision. The client sits facing the examiner approximately 2 feet away. The eyes of the client and the examiner should be at the same level. Both the examiner and the client cover the eyes directly opposite to one another and stare at each other's uncovered eye. A small object is brought from the peripheral visual field and tests the superior, temporal, inferior, and nasal field. The client states when he or she sees the object.

Test-Taking Strategy: Use the process of elimination. Eliminate option 3 because this option describes the test for color vision. Option 4 does not describe a confrontational test and addresses testing color. Visualize the process of testing as you read through options 1 and 2. This may assist you in selecting the correct option. If you had difficulty with this question, review this assessment test.

Level of Cognitive Ability: Application
Client Needs: Health Promotion and Maintenance
Integrated Concept/Process: Nursing Process/Implementation
Content Area: Adult Health/Eye
Reference: Jarvis, C. (2000). *Physical examination and health assessment* (3rd ed.). Philadelphia: W.B. Saunders, p. 308.

253. 1

Rationale: Because acetylcysteine has a pervasive flavor of rotten eggs, it must be disguised in a flavored ice drink and is preferably drunk through a straw to minimize contact with the mouth. Acetylcysteine is the antidote for acetaminophen. It is a solution that is also used as a mucolytic agent, administered via nebulization. It is not administered by the IV, IM, or SC route.

Test-Taking Strategy: Use the process of elimination. Knowing that the medication is a solution that is also used for nebulization treatments will assist you in selecting the option that indicates an oral route. Note that options 2, 3, and 4 are similar and indicate parenteral administration and option 1, the correct option, indicates oral administration. Review this medication if you had difficulty with this question.

Level of Cognitive Ability: Application
Client Needs: Physiological Integrity
Integrated Concept/Process: Nursing Process/Implementation
Content Area: Pharmacology
Reference: Hodgson, B., & Kizior, R. (2001). *Saunders nursing drug handbook 2001.* Philadelphia: W.B. Saunders, p. 11.

254. 2

Rationale: Side effects of baclofen include drowsiness, dizziness, weakness, and nausea. Occasional side effects include headache, paresthesia of the hands and feet, constipation or diarrhea, anorexia, hypotension, confusion, and nasal congestion. Paradoxical central nervous system excitement and restlessness can occur along with slurred speech, tremor, dry mouth, nocturia, and impotence.

Test-Taking Strategy: Use the process of elimination. Option 2 is the option that is most closely associated with a neurological disorder. If you had difficulty with this question, review the side effects related to baclofen.

Level of Cognitive Ability: Analysis
Client Needs: Physiological Integrity
Integrated Concept/Process: Nursing Process/Assessment
Content Area: Pharmacology

Reference: Hodgson, B., & Kizior, R. (2001). *Saunders nursing drug handbook 2001.* Philadelphia: W.B. Saunders, pp. 95-96.

255. 2

Rationale: Acetylsalicylic acid (aspirin) may be used to reduce the risk of recurrent transient ischemic attacks (TIAs) or stroke, or to reduce the risk of MI in clients with unstable angina or with a history of a previous MI. The normal dose for clients being treated with acetylsalicylic acid (aspirin) to decrease thrombosis and MI is 300 to 325 mg daily. Clients being treated to prevent TIAs are usually prescribed 1.3 g daily in 2 to 4 divided doses. Clients with rheumatoid arthritis are treated with 3.2 to 6 g daily in divided doses.

Test-Taking Strategy: Use the process of elimination. Read the question carefully. Note the key words *reduce the risk of MI.* This should indicate to you that the client is receiving the medication as a preventive measure, directing you to the lowest dose of medication. If you had difficulty with this question, review acetylsalicylic acid (aspirin) dosages.

Level of Cognitive Ability: Application
Client Needs: Physiological Integrity
Integrated Concept/Process: Nursing Process/Assessment
Content Area: Pharmacology
Reference: Hodgson, B., & Kizior, R. (2001). *Saunders nursing drug handbook 2001.* Philadelphia: W.B. Saunders, p. 76.

256. 4

Rationale: The TENS unit is a portable unit and the client controls the system for relieving pain and reducing the need for analgesics. It is attached to the skin of the body by electrodes. Hospitalization is not required.

Test-Taking Strategy: Use the process of elimination. Note the word *not* in the stem of the question. You should be directed to option 4, because it would not be a very cost effective pain management technique if the client required hospitalization. Review the principles related to the TENS unit if you had difficulty with this question.

Level of Cognitive Ability: Application
Client Needs: Health Promotion and Maintenance
Integrated Concept/Process: Teaching/Learning
Content Area: Pharmacology
Reference: Monahan, F., & Neighbors, M. (1998). *Medical-surgical nursing: Foundations for clinical practice* (2nd ed.). Philadelphia: W. B. Saunders, p. 892.

257. 4

Rationale: Ineffective individual coping may be evidenced by inability to meet basic needs, inability to meet role expectations, alteration in social participation, use of inappropriate defense mechanisms, or impairment of usual patterns of communication. Altered thought processes is evidenced by altered attention span, distractibility or disorientation to time, place, person, and events. Altered family process may exist when the family has difficulty adapting or responding to the changes or traumatic experience of the member in crisis.

Test-Taking Strategy: Use the data presented in the question to direct you to the correct option. Option 3 can be easily eliminated because the client is presently experiencing anxiety. Eliminate option 1, because there are no data in the question that addresses the family. Similarly, there are no data to suggest altered thought processes, so this option is eliminated also, leaving option 4 as the correct option. Review nursing diagnoses for the client experiencing anxiety if you had difficulty with this question.

Level of Cognitive Ability: Analysis
Client Needs: Psychosocial Integrity
Integrated Concept/Process: Nursing Process/Analysis
Content Area: Mental Health
Reference: Keltner, N., Schwecke, L., & Bostrom, C. (1999). *Psychiatric nursing* (3rd ed.). St. Louis: Mosby, p. 153.

258. 2
Rationale: Bubbling in the water seal compartment is caused by air passing out of the pleural space into the fluid in the chamber. Intermittent bubbling is normal. It indicates that the system if accomplishing one of its purposes, that is, removing air from the pleural space. Continuous bubbling during both inspiration and expiration indicates that an air leak exists. If this occurs, it must be corrected.

Test-Taking Strategy: Focus on the key words *intermittent bubbling* and *water seal compartment*. Recalling that intermittent bubbling is normal will direct you to option 2. If you are unfamiliar with chest tube drainage systems, review this content.

Level of Cognitive Ability: Analysis
Client Needs: Physiological Integrity
Integrated Concept/Process: Nursing Process/Implementation
Content Area: Adult Health/Respiratory
Reference: Potter, P., & Perry, A. (2001). *Fundamentals of nursing* (5th ed.). St. Louis: Mosby, p. 1175.

259. 1
Rationale: The nurse tilts the client's head slightly away and holds the otoscope upside down as if it were a large pen. The pinna is pulled up and back and the nurse visualizes the external canal while slowly inserting the speculum. Options 2, 3, and 4 are incorrect.

Test-Taking Strategy: Use the process of elimination. Note that the question addresses the adult client. Use basic knowledge regarding the administration of ear medications to select the correct option. In the adult, the pinna is pulled up and back. Review the procedure for performing an otoscopic examination if you had difficulty with this question.

Level of Cognitive Ability: Application
Client Needs: Health Promotion and Maintenance
Integrated Concept/Process: Nursing Process/Assessment
Content Area: Adult Health/Ear
Reference: Jarvis, C. (2000). *Physical examination and health assessment* (3rd ed.). Philadelphia: W.B. Saunders, pp. 355-356.

260. 2
Rationale: Cinobac is a urinary antiseptic and is administered with meals to decrease gastrointestinal side effects. The normal dosage is 1 gram per day administered in 2 to 4 divided doses for a period of 7 to 14 days.

Test-Taking Strategy: Use the process of elimination. Eliminate options 1 and 4 first because they are similar. From the remaining options, recalling that this medication is administered more than once daily will direct you to option 2. Review this medication if you had difficulty with this question.

Level of Cognitive Ability: Application
Client Needs: Health Promotion and Maintenance
Integrated Concept/Process: Teaching/Learning
Content Area: Pharmacology
Reference: Clark, J., Queener, S., & Karb, V. (2000). *Pharmacologic basis of nursing practice* (6th ed.). St. Louis: Mosby, p. 520.

261. 1
Rationale: The client with severe flail chest will have significant paradoxical chest movement. This causes the mediastinal structures to swing back and forth with respiration. This movement can affect hemodynamics. Specifically, the client's CVP rises, the filling of the right side of the heart is impaired, and the arterial blood pressure falls. This is referred to as mediastinal flutter.

Test-Taking Strategy: Use the process of elimination. Since the question makes no mention of hemorrhage or bleeding, hypovolemic shock is eliminated first. Knowing that these signs and symptoms are not compatible with fat embolism helps you eliminate that option next. From the remaining options, knowing that mediastinal shift is a result of tension pneumothorax helps you to choose mediastinal flutter as the correct option. Review the complications of a flail chest if you had difficulty with this question.

Level of Cognitive Ability: Analysis
Client Needs: Physiological Integrity
Integrated Concept/Process: Nursing Process/Assessment
Content Area: Adult Health/Respiratory
Reference: Black, J., & Matassarin-Jacobs, E. (1997). *Medical-surgical nursing: Clinical management for continuity of care* (5th ed.). Philadelphia: W. B. Saunders. p. 2527.

262. 2
Rationale: Cough is the most frequent symptom of lung cancer, which begins as nonproductive and hacking, and progresses to productive. In the smoker who already has a cough, a change in the character and frequency of cough usually occurs. Wheezing and blood-streaked sputum (hemoptysis) are later signs. Pain is a very late sign, and is usually pleuritic in nature. Hoarseness indicates that the affected tissue is in the upper airway.

Test-Taking Strategy: Use the process of elimination. Begin to answer this question by eliminating pain and hemoptysis, because it is reasonable that these would be later signs. To discriminate between cough and hoarseness, think about location. Hoarseness would indicate that the affected tissue is in the upper airway, while cough would indicate lower airway. Since the question is asking about lung cancer, which is lower airway, the answer must be cough. Review the frequent early symptoms of lung cancer if you had difficulty with this question.

Level of Cognitive Ability: Application
Client Needs: Physiological Integrity
Integrated Concept/Process: Nursing Process/Assessment
Content Area: Adult Health/Respiratory
Reference: Monahan, F., & Neighbors, M. (1998). *Medical-surgical nursing: Foundations for clinical practice* (2nd ed.). Philadelphia: W.B. Saunders, p. 696.

263. 3
Rationale: The initial nursing assessment of a client in a crisis state is to evaluate the physical condition of the client, the potential for self-harm, and the potential for harm to others. Once this has been determined and appropriate interventions have been initiated, the nurse would then proceed with the mental health interview.

Test-Taking Strategy: Use Maslow's Hierarchy of Needs theory to answer the question. Physiological needs take priority over other needs. Option 3 is the only option that addresses a

physiological need. Review care of a client in crisis if you had difficulty with this question.
Level of Cognitive Ability: Analysis
Client Needs: Physiological Integrity
Integrated Concept/Process: Nursing Process/Assessment
Content Area: Mental Health
Reference: Fortinash, K., & Holoday-Worret, P. (2000). *Psychiatric mental health nursing* (2nd ed.). St. Louis: Mosby, p. 598.
264. **3**
Rationale: Although frequency and intensity of bowel sounds will vary depending on the phase of digestion, normal bowel sounds are relatively high-pitched clicks or gurgles. Loud gurgles (borborygmi) indicate hyperperistalsis. Bowel sounds will be more high pitched and loud (hyperresonance) when the intestines are under tension, such as in intestinal obstruction. A swishing or buzzing sound represents turbulent blood flow associated with a bruit. Bruits are not normal sounds.
Test-Taking Strategy: Use the process of elimination. Normally, bowel sounds are audible in all four quadrants; therefore option 2 and option 4 can be eliminated. From the remaining options, use knowledge regarding normal findings to direct you to option 3. Review abdominal assessment if you had difficulty with this question.
Level of Cognitive Ability: Comprehension
Client Needs: Physiological Integrity
Integrated Concept/Process: Nursing Process/Assessment
Content Area: Adult Health/Gastrointestinal
Reference: Lewis, S., Heitkemper, M., & Dirksen, S. (2000). *Medical-surgical nursing: Assessment and management of clinical problems* (5th ed.). St. Louis: Mosby, p. 1025.
265. **4**
Rationale: The client presents a lethality potential if the client appears disorganized and impulsive. Clients at higher risk include those with a history of a dual diagnosis of mental illness and substance abuse, a personal or family history of suicide attempts, depression, alcoholism, or psychotic episodes. Having a plan, particularly if the method is immediate and available, makes the client a very high risk.
Test-Taking Strategy: Use the process of elimination. Noting the key words *a very high risk* should easily direct you to option 4. Also, note the key words *immediate plan* in the correct option. If you are unfamiliar with the risk factors associated with suicide, review this content.
Level of Cognitive Ability: Analysis
Client Needs: Psychosocial Integrity
Integrated Concept/Process: Nursing Process/Assessment
Content Area: Mental Health
Reference: Fortinash, K., & Holoday-Worret, P. (2000). *Psychiatric mental health nursing* (2nd ed.). St. Louis: Mosby, pp. 664-665.
266. **2**
Rationale: Lomotil is an antidiarrheal product, which decreases the frequency of stools, usually by reducing the volume of liquid in the stools. Options 1, 3, and 4 are not associated therapeutic effects of this medication.
Test-Taking Strategy: Use the process of elimination. Focus on the diagnosis presented in the question. Thinking about the clinical manifestations that occur in this condition will easily direct you to option 2. If you had difficulty with this question, review the therapeutic effect of Lomotil.

Level of Cognitive Ability: Analysis
Client Needs: Physiological Integrity
Integrated Concept/Process: Nursing Process/Evaluation
Content Area: Adult Health/Gastrointestinal
Reference: Wilson, B., Shannon, M., & Stang, C. (2000). *Nurses drug guide 2000.* Stamford, Conn.: Appleton & Lange, p. 467.
267. **4**
Rationale: Azulfidine is an antiinflammatory sulfonamide. It can cause photosensivity and the client should be instructed to avoid sun and ultraviolet light. It should be administered with meals if possible to prolong intestinal passage. The client needs to take the medication as prescribed and continue for the full length of treatment even if symptoms are relieved. Constipation is not associated with this medication.
Test-Taking Strategy: Use the process of elimination. Note the key words *need for further education.* Eliminate option 3 first because this is a general measure regarding medication therapy. Knowing that this medication is a sulfonamide will assist in eliminating options 1 and 2. Review client teaching points regarding this medication if you had difficulty with this question.
Level of Cognitive Ability: Analysis
Client Needs: Health Promotion and Maintenance
Integrated Concept/Process: Teaching/Learning
Content Area: Adult Health/Gastrointestinal
Reference: Hodgson, B., & Kizior, R. (2001). *Saunders nursing drug handbook 2001.* Philadelphia: W.B. Saunders, pp. 953-955.
268. **2**
Rationale: Fluid volume excess, related to the accumulation of fluid in the peritoneal cavity and dependent areas of the body, can occur in the client with cirrhosis. Fluids should be restricted, including fluids given with medications and meals. Sodium restriction will also aid in reducing fluid volume excess. Options 3 and 4 will not assist in reducing fluid volume excess.
Test-Taking Strategy: Note that the issue is to reduce fluid excess. Options 3 and 4 can be eliminated first because they are unrelated to this issue. Recalling that sodium will retain fluids will assist in eliminating option 1. Review care of a client with cirrhosis if you had difficulty with this question.
Level of Cognitive Ability: Application
Client Needs: Physiological Integrity
Integrated Concept/Process: Nursing Process/Planning
Content Area: Adult Health/Gastrointestinal
Reference: Monahan, F., & Neighbors, M. (1998). *Medical-surgical nursing: Foundations for clinical practice* (2nd ed.). Philadelphia: W. B. Saunders, p. 1190.
269. **1**
Rationale: Lactulose is an osmotic laxative. The desired effect is 2 to 3 soft stools per day with an acid fecal pH. Lactulose creates an acid environment in the bowel, resulting in a fall of the colon's pH from 7 to 5. This causes ammonia to leave the circulatory system and move into the colon. Diarrhea may indicate excessive administration of the medication. Options 3 and 4 do not determine that a desired effect has occurred.
Test-Taking Strategy: Use the process of elimination. Knowledge regarding the purpose and action of this medication is required to answer this question. Focusing on the client's diagnosis will assist in determining the action of this

medication. Review this important medication if you had difficulty with this question.

Level of Cognitive Ability: Analysis
Client Needs: Physiological Integrity
Integrated Concept/Process: Nursing Process/Evaluation
Content Area: Adult Health/Gastrointestinal
Reference: Ignatavicius, D., Workman, M., & Mishler, M. (1999). *Medical-surgical nursing across the health care continuum* (3rd ed.). Philadelphia: W.B. Saunders, p. 1477.

270. 2
Rationale: This medication binds with bile salts in the intestines to form a compound that is excreted in the feces. The client should be instructed to mix the medication with 3 to 6 ounces of water, milk, fruit juice, or soup. It should be administered just before meals. It is not administered via rectal suppository.
Test-Taking Strategy: Knowledge regarding the administration of this medication is required to answer this question. Recalling that this medication needs to be mixed in another substance will direct you to option 2. Review this medication if you had difficulty with this question
Level of Cognitive Ability: Application
Client Needs: Health Promotion and Maintenance
Integrated Concept/Process: Teaching/Learning
Content Area: Adult Health/Gastrointestinal
Reference: Hodgson, B., & Kizior, R. (2001). *Saunders nursing drug handbook 2001.* Philadelphia: W.B. Saunders, p. 216.

271. 4
Rationale: Viokase aids in the digestion of protein, carbohydrate, and fat in the gastrointestinal tract. It is used to treat steatorrhea associated with postgastrectomy syndrome following bowel resection. The nurse should record the number of stools per day and stool consistency to monitor the effectiveness of this enzyme therapy. If it is effective, the stools should become less frequent and less fatty. Options 1, 2, and 3 are incorrect.
Test-Taking Strategy: Use the process of elimination. Knowledge regarding the use and therapeutic effect of this medication is required to answer this question. Focusing on the client's diagnosis will assist in directing you to the correct option. If you are unfamiliar with this medication, review this content.
Level of Cognitive Ability: Analysis
Client Needs: Physiological Integrity
Integrated Concept/Process: Nursing Process/Evaluation
Content Area: Adult Health/Gastrointestinal
Reference: Hodgson, B., & Kizior, R. (2001). *Saunders nursing drug handbook 2001.* Philadelphia: W.B. Saunders, p. 787.

272. 3
Rationale: Expected outcomes for the client with PUD experiencing pain include: elimination of irritating foods from the diet, ability to take prescribed medications that will reduce pain, reporting that pain is relieved or prevented with medication, and an ability to sleep through the night without pain. The client who continues to be awakened by pain requires further modification of medication therapy, which may include adjustment of timing of histamine H_2-receptor antagonist, or an additional dose of antacid before the time when pain awakens the client.
Test-Taking Strategy: Use the process of elimination and note key words *expected outcomes* and *not met.* This tells you that the correct answer is an option that indicates insufficient pain management. This should easily direct you to option 3. Review care of a client with PUD if you had difficulty with this question.
Level of Cognitive Ability: Analysis
Client Needs: Physiological Integrity
Integrated Concept/Process: Nursing Process/Evaluation
Content Area: Adult Health/Gastrointestinal
Reference: Monahan, F., & Neighbors, M. (1998). *Medical-surgical nursing: Foundations for clinical practice* (2nd ed.). Philadelphia: W. B. Saunders, p. 1032.

273. 2
Rationale: The client is experiencing loss and is feeling hopeless. The most therapeutic response by the nurse is the one that attempts to translate words into feelings. In option 1, the nurse is voicing doubt. In option 3, the nurse is disagreeing with client, which implies that the nurse has passed judgment on the client's ideas or opinions. In option 4, the nurse uses sarcasm that gives advice and is nontherapeutic as a nursing response.
Test-Taking Strategy: Use the process of elimination and therapeutic communication techniques. Option 2 is the only option that addresses feelings. Review therapeutic communication techniques if you had difficulty with this question.
Level of Cognitive Ability: Application
Client Needs: Psychosocial Integrity
Integrated Concept/Process: Communication and Documentation
Content Area: Mental Health
Reference: Stuart, G.W., & Laraia, M.T. (1998). *Principles and practice of psychiatric nursing* (6th ed.). St. Louis: Mosby, p. 39.

274. 1
Rationale: Immediately following radical neck dissection, the client will have a wound drain in the neck attached to portable suction, which drains serosanguineous drainage. In the first 24 hours after surgery, the drainage may total 80 to 120 mL.
Test-Taking Strategy: Note the key words *immediate postoperative period.* Since the wound suction tube does not sit in the airway, option 4 is eliminated. Since serous drainage has no blood, this is not likely to be noted in the immediate postoperative period. Knowing that grossly bloody drainage indicates bleeding or hemorrhage, will direct you to option 1. Review normal expected assessment findings following radical neck dissection if you had difficulty with this question.
Level of Cognitive Ability: Application
Client Needs: Physiological Integrity
Integrated Concept/Process: Nursing Process/Assessment
Content Area: Adult Health/Respiratory
Reference: Smeltzer, S., & Bare, B. (2000). *Brunner & Suddarth's Textbook of medical-surgical nursing* (9th ed.). Philadelphia: Lippincott Williams & Wilkins, p. 820.

275. 4
Rationale: The sudden change in the depressed client's mood and affect may indicate that the client has come to a decision about suicide. The only way to be sure is to ask the client directly. Option 1 *assumes* a meaning of the behavior. Option 2 offers no different strategy than would be used with any client. Notifying others of your concern does nothing to address the problem directly.
Test-Taking Strategy: Use the process of elimination focusing on the issue, client safety. Remember, the only way to be sure

about a client's suicide intent, is to ask the client. Review care of the suicidal client if you had difficulty with this question.
Level of Cognitive Ability: Application
Client Needs: Physiological Integrity
Integrated Concept/Process: Nursing Process/Implementation
Content Area: Mental Health
Reference: Fortinash, K., & Holoday-Worret, P. (2000). *Psychiatric mental health nursing* (2nd ed.). St. Louis: Mosby, p. 664.

276. 1
Rationale: The client is placed in the left Sims' position for the procedure. This position takes the best advantage of the client's anatomy for ease in introducing the colonoscope. The other options are incorrect.
Test-Taking Strategy: Use the process of elimination and concepts related to gastrointestinal (GI) anatomy to answer this question. The correct option identifies the same procedure used for giving the client an enema while lying down. When answering factual questions such as these, remember the guiding principles and attempt to visualize the procedure to help you select the correct option. Review this procedure if you had difficulty with this question.
Level of Cognitive Ability: Application
Client Needs: Physiological Integrity
Integrated Concept/Process: Teaching/Learning
Content Area: Adult Health/Gastrointestinal
Reference: Monahan, F., & Neighbors, M. (1998). *Medical-surgical nursing: Foundations for clinical practice* (2nd ed.). Philadelphia: W. B. Saunders, p. 975.

277. 3
Rationale: The client with TB should wash the hands carefully after each contact with respiratory secretions. The client should cover the mouth and nose when laughing, sneezing, or coughing. Used tissues are discarded in a plastic bag. Oral care is done as for any other client.
Test-Taking Strategy: Focus on the issue of the question. Note that the question specifically asks for information about handling and disposal of secretions. The only option that addresses this issue is option 3. Review home care instructions for the client with TB if you had difficulty with this question.
Level of Cognitive Ability: Analysis
Client Needs: Health Promotion and Maintenance
Integrated Concept/Process: Teaching/Learning
Content Area: Adult Health/Respiratory
Reference: Ignatavicius, D., Workman, M., & Mishler, M. (1999). *Medical-surgical nursing across the health care continuum* (3rd ed.). Philadelphia: W.B. Saunders, p. 677.

278. 1
Rationale: Ultrasound of the gallbladder is a non-invasive procedure and is frequently used for emergency diagnosis of acute cholecystitis. The client does not need to be NPO for 24 hours but may be instructed to avoid carbonated beverages for 48 hours before the test to help decrease intestinal gas. It is a painless test and does not require the administration of oral tablets as preparation.
Test-Taking Strategy: Use the process of elimination and attempt to visualize this procedure in selecting the correct option. If you are unfamiliar with this test, review this content.
Level of Cognitive Ability: Application
Client Needs: Health Promotion and Maintenance
Integrated Concept/Process: Teaching/Learning
Content Area: Adult Health/Gastrointestinal

Reference: Monahan, F., & Neighbors, M. (1998). *Medical-surgical nursing: Foundations for clinical practice* (2nd ed.). Philadelphia: W. B. Saunders, p. 976.

279. 1
Rationale: The nurse who obtains a positive Mantoux reading calls the physician immediately. The physician would order a chest x-ray evaluation to rule out whether the client has clinically active tuberculosis (TB), or old, healed lesions. Sputum culture would be done next as indicated to confirm the diagnosis of active TB. The client can be placed on TB precautions prophylactically until a final diagnosis is made.
Test-Taking Strategy: Note the key words *highest priority.* Since the nurse may not order diagnostic tests, eliminate option 2 first. Likewise, option 4 can be eliminated, since calling employee health service is of no benefit to the client. From the remaining options, notifying the physician should have a higher priority than the documentation, even though they may both be done in the same narrow time period. Note that the question asks for the highest priority, not the first nursing action. Review the implications related to a positive Mantoux test if you had difficulty with this question.
Level of Cognitive Ability: Application
Client Needs: Safe, Effective Care Environment
Integrated Concept/Process: Nursing Process/Implementation
Content Area: Adult Health/Respiratory
Reference: Ignatavicius, D., Workman, M., & Mishler, M. (1999). *Medical-surgical nursing across the health care continuum* (3rd ed.). Philadelphia: W.B. Saunders, p. 676.

280. 3
Rationale: Medications known to lower cyclosporine levels include phenytoin, phenobarbital, rifampin, and trimethoprim-sulfamethoxazole. Cyclosporine levels should be monitored and the dosage adjusted in clients taking these medications.
Test-Taking Strategy: Use the process of elimination and knowledge regarding the medications that lower cyclosporine levels to answer this question. If you are unfamiliar with these medications, review this content.
Level of Cognitive Ability: Analysis
Client Needs: Physiological Integrity
Integrated Concept/Process: Nursing Process/Analysis
Content Area: Pharmacology
Reference: Lehne, R. (1998). *Pharmacology for nursing care* (3rd ed.). Philadelphia: W.B. Saunders, p. 729-730.

281. 1
Rationale: Exercising 3 to 4 hours every day is excessive physical activity and unrealistic for a sixteen-year-old. The nurse needs to further assess this statement immediately to find out why the client feels the need to exercise this much to maintain her figure. Although it's unfortunate that her best friend had this disease, it is not considered a major threat to this client's physical well-being. A weight that exceeds 15% below the ideal weight is most significant with anorexia nervosa. It is not considered abnormal to check weight every day. Many clients with anorexia nervosa check their weight close to 20 times a day.
Test-Taking Strategy: Note the key word *priority* in the stem of the question. Use the process of elimination. Eliminate options 3 and 4 first because these client statements are not significant or abnormal. From the remaining options, knowledge regarding the manifestations associated

with anorexia nervosa will direct you to option 1. Review these significant manifestations if you had difficulty with this question.

Level of Cognitive Ability: Analysis
Client Needs: Psychosocial Integrity
Integrated Concept/Process: Nursing Process/Analysis
Content Area: Mental Health
Reference: Leahy, J., & Kizilay, P. (1998). *Foundations of nursing practice: A nursing process approach.* Philadelphia: W.B. Saunders, p.763.

282. 3

Rationale: Stir-fried vegetables are allowed for strict vegetarians. A chocolate milkshake is not an appropriate choice because dairy products, such as milk, are not allowed. Because the wheat toast is buttered, it is also not allowed because butter is a dairy product. Strict vegetarians do not eat eggs. Foods that are eaten by a client that is a strict vegetarian include grains, fruits, and vegetables.

Test-Taking Strategy: Note the key words *strict vegetarian* in the question. Note the relationship between this type of diet and the food item in the correct option. Review foods that can be included in a strict vegetarian diet if you had difficulty with this question.

Level of Cognitive Ability: Application
Client Needs: Physiological Integrity
Integrated Concept/Process: Nursing Process/Planning
Content Area: Fundamental Skills
Reference: Leahy, J. & Kizilay, P. (1998). *Foundations of nursing practice: A nursing process approach.* Philadelphia: W.B. Saunders, p. 748.

283. 2

Rationale: Because of the risk of anaphylaxis during the administration of cyclosporine by IV, epinephrine and oxygen must be immediately available for use. An oral airway or a suction machine is not the priority item and it is not necessary to have a code cart at the bedside.

Test-Taking Strategy: Use the process of elimination. Knowledge that cyclosporine administered by IV can cause anaphylaxis will assist in directing you to option 2. Review care of a client receiving this medication by the IV route if you had difficulty with this question.

Level of Cognitive Ability: Application
Client Needs: Physiological Integrity
Integrated Concept/Process: Nursing Process/Planning
Content Area: Pharmacology
Reference: Lehne, R. (1998). *Pharmacology for nursing care* (3rd ed.). Philadelphia: W.B. Saunders, p. 731.

284. 1

Rationale: When administering Cyclosporine by IV, 1 mL of concentrate is diluted in 20 to 100 mL of 0.9% sodium chloride or 5% dextrose. The initial dose is 5 to 6 mg/kg (⅓ the oral dose) administered over 2 to 6 hours. The solution should be protected from light.

Test-Taking Strategy: Use the process of elimination. Note the key word *inappropriate.* Note that option 1 identifies administering the medication by IV bolus in a small amount of diluent. Review this medication and its administration by the IV route if you had difficulty with this question.

Level of Cognitive Ability: Application
Client Needs: Physiological Integrity
Integrated Concept/Process: Nursing Process/Implementation

Content Area: Pharmacology
Reference: Hodgson, B., & Kizior, R. (2001). *Saunders nursing drug handbook 2001.* Philadelphia: W.B. Saunders, p. 273.

285. 1

Rationale: Orthoclone is a monoclonal antibody. Upon binding to the CD3 site, the antibody blocks all T cell function. Options 2, 3, and 4 are not actions of this medication.

Test-Taking Strategy: Knowledge regarding the action of this medication is required to answer this question. Review the specific action of this medication if you had difficulty with this question.

Level of Cognitive Ability: Analysis
Client Needs: Physiological Integrity
Integrated Concept/Process: Nursing Process/Analysis
Content Area: Pharmacology
Reference: Clark, J., Queener, S., & Karb, V. (2000). *Pharmacologic basis of nursing practice* (6th ed.). St. Louis: Mosby, p. 462.

286. 4

Rationale: Brompheniramine is an antihistamine, which provides relief of symptoms caused by allergy. Antihistamines should be discontinued for at least 3 days (72 hours) before allergy skin testing to avoid false-negative readings. This client should have the appointment rescheduled for 3 days after discontinuing the medication.

Test-Taking Strategy: Use the process of elimination. Recall that this medication is an antihistamine and that antihistamines reduce the allergic response by virtue of their action. With this in mind, option 1 is eliminated first. Options 2 and 3 are also eliminated because the medication would still interfere with the test results. Review client instructions regarding skin testing if you had difficulty with this question.

Level of Cognitive Ability: Analysis
Client Needs: Physiological Integrity
Integrated Concept/Process: Nursing Process/Analysis
Content Area: Pharmacology
Reference: Wilson, B., Shannon, M., & Stang, C. (2000). *Nurses drug guide 2000.* Stamford, Conn.: Appleton & Lange, p. 172.

287. 3

Rationale: Acetylcystine can be given orally or by nasogastric tube to treat acetaminophen overdose, or it may be given by inhalation for use as a mucolytic. Before giving the medication as an antidote to acetaminophen, the nurse assures that the client's stomach is empty through emesis or gastric lavage. The solution is diluted in cola, water, or juice to make the solution more palatable. It is then administered orally or by nasogastric tube.

Test-Taking Strategy: Use the process of elimination. Begin to answer this question by eliminating options 1 and 2. This medication is not given by the inhalation route to treat acetaminophen overdose, and acetylcystine is the antidote (to acetaminophen). To discriminate between the last two options, it is necessary to know either of two things. First, knowing that the solution must be diluted directs you to option 3. Second, knowing that the stomach must be emptied for maximal effect of the antidote also directs you to option 3. Review administration of the medication if you had difficulty with this question.

Level of Cognitive Ability: Analysis

Client Needs: Physiological Integrity
Integrated Concept/Process: Nursing Process/Assessment
Content Area: Pharmacology
Reference: Deglin, J., & Vallerand, A. (2001). *Davis's drug guide for nurses* (7th ed.). Philadelphia: F.A. Davis, pp. 7-9.

288. 3
Rationale: Naloxone hydrochloride is an antidote to opioids, and it may also be given to the postoperative client to treat respiratory depression. When given to the postoperative client for respiratory depression, it may also reverse the effects of analgesics. Therefore the nurse must assess the client for a sudden increase in the level of pain experienced.
Test-Taking Strategy: Use the process of elimination. Recall that this medication is an antidote to narcotic analgesics, and that it would likely cause sudden pain in the postoperative client, or return of pain in clients who receive narcotic analgesics. If you had difficulty with this question, review this medication.
Level of Cognitive Ability: Application
Client Needs: Physiological Integrity
Integrated Concept/Process: Nursing Process/Assessment
Content Area: Pharmacology
Reference: Deglin, J., & Vallerand, A. (2001). *Davis's drug guide for nurses* (7th ed.). Philadelphia: F.A. Davis, p. 841.

289. 1
Rationale: The signs and symptoms described in the question are consistent with perforation of the ulcer, which then progresses to peritonitis if the perforation is large enough. The client with intestinal obstruction would most likely complain of abdominal pain, distention, and nausea and vomiting. The client with hemorrhage would be vomiting blood or coffee-ground material, or would be expelling black, tarry, or bloody stools. Intractability is a term that refers to continued symptoms of a disease process, despite ongoing medical treatment.
Test-Taking Strategy: Use the process of elimination. Focus on the signs and symptoms presented in the question to direct you to option 1. Review the signs of perforation if you had difficulty with this question.
Level of Cognitive Ability: Analysis
Client Needs: Physiological Integrity
Integrated Concept/Process: Nursing Process/Assessment
Content Area: Adult Health/Gastrointestinal
Reference: Monahan, F., & Neighbors, M. (1998). *Medical-surgical nursing: Foundations for clinical practice* (2nd ed.). Philadelphia: W. B. Saunders, p. 1029.

290. 3
Rationale: The client with an ileostomy is prone to dehydration due to the location of the ostomy and should not take laxatives. This will compound the potential risk for the client. Clients are at risk for deficiency of iron, folate, and cyanocobalamin, and should receive these as supplements if necessary.
Test-Taking Strategy: Use the process of elimination and note the key word *contraindicated*. Recalling that dehydration is an important risk for ileostomy clients, and knowing what can trigger episodes of dehydration will direct you to option 3. Review care of a client with an ileostomy if you had difficulty with this question.
Level of Cognitive Ability: Analysis
Client Needs: Physiological Integrity
Integrated Concept/Process: Nursing Process/Assessment

Content Area: Adult Health/Gastrointestinal
Reference: Monahan, F., & Neighbors, M. (1998). *Medical-surgical nursing: Foundations for clinical practice* (2nd ed.). Philadelphia: W. B. Saunders, p. 1013.

291. 2
Rationale: Serosanguineous drainage with a small amount of bile is expected from the Penrose drain for the first 24 hours. Drainage then decreases and the drain is removed usually within 48 hours. The physician does not need to be notified. A sterile dressing covers the site and should be changed to prevent infection and skin excoriation.
Test-Taking Strategy: Use the process of elimination. Eliminate options 3 and 4 first because they are similar. Knowledge of the normal expected findings following cholecystectomy will easily direct you to option 2. Review these expected findings if you had difficulty with this question.
Level of Cognitive Ability: Application
Client Needs: Physiological Integrity
Integrated Concept/Process: Nursing Process/Implementation
Content Area: Adult Health/Gastrointestinal
Reference: Monahan, F., & Neighbors, M. (1998). *Medical-surgical nursing: Foundations for clinical practice* (2nd ed.). Philadelphia: W. B. Saunders, p. 1114.

292. 1
Rationale: The nurse ensures that all system connections are securely taped to prevent accidental disconnection, and that an occlusive dressing is maintained at the chest tube insertion site. Drainage is noted and recorded every hour in the first 24 hours after insertion and every 8 hours thereafter. The system is kept below the level of the waist. Assessment for crepitus is done once every 8 hours. Sterile water is only added to the suction control chamber as needed to replace evaporation losses. Continuous bubbling in the water seal chamber indicates an air leak in the system, and requires immediate investigation and correction.
Test-Taking Strategy: Note that each options has two parts. In order for the option to be correct, both parts of the answer must be correct. Knowing this, eliminate options 3 and 4 first. Water only needs to be added as needed and there should not be continuous bubbling in the water seal. Knowing that chest tube assessment is done at least every 8 hours, helps you to select option 1. Review the assessment measures required in the care of a client with a chest tube if you had difficulty with this question.
Level of Cognitive Ability: Application
Client Needs: Physiological Integrity
Integrated Concept/Process: Nursing Process/Implementation
Content Area: Adult Health/Respiratory
Reference: Ignatavicius, D., Workman, M., & Mishler, M. (1999). *Medical-surgical nursing across the health care continuum* (3rd ed.). Philadelphia: W.B. Saunders, p. 654.

293. 3
Rationale: HBIG and the vaccine are given to infants with perinatal exposure to prevent hepatitis and achieve lifelong prophylaxis and is administered within 12 hours of birth. Immune Globulin (IG) is given to prevent hepatitis A.
Test-Taking Strategy: Focus on the issue, a mother with hepatitis B. Knowledge of the different types of pre- and post-exposure prophylaxis for hepatitis A and B is needed to answer this question. If you had difficulty with this question, review content associated with hepatitis immunization.

Level of Cognitive Ability: Analysis
Client Needs: Safe, Effective Care Environment
Integrated Concept/Process: Nursing Process/Implementation
Content Area: Adult Health/Gastrointestinal
Reference: LeMone, P., & Burke, K. (2000). *Medical-surgical nursing: Critical thinking in client care* (2nd ed.). Upper Saddle River, N.J.: Prentice-Hall, p. 523.

294. 3
Rationale: A replacement tube of the same size and an obturator is kept at the bedside at all times in case the tracheostomy tube is dislodged. Additionally, a curved hemostat that could be used to hold the trachea open if dislodgment occurs should also be kept at the bedside. An oral airway and epinephrine would not be needed.
Test-Taking Strategy: Use the process of elimination. Eliminate option 4 first because a tracheostomy set of the next larger size would not be appropriate for the client. Next eliminate option 2 because it is unrelated to the issue of the question. From the remaining options, recall that the airway has been altered because of the tracheostomy, so an oral airway would not be necessary. Remember that a replacement tube and an obturator should be kept at the bedside of a client with a tracheostomy, along with a curved hemostat, at all times. Review care of a client with a tracheostomy if you had difficulty with this question.
Level of Cognitive Ability: Application
Client Needs: Physiological Integrity
Integrated Concept/Process: Nursing Process/Planning
Content Area: Adult Health/Respiratory
Reference: Monahan, F., & Neighbors, M. (1998). *Medical-surgical nursing: Foundations for clinical practice* (2nd ed.). Philadelphia: W.B. Saunders, p. 566.

295. 4
Rationale: When the high pressure alarm sounds on a ventilator, it is most likely due to an obstruction. The obstruction can be caused by the client biting on the tube, kinking of the tubing, or mucus plugging requiring suctioning. Options 1 and 2 would cause the low pressure alarm to sound. Option 3 delays necessary treatment.
Test-Taking Strategy: Use the process of elimination. Note the key words *high-pressure alarm* in the question. Recalling that that the high pressure alarm indicates a possible obstruction will assist in directing you to the correct option. Review nursing interventions related to care of a client on a ventilator if you had difficulty with this question.
Level of Cognitive Ability: Application
Client Needs: Physiological Integrity
Integrated Concept/Process: Nursing Process/Implementation
Content Area: Adult Health/Respiratory
Reference: Ignatavicius, D., Workman, M., & Mishler, M. (1999). *Medical-surgical nursing across the health care continuum* (3rd ed.). Philadelphia: W.B. Saunders, p. 705.

296. 1
Rationale: With normal breathing, the water level rises with inspiration and falls with expiration. The opposite, falls with inspiration and rises with expiration, occurs when the client is on positive pressure mechanical ventilation. This is an expected normal occurrence in a chest tube drainage system, therefore no action is necessary.
Test-Taking Strategy: Use the process of elimination. Recalling that a fluctuating water level is expected in the water seal chamber will assist in directing you to option 1. Review chest tube drainage systems if you had difficulty with this question.
Level of Cognitive Ability: Analysis
Client Needs: Physiological Integrity
Integrated Concept/Process: Nursing Process/Implementation
Content Area: Adult Health/Respiratory
References: Monahan, F., & Neighbors, M. (1998). *Medical-surgical nursing: Foundations for clinical practice* (2nd ed.). Philadelphia: W.B. Saunders, p. 578.

297. 3
Rationale: If constant bubbling occurs in the water seal chamber it may indicate a leak in the system. From the options provided, the most appropriate is to notify the physician.
Test-Taking Strategy: Note the key words *constant bubbling in the water seal chamber.* Visualize this drainage system to answer the question. Knowing that this is an unexpected occurrence, and may indicate a potential complication with the chest tube drainage system will assist in directing you to option 3. If you had difficulty with this question or are unfamiliar with the care to the chest tube drainage system, review this content.
Level of Cognitive Ability: Analysis
Client Needs: Physiological Integrity
Integrated Concept/Process: Nursing Process/Implementation
Content Area: Adult Health/Respiratory
Reference: Ignatavicius, D., Workman, M., & Mishler, M. (1999). *Medical-surgical nursing across the health care continuum* (3rd ed.). Philadelphia: W.B. Saunders, p. 654.

298. 1
Rationale: A common side effect of this medication is agranulocytopenia and anemia. The nurse carefully monitors CBC results for these changes. With early infection or in the client who is asymptomatic, CBC levels are monitored monthly for 3 months, then every 3 months thereafter. In clients with advanced disease, they are monitored every 2 weeks for the first 2 months, and then once a month if the medication is tolerated well.
Test-Taking Strategy: Recalling that AZT causes agranulocytopenia and anemia will direct you to option 1. Review the adverse effects of this medication if you had difficulty with this question.
Level of Cognitive Ability: Analysis
Client Needs: Physiological Integrity
Integrated Concept/Process: Nursing Process/Assessment
Content Area: Adult Health/Immune
Reference: Hodgson, B., & Kizior, R. (2001). *Saunders nursing drug handbook 2001.* Philadelphia: W.B. Saunders, pp. 1067-1069.

299. 2
Rationale: The bacille Calmette-Guérin vaccine is routinely given in many foreign countries to enhance resistance to TB. The vaccine uses attenuated tubercle bacilli, so the client will always test positive on skin testing. This client needs to be evaluated for TB with a chest x-ray evaluation.
Test-Taking Strategy: Use the process of elimination. Recalling that the BCG vaccine contains attenuated tubercle bacilli will direct you to option 2. Review the characteristics of this vaccine if you had difficulty with this question.
Level of Cognitive Ability: Analysis
Client Needs: Physiological Integrity

Integrated Concept/Process: Nursing Process/Analysis
Content Area: Adult Health/Respiratory
Reference: Ignatavicius, D., Workman, M., & Mishler, M.
(1999). Medical-surgical nursing across the health care continuum
(3rd ed.). Philadelphia: W.B. Saunders, p. 676.

300. **4**
Rationale: The client taking a single daily dose of theophylline,
a xanthine bronchodilator, should take the medication early
in the morning. This enables the client to have maximal
benefit from the medication during daytime activities. Additionally, this medication causes insomnia. The client should
take in at least 2 liters of fluid per day to decrease viscosity of
secretions. The client should check with the physician before
changing brands of the medication, because there may be
different levels of bioavailability. The client also checks with

the physician before taking OTC cough, cold, or other
respiratory preparations with theophylline because they could
have interactive effects, increasing the side effects of theophylline and causing dysrhythmias.
Test-Taking Strategy: Use the process of elimination. Note the
key words needs further information. Use of basic medication
administration principles will direct you to option 4. Review
client teaching points related to this medication if you had
difficulty with this question.
Level of Cognitive Ability: Analysis
Client Needs: Health Promotion and Maintenance
Integrated Concept/Process: Nursing Process/Evaluation
Content Area: Pharmacology
Reference: Wilson, B., Shannon, M., & Stang, C. (2000). Nurses
drug guide 2000. Stamford, Conn.: Appleton & Lange, p. 1350.

REFERENCES

Altman, G., Buchsel, P., & Coxon, V. (2000). Delmar's Fundamental & advanced nursing skills. Albany, NY: Delmar.

Ashwill, J., & Droske, S. (1997). Nursing care of children: Principles and practice. Philadelphia: W.B. Saunders.

Ball, J., & Bindler, R. (1999). Pediatric nursing: Caring for children (2nd ed.). Stamford, Conn.: Appleton & Lange.

Beare, P., & Myers, J. (1998). Adult health nursing (3rd ed.). St. Louis: Mosby,

Black, J., & Matassarin-Jacobs, E. (1997). Medical-surgical nursing: Clinical management for continuity of care (5th ed.). Philadelphia: W. B. Saunders.

Bowden, V., Dickey, S., & Greenberg, C. (1998). Children and their families: The continuum of care. Philadelphia: W.B. Saunders.

Clark, J., Queener, S., & Karb, V. (2000). Pharmacologic basis of nursing practice (6th ed.). St. Louis: Mosby.

Cleveland, L., Aschenbrenner, D., Venable, S., & Yensen, J. (1999). Nursing management in drug therapy. Philadelphia: Lippincott.

Corbett, J. (2000). Laboratory tests and diagnostic procedures (5th ed.). Upper Saddle River: N.J.: Prentice-Hall.

Craven, R., & Hirnle, C. (2000). Fundamentals of nursing: Human health and function (3rd ed.). Philadelphia: Lippincott.

Deglin, J., & Vallerand, A. (2001). Davis's drug guide for nurses (7th ed.). Philadelphia: F.A. Davis.

Fischbach, F. (2000). A manual of laboratory & diagnostic tests (6th ed.). Philadelphia: Lippincott Williams & Wilkins.

Fortinash, K., & Holoday-Worret, P. (2000). Psychiatric mental health nursing (2nd ed.). St. Louis: Mosby.

Giger, J., & Davidhizar, R. (1999). Transcultural nursing: Assessment & Intervention (3rd ed.). St. Louis: Mosby.

Gorrie, T., McKinney, E., & Murray, S. (1998). Foundations of maternal-newborn nursing (2nd ed.). Philadelphia: W.B. Saunders.

Grodner, M., Anderson, S., & DeYoung, S. (2000). Foundations and clinical applications of nutrition: A nursing approach. St. Louis: Mosby.

Gutierrez, K. (1999). Pharmacotherapeutics: Clinical decision-making in nursing. Philadelphia: W.B. Saunders.

Harkreader, H. (2000). Fundamentals of nursing: Caring and clinical judgment. Philadelphia: W.B. Saunders.

Hodgson, B., & Kizior, R. (2001). Saunders nursing drug handbook 2001. Philadelphia: W.B. Saunders.

Ignatavicius, D., Workman, M., & Mishler, M. (1999). Medical-surgical nursing across the health care continuum (3rd ed.). Philadelphia: W.B. Saunders.

Jarvis, C. (2000). Physical examination and health assessment (3rd ed.). Philadelphia: W.B. Saunders.

Keltner, N., Schwecke, L., & Bostrom, C. (1999). Psychiatric nursing (3rd ed.). St. Louis: Mosby.

Kozier, B., Erb, G., Berman, A., & Burke, K. (2000). Fundamentals of nursing: Concepts, process, and practice (6th ed.). Upper Saddle River, N.J.: Prentice-Hall.

Kuhn, M. (1998). Pharmacotherapeutics: A nursing process approach (4th ed.). Philadelphia: F.A. Davis.

Ladewig, P., London, M., & Olds, S. (1998). Maternal-newborn care: The nurse, the family, and the community (4th ed.). Menlo Park, Calif.: Addison-Wesley Longman.

Leahy, J., & Kizilay, P. (1998). Foundations of nursing practice: A nursing process approach. Philadelphia: W.B. Saunders.

Lehne, R. (1998). Pharmacology for nursing care (3rd ed.). Philadelphia: W.B. Saunders.

LeMone, P., & Burke, K. (2000). Medical-surgical nursing: Critical thinking in client care (2nd ed.). Upper Saddle River, N.J.: Prentice-Hall.

Lewis, S., Heitkemper, M., & Dirksen, S. (2000). Medical-surgical nursing: Assessment and management of clinical problems (5th ed.). St. Louis: Mosby.

Lowdermilk, D., Perry, S., & Bobak, I. (2000). Maternity & women's health care (7th ed.). St. Louis: Mosby.

Luckmann, J. (1997). Saunders manual of nursing care. Philadelphia: W.B. Saunders.

Maher, A., Salmond, S. & Pellino, T. (1998). Orthopaedic nursing (2nd ed.). Philadelphia: W.B. Saunders.

Monahan, F., & Neighbors, M. (1998). Medical-surgical nursing: Foundations for clinical practice (2nd ed.). Philadelphia: W.B. Saunders.

Olds, S., London, M., & Ladewig, P. (2000). Maternal-newborn nursing: A family and community-based approach (6th ed.). Upper Saddle River, N.J.: Prentice-Hall Health.

Phipps, W., Sands, J., & Marek, J. (1999). Medical-surgical nursing: Concepts & clinical practice (6th ed.). St. Louis: Mosby.

Potter, P., & Perry, A. (2001). Fundamentals of nursing (5th ed.). St. Louis: Mosby.

Purnell, P., & Paulanka, B. (1998). Transcultural healthcare: A culturally competent approach. Philadelphia: F.A. Davis.

Rocchiccioli, J., & Tilbury, M. (1998). Clinical leadership in nursing. Philadelphia: W.B. Saunders.

Salerno, E. (1999). Pharmacology for health professionals. St. Louis: Mosby.

Sherwen, L., Scoloveno, M.A., & Weingarten, C. (1999). Maternity nursing: Care of the childbearing family (3rd ed.). Stamford, Conn.: Appleton & Lange.

Smeltzer, S., & Bare, B. (2000). *Brunner & Suddarth's Textbook of medical-surgical nursing* (9th ed.). Philadelphia: Lippincott Williams & Wilkins.

Smith, S., Duell, D., & Martin, B. (2000). *Clinical nursing skills: Basic to advanced skills* (5th ed.). Upper Saddle River, N.J.: Prentice-Hall Health.

Stuart, G.W., & Laraia, M.T. (1998). *Principles and practice of psychiatric nursing.* (6th ed.). St. Louis: Mosby.

Varcarolis, E. (1998). *Foundations of psychiatric mental health nursing* (3rd ed.). Philadelphia: W.B. Saunders.

Wilson, B., Shannon, M., & Stang, C. (2000). *Nurses drug guide 2000.* Stamford, Conn.: Appleton & Lange.

Wong, D. (1999). *Whaley & Wong's Nursing care of infants and children* (6th ed.). St. Louis: Mosby.

Yoder-Wise, P. (1999). *Leading and managing in nursing* (2nd ed.). St. Louis: Mosby.

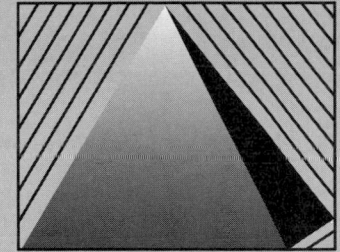

General Bibliography

Altman, G., Buchsel, P., & Coxon, V. (2000). *Delmar's fundamental & advanced nursing skills*. Albany, N.Y.: Delmar.

Ashwill, J., & Droske, S. (1997). *Nursing care of children: Principles and practice*. Philadelphia: W.B. Saunders.

Ball, J., & Bindler, R. (1999). *Pediatric nursing: Caring for children* (2nd ed.). Stamford, Conn.: Appleton & Lange.

Ball, J., & Bindler, R. (1999). *Quick reference to pediatric clinical skills*. Stamford, Conn.: Appleton & Lange.

Beare, P., & Myers, J. (1998). *Adult health nursing* (3rd ed.). St. Louis: Mosby.

Black, J., & Matassarin-Jacobs, E. (1997). *Medical-surgical nursing: Clinical management for continuity of care* (5th ed.). Philadelphia: W.B. Saunders.

Bowden, V., Dickey, S, & Greenberg, C. (1998). *Children and their families: The continuum of care*. Philadelphia: W.B. Saunders.

Clark, M.J. (1999). *Nursing in the community: Dimensions of community health nursing* (3rd ed.). Stamford, Conn.: Appleton & Lange.

Clark, J., Queener, S., & Karb, V. (2000). *Pharmacologic basis of nursing practice* (6th ed.). St. Louis: Mosby.

Cleveland, L., Aschenbrenner, D., Venable, S., & Yensen, J. (1999). *Nursing management in drug therapy*. Philadelphia: Lippincott.

Corbett, J. (2000). *Laboratory tests and diagnostic procedures* (5th ed.). Upper Saddle River, N.J.: Prentice-Hall.

Craven, R., & Hirnle, C. (2000). *Fundamentals of nursing: Human health and function* (3rd ed.). Philadelphia: Lippincott.

Deglin, J., & Vallerand, A. (2001). *Davis's drug guide for nurses* (7th ed.). Philadelphia: F.A. Davis.

Elkin, M., Perry, A., & Potter, P. (2000). *Nursing interventions and clinical skills* (2nd ed.). St. Louis: Mosby.

Fischbach, F. (2000). *A manual of laboratory & diagnostic tests* (6th ed.). Philadelphia: Lippincott Williams & Wilkins.

Fortinash, K., & Holoday-Worret, P. (2000). *Psychiatric mental health nursing* (2nd ed.). St. Louis: Mosby.

Giger, J., & Davidhizar, R. (1999). *Transcultural nursing: Assessment & Intervention* (3rd ed.). St. Louis: Mosby.

Gorrie, T., McKinney, E., & Murray, S. (1998). *Foundations of maternal-newborn nursing* (2nd ed.). Philadelphia: W.B. Saunders.

Grodner, M., Anderson, S., & DeYoung, S. (2000). *Foundations and clinical applications of nutrition: A nursing approach*. St. Louis: Mosby.

Gutierrez, K. (1999). *Pharmacotherapeutics: Clinical decision-making in nursing*. Philadelphia: W.B. Saunders.

Harkreader, H. (2000). *Fundamentals of nursing: Caring and clinical judgment*. Philadelphia: W.B. Saunders.

Hodgson, B., & Kizior, R. (2001). *Saunders nursing drug handbook 2001*. Philadelphia: W.B. Saunders.

Ignatavicius, D., Workman, M., & Mishler, M. (1999). *Medical-surgical nursing across the health care continuum* (3rd ed.). Philadelphia: W.B. Saunders.

Jarvis, C. (2000). *Physical examination and health assessment* (3rd ed.). Philadelphia: W.B. Saunders.

Johnson, M., Bulechek, G., Dochterman, J., Maas, M., Moorhead, S. (2001). *Nursing diagnoses, outcomes, and interventions*. St. Louis: Mosby.

Karch, A. (2000). *Focus on nursing pharmacology*. Philadelphia: Lippincott.

Kee, J., & Marshall, S. (2000). *Clinical calculations: With applications to general and specialty areas* (4th ed). Philadelphia: W.B. Saunders.

Keltner, N., Schwecke, L., & Bostrom, C. (1999). *Psychiatric nursing* (3rd ed.). St. Louis: Mosby.

Kozier, B., Erb, G., Berman, A., & Burke, K. (2000). *Fundamentals of nursing: Concepts, process, and practice* (6th ed.). Upper Saddle River, N.J.: Prentice-Hall.

Kuhn, M. (1998). *Pharmacotherapeutics: A nursing process approach* (4th ed.). Philadelphia: F.A. Davis.

Ladewig, P., London, M., & Olds, S. (1998). *Maternal-newborn care: The nurse, the family, and the community* (4th ed.). Menlo Park, Calif.: Addison-Wesley.

Leahy, J., & Kizilay, P. (1998). *Foundations of nursing practice: A nursing process approach*. Philadelphia: W.B. Saunders.

Lehne, R. (1998). *Pharmacology for nursing care* (3rd ed.). Philadelphia: W.B. Saunders.

LeMone, P., & Burke, K. (2000). *Medical-surgical nursing: Critical thinking in client care* (2nd ed.). Upper Saddle River, N.J.: Prentice-Hall.

Lewis, S., Heitkemper, M., & Dirksen, S. (2000). *Medical-surgical nursing: Assessment and management of clinical problems* (5th ed.). St. Louis: Mosby.

Lindeman, C., & McAthie, M. (1999). *Fundamentals of contemporary nursing practice*. Philadelphia: W.B. Saunders.

Lowdermilk, D., Perry, S., & Bobak, I. (2000). *Maternity & women's health care* (7th ed.). St. Louis: Mosby.

Luckmann, J. (1997). *Saunders manual of nursing care*. Philadelphia: W.B. Saunders.

Lueckenotte, A. (2000). *Gerontologic nursing* (2nd ed.). St. Louis: Mosby.

Maher, A., Salmond, S., & Pellino, T. (1998). *Orthopaedic nursing* (2nd ed.). Philadelphia: W.B. Saunders.

Monahan, F., & Neighbors, M. (1998). *Medical-surgical nursing: Foundations for clinical practice* (2nd ed.). Philadelphia: W.B. Saunders.

Olds, S., London. M., & Ladewig, P. (2000). *Maternal-newborn nursing: A family and community-based approach* (6th ed.). Upper Saddle River, N.J.: Prentice-Hall Health.

Peckenpaugh, N., & Poleman, C. (1999). *Nutrition essentials and diet therapy* (8th ed.). Philadelphia: W.B. Saunders.

Phipps, W., Sands, J., & Marek, J. (1999). *Medical-surgical nursing: Concepts & clinical practice* (6th ed.). St. Louis: Mosby.

Potter, P., & Perry, A. (2001). *Fundamentals of nursing* (5th ed.). St. Louis: Mosby.

Purnell, P., & Paulanka, B. (1998). *Transcultural healthcare: A culturally competent approach.* Philadelphia: F.A. Davis.

Riley, J. (2000). *Communication in nursing* (4th ed.). St. Louis: Mosby.

Rocchiccioli, J., & Tilbury, M. (1998). *Clinical leadership in nursing.* Philadelphia: W.B. Saunders.

Salerno, E. (1999). *Pharmacology for health professionals.* St. Louis: Mosby.

Sherwen, L., Scoloveno, M.A., & Weingarten, C. (1999). *Maternity nursing: Care of the childbearing family* (3rd ed.). Stamford, Conn.: Appleton & Lange.

Smeltzer, S., & Bare, B. (2000). *Brunner & Suddarth's textbook of medical-surgical nursing* (9th ed.). Philadelphia: Lippincott Williams & Wilkins.

Smith, S., Duell, D., & Martin, B. (2000). *Clinical nursing skills: Basic to advanced skills* (5th ed.). Upper Saddle River, N.J.: Prentice-Hall Health.

Spector, R. (2000). *Cultural diversity in health & illness* (5th ed.). Upper Saddle River, N.J.: Prentice-Hall.

Spratto, G., & Woods, A. (2001). *PDR nurse's drug handbook.* Montvale, N.J.: Medical Economics.

Stuart, G.W., & Laraia, M.T. (1998). *Principles and practice of psychiatric nursing.* (6th ed.). St. Louis: Mosby.

Swanson, J., & Nies, M. (1997). *Community health nursing: Promoting the health of aggregates* (2nd ed.). Philadelphia: W.B. Saunders.

Varcarolis, E. (1998). *Foundations of psychiatric mental health nursing* (3rd ed.). Philadelphia: W.B. Saunders.

Wilson, B., Shannon, M., & Stang, C. (2000). *Nurses drug guide 2000.* Stamford, Conn.: Appleton & Lange.

Wong, D. (1999). *Whaley & Wong's Nursing care of infants and children* (6th ed.). St. Louis: Mosby.

Yoder-Wise, P. (1999). *Leading and managing in nursing* (2nd ed.). St. Louis: Mosby.

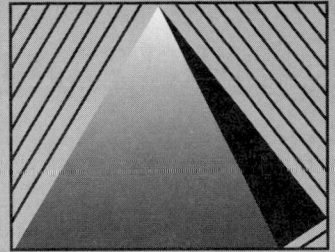

Index